The New Look

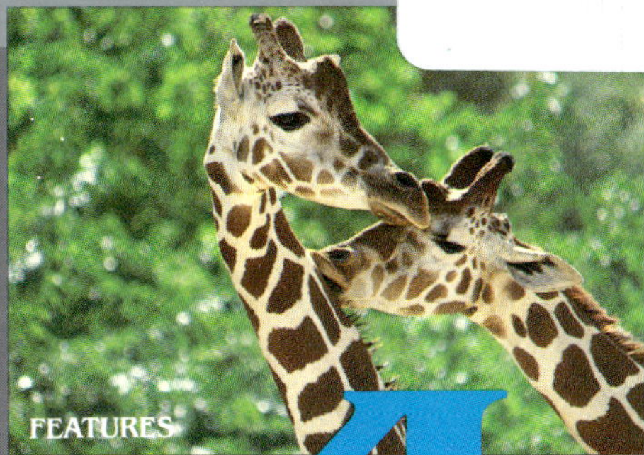

AGFA

XT 320® High Speed and XT 125® Color Negative Films

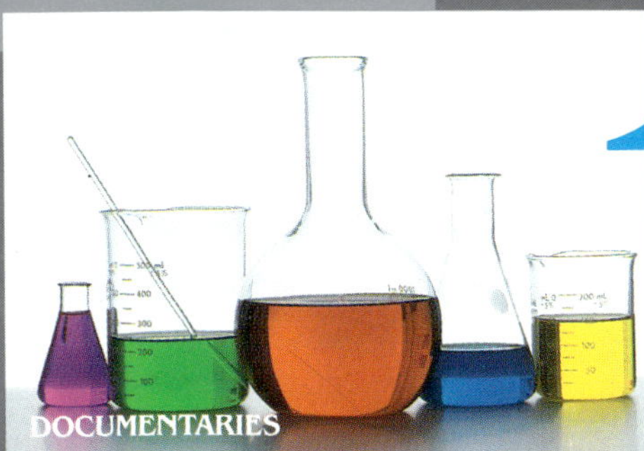

AGFA XT Films — The product of AGFA's new twin crystal technology will give you better color, sharper reproduction, finer grain.

You will see the difference!

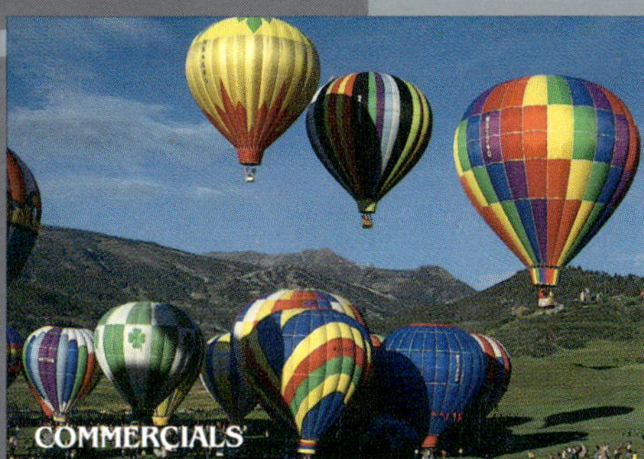

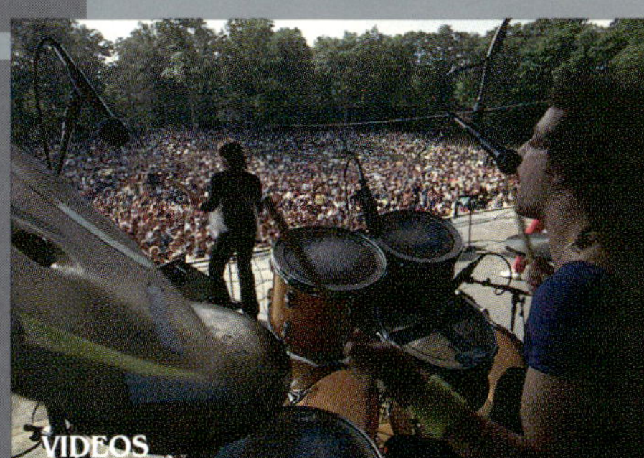

AGFA-GEVAERT, INC.
Motion Picture Products Division

East of the Mississippi:
100 Challenger Road, Ridgefield Park, NJ 07660
(201) 440-2500 or (212) 563-5500

West of the Mississippi:
1801 Century Park East, Los Angeles, CA 90067
(213) 552-9622
1633 Old Bayshore Highway, Burlingame, CA 94010
(415) 692-2432

AGFA-GEVAERT N.V., B-2510 Mortsel, Belgium

AGFA

NEW YORK
BEVERLY HILLS
NASHVILLE
LONDON
ROME
SYDNEY
MUNICH

WILLIAM MORRIS AGENCY, INC.

The Agency Of The Entertainment World

NEW YORK—1350 Avenue Of The Americas, New York, N.Y. 10019 • (212) 586-5100, Telex 620165
BEVERLY HILLS—151 El Camino, Beverly Hills, Calif. 90212 • (213) 274-7451, (213) 272-4111, Telex 673102
NASHVILLE—2325 Crestmoor Road, Nashville, Tenn. 37125 • (615) 385-0310, Telex 554472
LONDON—31/32 Soho Square, London W1V 5DG England • Phone 01-434-2191
Cable Address—"Willmorris London," Telex 851-27928
*ROME—Giosué Carducci 10-00187 Rome, Italy • Phone: 48-69-61
Telex 843-625614, *Cable Address*—"Willmorris Rome".
*MUNICH—Lamontstrasse 9, 8 Munich 80 • Telex "Alcap/Willmorris D"
*SYDNEY—55 Victoria Street, Potts Point, NSW 2011 • Phone: 02-356-4144

*Corresponding Offices

1987

INTERNATIONAL TELEVISION & VIDEO ALMANAC

32nd Edition

Editor: RICHARD GERTNER

Associate Editor: WILLIAM PAY

Video Editor: JANE KLAIN

Quigley Publishing Company, Inc.

New York • London

(212) 247-3100 (0268 417055)

Foreword

With this volume, the 32nd edition, the INTERNATIONAL TELEVISION ALMANAC acquires a new name: TELEVISION & VIDEO ALMANAC, reflecting the introduction of extensive data on the important and burgeoning home video market. That business has grown in the space of a very few years to staggering heights which are indicated in these statistics: 28,500,000 U.S. video cassette recorder households in 1986 (compared to 1,850,000 in 1980) and annual sales of 62,000,000 pre-recorded video cassettes to retailers in 1986 (compared to 3,000,000 in 1980). This newly renamed ALMANAC supplies the who, what, when and where of home video, along with the other departments in the television fields it has covered now for over three decades.

—RICHARD GERTNER

32nd Edition
INTERNATIONAL
TELEVISION
& VIDEO
ALMANAC
For 1987
ISSN: 0539-0761
ISBN: 0-900610-37-9

PRINTED IN THE UNITED STATES OF AMERICA

Table of Contents

THE YEAR IN REVIEW 8-A
STATISTICS 12-A
EMMY AWARD WINNERS 26-A
INDEX OF SUBJECTS 17-A
INDEX OF ADVERTISERS 30-A
WHO'S WHO 1–300
SERVICES 301–339
HOME VIDEO 341–455
- STATISTICS 341–352
- PRODUCERS 353–356
- PRODUCTION COMPANIES 357–380
- WHOLESALE DISTRIBUTORS 381–396
- MAJOR VIDEO RETAIL STORES 397–409
- EQUIPMENT MANUFACTURERS 411–418
- CONSUMER AND TRADE PUBLICATIONS 419–423
- TRADE ASSOCIATIONS 425–427
- VIDEO SERVICES 429–450
- HOME VIDEO WORLD MARKET 451–455

COMPANIES 456–472
CABLE TELEVISION 473–481
PRODUCERS-DISTRIBUTORS 482–499
STATIONS 500–565
ADVERTISING AGENCIES-STATION REPRESENTATIVES 566–572
PROGRAMS 573–590
ORGANIZATIONS 591–604
THE PRESS 605–611
THE INDUSTRY IN GREAT BRITAIN & IRELAND 612–637
THE WORLD MARKET 638–652

The Year in Review

As it had in the 1984–85 television season and in decades before, network TV continued to dominate the American television market in attracting an overall audience in 1985–86. Signs of erosion in that position were more ominous than ever from the competition, however: cable and home video.

The number of basic cable households increased by one million in the first six months of 1986, making the total 41 million. The number of U.S. videocassette recorder households had ballooned to 28 and a half million in the same period—a six-months growth of 21.3%. The number of pay TV subscribers also rose—standing at 22,800,000 at the end of June, 1986. (For further information about developments in the home video field see that section in this book under the heading of "Statistics.")

Not very encouraging news for the networks, two of which—ABC and NBC—were undergoing changes in ownership, while the other, CBS, was in upheaval due to a decline in net income in 1985 a staggering 87%. Along with its other troubles CBS was supplanted by NBC as leader in the 1985–86 ratings race (figures compiled by the A.C. Nielsen Company.) And ABC was third again.

1986 saw formal completion of the takeovers of ABC and NBC which had been set into motion the year before. Capital Cities Communications officially acquired ABC and the merged company's name was changed to Capital Cities/ABC, Inc. General Electric Corporation purchased RCA (for $6.28 billion), among the divisions of which is the National Broadcasting Company, operator of the NBC-TV network.

All three networks had important changes in top management in 1986. At NBC Robert Wright replaced Grant A. Tinker as chief executive officer, although Wright was not given Tinker's chairman title, that being taken by John F. Welch of GE. Instead Wright was named president as well as CEO. At ABC Daniel B. Burke replaced Frederick J. Pierce as president and chief operating officer.

Over at CBS there was no takeover by another company, but the network's largest stockholder, Laurence A. Tisch, was instrumental in bringing about the resignation of Thomas H. Wyman as chairman, president and chief executive officer. Until Wyman could be replaced, CBS' founder William Paley returned to active duty as acting chairman of the board. Tisch was named acting CEO.

This turnaround at the top followed the elimination of 700 jobs at the CBS Broadcast Group in 1986 in a drastic move to cut costs as sharply as possible.

At ABC the company laid off hundreds of employees after the merger in January. NBC, the new top-rated network, was also examining cost problems; but there was no wholesale rolling of heads before the new season began.

NBC's triumph in the ratings was its first in three decades of such tallying by Nielsen. It had tied CBS in prime-time ratings in 1969–70 and 1970–71, and ABC had led in three seasons, but the rest of the time CBS had reigned as king. NBC finished the 1985–86 season with a 17.5 rating, an increase of 8% over last season's 16.2 mark. CBS slipped from 16.9 to 16.7. NBC also led in every age-group division except for adults over 55, which remained the province of CBS.

The top ten shows for 1985–86, in order, were: "The Cosby Show" (NBC); "Family Ties" (NBC); "Murder, She Wrote" (CBS); "60 Minutes" (CBS); "Cheers" (NBC); "Dallas" (CBS); "Dynasty" (ABC); "The Golden Girls" (NBC); "Miami Vice" (NBC); and "Who's The Boss?" (ABC).

The list breaks down to five comedies, two soap operas, one action-adventure, one mystery, and one "news" program.

MGM/UA Communications Co.

Top-rated movies-made-for-TV of the 1985–86 season were "Return to Mayberry" and "Perry Mason Returns"—sequels in a way to long-gone prime-time series (but still available in syndication). NBC led in the TV-movies field with 11 out of the first 20 rated as most popular; CBS had nine; ABC none. The latter network, however, had the number one mini-series of the season: "North and South."

The major networks will have a new competitor in the 1986–87 season with the launching of a "fourth network" by 20th Century Fox: the Fox Broadcasting Company. Broadcasting commenced in October with "The Late Show Starring Joan Rivers" and more programs were slated to follow.

Predictably, it is comedy which leads in the new network programming for 1986–87. There are 28 such shows slated (for details of the line-up see the "Programs" section in this book). There are some new action-adventure series, too, but no new soap operas. "Dallas," number one in the 1984–85 season, fell to sixth place in 1985–86, and "Dynasty" dropped from second to seventh. "Knots Landing" slipped from ninth to 18th and "Falcon Crest" was kicked out of the top ten and landed at 24th.

In daytime scheduling a significant program development came with the decision of CBS to end production of its low-rated "CBS Morning News" by its News Division and turn the valuable early A.M. time period over to a two-hour show to be produced by a company unit that is not part of either the Entertainment or the News Division. This program started the first of 1987.

The creation of the new production unit is a watershed in the history of CBS News—long held in high esteem as the best in the industry. How the new show does will be closely watched by the industry.

STATISTICS

Network and Station Operations

There were 924 commercial stations operating in the United States as of January, 1986 located in over 450 markets and serving some 85,900,000 families.

GROWTH OF COMMERCIAL TELEVISION STATIONS

	1960	**1965**	**1970**	**1975**	**1980**	**1985**	**1986**
Total	515	569	677	706	734	883	924
VHF	440	481	501	514	516	520	522
UHF	75	88	176	192	218	363	402

VIEWING HABITS

TELEVISION USAGE

Number of TV homes	85,900,000
Number of color TV homes	80,100,000
Homes with two or more sets	48,700,000

	1950	**1970**	**1985**
Avg. Hours per Home	4 hrs. 35 min.	5 hrs. 56 min.	7 hrs. 10 min.

COMMERCIAL TELEVISION STATIONS

	1986	**1975**	**1965**	**1955**
Total	924	706	569	411
VHF	522	514	481	297
UHF	402	192	88	114

COLOR TELEVISION

	1960	**1975**	**1986**
Homes	340,000	48,500,000	80,100,000
Per Cent of TV Home	0.7	70.8	93

Source: A. C. Nielsen

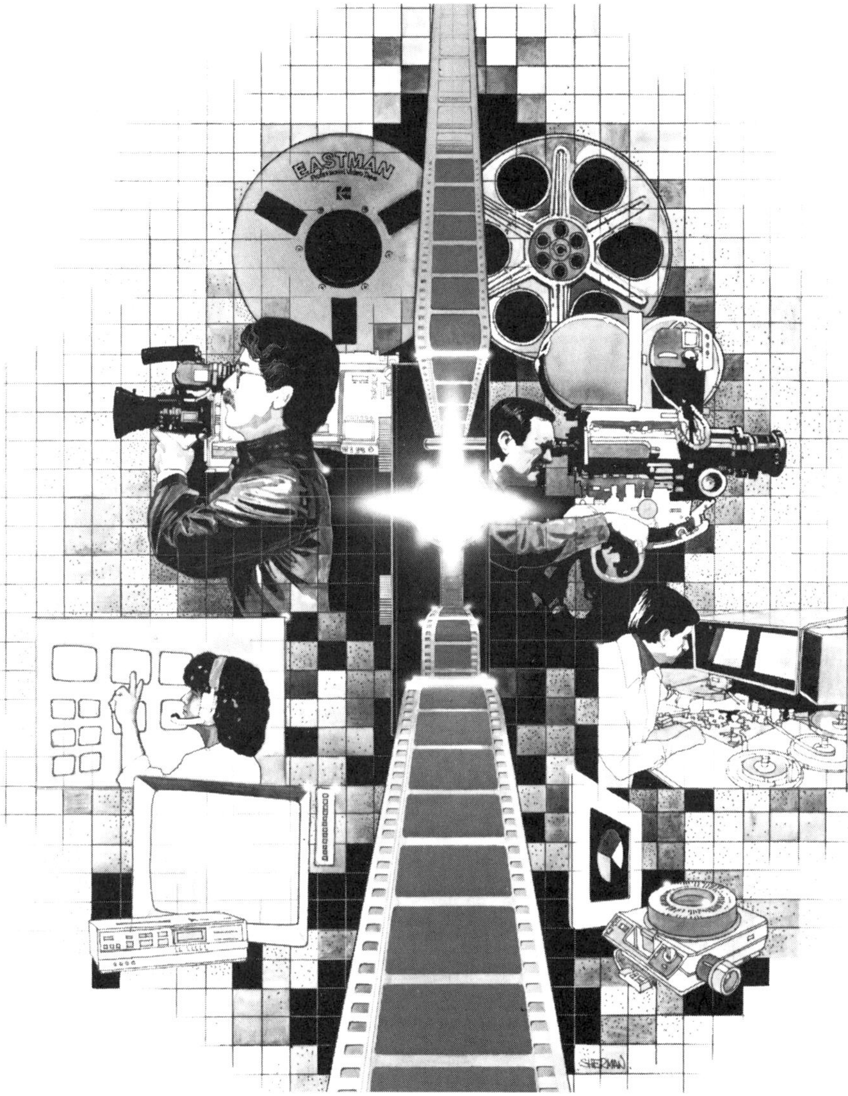
EASTMAN

A BREAKDOWN OF TELEVISION VIEWERS

	Avg. Viewing Time Per TV Time Per Day (Hours and Minutes)
Total U.S.	7:48
By Household Income	
Under $15,000	7:59
$20,000 and over	7:45
$30,000 and over	7:39
$40,000 and Over	7:42
By Age of Lady of House	
18–34	7:58
35–54	8:30
55 and Over	7:42
By Household Size	
1 person	6:02
2 persons	7:02
3 persons	9:15
4 or more	9:37
By Education of Head of House	
Under 4 Yrs. H.S.	8:17
4 Yrs. H.S.	8:22
1+ Yrs. College	6:57
4+ Yrs. College	6:32
By Territory	
Northeast	7:58
East Central	8:35
West Central	7:21
South	7:52
Pacific	7:18
By County Size	
A	7:48
B	8:06
C & D	7:32

Source: A. C. Nielsen

TOTAL ADVERTISING VOLUME

	Millions of Dollars			
	1984	1985	% Change	% of Total
Total Advertising	$87,820	$94,750	+ 7.9	100.0
TELEVISION	19,498	20,533	+ 5.3	21.7
Newspapers	23,522	25,170	+ 7.0	26.5
Magazines	4,932	5,155	+ 4.5	5.4
Radio	5,817	6,490	+11.6	6.9
Outdoor	872	945	+ 8.3	1.0
Business Papers	2,270	2,375	+ 4.6	2.5
All Others	30,909	34,082	+10.3	36.0

Source: McCann-Erickson 5/86

NATIONAL ADVERTISING INVESTMENTS IN MAJOR MEDIA

	Millions of Dollars			
	1984	1985	% Change	% of Total
TELEVISION	$14,414	$14,819	+ 2.8	52.9
Network	8,526	8,258	− 2.8	29.6
Spot	5,488	6,004	+ 9.4	21.4
Syndicated Barter	400	530*	+32.5	1.9
Newspapers	3,081	3,352	+ 8.8	11.9
Magazines	4,932	5,155	+ 4.5	18.4
Radio (Network & Spot)	1,517	1,700	+12.1	6.1
Outdoor	562	610	+ 8.3	2.2
Business Papers	2,270	2,375	+ 4.6	8.5
Total Major Media	$26,776	$28,011	+ 4.6	100.0

Source: McCann-Erickson 5/86
*TvB estimate

LOCAL ADVERTISING INVESTMENTS IN MAJOR MEDIA

	Millions of Dollars			
	1984	1985	% Change	% of Total
TELEVISION	$ 5,084	$ 5,714	+ 9.4	17.5
Newspapers	20,441	21,818	+ 6.7	66.8
Retail	12,784	13,442	+ 5.1	41.2
Classified	7,657	8,376	+ 9.4	25.6
Radio	4,300	4,790	+11.4	14.7
Outdoor	310	335	+ 8.3	1.0
Total Major Media	$30,135	$32,657	+ 8.4	100.0

Source: McCann-Erickson 5/86

LEADING LOCAL TV CATEGORIES

	add (000)		
	1984	1985	% Change
1. Restaurants & Drive-Ins	$577,598.6	$671,970.5	+16
2. Auto Dealers*	257,027.5	311,211.7	+21
3. Food Stores & Supermarkets	243,865.1	259,028.5	+ 6
4. Banks, Savings & Loans	197,538.5	195,283.9	− 1
5. Furniture Stores	164,865.7	186,999.9	+13
6. Department Stores	167,504.1	186,191.9	+11
7. Radio Stations & Cable TV	128,577.5	134,482.4	+ 5
8. Appliance Stores	85,586.4	121,883.1	+42
9. Amusements & Entertainment	104,482.0	121,496.5	+16
10. Discount Department Stores	92,576.5	114,816.4	+24

Source: BAR *Dealer Associations Not Included

LENGTH OF COMMERCIALS

Commercial Length	Non-Network 1983	1984	1985
10 seconds	6.0%	5.8%	5.5%
15 seconds	—	0.4	1.3
20 seconds	0.1	0.1	0.1
30 seconds	87.8	88.2	88.0
45 seconds	1.2	0.7	0.6
60 seconds	2.9	2.8	2.7
90 sec. or more	2.0	2.0	1.8
	100%	100%	100%

Commercial Length	Network 1983	1984	1985
10 seconds	0.9%	1.0%	1.3%
15 seconds	0.2	5.2	10.1
20 seconds	—	—	0.8
30 seconds	93.8	89.2	83.5
45 seconds	2.9	2.0	1.7
60 seconds	1.8	2.1	2.2
90 sec. or more	0.4	0.5	0.4
	100%	100%	100%

Source: BAR

TELEVISION SET SALES 22,500,000 IN 1985

	Total	Color	Monochrome
1975	10,637,000	6,219,000	4,418,000
1980	18,532,000	11,803,000	6,729,000
1981	18,479,000	12,423,000	6,056,000
1982	16,406,000	11,484,000	4,922,000
1983	19,681,000	14,034,000	5,647,000
1984	22,384,000	17,190,000	5,194,000
1985*	22,500,000	18,000,000	4,500,000

Source: EIA, Domestic & Imports *preliminary

CABLE TV OPERATING SYSTEMS AND SUBSCRIBERS

	1960	1965	1970	1975	1980	1985
Operating Systems	640	1,325	2,490	3,366	4,048	6,600
Subscribers (millions)	0.7	1.3	4.5	9.8	15.5	37.3
% of TV Homes	1.4%	2.4%	7.6%	14.3%	20.5%	43.7%

Source: Television Digest

ALPHABETICAL INDEX OF SUBJECTS

A

ABC Pictures International 483
ABC Video Enterprises 359
AEF Entertainment 359
AFP Distributors, Inc. 483
A & M Video 359
A M Productions Home Video 359
ANE Home Video 359
A.P.A. 483
ARC Video, Inc. 359
AVG Inc./SQN Corp. 359
AVS, Inc. 359
Academy Film Productions, Inc. 483
Academy Home Entertainment, Inc. 359
Academy of TV Arts and Sciences Awards
1985–86 .... 26-A
Acorn Sports, Inc. 359
Active Home Video 359
Admit One Video Presentations 359
Adventures in Cassettes 359
Advertising Agencies
Great Britain 632
U.S. 320
Aero/Space Visuals Society 359
Agriculture, Dept. of 337
Air Force, Dept. of the 337
Alamance Co. 359
Alameda County Office of Education 359
Alan Enterprises 483
Alden Films 483
Allend'or Productions, Inc. 483
All Seasons Entertainment 359
Lewis Allen/Peter Newman Prods. 359
Almi Television 483
Alpine Film & Video Exchange 359
Alti Corporation 360
American Broadcasting Companies, Inc. 457
American Cablesystems Corp. 475
American Educational Films 360
American Film Productions, Inc. 483
American Home Video Library 360
American Humanist Association 360
American National Enterprises, Inc. 360
American Red Cross 360
American Sports Network, Inc. 360
American TV & Communications Corp. 475
American Video 360
American Video Works 360
Amrit Productions, Inc. 360, 483
Amstar Prods. 360
Animals and Trainers 311
Animation 311
Animated Productions, Inc. 483
Anti-Defamation League of B'Nai B'rith 360
Morris Anton Associates 360
Appalshop, Inc. 360
Arlington Movie Studios 483
Armour Prods. 360
Army, Dept. of the 337
Army and Air Force Motion Picture Service ... 337
Artmusic, Inc. 360
Arts & Entertainment Network 478
Artzco Productions, Inc. 483
Asia Society 360
Associated Press, The 478, 483
Associations, U.S. 591
British 635
Astoria Pictures Corp. 483
Atlantic Film 360
Atlantic Television 483
Atlantis Prods., Inc. 360
Audio Productions 483
Aura Prods. 360
Aurora General Entertainment 483
Avant Communications, Inc. 361
Award and Poll Winners 26-A

B

BBC Television Enterprises 483
BBI 484
BFA Educational Media. 361
Baffico/Breger Video 361
Bandera Enterprises, Inc. 361
Banner Associates, Inc., Bob 484
Barbre Productions Inc. 484
Barnholtz Organization 361
Baron, Robert & Associates 484
Barr Films 361
Barry, Ben & Associates 484
Barry & Enright Prods. 484
Beck, Alexander Films 484
Norman Beerger Prods. 361
Behrens Co. 484
Best Film & Video Corp. 361, 484
Biographies 1–300
Black Entertainment Network 478
Blackhawk Films, Inc. 361
Blackstone, Milton, Associates 484
Michael Blackwood Prods. 361
Blair Entertainment 484
Les Blank's Flower Films & Video 361
Bodacious Films 361
Book-of-the-Month Club, Inc. 361
Bookshelf Video 361
Borden Prods. 484
Bosustow Prods. 361
Braverman Productions 484
Bray Studios 484
Brickyard, Ltd. 484
Britannica Video 361
British (see Great Britain)
British Broadcasting Corp. 457
Broadcast Quality, Inc. 361
Broadman 361

Brooklyn College 361
Brown, Barry, Brillig Prod., Inc. 484
Budget Video, Inc. 355
Bullfrog Films 361
Buena Vista International 484

C

CBS/Fox Video 355
CBS, Inc. 460
CBS Video Club/CBS Video Library 362
CBS Worldwide Enterprises 362
CC Studios/Children's Circle 362
CVI/Cirace Video Intl. 362
Cable News Network 478
Cable Satellite Public Affairs Network 478
Cable Television 474
Cable TV Co. 475
Cable Video 362
Cablevision Systems Development Co. 475
Calypso Video, Inc. 362
Camelot Entertainment 484
Campaign Coaches of Long Island 485
Campus, Steve, Prods. 485
Candlelight Studios 362
Cannell Prods. 485
Cape Cod Writers Conference 362
Capital Cities/ABC, Inc 457
Capital-Cities Cable, Inc. 457
Caravatt Communications 362
Cardinal Communications, Inc. 475
Carlson, George & Associates 485
Carthay Sound Stage 485
Castle Hill TV 485
Catholic TV Network/Bay Area Dioceses 362
Centerpoint Productions 485
Centron Films 362
Doris Chase Productions 362
Children's Television Workshop 461
Children's Video Library 362
Christ for the Nations 362
Christian Broadcasting Network 478
Christian Media 362
Chronicle Video Cassettes 362
Churchill Films, Inc. 362
Cinecraft, Inc. 485
Cinema Guild 363
Cinema Products 363
Cinema Shares Int'l. TV 485
Cinemagreats 363
Cinemax 478
Cinetudes Film Productions 485
Cineworld Corp. 485
Circle Video Prods. 363
City Film Productions, Inc. 485
Clark, Dick Co. 485
Classic Family Entertainment 363
Coast Prods. 485
Coast Special Effects 485
Coast Telecourses 363
Colbert Television 485
Color Leasing, Inc. 363
Columbia Pictures Television 461, 478, 485
Columbia School of Biblical Education 363
Comcast Cable 475
Comet Video 363
Comex Systems 363
Communication Comm. of Nat'l. Churches of Christ 485
Communicorp, Inc. 363
Companies 456
Company of Artists Productions, Inc. 485
Compuvid 363
Concepts Unlimited 363
Concordia Publishing House 363
Condor Pictures, Inc. 485
Consultants 312
Contempo Communications, Inc. 486
Continental Cablevision 475
Continental Video, Inc. 363
Cooper Wireless Cable 478
Coproducers Corp. 486
Corinthian Broadcasting Corp. 462
Cornell University Audio Visual Center 363
Coronet Films 363
Corporation for Entertainment & Learning 486
Corradine, Tom J., & Associates 486
Costumes and Uniforms 312
Courier Prods. 363
Cox Cable Communications 475
Cox Film Enterprises 486
Covenant Video 363
Craven, Thomas Film Corporation 486
Creative Tax Planning Assn. 364
Creative Visions Video 364
Crosby, Bing, Enterprises 486
Crossover Programming Co. 486
Crown Video 364
Crystallus Films 364
Crystal Pictures 486
A.S. Csaky Motion Picture & Video Prods. 364
Cummings Productions, Inc. 486
Cunningham Dance Foundation 364
Custom Films/Video 364
Cutting Rooms 312
Cycle Vision Tours 364
Czar Prods., Inc. 364

D

Damon & Grace Corp. 364
Dawn's Video 364
Daya, Inc. 364
Defense, Dept. of 337
DeLuz Video 364
Department of the Army, Radio and TV 337
Depicto Films, Inc. 486
Development Communications, Inc. 364
Dial Prods. 364
Digital Touch Ltd. 364
Direct Broadcast Programs, Inc. 364
Direct Video 364
Discount Video Tapes, Inc. 364
Disney Channel 478
Disney Home Video 356

Disney, Walt, Productions 462, 486
Distributors, Home Video 381
Dobovan Prods. 364
Double Vision Video Prods. 364
Documentary Films, Inc. 486
Dubie-Do Productions 486
Dudkowski-Lynch Associates 364
Dunn, Cal, Studios 486

E

EDC Publishing 364
ESPN 478
Eagle Prods., Ltd. 364
Eastman Kodak Company 462
Echo Prods. Ltd. 365
Echo Film Prods. 365
Educational Cable Consortium, Inc. 365
Educational Dimensions Group 365
Educational Video, Inc. 365
Edwards, Ralph, Productions 486
Electronic University 365
Embassy Communications 463, 486
Embassy Home Entertainment 355
Empire Television 486
Emory Medical TV Network 365
Enter-Tel, Inc. 365
Environmental Video, Inc. 365
Epic Pictures 365
Episcopal Radio-TV Foundation 365
Equinox Entertainment Corp. 365
Equipment, Lighting 315
Esquire Publishing Corp. 365
Event Video 365
Everything Video 365
Eye Contact, Inc. 365

F

FFH Video 365
FJC-Intellimedia, Inc 365
Family Films 486
Family Home Entertainment 365
Faye Productions 487
Fedderson, Don, Productions 487
Federal Communications Commission 337
Federal Trade Commission 337
Ferde Grofe Films 366
Festival Films 366
Filmack Studios 487
Film Carriers 313
Film Company, The 487
Film Exchanges 302
Film/Jamel Prods. 487
Film Laboratories 307
Film Libraries, Stock-Shot 310
Film Processing, Raw Stock and Storage 307
Film Storage Vaults 310
Films Five, Inc. 487
Films Made for TV 583
Fima Noveck Productions 487
Financial News Network 479
Format Productions, Inc. 487
Four Point Entertainment 366
Four Star International 487
Fox Broadcasting Co. 463
Fox/Lorber Associates 366
Frank, Sandy Film Syndication 487
Freewheelin' Films Ltd. 366
Fries Distribution Co. 487

G

GN Communications, Ltd. 366
Gateway Films, Inc. 366
Galaxie Productions, Inc. 487
Genesis Project, Inc. 366
Gilson International 487
Glen Glenn Sound Co. 487
Glenar Studios 487
Glenn Video Vistas 366
Global Village 366
Gold, Melvin L., Enterprises 487
Golden Bay Video 366
Golden Classics Media 366
Golden Productions 366
Goodson-Todman Productions 487
Gorgon Video 366
Gospel Films, Inc. 366
Gospel Video 366
Goulding-Elliott-Greybar Productions 487
Government Film Bureaus 337
Granada TV International 366, 487
Grand Award Video 366
Grant, Sherry Enterprises 487
Grass Roots Network 366
Gravity Sports Films 366
Gray-Schwartz Enterprises 487
Great Britain & Ireland
  Advertising Agencies 632
  Associations 635
  Camera Equipment 627
  Costume Suppliers 632
  Equipment Manufacturers 637
  Government Units & Program
    Contractors 616
  Laboratories 628
  Libraries, Film & Music 628
  Market Research 629
  News Film Services 632
  Producers and Distributors 620
  Services for Producers 627
  Studios 630
  Recording Studios 629
  Titling—Special Effects 630
  Year in Review 613
Great Mountain Prods. 366
Greatest Fights of the Century Inc. 488
Green Mountain Post Films 367
Group W Cable 475
Group W. Prods. 488
Leo. A. Gutman, Inc. 488
Guymark Studios 488

H

HBO/Cannon Video 355
H-R Prods. 488
Ham Mastertapes 367
Handel Film Corp. 488
Hanna-Barbera Prods. 488
Harmon, Larry Pictures 488
Harmony Gold 488
Harmony Vision 367
Harris-Tuchman Prods., Inc. 488
Harriscope Broadcasting Corporation 488
Hartley Film Foundation 367, 488
Health and Human Services, Dept. of 337
Health Media of America 367
Henley, Arthur, Productions 488
Henwood Cinema Video 367
Heritage Communications 475
Hewlett-Packard 367
Alfred Higgins Prods., Inc. 367
High Gate Pictures 367
Don L. Higley & Associates 367
Hollywood Home Theatres 367
Hollywood Intl. Film Corp. of America 367
Home Box Office 479
Home Entertainment Productions 479
Home Theatre Network 479
Home Video
- Consumer and Trade Publications 419
- Equipment Manufacturers 419
- Major Video Retail Stores 397
- Producers 353
- Services 429
- Statistics 341
- Trade Associations 425
- Wholesale Distributors 381
- World Market 451

Hot Licks Prods., Inc. 367
Houghton Mifflin Co. 367
How To Video Corp. 367
Hyde Park Media 367

I

IATSE (International Alliance of Theatrical Stage Employees & Moving Picture Operators of the U.S. & Canada) (AFL-CIO) 596
IRS Video 367
ITC Entertainment 488
Icarus Films 367
Image Magnetic Associates 367
Images Video & Film Archive 367
Imperial Video Corp. 367
Impulse Entertainment 368
Increase Video 368
Independent-International Pictures 489
Innovations in Video 368
Instant Replay Video Magazine 368
Instructional Video Cassette Corp. 368
Intercollegiate Video Clearing House 368
Interior, Dept. of the 337
Interlingual TV, K.K. 489
International Creative Management 463
International Film Bureau Inc. 489
International Film Exchange 489
International Historic Films 368
International Marketing Services 368
International Motion Picture Almanac (see Quigley Publishing Co.) 606
International Sunday School Lesson 368
International Television & Video Almanac (see Quigley Publishing Co.) 606
Ivy Films 368

J

JEF Films 368
JMJ Prods. 368
Stefaan Janssen Studio 368
Johansen Video Prods. 368
Justice, Dept. of 337

K

K-Video Prods 368
Kalmbach Publishing Co. 368
Karl/Lorimar Home Video, Inc 355
Kartes Prods., Inc. 368
Keach, Stacy, Prods. 489
Keep the Faith, Inc. 368
Allan Keith Prods., Inc. 368
Kempner, Inc. 489
Kennen Publishing 369
Key Video 355
Killiam Shows, Inc. 489
King Features Entertainment, Inc. 489
King International Corp. 489
King of Video 369
King World Prods. 489
Klein, Walter J. Co. Ltd. 369, 489
Kultur Intl. Films Ltd. 369

L

LBS Communications 489
Landsburg, Alan, Prods. 489
Lane, Don Pictures, Inc. 489
Laufman & Co. 490
Lawrence, Robert, Productions, Inc. 490
Learn, Inc. 369
Learning Corp. of America 369
Legalvision, Inc. 369
Leisure Time Products/3M 369
Leonard, Herbert B., Productions, Inc. ... 490
Liberty Studios Inc. 490
Library of Congress 337
Life Video Gospel Assn. 369
Lifetime 479
Lightning Video 355
Ligonier Valley Student Center 369
Literary and Talent Agencies 319
The Little Red Filmhouse 369

Llamavision 369
Lorimar-Telepictures Television 463, 490
Lott Video Productions, Inc. 490

M

MCA Television 464, 490
MCA Distributing Group 355
MGM/UA Communications Co. 464
MGM/UA Home Entertainment Group 355
MGM/UA Television Productions
& Distribution 464, 491
MGS Services 491
MMI Video Inc. 369
MPI Home Video 369
MPO Videotronics, Inc. 491
MRC Films & Video 491
MTM Enterprises 465
MTV Networks 479
Macmillan Video 369
Madison Square Garden TV 491
Magic Window 369
Magna Systems, Inc. 369
Magnavox Consumer Electronics 465
Magnum Entertainment 370
Mercedes Maharis Prods. 370
Major League Baseball Prods. 370
Maljack Prods., Inc. 370
Manley Productions, Inc. 491
Manson Intl./Manson TV 491
Manta Film Prods., Ltd. 370
Marathon International Productions, Inc. 491
Market Place, The 370
Market W Prods., Inc. 370
Mass Media Video Ministries 370
Master Arts Video 370
MasterVision 370
Mattingly Prods., Ltd. 370
Cameron McKay Prods., Inc. 370
Medallion Prods. 370
Medallion TV Enterprises, Inc. 491
Media Bus, Inc. 370
Media Concepts, Inc. 370
Media Home Entertainment 355
Mediacast TV 370
Meeting House Prods. 370
Metacom Audio Publishing Group 370
Metro Video Prods. 370
Metropolitan Museum of Art 371
Midnight Video 371
Midwest Video Corp. 476
Mike Milkovich Enterprises 371
Milner-Fenwick, Inc. 491
Mindware Video Programming 371
Mode-Art Pictures, Inc. 491
Modern Satellite Network 479
Modern Sound Pictures, Inc. 491
Modern Talking Picture Service 465, 491
Arthur Mokin Prods., Inc. 371
Monterey Home Video 371
Morcraft Films, Inc. 371
Morris, William, Agency, Inc. 471
Morris Video 371
Mossman Williams Prods. 371
Motion Picture Almanac (publication) 606
Motion Picture Service Co. 491
Motor Cycle Video 371
Movie Buff Video 371
Movie Merchants 371
Movietonews, Inc. 491
Multi-Video Inc. 371
Multimedia Entertainment 491
Muppet Home Video 371
Music Media 371
Music, Music Libraries and Music Cutting 315

N

NBC Intl. Ltd. 491
NFL Films 371
NSI Video 371
NTSC Video Co., Inc. 371
Nashville Network 479
National Broadcasting Co. 465
National Film Board of Canada 371
National Geographic TV 371
National Golf Foundation 371
Natural Reflections Video 372
Nebulae Prods. 372
Sara Needham Gallery 372
Networks 456
New Age Video, Inc. 372
New Breed Music 372
NewChannels Corp. 476
Newhouse Broadcasting 476
New Liberty Films 372
New Mode Media 372
New Orleans Video Access Center 372
New Video Center, Inc. 372
New World TV 491
New World Video 355
New York Times Prods. 372
Nightingale-Conant Corp. 372
Northeast Prods., Inc. 372
Nostalgia Merchant 355
Nova Video Art 372

O

Ocean Video Inc. 372
Odyssey Productions, Inc. 492
Okun, Lillian Productions 492
O'Neill and Jeffries Film Prods. 372
Optical Programming Associates 372
Organizations
Great Britain 635
U.S. 591
World Market 639
Original Face Video 372
Orion Home Entertainment Corp. 467
Orion Pictures Television 492
Owensby Studios 492

P

P.A.T. Film Services, Inc. 492
Pacific Arts Video Records 372
Pakula Productions 492
Paragon Video Prods. 372
Paramount Home Video 356
Paramount Television & Video
  Distribution Division 468, 492
Parent's Magazine Enterprises 372
Parker, Tom TV 492
Pat Film & Video Services 372
Pathe Pictures 492
Peak Performance, Inc. 373
Pearson, John, Int'l. 492
Pelican Films 373
Penguin Video Prods. 373
Phipps and Co. Prods. 373
Phoenix Films, Inc. 373
Pohlman Film Production 492
Pola Prods., Inc. 373
Poll and Award Winners 26-A
Polygram Video Music U.S. 373
Post-Newsweek Cable 476
Premier Film & Recording Corp. 492
Press, The
  Newspaper Listing 609
  Trade Publications 605
Prime Cable Corp. 476
Prime T.V. Films, Inc. 493
Prince Leopard Film Prods., Inc. 373
Prism 356, 479
Producers Consortium 373
Producers Intl. Corp. 373
Programs
  Films Made for TV 583
  Network 574
  Syndicated 579
Program Syndication Services 493
Progress Research, Inc. 373
Properties and Scenery 316
ProServ TV 493
Public Access Producers Assn. 373
Public Broadcasting Service 468
Public Production Group 373
Publications
  Home Video 419
  Trade 606
Publicity Representatives 320
PyraVid Intl. 373

Q

Quadrus Media Ministry, Inc. 373
Quality Program Sales 493
Quigley Publishing Company 606

R

RCA/Columbia Pictures Home Video 356
RCA Corp. 468
RCA Videodiscs 373
RICON Enterprises 373
RKM Video Publishing Co. 373
RKO General, Inc. 469
RKO Home Video 356
RMI Media Prods., Inc. 373
Radio and Television Packagers, Inc. 493
Ragsdale, Carl Associates, Ltd. 493
Rainbow Programming Services 479
Random House 373
Rasky, Harry, Productions, Inc. 493
Ravenswood Prods. 374
Reader's Digest 374
Redlin, Productions, Inc. 493
Reeves Corporate Services 374
Rego Irish Records & Tapes, Inc. 374
Rental Studios and Production Facilities 316
Republic Pictures 356, 469, 493
Research, Market
  British 629
  U.S. 315
Research Press 374
Retail Stores, Home Video 397
Reuters News-View 479
Rhapsody Films 374
Rhino Video 374
Ed Rich Prods., Inc. 374
Ring-Ting-a-Ling Prods. 493
Riviera Productions 493
Rizzoli/A.C. Video 374
Rocky Mountain Motion Pictures 374
Rodale Press, Inc. 374
Roffman, Richard H., Associates 493
Rogers U.S. Cablesystems, Inc. 476
Rourke, Jack, Productions 493
Ruby-Spears Enterprises 493

S

SFM Entertainment 494
Sagebrush Prods. 374
Sammons Communications 476
Satori Entertainment Corp. 479
Saturn Prods., Inc. 374
Scenery and Properties 316
Schaefer-Karpf 494
Screening Rooms 316
Sea-TV 374
See Hear Industries 374
Select-a-Tape 374
Self Improvement Video, Inc. 374
Serendipity Communications 374
Service Electric Cable TV 476
Services
  Advertising Representatives 320

Animals and Trainers 311
Animation 311
Camera Sales, Rentals, Repairs 311
Colorization by Computer 312
Completion Guarantees and Bonding 312
Consultants 312
Costumes & Uniforms 312
Cutting Rooms 312
Editing Equipment 313
Film Carriers 313
Film Exchanges 302
Film Storage 310
Government Film Bureaus 337
Home Video 429
Laboratories 307
Lighting Equipment 315
Market Research 315
Merchandisers 315
Music, Music Libraries, Music Cutting 315
Photo Reproduction Labs 308
Properties and Scenery 316
Publicity Representatives 320
Raw Stock Manufacturers 310
Rental Studios and Production Facilities 316
Screening Rooms 316
Slides-Telops 317
Sound and Recording Services 317
Stock-Shot Film Libraries 310
Stop Watches 318
Talent and Literary Agencies 319
Trailer Distributors 318
Sherwood Video Production Co. 374
Shokus Video 374
Showtime/The Movie Channel 479
Single Concept Films 375
Slesinger, Stephen, Inc. 494
Snoopy's Home Video Library 375
Society of Manufacturing Engineers 375
Sonoma Video Prods. 375
Sony Corp. of America 469
Sony Video Communications 356
Sony Video Software 375
Southbrook Entertainment 494
Spalla, Rick, Video Productions 494
Spanish International Network 469, 480
Spectradyne 480
Spectrum Video 375
Spelling Productions, Aaron 494
Sperry Corp. Information Group 375
Sports Films & Talents, Inc. 375
Sports World Cinema 375
Spotlight Video 375
Star Video Prods. 375
Stations
U.S. and Territories & Possessions 500
World Market 639
Statistics 12-A
Stop Watches 318
Storer Cable 476
Martha Stuart Communications, Inc. 375
Sun Video 375
Sun West Video Services 375
Supervideo 375
Survival Anglia Ltd. 494
SyberVision Systems, Inc. 375
Syndistar, Inc. 375

T

TFI 494
TV Collector 375
TV Sports Scene, Inc. 376
Taffner, Ltd 494
Taft Broadcasting Co. 469
Taft Entertainment Co. 469
TeleCable Corp. 476
Telecine Film Studios 494
Telecine Spanish Video 376
Tele-Communications, Inc. 476
Telefilm Co., Inc./Saturn Prods. 376
Telemated Motion Pictures 494
Telemount Pictures, Inc. 494
TelePrompTer Corporation 476
Telequest, Inc. 376
Television & Video Almanac (publication) 606
Teleworld, Inc. 494
Telic 494
Telstar, Inc. 376
Tempo TV Network 480
Terr, Michael, Inc. 494
Texas Community Antennas Group 476
Thomas Productions, Bob 495
3M Co./Leisure Time Products 376
Thriller Video 376
Times Mirror Cablevision 476
Titus Productions, Inc. 495
Tobias, Herb, & Associates, Inc. 495
Touchstone Home Video 376
Tournament Video Tapes 376
Tower Productions 495
Trade Publications 605
Trailer Distributors 318
Transvue TV Int'l. 495
Trans World Entertainment 456
Tribune Entertainment 495
Trinity Broadcasting 480
Turn of the Century Fights, Inc. 495
Twentieth Century-Fox Telecommunications, Inc. 480
Twentieth Century-Fox Television, Inc. 469, 495
Two Star Films, Inc. 376
Twyman Films 495

U

UACC Midwest 476
UC Video 376
UPA Productions of America 495
USA Cable Network 480
USA Home Video 356
Understanding Personal Computers 376

Unicorn Video, Inc. 376
United Artists Cablevision Corp. 376
United Entertainment, Inc. 376
United Press International 495
United States Prods. 495
Universal Television 470, 495
Upswing Artists Management Ltd. 376

V

VCI Home Video 377
VC II Home Video 377
VCL Communications, Inc. 377
VIP Video 377
Valiant International Pictures 496
Van Dam Prods. 377
Van Praag Productions 496
Vanguard Video 377
Vencompass, Inc. 377
Veritas Prods. 496
Versatile Television Productions, Inc. 496
Vestron Video 356
Viacom Cable 477
Viacom International 496
Vidcrest 377
Video Action 377
Video Aided Instruction, Inc. 377
Video Arts Intl., Inc. 377
Video Associates 377
Video City Prods. 377
Video Craft 377
Video Dynamics 377
Video Educational Systems 377
Video Gems 377
Video Image, Inc. 378
Video Intl. Publishers, Inc. 378
Video Knowledge, Inc. 378
Video Latino 378
Video Library 378
Video Library of Arts 378
Video Naturals Co. 378
Video Presentation, Inc. 378
Video Reel, Inc. 378
Video Research 378
Video Sports Prods. 378
Video Tech 378
Video Travel, Inc. 378
Video Unlimited, Inc. 378
Video Visa, Inc. 378
Video Vision Associates, Inc. 378
Video Yesteryear 378
Videoamerica 356
Videodisc Publishing, Inc. 378
Videofashion 379
Videograph 379
Videologue Marketing Corp. 379
Videotakes, Inc. 379
Vidmark 379
Vidistrib, Inc. 496
Viking Films Inc. 496
Vision Cable Communications 477
Vision Prods. 379
Vision Prods. Ltd. 379

W

WTBS (Turner) 480
WW Entertainment 496
Wade, Rogers, Productions, Inc. 496
Warner Bros. Television 470, 496
Warner Amex Cable Communications 477
Warner Home Video 356
Weather Channel 480
Weiss Global Enterprises 379, 497
Western Communications 477
Western Film & Video, Inc. 379
Western Publishing Co., Inc. 379
Westlamb Associates 379
Weston Woods Studios, Inc. 379
Who's Who 1–300
Wild Wing Prods. 379
Wilderness Video 379
William Morris Agency 471
Wade Williams Prods. 379
Windward Video 379
Wizard Video, Inc. 379
Wombat Prods. 379
Wonderland Video 380
Wooden Boat Publications, Inc. 380
World Market, The 645
World Video Home Video 380
World Research, Inc. 380
World Video Enterprise, Inc. 380
World Video Pictures 380
Worldvision Enterprises 497
Worldvision Home Video, Inc. 380
Worldwide TV News 498
Wright, Carter Enterprises 498
Wrightwood Entertainment 499

X

Xerox Information Resources Group 380

Z

Z Channel 480
Zenith Electronics Corporation 472
Ziv International 499

Emmy Award Winners

ACADEMY OF TELEVISION ARTS AND SCIENCES

1985–86 TELEVISION ACADEMY AWARDS Categories and Areas of Achievement For the Emmy Award FOR THE PERIOD FROM July 1, 1985 THROUGH June 30, 1986

OUTSTANDING COMEDY SERIES
The Golden Girls Paul Junger Witt, Tony Thomas (executive producers); Paul Bogart (supervising producer); Paul Junger Witt, Tony Thomas, Kathy Speer, Terry Groissman (producers); Marsha Posner Williams (co-producer).

OUTSTANDING DRAMA SERIES
Cagney & Lacey, Barney Rosenzweig (executive producer); Liz Coe (supervising producer); Ralph Singleton, Patricia Green, Steve Brown (producers); P. K. Knelman (co-producer), CBS.

OUTSTANDING MINISERIES
Peter the Great, Marvin J. Chomsky (producer); Konstantin Theoren (line producer), NBC.

OUTSTANDING VARIETY, MUSIC OR COMEDY PROGRAM
The Kennedy Center Honors: A Celebration of the Performing Arts, Nick Vanoff, George Stevens Jr. (producers), CBS.

OUTSTANDING DRAMA/COMEDY SPECIAL
Love Is Never Silent, Marian Rees (executive producer); Juliana Fjeld (co-executive producer), NBC.

OUTSTANDING CHILDREN'S PROGRAM
Anne of Green Gables—Wonderworks, (series); Kevin Sullivan, Lee Polk (executive producers); Kevin Sullivan, Ian McDougall (producers), PBS.

OUTSTANDING LEAD ACTOR IN A COMEDY SERIES
Michael J. Fox, "Family Ties," NBC.

OUTSTANDING LEAD ACTOR IN A DRAMA SERIES
William Daniels, "St. Elsewhere," NBC.

OUTSTANDING LEAD ACTOR IN A MINISERIES OR SPECIAL
Dustin Hoffman, "Death of a Salesman," CBS.

OUTSTANDING LEAD ACTRESS IN A COMEDY SERIES
Betty White, "The Golden Girls," NBC.

OUTSTANDING LEAD ACTRESS IN A DRAMA SERIES
Sharon Gless, "Cagney & Lacey," CBS.

OUTSTANDING LEAD ACTRESS IN A MINISERIES OR SPECIAL
Marlo Thomas, "Nobody's Child," NBC.

OUTSTANDING SUPPORTING ACTOR IN A COMEDY SERIES
John Larroquette, "Night Court," NBC.

OUTSTANDING SUPPORTING ACTOR IN A DRAMA SERIES
John Karlen, "Cagney & Lacey," CBS.

OUTSTANDING SUPPORTING ACTOR IN A MINISERIES OR SPECIAL
John Malkovich, "Death of a Salesman," CBS.

OUTSTANDING SUPPORTING ACTRESS IN A COMEDY SERIES
Rhea Perlman, "Cheers," NBC.

OUTSTANDING SUPPORTING ACTRESS IN A DRAMA SERIES
Bonnie Bartlett, "St. Elsewhere," NBC.

OUTSTANDING SUPPORTING ACTRESS IN A MINISERIES OR A SPECIAL
Colleen Dewhurst, "Between Two Women," ABC.

OUSTANDING INDIVIDUAL PERFORMANCE IN A VARIETY OR MUSIC PROGRAM
Whitney Houston, "The 28th Annual Grammy Awards," CBS.

OUSTANDING GUEST PERFORMER IN A COMEDY SERIES
Roscoe Lee Browne, "The Cosby Show," NBC.

OUTSTANDING GUEST PERFORMER IN A DRAMA SERIES
John Lithgow, "Amazing Stories," NBC.

OUTSTANDING INDIVIDUAL ACHIEVEMENT—CLASSICAL MUSIC/DANCE PROGRAMMING—PERFORMING
Placido Domingo, "Cavalleria Rustiana," "Great Performances," PBS.

OUTSTANDING DIRECTING IN A COMEDY SERIES
Jay Sandrich, "The Cosby Show," "Denise's Friend," NBC.

OUTSTANDING DIRECTING IN A DRAMA SERIES
Georg Stanford Brown, "Cagney & Lacey," "Parting Shots," CBS.

OUTSTANDING DIRECTING IN A VARIETY OR MUSIC PROGRAM
Waris Hussein, "Copacabana," CBS.

OUTSTANDING DIRECTING IN A MINISERIES OR A SPECIAL
Joseph Sargent, "Love Is Never Silent," "Hallmark Hall of Fame," NBC.

OUTSTANDING WRITING IN A COMEDY SERIES
Barry Fanaro, Mort Nathan, "The Golden Girls," "A Little Romance," NBC.

OUTSTANDING WRITING IN A DRAMA SERIES
Tom Fontana, John Tinker, John Masius, "St. Elsewhere," "Time Heals," NBC.

OUTSTANDING WRITING IN A VARIETY OR MUSIC PROGRAM
David Letterman, Steve O'Donnell, Sandy Frank, Joe Toplyn, Chris Elliott, Matt Wickline, Jeff Martin, Gerard Mulligan, Randy Cohen, Larry Jacobson, Kevin Curran, Fred Graver, Merrill Markoe, "Late Night With David Letterman Fourth Anniversary," NBC.

OUTSTANDING WRITING IN A MINISERIES OR A SPECIAL
Ron Cowen, Daniel Lipman (teleplay), **Sherman Yellen,** "An Early Frost," NBC.

OUTSTANDING ACHIEVEMENT IN MUSIC COMPOSITION FOR A MINISERIES OR A SPECIAL
Laurence Rosenthal, "Peter the Great," Part I, NBC.

OUTSTANDING TECHNICAL DIRECTION/ELECTRONIC CAMERAWORK/VIDEO CONTROL FOR A SERIES
For a single episode of a regular series
Gerry Bucci (technical director), **Randy Baer, Dale Carlson, Steve Jones, Donna J. Quante** (camerapersons), **Victor Bagdadi** (senior video control), "The Golden Girls," pilot, NBC.

OUTSTANDING CLASSICAL PROGRAM IN THE PERFORMING ARTS
Wolf Trap Presents the Kirov: Swan Lake, Michael B. Styer (executive producer), Phillip Byrd (senior producer), John T. Potthast (producer), PBS.

OUTSTANDING INFORMATIONAL SERIES
Laurence Olivier—A Life, Nick Evans, Nick Elliott (executive producers), Bob Bee (producer), PBS; **Planet Earth,** Thomas Skinner (executive producer), Gregory Andorfer (series producer); Georgann Kane (coordinating producer), PBS.

OUTSTANDING INFORMATIONAL SPECIAL
W. C. Fields Straight Up, Robert B. Weide (executive producer); Ronald J. Fields (co-producer), PBS.

OUTSTANDING ANIMATED PROGRAM
Garfield's Halloween Adventure, Jay Poynor (executive producer).

OUTSTANDING INDIVIDUAL ACHIEVEMENT—INFORMATIONAL PROGRAMMING—DIRECTING
David Heeley, "The Spencer Tracy Legacy: A Tribute by Katharine Hepburn," PBS.

OUTSTANDING INDIVIDUAL ACHIEVEMENT—CLASSICAL MUSIC/DANCE PROGRAMMING—DIRECTING
Franco Zeffirelli, "Cavalleria Rusticana," PBS.

OUTSTANDING ACHIEVEMENT IN CHOREOGRAPHY
Walter Painter, "Sylvia Fine Kaye's Musical Comedy Tonight," "Great Performances," PBS.

OUTSTANDING INDIVIDUAL ACHIEVEMENT—INFORMATIONAL PROGRAMMING—WRITING
John L. Miller, "The Spencer Tracy Legacy: A Tribute by Katharine Hepburn," PBS.

OUTSTANDING INDIVIDUAL ACHIEVEMENT—CLASSICAL MUSIC/DANCE PROGRAMMING—WRITING
John Ardion, "Gala of Stars 1986," PBS.

OUTSTANDING CINEMATOGRAPHY FOR A SERIES
John McPherson, ASC, "Amazing Stories," "The Mission," NBC.

OUTSTANDING CINEMATOGRAPHY FOR A MINISERIES OR A SPECIAL
Sherwood Woody Omens, ASC, "An Early Frost," NBC.

OUTSTANDING ART DIRECTION FOR A SERIES

Jacqueline Webber (art director), **Norman Rockett** (set decorator), "St. Elsewhere," NBC.

OUTSTANDING ART DIRECTOR FOR A VARIETY OR MUSIC PROGRAM

Roy Christopher (production designer). "The 58th Annual Academy Awards," ABC.

OUTSTANDING ART DIRECTION FOR A MINISERIES OR A SPECIAL

Tony Walton (production designer), **John Kasarda**(art director), **Robert J. Franco** (set decorator), "Death of a Salesman," CBS.

OUTSTANDING ACHIEVEMENT IN MUSIC COMPOSITION FOR A SERIES (Dramatic Underscore)

Arthur B. Rubinstein, "Scarecrow & Mrs. King," "We're Off to See the Wizard," CBS.

OUTSTANDING ACHIEVEMENT IN MUSIC DIRECTION

Ian Fraser (music director), **Ian Fraser, Lanny Meyers, Tommy Newsom, Glen Roven, Larry Schwartz, Torrie Zito** (principal arrangers); "The 1986 Tony Awards," CBS.

OUTSTANDING ACHIEVEMENT IN MUSIC AND LYRICS

Larry Grossman (composer), **Buz Kohan** (lyricist), "Andy Williams and the NBC Kids Search for Santa," NBC.

OUTSTANDING COSTUME DESIGN FOR A SERIES

Alfred E. Lehman, "Murder, She Wrote," "Widow, Weep for Me," CBS.

OUTSTANDING COSTUME DESIGN FOR A VARIETY OR MUSIC PROGRAM

Bill Hargate, "Sylvia Fine Kaye's Musical Comedy Tonight III—Great Performances," PBS.

OUTSTANDING COSTUME DESIGN FOR A MINISERIES OR A SPECIAL

Ella Maklakova (U.S.S.R.), **Sibylle Ulsamer** (Italy), "Peter the Great," Part I, NBC.

OUTSTANDING ACHIEVEMENT IN COSTUMING FOR A SERIES

Susan Smith-Nashold (costume supervisor), **Robert M. Moore** (costumes); **Charles Drayman, Ann Windsor, Kathy O'Rear** (costumers), "St. Elsewhere," NBC.

OUTSTANDING ACHIEVEMENT IN COSTUMING FOR A MINISERIES OR SPECIAL

For a single episode of miniseries or for a special

Joie Hutchison (Women's Costume Supervisor), **Pat McGrath** (Men's Costume Supervisor), **Vicki Sanchez** (Women's Costumer), "North and South, Book I, Part IV," ABC.

OUTSTANDING ACHIEVEMENT IN MAKEUP FOR A SERIES FOR A SINGLE EPISODE OF A REGULAR SERIES

Rod Wilson, "Airwolf—The Horn of Plenty," CBS.

OUTSTANDING ACHIEVEMENT IN MAKEUP FOR A MINISERIES OR A SPECIAL

For a single episode of a miniseries or for a special

Del Acevedo, Paul Stanhope and **Peter Owen,** "Second Serve," CBS.

OUTSTANDING ACHIEVEMENT IN HAIR STYLING FOR A SERIES FOR A SINGLE EPISODE OF A REGULAR SERIES

Bernadette Parker, "Amazing Stories—Gather Ye Acorns," NBC.

OUTSTANDING ACHIEVEMENT IN HAIRSTYLING FOR A MINISERIES OR A SPECIAL

K. G. Ramsey, "Second Serve," CBS.

OUTSTANDING EDITING FOR A SERIES

Neil Mandelberg, "Moonlighting—The Dream Sequence Always Rings Twice," ABC.

OUTSTANDING EDITING FOR A MINISERIES OR A SPECIAL

Jerrold L. Ludwig, A.C.E., "An Early Frost," NBC.

OUTSTANDING EDITING FOR A SERIES

Henry F. Chan, "The Cosby Show—Full House," NBC.

OUTSTANDING EDITING FOR A MINISERIES OR SPECIAL MULTICAMERA PRODUCTION

Pam Marshall, "American Bandstand's 33⅓ Celebration," ABC.

OUTSTANDING SOUND EDITING FOR A SERIES

For a single episode of a regular series.

Richard Anderson (supervising sound editor), **Wayne Alwine, James Christopher, George Frederick, John Stacy, Bert Weinstein** (sound editors), **Lettie Odney** (ADR editor), **Ken Wannberg** (music editor), "Amazing Stories," "The Mission," NBC.

OUTSTANDING SOUND EDITING FOR A MINISERIES OR A SPECIAL

For a single episode of a miniseries or for a special.

David R. Elliott (supervising sound editor), **Dino Di Muro, Mark Friedgen, Mike Graham, Larry Kemp, Joe Mayer, Joe Melody, Stewart Nelson, Eric Scott, Rusty Tinsley, Scot Tinsley, Bill Williams** (sound editors), **Russ Tinsley** (ADR editor), **Daniel A. Carlin** (music editor), "Under Seige," NBC.

OUTSTANDING SOUND MIXING FOR A COMEDY SERIES OR A SPECIAL

(For a single episode of a comedy series or for a special; Emmy(s) to a maximum of four mixers. Pre-production, production, and re-recording mixers are all eligible.)

Michael Ballin, Robert Douglas, Douglas Grey, Thomas Huth, "Cheers," "Fear Is My Co-Pilot," NBC.

OUTSTANDING SOUND MIXING FOR A DRAMA SERIES

For a single episode of a drama series

William Gazecki, Andy McDonald, Bill Nicholson, Blake Wilcox, "St. Elsewhere," "Time Heals Part 2," NBC.

William Gazecki, Andy McDonald, Bill Nicholson, Blake Wilcox, "St. Elsewhere," "Time Heals Part 2," NBC.

OUTSTANDING SOUND MIXING FOR A VARIETY OR MUSIC SERIES OR A SPECIAL

For a single episode of a live or recorded variety or music series or for a special.

Tom Ancell, David E. Fluhr, "Mr. Previn Comes to Town," PBS.

OUTSTANDING SOUND MIXING FOR A DRAMA MINISERIES OR A SPECIAL

For a single episode of a miniseries or special.

David E. Campbell, CAS, John T. Reitz, CAS, Gregg C. Rudloff, CAS, Keith A. Wester, CAS, "An Early Frost," NBC.

OUTSTANDING TECHNICAL DIRECTION/ELECTRONIC CAMERA/VIDEO CONTROL FOR A MINISERIES OR A SPECIAL

Gene Crowe, Harry Tatarian (technical directors), **Toby Brown, Ed Chaney, Mike Denney, Larry Heider, Pat Kenney, Bob Keys, Dave Levisohn, Wayne Orr, Hector Ramirez, Ron Sheldon** (camerapersons), **John Palacio, Keith Winikoff** (senior video control), "Neil Diamond . . . Hello Again," CBS.

OUTSTANDING LIGHTING DIRECTION (ELECTRONIC) FOR A SERIES

For a single episode of a regular series.

Bob Dickinson, "Solid Gold," episode # 283, SYN.

OUTSTANDING LIGHTING DIRECTION (ELECTRONIC) FOR A MINISERIES OR A SPECIAL

For a single episode of a miniseries or for a special.

Marilyn Lowey, John Rook, Kim Killingsworth, "Neil Diamond . . . Hello Again," CBS.

OUTSTANDING SPECIAL VISUAL EFFECTS

Phil Tippet, "Dinosaur!" CBS; **Michael McAlister,** "Ewoks: The Battle for Endor," ABC.

OUTSTANDING GRAPHICS AND TITLE DESIGN

Betty Green, "Stingray," NBC.

1985–86
TELEVISION ACADEMY AWARDS
Categories and Areas of Achievement
For the Emmy Award for Daytime Programs
FOR THE PERIOD FROM March 6, 1985 THROUGH March 5, 1986

OUTSTANDING DRAMA SERIES

William J. Bell, H. Wesley Kenney (executive producers), **Edward Scott, Tom Langan** (producers), "The Young and the Restless," CBS.

OUTSTANDING GAME-AUDIENCE PARTICIPATION SHOW

Bob Stewart (executive producer), **Anne Marie Schmitt** (producer), "The $25,000 Pyramid," CBS.

OUTSTANDING CHILDREN'S SERIES

Dulcy Singer (executive producer), **Lisa Simon** (producer), "Sesame Street," PBS.

OUTSTANDING CHILDREN'S SPECIAL

Frank Doelger, Mark Gordon (executive producers), **Alan C. Blomquist** (producer), "The War Between the Classes," CBS.

OUTSTANDING LEAD ACTRESS, DRAMA SERIES:

Erika Slezak, "One Life to Live," ABC.

OUTSTANDING LEAD ACTOR, DRAMA SERIES

David Canary, "All My Children," ABC.

OUTSTANDING SUPPORTING ACTRESS, DRAMA SERIES

Leann Hunley, "Days of Our Lives," NBC.

OUTSTANDING SUPPORTING ACTOR, DRAMA SERIES

John Wesley Shipp, "As the World Turns," CBS.

OUTSTANDING INGENUE, DRAMA SERIES

Ellen Wheeler, "Another World," NBC.

OUTSTANDING YOUNGER LEADING MAN, DRAMA SERIES
Michael E. Night, "All My Children," ABC.
OUTSTANDING GAME SHOW HOST
Dick Clark, "The $25,000 Pyramid," CBS.
OUTSTANDING TALK-SERVICE SHOW HOST
Phil Donahue, "Donahue," syndicated.
OUTSTANDING DRAMA SERIES DIRECTING TEAM
Dennis Steinmetz, Rudy Vejar, Frank Pacelli (directors), **Randy Robbins, Betty Rothenberg** (associate directors), "The Young and the Restless," CBS.
OUTSTANDING DRAMA SERIES WRITING TEAM
William J. Bell (head writer), **Kay Alden, John F. Smith, Sally Sussman, Eric Freiwald, John Randall Holland, Meg Bennett, Enid Powell** (writers), "The Young and the Restless," CBS.
OUTSTANDING ANIMATED PROGRAM
Jim Henson, Margaret Loesch, Lee Gunther (executive producers), **Bob Richardson** (producer), **Hank Saroyan** (director), **Jeffrey Scott** (writer), "Jim Henson's Muppet Babies," CBS.
OUTSTANDING TALK-SERVICE PROGRAM
Patricia McMillen (executive producer), **Gail Steinberg** (senior producer), **Lorri Antoszi Benson, Janet Harrell, Marlaine Selip, Susan Sprecher** (producers), "Donahue," syndicated.
OUTSTANDING SPECIAL CLASS PROGRAM AREA
Helen Marmor (executive producer), **Randoph Wands, Jennie Tong** (producers), "Chagall's Journey," NBC; **John Goberman** (producer), "Live From Lincoln Center: Chamber Music Society of Lincoln Center with Irene Worth and Horacio Gutierrez," PBS.
OUTSTANDING PERFORMER, IN CHILDREN'S PROGRAMMING
Pearl Bailey, "Cindy Eller: A Modern Fairy Tale," ABC.
OUTSTANDING GAME SHOW DIRECTING
Dick Carson, "The Wheel of Fortune," NBC.
OUTSTANDING TALK/SERVICE SHOW DIRECTING
Russel F. Morash, "This Old House," PBS.
OUTSTANDING DIRECTING IN CHILDREN'S PROGRAMMING
Martin Sheen, "Babies Having Babies" ("CBS Schoolbreak Special"), CBS.
OUTSTANDING WRITING IN A CHILDREN'S SERIES
Norman Stiles, Sara Compton, Tom Dunsmuir, Judy Freudberg, Tony Geiss, Emily Kingsley, David Koar, Sonia Manzand, Jeff Moss, Mark Saltzman, Nancy Sans, Luis Santeiro, Cathy Rosenberg Turow, "Sesame Street," PBS.
OUTSTANDING WRITING IN A CHILDREN'S SPECIAL
Jeffrey Auerbach, Kathryn Montgomery, "Babies Having Babies" ("CBS Schoolbreak Special"), CBS.
OUTSTANDING SPECIAL CLASS WRITING AREA
Catherine Faulkner, "Chagall's Journey," NBC.
OUTSTANDING ART DIRECTION/SET DECORATION/SCENIC DESIGN
Victor Dinapoli (art designer), **Nat Monsioi** (set decorators), "The Price Is Right," CBS.
OUTSTANDING TECHNICAL DIRECTION/ELECTRONIC CAMERA/VIDEO CONTROL
Dick Holden (technical director/electronic camera), "This Old House," PBS.
OUTSTANDING CINEMATOGRAPHY
Elswitt Robert, "The War Between the Classes" ("CBS Schoolbreak Special").
OUTSTANDING MUSIC DIRECTION AND COMPOSITION
Michael Franks (music director/composer), "Are You My Mother?" ("ABC Afterschool Special"), ABC.
OUTSTANDING GRAPHICS AND TITLE DESIGN
James Castle, "New Love American Style," ABC.
OUTSTANDING MAKEUP AREA
Larry Abbott, "No Greater Gift" ("ABC Afterschool Special"), ABC.
OUTSTANDING LIVE & TAPE SOUND MIXING AND SOUND EFFECTS FOR A DRAMA SERIES
Scott A. Millan (preproduction & production mixer), **Tommy Persson** (production mixer), **Rafael O. Valentin, Donald D. Henderson** (postproduction mixers), **Larry Mabbiore, Peter Romano** (sound effects technicians), "The Young and the Restless," CBS.
OUTSTANDING LIGHTING DIRECTION FOR A DRAMA SERIES
Frank Olson, Jeme Youte, Hal Anderson, Lincoln John Stulik, "As the World Turns," CBS.
OUTSTANDING COSTUME DESIGN FOR DRAMA SERIES
David Danble, Nanzi Adzima, Bud Santora, "Guiding Light," CBS.
OUTSTANDING LIGHTING DIRECTION
Carl Gibson, "Kids, Incorporate," syn.
OUTSTANDING COSTUME DESIGN
Bill Kellard (live action), **Caroly Wilcox, Richard Termine, David Valasquez, Robert Flanagan** (Muppets), "Sesame Street," PBS.
OUTSTANDING ART DIRECTION/SET DECORATION/SCENIC DESIGN FOR A DRAMA SERIES
Sy Tomashoff (art director), **Jay Garvin** (set decorator), "Capitol," CBS.
OUTSTANDING TECHNICAL DIRECTION/ELECTRONIC CAMERA/VIDEO CONTROL FOR A DRAMA SERIES
Rick Labbold, Chuck Guzzi (technical directors), **Gorm Erickson, Pat Kenney, Bob Welsh, Ted Morales, Toby Brown, Paul Johnson** (camera personnel), **Roberto Bosio, Janice Bendiksen** (senior video control), "Capitol," CBS.
OUTSTANDING MUSIC DIRECTION AND COMPOSITION FOR A DRAMA SERIES
Jill Diamond, Rae Kraus (music directors), **Billy Chinnock, Patricia Stotter, James Lawrence** (composers) "Search for Tomorrow," NBC.
OUTSTANDING MAKEUP FOR A DRAMA SERIES
Pam P. K. Cole (head makeup artist), **Diane Lewis, Donna Messina, Catherine McCann Davison, Sundi Martino, Becky Bowen,** "General Hospital," ABC.
OUTSTANDING HAIRSTYLING FOR A DRAMA SERIES
Linda Librizzi Williams, Ralph Stanzione, "Guiding Light," CBS.
OUTSTANDING HAIRSTYLING AREA
Sherry Baker, "Pippi Longstocking," ABC.
OUTSTANDING VIDEO TAPE EDITING
Stuart Pappe, "Babies Having Babies" ("CBS Schoolbreak Special"), CBS.
OUTSTANDING LIVE & TAPE SOUND MIXING AND SOUND EFFECTS
Mark Bovos (production mixer), **Tom Huth** (postproduction mixer), **Mike Mitchel** (sound effects technician), "Babies Having Babies," ("CBS Schoolbreak Special"), CBS.
OUTSTANDING FILM EDITING
Harvey Greenstein, Wally Katz, Douglas W. Smith, "3-2-1 Contact," PBS.
OUTSTANDING FILM SOUND EDITING
David Gelfand (supervising editor), **Laura Civiello** (sound editor), **David Gelfand** (supervising music editor), "Don't Touch," ("ABC Afterschool Special"), ABC.
OUTSTANDING FILM SOUND MIXING
Petur Hliddal (production mixer), **Thomas Fleischman** (recording mixer), "Can a Guy Say No?" ("ABC Afterschool Special"), ABC.

WINNERS FOR TV JOURNALISM:

OUTSTANDING COVERAGE OF A SINGLE BREAKING NEWS STORY (PROGRAMS)
Mexican Earthquake (9/23/85) (Evening News), Lane Vernardos, exec. producer; David Browning, Tom Bettag, sr. producers; Dan Rather, reporter-correspondent, CBS; **Crash of Delta** (8/2/85) ("Nightline"), Richard N. Kaplan, exec. producer; William Moore, Robert Jordan, sr. producers; Robert LeDonne, Steve Lewis, Tara Sonenshine, Heather Vincent, Kyle Gobson, producers; James Walker, Ted Koppel, reporter-correspondents, ABC; **Colombian Volcano** (11/15/85) ("Nightline"), Richard N. Kaplan, exec. producer; William Moore, Robert Jordan, sr. producers; Sergio Guerrero, Monica Harari Schnee, producers; Ted Koppel, reporter-correspondent, ABC.
COVERAGE OF A SINGLE BREAKING NEWS STORY (SEGMENTS)
In the Fire's Path (7/11/85) ("20/20"), David Doss, producer; Ken Kashiwahara, reporter-correspondent, ABC; **A Bank Fails** (12/4/85) ("Evening News"), Lane Vernardos, exec. producer; Linda Mason, sr. producer; Lance Heflin, prod.; Jane Byrant Quinn, reporter, CBS; **Trojan Horse** (12/4/85) ("Evening News"), Michael Gavshon, producer; Allan Pizzey, reporter, CBS.
OUTSTANDING BACKGROUND/ANALYSIS OF A SINGLE CURRENT STORY (PROGRAMS)
In South Africa (3/8,19,22/85), Richard N. Kaplan, exec. producer, William Moore, Robert Jordan, Betsy West, sr. producers; Lionel Chapman, Terry Irving, Steve Lewis, Tara Sonenshine, producers; Kenneth Walker, Jeff Greenfield, reporters, ABC; **Acid Rain: New Bad News** (4/2/85) ("Nova"), John Angier, producer-reporter, PBS; **Men Who Molest** (4/16/85) ("Frontline"), Rachel V. Lyon, producer; Bobbie Birleffi, reporter, PBS.
OUTSTANDING BACKGROUND/ANALYSIS OF A SINGLE CURRENT STORY (SEGMENTS)
Schizophrenia (12/1/85) ("60 Minutes"), Allan Maraynes, producer; Ed Bradley, reporter, CBS; **Farm Suicide** (2/13/85) ("MacNeil/Lehrer"), Les Crystal, exec. producer; Mike Joseloff, Joe Quinlan, producers; Kwame Holman, correspondent; Marie MacLean, reporter, PBS; **Vietnam Remembered** (4/19,22,25/85) ("World News Tonight"), Sally V. Holm, producer, Richard Threlkeld, correspondent, ABC; **Ronald Reagan: The Movie** (12/15/85) ("60 Minutes"), Suzanne St. Pierre, producer; Morley Safer, correspondent, CBS.
INVESTIGATIVE JOURNALISM (PROGRAMS)
Retreat from Beirut (2/26/85) ("Frontline"), David Fanning,

exec. producer; Sherry Jones, sr. producer; Nancy Gross, producer; William Greider, correspondent, PBS.

INVESTIGATIVE JOURNALISM (SEGMENTS)

Mob Gas (12/3,4/85) ("Nightly News"), Brian Ross, Ira Silverman, producers; Brian Ross, reporter, NBC; **International Christian Aid Investigation** Charles Stuart, sr. producer; Peter Lance, reporter, ABC; **Military Medicine** (1/10/85), Chuck Collins, producer; Mark Nykanen, reporter, NBC.

OUTSTANDING INTERVIEW/INTERVIEWER(S) (PROGRAM)

The Times of Harvey Milk (11/13/85), Robert Epstein, Richard Schmiechen, producers; Harvey Fierstein, interviewer, PBS.

OUTSTANDING INTERVIEW/INTERVIEWER(S) (SEGMENTS)

Liz Carpenter: A Conversation With Bill Moyers ("Sunday Morning"), Lindsay Miller, producer; Bill Moyers, interviewer, CBS.

OUTSTANDING COVERAGE OF CONTINUING NEWS STORY (SEGMENTS)

AIDS: Chapter One (2/12/85) ("Nova"), Paula S. Apsell, executive producer; Thea Chalow, producer, PBS.

OUTSTANDING COVERAGE OF A CONTINUING NEWS STORY (PROGRAMS)

Children in Poverty (10/21, 22/85) ("World News Tonight"), Richard O'Regan, Susan Aasen, producers; Karen Burnes, reporter, ABC; **Africa: Struggle for Survival** (7/16,22,26/85), ("CBS Evening News With Dan Rather"), Martin Koughan, producer, Bill Moyers, reporter, CBS; **Vietnam Now** (4/22,23,24/85) ("CBS Evening News With Dan Rather"), Lane Vernardos, exec. producer; Linda Mason, sr. producer; Bob Anderson, producer; Bob Simon, reporter, CBS.

SPECIAL CLASSIFICATION FOR OUTSTANDING PROGRAM/ ACHIEVEMENT (PROGRAMS)

The Skin Horse (10/16/85), Nicki Green, exec. producer; Nigel Evans, Sue Ducat, producers, PBS; **The Times of Harvey Milk** (11/13/85), Robert Epstein, Richard Schmiechen, producers, PBS.

SPECIAL CLASSIFICATION FOR OUTSTANDING PROGRAM ACHIEVEMENT (SEGMENTS)

Paul Host (12/15/85) ("America Today"), Joan Steffend, co-producer, reporter-correspondent, PBS; **Bicycle Messengers** (5/10//85) ("On the Road"), Bernard Birnbaum, sr. producer; Cathy Lewis, producer, Charles Kuralt, reporter-correspondent, CBS.

OUTSTANDING INFORMATIONAL, CULTURAL OR HISTORICAL PROGRAMMING (FOR PROGRAMS)

My Heart, Your Heart (2/27/85) ("MacNeil/Lehrer Newshour"), Lawrence Pomeroy, producer; Jim Lehrer, reporter-correspondent, PBS; **Hiroshima Remembered** (8/6/85) Laurie Toth, producer; Gail Harris, reporter-correspondent, PBS; **The Lifer and the Lady** (2/5/85) ("Frontline"), John Kastner, producer PBS; **A Class Divided** (3/26/85) ("Frontline"), David Fanning, exec. producer; William Peters, producer; Charlie Cobb, correspondent, PBS.

OUTSTANDING INFORMATIONAL, CULTURAL OR HISTORICAL PROGRAMMING (FOR SEGMENTS)

Music Man (12/30/85) ("American Almanac"), Linda Ellman, producer, Lucky Severson, correspondent, NBC; **The Beeb** (9/15/85) ("60 Minutes"), John Tiffin, producer; Morley Safer, reporter-correspondent, CBS; **Julia** (3/10/85) ("60 Minutes"), Don Hewitt, exec. producer; Philip Scheffler, sr. producer; Marti Galovic Palmer, producer, CBS.

OUTSTANDING INDIVIDUAL ACHIEVEMENT IN NEWS AND DOCUMENTARY PROGRAMMING—WRITERS

Perry Wolff, Elena Mannes, "Whose America Is It?" (9/3/85) ("CBS Reports"), CBS; **Marshall Frady, Judy Crichton, John Fielding, Christopher Isham, Phil Lewis, Steve Singer, Andrew Schlesinger, Peter Bull,** "The Fire Unleashed" (6/6/85), ABC.

OUTSTANDING INDIVIDUAL ACHIEVEMENT IN NEWS AND DOCUMENTARY PROGRAMMING—DIRECTORS

Elena Mannes, "Whose America Is It?" (9/3/85) ("CBS Reports"), CBS; **Paul Wagner, Marjorie Hunt,** "The Stone Carvers" (7/4/85), PBS; **Harry Rasky,** "Homage to Chagall—The Colours of Love" (7/15/85), PBS.

OUTSTANDING INDIVIDUAL ACHIEVEMENT IN NEWS AND DOCUMENTARY PROGRAMMING—CINEMATOGRAPHERS

Belinda Wright, Stanley Breeden, "Land of the Tiger: A National Geographic Special" (1/16/85), PBS.

OUTSTANDING INDIVIDUAL ACHIEVEMENT IN NEWS AND DOCUMENTARY PROGRAMMING—ELECTRONIC CAMERAPERSONS: VIDEOGRAPHERS (STUDIO & LOCATION)

Michael Watson, "3 Segments: Desert, Winter Calving, Colorado Gold" (8/4, 3/24, 10/27/85) ("America Today"), PBS; **Isadore Bleckman,** "Bicycle Messengers" (5/10/85) (5/10/85) ("CBS Evening News, On the Road"), CBS.

OUTSTANDING INDIVIDUAL ACHIEVEMENT IN NEWS AND DOCUMENTARY—SOUND

Joan Franklin, sound editor; **Alan Berliner, Albee Gordon,** sound recordist, "The Slave Ships of the Sulu Sea" (10/31/85) ("20/20"), ABC; **Belinda Wright,** "Land of the Tiger: A National Geographic Special" (1/16/85), PBS.

OUTSTANDING INDIVIDUAL ACHIEVEMENT IN NEWS AND DOCUMENTARY PROGRAMMING—FILM EDITORS & FILM POSTPRODUCTION EDITORS

Annamaria Szanto, "The Precious Legacy" (2/22/85), PBS; **Deborah Hoffmann, Robert Epstein,** "The Times of Harvey Milk" (11/13/85), PBS.

OUTSTANDING INDIVIDUAL ACHIEVEMENT IN NEWS AND DOCUMENTARY PROGRAMMING—TAPE EDITORS: VIDEOTAPE EDITORS AND VIDEOTAPE POSTPRODUCTION EDITORS

Jess Bushyhead, videotape editor, "The Music Man" (12/30/85) ("American Almanac"), NBC; **Jess Bushyhead,** videotape editor, "The Year 1985 in Review" (12/31/85) ("Today"), NBC.

OUTSTANDING INDIVIDUAL ACHIEVEMENT IN NEWS AND DOCUMENTARY PROGRAMMING—TITLE SEQUENCES

John Ridgway, art director, **Craig Rice, Teri Freedman, Ron Clark, Harry Marks,** "Entertainment This Week" (6/8/85), syn.

OUTSTANDING INDIVIDUAL ACHIEVEMENT IN NEWS AND DOCUMENTARY PROGRAMMING—MUSIC COMPOSERS

Lyn Murray, "Miraculous Machines" ("PBS National Geographic Special"), PBS.

INDEX OF ADVERTISERS

A

Agfa-Gevaert, Inc. 1-A

B

Bookcrafters, Inc. 653
Brookhaven Press .... 25-A, 340, Third Cover

D

Ducommun, M. Company 5-A

E

Eastman Kodak 13-A

F

Filmtreat International 309

M

MGM/UA Communications Co. 9-A
Morris, William Agency 2-A

R

Rank Film Laboratories 11-A
Rank Organisation, The 7-A

S

Silvercup Studio Associates .... Back Cover

W

Will Rogers Institute 654
Worldvision Enterprises, Inc. ...... Second Cover

Who's Who

In MOTION PICTURES and TELEVISION

A

AAMES, WILLIE: Actor. r.n. William Upton. b. California, July 15, 1960.
PICTURES: Hog Wild, Scavenger Hunt, Zapped!, Cut and Run.
TELEVISION: We'll Get By, Courtship of Eddie's Father, The Odd Couple, Swiss Family Robinson, Wait Til Your Father Gets Home, Eight is Enough, etc.

AARON, PAUL: Director. Bdwy. shows include Salvation, Paris Is Out, '70 Girls '70, Love Me Love My Children, etc.
PICTURES: A Different Story, A Force of One, Deadly Force.
TELEVISION: The Miracle Worker, Thin Ice, Maid in America, When She Says No.

AARON, ROY H.: Executive. Attorney in L.A. law firm of Pacht, Ross, Warne, Bernhard & Sears. Joined Plitt Companies in 1978 as snr. v.p. & gen. counsel. In 1980 named pres. & chief operating officer of Plitt Theatres, Inc. and related Plitt companies.

ABARBANEL, SAM X.: Producer, writer, publicist. b. Jersey City, N.J. Mar 27, 1914. e. Cornell U & U. of Illinois, B.S. 1935. Newspaperman Chicago before joining N.Y. exploitation dept. Republic, then to studio as ass't. publicity director. World War II in Europe with 103rd Div. After war independent publicist and producer. Co-prod. Argyle Secrets, 1948. Co-wrote orig. s.p., co-produced U.A.'s Prehistoric Women, 1950. Exec. Prod. U.A.'s Golden Mistress. In 1963 to Spain as associate prod. MGM's Gunfighters of Casa Grande, and Son of Gunfighter. Formed own co. in Spain, 1966. Produced Narco Men. Co-authored, prod. Last Day of War. Orig. & co-s.p. Avco's Summertime Killer, 1972.

ABEL, WALTER: Actor, b. St. Paul, Minn., 1898; e. Amer. Acad. Dram. Art, N.Y. Role in touring co. of N.Y. prod. "come Out of the Kitchen," then stock, vaudeville; stage mgr. touring cos. Minnie Maddern Fiske & others; on Broadway in "A Square Peg," "Long Watch"; m.p. sound debut in "Three Musketeers" 1935.
PICTURES INCLUDE: Witness Chair, Racket Busters; Arise, My Love; Holiday Inn, Star Spangled Rhythm, 13 Rue Madeleine, Kid from Brooklyn, Hal Roach Comedy Carnival, So This Is Love, Island in the Sky, Night People, Indian Fighter, The Steel Jungle, Bernadine, Raintree County, Handle with Care, Mirage.

ABELES, ARTHUR: Chairman, Filmarketeers, Ltd. b. 1914. Educated Duke University, Columbia University, U.S. 1939–1941: general manager, West Indies, Warner. 1941. assistant general manager, Brazil, Universal. 1942–5: general manager, Uruguay, Warner. 1945–7: supervisor, Argentina, Chile, Uruguay, Paraguay, Warner. 1948–68: Managing director, Warner Bros. Pictures, Warner Theatre, Warner Bros. Production; Director Henderson Film Laboratories; Vice-pres., Warner Bros. Intl. in chg. of Europe, the Near East and North Africa. 1968–70; Managing director, Universal Pictures Ltd. Vice-president Universal International in charge of U.K., Continent and Middle East. 1970–7: Co-chairman, Cinema International Corporation. 1978: Chairman, Filmarketeers, Ltd.-Filmbond Services (London) Ltd.

ABEND, SHELDON: Executive. b. New York, N.Y. June 13, 1929. Maritime Labor-Rel. Negotiator, 1954–56; chmn., Maritime Union, 1954–56; head, exec. dir. Research Co. rep. estates decreased authors, est. 1957. indep. literary negotiator, C&C films, A.A.P., RKO General Inc., David O. Selznick, 1959–65; pres. American Play co. Inc., Century Play Co. Inc., 1961–72; est. Million Dollar Movie Play Library, 1962; pres. American Literary Consultants est. 1965; exec. v.p. Chantec Enterprises Inc. 1969–72. Marketing Literary Consultant for Damon Runyon Estate. Copyright analyst and literary rights negotiator, United Artists Corp. Founder and chrm. of Guild for Author's Heirs, 1970–72, Literary negotiator and prod. consultant for Robert Fryer, 1972. Founder of the Copyright Royalty Co. for Authors' Heirs, 1974; copyright consultant for Films, Inc. 1975; literary agent for Bway. play, Chicago, 1975. Owner of 53 classic RKO motion pictures for the non-theatrical markets. Distributed by Films, Inc. Revived publishing of Damon Runyon stories in quality paperback in conjunction with Runyon-Winchell cancer fund. Published six mystery stories written by Cornell Woolrich—all of which were produced by Alfred Hitchcock for TV & motion pictures, 1976. 1978–assoc. prod. of film, Why Would I Lie?; Originator of Million Dollar Movie Book Theatre and Million Dollar Movie Sound Track Co., 1980; assoc. prod. of Bdwy. revival, Shanghai Gesture, 1981. Published thru Ballantine five Cornell Woolrich books owned by S. Abend, 1982–83; Co-authored book. The Guardians; 1985, published through William Morrow, Romance of the Forties by Damon Runyon, 1986; 1985, founded American Concerts, Inc. and American Theatre Collections, Inc. Pres. of both.

ABRAHAM, F. MURRAY: Actor. b. Oct. 24, 1940. Attended Univ. of (1959-61); trained for stage at Herbert Berghof Studio with Uta Hagen. Stage debut in Los Angeles in The Wonderful Ice Cream Suit, 1965. New York debut in Fantasticks, 1966. Film debut in Serpico, 1974.
PICTURES: The Sunshine Boys, All the President's Men, The Big Fix, Scarface, Amadeus. (AA-best actor).
TELEVISION: Love of Life, Kojak, Marco Polo, How to Survive a Marriage, All in the Family, Dream West, etc.

ABRAHAMS, GARY: Executive. e. Univ. of Arizona (BA); in 1968 joined Paramount TV as asst. to v.p.; 1974–75, asst. to prod., The Movies; 1971–78, assoc. dir., Los Angeles Intl. Film Exposition (Filmex); 1978, joined Marble Arch Productions, as exec. asst. to pres.; named dir. of corporate relations & merchandising, 1979; project coordinator, Los Angeles Film Center, 1981. v.p., Cable Programming, Interscopr Communications, 1982; dir. of development, American Cinematheque, 1984.

ABRAHAMS, JIM: Producer-Writer-Director. b. Milwaukee, WI, May 10, 1944. e. Univ. of Wisconsin. 1979, with friends David and Jerry Zukor, opened the Kentucky Fried Theatre in Madison—a multimedia show specializing in live improvisational skits mixed with videotaped and film routines and sketches, with the threesome writing and appearing in most. Opened new theatre in Los Angeles in 1972 and developed large following. Trio wrote script for first film, The Kentucky Fried Movie, followed by Airplane! (1980) which they also wrote and jointly directed and served as executive producers.
PICTURES: Top Secret! (co-dir., co-s.p.); Ruthless People (co-dir.)

ABRAHAMS, MORT: Producer. b. New York, N.Y., exec. prod. Producers Showcase, NBC-TV June 1956–57; Suspicion, 1958; dir. programming, prod., NTA, 1958–1960; exec. prod. Cooga Mooga Prod. Inc., 1960–1961. Producer: Target, The Corruptors 1961, Route 66, 1962–63; writer T.V. Shows, 1963–64; prod., Kraft Suspense Theatre, 1965; prod., Man from U.N.C.L.E., 1965–66; Executive Vice-President, AJAC Prod. 1966. Assoc. prod. "Doctor Doolittle," "Planet of the Apes," "Goodbye, Mr. Chips." Prod., "The Chairman." Assoc. producer & writer, "Beneath the Planet of the Apes"; 1969, Vice President in charge of production, Rastar Prods.: 1971–74 exec. prod. American Film Theatre & v.p. Ely Landay Org. in chg. West Coast prod. exec. prod. on Luther, Homecoming, Man in the Glass Booth; 1977–78, exec. prod., The Greek Tycoon, Hopscotch, exec. prod., 1980; exec. in chg. prod., The Chosen, Beatlemania, 1981; exec. prod., The Deadly Game; 1982, exec. prod. Separate Tables, Mr. Halpern and Mr. Johnson; prod., Arch of Triumph (CBS); exec. prod., The Holcraft Covenant (Thorn-EMI); v.p., World Media Prods. Inc.

ACKERMAN, BETTYE: Actress. b. Cottageville, S.C., Feb. 28, 1928. e. Columbia Univ., 1948–52. Taught dancing 1950–54.
PLAYS INCLUDE: No Count Boy (1954), Tartuffe (1956), Sophocles' Antigone, and "Oedipus at Colonus" (1956). The Merchant of Venice (1971).
PICTURES INCLUDE: Face of Fire (1959), Companions in Nightmare, Rascal.
TV: Alcoa Premiere, Hitchcock, Perry Mason, Breaking Point, Dr. Maggie Graham on Ben Casey series for five yrs., Hope-Chrysler Theatre, Bonanza, FBI Story, Mannix, Ironsides, "Medical Center," regular on "Bracken's World," Colombo, Sixth Sense, Heat of Anger, Return to Peyton Place, (6 months 1972) Rookies, Barnaby Jones, Police Story, Gunsmoke, Harry O, Streets of San Francisco, S.W.A.T., Petrocelli, Wonder Woman, Police Woman, Chips, 240-Robert, The Waltons, Dynasty, Falcon Crest, Me and Mom, Trapper John M.D.
LP RECORDS: Salome & School for Scandal.

ACKERMAN, HARRY S.: Executive. b. Albany, N.Y., Nov. 17, 1912, e. Dartmouth Coll. Began as writer, actor, producer. Joined Young & Rubicam adv. agcy. 1936; became v.p. of program operations, 1946. Exec. prod. CBS, 1948. Dir. of network programs—Hollywood, June, 1948; v.p. charge network radio programs, 1950; v.p. chge. network TV programs CBS-TV, Hollywood, June, 1951; exec. dir. spec. progs. CBS network, 1956; formed independent company 1957; v.p. and exec. prod. Screen Gems Inc., 1958–1973; pres. Harry Ackerman Prods. nat'l. pres., Academy TV Arts and Sciences, two terms; now pres., Harry Ackerman Prods.

ACKLAND, JOSS: Actor. b. London, England, Feb. 29, 1928. Member of old Vic; toured Russia and U.S. with them. Over 400 TV appearances.
PICTURES INCLUDE: Seven Days to Noon, Royal Flash, Crescendo, The House That Dripped Blood, Villain, England Made Me, The Black Windmill, Great Expectations, The Greek Tycoon, Someone is Killing the Great Chefs of Europe, Saint Jack, The Apple, Rough Cut, Lady Jane.

ADAM, KEN: Art dir. b. Berlin, Germany, 1921. e. St. Pauls School, London, and London Univ., student of architecture. 6 years war service as RAF pilot. Ent. m.p. ind. as draughtsman 1947. Art dir. Around the World in 80 Days, Trials of Oscar Wilde, Dr. No, Sodom and Gomorrah, Dr. Strangelove, Goldfinger, Thunderball, Ipcress File, You Only Live Twice, Funeral in Berlin, Chitty Chitty Bang Bang, Goodbye Mr. Chips, The Owl and the Pussycat, Diamonds Are Forever, Sleuth, The Last of Sheila, Barry Lyndon, Salon Kitty, 7% Solution, The Spy Who Loved Me, Moonraker, King David, Agnes of God.

ADAMS, BROOKE: Actress. b. New York City. e. High School of Performing Arts; Institute of American Ballet; Lee Strasberg. Made professional debut at age of six in Finian's Rainbow. Worked steadily in summer stock and TV until age 18. After hiatus resumed acting career.
PICTURES: Car Wash, Days of Heaven, Invasion of the Body Snatchers, Cuba, a Man, a Woman and a Bank, Utilities, The Dead Zone, Almost You, Key Exchange.
TELEVISION: James Dean: Portrait of a Friend, The Last of the Belles, The Lords of Flatbush, The Daughters of Joshua Cabe, Murder on Flight 502, The Bob Newhart Show, Police Woman, Lace, Special People, Lace II.

ADAMS, DON: Actor. b. New York City, Apr. 13, 1926. Won Arthur Godfrey talent contest. Was nightclub impressionist before starting in TV.
PICTURE: The Nude Bomb.
TELEVISION: Bill Dana Show, Get Smart, The Partners, Hooray for Hollywood, Don Adams Screen Test, Three Times Daley, Billy.

ADAMS, EDIE: Actress, singer. r.n. Edith Adams Kovacs. b. Kingston, Pa., April 16, 1931. e. Juilliard School of Music, Columbia School of Drama.
STAGE: Wonderful Town, 1952–54; Lil Abner, 1956–57.
TV: The Chevy Show, 1958: Take a Good Look, 1960–61; Here's Edie, 1962–63; Movie: Ernie Kovaks' Between the Laughter.
PICTURES INCLUDE: The Apartment, Mad, Mad, Mad, Mad World, Call Me Bwana, Under the Yum, Yum Tree, Love With A Proper Stranger, Lover Come Back, The Best Man, Maid in Paris, The Honey Pot, Up in Smoke.

ADAMS, GERALD DRAYSON: Writer. b. Winnipeg, Manitoba; e. Oxford University. Export exec. 1925–30; literary agt. 1931–45. Member: Screen Writers' Guild.
PICTURES INCLUDE: (jt. orig. screen story) Magnificent Rogue, (jt. s.p.) Plunderers, (s.p.) Gallant Legion, (jt. s.p.) Big Steal; collab. story, Dead Reckoning; Orig. s.p. Battle of Apache Pass, Son of Ali Baba, Flaming Feather, Flame of Araby; collab. s.p. Lady from Texas, Steel Town, Untamed, Frontier; story, collab. s.p., Duel at Silver Creek; st., s.p., Princess of the Nile, Three Young Texans, Gambler from Natchez; st., Wings of the Hawk, Between Midnight and Dawn; st., adapt., Taza son of Cochise; collab. s.p. story, Gambler from Natchez, Chief Crazy Horse, s.p. Golden Horde; adapt. s.p. Prince Who Was a Thief; orig. s.p., Sea Hornet; s.p., Three Bad Sisters; orig., s.p., Duel on the Mississippi; orig. Black Sleep, s.p., War Drums; story, collab. s.p., Gun Brothers; story, Affair in Reno; story, s.p., Frontier Rangers; story, s.p., Gold, Glory & Custer; orig. story, collab. s.p., Kissin Cousins. Orig. s.p. Harem Scarem.
TV: Maverick, G.E. Theatre, Northwest Passage, Broken Arrow, Cheyene, 77 Sunset Strip.

ADAMS, JULIE: Actress. r.n. Betty May Adams. b. Waterloo, La., Oct. 17, 1928; e. Jr. Coll., Little Rock, Ark., m. Ray Danton, Actor; Coll. dramatic; m.p. debut in Red Hot and Blue, Bright Victory; as Betty Adams in: The Dalton Gang, Marshal of Heldorado, West of the Brazos; since in Hollywood Story, Finders Keepers, Bend of the River, Treasure of Lost Canyon, Horizons West, Lawless Breed, Mississippi Gambler, Man from the Alamo, Wings of the Hawk, Star of Tomorrow, 1953.
PICTURES INCLUDE: Tickle Me, The Last Movie, MCQ, The Wild McCullochs, Killer Force, The Fifth Floor.
TV: Go Ask Alice, Capitol.

ADDISON, JOHN: Composer. b. West Chobham (Surrey) Eng., March 16, 1920; e. Wellington and Royal Coll. of Music. Entered m.p. ind. in 1948, Professor, Royal College of Music.
PICTURES INCLUDE: (Music scores) The Honey Pot, Torn Curtain, A Fine Madness, I Was Happy Here, The Loved One, Guns At Batasi, The Uncle, Girl With Green Eyes, Tom Jones, The Loneliness of the Long Distance Runner, A Taste of Honey, The Charge of the Light Brigade, Smashing Time, Start The Revolution Without Me, Country Dance (in U.S., Brotherly Love), Forbush and the Penguins, Sleuth, Luther, Dead Cert, Ride A Wild Pony, Seven-Per-Cent Solution, Swashbuckler, Joseph Andrews, A Bridge Too Far, The Pilot, High Point, Strange Invaders, Grace Quigley, Code Name: Emerald.
BALLETS INCLUDE: Carte Blanche (at Sadler Wells and Edinburgh Festival).
PLAYS INCLUDE: The Entertainer, The Chairs, Luther, Midsummer Nights Dream, The Broken Heart, The Workhouse Donkey, Hamlet, Semi-Detached, The Seagull, Saint Joan of the Stockyards, Listen to the Mockingbird, Cranks (revue), Antony & Cleopatra, I Claudius, Twelfth Night, Bloomsbury.
TV: Sambo and the Snow Mountains, Detective, Hamlet, The Search for Ulysses, Way of the World, Back of Beyond, Black Beauty, The Bastard, Deadly Price of Paradise, Centennial, Pearl, Love's Savage Fury, Like Normal People, The French Atlantic Affair, Nero Wolfe, Mistress of Paradise, Eleanor First Lady of The World, Charles and Diana: A Royal Love Story, Mail Order Bride, Ellis Island, Murder She Wrote, Thirteen at Dinner, Dead Man's Folly, Mr. Boogedy.
STAGE MUSICALS: The Amazons, Popkiss.

ADELMAN, GARY: Executive. e. Calif. State Univ., Long Beach State. 1969, asst. dir. on feature, The Masterpiece; assoc. prod. on The Candy Snatchers. Produced first feature film, The Severed Arm, 1974. Assisted Winston Hock in development of 3-D process, 1975. 1976–82, pres. & COO of Monarch Prods. Post-prod. consultant for Jerry Gross Organization. 1983, founder and partial owner of New Image Releasing, Inc., new prod. & dist. co. Holds post of secty./treas.

ADELMAN, JOSEPH A.: Executive. b. Winipeg, Manitoba, Canada, Dec. 27, 1933. e. New York University, B.A., 1954; Harvard Law School, J.D., 1957, graduated cum laude, Attorney, United Artists Corp., New York, 1958; named west coast counsel, Hollywood, 1964; named executive assistant to the vice-president in charge of production 1968; named vice-president, west coast business and legal affairs, 1972; named executive vice-president, Association of Motion Pictures and Television Producers, 1977. Admitted to New York, California and U.S. Supreme Court bars; member, Phi Beta Kappa; American Bar Association; Los Angeles Copyright Society; Academy of Motion Picture Arts and Sciences; legislative liaison committee, Motion Picture Association of America; board of directors, AMPTP, 1969– ; board of trustees, Theatre Authority, 1970– .

ADELSON, MERV: Producer. b. Los Angeles, Oct. 23, 1929. e. UCLA. Bd. chmn., Lorimar Productions.
PICTURES INCLUDE: Twilight's Last Gleaming, The Choirboys, Who Is Killing the Great Chefs of Europe?, Avalanche Express, The Big Red One.
TELEVISION: The Waltons, Eight Is Enough, Dallas, Kaz, The Waverly Wonders, Knots Landing, Sybil, A Man Called Intrepid, The Blue Knight, Helter-Skelter.

ADJANI, ISABELLE: Actress. B. Germany, June 27, 1955.
PICTURES: The Slap, The Story of Adele H., The Tenant, Faustine, Barocco, The Driver, Nosferatu—The Vampire, The Bronte Sisters, Quartet, Next Year If All Goes Well, One Deadly Summer, Subway, Ishtar.

ADLER, BOB: Actor, r.n. Robert Fick Adler. b. Hoboken, N.J., Mar. 24, 1906. Ranch Foreman, polo player, horse trainer, riding instructor; horseman in D. W. Griffiths "America" 1924, and others; in many Westerns since; member 20th-Fox Stock Co. from 1944.
PICTURES INCLUDE: My Darling Clementine, Smoky, Captain from Castile, Green Grass of Wyoming, Yellow Sky, Broken Arrow, Two Flags West, Lure of the Wilderness, Inferno, Hell and High Water, Prince Valiant, Broken Lance, Violent Saturday, Untamed, The Tall Men, Bottom of the Bottle, Proud Ones, The Silver Ship, Valerie, Fury at Showdown, Yellow Sky, Rope Law, Untamed, Rios Conchos, Whiskey Renegades, Stagecoach, Bandalero, The Undefeated.
TV: Flicka, Broken Arrow, Have Gun Will Travel, Cheyenne, Laramie, Rawhide, Bonanza, Daniel Boone, Gunsmoke, Batman, Judd, Big Valley, Lancer, Outcasts, Land of the Giants, Medical Center.

ADRIAN, IRIS: Actress, r.n. Iris Adrian Hostetter. b. Los Angeles, May 29, 1913; p. prof. Dancer, on stage N.Y. and abroad in "Follies of 1931"; m.p. debut in MGM two-reel color films.
PICTURES INCLUDE: Smart Woman, Out of the Storm, Paleface, Sky Dragon, There's a Girl in My Heart, Tough Assignment, Once a Thief, Always Leave Them Laughing, Stop That Cab, My Favorite Spy, Highway Magnet, Fast & The Furious, Crime Wave, Devil's Harbor, Carnival Rock, The Buccaneer, Blue Hawaii, The Errand Boy, Fate is the Hunter, That Darn Cat, The Odd Couple, The Love Bug.

AGAR, JOHN: Actor. b. Chicago, Ill., Jan 31, 1921. In service World War II. Has appeared in Fort Apache, Adventure in Baltimore.
PICTURES INCLUDE: I Married a Communist, Sands of Iwo Jima, She Wore a Yellow Ribbon, Breakthrough, Magic Carpet, Along the Great Divide, Woman of the North Country, Man of Conflict, Bait, Rocket Man, Shield for Murder, Golden Mistress, Revenge of the Creature, Hold Back Tomorrow, Tarantula, Star in the Dust, Joe Butterfly, St. Valentine's Day Massacre, Waco, Johnny Reno, Women of the Prehistoric Planet.

AGUTTER, JENNY: Actress. b. Taunton, England, 1952. e. Elmhurst Ballet School. m.p. debut East of Sudan, 1964. Emmy for best supporting actress, 1971; Variety Club of Grt. Britain Most Promising Artiste Award 1971; BAFTA best supporting actress award for Equus, 1976.
PICTURES: Ballerina, Gates of Paradise, Star!, I Start Counting, Walkabout, The Railway Children, War of Children, Logan's Run, The Eagle Has Landed, The Man in the Iron Mask, Equus, Dominique, Clayton & Catherine, The Riddle of the Sands, Sweet William, The Survivor, Amy, The American Werewolf, Secret Places.
PLAYS: School for Scandal, Rooted, Arms and the Man, The Ride Across Lake Constance, The Tempest, Spring Awakening, Hedda, Betrayal, 1982–83 Member, Royal Shakespeare Co.—King Lear, Arden of Taversham, The Body.
TELEVISION: The Great Mr. Dickens, The Cherry Orchard, The Snow Goose, As Many as Are Here Present, A House in Regent Place, There's Love and Dove, Kiss Me and Die, A Legacy, The Waiting Room, Six Million Dollar Man, School Play, The Mayflower, Voyage of the Pilgrims, Beulah Land, Love's Labor Lost.

AIELLO, DANNY: Actor. b. June 20, 1933. On Broadway before entering films.
PICTURES: Blood Brothers, Fingers, Defiance, Hide in Plain Sight, Ft. Apache, the Bronx, Chu Chu and the Philly Flash, The Purple Rose of Cairo, Key Exchange, The Protector.
TELEVISION: Family of Strangers, Lady Blue.

AIMEE, ANOUK: Actress. b. April 27, 1934. Paris, France. r.n. Francoise Dreyfus. Studied, Bauer-Therond dramatic school, Paris. Debut: 1946. La Maison Sous La Mer.
FILMS INCLUDE: Les Amants De Verone, The Golden Salamander, Le Rideau Cramoisi, Nuit D'Orage, La Bergere et Le Ramoneur (Cartoon), Mauvais Rencontres, Nina, Stresemann, Tous Peuvent Me Tuer, Pot Bouille, Modigliani of Montparnasse, Le Tete Contres Les Murs, Les Dragueurs, La Dolce Vita, Le Farcuer, Lola, Les Amours De Paris L'Imprevu, 8½, Sodom and Gomorrah, La Fuga, A Man and a Woman, Un Soir, Un Train, The Appointment, The Model Shop, Justine, The Mandarians, Tragedy of a Ridiculous Man, Leap into the Void.

AKINS, CLAUDE: Actor. b. Nelson, Ga., May 25, 1918. e. Northwestern Univ. Worked as salesman in Indiana before joining Barter Theatre for season. Came to New York; appeared in The Rose Tattoo. Spent several seasons with touring cos.
PICTURES INCLUDE: From Here to Eternity, The Caine Mutiny, Skyjacked, Flap, Devil's Brigade, Inherit the Wind, The Great Bank Robbery.
TV: Police Story, Cannon, McCloud, Marcus Welby, M.D., Mannix, The Streets of San Francisco, Movin' On, The Rhinemann Exchange, Mini-Series: Dream West.

AKTER, MAHMOOD ALI KHAN: Producer-Distributor-Exhibitor: b. Hyderabad Deccan, India, Apr. 12, 1926. Graduate of Arts. Formerly with Columbia Films of Pakistan Ltd., gen. mgr., Hussein & Co. controlling film dist. of United Artists Corp., Selznick Intl., London Films, Pathe Overseas. Participant foreign leaders prog. of Intl. Educational Exchange Service of U.S.A. State Dept.; mgr., Paramount Films of Pakistan, Ltd., 1959–64; mgr. dir., General Film Distributors, Lahore. Chm., Motion Picture Importer's Group, Lahore, Mgr. dir., Pak Boor Corp.

ALBECK, ANDY: Executive. Pres & chief exec. officer, United Artists Corp. b. U.S.S.R., Sept. 25, 1921. Industry career began in 1939 with Columbia Pictures Intl. Corp. 1947, Central Motion Picture Exchange. 1949, Eagle Lion Classics, Inc. Joined UA in 1951 in intl. dept., functioning in the area of operations. After filling a number of key posts, named asst. treas. in 1970. In 1972 became v.p. of UA and its subsidiary, UA Broadcasting, Inc. 1973, appt. pres. of UA Broadcasting and in 1976 named snr. v.p.—operations. Named UA Corp. pres. & chief exec. officer in 1978. Retired, 1981.

ALBERGHETTI, ANNA MARIA: Singer, actress. b. Pesaro, Italy, May 15, 1936; d. Daniele Alberghetti, cellist. Concert debut in 1948 in Pesaro, then toured Italy, Scandinavia, Spain; Am. debut Carnegie Hall, 1950, sang with N.Y. Philharmonic Society, Phila. Symphony, on television. Screen debut in The Medium, 1950; then Here Comes Groom, Stars Are Singing, Last Command, 10,000 Bedrooms, Cinderfella. Star: Carnival. Broadway stage. Winner Antoinette Perry (Tony) Award for best actress.
TV: Toast of the Town, Cavalcade of Stars, Arthur Murray Show, Bob Hope, Eddie Fisher, Red Skelton, Dinah Shore, Desilu Playhouse, G.E. Theatre, Chevy Show, Dupont Show, Voice of Firestone, Colgate Hour, Climax, Loretta Young, Ford Jubilee, Perry Como.

ALBERT, EDDIE: Actor. r.n. Eddie Albert Heimberger. b. Rock Island, Ill. Apr. 22, 1908, e. U. Minn., Radio NBC.
BROADWAY: Brother Rat, Say Darling, The Music Man, Room Service, The Boys from Syracuse, Seven Year Itch, You Can't Take It With You, Our Town, No Hard Feelings, Reuben Reuben, Miss Liberty.
PICTURES INCLUDE: Brother Rat, Four Wives, Angel from Texas, Dispatch from Reuter's, Rendezvous With Annie, Perfect Marriage, Smash-Up, The Story of a Woman, Time Out of Mind, Hit Parade of 1947, Dude Goes West, You Gotta Stay Happy, Fuller Brush Girl, You're in the Navy Now, Carrie, Meet Me After the Show, Actors and Sin, Roman Holiday, Girl Rush, I'll Cry Tomorrow, Oklahoma Attack, Teahouse of the August Moon, Orders to Kill, Gun Runners, Roots of Heaven, The Young Doctors, The Longest Day, Captain Newman, The Heartbreak Kid, Miracle of the White Stallions, Seven Women, McQ, The Take, The Longest Yard, Escape to Witch Mountain, The Devil's Rain, Hustle, Birch Interval, Foolin' Around, Yesterday, The Concorde-Airport 79, The Border, Ladyfingers, How to Beat the High Cost of Living, Take This Job and Shove It, Yes, Giorgio, Bless 'em All, Dreamscape;, Stitches, Head Office.
TV: Green Acres, Switch!, The Yeagers, Benjamin Franklin, The Borrowers, Killer Bees, Nutcracker, Anything Goes, Crash, The Word, Evening in Byzantium, Pirates Key, Living in Paradise, Oklahoma Dolls, The Plan, Peter and Paul, The Fall Guy, Goliath Awaits, Concord, Beyond Witch Mountain, Rooster, Love Boat, Rhode Island Demon Murder, Coalfire, In like Flynn, Dress Gray.

ALBERT, EDWARD: b. Los Angeles, Feb. 20, 1951. e. UCLA. Son of actor Eddie Albert and actress Margo. Was prod. asst. on Patton in Spain. Has appeared with father on radio and TV shows. Is photographer and has exhibited work in L.A.
PICTURES INCLUDE: Butterflies Are Free (debut), Forty Carats, Midway, The Domino Principle, The Greek Tycoon, When Time Ran Out, A Time To Die, Ellie, Getting Even.
TELEVISION: Yellow Rose, The Last Convertible.

ALBRIGHT, LOLA: Actress. b. Akron, Ohio, July 20, 1925; e. Studied piano 12 years. Switchboard operator and stenographer NBC; stenographer with WHAM and bit player; photographers' model. screen debut in "The Pirate" 1948.
PICTURES INCLUDE: Easter Parade, Girl from Jones Beach, Tulsa, Champion, Good Humor Man, Bodyhold, When You're Smiling, Sierra Passage, Killer That Stalked New York, Arctic Flight, Silver Whip, Treasure of Ruby Hills, Magnificent Matador, Beauty on Parade, Tender Trap, A Cold Wind in August, Kid Galahad, Lord Love a Duck, Where Were You When the Lights Went Out?, The Impossible Years, The Money Jungle.

ALCAINE, JOSE LUIS: Cinematographer. b. Tangier, Algeria, Dec. 26, 1938. e. Spanish Cinema School, Madrid. After graduation joined Madrid's Studio Moros doing commercials.
PICTURES INCLUDE: El Puente, El Sur, Taseo, Rustlers' Rhapsody, etc.

ALDA, ALAN: Actor. b. New York City, Jan. 28, 1936. e. Fordham. f. Robert Alda. Studied at Cleveland Playhouse; performed with Second City, then on TV in That Was The Week That Was; Broadway credits include The Owl and The Pussycat, Purlie Victorious, Fair Game For Lovers (Theatre World Award), The Apple Tree (Tony Award nomination).
PICTURES INCLUDE: Gone Are The Days, The Moonshine War, Jenny, The Mephisto Waltz, Paper Lion, To Kill a Clown, Same Time Next Year, California Suite, The Seduction of Joe Tynan (also dir.), The Four Seasons (actor, dir., s.p.), Sweet Liberty (also s.p., dir.).
TV: M*A*S*H, The Glass House.

ALDON, MARI: Actress. b. Toronto, Canada, Nov. 17, 1930. e. Central High, Toronto. A.T.C.L. of Trinity College, London, England: With Canadian ballet six yrs.; nat'l co. of Streetcar Named Desire, sang on radio; m.p. debut in Distant Drums; since in The Tanks Are Coming, This Woman Is Dangerous, Tangier Incident, Barefoot Contessa, Race for Life, Summertime.

ALDREDGE, THEONI V.: Costume Designer. b. Salonika, Greece. On Bdwy. (Timon of Athens, Two Gentlemen of Verona, A Chorus Line, Annie, 42nd Street, etc.) as well as theatrical films.
PICTURES INCLUDE: You're A Big Boy Now, Last Summer, I Never Sang for My Father, The Great Gatsby, The Fury, Eyes of Laura Mars, The Champ, The Rose, Rich and Famous, Annie, Ghostbusters.

ALEXANDER, JANE: Actress. b. Boston, Oct. 28, 1939. e. Sarah Lawrence Coll., Univ. Edinburgh. Stage career includes appearances on Bdwy., at Arena Stage, Washington, and Shakespeare Festival at Stamford, Conn.
PICTURES: The Great White Hope, A Gunfight, The New Centurions, All the President's Men, The Betsy, Night Crossing, Testament, City Heat, Square Dance, Sweet Country.
TELEVISION: Welcome Home, Johny Bristol, Miracle on 34th St., Death Be Not Proud, Eleanor and Franklin, Eleanor and Franklin: The White House Years, Playing for Time, When She Says No, Calamity Jane, Malice in Wonderland, Blood & Orchids.

ALEXANDER, RALPH: Executive. Began career with Universal Pictures in sales, 1949; various sls. jobs with 20th Century Fox and Lorimar. 1981–82, v.p., theatrical foreign sls., Filmway Pictures; 1982–84, v.p., sls, for Latin America & Southeast Asia, Embassy Pictures Intl. 1984, exec. v.p., multi-media foreign sls. for Robert Meyers Intl. Nov., 1985, joined Dino De Laurentiis Corp. as intl. sls. dir. in chg. all foreign sls. theatrical and ancillary rights except tv. 1986, promoted to v.p., intl. sls., DEG.

ALGAR, JAMES: Prod.-writer-director. b. Modesto, Calif. June 11, 1912. e. Stanford U.; B.A., M.A. Journalism. Entire career since 1934. Walt Disney Prods. Animator: Snow White; Director: Fantasia, Bambi, Wind in the Willows, Ichabod & Mr. Toad.
DOCUMENTARIES: war. health. True-Life Adventures: Seal Island, The Living Desert, Vanishing Prairie, The African Lion, Secrets of Life.
FEATURE CREDITS: Ten Who Dared, The Incredible Journey, Gnome-Mobile, White Wilderness, Rascal, The Legend of Lobo, The Jungle Cat, Run, Cougar, Run.
TELEVISION CREDITS: Producer: Run Light Buck, Run, The Not So Lonely Lighthouse Keeper, One Day on Beetle Rock, Wild Heart, Along the Oregon Trail, The Best Doggoned Dog in the World, One Day at Teton Marsh, Solomon, the Sea Turtle, Manado the Wolverine, Wild Geese Calling, Two Against the Arctic, Bayou Bay, Secrets of the Pond, Boy Who Talked to Badgers, Big Sky Man. Wrote and co-produced Great Moments with Mr. Lincoln; New York World's Fair; Circarama, America the Beautiful, Circle Vision 1958 Brussels World's Fair, Disneyland, Hall of Presidents, Disney World, Florida.
Shares in nine Oscars.

ALIN, MORRIS: Editor, writer, publicist, lyricist. e. College of the City of New York came into the M.P. industry, auditor of Hunchback of Notre Dame, roadshow oper., 1924; asst. sls. prom. mgr. Universal, 1926–27; slsmn., Universal, 1927; assoc. editor. The Distributor, MGM publication, 1927; editor, 1928–33; writer, publicist, MGM Studio, 1933–34; writer, publicist, Hollywood, New York, 1935–38; rej. Universal. 1938, editor, Progress: (Univ. publication); Twice winner of award, International Competition on Industrial Journalism; Senior publicist and Progress editor, Universal, 1961–67; editor Enterprise Press, 1968; member, executive Enterprise Press 1973; American Guild of Authors and Composers, American Society of Composers, Authors and Publishers, National Academy of Popular Music, and Motion Picture Pioneers.

ALLAN, TED: b. Clifton, Ariz., Comm. artist, actor SAG 1945, cameraman; photo training at Technicolor, Consolidated, MGM labs.; portrait photog., MGM, 20th-Century Fox, Selznick; created own film studio, 1952, prod. M.P. features, TV series, & pilots; Dir. of photog. 1956; 2 yr. contract Sinatra Enter.; 9 yrs. head CBS Cam. Dept. Hollywood; 3 yrs. 20th Cen. Fox, Pub-Stills & Featurettes for Von Ryan's Express, Fantastic Voyage, Sand Pebbles, Dr. Doolittle, The Detective, Lady in Cement, Tora, Tora, Tora. Featurettes for Universal: Seven Per Cent Solution, Hindenburg, Rollercoaster, Two Minute Warning, Gray Lady Down, The Promise, Dracula, Same Time Next Year.

ALLAND, WILLIAM: Producer. b. Delmar, Del., March 4, 1916. e. Baltimore. Acted in semi-professional groups; with Orson Welles' Mercury Theatre as actor, stage mgr.; asst. prod. Mercury Theatre radio series; ac., dialogue dir., Citizen Kane; act., Macbeth; U.S. Air Force, World War II; then radio writer; prod., Universal, 1952.
PICTURES INCLUDE: The Raiders, Flesh and Fury, Stand At Apache River, It Came From Outer Space, Creature From The Black Lagoon, Johnny Dark, This Island Earth, Dawn At Socorro, Four Guns To The Border, Chief Crazy Horse, Revenge Of The Creature, Tarantula, Creature Walks Among Us, Gun for a Coward, Land Unknown, Deadly Mantis, Mole People, Raw Wind in Eden, The Lady Takes a Flyer, As Young As We Are; Paramount, The Party Crashers, Colosus of New York, The Space Children; Allied Artists, Look In Any Window, The Lively Set.

ALLEN, DAYTON: Performer. b. New York, N.Y., Sept. 24, 1919. e. Mt. Vernon H.S. Motion picture road shows, 1936–40; disc jockey, WINS, N.Y., 1940–41; writer, vaudeville comedy bits, 1941–45; then radio comic, puppeteer and voices; TV since 1948; film commercials; shows include Oaky Doky, Bonny Maid Varieties, Howdy Doody, Jack Barry's Winky Dink, Abe Lincoln in Illinois, The Circle of Chalk, The Steve Allen Show.

ALLEN, DEDE: Film Editor. b. 1924. Once a messenger at Columbia Pictures, moved to editing dept., then to commercials and features.
PICTURES INCLUDE: Odds Against Tomorrow (1959), America, America, Bonnie and Clyde, Rachel Rachel, Alice's Restaurant, Little Big Man, Serpico, Dog Day Afternoon, Slapshot, The Wiz, Reds, Harry and Son, Mike's Murder, The Breakfast Club, Off Beat.

ALLEN, HERB: Producer. b. San Francisco, Calif., Dec. 24, 1913. e. U. of San Francisco, Pasadena Playhouse. Radio actor, anncr., Los Angeles, San Francisco; m.c., packager. Meet the Champ, children's TV show; asso. prod., Bob Crosby Show; prod., Johnny Carson show. CBS-TV.

ALLEN, IRVING: Dir., Prod. b. Poland, Nov. 24, 1905; e. Georgetown U., Ph.B. 1926. Film ed. Universal, Paramount, Republic 1929–40; shorts dir. RKO & Warner 1941–42; Academy Award 1942 for ed. short subject "Forty Boys and a Song"; U.S. Signal Corps officer 1942–45; debut as dir. "Strange Voyage" 1945; Academy Award 1947, prod. "Climbing the Matterhorn," best two-reel short. Exec. prod., Warwick Films.
PICTURES INCLUDE: Avalanche, Strange Voyage, High Conquest, 16 Fathoms Deep, Man on the Eiffel Tower, New Mexico, Slaughter Trail, (prod.): Paratrooper, Hell Below Zero, The Black Knight, Prize of Gold, Cockleshell Heroes, Safari, Zarak, Pickup Alley, Fire Down Below, High Flight, No Time to Die, The Man Inside, Bandit of Zhobe, Idol on Parade, Adamson of Africa, Jazz Boat, In the Nick, Let's Get Married, The Trials of Oscar Wilde, The Hellions, The Long Ships, Ghengis Khan, The Silencers, Murderers Row, The Ambushers, Hammerhead, The Wrecking Crew, The Desperados, Run Wild, Run Free, Cromwell, Eyewitness, The Story of a Racehorse.

ALLEN, IRWIN: Producer. b. New York, N.Y. e. Columbia U., CCNY, journalism & adv. ed., Hollywood; radio prod. dir., daily Hollywood program, 11 yrs.; radio & literary dir., own agency; then M.P. prod.
PICTURES INCLUDE: Double Dynamite, Girl in Every Port (co-prod.); assoc., prod., Where Danger Lives; prod., Dangerous Mission, The Animal World; prod., co-writer, director, The Story of Mankind; prod., writer, director, Sea Around Us (Academy Award), prod., co-writer, The Big Circus; prod., co-writer, director, The Lost World, Voyage to the Bottom of the Sea, Five Weeks in a Ballon; prod., director action sequences, The Poseidon Adventure, The Towering Inferno. The Swarm (prod.-dir.); Beyond the Poseidon Adventure (prod.-dir.); When Time Ran Out (prod.).
TV: Creator-prod., Voyage to the Bottom of the Sea, Lost in Space, Land of the Giant, The Time Tunnel, Adventures of the Queen, Swiss Family Robinson, Flood, Fire, The Return of Captain Nemo, Hanging by a Thread, Cave-In, Night the Bridge Fell Down, Memory of Eva Ryker. Producer: Code Red, Alice in Wonderland.

ALLEN, JAY PRESSON: Writer-Producer. b. Ft. Worth, TX, March 3, 1922. Wrote play, Prime of Miss Jean Brodie, produced on Bdwy. and also for theatrical films and TV. Wrote Forty Carats for stage.
PICTURES: Marnie, Prime of Miss Jean Brodie, Travels

with My Aunt, Cabaret, Funny Lady, Just Tell Me What You Want, It's My Turn also exec. prod.), Prince of the City (exec. prod.), Deathtrap (exec. prod.).

ALLEN, KAREN: Actress. b. Carrollton, Ill. e. George Washington Univ., Univ. of Maryland. Auditioned for theatrical company in Washington, D.C. and won a role in Saint, touring with it for 7 months. Spent several years with Washington Theatre Laboratory Co. Moved to N.Y., acting in student films at NYU and studying acting with Lee Strasberg at Theatre Institute. Major film debut in National Lampoon's Animal House in 1978.
PICTURES: Manhattan, The Wanderers, Cruising, A Small Circle of Friends, Raiders of the Lost Ark, Shoot the Moon, Split Image, Strange Invaders, Until September, Starman.
TELEVISION: Circle of Children, Part II.

ALLEN, LEWIS: Director. b. Shropshire, England, Dec. 25, 1905; e. Tettenhall Coll., Staffs, Eng. Exec. in chg. of N.Y. & London prod. for Gilbert Miller; actor & stage dir. N.Y. & England; dir. (N.Y.) Laburnum Grove, Amazing Doctor Clitterhouse, Ladies & Gentlemen; (London) The Women, studied m.p. prod. at Paramount 2 yrs.; apptd. dir. with debut of "The Uninvited" 1943.
PICTURES INCLUDE: Appointment With Danger, Suddenly, Another Time Another Place, The Lorelei.

ALLEN, MEL: TV commentator b. Birmingham, Ala., Feb. 14, 1913. e. U. Alabama, A.B. 1932, U. Alabama Law School LL.B. 1936. Started as sportscaster in Birmingham, while in law school; speech instructor in U. Ala. 1935–37; to N.Y. 1937, as staff announcer CBS to 1943; served in U.S. Army World War II in infantry until the war ended, then before discharge was transferred to work on NBC Army Hour; sportscasting throughout U.S., joined N.Y. Yankees, 1946, concurrently narrating many shorts incl. How to Make a Yankee, appearing on radio & video and in Babe Ruth Story; sports commentator Fox Movietonews; voted best sportscaster in Motion Picture Daily-Fame radio. TV polls; Monitor, NBC; NCAA TV College Football, NBC; World Series (1938–1964), CBS-NBC; Rose Bowl (1951–1962), NBC; Sports Broadcasters Hall Of Fame.

ALLEN, NANCY: Actress. b. New York City, June 24.
PICTURES: The Last Victim, The Last Detail, Carrie, I Wanna Hold Your Hand, Home Movies, 1941, Dressed to Kill, Blow Out, The Buddy System, Not for Publication, Terror in the Aisles.
TELEVISION: Movie: The Gladiator.

ALLEN, REX: Actor. b. Wilcox, Ariz., Dec. 31, 1922; e. Wilcox H.S. 1939. Vaudeville & radio actor; WLS, Chicago, 5 yrs.; was rodeo star appearing in shows through USA.
PICTURES INCLUDE: Arizona Cowboy, Hills of Oklahoma, Under Mexicali Stars, Thunder in God's Country, Rodeo King & The Senorita, I Dream of Jeanie, Last Musketeer, South Pacific Trail, Old Overland Trail, Down Laredo Way, Phantom Stallion, For the Love of Mike, Tomboy and the Champ; narr., Walt Disney.
TV: Perry Como Special; commercials, Wonderful World of Color (NBC) Frontier Doctor.
RECORDINGS: Crying in The Chapel, Don't Go Near the Indians, Warner Bros. Records. 1966 Radio Man of the Year; 1966 Cowboy Hall of Fame.

ALLEN, ROBERT: Actor. e. Dartmouth Coll. Began film career in 1926.
PICTURES INCLUDE: Love Me Forever, Party Wire, Winter Carnival, Crime and Punishment, Pride of the Marines, Black Room Mystery, Death Flies East, Air Hawks, Bob Allen Ranger Series, Craig's Wife, Awful Truth, Lady of Secrets, Keep Smiling, Meet the Girls, Everybody's Baby, The City, Winner Take All, Fire-Away, Pie In The Sky.
PLAYS INCLUDE: Blessed Event, Popsy, Kiss Them for Me, Show Boat, I Killed the Count, Auntie Mame, A Few Wild Oats, Time Out for Ginger.
TV: Kraft, Armstrong Theatre, Philco, The Web, Suspense, Ethel & Albert, Danger, Lux Playhouse, Pulitzer Prize Playhouse, Lamp Unto My Feet.

ALLEN, STEVE: Performer. b. New York, N.Y., Dec 26, 1921. U.S. Army 1942; radio shows, Los Angeles; TV, N.Y., 1950; shows include: What's My Line, Steve Allen Show, Tonight, I've Got a Secret, Meeting of Minds, Laughback.
PICTURES INCLUDE: Down Memory Lane, Warning Shot, I'll Get By, Benny Goodman Story, College Confidential.
COMPOSER OR LYCRICIST: This Could Be the Start of Something Big, Pretend You Don't See Her, South Rampart St. Parade, Picnic, .Houseboat, On the Beach, Sleeping Beauty, Bell, Book and Candle, Gravy Waltz, Impossible.
AUTHOR: Fourteen For Tonight, Steve Allen's Bop Fables, The Funny Men, Wry On the Rocks, The Girls on the Tenth Floor, The Question Man, Mark It and Strike It, Not All of Your Laughter, Not All of Your Tears, Bigger Than a Breadbox, A Flash of Swallows, The Wake, Princess Snip-Snip and the Puppykittens, Curses, Schmock-Schmock!, Meeting of Minds, Ripoff, Meeting of Minds-Second Series, Rip-off, Explaining China, The Funny People, Talk Show Murders, Beloved Son: Story of the Jesus Cults, More Funny People, How To Make a Speech, How To Be Funny.

ALLEN, WOODY: Actor, Director, Writer. r.n. Allen Stewart Konigsberg. b. New York City, 1935. Began writing comedy at age 17, contributing to various magazine and top TV comedy shows.
STAGE: Author of Play It Again, Sam; Don't Drink The Water.
PICTURES INCLUDE: What's New Pussycat? (story, screenplay, actor); Casino Royale (actor); What's Up Tiger Lily? (dubbed scr., act.); Take the Money and Run (co-story, co-scr., dir., act.); Bananas (scr., dir., act.); Everything You Always Wanted to Know About Sex* But Were Afraid to Ask (scr., dir., act.); Sleeper, (scr., dir., act.); Love and Death (s.p., act.); The Front (act.), Annie Hall (co. s.p., dir., act.); Interiors (s.p., dir.); Manhattan (co.-s.p., dir., act.); Stardust Memories (s.p., dir., act.); A Midsummer Night's Sex Comedy (s.p., dir.). Zelig (s.p., dir., act.), Broadway Danny Rose (s.p., dir., act.); The Purple Rose of Cairo (dir., s.p.); Hannah and Her Sisters (dir., s.p., actor).

ALLISON, FRAN: Performer. b. LaPorte City, Iowa; m. Archie Levington; e. Coe College, Cedar Rapids; sch. teacher, Iowa; started radio career as songstress Iowa Sta., 1934; starred in numerous programs, Chicago, 1937; Aunt Fanny of Breakfast Club; Fran of Kukla, Fran and Ollie on TV since 1947. Numerous commercials, daily TV variety show, 1958; Fac. mem., Careers Acad. Milwaukee.

ALLYSON, JUNE: Actress. r.n. Ella Geisman. b. Westchester, N.Y., Oct. 7, 1917. Started as chorus girl in school; m.p. debut in Best Foot Forward (1943). Voted one of ten best money-making stars in m.p. Herald-Fame poll, 1955.
BROADWAY INCLUDES: Best Foot Forward, 40 Carats, National Company, No No Nanette.
PICTURES INCLUDE: Girl Crazy, Thousands Cheer, Meet the People, Two Girls and a Sailor, Secret Heart, Reformer and Redhead, Right Cross, Too Young to Kiss, Girl in White, Battle Circus, Remains to be Seen, The Stratton Story, Little Women, Executive Suite, Glenn Miller Story, Woman's World, Strategic Air Command, The Strike, McConnell Story, You Can't Run Away From It, Opposite Sex, Interlude, My Man Godfrey, Stranger In My Arms, They Only Kill Their Masters, That's Entertainment!
TV: The June Allyson Show, Movie-of-the-Week: See the Man Run, 20th Century Follies.

ALMENDROS, NESTOR: Cinematographer. b. Barcelona, Spain, 1930. Worked with numerous directors in Europe—notably Eric Rohmer and Francois Truffaut—before coming to U.S.
PICTURES INCLUDE: La Collectionneuse, My Night at Maud's, Clare's Knee, Love in the Afternoon, Perceval Le Gallois, The Wild Child, The Man Who Loved Women, The Story of Adele H., The Last Metro, Days of Heaven (Oscar, 1978), Goin' South, Madame Rosa, Kramer Vs. Kramer, The Green Room, Love on the Run, The Valley, The Blue Lagoon, Still of the Night, Places in the Heart.

ALMOND, PAUL: Producer-Director-Writer. b. Montreal, Canada, April 26, 1931; e. McGill U., Balliol Coll., Oxford. 1954–66 produced and directed over a hundred television dramas in Toronto, London, N.Y., and Hollywood; prod., dir., s.p., Isabel 1968, Act of the Heart 1970; Etrog (dir.; best Canadian feature); Journey 1972; Ups and Downs, 1982.

ALONSO, MARIA CONCHITA: Actress-Singer. b. Cuba, 1957. Family moved to Venezuela when she was five. 1971, Miss Teenager of the World. 1975, Miss Venezuela. Appeared in four feature films and 10 soap operas before coming to U.S. Recorded several albums as singer.
PICTURES: Moscow on the Hudson, Touch and Go, A Fine Mess.

ALTERMAN, JOSEPH GEORGE: Executive. b. New Haven, Conn., Dec. 17, 1919. e. Wesleyan Univ., B.A., 1942; Institute for Organization Management, Yale Univ. 1957–59; exec. assist., SoundScriber Corp., 1945–48; district mgr., Industrial Luncheon Service, 1948–55; asst. secretary and admin. Secretary, Theatre Owners of America, 1955; Exec. dir. and vice pres., Natl. Assn. of Theatre Owners, 1966; Exec. v.p. COMPO., 1970.

ALTMAN, ROBERT: Director, writer, producer. b. Kansas City, Mo., Feb. 20, 1925. e. U. of Mo. Worked as Director for Dean Story; dir., Countdown, That Cold Day in the Park, M.A.S.H.; s.p. and dir., McCabe & Mrs. Miller, Brewster McCloud, Images, The Long Goodbye, Thieves Like Us, California Split, Nashville, Buffalo Bill and the Indians, The Late Show (prod.) Welcome to L.A. (prod.), Three Women (prod., dir., s.p.); A Wedding (prod., dir.); Remember My Name (prod.); Quintet (prod., dir.); A Perfect Couple (prod., dir.); Rich Kids (prod.); Health (prod., dir., s.p.), Popeye (dir.); Come Back to the Five & Dime, Jimmie Dean, Jimmie Dean (co-prod., dir.): Streamers (co-prod., dir.).

TV: Wrote, prod. and dir., Roaring Twenties, Bonanza, Bus Stop, Combat, Kraft Theatre and pilots for The Gallant Men and The Long Hot Summer.

ALTON, JOHN: Cinematographer. b. Oct. 5, 1901, Hungary. Laboratory technician, MGM 1924; Paramount cameraman 1928; sent to Paris, France, chg. camera dept., 1931; installed studios for Lumiton & Sono Film (South America); writer, photographer & dir. many Spanish pictures; returned to U.S. 1937, cinematographer Hollywood; served in U.S. Signal Corps as Capt., World War II. Books include: Painting With Light, Photography and Lighting in General; received Sintonia Medal for best photography in Argentina, 1937. Academy Award best color photog. American in Paris ballet, 1951.
PICTURES INCLUDE: Witness to Murder, Big Combo, Catered Affair. Member: ASC, AMPAS.

ALVIN, JOHN: Actor. r.n. John Alvin Hoffstadt; b. Chicago, Oct. 24, 1917; e. Pasadena (Calif.) Playhouse. On radio Chicago & Detroit; on N.Y. stage "Leaning on Letty," "Life of the Party," Screen debut 1944 in "Destination Tokyo."
PICTURES INCLUDE: Missing Women, Two Guys from Texas, Bold Frontiersman, Train to Alcatraz, Shanghai Chest, Carrie, April In Paris, Torpedo Alley, Somewhere in Time.

AMATEAU, ROD: Director. b. New York, N.Y., Dec. 20, 1927. Staff writer, CBS radio; stage mgr., Lux Radio Theatre; U.S. Army, 1941; junior writer, 20th Century-Fox; then test dir., second unit dir.; TV dir., numerous shows including Schlitz Playhouse of Stars, Four Star Playhouse, General Electric Theatre, Private Secretary, Dennis Day Show, Lassie, Ray Milland Show, Bob Cummings Show, dir. & prod. Burns & Allen Show, Dobie Gillis.
PICTURES INCLUDE: The Statue, Where Does It Hurt?, The Wilby Conspiracy, Drive-In, Lovelines.

AMECHE, DON: Actor. b. Kenosha, Wis., 1908; e. Columbia Coll., U. Wisconsin. In stock; on radio; m.p. debut 1936. In television from 1951; on Broadway in Silk Stockings, 1955; International Show Time.
PICTURES INCLUDE: Sins of Man, Ladies in Love, Ramona, You Can't Have Everything, Alexander's Ragtime Band, Swanee River, Four Sons, That Night in Rio, Kiss the Boys Goodbye, So Goes My Love, That's My Man, Sleep My Love, Slightly French, A Fever in the Blood, Ring Around the World, Picture Mommy Dead, Suppose They Gave a War & Nobody Came, The Boatniks, Trading Places, Cocoon.
TELEVISION: A Masterpiece of Murder.

AMES, LEON: Actor. r.n. Leon Wycoff. b. Portland, Ind., Jan. 20, 1903. Aviator; with Champlin Players, Lansford, Pa., in stock and on stage; plays include: Tobacco Road, Male Animal, Land Is Bright; m.p. debut in "Murders in the Rue Morgue," 1932; owner & vice-pres. Studio City Ford Co.
PICTURES INCLUDE: Meet Me in St. Louis, Thirty Seconds Over Tokyo, Yolanda and the Thief, Merton of the Movies, On an Island With You, Velvet Touch, Date With Judy, Battleground, Ambush, Big Hangover, Little Women, Dial 1119, Happy Years, Alias a Gentleman, Watch the Birdie, Cattle Drive, On Moonlight Bay, It's a Big Country, Angel Face, By the Light of the Silvery Moon, Let's Do It Again, Sabre Jet, Peyton Place, From the Terrace, Absent Minded Professor, Son of Flubber, Misadventures of Merlin Jones, The Monkey's Uncle, On a Clear Day You Can See Forever, Tora! Tora! Tora!, Testament.
Under contract CBS TV; Life with Father, Father of the Bride, Mr. Ed.

AMES, LOUIS B.: Executive. b. St. Louis, Mo. Aug. 9, 1918; e. Washington U., St. Louis; m. Jetti Preminger; began as music consultant and staff director of musical programs for NBC; music dir. 1948, WPIX; 1951 apptd. program mgr., WPIX; assoc. prod., Today, NBC TV, 1954; feature editor Home, 1957; Adm.-prod. NBC Opera, 1958; dir. cultural prog. N.Y. World's Fair, 1960–63; dir. RCA Pavillion, N.Y. World's Fair, 1963–65; 1966 dir., Nighttime, TV; 1969, dir. of Programming N.W. Ayer & Sons, Inc. 1973 Mgr. Station Services, Television Information Office. NYC.

AMSTERDAM, MOREY: Prod., Writer, Composer, Musician, Actor. b. Chicago, Ill., Dec. 14, 1914. e. U. of Calif., Berkeley. Boy soprano. Radio KPO, 1922; night-club performer, Chicago, 1929; comedian, singer, musician. Rube Wolf Orchestra; comedian, Optimistic Doughnut Program, 1930; writer, vaudeville; comedian, writer, Al Pearce Gang, 1932; writer, MGM, 1937; co-writer, radio shows; m.p. Columbia, Universal; writer, performer, USO Shows, 1942–43; owner, performer, the Playgoers-club; v.p. American International Pictures.
TV: Stop Me If You've Heard This One, Broadway Open House, Morey Amsterdam Silver Swan Show, Dick Van Dyke Show. Exec. Star-prod. Can You Top This.
PICTURES INCLUDE: Don't Worry . . . We'll Think of a Title, Machine Gun Kelly, Murder, Inc.
SONGS: Rum and Coca Cola, Why Oh Why Did I Ever Leave Wyoming, Yak A Puk, etc.

AMYES, JULIAN: TV Producer-Director and Film Director. Early career, stage producer, actor, film actor. Films Incl. A Hill in Korea. Recent TV productions: No Man's Land, Great Expectations. Formerly Head of Drama, (Granada TV) and Director, Granada TV Board.

ANDERSON, DAPHNE: Actress. b. London, Eng., April 27, 1922; e. Kensington High School. Stage debut in pantomime chorus 1937; screen debut in Trottle True 1948.
PICTURES INCLUDE: Cloudburst, Beggar's opera, Hobson's Choice, A Kid for Two Farthings, The Prince and the Showgirl, No Time for Tears, Snowball, Stork Talk, Captain Clegg, The Launching, I Want What I Want.
TV: Silas Marner (Serial), Gideon's Way (Serial), Dr. Finlay's Casebook, Happy Family, The Imposter, The Harry Worth Show, The Whitehall Worrier, The Suede Jacket, Casanova, Haunted Series, Thirty Minute Theatre, Justice is a Woman, Paul Temple, Today, 2 Cars.

ANDERSON, GERRY: Hon. F.B.K.S., Producer, b. London, 1929. Ent. ind. 1946. Chmn./man. dir. Gerry Anderson Productions, Ltd. Over 320 pictures produced for TV worldwide. 1981 Co-founded Anderson Burr Pictures. 1982 commenced production on Terrahawks in association with London Weekend Television; second series, Terrahawks, 1984; Space Pilot pilot for series in assoc. with TVS, 1985–6.

ANDERSON, J. WAYNE: Executive. b. Clifton Forge, VA, Feb. 19, 1947. e. USA Signal School (1965–67); USN Service Schools (1967). USMC, 1965–69; opened 1st military 35mm m.p. theatre, DaNang, Vietnam, 1967–69; dist. mgr., R/C Theatres, 1971–75; v.p., 1976–83; pres. of opns., 1983–present.
MEMBER: Nat. Assn. of Theatre Owners technical advancement committee, 1981–present; Huntsman Condo bd. dir., 1979–83; pres., Huntsman, 1982–83.

ANDERSON, JUDITH: Actress. b. Adelaide, Australia, Feb. 10, 1898. Stage debut (Sydney) in "Royal Divorce" 1915; on New York stage & in stock 1918; toured 1920; m.p. debut in "Blood Money" 1933. Entertained U.S. Armed Forces overseas, World War II; received Donaldson Award 1948, New York Critics Award 1948, American Academy of Arts & Sciences Award for Best Speech 1948. N.Y. stage, 1952, In the Summer House, 1953.
PLAYS INCLUDE: Dear Brutus, Cobra, Dove, Strange Interlude, Old Maid, Mourning Becomes Electra, Macbeth, Medea.
PICTURES INCLUDE: King's Row, Rebecca, Laura, Spector of the Rose, Diary of a Chambermaid, Strange Love of Martha Ivers, Red House, And Then There Were None, Tycoon, Pursued, Salome, Come of Age, Cinderfella, Cat on a Hot Tin Roof, A Man Called Horse, Star Trek III.

ANDERSON, LINDSAY: director (cinema & theatre) and writer. b. Bangalore, India, 1923. e. Cheltenham College and Wadham College, Oxford (classical scholar). Ent. Ind. 1948 as writer-director in charge industrial film prod., also contributing editor independent film quarterly Sequence. Wrote Making a Film 1951; About John Ford (1981). Principal doc. films; O. Dreamland, Thursdays Children (collab. s.p. & dir.) Guy Brenton: Hollywood Short Subject Award, 1954, Three Installations, Pleasure Garden, Wakefield Express, Every Day Except Christmas (Venice Grand Prix, 1957), March to Aldermaston. Founder mem. Free Cinema group. National Film Theatre 1956/9. Recent Doc.: The Singing Lesson (Documentary Studio, Warsaw).
TV INCLUDES: Five episodes Robin Hood series, commercials, 1959–75. 1978 Dir. The Old Crowd.
PLAYS INCLUDE: The Long and the Short and the Tall, Billy Liar, The Fire Raisers, Diary of a Madman, Sergeant Musgraves Dance, The Cherry Orchard, Inadmissible Evidence (At Contemporary Theatre, Warsaw), In Celebration, The Contractor Home, The Changing Room, Artistic director, Royal Court theatre 1969–70. Associate, 1970–76. The Farm, Life Class, What the Butler Saw, The Sea Gull, The Bed Before Yesterday; 1977: The Kingfisher; 1978: Alice's Boys; 1980: Early Days; 1981: Hamlet; 1983: The Cherry Orchard; 1984: Playboy of the Western World; 1986: In Celebration (N.Y.); Hamlet (Washington, DC).
PICTURES INCLUDE: This Sporting Life, 1963; The White Bus, 1966; If. . ., 1968; O Lucky Man!, 1973, In Celebration, 1975; Britannia Hospital, 1982; If You Were There, 1985.

ANDERSON, LONI: Actress. b. St. Paul, MN, Aug. 5. e. Univ. of Minn. Taught school before acting.
TELEVISION INCLUDES: WKRP in Cincinnati, Three on a Date, Christmas in Opryland, Shaun Cassidy Special, Bob Hope specials, etc. Movie 2: The Jayne Mansfield Story, A Letter to Three Wives.
PICTURE: Stroker Ace.

ANDERSON, MELISSA SUE: Actress. b. Berkeley, CA, Sept. 26, 1962. Took up acting at suggestion of a dancing teacher. Did series of commercials; guest role in episode of Brady bunch; episode of Shaft. Gained fame as Mary Ingalls on Little House on the Prairie series.
TELEVISION: Very Good Friends, James at 15, The Loneliest Runner, First Affair.

ANDERSON, MICHAEL: Director. b. London, England, 1920; e. France, Germany, Spain. Ent. m.p. industry as actor, 1936; asst. dir., unit manager on such films as In Which We Serve, Pygmalion, French Without Tears; Army service 1942–46; Co-dir., Private Angelo, 1949; since dir. Waterfront, Hell Is Sold Out, Night Was Our Friend, Will Any Gentleman?, The Dam Busters, 1984, Around the World in 80 Days, Yangtse Incident (Battle Hell), Chase A Crooked Shadow, Shake Hands with the Devil, The Wreck of the Mary Deare, All the Fine Young Cannibals, The Naked Edge, Flight From Ashiya, Monsieur Cognac, Operation Crossbow, The Quiller Memorandum, Shoes of the Fisherman, Pope Joan, Dr. Savage, Conduct Unbecoming, Logan's Run, Orca, Dominique, The Martian Chronicles, Bells, Apple and Pair, Separate Vacations, Vengeance.

ANDERSON, MICHAEL, JR.: Actor. b. London, 1943. son of dir. Michael Anderson. ent. films as child actor, 1954.
TV: Queen's Champion, Ivanhoe, The Monroes.
PICTURES INCLUDE: Tiger Bay, The Moonraker, The Sundowners, Reach For Glory, In Search of the Castaways, Play It Cool, Greatest Story Ever Told, Dear Heart, Major Dundee, The Glory Days, The Sons of Katie Elder, Logan's Run, The Martian Chronicles, Love Leads the Way.

ANDERSON, RICHARD: Actor. b. Long Branch, N.J., Aug. 8, 1926. U.S. Army, World War II. Began acting career in summer theatre in Santa Barbara and Laguna Playhouse where spotted by MGM executives who signed him to six-yr. contract. Appeared in 26 films for MGM before leaving studio.
PICTURES INCLUDE: 12 O'Clock High, The People Against O'Hara,, The Story of Three Loves, Escape from Fort Bravo, Forbidden Planet, The Long Hot Summer, Compulsion, Seconds, Paths of Glory, Tora! Tora! Tora!, Along Came a Spider, Macho Callahan, Doctors' Wives, Play It as It Lays, The Honkers, Stone, Redneck America.
TV: Bus Stop, Perry Mason, 12 O'Clock High (all regular), Ironside, The Big Valley, Mannix, My Friend Tony, The Mod Squad, Land of the Giants, The FBI, Gunsmoke. Series: The Six Million Dollar Man, The Bionic Woman.

ANDERSON, ROLAND: Art director. In 1933 collab. with Hans Dreier on "This Day and Age," Par. Since then collaborated in art direction on many productions, including Lives of a Bengal Lancer, Hands Across the Table, Give Us This Night, Till We Meet Again, The Buccaneer, Union Pacific, North West Mounted Police, Love Thy Neighbor, The Crystal Ball, Story of Dr. Wassel, Road to Utopia, Let's Dance, Branded, Carried, Son of Paleface, Just For You, Here Come the Girls, White Christmas, Country Girl, We're No Angels, Court Jester.

ANDERSON, SYLVIA: Producer/Writer. (Pinewood Studios). b. London. e. London Univ. Entered m.p. ind. 1960.
TV: Thunderbirds; etc.
PICTURES INCLUDE: UK rep. for Home Box Office of America. First published novel Love and Hisses.

ANDERSON, WILLIAM H.: Producer; Member of Bd. of Dir. Walt Disney Productions. b. Utah, October 12, 1911. e. Compton College. Firestone Rubber Co.; Universal Credit Co.; Walt Disney Prods. 42 years.
PICTURES INCLUDE: Old Yeller, Swiss Family Robinson, Happiest Millionaire, The Computer Wore Tennis Shoes, Barefoot Executive, $1,000,000 Duck, Superdad, Strongest Man In The World, Apple Dumpling Gang, Treasure of Matecumbe, Shaggy D.A.
TV: Zorro Series 1958–1959 (20 half-hour segments); 1959–1960 (38 half-hour segments), Wonderful World of Disney: Zorro, Texas John Slaughter, Daniel Boone, The Swamp Fox, Pop Warner Football (1960–1961), Johnny Shiloh, Mooncussers, 1962–1963; Bristle Face, The Scarecrow of Romney Marsh (1963–1964); the Legend of Young Dick Turpin (1965–1966); Willie and the Yank (1966–1967); A Boy Called Nuthin', The Young Loner (1967–1968); The Wacky Zoo of Morgan City (1970–1971); The Mystery of Dracula's Castle (1972–1973); The Bull From the Sky, co-producer; 1975–1976; Great Sleeping Bear Sled Dog Race, co-producer (1976–1977).

ANDERSSON, BIBI: Actress. b. Stockholm, 1935. e. Royal Dramatic Theatre School.
PICTURES INCLUDE: (for director, Ingmar Bergman) Smiles of a Summer Night, 1955; The Seventh Seal, Wild Strawberries, Brink of Life, The Magician, The Devil's Eye, Not to Mention All these Women, Persona; other films: My Sister, My Love Le Vio A Passion, Black Palm Trees, Story of a Woman, Duel at Diablo, The Kremlin Letter, The Passion of Anna, I Never Promised You a Rose Garden, Quintet, The Concord: Airport '79, Enemy of the People.

ANDES, KEITH: Actor. b. Ocean City, N.J., July 12, 1920. e. Temple U., Oxford. Radio work; on Broadway in Winged Victory, Kiss Me Kate, Maggie.
PICTURES INCLUDE: Farmer's Daughter, Clash By Night, Blackbeard the Pirate, Split Second, Life at Stake, Second Greatest Sex, Away All Boats, Pillars of the Sky, Back from Eternity, Damn Citizen, Surrender, Hells Bloody Devils, And Justice for All.
TV: This Man Dawson, Glynis.
BROADWAY: Wildcat.

ANDRESS, URSULA: Actress. b. Berne, Switzerland, 1936. M.p. Hollywood, 1955.
PICTURES INCLUDE: Dr. No, Four For Texas, Fun in Acapulco, Toys For Christmas, She, Tenth Victim, What's New Pussycat?, Chinese Adventures in China, Casino Royale, The Southern Star, Perfect Friday, The Red Sun, Scaramouche, Clash of the Titans.
TELEVISION: Peter the Great.

ANDREWS, ANTHONY: Actor. b. London, England, 1948.
PICTURES: Operation Daybreak, Under the Vocano, The Holcroft Covenant, etc.
TELEVISION: Romeo and Juliet, QB VII, Upstairs Downstairs, Danger UXB, Brideshead Revisited, Ivanoe, The Scarlet Pimpernel, Sparkling Cyanide, A.D.

ANDREWS, DANA: Actor, b. Collins, Miss., Jan. 1, 1912: e. Sam Houston Coll.; Pasadena Community Playhouse. Account with Gulf Refining Co., 1930; chief accountant Tobins, Inc., 1931; acted with Pasadena Playhouse 3 yrs.; m.p. debut in "The Westerner" 1939; Vice Pres. Screen Actor's Guild, 1962–63, Pres. 1964–66.
PICTURES INCLUDE: Best Years of Our Lives, Iron Curtain, Foolish Heart, Forbidden Street Bway play, Two for the See-Saw, Laura, Edge of Doom, Where Sidewalk Ends, Sealed Cargo, The Frogmen, I Want You, Assignment—Paris, Elephant Walk, Duel in the Jungle, Three Hours to Kill, Smoke Signal, Strange Lady in Town, While the City Sleeps, Commanche, Beyond a Reasonable Doubt, Spring Reunion, Night of the Demon, Zero Hour, Enchanted Island, The Fear Makers, The Crowded Sky, Madison Avenue, The Satan Bug, Crack in The World, In Harm's Way, Battle of the Bulge, Devil's Brigade, The Loved One, Innocent Bystander, The Last Tycoon, Airport, 1975, Born Again.
TV: Alas Babylon; G.E., The Playoff; Barbara Stanwyck; Dupont, Mutiny; 4 Star, Crazy Sunday; Checkmate, Alcoa, The Boy Who Wasn't Wanted; Twilight Zone, No Time Like The Past; Dick Powell, Last of the Big Spenders; Alcoa, The Town That Died, Bob Hope Chrysler, A Wind of Hurricane Force, Bright Promise (movie), Shadow in the Streets, One Small Step Forward (series), The Right Hand Man (Playhouse 90) Ike (ABC movie).
DINNER THEATRE: The Marriage-Go-Round; The Best of Friends, Angel Street, The Gang's All Here, Any Wednesday, A Man for All Seasons.

ANDREWS, EAMONN: C.B.E. Announcer and commentator. b. Dublin, Ireland, Dec. 19, 1922. e. Irish Christian Brothers (Dublin), Radio, vaudeville and legit. stage experience in Dublin; TV with BBC 1950; quiz master on several programs, sports com., columnist, author, playwright; Founder, chairman, Irish Television Authority; ABC-TV, 1964–67; Eamonn Andrews Show, and World of Sport, Thames TV's daily, Today, This Is Your Life, Time For Business, Top of the World, What's My Line.

ANDREWS, HARRY: CBE, Actor. b. Tonbridge, Kent, England, 1911. First stage appearance. Liverpool, 1933. London stage 1935, "Worse Things Happen at Sea," to U.S., 1936, "Hamlet." Army Service 1939–45. Screen debut 1952, The Red Beret.
PICTURES INCLUDE: The Black Knight, The Man Who Loved Redheads, A Hill in Korea, Alexander the Great, Moby Dick, Ice Cold in Alex, Devil's Disciple, Solomon and Sheba, In the Nick, Circle of Deception, Cleopatra, The Best of Enemies, Reach For Glory, The Inspector, Barraba, 55 Days at Peking, The Snout, The System, The Hill, The Agony and the Ecstasy, The Sands of the Kalahari, The Deadly Affair, A Dandy in Aspic, The Charge of the Light Brigade, The Night They Raided Minsky's, The Seagull, A Nice Girl Like Me, Too Late the Hero, The Gaunt Woman, Country Dance (in U.S. Brotherly Love), Entertaining Mr. Sloane, Wuthering Heights, I Want What I Want, Nicholas and Alexandra, The Nightcomers, The Ruling Class, Man of La Mancha, Theatre of Blood, The Mackintosh Man, Man at the Top, The Skyriders, The Blueblrd, The Passover Plot, The Prince and The Pauper, Equus, Superman, The Medusa Touch, The Big Sleep, Death on the Nile, SOS Titanic, Curse of King Tut's Tomb, Seven Dials Mystery, The Sound Machine, A Question of Guilt.
TV: Affair of Honour, Clayhanger, Two Gentle People,

Leo Tolstoy, A.J. Wentworth B.A., Lent, Dynasty, Return of Sherlock Holmes, Inside Story.

ANDREWS, JULIE: Actress, Singer. b. Walton-on-Thames. Eng., Oct 1, 1935 debut, Eng. Starlight Roof Revue; pantomime of Cinderella.
PLAYS: The Boy Friend, My Fair Lady, Camelot.
PICTURES INCLUDE: Mary Poppins, The Americanization of Emily, The Sound of Music, Hawaii, Torn Curtain, Thoroughly Modern Millie, Star!, Darling Lili, The Tamarind Seed, "10," "S.O.B," Victor/Victoria, The Man Who Loved Women, That's Life.
TV: High Tor, Julie and Carol at Carnegie Hall, The Andy Williams Show, The Julie Andrews Show, An Evening with Julie Andrews and Harry Belafonte, The World of Walt Disney, Julie and Carol at Lincoln Center, Julie Andrews Hour (ABC Television series 1972–73); Julie on Sesame Street, 1973; Julie Andrews' Christmas Special, 1973; Julie and Dick in Covent Garden, 1974; Julie Andrews and Jackie Gleason Together, 1974; Julie Andrews—My Favorite Things, 1975.
AUTHOR: Mandy, Last of the Really Great Whangdoodles, 1973.

ANDRIEUX, ROGER: Director Writer. b. France, Aug. 24, 1940. Began in French theatre, went to UCLA, took his MFA, made several short subjects as well as his first feature film in English.
PICTURES INCLUDE: Mr. Brown (s.p., dir.); Bonjour Amour (co-s.p., dir.); La Petite Sirene (s.p., dir., prod.).

ANGEL, HEATHER: Actress. b. Oxford, England, Feb. 9, 1909; e. Wycombe Abbey School. On stage 1926–30; British m.p. debut in "City of Song" 1939; U.S. m.p. debut in "Pilgrimage" 1932.
PICTURES INCLUDE: Hound of the Baskervilles, After Office Hours, Berkeley Square, Charlie Chan's Greatest Case, Orient Express, Springtime, for Henry, Informer, Three Musketeers, Last of the Mohicans, Bulldog Drummond series, Pride and Prejudice, That Hamilton Woman, Suspicion, Lifeboat, In the Meantime Darling, Saxon Charm, Alice in Wonderland, Peter Pan.
TV: Family Affair.

ANGERS, AVRIL: Actress, comedienne, singer. b. Liverpool, Eng., April 18; Stage debut at age of 14; screen debut in 1947 in Lucky Mascot.
PICTURES INCLUDE: Miss Pilgrim's Progress, Don't Blame the Stork, Women Without Men, Green Man, Devils of Darkness, Be My Guest, Three Bites of the Apple, The Family Way, Two a Penny, The Best House in London, Staircase, There's a Girl in My Soup, Forbush and the Penguins, Gollocks (1973), Confessions of a Driving Instructor, Dangerous Davies.
TV: How Do You View, Friends and Neighbors, Dear Dotty, Holiday Town, Charlie Fainsbarn Show, Arthur Askey Show, All Aboard, The Gold Hunter, Bob Monkhouse Show, Before The Fringe, Hudd, Coronation Street, Dick Emery Show, Dad's Army, Bright Boffins, The More We Are Together, The Millionairess, Liver Birds, Looks Familiar, No Appointment Necessary, The Songwriters, All Creatures Great and Small, Coronation Concert, Minder, Smuggler, Just Liz, Give Up a Clue, Are You Being Served.
PLAYS INCLUDE: The Mating Game; Musical, Cockie; Murder at the Vicarage, Little Me, Norman, Is That You?, Blithe Spirit, Oklahoma!, Gigi, The Killing of Sister George.

ANHALT, EDNA: Associate producer, writer. b. New York, N.Y., Apr. 10, 1914; e. Kathryn Gibbs Sch., 1932; U. doc. films; prod. mgr., Rockefeller Found. films.
PICTURES INCLUDE: (Orig. story, collab., assoc. prod., s.p.) Strange Voyage, Avalanche, Younger Brothers, Return of Frontiersman, Embraceable You, Sierra, The Sniper, My Six Convicts, Eight Iron Men, Member of the Wedding, Three Lives, The Big Kill, Not as a Stranger, Pride and the Passion, Girls, Girls, Girls, Decision at Delphi.
Academy Award, orig. story collab., Panic in the Streets.
Member: Acad. of M.P. Arts & Sciences; S.W.G.

ANHALT, EDWARD: Writer. b. New York, N.Y. Academy Award. orig. story collab., Panic in the Streets.
PICTURES INCLUDE: The Young Savages, Academy Award, screenplay, Becket, In Enemy Country, Boeing-Boeing, The Young Lions, Day of the Guns, Not As a Stranger, Madwoman of Chaillot, Member of the Wedding, Boston Strangler, Jeremiah Johnson, Q B VII (TV), Luther, Escape to Athena.

ANNAKIN, KENNETH: Director, writer. b. Yorkshire, England. Graduated through Experimental Theatre and Documentary. Films incl: Across The Bridge, Swiss Family Robinson, Very Important Person, The Longest Day, The Fast Lady, The Informers, Those Magnificent Men In Their Flying Machines, Battle Of The Bulge, The Long Duel, Monte Carlo Or Bust, Call Of The Wild, Paper Tiger, The Fifth Musketeer, The Pirate Movie.

ANN-MARGRET: Actress, singer. b. Stockholm, Sweden, April 28, 1941. e. grad., New Trier High School, Winnetka, Ill., attended Northwestern University. Radio shows, toured with band; worked with George Burns, Sahara, Las Vegas. TV debut, Jack Benny Show, April, 1961.
PICTURES INCLUDE: debut, Pocketful of Miracles, State Fair, Bye, Bye Birdie, Viva Las Vegas, Kitten With a Whip, Bus Riley's Back in Town, Once A Thief, Cincinnati Kid, The Swinger, Stagecoach, Murderer's Row, The Pleasure Seekers, Made in Paris, The Tiger and the Pussycat, C. C. & Company, Carnal Knowledge, RPM, The Outside Man, The Train Robbers, Tommy, The Last Remake of Beau Geste, The Twist, Joseph Andrews, The Cheap Detective, Magic, The Villain, Middle Age Crazy, Lookin' To Get Out, The Return of the Soldier, Twice in a Lifetime, 52 Pick-up.
TELEVISION: Movies: Who Will Love My Children?, A Streetcar Named Desire.

ANSARA, MICHAEL: Actor. b. Lowell, Mass., April 15, 1927. e. Pasadena Playhouse. Served in U.S. Army; then summer stock, little theatre, road shows.
PICTURES INCLUDE: The Robe, Julius Caesar, Sign of the Pagan, Bengal Brigade, Soldiers Three, Only the Valiant, New Orleans Uncensored, Diane, Lone Ranger, Sol Madrid, Daring Game,The Bears And I, Mohammad, Messenger of God, The Manitou, Gas.
TV: Broken Arrow, Law of the Plainsman, Westerner, Centennial.

ANSPACH, SUSAN: Actress. b. New York City. e. Catholic University (Washington, D.C.) After school returned to N.Y. and in 3 years had performed in 11 off-Bwy. and moved to Los Angeles and entered films.
PICTURES INCLUDE: Five Easy Pieces, The Landlord, Play It Again Sam, Blume in Love, The Big Fix, Running, The Devil and Max Devlin, Gas, Misunderstood.
TELEVISION: Yellow Rose, Space.

ANTHONY, TONY: Actor-producer-writer. b. Clarksburg, West Virginia. e. Carnegie Mellon.
PICTURES INCLUDE: Force of Impulse, Pity Me Not, The Wounds of Hunger, A Stranger in Town, The Stranger Returns, A Stranger in Japan, Come Together, Blindman, Pete Pearl and the Pole, Let's Talk About Men, Get Mean, The Boy Who Owned a Melephant, Treasure of the Four Crowns, Comin' at Ya.

ANTON, SUSAN: Actress. b. Oak Glen, CA, Oct. 12, 1951. e. Bernardino Coll. Worked in night clubs and did song recordings. Film debut, Golden Girl, 1979.
TELEVISION: The Cliffhangers, Presenting Susan Anton.

ANTONIONI, MICHELANGELO: Director. b. Ferrara, Italy, Sept. 29, 1913. e. Bologna University. Film critic on local paper, then script writer and asst. director. First films as a director were documentaries, including: Gente del Po (1947) and N.U. First feature Love Story, 1950; since The Lady Without Camelias, Love in a City, I Vinti, The Friend, The City, L'Avventura, The Night, The Eclipse, The Red Desert, Blow-Up, Zabriskie Point, The Passenger.

ANTONOWSKY, MARVIN: Executive. b. New York City, Jan. 31, 1929. e. N.Y. City College, BBA & MBA. Joined Kenyon and Eckhart in 1957 for which was media research dir.; named marketing v.p. With Norman, Craig, & Kummel as v.p., mktg. services. 1965, became v.p. in chg. of media research and spot buying at J. Walter Thompson. In 1969 joined ABC-TV as v.p. in chg. research. Left to become v.p. in chg. of programming at NBC-TV. 1976, sr. v.p., Universal-TV. 1979, joined Columbia Pictures as pres., mktg. & research. Rejoined MCA/Universal Pictures as pres, mktg., Nov. 1983.

ANTONY, SCOTT: Actor. b. Gosforth, Newcastle-upon-Tyne, England. e. Leeds Univ. Rec'd scholarship at Royal Academy of Dramatic Art. Ken Russell found him there and gave him role in Savage Messiah (1972). Has done much TV work in Britain.
PICTURES INCLUDE: Savage Messiah, The Mutations, Dead Cert.

ANZARUT, RAYMOND: Executive producer. b. Lebanon, 1912. e. French Lyceum, Alexandria, Egypt and Paris. Entered film industry 1941 on Jeannie. Subsequently worked on The Day Will Dawn, Talk About Jacqueline, Secret Mission, On Approval. Prod. asst. on They Met in the Dark. Prod. mgr. Flight from Folly. Prod. mgr. in Egypt on Caesar and Cleopatra in 1945. With Marcel Hellman as prod. mgr. on Meet Me at Dawn. Prod. mgr. Swiss location, Scott of the Antarctic; prod. mgr. of Wessex Film Productions Ltd. on Esther Waters, Once a Jolly Swagman, All Over the Town, Mr. Prohack, The Wooden Horse, Gen. prod. mgr. on The Grand Design (six technicolor two-reelers on European Recovery for E.C.A.). Appointed gen. mgr. of Wessex 1950. Appointed prod. & admin. head, E.C.A. Motion Picture Section, Paris, 1952. Then with Coronado (Sea Devils), Carol Reed 1–1 British Lion (Man Between), Watergate-

British Lion (An Inspector Calls) 1953. British Lion-London Films (The Man Who Loved Redheads), David Lean-Lopert Films Inc. (Summer Madness) 1954, London Films (Storm Over the Nile) 1955, Sailor Beware 1955, Dry Rot 1956, Esther Costello 1956–57. Assoc. prod. on The Silent Enemy 1957, Room at the Top, 1958, Our Man in Havana, 1959, 1960; prod. sup. Mysterious Island (Charles Schneer 1–1 Columbia), 1961; Lolita, 1962; The War Lover, Lord Jim. Reconnaissance of South-East Asia, setting up and filming in Hong Kong and Cambodia. Decorated by Prince Sihanouk of Cambodia; prod. sup., Scene Nun, Take One. Assoc. prod. The Hill, 1966–67; The Dirty Dozen. Exec. prod. for Warner Bros. Seven Arts Prods. Ltd. London, May 1967–Sept. 1969 when Company was taken over by Kinney. Re-joined Ken Hyman in Nov., 1969 (Inter-Hemisphere Productions Ltd.) as prod. exec., 71/72 preparing projects for Universal Pictures Ltd. 1972 with Kenneth Hyman reverted to indep. prod. and helped prepare Emperor of the North Pole, in London. Organized and supervised all London filming for Gaumont International (Paris). Le Silencieux. 1973: preparing the Heights of Aervos for Inter-Hemisphere Productions. Organized and supervised Eng. loc. for La Gifle. Rejoined Inter-Hemisphere Prod., 1975–76.

APFEL, EDWIN R.: Executive. b. New York, N.Y., Jan. 2, 1934. e. Franklin and Marshall College, B.A., 1955. copywriter and account executive, Donahue and Coe, 1955–60; adv. publicity dept., Metro-Goldwyn-Mayer, 1960–62; dir. of adv. and creative services, MGM, Verve Records, 1962–63; dir. of adv., Embassy Pictures 1963–65; Advertising Writer, Consultant, 1965.

APPELBOOM, MAX: Producer. b. Amsterdam, Holland, March 7, 1924. e. art schools in Holland, Belgium and France. Started in the motion picture businness in 1946 with J. Arthur Rank, then to RKO Radio Pictures. Worked from 1953–56 in Hollywood as writer, director and producer. Returned in 1956 to his home base, Amsterdam. Now pres. Max Appelboom Producties, Inc. and Appletree Filmproductions Inc.
PICTURES INCLUDE: Floris, Monkey Business, Will O' The Wisp, Water For Waterland, The Bearboat, Gangrene, The Buggy Man and The New Adventures of Heidi.

APTED, MICHAEL: Director. Broke into show business at Granada TV in England in early 1960s as trainee, researcher, and finally director. By 1965 was producer-director for local programs and current affairs; then staff drama dir. for TV series, plays and serials. In late 1960s left Granada to free-lance.
PICTURES INCLUDE: Triple Echo, Stardust, The Squeeze, Agatha, Coal Miner's Daughter, Continental Divide, Gorky Park, Firestarter, Firstborn, 7 Up, 28 Up, Critical Condition.
TELEVISION: Poor Girl, High Kampf, Highway Robbery, Kisses at 50, The Collection (won Intl. Emmy Award for last).

ARBEID, BEN: Producer. Films incl: The Barber of Stamford Hill, Children of the Damned, Private Potter, The Jokers, Hoffman; The Hireling, Columbia Grand Prix—Cannes, Eagles Wing, Enigma.

ARCHER, ANNE: Actress. Daughter of actress Marjorie Lord and actor John Archer. Married Terry Jastrow, actor and TV network sports producer-director.
PICTURES INCLUDE: The All-American Boy, Honkers, Cancel My Reservation, Trackdown, Lifeguard, Paradise Alley, Hero at Large, Green Ice, Waltzing Across Texas, The Naked Face, Too Scared To Scream, The Check Is in the Mail.
TELEVISION: The Pirate (mini-series), The Blue Knight, Seventh Avenue, The Sky's No Limit.

ARCHER, JOHN: Actor. r.n. Ralph Bowman, b. Osceola, Neb., May 8, 1915; e. U. So. Calif. Won Jesse L. Lasky "Gateway to Hollywood" talent quest; m.p. debut in "Flaming Frontiers" 1938; on N.Y. stage also.
PICTURES INCLUDE: White Heat, After Nightfall, Destination Moon, Big Trees, Yank in Indo-China, Sound Off, Rodeo, Sea Tiger, The Stars Are Singing, Dragon's Gold, No Man's Woman, Emergency Hospital.

ARCHER, ROBERT V.: Executive. Joined Paramount Pictures in 1967 as adm. asst. to v.p. of facilities and TV prod. In 1975 named dir. of studio admin. 1977 promoted to dir. of studio operations and admin., responsible for prod. servicing and admin. depts. of studio.

ARCHERD, ARMY: Columnist-TV Commentator. r.n. Armand Archerd, b. N.Y., Jan. 13. ed. UCLA Grad. '41, US Naval Academy Post Graduate School, 1943. Started as usher at Criterion Theatre, N.Y., while in high school. After grad. UCLA, worked at Paramount studios before entering Navy, Lt., joined AP Hollywood bureau 1945, Herald-Express, Daily Variety as columnist, 1953. M.C. Hollywood premieres and Academy Awards. President, founder Hollywood Press Club, awards from Masquers, L.A. Press Club, Hollywood Foreign Press Club, and "Newsman of the Year" award from Publicists Guild, 1970; "Movie Game" TV Series; People's Choice, co-host.

ARDEN, EVE: Actress. r.n. Eunice Quedens. b. Mill Valley, Calif., 1912. Appeared with Alcazar stock co., Bandbox Repertory Theatre; Broadway debut in "Ziegfeld Follies of 1936" also in "Ziegfeld Follies of 1938" and Let's Face It, Night And Day, Cover Girl, Voice of the Turtle, Goodbye, My Fancy, We're Not Married, Our Miss Brooks, Anatomy of a Murder, Dark at the Top of the Stairs, Sergeant Deadhead, The Strongest Man in the World, Grease, Grease 2.
TV: Our Miss Brooks, The Eve Arden Show, The Mothers-in-Law.
STAGE: Mame, Hello Dolly, Butterflies Are Free.

ARDEN, MARY: Actress. b. Litchfield, Mich., Dec. 9, 1910. e. Northwestern U., Anne Wolters School of Speech & Drama. Appeared in stock; radio, March of Time, Lux.
PICTURES INCLUDE: Jealousy, Youth Aflame, Missing Corps, Father Take a Wife, Best Years of Our Lives.
TV: Playhouse 90, Climax, Studio One.

ARKIN, ALAN: Actor-Director, b. New York City, March 26, 1934. e. Los Angeles City College, Los Angeles State College, Bennington (Vt.) College. Member folk singing group The Tarriers; off-Broadway, Second City, Man Out Loud, From the Second City; Broadway, Enter Laughing, Luv. Dir. Little Murders, White House Murders.
PICTURES INCLUDE: The Russians Are Coming, The Russians Are Coming, Wait Until Dark, The Heart is a Lonely Hunter, Pope, Catch 22, Deadhead Miles, Last of the Red Hot Lovers, Freebie and the Bean, Rafferty and the Gold Dust Twins. Director: Little Murders, Hearts of the West, 7½ Per Cent Solution, The In-Laws, Simon, Chu Chu and the Philly Flash, The Return of Mr. Invisible, Joshua Then and Now, Bad Medicine, Big Trouble, Full Moon High.
TELEVISION: A Deadly Business.

ARKOFF, SAMUEL Z.: Producer, Motion Picture Executive. Chairman & President of the Samuel Z. Arkoff Company (formed 1980) and Arkoff Int'l. Pictures (formed 1981). b. Fort Dodge, Ia., June 12, 1918. e. U. of Colorado, U. of Iowa & Loyola U. Law School. m. Hilda Rusoff. USAF Cryptographer World War II. Co-founder American Releasing, 1954, and American International Pictures, 1955. President and Chairman of the Board American International Pictures until 1979. Named with partner James H. Nicholson as Producers of the Year in 1963 by Allied States Association of Motion Picture Theatre Owners and in 1964 as Master Showmen of the Decade by the Theatre Owners of America. Also named Producers of the Year at the Show-A-Rama VIII, and in 1966 and 1967 voted among top ten producers in exhibitor ratings by the independent theatre owners. In Rome in 1970 honored by President of the Republic of Italy with decree naming him Commendatore of the Order of Merit. In 1971 he and Nicholson named Pioneers of the Year by the Foundation of the Motion Picture Pioneers, Inc. Since appointment in 1973, has served as International vice pres. of Variety Clubs International. Vice pres., Permanent Charities Committee. Appointed Member of the Board of Trustees of Loyola Marymount Univ., Los Angeles, in 1979. Honored by a retrospective on 25th anniversary of AIP at museum of Modern Art, July–Sept., 1979.
PRODUCTION CREDITS: On more than 200 pictures including Amityville Horror, Dressed to Kill, How to Beat the High Cost of Living, The Earthling, Love at First Bite, Meteor, California Dreaming, Force Ten from Navarone, The House of Usher, Pit and the Pendulum, Tales of Terror, Master of The World, Premature Burial, Panic in the Year Zero, The Raven, Beach Party, Haunted Palace, Comedy of Terrors, Bikini Beach, Masque of the Red Death, Muscle Beach Party, Pajama Party Tomb of Ligeia, Wild Anges, Devil's Angels, The Trip, Three in the Attic, Wild in the Streets, The Oblong Box, Scream and Scream Again, Murders in the Rue Morgue, Cry of the Banshee, Bloody Mama, Wuthering Heights, Dr. Phibes, Frogs, Blacula, Dillinger, Heavy Traffic, Hennessy, Cooley High, Food of the Gods, Futureworld, Great Scout and Cathouse Thursday, Land that Time Forgot, People That Time Forgot, At The Earth's Core, Island of Dr. Moreau, and A Winning Season.

ARLEDGE, ROONE: Executive. b. Forest Hills, N.Y., July 8, 1931. e. Columbia Univ. Entered industry with Dumont Network in 1952; joined U.S. Army, 1953, serving at Aberdeen Proving Ground in Maryland, where produced and directed radio programs. Joined NBC in 1954 where held various production positions. In 1960 went to ABC TV; 1964, named v.p. in chg. of ABC Sports. Created ABC's Wide World of sports in April, 1961. Named pres. of ABC News in 1968; pres. of ABC News and Sports, 1977. Hold four George Foster Peabody Awards for sports reporting; 19 Emmy awards.

ARLING, ARTHUR E.: Cinemotographer. b. Missouri, Sept. 2, 1906; e. N.Y. Institute of Photography. Entered m.p. Fox studio 1927 as asst. cameraman, 2nd cameraman 1931; operative cameraman on "Gone With the Wind" which won the Academy Award for technicolor photography 1939. Lt. Comdr. U.S.N.R., World War II; received Academy Award as dir. of Photography on "The Yearling" 1946. Member: Amer. Soc. of Cinematographers.
PICTURES INCLUDE: Homestretch, Captain from Castile, Mother Was A Freshman, You're My Everything, Wabash Avenue, My Blue Heaven, Call Me Mister, Belles on their Toes, The Glass Slipper, Three for the Show, Love Me or Leave Me, I'll Cry Tomorrow, Ransom, Great American Pastime, Tammy & the Bachelor, Pay the Devil, Story of Ruth, Pillow Talk, Lover Come Back, Notorious Landlady, Boys Night Out, My Six Loves.

ARMOUR, REGINALD: Foreign dist., prod. b. Chicago, Ill. Nov. 28, 1905; e. Edinburgh, Scotland. Exec. RCA Victor Co. to 1933; estab. exch. India, Burma, Ceylon RKO Radio; Far East gen. mgr.; European gen. mgr. (Paris) 1937; exec. asst. to pres. RKO 1941; asst. gen. mgr. RKO studios 1942; British & European rep. Walt Disney Prod. 1942; financial field (N.Y.) 1943; exec. vice-pres. Richard Condon, Inc. 1944; with overseas br. OWI 1945; foreign rep. Columbia Internatl. Corp. (N.Y.) 1945–49; joined Republic Pictures Internatl. Corp. 1949; apptd. v.p., 1950; supvr., Europe & Near East for Republic 1952, exec. v.p. Republic Pictures International (Great Britain) and man. dir. Republic Prod. (Gt. Brit.) Ltd.; exec. v.p. Republic Pictures International Corp., 1955; pres., The Dorsey Corp., 1960; Vice Chmn., The Dorsey Corp., 1964; pres., SOS Photo-Cine-Optics, Inc., 1965; pres. F&B/Ceco of Calif. Inc., 1967; pres. Instant Protection Systems, Inc., 1971. Exec. V.P. and Treas. The Quedo Corporation and International Producers Services, Inc. 1973; 1974, V.P. & Treas. Dyna-Soar, Inc.; 1977, exec. v.p. & treas., Two Feathers Prods.; 1981, pres., Armour Enterprises, Inc.; 1985, pres., Group Media Prods., Inc.

ARMSTRONG, BESS: Actress. b. Baltimore, MD, Dec. 11, 1953. e. Brown Univ.
PICTURES: The Four Seasons, Jekyll and Hyde Together Again, High Road to China, Jaws 3-D, The House of God, Nothing in Common.
TELEVISION: On Our Own, Getting Married, Lace, etc.

ARMSTRONG, GILLIAN: Director. b. Melbourne, Australia, 1950. e. Swinburne Coll. Did numerous shorts (Storytime, Old Man and Dog, One Hundred a Day, etc.) and documentaries (A Time and a Place, Tassie Wood, etc.) before turning to features.
PICTURES: My Brilliant Career, Starstruck, Mrs. Soffel.

ARMSTRONG, GORDON: Executive, b. East Orange, N.J., Nov. 26, 1937. e. Arizona State Univ., graduate studies at N.Y.U. Entered ind. as newspaper contact for MGM (1960–63); with Allan, Foster, Ingersoll and Weber 1963–70 as acct. exec.; joined 20th Century-Fox in 1970 as nat. pub. dir. In 1975 appt. dir. of adv.-pub.-promo. for Dino De Laurentiis Corp. In 1978, became vice pres., worldwide marketing for the company; 1980, named v.p., adv.-pub.-prom., Universal Pictures; 1984, named exec. v.p., mktg. MCA Recreation.

ARNALL, ELLIS GIBBS: Lawyer, Exec. b. Newnan, Ga. Mar. 20, 1907; e. Mercer U.; U. of South, A.B. 1928 D.C.L. 1947; U. of Georgia LL.B. 1931; Atlanta Law School, LL.D. 1941; Piedmont Coll., LL.D 1943; Bryant Coll., LL.D. 1948; Georgia state representative from Coweta County, 1936–38; asst. Attorney-General (Ga.) 1938–42; Attorney-General (Ga.) 1942–43; Governor of Ga. 1943–47; pres. Dixie Life Insurance Co.; pres., Columbus National Life Insurance Co. senior mem. law firm Arnall, Golden & Gregory; pres. Georgia State Jr. Chamber of Commerce 1939; trustee U. of South; author of "The Shore Dimly Seen" 1946. "What The People Want" 1948; member U.S. Natl. Com. on UNESCO; member U.S. delegation to 4th annual conference UNESCO, Paris, France, 1949. Member: SIMPP (Pres. 1948); 1952 on leave as dir. Office of Price Stabilization, Washington; back to SIMPP, Sept. 1952; pres. Ind. Film Prod. Export Corp., 1953; member bd. of dir., exec. com., U.S. Nat. Comm. for UNESCO, 1964–65, trustee, Mercer Univ. 1964–68; chair. bd. Coastal States Life Insurance Co., chair. bd. National Association of Life Companies. Member Academy Motion Picture Arts & Sciences; vice chm., Sun Life of America Group, Inc.

ARNAZ, DESI: Actor, b. Santiago, Cuba, Mar. 2, 1917. e. Colegio Dolores, Jesuit Prep School, Santiago; at the age of 17 was the vocalist with a band at Miami Beach, Fla.; later with own rhumba band; played in N.Y. night clubs; on stage in "Too Many Girls;" m.p. debut in "Too Many Girls" 1940; served as Staff Sgt. U.S. Army Medical Corps 3 years; musical dir. Bob Hope show 1946–47. Indep. prod.-owner, Corona Breeding Farm.
PICTURES INCLUDE: Father Takes A Wife, Four Jacks and a Jill, Navy Comes Through, Bataan, Cuban Pete, Long Long Trailer, Holiday in Havana; (actor-prod.) Forever Darling, The Escape Artist.
TV: (Actor-exec. prod.) I Love Lucy TV films, The Lucille Ball-Desi Arnaz Show; Pres. Desilu Productions, Inc., 1962; Pres. Desi Arnaz Prod. Inc., 1965; Prod. The Mothers-in-Law.

ARNAZ, JR., DESI: Actor-Singer, b. Jan. 19, 1953. Son of Lucille Ball and Desi Arnaz. Began appearing on I Love Lucy show on TV in infancy and on various Lucy shows since. Gained fame as rock singer and musician with the Dino, Desi and Billy group. Film debut in Red Sky at Morning in 1972.
PICTURES INCLUDE: Red Sky at Morning, Marco, She Lives (tv), Joyride, A Wedding, House of the Long Shadows.

ARNAZ, LUCIE: Actress. b. Los Angeles, July 17, 1951. Daughter of Lucille Ball and Desi Arnaz. On Broadway in Bye, Bye Birdie, Goodbye Charlie, Lil Abner, They're Playing Our Song, etc.
PICUTRES: Billy Jack Goes to Washington, The Jazz Singer, Second Thoughts.
TELEVISON: Here's Lucy, The Black Dahlia, The Mating Season.

ARNAUD, LEO: Composer, arranger, conductor. b. Lyons, France, July 24, 1904: e. Ormesson Music Acad., Ph.D. Faculty mem. & symph. cond., Ormesson Music Acad., 1922–27; mus. dir. & arr. in France & England, 1927–30; Fred Waring Orch., U.S., 1931–35; arr. vocal coach, comp., mus. dir., MGM, 1936–44; U.S. Armed Forces, 1945 dir. many orch. including; L.A. Concert Band, American Legion Band, Hollywood String Orch., Beverly Hills, Symph. Orch.; free-lance mus. dir., comp., arr. since 1945.
PICTURES INCLUDE: One Touch of Venus, Easter Parade, Date With Judy, Three Little Words, Lovely to Look At, Stars & Stripes Forever, Rose Marie, Seven Brides for Seven Brothers.

ARNELL, PETER: Producer. b. Bridgeport, Conn., e. U. of Mich., A.B. Pub. dir., prog., WJLS, Beckley, W.Va.; m.c. & disc jockey, WPEN, Philadelphia; actor, announcer, N.Y.; creator of Rate Your Mate, Name's the Same; creator & prod. of Wheel of Fortune, Balance Your Budget, I'll Buy That, Take a Guess, What's in a Word? prod. Chance of Romance, Take a Good Look, Celebrity Talent Scouts, Face the Facts, Talent Scouts, Take My Word, Ernie Kovacs' Take a Good Look.

ARNESS, JAMES: Actor. b. Minneapolis, Minn., May 26, 1923. e. Beloit College. Served in U.S. Army; worked in advertising, real estate; m.p. debut in Farmer's Daughter.
PICTURES INCLUDE: Battleground, Hell Gate, Man from Texas, People Against O'Hara, Iron Man, The Thing, Big Jim McLain, Horizon's West, Lone Hand, Island in the Sky, Veils of Bagdad, Hondo, Her Twelve Men, Them, Many Rivers to Cross, Flame of the Islands, Sea Chase.
TV SHOWS: Gunsmoke, How the West Was Won, McLain's Law.

ARNOLD, DANNY: Writer, actor. r.n. Arnold Rothman; b. New York, N.Y., Jan. 23, 1925. Appeared in summer stock, night clubs, vaudeville; entered m.p. ind. as sound effects ed., Columbia, 1944–46; then legit., night clubs, vaudeville, 1946–50. Appeared in m.p. Breakthrough, Inside the Walls of Folsom Prison, Sailor Beware, Jumping Jacks, Scared Stiff, Stars Are Singing,; featured on Martin and Lewis TV show 2 yrs., and wrote their Comedy Hours to 1953.
PICTURES INCLUDE: collab. s.p., story, The Caddy; collab., s.p., Desert Sands: story, s.p., Fort Yuma, story, s.p. Rebel in Town; s.p., Outside the Law. Writer-TV, Tennessee Ernie Ford Show.

ARNOLD, EDDY: Singer. b. Henderson, TN, May 15, 1918. Radio performer, Nashville, Tenn.; recording star since 1946; records include That's How Much I Love You, Anytime; star of Eddy Arnold Show, ABC-TV.

ARNOLD, JACK: Producer, Director. b. New Haven, Conn., Oct. 14, 1916; e. Ohio State U., Amer. Acad. of Dramatic Arts. Actor on B'way, Brit. m.p.; U.S. Air force, 1942–45; prod. 25 documentary films for State Dept., Army & private industry including With These Hands; dir., 1952.
PICTURES INCLUDE: The Mouse That Roared, Bachelor in Paradise, Global Affair, The Incredible Shrinking Man, It Came From Outer Space, The Creature from the Black Lagoon, Girls in The Night, Revenge of The Creature, The Tattered Dress, Glass Web, Man in The Shadow, Man From Bitter Ridge; dir. story; Tarantula, Red Sundown, Decision at Durango, Outside The Law, Pay The Devil, No Name On The Bullet, The Lady Takes A Flyer, The Lively Set, High School Confidential. Producer, Universal 1956; dir., Black Eye, 1974, Swiss Conspiracy, 1975.

ARNOUL, FRANCOISE: Actress. r.n. Francoise Gautsch. b. Algeria, 1931. Studied acting in Paris; m.p. debut in 1949.
PICTURES INCLUDE: Companions of the Night, Sheep

Has Five Legs, The Bed, Inside a Girl's Dormitory, Tempest in the Flesh, Only the French Can (French CanCan).

ARNOW, TED J.: Executive. b. Brooklyn N.Y. e. St. Johns Univ. Washington and Lee Univ. Served as dir. of recreation for 262nd General Hospital in Panama. Veteran of over 50 yrs. in amusement industry. Is v.p. for adv., pub., & promo, for Loew's Theatres. Member: Motion Picture Pioneers, Variety Clubs, Will Rogers Hospital; former pres. of AMPA (Assoc. M.P. Advertisers).

ARQUETTE, ROSANNA: Actress. b. 1960. Granddaughter of humorist Cliff Arquette (Charlie Weaver). Film debut as bit player in S.O.B., 1981.
PICTURES: Baby, It's You, The Aviator, Desperately Seeking Susan, After Hours, Silverado, Lies, 8 Million Ways To Die, Nobodys' Fool.
TELEVISION: The Executioner's Song, Johnny Belinda, Survival Guide.

ARTHUR, BEATRICE: Actress. b. New York City, May 13, 1923. Franklin Institute of Sciences & Art. m. Gene Saks. Studied with Erwin Piscator at New School for Social Research; first stage role as Lysistrata; professional stage debut in Dog Beneath the Skin, 1947, followed by Gas, Yerma, No Exit, Six Characters in Search of an Author. The Owl and the Pussycat, etc.; stock appearances include Personal Appearance, Candlelight, Love or Money, The voice of the Turtle; recent N.Y. stage includes Ullysses in Nighttown, Chic, Mame (Tony award), Fiddler on the Roof.
PICTURES INCLUDE: That Kind of Woman, Lovers and Other Strangers, Mame, History of the World—Part I.
TV: Numerous guest appearances; Maude.

ARTHUR, EDWARD B.: Executive. b. New York City, Sept. 30, 1915. e. San Jose State Coll.; Los Angeles Jr. Coll. Engaged in operation management, purchasing of films etc. in Calif., N.Y., Missouri, Illinois; served in armored div. World War II, 1st Lt., at close of war Special Service unit (Germany) in chg. of distribution of films to service units; resumed his post as gen. mgr. Arthur Enterprises, Inc. which he had joined in 1935; named pres. St. Louis Amusement Co., 1946. Member: Variety Club.

ARTHUR, JEAN: Actress b. New York City, Oct. 17, 1908. On stage; minor roles. m.p. debut as lead in "Warming Up" 1928.
PICTURES INCLUDE: Canary Murder Case, Mysterious Dr. Fu Manchu, Whirlpool, Mr. Deeds Goes to Town, You Can't Take It With You, Too Many Husbands, Talk of the Town, Lady Takes a Chance, Impatient Years, Foreign Affair, Shane.
N.Y. STAGE: Peter Pan, 1950.
TV: The Jean Arthur Show.

ARTHUR, ROBERT: Actor, r.n. Robert Arthaud. b. Aberdeen, Wash., June 18; e. U. Washington (U.S. Navy training program). Won H.S. radio announcing contest; prof. announcer & disc jockey; m.p. debut in "Roughly Speaking" 1945.
PICTURES INCLUDE: Nora Prentiss, Sweetheart of Sigma Chi, Devil on Wheels, Mother Wore Tights, 12 O'Clock High, September Affair, Air Cadet, Big Carnival, On the Loose, Belles on Their Toes, Just For You, The Ring, Young Bess, Take the High Ground, Return from the Sea, Top of the World, Desperados Are in Town, The System, Green Grass of Wyoming, Switchblade, Hellcats of the Navy, Young and Wild, Yellow Sky, Mother is a Freshman.

ARTHUR, ROBERT: Producer, b. New York City, Nov. 1, 1909; e. Southwestern U., U. Southern Calif. Oil operator 1929–36; joined MGM as writer 1937. Served in the United States Army 1942–45.
PICTURES INCLUDE: (prod.) Buck Private Come Home, For the Love of Mary, Mexican Hayride, Abbott and Costello in Foreign Legion, Louisa, Wistful Widow of Wagon Gap, Abbott & Costello Meet Frankenstein, Francis, Golden Horde, Starlift, Story of Will Rogers, The Big Heat, The Black Shield of Falworth, Ricochet Romance, The Long Gray Line, Francis in the Haunted House, Day of Fury, Pillars of the Sky, Kelly and Me, Mr. Cory, Midnight Story, Man of a Thousand Faces, A Time to Love and a Time to Die, The Perfect Furlough, Operation Petticoat, The Great Impostor, Come September, Lover, Come Back, The Spiral Road, That Touch of Mink, For Love of Money, The Brass Bottle, Captain Newman, M.D., Bedtime Story, Father Goose, Shenandoah, Blindfold, A Man Could Get Killed, Hellfighters, Sweet Charity.

ARTZ, BOB: Theatre Executive. b. Spokane, WA, Aug 21, 1946 e. B.T.A. Pasadena Playhouse College of Theatre Arts. Began in 1968 as doorman; then asst. mgr to mgr. with National General Theatre Corporation. Joined Plitt Theatres in 1978 as dist. mgr and ad director—presently ad/pub director—West Coast for Plitt Theatres.
MEMBER: Variety Club, Life Member: Pasadena Playhouse Alumni & Assoc.

ASH, RENE: Producer. b. Brussels, Belgium, March 14, 1939; e. U. of Omaha. member of the Publicists Guild since 1968; Eastern Vice President of Pub Guild since 1973; Author of The Film Editor in Motion Pictures & Television; employed with I.A.T.S.E. 1968–1979, prior to which was assoc. editor, Greater Amusements; various articles published in foreign film magazines; editor-in-chief, Backstage; 1979–80; est. Ash, Inc., pres., Cinereal Pictures Nov., 1984–Oct, 1985; exec. v.p., Eagle Films Corp., since Nov., 1985.

ASHBY, HAL: Director. b. Ogden, Utah. e. Utah State Univ. Began career as film editor. Worked with Norman Jewison on The Cincinnati Kid, The Russians Are Coming, The Russians Are Coming, In the Heat of the Night (AA) and also as assoc. prod on The Thomas Crown Affair and Gaily, Gaily, Directing debut, The Landlord, 1970.
PICTURES INCLUDE: Harold and Maude, The Last Detail, Shampoo, Bound for Glory, Coming Home, Second Hand Hearts, Lookin' To Get Out, The Slugger's Wife, 8 Million Ways To Die.

ASHER, JACK: Producer, dir. of photography. b. London, 1916. Ent. m.p. ind. 1930 as asst. cameraman for Gainsborough camera operator 1935; 1940 returned to Gainsborough as camera operator; dir., photography Gainsborough 1961. Many films since; 1961 Co. prod. with brother Robert, She'll Have to Go; dir. of photo., Scarlett Blade, Stitch in Time; dir., photo., The Intelligence Men, dir. photog., The Early Bird, 1965.

ASHER, JANE: Actress. Born London, England, 1946. She has acted in many films and TV plays. Films: Greengage Summer, Masque Of The Red Death, Alfie, Deep End, Henry The Eighth and His Six Wives, Runners, Dream Child.
TELEVISION: Brideshead Revisited, Voyage Round My Father, East Lynne.

ASHLEY, ELIZABETH: Actress. b. Aug. 30, 1939. Success on stage in 1960 with role in Take Her, She's Mine, winning Tony Award. Next starred in Barefoot in the Park.
PICTURES INCLUDE: The Carpetbaggers, Ship of Fools, The Third Day, The Marriage of a Young Stockbroker, Paperback Hero, Golden Needles, Rancho DeLuxe, 92 in the Shade, Great Scout and Cathouse Thursday, Coma, Windows, Captured, Paternity, Split Image.
TELEVISION: Stagecoach.

ASHLEY, JOHN: Actor. r.n. John Atchley. b. Kansas City, Mo., Dec. 25, 1934; e. Oklahoma State U., BA 1956. Career started in Tulsa Little Theatre, 1956; screen debut, 1957, Dragstrip Girl; later: Motorcycle Gang, Suicide Battalion.
TV: Men of Annapolis, Sheriff of Cochise, Frontier Doctor; Matinee Theatre, Jefferson Drum.

ASHLEY, TED: executive b. Brooklyn, N.Y. Aug. 3, 1922. e. City College of N.Y. School of Business Administration. 1937–39. With William Morris Agency, agent. 1939–46; formed Ted Ashley Associates, 1946; pres. Ashley Famous Agency, 1954; director and chairman of executive committee of Warner Communications Inc., 1967 to 1974; chairman of bd. and chief exec. officer, Warner Bros. 1969–75; chm. & co-CEO, 1976–80; 1981, sr. consultant, Warner Communications; 1982–84, vice chm. of bd., WC.

ASNER, EDWARD: Actor. b. Nov. 15, 1929, Kansas City, Kans. e. Univ. of Chicago, where affilliated with campus acting group. Served two years with U.S. Army in France. Returned to Chicago to join Playwright's Theatre Club. Moved to N.Y.C.; Broadway debut in Face of a Hero. Appeared off-Broadway, in stock, and with American Shakespeare Festival. In 1961 moved to Hollywood to become active in films and TV.
PICTURES INCLUDE: Peter Gunn, The Slender Thread, The Satan Bug, Kid Galahad, The Wrestler, Fort Apache, The Bronx, Daniel.
TELEVISION: Medical Center, Name of the Game, Mod Squad, Ironside, The Mary Tyler Moore Show (regular), Rich Man, Poor Man, Lou Grant, Off the Rack. Movies: Hey, I'm Alive, Anatomy of an Illness, Vital Signs. Mini-series: Tender is the Night.

ASSANTE, ARMAND: Actor. b. New York City, Oct. 4, 1949. e. AADA. Appeared with regional theatre groups and off-Bdwy. On Bdwy. in Boccaccio, Comedians, Romeo and Juliet, etc.
PICTURES: Lords of Flatbush, Paradise Alley, Prophesy, Little Darlings, Love and Money, Private Benjamin, I, the Jury, Unfaithfully Yours, Belizaire the Cajun.
TELEVISION: Human Feelilngs, Lady of the House, The Pirate, Sophia Loren—Her Own Story, Why Me?, Evergreen, A Deadly Business.

ASSEYEV, TAMARA: Producer. Began career as asst. to Roger Corman, working on 8 films with him. In 1967 started to produce films independently. In 1972 met Alex (Alexandra) Rose and later began co-producing films with her, starting with Drive-In, released by Columbia.

PICTURES INCLUDE: The Wild Racers, Paddy, The Arousers, The History of Atlantic Records, Co-produced with Ms. Rose: Drive-In, I Wanna Hold Your Hand, Big Wednesday, Norma Rae.

ASTAIRE, FRED: Dancer, actor, b. Omaha, Neb. May 10, 1900; e. at home; sister: Adele Astaire, dancer. Brother-sister dance team formed 1907; vaudeville debut 1908; Broadway shows include, Over the Top, Passing Show if 1918, Apple Blossoms, For Goodness Sakes, Lady Be Good, Smiles, Funny Face, Gay Divorcee, Bandwagon; team dissolved 1932; m.p. debut in Dancing Lady 1933; voted Money-Making Star in Motion Picture Herald-Fame Polls 1935–36–37; served with U.S.O. overseas World War II.
PICTURES INCLUDE: Flying Down to Rio, Gay Divorcee, Roberta, Top Hat, Swing Time, Carefree, Story of Vernon and Irene Castle, Holiday Inn, Sky's the Limit, Ziegfeld Follies, Blue Skies, Easter Parade, Special Academy Award for "raising standards of all musicals," 1949. TV specials. Won 9 Emmy Awards, 1958 (An Evening with Fred Astaire) 1959, Another Eve, with Fred Astaire; 1960 Astaire Time; Alcoa Premiere, 1962, Barkleys of Broadway, Let's Dance, Three Little Words, Royal Wedding Belle of New York, Band Wagon, Daddy Long Legs, Funny Face, Silk Stockings, On the Beach, The Pleasure of His Company, Notorious Landlady, Finians Rainbow, 1967, Midas Run, 1968. The Towering Inferno, 1974, That's Entertainment, Part Two, 1976, The Purple Taxi, Ghost Story.
TV: Fred Astaire Show, 1968, It Takes A Thief, A Family Upside Down, Man in the Santa Claus Suit.

ASTIN, JOHN: Actor. b. Baltimore, Md. March 30, 1930. e. Washington and Jefferson College, Washington Drama School, Johns Hopkins U., grad. B.A., U. of Minnesota Graduate School; first prof. job., off broadway, Threepenny Opera; Broadway debut, Major Barbara; dir., co-prod., A Sleep of Prisoners, Phoenix Theatre; during 1955–59, did voices in cartoons, commercials; I'm Dickens . . . He's Fenster, as Harry Dickens, The Adams Family.
STAGE SHOWS INCLUDE: The Cave Dwellers, Ulysses in Nighttown, Tall Story.
PICTURES INCLUDE: West Side Story, That Touch of Mink, Candy, Viva, Max!, Bunny O'Hare, Get to Know Your Rabbi, Every Little Crook and Nanny, Freaky Friday.

ASTOR, MARY: Actress, r.n. Lucille V. Langhanke; b. May 3, 1906; e. Kenwood-Loring School (Chicago). Beauty contest winner 1920; m.p. debut in "Beggar's Maid" 1920; radio m.c. 2½ yrs.; on stage in: Among the Married, Tonight at 8:30, Male Animal.
PICTURES INCLUDE: (silent) Don Juan, Bright Shawl, Beau Brummel; (sound) Lost Squadron, Jennie Gerhardt, Easy to Love, Man With Two Faces, Listen Darling, Dodsworth, Maltese Falcon, Across the Pacific, Meet Me in St. Louis, Fiesta, Cynthia, Cass Timberlane, Desert Fury, Act of Violence, Little Women, Any Number Can Play, Kiss Before Dying, Return to Peyton Place, Youngblood Hawke, Hush, Hush Sweet Charlotte.

ATHERTON, WILLIAM: b. New Haven, Conn., 1949. While in high school became youngest member of Long Wharf Theatre Co. Given scholarship to Pasadena Playhouse; then switched to Carnegie Tech School of Drama in 1965. In college years toured with USO prods. in Europe and in stock and industrial shows. Came to N.Y. where first prof. job was in nat'l. co. of Little Murders.
PICTURES INCLUDE: The New Centurions, The Sugarland Express, The Day of the Locust, The Hindenburg, Looking for Mr. Goodbar, Real Genius.
PLAYS: The House of Blue Leaves, The Basic Training of Pavlo Hummel, The Sign in Sidney Brustein's Window.
TELEVISION: Centennial, Malibu.

ATKINS, CHRISTOPHER: Actor. b. Rye, NY, Feb. 21, 1961. e. Dennison Univ., Ohio. Early modelling jobs; theatrical film debut in The Blue Lagoon (1980).
PICTURES: The Pirate Movie, A Night in Heaven.
TELEVISION: Movie: Raid on Short Creek. Series: Dallas.

ATTENBOROUGH, DAVID: Broadcaster. b. London, May 8, 1926; e. Wyggeston School, Leicester; Clare College, Cambridge, early career, editor in educational publishing house, ent. BBC-TC Sept. 1952. Prod. Zoo Quest series, Travellers Tales, Adventure and other prog., travel, Eastward with Attenborough, The Tribal Eye, Life on Earth, exploration natural History and anthropology. Controller BBC-2, 1965–68; Dir. of Prog. BBC-TV, 1969–72.

ATTENBOROUGH, RICHARD: Actor, producer, director. b. Cambridge, Eng., Aug. 29, 1923; m. 1945 Sheila Beryl Grant Sim. Wyggeston Grammar School, Leicester. Leverhulme Scholarship to Royal Academy of Dramatic Art, 1941 (Bancroft Medal). First stage appearance Ah Wilderness, 1941. London debut in Awake and Sing, 1942. First film appearance in In Which We Serve, 1942. Appeared in The Little Foxes, Piccadilly Theatre, 1942; Brighton Rock, Garrick Theatre 1943. Joined R.A.F. 1943; seconded to R.A.F. Film Unit, 1944, and appeared in Journey Together; demobilised, 1946. Returned to stage, Jan. 1949, in The Way Back (Home of the Brave), To Dorothy, A Son, 1950; Sweet Madness, 1952; The Mousetrap, 1952–54; Double Image, 1956–1957; The Rape of the Belt, 1957–1958.
PICTURES INCLUDE: School for Secrets (Secret Flight), The Man Within (The Smugglers), Dancing with Crime, Brighton Rock (Young Scarface), London Belongs to Me (Dulcimer Street), The Guinea Pig, The Lost People, Boys in Brown, Morning Departure (Operation Disaster), Hell is Sold Out, The Magic Box, Gift Horse (Glory at Sea), Father's Doing Fine, Eight O'Clock Walk, The Ship That Died of Shame, Private's Progress, The Baby and the Battleship, Brothers-in-Law, The Scamp, Dundirk, The Man Upstairs, Sea of Sand, Danger Within, I'm All Right Jack, Jetstorm, S.O.S. Pacific; 1959 formed Beaver Films with Bryan Forbes and appeared in and co-produced The Angry Silence; formed Allied Film Makers and appeared in their first film The League of Gentlemen; produced Whistle Down The Wind, appeared in Only Two Can Play, All Night Long, The Dock Brief (Trial & Error); produced The L-Shaped Room, appeared in The Great Escape, appeared in and produced Seance on a Wet Afternoon; appeared in The Third Secret, 1963; Guns at Batasi, 1964; The Flight of the Phoenix, 1965; The Bliss of Mrs. Blossom, Only When I Larf, 1968. Prod. and dir.: Oh! What a Lovely War, 1968. Appeared in The Last Grenade, A Severed Head, Loot, and made quest appearances in The Magic Christian and David Copperfield, 1969, 10 Rillington Place, 1970, Young Winston, 1972 appeared in Rosebud, Ten Little Indians, Brannigan. Conduct Unbecoming 1974, directed A Bridge Too Far, 1976. Appeared in The Chess Players, 1977; dir. Magic, 1978, actor, The Human Factor, 1978; Gandhi (prod.-dir.), 1982; A Chorus Line (dir.), 1985.

ATTERBURY, MALCOLM: Actor. b. Philadelphia, Pa. Feb. 20, 1907, e. Hill School, Pa. Radio editor, Phila. Ledger; prog. mgr., gen. mgr., performer, Phila. Ledger radio station, WHAT, 7 yrs.; concert, vaudeville, Schubert musicals, 7 yrs.; Tamarack Playhouse, 5 yrs.; owned, oper., Albany Playhouse, 6 yrs.; conducted thea. seminars, Skidmore, R.P.I., College of St. Rose.
TV: Hallmark Hall of Fame, Lux Video Thea., Playhouse 90, Studio One, G.E. Theatre, Cheyenne, Perry Mason, Gunsmoke, 77 Sunset Strip, Alfred Hitchcock Presents, Route 66, The Defenders, The Untouchables, Dr. Kildare, Profiles In Courage, Fugitive, FBI, Hazel, Bonanza, Voyage to the Bottom of the Sea, Judd.
PICTURES INCLUDE: Dragnet, Storm Center, Crime in the Streets, Reprisal, Crime of Passion, Toward the Unknown, No Time for Sergeants, Rio Bravo, North by Northwest, Wild River, From the Terrace, Summer and Smoke, Advise and Consent, The Birds, The Chase, Hawaii.
BROADWAY: One Flew Over the Cuckoo's Nest.

ATTWOOLL, HUGH: Assoc. Producer. b. 1914. Ent. films 1928.
PICTURES INCLUDE: The Castaways, The Horse Without A Head, Three Lives or Thomasina, Dr. Syn, The Moonspinners, The Legend of Young Dick Turpin, The Fighting Prince of Donegal, Only When I Larf, Guns in the Heather, David Copperfield, Kidnapped, Diamonds on Wheels, Persecution, One of our Dinosaurs Is Missing, Escape From The Darkness, Harness Fever, Candleshoe, The Spaceman and King Arthur, Watcher in the Woods, The London Connection.

ATWATER, GLADYS: Writer. Has written many m.p. scripts; member of writing team with Robert Bren since 1939; v.p. Bremex, Inc., writings include: (collab. orig.) Man Who Found Himself: (collab. orig. story) Argentine Nights, First Yank into Tokyo, in Old California; (collab. s.p.) Criminal Lawyer, Crashing Hollywood, This Marriage Business, Crime Ring; (collab. story) El Paso, Tag for Murder, Blood on the Shrine, Legacy in Nylons, Aztec Dagger, Female Menagerie. Collab. story, s.p., Great Sioux Uprising, Siege at Red River; collab. s.p., Overland Pacific; collab. stor. Naked Alibi, Treasure of Pancho Villa; TV: Lone Wolf in Mexico, Stolen Train, Casey Jones series, Winds of the Four Seasons, collab. s.p.; collab. s.p. orig. story The Hawaiians.

AUBERJONOIS, RENE: Actor. b. New York City, June 1, 1940. On Bdwy. in Dark of the Moon, Beyond the Fringe, Charley's Aunt, A Cry of Players, Coco, Tricks, The Ruling Class.
PICTURES INCLUDE: Brewster McCloud, McCabe and Mrs. Miller, Pete 'n Tillie, Hindenberg, King Kong, Eyes of Laura Mars, Where the Buffalo Roam; 3:15.
TELEVISION: Benson.

AUBREY, JAMES T., JR.: Executive. b. La Salle, Ill., Dec. 14, 1918. e. Princeton U., 1941, m. Phyllis Thaxter, U.S. Air Force, 1941–45; salesman, Street and Smith, Conde Nast Pub., 1946–47; account exec. KNX, Los Angeles, 1948; account exec., KNXT, 1951; sales mgr., then gen. mgr., KNXT and CTPN, 1952. Man. network prog., Hollywood CBS-TV, 1956; V.P. programs and talent, ABC-TV 1957;

v.-p. CBS. 1958; exec. v.p. CBS-TV, 1959; pres. CBS-TV, 1959. In 1969–73 MGM pres.; now indep. prod.
PICTURES INCLUDE: Futureworld (prod.), The Hunger.

AUDRAN, STEPHANE: Actress. b. France, 1938. Ex-wife of French star Jean-Louis Trintignant; now married to director Claude Chabrol.
PICTURES INCLUDE: Les Cousins (debut under direction of Chabrol), The Champagne Murders, Les Biches, La Femme Infidele, The Beast Must Die, The Lady in the Car, Le Boucher, Without Apparent Motive, Dead Pigeon on Beethoven Street, The Discreet Charm of the Burgeoisie, The Devil's Advocate, The Blackbird (American film debut), Silver Bears, Blood Relatives.
TELEVISION: Mistral's Daughter, The Blood of Others, The Sun Also Rises.

AUERBACH, NORBERT T.: President & Chief Executive Officer, United Artists Corp. b. Vienna, 1923. Educated in U.S. and served with U.S. Army Intelligence in Europe during World War II. Joined m.p. business in 1946 after graduation from U.C.L.A. (business admin.). First asst. dir. at Service Studios in Calif. Moved to N.Y. to join domestic sales dept. of Film Classics. Left for position with Columbia Pictures in foreign dept. In 1950 assigned to Paris office, where remained for over decade, except for 18 mos. in Portugal as mgr. Returned to Paris in 1953 and filled number of exec. sls. positions for Columbia, ultimately rising to continental mgr. 1961, left Columbia to produce films in France. Resumed career in dist., this time at Paris office of United Artists, becoming continental mgr. In 1966 returned to production to make The Thief of Paris. 1967, joined Seven Arts Prods. heading theatrical and TV sls. operations in Paris. When Seven Arts acquired Warner Bros., he became continental sls. mgr. for Warners in Paris. 1968, set up European prod. and dist. org. for CBS Cinema Center Films, operating from London. 1972, moved to L.A. as v.p., foreign mgr. for CCF. Returned to London in 1973 to be consultant in prod, and dist. Rejoined UA in 1977 as sls. mgr. for Europe and the Middle East. Named snr. v.p. & foreign mgr. in 1978. Named pres. & COO, Jan. 1981; pres., CEO, Feb. 1981. Co-pres., United Int'l Pictures, London, till 1982. In 1983 formed Packaging and financing Co., Eliktra, Inc. 1982, acting pres. and chief exec. officer of Almi Distribution Corp, Now Almi consultant.

AUMONT, JEAN PIERRE: Actor. b. Paris, 1913. e. Conservatoire of Drama. Roles French stage and films. U.S. pictures: Assignment in Brittany, Cross of Lorraine, In 1943 enlisted Free French Army.
PICTURES INCLUDE: Heartbeat, Siren of Atlantis, Affairs of a Rogue, Wicked City, Lili, Life Begins Tomorrow, Gay Adventure, Charge of the Lancers, Hilda Crane, Enemy General, The Devil at 4 O'Clock, Castle Keep, Cauldron of Blood, Day for Night, Mahogany, Catherine & Co., Sweet Country.
STAGE: Tovarich, Incident at Vichy, Carnival, Camino Real.
TELEVISION: Sins.

AURELIUS, GEORGE M.: Executive. b. Grasston, Minn., Sept. 16, 1911; e. U. of Minnesota. Ent. m.p. ind. 1927 as usher Finkelstein & Ruben, St. Paul; asst. mgr. 1929–30; to Warner Theatres, New York 1931; man. Moss' Broadway; Minnesota Amusement Co. 1932–41; city mgr. Publix-Rickards-Nace. Paramount-Nace Theatres, Tucson, Ariz. 1941–46; V.P. ABC Theas. of Arizona, Inc. 1949–67; pres. ABC North Central Theatres, Inc., 1967–1972; V.P. ABC Intermountain Theatres, Inc., V.P. ABC Theatres of California, Inc. 1972–1974; Mgmt. Consulting and ShoWest Convention & Trade Show since 1975, named exec. dir., 1979. Retired 1985.

AURTHUR, ROBERT ALAN: Writer-producer. b. New York, N.Y., June 10, 1922. e. Univ. of Pennsylvania, BA, 1942. U.S. Marine Corps., 1942–46; author: History of the Third Marine Division, Inf. Journal Press, 1946; short story writer, The New Yorker, Harpers, Esquire, Sat. Eve. Post, etc. 1946–50; novel: The Glorification of Al Toolum; Rinehart, 1951; partner, Circle Records, 1947–50; freelance TV dramatist, 1951–58, vice-pres., Talent Associates-Paramount Ltd., 1961; pres., Edgewater Prods. Monthly column "Hanging Out" Esquire Magazine 1972, NYU School of Arts, Instructor screenplay writing, 1975; Delegate to Moscow Film Festival, International Writers Guild Symposium, Leningrad, 1975.
TV INCLUDES: script ed., Philco Playhouse, Mr. Peepers, assoc. prod., Philco Playhouse, then prod.; prod., Sunday Showcase, NBC, Years of Decision, pilots: Inside Danny Baker, The Laughmakers, ABC. Head of new prog. dev. United Artists-TV, 1963–64.
PICTURES INCLUDE: screenwriter. Warlock, The Mountain Is Young; writer, co-prod., Edge of the City; s.p. Lilith, s.p. Grand Prix, For the Love of Ivy, s.p. and dir. The Lost Man, Indians (s.p.), Ending (s.p.).
BROADWAY: Author, A Very Special Baby, Kwamina, Carry Me Back to Morningside Heights.

AUSTIN, BUD: Executive. r.n. Harold M. b. New York, N.Y. e. Univ. of North Carolina, New York U., Pres. Austin Productions 1971; U.S. Army 1942–46; pres., Donna Hale Corp. 1948; pres., Lindley Corp. 1949; nat'l. sls. mgr. Official Films, 1950–53; vice-pres., Telefilm Ent., 1954; vice-pres. NTA, 1955; pres. Austin Television Prods., 1956; 1956–65, sr. exec. v.p., Goodson-Todman Prods.; exec. vice-pres., Filmways, Inc., 1965; 1973, Vice President Creative Services and Marketing Paramount Pictures Corp. Executive Producer, Elaine May film "Mikey and Nicky," Executive Producer and Creator "Take Five" for CBS-TV; 1973–76, chief exec. officer, Paramount TV; pres., Bud Austin Productions. 1979, prod., Perfect Gentlemen; exec. prod., Whew (TV game show); 1980, creative consultant, Universal TV. On bd. of dir., Producers Guild of America; chm. Cable Committee. Prod.: Still the Beaver; exec. prod.: Johnny Dangerously (20th-Fox).

AUSTIN, JOHN: Producer. b. Australia, 1923; Asst. Dir. of Entertainment for American Red Cross, 1942–45; assoc. West Coast rep. of Rodgers & Hammerstein, 1945–47; with Ministry of Info., Gov't of India, 1947–48; prod. TV films in Europe, 1949; shows include Intrigue, International Rendezvous, International Affair; prod. film Lasca. Since 1954, representative of leading foreign newspapers in Hollywood as correspondent for the entertainment industry. 1974–1977 West Coast editor, Screen International. 1977–1981, international editor, The Hollywood Reporter. President: Inter-Global Film Consultants. Since 1982, vice president, editor in chief, Film News-International for VPA, Inc. Consultant to foreign producers on U.S. marketing and advertising techniques.

AUSTIN, RAY: Director-Writer-Producer. b. London, England, Dec. 5, 1932. Has written, produced and directed many TV series, specials and movies.
TELEVISION: Director of series: Avengers, The Champions, Department S, Randall & Hopkirk, Ugliest Girl in Town, Journey into the Unknown, Magnum P.I., Simon and Simon, House Calls, Kings Crossing, Fall Guy, Time Street, Spencer for Hire. Writer: Randall & Hopkirk, Department S. Producer-Director: The Perfumed Garden. Director: It's the Only Way To Go, Fun and Games, Space 1999, New Avengers, Hawaii Five-O, Sword of Justice, Webb, Barnaby Jones, Hardy Boys, Wonder Woman, Salvage, B.G. and the Bears, Hart to Hart, The Yeagers, Man Called Sloane, From Here to Eternity, Bad Cast, Westworld, Tales of the Gold Monkey, The Return of the Man from UNCLE. Director-Writer: Black Beauty, Zany Adventures of Robin Hood (CBS), The Master (NBC), Hart to Hart (ABC series) V (CBS), Air Wolf.
PICTURES: Virgin Witches, House of the Living Dead.

AUTANT-LARA, CLAUDE: Director. Began career as scenic designer for French films in early 1920s; then asst. director; first solo venture experimental film, 1923; in Hollywood, 1930–32. dir. parlor Bedroom and Bath, Incomplete Athlete.
PICTURES INCLUDE: Devil in the Flesh, Seven Deadly Sins (seq.), Red Inn, Oh Amelia, Game of Love, Red and the Black.

AUTEN, H. WILLIAM: Executive. b. Cardiff, Wales, Mar. 7, 1921; e. Neville House, Eastbourne; U. Coll. School of London. With sales dept., Warner Bros. (London) 1939; served as Major on Brit. Army Staff 1939–47, including custodianship of UFA, GMBH 1945–46; European & Near Eastern mgr. United Artists 1948; asst. foreign mgr. Eagle Lion Films, Inc. (N.Y.) 1948–49; founder & pres. Benagoss Productions, Inc. June, 1949, to produce and finance pictures; org. Ballentine Pict., 1951.

AUTRY, GENE: Actor. b. Tioga, Tex., Sept. 29, 1907. Railroad telegrapher at Sapulpa, Okla., 1925; became radio singer and recording artist (Columbia Records) 1928; screen debut 1934 at Mascot Pictures (later became Republic) as screen's first singing cowboy. Starred in 89 feature films and 91 half hour TV films, The Gene Autry Show, 1950–1955. Formed Flying A Productions, produced Annie Oakley, The Range Rider, Buffalo Bill, Jr. and Adventures of Champion TV series. Wrote or co-wrote and recorded over two hundred songs, has 9 Gold Records, including all-time best seller, Rudolph the Red-Nosed Reindeer. Voted top money making Western star 1937–42, and in top Western stars 1936, 1946–54; first Western star to be in top ten money makers from 1938 to 1942. Served in U.S.A.A.F. as flight officer, 1942–45; on USO tour overseas 3 mos.; immediately therafter resumed radio career with former sponsor, the Wm. Wrigley Co., formed Gene Autry Productions, Inc., star of Madison Square Garden Rodeo first in 1940; composed & recorded song "Here Comes Santa Claus"; owner radio & TV stations, and California Angels ball team.

AVAKIAN, ARAM: Director. b. N.Y.C. Was still photographer and editor before becoming director with The End of the Road.

PICTURES INCLUDE: Cops and Robbers, 11 Harrowhouse.

AVALON, FRANKIE: Entertainer. r.n. Francis Thomas Avalone. b. Phila., Sept. 18, 1940; e. South Phila. High. Trumpet Prodigy age 9 yrs; Recording contract, Chancellor Records, Inc., 1957; Gold Record, Venus 1959; Gold Album, Swingin' on a Rainbow, 1959; Night Clubs.
TV: Ed Sullivan, Perry Como, Pat Boone, Arthur Murray, Dick Clark Shows, Milton Berle, Golden Circle Spectacular; Dinah Shore Show, Steve Allen Show.
PICTURES INCLUDE: Guns of the Timberland, The Alamo, Voyage to the Bottom of the Sea, Sail a Crooked Ship, Panic in the Year Zero, Bikini Beach, Beach Blanket Bingo, Jet Set, I'll Take Sweden, Sgt. Deadhead, The Take, Grease.

AVEDON, DOE: Actress. b. Old Westbury, N.Y. Bookkeeper; then actress.
BROADWAY: Young and the Fair, My Name is Aquilon.
PICTURES INCLUDE: High and the Mighty, Deep In My Heart, The Boss.
TV: Big Town.

AVILDSEN, JOHN G.: Director-Cinematographer-Editor. b. Chicago. e. N.Y. Univ. After service in Army made film with friend, Greenwich Village Story, then joined ad agency to write and produce film commercials. Entered m.p. industry as ass't. cameraman on Below the Hill, followed with prod. mgr. job on Italian film made in U.S. Then made first theatrical short, Smiles. Arthur Penn hired him as prod. mgr. on Mickey One. Produced, photographed and edited a short, Light, Sound, Diffuse. Returned to industry to make films for ad agencies before resuming theatrical career.
PICTURES INCLUDE: Turn on to Love (1st feature, dir., photo.), Out of It (dir., photo.), Sweet Dreams (dir., photo, editor), Guess What We Learned in School Today? (dir., photo editor), Joe (dir., photo.), Cry Uncle (dir., photo., editor), Save The Tiger (dir.), W. W. and the Dixie Dancekings (dir., editor), Inaugural Ball (dir.), Rocky (dir.); Slow Dancing in the Big City (dir., editor, operator), The Formula (dir., editor), Neighbors (dir. and supv. editor); Traveling Hopefully (documentary, 1982) (dir.); A Night in Heaven (dir., editor, operator). 1983; The Karate Kid (dir., editor), 1984; Happy New Year (dir.), 1986; The Karate Kid: Part II. (dir., editor), 1986.

AVNET, JON: Producer. e. Sarah Lawrence Coll. Began career as director of off-Bdwy. prods. Produced and directed low-budget film, Confusion's Circle, which brough a directing fellowship at American Film Institute. There produced and directed Thursday Night Woman. Joined Weintraub/Heller Prods. as assoc. prod., where met Steve Tisch, with whom formed Tisch/Avnet Prods.
PICTURES: Outlaw Blues, Risky Business, Deal of the Century.
TELEVISION: Homeward Bound, No Other Love, Prime Suspect, Something So Right.

AXELROD, GEORGE: Playwright, writer, prod., dir. b. New York, N.Y., June 9, 1922, stage mgr., actor, summer stock, 1940–41; radio writer, 1941–52; writer, novels: Beggar's Choice, Blackmailer; co-writer, night club musical: All About Love, 1951.
BROADWAY: The Seven Year Itch, Will Success Spoil Rock Hunter?, Visit to a Small Planet, Once More With Feeling, Goodbye Charlie.
PICTURES INCLUDE: Phifft, The Seven Year Itch, Bus Stop, Breakfast at Tiffany's, The Manchurian Candidate. Paris When It Sizzles, How to Murder Your Wife, Lord Love a Duck, The Secret Life of an American Wife (prod., s.p.).

AXELROD, JONATHAN: Writer. b. N.Y.C. July 9, 1948. Stepson of writer George Axelrod. Started as on-set "gofer" before writing screen plays.
PICTURES INCLUDE: The Dirty Movie, Every Little Crook and Nanny.

AYKROYD, DAN: Actor-Writer. b. Ottawa, Canada. July 1, 1952. Performed and recorded with John Belushi as the Blues Brothers. On TV in Coming up Rosie (Canada). Saturday Night Live., s writer and performer.
PICTURES INCLUDE: M. Mike's Mondo Video. Love at First Sight, 1941, The Blues Brothers, Neighbors, Doctor Detroit, Trading Places, Twilight Zone—The Movie, Ghostbusters, Nothing Lasts Forever, Into the Night, Spies Like Us.

AYRES, GERALD: Producer–Writer. e. Yale Univ., where had four plays produced. Became Broadway play doctor and then joined Columbia Pictures as freelance reader. Named story editor; exec. ass't. to v.p. Mike Frankovich; then v.p. in chg. creative affairs in Hollywood. Left in 1970 to become independent. Formed Acrobat Films.
PICTURES INCLUDE: Cisco Pike, The Last Detail, Rich and Famous (s.p. only), Foxes (also s.p.).

AYRES, LEW: Actor. b. Minneapolis, Minn., Dec. 28, 1908. Toured Mexico with own orchestra; played with Henry Halstead's Orchestra; screen debut in The Sophomore, "The Kiss" 1929; served as medical corpsman & asst. chaplain World War II.
PICTURES INCLUDE: All Quiet on the Western Front, Common Clay, Doorway to Hell, Okay America, State Fair, Dr. Kildare series; (dir.) Hearts of Bondage, Dark Mirror, Unfaithful, Johnny Belinda, The Capture, New Mexico, No Escape, Donovan's Brain, The Carpetbaggers, Advise and Consent, Altars to the East (dir-nar. star-prod.), Last Generation, 1971, Biscuit Eater, The Man, Battle for the Planet of the Apes, Damien-Omen II, Battlestar Galactica.
TELEVISION: Under Siege.

AZZATO, ANTHONY: Executive; b. New York City, Oct. 7, 1912. e. Fordham Univ., City Col. of New York; production supervisor, film editor, director, documentary and comm. films, 1938–48; Sound Masters, Inc.; U.S. Army Signal Corps, 1942–46; film editor, Paramount, 1932–42; appt'd director of film programs, WPIX, 1948; also film program consultant, KLAC, Los Angeles; dir. of station relations, National Telefilm Assoc. 1956, v.p., Swan & Mason Adv., 1961; v.p., Sales, Teledynamics Corp.; v.p. Teledynamics Corp.

B

BABCOCK, DWIGHT V.: Writer. b. Ida Grove, Ia., Feb. 19, 1909. e. Modesto Jr. Coll. Author short stories, novelist. First Screenplay at Universal, 1943. 26 screen credits since at various studios. TV, free lance, includes 100 produced teleplays; co-author, Chautauqua.

BACALL, LAUREN: Actress. b. New York City, Sept. 16, 1924; e. American Acad. Dram. Arts. m. late Humphrey Bogart, actor. Fashion model; on stage, plays include: Johny Two-by-Four, Franklin Street; m.p. debut in "To Have and Have Not" 1944.
BROADWAY: Cactus Flower, Goodbye Charlie, Applause (Tony Award, Best Actress in musical), Woman of the Year.
PICTURES INCLUDE: Big Sleep, Confidential Agent, Dark Passage, Key Largo, Young Man with a Horn, Bright Leaf, How to Marry a Millionaire, Woman's World, Cobweb, Blood Alley, Written on the Wind, Designing Woman, Flame Over India, Shock Treatment, Gift of Love, Sex and the Single Girl, Harper, Murder on the Orient Express, The Shootist, Health, The Fan.
TV: Applause

BACHARACH, BURT: Composer-Conductor-Arranger. b. Kansas City, MO, May 12, 1928. e. McGraw Univ. Mannes School of Mucis, Music Academy of the West. Has conducted for Marlene Dietrich, Vic Damone, etc.
PICTURES INCLUDE: What'S New Pussycat?, Casino Royale, Butch Cassidy and the Sundance Kid, Lost Horizon, Arthur.
TELEVISION: Burt Bacharach Special.

BACK, LEON B.: Exhibiter. b. Philadelphia, Pa., Oct. 23, 1912; e. Johns Hopkins U., B.E., 1932; U. of Baltimore, LL.B., 1933. Entered m.p. ind. as mgr. for Rome Theatres, Inc., Baltimore, Md., 1934; booker, asst. buyer, 1936; asst. to gen. mgr. 1939; U.S. Navy, 1944–46; v.p., gen. mgr., Rome Theatres, 1946; Allied MPTO of Md. 1952–55; nat'l dir. Allied States, 1952–55; nat'l secy. 1954, Pres. NATO of Maryland 1969–80, Pres. USO Council, Greater Baltimore 1969–75; Chariman board of trustees, Employees Benefit Trust for Health & Welfare Council of Central Maryland, 1970–79.

BACKE, JOHN DAVID: Executive. b. Akron, OH, July 5, 1932. e. Miami U (BS, 1954); Xavier U. (MBA, 1961). Various managerial positions in engineering, financing and marketing functions, Gen. Electric Co., 1957–66; v.p., dir. mktg., Silver Burdett Co., div. Gen. Learning Corp., 1966–68; pres., 1968–69; exec. v.p., Gen. Learning Corp., 1969; pres., chief exec. officer, 1969–73; pres., CBS Pub. Group, 1973–76; v.p., dir., CBS, Inc. 1973–76; pres., chief exec. officer, mem. fin. comm., dir., 1976–80; now. chm., Tomorrow Entertainment, Inc., and chm., Backe Communications, Inc.

BACKUS, JIM: Actor. b. Cleveland, Ohio, Feb. 25, 1913; e. Amer. Acad. of Dram. Arts. Began in stock & vaudeville; radio announcer; radio actor on Ilum On stage in Hitch your Wagon; m.p. debut in Easy Living, Abner, Alan Young show & own shows.
PICTURES INCLUDE: Half Angel, His Kind of Woman, Bright Victory, Hollywood Story, Man With a Cloak, Iron Man, Here Come the Nelsons, I'll See You in My Dreams, Deadline, U.S.A., Androcles and the Lion, Don't Bother to Knock, Pat and Mike, Above and Beyond, I Love Melvin,

Angel Face, Geraldine, Human Jungle, Francis in the Navy, Rebel Without a Cause, Square Jungle, Meet me in Las Vegas, The Wonderful World of the Brothers Grimm, Critics Choice, Six Loves, Boys' Night Out, The Horizontal Lieutenant, Zoto!, Hello Down There, Pete's Dragon.
TV: I Married Joan, Gilligan's Island.
RECORDINGS: Delicious, Cave Man.
BOOKS: Rocks On the Roof, Back to Backus, What Are You Doing After the Orgy.

BACON, KEVIN: Actor. b. Philadelphia. Studied at Manning St. Actor's Theatre. Apprentice at Circle-in-the Square in N.Y. Bdwy. debut in Slab Boys with Sean Penn. Film debut in National Lampoon's Animal House (1978).
PICTURES: Friday the 13th, Hero at Large, Only When I Laugh, Diner, Footloose, Quicksilver, Rites of Summer.
TELEVISION: Movies: The Gift, Enormous Changes at the Last Minute. Series: Search for Tomorrow, Guiding Light.

BADHAM, JOHN: Director. b. England. Raised in Alabama; schooled at Yale, where acquired 2 degrees. Landed first job in Universal Studio mailroom; later was Universal Tour guide and assoc. prod. to Steven Spielberg. Made film trailers. Started directing movies for TV which led to theatrical debut with The Bingo Long & Travelling All-Stars and Motor Kings.
PICTURES: Saturday Night Fever, Dracula, Whose Life Is It Anyway?, Blue Thunder, War Games, Short Circuit.
TELEVISION: The Law, Isn't it Shocking?, etc.

BAER, JOHN G.: Executive—Engineer. b. New York City, May 8, 1934. e. Univ. of Tenn. at Chattanooga (B.S., physics, 1955). Joined Bausch and Lomb, Inc., as optical and mechanical engineer, 1957–67; director of research and development, 20th Century-Fox, New York, 1967–72; sales/engineering, Century Projector Corp., named pres. & chief exec. officer, Jan. 1, 1975.
MEMBER: Optical Society of America; Society of American Magicians; Intl. Brotherhood of Magicians; Magic Circle (London); 25–30 Club (honorary). Fellow of SMPTE and dir. Theatre Equip. Assn. Chm., PH-22 (motion picture) American Natl. Standards Institute U.S. delegate to Intl. Standards Organization. Elected mayor West Windsor Township, N.J., 1977.

BAILEY, JOSEPH W.: Attorney, producer. b. Columbia City, Ind., Dec. 13, 1910; e. U. of Chicago, PHB, 1928–31, U. of Chicago Law Sch., J.D., 1931–34. Practicing atty. at law, Chicago, Oct., 1934–June, 1940; with Louis G. Cowan to Apr. 1942; U.S. Navy, 1942–46; v.p. & treas., Louis G. Cowan, 1946–49; mgr., radio-TV dept., Grey Adv. Agency, 1949; exec. prod., Robert Montgomery Show & mgr., John Gibbs literary & talent agency, 1950–57; Prod. v.p. Ziv-United Artists, Inc. 1957–61. Resigned June 1961 to become partner in firm, Bronstein, Van Veen & Bailey; in practice of law specializing in allied field of TV, motion pictures and the theatre.

BAILEY, PEARL: Entertainer. b. Newport News, Va., March 29, 1918; e. Philadelphia and Washington, D.C. Career started when 15 years old, winner of amateur stage contest; toured mining towns of Pennsylvania as dancer; dancer and singer in vaudeville with Noble Sissle's band; stage acting debut in St. Louis Woman (won Donaldson Award, best newcomer of 1946); many night club appearances and TV shows; screen debut 1947, Variety Girl.
PLAYS INCLUDE: Arms and the Girl, Bless You All, House of Flowers, Hello Dolly.
PICTURES INCLUDE: Carmen Jones, Isn't it Romantic, That Certain Feeling, St. Louis Blues, Porgy and Bess, All the Fine Young Cannibals, The Landlord, Last Generation, Norman, Is That You?

BAILEY, ROBIN: Actor. b. Hucknail (Nottingham) Eng., Oct. 5, 1919. e. Henry Mellish School, Nottingham.
STAGE: Barrets of Wimpole Street, Theatre Royal, Nottingham, 1938; Screen debut, School for Secrets, 1946.
PICTURES INCLUDE: Private Angelo, Portrait of Clare, His Excellency, Gift Horse, Folly to be Wise, Single Handed, Sailor of the King, The Young Lovers, For Better or Worse, Catch Us If You Can, The Whisperers, Spy With A Cold Nose, You Only Live Twice, The Eliminator, Blind Terror, Down by the Riverside, Nightmare Rally, The Four Feathers.
TV: Olive Latimer's Husband, Seven Deadly Sins, The Power Game, Public Eye, Person To Person, Troubleshooters, Armchair Theatre, Split Level, The Newcomers, Discharge of Trooper Lusby, Brett, Owen M.D., Solidarity, General Hospital, Murder Must Advertise, Vienna 1900, Justice, The Pallisers, The Couch, Way of the World, Upstairs, Downstairs, Walk with Destiny, North and South, A Legacy, I Didn't Know You Cared, Punch Review, Play for Today, The Velvet Glove, Crown Court, Took and Co., The Good Companions, Cupid's Darts, Sorry, I'm a Stranger Here Myself, Call My Bluff, Jane, Potter, Tales from a Long Room, Sharing Time, Bleak House, Charters and Caldicott, Looks Familiar, On Stage.

BAKER, CARROLL: Actress. b. Johnstown, Pa., May 28, 1931. e. schools there and St. Petersburg (Fla.) Junior Coll. Career started as dancer in night clubs. Actors' Studio N.Y. Stage debut: Escapade, Then, All Summer Long; screen debut; Easy to Love.
PICTURES INCLUDE: Giant. Starred in Baby Doll, But Not for Me, The Miracle, Bridge to the Sun, Something Wild, How the West Was Won, The Carpetbaggers, Station Six Sahara, Sylvia, Cheyenne Autumn, Mister Moses, Harlow, The Sweet Body of Deborah, Paranoia, Andy Warhol's Bad, Watcher in the Woods, Star '80, Native Son.
TELEVISION: Hitler's S.S.: Portrait in Evil.

BAKER, DON: Theatre Executive. b. St. Louis, Mo., Dec. 16, 1931. e. St. Louis Univ. V.P., adv.-prom., Loews Theatres, New York. Member NATO, bd. dir. & nat'l. chm. adv. comm., 1972–present; mem. bd. of dir., Will Rogers Memorial Fund, 1974; pub. chm., Variety Clubs Intl. in Western Hemisphere; Commissioner, N.J. Film & TV Development Commission.

BAKER, GEORGE: Actor–Writer. b. Varna, Bulgaria, April 1, 1931, e. Lancing College, Sussex. Stage debut Deal Repertory Theatre, 1946. Film debut The Intruder, 1953.
PICTURES INCLUDE: Dam Busters, Ship That Died Of Shame, Woman For Joe, Extra Day, Feminine Touch, A Hill In Korea, No Time for Tears, These Dangerous Years, Tread Softly Stranger, Lancelot and Guinivere, Curse of the Fly, Mister Ten Per Cent, Goodbye Mr. Chips, Justine, The Executioner, On Her Majesty's Secret Service, A Warm December, The Fire Fighters, The Spy Who Loved Me, Thirtynine Steps, A Nightingale Sang in Berkeley Square, Hopscotch, North Sea Hijack.
TV FILM: Fan Show, Ron Raudell's programme 1956, Guinea Pig, Death of a Salesman, The Last Troubadour, The Square Ring, Nick of the River, Mary Stuart, Probation Officers, Far Away Music, It Happened Like This, Boule de Suif, Maigret, Zero One, Rupert Henzau, Miss Memory, Any Other Business, The Navigators, Common Ground, Alice, The Queen and Jackson, The Big Man Coughed and Died, Up and Down, Call My Bluff, The Baron, St. Patrick, Love Life, Seven Deadly Virtues, The Prisoner, The Sex Games, Z Cars, Paul Temple, Candida, Fenn Street, Man Outside, The Persuaders, Main Chance, Ministry of Fear, Voyage in the Dark, Dial M for Murder, Zodiac, The Survivors, I, Claudius, Print Out, Goodbye, Darling, Chinese Detective, Triangle, Minder, Hart to Hart, Goodbye Mr. Chips, Woman of Substance. Writer: The Total Spring, Imaginary Friends, The Bird Fancier, Robin of Sherwood, Time after Time, If Tomorrow Comes, Coast to Coast, Dead Head, The Canterville Those, Room at the Bottom.
WRITER: The Fatal Spring, Imiginary Friends, Going for Broke, The Marches of Wales, The Hopkins, Just a Hunch.

BAKER, J. EDWIN: Executive. b. Detroit, Mich., June 27, 1914. e. St. John's Coll. m. Marjorie R. Baker, actress. In 1935 produced Asylum of Horrors, stage show featuring the Frankenstein Monster (in person), which is still playing dates after 40 years. Known professionally as Dr. Silkini. In 1960 organized Intl. Artists Pictures, of which he is pres., to produce films.
PICTURES INCLUDE: Phycoscope, Magic Land of Mother Goose, Santa Visits Mother Goose Land, Vampire's Coffin, Teenage Tramp, Aztec Mummy.

BAKER, JOE DON: Actor. b. Groesbeck, TX, Feb. 12, 1936. Began career on N.Y. stage, impressing critics in Marathon 33 and Blues for Mr. Charlie. Film debut, Cool Hand Luke, 1967.
PICTURES INCLUDE: Guns of the Magnificent Seven, Adam at Six A.M., The Wild Rovers, Welcome Home, Soldier Boys, Junior Bonner, Walking Tall, Charley Varrick, The Outfit, Golden Needles, Mitchell, Framed, Wacko, The Natural, Fletch, Getting Even.

BAKER, ROBERT S.: Producer. b. London, 1916. Entered industry 1937 as assistant director. 1939–46: Army Film Unit. Produced 50 films including, Crossplot, Sea of Sand.
TELEVISION: Produced: The Saint (1962–9), Gideon's Way. Directed: The Treasure of Monte Cristo, Hellfire Club, The Siege of Sidney Street, Jack the Ripper, Producing The Persuaders! 1976–8: Return of the Saint. Devised: Return to Treasure Island.

BAKER, ROY: Prod.-Dir. b. London e. Lycee Corneille, Rouen; City of London School. Asst. dir. with Gainsborough 1934–40; served in Army 1940–46.
PICTURES INCLUDE: Operation Disaster, Don't Bother to Knock, Inferno, One That Got Away, A Night to Remember, The Singer Not the Song, Flame in the Streets, Quartermass and the Pit, The Anniversary, Vampire Lovers, Dr. Jekyll and Mr. Hyde, Asylum (Paris Grand Prize), Seven Golden Vampires.
TV: The Human Jungle, The Saint, Gideon's Way, The Baron, The Avengers, The Champions, Department S., The Persuaders, Danger UXB, Minder.

BAKSHI, RALPH: Animator-Writer-Director. b. New York City.
PICTURES: Fritz the Cat, Heavy Traffic, Coonskin, Wizards, The Lord of the Rings, Hey, Good Lookin', American Pop, Fire and Ice.

BALA, JOHN: Executive. e. Yale, Harvard, UCLA Graduate School Management. After schooling joined Rand Corp. to work in public-policy research for 4 years; then to 20th Fox as mgr. of financial analysis in corporate development dept. 1982–83, dir. of finance & research for Times-Mirror Videotex Services. Dec. 1983, joined 20th-Fox as v.p. of worldwide mkt. research.

BALABAN, A. J.: Theatre executive. b. Chicago, Apr. 18, 1889. In 1907 entered m.p. exhibition as operator of M.s. Nickelodeon Kedzie Theatre, Chicago; owned Movie Inn, restaurant with booths named for stars 1915; co-founder Balaban & Katz Corp. 1917; upon affiliation of B & K with Paramount named dir. of entertainment, then vice-pres.; abroad 9 yrs. returned to U.S. as circuit exhibitor 1935; gen. mgr. Roxy Theatre, N.Y., 1942; res. Jan 1, 1952, now consultant for 3 years; holds interest in Esquire, Carnegie theat., Chicago, with Harry and Elmer, brothers. Member: M.P. Pioneers, Jewish Theatrical Guild, French-American Club.

BALABAN, BOB: Actor. b. Chicago. Began working with Second City troupe while still in high school. Attended Colgate and New York Univ. while appearing on Bdwy. in Plaza Suite.
PICTURES: Catch 22, Midnight Cowboy, Girlfriends, Close Encounters of the Third Kind, Report to the Commissioner, Altered States, Prince of the City, Absence of Malice, Whose Life Is It Anyway?, 2010.
STAGE: You're a Good Man, Charlie Brown, The Inspector General, Who Wants to Be the Lone Ranger?, The Basic Training of Pavlo Hummel, The Children, The White House Murder Case.

BALABAN, ELMER: President H. & E. Balaban Corp., Chicago, Ill. e. U of Pa., 1931. With Paramount Publix 1931; Balaban & Katz, 1933; then H. & E. Balaban Corp. Pres., Plains Television; interest in WTVO, Rockford, Ill.; interest in WHNB, Hartford, Conn. and numerous cable-TV systems.

BALDWIN, ALEC: Actor. Started career in daytime tv on The Doctors while appearing on stage in A Midsummer Night's Dream, Summertree, The Wager, etc. Moved to L.A. where cast in tv pilots, series and movies. Theatrical film debut in Forever Lulu (1986). On Bdwy. stage in Loot (1986).
TELEVISION: Knots Landing (series), Dress Gray (movie).

BALIN, INA: b. Bklyn, N.Y. e. Forest Hills High; Part time drama, psychology courses. N.Y. Univ. Comm. model, salesgirl, receptionist. Prof. debut, Perry Como Show. Off-Bway, summer stock, Compulsion, Majority of One. N.Y. Stage. Film debut, The Black Orchid. TV and Broadway. Toured Europe 1961. Int'l Star of Tomorrow. Hollywood Foreign Press Golden Globe Award.
PICTURES INCLUDE: From the Terrace, Young Doctors, The Comancheros, The Greatest Story Ever Told, The Patsy, Charro!, The Projectionist.
TV: American Heritage, Stoney Burke, Adventures in Paradise, Kraft Theatre, The Lieutenant, Bonanza, The Loner, Voyage to the Bottom of the Sea, Run for Your Life.

BALL, LUCILLE: Actress. b. Jamestown, N.Y., Aug. 6, 1911. e. Chautaqua Inst. Music; John Murray Anderson Dram. School, p. Desiree Ball, concert pianist. Hattie Carnegie model, stage debut in "Rio Rita"; on Broadway in "Hey Diddle, Diddle," "Dream Girl," "Wildcat;" m.p. debut in "Roman Scandals"1933; entertained in Hollywood Canteen World War II; Voted most promising star in Motion Picture Daily's TV poll, 1951; best performer, 1952; best comedy team, 1954; best comedienne 1952, 54–55, 57; pres. Desilu Prod., Inc.; exec. prod., The Lucy Show; pres. Lucille Ball Prods., 1967.
PICTURES INCLUDE: Roberts, Stage Door, Big Street, Du Barry Was a Lady, Easy to Wed, Ziegfeld Follies, Lured, Sorrowful Jones, Easy Living, Miss Grant Takes Richmond, Fuller Brush Girl, Fancy Pants, Magic Carpet, Long Long Trailer, Forever Darling, Facts of Life, Critics Choice, Yours, Mine and Ours, Mame.
TV: I Love Lucy, The Lucy Show, Here's Lucy, Movie: Stone Pillow.

BALLARD, LUCIEN: Cinematographer. b. Miami, Okla., May 6, 1908; e. U. Okla., U. Pa. Started with Paramount as asst. cinematographer & cutter; since operative cinematographer.
PICTURES INCLUDE: Will Penny, The Party, How Sweet It Is!, The Wild Bunch, True Grit, The Ballad of Cable Hogue.

BALSAM, MARTIN: Actor. b. Nov. 4, 1919, N.Y.
PICTURES INCLUDE: On the Waterfront, 1954. Twelve Angry Men, Time Limit, Marjorie Morningstar, Al Capone, Middle of the Night, Psycho, Ada, Breakfast at Tiffany's, Cape Fear, Who's Been Sleeping in My Bed?, The Carpetbaggers, Youngblood Hawke, Seven Days in May, Harlow, The Bedford Incident, A Thousand Clowns, After the Fox, Hombre, 2001: A Space Odyssey, Trilogy, Catch 22, The Anderson Tapes, The Stone Killer, Summer Wishes, Winter Dreams, The Taking of Pelham 1,2,3, Murder on the Orient Express, Mitchell, All The President's Men, Two-Minute Warning, The Sentinel, Silver Bears, Cuba, The Goodbye People, St. Elmo's Fire, Death Wish, The Delta Force, Whatever It Takes.

BALTER, ALLAN: Executive. b. Detroit, Mich., August 28, 1925. e. Univ. of Michigan, B.A. Asst. casting dept., 20th Century-Fox Film Corp. 1950–53; mgr., Encino theatre, 1953–54; asst. casting dept., MGM Studios, 1954–55; editor, Action mag., 20th Century-Fox house-organ 1955–56; trade planter, 20th Century-Fox publicity, 1956–57; unit publicist, Bryna Prods. (UA) 1957–58; unit publicist, 20th Century-Fox, 1958–62; dir. of pub., adv., Daystar Prods.

BANCROFT, ANNE: Actress. r.n. Anne Italiano; b. N.Y.C., Sep. 17, 1931; e. American Academy of Dramatic Arts. Acting debut on TV, Studio One; many TV shows; film debut, Don't Bother to Knock.
PICTURES INCLUDE: Tonight We Sing, Treasure of the Golden Condor, Kid from Left Field, Demitrius and the Gladiators, Gorilla at Large, The Raid, Life in the Balance, New York Confidential, The Brass Ring, Naked Street, Last Frontier, Girl in the Black Stockings, Restless Breed, The Miracle Worker, The Pumpkin Eater (1964), Slender Thread, The Graduate (1967), Young Winston (1972), The Prisoner of Second Avenue, The Hindenburg, The Turning Point, Fatso (also dir. & s.p.), The Elephant Man, To Be Or Not To Be, Garbo Talks, Agnes of God, 'night Mother, 84 Charing Cross Road.
PLAYS: Two For the Seasaw, The Miracle Worker, Mother Courage, The Devils, A Cry of Players.

BAND, ALBERT: Producer-director. b. Paris, France, May 7, 1924; e. Lyceum Louis le Grand, won French-English Literature Prize 1938; entered film industry as cutter Pathe Lab.; prod. ass't to John Huston at MGM; first screen credit adaptation Red Badge of Courage novel; first direction. The Young Guns, Allied Artists; formed Maxim Productions, Inc., Sept. 1956; prod.-dir. Killer on the Wall for United Artists. 1958 prod.-dir. Face of Fire; 1962 dir. The Avenger; 1963 dir. Grand Canyon Massacre; 1965 prod.-dir. The Tramplers; 1966 prod. The Hellbenders. Recently formed Albert Band Intl. Prods., Inc.
PICTURES INCLUDE: A Minute to Pray, A Second to Die, Little Cigars, Dracula's Dog, She Came to the Valley, Metalstorm, The Destruction of Jared, Swordkill.

BANNEN, IAN: Actor. b. Airdrie, Scotland, 1928. Early career Shakespeare Memorial Theatre, Stratford-on-Avon.
STAGE: A View From the Bridge, The Iceman Cometh, Long Days Journey Into Night, Sergeant Musgrave's Dance. Royal Shakespeare Thea. Co. 1961–62. The Iceman Cometh, 1974. Hedda Gabler, 1977. Translations, 1981 (Drama Critics Award); Riverside Mermaid Theatres, 1983; Moon for the Misbegotten (London, Boston Bdwy.).
PICTURES INCLUDE: Carlton-Browne of the F.O., Man in Cocked Hat, Macbeth, Station Six Sahara, Mister Moses, The Hill, Flight of the Phoenix, (nominated for AA), Sailor From Gibraltar, Penelope, Too Late the Hero, The Deserter, Jane Eyre, Fright, The Offence (BAFTA nomination), The Macintosh Man, Bite the Bullet, Watcher in the Woods, Eye of the Needle, Night Crossing, Ghandi, Gorky Park, Defense of the Realm, Lamb, Attempt on the Pope.
TV: Johnny Belinda, Tinker, Tailor, Soldier, Spy, Cousin Phillis.

BANNER, BOB: Producer-director. b.. Ennis, Tex., Aug. 15, 1921; e. Southern Methodist Univ., B.A., 1939–43, Northwestern Univ., M.A., 1946–48. U.S. Naval Reserve 1943–46; faculty, Northwestern Univ., 1948–50; staff dir., NBC-TV in Chicago, 1949–50; dir., Garroway at Large, 1949–50; prod. & dir., Fred Waring Show, 1950–53; dir. Omnibus. Metropolitan Opera Prod., 1953; Nothing But the Best (prod. dir.) NBC, 1953; Omnibus, CBS, 1953–54; Dave Garroway Show, NBC, 1953–54; (prod. dir) Dinah Shore Show, 1954–57; exec. prod. Garry Moore Show; exec. prod. Candid Camera TV show; exec. prod., Carnegie Hall Salutes Jack Benny, 1961; exec. prod., Julie & Carol at Carnegie Hall, 1962; exec. prod., Carol & Co., 1963; Jimmy Dean Show, 1963–66; Calamity Jane, Once Upon A Mattress, '64; The Entertainers, '65; Carol × 2, '66; Kraft Summer Music Hall, '66, 1966 Carol & Co., Ice Follies, Carol Burnett Show, 1969, Peggy Fleming at Madison Square Garden, 1967; John Davidson at Notre Dame, Here's Peggy Fleming, 1971; Peggy Fleming at Sun Valley, The American West of John Ford, 1971; Love! Love! Love!—Hallmark Hall of Fame, 1972; To Europe With Love, 1972.
PICTURES INCLUDE: Warning Shot (for TV), My Sweet Charlie, Mongo's Back in Town, 1971.
TELEVISION: Movies of the week: The Last Survivors, Journey From Darkness. Special: Peggy Fleming Visits the Soviet Union. Game Show: Almost Anything Goes. Specials: Perry Como's Lake Tahoe Holiday '75, Perry Como's

Christmas In Mexico '75, Perry Como's Hawaiian Holiday '76, Perry Como's Spring In New Orleans '76. Daily Variety Series: Don Ho Show '76; Perry Como Las Vegas Style '76, Perry Como's Christmas in Austria '76, Jr. Almost Anything Goes '76, All-Star Anything Goes '77, Peggy Fleming and Holiday on Ice at Madison Square Garden '76; Julie Andrews, One Step Into Spring '78; Leapin' Lizards, It's Liberace '78; Perry Como's Easter By The Sea '78.

BAR, JACQUES JEAN LOUIS: Executive. Producer. b. Chateauroux, France, Sept. 12, 1921; e. Lycees Lakanal and Saint Louis, France. Formed Cinema-Theatre d'Avallon, 1944; Cite-Films S.A., 1947; Spira in assoc. with MGM, 1961; first Hollywood film, co-prod. Scratch A Thief, 1964; prod. 43 pictures in France, Spain, Italy, Switzerland, Japan and Brazil, 1948–64.
PICTURES INCLUDE: Where the Hot Wind Blows, Bridge to the Sun, Riffifi in Tokyo, A Very Private Affair, Swordsmen of Siena, Monkey in Winter, The Turfist, Any Number Can Win, The Day and the Hour, Joy House, Guns for San Sebastian.

BARAGREY, JOHN: Actor. b. April 15, 1919; e. U. of Alabama, 1939.
PICTURES INCLUDE: Loves of Carmen, Shockproof, Pardners, The Fugitive Kind.
BROADWAY: The Enchanted, Royal Family, Richard III, The Devils, The Grass Harp, Murderous Angels.
TV: Studio One, Suspense, Television Playhouse, Danger, Kraft Theatre, You Are There, U.S. Steel Hour, Robert Montgomery Playhouse, Omnibus, Climax, Hitchcock Presents, G.E. Theatre, Suspicion, Schlitz Playhouse, Playhouse 90, Cimarron City, American Heritage, The Defenders.

BARBER, ARNOLD: Executive. b. London, England. Career in m.p. ind. started with RKO. Subsequently with AB-Pathe following war service until appointment with Warner-Pathe Dist. which led him through sales exec. positions until he headed company. Formed Sotia-Barber Distributors Ltd. in 1970. Now man. dir. Barber Intl. Films, Ltd.

BARBERA, JOSEPH R.: Executive. b. N.Y.C. e. N.Y. Univ., American Institute of Banking. After schooling joined Irving Trust Co. in N.Y.C.; started submitting cartoon drawings to leading magazines selling one to Collier's. Left banking to seek career in cartooning. Joined Van Buren Associates as sketch artist, later going to work in animation dept. of MGM Studios. At MGM met Willaim Hanna, who became his lifelong business associate. Made first animated short together in 1938, starting the famous Tom & Jerry series which they produced for 20 years. Left MGM in 1957 to form Hanna-Barbera Productions to make cartoons for TV. Series have included Yogi Bear, Huckleberry Hound, The Flintstones. Hanna-Barbera became a subsidiary of Taft Bdg. Co. in 1968 with both men operating studio under long-term agreements with Taft. Barbera is pres. until 1980. Company entered theatrical production with Charlotte's Web in 1973. 1982: Heidi's Song.

BARBOUR, ALAN G.: Writer, editor, publisher. b. Oakland, Calif., July 25, 1933. ed. e. Rutgers University, m. Catherine Jean Callovini, actress, teacher, American Academy of Dramatic Arts, American Mime Theatre. U.S. Army, worked as computer programmer. Formed Screen Facts Press in 1963, Screen Facts Magazine. Compiled, edited: The Serials of Republic, The Serials of Columbia, Great Serial Ads, The B Western, Serial Showcase, Hit the Saddle, The Wonderful World of B-Films, Days of Thrills and Adventure, Serial Quarterly, Serial Pictorial, Karloff—A Pictorial History, Errol Flynn—A Pictorial Biography, A Pictorial History of the Serial, A Thousand and One Delights, Cliffhanger, The Old-Time Radio Quiz Book, Direct. Mktg. Div., RCA Records. Mgr., A & R RCA Video Club.

BARBOUR, MALCOLM: Executive. b. London, England, May 3, 1934; e. Radley College, Oxford, England, Columbia Coll. At N.B.C. was press info. asst., 1958–59; asst. magazine ed., 1959–62; assoc. mag. ed., 1962–64; sr. mag. ed., 1964–65; mgr. of magazine pub., National Broadcasting Company, 1965–67; pub. mgr., Buena Vista, 1967–68; Eastern story ed., Walt Disney Prod., 1968–69; dir. of adv. & pub. relations, Buena Vista, 1969.

BARDOT, BRIGITTE: Actress. b. Paris, France, 1934. Model.
PICTURES INCLUDE: Le Trou Normand, Un Acte D'Amour, Helen of Troy, Le Fils De Caroline Cherie, Les Grandes Moneuvres, Doctor at Sea, En Effeuillant La Marguerite, The Bride Is Much Too Beautiful, Moonlight Jewelers, La Femme et Le Pantin, Will You Dance With Me, Manina, La Fille Sans Voiles, Si Versailles M'Etait Conte, Trahi, Futures Vedettes, La Lumiere D'En Face, Une Sacre Gamine, And God Created Woman, Le Parisienne, En Cas De Malheur, Love Is My Profession, Babette Goes to War, La Verite Contempt, A Very Private Affair, Two Weeks in September, Viva Maria, Shalako, Spirits of the Dead, Les Femmes.

BARE, RICHARD L.: Producer, director. b. Turlock, Calif. Dir. or Warner: Smart Girls Don't Talk, Flaxy Martin, This Side of The Law, House Across The Street, Return of Frontiersman; SDG Best Dir. TV award, 1959; author, The Film Director (Macmillan), 1971.
TV: 77 Sunset Strip, Maverick, 1956, So This is Hollywood (1955-NBC), The Islanders (1960), Dangerous Robin (1961), This Rebel Breed, Twilight Zone, Bus Stop (1962), Adventures in Paradise, The Virginian (1963), Kraft Theatre, Run For Your Life, Green Acres Series (186 episodes-1969), Farraday and Son, 1974; Westwind (NBC) 1976.
PICTURES INCLUDE: Wrote, directed and produced Wicked, Wicked, MGM, 1973; Story of Chang & Eng, 1984; City of Shame, Fox, 1985; Sudden Target, AM Entertainment, 1986.

BAREN, HARVEY M.: Executive. b. New York City, Nov. 25, 1931. e. N.Y. State U. Served in U.S. Army, 1952–54; United Artists Corp., 1954–59 (contract dept., print dept., booker—N.Y. branch); asst. to general sls. mgr., Magna Pictures Corp., 1959–61; road show mgr., national sales coordinator, 20th Century-Fox, 1961–71; asst. general sales manager, Allied Artists Pictures, 1971–79; v.p., gen. sls. mgr., Nat'l. Screen Service, 1978–79; v.p., gen. sls. mgr., Cannon Pictures, 1979–80. 1980, pres. of Summit Feature Distributors; 1983, exec. V.P., dir., MGM/UA Classics.

BARI, LYNN: Actress. r.n. Marjorie Bitzer; b. Roanoke, Va., 1917. First Screen appearance as dancing girl in Dancing Lady (MGM). Became Fox contract player 1934.
PICTURES INCLUDES: Shock, Margie, Home Sweet Homicide, Nocturne, Amazing Mr. X, Kid from Cleveland, I'd Climb Highest Mountain, On the Loose, Sunny Side of the Street, Has Anybody Seen My Gal, I Dream of Jeanie, Francis Joins the Wacs, A&C Meet the Keystone Kops, Women of Pitcairn Island, Damn Citizen, Trauma.

BARKER, ROBERT WILLIAM: TV Host. b. Darrington, Wash., Dec. 12. e. Springfield Central H.S., Drury Coll. News writer, announcer, disc jockey KTTS until 1949. News editor, staff announcer, Station WWPG; wife, Dorothy Jo. Emcee Truth or Consequences, 1956. Pres. Bob Barker Prod., Inc., M.C. Miss USA Pageant, CBS-TV, since 1967, M.C. Miss Universe Pageant, CBS-TV since 1967, M.C. Rose Parade, since 1970. Prod.-M. C. Pillsbury Bakeoff, since 1970 CBS. Prod. Lucky Pair, syndicated, M.C. Price Is Right-CBS, 1972; Narrator, 500 Festival Parade, Indianapolis 1969–81.

BARKETT, STEVE: Actor-Director-Producer-Film Editor. b. Jan. 1, 1950, Oklahoma City, Okla. Exhibited and scored over 52 feature length classic silent films prior to coming to Los Angeles in 1970. Executive in several nontheatrical releasing companies including Independent Film Associates. Established the Nautilus Film Company in 1978.
PICTURES INCLUDE: Actor: The Egyptians are Coming, Corpsegrinders, Cruise Missile. Films as Actor, Director, Producer: The Movie People, Night Caller, The Aftermath. Actor-Director-Writer: Judgment Day.

BARKIN, ELLEN: Actress. b. Bronx, NY, 1959. e. Hunter Coll.
PICTURES: Diner, Buckaroo Banzai, Harry and Son, Desert Bloom
TELEVISION: Act of Vengence.

BARLOW, PHIL: Executive. Began career with National General Theatres in 1961 in Salt Lake City; later transferred to Los Angeles as Southern Calif. div. buyer. Worked as buyer for NGT and Syufy Theatres in San Francisco. Joined General Cinema Corp. in NYC as natl. coordinator of film. Served 10 years as v.p. with Edwards Theatre Circuit, being named sr. v.p. in January, 1985. Left to join Buena Vista Dist. Co. as v.p. & gen. sls. mgr.

BARNES, BILL: Producer-Manager. b. Wilson, N.C., Jan 28, 1939. e. Univ. of N.C., Chapel Hill, BA. Radio, TV, Motion Pictures. Casting dir. and story ed. for Otto Preminger 1962–1969; motion picture agent with IFA in 1970 and merged into Intl. Creative Management; joined Producer Circle Co., Jan. 1979 as v.p., creative affairs. Formed own personal mgt. co., 1983.

BARNETT, GABRIEL: Graduate U.S.C. 1925 with B.L.L., publisher of theatre programs and commercial film advertising. Established in 1938. Creator of the Barnett theatre clock. Now engaged in producing intermission music for motion picture theatres.

BARON, MARK: Executive. Pub./mktg. career at Factors Etc., McFadden, Strauss & Irwin before joining Columbia Pictures as sr. exec. liaison to Coca-Cola Co., coordinating mktg. programs between parent co. and feature film div. Worked as dir. of pub./promo. on Annie & Gandhi. Left to go to Stone/Halinan Associates as exec. v.p., mktg./admin. 1985, formed own mktg./consulting firm specializing in independent film producers before joining Warner Bros. as v.p., pub., coordinating overall pub. & promo. efforts on specific WB film projects.

BARR, ANTHONY: Producer, director, actor. r.n. Morris Yaffe. b. St. Louis, Mo., March 14, 1921. e. Washington Univ., B.S. 1942. Actor, asst. stage mgr., 1944–46; stage mgr., Katherine Dunham Dancers, 1946–47; teacher, actor, dir. in chg. Film Actors' Workshop, Professional Theatre Workshop, Hollywood; v.p. current prime time series, ABC-TV; v.p., current dramatic program production, CBS-TV; v.p., CBS Entertainment Prods.
BROADWAY: Jacobowsky and the Colonel, Winters' Tale, Embezzled Heaven.
PICTURES INCLUDE: (actor) People Against O'Hara, Border Incident, The Hollywood Story, The Mozart Story, (co-prod.) Dime With A Halo.
TV: (dir.) Art Linkletter's Houseparty, About Faces (ABC-TV), (assoc. dir.) Climax, Shower of Stars, (prod.) Climax, Summer Studio One, (assoc. prod. CBS-TV) Climax, Playhouse 90, Pursuit, G.E. Theatre, The Law and Mr. Jones, Four-Star.
BOOK: Acting for the Camera, 1982.

BARRETT, JAMES LEE: Screen writer, producer. b. Charlotte, N.C., Nov. 19, 1929. e. Anderson Jr. College, Furman Univ., Penn State Univ., Art Students League. U.S. Marine Corps.
PICTURES INCLUDE: The D.I. (Marine Corps Combat Correspondents Award), The Greatest Story Ever Told, The Truth About Spring, Shenandoah, The Green Berets, Bandolero, The Undefeated, tick . . . tick . . . tick, The Cheyenne Social Club, Fools' Parade, Something Big, Smokey and the Bandit, Wild Horse Hank.
STAGE: Shenandoah (Tony Award) best musical book, 1974–75; Theatre Club annual award.
TV: The Awakening Land, Parts I and II (Certificate of Commendation, American Women in Radio and Television), Stubby Pringles' Christmas (Humanitas Nomination), The Day Christ Died, Belle Starr, Angel City, Mayflower: The Pilgrim Experience, You Are the Jury, Big Bad John, The Defiant Ones, Stagecoach, Vengeance.
SERIES: Created Our House.

BARRETT, RONA: News Correspondent e. N.Y. Univ. (communications major) created the column, Rona Barrett's Young Hollywood, which led to featured column in 1960 in Motion Picture Magazine and a nationally syndicated column distributed to 125 newspapers by the North American Newspaper Alliance. Turned to TV; initial appearances on ABC Owned Stations in 5 cities, providing two-minute reports for local newscasts. This resulted in a network morning program, co-hosted by Joanna Barnes, called Dateline Hollywood. In 1969 she created first daily syndicated TV news segment for Metromedia. 1975, became arts and entertainment editor for ABC's Good Morning America. 1980, joined NBC News. Then publisher and exec. editor, newsletter, The Rona Barrett Report. 1985, pres., Rona Barrett Communications, Inc., sr. corresp., Entertainment Tonight; Mutual Radio Network.

BARRIE, GEORGE: Executive. b. Brooklyn, N.Y. Feb. 9, 1918. e. N.Y.U. Left school to embark on business career, beginning with soda fountain concessions in drugstores. Played in dance band and later became booker for bands. Turned to beauty products, forming co. Caryl Richards. In 1963 acquired Faberge, merging it with own firm. Entered leisure time field with records, books, films and TV.
PICTURES INCLUDE: A Touch of Class, Night Watch, Welcome to Arrow Beach, Book of Numbers, Hang-Up, Miracles Still Happen, Hugo the Hippo, Whiffs, Thieves.

BARRIE, MONA: Actress. b. London, England, Dec. 18, 1909. On stage Australia, England (Hay Fever, Bitter Sweet Autumn Crocus, others). From 1933 on screen.
PICTURES INCLUDE: Devil's Mask, Just Before Dawn, Secret of the Whistler, I Cover Big Town, Cass Timberlane, When a Girl's Beautiful, The First Time, Strange Fascination.

BARRON, ARTHUR RAY: Executive. b. Mt. Lake, Minn., July 12, 1934. e. San Diego State College, 1956–60; B.S. Accounting. Certified public acc't, Calif., 1960. Lybrond, Rans Bros. and Montgomery, 1960–63; Desilu Productions, Inc., 1963–67; v.p. finance and administration, Paramount Television, 1967–70 v.p. Finance, Paramount Pictures Corp., 1970; senior v.p. finance and administration, 1971; exec. v.p., finance & admin., 1974; exec. v.p. 1980; exec. v.p., Gulf & Western Industries, entertainment & communications group, 1983; promoted to pres., 1984.

BARRY, DONALD (Red): Actor, r.n. Donald Barry de Acosta; b. Houston, Tex.; e. Tex. Sch. Mines. In 1936 in "Night Waitress" (RKO Radio), thereafter to 1939 in number of feature pictures, including "The Woman I Love," "Sinners in Paradise," "The Crowd Roars." From 1939 in Westerns, attaining wide popularity as Republic Western star. Entertained troops overseas. Voted one of first ten Money-Making Western Stars in Motion Picture Herald-Fame Polls 1942, 1943, 1944.
PICTURES INCLUDE: Jesse James' Women, Untamed Heiress, Twinkle in God's Eye, I'll Cry Tomorrow, Seven Men From Now, Shalako, The Shakiest Gun in the West, Orca, The Swarm.

BARRY, GENE: Actor. r.n. Eugene Klass; b. New York, N.Y., June 14, 1921; e. New Utrecht H.S. Bklyn. Appeared in little & summer theatre.
BROADWAY: Rosalinda, Catherine Was Great, Happy Is Larry, Bless You All, La Cage Aux Folles.
PICTURES INCLUDE: Atomic City, Girls of Pleasure Island, War of the Worlds, Those Redheads from Seattle, Alaska Seas, Red Garters, Naked Alibi, Soldier of Fortune, Purple Mask, Houston Story, Back from Eternity, China Gato, 27th Day, Maroc 7.
TV: Bat Masterson, Burke's Law, The Name of the Game.

BARRY, JOHN: Composer, arranger, conductor. b. York, England, 1933. Artist and prod., CBS Records.
TV: Elizabeth Taylor in London, Sophia Loren in Rome.
PICTURES INCLUDE: Beat Girl, Never Let Go, The Amorous Prawn, From Russia With Love, Seance On a Wet Afternoon, Zulu, Goldfinger, The Ipcress File, The Knack, King Rat, Born Free, Thunderball, The Chase, The Wrong Box, The Quiller Memorandum, The Whisperers, Deadfall, Petulia, You Only Live Twice, The Lion in Winter, Midnight Cowboy, The Appointment, The Tamarind Seed, The Dove, The Day of the Locust, Robin and Marian, King Kong, The Deep, The Betsy, Moonraker, The Black Hole, Somewhere in Time, Hammett, Frances, Mike's Murder, Until September, The Cotton Club, A View to a Kill, Jagged Edge, Out of Africa., Howard the Duck.

BARRY, MICHAEL: Executive. b. May 15, 1910. Theatre & film dir., TV as BBC prod., 1938; during war in Royal Marines; rejoined TV as writer, prod., 1946; wrote and prod. Promise of Tomorrow, Passionate, Pilgrim, Shout Aloud Salvation; head of TV Drama Dept. June 1951. Awarded O.B.E. June, 1956. Programme Controller Telefis Eireann, Sept. 1961.

BARRYMORE, CHAUNCEY: Actor-Writer. b. Great Smokey Mts., July 7, 1946. Studied acting and playwriting in New York at American Stanislavski Institute & The New School for Social Research. Author of book, Revelations.
PICTURES INCLUDE: It's My Turn, Forever One, Stardust Memories, Smorgasboard, Forbidden Love, Star 80, Space Raiders, Prince of the City, etc.
TELEVISION: Many series, including Cagney & Lacey, Lottery, Another World. Movies: Shiek-of-Miramar, Will There Be a Morning?, The Day After, etc.

BARRYMORE, DREW: Actress. b. Los Angeles, Feb. 22, 1975. Daughter, John Barrymore, Jr.
PICTURES: Altered States, E.T.: The Extra Terrestrial, Firestarter, Irreconcilable Differences, Cat's Eye.
TELEVISION: Suddenly Love, Bogey, Disneyland's 30th Anniversary, Night of 100 Stars II.

BARRYMORE, JOHN BLYTH, JR.: Actor. b. Beverly Hills, Calif., June 4, 1932. e. St. John's Military Acad., various public and private schools; p. late John Barrymore, Delores Costello (Mrs. John Vruwink). Debut in The Sundowners; many TV appearances.
PICTURES INCLUDE: High Lonesome, Big Night, Thunderbirds, While the City Sleeps, Shadow on the Window, War of The Zombies, Never Love A Stranger, The Night They Killed Rasputin, High School Confidential.

BART, PETER: Executive. e. Swarthmore College and The London School of Economics. Served eight years as correspondent for The New York Times and wrote for such magazines as Harper's, The Atlantic Saturday Review, etc. Joined Paramount Pictures in 1965. Named exec. ass't. to Robert Evans, exec. in charge of world-wide production. Appointed v.p. prod. Resigned post in 1973 to develop and produce own films for Para. Appointed pres. Lorimar Films, 1978. Resigned, 1979, to be independent producer 1983, joined MGM as snr. v.p., prod., m.p. div. Resigned, 1985, to be indep. prod. Novels: Author-Thy Kingdom Come (1983); Destinies (1979).
PICTURES INCLUDE: Islands in the Stream, Fun with Dick and Jane (both co-prod.), Revenge of the Nerd (exec. prod.); Youngblood (co-prod.).

BARTHOLOMEW, FREDDIE: Actor. b. London, Eng., Mar. 28, 1924. Stage debut 1927; m.p. debut U.S. in "David Copperfield" 1935.
PICTURES INCLUDE: Anna Karenina, Lloyds of London, Little Lord Fauntleroy, Devil Is a Sissy, Lord Jeff, Captains Courageous, Kidnapped, Swiss Family Robinson, Naval Academy, Yank at Eton, Junior Army, The Town Went Wild, St. Benny the Dip.

BARTKOWIAK, ANDRZEJ: Cinematographer. b. Lodz, Poland, 1950. Attended Polish Film School. Moved to US in 1972,

gaining experience in TV commericals and low-budget features. Protege of Sidney Lumet, for whom did four pictures.
PICTURES: Prince of the City, Deathtrap, The Verdict, Daniel, Terms of Endearment, Prizzi's Honor.

BARTLETT, HALL: Producer, Director, Writer. b. Kansas City, Mo., Nov. 27, 1925; e. Yale U., B.A. 1942. U.S. Naval Reserve 1942–47; formed Hall Bartlett Productions, 1952; prod. Navajo (winner of 27 nat'l awards & Festival of Brit. Award at Edinburgh); prod., s.p. Crazy-legs (winner of 9 nat'l awards, including Parents Mag. Gold Medal); prod., dir., s.p. Unchained (winner of Parents Mag. Gold Medal, Brotherhd. award of Nat. Con. of Christians and Jews); theme song, Unchained Melody, most pop. song of '55; prod., dir., s.p. Durango; prod. dir. s.p. Zero Hour, All the Young Men, Sol Madrid, photog., prod., Changes, prod. dir. Winner of the Sans Sebastian Festival, The Sandpit Generals, prod., dir., writer; winner of Grand Prize of VII International Film Festival of Moscow. Producer, director Jonathan Livingston Seagull; Producer, director, Cleo Laine Special, Zubin Mehta Special; producer, director, The Children of Sanchez; prod., dir., s.p.: Comeback, Love Is Forever.

BARUCH, ANDRE: Annoucer, commentator. b. Paris, France. e. Pratt Institute, Brooklyn, N.Y.; Columbia U.; Beaux Arts. Commercials for American Character, BC Headache Powder, Transogram Helene Curtis, Drajel, Lorillard; Prod. dir. for national sales conventions; TV, film prod. Helizer, Waring & Wayne, Inc.

BARUCH, RALPH M.: Executive. b. Paris, France, Aug. 5, 1923. e. The Sorbonne, Administrative aide, SESAC, Inc. 1944–48; account exec., DuMont Television Network, 1948–52; Eastern sales mgr., Consolidated Television Films, 1953–54; account exec., CBS Films, 1954; account supervisor, 1957; dir. international sales, 1959; v.p., CBS Enterprises, 1961–70; pres., Viacom Enterprises, 1971; pres., Viacom International, 1979; named chm. & chief exec. officer, Viacom International; pres., International Radio & Television Society; chmn., Rewrite Committee (Communications Act), NCTA; former member of the board of directors and former chmn., Pay Cable Committee, NCTA; chm., NCTA Public Policy Planning Committee; gov. (New York), fellow of International Council of the National Academy of Television Arts & Sciences.

BARWOOD, HAL: Writer-Producer. e. Univ. of S. Calif. School of Cinema. Writes scripts in collaboration with Matthew Robbins, Barwood branching out into producing with Corvette Summer in 1978.
PICTURES INCLUDE: Scripts, all with Robbins: The Sugarland Express, The Bingo Long Traveling All-Stars and Motor Kings, Corvette Summer (also prod.), Dragonslayer (also prod.).

BARYSHNIKOV, MIKHAIL: Dancer-Actor. b. Riga, Latvia, Jan. 27, 1948. Joined Korov Ballet, Leningrad; defected to U.S. With American Ballet Theatre, New York City Ballet Company.
PICTURES: The Turning Point, That's Dancing!, White Nights.
TELEVISION: Baryshnikov at the White House, Bob Hope on the Road to China, Baryshnikov on Broadway, AFI Salute to Fred Astaire, Baryshnikov in Hollywood, AFI Salute to Gene Kelly, etc.

BASCH, BUDDY: Print Media Syndicater-Publicist-Producer. b. South Orange, N.J., June 28, 1922. e. Columbia Univ. Began career as "Youngest Radio Editor in U.S." at 15, since written for national mags, syndicates, wire services, and newspapers. Edited and published "Top Hit Club News"-7 years. Joined Donahue and Coe 1940 on m.p. accounts, U.S. Army in Europe 1942–45. 1945 until 1967: own publicity and promotion office, working on m.p. company accounts and stars such as Burl Ives, Dinah Shore, Tony Martin, Danny Kaye, Peter Lorre, Tony Bennett, Gloria De Haven, McGuire Sisters, Rhonda Fleming, Sammy Davis, Jr., Anna Maria Alberghetti, Polly Bergen, Meyer Davis, The Beatles, Glenn Miller and Tommy Dorsey Orchestras. Produced many shows for radio, TV and stage in New York, Newark, Chicago, Hartford. Asst. to publisher, The Brooklyn Eagle 1962. 1966 formed Buddy Basch Feature Syndicate, covering assignments on show business, travel and general subjects for N.Y. Daily News, A.P., Travel/Holiday, Frontier Magazine, Kaleidoscope, True, United Features, Gannett Westchester-Rockland Newspapers, Bergen (N.J.) Record, Argosy, N.A.N.A., Womens' New Service, Today Magazine, Christian Science Monitor, New York Post, Inflight Magazine, Deseret News, California Canadian, etc.

BASINGER, KIM: Actress. Began career as model in New York; started in TV series, Dog and Cat. Pursues singing career under the nom-de-chant, Chelsea.
PICTURES: Never Say Never Again, Mother Lode, The Man Who Loved Women, The Natural, 9½ Weeks, Fool for Love.
TELEVISION: Movies: From Here to Eternity, Katie: Portrait of a Centerfold.

BASS, SAUL: Director-Producer. b. New York City May 8, 1920. e. Arts Students League. Pres. of, Saul Bass/Herb Yager & Assoc. Has directed short films, m.p. titles/prologues/epilogues, TV show openings, TV commercials. Directorial feature debut in 1974 with Phase IV.
PICTURES INCLUDE: (shorts), The Searching Eye, From Here to There, Why Man Creates (Academy Award); Notes on the Popular Arts (AA nomination), The Solar Film (AA nomination), Bass on Titles, Quest; (titles) Carmen Jones, The Man With The Golden Arm, Anatomy of a Murder, Vertigo, Psycho, Around the World in 80 Days, West Side Story, That's Entertainment II.

BATCHELOR, JOY: Director. b. Watford (Eng), May 12, 1914. e. Grammar School & Art School. Early career, illustrator & Designer. Entered m.p. in 1935 & is connected with the production of over 500 cartoon films. Co-director, co-prod., collab. s.p., Animal Farm, first British full length color feature cartoon; dir. Dam the Delta, The Colombo Plan, The Commonwealth, Ruddigore, The Five, Wotdot, Contact, Ass and the Stick. Christmas Feast, Carry on Milkmaids.

BATES, ALAN: Actor. b. Allestree, Derbyshire England, Feb. 17, 1934.
TV APPEARANCES: The Thug, A Memory of Two Mondays, The Jukebox, The Square Ring, The Wind and the Rain, Look Back in Anger, Three on a Gasring, Duel for Love, A Hero for Our Time, Plaintiff & Defendant, Two Sundays, The Collection, The Mayor of Casterbridge, The Trespasser, Very Like a Whale, Voyage Round My Father, An Englishman Abroad, Separate Tables, Dr. Fischer of Geneva, One for the Road.
STAGE: On London and New York stage. The Caretaker, Long Days Journey Into Night, Poor Richard, In Celebration, Hamlet, Butley, The Taming of the Shrew, Life Class, Otherwise Engaged, The Seagull, Stage Struck, A Patriot for Me, One for the Road, Victoria Station, Dance of Death, Yonadab.
PICTURES INCLUDE: The Entertainer, Whistle Down the Wind, A Kind of Loving, The Caretaker, Nothing But the Best, Zorba The Greek, Georgy Girl, King of Hearts, Three Sisters, Far From the Madding Crowd, The Fixer, Women in Love, Joe Egg, The Go Between, Impossible Object, Butley, In Celebration, Royal Flash, An Unmarried Woman, The Shout, Rose, Nijinsky, Quartet, The Return of the Soldier, The Wicked Lady, Duet for One.

BATTY, PETER: Producer, director, writer. b. Sunderland, England, 1931. e. Bede Grammar School and Queen's College, Oxford. Feature-writer both sides Atlantic 1954–58. Joined BBC TV 1958 dir. short films. Edited Tonight programme 1963–4. Exec. prod. ATV 1964–68. Awarded Grand Prix for doc. at 1965 Venice and Leipzig festivals. Official entries 1970 and 1971 San Francisco and Melbourne festivals. Own company since 1968 prod. TV specials, series, commercials.
TV PRODUCTIONS INCLUDE: The Quiet Revolution, The Big Freeze, The Katanga Affair, Sons of the Navy Man, The Fall and Rise of the House of Krupp, The Road to Suez, The Suez Affair, Battle for the Desert, Vietnam Fly-In, The Plutocrats, The Aristocrats, Battle for Cassino, Battle for the Bulge, Birth of the Bomb, Search for the Super, Operation Barbarossa, Farouk: Last of the Pharaohs, Superspy, Spy Extraordinary, Sunderland's Pride and Passion, A Rothschild and His Red Gold, The World of Television, The Story of Wine, The Rise and Rise of Laura Ashley, The Gospel According to Saint Michael, Battle for Warsaw, Battle for Dien Bien Phu, Nuclear Nightmares. A Turn Up In A Million, Il Poverello, Swindle!, The Algerian War, Fonteyn and Nureyev: The Perfect Partnership. Contributed 6 episodes to Emmy-winning WORLD At WAR series.

BAUER, HARALD P.: Executive. b. Berlin, Mar. 16, 1928 e. MA. Pol. Sci./Int. Law. Joined Associated Press 1950, foreign correspondent; 1970, appointed regional mgr. Joined United Press International 1971 as regional mgr. (Southwest U.S.); 1974, appointed gen. mgr. for Unicom Economic News Service; 1978 appointed gen. exec. for Europe; 1981, appointed v.p. for news and information services and corporate development; 1983, joined United International Pictures as pres.,—Pay-TV Group; 1985, v.p. & gen. mgr., United Media, New York.

BAUER, STEVEN: Actor. b. Cuba, 1956. Moved with family to Miami at age 3. e. Miami Dade Jr. Coll. where studied acting. Breakthrough came with selection for role in Que Pasa U.S.A.? for Public TV. Signed by Columbia TV and moved to California.
PICTURES: Scarface, Thief of Hearts, Running Scared.
TELEVISION: Series: The Rockford Files, Doctors Private Lives, From Here to Eternity, Hill Street Blues, One Day

at a Time. Movies: She's in the Army Now, Nichols and Dymes, An Innocent Love, etc.

BAUM, MARTIN: Executive. b. New York, N.Y. March 2, 1924; president, ABC Pictures; previously partner Baum & Newborn Theatrical Agency; head of West Coast office General Artists Corp., head of m.p. dept., Ashley Famous Agency; President of Martin Baum Agency; sr. exec. v.p. Creative Management Associations; president Optimus Productions, Inc., producing Bring Me the Head of Alfredo Garcia, The Wilby Conspiracy, and The Killer Elite. Partners with Michael Ovitz, Ron Meyer, Rowland Perkins, Bill Haber in Creative Artists Agency, Inc.

BAUMGARTEN, CRAIG: Executive. Partner in independent prod. co., New America Cinema. Joined Paramount Picutres as prod. exec.; named v.p., prod. In 1980 went to Keith Barish Prods., of which was pres. three years. In 1983 appt. exec. v.p. & exec. asst. to the pres. & CEO, Columbia Pictures. Resigned 1985; joined Lorimar Motion Pictures as pres.

BAUMSTONE, HAROLD: Executive. b. New York City, June 27, 1911; e. U. No. Carolina, B.A. 1932; prod. & distrib. of short subjects; pres., Institutional Cinema Inc., National 16mm Film Exchange, now representing Columbia Pictures, Warner Bros., American International and ind. prod. Exclusive distributor for 16mm markets for foreign films.

BAXTER, BILLY: Executive. b. N.Y.C., Feb. 8, 1926. e. Holy Cross, 1948. Mgr., Ambassador Brokerage Group, Albany, 1957–58; Bill Doll & Co., 1959–63; organ., prod., radio show, Earl Wilson Celebrity Column, 1962; prod. Bwy show, Mandingo, with Franchot Tone, 1962; dir. of promotion, spec. events, Rumrill Ad Agency, 1963–64; dir. of promotion, exploitation, Landau Co., 1964–65; dir. of adv. and pub., Rizzoli Co., 1965; resigned, Rizzoli, 1966. Consultant on special events to the Philip Morris Corp. and American Express. Coproducer on movies Love and Anarchy, Daughters-Daughters, Outrageous, One Man, Dawn of the Dead. Produced Diary of the Cannes Film Festival with Rex Reed, 1980.

BAXTER, KEITH: Actor. b. April 29, 1933, Monmouthshire, South Wales. e. Wales, entered Royl Academy of Dramatic Arts in 1951. 1952–55 in national service; returned to RADA. Did years of repertory work in Dublin, Croydon, Chichester, London's West End, and New York. Biggest stage hit in Sleuth, both London and N.Y.
PICTURES INCLUDE: The Barretts of Wimpole Street, Peeping Tom, Chimese at Midnight, With Love in Mind, Ash Wednesday.
TELEVISION: For Tea on Sunday, Hold My Hand Soldier, Saint Joan.

BAXTER, STANLEY: Actor. b. Glasgow, Scotland, 1928. e. Hillhead High School, Glasgow. Principal comedian in Howard & Wyndham pantomimes. Summer revues. Televised regularly on BBC-TV, and also frequent broadcaster. M.P. debut 1955 in Geordie.
STAGE: The Amorous Pawn, On the Brighter Side, 1961, Chase Me Comrade, in Australia, 1965; Cinderella. 1966–68, What the Butler Saw; 1969; Phil The Fluter, 1969–70. Mother Goose Pantomime seasons 1970/71, 71/72, 72/73, 73/74. Jack & The Beanstalk, 75/76/77/78. Cinderella 79/80 81/82; Mother Goose, 82/83/84/85.
PICTURES INCLUDE: Very Important Person, Crooks Anonymous, The Fast Lady, Father Came Too Joey Boy.
TV: Baxter on (Series) 1964; The Confidence Course 1965, The World of Stanley Baxter, 1966; Stanley Baxter Show, 1967, Stanley Baxter Show, 1968, 1971, Time for Baxter, 1972, The Stanley Baxter Big Picture Show, 1973. The Stanley Baxter Moving Picture Show, 1974. Part III, 1975. "Stanley Baxter's Christmas Box," 1976. Bing Crosby's Merrie Olde Christmas, 1977. Stanley Baxter's Greatest Hits, 1977. Baxter on Television, 1979, Stanley Baxter Series, 1981, The Stanley Baxter Hour, 1982; Children's Royal, 1984; Stanley Baxter's Christmas Hamper, 1985.

BEAL, JOHN: Actor, r.n. J. Alexander Bliedung. b. Joplin, Mo., Aug. 13, 1909; e. Wharton School, Pa. U. On Broadway in: Another Language, She Loves Me Not, Petrified Forest, etc: m.p. debut in "Another Language" 1933; serves in U.S.A.A.F. World War II.
PICTURES INCLUDE: Little Minister, Les Miserables, We Who Are About to Die, Man Who Found Himself, Arkansas Traveler, Cat and the Canary, Great Commandment, Doctors Don't Tell, Atlantic Convoy, Edge of Darkness; Stand By, All Networks, Key Witness, Madame X, Double Wedding, Beg, Borrow or Steal, Port of Seven Seas, Alimony, Song of Surrender, Chicago Deadline, My Six Convicts, Remains to Be Seen, The Vampire, The Sound and the Fury, That Night, Ten Who Dared, Amityville 3-D.

BEAN, ORSON: Actor. b. Burlington, VT, July 22, 1928. Performed in nightclubs as comic and on Broadway (School for Scandal, Will Success Spoil Rock Hunter?, Subways Are for Sleeping, Roar of the Grease Paint; the Smell of the Crowd, Ilya Darling, etc.)
PICTURES INCLUDE: Lola, Skateboard, Forty Deuces.

BEATTY, NED: Actor. Worked at Barter Theatre in Virginia for seven years, appearing in over 70 plays. First N.Y. performance in The Great White Hope.
PICTURES: Deliverance (debut), Nashville, W.W. and the Dixie Dance Kings, Exorcist II: The Heretic, Network, The Great Georgia Bank Hoax, Superman, Promises in the Dark, Hopscotch, The Incredible Shrinking Woman, Superman II, The Toy, Touched, Stroker Ace, Back to School.
TELEVISION: The Last Days of Pompeii, Celebrity, Robert Kennedy and His Times.

BEATTY, ROBERT: Actor. b. Hamilton, Ont., Canada, Oct. 19, 1909. e. U. Toronto. London stage debut: Idiot's Delight, 1938. On screen first in Suspected Persons, 1942.
PICTURES INCLUDE: San Demetrio London, It Happened One Sunday, Appointment with Crime, Ood Man Out, Green Fingers, Against the Wind, Another Shore, Portrait from Life, Her Favorite Husband, Captain Horatio Hornblower, Calling Bulldog Drummond, Magic Box, Wings of Danger, The Gentle Gunman, The Oracle, The Net (Project M.7), Man on the Tightrope, Broken Horseshoe, The Square Ring, Albert RN (Break to Freedom), Loves of Three Women, Out of the Clouds, Portrait of Alison (Postmark for Danger),Tarzan and the Lost Safari, Something of Value, Time Lock, The Shakedown, The Amorous Prawn, Stanley Kubrick's 2001, Where Eagles Dare, Sitting Target, Pope Joan, The Pink Panther Strikes Again, Golden Rendezvous, Superman III, The Highlander.
TV: Weekly guide, Saturday Night Out, Dial 999 series, The Human Jungle (Series), Court Martial Series, Time Lock, Man at the Top, The Venturers, Thriller, Jesus of Nazareth, Blake's Seven, Park Ranger, The Martian Chronicles, Walk with Destiny, Suez, The Rose, Medallion, Tales of the Unexpected, Murder of a Moderate Man, Murder on the Orient Express.

BEATTY, WARREN: Actor. b. Richmond, Va., March 30, 1938. e. Northwestern U.; small roles on television; Compulsion, winter stock. North Jersey Playhouse; Broadway debut, A Loss of Roses.
PICTURES INCLUDE: Splendor in the Grass, The Roman Spring of Mrs. Stone, All Fall Down, Lilith, Mickey One, Promise Her Anything, Kaleidoscope; prod. & starred in Bonnie and Clyde, The Only Game in Town, McCabe and Mrs. Miller, Dollars, The Parallax View, Shampoo (producer, co-author, star), The Fortune, Heaven Can Wait (star, prod., co-dir., co-s.p.), Reds (star, prod., dir., co-s.p.), Ishtar (prod., star).

BEAUMONT, HUGH: Actor. b. Lawrence, Kan., Feb. 16, 1909. e. U. of Chattanooga; U.S.C.
PICTURES INCLUDE: Michael Shayne series, PRC; Blue Dahlia, Guilt of Janet Ames, Counterfeiters, Last Outpost, Lost Continent, Phone Call from a Stranger, Wild Stallion, Night Without Sleep, The Mississippi Gambler, Hell's Horizon.

BECK, ALEXANDER J.: Executive. b. Ung. Brod, Czechoslovakia, Nov. 5, 1926. e. Charles Univ. Prague, NYU. Owns 500 features and westerns for foreign distribution and library of 1400 shorts. Importer and exporter; Pres., chairman of bd. Alexander Beck Films, 1955; formed Albex Films and A.B. Enterprises, 1959; formed & pres., Beckman Film Corp., 1960; formed Alexander Beck Productions, 1964. Sept. '69 formed Screencom Int'l Corp., 1986, formed Beck Intl. Corp.

BECK, JACKSON: Actor-announcer-narrator. b. N.Y.C. TV and radio commercials, children's records, comm. & industrial films; Narrator.

BECK, JOHN: Actor. b. Chicago. Acted with mid-western theatre groups; had basic training in scores of TV series. Theatrical debut in Three in the Attic.
PICTURES INCLUDE: Three in the Attic, Mrs. Pollifax, Spy, Lawman, Pat Garrett and Billy the Kid, Sleeper, Deadly Honeymoon, Rollerball, Paperback Hero, The Big Bus, Audrey Rose, The Other Side of Midnight.
TV: Guest star roles on Bonanza, Mannix, Hawaii Five-O, etc.

BECK, MICHAEL: Actor. b. Memphis, TN. e. Millsap College on football scholarship (quarterback). Became active in college theatre. In 1971 went to London, England to attend Central School of Speech and Drama; studied 3 years, following which toured England with repertory companies for 2 years. Returned to U.S.; cast as lead in independent film, Madman (shot in Israel in 1977).
PICTURES: Madman, The Warriors, Xanadu, Megaforce, The Golden Seal.
TELEVISION: Holocaust, Mayflower: The Pilgrim Adventure, Alcatraz: The Rock, Clarence Carnes, Celebrity, Rearview Mirror.

BECK, MYER P.: Sales, prod. rep. b. Meriden, Conn.; e. N.Y.U. School of Journalism. Newspaperman; publicist; publicity dir. United Artists; eastern mgr. Russell Birdwell Associates; formed own sls. prod. rep. office 1945, repr. Albert R. Broccoli; Jerome Hellman Productions, Stanley Kramer Pictures Corp.

BEDELIA, BONNIE: Actress. b. New York City, March 25, 1946. e. Hunter Coll.
PICTURES: The Gypsy Moths, They Shoot Horses Don't They?, Lovers and Other Strangers, The Big Fix, Heart Like a Wheel, The Boy Who Could Fly, Death of an Angel, Violets Are Blue.
TELEVISION: Hawkins on Murder, A Question of Love, Salem's Lot, Fighting Back, Alex: The Life of a Child, etc.

BEERY, NOAH, JR.: Actor. b. New York City, Aug. 10, 1916; son of Noah Beery, screen actor; e. Urban and Harvard Mil. Acad. Travelled with parents in stock company. Appeared as child in Mark of Zorro 1920.
PICTURES INCLUDE: Father and Son, Road Back, Only Angels Have Wings, Doolins of Oklahoma, Davy Crockett, Indian Scout, Last Outpost, Savage Horde, Rocketship XM, Two Flags West, Tropic Zone, Cimarron Kid, Wagons West, Story of Will Rogers, Wings of the Hawk, War Arrow, The Yellow Tomahawk, Black Dakotas, White Feather, Jubal, Fastest Gun Alive, Journey to Shiloh, Heaven With A Gun, Walking Tall, The Spikes Gang, The Best Little Whorehouse in Texas.
TELEVISION: Yellow Rose.

BEICH, ALBERT: Writer. b. Bloomington, Ill., June 25, 1919. e. McGill U. Radio writer.
PICTURES INCLUDE: You Can't Beat the Law, Girls in Chains, Gangs of the Waterfront, Gay Blades, Bridge Goes Wild, Key to the City, Yellow Cab Man, The Milkman, Lieutenant Wore Skirts.

BEJTMAN, VINCENT: Executive. b. Poland. Started career producing entertainment films in native land. Came to U.S. during war. Named pres. of PIC Films, Inc., financed by Polish govt.-in-exile in London and the British Information Center. Company produced over 30 films depicting Poland participation in World War II. Formed Cine Classics Films, Inc. specializing in import of foreign films for U.S. market, including Rules of the Game, Zero De Conduit, etc. Produced documentaries (The Great Betrayal, Last Days of Warsaw.) Co-produced Naked Amazon. Now pres. of Vee Bee Productions, Inc. and involved in American-European co-production.

BELAFONTE, HARRY: Actor, singer. b. New York City, March 1, 1927. Professional debut; Royal Roost nightclub, N.Y., Village Vanguard, 1950. Broadway debut: John Murray Anderson's Almanac, 1953.
SHOWS INCLUDE: Three for Tonight, A Night With-Belefonte.
PICTURES INCLUDE: Bright Road, Carmen Jones, Island In The Sun, Odds Against Tomorrow, The World, The Flesh & The Devil, The Angel Levine, Buck and the Preacher, Uptown Saturday Night (prod., star).

BELFER, HAL B.: Exec. Producer-Director-Choreographer. b. Los Angeles, Feb. 16. e. Univ of So. Calif. (cinematography); Univ. of Calif. (writing). Head of choreography dept. at 20th Century-Fox. Head of choreography dept. at Universal Studios. Dir. of entertainment, in Las Vegas, Riviera and Flamingo Hotels. Prod., musical shows for Mexico City, Aruba, Puerto Rico, Montreal, Las Vegas. Dir., TV commercials and industrials. H.R. Pufnstuf TV series. Theatricals: Over 150 features. Producer-Director-Choreographer, Premore, Inc. Develop TV specials and sitcom, tape and film. Exec. prod., Once Upon a Tour and Dora's World, Rose on Broadway, Secret Sleuth, Inn by the Side of the Road, Imagine That!. Special staging "Tony The Pony" Series and prod., segment of What a Way to Run a Railroad; TV specials. Talent development programs, Universal Studios, 20th Century-Fox. Personal management and show packager; 1982, exec. prod., Enchanted Inn (TV Special), Cameo Music Hall I, Stage mgr.: Promises Promises, A Chorus Line (Sahara Hotel, Las Vegas).

BEL GEDDES, BARBARA: Actress. r.n. Barbara Geddes Lewis. b. New York City, Oct 31, 1922; p. Norman Bel Geddes, scenic designer. Stage debut in "Out of the Frying Pan"; toured USO camps in "Junior Miss" 1941; screen debut in "The Long Night" 1946; Star of Tomorrow, 1949. N.Y. Stage: The Moon is Blue, Cat on a Hot Tin Roof, Mary, Mary, Everything in the Garden. On TV in Dallas.
PICTURES INCLUDE: I Remember Mama, Blood on the Moon, Caught, Panic in Streets, Fourteen Hours, The Five Pennies, Five Branded Women, By Love Possessed, Summertree, The Todd Killings.

BELL, TOM: Actor. b. Liverpool, England, 1932. Early career in repertory and on West End stage. First TV appearance in Promenade.
TV: No Trams to Lime Street, Love On the Dole, A Night Out, Cul de Sac, The Seekers, Long Distance Blue, The Virginian. Film debut 1960 in Payroll.
PICTURES INCLUDE: The Kitchen, H.M.S. Defiant, Prize of Arms, L-Shaped Room, Rebels Against the Light, Ballad in Blue, He Who Rides a Tiger, In Enemy Country, The Long Days Dying, Lock Up Your Daughters.

BELLAMY, EARL: Prod. Dir. b. Minneapolis, Minn., March 11, 1917. e. L.A. City Coll. Universal Studios.
PICTURES: Fluffy, Gun Point, Munsters Go Home, Sidewinder, Speedtrap.
TV: Bachelor Father, Wells Fargo, Lone Ranger, Alcoa Premiere, Arrest and Trial, The Virginian, The Crusaders, Schlitz Playhouse, Heinz, Rawhide, The Donna Reed Show, Andy Griffith Show, Wagon Train, now president, The Bellamy Productions Co., Laramie, Laredo, I Spy, Mod Squad, Medical Center.

BELLAMY, RALPH: Actor. b. Chicago, Ill., June 17, 1905. Stock and repertory, 1922–30; pres. Actors Equity, 1952; council, Lambs, 1952; TV includes major live and film dramatic shows, voted many TV awards.
BROADWAY: Town Boy, Roadside, Tomorrow the World, State of the Union, Detective Story.
PICTURES INCLUDE: Great Impersonation, Lady on a Train, Guest in the House, Delightfully Dangerous, Court Martial of Billy Mitchell, Sunrise at Campobello, The Professionals, Rosemary's Baby, Oh, God!, Trading Places.
TELEVISION: Space

BELLFORT, JOSEPH: b. New York. e. New York U., B'klyn Law Sch. Joined RKO Service Corp., Feb., 1930; trans. to RKO Radio Pictures, legal dept., May 1942; joined RKO Fgn. dept., Oct., 1944, handled Far Eastern division, Dec. 1946; then asst. to European gen. mgr.; gen. European mgr., 1949–1958; gen. sales mgr. National Screen Service, 1959; home office sup., Europe & Near East, 20th Century-Fox, 1963; home office intl. mgr., 20th Century-Fox, 1966. Ass't v.p. and foreign mgr. 20th Cent.-Fox, 1967; vice president 20th Century-Fox, Int. Corp. & Inter-America, Inc. 1968; named sr. v.p., 1975. Resigned from Fox, 1977, to become v.p., Motion Picture Export Assn. of America in New York. Retired 1983.

BELLOCCHIO, MARCO: Director-Writer. b. Italy, 1939.
PICTURES: Fists in the Pocket, China Is Near, Leap into the Void, Vacations in Val Trebbia, The Eyes The Mouth, Henry IV.

BELMONDO, JEAN-PAUL: Actor. b. Neuilly-sur-Seine, France, April 9, 1933. e. private drama school of Raymond Girard, and the Conservatoire d'Art Dramatique. Formed a theater group with Annie Girardot and Guy Bedos.
THEATRE INCLUDE: Jean Marais' production of Caesar and Cleopatra, Treasure Party. Oscar, 1958.
PICTURES INCLUDE: A Pied, A Cheval et En Voiture (By Foot, Horse and Car), Look Pretty and Shut Up, Drole de Dimanche, Les Tricheurs, Les Copains du Dimanche, Charlotte et Son Jules, A Double Tour, Breathless, Classe Tous Risques, Moderato Cantabile, La Francasie et l'Amour, Les Distractions, Mademoiselle Ange, La Novice, Two Women, La Viaccia, Une Femme Est Une Femme, Leon Morin, Pretre, Les Amours Celebres, Un Singe en Hiver, Le Doulos, L'Aine des Ferchaux, La Mer A Boire, Banana Peel, That Man From Rio, Cent Mille Dollars au Soleil, Echappement Libre, La Chasse a l'Homme, Dieu a Choisi Paris, Weekend a Zuydcocte, 100,000 Dollars au Soleil, Par Un Beau Matin d'Ete, Up to His Ears, Is Paris Burning?, The Thief of Paris, Tender Scoundrel, Pierrot le Fou, The Brain, Love Is a Funny Thing, Mississippi Mermaid, Borsalino, Inheritor, Stavisky, Fear Over the City.

BENDHEIM, III, SAM: Executive. b. Richmond, Va., June 15, 1935. e. Washington & Lee Univ. Joined Neighborhood Theatre, Inc., 1958 as exec. trainee. Was dir. of adv. (1960–63); bd. member, ass't. treas. (1962); ass't to gen. mgr. (1963–67) v.p. (1967). Member: NATO of Virginia; former pres. & chm., NATO of Virginia; bd., pres. advisory council, exec. comm., NATO; bd., Foundation of Motion Picture Pioneers; general partner, Neighborhood Booking & Buying Service.

BENDICK, ROBERT: b. New York City Feb. 8, 1917; e. New York U., White School Photography; U.S Airforce, World War II. Documentary and still cameraman before joining CBS Television as cameraman and dir., 1940; rejoined CBS Television as dir. special events, 1946; promoted dir. news & special events; acting program dir. 1947; res. Oct. '51. Collab with Jeanne Bendick on Making the Movies, Electronics for Young People, Television Works Like This, Filming Works Like This, 1971; Prod. Peabody Awardwinning U.N. show. The U.N. in Action; v.p., Cinerama Prod., co-prod. This Is Cinerama; co-dir., Cinerama Holiday; prod. Dave Garroway Show Today, prod., Wide Wide World 1955–56, NBC prod. dir. C.V. Whitney Pict., June, 1956; Merian C. Cooper Ent., 1957; prod. NBC, 1958. Prod.; Garroway Today Show, Bob Hope 25 Yrs. of Life Show,

1961; Bell Telephone Threshold Science Series, Groucho Marx, Merrily We Roll Along, US Steel Opening New York World's Fair, 1964. Prod. First Look Series 1965 (Ohio St. Award); prod. & dir. American Sportsman, ABC; prod., pilot, Great American Dream Machine (NET) Emmy Award, 1971 and 1972; 1975, Co-exec. prod., Dick Cavett—Feeling Good. pres. Bendick Assoc. Inc.,; prod. of education audio-visual systems, Bd. of Governors, N.Y. Academy of TV Arts and Sciences. 1976, co-author with Jeanne Bendick, TV Reporting. Consultant, Warner Qube Cable Co.; 1978, produced/directed, Fight for Food (PBS). Program consultant to Times-Miror Cable Co., L.A. Produced segment ABC 20/20.

BENEDEK, LASLO: Director b. Budapest, Hungary, Mar. 5, 1907; e. U. Vienna; Psycho-Analytic Clinic. Writer & photographer while in coll.; cameraman Budapest; first asst. cameraman several studios; cameraman UFA & Terra; film cutter; cutter & asst. prod. to Joe Pasternak; to Paris as cutter, then Engl dial. on "Antonia"; writer (England) 2 yrs.; montage dir. MGM 1937; writer (Mexico); assoc. prod. (Hollywood) on musicals; contract dir. MGM; Stanley Kramer Co., Col.; 1976–80, Chairman of Graduate Film Program, New York University. 1983, visiting professor, Annenberg School of Communication, Univ. of P.A. 1984, Film & TV Academy, Munich, Germany. Production advisor, S. Carolina ETV.
PICTURES INCLUDE: Kissing Bandit, Port of New York, Death of a Salesman, Storm Over Tibet, Wild One, Bengal Brigade; Sons, Mothers and a General, Affair in Havana, Moment of Danger, Recours en Grace, Namu, The Killer Whale, A Daring Game, The Night Visitor.
TV: 4 Star Playhouse, Dupont Theatre, Stage 7, Loretta Young Show, Telephone Time, Perry Mason, Naked City, Untouchables, Outer Limits.
STAGE: Belial, Twelfth Night.

BENEDICT, DIRK: Actor. b. Helena, Mont. r.n. Dirk Niewoehner. e. Whitman College, Walla Walla, Wash. Enrolled in John Fernald Academy of Dramatic Arts, Rochester, Mich., after which had season with Seattle Repertory Theatre; other in summer stock at Ann Arbor, Mich. Broadway debut, 1970, Aberlard and Heloise. Film debut, Georgia, Georgia, 1972.
PICTURES INCLUDE: Ssssss, W, Battlestar Galactica, Scavenger Hunt.
TELEVISION: Hawaii Five-O (one episode), Chopper One (series), Battlestar Galactica (series); The A Team (series).

BENJAMIN, RICHARD: Actor. b. New York, N.Y., May 22, 1939; e. Northwestern U. Plays; Central Park productions of The Taming of the Shrew, As You Like It; toured in Tchin Tchin, A Thousand Clowns, Barefoot in the Park, The Odd Couple. Broadway debut in Star Spangled Girl, 1966. Directed London productions of Barefoot in the Park. TV series, He and She, with wife Paula Prentiss, 1967.
PICTURES INCLUDE: Goodbye, Columbus, Catch 22, Diary of a Mad Housewife, The Marriage of a Young Stockbroker, The Steagle, Portnoy's Complaint, The Last of Sheila, Westworld, The Sunshine Boys, Love at First Bite, Scavenger Hunt, The Last Married Couple in America, How to Beat the High Cost of Living, First Family, Director: My Favorite Year, Racing with the Moon, City Heat, The Money Pit.

BENNET, SPENCER G.: Director. b. Brooklyn, N.Y., Jan. 5, 1893. e. Manual Training H.S., Brooklyn, N.Y.; played stunt and thrill parts; asst. dir., Pathe; prod., dir., from 1925–64. Retired.
CREDITS INCLUDE: Play Ball (serial), The Green Archer (serial), Snowed in (serial), The Fighting Marine (serial) and many other serials and westerns. Submarine Seahawk, Atomic Submarine, Bounty Killer, Requiem For a Gunfighter.

BENNETT, BRUCE: Actor. r.n. Herman Brix. b. Tacoma, Wash., 1909; e. U. Washington.
PICTURES INCLUDE: My Son is Guilty, Lone Wolf Keeps a Date, Atlantic Convoy, Sabotage, Underground Agent, More the Merrier, Sahara, Man I Love, Stolen Life, Nora Prentiss, Cheyenne, Treasure of Sierra Madre, Dark Passage, Smart Girls Don't Talk, Second Face, Great Missouri Raid, Last Outpost, Angels in the Outfield, Sudden Fear, Dream Wife, Dragonfly Squadron, Robbers Roost, Big Tipoff, Hidden Guns, Bottom of the Bottle, Strategic Air Command.

BENNETT, CHARLES: Writer, director. b. Shoreham, England. British Army. Contract, Universal, 1937; wrote British Ministry of Information, WW II; dir. s.p. over 50 TV shows, including Cavalcade of America, Schilitz Playhouse, The Christophers, Four Star.
PLAYS INCLUDE: Blackmail, The Last Hour, Sensation, The Danger Line, Page From a Diary, The Return, After Midnight.
PICTURES INCLUDE: Blackmail, The 39 Steps, Secret Agent, The Man Who Knew Too Much (orig.), Sabotage, The Girl Was Young, Balalaika, The Young in Heart, Foreign Correspondent, Reap the Wild Wind, Joan of Paris, They Dare Not Love, The Story of Dr. Wassell, Unconquered, Ivy, Sign of the Ram, Kind Lady, The Green Glove, Dangerous Assignment, Madness of the Heart (dir.), The Big Circus, The Lost World, Voyage to the Bottom of the Sea, Five Weeks in a Balloon.

BENNETT, HARVE; Producer. r.n. Harve Fischman. b. Chicago, Ill., Aug. 17, 1930. e. U.C.L.A. Quiz Kids radio show, 5 yrs.; newspaper columnist, drama critic; freelance writer; Assoc. prod., CBS-TV; free-lance TV writer; prod. of special events. CBS-TV; dir., Television film commercials; program exec., ABC, vice pres., programs west coast—ABC-TV; prod.-writer, Mod Squad. Creator-writer, The Young Rebels, Screen Gems; exec. prod., Six Million Dollar Man, Bionic Woman, Rich Man, Poor Man, Universal Studios; Pres., Bennett-Katleman. Productions at Columbia Studios, and exec. prod. on American Girls series (CBS), From Here to Eternity (NBC), Salvage 1 (ABC). Joined Paramount's Motion Picture Group, acting as exec. prod. & co-author of Star Trek II: The Wrath of Khan; prod. & author of Star Trek III: The Search for Spock. 1984, entered long-term deal with Para.

BENNETT, JILL: Actress. b. Penang (Federated Malay Straits), Dec. 24, 1931. Stage debut at Stratford-on-Avon, 1948; screen debut 1952 in Moulin Rouge.
PICTURES INCLUDE: Hell Below Zero, The Criminal, Extra-Day, Lust For Life, The Skull, The Nanny, Charge of Light Brigade, Inadmissible Evidence, I Want What I Want, Quilp, Full Circle, For Your Eyes Only, Britannia Hospital, Lady Jane.
TV: The Heiress, Trilby, Jealousy, A Midsummer Night's Dream, The Three Sisters, Glimpse of the Sea, Return to the Sea, The Book Bag (Somerset Maugham Series), It's Only Us, The Parachute, Hotel in Amsterdam, Speaking of Murder, Intent to Murder, Jill and Jack, Almost A Vision, Hello Lola, The Old Crowd, Orient Express (French TV), The Aerodrome, Poor Little Rich Girls (series), Country, Paradise Postponed, Worlds Beyond.

BENNETT, JOAN: Actress. b. Palisades, N.J., Feb. 27, 1910; e. St. Margaret's Boarding School, Waterbury, Conn.; L'Ermitage, Versailles, France; member of famous Bennett acting family; m. Walter Wanger, prod. On stage with father, Richard Bennett in "Jarnegan"; m.p. debut in "Bulldog Drummond" 1929; vice-pres. & treas. Diana Prods. 1945.
PICTURES INCLUDE: Three Live Ghosts, Disraeli, Moby Dick, Little Women, Pursuit of Happiness, Mississippi, Woman in the Window, Secret Beyond the Door, Man Who Reclaimed His Head, Hollow Triumph, Scar, Reckless Moment, For Heaven's Sake, Father of Bride, Father's Little Dividend, The Guy Who Came Back, Highway, Dragnet, We're No Angels, There's Always Tomorrow, Navy Wife, Desire in the Dust, Suspiria.
TV: Starring in ABC Dark Shadows.

BENSON, HUGH: Producer. b. New York. Sept. 7, 1917. e. New York public schools. Six yrs. infantry, then Air Force. Three yrs. European Theatre of War, As master sergeant, Air Force, two yrs., non com in chg. of soldier units under, prod.-dir., Joshua Logan. Joined Blaine-Thompson Advertising Agency as dir. of public relations; assist. to producers, Ed Sullivan and Marlo Lewis, Ed Sullivan Show, 1947–50; dir. television, public relations, Roy Dunstine Agency, 1951; hd. of radio, television promotion, publicity dept., Warner Bros., June, 1955; appointed assist. to Steve Trilling, vice-pres. and exec. associate of Jack L. Warner, 1956; exec. asst. to William T. Orr, Warner v.p. in chg. of production, 1956; prod., United Artists, 1963; exec. asst. to William T. Orr, Warner Bros., 1964–65. Exec. Prod., Screen Gems, 1966, Prod., Cinema Center Films, 1969–71, prod., MGM, 1972; appointed exec. prod., MGM Television, 1972. 1975 indep. prod. On staff Col.-tv, 1975, pilots and long form.
PICTURES: Nightmare Honeymoon (prod.), Logan's Run (assoc. prod.), Billy Jack Goes to Washington (prod.).
TELEVISION: Contract On Cherry St. (prod.) Child Stealers, Goldie and the Boxer, A Fire in the Sky, Confessions of a Lady Cop, The Dream Merchants, Goldie and the Boxer Go to Hollywood, Goliath Awaits, The Blue and the Gray (prod.), Hart to Hart (prod.), Master of Ballentrae (sup. prod.); 1985: Anna Karenina, The Other Lover, I Dream of Jeannie 15 Yrs. Later, Miracle of the Heart: A Boy's Town Story, Crazy Like a Fox (all prod.).

BENSON, LEON: Producer-Director. g. Cincinnati, Ohio, Nov. 9. e. New York University, University of Cincinnati. Advertising Dept. Paramount, 1938, head of Trailer Dept., 1940. U.S. Army Air Corps, 1942–46, Major, First head of TV Dept. L.A. office of J. Walter Thompson Co., 1946–51. Head of Story Dept. Ziv TV, 1951; prod. and dir. West Point, 1955–56; Sea Hunt, 1956–60; Ripcord, 1960–62. Prod.-Dir. Flipper TV series, 1963–64. Under contract, Universal, 1965–66, prod.-dir. episodes, Kraft Suspense Theatre, The Virginian, dir. episodes, Chrysler Theatre, Laredo. Prod. Tarzan TV series, 1966. Under contract,

NBC Prods., 1967–70, as staff dir. Bonanza, High Chaparral. Prod. theatrical feature, Chosen Survivors, 1973. Also dir. Owen Marshall, Counsellor at Law, Mission Impossible, The Eleventh Hour, Ben Casey, Wild Wild West, Rat Patrol, The Lieutenant, Outer Limits, The Loner, Empire.

BENSON, ROBBY: Actor. b. Dallas, 1957. Father, Jerry Segal, is writer, and mother, Ann Nelson, veteran of Dallas stage and natl. summer stock. Robby appeared on Broadway in The King and I at age five. Also worked 6 mos. in soap opera, Search for Tomorrow. Big break in feature films in Jeremy. Co-wrote screenplay of One on One (1977) with father and starred in film.
PICTURES: Jeremy, Jory, The Godfather—Part II, Ode to Billy Joe, Lucky Lady, One on One, The End, Ice Castles, Walk Proud, Die Laughing (also prod., co-s.p.), Tribute, The Chosen, Running Brave, Harry and Son.
TV: The Death of Richie, Remember When, Virginia Hill, All the Kind Strangers, Death Be Not Proud.
STAGE: Zelda, The Rothschilds.

BENTLEY, JOHN: Actor. b. Warwickshire, Eng. Dec. 2, 1916. e. King Edward's Grammar Sch., Birmingham. Radio debut, 1933; Alexandra & Birmingham Rep. Cos. in 1934; stage debut in New Faces, London, 1940; m.p. debut in Hills of Donegal, 1946.
PICTURES INCLUDE: Calling Paul Temple, Paul Temple's Triumph, Happiest Days of Your Life, Torment, She Shall Have Murder, Salute the Toff, Hammer the Toff, Woman's Angie, Lost Hours, Tread Softly, Black Orchid, Paul Temple Returns, River Beat, Double Exposure, Scarlet Spear, Golden Ivory, The Flaw, Profile, Last Appointment, Confession, Deadliest Sin, Flight from Vienna, Strangehold, Blind Man's Bluff, Dial 999, Way Out, Escape in the Sun, Istanbul, Submarine Seahawk, The Singer Not the Song, Mary Had a Little, The Sinister Man, An Helligen Wassern, The Fur Collar, The Shadow of Treason.
TV: Strictly Personal, African Patrol, Crossroads, Armchair Theatre, Any Other Business, Misfire, Time Out of Mind.

BENTON, ROBERT: Writer-Director. b. Waxahachie, Texas, 1932. e. Univ. of Texas (B.A.); Was art director at Esquire Magazine where he met David Newman, a writer-editor, and formed writing partnership. All writing credits shared with Newman. Benton made directorial debut with Bad Company (1972).
PICTURES INCLUDE: Bonnie and Clyde, There Was a Crooked Man, What's Up, Doc?, Bad Company (also directed) The Late Show (written and directed solo), Superman (with Mario Puzo and Tom Mankiewicz), Money's Tight, Bad Company (also dir., solo); Superman (co.-s.p.); Kramer vs. Kramer (dir. s.p.); Still of the Night (dir., s.p.); Places in the Heart (dir., s.p.).
STAGE: It's a Bird . . . It's a Plane . . . It's Superman (libretto), Oh! Calcutta (one sketch).

BERCUTT, MAX: Executive. b. Omaha, Neb., Oct. 14, 1910. e. U. of Southern California, 1933. Pres., Paris-American Guide Services, Paris, France; publicist David O. Selznick Prod.; U.S. Navy officer World War II; Warner Bros. field rep.; assistant to exec. vice-pres.; director of publicity, Warner Bros. Seven Arts Studio; resigned, September, 1969. Formed Max Bercutt Co., Jan. 1970.

BERENGER, TOM: Actor. b. Chicago, May 31, 1950. e. Univ. of Missouri (drama dept.) Acted in regional theatres and off Bdwy. Plays include The Rose Tattoo, Electra, Streetcar Named Desire, End as a Man. Film debut in the Sentinel (1977).
PICTURES: Looking for Mr. Goodbar, In Praise of Older Women, Butch and Sundance: The Early Days, The Dogs of War. The Big Chill, Eddie and the Cruisers, Beyond the Door, Fear City, Firstborn, Rustler's Rhapsody.
TELEVISION: One Life to Live (series), Johnny We Hardly Knew Ye, Flesh and Blood, If Tomorrow Comes.

BERESFORD, BRUCE: Director-Writer. b. Australia, 1949.
PICTURES INCLUDE: The Adventures of Barry McKenzie, Barry McKenzie Holds His Own (also prod.), Side by Side, Don's Party (d. only), The Getting of Wisdom (d. only), Breaker Morant, The Club (d. only), Puberty Blues (d. only); King David (d. only), Crimes of the Heart.

BERG, JEFF: Executive. b. Los Angeles, May 26, 1947. e. Univ. Calif., Berkeley, (BA 1969). V.p., head lit. div., Creative Mgt. Associates, Los Angeles, 1969–75; v.p., m.p. dept., International Creative Associates, 1975–80; pres., 1980-–. Dir., Joseph Intl. Industries.

BERGEN, CANDICE: Actress. b. Beverly Hills, Calif., May 9, 1946. e. U. of Pennsylvania. Modeled during college; m.p. debut, The Group, 1965; free lance photo-journalist.
PICTURES INCLUDE: The Group, The Sand Pebbles, The Day the Fish Came Out, Live for Life, The Magus, The Adventurers, Getting Straight, Soldier Blue, Carnal Knowledge, The Hunting Party, T. R. Baskin, 11 Harrowhouse, Bite the Bullet, The Wind and the Lion, The Domino Principle, A Night Full of Rain, Olivers' Story, Starting Over, Rich and Famous, Gandhi, Stick.
TELEVISION: Hollywood Wives, Arthur the King, Murder: By Reason of Insanity.

BERGEN, POLLY: Singer, actress. b. Knoxville, Tenn., July 14, 1930. e. Compton Jr. Coll., Calif. Prof. debut radio at 14; in light opera, summer stock; sang with orchestra and appeared in night clubs; Columbia recording star; Emmy Award, best actress, 1957–58; pres. The Polly Bergen Co.; on stage, John Murray Anderson's Almanac, Champagne Complex, First Impressions.
TV: G.E. Theatre, Schlitz Playhouse, Playhouse 90, Studio One, Perry Como, Ed Sullivan Show, To Tell the Truth, Polly Bergen Show, Bob Hope Show, Bell Telephone, Wonderful World of Entertainment, Dinah Shore Show, NBC, CBS specials, Dean Martin Show, Andy Williams Show, Red Skelton Show, Mike Douglas Show.

BERGER, BENJAMIN N.: Executive. b. Poland, Mar. 5, 1896. Pres. Berger Amusement Co.; won decision in Fed. Court against payment to ASCAP for theatre seat tax.

BERGER, HELMUT: Actor. b. Salzburg, 1942. e. Feldkirk College and Univ. of Perugia. First film, small role in Luchino Visconti's The Witches (Le Streghe)in 1966.
PICTURES INCLUDE: The Young Tigers, The Damned, Do You Know What Stalin Did To Women?, The Garden of the Finzi-Continis, Dorian Gray, A Butterfly with Bloody Wings, The Greedy Ones, The Strange Love Affair, Ludwig, Ash Wednesday, Conversation Piece, The Romantic Englishwoman, Orders to Kill, Madame Kitty, Merry-Go-Round, Code Name: Emerald.

BERGER, RICHARD L.: Executive. e. UCLA. In 1964 joined acct. dept., 20th Century-Fox; promoted to exec. position in Fox-TV. Was dir. of programming, then v.p. of programs. Appt. asst. v.p. prod. 20th-Fox. Left in 1975 to join CBS-TV as v.p. dramatic development. Returned to 20th-Fox in 1977 as v.p., domestic prod., 20th Century-Fox Pictures. Joined Warner Bros. Prods.; resigned 1984. Named sr. v.p., United Artists Corp., promoted to pres.

BERGERAC, JACQUES: Actor. b. Biarritz, France. Career includes Five Minutes With Jacques Bergerac on radio; in the theatre, on tour in Once More With Feeling; on most major network TV shows.
PICTURES INCLUDE: Twist of Fate, The Time is Now, Strange Intruder, Come Away With Me, Les Girls, Gigi, Man and His Past, Thunder in the Sun, Hypnotic Eye, A Sunday in Summer, Fear No More, Achiles, A Global Affair, Taffy and the Jungle Hunter, The Emergency Operation, Lady Chaplin, The Last Party, One Plus One.

BERGMAN, ALAN: Songwriter. b. New York City, Sept. 11, 1925. e. Univ. of North Carolina, UCLA. M., Marilyn Bergman with whom collaborates.
PICTURES INCLUDE: In the Heat of the Night, The Thomas Crown Affair, Happy Ending, Gaily, Gaily, Pieces of Dreams, Sometimes a Great Notion, The Way We Were, A Star Is Born, John and Mary, Life and Times of Judge Roy Bean, The One and Only, Same Time Next Year, And Justice for All, The Promise, A Change of Seasons, Yentl.
TELEVISION: Queen of the Stardust Ballroom, Sybil, and themes for Maude, Good Times, Alice, Nancy Walker Show, etc.

BERGMAN, INGMAR: Writer-director. b. Uppsala, Sweden, July 14, 1918. e. Stockhom U. Directed university play prods.; wrote & dir. Death of Punch, 1940; first theatrical success, dir., Macbeth, 1940; writer-director, Svensk Film-industri, 1942-present; first s.p, Frenzy, 1943; first directorial assignment, Crisis, 1946; chief prod., Civic Malmo, 1956–60.
PICTURES INCLUDE: Kris, 1946 Det Regnar Pa Var Karlek, Skepp Till Indialand, Night is My Future, Port of Call, The Devil's Wanton, Three Strange Loves, Till Gladje, Summer Interlude (Illicit Interlude), High Tension, Bris (soap ads), Secrets of Women, Monika, The Naked Light, A Lesson in Love, Dreams, Smiles of a Summer Night, Sista Paret Ut, The Seventh Seal, Wild Strawberries, Brink of Life, The Magician, The Virgin Spring, The Devil's Eye, Through a Glass Darkly, Winter Light, The Silence, All These Women, Persona, Hour of the Wolf, Shame, The Passion of Anna, Cries and Whispers, Scenes from a Marriage, Face to Face, The Serpent's Egg, Autumn Sonata, Life of the Marionettes, Fanny and Alexander, After the Rehearsal.

BERGMAN, MARILYN: Songwriter. b. New York City, Nov. 10, 1929. e. New York Univ. M. Alan Bergman with whom collaborates. See credits under his name.

BERLE, MILTON: Actor. r.n. Milton Berlinger; b. New York City, July 12, 1908; e. Professional Children's Sch., N.Y. in vaudeville; on N.Y. stage (Ziegfeld Follies 1936, Life Begins at 8:40, etc.): night clubs; concurrently on radio & screen.
TV: Star of own NBC show; Texaco Star Theatre,

1948–54, Kraft Music Hall TV Show, 1958–59, Jackpot Bowling, 1960–61, Doyle Against the House, Dick Powell Show, 1961, Chrysler TV special, 1962, The Milton Berle Show, 1966.
PICTURES INCLUDE: Tall, Dark and Handsome, Sun Valley Serenade, Over My Dead Body, Margin for Error, Always Leave Them Laughing, Let's Make Love, It's a Mad Mad Mad World, The Happening, Who's Minding the Mint, Where Angels Go . . . Trouble Follows, Can Hieronymus Merkin Ever Forget Mercy Humppe and Find True Happiness?, Lepke, Broadway Danny Rose.

BERLIN, IRVING: Composer. r.n. Israel Baline. b. Russia, May 11, 1888. To New York, 1893. As youth, singing waiter in N.Y.; early began writing songs. One of first successes, Alexander's Ragtime Band. Entered music pub.; member Waterson, Berlin & Snyder. W.W.I, sgt. inf. U.S. Army. Composer many indiv. and stage musical songs. In 1937 wrote songs for screen prod. Top Hat (RKO); in 1942 prod. stage musical This Is the Army for U.S. Army Fund; in 1943 assoc. with Warner Bros. in prod. film version. Member: Lambs, Friars (N.Y.); pres. Irving Berlin Music Corp., music pub.
PICTURES INCLUDE: Follow the Fleet, On the Avenue, Carefree, Alexander's Ragtime Band, Second Fiddle, Holiday Inn, Blue Skies, Easter Parade, Annie Get Your Gun, Call me Madam, White Christmas, There's No Business Like Show Business.

BERLINGER, WARREN: Actor, b. Brooklyn, N.Y., Aug. 31, 1937. e. Col. Univ.
STAGE: Annie Get Your Gun, The Happy Time, Bernardine, Take A Giant Step, Anniversary Waltz, Roomful of Roses, Blue Denim, Come Blow Your Horn, How To Succeed in Business Without Really Trying, (London) Who's Happy Now?, California Suite, 77–78 tour.
PICTURES INCLUDE: Teenage Rebel, Three Brave Men, Blue Denim, Because They're Young, Platinum High School, The Wackiest Ship in the Army, All Hand on Deck, Billie, Spinout, Thunder Alley, Lepke, The Four Deuces, I Will . . . I Will . . . For Now, Harry and Walter Go to New York, The Shaggy D.A., The Magician of Dublin, The Cannonball Run, The World According to Garp.
TV: Secret Storm (serial), Alcoa, Goodyear, Armstrong, Matinee Theatre, Joey Bishop Show, The London Palladium, Kilroy, Billie, Bracken's World, The Funny Side (NBC 1971–72); Touch of Grace, (ABC-TV 1972–73); The Most Wanted Woman, The Other Woman.

BERMAN, MONTY: producer/cinematographer. b. London, England.
PICTURES INCLUDE: Voice of Merill, Tiger by the Tail, Blood of the Vampire, The Trollenberg Terror, Sea of Sand, Jack The Ripper, Flesh and the Fiends, The Siege of Sidney Street, Hellfire Club, Treasure of Monte Cristo, What a Carve Up.
TV: The Saint, Gideon's Way, The Baron, The Champions, Department S. Randall & Hopkirk (Deceased), Jason King, The Adventurer, Secret of Storm Mountain.

BERMAN, MONTY M.: Film and theatrical costumier. b. London, England, 1912. Personally costumed films and shows since 1931. Squad Leader RAF 1940–45; Bomber Command, M.B.E. Since war has costumed major films and shows and numerous TV prod.
PICTURES INCLUDE: Doctor Zhivago, Tom Jones, Longest Day, My Fair Lady, Oliver, Cromwell, Patton, Fiddler on the Roof, A Bridge Too Far, The Other Side of Midnight, Julia, The Slipper And The Rose, A Little Night Music, Star Wars, Superman, James Bond Films, The Four Musketeers, Mommie Dearest, Raiders of the Lost Ark, Chariots of Fire, Superman II and III, Gandhi, Yentl, The Dresser, Indiana Jones and The Temple of Doom, Cotton Club, Out of Africa.

BERMAN, PANDRO S.: Producer. b. Pittsburgh, Pa. Mar. 28, 1905. Son of late Harry M. Berman, gen. mgr. Universal, FBO. Asst. dir. film ed., FBO; film & title ed. Columbia Studios; chief film ed. RKO, later asst. to William Le Baron & David Selznick; became prod. 1931 (RKO). A Champion of Champions Producers in Fame ratings. Joined MGM 1940.
PICTURES INCLUDE: What Price Hollywood, Symphony of Six Million, Bachelor Mother, The Gay Divorcee, Of Human Bondage, Morning Glory, Roberta, Alice Adams, Top Hat, Winterset, Stage Door, Vivacious Lady, Gunga Din, Hunchback of Notre Dame, Ziegfeld Girl, Honky Tonk, Seventh Cross, National Velvet, Dragon Seed, Portrait of Dorian Grey, Love Affair, Undercurrent, Sea of Grass, Three Musketeers, Madame Bovary, Father of the Bride, Father's Little Dividend, Prisoner of Zenda, Ivanhoe, All the Brothers Were Valiant, Knights of the Round Table, Long, Long Trailer, Blackboard Jungle, Bhowani Junction, Something of Value, Tea and Sympathy, Brothers Karamazov, Reluctant Debutante, Butterfield 8, Sweet Bird of Youth, The Prize, A Patch of Blue, Justine, Move.

BERNARD, JUDD: Writer-producer. b. Chicago, Ill., stage, The World of Carl Sandberg.
PICTURES INCLUDE: Double Trouble, Point Blank, Blue, Fade In, Negatives, The Man Who Had Power Over Women, Deep End, Glad All Over, and Now For Something Completely Different, The Marsailles Contract, Inside Out, The Class of Miss MacMichael, Enter the Ninja, The Playboy Guide to Amsterdam.

BERNARD, MARVIN A.: Executive. b. New York City, Oct. 1, 1934. e. N.Y.U. Associated with Rapid Film Technique, Inc., 1949–63: developed technological advances in film preservation, responsible for public underwriting; 1964–69; real estate sales & investments in Bahamas, then with Tishman Realty (commercial leasing div.); v.p. and operating head of International Film Treat 1970–1973; authored film damaged control chart, a critical analysis of film care and repair—1971; 1973-elected to and for inclusion in 1973–74 edition of Who's Who, because of his expertise in the field of motion picture film rejuvenation; for more than two decades; founded Filmlife Inc. with latest mechanical and technical advancement in field of film rejuvenation 1973–75 bd. chrmn, and chief operating officer of Filmlife Inc., motion picture film rejuvenation company. Feb. 1975 elected President in addition to remaining bd. chairman.

BERNHARD, HARVEY: Producer. b. Seattle, Wash., March 5, 1924. e. Stanford Univ. In real estate in Seattle, 1947–50; started live lounge entertainment at the Last Frontier Hotel, Las Vegas, 1950. Partner with Sandy Howard, 1958–60; v.p. in chg. prod., David L. Wolper Prods., dividing time between TV and feature films, 1961–68; with MPC, v.p., chg. prod., 1968–70. Now pres. of Harvey Bernhard Ent., Inc.
PICTURES INCLUDE: The Mack (1973), The Omen (1976), Damien—Omen II (1978), The Final Conflict (1981), The Beast Within (1981), Ladyhawke (exec. prod., 1984), Goonies (prod., 1985), Lost Boys (1986).

BERNSTEIN, Baron cr 1969 (Life Peer) of Leigh; Sidney Lewis Bernstein LLd; Chairman; Granada Group PLC from 1934–79. Pres. since 1979. (Granada Television, Granada Theatres, Granada TV Rental, Granada Motorway Services, Novello & Co). b. 30 Jan. 1899. A founder, Film Society, 1924. Films Adviser, Min. of Inf. 1940–45; Liason, British Embassy, Washington 1942; Chief, Film Section SHAEF 1943–45. Lecturer on Film and International Affairs, New York Univ. and Yale. Governor, Sevenoaks School. Member, Resources for Learning Committee, Nuffield Foundation, Member: Jerusalem Committee. Address: 36 Golden Square, London, W1.

BERNSTEIN, BOB: Executive. Began public relations career 1952 at DuMont TV Network, followed by 2 yrs. as press agent for Liberace. With Billboard Magazine as review editor 3 yrs. Joined Westinghouse Bdg. Co. as p.r. director 1959. In 1963 named p.r. director for Triangle Publications, serving in various capacities to 1971. Joined Viacom Intl. as director of information services. In 1975 formed own co., March Five Inc., p.r. and promotion firm.

BERNSTEIN, ELMER: Composer-conductor. b. New York, N.Y. Apr. 4, 1922. Scholarship, Juilliard. e. Walden School, New York U., U.S Army Air Force radio unit. After war 3 yrs. recitals, musical shows, United Nations radio dept; pres., Young Musicians Found.; 1st v.p. Academy of Motion Picture Arts & Sciences; co-chairman music branch. Music dir. Valley Symphony. Recording: United Artists. More than 90 major films. Pres. of Composers & Lyricists Guild of America past 5 years.
PICTURES INCLUDE: The Ten Commandments. Man With the Golden Arm, The Great Escape, To Kill a Mockingbird (received ten Academy Award nominations and Oscar, 1967), The Carpetbaggers, The Magnificent Seven, Birdman of Alcatraz, Walk on the Wild Side, Hallelujah Trail, The Reward, Seven Women, Cast A Giant Shadow, Hawaii, Thoroughly Modern Millie, True Grit, Cahill, U.S. Marshall, McQ., Gold, The Trial of Billy Jack, Report to the Commissioner, From Noon Till Three, Sarah, The Shootist, Bloodbrothers, Meatballs, Airplane!, Going Ape, The Chosen, Five Days One Summer, Airplane II: The Sequel, Spacehunter, Spies Like Us, Legal Eagles, Three Amigos.
TV: Hollywood: The Golden Years (special), The Race for Space; Parts I & II (special), D-Day (special), The Making of the President—1960 (special), won Emmy Award), Hollywood and the Stars (special), Voyage of the Brigantine Yankee (special), Crucification of Jesus (special), Julia series, Owen Marshall series, Ellery Queen series, Serpico series, Gulag.

BERNSTEIN, JACK B.: Producer. b. New York City May 6, 1937. e. Univ. of City of NY (BA, sociology). U.S. Army-Europe, 1956–58; research bacteriologist, 1959–61. Entered industry in 1962 with S.I.B. Prods., Paramount, as v.p. & gen. mgr.; 1964–66, v.p. & gen. mgr. C.P.I. Prods, 1966–73 prod. mgr. & asst. dir., free lance. 1973–1982,

assoc. prod. & exec. prod. at several studios. 1983–86, v.p. worldwide prod., Walt Disney Pictures. Member: DGA, Friars, Academy of MP Arts & Sciences; Academy of TV Arts & Sciences.
PICTURES: Assoc. Prod.: The Other Side of Midnight, The Fury, Butch & Sundance, The Early Days, Six Pack, Unfaithfully Yours. Exec. Prod.: North Dallas Forty, Monsignore, The Beast Within. Co-producer: Wildfire

BERNSTEIN, JAY: Producer—Personal Manager. b. Oklahoma City, OK, June 7, 1937. e. Pomona Coll. 1963–76, pres. of Jay Berstein Public Relations, representing over 600 clients, including William Holden, Sammy Davis, Jr., Sally Field, Burt Lancaster, James Caan, Faye Dunaway, George Burns, Milton Berle, Virginia Mayo, Jayne Mansfield, Richard Pryor, Claire Trevor, O.J. Simpson, George Segal, Dionne Warwick, etc. Formed Jay Berstein Enterprises, acting as personal manager for Farrah Fawcett, Suzanne Somers, Kristy McNichol, Susan Hayward, Donald Sutherland, Bruce Boxleitner, Robert Conrad, Susan Saint James, Robert Blake, William Shatner, Linda Evans, Cicely Tyson, etc. Past pres., Bernstein-Thompson Entertainment Complex, entertainment and personal mgt. firm.
PICTURES: Executive producer of Sunburn, Nothing Personal.
TELEVISION: Executive producer for movies, The Return of Mike Hammer, Mickey Spillane's Margin for Murder; Wild, Wild, West, Revisted; More Wild, Wild West. Murder Me, Murder You, More Than Murder. Series: Bring 'Em Back Alive, Mike Hammer, Houston Knights (series).

BERNSTEIN, WALTER: Director-Writer. b. New York City. e. Dartmouth, Wrote for New Yorker Magazine; in World War II was roving correspondent for Yank Magazine. Returned to New Yorker after war. Wrote TV scripts; published book Keep Your Head Down (collection of articles).
PICTURES INCLUDE: Writer: The Molly McGuires, The Money Trap, Fail Safe, Paris Blues, Heller in Pink Tights, Semi-Tough, The Front, An Almost Perfect Affair, Yanks, Little Miss Marker. Director: Little Miss Marker (debut).

BERRY, JOHN: Director. b. N.Y.C., 1917. Directed films in Hollywood mid and late '40s; went abroad during McCarthy era in U.S. where worked in French film industry. Later went to London to do stage work, acting as well as directing. Returned to U.S. to do stage work; returned to Hollywood to do TV.
PICTURES INCLUDE: Cross My Heart, From This Day Forward, Miss Susie Slagle's, Casbah, Tension, He Ran All the Way, Ca Va Barder, The Great Lover, Je Suis un Sentimental, Tamango, On Que Mambo, Maya, Thieves.
TV: One Drink at a Time, Farewell Party, Mr. Broadway, etc.

BERRY, KEN: Actor. b. Moline, IL, Nov. 3.
PICTURES INCLUDE: Two for the Seesaw, Hello Down There, Herbie Rides Again, The Cat from Outer Space.
TELEVISION: The Reluctant Heroes, Wake Me When the War Is Over, Ken Berry Show, Mayberry RFD, F. Troop, Mama's Family.

BERTINELLI, VALERIE: Actress. b. Wilmington, Del., April 23, 1960. Dramatic training at Tami Lynn Academy of Artists in California. Made early TV appearances in the series, Apple's Way, in commercials, and in public service announcements. Recently started own production company to acquire properties for self.
TELEVISION: Movies: Young Love. First Love, The Promise of Love, The Princess and the Cabbie, I Was a Mail Order Bride, The Seduction of Gina, Shattered Vows, Rockabye, Silent Witness. Specials: The Secret of Charles Dickens, The Magic of David Cooperfield, etc. Series: One Day at a Time.
PICTURE: Number One with a Bullet.

BERTOLUCCI, BERNARDO: Director-Writer, b. Parma, Italy, March 16, 1941. e. Rome University. Son of Attilio Bertolucci poet and film critic. First worked in films at age of 20 as asst. dir. to Pier Paolo Pasolini on latter's first film Accattone: in 1962 made debut film, The Grim Reaper, from script by Pasolini.
PICTURES INCLUDE: Before the Revolution, Partner, Love and Rage (one episode: Agony). The Spider's Strategem, 1900, Luna, Tragedy of a Ridiculous Man.

BESMAN, MICHAEL: Executive. e. U.C.L.A. (BA in film studies). Gained first experience in m.p. industry as asst. to director Michael Wadleigh during post-production work on Wolfen. Served as asst. to prod. Aaron Russo in developing new projects, including Trading Places. 1983, joined Paramount Pictures as researcher for story dept. Named creative exec. with studio prod. dept. 1985, promoted to exec. dir., production, for Paramount M.P. Group.

BEST, BARBARA: Publicist. b. San Diego, Calif., Dec. 2, 1921. e. U.S.C., A.B., 1943. Pub., 20th Century-Fox, 1943–49; reporter, San Diego Journal, 1950 Stanley Kramer Co. 1950–53; own agency, Barbara Best & Associates, 1953–66; 1966 exec. v.p. Jay Bernstein Public rel.; Freeman and Best, 1967–74; Barbara Best Inc. personal management, current.

BEST, JAMES: Actor. b. Corydon, Ind., July 26, 1926. Magazine model; on stage; in European roadshow cast of "My Sister Eileen"; served as M.P. with U.S.A.A.F., World War II; m.p. debut in Comanche Territory, 1949.
PICTURES INCLUDE: Winchester 73, Air Cadet, Cimarron Kid, Steel Town, Ma & Pa Kettle At the Fair, Francis Goes to West Point, Seminole, The President's Lady, City of Bad Men, Column South, Riders to the Stars, The Raid, Caine Mutiny, Return from the Sea, The Left-Handed Gun, They Rode West, Seven Angry Men, Come Next Spring, Baby, The Rack, Sounder, Ode to Billy Joe, The End, Hooper, Rolling Thunder.

BETHUNE, ZINA: Actress, dancer, singer. B. New York, 1950. B'way: Most Happy Fella, Nutcracker. New York City Ballet (Balanchine), Zina Bethune & Company Dance Theatre, The Bethune Ballet.
PICTURES: Sunrise At Campobello, Who's That Knocking At My Door. National Tours: Sweet Charity, Carnival, Oklahoma, Damn Yankees, Member of the Wedding, The Owl & The Pussycat.
TV: The Nurses, Lancer, Cains Hundred, Naked City, Route 66, Little Women, Judy Garland Show, Jackie Gleason Show, Gunsmoke, Dr. Kildare, Emergency, Planet of The Apes, Police Story, Chips, Hardy Boys, The Gymnast.

BETTGER, LYLE: Actor b. Philadelphia, Pa., Feb. 13, 1915; m. Mary Rolfe, actress; e. Haverford School, Phila., Amer. Acad. Dramatic Art, N.Y.C. Started in summer stock; in road cos. of Brother Rat, Man Who Came to Dinner.
STAGE: John Loves Mary, Love Life, Eve of St. Mark.
PICTURES INCLUDE: No Man of Her Own, Union Station, First Legion, Greatest Show on Earth, Sea Chase, Gunfight at OK Corral, Johnny Reno, Nevada Smith, Return of The Gunfighter, The Hawaiians, Carnival Story, The Seven Minutes.
TV: Court of Last Resort, Grand Jury, Hawaii 5-0, Police Story.

BEVILLE, HUGH M., Jr.: Executive; b. April 18, 1908; e. Syracuse U. and NYU (MBA); to NBC 1930 statistician, Chief Statistician; Research mgr., dir., research; U.S. Army 1942–46; dir. of research and planning for NBC, v.p., planning and research, 1956; v.p., Planning, 1964; Consultant, 1968; Professor Business Admin., Southampton College, 1968. Exec. dir., Broadcast Rating Council, 1971–82, author-consultant, contributing editor, TV/Radio Age, 1982–85. Columnist, Electronic Media; author, Audience Ratings; Radio, Television, Cable, 1985.

BEY, TURHAN: Actor. b. Vienna, Austria, March 30. Made U.S. m.p. debut in 1941.
PICTURES INCLUDE: Footsteps in the Dark, Burma Convoy, Bombay Clipper, Drums of the Congo, Destination Unknown, White Savage, Dragon Seed, Arabian Nights, Bowery to Broadway, Night in Paradise, Out of the Blue, Amazing Mr. X, Parole, Inc., Adventures of Casanova, Song of India, Prisoners of the Casbah, Stolen Indentity.

BEYMER, RICHARD: Actor, r.n. George Richard Beymer, Jr., b. Avoca, Iowa, Feb. 21, 1939, e. N. Hollywood H.S., Actors Studio. Performer, KTLA, Sandy Dreams, Fantastic Studios, Inc., 1949, Playhouse 90.
PICTURES INCLUDE: Indiscretion of an American Wife, So Big, Johnny Tremaine, The Dairy of Anne Frank, High Time, West Side Story, Bachelor Flat, Five Finger Exercise, Hemingway's Adventures of a Young Man, The Longest Day, The Stripper, Cross Country.

BIBAS, FRANK PERCY: Executive. b. New York City, 1917; e. Brown & Columbia Universities; Capt., Army Air Corps, World War II. Entered m.p. ind. adv. dept., Donahue & Coe; later pub. dept. American Display, thence to dist. dept., National Screen Service. In 1945 joined Casanave-Artlee Pictures Inc.; apptd. vice-pres. in charge of sales 1946 (dist. Selznick reissues in U.S.); vice-pres. Casanave Pictures, Inc. & Sixteen M.M. Pictures Inc., from 1949 mgr. m.p. dept., McCann-Erickson ad agency; joined Roland Reed TV Inc., v.p., prod., 1955. Prod-dir. with Hal Roach Studios, 1957. 1961 to present N.Y.C. partner, Bibas-Redford Inc. Production Co. 1962 won Academy Award for "Project Hope," documentary. Member: S.M.P.T.E., Acad. of TV Arts and Sciences, Directors Guild of America.

BICK, JERRY: Producer. b. New York City. e. Columbia Univ., Sorbonne. m. actress Louise Fletcher. Taught English at Univ. of Ga. and was radio sports announcer in Savannah, Ga., before entering firm industry in pub. dept. of MGM, N.Y. Opened own literary agency in Hollywood representing film, TV writers. Began career as producer in London; debut film, Michael Kohlhaas (1969), made in Czechoslovakia.
PICTURES INCLUDE: The Long Goodbye, Thieves Like

Us, Russian Roulette, Farewell My Lovely, The Big Sleep, Against; All Odds (exec.), Swing Shift.

BIEHN, MICHAEL: Actor. b. Nebraska, 1957. At 18 years moved to Los Angeles and studied acting. First professional job in 1977 in TV pilot for Logan's Run.
PICTURES INCLUDE: Coach, Hog Wild, The Fan, The Lords of Discipline, The Terminator, Aliens.
TELEVISION: Pilots for James at Fifteen and The Runaways; several movies-of-the-week, ABC Afternoon Specials. Series: Police Story, Family. Movies: China Rose, Deadly Intentions.

BIEN, WALTER H.: Producer. b. San Francisco, April 16, 1923; e. UCLA, 1944. Entered m.p. ind. as film editor, MGM, 1943, Monogram, 1946; Eagle Lion, 1948; formed TV production company 1950, prod. live shows in L.A. area; Universal TV comm. dept., 1954; Warner Bros., to start comm. & ind. div., 1956; exec. prod. in chg. TV comm.& ind. films div., prod. Bell System Science Series; pres., SIB Productions, Inc., SIB-Tower 12.

BILBY, KENNETH W.: Executive. b. Salt Lake City, Utah, Oct. 7, 1918. e. Columbia U., U. of Ariz., B.A. With N.Y. Herald-Tribune, 47–50; author, New Star in the Near East, 1950; pub. rel. rep. to RCA Victor, Camden, New Jersey, 1950–54; exec. v.p. National Broadcasting Co., N.Y., 1954–60; v.p. public affairs, RCA, 1960–62, exec. v.p., 1962–75; exec. v.p. corporate affairs, 1976–present.

BILIMORIA, N. M.: Distributor. b. Oct. 7, 1922, Partner in M. B. Bilimoria & Son, Bombay; dir. Dominion Films (P) Ltd. Bombay; Modern Films Private Ltd., Bombay; Partner, Bilimoria & Lalji, Calcutta; Distrbutors Combine, Bombay; Bilimoria & Chhotubhai, Delhi; Moti Talkies, Delhi; Agent: Union Carbide India Ltd., Calcutta and Union Carbide International Co., N.Y.

BILL, TONY: Actor-Producer. b. San Diego, Ca. e. Notre Dame. Began career in films in 1963 acting in Come Blow Your Horn. In 1971 founded Bill/Phillips Prods. with Julia and Michael Phillips. Left in 1973 to be independent.
PICTURES INCLUDE: Actor: You're a Big Boy Now, Castle Keep, Shampoo, Heartbeat. Co-producer: Deadhead Miles, Steelyard Blues, The Sting. Prod.: Hearts of the West, Harry and Walter Go to New York, Boulevard Nights (exec. prod.); Going in Style (co-prod.). Director: My Bodyguard, Six Weeks.

BILLITTERI, SALVATORE: Executive. b. Belleville, N.J., March 21, 1921. e. Fordham U.: U.S. Air Force, 1943–45; ent. m.p. ind., doorman in N.Y. theatre, 1939; theatre mgr., 1947; film slsman, Casolaro Film Distributing Co., 1947–51; co-owner many foreign films; film editor, I.F.E., 1951; head of editing, prod. dept., Titra Sound Corp., 1956; head of east coast production, American International Pictures, 1961; dir. Post Prod., 1970; named v.p. 1974, sr. v.p. of Filmways Pictures, 1980; sr. v.p., post production, Orion Pictures Dist. Corp., 1982.

BINNS, EDWARD: Actor. b. Penn. Broadway debut in Command Decision, 1947. Has since appeared in TV, theatre, m.p. and commercial voice-overs.
PICTURES INCLUDE: Fail-Safe, Twelve Angry Men, Compulsion, Patton, The Americanization of Emily, Judgment at Nuremburg, Lovin' Molly, Night Moves, Oliver's Story.
TV: Kraft Theatre, Studio One, Danger, Brenner (series), The Defenders, The Nurses, It Takes a Thief (series).
STAGE: Detective Story, Caligula, The Caine Mutiny Court Martial, A Touch of the Poet.

BIONDI, JR. FRANK J.: Executive. b. 1945. President of Home Box Office, then chm. & chief exec. off. Resigned 1984 to join Coca-Cola Co. as exec. v.p., entertainment business arm.

BIRCH, WILLIAM: Cinematographer. b. Chicago, Ill., Mar. 1, 1918. Asst., Movietonews, 1937–40; army signal corp, 1940–44; head of midwestern bureau, did camera, NBC News & Document.; established own service; estab. William Birch & Assoc. Inc.
Won two Emmys, cameraman of the yr., Nat. Headliners Award.

BIRMINGHAM, PAUL A.: Executive. b. Burbank, Calif., Feb. 12, 1937. e. University of Calif., Univ. of South. Calif.; sr., v.p. studio operations and admin., Paramount Pictures.

BIRNEY, DAVID: Actor. b. Washington, D.C., April 23, 1940. e. Dartmouth, UCLA. m. actress Meredith Baxter Birney. Following college and the Army went to N.Y. where appeared in Lincoln Center prod. of Summertree. Appeared for two yrs. on TV daytime series, Love is a Many Splendored Thing, doing other stage roles in same period.
PICTURES INCLUDE: Trial by Combat, Oh, God, Book II.
TV: Bridget Loves Bernie (series), Police Story (segments), The Adams Chronicles, Serpico (series), Master of the Game.

BIROC, JOSEPH F.: Cinematographer. b. New York, N.Y., Feb. 12, 1903. e. Emerson H.S., Union City N.J.
PICTURES INCLUDE: Bwana Devil, Glass Wall, Tall Texan, Vice Squad, Donovan's Brain, Appointment in Honduras, Down Three Dark Streets, Lone Wolf, T-Men in Action, Man Behind the Badge, Dear Phoebe, Nightmare, Tension at Table Rock, Attack, Black Whip, Run of the Arrow, Ride Back, Garment Jungle, China Gate, Ice Palace, FBI Story, 13 Ghosts, Home Before Dark, Operation Eichmann, Devil at 4 O'clock, Gold of the Seven Saints, Reprieve, Opium Eaters, Hitler, Sail a Crooked Ship, Bye Bye Birdie, Toys in the Attic, Promises-Promises, Under the Yum-Yum Tree, Viva Las Vegas, Kitten With a Whip, Ride the Wild Surf, Renegade Posse, Gunfight at Commanche Pass, Hush . . . Hush Sweet Charlotte, I Saw What You Did, Flight of the Phoenix, The Russians are Coming, The Russians are Coming, The Swinger, Warning Shot, Enter Laughing, Who is Minding the Mint, Garden of Cucumbers, The Killing of Sister George, What Ever Happened to Aunt Alice?, Too Late the Hero, Mrs. Polifax Spy, Excape from the Planet of the Apes, The Organization, The Grissom Gang, Cahill, U.S. Marshall, The Longest Yard, The Towering Inferno, Hustle, The Duchess And The Dirtwater Fox, The Choirboys, Beyond the Poseidon Adventure, Airplane!, Hammet, All the Marbles.
TV: Four Star Theatre, Readers Digest, Superman, Richard Diamond, Alcoa Theatre, Grindl, Solo, Ghost Breakers, Take Her She's Mine, Heaven Help Us, Hardy Boys, Brian's Song, Gidget Gets Married, Ghost Story, Thursdays Game, Lonely Hearts "555," Family Upside Down, S.S.T. Death Flight, Little Women, Scruples, The Gambler, A Death in California, A Winner Never Quits, Outrage.
TV PILOTS: Wonder Woman, Honky Tonk, The Moneychangers, Washington, D.C., Clone Master, Desperate Lives, Casablanca, Another Jerk, House Detective, Hell Town U.S.A., Flag

BISHOP, JULIE: Actress. b. Denver, Colo., Aug. 30, 1917. e. Westlake, Kenwood, Schools for Girls (Former screen name Jacqueline Wells); m.p. debut 1941.
PICTURES INCLUDE: Nurse's Secret, International Squadron, Steel Against the Sky, Lady Gangster, Busses Roar, Cinderella Jones, Murder in the Music Hall, Idea Girl, Strange Conquest, Last of the Redmen, High Tide, Deputy Marshal, Threat, Sands of Iwo Jima, Westward the Women, Sabre Jet, High and the Mighty, Headline Hunters.

BISSET, JACQUELINE: Actress. b. Weybridge, England, September 13, 1944. e. French Lyee, London. After photographic modeling made film debut in The Knack.
PICTURES INCLUDE: Two For The Road, The Sweet Ride, The Detective, Bullitt, The First Time, Airport, The Grasshopper, The Mephisto Waltz, Believe in Me, Stand Up and Be Counted, The Thief Who Came to Dinner, Murder on the Orient Express, End of the Game, The Spiral Staircase, St. Ives, Sunday Woman, The Deep, The Greek Tycoon, Who Is Killing the Great Chefs of Europe?, When Time Ran Out, Rich and Famous, Inchon, Class, Under the Volcano.
TELEVISION: Choices.

BIXBY, BILL: Actor. b. San Francisco, Calif., Jan. 22, 1934. e. Univ. of Calif., Berkeley. Worked in indust. films. Gen. Motors, Chrysler.
TV: Dobie Gillis, Danny Thomas Show, Joey Bishop Show, Andy Griffith Show, My Favorite Martian, Eddie's Father, The Hulk, Goodbye Beantown, International Airport.
STAGE: Fantasticks (nat'l company), Under the Yum Yum Tree.
PICTURES INCLUDE: Lonely Are the Brave, Irma La Douce, Yum Yum Tree, Ride Beyond Vengeance, This Way Out Please.

BLACK, ALEXANDER F.: Publicist. b. New Rochelle, N.Y., Dec. 27, 1918. B.A. Brown U., 1940. Joined Universal 1941. U.S. Navy 1942–45, Lt. Sr. Grade. Rejoined Universal 1946 serving in various capacities in Foreign Department, becoming Director of Foreign Publicity for Universal International Films, Inc. in 1967; 1974, named exec. in chg. intl. promotion for MCA-TV.

BLACK, KAREN: Actress. b. Park Ridge, Ill., 1943. e. Northwestern Univ. Left school for New York to join the Hecscher House, where she appeared in several Shakespearean plays. In 1965 starred in Playroom, which ran only 1 mth. but won her a nom. as best actress of season by N.Y. drama critics. Made m.p. debut in 1966 in You're a Big Boy Now.
PICTURES INCLUDE: Easy Rider, Five Easy Pieces, Drive, He Said, A Gunfight, Born To Win, Portnoy's Complaint, The Pyx, Rhinoceros, The Outfit, The Great Gatsby, Airport 1975, Law and Disorder, Day of the Locust, Nashville, Family Plot, Crime and Passion, Burnt Offerings, Capricorn One, Because He's My Friend, In Praise of Older Women, The Rip-off, Greed, Danny Travis, Chanel Solitaire, Come Back to the Five and Dime, Jinmie Dean, Jinmie Dean,

Growing Pains, Martin's Day, Cut and Run, Invaders from Mars.
STAGE: Happily Never After, Keep It in the Family.

BLACK, STANLEY: Composer, conductor, musical director. Resident Conductor, BBC, 1944–52. Musical Director 105 feature films and Pathe Newsreel music: Music dir. Associated British Film Studios 1958–64. Guest Conductor Royal Philharmonic Orchestra and London Symphony. Orchestra; many overseas conducting engagements including (1977) Boston Pops and Winnipeg Symphony. Associated Conductor Osaka Philharmonic Orchestra. Exclusive recording contract with Decca Record Co. since 1944.
PICTURES INCLUDE: Crossplot, The Long, The Short and The Tall, Rattle of a Simple Man, The Young Ones, Hell is a City, Top Secret, etc., 1977 Valentino.

BLACK, THEODORE R.: Attorney, b. New Jersey, Aug. 11, 1906; e. Harvard, B.A. 1927, LL.B., 1930 (Sigman Alpha Mu Frat.). Formerly General Counsel, bd. member, Republic Pictures Corp. Member: Nat'l Panel of Arbitrators, American Arbit. Assn., Bd. N.Y. Ethical Culture Society.

BLACKMAN, HONOR: Actress. b. London, Eng. Stage debut. The Gleam 1946. Screen debut, Fame Is the Spur.
TV: African Patrol, The Witness, Four Just Men, Probation Officer series, Top Secret, Ghost Squad, Invisible Man, The Saint, The Avengers series.
PICTURES INCLUDE: Quartet, Daughter of Darkness, A Boy A Girl and a Bike, Diamond City, Conspirator, So Long at the Fair, Set a Murderer, Green Grow the Rushes, Come Die My Love, Rainbow Jacket, Outsiders, Delavine Affair, Three Musketeers, Breakaway, Homecoming, Suspended Alibi, Dangerous Drugs, A Night to Remember, The Square Peg, A Matter of Who, Present Laughter, The Recount, Serena, Jason & The Golden Fleece, Goldfinger, The Secret of My Success, Moment to Moment, Life at the Top, A Twist of Sand, Shalako, Struggle for Rome, Twinky, The Last Grenade, The Virgin and the Gypsy, Fright, Something Big, Out Damned Spot, Ragtime, Summer, Cat and the Canary.

BLAINE, VIVIAN: Actress. r.n. Vivian S. Stapleton. b. Newark, N.J., Nov. 21, 1924; e. South Side H.S., Newark. Singer with various bands in New Jersey 1937–39, thereafter night clubs; 20th-Fox contract 1942. Personal appearance on Great Britain stage from 1947; co-starred Guys and Dolls N.Y. stage and London stage; Hatful of Rain, N.Y. stage; Guys and Dolls film 1955.
Member: Academy of M.P. Arts & Sciences, A.F.R.A., Equity, S.A.G., A.G.V.A.
PICTURES INCLUDE: He Married His Boss, Thru Different Eyes, Greenwich Village, Something for the Boys, Nob Hill, State Fair, Three Little Girls in Blue, If I'm Lucky, Skirts Ahoy, Public Pigeon No. 1.

BLAIR, BETSY: Actress. r.n. Betsy Boger. b. New York, N.Y., Dec. 11.
BROADWAY: Beautiful People, Richard II, actress in little theatre groups.
PICTURES INCLUDE: Another Part of the Forest, Kind Lady, Othello, Marty, Halliday Brand, A Delicate Balance.
TV: Appearances on U.S. Steel Hour, Ford Theatre, Philco, Kraft.

BLAIR, JANET: Actress. b. Blair, Pa., April 23, 1921. With Hal Kemp's Orchestra; on tour South Pacific play, 1950–52.
PICTURES INCLUDE: Three Girls About Town, Blondie Goes to College, Two Yanks in Trinidad, Burn Witch Burn, Broadway, My Sister Eileen, Something to Shout About, Once Upon a Time, Tars and Spars, Gallant Journey, Fabulous Dorseys, I Love Trouble, Black Arrow, Fuller Brush Man, Public Pigeon No. 1, Boys Night Out, The One and Only, Genuine, Original Family Band.

BLAIR, LARRY: Actor. r.n. Larry Bess. b. Newark, N.J., June 27, 1935; f. Herman Bess, NYC radio executive. e. public and private schools, Newark and Asbury Park, N.J. Began in showbusiness, age 13 as D.J. and actor in NYC; 1954–55, production assistant, WABC-TV, NYC; 1955–62, associate director and director, WNEW-TV, NYC; 1962–71, D.J., newscaster with WFIL, Phila., WTIC (Hartford), WHN, WMCA, NYC. 1971 to present, commercial spokesman, narrator and actor.

BLAIR, LINDA: Actress. b. St. Louis, Jan. 22, 1959. Model and actress on TV commercials before going into films.
PICTURES: The Sporting Club, The Way We Live Now, The Exorcist, Airport '75, Sweet Hostage, Exorcist II: The Heretic, Hell Night, Chained Heat, Night Patrol, Savage Streets, Savage Island.
TELEVISION: Born Innocent, Sarah T.—Portrait of a Teenage Alcoholic, Victory at Entebbe.

BLAKE, AMANDA: Actress. r.n. Beverly Louise Neill; b. Buffalo, N.Y., Feb. 20, 1931. Telephone operator; in m.p. 1950.
PICTURES INCLUDE: Battleground, Stars in My Crown, Counterspy Meets Scotland Yard, Scarlet Angel, Cattle Town, Lili, Sabre Jet, Miss Robin Crusoe, About Mrs. Leslie, Adventures of Hajji Baba, Star Is Born, Glass Slipper, High Society.
TV: Double Exposure; Schlitz Playhouse, General Electric Theater, Four Star Playhouse, Cavalcade of America, Lux Video Playhouse, My Favorite Husband, Professional Father, The Red Skelton Show, Climax, Gunsmoke.

BLAKE, DAVID M.: Producers' Representative. b. Trincomalee, Ceylon, April 19, 1948. Ent. m.p. ind. 1968 British Lion Films, London. Lion Int'l. Films, O'Seas Division. Appointed 1970 U.S. representative. New York. British Lion Films, Shepperton Studios, Lion TV.

BLAKE, ROBERT: Actor. b. Nutley, N.J., Sept. 18, 1933. m. actress Sondra Kerry. Started as Hollywood stunt man in Rumble on the Docks and The Tijuana Story. First acting job was in the Gallery Theater in Hatful of Rain.
PICTURES INCLUDE: Town Without Pity, Pt-109, The Greatest Story Ever Told, The Connection, This Property is Condemned, In Cold Blood, Tell Them Willie Boy is Here, Corky, Electra-Glide in Blue, Busting, Second Hand Hearts, Coast to Coast.
TV: Baretta, Blood Feud, Hell Town (also s.p.).

BLAKELY, SUSAN: Actress. b. Germany, where father was stationed in Army. Studied at Univ. of Texas. m. writer Todd Merer. Became top magazine and TV commercial model in N.Y. Film acting debut in Savages.
PICTURES INCLUDE: The Lords of Flatbush, The Way We Were, The Towering Inferno, Report to the Commissioner, Shampoo, Capone, The Concorde—Airport '79.
TELEVISION: Rich Man, Poor Man. Movies: Secrets, The Heart of a Champion, International Airport, Blood & Orchids, The Annihilator.

BLANC, MEL: Executive, voice specialist. r.n. Melvin Jerome Blanc. b. San Francisco, Calif., May 30, 1908. e. Lincoln H.S., Portland, Ore., 1918–21. musician, NBC Radio, San Francisco, 1928; orchestra conductor, Orpheum theatre, Portland, Ore., 1931; free lance, violin, tuba, bass player, 1925–30; voices on Warner Bros. Cartoons, Bugs Bunny, Porky Pig, Daffy Duck, etc. since 1937; running characters, Jack Benny Show, Radio & TV since 1940.
In radio: Point Sublime, 1942–44; Judy Canova Show, 1940–48; Burns and Allen; Jack Carson Show; Abbott and Costello; Dagwood and Blondie; Al Pierce Show, 1938–50; Chairman of the Board, Blanc Communications Corp., 1960–63.
TV: The Bugs Bunny Show, The Porky Pig Show, The Munsters, Flintstones, Speed Buggy Animated Show (Hanna Barbera).

BLANCO, RICHARD M.: Executive, b. Brooklyn, N.Y., e. electrical engineering, Wentworth Institute. J.C., 1925–27; bus. admin., Univ. of Calif., 1939–40; U.S. Govt. College, 1942. Superv. Technicolor Corp., 1931–56; organ. and oper. Consumer Products, Kodachrome film process., Technicolor, 1956–62; dir. of MP Govt. and theatr. sales, N.Y. and Washington, D.C. 1963–65; gen. mgr. of Technicolor Florida photo. operations at Kennedy Space Center., prod. document and educ. films for NASA, 1965; VP of TV division, Technicolor Corp. of America; 1967 elected corporate v.p. Technicolor, Inc.; 1971 pres., Technicolor Graphic Services, Inc.; 1974, elected chm. of bd. of Technicolor Graphic Services; 1977, elected to board of directors of Technicolor Inc.

BLANE, RALPH: Composer. b. Broken Arrow, Okla., July 26, 1914. e. Northwestern U. Started as singer, then vocal arranger for Broadway shows; appeared on NBC radio. Formed partnership with Hugh Martin, wrote Best Foot Forward; m.p. composer since 1939.
PICTURES INCLUDE: Best Foot Forward, Meet Me in St. Louis, My Dream Is Yours, One Sunday Afternoon, My Blue Heaven, Friendly Island, Skirts Ahoy, French Line, Athena, Girl Rush, The Girl Most Likely, Who is Sylvia?, Ziegfeld Follies, Broadway Rhythm, Abbott and Costello in Hollywood, Easy to Wed.
TV: The Great Quillow. 1961; same in color for NBC, 1963.
BROADWAY: Three Wishes for Janie, Tattered Tom, Something About Anne, Don't Flash Tonight.

BLANK, MYRON: Circuit executive. b. Des Moines, Ia. Aug. 30, 1911; son of A.H. Blank, circuit operator; e. U. Mich. On leaving coll. joined father in operatin Tri-States and Central States circuits. On leave 1943–46 in U.S. Navy, officer in charge visual educ. Now pres. Central States Theatre Corp.; pres. TOA, 1955; chmn. bd. TOA Inc. 1956–57; exec. chm. of NATO. Pres. of Greater Des Moines Comm.; treas., Iowa Methodist Medical Center; board, Iowa Des Moines Natl. Bank.; pres., Iowa Phoenix Corp., recipient of Brotherhood Award of National Conference of Christians & Jews; board, Simpson College; chm., Blank Park Zoo.

BLATTNER, GERRY: Producer. b. Liverpool, 1913. Ent. industry 1928. Blattner Studios, Boreham Wood. Studies include

Berlin Research Labs, 1930. Studio mgr., British National Studios, 1936. Gen. mgr., British Lion Studios, Isleworth and Shepperton studios. Joined board of Warner Bros. First National Prods., 1946–67. Was exec. in charge of Warner Bros. European Prods. Started own indep. prod. co. in Nov. 1967.
PICTURES INCLUDE: The Crimson Pirate, Helen of Troy, The Nun's Story, Indiscreet, The Sundowners.

BLATTNER, ROBERT: Executive. b. Dover, DE, March 5, 1952. e. Harvard Coll. (BA, 1974); Harvard Bsn. Schl. (MBA, 1976). 1980–81, dir. sls., Columbia Pictures Home Entertainment; 1981–82, promoted to v.p. & gen. mgr.; 1982–83, v.p., gen. mgr., RCA/Columbia Pictures Home Video; named pres., 1983.

BLATTY, WILLIAM PETER: Writer-Producer. Novelist who wrote John Goldfarb, Please Come Home (filmed) and Twinkle, Twinkle, Killer Kane before biggest success with The Exorcist, which became a 55-week best-selling book. He wrote s.p. and functioned as prod. on film version.
PICTURES INCLUDE: A Shot in the Dark (s.p.), What Did You Do in the War, Daddy? (s.p), The Great Bank Robbery, Darling Lilli (co. s.p.), The Exorcist (s.p., prod.), The Ninth Configuration (s.p., prod. dir.).

BLAU, MARTIN: Executive. b. N.Y.C., June 6, 1924. e. Ohio U., 1948. Employed on newspapers in Ohio, Tex., W. Va., Pub. dept., Columbia Pictures, 1951; asst. pub. mgr. 1959; pub. mgr., Columbia Internat'l, 1961; admin. asst. to v.p. of adv. & pub. Columbia Pictures, 1966. Dir. adv. and publicity, Columbia Pictures International, 1970; v.p., 1971; sr. v.p., 1985.

BLAUSTEIN, JULIAN: Producer. b. New York City, May 30, 1913. e. Harvard 1933. Ent. m.p. ind. as reader for Universal 1935; asst. story ed. 1935–36; story ed. 1936–38; in chg. story dept. Music Corp. of America 1938–39; story ed. Paramount 1939–41; Signal Corps Photo. Center 1941–46; edit. supervisor of Selznick 1946–48; to 20th-Fox as prod. 1949; apptd. exec. prod. 20th Cent.-Fox, 1951 to Dec. 1952.
PICTURES INCLUDE: Broken Arrow, Mister 880, Half Angel, Just One More Chance, Take Care of My Little Girl, Day the Earth Stood Still, Outcasts, Don't Bother to Knock, Desiree, The Racers, Storm Center, Cowboy, Bell Book and Candle, The Wreck of The Mary Deare, Two Loves, The Four Horsemen of the Apocalypse, Khartoum.

BLEAK, JANINE: Executive. e. Univ. of So. Calif. business school; degree in mktg. & finance. Natl. media supr. with West Coast office of J. Walter Thompson. 1985, joined Warner Bros. as media mgr.

BLEES, ROBERT: Writer-Producer. Phi Beta Kappa, Dartmouth. Time and Life Magazines. Exec. boards of Writers Guild, Producers Guild.
PICTURES INCLUDE: Magnificent Obsession, Autumn Leaves, The Glass Web, James Cain's Love's Lovely Counterfeit.
TV: Producer of Combat!, Bonanza, Bus Stop, Kraft Theater. Writer also of Alfred Hitchcock, Cannon, Barnaby Jones, Harry O, Columbo, Flamingo Road, Magnum.

BLEIER, EDWARD: Executive. b. N.Y., N.Y., October 16, 1929. e. Syacuse University, 1951, C.U.N.Y. Graduate Courses. Reporter: Syracuse Herald Journal, Long Island Daily Press 1947–50. Sportscaster: WNEW, N.Y.; WSYR, Syracuse, 1947–50. American Broadcasting Company, 1952–57; 1959–68. Vice President in charge of Public Relations & Planning (Marketing, Advertising, Publicity), Broadcast Div. Vice President in chg. of daytime Programming & Sales, ABC-TV Network; vice pres./gen. mgr. sales, ABC-TV Network; Account Executive, ABC-TV Network & WABC-TV. Vice Pres. Radio-Television-Film, Tex McCrary, Inc. 1958; Program Service Manager, DuMont Television Network, 1951; U.S. Army Psy. War School; Ex-chm., TV Committee, NASL; ex-Trustee, NATAS; founder-director & vice-chm., International TV Council (NATAS); pres., IRTS; ATAS; guest professor: several universities. Pres., pay-tv & network features, Warner Bros.

BLENDER, LEON PHILIP: Executive. b. Kansas City, Mo., Feb. 15, 1920; e. Kansas State Co., 1941. 20th Century-Fox Dist. Co., 1947–51; Kranz-Levin pictures, 1951–56. gen. sls. mgr. American International Film Dist. Corp., 1956–57; v.p. 1960; American Intl. Pictures, senior v.p., sales dist., later exec. v.p. sales and distribution; 1979, exec. v.p. sales & distribution, Film Ventures Intl.; 1983, exec. v.p., world-wide dist., Summa Vista Pictures.

BLOCH, ROBERT: Writer. b. Chicago, Ill., April 5, 1917; novelist short-story writer; 50 published books, incl. Psycho, Psycho II, The Night of the Ripper, etc.; wrote radio series, Stay Tuned for Terror, adapting own stories; national pres., Mystery Writers of Amer. (1970–71); entered films, 1960.
PICTURES INCLUDE: The Couch, Cabinet of Caligari, Straitjacket, The Night-Walker, The Psychopath, The Deadly Bees, (collab.) Torture Garden, The House That Dripped Blood, Asylum. (Films adapted from published work). Psycho, The Skull.
TV: Features: The Cat Creature, The Dead Don't Die. Approx. 70 credits on Hitchcock, Thriller, Star Trek, etc.

BLOCK, WILLARD: Executive. b. New York, N.Y., March 18, 1930. e. Columbia College, Columbia University Law School, 1952. Counter-Intelligence Corps., U.S. Army, 1952–54, account exec., Plus Marketing, Inc. 1954–55; joined sales staff, NBC Television Network, 1955–57; sales staff, CBS Enterprises, Inc., 1957; international sales mgr, 1960; dir., international sales, 1965; v.p., 1967; v.p., Viacom Enterprises, 1971; pres., 1972; v.p. MCA-TV, 1973; v.p., gen. mgr., Taft, H-B International, Inc.; pres. Willard Block, Ltd.; 1979, named pres., Viacom Enterprises; 1982, pres. Viacom Worldwide Ltd.

BLOOM CLAIRE: Actress. b. London, Eng., Feb. 15, 1931; e. Badminton School (U.S.A.). Stage debut at Playhouse, Oxford, Sept., 1947; Old Vic seasons, etc.; screen debut in Limelight, 1951.
PICTURES INCLUDE: Innocents in Paris, Limelight, The Man Between, Richard III, Alexander the Great, The Brothers Karamazov, Look Back in Anger, The Royal Game, The Wonderful World of the Brothers Grimm, The Chapman Report, The Haunting, Alta Infidelita, Il Maestro di Vigenuono, The Outrage, The Spy Who Came In From the Cold, Charley, The Illustrated Man, Three Into Two Won't Go, A Severed Head, Red Sky at Morning, A Doll's House, Islands In The Stream, Clash of the Titans, Always, Deja Vu.
TV: Misalliance, (Playhouse90), Anna Karenina, Wuthering Heights, Ivanov, Wessex Tales, An Imaginative Woman, A Legacy, In Praise of Love, The Orestaia, Henry VIII, Brideshead Revisited, Hamlet, Cymbeline, King John, Ann and Debbie, Ellis Island, Florence Nightingale, The Ghost Writer, Time and the Conways, Shadow Lands, Liberty.

BLOOM, VERNA: Actress. b. Lynn, Mass. e. Boston Univ. Studied drama at Uta Hagen-Herbert Berghof School. Performed with small theatre groups all over country; then started repertory theatre in Denver. Appeared on Broadway in Marat/Sade (played Charlotte Corday). Film debut, Medium Cool, 1969.
PICTURES INCLUDE: The Hired Hand, High Plains Drifter, Badge 373, National Lampoon's Animal House, After Hours.

BLOOM, WILLIAM: Producer. b. New York, N.Y., Feb. 28, 1915. e. U. of Pa., BA, 1935. Story dept., Columbia, N.Y., 1936; U.S. Army Signal Corps, 1941–45; asst. to Ender Bohem, Columbia, Hollywood; then prod. and asst. to B.B. Kahane, 1947–51; asst. to Julian Blaustein, Fox, 1951; prod., 1952.
PICTURES INCLUDE: Glory Brigade, Inferno, On the Threshold of Space.

BLOOMER STEPHEN J.: Exhibitior. b. Belleville, IL Nov. 12, 1947. e. No. Ill. Univ. (BS in ED, 1969). Elementary school band director, 1969–75; insurance sales, NY Life Insurance Co., 1975–77; asst. mgr., NY Life, 1977–1979; joined BAC Theatres Jan., 1979 as warehouse mgr.; Nov. 1979, named gen. mgr.

BLUM, HARRY N.: Executive. b. Cleveland, Oh., Oct. 3, 1932. e. Univ of Mich. (BBA, LLB). Was attorney in Ohio, toy & hobby industry executive, management consultant, and venture capital and investment manager before entering industry. Now heads The Blum Group, entertainment financing, Packaging, production and international marketing Co.
PICTURES INCLUDE: Executive Action (assoc. prod.); The Land That Time Forgot (assoc. prod.); At the Earth's Core (exec. prod.); Drive-In (assoc. prod.) Diamonds (exec. prod.); The Bluebird (assoc. prod.); Obsession (prod.); Skateboard (prod.); The Magician of Lublin (exec. prod.); Duran Duran—Arena (exec. prod.).

BLUMENSTOCK, SID: Ad. exec. New York City. Publicity dir. Warner Bros. Atlantic City theatres 1934–38; joined 20th Fox adv. dept. 1938; asst. exploitation mgr. 1944–49; advertising mgr. Paramount 1949; asst. nat'l. dir. adv. pub., exploit, 1951–58; MPH Coord. 1959 Academy telecast; v.p. Embassy Pictures, 1959; v.p. Chas. Schlaifer Agency, Hollywood, October, 1959–62; v.p. Safranski Prod., Inc.; adv. dir., Embassy Pictures, 1964–67; Walter Reade Org., 1967–70 Levitt-Pickman Film Corp., adv. dir., 1971–72.

BLUMOFE, ROBERT F.: Producer. b. New York, N.Y. e. Columbia Coll., A.B. Columbia U. Sch. of Law. J.D. v.p., West Coast oper., U.A., 1953–66; independent prod., pres. RFB Enterprises, Inc; American Film Institute, director, AFI-West, Sept. 1, 1977–81. Now indep. prod.

BLYTH, ANN: Actress. b. Mt. Kisco, N.Y., Aug. 16, 1928; e. New Wayburn's Dramatic School. On radio in childhood; with San Carlos Opera Co. 3 years; Broadway debut in "Watch on the Rhine"; on tour.
PICTURES INCLUDE: Chip Off the Old Block, Merry

Monahans, Brute Force, Swell Guy, Mr. Peabody and the Mermaid, Woman's Vengeance, Mildred Pierce, Free for All, Top o' the Morning, Our Very Own, Great Caruso, Katie Did It, Thunder on the Hill, I'll Never Forget You, Golden Horde, One Minute to Zero, World in His Arms, Sally and Saint Anne, All the Brothers Were Valiant, Rose Marie, The Student Prince, King's Thief, Kismet, Buster Keaton Story, Jazz Age, Slander, The Helen Morgan Story.

BOASBERG, CHARLES: Sales executive. b. Buffalo, N.Y., Aug. 20, 1906; e. Cornell U., A.B. 1927; RKO salesman, Buffalo 1930; br. mgr. Buffalo 1937; dist. mgr., Cleveland 1940; Metropolitan dist. mgr., N.Y.C. 1944; apptd. north south div. mgr. 1947. Named gen. sales mgr., dir., RKO Pict., Oct., 1952; v.p., gen. mgr. Dist. Corp. of America, 1954–55; joined Paramount, 1955, in chg. world wide sales of the Ten Commandments, gen. sls. mgr., pres. Warner Bros. Dist. Corp., Jan. 1958. Res., July, 1962; domestic gen. sls. mgr. & v.p., Paramount Film dist. Corp., 1962; pres., Paramount Film Dist. Corp., 1963, and V.P. Paramount Pictures, Inc. 1967; v.p. National General Corporation, 1968; pres. Nat'l Gen'l Pictures Corp., 1969. In 1964 formed Boasberg/Goldstein, consultants to film producers, now Charles Boasberg, Inc.

BOCHNER, HART: Actor. b. Toronto, 1956. e. Univ. San Diego. Debut, Islands in the Stream (1977).
PICTURES: Breaking Away, Terror Train, Rich and Famous, Supergirl, The Wild Life.
TELEVISION: The Sun Also Rises.

BOCHNER, LLOYD: Actor. b. Canada, July 29, 1924.
PICTURES: Drums of Africa, The Night Walker, Sylvia, Tony Rome, Point Blank, The Detective, The Horse in the Gray Flannel Suit, Tiger by the Tail, Ulzana's Raid, The Man in the Glass Booth, Hot Touch, The Lonely Lady, Louisiana.
TELEVISION: A Fire in the Sky, Greatest Heroes of the Bible, The Golden Gate Murders, Dynasty, Mazes & Monsters, etc.

BODE, RALF: Cinematographer. b. Berlin, Germany. Attended Yale where was actor with drama school and acquired degree in directing. Received on-job training teaching combat photography and making films for Army at Ft. Monmouth. First professional job in films was gaffer on Harry, followed by long association with director John G. Avildsen, for whom served as gaffer and lighting designer on Guess What We Learned in School Today, Joe, and Cry Uncle. Later served as dir. of photography for Avildsen on Inaugural Ball and as East Coast dir. phot. for Rocky.
PICTURES INCLUDE: Saturday Night Fever, Slow Dancing in the Big City, Gorky Park, Violets Are Blue.
TELEVISION: PBS Theatre in America, working as lighting designer and dir. of photo. Also many TV commercials.

BOEHM, SIDNEY: Writer. b. Philadelphia, Pa., Apr. 4, 1908; Lehigh U. 1935–29. m. Ellen Kasputis. Reporter, N.Y. Journal-American & I.N.S., 1930–45.
PICTURES INCLUDE: Union Station, Big Heat, Atomic City, Six Bridges To Cross, The Raid, Rogue Cop, The Savage, Violent Saturday, Hell on Frisco Bay, Tall Men, Bottom of the Bottle, Revolt of Mamie Stover, Woman Obsessed, Seven Thieves, Sylvia, Rough Night in Jericho.

BOETTICHER, BUDD: Producer, director, writer. r.n. Oscar Boetticher, Jr. b. Chicago, Ill., July 29, 1918. e. Ohio State U. bull fighter; then technical dir., "Blood and Sand," 1941; asst. dir., Hal Roach studios and Columbia 1941–44; became feature director at Columbia in 1944; dir. Eagle Lion, 1946; dir., Universal; independ. prod., 1954.
PICTURES INCLUDE: Behind Locked Doors, Assigned to Danger, Black Midnight, Killer Shark, Wolf Hunters, Bullfighter and the Lady, Cimarron Kid, Bronco Busters, Red Ball Express, Horizons West, City Beneath the Sea, Seminole, Man from the Alamo, Wings of the Hawk, East of Sumatra, Magnificent Matador, Killer Is Loose, Seven Men From Now, Decision at Sundown, The Tall T, Buchanan Rides Alone, Ride Lonesome Westbound, The Rise and Fall of Legs Diamond, Comanche Station, The Carlos Arruza Story.

BOFFETY, JEAN: Cinematographer. Born in France.
PICTURES INCLUDE: Act of the Heart, Journey, Les Choses De La Vie, Cesar and Rosalie, Thieves Like Us.

BOGARDE, DIRK: Actor. b. Hampstead, London, Eng., March 28, 1921. e. Allen Glens College, Glasgow & University College, London. Started theatrical career with Amersham Repertory Co., then London stage; in Army in World War II; screen debut in Esther Waters Films. Top ten British star, 1953–54, 1956–64; number one British money-making star 1955, 1957, 1958, 1959; Variety Club Award—Best Performance 1961–64. British Academy Award, Darling, 1966.
PICTURES INCLUDE: Quartet, Once a Jolly Swagman, Mr. Prohack, Blue Lamp, Five Angles on Murder, Gentle Gunman, So Long at the Fair, Blackmailed, Woman in Question, Hunted (Stranger in Between), Penny Princess, Desperate Moment, They Who Dare, The Sleeping Tiger, Doctor in the House, For Better or Worse, The Sea Shall Not Have Them, Simba, Doctor at Sea, Appointment in London, Cast a Dark Shadow, Doctor At Large, Spanish Gardener, Ill Met by Moonlight, Campbell's Kingdom, A Tale of Two Cities, The Wind Cannot Read, The Doctor's Dilemma, Libel, The Angel Wore Red, Song Without End, The Singer Not The Song, Victim, H.M.S. Defiant, The Password Is Courage, I Could Go on Singing, The Mind Benders, The Servant (British Academy Award 1964), Hot Enough for June, Doctor Distress, The High Bright Sun, King and Country, Darling . . . , Modesty Blaise, Accident, Our Mother's House, Sebastion, The Fixer, Justine, Oh What a Lovely War, The Damned, Death in Venice, Le Serpent, The Night Porter, Permission to Kill, Providence, A Bridge Too Far, Despair.
TV: (USA) The Little Moon of Alban, Hallmark, 1964. Blythe Spirit, Hallmark, 1966, Upon This Rock, The Patricia Neal Story.

BOGART, PAUL: Director. b. New York, N.Y. Nov. 21, 1919.
FILMS INCLUDE: Marlowe, Hall of Anger, Skin Game, Class of '44, Mr. Ricco, Oh, God! You Devil.
TV: (Specials) Ages of Man, Mark Twain Tonight, The Final War of Ollie Winter, Dear Friends, Secrets, The House Without a Christmas Tree, Look Homeward Angel, The Country Girl, Double Solitaire, The Thanksgiving Treasure, Tell Me Where it Hurts, The Adams Chronicles.

BOGDANOVICH, PETER: Director, producer, writer, actor. b. Kingston, N.Y., July 30, 1939 e. Collegiate School, Stella Adler Theatre School, N.Y. 1954–58. Stage debut, N.Y. Shakespeare Festival, Amer. Shakespeare Festival, others, 1955–58. Off-Bway: dir.-co. prod. The Big Knife, 1959, Camino Real, Ten Little Indians, Rocket to the Moon, 1961, dir.-prod. Once in a Lifetime, 1964. Film critic and feature writer, general publications, 1958–85, Monographs for Museum of Modern Art Film Library on Orson Welles, Alfred Hitchcock, Howard Hawks, 1961–63. Books: John Ford, (U. of Calif. Press), Fritz Lang in America (Praeger), 1969; Allan Dwan—The Last Pioneer (Praeger), 1971; Pieces of Time (Arbor House), 1973, enlarged 1985; The Killing of the Unicorn: Dorothy Stratten 1960–1980 (Morrow), 1984. Second-unit dir.-writer, The Wild Angels (Roger Corman-Amer. International), 1966. Dir.-prod.-writer-actor, Targets (Saticoy Prods. Para.), 1968. Dir.-writer, The Last Picture Show (BBS Prods. Col.) 1971, dir.-writer, Directed by John Ford (AFI-Calif. Arts Comm.), 1971; dir.-prod.-writer, What's Up Doc?, (Saticoy Prod.-WB), 1972; dir.-prod. Paper Moon (Saticoy Prod.-Directors Company-Para.), 1973; dir.-prod., Daisy Miller (Copa De Oro Prod. Directors Company-Para.), 1974; dir.-prod.-writer At Long Last Love (Copa De Oro Prod.-20th Century-Fox), 1975; dir.-writer Nickelodeon (Chartoff-Winkler Prod.-Col.), 1976; dir.-writer-actor, Saint Jack (Copa de Oro-Orion-New World), 1979; dir.-writer, They All Laughed, 1981 (Moon Pictures—PSO—Time/Life), 1981; dir., Mask (Marstar-Universal), 1985.

BOHEM, ENDRE: Producer, writer. b. Hungary, e. U. Vienna. Exec. Asst. to E. Mannix, MGM and Harry Cohen, Columbia. Prod. shorts series: Passing Parade, Nostradamus, What do You Think, Crime Does Not Pay, Tell Tale Heart.
PICTURES INCLUDE: Night Has a 1000 Eyes, The Redhead and the Cowboy, Alias Nick Beal, Streets of Laredo, Postal Inspector, Wonder of Women, Thirst, House With a 1000 Candles, Two Wise Maids, Little Orphan Annie, Lord Jeff, Crime of the Century, Twin Stars, Bengazi.
TV: Revlon Mirror, Ford Theatre, Rawhide.

BOLGER, RAY: Actor, dancer. b. Dorchester, Mass., Jan. 10, 1906; e. O'Brien Dancing School, Boston. Bank clerk; vacuum salesman; accountant & student Russakoff's Ballet School; with insurance co.; stage debut with Bob Ott's Musical Comedy repertory touring New England; in dance team Sanford & Bolger; prod. two-reel M.P. Toured South Pacific with USO, World War II; m.p debut in "Great Ziegfeld" 1936; Own TV show, ABC, 1954–55.
SHOWS INCLUDE: Passing Show of 1926, Heads Up, Scandals of 1931, Life Begins at 8:40, On Your Toes, By Jupiter; N.Y. stage, Three to Make Ready, Where's Charley?, All American, Come Summer.
PICTURES INCLUDE: Rosalie, Wizard of Oz, Sunny, Four Jacks and a Jill, Look for the Silver Lining, Make Mine Laughs, Where's Charley?, April in Paris, Babes in Toyland, The Runner Stumble.

BOLOGNA, JOSEPH: Actor-Writer. m. actress-writer Renee Taylor. b. Brooklyn, N.Y. e. Brown Univ., Providence, R.I. Service in Marine Corps and on discharge joined ad agency, becoming director-producer of TV commercials. Collaborated with wife on short film, 2, shown at 1966 N.Y. Film Festival. Together they wrote Lovers and Other Strangers, Bdwy. play, in which both also acted. Wrote s.p. for film version. Both wrote and starred in Made for Each Other, and created and wrote TV series, Calucci's Dept.

PICTURES INCLUDE: Lovers and Other Strangers (co.-s.p.), Made for Each Other (co.-s.p., star), Cops and Robbers (actor), Mixed Company (actor), The Big Bus (actor), Chapter Two (actor), My Favorite Year (actor), Blame It on Rio (actor), The Woman in Red (actor), Transylvania 6-5000 (actor).
TV: Calucci's Dept. (co.-s.p.), Honor Thy Father (movie—actor), Copacabana, A Time To Triumph. Mini-Series: Sins.

BOLT, ROBERT: Writer, b. Sale, England, 1924. Ent. m.p. ind. 1961.
PICTURES INCLUDE: Lawrence of Arabia, Dr. Zhivago, A Man For All Seasons (play and film), Ryan's Daughter, Dir. own s.p. Lady Caroline Lamb, The Bounty.

BOND, ANSON: Producer, writer. b. Cleveland, Ohio, Mar. 21, 1914; p. Charles Anson Bond, founder, Bond Clothing Co. & Bond Stores, Inc. e. Yale Prep. & pre-legal, Stuyvesant Sch., Warrenton, Va. Washington corr., 30 Ohio newspapers, 1930–33; asst. to pres., C.W. Hord Co., N.Y. 1933–36; apprenticeship in m.p. prod. 1936–39; dir., prod., writer. U.S. armed forces, 1940–45; head pub. firm, Bond-Charteris, prod. radio program. The Saint; publ. Craig Rice Crime Digest & Movie Mystery Magazine.
PICTURES INCLUDE: The Judge, Not Wanted, Vicious Years, (co-prod.) Journey Into Light, Japanese War Bride, China Venture.

BOND, DEREK: Actor, Scriptwriter. b. Glasgow, Jan. 26, 1920; e. Haberdasher' Askes School, London. Stage debut in "As Husbands Go" 1937; served in Grenadier Guards H.M. Forces 1939–46, awarded Military Cross; m.p. debut in "Captive Heart" 1946; author of Unscheduled Stop, Two Young Samaritians, Ask Father Christmas, Packdrill, Double Strung, Order to Kill, The Riverdale Dam, Sentence Deferred, The Mavroletty Fund. Many TV appearances.
PICTURES INCLUDE: Nicholas Nickleby, Joanna Godden, Uncle Silas, Scott of the Antarctic, Marry Me, Poets Pub, Weaker Sex, Broken Journey, Christopher Columbus, Tony Draws a Horse, Quiet Woman, Hour of Thirteen, Distant Trumpet, Loves's A Luxury, Trouble in Store, Svengali, High Terrace, Stormy Crossing, Rogues Yarn, Gideon's Day, The Hand, Saturday Night Out, Wonderful Life, Press For Time, When Eight Bells Toll, Intimate Reflections.

BONET, NAI: Actress—Producer. Worked in entertainment field since age of 13, including opera, films, TV, stage, night clubs and records.
PICTURES INCLUDE: Actress: The Soul Hustlers, The Seventh Veil, Fairy Tales, The Soul of Nigger Charlie, The Spy with the Cold Nose, John Goldfarb Please Come Home, etc. Wrote and starred in Nocturna and Hoodlums.
TELEVISION: Johnny Carson Show, Merv Griffin Show, Joe Franklyn Show, Beverly Hillbillies, Tom Snyder Show.

BONO, SONNY: Singer-Actor-Director-Writer. b. Detroit, Mich. Feb. 16, 1940. r.n. Salvatore Bono. Started writing songs at age 16; entered record business with Specialty Records as apprentice prod. Became ass't. to Phil Spector, rock music prod. and did background singing. Has recorded albums with former wife Cher and made two feature films, and formed nightclub act with her. CBS comedy-variety series began as summer show in 1971 and made regular later that year.
PICTURES INCLUDE: Good Times, Chastity (prod., s.p.), Escape to Athena, Airplane II: The Sequel, Special Delivery, Troll.
TELEVISION: Sonny & Cher Comedy Hour, Sonny Comedy Revue.

BOOKE, SORRELL: Actor. b. Buffalo, NY, Jan. 4, 1930. e. Columbia Univ. Joined summer stock company in Charleston, West Virginia, and later in Provincetown, Mass. After stint with armed forces returned to New York and off-Bdwy. plays. Bdwy. debut in The Sleeping Prince, followed by appearances in over 100 plays.
PICTURES: What's Up Doc?, Freaky Friday, etc.
TELEVISION: Series; Route 66, Soap, What's Happening!, The Dukes of Hazzard, etc.

BOOKMAN, ROBERT: Executive. b. Los Angeles. e. University of California, Yale Law School. Motion picture literary agent, IFA 1972–74, ICM 1974–79. 1979 joined ABC Motion Pictures as v.p., worldwide production; 1984, Columbia Pictures, exec. v.p., world-wide prod.

BOONE, JR., ASHLEY A.: Executive. b. 1939. e. Brandeis Univ. Started career at United Artists in adv./pub.; later with Cinema Center Films; adm. asst., Motown Records; assoc. prod. for Sidney Poitier's E & R Productions. Joined 20th-Fox in 1972 in sls. dept.; advanced to sr. sls. & mktg. postitions in feature film operation. In 1979 appt. pres. of 20th-Fox Distribution & Marketing. Joined Ladd Co., v.p. in chg. dist. & mktg., 1983; Pres., Columbia Pictures Mktg. & Dist. Group, 1984. Resigned 1985 but remained special mkt. consultant. 1986, joined Lorimar Pictures as pres., mktg. & dist.

BOONE, PAT: Singer. b. Jacksonville, Fla., June 1, 1934. e. David LipsComb College, No. Texas State Coll., grad. magna cum laude, Columbia U. Winner of Ted Mack's TV show; joined Arthur Godfrey TV show, 1955. m.p. debut in Bernadine. Most promising new male star, M.P.D.-Fame Poll 1957.
AUTHOR: Twixt Twelve and Twenty, and Between You & Me and the Gatepost. One of top ten moneymaking stars M.P. Herald-Fame Poll, 1957; wrote book, The Real Christmas.
RECORDINGS: Ain't That a Shame, I Almost Lost My Mind, Friendly Persuasion, Love Letters in the Sand, April Love, Tutti Frutti, Speedy Gonzales, Days of Wine & Roses, Moody River.
PICTURES INCLUDE: Bernadine, April Love, Mardi Gras, Journey to the Center of the Earth, All Hands on Deck, State Fair, The Main Attraction, The Yellow Canary, The Horror of It All, The Perils of Pauline, The Cross and the Switchblade.

BOORMAN, JOHN: Producer, director. b. London, England. Wrote film criticism at age of 17 for British publications; served in National Service in Army; joined independent Television News as film editor; prod. documentaries for Southern Television; joined BBC, headed BBC Documentary Film Unit.
PICTURES INCLUDE: Catch Us If You Can, Point Blank, Hell In the Pacific, Leo The Last, Deliverance, Zardoz, Exorcist II: The Heretic, Excalibur (prod., dir., s.p.), The Emerald Forest (prod., dir.).

BOOTH, JAMES: Actor, Scriptwriter. b. Croydon, England, 1931. Early career with R.A.D.A., Old vic and Theatre Workshop; on West End stage: Fings Aint Wot They Used To Be. Subsequently: King Lear, Comedy of Errors, A Thousand Clowns, The Fire Raisers, The Entertainer, The Recruitng Officer, Travesties, The Tempest.
PICTURES INCLUDE: Trials of Oscar Wilde, Sparrows Can't Sing, The Hellions, French Dressing, Zulu, 90 Degrees in the Shade, Secret of My Success, Bliss of Mrs. Blossom, Boomerang, The Man Who Had Power Over Women, Darker Than Amber (1969), Macho Callaghan (1970), Revenge, Percy's Progress, Brannigan, Robbery, Penny Gold, Airport 77.
TV: The Ruffians, The Great Gold Bullion Robbery, Stray Cats and Empty Bottles, Them.

BOOTH, MARGARET: Film Editor. b. Los Angeles, 1898. Awarded honorary Oscar, 1977.
PICTURES INCLUDE: Why Men Leave Home, Husbands and Lovers, Bridge of San Luis Rey, New Moon, Susan Lenox, Strange Interlude, Smilin' Through, Romeo and Juliet, Barretts of Wimpole Street, Mutiny on the Bounty, Camille, etc. Supervising editor on Own and the Pussycat, The Way We Were, Funny Lady, Murder by Death, The Goodbye Girl, California Suite, The Cheap Detective (also assoc. prod.), Chapter Two. Editor: Annie. Exec. Prod.: The Slugger's Wife.

BOOTH, SHIRLEY: Actress. b. New York, N.Y., Aug. 20, 1907. Joined Poli Stock Co., Hartford, Conn., at 12; Broadway debut in Hell's Bells, 1925; on radio in Duffy's Tavern; m.p. debut in Come Back Little Sheba (Academy Award, Best Actress, 1952).
PLAYS: After Such Pleasures, 3 Men on a Horse, Philadelphia Story, My Sister Eileen, Tomorrow the World, Goodbye My Fancy, Come Back Little Sheba, A Tree Grows in Brooklyn, Time of the Cuckoo, The Desk Set, Look to the Lillies, Miss Isobel, Juno, Colettes Second String, Glass Menagerie.
PICTURES INCLUDE: About Mrs. Leslie, Hot Spell, The Matchmaker.
TV: Perle Mesta Story, Hazel, A Touch of Grace.

BOOTHE, POWERS: Actor. b. Snyder, TX, 1949. On Broadway in Love Star.
TELEVISION: Skag, Guyana Tragedy–The Story of Jim Jones, Philip Marlowe Series (HBO).
PICTURES INCLUDE: Cruising, Southern Comfort, A Breed Apart, The Emerald Forest, Extreme Prejudice.

BORCHERS, CORNELL: Actress. b. Heydekrug, Germany, March 16; e. Gottingen U. Berlin actors school, m. Dr. Anton Schelkopf.
PICTURES INCLUDE: (German) Martina, Das ewige Spiel, Haus des Lebens, Schule fur Ehegluck; (English) Big Lift, Divided Heart, Oasis, Never Say Goodbye, Istanbul, Alone Together.

BORGE, VICTOR: Comedian, pianist. b. Copenhagen, Denmark, Jan. 3, 1909. Child prodigy at age 10. Later bacame humorous concert artist. Wrote and starred in musical plays and films in Denmark. Fled Nazis in 1941, came to America.
Appeared on Bing Crosby radio show. Concert and Nightclub tours. TV variety shows. One-man Broadway show. Comedy in Music. 1953, three-year run. Second edition in 1964. World tour. One-man TV show.

BORGINE, ERNEST: Actor. b. Hamden, Conn., Jan. 24, 1918. e. Randall School of Dramatic Art, Hartford. Served in U.S. Navy; then little theatre work, stock companies; on Broadway in Harvey, Mrs. McThing; many TV appearances; m.p. debut in Whistle at Eaton Falls.
PICTURES INCLUDE: The Mob, China Corsair, From Here to Eternity, Demetruis & the Galdiators, Johnny Guitar, Vera Cruz, Bad Day at Black Rock, Marty (Acad. Award best actor 1955), Run for Cover, Violent Saturday, Last Command, Square Jungle, Catered Affair, Jubal, Best Things in Life are Free, Three Brave Men, Pay or Die, Go Naked in the World, Rabbit Trap, 10 Years a Counterspy, Summer of the Seventeenth Doll, Barabbas, Chuka, The Dirty Dozen, The Wild Bunch, The Adventurers, Suppose They Gave a War and Nobody Came?, A Bullet for Sandoval, Bunny, O'Hare, Hannie Caulder, The Revengers, Legend of Lylah Clare, The Poseidon Adventure, The Emperor of the North, Law and Disorder, The Devil's Rain, Hustle, Shoot, The Greatest, Crossed Swords, Convoy, The Black Hole, When Time Ran Out, Escape from New York, Deadly Blessing, The Graduates of Malibu High.
TV: Philco Playhouse, General Electric Theater, Wagon Train, Laramie, Zane Grey Theater, Alcoa Premiere, McHale's Navy, Blood Feud, Last Days of Pompeii, The Dirty Dozen: The Next Mission.

BORODINSKY, SAMUEL: Executive. b. Brooklyn, NY, Oct. 25, 1941. e. Industrial School of Arts & Photography. Expert in film care and rejuvenation. Now exec. v.p., Filmtreat International Corp. Previously with Modern Film Corp. (technician) and Comprehensive Filmtreat, Inc. & International Filmtreat (service manager).

BOSLEY, TOM: Actor. b. Chicago, Oct. 1, 1927. e. DePaul Univ. Had roles on radio in chicago and in stock productions before moving to New York. Appeared off-Bdwy and on road before signed to play lead in Fiorello! for George Abbott on Bdwy. First actor to win Tony, Drama Critics, ANTA and Newspaper Guild awards in one season for that role. Has since done many plays, movies and TV appearances.
PICTURES: Love with the Proper Stranger, The World of Henry Orient, Divorce, American Style, Yours, Mine & Ours, The Secret War of Harry Frigg, Mixed Company, Gus.
TELEVISION: Series: Debbie Reynolds Show, Sandy Duncan Show, Happy Days, Movies: The Girl Who Came Gift Wrapped, Death Cruise, The Night the Martians Landed, Love Boat. Specials: Testimony of Two Men, The Bastard.

BOSTICK, ROBERT L.: b. Waynesboro, Georgia, Oct. 25, 1909. e. Georgia Tech, Atlanta (ME, Eng.) 1932. Started with National Theatre Supply, Atlanta, salesman, Memphis, 1933; br. mgr. 1937; br. mgr. Dallas, 1942; Vice Pres., Southern Division Mgr., 1952; retired 1968. Chief Barker Variety Club Tent 20, Memphis 1950–51. Since 1957, has served as International Rep., International Ambassador-at-Large, and International Vice Pres. for Variety Clubs International. Since 1968, owner & operator of theatres in Memphis and Charlotte areas.

BOSTWICK, BARRY: Actor. b. San Mateo, CA, Feb. 24, 1945. On Broadway in Grease, The Knew What They Wanted, The Robber Bridegroom, etc.
PICTURES: Movie Movie, Megaforce, etc.
TELEVISION: Movies: Scruples, Moviola—The Silent Lovers, Foul Play, Summer Girl, An Uncommon Love, George Washington, A Woman of Substance, Deceptions, Betrayed by Innocence, etc.

BOSUSTOW, NICK: Producer. b. Los Angeles, Calif., March 28, 1940. e. Menlo College, Calif. Administration. MCA, International sales, 1963. Pres., Stephen Bosustow Productions, 1967; pres., ASIFA-West; Academy Award '70 best short, Is it always right to be right?; 1973 Academy Award nomination, The Legend of John Henry. The Incredible Book Escape, Misunderstood Monsters, A Tale of Four Wishes, Wrong Way Kid (TV specials). 1977, pres., Bosustow Entertainment, Inc.

BOSUSTOW, TED: Producer-Director-Editor. b. Hollywood, Calif., Feb 18, 1938. e. UCLA Cinema in Westwood, La Sorbonne, Paris.
PICTURES INCLUDE: Beware of Thin Ice, Big Boys Don't Cry, Avati and the Mezzotint. Edited short, Is It Always Right to Be Right? (AA, 1971).
TELEVISION: About a Week (community affairs series; Emmy award).

BOTTOMS, JOSEPH: Actor. b. Santa Barbara, Calif. April 22, 1954. Did plays in jr. high school in Santa Barbara and then with community theatre. Made m.p. debut in The Dove (1974).
PICTURES INCLUDE: Crime and Passion, King of the Mountain, Blind Date.
TV: Owen Marshall, Winesburg, Ohio, Celebrity.

BOTTOMS, SAM: Actor. b. Santa Barbara, CA, Oct. 17, 1955. Brother of Timothy and Joseph Bottoms.
PICTURES: The Last Picture Show, Class of '44, Zandy's Bride, The Outlaw Josey Wales, Apocalypse Now, Up from the Depths, Bronco Billy.
TELEVISION: Savages, Greatest Heroes of the Bible, East of Eden, Desperate Lives.

BOTTOMS, TIMOTHY: Actor. b Santa Barbara, Calif., Aug. 30, 1951. Early interest in acting; was member of S.B. Madrigal Society, touring Europe in 1967. Sang and danced in West Side Story local prod.
PICTURES INCLUDE: Johnny Got His Gun (debut), The Last Picture Show, Love and Pain, The Paper Chase, The White Dawn, The Crazy World of Julius Vrooder, Seven Men at Daybreak, A Small Town in Texas, Rollercoaster, The Other Side of the Mountain: Part II, Hurricane, Hambone and Hillie, Invaders from Mars.

BOUDOURIS, A: Executive. b. Toledo, Ohio, Jan. 31, 1918. e. U. of Toledo, 1945–47, USN, radio-radar, 1941–45; carrier pilot. Service, installation, projection equip., 1934–36; Strong Electric, 1936–41; Pres., Theatre Equip. Co., 1945–65; Theatre Operating Co., since 1947; pres. Eprad, Inc., 1949, bd. chmn., 1980. Member (ex-chm.) or NATO'S Technical Advisory Comm., Pres. NATO of Ohio, NATO representative on American National Standards Committee; now Vice Pres. NATO. Chairman, NATO Statistical Committee; Member, Projection Practices and Sound Comm. of SMPTE; NATO Representative International Standards Organization (Geneva), Member National Electrical Code Committee Panel #15. Recipient, SMPTE Fellowship Award, 1980.

BOULTING, ROY: Producer, director. b. Bray, Buckinghamshire, England, Nov. 21, 1913. e. McGill U., Montreal. Capt., Brit. Army, World War II. Dir. Charter Film, Charter Film Prod. Ltd. London; dir. British Lion Films, Ltd., 1958.
PICTURES INCLUDE: Inquest, Trunk Crime, Pastor Hall, Thunder Rock, Desert Victory, Burma Victory, Fame is the Spur, Brighton Rock, Guinea Pig, Seven Days to Noon, Lucky Jim, High Treason, Singlehanded (Sailor of the King), Seagulls Over Sorrento (Crest of the Wave), Josephine and Men, Private's Progress, Run for the Sun, Brothers in Law, Happy Is the Bride, Carlton-Browne of the F.O., I'm All Right Jack, The Risk, The French Mistress, Heavens Above! Rotten to The Core, The Family Way, Twisted Nerve, There's a Girl in My Soup, Soft Beds, Hard Battles, 1977, co-author with Leo Marks of play, Favourites, Danny Travis, 1978; The Last Word, 1979.

BOWERS, WILLIAM: Writer, producer. b. Las Cruces, New Mexico, Jan. 17, 1916; e. U. Mo. Playwright (Where Do We Go From Here, Back to Eden). Reporter, feature writer, N.Y. World-Telegram: then N.E.A. Hollywood corresp.; later radio scripts (Helen Hayes Theat., etc.). Began screen writing 1942 with collab. s.p. My Favorite Spy.
PICTURES INCLUDE: Alias Jesse James, Imitation General, The Law and Jake Wade, The Sheepman, My Man Godfrey, The Best Things in Life, Tight Spot, Split Second, The Gunfighter, The Web, Support Your Local Sheriff.

BOWIE, DAVID: Singer/Actor. b. Brixton, South London, England, Jan. 8, 1947. r.n. David Robert Jones.
PICTURES: The Man Who Fell to Earth, Just a Gigolo, The Hunger, Merry Christmas, Mr. Lawrence, Into the Night, Absolute Beginners (act., music), Labyrinth (act., music).

BOX, BETTY: OBE. Producer. b. Beckenham, Kent. Assisted Sydney Box in prod. 200 propaganda films in World War II. Assoc. prod. Upturned Glass.
PRODUCTIONS INCLUDE: Dear Murderer, When the Bough Breaks, Miranda, Blind Goddess, Huggett Family series. It's Not Cricket, Marry Me, Don't Ever Leave Me, So Long At the Fair, The Clouded Yellow, Appointment With Venus (Island Rescue). Venetian Bird (The Assassin), A Day to Remember, Doctor in the House, Mad About Men, Doctor at Sea, The Iron Petticoat, Checkpoint, Doctor at Large, Campbell's Kingdom, A Tale of Two Cities, The Wind Cannot Read, The 39 Steps, Upstairs and Downstairs, Conspiracy of Hearts, Doctor in Love, No Love for Johnnie, No, My Darling Daughter, A Pair of Briefs, The Wild and the Willing, Doctor in Distress, Hot Enough for June (Agent 8¾), The High Bright Sun, (McGuire Go Home), Doctor in Clover, Deadlier Than the Male, Nobody Runs Forever, The High Commissioner, Some Girls Do, Doctor in Trouble, Percy, The Love Ban, Percy's Progress.

BOXLEITNER, BRUCE: Actor. b. Elgin, IL, May 12, 1950. After high school enrolled in Chicago's Goodman Theatre, staging productions in the city and working with lighting and set design in addition to acting. Theatrical film debut in The Baltimore Bullet (1980).
TELEVISION: Series: How the West Was Won, The Macahans, Bring 'Em Back Alive, Scarecrow and Mrs. King. Movies: Happily Ever After, Kenny Rogers as The

Gambler, The Gambler, Part II, Kiss Me, Kill Me, Fly Away Home, Kenny Rogers as The Gambler: The Adventure Continues, Passion Flower, etc. Mini-Series: The Last Convertible, Bare Essence, East of Eden.
PICTURES: The Baltimore Bullet, Tron.

BOYARS, ALBERT: Executive. b. N.Y.C. Aug. 11,: e. N.Y.U.: U.S. Navy, 1941–45. David O. Alber Assoc., 1945–51: Greater N.Y. Fund, Robert S. Taplinger Assoc., Michael Myerberg Prod., 1951–54: pub. rel. dir., Transfilm-Caravel Inc., and parent co. Buckeye Corp., 1954–63: director spec. projects in adv-pub-exploit. M-G-M, 1963–64; dir. of adv. & pub. Trans-Lux Corp., 1964, v.p. of adv. and pub. rel., Trans-Lux Multimedia Corp., 1976. Under his marketing aegis are the attractions The New York Experience, The Space Works, and The Seaport Experience.

BOYER, PHIL: TV Executive. b. Portland, Oreg. e. Sacramento State Univ. Began broadcasting career as 12-year-old in Portland, establishing nation's first youth radio facility— a 5-watt facility in the basement of his home. At 16 began working at KPDQ, Portland; two years later joined KPTV, Portland, as announcer. In 1960 joined KEZI-TV, Eugene, Oreg., heading prod. and prog. depts. In 1965 named staff prod.-dir. for KCRA, TV, Scramento, Calif., becoming prod. mgr. in 1967 and prog. mgr. in 1969. In 1972 joined KNBC-TV, Los Angeles, as prog. dir. In 1974 named v.p., programming, of ABC Owned Television Stations; 1977, v.p.-gen. mgr., WLS-TV, Chicago; 1979, v.p.-gen. mgr. of WABC-TV, New York.

BOYETT, ROBERT LEE: Producer. e. Duke Univeristy (B.A.) and Col. Univ. (Master's in mkt.). Began career in media and mkt. research at Grey Advertising, Inc. Was program development consultant for PBS. In 1973 joined ABC as dir. of prime time series TV, East Coast. In 1975 named ABC TV v.p. & asst. to v.p. programs for West Coast. In 1977 joined Paramount Pictures in newly created position of v.p., exec. asst. to pres. & chief operating officer. 1979, joined Miller-Milkis–Boyett Productions to produce for Paramount Television.

BOYLE, BARBARA D.: Executive. b. New York City, Aug. 11, 1935. e. Univ. of Calif., Berkeley (BA, 1957); Univ. of Calif., L.A. (JD, 1960). Named to bar: Calif., 1961; N.Y., 1964; Supreme Ct., 1964. Atty. in busn. affairs dept. & corp. asst. secty., American Intl. Pictures, Los Angeles, 1969–65; partner in law firm, Cohen & Boyle, L.A., 1967–74; exec. & gen. counsel, COO, New World Pictures, L.A., 1974–82. Sr. v.p. prod., Orion Pictures, L.A., 1982–85; exec. v.p., prod., RKO Pictures, L.A., 1986–present. Co-chmn., Entertainment Law Synposium Advisory Committee, UCLA Law School, 1979–80.
MEMBER: Academy of Motion Picture Arts & Sciences, Women in Film (pres., 1977–78), Women Entertainment Lawyers Assn., California Bar Assn., N.Y. State Bar Assn.

BOYLE, PETER: Actor. b. Philadelphia, 1933. e. LaSalle College. Was monk in Christian Bros. order before leaving in early 60s to come to N.Y. Acted in off-Broadway shows and joined The Second City in Chicago. Also did TV commercials.
PICTURES INCLUDE: Joe (debut), T.R. Baskin, The Candidate, Steelyard Blues, Slither, The Friends of Eddie Coyle, Kid Blue, Crazy Joe, Young Frankenstein, Swashbuckler, F.I.S.T., Brinks' Job, Hardcore, Beyond the Poseidon Adventure, Where the Buffalo Roam, In God We Trust, Outland, Hammett, Yellowbeard, Johnny Dangerously, Turk 182.

BOYLE, WILLIAM NEAL (Billy): Producer. b. London, England; e. Rothschild Grammar School. Ent. m.p. 1927 with British International Pictures on set design & construction. Subsequently con. manager, first asst. Dir., Pro. & Loc.; several American and British Cos.; Produced 17 pictures for Republic Pictures International; Productions Controller, Dudley Pictures International-Hollywood; United Artists. Paramount Pictures. dir., W.N.B. Prods., 1966. Incorporated Films and W.N.B. Prods., 1970, W.N.B. World Locations, 1971, TV series.
PICTURES INCLUDE: Demi Paradise, Tawny Pipit, Good Time Girl, Man Within, Quartet, Trio, Encore, So Long at The Fair, Highly Dangerous, Holiday Camp, Easy Money, Lady of Vengeance, High Hell, African Story (World locations).

BRABOURNE, THE LORD: Producer. b. London, Nov. 9, 1924.
PRODUCTIONS INCLUDE: Harry Black, Sink the Bismarck, H.M.S. Defiant, Othello, The Mikado, Up the Junction, Romeo and Juliet, Dance of Death, Tales of Beatrix Potter, Murder on the Orient Express, Death On The Nile, Stories from a Flying Trunk, The Mirror Crack'd, Evil Under the Sun, A Passage to India, Little Dorrit.

BRACKEN, EDDIE: Actor. b. New York City, Feb. 7, 1920: e. Prof. Children's School for Actors, N.Y.C.: m. Connie Nickerson, actress. Vaudeville & night club singer: stage debut in "Lottery" 1930; m.p. debut in "Life with Henry" 1940.
PLAYS: Lady Refuses, Iron men, So Proudly We Hail, Brother Rat, What A Life, Too Many Girls, Seven Year Itch, Shinbone Alley, Teahouse of the August Moon, You Know I Can't Hear You when The Water's Running, The Odd Couple, Never Too Late, Sunshine Boys, Hotline to Heaven, Hello, Dolly, Damn Yankees, Sugar Babies, Show Boat.
PICTURES INCLUDE: Fleet's In, Happy Go Lucky, Sweater Girl, Star Spangled Rhythm, Young and Willing, Hail the Conquering Hero, Miracle of Morgan's Creek, Girl From Jones Beach, Summer Stock, Two Tickets to Broadway, About Face, We're not Married, Slight Case of Larceny, National Lampoon's Vacation.
TV: Masquerade Party, Murder She Wrote, Blacks' Magic, Amazing Stories, Tales of the Dark Side.

BRADEN, WILLIAM: Executive/Producer. b. Alberta, Canada, 1939. e. Vancouver, British Columbia. Began career as stuntman in Hollywood, and has worked in all aspects of industry for 23 years. Worked for Elliott Kastner as prod. executive with offices at Paramount and with Jeffrey Bloom, of Feature Films, Inc., as prod. and v.p. in chg. of prod. before joining, Dunatai Corp., as head of film and t.v. prod., now indep. prod.
PICTURES: Pyramid (assoc. prod., prod. supv.), Russian Roulette (prod. exec.) 92 in the Shade (prod. exec.), Breakheart Pass (prod. exec.), Dogpound Shuffle (asst. dir., prod. supv.); Dublin Murders (supvr. re-edit); He Wants Her Back (prod.); Goldengirl (prod. exec.); Running Scared (prod.); Death Valley (asst. dir.); The Seduction (prod. exec.); Slapstick (prod. exec.).
TELEVISION: Requiem for a Planet (series, prod./creator); Nothing Great is Easy (special, exec. prod.); King of the Channel (special, exec. prod.); I Believe (special, prod.); If My People . . . (special, prod.), Jude (pilot, prod.). America: Life in the Family (dir./prod.) Also various Movies of the Week for networks.

BRADLEY, BILL: Performer, r.n. William M. Silbert. b. Jan. 1, 1921, Detroit, Mich.; e. Univ. of Detroit, So. Methodist; Disc jockey, m.c., many radio-TV shows, Detroit; panelist, Songs for Sale, CBS-TV, 1952; emcee, Bill Silbert show, Let's Go Bowling WABD-DuMont TV, 1952–53; Bill Silbert Show. WMGM radio; announcer, Red Buttons Show, NBC-TV; Philco Phonorama Time, Mutual; m.c., National Radio Fan Club, NBC; Magazine of the Air, Mutual, KLAC Hollywood, Bill Bradley Show; KTLA, Hollywood, M.C. Crime Story, Greet the People, Ad Lib, Hollywood Diary. Sales mgr., KLOS, Los Angeles.
PICTURES INCLUDE: Bundle of Joy, Thunderjets, The Alligator People, Young Jesse James, Lost Missile, Breakfast at Tiffanys, Return to Peyton Place, Looking for Love, Goonies.
TV: Bronco, 77 Sunset Strip, Hawaiian Eye, Sugarfoot, Combat, Adventures in Paradise, Police Station, Michael Shayne, Roarings 20's, The Outlaws, Breaking Point, The Fugitive, Bill Dana Show, My Living Doll, Joey Bishop Show, Ben Casey, Bing Crosby Show. Many commercials, Mannix, Wild Wild West, Name of the Game.

BRADY, FRANK L.: Theatre Executive. b. Columbus, Ga., Jan. 11, 1914. Former pres., Martin Theatres.

BRAEDEN, ERIC: Actor. b. Kiel, Germany. r.n. Hans Gudegast.
PICTURES: Colossus, The Forbin Project, The Law and Jake Wade, The Ultimate Thrill, Morituri, Escape from the Planet of the Apes, Lady Ice, A Hundred Rifles, Herbie Goes to Monte Carlo.
TELEVISION: The Young and the Restless (series).

BRAND, NEVILLE: Actor. b. Kewanee, Ill., Aug. 13, 1921. e. high sch., Kewanee. U.S. Army, 10 yrs to 1946; studied acting in N.Y.: M.P. debut in D.O.A.
PICTURES INCLUDE: Halls of Montezuma, Only the Valiant, The Mob, Flame of Araby, Stalag 17, Charge at Feather River, Man Crazy, Gun Fury, Riot in Cell Block 11, Long Gun, Prince Valiant, Return from the Sea, Fury at Gunsight Pass, The Prodigal, Return of Jack Slade, Bobby Ware Is Missing, Mohawk, Raw Edge, The Adventures of Huckleberry Finn, The Desperadoes, Three Guns for Texas, Birdman of Alcatraz, That Darn Cat, Scalawag, Cahill, U.S. Marshall, The Deadly Trackers, Psychic Killer, Evils of the Night.
TV: Laredo, The Captain and the Kings.

BRANDO, JOCELYN: Actress. b. San Francisco, Calif. e. Lake Forest Coll.; m.p. debut in The Big Heat; on B'way in Mr. Roberts, Desire Under the Elms, Golden State.
PICTURES INCLUDE: China Venture, Ten Wanted Men, Mommie Dearest.

BRANDO, MARLON: Actor. b. Omaha, Neb., April 3, 1924. e. Shattuck Military Acad., Faribault, Minn. Studied Dramatic Workshop, New York; played stock Sayville, Long Island, m.p. screen debut. The New state debut: I Remember Mama, then Truckline Cafe, Candida, A Flag is Born, Street Car Named Desire.

PICTURES INCLUDE: Streetcar Named Desire, Viva Zapata, Julius Caesar, Wild One, On the Waterfront (Acad. Award best actor, 1954). One of top ten Money-Making Stars, M.P. Herald-Fame poll, 1954–55. Guys and Dolls, Teahouse of the August Moon, Sayonara, The Young Lions, Mutiny on the Bounty, One-Eyed Jacks, The Ugly American, Bedtime Story, The Saboteur, Code Name, Morituri, The Fugitive Kind, The Chase, Appaloosa, The Countess From Hong Kong, Reflections in A Golden Eye, Night of the Following Day, Candy, Burn!, The Nightcomers, The Godfather, Last Tango in Paris, The Missouri Breaks, Superman, The Formula.

BRANDT, JANET: Actress. b. New York City. Acting debut at 6 years old with Yiddish Theater. Over 100 stage appearances in New York where she studied with Martha Graham and with Michael Chekov. Lectured on Shakespeare at the Strasberg Institute in L.A.
PICTURES INCLUDE: Actress: Cold Wind in August, Kotch, Mad Adventures of Rabbi Jacob, Sheila Levine, Semi-Tough, Dialogue Director: Battle of the Bulge, El Cid, Phaedre, View from the Bridge, King of Kings, etc.
TV: Actress: Odd Couple, Mannix, Lou Grant, etc.

BRANDT, RICHARD PAUL: Executive. b. New York, N.Y., Dec. 6, 1927; e. Yale U., (BS, Phi Beta Kappa), chief exec. off. & chm. Trans Lux Corp.; chm., Brandt Theatres; dir., American Book-Stratford Press, Inc.; dir., Presidential Realty Corp., member President's Advisory Council, National Association of Theatre Owners; chm., bd. of trustees, American Film Institute; trustee: American Theatre Wing.

BRANDY, HOWARD: Executive. b. Brooklyn N.Y., 1929. e. Emory Univ. Served with Marine Corps in Korean War. Worked as N.Y. press agent; in 1956 went with NBC. Was columnist for Hollywood Reporter in Las Vegas then went back into publicity as asst. exec. for Rogers and Cowan. Started own business; clients included Frankie Avalon, Fabian, Monkees, Fifth Dimension, Johnny Cash, etc. Joined Commonwealth United in London working for co. 5 yrs. before it folded. Entered film prod.
PICTURES INCLUDE: Blood from the Mummy's Tomb, The Take.

BRANSON, WALTER E.: Western division sales manager, RKO Pictures Corp. e. U. of Nebraska. Booker for Pathe, Omaha, 1922–24; then salesman in South Dakota; city salesman, br. mgr., Omaha, 1925–27; br. mgr.; Des Moines, 1927–28; St. Louis, 1928–29; to Pathe h.o. as western sales mgr.; br. mgr. Chicago, 1931; midwest dist. mgr., 1932; Midwest dist mgr., 1932–41; Western sales mgr., Aug., 1954; v.p. in charge of world-wide distribution 1955; exec. asst. to pres., National Screen Service, 1960; v.p. distrib., National Screen Service, 1960; v.p. distrib., National Screen Service, 1963; v.p. in charge of prod., National Screen Service, 1966.

BRASLOFF, STANLEY H.: Producer, director. b. Philadelphia, Pa., July 23, 1930. In U.S. Army was entertainment dir., Heidelberg military post, 1948–50; prod., dir. & acted for various little theatre & summer stock groups, 1950–60; created, wrote, co-prod., dir. & starred in "Time For Teens" TV show (Chicago); formed VCS Pictures Ltd.,prod. & dir. "Two Girls for a Madman," 1967; formed SHB Productions, Inc., prod. "Nightmare at Ghost Beach," 1968; wrote, co-prod, & dir. "Toys Are Not for Children," 1971.

BRAUDY, SUSAN: Executive. e. Bryn Mawr College; taught writing at Brooklyn College (1974). 1970–72, editor and writer at Newsweek; same post at Ms. Magazine, 1973–78. Worked in 1978 for producer Alberto Grimaldi. Has published numerous articles in New York Magazine, New Journal (Yale), The Atlantic, Village Voice, etc. In 1981 appt. Warner Bros. v.p., east coast production. 1981, novel, Who Killed Sal Mineo?, published.

BRAUER, LE ROY: Executive. b. Cincinnati, Ohio, Sept. 30, 1902, e. Col. U. Salesman, Cincinnati Standard Film Service, 1919. Universal, 1921–46, as salesman, branch mgr., Supvsr., China, Japan; br. mgr. New Orleans, other cities, then sales mgr., Europe, Middle East and India. Columbia Pictures, Intl. Corp. 1949–1951. Man. dir. Australia, 1951; chmn. bd., Exotic TV Film Distribs. Pty. Ltd.

BRAUNSTEIN, GEORGE GREGORY: Producer. b. New York City, May 23, 1947. e. Culver Military Academy, Univ. of CA (b.a. biology, chemistry—1970). Father is Jacques Braun-
stein (Screen Televideo Prods. At War with the Army, Young Lions, etc.). 1971, co-founder of The Crystal Jukebox—record productions, music management, music publishing co. Produced 12 hit albums for Decca Records of England and London Records, U.S.A. Entered m.p. production in 1975–76 producing Train Ride to Hollywood for Taylor-Laughlin Co., Pres. of Solar Survival Film Corp. 1981; dir. of acquisitions for Media Home Entertainment (video cassettes), 1980–82.
FILMS: Train Ride to Hollywood, Fade to Black, Surf II.

BRAVERMAN, CHARLES: Producer-Director. b. Los Angeles, Calif., March 3, 1944; e. L.A. City Coll., U. of S. Cal. (BA); m. Kendall Carly Browne, actress. Child actor, 1950–57. Two time Emmy winner.
TV: An American Time Capsule, The Smothers Brothers Racing Team Special, How to Stay Alive, David Hartman . . . Birth and Babies, Breathe a Sigh of Relief, The Television Newsman, Getting Married, The Making of a Live TV Show, Televisionland, Nixon: Checkers to Watergate, Braverman's Condensed Cream of Beatles, Two Cops, Peanuts to the Presidency: The Jimmy Carter Campaign; The Making of Beatlemania, Willie Nelson Plays Lake Tahoe, Tony Bennett Sings, What's Up, America?, The Big Laff Off, Engelbert at the MGM Grand, Oscar's First 50 Years, Frankie Valli Show, The Sixties, Showtime Looks at 1981, Roadshow, Kenny Rodger's America; St. Elsewhere; DTV (Disney Channel); Crazy Like a Fox; Dreams; The Richard Lewis Special; Prince of Bel Air, Brotherhood of Justice (both ABC movies).
PICTURES: Dillinger, Soylent Green, Same Time Next Year (all montages, titles), Can't Stop the Music (titles), Hit and Run (prod./dir.).

BRAVERMAN, MILLICENT: Adv. agency president (Braverman-Mirisch Inc.) KFAC AM & FM, syndicated radio Los Angeles commentator on books, literary critic, publishing specialist, b. New York City, B-M. Inc. founded 1963 to date. General advertising, print and broadcast media nationally.

BRAY, PAUL JR.: e. Rensselaer Polytechnic Institute. Experienced airline transport pilot and instrument flight instructor. Writer and director specializing in motion picture scripts and productions on all phases aviation, engineering and electronic from theoretical to practical industrial personnel training, and for Armed Forces and Vocational-Technical school instruction.

BRAZZI, ROSSANO: Actor. b. Bologna, Italy, 1916. e. U. of Florence. Started career on Italian stage; has appeared in numerous Italian pictures. On US-TV in The Far Pavillions.
PICTURES INCLUDE: (U.S.) Little Women, Three Coins in the Fountain, Barefoot Contessa, Summertime, South Pacific, Light in the Piazza, The Battle of Villa Fiorita, Rome Adventure, Dark Purpose, The Christmas That Almost Wasn't, The Bobo, Woman Times Seven, Krakatoa, East of Java, The Adventurers, Psychout for Murder, The Great Waltz, The Final Conflict, Fear City.

BREACHER, HAROLD: Executive. b. June 17, 1910. e. University of Calif, at L.A., B.A.; Univ. of Southern Calif., LL.B.; Univ. of South Calif., JD. Attorney at Law, 7 years. Bergerman-Breacher Motion Picture Agency, part owner. William Morris Agency, exec. agent; Famous Arts Agency, head Television Dept.; Ashley-Famous Agency, exec. packaging agent; United Artists Pictures Corp., head of sales & distribution United Kingdom, Europe, Middle East and Africa (TV); director, sales, U.K., Europe, Middle East & South Africa, Warner Bros. Television.

BRECHER, IRVING: Writer. b. New York City, Jan. 17, 1914. Yonkers Herald reporter; network programs writer for Milton Berle, Willie Howard, Al Jolson, etc., m.p. writer since 1937.
PICTURES INCLUDE: (collab. s.p.) Shadow of the Thin Man, Best Foot Forward, Meet Me in St. Louis; (collab, adapt.) Summer Holiday: (s.p.), Go West, At the Circus, Du Barry Was a Lady, Yolanda and the Thief, Life of Riley, Somebody Loves Me, Cry for Happy, Bye Bye Birdie, Sail a Crooked Ship.
TV: The Peoples Choice, The Life of Riley.

BREGMAN, MARTIN: Producer-Writer. b. New York City, May 18, 1926. e. Indiana Univ. & NYU.
PICTURES INCLUDE: Serpico, Dog Day Afternoon, The Next Man, The Seduction of Joe Tynan, S*H*E, Simon, The Four Seasons, Venom, Scarface, Sweet Liberty.

BREN, ROBERT J.: Producer, writer. b. Guanajuato, Mex. Film writing debut with "Looking for Trouble" 1934; in U.S. Signal Corps, World War II, also co-ordinator Inter-American Affairs as m.p. program office head, N.Y.C. & Wash. D.C.
PICTURES INCLUDE: This Marriage Business, Crime Ring, Parents on Trail, American Empire, Underground Agent, Charter Pilot, In Old California, Gay Senorita, Five Little Peppers and How They Grew, prod. First Yank into Tokyo, assoc. prod. El Paso, Overland Pacific; Naked Alibi, Treasure of Pancho Villa, The Great Sioux Uprising, Siege at Red River, Without Orders, Maltrata (O.S., S.P., producer) for Bremex Corp., Mexico; Cajeme (O.S., S.P., producer) for Bremex, S.A., Mexico.
TV: Lone Wolf in Mexico, Stolen Train, Casey Jones series. Formed Bremex, indep. picture co., 1963; collab. s.p., Winds of the Four Seasons; collab. s.p., orig. story, The Hawaiians, 1967. Wrote & collaborated on Blood On the Shrine, Legacy in Nylons, Aztec Dagger, Female Menagerie, Tag for Murder.

BRENNAN, EILEEN: Actress. b. Los Angeles, Sept. 3, 1935. Daughter of silent film actress Jean Manahan. e.

Georgetown Univ. American Academy of Dramatic Arts (N.Y.). Big break came with lead in off-Bdwy. musical, Little Mary Sunshine.
PICTURES INCLUDE: Divorce, American Style, The Last Picture Show, Scarecrow, The Sting, Daisy Miller, At Long Last Love, Hustle, Murder by Death, The Cheap Detective, Private Benjamin, Clue.
STAGE: The Miracle Worker (tour), Hello, Dolly! (Bdwy.), and revivals of The King and I, Guys and Dolls, Camelot, Bells Are Ringing, etc. Did one-women revue, An Evening with Eileen Brennan.
TELEVISION: Private Benjamin, Off the Rack.

BRENNER, JOSEPH: Executive. b. Brooklyn, N.Y., Oct. 27, 1918; e. Brooklyn Coll. Started as usher, 1935, becoming mgr., Rogers Theatre, 1936; salesman, Eagle Lion Films, 1946; Screen Guild Prods., 1948; sales mgr., Ellis Films, 1949; formed Joseph Brenner Associates, 1953.

BRESSON, ROBERT: Writer-Director. b. France, Sept. 25, 1907.
PICTURES: Les Anges du Peche, Les Dames du Bois de Boulogne, Le Journal d'un Cure de Campagne, Pickpocket, The Trial of Joan of Arc, Au Hazard Balthasar, Mouchette, Une Femme Douce, Lancelot du Lac, Le Diable Probablement, De Weg Naar Bresson.

BREST, MARTIN: Director. b. Bronx, New York, 1951. e. NY Univ. School of Film. Made award-winning short subject, Hot Dogs for Gauguin. Accepted into fellowship program at American Film Institute, making first feature, Hot Tomorrows, as AFI project.
PICTURES: Going in Style, Beverly Hills Cop.

BREWER, ROY M.: b. Cairo, Neb., Aug. 9, 1909. Was projectionist 1925; chief projectionist, Capitol Theatre, Grand Island, Neb. 1927–39; pres. Nebraska State Fed. of Labor 1933; active in Nebraska labor movement in this period; NRA labor compliance officer for Nebraska 1934–35; campaigned for U.S. Senator George W. Norris in chg. campaign hdqts. 1936; re-elected pres. Nebraska State Federation of Labor 1937; covered legislature for Federation 1939, 1941, 1943; chief, plant & community facilities service War Prod. Bd. Washington 1943–45; apptd. specl. internl. rep. LATSE 1945; then made internl. rep. in Hollywood, rep. Richard F. Walsh, LATSE pres.; exec. ass't Steve Broidy, Allied Artists president, October, 1953; mgr. of br. oper., 1955; apptd. admin. sls. asst. to Edward Morey, vice-pres., Allied Artists, 1962; mgr. prod. dev., 1965. Member: Hollywood AFL Film Council, M.P. Ind. Council, M.P. Alliance, Pres, Pern Char. Committee 1965 Studio mgr. and prod. rep. for West Coast.

BRIAN, DAVID: Actor. b. New York City, Aug. 5, 1914; e. C.C.N.Y. Doorman; chorus boy stage debut in New Moon.
STAGE: You Said It, Bittersweet, Princess Charming, Let 'Em Eat Cake, Crazy Quilt, Beat the Band, Candle in the Wind. By Jupiter and night club singer & dancer; in vaudeville; m.c. in South American night club; served as instructor in U.S. Coast Guard 1942–45; m.p. debut 1949, in Flamingo Road.
PICTURES INCLUDE: Intruder in the Dust, Beyond the Forest, Breakthrough, Damned Don't Cry, Inside Straight, Forth Worth, Inside Walls of Folsom Prison, This Woman is Dangerous, Springfield Rifle, Million Dollar Mermaid, Ambush at Tomahawk Gap, Perilous Journey, Dawn at Socorro, High and the Mighty, Timberjack, Fury at Gunsight Pass, The Rabbit Trap, The Seven Minutes.
TV: Mr. District Attorney.

BRICKMAN, PAUL: Writer/Director. b. Highland Park, IL. e. Claremont Men's college, So. Calif. Worked as camera asst., then story analyst at Paramount, Columbia, and Universal. Debut script: Citizen's Band (1977; also called Hard To Handle). Debut as director with Risky Business (1983).
PICTURES: The Bad News Bears in Breaking Training (s.p.), Risky Business, (dir., s.p.), Deal of the Century (s.p.).

BRIDGES, BEAU: Actor. b. Hollywood, Calif., Dec. 19, 1941. f. Lloyd Bridges; e. U.C.L.A., U. of Hawaii. After several feature film bit parts and more than 80 TV credits, made screen feature debut in The Incident.
PICTURES INCLUDE: For Love of Ivy, Gaily, Gaily, The Landlord, Adam's Woman, The Christian Licorice Store, Hammersmith Is Out, Child's Play, Your Three Minutes Are Up, Lovin' Molly, The Other Side of the Mountain, Dragonfly, Swashbuckler, Two Minute Warning, Greased Lightning, Norma Rae, The Runner Stumbles, Honky Tonk Freeway, Night Crossing, Love Child, The Hotel New Hampshire.
TV: Ensign O'Toole, Sea Hunt, Ben Casey, Dr. Kildare, Mr. Novak, Combat, Eleventh Hour, Space, A Fighting Choice, Outrage.

BRIDGES, JAMES: Actor-Writer-Director. b. Paris, Ark., Appeared as an actor in 50 TV shows and five feature films. Has written 16 plays and is published in New Theatre for Now, 18 hour Hitchcock Shows and one Great Adventure, Go Down Moses. Worked as writer on 14 features. As director, worked in New York, Edinburgh Festival, Mark Taper and Ahmanson in LA.
PICTURES INCLUDE: The Appaloosa (A.P.), Forbin Project (s.p.), The Baby Maker (s.p., dir.), The Paper Chase (s.p., dir.); September 30, 1955 (s.p., dir.); The China Syndrome (dir., co-s.p.); Urban Cowboy (co-s.p., dir.), Mike's Murder (d., s.p.); Perfect (prod., d., s.p.).

BRIDGES, JEFF: Actor. b. Los Angeles, 1951. Made acting debut at eight in the TV Sea Hunt series of his father, Lloyd Bridges. Acted also in Lloyd Bridges Show. At 14 toured New England with father in stock production Anniversary Waltz. Studied acting with Uta Hagen in New York. Brother of actor Beau Bridges.
PICTURES: The Last Picture Show, Fat City, Bad Company, Lolly Madonna (XXX), The Last American Hero, The Iceman Cometh, Thunderbolt and Lightfoot, Rancho Deluxe, Hearts of the West, Stay Hungry, King Kong, Somebody Killed Her Husband, Winter Kills, Heaven's Gate, Cutter and Bone, Tron, Kiss Me Goodbye. Against All Odds, Starman, Jagged Edge, 8 Million Ways To Die, The Morning After.

BRIDGES, LLOYD: Actor. b. San Leandro, California, January 15, 1913. Went into stock from college dramatics.
PICTURES INCLUDE: Miss Susie Slagles's, Abilene Town, Canyon Passage, Ramrod, Trouble with Women, Hideout, Calamity Jane and Sam Bass, Trapped, Rocketship XM, Try and Get Me, Colt .45, Three Steps North, Whistle at Eaton Falls, Last of the Comanches, High Noon, Plymouth Adventure, Tall Texan, Kid from Left Field, City of Bad Men, Limping Man, Pride of the Blue Grass, Deadly Game, Apache Woman, Wichita, Wetbacks, The Rainmaker, Daring Game, The Goddess, The Happy Ending, Silent Night, Lonely Night, Airplane!
TELEVISION: Sea Hunt, The Loner, Movieola, The Blue and the Gray, George Washington, Dress Gray, North & South Book II.

BRIEN, LIGE: Executive, b. Pittsburgh, Pa., Mar. 23; e. U. Pittsburgh, B.A. Asst. theatre mgr. 1937; theatre mgr. (Pa.); winner of many prizes for publicity, exploitation, grosses; winner of M.P. Herald Bronze Grand Award 1939, Silver Award 1944 & War Showmanship Award; press-book ed. PRC Pictures 1945, appt'd exploitaton mgr., 1946; since exploit. mgr. Eagle Lion Classics; to U.A. as dir., spcl. events, April, 1951. Pres. AMPA, 153–54; asst. exploitation mgr., 20th Fox, 1960; nat'l dir. mdsg., Paramount Pictures, 1961–65; Expl. Dir., Seven Arts Pictures. (Warner Bros.). Exploitation liaison between Hollywood studio and New York offices, 1982, started new co., Golden Triangle Promotions.

BRIGHT, RICHARD S.: Executive. b. New Rochelle, N.Y., Feb. 28, 1936. e. Hotchkiss School (1953–54); Wharton School of Finance, Univ. of Penna. (1954–58). With U.S. Army Finance Corp., 1959–60. Was corporate exec. prior to founding in 1973 Persky-Bright Organization, private investment group to finance films. Now bd. chm., Persky-Bright Productions, Inc.; adjunct professor at Columbia Univ. School of Fine Arts.
PICTURES INCLUDE: Last Detail, Golden Voyage of Sinbad, For Pete's Sake, California Split, The Man Who Would Be King, Funny Lady, The Front, and Equus. Financing/production services for: Hard Times, Taxi Driver, Missouri Breaks, Bound for Glory, Sinbad and the Eye of the Tiger, Hair, Still of the Night. Executive Producer: Tribute.
TELEVISION: The President's Mistress (co-produced), a CBS Television feature.
STAGE: A History of the American Film (1978); Album (Off-Broadway Co-produced) 1980; Currently preparing with James Nederlander for Broadway, Dennis The Menace.

BRIGHTMAN, HOMER H.: Writer b. Port Townsend, Washington. e. at the Washington State Nautical School-ship. Apprentice at 14, spent 10 years at sea as 2nd and 3rd officer; claims dept., Dollar Steamship Lines Shanghai, Hong Kong, Singapore: Academy Award for short Lend a Paw 1939; assoc. Walt Disney Prod. 13 years; created It's A Dog's Life, TV show; animated cartoon shorts for MGM, Walter Lantz, U.P.A.
PICTURES INCLUDE: Saludos Amigos, Three Caballeros, Make Mine Music, Fun and Fancy Free, Melody Time, Cinderella. Writer (collab.) TV shorts.

BRINKLEY, DAVID: TV News Correspondent. b. Wilmington, N.C., July 10, 1920. Started writing for hometown newspaper; attended Univ. of N.C., Vanderbilt University. Joined United Press before entering Army, World War II. After discharge in 1943 joined NBC News in Washington as White House corr. Co-chm. for many years with late Chet Huntley on NBC Nightly News. Now delivers personal reports (David Brinkley's Journal) on same program.

BRISKIN, MORT: Producer-Writer. b. Oak Park, Ill. e. Univ. of So. Calif. Attended Harvard and Northwestern law schools, being admitted to the Bar at 20. Practiced law before entering m.p. industry in management with such stars as Mickey Rooney. Turned to production and also wrote screenplays for 16 of his 29 films. Created nine TV series and was prod. or exec. prod. of some 1,350 TV segments of which he wrote more than 300.

PICTURES INCLUDE: The River, The Magic Face, No Time for Flowers, The Second Woman, Quicksand, The Big Wheel, The Jackie Robinson Story, Ben, Williard, Walking Tall, Framed.

TV: Sheriff of Cochise, U.S. Marshal, The Texan, Grand Jury, The Walter Winchell File, Official Detective, Whirlybirds.

BRITTANY, MORGAN: b. Hollywood, CA, Dec. 5, 1951. r.n. Suzanne Cupito.

PICTURES: Marnie, The Birds, Gypsy, Gable and Lombard, etc.

TELEVISION: Series: Dallas. Movies: Amazing Howard Hughes, Delta County, Going Home Again, The Dream Merchants, Moviola, etc.

BRITTON, TONY: Actor, b. Birmingham, England, 1924; e. Thornbury Grammar School, Glos. Early career as clerk and in repertory; TV debut, 1952, The Six Proud Walkers (serial), m.p. debut, 1955 in Loser Takes All.

PLAYS INCLUDE: The Guv'nor, Romeo and Juliet, The Scarlet Pimpernel, The Other Man, The Dashing White Sergeant, Importance of Being Earnest, An Ideal Husband, School for Scandal, A Dream of Treason, That Lady, The Private Lives of Edward Whiteley, Affairs of State, The Night of The Ball, Gigi, The Seagull, Henry IV Part 1, Kill Two Birds, Cactus Flower, A Woman of No Importance, The Boston Story, Lady Frederick, My Fair Lady, Move Over Mrs. Markham, No No Nanette, Dame of Sark, The Chairman.

PICTURES INCLUDE: Birthday Present, Behind the Mask, Operation Amsterdam, The Heart of a Man, The Rough and the Smooth, The Risk, The Horsemasters, Stork Talk, The Break, There's a Girl in My Soup, Forbush and The Penguins, Sunday Bloody Sunday, Night Watch, The Day of the Jackal.

TV: Melissa series, Father Dear Father series, The Man Who Understood Women, Ooh La La, Call My Bluff, The Nearly Man.

BROADNAX, DAVID: Producer-Writer-Actor. b. Columbus, GA, Dec. 16. PICTURES: The Landlord (act.), Come Back Charleston Blue (act.), Sharpies (prod., co-s.p., act.), Zombie Island Massacre (prod., act., original story).

TELEVISION: As the World Turns, Another World, Edge of Night, Love Is a Many Splendored Thing, Search for Tomorrow.

BROCCOLI, ALBERT: Producer. b. New York City, April 5, 1909, e. C.C.N.Y. Agriculturist in early years; entered m.p. ind. as asst. director, 20th Century-Fox, 1938.

PRODUCTIONS INCLUDE: Red Beret (Paratrooper), Hell Below Zero, Black Knight, Prize of Gold, Cockleshell Heroes, Safari, Zarak, Pickup Alley, Fire Down Below, Odongo, High Flight, No Time to Die, The Man Inside, Idle on Parade, Adamson of Africa, Bandit of Zhobe, Jazz Boat, In the Nick, Let's Get Married, The Trials of Oscar Wilde, Johnny Nobody, Carolina, Dr. No, Call Me Bwana, From Russia With Love, Goldfinger, Thunderball, You Only Live Twice, Chitty Chitty Bang Bang, On Her Majesty's Secret Service, Diamonds Are Forever, Live and Let Die, The Man With The Golden Gun, The Spy Who Loved Me, Moonraker, For Your Eyes Only, Octopussy, A View to a Kill.

BROCKMAN, MICHAEL: Executive. e. Ithaca Coll. Joined ABC as v.p., daytime programming, ABC Entertainment, 1974; later v.p., tape prod. operations and admin. Left to become v.p., daytime programs, NBC Entertainment, 1977.

BRODERICK, MATTHEW: Actor. Theatrical film debut in Max Dugan Returns. (1983).

PICTURES: WarGames, Ladyhawke, 1918, On Valentine's Day, Ferris Bueller's Day Off, Project X.

STAGE: Brighton Beach Memoirs (Tony Award), Biloxi Blues.

TELEVISION: Master Harold . . . and the Boys.

BRODKIN, HERBERT: Producer. b. New York, N.Y., Nov. 9, 1912. e. Michigan U., Yale Drama School, U.S Army, World War II; then scenery designer, prod. mgr., dir., summer stock; designer, dir., prod. mgr., Broadway theatres; prod. exec., Paramount, Universal; prod., designer, Charlie Wild Private Detective, CBS-TV; prod., ABC, 1951.

TV: Album, TV Hour, Motorola TV Hour, Center Stage, Elgin Hour, Goodyear Playhouse, Alcoa Hour, Sebastian.

BRODNEY, OSCAR: Writer, Producer. b. Boston, Mass., e. Boston U., LLB, 1927; Harvard, LLM, 1928. Atty., Mass. Bar, 1928–35.

PICTURES INCLUDE: She Wrote the Book, If You Knew Susie, Are You With It?, For the Love of Mary, Mexican Hayride, Arctic Manhunt, Yes Sire, That's My Baby, Double Crossbone, Gal Who Took the West, South Sea Sinner, Comanche Territory, Harvey; story, Frenchie, Francis Goes to the Races, Little Egypt, Francis Covers the Big Town, Willie & Joe Back at the Front, Scarlet Angel, Francis Goes to West Point, Walking My Baby Back Home, Sign of the Pagan, Glenn Miller Story, Black Shield of Falworth, Captain Lightfoot, The Spoilers, Purple Mask, Lady Godiva, Day of Fury, Star in the Dust, Tammy and the Bachelor, When Hell Broke Loose, Bobkins, Tammy Tell Me True, The Right Approach, All Hands on Deck, Tammy and the Doctor, The Brass Bottle, I'd Rather Be Rich.

BRODSHAUG, MELVIN: Producer. b. Davenport, N.D., May 22, 1900; e. No. Dakota State University, B.S., 1923; Litt.D. 1958 Chicago U., M.A. 1927, Columbia U., Ph.D. 1931; Supt. of Schools, Arnegard, N.D. 1923–28; research assoc. Erpi Classroom Films 1930; apptd. dir. research Encyclopedia Britannica Films Inc., apptd. vice-pres. 1945, in chg. of product development; apptd. member bd. dir. 1951, Dean of Boston U. Sch. of Public Relations & Communications, 1954–62,dir., Boston U film library, 1962–65. Prof. and consultant, Norfolk State Coll., Va., 1965–70; independent educational film producer 1970.

BRODSKY, JACK: Producer. b. Brooklyn, N.Y. e. George Washington High School. Writer for N.Y. Times; joined 20th-Fox publicity in N.Y. in 1956. Left in 1961 to head national ad-pub for Filmways. Joined Rastar Productions to work on "Funny Girl"; later named v.p. in charge of prod. In 1976 named v.p. in chg. film prod. prom., Rogers & Cowan; 1978, Columbia Pictures v.p., adv., pub., promo.; 1979, named exec. v.p. of Michael Douglas' Big Stick Productions; 1983; joined 20th-Fox as exec. v.p., worldwide adv., pub., exploit. Resigned 1985 to resume career as producer.

PICTURES INCLUDE: Little Murders, Everything You Always Wanted To Know About Sex (exec. prod.), Summer Wishes, Winter Dreams, Jewel of the Nile.

AUTHOR: The Cleopatra Papers, with Nat Weiss.

BROKAW, NORMAN R.: Executive. b. April 21, 1927, New York City. Joined William Morris Agency as trainee, in 1943, junior agent, 1948; sr. agent, company exec. in m.p. and TV, 1951; 1974, v.p., William Morris Agency, World Wide all areas. 1981, named exec. v.p. & member of board, William Morris Agency, worldwide; 1986, named co-chm. of bd., WMA, worldwide. Member Academy of TV Arts & Sciences, Academy M.P. Arts & Sciences. Member bd. of dir. of Cedars-Sinai Medical Center, Los Angeles; pres., The Betty Ford Cancer Center. Clients include President and Mrs. Gerald R. Ford.

BROKAW, TOM: TV Host—Anchorman. b. 1940. e. Univ. of So. Dakota. Joined KMTV, NBC affiliate in Omaha, in 1962; 1965, joined WSB-TV, Atlanta. Worked in L.A. bureau of NBC News, anchored local news shows for KNBC, NBC station (1966–73). In 1973 named NBC News' White House correspondent; was anchorman of NBC Saturday Night News. Named host of Today show in August, 1976. In 1982 co-anchor, NBC Nightly News.

BROLIN, JAMES: Actor. b. Los Angeles, July 10, 1942. e. UCLA. Debut in Bus Stop (TV series); named most Promising Actor of 1970 by Fame and Photoplay magazines.

PICTURES INCLUDE: Take Her She's Mine, Goodbye, Charlie, Von Ryan's Express, Morituri, Our Man Flint, The Boston Strangler, Skyjacked, West World, Gable and Lombard, The Car, Capricorn One, The Amityville Horror.

TV: The Monroes, Marcus Welby, M.D., (Emmy award), Short Walk to Daylight, Class of '63, Hotel, Beverly Hills Cowgirl Blues.

BROMFIELD, JOHN: Actor. r.n. Farron Bromfield; b. South Bend, Ind., June 11, 1922; e. St. Mary's College. College football star. Served in U.S. Navy, medical discharge; worked as tuna fisherman. Film debut in Harpoon, 1948; under contract to Hal Wallis.

PICTURES INCLUDE: Sorry Wrong Number, Harpoon, Rope of Sand, Hold That Line, Flat Top, Easy to Love, Ring of Fear, Black Dakotas, Revenge of the Creature, Big Bluff, Three Bad Sisters, Manfish, Crime Against Joe, Quincannon Frontier Scout, Hot Cars.

BROMHEAD, DAVID M.: Executive. b. Teaneck, NJ, Jan. 7, 1960. e. Leighton Park School, Reading, England, (1973–78). Overseas sls. exec., Rank Film Dist., 1980; joined New World Pictures, 1984, dir. intl. dist.; named dir., TV dist., 1986.

BROMHEAD, MICHAEL: Executive. b London, England, May 30, 1924. e. Charterhouse and St. John's College, Cambridge, RAF pilot during war, Ent. m.p. ind. 1947, with Eagle-Lion; resigned, 1950. Appt. overseas man. Independent Film Dist.; dir. One World Film Dist. 1953; dir. Lion International Films, 1955; New York rep. Lion International, 1958; pres., Lion International Films, Inc., 1959; general manager Lion International Films, 1962; dir. London Independent Producers, Ltd.; man. dir., Alliance Intl. Film Distribs., Ltd., 1966. Dir. EMI Film Dist., 1970. Dir., gen. mgr., 1971; appt. dir. overseas dist., 1975; dir., EMI Film Theatre

Corp., man. dir., Thorn. EMI Film Dist. Ltd., 1979; v.p., mktg. & dist., Thorn EMI Screen Entertainment, Inc., 1984.

BRON, ELEANOR: Actress. Started career in Establishment Club, London, and on American tour. Leading lady on British TV show Not So Much A Programme, More a Way of Life.
PICTRUES INCLUDE: Help, Alfie, Two For The Road, Bedazzled, Women in Love, The Millstone.
THEATRE: The Doctor's Dilemma, Howard's End, The Prime of Miss Jean Brodie.

BRONDFIELD, JEROME: b. Cleveland, O., Dec. 9, 1913; e. Ohio State U., 1936. Reporter, ed. on Columbus Dispatch, Associated Press, story ed., script head, RKO Pathe, Oct., 1944; writer, dir. & supvr. of many doc. shorts incl. This Is America series; TV writer; short story writer; collab. s.p., Below the Sahara; s.p. Louisiana Territory; doc. film writer; Author, Woody Hayes, The 100-Yard War, Knute Rockne, The Man & the Legend.

BRONSON, CHARLES: Actor. b. Penn., 1920. m. Jill Ireland, actress. Worked as a coal miner. Starred on his own TV series Meet McGraw.
PICTURES INCLUDE: Red Skies of Montana, Pat and Mike, House of Wax, Drumbeat, Vera Cruz, Jubel, Lonely Are the Brave, Machine Gun Kelly, Never So Few, A Thunder of Drums, The Magnificent Seven, The Great Escape, The Sandpiper, The Battle of the Bulge, Pancho Villa, The Dirty Dozen, This Property is Condemned, Once Upon a Time in the West, Goodbye, Friend, Rider in the Rain, You Can't Win Em All, Someone Behind the Door, Red Sun, Chato's Land, The Mechanic, The Valachi Papers, The Stone Killer, Mr. Majestyk, Death Wish, Breakout, Hard Times, Breakheart Pass, From Noon Till Three, St. Ives, The White Buffalo, Telefon, Borderline, Caboblanco, Death Hunt, Death Wish II, The Evil That Men Do, Death Wish 3, Murphy's Law.
TELEVISION: Act of Vengeance.

BRONSTON, SAMUEL: Producer. b. Russia; e Sorbonne, Paris. Film distributor, Paris; prod. exec. Columbia Studios, Hollywood; Martin Eden, City Without Men, Producer, Columbia Pictures; resigned to form Samuel Bronston Pict., Inc.; exec. prod. Jack London, A Walk in the Sun. color documentaries produced first time in Vatican; prod. John Paul Jones 1959; Received U.S. Navy Meritorious Pub. Serv. Citation; pres. Samuel Bronston Productions; 1960 prod. King of Kings, El Cid; 1962, 55 Days at Peking; 1963. The Fall of the Roman Empire; prod. Circus World, 1964, Condor Award, Society for Pan American Culture—for El Cid, 1962 (Award shared with Stanford University), The Hollywood Foreign Press Association Golden Globe for the achievement of his outstanding production of El Cid, 1962, Italian Order of Merit with Medal of Commendatore. Grand Cross of Merit by the Equestrian Order of the Knights of the Holy Sepulchre. (The highest honor of the Catholic Church), The Encomienda of the Order of the Great Cross of Isabel la Catolica. President Samuel Bronston Studios, Madrid, Spain.

BROOK, PETER: Director. b. London, England, March 21, 1925. e. Magdalen Coll., Oxford. Gained fame as stage director before doing films. (Man and Superman, Marat/Sade, A Midsummer Night's Dream, etc.)
PICTURES INCLUDE: The Beggar's Opera, Moderato Cantabile, Lord of the Flies, Marat/Sade, Tell Me Lies, King Lear, Meetings with Remarkable Men.

BROOKE, PETER R.: Writer. b. Berlin, Germany, April 12, 1929. e. Germany, Switzerland, England. With Warner Bros., 1944–46, mail room, pub.. dept., then asst. casting dir.; contract writer, Robert Riskin Prod., Paramount; then free lance; radio writer many shows; TV writer for Teevee Prod., Celebrity Playhouse, Science Fiction Theatre; staff writer, Universal Pictures; left Universal to join Excelsior under new banner of Warbrook Inc. as writer-producer.
PICTURES INCLUDE: Basketball Fix, Sweet Violence orig., Outside the Law.
TV: Sea Hunt, 77 Sunset Strip, Sugar Foot, The Fugitive, Six Million Dollar Man.

BROOKS, DICK: Executive, b. New York, N.Y., e. U. of Georgia; reporter, Atlanta (Ga.) Journal; sports ed. Gainesville Times; correspondent, Pacific Stars & Stripes; entered m.p. industry as staff writer, 20th Century-Fox pub. dept; nat'l pub. dir, Seven Arts Productions, Paramount pub. mgr.; nat'l pub. dir. 20th Century-Fox; adv-pub. dir, Rastar Prods; Warner Bros. pub. dir; formed Dick Brooks Unlimited, Beverly Hills entertainment p.r. company 1980.

BROOKS, JAMES L.: Director-Producer-Writer. b. North Bergen, NJ. e. NY Univ. Copyboy for CBS News, NY; promoted to newswriter. 1965 moved to L.A. to work for David Wolper's documentary prod. co. 1969 conceived idea for series, Room 222; formed partnership with fellow writer Allan Burns. Together they created Mary Tyler Moore Show in 1970. 1977, established prod. co. on Paramount lot with other writers, producing and creating the series, The Associates and Taxi.
PICTURES: Starting Over (s.p.); Terms of Endearment (dir., prod., s.p.).

BROOKS, JOSEPH: Producer-Director-Writer-Composer-Conductor. Well-known for composing music for TV commercials before turning to producing, directing, writing and scoring theatrical feature, You Light Up My Life, in 1977. Winner of 21 Clio Awards (made by adv. industry); created music for 100 commercials. Has also composed for theatrical films.
PICTURES INCLUDE: Scores: The Garden of the Finzi Continis, Marjoe, Jeremy, The Lords of Flatbush. Produced, directed, wrote, and composed, arranged and conducted music for You Light Up My Life. Produced, directed, wrote starred in and composed music for If Ever I See You Again.

BROOKS, MEL: Writer-Director-Actor. b. Brooklyn, 1926. m. actress Anne Bancroft. As child did impressions and was amateur drummer and pianist. First appearance as actor in Golden Boy in Redbank, N.J. Was also director and social director in the Catskills. Became writer for Sid Caesar on TV's Broadway Review and Your Show of Shows, writing for latter for decade. Teamed with Carl Reiner for comedy record album, 2000 Year Old Man and The 2000 and 13 Year Old Man.
PICTURES INCLUDE: The Critic (short, s.p.-narrator), The Producers, The Twelve Chairs, Blazing Saddles, Young Frankenstein, Silent Movie, High Anxiety (prod., dir., s.p.). History of the World—Part 1 (prod., dir., s.p., actor, composer), To Be Or Not To Be (prod., actor).
TV: Get Smart (writer), When Things Were Rotten (creator).
STAGE: Shinbone Alley, All-American (books for musicals).

BROOKS, RICHARD: Writer, director. b. Philadelphia, May 18, 1912; e. Temple Univ.; Radio writer, narrator and commentator, NBC. Author of several short stories. Novels, Brick Fox Hole, Boiling Point, The Producer.
PICTURES INCLUDE: Swell Guy, Brute Force, To the Victor, Crossfire, Key Largo, Mystery Street, Storm Warning, Deadline U.S.A., Battle Circus, Take The High Ground, Flame and the Flesh, Last Time I Saw Paris, Blackboard Jungle, Last Hunt, Catered Affair, Something of Value, The Brothers Karamazov, Cat on A Hot Tin Roof, Elmer Gantry (Academy Award for s.p. 1961); Sweet Bird of Youth, writer, Lord Jim, The Professionals, In Cold Blood, The Happy Ending, Dollars, Bite the Bullet, Looking for Mr. Goodbar, Wrong Is Right (also prod.), Fever Pitch (also prod.).

BROSNAN, PIERCE: Actor. b. Ireland, May 16, 1953. On stage in London (Wait Until Dark, The Red Devil Battery Sign, etc.)
PICTURES: The Mirror Crack'd, The Long Good Friday, Nomads.
TELEVISION: Murphy's Stroke, The Manions of America, Nancy Astor, Remington Steele.

BROUGHTON, BRUCE: Composer. b. Los Angeles, Mar. 8, 1945. e. Univ. of So. Calif. (BM, 1967). Music supvr., CBS-TV, 1967–77. Since then has been freelance composer for TV and films. Member: Academy of TV Arts & Sciences; Society of Composers & Lyricists, Academy of Motion Picture Arts & Sciences. Nominated 11 times for Emmy; won in 1981 for Buck Rogers, in 1983 for Dallas and in 1984 for Dallas and The First Olympics. Nominated in 86 for Oscar for Silverado.
TELEVISION: Series: Hawaii Five-O, Gunsmoke, Quincy, How the West Was Won, Logan's Run, The Oregon Trail, Buck Rogers, Dallas. Movies: The Paradise Connection, Desperate Voyage, The Return of Frank Cannon, Desperate Lives, Killjoy, One Shoe Makes It Murder, The Master of Ballantrae, MADD, The Candy Lightner Story, Cowboy. Mini-Series: The Blue and the Gray, The First Olympics–Athens: 1896.
PICTURES: The Prodigal, The Ice Pirates, Silverado, Young Sherlock Holmes, Sweet Liberty, The Boy Who Could Fly.

BROUMAS, JOHN G.: Exec. b. Youngstown, O. Oct. 12, 1917, e. Youngstown, O. usher, Altoona Publix Theatres, 1933, usher to asst. mgr., Warner Thea. 1934–39; mgr. Grand 1939–40; mgr. Orpheum 1940–41. WW-II active, Officer Chemical Corps, past commander 453rd Chem. Grp. (Reserve); Member Reserve Officers Assoc.; Gen. mgr. Pitts & Roth Theatres 1946–54; President, Broumas Theatres; bd. govnrs., Variety Club, Tent No. 11, 1959–73; Wash., first asst. chief barker, 1964 & 1971; chief barker, 1965–1966, 1972 V.P.T.O.A. 1965; V.P. NATO, 1969; past pres. & bd. chmn. Maryland Theatre Owners; bd. of directors of NATO of Va., Md., D.C.; pres., Broumas Theatre Service; bd. chmn., Showcase Theatres; mem. bd., Foundation of Religious Action (FRASCO). Mem. Nat'l Immigration Comm. Founder of John G. Broumas Scholarship for Drama at Youngstown State Univ.; past pres. & Board Chairman Maryland Theatre Owners; v.p. & bd. of dir.—Virginia

Theatre Owners bd. of dir. NATO of D.C.; pres. B.C. Theatres; Sponsor of Andre G. Broumas Memorial Award—West Point; pres., McLean Theatre Corp.; member, Motion Picture Pioneers; sponsor, Broumas Scholastic and Athletic Scholarship for AHEPA Wash. D.C. area; director, McLean Bank McLean, Va.; honorary member, West Point Class 1954; Secretary-Treasurer, Tenley Circle Twin Theatre Corp.; President, Cinema Mgt. Corp; Director: Motion Picture Pioneers; Advisory Council: Will Rogers Memorial Hospital; Chief Barker: Washington, D.C. Variety Club, Tent #11, 1978–79 and bd. chmn., 1980; Life Patron, Variety Clubs Int'l., 1978; AHEPA Humanitarian Award, 1981; Dept. of Army, Patriotic Civilian Service Medal, 1982; WOMPI "good guy" award, 1974; Gold Medal for distinguished service to m.p. industry, 1978; bd. chm., Tantaloon Country Club, Oxon Hill, MD.; Chm. bd., McLean Bank.

BROWN, BLAIR: Actress. b. Washington, D.C., 1948. e. Pine Manor.
PICTURES: The Choirboys, One-Trick Pony, Altered States, Continental Divide, Flash of Green.

BROWN, BRYAN: Actor. b. Australia. Began acting professionally in Sydney. Worked in repertory theatres in England with the National Theatre of Great Britain. Returned to Australia to work in films while continuing stage work with Theatre Australia. Theatrical film debut, Love Letters from Teralba Road (1977).
PICTURES: The Irishman, Weekend of Shadows, Newsfront, Third Person Plural, Money Movers, Palm Beach, Cathy's Child, The Odd Angry Shot, Breaker Morant, Blood Money, Stir, Winter of Our Dreams, Far East, F/X, Tai-Pan.
TELEVISION: Mini-series: Against the Wind, A Town Like Alice, The Thorn Birds.

BROWN, CLARENCE: Director. b. Clinton, Mass., May 10, 1890; e. U. Tenn. Aviator, U.S. Army, World War I. Engineer, automobile industry; formed Brown Motor Co., Birmingham, Ala. To Hollywood 1915 as asst. to dir. Maurice Tourneur for whom he directed his first picture. The Great Redeemer. Joined MGM 1924. Launched Greta Garbo as star in Flesh and the Devil; other pictures with Garbo are Woman of Affairs, Anna Christie, Romance, Inspiration, Anna Karenina, Conquest.
PICTURES INCLUDE: The Eagle, Kiki, Night Flight, Sadie McKee, Ah, Wilderness!, Wife vs. Secretary, The Gorgeous Hussy, Of Human Hearts, Idiot's Delight, Edison the Man, The Human Comedy, White Cliffs of Dover, National Velvet, Letty Lynton, Possessed, Trial of '98, The Rains Came, The Human Comedy, Song of Love, Intruder in the Dust, To Please a Lady, Angels in the Outfield, When in Rome, The Yearling, Plymouth Adventure, The Secret Garden, Never Let Me Go.

BROWN, DAVID: Executive and Producer. b. New York, N.Y., July 28, 1916; e. Stanford U., A.B., 1936; Columbia U. (school of Journalism), M.S., 1937. Apprentice reporter, copy-editing, San Francisco News & Wall St. Journal, 1936; night ed. asst. drama critic, Fairchild Publications, N.Y., 1937–39; edit. dir. Milk Research Council, N.Y., 1939–40; assoc. ed., Street & Smith Publ., N.Y., 1940–43; assoc. ed., exec. ed., then ed.-in-chief, Liberty Mag., N.Y., 1943–49; edit. dir., nat'l education campaign, Amer. Medical Assn., 1949; assoc. ed., man. ed., Cosmopolitan Mag., N.Y., 1949–52; contrib. stories & articles to many nat'l mags.; man. ed., story dept., 20th-Fox, L.A., Jan., 1952; story ed. & head of scenario dept., May, 1953–56; appt'd. member of exec. staff of Darryl F. Zanuck, 1956; mem. of exec. staff, 20th-Fox studios, and exec. studio story editor, 1956–1960; Prod. 20th-Fox Studios, Sept. 1960–62; Editorial v.p. New American Library of World Literature, Inc., 1963–64; exec. story opers., 20th Century-Fox, 1964–67; vp. dir. of story operations, 1967; exec. vice-pres., creative operations and members, Board of Directors, 1969–71. Exec. v.p., member board of directors Warner Bros., 1971–1972; partner and director, The Zanuck/Brown Co., 1972; mbr., bd. of trustees, American Film Institute, 1972–80.
FILMS INCLUDE: The Sugarland Express, The Black Windmill, Sssssss, The Eiger Sanction, The Sting, MacArthur, Jaws, Jaws 2, Willie Dynamite, The Girl from Petrovka, The Island, Neighbors, The Verdict, Cocoon, Target.

BROWN, HAROLD: Executive. Pres., International Picture Show Co. since Dec., 1980. Previously pres., American International TV; v.p. & bd. mbr., American International Pictures (now Filmways).

BROWN, HARRY: Writer. b. Portland, Me., April 30, 1917. e. Harvard. With The New Yorker 1940; U.S. Army 1941–45.
PICTURES INCLUDE: (collab:) True Glory 1944, Walk in the Sun 1945, The Other Love, Arch of Triumph 1947; Wake of Red Witch, Man on Eiffel Tower, Sands of Iwo Jima (s.p.), Kiss Tomorrow Goodbye, Only the Valiant, Bugles in Afternoon, Place in the Sun (orig. story;) Academy Award collab., Apache Drums, The Sniper, Eight Iron Men, All the Brothers Were Valiant, Many Rivers to Cross, Virgin Queen, D-Day the Sixth of June, Between Heaven and Hell, Ocean's 11, El Dorado.

BROWN, HENRY: Executive. b. New York, N.Y., Feb. 18, 1899; e. C.C.N.Y., 1920; Columbia University, 1923. pres., Lakewood Amusement Corp.; pres., Atlas TV Corp.; pres. Capt. Zero Prods., Inc.

BROWN, HINMAN: M.P. Producer & director, b. N.Y.C. July 21, 1910; e. C.C.N.Y., St. Lawrence Univ. Radio & TV package prod. since 1927 include: Inner Sanctum, Thin Man, Bulldog Drummond, Dick Tracy, Terry and the Pirates, Joyce Jordan MD, Grand Central Station, CBS Radio Mystery Theatre, pres. Production Center, Inc.
PICTURES INCLUDE: That Night, Violators, The Stars Salute, The Price of Silence, The Road Ahead.

BROWN, HOWARD C.: Executive. b. Newport, N.H., Aug. 15, 1901. e. Boston U. Assoc. with Technicolor Motion Picture Corp., Before org. Colorart Pictures, 1926. Merged with Synchrotone Pictures & Kennedy Pictures, 1929, forming Colorart Synchrotone Corp. In 1930 org. Brown-Nagel Productions. Since 1933 has produced numerous shorts. Sales mgr., Cinecolor, 1936–37; pres. Howard C. Brown Co. 1937–1938. Sales mgr., Trimble Laboratories, Inc. 1947; formed Howard C. Brown Productions 1948, to release for United Artists. Prod. Kangaroo Kid; prod. Mating Urge, inter-nations, documentary; 1969, Film Exporter.

BROWN, JIM: Actor. b. St. Simons Island, Feb. 17, 1936. e. Manhasset H.S., Syracuse U. For nine years played football with Cleveland Browns; in 1964 won Hickock Belt as Professional Athlete of the year; founder, Black Economic Union.
PICTURES INCLUDE: Rio Conchos, The Dirty Dozen, Ice Station Zebra, The Split, Riot, Dark Of The Sun, 100 Rifles, Kenner, Tick . . . Tick . . . Tick, The Grasshopper, Slaughter, Slaughter's Big Rip-Off, I Escaped from Devil's Island, The Slams, Three the Hard Way, Take a Hard Ride.

BROWN, TOM: Actor. b. New York City, Jan. 6, 1913; son of Harry Brown, actor-producer, and Marie Francis, actress; e. N.Y. Prof. Children's School. On radio, then dram. stage (Neighbors, Many a Slip, Pardon My Glove, etc.). Screen debut in A Lady Lies, 1929.
PICTURES INCLUDE: Buck Privates Come Home, Duke of Chicago, Operation Haylift, Fireman Save My Child.
TV: General Hospital.

BROWN, WILLIAM: Executive. b. Ayr, Scotland, June 24, 1929. e. Ayr Academy, University of Edinburgh, where graduated Bachelor of Commerce 1950. Served to Lieutenant, Royal Artillery, 1950–52. Sales mgr. for Scotland Television Ltd. in London, England, 1958 to 1961, sales director 1961 to 1963. Deputy mng. dir. of Scottish Television Ltd. at Glasgow 1963–66, mng. dir. in 1966. Deputy chm. and mng.-dir. of STV from 1974. Director, independent TV Publications, London, England, 1968. On board of directors for Scottish National Orchestra, 1973. Member of Independent TV Companies Association, and chairman of same 1978–80. Holds C.B.E. honor from British Royalty.

BROWN, WILLIAM H., JR.: Director, concert mgr., Juilliard School of Music, 1946; TV prod., Young and Rubicam, 1948; dir., Life with Father, Climax, CBS-TV, 1954, Studio One 1955; prod. Paramount Television, 1958; Exec. prod., Shirley Temple Show, NBC, 1960; TV prod., Norman, Craig and Kummel, 1962; Compton, 1963; Post-Keyes-Gardner, 1965; Free lance, 1967.

BROWN, WILLET HENRY: Executive. Assist. gen. mgr., Don Lee, Inc., 1932–33; exec. v.p. Don Lee Broadcasting System, Hollywood, 1938–48; pres. Don Lee Broadcasting System, 1949–58; consultant, R.K.O. General Inc.: pres. Don Lee, Inc. pres. Laurie Leasing Corp.: pres. Pacific States Invest. Corp.: pres. Hillcrest Motor Company: pres., KGB INC, KGB-AM and KGB-FM, San Diego, Calif.: pres. bd. and dir. of KXOA, Inc., KXOA, AM and KXOA-FM, Sacramento, Calif.; gen. partner, Brown Bdcstng. Co., operating KYNO FM & AM, Fresno and KKAT-FM, Salt Lake City.

BROWNE, CORAL: Actress. b. Melbourne, Australia, July 23, 1913. Wife of Vincent Price. Theatre includes Mated, The Golden Gander, Death Asks a Verdict, The Man Who Came to Dinner, The Rehearsal, Lady Windermere's Fan, What the Butler Saw, The Waltz of the Toreadors, etc.
PICTURES: The Amateur Gentlemen, Pygmalion, The Prime Minister, Quartet, Madeleine, All at Sea, Rooney, The Ruling Class, The Killing of Sister George, The Drowning Pool, American Dreamer, Dreamchild, etc.
TELEVISION: Time Express, An Englishman Abroad, etc.

BROWNE, ROSCOE LEE: Actor, director, writer. b. Woodbury, N.J., 1925. e. Lincoln University, Pa. Post graduate studies in comparative literature and French at Middlebury College, Vermont, and Columbia U., N.Y. Taught French and lit. at Lincoln U. until 1952. National sales rep. for Schenley

Import Corp. 1946–56; he was one of the United States' international track stars and a member of ten A.A.U. teams. He was twice American champion in the 1000-yard indoor competition, twice all-American and, in 1951 in Paris, ran the fastest 800 meters in the world for that year. Professional acting debut, 1956, in Julius Caesar at the N.Y. Shakespeare Festival; published poet and short story writer.

BROADWAY: The Ballad of the Sad Cafe, The Cool World, General Seeger, Tiger, Tiger Burning Bright!, The Old Glory. Star and dir. A Hand is On The Gate; off Broadway; The Blacks, Aria da Capo.

PICTURES INCLUDE: The Comedians, Uptight, The Liberation of L. B. Jones, The Cowboys, World's Greatest Athlete, Superfly T.N.T., Logan's Run, Twilight's Last Gleaming, The Fifth Door.

TELEVISION: Space.

BROWNING, KIRK: TV Director; b. N.Y.C., Mar. 28, 1921; e. Brooks School, Andover, Mass., Avon Old Farms, Avon, Conn., and Cornell Univ.; 1940, reporter to News-Tribune in Waco, Texas; with American Field Service, 1942–45; adv. copywriter for Franklin Spier, 1945–48; became floor manager NBC-TV 1949; app't asst. dir. NBC-TV Opera Theatre in 1951 directing NBC Opera Theatre, TV Recital Hall, and Toscanini Simulcasts.

BRUCE, BRENDA: Actress. b. Manchester, England, 1922, e. privately. London stage debut, 1066 And All That; On screen 1944; Millions Like Us; TV Best Actress Award 1962.

PICTURES INCLUDE: Night Boat to Dublin, I see A Dark Stranger, They Came To A City, Carnival, Piccadilly Incident, While The Sun Shines, When The Bough Breaks, My Brother's Keeper, Don't Ever Leave Me, The Final Test, Law and Disorder, Behind the Mask, Peeping Tom, Nightmare, The Uncle.

BROADWAY: Gently Does it (1953),This Year Next Year, Happy Days, Woman In A Dressing Gown, Victor Eh!, Merry Wives of Windsor, The Revenger's Tragedy, Little Murders, Winters Tale, Pericles, Twelfth Night, Hamlet.

TV Appearances: Mary Britton series, Nearer to Heaven, Wrong Side of the Park, The Lodger, The Monkey And the Mohawk, Love Story, A Piece of Resistance, Give the Clown His Supper, Knock on Any Door, The Browning Version, Death of a Teddy Bear, Softly, Softly, The Girl, Happy, Family at War, Budgie.

BRUCE, GEORGE: Writer. b. Danville, Pa., Sept. 15, 1898; e. priv. Aviator, 1919–27; then free lance writer; mag. pub. From 1937 sole author or collab. s.p.

PICTURES INCLUDE: She's No Lady, The Crowd Roars, Navy Blue and Gold, Duke of West Point, King of the Turf, South of Pago Pago, Man in Iron Mask, Son of Monte Cristo, Corsican Brothers, Two Years Before the Mast, Miss Annie Rooney, Fiesta, Killer Mc Coy, Walk A Crooked Mile, Rogues of Sherwood Forest, Lorna Doone, Valentino, The Brigand, Kansas City, Confidential, Fury in Paradise, Solomon and Sheba.

BRUCKHEIMER, JERRY: Producer. b. Detroit. e. Univ. Arizona. Was adv. agency exec. in TV commercials before becoming producer of films. 1983, formed Simpson/Bruckheimer Prods. with Don Simpson and entered into deal with Paramount Pictures to produce.

PICTURES: Assoc. Prod.: Culpepper Cattle Company, Rafferty and the Gold Dust Twins. Producer: Farewell My Lovely, March or Die, Defiance, American Gigolo, Thief, Cat People (exec. prod.), Young Doctors in Love, Flashdance, Thief of Hearts, Beverly Hills Cop, Top Gun.

BRUCKNER, SIDNEY THOMAS: Executive. b. New York City, May 28, 1914; e. C.C.N.Y., B.B.A. 1931; Columbia U., post-graduate study 1931–32. Textile Buyer (partner) 1931–35; joined Columbia Pictures Intern. Corp. as home office rep., covered all countries south of U.S. 1935–38 and 1940–42, covered Europe with hdqtrs in England and Paris 1938–40; apptd. prod. supervisor (Mexican prod.) 1943; res. 1950; ind. prod., 1950, of Mexican films, American TV films; pres. Prod. Espada S.A.; technical advisor, Garden of Evil, Tall Men; prod. 19 TV shows, Capt. David Grief. Spanish/English dubbing of features, TV films, commercials. Mem. prod. Guild (Mexico), Variety Club (Mexico), American Club, Am. Soc.

BRUNING, RICHARD R.: Executive. b. Kansas City, Mo. e. Yale University, Harvard Business School. Asst. treas. Transamerica Corp., parent corp. of United Artists, from 1972. In 1979 named treas. of UA. 1980, named v.p. and treas. of UA Corp.

BRUSKI, NATALIO: Writer, Journalist, Buenos Aires. b. Buenos Aires, B.A. Argentina, Aug. 9, 1906; p. non-professionals; e. high school graduate; married; Had commercial career before entering m.p. ind. In 1932, mgr. Coliseo Theatre. In 1933, mgr. Govena Theatre. In 1934, film critic. La Pelicula, show business professional organ. In 1939; founded own trade paper, Cine-Prensa, since 1951, publicity mgr. for Columbia Pictures. Buenos Aires corresp., Quigley Publication since 1931.

BRUSSEAU, WILLIAM E.: Executive. b. Detroit, Mich. June 6, 1926. e. Engineering, Lawrence Institute of Technology, 1942–44; theatre arts UCLA, 1948; m.p. prod., USC, 1948–50. Joined staff engaged in producing documentaries; prod. films, science, industry, medical profession and the military. gen. doc., TV in Europe, Africa, Middle East, Far East, Latin America, U.S.; formed & pres. Westminster Films, 1950.

PICTURES INCLUDE: Mr. Texas, orig. story, A Cry in the Night, Skidrow, Stop Gap. The Glass Mountain, Dream of Paradise, Flamingo Feather, Shackleton.

BRYAN, DORA: Actress. b. Southport (Lancashire), Eng. e. Council School. Stage debut 1935. Screen debut Fallen Idol, 1948.

PICTURES INCLUDE: No Room at the Inn, Once Upon a Dream, Blue Lamp, Cure for Love, Now Barabas, The Ringer, Women of Twilight, The Quiet Woman, The Intruder, You Know What Sailors Are, Mad About Men, See How They Run, Cockleshell Heroes, Child in the House, Green Man, Carry on Sergeant, Operation Bullshine, Desert Mice, The Night We Got the Bird, A Taste of Honey.

BRYON, CHARLES ANTHONY: Producer. b. Constantinople, December 15, 1919. e. University of Paris, Harvard; Army Air Force 1942–1947. With UNESCO in Paris; NBC-International produced and wrote foreign programs for Dept. of State; public relations ECA mission to France. Film industry 1952 as director of public relations, research, Louis de Rochemont Associates, European prod. Cinerama Holiday; Dragon Prod., 1959, pres., exec. prod. of: The Silken Affair, Chase a Crooked Shadow, etc.

BRYON, KATHLEEN: Actress. b. London, England, Jan. 11, 1922; e. London U., Old Vic. co. student 1942. Screen debut in Young Mr. Pitt 1943.

PICTURES INCLUDE: Silver Fleet, Black Narcissus, Matter of Life and Death, Small Back room, Madness of the Heart, Reluctant Widow, Prelude to Fame, Scarlet Thread, Tom Brown's Schooldays, Four Days, Hell Is Sold Out, I'll Never Forget You, Gambler and the Lady, Young Bess, Night of the Silvery Moon, Profile, Secret Venture, Hand in Hand, Night of the Eagle, Hammerhead, Wolfshead, Private Road, Twins of Evil, Craze, Abdication, One of Our Dinosaurs Is Missing, The Elephant Man, From a Far Country.

TV: The Lonely World of Harry Braintree, All My Own Work, Emergency Ward 10, Probation Officer, Design for Murder, Sergeant Cork, Oxbridge 2000, The Navigators, The Worker; Hereward the Wake, Breaking Point, Vendetta, Play To Win, Who is Sylvia, Portrait of a Lady, Callan, You're Wrecking My Marriage, Take Three Girls, The Confession of Mariona Evans, Paul Temple, The Worker, The Moonstone, The Challengers, The Golden Bowl, The Edwardians, The New Life, Menance, The Rivals of Sherlock Holmes, the Brontes, On Call, Edward VII, Sutherland's Law, Crown Court, Anne of Avonlea, Heidi, Notorious Woman, General Hospital, North & South, Angelo, Within these Walls, Jubilee, Z Cars, Tales from the Supernatural, Secret Army, An Englishman's Castle, The Professionals, Forty Weeks, Emmerdale Farm, Blake Seven, The Minders, Together, Hedda Gabler, Nancy Astor, God Speed Co-operation, Take Three Women, Reilly.

BUCHHOLZ, HORST: Actor. b. 1933. e. High School. In radio and stage plays. Film debut. Marianne (French) 1955.

PICTURES INCLUDE: Himmel Ohne Sterne (No Star in the Sky), Robinson Must Not Die, Mon Petit, The Confessions of Felix Krull, Tiger Bay, Fanny One, Two, Three, Nine Hours to Rama, The Empty Canvas, The Great Waltz, Cervantes, Sahara, Code Name: Emerald.

TV: Raid on Entebbe, Crossings.

BUCK, JULES: Producer. b. St. Louis, Mo., July 30, 1917. Asst. to prod., The Killers; assoc. prod., Brute Force, Naked City, We Were Strangers; prod., Love Nest, Fixed Bayonets, Treasure of the Golden Condor, O.S.S., TV series; prod., The Day They Robbed the Bank of England, Great Catherine; formed Keep Films with Peter O'Toole. Co-prod., Under Milkwood. Prod., The Ruling Class. Exec. Prod., Man Friday. Prod., The Great Scout and Cathouse Thursday.

BUCKLEY, DON: Executive. In ad dept. United Artists Theaters; left to join Grey Advertising Agency, where was acct. exec. on Warner Bros. acct. Joined WB in 1980 as New York adv. mgr.; 1986, promoted to east. dir. of adv./promo. for WB.

BUCKNER, ROBERT H.: producer, writer b. Crewe Va., May 28, 1906; e. U. Va.: Edinburgh (Scotland) U. Newspaper corresp. New York World. 1926–27 in England: instructor, Belgian Mil. Acad. 1927–28: with Alfred A. Knopf, Inc., Doubleday, Doran, N.Y., pub., 1928–33; corresp. in Russia, Scandinavia, 1933–35; contrib. fiction, Amer. & Brit. mags., 1926–36. Author & collab. many s.p.

PICTURES INCLUDE: Gold Is Where You Find It, Jezebel, Dodge City, Virginia City, Knute Rockne, Santa Fe Trial,

Dive Bomber, Yankee Doodle Dandy, Desert Song. In 1943 prod. Gentleman Jim, Mission to Moscow, Desert Song. A Champion of Champion Producer in Fame ratings. (See Index). The Gang's All Here, Cheyenne, Life with Father, prod. Rogue's Regiment. Sword in the Desert; Free For All, Deported, Bright Victory, The Man Behind the Gun, Safari.

BUJOLD, GENEVIEVE: Actress. b. Montreal, July 1, 1942, e. Montreal Conservatory of Drama. m. TV Director Paul Almond. Worked in a Montreal cinema as an usherette; American TV debut: St. Joan.
STAGE: The Barber of Seville, A Midsummer Night's Dream, A House . . . A Day.
PICTURES INCLUDE: La Guerre est Finie, La Fleur de L'Age, Entre La Mer et L'eau Douce, King of Hearts, The Thief, Isabel, Anne of The Thousand Days, The Act of the Heart, The Journey, Earthquake, Swashbuckler, Obsession, Alex and the Gypsy, Another Man, Another Chance, Coma, Murder by Decree, The Last Flight of Noah's Ark, Monsignore, Tightrope, Choose Me, Trouble in Mind.
TV: Anthony and Cleopatra.

BURGER, HENRY: Executive. b. Pittsburgh, Pa., Mar. 26, 1915. Asst. mgr. and mgr., various theatres in Pittsburgh and W. Va.; asst. ad. pub. mgr., Pittsburgh Zone Warner Bros. Theatres, 1942; ad., pub. mgr., 1948; district mgr., Stanley Warner Theatres, Erie district, 1951; district mgr., Pittsburgh City Theaters, zone ad. pub. mgr., 1953; Zone mgr., Stanley Warner Midwest-Zone Theatres, 1962; nat. adv. pub. dir., Stanley Warner Theatres, 1965; zone manager, 1967.

BURKE, ALFRED, Actor. b. London, England, 1918. Ent. films 1954.
PICTURES INCLUDE: The Angry Silence, Moment of Danger, The Man Inside, The Man Upstairs, No Time To Die, Law and Disorder, Yangtse Incident, Interpol, Bitter Victory.
TV: The Crucible, Mock Auction, Parole, No Gun, No Guilt, The Big Knife, Parnell, The Strong Are Lonely, Home Of The Brave, The Birthday Party, The Watching Eye, Public Eye series.

BURKE, PAUL: Actor. b. New Orleans, La., July 21, 1926, e. Prep Schools, N.O., Pasadena Playhouse.
TV: Five Fingers, Harbor Master, Noah's Ark, Naked City, Playhouse 90, Studio One, Medic, Frontier, Men in Space, Man and the Challenge, Target, M-Squad, Black Saddle, Philip Marlowe, Martin Kane, Line Up, Dragnet, Man Without a Gun, Tightrope, Panic, Highway Patrol, Men of Annapolis, Flight, Naked City, 12 O'Clock High.
PICTURES INCLUDE: Once You Kiss a Stranger, Daddy's Gone A-Hunting, Valley of the Dolls.

BURKS, J. COOPER: Executive. b. Pilot Point, Texas, April 26, 1919. e. Oklahoma City University Oklahoma City Law School, American Institute of Banking (Special Finance Courses), U.S. Navy Schools at Wesleyan College, Middletown, Conn. University of North Carolina, Chapel Hill, N.C., Virginia Polytechnic Institute, Blacksburg, Va. Military: Commander USNR-Ret. WWII PT Boats, North Atlantic then as Naval Aviator—latter part WWII and Korean War. Business experience: Prior to theatre business, was in banking & construction business. Formed present company March, 1970. Now president at chairman of the board of AATI (American Automated Theatres, Inc.) in Oklahoma City. Military Affiars Committee, Chamber of Commerce, Life Member-Navy League.

BURLINSON, JOHN J., JR.: Executive. b. New York, N.Y., Dec. 26, 1930. e. Collegiate Sch. N.Y., Fordham U.; dir. promotion and adv., Henry Regnery Co. (book publishers). 1960; sls. mgr. Regnery, 1962; N.Y. rep., U.S. Press Association, 1963; v.p., Quigley Publishing Co., N.Y., 1964. Ad Dir. Better Theatres Theatre vending; adv. mgr. Motion Picture Daily, 1966; National Screen Service Corp. 1970, dir. inter-corporate promotion. 1972; dir. of admin., National Theatre Supply; 1974, gen. mgr., NTS; 1977, v.p. & gen. mgr., EPRAD, Inc.; 1980, named pres., EPRAD; 1983, dir., mktg., sls., adv., Strong International. Elected exec. dir. & treasurer of TESMA in 1967. Co-director NATO/NAC/TESMA Trade Show; sec. & dir., M.P. Pioneers, 1970; hon. dir. TESMA, 1971; member SMPTE, Variety Club. 1972; Vice President Equipment Assoc.; 1974; bd. mem. TEA and Conference chm.; 1982: TEA secty.; Chm. annual NY Variety Golf Tournament 1972–75; vice chairman, Motion Picture Div., Catholic Charities of NY, 1972–75. In 1984 named exec. dir., Variety Clubs Intl.

BURNETT, CAROL: Actress-comedienne-singer; b. San Antonio, Apr. 26, 1936; Jody and Louise (Creighton) Burnett; e. Hollywood H.S., UCLA. m. Joseph Hamilton, 1963; children-Carrie Louise, Judy Ann, Erin Kate. Introduced comedy song, I Made a Fool of Myself Over John Foster Dulles, 1957; Broadway debut in Once Upon a Mattress, 1959; regular performer Garry Moore TV show, 1959–62; appeared several CBS-TV spls., 1962–63, Broadway play Fade Out-Fade In, 1964, play Plaza Suite, 1970, film Pete 'n Tillie, 1972, musical play I Do, I Do, 1973; Same Time Next Year, 1977; Film Front Page, club engagements Harrah's Club, The Sands, Caesar's Palace; star Carol Burnett Show, CBS-TV. CBS-TV Spec. "6 Rooms Riv Vu" 74; "Twigs" The Grass Is Always Greener, Friendly Fire, The Tenth Month. 75. Films: The Front Page, A Wedding (best actress, San Sebastian Film Festival), Health, The Four Seasons, Chu Chu and the Philly Flash, Annie, Between Friends (HBO). Recipient outstanding comedienne award Am. Guild Variety Artists, 5 times; 5 Emmy awards for outstanding variety performance Acad. TV Arts and Scis., TV Guide award for outstanding female performer 1961, 62, 63; Peabody award, 1963; Golden Globe award for outstanding comedienne of year Fgn. Press Assn.; Woman of Year award Acad. TV Arts and Scis. One of the world's 20 most admired women voted in poll conducted by George Gallup (1977). First Annual National Television Critics Award for Outstanding Performance, 1977

BURNETT, W.R.: Writer. b. Springfield, Ohio, Nov. 25, 1899; e. Miami Mil. Inst., Ohio State U. Novelist (Little Caesar, Dark Hazard, Iron Man). Author of collab. s.p. including Scarface, Heart of a City, Whole Town's Talking, Dr. Socrates, High Sierra, Wake Island, This Gun for Hire, Yellow Sky, Belle Starr's Daughter, Asphalt Jungle, Vendetta, Iron Man, I Died a Thousand Times, The Racket, Dangerous Mission, Captain Lightfoot, Illegal.

BURNS, GEORGE: Actor. r.n. Nathan Birnbaum; b. New York City, Jan. 20, 1896. In vaudeville as singer in children's quartet, later as roller skater, then comedian; formed team Burns & (Gracie) Allen 1925; m. partner 1926. Team many years on Keith and Orpheum vaudeville circuits, then on screen in Paramount short subjects, on radio in England; in 1930 began long career Amer. radio. Feature picture debut 1932 in The Big Broadcast.
PICTURES INCLUDE: International House, Love in Bloom, College Swing, Honolulu, Two Girls and A Sailor, The Sunshine Boys, Oh, God, Just You and Me, Kid, Oh, God! Book II, Oh, God! You Devil.
TV: Co-star Burns & Allen show, CBS-TV.

BURNS, RALPH: Composer-Musical Conductor.
PICTURES: Lenny, Cabaret (AA), Lucky Lady, New York, New York, Movie, Movie, All That Jazz (AA), Urban Cowboy, Jinxed, Annie, My Favorite Year, Star 80, Perfect, etc.
TELEVISION: Baryshnikov on Broadway, Liza and Goldie Special (both Emmy awards), etc.

BURR, RAYMOND: Actor. b. New Westminster, B.C., Canada, May 21, 1917; e. Stanford U., U. of Calif., Columbia U., U. of Chungking. Forestry svce.: appeared on stage in many countries in Night Must Fall, Mandarin, Crazy with the Heat, Duke in Darkness; dir., Pasdena Community Playhouse, 1943; on radio.
PICTURES INCLUDE: Pitfall, Raw Deal, Key to the City, His Kind of Woman, Place in the Sun, New Mexico, Meet Danny Wilson, Mara Maru, Horizons West, Blue Gardenia, Fort Algiers, Casanova's Big Night, Gorilla at Large, Khyber Patrol, Rear Window, Passion, They Were So Young, You're Never Too Young, A Man Alone, Count Three and Pray, Please Murder Me, Godzilla King of the Monsters, Great Day in the Morning, Secret of Treasure Mountain, Cry in the Night, P.J., Airplane II: The Sequel.
TV: Perry Mason series, CBS-TV, 1957. Ironside series, CBS, 1970, Centennial (1978). Movies: Perry Mason Returns.

BURRELL-DAVIS, DEREK: Freelance producer, director with own company "B.D. Productions": b. York 1918 entered m.p. 1946 with J. Arthur Rank Org. 1950 joined B.B.C. T.V. as stage manager then producer. 1951 producer North Region. 1955 returned London, senior producer then executive producer. 1970 editor in charge B.B.C. T.V. O.B. entertainment progs. 1971 Head of Network Production Centre Manchester. 1977 left B.B.C. to freelance. Responsible for wide range of television productions covering sport, features and entertainment in U.K. and Europe.

BURRILL, TIMOTHY: Producer, Executive. b. North Wales, 1931. e. Eton College, Sorbonne Univ. Paris, Grenadier Guards 2 yrs, then London Shipping Co. Ent. m.p. ind. as resident prod. mgr. Samaritan Films working on shorts, commercials, documentaries, 1954. Ass't. dir. on feature films: The Criminal, The Valiant Years (TV series), On The Fiddle, Reach for Glory, War Lover, Prod. mgr: The Cracksman, Night Must Fall, Lord Jim, Yellow Rolls Royce, The Heroes, Of Telemark, Resident producer with World Film Services. 1968–1969: Privilege, Oedipus The King, 1969–1970: A Severed Head, Three Sisters, 1970 produced two films on pop music for Anglo-EMI. 1971 assoc. prod. Macbeth. 1972 first production administrator National Film School in U.K. 1973 Prod. Alpha Beta. 1974 Post production administrator The Three Musketeers. 1974: Prod. TV Special The Canterville Ghost; 1975; Assoc. Prod, That Lucky

Touch; 1976: UK Administrator, The Prince and the Pauper; 1977: North American Production controller, Superman 1; 1974–1983 Council Member of BAFTA: Co-produced Polanski's Tess; 1979–80 Managing Director Allied Stars (Breaking Glass, Chariots of Fire); 1981 co-produced NYSF Prod. Pirates of Penzance; 1979–80 V. Chmn. Film BAFTA; 1980–1983 Chmn. BAFTA: 1981 Gov. National Film School, Executive BFTPA Mbr. Cinematograph Films Council. 1982 Gov National Theatre; 1982 Produced Supergirl, The Fourth Protocol.

BURROWS, JOHN, H.: Producer. b. Brooklyn, N.Y., September 4, 1924. e. Yale, New York U. Law with interruption for service. U.S. Navy, World War II, lieut., son of George D. Burrows, vice-president Allied Artists, started film career as salesman for AA later joining studio; asst. prod. Lindsley Parsons Productions.

BURROWS, ROBERTA: Executive. e. Brandeis Univ; Academia, Florence, Italy. Career includes post as dir. of pub. for Howard Stein Enterprises and with Rogers & Cowan and Billings Associates. Joined Warner Bros. as sr. publicist 1979; named eastern pub. dir., 1986.

BURRUD, BILL: Exec. b. Los Angeles, Calif., Jan. 12, 1925. e. U. of Southern Calif., B.S.; Harvard Bus. School, ent. ind. as child actor; U.S. Navy, W.W. II; formed Bill Burrud Prods., 1954.

TV: Animal World, World of the Sea, Safari to Adventure, Challenging Sea, Secret World of Reptiles, Vanishing Africa, The Great American Wilderness, Predators of the Sea, Creatures of the Amazon, The Amazing Apes, The Amazing World, Animals Are The Funniest People.

BURSTYN, ELLEN: Actress. b. Detroit, Dec. 7, 1932. Majored in art; was fashion model in Texas when 18. Moved to Montreal as dancer; then N.Y. to do TV commercials, appearing for a year on the Jackie Gleason show. In 1957 turned to dramatics and won lead in show, Fair Game. Then went to Hollywood to do TV and films. Returned to N.Y. to study acting with Lee Strasberg; worked in TV serial, The Doctors.

PICTURES INCLUDE: For Those Who Think Young, Goodbye, Charlie, Tropic of Cancer, Alex in Wonderland, The Last Picture Show, The King of Marvin Gardens, The Exorcist, Harry and Tonto, Alice Doesn't Live Here Anymore, Providence, A Dream of Passion, Same Time Next Year, Resurrection, Silence of the North, The Ambassador, Twice in a Lifetime.

TELEVISION: Surviving, Act of Vengeance, Into Thin Air.

BURTON, BERNARD: Producer. Started as film ed.; prod. "Vagabond Lady" 1935.

PICTURES INCLUDE: She Gets Her Man, Fighting Youth, Invisible Ray, Showboat, When Love is Young, One Hundred Men and a Girl, You're a Sweetheart, Midnight Intruder, Little Tough Guy, Three Smart Girls Grow Up, Spring Parade, Moonlight in Havana, Get Help to Love, Gentleman Joe Palooka, Fighting Mad, Smart Woman, Underworld Story, Cry Danger, The Highwayman, Triple Cross, Beast from 20,000 Fathoms.

BURTON, LEVAR: Actor. b. Landstuhl, Germany, Feb. 16, 1957. e. Univ. of So. Calif. Signed to play role of Kunta Kinte in TV series, Roots, while still in school. Appears frequently on public TV, hosts children's show, Bebop, (PBC).

PICTURES: Looking for Mr. Goodbar, The Hunter.

TELEVISION: Roots, Billy: Portrait of a Street Kid, Battered, The Ron LeFlore Story, Dummy.

BUSCH, H. DONALD: Exhibitor. b. Philadelphia, PA Sept. 21, 1935. e. Univ. of PA (physics, math, 1956; law school, 1959). Since 1960 practiced law, anti-trust & entertainment. 1984, named pres., Budco Theatres, Inc. Since 1975, pres., Busch, Grafman & Von Dreusche, P.C.

MEMBER: Suburban General Hospital (dir.); Rainbow Fund (dir.); NATO (dir.); Philadelphia All-Star Forum (dir.); Montgomery County Bar Assn. (dir.). Former posts: dir. & pres., Abington Pa. School Board (1974–77); dir., Sports Legends, Inc. (1972–84).

BUSCH, NIVEN: Writer. b. New York City, N.Y., Apr. 26, 1903; e. Princeton U.; p. Briton Niven Busch, former v-p Lewis J. Selznick Enterprises; Exec. prod., Samuel Goldwyn Productions; m. Phyllis Cooper, 1936; children: Peter, Briton, Terence, Mary Kelly, Joseph, Nicholas, and Eliza. m. Carmencita Baker, 1956. div. 1969, m. Suzanne de Sanz 1973. Assoc. ed. Time mag., 1923–31; assoc. ed. & contrib. New Yorker, 1927–31; numerous articles, many national magazines. Regents professor, Univ. of Calif. 1971–78. Special lectures on film.

AUTHOR: Books: Twenty One Americans, Carrington Incident, Duel in the Sun, They Dream of Home, Day of the Conquerors, The Furies, The Hate Merchant, The Actor, California Street, The San Franciscans, The Gentlemen from California, The Takeover, No Place for a Hero, Continent's Edge.

PICTURES INCLUDE: The Crowd Roars, In Old Chicago, The Westerner, The Postman Always Rings Twice, Duel in the Sun, Till the End of Time, Pursued, Moss Rose; prod., The Capture, Distant Drums, Man from the Alamo, Moonlighter, Treasure of Pancho Villa, Moss Rose, He Was Her Man, The Angels Wash Their Face, Big Shakedown, Little Miss Pinkerton, Regents professor, Univ. of Cal., Irvine, 1971–75. San Diego, 1974; Lecturer Berkeley, 1977. Lecturer, Princeton, 1985, Ferris Teaching Fellow, Princeton, 1986.

BUSEY, GARY: Actor—Musician. b. Goose Creek, TX, June 29, 1944.

PICTURES INCLUDE: Last American Hero, Lolly Madonna, Gumball Rally, Alex and the Gypsy, A Star Is Born, The Buddy Holly Story, Straight Time, Big Wednesday, Foolin' Around, Carny, D.C. Cab, The Bear, Silver Bullet.

TELEVISION: Bloodsport, The Execution of Private Slovik.

BUTLER, DAWS: Actor (Voice), r.n. Charles Dawson Butler. b. Toledo, Nov. 16, 1916. With Time for Beany, 1948–53. Host (voice) of Off to See the Wizard TV program. From 1953 to present, various cartoon voices, including: Yogi Bear, Huckleberry Hound, Quick Draw McGraw, Loopie DeLoop, Chilly Willy, Peter Potamus, Mr. Jinx.

BUTTERFIELD, ELIZABETH: Production Manager. b. London, England e. London. Extensive theatrical experience as stage manager for The Old Vic Company (Michael Benthall, Tyrone Guthrie) and Donald Wolfit Company. Emigrated to Canada in 1957. Television experience includes: Quentin Durgens M.P. and Whiteoaks Of Jaina for C.B.C., Seaway, Ind.

PICTURES INCLUDE: A Fan's Notes, Warner Bros. 1971; Sunday In The Country, Quadrant, 1973; It Seemed Like A Good Idea At The Time, Quadrant, 1975; Find the Lady, Quadrant, 1976; Running, Buena Vista, 1978; Middle Age Crazy, Torment, 1979.

BUTTOLPH, DAVID: Music director.

PICTURES INCLUDE: Phantom of Rue Morgue, Secret of the Incas, Bounty Hunter, Long John Silver, Jump Into Hell, Target Zero, Lone Ranger, Steel Jungle, Santiago, Burning Hills, Cry in the Night.

BUTTONS, RED: Performer. r.n. Aaron Chwatt; b. N.Y.C., Feb. 5, 1919. Singer at the age of 13; comic, Minsky's. U.S. Army, 1943; in Army and film version of Winged Victory.

TV: Vickie, Wine, Women and Song, Barefoot Boy With Cheek, Hold It. Many TV appearances; star of Red Buttons Show CBS-TV, 1953; Best Comedian award 1953; NBC-TV, 1954; on screen in Sayonara (Academy Award best actor in supporting role 1957).

PICTURES INCLUDE: Imitation General, The Big Circus, Five Weeks in a Balloon, Harlow, They Shoot Horses Don't They, Who Killed Mary What's 'er name?, The Poseidon Adventure, Gable and Lombard, Viva, Knievel!, Movie Movie, When Time Ran Out.

BUTTS, R. DALE: Composer. b. Lamasco, Ky., March 12, 1910; e. Louisville Conservatory of Music. Started in vaudeville at 16, later playing, arranging for dance bands; staff arranger, pianist, radio stations; to Republic Pictures, 1944.

PICTURES INCLUDE: The Plunderers, Too Late for Tears, House by the River, Sea Hornet, The Outcast, Geraldine, Shanghai Story, Hell's Outpost, Santa Fe passage, Fighting Chance, No Man's Woman, Headline Hunter's, Lay That Rifle Down, Double Jeopardy, City of Shadows, Terror at Midnight, Stranger at My Door, Dakota Incident.

BUXBAUM, JAMES M.: Executive, producer, writer. b. Jamaica N.Y., March 8. e. Harvard, B.A., 1949, Columbia Law School, LL.B., 1955, spec. studies, The Hague Acad., Netherlands, 1953. Story ed. ZIV, Ivan Tors' Sea Hunt series, then assoc. prod., ZIV-CBS, Ivan Tors' Aquanauts series, story ed., 1957–60. Attorney, Wm. Morris Agency, 1962–63. Joined Ivan Tors Films, Inc. as v.p., prod. and wrote many episodes of Flipper series, 1964; exec. v.p. Ivan Tors Miami Studios, 1967–69; exec. v.p. Ivan Tors Films, Inc. 1968–69. Gen. mgr. Amer. Film Institute Center, Bev erly Hills, 1969. Member: State Bar of Calif., Amer. Bar Assoc. Exec. in charge of prod. for Island of the Lost.

BUZZI, RUTH: Actress. b. Wequetequak, CT, July 24, 1939. e. Pasadena Playhouse. Launched TV career on Garry Moore Show as comedy partner of Dom DeLuise. Created character Gladys Ormphby with Artie Johnson on TV's Laugh-In.

PICTURES INCLUDE: Freaky Friday, The Apple Dumpling Gang Rides Again, The Villain, Chu Chu and the Philly Flash, Easter Sunday.

TELEVISION: The Entertainers, The Donny & Marie Show (semi-regular), Rowan & Martin's Laugh-In, The Dean Martin Show, The Dean Martin Roasts, The Tonight Show, Kroft's Superstars, Rhoda (recurring role), Gladys and Tyrone (cartoon show, partial creator and voice of character) etc.

STAGE: Sweet Charity (Broadway), The Ruth Buzzi Show (Las Vegas), Pasadena Playhouse Theatre, and summer stock.
AWARDS: 4 Grammy nominations; Golden Globe winner, AGVA Variety Artist of the Year, 1977, Rhode Island Hall of Fame, Presidential Commendation for outstanding artist in the field of entertainment, 1980.

BYGRAVES, MAX: Comedian, actor. b. London, Eng., October 16, 1922. e. St. Joseph's R.C. School, Rotherhithe. After RAF service, touring revues and London stage, M.P. debut 1949 in Skimpy in The Navy. TV debut in 1953, with own show.
TV: Roamin Holiday series.
PICTURES INCLUDE: Tom Brown's Schooldays, Charlie Moon, A Cry from the Streets, Boobikins, Spare the Rod, Autobiograph "I Wanna Tell you A Story" Pub. 1976.
NOVEL: The Milkman's on His Way, pub. 1977. Received OBE New Year's Honours 1983.

BYRD, CARUTH C.: Production Executive. b. Dallas, Texas, March 25, 1942. Multi-millionaire businessman, chm. of Caruth C. Byrd Enterprises, Inc., who entered entertainment industry forming Communications Network Inc. in 1972, producer of TV commercials. Was principal investor in film Santee (1972) and in 1973 formed Caruth C. Byrd Prods. to make theatrical features. 1983, chrm., Lone Star Pictures.
PICTURES INCLUDE: Allan and Murph the Surf, The Monkeys of Bandapur (both exec. prod.).

BYRD, JOHN: Writer, director, producer. Entered m.p. industry 1934 via scenario dept. Rock Studios, Elstree; visited Hollywood to study requirements of U.S. market, 1939; 1940–45 B.B.C. War Correspondent, 1945–46 Riverside Studios, 1947–8 British National Studios.
PICTURES INCLUDE: Murder in Reverse, World Owes Me a Living, Waltz Time. 1949 formed own org. prod. bus. TV films. Prod. films in South Africa, Uganda, Kenya, Portugal and Mexico. Filming Durgapur Steelworks project, India, 1961; Steel Strides Ahead. Concerning Colour, Design for Tall Building, Jungle to Steel Town, Steelworks in Action, 1962–4; Dryer Felt Loom, Bridging the Highways, 1965; Filming in Afghanistan, 1966; Filming in South Africa, 1967; Built from Top, 1968; Building With Steel and Plastics, 1969; The Desert Will Yield, 1970; Long Sea Outfall, One Steelworks, One Contract, Highweld Process. 1971: Go-Con Process, Mechanical Handling, 1972. Undersea Tunnel to Hong Kong. 1973: Contract 1306—Zambia, Bridge Across the Avon; 1974 filming for British Steel Corp.
OTHER PICTURES: Murder in Reverse, World Owes Me a Living, Waltz Time. 1974–5 Anchor Project for British Steel Corporation. 1976–77 Filming in Mexico AHMSA Steelworks project. 1977, More Steel for Mexico; 1978, Filming in South Africa; 1979–80, Filming in France & Spain; 1982, Filming Construction of Humber Bridge; 1983–84, New Zealand on steel development project. 1984, Better Coal for Kellingly; 1985, SCAW Metals Project; 1986, SAPPI Paper Mill Project.

BYRNES, EDWARD: Actor. b. New York, N.Y., July 30, 1933. e. Harren H.S.; prof. debut, Joe E. Brown's Circus Show; appeared on stage in Tea and Sympathy.
PICTURES INCLUDE: Periscope, Marjorie Morningstar, Secret Invasion, Wicked, Wicked, Star Wars, Grease.
TV: Matinee Theatre, Crossroads, Jim Bowie, Wire Service, Navy Log, Oh Susanna!, 77 Sunset Strip.

BRYON, CHARLES ANTHONY: Producer. b. Constantinople, December 15, 1919. e. University of Paris, Harvard; Army Air Force 1942–1947. With UNESCO in Paris; NBC-International produced and wrote foreign programs for Dept. of State; public relations ECA mission to France. Film industry 1952 as director of public relations, research, Louis de Rochemont Associates, European prod. Cinerama Holiday; Dragon Prod., 1959, pres., exec. prod. of: The Silken Affair, Chase a Crooked Shadow, etc.

BYRON, WARD: TV Prod.-writer-dir. b. N.Y.C., June 2, 1910. e. New York. Orchestra leader, 1929–32; radio prod., writer, 1932–39. Ent. TV as asst. to prog. dir. of ABC; writer & producer of Paul Whiteman show in 1950; The Ameche-Langford Show; app'td exec. prod. of ABC-TV in 1950. Exec. prod., Canadian TV Young & Rubicam, 1955–57. Freelance writer prod., TV Specials & film series, v.p. gen, mgr. Trans-Nat'l Communications O'way Recording Studios; 1970, v.p. & sec. International Coproductions, motion picture distributors. Named pres. in 1979. Currently lecturing on early radio and TV.

BYRUM, JOHN: Writer—Director. b. Winnetka, Ill., March 14, 1947. e. N.Y. Univ. Film School. First job as "go-fer" on industrial films and cutting dailies for underground filmmakers. Went to England where wrote 1st s.p., Comeback. From 1970–73 was in N.Y.C. writing and re-writing scripts for low-budget films.
PICTURES INCLUDE: Mahogany (s.p.), Inserts (s.p., dir.) Harry and Walter Go to New York (story, s.p.), Heart Beat (s.p. dir.), Sphinx (s.p.), Scandalous (co.-s.p.), The Razor's Edge (co-s.p., dir.), The Whoopee Boys (dir.).

C

CAAN, JAMES: Actor. b. Bronx, N.Y., March 26, 1940; e. Hofstra Coll.: Appeared off-Broadway in La Ronde, 1961.
PICTURES INCLUDE: Lady in a Cage, The Glory Guys, Red Line 7000, Eldorado, Games, Journey to Shiloh, Submarine XQ/⅛, Rain People, Rabbit, Run, Brian's Song (TV), The Godfather, Slither, Cinderella Liberty, Freebie and the Bean, The Gambler, Godfather II, Funny Lady, Rollerball, The Killer Elite, Harry and Walter Go To New York, Silent Movie, A Bridge Too Far, Another Man, Another Chance, Comes a Horseman, Chapter Two, Hide in Plain Sight (also dir.), Thief, Kiss Me Goodbye.

CACOYANNIS, MICHAEL: producer, director, writer. b. Cyprus, June 11, 1922. Studied law in London, admitted to bar at age 21. Became a producer of BBC's wartime Greek programs while attending dramatic school. After acting on the stage in England, left in 1952 for Greece, where he made his first film, Windfall in Athens, with his own original script. While directing Greek classical plays, he continued making films.
PICTURES INCLUDE: Stella, The Girl in Black, A Matter of Dignity, Our Last Spring, The Wastrel, Electra, Zorba the Greek, The Day the Fish Came Out, The Trojan Women, Sweet Country.

CADELL, JEAN: Actress. b. Edinburgh, Scotland, Sept. 13, 1884; e. Edinburgh & Paris. Early prof. stage appearances on tour in Gt. Brit., beginning in London 1906 (The Inspector General); with Sir George Alexander's co. in Eng.; later numrous London, N.Y. prods.
PICTURES INCLUDE: Madeleine, Reluctant Widow, No Place for Jennifer, Obsessed, Whisky Galore, Meet Mr. Lucifer, Little Hut, The Surgeon's Knife, Rockets Galore, Upstairs and Downstairs, A Taste of Money, V.I.P.
TV: Whiteoakes, Arsenic and Old Lace, Doomsday for Dyson, Mary Rose, Eustace Diamonds (serial).

CAESAR, IRVING: Author, composer, publisher. b. New York, N.Y., July 4, 1895, e. C.C.N.Y. Abroad with Henry Ford on Peace Ship, World War I; songwriter since then, several songs with George Gershwin, songwriter for stage, screen and radio, including Swanee, Tea for Two, Sometimes I'm Happy, I want to Be Happy, Lady Play Your Mandolin, Songs of Safety, Songs of Friendship, Songs of Health and Pledge of Allegiance to the Flag.

CAESAR, SID: Performer. b. Yonkers, N.Y. Sept. 8, 1922. Musician. Joined Coast Guard in 1942. Appeared in "Tars and Spars." Signed for Broadway Revue by Max Liebman, 1949. Star of Your Show of Shows on NBC-TV 1950–54; star of Caesar's Hour, 1954–1957; voted best comedian (tied) in M.P. Daily's TV poll, 1951. Best Comedian, 1952; Best Comedy Team (with Imogene Coca), 1953; 5 Emmy Awards 1957; Sylvania Award, 1958. Sid Caesar Invites You, 1958; Formed Shelbrick Corp., TV, 1959; TV series As Caesar Sees It, 1962; Bway Play: Little Me, 1962–64; The Sid Caesar Show, 1963–64. Movie 1984: Found Money
PICTURES INCLUDE: It's a Mad, Mad, Mad, Mad World, The Spirit is Willing, The Busy Body, Guide for the Married Man, Ten from Your Show of Shows, Airport 1975, Silent Movie, Grease, The Cheap Detective, History of the World—Part I, Over the Brooklyn Bridge, Cannonball Run III.

CAGE, NICOLAS: Actor. b. Long Beach, CA, 1965. First starring role in Valley Girl (1983).
PICTURES: Rumble Fish, Racing with the Moon, The Cotton Club, Birdy. The Boy in Blue, Raising Arizona, Peggy Sue Got Married.

CAGNEY, WILLIAM J.: Producer. b. New York; brother of James Cagney, actor. e. City Coll., N.Y. (law student). Adv. rep., Fairchild Publications. From 1933 on screen in Ace of Aces, Lost in the Stratosphere, Stolen Harmony, etc. Became talent agent, Hollywood, then in 1940 joined Warner Bros. as assoc. prod. (The Strawberry Blonde), The Bride Came C.O.D., Captains of the Clouds, Yankee Doodle Dandy, etc.). In 1942 org. (with James C.) Cagney Prods.: pres. Cagney Prod.
PICTURES INCLUDE: Blood on the Sun, Johnny Come Lately, Time of Your Life, Kiss Tomorrow Goodbye, Only the Valiant, Bugles in the Afternoon, A Lion Is in the Streets.

CAHN, SAMMY: Lyricist, Producer. b. New York, N.Y. June 18, 1913; e. Seward Park H.S. Org. dance band with Saul Chaplin; collab. song writer for shows. m.p.
PLAYS INCLUDE: High Button Shoes, Skyscraper, Walking Happy many songs, 30 Acad. Award Nominations, Four Oscars for 3 Coins in Fountain, All The Way, High Hopes, and Call me Irresponsible! Only TV Emmy ever

given a song "Love & Marriage" From the TV award winning "Our Town".
PICTURES INCLUDE: Anchors Aweigh, 3 Coins in Fountain, Romance on High Seas, Some Came Running, Robin & Seven Hoods, The Tender Trap, Pocketfull of Miracles, Thoroughly Modern Millie. 1972, inducted into Songwriters' Hall of Fame.

CAIN, SUGAR: Actress. r.n. Constance McCain. b. Jerome, Ariz., Mar. 13. e. Univ. Washington, B.A., radio-drama; Colo. Woman's Col., A.A., journalism; Columbia Univ., grad TV. MP. Reg. on radio serials. Hopalong Cassidy, Clyde Beatty Show, Night club act, Mexico; appeared TV, Hollywood & N.Y. Plays include: nat. tours, Pajama Tops, In One Bed, Idiots Delight, Streetcar Named Desire, The Rainmaker, Dead End, Druid Circle.
PICTURES INCLUDE: Breakstone Affair, Life with Edmer, I've Been Here Before, Monster from 20,000 Fathoms, Dalton Women, I Shot Billy the Kid, Hostle Country, Dalton Gang, Africa Screams; Sporting Club, Apple Man, Klute, Panic in Needle Park, The French Connection, Effect of Gamma Rays, Summer Wishes, Winter Dreams; Dir.-writer, m.p. short, Rama.

CAINE, MICHAEL: Actor. b. London, Eng., March 14, 1933.
TV: The Compartment, The Playmates, Hobson's Choice, Funny Noises With Their Mouths, The Way With Reggie, Luck of the Draw, Hamlet, The Other Man.
PICTURES INCLUDE: Zulu, Ipcress File, Alfie, The Wrong Box, Gambit, Funeral in Berlin, Hurry Sundown, Billion Dollar Brain, Deadfall, The Magus, Play Dirty, Italian Job, The Battle of Britain, Too Late the Hero, Get Carter, Kidnapped, Zee and Company, Pulp, Sleuth, The Black Windmill, The Destructors, The Wilby Conspiracy, Peepers, The Romantic Englishwoman, The Man Who Would Be King, Harry and Walter Go to New York, The Eagle Has Landed, A Bridge Too Far, The Silver Bears, The Swarm, Ashanti, California Suite, Beyond the Poseidon Adventure, The Island, Dressed to Kill, The Hand, Victory, Deathtrap, The Jigsaw Man, Educating Rita, Beyond the Limit, Blame It on Rio, Water. The Holcroft Covenant, Hannah and Her Sisters, Sweet Liberty, Half Moon Street.

CALHOUN, RORY: Actor. r.n. Francis Timothy Durgin. b. Los Angeles, Calif., Aug. 8, 1923, e. Santa Cruz H.S. Worked as logger, miner, cowpuncher, for firefighter; m.p. debut in Something for the Boys, 1944.
PICTURES INCLUDE: Sunday Dinner for a Soldier, Nob Hill, Great John L, Red House, Adventure Island, That Hagen Girl, Sand, Massacre River, Ticket to Tomahawk, County Fair, I'd Climb the Highest Mountain, Rogue River, Meet Me After the Show, With a Song in My Heart, Way of a Gaucho, The Silver Whip, Powder River, How to Marry a Millionaire, River of No Return, Yellow Tomahawk, Bullet Is Waiting, Dawn at Socorro, Four Guns to the Border, The Looters, Ain't Misbehavin', Shotgun, Domino and Actor; actor, Treasure of Pancho Villa, The Spoilers, Red Sundown, Raw Edge, Flight to Hongkong, Utah Blaine, Big Caper, Finger On the Trigger, Young Fury, Black Spurs, Adventures of Marco Polo, Colossus of Rhodes, Angel, Avenging Angel.
TV: The Texans, The Blue and the Gray, Capitol.

CALLAN, MICHAEL: Actor, singer, dancer. b. Philadelphia, Pa. 1935. Singer, dancer, Philadelphia night clubs; to New York in musicals, including The Boy Friend and West Side Story; dancer Copacabana; in short-run plays, Las Vegas: 5 month run starred in That Certain Girl. Guest starred on major dramatic TV shows and Occasional Wife (series, star).
PICTURES INCLUDE: debut, They Came to Cordura, The Flying Fontaines, Because They're Young, Pepe, Mysterious Island, Gidget Goes Hawaiian, 13 West Street, Bon Voyage, The Interns, The Victors, The "New" Interns, Cat Ballou, Frasier, The Sensuous Lion, Lepke, The Photographer, The Cat and The Canary (1977), Record City (1977); The Donner Party (1978).
TELEVISION: Blind Ambition, Scruples.

CALLEY, JOHN: executive. b. New Jersey, 1930. Dir. of night time programming, dir. programming sales, NBC, 1951–57; prod. exec. and TV prod. Henry Jaffe Enterprises, 1957; v.p. in charge of Radio and Television, Ted Bates Advertising Agency, 1958; joined Filmways, Inc., 1960; exec. v.p. and prod. to 1969; exec. v.p. chg. world-wide prod. Warner Bros.; Pres., W.B. from Jan. 6, 1975; vice chm. bd., 1977. Now consultant.
PICTURES INCLUDE: Wheeler Dealer, The Americanization of Emily, Topkapi, The Cincinnati Kid, Loved One, Don't Make Waves, Ice Station Zebra, Catch-22.

CALLOW, EVERETT C.: Publicist. b. Perth Amboy, N.J. e. St. John's Coll. On ed. staff N.Y. World; service staff chief Paramount Thea., N.Y., 1926; mgr. Keith & Albee Theas., Phila., 1928; mgr. Stanley Theatre, Phila., 1929–31; dist. theatre mgr. various dists. in N.J., Pa. & Del.; apptd. dir. of adv. & publicity Warner Bros., Phila. zone, 1939; winner Quigley Silver Award, 1940; Lt. Col. U.S.M.C., 1943; returned to Warner post after war; 1950–51, internat'l dir. adv., pub., Cinerama, Feb., 1954. Member: American Legion Variety Post 713 (past commdr.); Military Order of Foreign Wars of U.S.; Adv. pub. dir., National Screen Service, 1965; VP in charge of adv. and pub. sales. TV, Foreign; pres. United Screen Arts, Inc. 1966; world wide dist. and adv. and production. Presently consultant.

CALVET, CORINNE: Actress. r.n. Corinne Dibos. b. Paris, France, April 30, 1926. e. U. of Paris School of Fine Arts; French stage and radio. Screen debut in France; La Part de L'Ombre, Nous Ne Sommes Pas Maries, Petrus. American screen debut: Rope of Sand.
PICTURES INCLUDE: When Willie Comes Marching Home, My Friend Irma Goes West, Quebec, On the Riviera, Peking Express, Thunder in the East, Sailor Beware, What Price Glory? Powder River, Flight to Tangier, The Far Country, So This Is Paris, Bluebeard's Ten Honeymoons, Adventures of a Young Man, Pound.

CAMERON, JOANNA: Actress—Director. b. Sept. 20, Aspen, Colo. r.n. Patricia Cameron, e. Univ. of Calif., Sorbonne. Pasadena Playhouse, 1968. Guinness Record: Most network programmed TV commercials. Prod., dir., documentary, Razor Sharp, 1981.
PICTURES INCLUDE: How To Commit Marriage (debut), P.S., I Love You, Pretty Maids All in a Row.
TV: Features: The All-American Beauty Contest, It Couldn't Happen to a Nicer Guy, High Risk. Other: The Survivors, Love American Style, Daniel Boone, Mission Impossible, The Partners, Search, Medical Center, Isis, Name of the Game, The Bold Ones, Marcus Welby, Petrocelli, Columbo, Switch, Bob Hope Special, Bob Hope 25th NBC Anniversary Special, Westwind, MacMillian, Spiderman, Swan Song, Johnny Carson, numerous commercials. Director: Various commercials, CBS Preview Special, closed circuit program host U.S.N., all TV equiped ships—actress and director, Razor Sharp (prod., div.), 1982.

CAMP, COLLEEN: Actress. b. San Francisco. Performing since age of three. TV debut on The Dean Martin Show; feature film debut, Battle for the Planet of the Apes (1973).
PICTURES: Smile, Funny Lady, Apocalypse Now, They All Laughed, The Seduction, Smokey and the Bandit III, Valley Girl, The Joy of Sex, Police Academy II, D.A.R.Y.L., Doing Time, Clue, Doin' Time.
TELEVISION: Magnum P.I., Dukes of Hazzard, WKRP in Cincinnati, Dallas, etc.

CAMPAGNOLA, GINO: Executive. Joined Paramount Pictures in 1975; held various sales positions, including v.p., sls. admin. In 1980 named v.p., asst. gen. sls. mgr.; now sr. v.p.

CAMPANELLA, TOM: Executive. Joined Paramount Pictures 1968 as asst. business mgr.; later worked for corporate div. and Motion Picture Group. Named exec. dir., natl. adv. 1979, made v.p., natl. adv. 1984, appt. sr. v.p., adv., for M.P. Group. of Paramount.

CAMPBELL, GLEN: Actor, singer. b. Delight, Ark., April 22, 1936. After forming local band became guitarist in Hollywood; records won two Grammy awards, 1967.
PICTURES INCLUDE: True Grit, Norwood.

CAMPBELL, MAE E.: Actress. b. March 19, St. Louis, Mo. Studied with the Actors Studio and Lee Strasberg.
PICTURES INCLUDE: The Old Boyfriends; two industrial films for the Veterans Administration Hospital.

CAMPBELL, ROBERT MAURICE: Producer, director. b. Detroit, Mich., Feb. 16, 1922. e. Mich. Conservatory of Music. Detroit Inst. of Musical Arts, American Theatre Wing. Featured player. assoc. dir., Detroit stage prod.; numerous radio appearances; pub. relations, U.S. Coast Guard, World War II; since 1946 dir., off-Broadway show; dir.-prod., Springer Pictures, Inc.; TV show: All-Star News; exec., Visual Transcriptions, Inc.; prod. Jazz Dance (Robert J. Flaherty Award, Edinburgh Film Festival Merit Award); co-author, prod. designer, See No Evil.

CAMPBELL, WILLIAM: Actor. b. Newark, N.J.; e. Feagin School of Drama Appeared in summer stock. B'way plays; m.p. debut in The Breaking Point; then in People Against O'Hara, Holiday for Sinners, Battle Circus, Code Two, Big Leaguer, Escape from Fort Bravo, High and the Mighty, Man Without a Star, Cell 2455 Death Row, Battle Cry, Running Wild, Backlash, Pretty Maids All in a Row, Black Gunn.

CANALE, GIANNA MARIA: Actress. b. Reggio Calabria, Italy, Sept. 12, e. Florence. Debut in Mysterious Knight.
PICTURES INCLUDE: Kiss of a Dead Woman, Count Orgolino, Son of D'Artagnan, Go for Broke, Adventure in Algiers, Eternal Chain, Theodora Slave Empress, Madame DuBarry, The Whole Truth.

CANBY, VINCENT: Journalist-Critic. b. Chicago, July 27, 1924. e. Dartmouth Coll. Navy officer during World War II. Worked on newpapers in Paris and Chicago. Joined Quigley Publications in 1951 in editorial posts on Motion Picture Herald. Reporter for Weekly Variety 1959–1965. Joined New York Times film news staff, 1965; named film critic, 1969.

CANDY, JOHN: Actor-Writer. b. Toronto, Canada, 1951. Began acting in 11th grade and continued while studying journalism at Centennial Community College, Toronto. First professional job as member of children's theatre group; performed in satirical review, Creeps. Had roles in several low-budget Canadian films before joining in 1972 Chicago's Second City Theatre for two years. Returned to Toronto to join Second City group there, which evolved into SCTV television series. Contributed as both performer and writer, earning two Emmy Awards (writing) when show picked up by NBC.
PICTURES: Faceoff, 1941, The Blues Brothers, Stripes, National Lampoon's Vacation, Splash, Brewster's Millions, Volunteers, Summer Rental, Armed and Dangerous, The Little Shop of Horrors.

CANFIELD, ALYCE: Writer. b. Los Angeles. e. U. of Calif. Magazine writer; author Mervyn LeRoy book It Takes More Than Talent; in collab. with Howard Duff original story for Models, Inc.; story Journey Into Fire, Assignment for Murder; s.p. for latter in collab. with Jerry Jerome; creator, exec. prod. Ziv TV series, Underground, USA.

CANNELL, STEPHEN J.: Writer-Producer. b. Los Angeles, CA, Feb. 5, 1942. Heads own TV prod. co.
TELEVISION: The Rockford Files, The Jordan Chance, The Duke, Stone, 10 Speed and Brownshow, Nightside, Midnight Offerings, The Greatest American hero, The Quest, The A-Team, Hardcastle and McCormick, The Rousters, Riptide, Hunger, Brothers-in-Law, etc.

CANNON, DYAN: Actress. b. Tacoma, Wash. January 4, 1937. e. U. of Washington. Studied with Sanford Meisner. Modelled.
TV: Playhouse 90, Movies: Diane's Adventure, Lady of the House, Master of the Game, Arthur the King, Jenny's War.
BROADWAY: The Fun Couple, Ninety-Day Mistress.
ROAD TOUR: How to Succeed in Business Without Really Trying.
PICTURES INCLUDE: Bob and Carol and Ted and Alice (Academy Award nomination), Doctors' Wives, The Anderson Tapes; The Love Machine; The Burglars, Such Good Friends, Shamus, The Last of Sheila, Child Under a Leaf, Heaven Can Wait, Revenge of the Pink Panther, Coast To Coast, Honeysuckle Rose, Deathtrap.

CANNON, JUDY: Actress. b. Santa Fe, N.M., June 16, 1938. e. Santa Monica City College, 1957; teenage Adrian model, 1954–56; toured as band singer, Orlo Wagner Orchestra, 1957; appeared in: The Little Hut, Girls of Summer, Made in Japan, Los Angeles Little Theatre, 1959–61; midwest musical comedy tour group, 1962; m.p. debut, Lullaby, 1963; Critics Choice, '63; A Comedy Tale of Fanny Hill, 1964.
TV: Smothers Bros. Show, Man From U.N.C.L.E., Chrysler Theatre, Run For Your Life, The Road West, My Three Sons, Death Valley Days.
PICTURES INCLUDE: More, 1970.

CANNON, WILLIAM: Writer, Producer, Director. b. Toledo, Ohio, Feb. 11, 1937. e. Columbia Coll., B.A., 1959, M.B.A., 1962. Dir. Off-B'way, Death of a Salesman, Pirates of Penzance, 1960. Wrote, prod., dir., Square Root of Zero, Locarno and San Francisco Film Festivals, 1963–65; Distrib., Doran Enterprises, Ltd; author, Skidoo, (Par-Otto Preminger), 1968, Brewster McCloud, (MGM), 1970; HEX (20th Century Fox) 1974; Knots Landing, 1982; Heaven on Earth, 1984; Author, Novel, The Veteran (E.P. Dutton) 1974; Publisher, Highlife and Movie Digest, 1978.

CANTON, ARTHUR H.: Executive, Blowitz & Canton Co. Inc. b. New York. e. N.Y. University, Columbia University, Capt. USAF. Pres., Canton-Weiner Films, indep. foreign films importers, 1947; MGM Pictures, eastern div. publicity manager, executive liaison, advertising-publicity, Independent Productions; public relations executive, v.p.; pres., Blowitz, Thomas & Canton Inc., 1964; pres., Arthur H. Canton Co. Inc.; prod. exec., Warner Bros., 1968–70; advertising-publicity v.p., Columbia Pictures, 1971; executive v.p. of advertising and publicity, Billy Jack Productions, 1974–76. Cofounder of Blowitz & Canton Co. Inc., 1976, chairman of the board. Now pres. of Arthur H. Canton Co. Member Academy of Motion Picture Arts and Sciences, Variety Clubs International, Film Information Council; Friars Club (bd. of dir.) 1985, m.p. producer.

CANTON, MARK: Executive. b. New York City June 19, 1949. e. UCLA, 1978, v.p., m.p. devlp., MGM; 1979, exec. v.p., JP Organization; 1980, v.p. prod., Warner Bros.; named sr. v.p., 1983 and pres. w-w theatrical prod. div., 1985.

CANUTT, YAKIMA: Director. b. Colfax, Wash., Nov. 29, 1895. World's Champion All-around Rodeo, 1917–24. From 1924 in pictures; stunt man, double, asst. dir.; dir. Republic Pictures, Hollywood, 1944.
PICTURES INCLUDE: Angel and the Badmen, Oklahoma Badlands, Carson City Raiders, Sons of Adventure, G-Men Never Forget, Dangers of the Canadian Mounted, Adventures of Frank and Jesse James, Lawless Rider.

CAPRA, FRANK: Producer, Director. b. Palermo, Sicily, Italy, May 18, 1897; e. Manual Arts H.S.; Calif. Inst. of Tech., B.Sc., 1918 dir., The Strong Man, Long Pants, Platinum Blonde, American Madness, Bitter Tea of General Yen, Lady for a Day, Broadway Bill, It Happened One Night, 1934; Mr. Deeds Goes to Town, 1936; You Can't Take It With You, 1938, Lost Horizon, Mr. Smith Goes to Washington, Meet John Doe, Arsenic and Old Lace, It's a Wonderful Life, State of the Union, Riding High, Here Comes the Groom, A Hole in the Head, Pocketful of Miracles; prod., dir., Why We Fight Series, U.S. Army; pres. Academy of Motion Picture Arts and Sciences, 1935–39; pres., Directors Guild of America, 1938–40, 1959. 1964 Prod. & Dir. Rendezvous in Space. During the years 1952–1956 produced and directed four educational science films: Our Mr. Sun, Hemo The Magnificent, Strange Case of Cosmic Rays and Unchained Goddess.

CAPRA, FRANK JR: Executive. Son of famed director Frank Capra. Served in various creative capacities on TV series (Zane Grey Theatre, Gunsmoke, The Rifleman, etc.). Associate producer on theatrical films (Planet of the Apes, Play It Again Sam, Marooned, etc.). Joined Avco Embassy Pictures in March, 1981, as v.p., worldwide production. In July, 1981, became pres. of A-E. Resigned May, 1982. Now with Pinehurst Industry Studios, North Carolina.
PICTURES INCLUDE: Producer: Born Again, The Black Marble, An Eye for an Eye.

CAPSHAW, KATE: Actress. b. Ft. Worth, TX. e. Univ. of Missouri. Taught school before moving to New York to try acting. Success came on TV before theatrical debut in A Little Sex, 1981.
PICTURES: Indiana Jones and the Temple of Doom, Best Defense, Dreamscape, Windy City, Power, SpaceCamp.
TELEVISION: The Edge of Night, Missing Children: A Mother's Story, etc.

CAPUCINE: Actress. r.n. Germaine Lefebvre. b. Toulon, France, January 6. e. attended schools at Saumur, France, B.A. Photographer's model, Paris. Came to N.Y. to model. Signed contract, Famous Artists.
PICTURES INCLUDE: debut, Song Without End, North To Alaska, Walk On the Wild Side, The Lion, The 7th Dawn, What's New Pussycat?, The Honey Pot, Fraulein Doktor, Fellini's Satyricon, Red Sun, Arabian Adventure, Trail of the Pink Panther.
TELEVISION: Sins.

CAPUTO, GEORGE: Executive. b. Genoa, Italy, Oct. 24, 1916. e. Lycee de Nice (France) 1930, Sorbonne, Paris, 1934. Partner, gen. mgr., Caputo & Co., Colombia, S.A.; pres., Master Films Dist., Inc., 1950; pres., Fiesta Tele-Cinema, S.A.; pres. International Sound Studios Inc.; pres., Fall River Investments S.A.; acquired Latin America and South America rights in perpetuity to full RKO package feature films library, 1961.

CARA, IRENE: Singer-Actress. b. New York City, Mar. 18, 1959. Off-Bdwy. shows include The Mr. Nobody Knows, lotta, etc. On Bdwy. in Maggie Flynn, Ain't Misbehaving', Via Galactica, etc.
PICTURES: Aaron Loves Angela, Sparkle, Fame, D.C. Cab, City Heat, Certain Fury, Killing 'em Softly,
TELEVISION: Roots—The Next Generation, Guyana Tragedy, For Us the Living, Tribute to Martin Luther King, Jr., etc.

CARDIFF, JACK: Director. b. Yarmouth, England, September 18, 1914. Early career as child actor, later cinematographer on Stairway to Heaven, Black Narcissus, Red Shoes, Scott of the Antarctic, Black Rose, Under Capricorn, Pandora and the Flying Dutchman, African Queen, Magic Box, The Brave One, War and Peace, The Vikings; started as dir. 1958.
PICTURES INCLUDE: Intent to Kill, Beyond This Place, Scent of Mystery, Sons and Lovers, Fanny, My Geisha, The Lion, The Long Ships, Young Cassidy, The Liquidator, Dark of the Sun, The Girl on the Motorcycle, Penny Gold, The Mutations, Ride A Wild Pony, The Prince and The Pauper, Behind the Iron Mask, Death on the Nile, The Dogs of War and Ghost Story (Cinematographer), The Wicked Lady, Scandalous, The Far Pavilions, The Last Days of Pompeii, Cat's Eye, Conan the Destroyer, Blue Velvet.

CARDINALE, CLAUDIA: Actress. b. Italy, 1939.
PICTURES INCLUDE: Persons Unknown, 1958; Upstairs and Downstairs, Il Bell' Antonio, Rocco and His Brothers, Cartouche, The Leopard, Eight and a Half, The Pink

Panther, Circus World, Of A Thousand Delights, Blindfold, Last Command, The Professionals, Don't Make Waves, The Queens, The Red Tent, Conversation Piece, Escape to Athena, Immortal Bachelor.
TELEVISION: Princess Daisy.

CAREY, HARRY JR.: Actor. b. Saugus, Calif., May 16, e. Newhall, Cal., public school, Black Fox Military Acad., Hollywood; m. Marilyn Fix. two children, Steven and Melinda; Summer stock, Skowhegan, Me., with father; page boy, NBC, New York; U.S. Navy 1941–46; Screen debut: Pursued, then Red River, Moonrise.
PICTURES INCLUDE: Three Godfathers, She Wore a Yellow Ribbon, Wagonmaster, Rio Grande, Copper Canyon, Warpath, Wild Blue Yonder, Monkey Business, San Antone, Island in the Sky, Gentlemen Prefer Blondes, Beneath the 12-Mile Reef, Silver Lode, The Outcast, Long Gray Line, Mister Roberts, House of Bamboo, Great Locomotive Chase, The Undefeated Big Jake, Something Big, One More Train To Rob, The Long Riders, Endangered Species, Mask.

CAREY, MACDONALD: Actor. b. Sioux City, Iowa, March 15, 1913; e. Phillip Exeter Acad., U. Wis., U. Iowa. On stage (stock); in radio serials. On B'way in Anniversary Waltz; m.p. debut in 1942.
PICTURES INCLUDE: Dr. Broadway, Take a Letter Darling, Wake Island, Suddenly It's Spring, Variety Girl, Dream Girl, Hazzard, Streets of Laredo, Song of Surrender, South Sea Sinner, Copper Canyon, Great Missouri Raid, Mystery Submarine, Excuse My Dust, Meet Me After the Show, Let's Make It Legal, Cave of the Outlaws, My Wife's Best Friend, Count the Hours, Outlaw Territory, Fire Over Africa, Stranger At My Door, American Gigolo.
TV: Days of our Lives, Roots.

CAREY, PHIL: Actor. b. Hackensack, N.J., July 15, 1925; e. Mohawk U., U. of Miami, U.S. Marines; New England stock; m.p. debut in Operation Pacific.
PICTURES INCLUDE: Inside the Walls of Folsom Prison, This Woman Is Dangerous, Springfield Rifle, Calamity Jane, Gun Fury, The Nebraskan, Massacre Canyon, Outlaw Stallion, They Rode West, Pushover, The Long Gray Line, Wyoming Renegades, Mister Roberts, Count Three and Pray, Three Stripes in the Sun, The Time Traveler, Once You Kiss a Stranger, Three Guns for Texas, The Seven Minutes. TV: Laredo.

CARISCH, GEORGE: Exhibitor. b. Minneapolis, MN DEc. 12, 1935. e. Hamline Univ. (BS); Univ. of Minnesota (BEE). Chm., Carisch Theatres, Inc.

CARLIDGE, WILLIAM: Executive. b. Fenton, Eng., May 2, 1910. e. Grafton Boys' School. Entered m.p. ind. in 1930 as mgr. Ilford Hippodrome; circuit mgr. Union Cinemas, 1935; supervisor for Northern Ireland. Associated British Cinemas Ltd., 1947; first regional controller for Northern Region, personal asst. to man. dir. 1949; gen. man. Associated British Cinemas Ltd. 1951; dir. 1955; asst. man. dir. 1959; Board of Associated British Corp., 1964, now known as EMI Film and Theatre Corp.

CARLINO, LEWIS JOHN: Writer. b. N.Y.C., Jan. 1, 1932. e. USC. Early interest in theatre, specializing in writing 1-act plays. Winner of Obie award (off-Bdwy. play). Won Rockefeller Grant for Theatre, the Int'l. Playwriting Competition from British Drama League, Huntington Hartford Fellowship.
PICTURES INCLUDE: Seconds, The Brotherhood, The Fox (co-s.p.), The Mechanic, The Sailor Who Fell From The Sea, (s.p., dir.), I Never Promised You a Rose Garden (co. s.p.), The Ace (s.p., dir.), Resurrection (s.p.), Class (dir.).
PLAYS: Cages, Telemachus Clay, The Exercise, Double Talk, Objective Case, Used Car for Sale, Junk Yard.

CARLISLE, ROBERT: Producer. b. Los Angeles, Calif., Sept. 19, 1906. Cutter, Metro; Universal; John Stahl; Columbia; film ed. in chf. Columbia; prod. short subjects with Jerry Fairbanks including: Popular Science, Unusual Occupations, Speaking of Animals (two Academy of M.P. Arts & Sciences awards); prod. industrials for Dupont, Union Pacific RR; trophy at Italy's Cortina Sports Film Festival for ski film, 1957; prod. and dir. films on world affairs for Dept. of Defense; prod. Wondsel, Carlisle & Dunphy, Inc., 1957.

CARLTON, RICHARD: Executive. b. New York City, Feb. 9, 1919. e. Columbia U., Pace Inst. Columbia Pictures 1935–41; U.S. Army 1941–45; National Screen Serv. 1945–51; Sterling Television 1951–54; U.M. & M. TV Corp. 1955; v.p. in charge of sales, Trans-Lux Television Corp., 1956; exec. vice-pres., Television Affiliates Corp., 1961; exec. v.p. Trans-Lux Television Corp.; v.p. Entertainment Div. Trans-Lux Corp., 1966. Pres., Schnur Appel, TV, Inc. 1970; Deputy Director, American Film Institute, 1973. Pres., Carlton Communications Corporation, 1982; exec. dir., International Council, National Academy of Television Arts and Sciences, 1983.

CARMEN, JEAN: See Jean Carmen Dillow.

CARMICHAEL, IAN: Actor. b. Hull, England, June 18, 1920. e. Scarborough College, Bromsgrove School, Stage debut; R.U.R. 1939. Film debut: Bond Street, one of the top ten British money making stars M.P.H.—Fame Poll 1957, 1958.
TV: New Faces, Twice Upon a Time, Passing Show, Tell Her The Truth, Lady Luck, Give My Regards to Leicester Square, Jill Darling, Don't Look Now, Regency Room, Globe Revue, Off the Record, Here and Now, The Girl at the Next Table, Gilt and Gingerbread, The Importance of being Earnest, Simon and Laura, 90 Years On, The World of Wooster, The Last of the Big Spenders, The Coward Revue, Odd Man In, Bachelor Father, Lord Peter Wimsey, Alma Mater, Comedy Tonight, Song by Song, Country Calendar, Down at the Hydro.
PICTURES INCLUDE: Trottie True, Mr. Prohack, Time Gentlemen Please, Meet Mr. Lucifer, Betrayed, Coldits Story, Storm Over the Nile, Simon and Laura, Private's Progress, Brothers in Law, Lucky Jim, Happy Is the Bride, The Big Money, Right, Left and Center, I'm Alright Jack, School for Scoudrels, Light Up the Sky, Double Bunk, The Amorous Prawn, Hide and Seek, Heavens Above, Smashing Time, The Magnificent Seven, Deadly Sins, From Beyond the Grave, The Lady Vanishes.

CARNEY, ART: Performer. b. Mt. Vernon, N.Y., Nov. 4, 1918. Many radio shows. U.S. Army, 1944–45; performer, Jackie Gleason's Honeymooners.
TELEVISION: Studio One, Kraft, Omnibus, Chevy Show, Playhouse 90, Dupont Show of the Month—"Harvey," Sid Caesar Show, Alfred Hitchcock Presents—"Safety for the Witness," Art Carney meets Peter and the Wolf," Playhouse 90—"Fabulous Irishman," "Charley's Aunt," "Velvet Alley," "Art Carney Meets the Sorcerer's Apprentice," The Sid Caesar-Art Carney Show, Our Town, Very Important People, Man in the Dog Suit, Call Me Back, Batman, Carol Burnett Show, Jonathan Winters Show, Tonight Show. Movies: The Night They Saved Christmas, A Doctor's Story, Terrible Joe Moran, Izzy and Moe.
PICTURES INCLUDE: Harry and Tonto, W. W. and the Dixie Dancekings, Won Ton Ton, The Late Show, Take This Job and Shove It, Better Late Than Never, Firestarter, The Naked Face.
STAGE: The Rope Dancers, Take Her She's Mine, (Bdwy.), The Odd Couple (Bdwy.), Lovers (Bdwy.), The Prisoner of Second Avenue (Bdwy.), Sunburn, Going in Style, Defiance, Roadie.

CARNEY, FRED: Producer, director. b. Brooklyn, N.Y., June 10, 1914; e. Mt. Vernon H.S., 1932. Actor on B'way & summer stock; prod. mgr. for radio show, Truth or Consequences; asst. to prod.-dir of Kraft TV Theatre, 3 yrs.; dir., Kraft, Pond's Show; creator-prod., Medical Horizons; dir., Lux Video Theatre; prod. commercials at Cunningham & Walsh. Assoc. Prod. Everybody's Talking for ABC-TV. Ass't. Exec. Dir., Hollywood Chpt., Nat'l. Acad. TV; Assoc. prod. 40th Acad. Award show, ABC-TV Arts & Sciences; currently acting in feature films and TV.

CARON, LESLIE: Dancer, actress. b. Paris, France. July 1, 1931. e. Convent of Assumption, Paris; Nat'l Conservatory of Dance, Paris. Did solo bit parts, then starred joined Ballet des Champs Elysees. In 1950, signed MGM lead film role in An American in Paris; since in Man with a Cloak, Glory Alley, Story of Three Loves, Lili, Glass Slipper, Daddy Long Legs, Gaby, Gigi, The Doctor's Dilemma, The Man Who Understood Women, The Subterraneans, Fanny, Guns of Darkness, The L Shaped Room, Father Goose, Promise Her Anything, A Very Special Favor, Is Paris Burning, Head of the Family, The Beginners, Madron, Chandler, Purple Night, Valentino.
TELEVISION: Master of the Game.

CARPENTER, CARLETON: Actor. b. Bennington, VT., July 10; e. Bennington H.S.; Northwestern U. (summer scholarship). Began career with magic act, clubs, camps, hospitals, New Eng.; then toured with carnival; first N.Y. stage appearance in Bright boy.
STAGE: Career Angel, Three To Make Ready, The Magic Touch, The Big People, Art of Dust, John Murray Anderson's Almanac. Appeared night clubs; radio; as model magazines, TV debut, Campus HoopLa show. Screen debut Lost Boundaries (alos wrote song for film, I Wouldn't Mind).
PICTURES INCLUDE: Summer Stock, Father of the Bride, Two Weeks With Love, Whistle at Eaton Falls, Fearless Fagan, Sky Full of Moon, Take the High Ground, Some of My Best Friends Are . . .

CARPENTER, JOHN: Director-Writer. b. Carthage, NY, Jan. 16, 1948. e. USC. Married to Adrienne Barbeau. At USC became involved in film short, Resurrection of Bronco Billy, which won Oscar as best live-action short of 1970. Also at USC began directing what ultimately became Dark Star, science fiction film that launched his career.
PICTURES: Assault on Precinct 13, Halloween (also music), Eyes of Laura Mars (s.p. only), The Fog (also music), Escape from New York (also music); Halloween II

(co-prod.); The Thing (dir.); Christine (dir., music); Starman (dir.); Big Trouble in Little China (dir., music).

CARPENTER, ROBERT L.: Executive. b. March 20, 1927, Memphis, Tenn. Joined Universal Pictures in 1949 as booker in Memphis exchange; promoted to salesman there in 1952 and branch mgr. in 1958. In 1963 named Los Angeles branch manager. In Dec., 1971 moved to New York to become asst. to general sales mgr. Named gen. sls. mgr. on April 16, 1972, replacing Henry H. Martin when latter became pres. of Universal. Left in 1982 to become consultant and producer's rep. 1984, joined Cannon Releasing Corp. as east. div. mgr.

CARR, ALLAN: Producer—Personal Manager. b. Highland Park, Ill. e. Lake Forest College, Northwestern Univ. First venture in show business as one of creators of Playboy Penthouse TV series. Produced plays at Civic Theatre, Chicago. Asst. to Nicholas Ray on King of Kings shot in Madrid. Became talent scout, launching Marlo Thomas in play, Sunday in New York, on West Coast. Other clients have included Ann-Margret, Peter Sellers, Nancy Walker, Marvin Hamlisch, Stockard Channing, Melina Mercouri, Franke Valli, etc. Served as creative consultant to Robert Stigwood Organisation in marketing and promotion of movie, Tommy. Presented Survive! with Stigwood.
PICTURES: Producer: The First Time, C.C. and Company, Grease (co-prod.), Can't Stop the Music (co-prod. co. s.p.), Grease 2 (co-prod.), Where the Boys Are (prod.).

CARR, ARNOLD: Publicist. b. Chicago, Ill., Aug. 9, 1931. e. Univ. of Missouri. Began public relations handling tour with Dimitri Mitropoulos, U.S. State Depart.; Columbia Broadcasting System; pub. dir., KABC-TV; Screen Gems; pub. rel. dir., Hanna-Barbera Prod.; formed own firm, 1962; partnered with Richard Carter 1964; resumed business under own name, Arnold Carr Public Relations.

CARR, JOHN: Ex. Producer-Director-Writer. b. West Virginia, Jan. 19, 1930. Now pres. of Pan-American Pictures Corp.
PICTURES: Sanitarium, Gretta (dir.); The Dark Side of Love, The Rebel's Mistresses, The Runaways, The Talisman (s.p.).

CARR, MARTIN: Producer-Director-Writer b. N.Y.C. Jan 20, 1932. e. Williams Coll. Worked for all three networks.
TELEVISION: PBS Smithsonian World (exec. prod.). For CBS produced, wrote and directed CBS Reports: Hunger in America, The Search for Ulysses, Gauguin in Tahiti, Five Faces of Tokyo, Dublin Through Different Eyes. For NBC produced, wrote and directed NBC White Paper: Migrant, NBC White Paper: This Child Is Rated X. Also directed drama, dance, music, opera specials and daytime serial for CBS-TV. ABC Close-Up. The Culture Thieves. PRS Global Paper: Waging Peace, ABC News 20/20; NBC, The Human Animal.
AWARDS: Winner of 5 Emmys; 3 Peabody awards; 2 Du-Pont Col. Journalism awards; Robert F. Kennedy award; Sidney Hillman award; Writers Guild Award.

CARR, THOMAS: Director; b. Philadelphia, Pa., July 4, 1907. On screen at 2½ yrs. for Lubin Co., Phil.; starred in Little Britches at 5 yrs., actor on stage, radio & screen until 1937; then became dialogue clerk, Republic Studios, advancing to script; asst. assoc. prod; assoc. prod. 1944; dir. 1945. Pictures include many westerns, Bobby Ware is Missing.

CARRADINE, DAVID: Actor. b. Hollywood, Oct. 8, 1940. f. John Carradine. e. San Francisco State. Began career in local repetory; first TV on Armstrong Circle Theatre and East Side, West Side; later TV includes Shane series and Kung Fu; N.Y. stage in The Deputy, Royal Hunt of The Sun.
PICTURES INCLUDE: Taggart, Bus Riley's Back in Town, Too Many Thieves, The Violent Ones, Heaven With a Gun, Young Billy Young, The Good Guys and the Bad Guys, Gallery of Horrors, The McMasters, Macho Callahan, A Gunfight, McCabe & Mrs. Miller, Boxcar Bertha, Death Race 2000, Bound for Glory, The Serpent's Egg, Gray Lady Down, The Long Riders, Cloud Dancer, The Winged Serpent, Lone Wolf McQuade, P.O.W. The Escape.
TELEVISION: Movies: Jealousy, The Bad Seed, Kung Fu: The Movie. Mini-series: North & South; Book II.

CARRADINE, JOHN: Actor. b. New York City., Feb. 5, 1908. On stage in Shakespearian roles. A Funny Thing Happened on My Way to the Forum. On screen from 1936.
PICTURES INCLUDE: Fallen Angel, House of Dracula, Captain Kidd, Face of Marble, House of Frankenstein, It's in the Bag, Private Affairs of Bel Ami, C-Man, Cassanova's Big Night, Thunder Pass, Johnny Guitar, The Egyptian, Stranger on Horseback, Hidden Guns, Court Jester, Desert Sands, The Kentuckian, Dark Venture, Black Sheep, The Good Guys and the Bad Guys, Boxcar Bertha, Everything You Always Wanted to Know About Sex*, The Shootist, The Last Tycoon, The Sentinel, Zorro, The Gay Blade, House of the Long Shadows, Evils of the Night.

CARRADINE, KEITH: Actor. b. San Mateo, Calif. Aug. 8, 1950. Son of actor John Carrradine, brother of David. e. Colorado State Univ. Got first break in rock opera "Hair." Screen debut in A Gunfight (1971).
PICTURES INCLUDE: McCabe and Mrs. Miller, Idaho Transfer, Emperor of the North, Thieves Like Us, Nashville, Lumiere, Welcome to L.A., The Duellists, Pretty Baby, Old Boyfriends, An Almost Perfect Affair, The Long Riders, Southern Comfort, Maria's Lovers, Choose Me, Trouble in Mind.
TELEVISION: Chiefs, Scorned and Swindled, A Winner Never Quits.

CARRADINE, ROBERT: Actor. b. San Mateo, CA, March 24, 1954. Son of John Carradine; brother of Keith and David Carradine.
PICTURES: The Cowboys, Mean Streets, Aloha Bobby and Rose, Jackson County Jail, The Pom Pom Girls, Cannonball, Massacre at Central High, Joyride, Orca, Blackout, Coming Home, The Long Riders, The Big Red One, Heartaches, Wavelength, Just the Way You Are, Number One with a Bullet, Revenge of the Nerds.
TELEVISION: Movies: Footsteps, Go Ask Alice, The Hatfields and the McCoys, The Survival of Dana, The Sun Also Rises.

CARRERA, BARBARA: Actress. Fashion model before film debut in The Master Gunfighter, 1976.
PICTURES: Embryo, The Island of Dr. Moreau, When Time Ran Out, Condorman, I the Jury, Lone Wolf McQuade, Never Say Never Again, Wild Geese II.
TELEVISION: Centennial, Matt Houston, Masada, etc.

CARRERAS, SIR JAMES K.C.V.O. M.B.E.: Chariman and chief executive. Hammer Film Productions Ltd. 1946–1973; past-president, Variety International; chairman, Royal Naval Film Corporation; Friends of the Duke of Edinburgh's Award Scheme; director, National Screen Service; trustee, Young Volunteer Force Foundation; vice-president, London Federation of Boys' Clubs; member of the council, Cinema and Television Benevolent Fund.

CARROLL, CARROLL: Writer, producer, b. New York, N.Y. m.p. critic, feature writer, N.Y. Sunday World; free lance writer, nat'l mags: radio writer, J. Walter Thompson, N.Y. 1932–36; West Coast, 1936–46; v.p., writer, prod., Ward Wheelock Co., West Coast, 1946–53. CBS, NBC, JWT, East Coast 1957–67. Now based in Hollywood.
SHOWS INCLUDE: (radio) Bing Crosby, Al Jolson, Rudy Vallee, Eddie Cantor, Burns & Allen, Joe Penner, Kraft Music Hall, Edgar Bergen, Frank Sinatra, Bob Crosby, Corliss Archer, Double or Nothing. Club 15; (TV) head writer, Bob Crosby Show; CBS-TV creative staff, 1953–55; General Electric Hour; Young & Rubicam TV, 1955; NBC-TV creative staff, 1956–57; ed. dept., J. Walter Thompson Co., 1957–67. Writer, prod., Chase & Sanborn 100th Anniv. Radio Show with Edgar Bergen, 1964; C & S 101. Anniv. Show with Fred Allen, 1965; 1966 NBC 40th Anniv. Show. Free-lance writer and adv. consultant, 1967–77. Book Reviewer for Variety and Columnist, "And Now a Word from . . ." in Variety, 1967–84.
AUTHOR: "None of Your Business or My Life with J. Walter Thompson," 1970. "My Life With . . ." 1978. Co-author with Henny Youngman "Take My Wife . . . Please!" Editoral consultant "Liberace." Editorial Consultant "Mike Douglas, My Story," Co-author with Ed McMahon, "Here's Ed." Co-author with Bob Hope: "I Never Left Home", "So This is Peace," Author, Carroll's First Book of Proverbs, or Life Is a Fortune Cookie.

CARROLL, DIAHANN: Actress-Singer. b. New York City, July 17, 1935. On Bdwy. in No Strings, Agnes of God, etc. Film debut in Carmen Jones, 1954.
PICTURES: Porgy and Bess, Goodbye Again, Paris Blues, Hurry Sundown, The Split, Claudine, etc.
TELEVISION: Series: Julia, Dynasty. Movies: I Know Why the Caged Bird Sings, Sister Sister, etc.

CARROLL, GORDON: Producer. b. Balt. Md., Feb. 2, 1928. e. Princeton U. Advtg. exec., Foote, Cone & Belding, 1954–58; Ent. industry, Seven Arts Prods., 1958–61; v.p., Staff Prod., Jalem Prods., 1966–1969; Independent Producer to present.
PICTURES INCLUDE: How to Murder Your Wife, Luv, Cool Hand Luke, The April Fools, Pat Garrett and Billy the Kid, Alien, Blue Thunder, Aliens.

CARROLL, LAURIE: Singer, actress. b. Cambridge, Mass., April 15, 1935. e. U.S.C. Actress in little theatre group, Los Angeles; on Broadway in Plain and Fancy.
TV: You Are There, Damon Runyon Theatre, Shower of Stars; feature singer, Johnny Carson Show, CBS-TV.

CARROLL, MADELEINE: Actress. b. West Bromwich, England, Feb. 26, 1906; e. Birmingham U., B.A. Taught school. Given leading role in Brit. "Guns of Loos" 1929; thereafter in many Brit. & U.S. (from 1934).

PICTURES INCLUDE: Young Woodley, Madame Guillotine, I Was a Spy, Thirty-Nine Steps, Case Against Mrs. Ames, General Died at Dawn, Lloyds of London, Prisoner of Zenda, Cafe Society, Convoy, Lady in Distress, My Favorite Blonde.

CARROLL, PAT: Performer. b. Shreveport, La., May 5, 1927. e. Immaculate Heart College, LA.; Catholic University, Wash., D.C. Joined U.S. Army in capacity of "civilian actress technician." Night club entertainer in N.Y., 1949.
TV: Red Buttons, George Gobel, Jimmy Durante and Mickey Rooney; Caesar's Hour, 1956. Bdwy.
STAGE: Catch a Star.

CARSON, JEANNIE: Actress. b. Yorkshire, England. Amer. Citizen, 1966, in musicals Ace of Clubs, Love from Judy; Ent. Motion Pictures in 1954 in As Long as They're Happy; Alligator Named Daisy, Mad Little Island.
TV: Best Foot Forward, Little Women, Berkeley Square, The Rivals, Frank Sinatra Show, Own TV Series, Hey Jeannie and Jeannie Carson Show. Toured in Sound of Music, Camelot, 110 in the Shade. Under contract to Decca.

CARSON, JOHNNY: Comedian. b. Corning, Ia., Oct. 23, 1925. e. U. of Neb. U.S. Navy service; with station KFAB, Lincoln, Neb.; WOW radio-TV, Omaha, 1948; announcer, KNXT, Los Angeles, 1950; then program, Carson's Cellar; quizmaster, Earn Your Vacation, 1954; writer for Red Skelton; star of Johnny Carson Show, CBS-TV; Who Do You Trust, ABC-TV; The Tonight Show Starring Johnny Carson, NBC-TV.

CARSTENSEN, VERN: Exec. b. Clinton, Ia., May 24, 1914. e. U. of Iowa, 1933–38.
RADIO: announcer, 1936–38, WSUI, Iowa City, WOC, Davenport, WHBF, Rock Island, CBS, Chicago; prog. dir., sls. prom., KROS, Clinton, 1939–42; U.S. Army, 1942–46, Armed Forces Radio Network, No. Africa, orig. Mobile Radio Station, Italy, Armed Forces Radio Service Hdqtrs., Hollywood, OIC overseas liaison; prod. mgr., Mayfair Transcription Co., 1946–51; exec. asst., Alan Ladd Enterprises Inc., 1951–58; assoc. prod., exec. coord., Jaquar Prods., 1958–61; v.p., sec., Eagle Animation Corp.; sec.-treas., Juggernaut Prods. Inc., 1962–64; exec. v.p. Dale Robertson Assoc., 1963; exec. v.p., United Screen Arts Inc. 1964–66; exec. v.p. Juggernaut, Inc. 1966–68, v.p. Entertainment Associates, Inc. 1968–70; v.p. Tommy Walker Productions 1970–73; pres. Center Features, Inc. 1973–1976; 1977–1978, exec. v.p., Justin & Assoc. Inc.; 1979–81, v.p. Great Rollerworks Corp.

CARTER, HELENA BONHAM: Actress. b. England, May 26, 1966. e. Westminster. Appeared on BBC in A Pattern of Roses; seen by director Trevor Nunn who cast her in Lady Jane (1986), theatrical film debut.
PICTURES: Lady Jane, A Room with a View.

CARTER, JACK: Actor, r.n., Jack Chakrin. b. New York, June 24, 1923. e. Brooklyn College, Feagin Sch. of Dram. Arts. Worked as comm. artist for adv. agencies. Debut Broadway in Call Me Mister, 1947; starred in TV Jack Carter Show. Seen on most major variety, dram. programs, incl. Ed Sullivan Show. Emmy nom. 1962 for Dr. Kildare seg. Played most major nightclubs. App. Broadway in Top Banana; Mr. Wonderful.
PICTURES INCLUDE: The Horizontal Lieutenant, Viva Las Vegas, The Extraordinary Seaman, The Resurrection of Zachary Wheeler.

CARTER, LYNDA: Actress. b. Phoenix, Ariz., July 24. e. Arizona State Univ. Wrote songs and sang professionally in Arizona from age of 15; later toured for 4 yrs. with rock 'n' roll band. Won beauty contests in Ariz. and became Miss World-USA in 1973. Dramatic training with Stella Adler and Charles Conrad.
TELEVISION: The New Adventures of Wonder Woman; numerous specials; Rita Hayworth Love Goddess (movie).

CARTER, MAURICE: Art director/designer. b. London, England, 1913. Grad. of The Royal Society of Art Masters. Early career as interior decoration designer. Ent. m.p. ind. 1934/5 Islington Studios, became art dir. 1938. Involved in development back projection. Has art dir. or designed over eighty features includ. Man in Grey, Becket, The Battle of Britain, Anne of the Thousand Days, Innocent Bystanders, The Land that Time Forgot, At The Earth's Core, The People That Time Forgot, The Great Train Robbery. Specializes in period subject and special effect. Three times nominated for American Academy awards and twice for British Film Academy awards. Founder of Guild of Film Art Directors.

CARTER, TRACY: Actress. r.n. Tracy Olsen b. Los Angeles Calif., Feb. 16, 1940. e. Hollywood Sch. of Drama, 1957–58; Pasadena Playhouse, 1958–61. Pianist, 15 years, Los Angeles Conservatory.
TV: Have Gun Will Travel, Ripcord, 77 Sunset Strip, Fred McMurray Show, The Deputy, June Allyson Show, Michael Shayne, Betty Hutton Show, Divorce Court, Kraft Suspense Theatre, Bonanza, Beauty Fair.
PLAYS: Desperate Hours, Look Back in Anger, Puss 'n Boots, The Thousand Dollar Mule, Taming of the Shrew, Richard III.
PICTURES INCLUDE: The Couch, Boy on the Run, Terrified, Dust Is My Tomorrow, Sweet Hell, I'll Love You Forever, Johnny Reno, Waco, Red Tomahawk, Journey to the Center of Time.

CARTIER, RUDOLPH: TV producer, director. b. Vienna, Austria, April 17, 1908. Stage designer, journalist, writer, film dir. and prod.; entered m.p. industry 1929. Joined BBC-TV drama dept., 1952; senior producer-director, 1953.
PICTURES INCLUDE: L'Aigion, Quatermass Experiment, Wuthering Heights, That Lady, Such Men Are Dangerous, Rebecca, Liebelei, Captain Banner, Nineteen Eighty-Four, The Creature, Moment of Truth, Midsummer Fire, Thunder Rock, Quatermass II, Devil's General, White Falcon, Maverling Affair, Arrow to the Heart, Fugitive, Cold Light, Saint of Bleecker Street, Dark Victory, Clive of India, Queen and the Rebels, Salome, Mother Courage, A Tale of Two Cities, Midsummer Night's Dream, Quatermass and the Pit, Tobias and the Angel, Roshomon, Adventure Story, Anna Karenina, Cross of Iron, Golden Fleece, The Liars, Carmen, Dr. Korczak and the Children, Sword of Vengeance, Aspern Papers, Anna Christie, Stalingrad, Respectable Prostitute, Lady of the Camellias, Midnight Men, July Plot, Wings of the Dove, Ironhand, Joel Brand Story, Gordon of Khartoum, Lee Oswald-Assassin, The Survivors, Level Seven, Firebrand, The Burning Bush, The Fanatics, The Rebel, Conversation at Night, An Ideal Husband, Rembrandt, The Bear, The Year of the Crow, The Proposal, Lady Windermere's Fan (1972), The Deep Blue Sea, Fall of Eagles (1974), Loyalties (1976).
TV: Winslow Boy, Gaslight, Sacrifice to the Wind, The Patriot, A Night Out, Death Has Many Faces, Attorney-General, The Consul, Aspern Papers, That Lady, Corinth House, The Savages, Alibi for James, Mr. Pickwick, The Spanish Civil War, In the Name of Conscience.

CASE, NELSON: Announcer. b. Long Beach, Calif, e. William and Mary Coll. Joined NBC, San Francisco, 1931, announcer, NBC, New York, 1934; freelance 1939; U.S. Navy, 1942–45; Lowell Thomas Show, 1946; TV announcer-host.
SHOWS: Pulitzer Prize Playhouse, Robert Mongomery Presents, Jackie Gleason Show, Omnibus, Red Buttons Show, Masquerade Party, Wide Wide World.

CASELLI, LAMAR: Director. b. San Francisco, Calif., June 16, 1921. e. U. of Wash.; U. of Calif. at L.A.; B.A., 1946; M.A. Telecommunications UCLA 1971; Pilot-Air Corps, 1943–45, legit actor & stage mgr., 1947–50; stg. mgr., assoc. dir. and dir., CBS-TV and NBC-TV, 1950–56; C.C. medical and industrial TV, 1955–63; staff dir., CBS-TV, The Last Word, Lamp Unto My Feet, Look Up and Live, 1957–58; F.L. dir., G.E. College Bowl, CBS-TV. NBC-TV, 1959–64; dir. Alumni Fun CBS-TV, 1964; 1965 Insight CBS-TV; Morning Star, serial NBC-TV; 1966 Young Marrieds, serial ABC-TV; 1967-present, prof., Loyola Univ., 1969, dir. film TV, Death Valley Days; 1970–71, also 1976–77 dir., General Hospital (ABC-TV serial), dir., This is the Life, synd. series, 1975–79.

CASS, PEGGY: Actress. b. Boston, May 21, 1924. On Broadway in Burlesque, Bernardine, Auntie Mame, Don't Drink the Water, Front Page, Last of the Red Hot Lovers, etc.
PICTURES: The Marrying Kind, Auntie Mame, Gidget Goes Hawaiian, The Age of Consent, Paddy, etc.
TELEVISION: The Hathaways, Garry Moore Show, To Tell the Truth, etc.

CASSAVETES, JOHN: Director, Actor. b. New York, N.Y., Dec. 9, 1929. e. Colgate College, N.Y. Acad. of Dramatic Arts. m. Gena Rowlands. Actor in stock co.; asst. stage mgr. for Broadway play Fifth Season; many TV credits including Omnibus, Elgin Playhouse.
PICTURES INCLUDE: Taxi, Night Holds Terror, Crime in the Streets, Edge of the City, Fever Tree, Shadows (dir.), Too Late Blues (dir., s.p.), A Child is Waiting (dir), Faces, Husbands (actor, s.p., dir.), Minnie & Moskowitz (s.p., dir.), Devil's Angels, The Dirty Dozen, Rosemary's Baby, Machine Gun McCann, Woman Under The Influence, (dir.), Mikey and Nicky, Killing of a Chinese Bookie (dir., s.p.); Two Minute Warning (actor); Opening Night, 1977 (s.p., dir.), The Fury (actor) 1978. Brass Target (actor) 1978, Gloria (s.p., dir.), Whose Life Is It Anyway? (actor); Tempest (actor); Marvin and Tige (actor); Love Streams (dir., co. s.-p., actor); Big Trouble (dir.).

CASSEL, ALVIN I.: Executive. b. New York City, July 26, e. Univ. of Mich., 1938 BA. Capt. in U.S. Army European Theatre, 1941–45. Surveyed Central Africa for MGM, 1946–50, then assumed duties as asst. mgr. for MGM South Africa. Continued with MGM in West Indies, 1950–51 and Philippines, 1951–57. In 1957 joined Universal as mgr./supvr. for Southeast Asia; back to MGM in 1963 as supvr.

S.E. Asia; 1967, with CBS Films as Far East supvr. In 1972 established Cassel Films to secure theatrical films for foreign distributors, principally in Far East, 1979, consultant for Toho-Towa co. of Japan and other Far East distributors.

CASSEL, JEAN-PIERRE: Actor. b. Paris, Oct. 27, 1932. began as dancer, attracting attention of Gene Kelly in Left Bank nightspot, who gave him film work. Appeared in plays before becoming established as leading French screen star.
PICTURES INCLUDE: Games of Love, The Gay Deceiver, Five Day Lover, The Vanishing Corporal, The Male Companion, A Woman Passed By, Is Paris Burning?, Those Magnificent Men in Their Flying Machines, The Killing Game, Oh! What a Lovely War, The Bear and The Doll, The Rupture, The Boat on the Grass, Baxter!, The Discreet Charm of the Bourgeoisie, The Three Musketeers, Le Mouton Enrage, Murder on the Orient Express, Who Is Killing the Great Chefs of Europe?

CASSIDY, DAVID: Actor. b. April 12, 1950. Son of Shirley Jones and late Jack Cassidy; brother of Shaun.
TELEVISION: The Partridge Family, Man Undercover, The Night the City Screamed.

CASSIDY, JOANNA: Actress. b. Camden, N.J., 1944. e. Syracuse Univ.
PICTURES: The Laughing Policeman, The Outfit, Bank Shot, Stay Hungry, Prime Time, The Late Show, Night Child, Stunts, The Glove, Our Winning Season, Night Games, Blade Runner, Club Paradise.
TELEVISION: 240–Robert, Reunion, The Children of Times Square, Pleasures.

CASSIDY, SHAUN: Actor/Singer/Composer. b. Los Angeles, Sept. 27, 1958. One of 3 sons of Shirley Jones and late Jack Cassidy. e. Bev. Hills high school. Began recording in 1976 and toured Europe and Australia, appearing on numerous TV shows. Has had several hit records.
TELEVISION: Hardy Boys Mysteries, numerous specials, talk shows.
PICTURES: Born of water (debut for Ameri. Film Inst.).

CASTELL, ANTONIO: Executive. b. Havana, Cuba, Dec. 9, 1911; e. U. of Havana; publicity dir., Cuba, 1937; motion picture exhibitor, 1937–48; distributor, Cooperative Cinematografica; owner dir., Alex and Atlas Films, up to 1961; distributor, Spanish pictures for the Americas.

CASTELLANO, RICHARD S.: Actor, Producer. b. New York City, September 4, 1933. e. Commerce H.S., Columbia U. Before acting career was owner of construction company and employed as construction consultant.
THEATRE: 1963: New Yiddish Theatre; 1965–66: starred off-Broadway in A View From The Bridge; 1966: on Broadway in The Investigation and That Summer That Fall; 1967: Stratford Shakespeare Company Festival; 1968: Mike Downstairs, Why I Went Crazy. Also on Broadway in Sheep On The Runway and Lovers and Other Strangers (Tony nomination).
PICTURES: A Fine Madness, Lovers and Other Strangers (Academy nomination), Night of the Juggler, The Godfather.
TELEVISION: NYPD, The Super, Incident on a Dark Street, Honor Thy Father, Joe and Sons, Gangster Chronicles.

CASTLE, WALTER H.: Cinematographer. b. Santa Ana, Calif., May 19, 1905, Engaged continuously in photographic work for 27 years with Fox Films Corp. and 20th Century-Fox Film corp., as director of photography; Walt Disney Prod., TV, Hardy Boys, American Dairy Story, Spin, Mickey Mouse Club, Our Friend the Atom, Saga of Andy Burnett; spec. effects for Trapeze.

CATES, GILBERT: Director-Producer. b. New York City, June 6, 1934. e. Syracuse Univ. Began TV career as guide at NBC studios in N.Y., working way up to prod. and dir. of game shows (Camouflage, Haggis Baggis, Mother's Day, etc.). Created Hootenanny and packaged and directed many TV specials.
PICTURES INCLUDE: The Painting (short), Rings Around the World, I Never Sang for My Father, Summer Wishes, Winter Dreams (dir. only); One Summer Love, (prod.-dir.), 1975; The Promise, 1978, The Last Married Couple in America, 1980; Oh, God!— Book II, 1980.
TELEVISION: International Showtime (1963–65 exec. prod.-dir.), Electric Showcase Specials ('65, dir.-prod.), To All My Friends on Shore ('72-dir.-prod.), The Affair ('73-dir.), After the Fall ('74-dir.-prod.), Johnny, We Hardly Knew Ye, (1976-prod.-dir.), The Kid from Nowhere (1981-prod.); Country Gold (1982–dir.); Hobson's Choice (1983–dir.); Burning Rage (1984-dir.); Consenting Adult (1985-dir.).
STAGE: Director: Tricks of the Trade, Voices, The Price (Long Wharf Theatre). Producer: Solitaire/Double Solitaire, The Chinese and Mr. Fish, I Never Sang for My Father, You Know I Can't Hear You When the Water's Running.

CATES, JOSEPH: Producer-Director. b. 1924. e. New York Univ. Brother of Gilbert Cates. One of first producers of live TV with Wish Upon a Star, 1947. Prod., Jackie Gleason Show, game shows, various specials. Films include Last Married Couple in America.

CATES, PHOEBE: Actress. b. NYC, 1964. Daughter of TV producer Joseph Cates. Dance prodigy and fashion model before launching acting career in Paradise. Studied with Actors Circle theatre group.
PICTURES: Paradise, Fast Times at Ridgemont High, Private School, Gremlins.
TELEVISION: Movies: Baby Sister, Lace, Lace II.

CAULFIELD, JOAN: Actress. b. Orange, N.J., June 1, 1922. e. Columbia U. Harry Conover model 1942–43; on stage 1943–44; screen debut in "Miss Susie Slagle's" 1945.
PICTURES INCLUDE: Dear Ruth, Variety Girl, Unsuspected, Sainted Sisters, Larceny, Pretty Girl, Lady Said No, Rains of Ranchipur, Buckskin.
TV: Sally, My Favorite Husband, CBS.

CAVANAUGH, ANDREW: Executive. Held positions with Norton Simon, Inc. and Equitable Life Insurance Co. before joining Paramount Pictures in 1984 as v.p., human resources. 1985, appt. sr. v.p., administration, mng. personnel depts. on both coasts. Also oversees corp. admin. function for Paramount.

CAVETT, DICK: Actor-Writer. b. Kearny. Nebr., Nov. 19, 1937. e. Yale Univ. Acted in TV dramas and Army training films, Was writer for Jack Paar, and his successors on the Tonight Show and had comedy writing assignments with Merv Griffin, Jerry Lewis, Johnny Carson. In 1967 wrote for self and appeared in night clubs. On TV starred in Where It's At (special on ABC Stage 67) and What's In (special). Began daytime series for ABC-TV in 1968, three-weekly series summer of 1969. Current program: The Dick Cavett Show.

CHABROL, CLAUDE: Director. b. 1930. One of the first directors involved in the French New Wave.
PICTURES INCLUDE: Le Beau Serge, The Cousins, Leda, Les Bonnes Femmes, Les Godelureaux, The Third Lover, Seven Capital Sins, Ophelia, Landru, Le Tigre Aime la Chair Fraiche, Marie-Chantal Contre le Docteur Kah, Le Tigre Se Parfume a la Dunamite, Paris vu par . . . Chabrol, La Ligne de Demarcation, The Champagne Murders, The Route to Corinth, Les Biches, Le Femme Infidele, This Man Must Die, Le Boucher, La Rapture, Ten Days' Wonder, Just Before Nightfall, Dr. Popaul, Les Noces Rouges, Nada, The Blood of Others (TV in U.S.), The Horse of Pride.

CHAFFEY, DON: Director. b. Hastings, England, 1917. Trained as artist; secured work in art dept. of Gainsborough Studios in early 40s. Eventually moved to Gaumont British International where directed first film, a documentary on dog-fish.
PICTURES INCLUDE: Times Is My Enemy, The Girl in the Picture, The Flesh is Weak, A Question of Adultery, The Man Upstairs, Danger Within, Dentist in the Chair, Greyfriars Bobby, Nearly a Nasty Accident, A Matter of Who, The Prince and the Pauper, Jason and the Argonauts, A Jolly Bad Fellow, One Million Years B.C., The Viking Queen, A Twist of Sand, Creature the World Forgot, The Three Lives of Thomasina, The Horse Without a Head, Ride a Wild Pony.

CHAIKIN, WILLIAM E.: Executive. b. Cleveland, Ohio, April 7, 1919. e. Ohio State Univ. (BS, journalism; MS political science). Was newspaper reporter and columnist for paper in Ohio, Indiana and Florida before joining 20th-Fox pub. dept. in 1945. And in pub. depts. of Republic and Eagle Lion Films. Later pres., Chaikin-Perret, p.r. firm. Became v.p. and treas. of Standard Capital, investment banking firm, where financed and supervised prod. of over 60 films. In 1963 named pres. and bd. chm. of Charter Title Insurance Co. in Los Angeles. Is member of the Board of Mariners Savings and Loan. Is mem. of bd. of Mariners Financial Corp., financial holding co. diversified building firm. From 1968–74 was v.p. in chg. of West Coast operations of Avco Embassy Pictures Corp. and asst. to James R. Kerr, pres. of Avco Corp. in July, 1974, assumed presidency of Avco Embassy Pictures Corp. to 1980.

CHAKERES, MICHAEL H.: Executive b. Ohio, Graduate of Wittenberg University; pres. and chm. of bd. of Chakeres Theatres of Ohio and Kentucky. U.S. Army AF 1942–45. Bd. of Dir.: National NATO, NATO of Ohio, Will Rogers Hospital, Motion Picture Pioneers, Society National Bank, Wittenberg University, Mercy Medical Center. Member: Variety Club, Masons, Scottish Rite, I.O.O.F. Order of AHEPA, Ohio Heart Ass'n., Rotary Club, City of Hope.

CHAKIRIS, GEORGE: Actor. b. Norwood, Ohio, Sept. 16, 1934. Entered m.p. industry as a dancer in There's No Business Like Show Business and Brigadoon; academy award for West Side Story. Starred in the Young Girls of Rocheford, The Big Cube.

CHALMERS, PATRICK: b. Aberdeenshire, Scotland, 1940. e. Fettes College, Edinburgh, Aberdeen School of Agriculture, and Durham University. Joined BBC in 1973 as radio producer and became television producer, 1975. Senior producer at Aberdeen 1970, helping with lauch of Radio Aberdeen. Has won awards for films at Berlin Film Festival. Head of Television, BBC Scotland, 1978.

CHAMBERLAIN, RICHARD: Actor. b. Los Angeles, May 31, 1935. Became TV star in Dr. Kildare series (1961–65). Theatrical film debut in 1962. A Thunder of Drums.
PICTURES INCLUDE: Twilight of Honor, Joy in the Morning, Petulia, The Madwoman of Chaillot, Julius Caesar, The Music Lovers, Lady Caroline Lamb, The Three Musketeers, The Towering Inferno, The Slipper and the Rose, The Last Wave, The Swarm, Murder By Phone, King Solomon's Mines.
TV: Hamlet (1970). Movies: F. Scott Fitzgerald and the Last of the Belles, The Count of Monte Cristo, Race to the Pole, Wallenberg: A Hero's Story, Mini-Series: Centennial, Shogun, The Thorn Birds, Dream West.

CHAMBERS, EVERETT: producer, director. b. Montrose, Calif.; Aug. 19, 1926. e. New School For Soc. Res., Dramatic Workshop, NYC. Entered industry as actor; worked with Fred Coe as casting dir. and dir., NBC, 1952–57; prod., dir. Run Across the River, indep. feature and The Kiss, short nominated for Acad. Award, 1958; prod. Johnny Staccato, MCA, 1959; prod., Tess of the Storm Country, 20th-Fox.
TV: Target: The Corrupters, Dick Powell Theater, Saints and Sinners (pilot), The New Lloyd Bridges Show, numerous pilots; prod., dir., co-author with Don Gordon, The Lollipop Cover, Chicago Film Fest. awards, Best Film, Best Actor, 365 episodes Peyton Place, prod. writer for Nightslaves-ABC Movie of the Week, exec. prod. Monty Nash, prod. staff producer ABC TV; produced movies of the week, Moon of the Wolf, Trouble Comes to Town, The Great American Beauty Contest, Can Ellen Be Saved?, The Girl Must Live, They Only Come Out at Night. Currently prod. of Columbo.

CHAMPION, JOHN C.: Director, producer, writer. b. Denver, Col., Oct. 13, 1923; e. Stanford U., Wittenberg Coll.; p. Lee R. Champion, Supreme Court Judge. Col. Entered m.p. in Fiesta; did some radio work; in stock at MGM briefly; co-pilot Western Air Lines, Inc., 1943; served in U.S. Army Air Force, air transport command pilot 1943–45; public relations officer AAF; writer & prod. for Allied Artists; v.p. prod. Commander Films Corp.: press. Champion Pictures, Inc.; prod., MGM, Warner, Para., Universal, Member: SAG, SWG, SIMPP, SPG; TV Academy, Prod. Writer, MIRISCH-U.A.; prod. TV Laramie series; created McHales Navy; author, novel, The Hawks of Noon, 1965; National Cowboy, Hall of Fame Award, 1976.
PICTURES INCLUDE: Panhandle, Stampede, Hellgate, Dragonfly Squadron, Shotgun, Allied Artists; Zero Hour, Paramount; The Texican, Columbia; Attack on the Iron Coast, Submarine X-1, The Last Escape, Mirisch-United Artists; Brother of the Wind, Sun International, dir-prod-writer, Mustang Country, Universal.

CHAMPION, MARGE: Dancer, actress. b. Los Angeles, Calif., Sept. 2, 1923. e. Los Angeles public schools; p. Ernest Belcher, ballet master; m. Gower Champion, dancer, actor. In Blossom Time, Student Prince for Los Angeles Civic Opera; Dark of the Moon. Beggar's Holiday in N.Y. Made debut with husband as dancing team, played many night clubs; m.p. Debut in Mr. Music; then signed by MGM; Fame Star of Tomorrow, 1952; on B'way in 3 for Tonight, 1955; toured, invitation to A March 1962.
PICTURES INCLUDE: Show Boat, Lovely to Look At, Everything I Have Is Yours, Give a Girl a Break, Three for the Show, Jupiter's Darling, The Swimmer, The Party, The Cockeyed Cowboys of Calico County.
TV: GE Theatre, Chevy Show, Telephone Hour, etc.

CHAN, DARLENE K.: Executive. e. UCLA. Worked as prod. asst. on various independent films, including pilot for Disney Channel. 1983, joined Paramount Pictures as creative executive. 1985, named exec. dir. of prod., Walt Disney Pictures.

CHANCELLOR, JOHN: TV Anchorman and News Reporter. b. Chicago, 1927. e. Univ. of Ill. Following military service joined Chicago Sun-Times (1948) and after two years moved to NBC News as Midwest corr. In 1948 assigned to Vienna bureau. Subsequently reported from London; was chief of Moscow bureau before appt. as host of Today program for one year (1961). Left NBC 1965–67 to become dir. of Voice of America. In recent yrs. anchorman for special coverage of moon landings, political conventions, inaugurations etc. Anchorman, NBC Nightly News, 1970–82. Now sr. commentator, NBC News, delivering news commentaries on NBC Nightly News.

CHANDLER, CHICK: Actor. b. Kingston, N.Y.
STAGE: Great Magoo, Best Man, Harvey, Our Town, Dinner at Eight, Star Dust, Show Boat, Maytime, Roberta, Firefly.
MUSICAL COMEDY: Pajama Game, Damn Yankees, Brigadoon. On screen from 1934.
PICTURES INCLUDE: Blood Money, Big Shot, Alexander's Ragtime Band, Mother Wore Tights, Time Out for Romance, Swanee River, Bride Came C.O.D., Battle Cry, Mad Mad Mad World, Lost Continent and over 100 more.
TV: Soldiers of Fortune, One Happy Family, Freelance major TV shows.

CHANNING, CAROL: Actress. b. Seattle, Jan. 31, 1923. e. Bennington Col. Long career on Broadway and road; most notably in Gentlemen Prefer Blondes, Lend an Ear, and Hello Dolly!
PICTURES: First Traveling Saleslady, Thoroughly Modern Millie, Skidoo.
TELEVISION: Svengali and the Blonde, Three Men on a Horse, Crescendo; many guest appearances.

CHANNING, STOCKARD: Actress. b. New York City, Feb. 13, 1944. Has performed in some 25 plays as well as small roles in two Hollywood films, leading to the starring role in the ABC Movie-of-the-Week, The Girl Most Likely To.
PICTURES INCLUDE: The Fortune, The Big Bus, Sweet Revenge, Grease, The Cheap Detective, The Fish That Saved Pittsburgh, Without a Trace, Heartburn, The Men's Club.
TELEVISION: Not My Kid.

CHAPIN, DOUG: Producer. Began career as actor; then switched to film production, making debut with When a Stranger Calls, 1979.
PICTURES: Pandemonium, American Dreamer.
TELEVISION: Movies: Belle Starr, Missing Pieces, Second Sight.

CHAPIN, SLOCUM: Executive. b. Quincy, Mass. May 12, 1913; e. Dartmouth College, 1936. With Broadcast Builders, Hanover, N.H.; sales prom., World Broadcasting System; sales exec., WOC, Davenport, Ia.; sales mgr., WKBN, Youngstown, O.; gen. mgr., WSTC, Stamford, Conn.; network sales staff, ABC, 1942–48; east. TV sales mgr., ABC, 1948–51; v.p. in charge of owned TV stations, ABC, 1951; sales vice pres., ABC-TV, 1954; V.P. client relations, 1957; v.p. sls., Western division 1959; v.p. sls. National division, 1963; v.p. exec. relations, 1964.

CHAPLIN, CHARLES S.: Executive. b. Toronto, Ont., Canada, June 24, 1911. Studied Law. Entered m.p. ind. 1930 as office boy with United Artists; then office mgr. booker, St. John, N.B., 1933; br. mgr. 1935; to Montreal in same capacity, 1941; named Canadian gen. mgr., June 11, 1945; resigned January 1962. Vice-pres. Canadian sls. mgr., Seven Arts Prod., 1962; chief exec. off., v.p., dir. TV sls., Europe-Africa, Middle East-Socialist countries, 1968–70; v.p., WB-Seven Arts, 1970–72; exec. v.p. intl. film dist., NTA (Canada) Ltd., Toronto Intl. Film Studios, 1972–80; pres., Charles Chaplin Enterprises, specializing in theatrical and TV sls. and prod. Member: B'nai Brith, Toronto Bd. of Trade, various charitable org., many trade assns., pres. Canadian M.P. Dist. Assn., Chmn. m.p. section Com. Chest, chmn. publ. rel. comm. & past-chmn., M.P. Industry Council; Natl. Board Council Christians & Jews, University of Haifa, etc.

CHAPLIN, GERALDINE: Actress. b. Santa Monica, CA. 1944. Daughter of Charles Chaplin. Starred in over 20 European productions, including seven with Spain's leading filmmaker, Carlos Saura.
PICTURES INCLUDE: Doctor Zhivago, Stranger in the House, I Killed Rasputin, The Hawaiians, Zero Population Growth, Innocent Bystanders, The Three Musketeers, Nashville, Buffalo Bill and the Indians, Welcome to L.A., Roseland, Remember My Name, The Mirror Crack'd.
TELEVISION: The Corsican Brothers, My Cousin Rachel.

CHAPLIN, SAUL: Musical director and producer. b. Brooklyn, N.Y. Feb. 19, 1912. e. NYU 1929–34. Wrote vaude. material, 1933–36; songwriter Vitaphone Corp.; other, 1934–40; Columbia, 1940–48; MGM, from 1948; songs include: Bei Mir Bist Du Schoen, Shoe Shine Boy, Anniversary Song.
PICTURES INCLUDE: Acad. Award, collab. best scoring of mus., American in Paris, 1951, 7 Brides for 7 Brothers, 1954; West Side• Story, 1961; mus. dir., Lovely to Look At, Give A Girl a Break, Kiss Me Kate, Jupiter's Darling; mus. supve. Interrupted Melody, High Society; assoc. prod. Les Girls; music assoc. prod. Merry Andrew; assoc. prod. Can Can, West Side Story, The Sound of Music; prod. Star, 1968; assoc. prod., The Man of La Mancha, 1972; co-prod. That's Entertainment, Part Two.

CHAPMAN, MICHAEL: Cinematographer. b. New York City, Nov. 21, 1935. Early career in N.Y. area working on documentatries before becoming camera operator for cinematographer Gordon Willis on The Godfather.
PICTURES: The Last Detail, White Dawn, Taxi Driver,

The Front, The Next Man, Fingers, The Last Waltz, Invasion of the Body Snatchers, Hard Cove, The Wanderers, Raging Bull.

CHAPMAN, TEDWELL: Playwright, journalist. b. Chicago, Ill., April 12, 1917. e De Paul University, Layola University, Columnist, Hollywood Feature Syndicate, editor, Tailwagger Magazine, Hoja de Lunes (weekly, Malaga, Spain).
CREDITS: Abroad With Two Yanks (collab. orig. story & s.p.), The Fabulous Suzanne (collab. orig. s.p.), The Flanagan Boy (collab. s.p.), Drop In Anytime (orig. s.p.), Forever Is a Long Time (TV, orig. story & s.p.), The Crowded Bed (TV, orig. s.p.), Twice Upon a Time (Stage), The Intriguing Stranger (Stage), Bedlam (Stage), The Shame of Cain (Stage, book & lyrics), South of Granada (Stage, book & lyrics).

CHARI, V.K.N.: Public relation counsel & Publicity advisor. b. Salem, 1913. Till 1956 publicity & pub. relations officer, Gemini Studios, Madras. Presently film publicity adviser to film studios and film producers. Editor: Advertiser's Vademecum, Indian Advertising Year Book, An Economic Guide to India, The Languages of India. Refer-india, etc. Hon. Genl. Secretary. The Indian Council of Public Affairs, Madras. Journalist & news correspondent, B44 First mainroad Sastrinagar, Madras 20.

CHARISSE, CYD: Dancer, actress. r.n. Tula Ellice Finklea. b. Amarillo, Tex., Mar. 8, 1923. m. Tony Martin, singer; e. Hollywood Prof. School. Toured U.S. & Europe with Ballet Russe; screen debut in "Something to Shout About," 1943. Elected Star of Tomorrow 1948.
PICTURES INCLUDE: Mission to Moscow, Three Wise Fools, Till the Clouds Roll By, On an Island with you, Words and Music, Kissing Bandit, Tension, East Side, West Side, Mark of the Renegade, Wild North, Singin' in the Rain, Sombrero, Band Wagon, Easy to Love, Brigadoon, Deep in My Heart, It's Always Fair Weather, Meet Me in Las Vegas, Silk Stockings, Black Tights, Two Weeks in Another Town, The Silencers, Maroc 7.

CHARLES, MARIA: Actress. b. London, England, Sept. 22, 1929. Trained at Royal Academy of Dramatic Art. London Stage Debut 1946 in Pick Up Girl. Subseq.
STAGE (London): Women of Twilight, The Boy Friend, Divorce Me, Darling!, Enter A Free Man, They Don't Grow on Trees, Winnie the Pooh, Jack the Ripper, The Matchmaker, Measure for Measure, Annie (1979–80).
PICTURES INCLUDE: Folly To Be Wise, The Deadly Affair, Eye of the Devil, Great Expectations, The Return of the Pink Panther, Cuba.
TELEVISION: The Likes of 'Er, The Moon and the Yellow River, Down Our Street, Easter Passion, Nicholas Nickleby, The Voice of the Turtle, The Fourth Wall, The Good Old Days, Turn Out the Lights, Angel Pavement, The Ugliest Girl in Town, Other Peoples Houses, Rogues Gallery, The Prince and the Pauper, Crown Court, Barmitzvah Boy, Secret Army, Agony.

CHARLESON, IAN: Actor. b. Aug. 11, 1949, Edinburgh, Scotland. e. Edinburgh Univ.; trained for stage at London Academy of Music and Dramatic Art.
PICTURES: Jubilee, Chariots of Fire, Ghandi, Ascendancy, Greystoke.
TELEVISION: Rock Follies, Churchill's People, The Paradise Run, Antony and Cleopatra, Something's Got to Give, Master of the Game, A Month in the Country, The Devil's Lieutenant.

CHARTERIS, LESLIE: Writer, producer. b. Singapore, 1907; e. Cambridge, Eng. Novelist; creator The Saint, protagonist of mystery novels and series of pictures based on them prod. by RKO from 1938 and by Julian Lesser from 1952.

CHARTOFF, ROBERT: Producer. b. N.Y.C. e. Union College (A.B.), Col. Univ. (LLB). Met Irvin Windler through mutual client at William Morris Agency (N.M.) and established Chartoff-Winkler Prods. All films co-produced with Winkler.
PICTURES INCLUDE: Double Trouble, Point Blank, The Split, They Shoot Horses Don't They?, The Strawberry Statement, Leo The Last, Believe in Me, The Gang That Couldn't Shoot Straight, The New Centurions, Up the Sandbox, The Mechanic, Busting, The Gambler, SPYs, Breakout, Nickleodeon, New York, New York, Valentino, Rocky, Comes a Horseman, Uncle Joe Shannon, Rocky II, Raging Bull, True Confessions, Rocky III, Right Stuff, Rocky IV.

CHASE, BRANDON: Producer-Director. President MPA Feature Films, Inc.; newscaster-news director NBC-TV 1952–57. Executive director Mardi Gras Productions, Inc. and member of Board of Directors. Now pres., Group I Films, Ltd., and V.I. Prods., Ltd.; pres., Group 2 Entertainment; owner, Video Vending Machine by Diebold.
PICTURES INCLUDE: The Dead One, The Sinner and the Slave Girl, Bourbon Street Shadows, Verdict Homicide, Face of Fire, Four for the Morgue, Mission To Hell, The Wanton, Harlow, Girl In Trouble, Threesome, Wild Cargo, The Depraved, Alice in Wonderland, The Models, Sensuous 3, The Four Of Us, Against All Odds, The Giant Spider Invasion, House of 1,000 Pleasures, The Rogue, Eyes of Dr. Chaney, Alligator, Crash!, Take All of Me, The Teasers, The Psychic, UFOs Are Real, The Actresses, The Sword and the Sorcerer.
TELEVISION: Wild Cargo (series prod.-dir.); This Strange and Wondrous World (prod.-dir.).

CHASE, CHEVY: Actor. b. New York City, Oct. 8, 1944. e. Bard College. Teamed with Kenny Shapiro and Lane Sarasohn while still in school to collaborate on material for underground TV, which ultimately became off-Broadway show and later movie called Groove Tube. Co-wrote and starred in Saturday Night Live on TV, winning 2 Emmys for outstanding continuing or single performance by a supporting actor in variety and music and as writer for show. Has exclusive contract as performer with NBC. Feature film debut in Foul Play in 1978.
PICTURES: Caddyshack, Seems Like Old Times, Under the Rainbow, Modern Problems, National Lampoon's Vacation, Deal of the Century, Fletch, National Lampoon's European Vacation, Spies Like Us, Three Amigos.

CHASE, STANLEY: Producer. b. Brooklyn, N.Y., May 3. e. NYU (B.A.); Columbia (post-grad.). M. actress/artist Dorothy Rice. Began career as assoc. prod. of TV show Star Time; story dept., CBS-TV; then produced plays off-Bdwy. and on Bdwy., winner Tony and Obie awards for Threepenny Opera. Joined ABC-TV as dir. in chg. programming; exec. consultant, Metromedia Producers Org.; prod. & exec. Alan Landsburg Productions. Formed Stanley Chase Productions, Inc. in 1975, which heads as pres.
PICTURES INCLUDE: To Hell with Heroes, Colossus: The Forbin Project; High-Ballin' (exec. prod.); Fish Hawk (exec. prod.); The Guardian (HBO).
TELEVISION: Inside Danny Baker (pilot); Al Capp special (prod., writer); Happily Ever After (pilot; prod., writer); Bob Hope Presents the Chrysler Theatre series; Jigsaw (pilot); Fear on Trial (Emmy nomination); Courage of Kavik (exec. prod.); An American Christmas Carol, Grace Kelly.
STAGE: Producer of following plays: Threepenny Opera, The Potting Shed, The Cave Dwellers, A Moon for the Misbegotten, Free and Easy.

CHASMAN, DAVID: Executive. b. N.Y., Sept. 28, 1925. e. School of Industrial Art, 1940–43; Academie De La Grande-Chaumiere, 1949–50. Monroe Greenthal Co., Inc. 1950–53; Grey Advertising Agency, Inc., 1953–60. Free lance consultant to industry 1950–60; worked on pictures for UA, 20th-Fox, Columbia, Samuel Goldwyn, City Film; Adv. mgr. United Artists, 1960; exec. dir. adv., United Artists, 1962; exec. production, United Artists, London, 1964; v.p. in prod. United Artists, 1969; v.p. of west coast operations, U.A. 1970; Senior Vice President in charge of Production, U.A. 1972; President, Convivium Productions Inc., 1974. Joined MGM; named exec. v.p.-worldwide theatrical prod.

CHATELAIN, DIDIER: Production Executive. b. Jan. 24, Paris, France. Educated Paris and Ploytechnic, London. Degree in Business Administration, Marketing & Advertising. Entered industry in 1970 joining Herman Cohen Productions in London and Hollywood, starting with the advertising & promotion of Crooks and Coronets, 1971; Trog, 1972, Today We Kill . . . Tomorrow We Die!, 1973; The Strangers Gundown, 1974. Assistant Producer, Craze, 1974. Now v.p., Cobra Media, Inc.

CHAUDHRI, AMIN QAMAR: Director, Cinematographer-Editor. b. Punjab, India, April 18, 1942. e. Hampstead Polytechnic, London, City U., N.Y. Pres., Filmart Enterprises Ltd. & Filmart Int'l. Ltd., Pres./CEO, Continental Film Group.
PICTURES INCLUDE: Director: Kashish, Sweet Vengeance, Khajuraho, Eternal, Urvasi, Konarak, Black Rodeo, The Land of Buddha, Love Generation, Producer: Deadly Vengeance, Producer/Director: Once Again, An Unremarkable Life, Seems Like Yesterday.
CINEMATOGRAPHY: Right On, Sweet Vengeance, The Hopefuls, The Wicked Die Slow, The Love Statute, Vice Girls, Ltd., Who Says I Can't Ride a Rainbow, Black Rodeo, Medium is the Message, Death of a Dunbar Girl, Kashish, Deadly Vengeance.
TELEVISION: Reflections of India (prod.-dir.).

CHER: Singer-Actress. b. El Centro, Calif. May 20, 1946. r.n. Cherilyn Sarkisian. Began singing with then husband Sonny Bono in 1965; first hit record, I Got You Babe, sold 3 million. Made two films and then debuted nightclub musical-comedy act in 1969. CBS comedy-variety series started as summer show in 1971; became regular following December.
PICTURES INCLUDE: Good Times, Chastity, Come Back to the Five and Dime, Jimmy Dean, Jimmy Dean, Silkwood, Mask.
TELEVISION: Sonny & Cher Comedy Hour, Cher.

CHEREN, ROBERT M.: Executive. b. Winthrop, MA, June 12, 1947. e. Graham Coll. (1967). 1968, joined 20th Century

Fox sales dept. in Boston; 1969, named branch mgr. 1975, transferred by Fox to Los Angeles as dist. mgr.; 1976, promoted to west. div. mgr. 1979, to Columbia Pictures as west, div. mgr.; 1981, joined Filmways (later Orion Pictures) as v.p. & gen. sls. mgr. 1984, named Orion exec. v.p., then pres., Orion Pictures Dist. Corp.
MEMBER: Academy of Motion Picture Arts & Sciences, Variety Club New York, Variety Club Tent 25 So. Calif.; Foundation of Motion Picture Pioneers.

CHERMAK, CY: Producer-writer. b. Bayonne, N.J., Sept. 20, 1929. e. Brooklyn College; Ithaca College.
TELEVISION: Produced Ironsides, The Virginian, The New Doctors, Amy Prentiss, Night Stalkers, Barbary Coast, CHIPS. TV movie: Murder at the World Series.

CHERTOK, HARVEY: Executive. b. New York, N.Y., Oct. 29, 1932. e. N.Y.U., grad. school, bus. admin. Merchandising mgr., National Telefilm Assocs., Jan. 1956–Aug. 1959; supv., adv., United Artists Associated, Aug. 1959–March 1961; dir., adv., sls. prom., publicity, Seven Arts Associated Corp., 1961–1968; prod., 7 Surprizes, 1964; 1968 TV v.p. advertising-publicity, Warner-7 Arts, co.-prod., The Great Charlie Chan (Golden Press) 1968; Pres. The Children's Movie of the Month, Inc., 1969–71; marketing consultant, United Artists Television, 1972–73; V.P.-special-projects, The American Film Theatre, Inc. 1973–75; v.p. adv., sls. pro., pub. for Time-Life Television, 1975; named v.p., adv./promo, Time Life-tv, 1978–81.

CHERTOK, JACK: Producer. b. Atlanta, Ga., July 13. Began career as script clerk, MGM; later asst. carmeraman, asst. dir., head of music dept., short subjects prod. Feature prod. MGM 1939–42 ("The Penalty," "Joe Smith, American," "Kid Glove Killer," "The Omaha Trail," "Eyes in the Night," etc.). In July 1942, apptd. Hollywood prod. chief, Co-Ord. Inter-Amer. Affairs, serving concurrently with regular studio work. Left MGM 1942 and prod. for Warner Bros. to late 1944; pres.: Produced The Corn is Green and Northern Pursuit for Warner Bros. Pres. Jack Chertok TV, Inc.

CHESTER, HALE.: Producer. b. Brooklyn, N.Y., Mar. 6, 1921. On N.Y. stage; film debut in "Crime School" 1937, followed by "Little Tough Guy" series. "Juvenile Court"; personal appearance tour of U.S. and Canada 1941–44; entered m.p. production 1944, doing a series of musical shorts. Member: IMPPA. Prod. Joe Palooka series begin with "Joe Palooka Champ" 1946, released via Monogram, Smart Woman; v.p. in chge. prod., Mutual Films Corp., 1951.
PICTURES INCLUDE: Joe Palooka in The Squared Circle, Underworld Story, The Highwayman, Triple Cross, Models, Beast from 20,000 Fathoms, Crashout, Bold and The Brave, The Weapon, The Haunted, School for Scoundrels, Two-Headed Spy, His and Hers, Hide and Seek, The Comedy Man, The Double Man, The Secret War of Harry Frigg.

CHETWYND, LIONEL: Executive, writer. b. London, England, 1940. Emigrated to Canada, 1948. B.A. (Economics, Sir George Williams Univ. Montreal), B.C.L.-McGill University, Montreal. Graduate Work-Law—Trinity College, Oxford. Admitted to Bar–Province of Quebec, 1968. C.B.C.—TV-Public Affairs and Talks, 1961–1965. CTV network 1965–67. Controller commercial TV and film rights, Expo '67. Freelance writer and consultant 1961–68. Joined Columbia Pictures Intern. New York July 1968, transferred to Columbia Pictures Corp. Ltd., London, Sept. 1968. Asst. man. dir. January 1969. Asst. man. dir. Columbia-Warner UK, 1971. Story and book for musical Maybe That's Your Problem, 1971–1973: s.p., Apprenticeship of Duddy Kravitz; The Guest Room (TV).

CHIKADA, TADASHI: Executive. b. Japan Nov. 20, 1919. e. Tokyo Foreign Language Univ. 1940–6 with Showa Tsusho in Japan and China; 1947–50 Izumi Sangyo, transferring to Nihon Eiga Shizai (Japan Movie Equipment Co.) which later became Toshiba Photo Phone Co.; appt. director and gen. mgr. of Trade Div. in 1972, and in 1974 director in charge of trade.

CHILTON, T. E.: Executive. b. Kent, England, 1929. Ent. m.p. ind. 1951 with J.F. Brockliss. 1953 Simplex Apro. 1955. Rank Percision Industries, then various appointments in equipment industry in Rank Organisation becoming Asst. Man. Dir. 1968, Man. Dir. 1971. Appt. man. dir. Rank Leisure Service 1973. Appt. chairman Rank Leisure Services, Rank Hotels, Rank Advertising Films, Rank Film Distributors, Pinewood Studios, 1976, dir. Rank Organisation 1976.

CHIN, ELIZABETH MAE: Executive. b. New York, N.Y. Nov. 2, 1938. e. George Washington H.S. 1956; C.C.N.Y., Business Administration 1960; Internal Auditor 1960; International trade and entrepreneur of international dairy franchise 1968. Entered motion picture industry in 1974 as agent for independent film distribution in theatrical and television. Presently, executive of Far East Enterprises, and Emcee World Associates, Inc. and Bergen Intl. Corp.

CHING, WILLIAM: Actor. b. St. Louis, Mo., Oct. 2, 1913. e. Spring Hills Coll. Radio Singer; on Broadway in Allegro.
PICTURES INCLUDE: Pat and Mike, Never Wave at a Wac, Give a Girl a Break, Scared Stiff, The Moonlighter, Tall Man Riding, Magnificent Matador.
TV: featured actor, Our Miss Brooks; NBC-TV.

CHINICH, JESSE: Exeuctive. b. Hoboken, N.J., Dec. 17, 1921; e. N.Y.U. Law S., L.L.B. 1938. Lawyer with Hovell, Clarkson and Klupt, 1938–41; U.S. Army, 1941–46; joined Paramount Theatres as film buyer, 1946–51; circuit supervisor, Rugoff & Becker, NYC, 1951–53; western div. sales mgr., Buena Vistra Film Dist., Co., 1953–61; Ass't gen. sales mgr. co-ordinator Cinema V Dist.; ass't sales mgr., Allied Artists; sales executive, special projects, Warner Bros. Dist. Corp. Now Publisher of weekly newsletters.

CHISSELL, NOBLE (KID): Actor. b. Indianapolis, Ind., Feb. 16, 1910; e. City Coll. of L.A., U.S. Merchant Marine, prof. boxer, prison officer, U.S. Navy Middleweight Boxing Champ 1932, World Marathon Dance Champion 1928, Champ Walkathoner 1934–35. Chairman/m.c. world famed Cauliflower Alley Club, co-ed boxing/wrestling group, since 1968. Middleweight Senior Olympic Skill Boxing Champ 1974–78 m.c. Burbank Easter Parade 1979–80. Nostalgic Movie/Boxing columnist, Hollywood Independent; boxing columnist, Official Boxing Record; Master of Ceremonies, Film Welfare League benefit Show, 1980.
STAGE: Cafe Frisco, All the Kings Men, J. Silverheel's Indian Pageant, Love in Upper Sandusky, Lower Depths, Meet the World, Twelfth Night.
PICTURES INCLUDE: Abe Lincoln in Illinois, Home in Indiana, Dillinger, Grand Canyon, Young At Heart, Guys and Dolls, Big Chase, Friendly Persuasion, Bonnie and Clyde, More Dead Than Alive, Hell Cats, Big Foot, They Shoot Horses, Don't They?, Mule Feathers, The Clones, Ex-Champ, Jealousy, The Leather-pusher, Song of Arizona, The Polygamist, The Traveling Executioner, Three in The Saddle, Arizona Mission, El Salvaje, Pistol Packing Mama, The Rebel Breed, etc.
TV: Marshall of Gunsight Pass, Colgate Comedy Hour, Life of Riley, It's a Great Life, Dragnet, Playhouse 90, Climax, People's Court, Gunsmoke, Gallagher-Disney Series, High Chaparral, To Tell the Truth, Dating Game, 20 Bob Hope Comedy Specials. Also, Minsky Follies 1975, Hollywood.

CHODOROV, EDWARD: Writer, dir. b. New York City, April 17, 1924. e. Brown U. Writer, dir., plays; Writer, prod., films.
PLAYS INCLUDE: Wonder Boy, Kind Lady, Cue for Passion, Those Endearing Young Charms, Decision, Common Ground, The Spa, Signor Chicago, Oh Men Oh Women, M. Lautrec, Erskine, Listen to the Mocking Bird, etc. Writer-prod. Warners, 20th, Col., MGM. Wrote Billy Rose Show ABC; writer dir., prod. Sam Spiegel, Horizon Pictures, 1961–63; Writer-prod.-dir. A.C.E. Prods. (London) 1964; Columbia, 1965; 20th-Fox, 1966–67; writer-producer, Warner-7 Arts, 1968, 1969; writer-dir., Dowling, Whitehead, Stevens, 1971–72; Cheryl Crawford Prods., 1973, Universal, 1974–75; Theatre Guild 1976; Instructor film/TV writing California State University 1976–78; New York University 1979; lecturer theatre at Actors & Directors Lab, Los Angeles 1980; instructor stage directing A&D Lab, 1980.

CHOMSKY, MARVIN J.: Director. b. Bronx, N.Y. Started in theatre business at early age as art dir. with such TV credits as U.S. Steel Hour, Playhouse 90, Studio One, etc. Later worked with Herb Brodkin who advanced him to assoc. prod. with such TV shows as The Doctors and The Nurses. Brought to Hollywood in 1965 as assoc. prod. for Talent Associates, producing series of TV pilots.
PICTURES INCLUDE: Evel Knievel, Murph the Surf, Mackintosh and T.J., Tank.
TV: The Wild, Wild West, Gunsmoke, Star Trek, Then Came Bronson, and many Movies of the Week: Holocaust, Victory at Entebbe, Roots, Attica, The Narobi Affair, Life and Times of Robert Kennedy, Evita, Peter the Great, The Deliberate Stranger.

CHONG, RAE DAWN: Actress. Daughter of comic Tommy Chong.
PICTURES: Quest for Fire, The Corsican Brothers, Beat Street, Choose Me, Commando, The Color Purple, Soul Man.
TELEVISION: Badge of the Assassin.

CHONG, TOMMY: Singer-Actor-Writer. b. Edmonton, Alta., Canada, May 24, 1938. Was guitar player with various Canadian rhythm and blues combinations, teamed with Richard Marin (Cheech) in improvisational group. Has made comedy recordings.
PICTURES: Cheech and Chong's Up in Smoke, Cheech and Chong's Next Movie, Cheech and Chong's Nice Dreams, Things Are Tough All Over, It Came from Hollywood, Still Smokin', The Corsican Brothers (also s.p., dir.), After Hours.

CHOOLUCK, LEON: Producer-Director. b. New York, March 19, 1920; e. CCNY, 1938. Production, distribution, editing with Consolidated Film Industries 1936–40; Army Pictorial Service as news photographer 1941–45; Indep. as ass. dir. and prod. mgr. 1946–56; prod. for Regal Films and Orbit Pro., 1957–58; dir. Highway Patrol, 1958. Various occupations on stage 1947–58; prod. mgr., Daystar Prods., ABC-TV series, Stoney Burke; prod. mgr., assoc. prod., Daystar Prods., 1962–63; prod. supv., Encyclopedia Britannica Films, in Spain, 1964; prod. supv., U.S. Pictures, Battle of the Bulge; loc. mgr., Three F Prods., assoc. prod. I Spy, TV Series, 1965–67. Vice Pres. Fouad Said Cinemobile Systems, 1969–70. Pres., The Society (film prod. org.).

PICTURES INCLUDE: Hell on Devil's Island, Plunder Road, Murder by Contract, City of Fear, The Fearmakers, Day of the Outlaw, Bramble Bush, Rise and Fall of Legs Diamond, Studs Lonigan, Three Blonds in His Life, El Cid, The Outer Limits, Midas Run, The Grissom Gang, Kotch, Payday, 1971; Three the Hard Way-'73–74; Take a Ride-'74–75, Apocalypse Now, Loving Couples. Produced Wonders of China for Disney Circlevision.

TELEVISION: Prod. supvr. 1974–76; NBC (2 hr.) Specials, Strange Homecoming, Michener's Dynasty, Judge Horton and the Scottsboro Boys, Pearl, A Rumor of War, Murder in Texas.

CHOW, RAYMOND: Producer. b. Hong Kong. e. St. John's University, Shanghai. Worked as journalist for Hong Kong Standard; then joined the U.S. Information Agency, establishing its Chinese radio station which broadcast to the Chinese mainland. In late 1950s joined Shaw Brothers as head of their publicity operations. In next 12 years became right-hand man of Run Run Shaw and head of production. In 1971 formed The Golden Harvest Group to produce Chinese-language films in Hong Kong. Two kung-fu films featuring Bruce Lee put Harvest into intl. market. Started English-language films in 1977, beginning with The Amsterdam Kill and The Boys in Company C.

FILMS: Lassiter, Cannonball Run II.

CHRISTIAN, LINDA: Actress. r.n. Blanca Rosa Welter. b. Tampico, Mex., Nov. 13, 1924, e. Mexico, Venezuela, Palestine, So. Africa, Holland, Italy; attended medical school in Palestine; Worked for British Censorship Bureau in Palestine; asst. to plastic surgeon; screen debut in Holiday in Mexico.

PICTURES INCLUDE: Green Dolphin Street, Tarzan and the Mermaids, The Happy Time, Battle Zone, Slave of Babylon, Athena, Thunderstorm, The VIPs.

CHRISTIANSEN, ROBERT W.: Producer. b. Porterville, CA. e. Bakersfield College. Spent 3 years in Marine Corps. Worked on Hollywood Reporter in circulation and advertising. Joined Cinema Center Films; prod. asst. on Monte Walsh and Hail Hero. Co-produced first feature in 1970, Adam at Six A.M., with Rick Rosenberg, with whom co-produced all credits listed.

PICTURES INCLUDE: Adam at Six A.M., Hide in Plain Sight.

TV: Features: Suddenly Single, The Glass House, A Brand New Life, The Man Who Could Talk to Kids, The Autobiography of Miss Jane Pittman, I Love You . . . Goodbye, Queen of the Stardust Ballroom, Born Innocent, A Death in Canaan, Strangers, Robert Kennedy and His Times, Kids Don't Tell, As Summers Die.

CHRISTIE, HOWARD J: Producer. b. San Francisco, Calif., Sept. 16, 1912. e. Berkeley, U. of Calif. Entered m.p. ind. following graduation from coll. in 1934, as actor; asst. dir. 1936–40; assoc. prod., 1942–44, Deanna Durbin pictures. Member: Screen Directors Guild, Screen Producers Guild, Delta Tau Delta, vice pres., Reeve M.C.A. Inc., 1961.

PICTURES INCLUDE: Lady on a Train, Because of Him I'll Be Yours, A & C Meet the Invisible Man, Golden Horde, Comin' Round the Mountain, Lost in Alaska, Against All Flags, Yankee Buccaneer, Seminole, Lone Hand, A & C Go To Mars, A & C Meet Dr. Jekyll and Mr. Hyde, Back to God's Country, Yankee Pasha, A & C Meet Keystone Kops, Smoke Signal, The Looters, Purple Mask, A & C Meet the Mummy, Price of Fear, Congi Crossing, Showdown at Abilene, Toy Tiger, Away All Boats, I've Lived Before, Wagon Train, The Raiders, Sword of Ali Baba, Senes, Laredo, Ride to Hangman's Tree, Journey to Shiloh, Nobody's Perfect, A Man Called Gannon.

TV: The Virginian.

CHRISTIE, JULIE: Actress. b. Chukua, Assam, India, July 14, 1941. e. Year in France followed by Drama School in England. TV debut in A for Andromeda. Birmingham Rep.; Royal Shakespeare Co.; East European and American tour, Starred (NY) in Uncle Vanya.

PICTURES INCLUDE: Fast Lady, Billy Liar, Young Cassidy, Darling, Dr. Zhivago, Farenheit 451, Far From the Madding Crowd, Petualia, In Search of Gregory, The Go-Between, McCabe and Mrs. Miller, Don't Look Now, Shampoo, The Demon Seed, Heaven Can Wait, The Return of the Soldier, Heat and Dust, Power, Miss Maggie.

CHRISTINE, VIRGINIA: Actress. b. Stanton, Iowa, March 5. e. UCLA Los Angeles, Calif.; has appeared in more than 400 motion pictures and television productions.

PICTURES INCLUDE: Mission to Moscow, Counter Attack, The Killers, Cover Up, The Men, Cyrano De Bergerac, Cobweb, High Noon, Not as a Stranger, Spirit of St. Louis, Three Brave Men, Judgment in Nuremberg, The Prize, Four For Texas, A Rage to Live, Guess Who's Coming to Dinner, Hail Hero, Daughter of the Mind.

TV: Dragnet, Abbot & Costello, Dangerous Assignment, Racket Squad, Superman, Schlitz Playhouse, Four Star Playhouse, The Whistler, Code 3, Ford Theatre, You Are There, Stage 7, Passport to Danger, Soldier of Fortune, Heinz Show, Anthology, Four Star Playhouse, Cavalcade of America, Alfred Hitchcock Presents, Father Knows Best, Crusader, Kellogg, Front Row Center, The Twisted Road, Matinee, Private Secretary, Fort Laramie, Big Town, Science Fiction, Frontier Detective, Lone Ranger, Jim Bowie, Wire Service, Whirlybirds, Gunsmoke, Las Vegas Story, Trackdown, The Thin Man, San Francisco Beat, Stranger In Town, T Men, Casey Jones, Climax, Mickey Spillane, The Millionaire, Behind Closed Doors, Target, Peter Gunn, Zane Grey Theatre, Wyatt Earp, Secret Mission, The Donna Reed Show, Wanted Dead Or Alive, Buckskin, Loretta Young Show, Starperformance, Rescue 8, Steve Canyon, State Trooper, Twilight Zone, General Electric Theatre, How to Marry A Millionaire, Rifle Man, June Allyson Show, Rawhide, M Squad, Coronado 9, Man From Black Hawk, Grand Jury, Riverboat, 77 Sunset Strip, Happy, The Thriller, Lawless Years, The Untouchables, Death Valley Days, Verdict Is Yours, Deputy, Perry Mason, Wagon Train, Mr. Ed, Maverick, The Shirley Temple Show, Asphalt Jungle, Harrigan and Son, Tales of Wells Fargo, Bronco, Line Of Duty, The New Breed, Going My Way, Stoney Burke, Bonanza, The Eleventh Hour, Ben Casey, The Virginian, The Fugitive, Day In Court, Hazel, Singing Nun, Billy The Kid, The Big Valley, The FBI, Laredo, A Man Called Shenandoah, Jericho, Judd for the Defense, The Invaders, Lancer, Nanny And The Professor.

STAGE: Hedda Gabler, Mary, Queen of Scots, Miss Julie, Desdemona.

CHRISTOPHER, JORDAN: Actor, musician. b. Youngstown, Ohio, 1941. e. Kent State U. Led rock 'n' roll group, "The Wild Ones." Broadway debut, Black Comedy, 1967.

PICTURES INCLUDE: Return of the Seven, The Fat Spy, The Tree, Pigeons, Brainstorm, Star 80.

CIANNELLI, LEWIS E.: Associate Producer. b. New York, Jan. 12, 1923 Univ. of Calif., 1941, Leland Stanford Univ.-AB 1947. Meschini Institute, Rome, 1950. World War II 1942–46. Acct. exec. adv. firm 1947–48. Actor: TV and motion pictures, 1948–50. Exec. asst. Industrie Cinematografiche Sociali, 1950, Director of Foreign Sls. I.C.S. and on board of A.N.I.C.A. 1953. Production exec. Lux Film, Rome 1953. Head of Production Republic Pictures, Italy 1954–55; assoc. prod. The Best of the Post; assoc. prod., exec. asst. Ponti & Girosi, That Kind of Women; Heller in Pink Tights, assoc. prod. NBC-TV; Ford Startime, Chevy Special Mexico, Rivak The Barbarian, The Americans, Outlaws.

PLAYS: OK Nero! Twin Trouble, The Bed.

CILENTO, DIANE: Actress. b. Queensland, Australia, 1934. e. Toowoomba. Went to New York and finished schooling and then American Acad. of Dramatic Art; first theatre job at 16; toured U.S. with Barter Co.; returned to London and joined Royal Acad. of Dramatic Art; several small parts and later repertory at Manchester's Library Theatre.

PICTURES INCLUDE: Angel Who Pawned Her Harp, Passing Stranger, Passage Home, Woman for Joe, Admirable Crichton, Truth About Women, Jet Storm, The Full Treatment, The Naked Edge, The Breaking Point, Once Upon A Tractor for UN, Hombre.

THEATRE: N.Y. stage: Tiger at the Gates, I Thank a Fool, The Third Secret, Tom Jones, The Rattle of a Simple Man, The Agony and the Ectasy, Hombre, Once Upon a Tractor, Negatives, The Four Seasons, The Bonne Soup, Heartbreak House. (NY), the Big Knife, Orpheus, Altona, Castle in Sweden, Naked, Marys, I've Seen You Cut Lemons.

TV: La Bell France (series), Court Martial, Blackmail, Dial M for Murder, Rogues Gallery, Rain, Lysistrata.

CIMINO, MICHAEL: Writer-Director. b. 1943. Protege of Clint Eastwood, who signed him to do s.p. for Magnum Force and then to write and direct Thunderbolt and Lightfoot, in both of which Eastwood starred.

PICTURES: The Deer Hunter, Heavens' Gate, Year of the Dragon.

CIPES, ARIANNE ULMER: Executive. b. New York City, July 25. Daughter of film director Edgar G. Ulmer. e. Royal Academy of Dramatic Arts, London, Univeristy of London; actress, then production and dubbing, Paris; CDC, Rome; Titra, New York; 1975–77, v.p., Best International Films (international film distributor), Los Angeles; 1977 co-founder and sr. v.p./sales & services of Producers Sales Organization, 1981, named exec. v.p., American Film Marketing Assn. 1982–83, pres. Founded AUC Films, consulting and international sales-producers rep.

CIPES, JAY H.: Executive. b. N.Y., Dec. 14. e. Cornell U. 1960–66, independent producer-packager-distributor European features for U.S. TV sales; 1967, producer, 20th Century-Fox TV; 1970, producer, Four Star TV; 1971, marketing exec.; Technicolor, Inc.; 1973, v.p., marketing, Technicolor, Inc.; 1979 sr. v.p., director worldwide marketing, Technicolor, Inc. professional film division.

CLAGETT, MANNING (TIM): Executive. b. Washington, D.C., Aug. 22, 1913. e. U. of Southern Calif,; U. of Calif., Los Angeles; Geo. Wash. U. Correspondent for Washington Herald, Washington Times-Herald 1937–41; Washington Star, 1941–48. Joined U.S. Merchant Marine 1943–44; corr., Washington Post 1945–46; own news bureau 1946–48. Assoc. Director of information, Motion Picture Assoc. of America, Washington, 1948–1958; dir. pub. rel. MPAA, 1953; dir. State Leg. Service, MPAA, 1956; v.p., 1961; special consultant, 1970.

CLARK, CANDY: Actress. b. Oklahoma. Was successful model in N.Y. before landing role in Fat City, 1972. Continues to model between films.
PICTURES INCLUDE: Fat City, American Graffiti, The Man Who Fell To Earth, Citizens Band, The Big Sleep, When You Comin' Back, Red Ryder, More American Graffiti, Blue Thunder, Amityville 3-D, Hambone and Hillie, Cat's Eye.

CLARK, DANE: Actor. b. New York City, Feb. 18, 1915; e. Cornell U., Johns Hopkins U. In radio series 2 yrs.; on N.Y. stage (Of Mice and Men, Dead End, etc.).
PICTURES INCLUDE: Glass Key, Sunday Punch, Pride of the Yankees, Tennessee Johnson, Action in the North Atlantic, Destination Tokyo, Very Thought of You, Hollywood Canteen, God Is My Co-Pilot, Her Kind of Man, That Way With Women, Deep Valley, Embraceable You, Moonrise, Whiplash, Without Honor, Backfire, Barricade, Never Trust a Gambler, Fort Defiance, Highly Dangerous, Gambler and the Lady, Go Man Go, Blackout, Paid to Kill, Thunder Pass, Port of Hell, Toughest Man Alive.
TV: No Exit, The Closing Door, Wire Service, Bold Venture (series).

CLARK, DICK: Performer. b. Mt. Vernon, N.Y. Nov. 30, 1929. Syracuse Univ. graduated 1951, summer announcer WRUN, Utica 1949, staff announcer WOLF, Syracuse 1950. After graduation 1951, took regular job with WOLF. Rejoined WRUN, Utica, then joined WKTV, Utica. Announcer WFIL Philadelphia 1952. Host of American Bandstand ABC-TV nationwide, the Dick Clark Beechnut Show, Dick Clark's World of Talent, The Object Is, Missing Links, Record Years, Years of Rock. Producer of TV shows, Where The Action Is, Swinging Country, Happening, Get It Together, Shebang, Record Years, Years of Rock. Author of Your Happiest Years, Random House . . . 1959, Author of Rock, Roll & Remember, T.Y. Crowell, 1976 and To Goof or Not to Goof, Bernard Geis, 1963. . . . Dick Clark's Easygoing Guide to Good Grooming, Dodd, Mead 1986 . . . The History of American Bandstand, Ballantine, 1986. Formed Dick Clark Productions 1956 . . . Business engaged in motion picture production: Because They're Young, The Young Doctors, Psychout, The Savage Seven, Killers Three, Elvis, the Movie, Remo Williams: The Adventure Begins. In-person concert division, marketing and communications division, cable TV programing department and radio division. Executive Producer of Dick Clark's Rockin' New Year's Eve, American Music Awards, Academy of Country Music Awards, TV Censored Bloopers, The Golden Globe Awards, TV's Censored Bloopers and Practical Jokes and TV Movies: Elvis, Man in the Santa Claus Suit, Murder in Texas, The Demon Murder, The Woman Who Willed a Miracle, Copacabana, Birth of the Beatles, You Are the Jury. Producer: Live Aid—An All-Star Concert for African Relief. Winner of 4 Emmys.

CLARK, GREYDON: Producer-Director-Writer. b. Niles, MI, Feb. 7, 1943. e. Western Michigan Univ. (B.A., theatre arts, 1963). Heads own company, World Amusement Corp., Sherman Oaks, CA.
PICTURES: Writer: Satan's Sadists, Psychic Killer. Director-Writer: Mothers, Fathers, & Lovers, Bad Bunch. Producer-Writer-Director: Hi-Riders, Angel's Brigade, The Warning.

CLARK, HILARY J.: Executive. e. Univer. of So. Calif (BA, 1976). Began industry career 1978 as ad-pub admin. in co-op adv. dept., Buena Vista Dist. Co. Promoted to mgr. of natl. field pub & promo. Acted as unit publicist on numerous films (Explorers, Sylvester, Swing Shift, Crossroads, etc.) before returning to BV 1986 as natl. pub. dir. for Walt Disney Pictures.

CLARK, JOHN L.: Executive. b. Owenton, Ky., Sept. 13, 1907; e. Univ. of Tenn. Talent scout, Brunswick Phono. Co.; mgr., WLW, Cincinnati; formed Transamerican Broad. & Tele. Corp. with Warner Bros.; prod. 50 TV films, 1941–44; created & prod. many radio & TV programs; pres. & sole owner, Transamerican.

CLARK, KENNETH: Journalist, executive. b. Dekalb, Ill., Aug. 1, 1899; e. U. Ill. Washington & foreign corresp. United Press, Internatl. News Service, Universal Service. Joined M.P. Prod. & Dist. Amer., 1936. Leave of absence 1942 to join U.S. Army; Maj., Lt. Col. and Col.; Returned to MPAA, Nov., 1945; v.p., 1953; exec. v.p., MPAA, 1962; v.p., MPEAA, 1953, Retired, 1984.

CLARK, PETULA: Actress and vocalist. b. Ewell, Surry, England, Nov. 15, 1932.
PICTURES INCLUDE: The Huggets, Dance Hall, White Corridors, The Card, Made In Heaven, Gay Dog, Runaway Bus, That Man Opposite, Finian's Rainbow, Goodbye Mr. Chips.

CLARK, SAMUEL H.: Exhibitor. b. Boston, Mass., Jan. 10, 1914. Owner, Music Suppliers, Boston, Mass.; founded Music Suppliers of New England, 1945; pres., ABC-Paramount Records Inc., 1955–65; v.p., head thea. operations, American Broadcasting-Paramount Theatres, Inc., Jan. 1965; dir., May, 1965.

CLARK, SUSAN: Actress. b. Canada, March 8, 1944. Trained at Royal Academy of Dramatic Arts in London. Made m.p. debut in Banning, 1967.
PICTURES INCLUDE: Coogan's Bluff, Madigan, Colossus: The Forbin Project, Tell Them Willie Boy Is Here, Skullduggery, Skin Game, Valdez Is Coming, Showdown, The Midnight Man, Night Moves, Airport 1975, The Apple Dumpling Gang, The North Avenue Irregulars, Murder by Decree, City on Fire, Promises in the Dark.
TELEVISION: Webster.

CLAYBURGH, JILL: Actress. b. NYC, April 30, 1944. Appeared on Broadway in Jumpers, Pippin, The Rothschilds, etc.
PICTURES INCLUDE: Portnoy's Complaint, The Thief Who Came to Dinner, Terminal Man, Gable and Lombard, Silver Streak, Semi-Tough, An Unmarried Woman, Starting Over, Luna, It's My Turn, First Monday in October, I'm Dancing As Fast As I Can, Hannah K, Where Are The Children?
TV: Griffin and Phoenix.

CLAYTON, JACK: Producer, director. b. 1921. Ent. m.p. 1935 as asst. dir. for London Films, Fox, Warner. Served H.M. Forces 1940–46. prod. man. Ideal Husband; assoc. prod. Queen of Spades, Flesh and Blood, Moulin Rouge, Beat the Devil, The Good Die Young, I am a Camera; prod. dir. Bespoke Overcoat, 1955, Venice Festival prize-winning film; prod. Sailors Beware, Dry Rot, Three Men in a Boat; dir. Room at the Top, The Innocents, The Pumpkin Eater; prod.-dir., Our Mother's House, 1967; The Great Gatsby, 1974; Something Wicked This Way Comes, 1982.

CLEESE, JOHN: Actor. b. Weston-Super-Mare, England, Oct. 27, 1939. e. Clifton Coll.; Cambridge. Member Monty Python's Flying Circus.
PICTURES: Interlude, The Best House in London, The Rise and Rise of Michael Rimmer, And Now for Something Completely Different, The Love Ban, Monty Python and the Holy Grail, The Life of Brian, The Great Muppet Caper, Time Bandits, Privates on Parade, Monty Python's The Meaning of Life, Yellowbeard, etc.
TELEVISION: Taming of the Shrew, Doctor in the House, Fawlty Towers, etc.

CLEMENS, BRIAN: Writer, producer, director. b. Croydon, England, 1931. Early career in advertising then wrote BBC TV play. Later TV filmed series as writer, script editor and features. Script editor "Danger Man"; Won Edgar Allen Poe Award for Best TV Thriller of 1962 (Scene of the Crime for U.S. Steel Hour). Various plays for Armchair Theatre; ATV Drama 70; Love Story. Writer and Producer of The Avengers (two Emmy nominations for Best Production 1967 and 1968), Winner two Edgar Allen Poe Awards, Cinema Fantastique Award for best Screenplay.
PICTURES INCLUDE: The Tell-Tale Heart, Station Six-Sahara, The Peking Medallion, And Soon The Darkness, The Major, and, When The Wind Blows, See No Evil, Dr. Jekyll and Sister Hyde, Golden Voyage of Sinbad, Watcher in the Woods, Stiff.
TV: Wrote and prod.: The New Avengers, The Professionals, Escapade (in US for Quinn Martin).

CLIFT, DENISON: Author and director. b. May 2, 1893; e. Stanford U. Editor, Overland Monthly and other publications; publicity expert, San Francisco, 1917. Scenario writer and dir. for Fox, Paramount, MGM; dir. Honor Among Men, Ports of Call, This Freedom, A Bill of Divorcement, Paradise, The Mystery of the Mary Celeste, etc. Dir. for British International, Ideal Films, Gainsborough Pictures and Hammer Prod., London. Author of novels, Guns of Galt, Man About Town, The Mighty Thing, I Belong to You. Author of the New York plays, The Woman Disputed, Scotland Yard; and London plays, The Moon Is Red and Gentle Rain.

CLORE, LEON: Producer. Co-prod.: Conquest of Everest, Virgin Island, Every Day Except Christmas (Grand Prix Venice), Apaches. Executive Producer: Time Without Pity. Producer: Sunday by the Sea. (Grand Prix Venice), Bow Bells, We Are the Lambeth Boys (Grand Prix Tours), Dispute (British Film Academy Award), I Want to Go to School, All Neat in Black Stockings, Morgan-A Suitable Case For Treatment, The French Lieutenant's Woman.

CLORK, HARRY: Writer. r.n. Clarke; b. Galveston, Tex. e. St. Paul's Academy Garden City, Long Island, N.Y. Was husband of late Nora Bayes, writer of her stage material; author several stage plays (Smiling Faces, The Milky Way, See My Lawyer) (collab., filmed in 1936 by Paramount); adapt. many plays for Shubert stage enterprises; radio writer. From 1935 writer many s.p. & adapt.

PICTURES INCLUDE: Thrill of Brazil, Mighty McGurk, Sainted Sisters, Painting the Clouds with Sunshine, Tea for Two, Ma and Pa Kettle at Waikiki, The Prisoner.

TV: Beulah, Life of Riley.

CLOSE, GLENN: Actress. b. Greenwich, CT. e. College of William and Mary. Professional debut at Phoenix Theatre, New York, in season of plays including Love for Love, The Member of the Wedding, Rules of the Game. Also accomplished musical performer (lyric soprano), appearing on Bdwy. in Rex and Barnum.

PICTURES: The World According to Garp (debut), The Big Chill, The Natural, The Stone Boy, Jagged Edge, Maxie.

TELEVISION: Movies: The Orphan Train, Too Far To Go, Something About Amelia.

CLOVER, DAVID: Actor. b. November 10.

TELEVISION INCLUDES: Policewoman, Police Story, McLaren's Raiders; Kate McShane; One Day At A Time; Delphi Bureau; On The Rocks; The Dick Cavett Special.

CLUG, A. STEPHEN: Executive. b. New York City, Apr. 2, 1929. e. Colgate Univ., Columbia Law School. Was special agent, U.S. Army Counter Intelligence Corps, Far East Command, 1951–4. Started with industry as branch mgr., Paramount Films of Indonesia, 1954; mgr. dir., Paramount Films of India, Ltd., supervising India, Burma, Pakistan, Persian Gulf, 1955–57; Far East supvr. for special handling, The Ten Commandments, 1957–8; co-ordinator world-wide program theatrical re-releases, Paramount Intl., 1958–9; mgr., dir., Paramount Films of Brasil, 1959–65; v.p. & exec. prod., Gold Dolphin Prods., Inc., N.Y., 1965–69; gen. mgr. & supvr. Central America/Caribbean areas, MGM Intl. Inc., Panama, 1969–71; gen. mgr., MGM Puerto Rico/supvr. Caribbean area/MGM Cinemas, 1971–3; dir. sls. & asst. continental supvr. for Europe, UK, Middle East, MGM Intl., Inc. 1973–79; v.p./sls. mgr., MGM Intl., headquartered in Paris, 79–82; joined MPEAA as v.p. and regional rep. for Far East and Australasia, headquarted in Singapore, 1982.

CLYDE, THOMAS: Producer. b. Battle, England, Ent. m.p. ind. 1949. After writ. dir. documentaries, with Ivan Foxwell as prod. mgr. The Intruder, Coldits Story; 1956 to Douglas Fairbanks, Ltd., prod. The Hostage, 1957 for own Company, Cavalcade Films, Ltd. Chase a Crooked Shadow; Moment of Danger, Follow That Horse, Guns of Darkness, Work Is a Four Letter Word.

COBE, SANDY: Executive, Producer-Distributor. b. New York City, N.Y., Nov. 30, 1928. e. Tulane Univ. (B. of A., fine arts). U.S. Army WW II & Korea, combat photographer; Loews Theatre Corp., theatre mgr., N.Y. Daily News, photographer; WPIX-TV, cinematographer; Artmark Pictures, N.Y., produced 11 features. Pepsicola, v.p., Pepco Special events, in charge of N.Y.'s World Fair operations and promotion. General Studios, exec. v.p., distribution; First Cinema Releasing Corp., pres. formed Sandy Cobe Productions, Inc., producer, packager, European features for U.S. theatrical & television. Pres., Intercontinental Releasing Corportion, domestic and foreign distribution of theatrical features.

MEMBER: Masons (Scottish-Rite 32nd), Shrine, Variety Clubs Tent 25, Academy of Television Arts and Sciences. Special commendations from: California State Senate, Los Angeles City Council, California State Assembly and County of Los Angeles.

PICTURES: Terror on Tour (prod.), Access Code (exec. prod.), A.R.C.A. D.E. (prod.).

COBE, SHARYON REIS: Executive. b. Honolulu, Hawaii. e. Univ. of Hawaii, Loyola Marymount Univ. Dancer Fitzgerald, & Sample, N.Y. United Air Lines, N.Y.; v.p., story editor, Gotham Publishing N.Y.; v.p., distribution-foreign sales, World Wide Film Distributors, L.A.; exec. v.p., Intercontinental Releasing Corp., L.A.

MEMBER: Women in Show Business, Ladies of Variety (lent 25).

PICTURES: Terror on Tour (prod. co-ordinator), Home Sweet Home (prod. mgr.), To All a Good Night (assoc. prod.), Access Code (co-prod.).

COBURN, JAMES: Actor. b. Laurel, Neb., Aug. 31, 1928. e. Los Angeles City College, where he studied drama. Served in U.S. Army. First acting role in coast production of Billy Budd. Later to New York, where he worked on TV commercials, then in teleplays on Studio One, GE Theatre, Robert Montgomery Presents. Summer stock in Detroit before returning to Hollywood. First film, 1959, was Ride Lonesome.

PICTURES INCLUDE: Foes of the Fugitive, The Magnificent Seven, Hell Is for Heroes, The Great Escape, Charade, The Americanization of Emily, The Loved One, Major Dundee, A High Wind in Jamaica, Our Man Flint, What Did You Do in the War, Daddy?, Dead Heat on a Merry-Go-Round, In Like Flint, Waterhole No. 3, Candy, Hard Contract, The Last of the Mobile Hot Shots, The Carey Treatment, The Honkers, Duck, You Sucker, The Last of Sheila, Harry in Your Pocket, A Reason to Live, A Reason to Die, The Internecine Project, Bite the Bullet, Hard Times, Sky Riders, The Last Hard Men, Midway, Cross of Iron, Firepower, The Big Bullet, Loving Couples, Looker, Martin's Day, Death of a Soldier.

TELEVISION: Draw!, Sins of the Fathers.

COCA, IMOGENE: Actress. b. Philadelphia, Nov. 18, 1908. p. the late Joe Coca, orchestra leader, and Sadie Brady, retired vaudevillian. At 11, debut tap dancer in New York vaudeville; solo dancer Broadway musicals; as comedienne, in New Faces of 1934; with husband, Bob Burton, in Straw Hat Revue in 1939, and others through 1942. New York night clubs, Cafe Society and Le Ruban Bleu, New York; Palmer House, Chicago; Park Plaza, St. Louis. 1949 to TV via Broadway Revue, evolved routines with Sid Caesar, Your Show of Shows, 1950–54. NBC-TV; Imogene Coca Show, 1954, 1955; Sid Caesar invites you, 1958, Glinda.

PICTURES INCLUDE: Under the Yum Yum Tree, Rabbit Test, National Lampoon's Vacation, Nothing Lasts Forever.

COCCHI, JOHN: Writer-Critic. b. Brooklyn, N.Y., June 19, 1939. e. Fort Hamilton High School, 1957; Brooklyn College, AAS, 1961. U.S. Army, 1963–65. Puritan Film Labs, manager,1967–9. Independent-International Pictures, biographer-researcher, 1969. Boxoffice Magazine, critic, reporter, columnist, 1970–79. Co-author: The American Movies Reference Book (Prentice-Hall). Contributor: Screen Facts, Film Fan Monthly, Films in Review. Actor in: The Diabolical Dr. Ongo, Thick as Thieves, Captain Celluloid VS. the Film Pirates. Worked on dubbing: Dirtymouth, 1970. Author, The Westerns, a Movie Quiz Book. Contributor to various books on films. Author, Second Feature (A History of the 'B' Movie). Now free lance writer, researcher, agent. Recent credits: researcher for American Movie Classics (Rainbow Programming Service); contributor to book, 500 Greatest American Sound Films. Consultant to Killiam Shows, Prof. Richard Brown, etc.

COCHRAN, RON: Producer, writer, narrator. b. Saskatchewan, Canada, Sept. 20, 1912. e. Parsons College U. of Fla. Newscaster for radio stations in Rock Island, Ill., Des Moines, St. Louis; special agent, FBI 1942–45; then returned to radio as news dir., dir. of news WCOP Boston 1945–51; joined CBS-TV news staff, 1951, in Washington; newscaster, Late News Show; news roundups, CBS radio; moderator, Capitol Cloakroom, Where Do You Stand, Man of the Week; CBS news staff, N.Y., 1954; newscaster. The Late News; moderator, Youth Takes a Stand, One O'clock Report, CBS-TV; In Person, CBS-Radio; News, ABC-TV, 1962; Ron Cochran With the News 1967; Pres., Ron Cochran Enterprises Inc., producer and syndicator or radio and television.

COCO, JAMES: b. Bronx, N.Y., Mar. 21, 1929. Became stage mgr. of touring children's theatre while still in teens. Was character actor in summer stock and off-Bdwy. prods. before appearing on Bdwy. in Man of La Mancha and The Last of the Red Hot Lovers.

PICTURES INCLUDE: A New Leaf, the Strawberry Statement, Tell Me That You Love Me, Junie Moon, Such Good Friends, Man of La Mancha, The Wild Party, Murder by Death, The Cheap Detective, Scavenger Hunt, Wholly Moses, Only When I Laugh, The Muppets Take Manhattan.

TELEVISION: Marcus Welby, M.D., The Flip Wilson Show, The Trouble With People, VD Blues, Calucci's Dept.

COEN, GUIDO: Producer and Executive Prod. series pictures for Fortress Films and Kenilworth Films.

PICTURES INCLUDE: One Jump Ahead, Golden Link, The Hornet's Nest, Behind the Headlines, Murder Reported, There's Always a Thursday, Date with Disaster, The End of the Line, The Man Without A Body, Woman Eater, Kill Her Gently, Naked Fury, Operation Cupid, Strictly Confidential, Dangerous Afternoon, Jungle Street, Strongroom, Penthouse, Baby Love, One Brief Summer, Burke and Hare, Au Pair Girls, Intimate Games, Twickenham Studios.

COHEN, CHARLES: Executive. b. Brooklyn, N.Y., Sept. 15, 1912; e. Brooklyn Coll. Pub. dept., MGM, 1931; U-I, 1948–50; 20th-Fox, 1950; assoc. adv. mgr.; eastern asst. adv. & pub. mgr. Allied Artists, 1955; home off. pub. mgr. Warner Bros., 1957. Eastern adv. mgr. 1958; eastern adv., pub. mgr., 1960; Exec. ass't to adv. pub. director, 1960; expl. dir., Embassy Pictures, 1961; nat. adv. & pub. dir., Cinema V Dist., 1964; Adv. & Pub. Dir., Sigma III, 1968; adv., pub. mgr., The Cannon Group, 1970, v.p., adv.-pub. rel. 1971; Adv.-Pub. Dir., U.A. Eastern Theatres, 1973–77 (retired). Since 1978, has served as volunteer writer for Variety Clubs International magazine, the Barker, and in the creation of institutional fund-raising ad campaigns for V.C.I. Co-author with Morton Sunshine of This is Variety, a brochure tracing the origins, development and accomplishments of Variety Clubs around the world.

COHEN, ELLIS A.: Producer-Writer. b. Baltimore, Md. Sept. 15, 1945. e. Balt. Jr. Coll. (A.A.). Since 1983 pres., Hennessey Entertainment, Ltd. 1980, pres. Ellis A. Cohen Prods., 1978, Director of TV Network Boxing Events, Don King Productions, Inc., NYC 1978, Account Exec., Solters & Roskin P.R. L.A. 1977, Prod., Henry Jaffe Enterprises, Inc., 1974–76 dir., worldwide pub./adv., William Morris Agency, 1963, talent coordinator, Cerebral Palsy Telethon, WBAL-TV, Baltimore; 1964, p.r. asst. Campbell-Ewald Adv. Agency, L.A.; 1966, and mgr., Hochschild Kohn Dept. Stores, Baltimore; 1968–69, asst. dir., p.r. entertainment, talent booking for Club Venus Night Club, Baltimore; 1968, created-edited The Forum Oracle, national entertainment mag. 1969–72, dir., p.r., Jewish Community Center of Baltimore; 1970, leave of absence to work as corr. in Israel, Denmark & London; 1972, dir., p.r. & adv., The Camera Mart, New York; 1972–74 creator & editor-in-chief, TV/New York Magazine, nationwide TV mag.; Producer, New York Area Emmy Awards Telecast (1973 & 1974), WOR-TV (prod.), chm., exec. prod. of TV Academy Celebrity drop-in luncheon series; 1972, talent coordinator Bob Hope's Celebrity Flood Relief Telethon. Member: Writers Guild of America, Producers Guild of America, Friars Club, Amer. Newspaper Guild, Intl. Press Corp., Israeli Press Corp., National Academy of TV Arts & Sciences, Academy of Television Arts & Sciences, Screen Arts Guild. Mayor Beame's Committee In The Public Interest for NYC; executive producer, 1976 Democratic National Convention Gala.
TELEVISION: Aunt Mary (Dec. 1979), a Hallmark Hall of Fame, 2-hr. movie special, CBS-TV (prod.-story by); New York Area Emmy Awards. Telecast; January 1973 WOR-TV (prod.) and January 1974, WOR-TV (prod.). First Steps (CBS movie, 1984); Love, May (CBS movie) (prod.); First Steps (CBS movie) (prod.).

COHEN, HERMAN: Producer, writer. b. Detroit, Mich. Age 12, usher, Detroit, Dexter theatre; chief of service, Detroit, Fox theatre; mgr., booker, Dexter Theatres; military service; house mgr., Fox theatre; sales mgr. Columbia Pictures, Detroit; prod., Realart, Jack Broder Productions, Hollywood; formed own prod. Co., 1953; owner, Fox and Cinderella Theatres, Detroit; prod. pictures for Columbia and Warner Bros. Currently heads Cobra Media, Inc.
PICTURES INCLUDE: River Beat, Magnificent Roughnecks, The Brass Legend, Target Earth, Crime of Passion, Horrors of the Black Museum, I was a Teenage Werewolf, I Was a Teenage Frankenstein, Blood of Dracula, How to Make a Monster, Konga, Headless Ghost, Black Zoo, A Study in Terror, Berserk, Crooks and Coronets, TROG, Craze.

COHEN, IRWIN R.: Exhibition Executive. b. Baltimore, Md., Sept. 4, 1924. Attended Massanutten Acacemy, Woodstock, Va., Member of alumni board of directors; attended University of Baltimore, bachelor of laws, 1948. Admitted to Maryland bar, 1948, partner law firm Cohen & Dackman since 1952. In exhibition 1938 to date. Founded R/C Theatres 1966, chief exec. officer 1966 to date. Member of Variety Club, Tent #11, Member of Board of Directors NATO of Maryland, past pres. NATO of Virginia 1975–77, past chmn. board NATO of Virginia 1977–79. Member of exec. comm. and member of board of directors National NATO. One of the founders, co-atny., and vice-chmn. of Key Federal Savings & Loan Association 1961 to date.

COHEN, LARRY: Writer-Director. b. Chicago, IL, April 20, 1947. e. Univ. of Wisconsin.
PICTURES: Writer: Carrie, God Told Me To, The American Success Company, The Jury. Writer-Director: The Winger Serpent (also prod.), Special Effects, Perfect Strangers, Full Moon High (also prod.).

COHEN, MILTON E.: Distributor. b. Chicago, Ill., e. University of Illinois. Entered motion picture industry as salesman. United Artists, Chicago, 1925–29; Columbia, Chicago, 1929–31; salesman, Detroit, 1931–38; sales mgr., RKO, Detroit, 1938; branch mgr., 1943; Eastern-Central dist. mgr., 1946; Eastern sales mgr., Eagle Lion Classics, 1948; genl. sales mgr., 1951; western & southern sales mgr., United Artist, 1951; Eastern & Southern sales mgr., 1952; supervisor, sales, Around The World In 80 Days, 1958; Eastern Canadian sales mgr., 1959; national dir., Roadshow Sales, 1961; retired. United Artists, 1969; exec. v.p. in charge of theatrical distrib. for Trans Globe Films, Inc., 1971.

COHEN, NATHAN: Executive. b. London, Eng., Dec. 23, 1905. Entered m.p. ind. as exhibitor 1930; into production and distribution 1942. Director: Thorn EMI Films Ltd. Nat Cohen Entertainments.

COHEN, ROB: Producer-Director. b. 1949. Formerly exec. v.p. in chg of m.p. and TV for Motown. Started as dir. of m.p. for TV at 20th Century-Fox. Joined Motown at age of 24 to produce films. Headed own production co. 1985, appt. pres., Keith Barish Prods.
PICTURES INCLUDE: Mahogany, Bingo, Long and the Traveling All-Stars, Scott Joplin, Almost Summer, Thank God It's Friday, The Wiz, A Small Circle of Friends (dir.), Scandalous (dir.), The Razor's Edge (prod.).
TELEVISION: Miami Vice (dir.).

COHN, ROBERT: Producer. b. Avon, N.J., Sept. 6, 1920; e. U. Michigan, B.A., '41; p. Jack Cohn. Joined Columbia as asst. dir. In World War II, as Signal Corps film cutter. Air Corps Training Lab. unit mgr., combat aerial m.p. camera man with 13th A.A.F. Awarded: DFC, Air Medal & 3 clusters, Purple Heart. Assoc. prod. "Lone Wolf In London" 1947; prod. "Adventures in Silverado" 1948, all Col. Headed Robert Cohn prod. unit at Columbia, pres. International Cinema Guild. Columbia European prod.: exec. Columbia Studios. Hollywood: formed Robert Cohn Prod.
PICTURES INCLUDE: Black Eagle, Rusty Leads the Way, Palomino, Kazan, Killer That Stalked New York, The Barefoot Mailman, Mission Over Korea, The Interns, The New Interns, The Young Americans.

COHEN, ROBERT B.: Executive. e. George Washington Univ. (BA), Southern Texas School of Law. 1980–84, atty. for Greenberg, Glusker, Fields, Clamans and Machtinger (LA). Was asst. gen. counsel for Columbia Pictures. Joined Paramount 1985 as sr. atty. for M.P. Group. to oversee legal functions for assigned feature films.

COLBERT, CLAUDETTE: Actress: r.n. Claudette Chauchoin. b. Paris, Sept. 13, 1907. e. public schools, Paris, New York; Art Students League (N.Y.). On N.Y. stage (debut, Wild Wescotts; following Marionette Man, We've Got to Have Money, Cat Came Back, Kiss in a Taxi, Ghost Train, The Barker, Dynamo, etc.). First screen role in Love O' Mike (silent); thereafter featured and starred in many prod. Academy Award best actress, 1934 (It Happened One Night, Columbia); voted one of ten best Money Making Stars in Fame Poll, 1935, 36, 47.
PICTURES INCLUDE: Cleopatra, I Cover the Waterfront, No Time for Love, Practically Yours, Since You Went Away, So Proudly We Hail, Guest Wife, Tomorrow is Forever, The Egg and I, Sleep My Love, Family Honeymoon, Bride for Sale, Three Came Home, The Secret Fury, Thunder on the Hill, Let's Make It Legal, Outpost in Malaya, Daughters of Destiny, Texas Lady, Parrish.
BROADWAY: Marriage Go Round, Irregular Verb to Love.

COLE, GEORGE: Actor. b. London, Eng., Apr. 22, 1925. e. Secondary Sch. Surrey. Stage debut in White Horse Inn, 1939; m.p. debut in Cottage to Let, 1941.
PICTURES INCLUDE: Henry V, Quartet, My Brother's Keeper, Laughter in Paradise, Scrooge, Lady Godiva Rides Again, Who Goes There (Passionate Sentry), Morning Departure (Operation Disaster), Top Secret (Mr. Potts Goes to Moscow), Happy Family, Will Any Gentleman, Apes of the Rock, The Intruder, Happy Ever After (Tonight's the Night), Our Girl Friday (Adventures of Sadie), Belles of St. Trinian's, Prize of Gold, Where There's a Will, Constant Husband, Quentin Durward, The Weapon, It's a Wonderful Life, Green Man, Bridal Path, Too Many Crooks, Blue Murder at St. Trinians, Don't Panic Chaps, Dr. Syn, One Way Pendulum, Legend of Young Dick Turpin, The Great St. Trinian's Train Robbery, Cleopatra, The Green Shoes, Vampire Lovers, Fright, The Bluebird.
TV: Life of Bliss, A Man of Our Times, Don't Forget To Write, The Good Life, Minder.

COLE, SIDNEY: Prod., dir., writer. b. London, England, 1908; e. Westminster City Sch.; London U., BSc. Began at Stoll Studios 1930; then various feature and documentary studios. Dir. Roads Across Britain. Spanish ABC. Behind the Spanish Lines. Ed. Gaslight. Mr. Pimpernel Smith, San Demetrio, London, Nine Men, etc.; tech. adviser First of the Few; writer and assoc. prod. They Came to a City, Return of the Vikings; assoc. prod Dead of Night, Loves of Joanna Godden, Against the Wind, Scott of the Antarctic, The Magnet, Man in the White Suit, Train of Events (co-dir.); Operation Swallow (Eng. adapt.); The Angel Who Pawned Her Harp (writer-prod.); s.p., North Sea Bus. Assoc. prod. Escapade; prod. Sword of Sherwood Forest; prod. s.p. The Kitchen; prod. We Are The Engineers, One in Five.
TV: prod. Adventures of Robin Hood, The Buccaneers, Sword of Freedom, The Four Just Men, Danger Man

(Secret Agent), Man In A Suitcase, Adventures of Black Beauty, Dick Turpin, Smuggler.

COLEMAN, DABNEY: Actor. b. Austin, TX, Jan. 3, 1932. A regular on the TV series, Mary Hartman, Mary Hartman.
PICTURES INCLUDE: This Property Is Condemned, The Slender Thread, The Scalphunters, The Other Side of the Mountain, The Black Streetfighter, Rolling Thunder, Viva Knievel, North Dallas Forty, Nothing Personal, How To Beat the High Cost of Living, Melvin and Howard, Nine to Five, On Golden Pond, Modern Problems, Young Doctors in Love, Tootsie, WarGames, Cloak and Dagger, The Man with One Red Shoe.
TELEVISION: Murrow.

COLEMAN, GARY: Actor. b. Zion, IL, Feb. 8, 1968. Gained fame as star of TV's Diff'rent Strokes.
TELEVISION: The Little Rascals, America 2-Night, Good Times, The Jeffersons, Diff'rent Strokes, Lucy Moves to NBC, The Big Show, etc. Movies: The Kid from Left Field, Scout's Honor, Playing with Fire.
PICTURES: On the Right Track, Jimmy the Kid.

COLEMAN, NANCY: Actress. b. Everett, Wash. Dec. 30, 1917. e. U. Wash. In radio serials; on New York stage (with Gertrude Lawrence, in Theatre Guild productiions, etc.). Desperate Hours, 1955; m.p. debut, 1941, Rep. Co. tour of Europe and So. Am.
PICTURES INCLUDE: Kings Row, Dangerously They Live, Gay Sisters, Desperate Journey, Edge of Darkness, In Our Time, Devotion, Violence, Mourning Becomes Electra, That Man from Tangier, Slaves.
TV: Valiant Lady Producers Showcase. Am. Theatre Guild.

COLEMAN, THOMAS J.: Executive. b. Connecticut, Apr. 13, 1950. e. Boston Univ. Pres., Twalzo Music Corp., 1972–73; v.p., natl. sls. mgr., United Intl. Pictures, 1973–74; founded Atlantic Releasing Corp., 1974; Atlantic Television, Inc., 1981. All Atlantic corps. consolidated into Atlantic Entertainment Group, 1986. Co. has distributed over 100 films and produced 30 features and TV movies.
PICTURES: (Producer or Exec. Prod.): Valley Girl, Alphabet City, Roadhouse, Night of the Comet, Starchaser, Teen Wolf, Extremities, The Men's Club, Modern Girls, Nutcracker, etc.

COLER, JOEL H.: Executive. b. Bronx, N.Y., 1931. e. Syracuse University (B.A., journalism). Married and has two daughters. Worked as adv. asst. NBC; acct. exec. Grey advertising. Joined 20th Century-Fox 1964 as adv. coordinator Fox Intl.; 1967, named intl. adv./pub. mgr. 1974, named v.p. dir., intl. adv./pub.

COLLERAN, BILL: Producer-Director. b. April 16; story department 20th Century-Fox 1945–46; Director Louis de Rochemont 1946–50; stage mgr. NBC 1951; Assoc. Dir. The Hit Parade 1952–53; Dir. The Hit Parade, various TV specs. 1954–56; Dir. Cinerama Windjammer 1956; TV Specs. Bing Crosby, Frank Sinatra, Debbie Reynolds 1957–60; various TV specs. 1960–65, Exec. Prod. Judy Garland Show, Dean Martin Show, 1965–66; Dir. Richard Burton's "Hamlet" film, Prod. "Popendipity" ABC-TV spec. various other TV specs. 1967–70; 1971–77 Various TV specials and series; 1978–83, prod., dir., writer for Hill-Eubanks Group and Little Joey, Inc.; 1984–86, dir. music video for Simba; developing film to TV projects for own production co.

COLLIN, REGINALD: Producer/director. Trained at the Old Vic Theatre School as actor. Directed in repertory, also pantomimes and summer shows. Entered television 1958. Producer ITV's First Arts Programme Tempo. Producer of Callan, Mystery And Imagination, Special Branch, Napoleon And Love. 1975: Producer/director two Armchair Cinemas, also documentary on the Royal Shakespeare Theatre. 1976: Vice-Chairman of the British Academy of Film and Television Arts. Chairman of the Awards Committee. 1977: Appt. first dir. of BAFTA.

COLLINS, JOAN: Actress. b. London, Eng., May 23, 1933. e. Francis Holland School (London). Made stage debut in A Dolls House, Arts Theatre 1946. Screen debut in I Believe in You, 1952. TV appearances include Dynasty.
PICTURES INCLUDE: I Believe in You, Judgment Deferred, Decameron Nights, Cosh Boy, The Square Ring, Turn the Key Softly, Our Girl Friday (Adventures of Sadie), The Good Die Young, Land of the Pharaohs, Virgin Queen, Girl in the Red Velvet Swing, Opposite Sex, Sea Wife, Island in the Sun, Wayward Bus, Stopover Tokyo, The Bravados, Rally Round the Flag Boys, Seven Thieves, Esther and the King, Warning Shot, Can Hieronymus Merkin Ever Forget Mercy Humpe and Find True Happiness?, The Executioner, Tales from the Crypt, The Bawdy Adventures of Tom Jones, Empire of the Ants, The Big Sleep, Sunburn, The Stud, The Bitch.
TELEVISION: Movies: The Cartier Affair, The Making of a Male Model, Her Life As a Man. Mini-Series: Sins

COLLINS, PAT: Performer. r.n. Patricia Colinaka Allan. b. Detroit, Mich., May 7, 1935. e. U. of Ill., 1953. District mgr., Yardley Created Prods., Chicago; played in various nightclubs, Chicago, Miami, Las Vegas, etc. Now on CBS Morning News.
PICTURE: Experiment in Nightmares.
TV (1963–65): Steven Allen, Bill Dana Show, No Time for Sergeants, Mike Douglas, Art Linkletter, Honey West.

COLLINS, STEPHEN: Actor. b. Hastings-on-Hudson, N.Y., 1948. Appeared off-Bdwy. in Joseph Papp production before acquiring role on Bdwy. in The Ritz.
PICTURES: All the President's Men, Between the Lines, The Promise, Star Trek, Fedora, Loving Couples, Brewster's Millions.
TELEVISION: The Waltons, Barnaby Jones, Tales of the Gold Monkey, Chiefs, Dark Mirror, Threesome.

COLT, MARSHALL: Actor. b. New Orleans, LA, Oct. 26. e. Tulane Univ. Did naval tour in Southeast Asia during Vietnam War. Acted in local stage productions in San Francisco (Hotel Universe, Who's Afraid of Virginia Woolf?, Zoo Story, etc.).
PICTURES: Bimbo (short), North Dallas Forty, Those Lips, Those Eyes.
TELEVISION: Series: Family, Paper Chase, Streets of San Francisco, Barnaby Jones, McClain's Law, Lottery! Movies: Colorado C-1, Sharon: Portrait of a Mistress, Once an Eagle, etc.

COLVILLE, JOHN: Producer, Director. Started in theatre. Worked in all departments before becoming Film Editor on Features, Documentaries, and Television Series for both BBC/ITV. Extensive experience in Greece, Singapore, Spain, Switzerland—now establishing new Unit, Studios, and Producing films in Nigeria.

COMDEN, BETTY: Writer. b. Brooklyn, N.Y., May 3, 1919. e. NYU. Nightclub performer, 1939–44; all writing in collab. with Adolph Green; writer book, sketches & lyrics for many Bway. shows including: On the Town, Billion Dollar Baby, Two On the Aisle, Wonderful Town, Peter Pan, Fade Out . . . Fade In.
PICTURES INCLUDE: Good News, On the Town, Barkleys of Broadway, Singin' in the Rain, Band Wagon, It's Always Fair Weather, What a Way to Go, Bells Are Ringing, Auntie Mame, Say Darling.
BROADWAY: Lyrics with Adolph Green—Do Re Mi. Collab. writing, Adolph Green, A Party; worked on Bells Are Ringing; book, lyrics, Subways Are For Sleeping; Show, Hallelujah, Baby! Book for show Applause. Tony Awards for: Wonderful Town, Hallelujah Baby, Applause.

COMO, PERRY: Singer. b. Canonsburg, Penn., May 18, 1912 p. Pietro and Lucille Travaglini Como; e. Canonsburg local schools. Barber at 15; joined Carlone Band, then Ted Weems in 1936; CBS sustaining show; played many night clubs, records for Victor. Screen debut, Something for the Boys, 20th Century Fox.
PICTURES INCLUDE: Doll Face, If I'm Lucky.
TV: Perry Como show. NBC-TV. Best Male vocalist M.P. Daily, TV poll, 1952–55; radio poll, 1954. Best Male vocalist M.P. Daily, TV Poll, 1956: best TV performer M.P.D.—Fame poll 1957. Interfaith Award, 1953; Emmy, Peabody, Christopher Awards, 1955–56; Knight Commander and Lady Com. (Mrs. Como) of Equestrian Order of Holy Sepulchre of Jerusalem; personality of the yr., Variety Club, 1956. Perry Como Kraft Music Hall, NBC-TV.

COMPTON, JOYCE: Actress. b. Lexington, Ky.; e. Tulsa U. Screen debut in Ankles Preferred.
PICTURES INCLUDE: If I Had a Million, Luxury Liner, Only Yesterday, Affairs of a Gentleman, Christmas in Connecticut, Danger Signal, Hitchhike to Happiness, Charlie Chan of Alcatraz, Exposed, Incident, Grand Canyon, Jet Pilot.

CONAWAY, JEFF: Actor. b. New York City, Oct. 5, 1950. Started in show business at the age of 10 when he appeared in Bdwy. production, All the Way Home. Later toured in Critics Choice before turning to fashion modeling. Toured with musical group, 3½, as lead singer and guitarist. Entered theatre arts program at N.Y. Univ. Film debut at 19 in Jennifer on My Mind.
PICTURES: The Eagle Has Landed, Pete's Dragon, I Never Promised You a Rose Garden, Grease.
TELEVISION: The Mary Tyler Moore Show, Happy Days, Movin' On, Barnaby Jones, Kojak, TV movies: Having Babies, Delta County, U.S.A., Breaking Up Is Hard to Do, The Making of a Male Model.
SERIES: Taxi.

CONDE, RITA: Actress. b. Cuba. r.n. Elizabeth Cleanor Conde Griffiths. Now American citizen. In numerous films and on TV in Hollywood and starred in Mexican film, El Ahijado de la Muerte.
PICTURES INCLUDE: Ride the Pink Horse, Two Roaming Champs, No Sad Songs for Me, Topaz, Change of Habit,

Barquero, World's Greatest Lover, Love at First Bite, etc.
TELEVISION INCLUDES: I Love Lucy, Zorro, I Spy, Thriller, Night Gallery, Ironside, Chico and the Man, Days of Our Lives, Capitol, etc.

CONDON, CHRIS J.: Producer-Director-Motion Equipment Designer. b. Chicago, Dec. 7, 1922. e. Davidson Institute, USC, U.S. Air Force 1943–46. Founded Century Precision Optics, 1948. Designed Athenar telephoto lenses, Century Super wide-angle lenses and Duplikins. Co-founded StereoVision International, Inc. 1969 specializing in films produced in new 3-D process.
FILMS PRODUCED: The Wild Ride, The Surfer, Girls, Airline, The New Dimensions, Member SMPTE. Lecturer and consultant on motion picture optics and 3-D motion picture technology.

CONLEY, DICK: Executive. r.n. Richard Glen. b. La Cygne, Kansas, Feb. 7, 1920. e. Lamar Union H.S., Lamar, Colorado. Atlas Theatre Corp., Denver, 1938–43; merchandising specialist, National General Corp., 1944–62; district mgr., Kansas City-St. Louis area, 1962–68; area superv. Kansas City-Omaha-Des Moines-St. Louis area; pres., Petite Amusement Corp., Kansas City.

CONN, ROBERT A.: Executive. b. Philadelphia, Pa., Jan. 16, 1926; e. Lehigh U. 1944; U. of Pa., 1948. 1st Lt. Army Security Agency, 1944–46, 1951–52; furniture dist., Philadelphia, 1948–51; band & act. dept., MCA, 1952–53; dir. of adv. & prom. Official Films N.Y. 1954; head of Official Films Philadelphia sales office serving Pennsylvania, Baltimore, Washington, Cleveland and Detroit, 1956. Eastern Reg. Sls. Mgr. Flamingo Films, 1957; acct. exec. Dunnan and Jeffrey, Inc., June, 1961; v.p., Dunnan and Jeffrey, Jan. 1962; pres., adv. mgr., Suburban Knitwear Co., 1963; exec. v.p. Rogal Travel Service, 1964–68. 1968–78, pres. RAC Travel, Inc., Jenkintown, Pa. and pres. Royal Palm Travel, Inc. Palm Beach, Florida, 1978; Rosenbluth Travel Service, 1979; v.p., natl. retail mktg., E.F. Hutton & Co. (N.Y.), 1983.

CONNELY, PAUL V.: Executive. b. Boston, Mass., June 11, 1923. e. Boston Coll., MA, 1951, B.S.B.A., 1949; Fordham Univ., 1951–54; Asst. professor of Economics, Manhattan Coll., 1950–54; treas., America Corp. (formerly Chespeake Industries), 1957–59; treas., dir., Pathe-America Dist. Co. Inc., Sutton Pictures Co.; vice-pres., dir., Pathe Labs., Inc.; pres., dir., Pathe-Deluxe of Canada, Ltd. 1959–65; pres. International Business Relations, 1965–67; v.p., treas., dir. Movielab, Inc., 1968; v.p.—finance, Tele-Tape Corp., 1970.

CONNERY, SEAN: Actor. b. Edinburgh, Scotland, Aug. 25, 1930. Stage debut South Pacific, 1953.
TV: Requiem for a Heavyweight, Anna Christie, Boy With the Meataxe, Women in Love, The Crucible, Riders to the Sea, Colombe, Adventure Story, Anna Karenina, Macbeth (Canadian TV).
PICTURES INCLUDE: The Longest Day, Dr. No, From Russia With Love, Marnie, Woman of Straw, Goldfinger, The Hill, Thunderball, A Fine Madness, You Only Live Twice, Shalako, The Molly Maguires, The Red Tent, The Anderson Tapes, Diamonds Are Forever, The Offence, Zardoz, Ransom, Murder on the Orient Express. The Wind and The Lion, The Man Who Would Be King, Robin and Marian. The Next Man, A Bridge Too Far, The Great Train Robbery, Meteor, Cuba, Outland, Time Bandits, Wrong Is Right, Five Days One Summer, Never Say Never Again, Highlander.
Prod. dir., The Bowler and the Bonnet (film doc.), I've Seen You Cut Lemons (London stage). Director of Tantallon Films Ltd. (First production: Something Like the Truth).

CONNOR, KENNETH: Actor. b. London, England. Ent. m.p. industry 1949 in The Lady Killers.
TV: Ted Ray Show, Show Called Fred, Charlie Farnabarn's Show, Alfred Marks Time, As You Like It, Dickie Valentine Show, Black and White Minstrel, Anne Shelton, Hi Summer, series Don't Say A Word, Room at the Bottom, On the Houses, Frankie Howard Reveals All, Allo Allo, Hi de Hi, That's My Boy.
PICTURES INCLUDE: Carry on Sergeant, Carry on Nurse, Carry on Constable, Watch Your Stern, Carry on Regardless, Nearly a Nasty Accident, What a Carve Up, Call Me a Cab, Carry on Cleo, Captain Nemo, Carry On Up The Jungle, Carry On Matron, Carry On Abroad, Carry on England, Carry On Emanuelle.

CONNORS, CHUCK: Actor. r.n. Kevin Joseph Connors. b. Brooklyn, N.Y., April 10, 1924; e. Adelphi Acad., Seton Hall Coll., U.S. Army 3 yrs., then prof. baseball player.
TV: Dennis Day Show, Four Star Playhouse, Star and the Story, Reader's Digest, Gunsmoke, West Point, Rifleman series, Roots, Yellow Rose.
PICTURES INCLUDE: Pat and Mike, Code Two, Trouble Along the Way, South Sea Women, Dragonfly Squadron, Naked Alibi, Human Jungle, Target Zero, Three Stripes in the Sun, Good Morning Miss Dove, Hold Back the Night, Hot Rod Girl, Tomahawk Trail, Walk the Dark Street, Geronimo, Kill Them All and Come Back Alive, Capt. Nemo and the Underwater City, Profane Comedy, The Deserter, Support Your Local Gunfighter, Soylent Green, 99 and 44/100ths Dead, Airplane II: The Sequel.

CONNORS, MIKE: Actor. b. Fresno, Cal., Aug. 15, 1925. r.n. Krekor Ohanian. e. UCLA. Film debut in Sudden Fear; other pictures include Sky Commando, Day of Triumph, Flesh and Spur, Seed of Violence, Harlow, Good Neighbor Sam, Where Love Has Gone, Avalanche Express, Too Scared to Scream.
TV: Tightrope, Mannix (Golden Globe award).

CONRAD, ROBERT: Actor, singer. r.n. Conrad Robert Falk; b. Chicago, Ill., March 1, 1935; e. public schools, Northwestern U.; prof. debut, nightclub singer. Formed Robert Conrad Production, 1966.
TV: Lawman, Maverick, 77 Sunset Strip, Hawaiian Eye (series), Wild Wild West (series), Baa, Baa, Black Sheep (series), Centennial (mini-series), A Man Called Sloane (series). Movies: Wild Wild West Revisited, More Wild Wild West, Breaking Up Is Hard To Do, Will: G. Gordon Liddy, Confessions of a Married Man, Hard Knox, Two Fathers' Justice, Assassin, Charley Hannah, The Fifth Missile.
PICTURES: Thundering Jets, Palm Springs Weekend, Young Dillinger, Murph the Surf, Sudden Death, The Women in Red, Wrong Is Right.

CONRAD, WILLIAM: Actor, Producer, Director. b. Louisville, Ky., Sept. 27, 1920. e. Fullerton College. Announcer-writer-director for L.A. radio station KMPC before becoming WW II fighter pilot in 1943; returned to radio drama as original Matt Dillon of Gunsmoke Series; m.p. debut in The Killers, 1946; later acting credits include 30, Body and Soul, Sorry, Wrong Number, East Side, West Side, The Naked Jungle; TV credits include This Man Dawson, Klondike (produced and directed), 77 Sunset Strip (producer), True (directed 35 episodes); as m.p. producer for Warner Bros. credits include: Two On a Guillotine, Brainstorm, An American Dream, A Covenant With Death, First To Fight, The Cool Ones, The Assignment.
RECENT TV: Acting credits include The Brotherhood of the Bell, The D.A., Conspiracy to Kill, O'Hara, U.S. Treasury, Cannon (series).

CONROY, THOMAS: Exec. r.n. Coleman Thomas Conroy. b. Camden, N.J., Nov. 3, 1924; e. Yale U., hd. prof. camera dept., Bell and Howell Inc., New York, 1951; hd. camera dept., Cinerama Inc., 1952–55; National Theatres Inc., 1955; hd. camera dept., Cinemiracle; v.p. prod., prod. supv., Cinerama, Inc. 1960. Developed Cinerama single-lens system; v.p., production, Shannon Prod., Inc., 1967.
PICTURES INCLUDE: This Is Cinerama, Cinerama Holiday, Seven Wonders of the World, Windjammer, The Wonderful World of The Brothers Grimm, How the West Was Won, The Best of Cinerama, The Golden Head.

CONTE, JOHN: Actor, singer. b. Palmer, Mass.; e. Lincoln h.s., Los Angeles. Actor, Pasadena Playhouse; radio anncr., m.c.; Armed Forces World War II.
THEATRE: On Broadway in Windy City, Allegro, Carousel, Arms and the Girl.
TV: John Conte's Little Show, Max Liebman Spectaculars and dramatic shows, host and star of NBC Matinee Theatre; (1955–58). TV Hour of Stars; Mantovani Welcomes You.
PICTURES INCLUDE: Debut in Man With the Golden Arm, The Carpetbaggers.
Pres. KMIR-TV, Channel 36, Desert Empire Television Corp., Palm Springs.

CONTI, BILL: Composer. b. Providence, Rhode Island, 1943. Studied piano at age 7, forming first band at age 15. e. Juilliard School of Music. Toured Italy with jazz trio where scored first film, Candidate for a Killing. Returned to U.S. to be music supvr. on Blume in Love. for Paul Mazursky.
PICTURES: Harry and Tonto, Rocky, Handle with Care, F.I.S.T., Slow Dancing in the Big City, The Big Fix, Uncle Joe Shannon, An Unmarried Woman, Hurricane, Paradise Alley, Rocky II, Golden Girl, A Man, A Woman, and A Bank, Gloria, Private Benjamin, For Your Eyes Only, Carbon Copy, Split Image, Bad Boys, The Right Stuff, Unfaithfully Yours, The Bear, Mass Appeal, Gotcha, Nomad, Big Trouble, Beer, F/X.
TELEVISION: Kill Me If You Can, Stark, etc.

CONTI, TOM: Actor. b. Paisley, Scotland, Nov. 22, 1941. Trained at Royal Scottish Academy of Music, Glasgow. Did repertory work in Scotland before going to London, appearing with Paul Scofield on stage in Savages (1973). Film debut in Galileo (1975). On Bdwy. stage in Whose Life Is It Anyway? (1980).
PICTURES: The Duellists, The Haunting of Julia (Full Circle), Merry Christmas, Mr. Lawrence, Reuben, Reuben, American Dreamer, Miracles, Saving Grace.
TELEVISION: The Glittering Prizes, The Wall, etc.

CONVERSE, FRANK: Actor. b. St. Louis, Mo., May 22, 1938. e. Carnegie Tech. Early training on stage in New York.

Active in repertory theatres. Two seasons with Amer. Shakespeare Fest.
PICTURES INCLUDE: Hurry Sundown, Hour of the Gun.
TV: Mod Squad, Medical Center, The Bold Ones, N.Y.P.D. (series) Coronet Blue (series), The Guest Room, Movin' On, The Widowing of Mrs. Holyrod. Movies: The Rowdyman, Shadow of a Gunman, Tattered Web, Dr. Cook's Garden.
STAGE: The Seagull, Death of a Salesman, Night of the Iguana, A Man for All Seasons, The House of Blue Leaves, First One Asleep Whistle, Arturo Ui.

CONVY, BERT: Actor. b. St. Louis, July 23, 1934. e. UCLA. Was professional baseball player before turning to acting. On Broadway in The Matchmaker, Billy Barnes Revue, Nine, etc.
PICTURES: Gunman's Walk, Susan Slade, Act One, Semi-Tough, Jennifer, Hero at Large, The Cannonball Run.
TELEVISION: Dallas Cowboys Cheerleaders, Ebony, Ivory and Jade, Man in the Santa Claus Suit. Host on game show, Tattletales, Love Thy Neighbor.

CONWAY, GARY: Actor. b. Boston, 1938. r.n. Gareth Carmody, e. UCLA. As college senior was chosen for title role in Teen-Age Frankenstein. After graduating served in military at Ford Ord, CA. In 1960 began contract with Warner Bros., doing bits for films and TV. Has also appeared on stage.
PICTURES INCLUDE: The Guns of Texas, Once is not Enough, The Farmer (also prod.).
TV: Burke's Law.

CONWAY, KEVIN: Actor. Gained rerputation on N.Y. stage, winning Obie for performance in When You Comin Back, Red Ryder? Also on and off Broadway in such plays as One Flew Over the Cuckoo's Nest, Of Mice and Men, Moonchildren, The Plough and the Stars, etc.
PICTURES INCLUDE: Slaughterhouse Five, Shamus, Portnoy's Complaint, F.I.S.T., Flashpoint.
TV: Johnny We Hardly Knew You, The Deadliest Season.

CONWAY, TIM: Actor. b. Dec. 15, 1933, Willoughby, Ohio. e. Bowling Green State Univ. After 2 yrs. Army service joined KWY-TV in Cleveland as writer-director and occasional performer. Comedienne Rose Marie discovered him and arranged audition for the Steve Allen Show on which he became regular. In 1962 signed for McHale's Navy, series. Also has done night club appearances.
PICTURES INCLUDE: McHale's Navy, The World's Greatest Athlete, The Apple Dumpling Gang, Gus, The Shaggy D.A., Cannonball Run II, The Longshot (also s.p.).
TV: The Steve Allen Show, The Gary Moore Show, McHale's Navy, guest appearances on Hollywood Palace and shows starring Carol Burnett, Red Skelton, Danny Kaye, Dean Martin, Cher, Doris Day, etc.

CONWAY, SHIRL: Actress. r.n., Shirl Conway Larson; b. Franklinville, New York, June 13, 1916; e. U. of Michigan, 1934–38. Singer, comedian, nightclubs.
PLAYS: Gentlemen Prefer Blondes, Plain and Fancy.
TV: The Doctors and The Nurses.

COOK, ELISHA, JR.: Actor. b. San Francisco, December 26, 1907; e. St. Albans, Chicago boarding school. Joined Frank Bacon in "Lightnin'," at the age of 14.
THEATRE: Appeared with Ethel Barrymore in "Kingdom of God," in "Henry, Behave," "Many a Slip," "Three Cornered Moon," in London in "Coquette." Played in vaudeville and summer stock companies. Appeared in "Chrysalis," then "Ah, Wilderness," Theatre Guild success. Signed by Par. in 1936: Two in a Crowd, U; Pigskin Parade, etc.
PICTURES INCLUDE: Up in Arms, Cassanova Brown, Cinderella Jones, Dillinger, The Big Sleep, The Long Night, Don't Bother to Knock, I the Jury, Shane, Thunder Over the Plains, Drum Beat, Outlaw's Daughter, Timberjack, Indian Fighter, The Killing, Voodoo Island, Rosemary's Baby, Welcome to Hard Times, Blacula, The Great Northfield, Minnesota Raid, Emperor of the North, Electra-Glide in Blue, The Outfit, The Black Bird, The Champ, Parny, Hammett.

COOK, FIELDER: Prod., dir. b. Atlanta, Ga., Mar. 9, 1923. e. Washington & Lee U., BA, 1947; U. of Birmingham, Eng., post grad., 1948. Doctor of Fine Arts (Hon) (1973) (W & L). USNR, 1944; 7th Amphibious Force, 1944–45, J. Walter Thompson Co., 1947–56.
TV FILMS/SPECIALS: Family Reunion (4 hrs.); Gauguin, The Savage (3 hrs.); John Updyke's Too Far To Go; Maya Angelou's I Know Why The Caged Bird Sings; My Luke And I—The Lou Gehrig Love Story; Judge Horton & The Scottsboro Boys; Beacon Hill (tape, 2 hr. pilot); Miles To Go Before I Sleep: This Is The West That Was; Miracle On 34th Street; The Homecoming (pilot, The Waltons); The Hands of Carmac Joyce; Sam Hill; Beauty And The Beast; Teacher, Teacher; The Rivalry; Valley Forge; The Price; Harvey; Goodbye, Raggedy-Ann (also exec.-prod.) Brigadoon (also prod.); Will There Ever Be a Morning?; Why Me?, Evergreen.
PICTURES INCLUDE: Patterns, Home Is the Hero, A Big Hand for the Little Lady, How to Save a Marriage and Ruin Your Life, Prudence and the Pill, Eagle In a Cage, From the Mixed Up Files of Mrs. Basil E. Frankweiler, Seize the Day, Too Far To Go.
PLAYS: A Cook For Mr. General, Maneuvers.
AWARDS: Various for (after 1956): Patterns, Project Immortality; Big Deal in Laredo; Teacher, Teacher; Ben Casey Pilot; The Price; Brigadoon; Judge Horton And The Scottsboro Boys; The Homecoming.

COOK, KWENAM DAVID: Exec. b. Seoul, Korea, Mar. 16, 1922. e. Waseda U., Tokyo, Japan. ROK national assemblyman (Congress) 1959–61. Pres. Korean Gymnastic Assoc. 1967–70. Chairman: Century Co., Ltd., Seoul, producers, distributors, exhibitors, and importers of films. Honorary consul general for Peru.

COOK, RICHARD: Executive. Began career 1971 as Disneyland sls. rep.; promoted 1974 to mgr. of sls. Moved to studio in 1977 as mgr., pay TV and non-theatrical releases. 1980, named asst. domestic sls. mgr., for Buena Vista; 1981 promoted to v.p. & asst. gen. sls. mgr.; 1984, promoted to v.p. & gen. sls. mgr., B.V.; 1985, appt. sr. v.p., domestic distribution.

COOKE, ALISTAIR: Journalist and Broadcaster. b. Eng., Nov. 20, 1908; e. Jesus Coll., Cambridge; Yale; Harvard. Film crit. of BBC 1934–37. London corr. NBC 1936–37. BBC commentator in U.S. since 1937. Chief Amer. corr., Manchester Guardian, 1948–72; English narrator, The March of Time, 1938–39; v.o. narrator, Sorrowful Jones, 1948; narrator, Three Faces of Eve, 1957; narrator, Hitler, 1973; Peabody award winner for International reporting, 1952, 1973–83; author, Douglas Fairbanks, Garbo & The Night Watchmen. A Generation on Trial, One Man's America, Christmas Eve, The Vintage Mencken, etc.; m.c. Omnibus, TV show, 1952–61; m.c. prod. U.N.'s International Zone, Emmy Award, 1958; m.c., Masterpiece Theatre since 1971. Writer & narrator, America: A Personal History of The United States, TV series BBC, NBC, PBS, for which 5 Emmy Awards, 1973; Franklin Medal, Royal Society of Arts, 1973; Knighted, KBE, 1973; America (book) 1973; Six Men, 1977; Talk About America, 1968; The Americans, 1979; Above London, 1980; Masterpieces, 1981; The Patient Has the Floor, 1986.

COOLIDGE, MARTHA: Director-Writer-Producer. b. New Haven, CT, 1946. e. Rhode Island School of Design. M. producer Michael Backes. Started directing short films while in school. Has produced, directed and written several documentaries which have won festival awards, including David: Off and On (American Film Festival), Old Fashioned Woman (CINE Golden Eagle Award).
PICTURES: Valley Girl, Joy of Sex, The City Girl.

COOPER, BEN: Actor. b. Hartford, Conn., Sept. 30. e. Columbia U. On stage in Life with Father, Theatre; numerous radio, TV appearances.
PICTURES INCLUDE: Woman They Almost Lynched, A Perilous Journey, Sea of Lost Ships, Flight Nurse, Fortune Hunter, Johnny Guitar, Hell's Outpost, Eternal Sea, Last Command, Fighting Chance, Headline Hunters, Rose Tattoo, Rebel in Town, Chartroose Caboose, Red Tomahawk, The Fastest Gun Alive, One More Train to Rob, Support Your Local Gunfighter.

COOPER, HAL: Director and Performer. b. Feb. 22, 1923; N.Y.C.; e. U. of Mich.; m. Marta Salcido; child actor in various radio prog. since 1932; featured Bob Emery's Rainbow House, Mutual, 1936–46; asst. dir. Dock St. Theatre, Charleston, S.C., 1946–48.
TV: Your Sch. Reporter, TV Baby Sitter, The Magic Cottage as writer and producer; dir., Valiant Lady, Search for Tomorrow, Portia Faces Life, CBS-TV; dir., assoc. prod. Kitty Foyle, NBC-TV; prod. dir. Indictment, Para. TV; assoc. prod. dir. The Happy Time, Para. TV; prod. dir. For Better or Worse, CBS-TV; dir., The Clear Horizon, CBS-TV; Assoc., prod., dir., Surprise Package, CBS-TV; dir., Dick Van Dyke Show; prod., dir., The Art Linkletter Show, The Object Is. Dir.: Death Valley Days, I Dream of Jeannie, That Girl, I Spy, Hazel, Gidget, Gilligan's Island, NYPD, Mayberry, Courtship of Eddie's Father, My World and Welcome to It, The Odd Couple, Mary Tyler Moore, All in the Family. Exec. prod., dir. Maude, 1972–78; Phyl and Mikky, 1980; Love, Sidney, 1982–83; Gimme a Break, 1983–85.

COOPER, JACKIE: Actor-Director-Producer. b. Los Angeles, Sept. 15, 1922. Began theatrical career at age of 3 as m.p. actor; was member of Our Gang comedies. First starring role in 1930 in Skippy. Worked at every major studio, always with star billing. At 20 enlisted in Navy. After three-yr. tour of duty went to N.Y. to work in live TV. Appeared on Broadway stage in Mr. Roberts and on natl. tour and in London. Directed as well as acted in live and filmed TV. Served as v.p. in chg. of TV prod., for Screen Gems, from 1964 to 1969, when resigned to return to acting, directing, producing.

PICTURES INCLUDE: Actor—Movietone Follies, Sunny Side Up, Skippy, Sooky, The Champ, When a Fellow Needs a Friend, Lumpy, Lost, The Bowery, Treasure Island, O'Shaughnessy's Boy, The Devil Is a Sissy, Gangster's Boy, Seventeen, Gallant Sons, Her First Beau, Syncopation, Stork Bites Man, Kilroy Was Here, Everything's Ducky, The Love Machine, Chosen Survivors, Superman, Superman II. Director: Stand Up And Be Counted.
TELEVISION: People's Choice (directed 71 segments; also starred), Hennesy (dir. 91 segments; also starred) 1975 series: Mobile Two (star). Movies: The Night They Saved Christmas (dir.), Izzy and Moe (dir.).

COOPERMAN, ALVIN: Producer. b. Brooklyn, N.Y. Started career with Lee & J. J. Shubert, 1939–51; color team, dev. color TV for FCC approval, 1953; prod. first color TV shows with mobile unit, 1954; developed & prod. first Wide Wide World, June 1955; mgr. program sls., NBC Network, 1955; exec. prod. Producers Showcase, Dodsworth, Rosalinda, 1956; prod. Jack and the Beanstalk, Festival of Music, 1957; dir. prog. NBC-TV, Apr. 1957; joined HJ Enterprises as prod. NBC-TV, The Shirley Temple Storybook, 1957; exec. prod. Screen Gems, 1958; prod. Du Pont Show, 1959; exec. prod. Roncom Prod. 1960; Prod., Untouchables, 1961–63; exec. dir., Shubert Thea. Ent. 1963; v.p., special programs, NBC, 1967–68; exec. v.p., Madison Square Garden Center, 1968–72; President Madison Square Garden Center, Inc.; Chairman of the Board Athena Communications Corporation.
TELEVISION: Producer: Romeo and Juliet, 1976 (Emmy Nominee); Pele's Last Game, 1977; The Fourth King, 1977; Amahl and the Night Visitors, 1978; Live from Studio 8H—A Tribute to Toscanini, 1980 (Emmy Award); Live from Studio 8H—An Evening with Jerome Robbins and The New York City Ballet, 1980 (Emmy Award); Live from Studio 8H—Caruso Remembered, 1982; "Ain't Misbehavin'", 1982 (Emmy Nominee, NAACP Image Award, Best TV Show of the Year); Pope John Paul II, 1984; My Two Loves, 1986.

COOTE, BERNARD: Producer, exec., ent. m.p. industry 1945. Denham Studios; 1951, joined Group 3, Ltd.; 1953, studio manager, Beaconsfield Studios; 1955, gen. man.; 1957, dir. prod. Ivanhoe TV series; 1958, prod. Violent Moment, dir. Shepperton TV Productions, Ltd.; Assoc. prod. TV series, The Third Man, Samson of the Circus, Voyage of Discovery; 1960–63, mgr. Shell Intntl. documentary film unit; 1963–65, dir. documentary films in Africa; 1965–67, freelance feature prod., Europe and Middle East; 1967–present, U.K. prod. supervisor, United Artists.

COPPOLA, FRANCIS FORD: Writer-Producer-Director. b. Detroit, April 7, 1939. e. Hofstra Univ. (BA 1958); UCLA (1958–68, masters cinema).
PICTURES INCLUDE: Director: Dementia 13, You're a Big Boy Now, Finian's Rainbow, The Rain People. Writer: Patton, This Property is Condemned, Reflections in a Golden Eye, The Rain People, Is Paris Burning?, The Great Gatsby. Writer-Producer-Director: The Conversation, The Godfather, The Godfather, Part II; Apocalypse, Now, The Outsiders. Producer: American Graffiti, THX 1138. Executive Producer: The Black Stallion, Hammett, The Escape Artist, The Black Stallion Returns, Mishima. Director-co-writer: One from the Heart, Rumble Fish, The Cotton Club.
TV: The People (movie of the week).

CORD, ALEX: Actor. b. Floral Park, L.I., Aug. 3, 1931. r.n.-Alexander Viespi. Early career in rodeo; left to become actor. Studied at Shakespeare Academy (Stratford, Conn.) and Actor's Studio (N.Y.). Spent two yrs. in summer stock; in 1961 went on tour with Stratford Shakespeare Co. Made m.p. debut in Synanon, 1965.
PICTURES INCLUDE: Stagecoach, The Scorpio Letters, The Prodigal Gun, The Brotherhood, Stiletto, The Dead Are Alive, Chosen Survivors, Sidewinder One, Grayeagle.
TELEVISION: Guest in many series; Genesis II (tf).

CORDAY, BARBARA: Executive. b. New York City, Oct. 15, 1944. m. Barney Rosenzweig, TV producer. Began career as publicist in N.Y. and L.A. Turned to writing for TV; named v.p., ABC-TV, in chg. of comedy series development. 1982–84, headed own production co. in association with Columbia Pictures TV. June, 1984 named pres., Columbia Pictures TV. Member: Caucus of Writers, Producers & Directors; Hollywood Womens Coalition.
TELEVISION: Writer: American Dream (pilot), Cagney and Lacey (series), etc.

COREY, JEFF: Actor. b. New York City, Aug. 10, 1914; e. Feogin Sch. of Dram. Art. On stage in Leslie Howard prod. of Hamlet, 1936; Life and Death of an American, 1938. Screen debut 1940 in All That Money Can Buy, In The Matter of J. Robert Oppenheimer and Hamlet-Mark Taper Forum, L.A. King Lear, Beverly Music Center '73.
PICTURES INCLUDE: Syncopation, The Killers, Ramrod, Joan of Arc, Roughshod, Black Shadows, Bagdad, Outriders, The Devil and Daniel Webster, My Friend Flicka, Canyon City, Singing Guns, Seconds, In Cold Blood, Golden Bullet, Boston Strangler, True Grit, Butch Cassidy and The Sundance Kid, Beneath the Planet of the Apes, Getting Straight, Little Big Man, They Call Me Mister Tibbs, Clear and Present Danger, High Flying Lowe, Catlow, Something Evil, Premonition, Shine, Rooster, Oh, God!, Butch and Sundance: The Early Days, Up River, Conan the Destroyer.
TV: The Untouchables, The Beachcomber, The Balcony, Yellow Canary, Lady in A Cage, Outer Limits, Channing, The Doctors and The Nurses, Perry Mason, Gomer Pyle, Wild, Wild West, Run for Your Life, Bonanza, Iron Horse, Judd for Defense, Garrisons Gorillas, Gunsmoke, Hawaii Five O, Star Trek, dir. The Psychiatrist, Night Gallery, Alias Smith and Jones, Sixth Sense, Hawkins, Owen Marshall, Police Story, Bob Newhart Show, Six Million Dollar Man, Doctors Hospital, Starsky and Hutch, Land of the Free (film), Kojak, McCloud, Captains Courageous (Bell Tel. Hr.), Bionic Woman, Barney Miller, One Day At a Time, The Pirate, Lou Grant, The Powers of Jonathan Starr, Cry for the Strangers, Today's FBI, Knots Landing, Archie Bunker's Place, Faerie Tale Theatre, Night Court, Helltown (series), Morning Star/Evening Star (series), New Love American Style.

CORMAN, GENE: Producer. b. Detroit, Mich., Sept. 24, 1927. e. Stanford Univ. Went to work for MCA as agent; left to produce his first feature film, Hot Car Girl. Partner with brother Roger in Corman Company and New World Distributors.
PICTURES INCLUDE: Attack of the Giant Leaches, Not of This Earth, Blood and Steel, Valley of the Redwoods, Purple Reef, Beast from Haunted Cave, Cat Burglar, Tobruk, You Can't Win 'Em All, The Intruder, Von Richthofen and Brown, I Escaped from Devil's Island, Secret Invasion, Vigilante Force, F.I.S.T. (exec. prod.), The Big Red One.

CORMAN, ROGER WILLIAM: Executive-Director, Producer, Writer, Distributor. b. Detroit, Michigan, April 5, 1926. e. Stanford U. 1947; Oxford U., England 1950; U.S. Navy 1944; 20th Century-Fox, production department, 1948, story analyst 1948–49; Literary agent, 1951–52; story, s.p., assoc. prod. Highway Dragnet. Formed Roger Corman Prod. and Filmgroup. Produced over 200 feature films and directed over 60 of them. Formed production-releasing company, organization, New World Pictures, Inc., 1970. Formed production co., New Horizons, 1984; distribution co., Concorde, 1985.
PICTURES INCLUDE: Five Guns West, 1953, House of Usher, Little Shop of Horrors, 1961; Pit and the Pendulum, The Intruder, Masque of the Red Death, Tomb of Ligeia, The Secret Invasion, The Wild Angels, The Trip, Bloody Mama, Von Richtofen and Brown, Gasss, St. Valentine's Day Massacre, Box Car Bertha, Big Bad Mama, Death Race 2000, Eat My Dust, Capone, Jackson County Jail, Fighting Mad, Thunder & Lightning, Grand Theft Auto, I Never Promised You A Rosegarden, Deathsport, Avalanche, Battle Beyond the Stars, St. Jack, Love Letters.

CORNFIELD, HUBERT: Director-Writer-Producer. b. Istanbul, Turkey. e. University of Pennsylvania. Actors' Studio, 1952–54. Story analyst Allied Artists 1954. Directed first picture 1955. Lives in Paris since 1964.
PICTURES INCLUDE: Sudden Danger, Lure of the Swamp, Plunder Road, The Third Voice, Pressure Point, The Night of the Following Day.

CORRADINE, TOM J.: Producer, distributor. b. Chicago, Ill., Nov. 14, 1924. e. parochial schools; theatre mgr., booker, 1944; ent. TV ind. as film dir., CBS, west coast, 1949; formed Associate Co., 1952; assoc. prod., TV, Wild Bill Hickock, Judge Roy Bean, Rendezvous with Adventure; formed Artists Productions, Inc., 1963. Dir. west coast operations Republic Film Corp., 1965. Reactivated co. of artists to prod. TV commercials and specials, 1968. V.P. charge of production and V.P. national sales, TVNATIONAL Releasing Corp., 1977; 1978, formed Videobrary Inc. to produce and distribute pre-recorded video tapes for the home consumer.
PICTURES INCLUDE: The Big Tipoff, Night Freight, Port of Hell, Highway Dragnet, Kroma.

CORRI, ADRIENNE: Actress. b. Glasgow, Scotland, Nov. 13, 1933. Ent. Royal Acad. of Dramatic Art at 13; parts in several stageplays including The Human Touch; m.p. debut in The River.
PICTURES INCLUDE: Quo Vadis, The Kidnappers, A Clockwork Orange, Lease of Life, Make Me An Offer, Feminine Touch, The Big Chance, Corridors of Blood, Doctor of Seven Dials, The Rough and the Smooth, Hellfire Club, The Tell-Tale Heart, Dynamite Jack, Doctor Zhivago, Epilogue to Capricorn, Rosebud. Numerous TV appearances.

CORT, BUD: Actor. New Rochelle, NY, March 29, 1950. e. NY Univ. School of the Arts. Stage debut in Wise Child,

Bdwy. Theatrical film debut in MASH, 1970. Television debut in The Doctors.
PICTURES: Brewster McCloud, Harold and Maude, Why Shoot the Teacher?, The Secret Diary of Sigmund Freud, Invaders from Mars, etc.
TELEVISION: Brave New World, Bernice Bobs Her Hair, Faerie Tale Theatre, etc.

CORT, ROBERT W.: Executive. e. Univ. of Pennsylvania (Phi Beta Kappa). Moved into feature production after having worked primarily in marketing/advertising. Joined Columbia Pictures as v.p., 1976; elevated to v.p., adv./pub./promo. Named exec. v.p. of mktg. for 20th-Fox, 1980. Moved into feature production as senior v.p., 1981. In 1983 named exec. v.p., prod., 20th-Fox Prods. 1984, joined Interscope Communications as pres., entertainment division.

CORTESA, VALENTINA: Actress. b. Milan, Italy, Jan. 1, 1925. Started career at 15 in Rome. Screen debut: La Cens Delle Beffe, 1941; brought to Hollywood by 20th Century-Fox, following picture, A Yank in Rome; experience on dramatic stage in variety of roles inc. Shakespeare, O'Neill, Shaw.
PICTURES INCLUDE: Cagliostro, Glass Mountain, House on Telegraph Hill, Thieves' Highway, Les Miserables, Secret People, Barefoot Contessa, Shadow of the Eagle, Magic Fire, The Legend of Lylah Clare, Juliet of the Spirits, Day for Night, When Time Ran Out.

CORTEZ, STANLEY: Dir. Photography. b. New York City, br. Ricardo Cortez, actor; e. N.Y.U. Began working with portrait photographers (Steichen, Pirie MacDonald, Bachrach, etc.), N.Y. Entered film industry with Paramount Pictures; to Hollywood as camera asst. and later second cameraman, various studios; pioneer in use of montage; Signal Corps World War II, Yalta, Quebec, etc. Received Film Critics of Amer. award for work on Magnificent Ambersons. Under personal contract to David O. Selznick, Orson Welles, Walter Wanger, David Wolper. Contributor Encyclopedia Britannica.
PICTURES INCLUDE: Man on the Eiffel Tower, Shark River, (A.A. nominee) Since You Went Away, (A.A. nominee), Bad Lands of Dakota, Magnificent Ambersons, Eagle Squadron, Powers Girl, Since You Went Away, Smash Up, Flesh and Fantasy, Captain Kidd, Secret Beyond the Door, Fort Defiance, Riders to the Stars, Black Tuesday, Night of the Hunter, Man from Del Rio, Three Faces of Eve, Top Secret Affair, Angry Red Planet, Dionosaurus, Back Street, Shock Corridor, Nightmare in the Sun, The Naked Kiss, Blue, The Bridge of Remagen, The Date, Another Man, Another Chance. Special sequences on Damien, Omen II, Day the World Ended, Le Bon Vivant.

CORWIN, BRUCE CONRAD: Exhibitor. b. June 11, 1940, Los Angeles, Calif.; e. Wesleyan U.; Pres., Metropolitan Theatres Corp.; chmn., Will Rogers Hospital area ind. campaigns; pres., Variety Boys Club; Board of Trustees American Film Institute; Board of Trustees U.C.L.A. Foundation; pres., Variety Club Tent 25; Mbr., L.A. Children's Museum.

CORWIN, NORMAN: Writer, producer, director. b. Boston, Mass., May 3, 1910. Sports ed. Greenfield, Mass. Daily Recorder, 1926–29; radio ed., news commentator, Springfield Republican & Daily News, 1929–36; prog. dir., CBS, 1938. Bok Medal "for distinguished services to radio," 1942; Peabody Medal, 1942; awarded grant by Amer. Acad. of Arts & Letters, 1942; Page One Award, 1944; Distinguished Merit Award, Nat'l Conf. of Christians & Jews, 1945; Unity Award, Interracial Film & Radio Guild, 1945; Wendell Willkie One World Flight Award, 1946; Met. Opera Award for modern opera in collab. Bernard Rogers, 1946; first award, Res. Comm. of U.N., 1950; Radio & TV first award, Nat'l Conf. of Christians & Jews, 1951; Honor Medal of Freedom Foundation for TV show, Between Americans, 1951; ent., Radio Hall of Fame, 1962. Hon. doctorate Columbia Col. of Comms., 1967; Valentine Davies Award, WGA, 1972; P.E.N. Award, 1986; author of Thirteen by Corwin, More by Corwin, Untitled & Other Plays; The Plot to Overthrow Christmas, Dog in the Sky, Overkill and Megalove, Prayer for the 70s. Holes in a Stained Glass Window, Trivializing America; lectured at various colleges; taught courses U.C.L.A., U.S.C., San Diego State U., regents lecturer, UC at Santa Barbara; Chairman, Creative Writing, USC-Isomata; U. of Alberta, U. of So. Col., Witswatersrand U., Rand Afrikaans U., So. Africa, Cantatas, The Golden Door, 55; Yes Speak Out Yes (commissioned by UN, 1968). Faculty, USC School of Journalism, 1980–. Industry Achievement Award, Broadcast Promotion Assn. 1984; Stasheff lecturer, Univ. Michigan, 1984; sect'y., M.P. Academy Foundation, 1985.
STAGE PLAYS: The Rivalry, The World of Carl Sandburg, The Hyphen, Overkill and Megalove, Cervantes. Together Tonight: Jefferson, Hamilton and Burr.
PICTURES INCLUDE: Once Upon a Time, Blue Veil, The Grand Design, Scandal in Scourie, Lust for Life, The Story of Ruth.
TV: Inside the Movie Kingdom, The FDR series, The Plot to Overthrow Christmas, Norman Corwin Presents (for Westinghouse), The Court Martial of General Yamashita, Network at 50 (CBS). Wrote and hosted Academy Leaders (PBS).
Chmn. Doc. Award Com., Motion Picture Academy 1965–86; elected to bd. of governors, 1980. Chm., writers' exec. comm., M.P. Academy; co-chmn. scholarship com., m.p. Academy; member, Film Advisory Bd.; L.A. County Museum; Norman Corwin Presents series; member, bd. of trustees, Advisory Board, Filmex, member, board of directors, WGA.

COSBY, BILL: Actor, comedian. b. Philadelphia, Pa., July 12, 1938. e. Temple U.; served in United States Navy Medical Corps. Started as night club entertainer. Has appeared many times on TV variety shows, in numerous one-nighters across the country, and concert tours.
TV: Emmy Award 1966, 1967, 1968: Best Actor in Dramatic Series—"I Spy," NBC-TV. Emmy Award, 1969; The First Bill Cosby Special, I Spy, The Bill Cosby Special, The Second Bill Cosby Special, The Bill Cosby Show, Fat Albert, Fat Albert and the Cosby Kids.
COMEDY ALBUMS: Bill Cosby Is A Very Funny Fellow . . . Right!; I Started Out As a Child; Why Is There Air?; Wonderfulness; Revenge; To Russell, My Brother, Whom I Slept With; 200 MPH; It's True, It's True; 8:15, 12:15.
SINGING ALBUMS: Silverthroat, Hooray for the Salvation Army Band. Grammy Award, 1964, 1965, 1966, 1967, 1969: Best Comedy Album.
RADIO: The Bill Cosby Radio Program.
PICTURES INCLUDE: Man and Boy, Uptown Saturday Night, Let's Do It Again, Mother, Jugs and Speed, A Piece of the Action, California Suite, The Devil and Max Devlin, Bill Cosby Himself.

COSLOW, SAM: Producer, song writer. b. New York City, Dec. 27, 1905. Writer popular songs, many for screen prod. (Cocktails for Two, Just One More Chance, Sing You Sinners, etc.). In 1941 formed RCM Prod., Inc., with James Roosevelt. Apptd. Paramount prod. 1944. Academy Award (with Jerry Bresler), best two-reel short, 1943 (Heavenly Music). In 1945 joined Mary Pickford Prods. as prod.
PICTURES INCLUDE: Out of This World, Copacabana, Dreaming Out Loud.

COSELL, HOWARD: Sports Commentator. b. Winston-Salem, N.C., 1920. Studied law and practiced. Broadcasting career began in 1953 when hired to host program on which N.Y. area Little Leaguers were introduced to baseball stars. In 1956 ABC hired him for ten five-minute sports shows on weekends. He dropped legal work to concentrate on sports reporting. Has had wide variety of roles in TV: commentator on ABC Monday Night Football, Monday Night Baseball, and various sports specials. Has hosted the Howard Cosell Sports Magazine for 4 yrs. and hosts 14 shows each week on American Contemporary Radio Network. Has guested on numerous prime-time TV shows.
PICTURES: Bananas, Sleeper, The World's Greatest Athlete.

COSMATOS, GEORGE P.: Director-Producer-Writer. b. Jan. 4, 1941. e. London Univ. Asst. dir., Exodus and Zorba the Greek.
PICTURES: Restless (co.-prod., s.p., dir.); Massacre in Rome (co-s.p., dir.); The Cassandra Crossing (co.-s.p., dir.); Escape to Athena (co-s.p., dir.); Rambo: First Blood Part II (dir.), Cobra (dir.).

COSTA-GAVRAS, HENRI: Director. b. Athens, Greece, 1933. e. Studied at the Sorbonne. Worked as second, then first assistant to Marcel Ophuls, Rene Calir, and Rene Clement, on Banana Peel, All the Gold in the World, The Thieves, 1964; dir. and wrote s.p. The Sleeping Car Murders. Second film Un Homme De Trop won prize at the Moscow Festival, 1966. Dir. and collab. s.p. Z (won Acad. Award, Best Foreign Lang. Film). L'Aveu (The Vow), State of Siege, Special Section, Missing (also co-s.p.); Hannah K. (also co.-s.p.).

COTES, PETER: F.R.S.A. Producer, dir., writer. Began early career as actor; stage debut Henry V, London 1926; debut as stage producer, 1942; founded Peter Cotes prods. 1946 and Peter Cotes Players 1948, prod., dir. numerous plays; prod. dir. for BBC: Same Sky, The Mask, Shadow of the Vine, Infinite Shoeblack, The Road, What the Public Wants; exec. prod., dir. Associated-Rediffusion, 1956; Sup. prod. TV series, London Playhouse. Dir. Woman in a Dressing Gown, Ashes in the Wind, Hungry God. Co. dir., Waterfront; dir., Young and the Guilty, The Right Person Publications; No, Star Nonsense, Little Fellow (Charles Chaplin), A Handbook for the Amateur Theatre, George Robey. Head prod. Channel 7, Melbourne, Australia 1961. dir. doc., Australian Snowy Mountains; setting, dir., plays London West End, Broadway, 1962–63; TV consultant, McCann-Erickson (London); prod., dir.
TV: The Offence, Winter in Ischia, Also stage prods. in London. Assoc. prod., The World of Wooster, TV series

for BBC, Prod. & Dir. West End Theatre, among others: Impossible Years, Staring At the Sun, Janie Jackson, (revival), Pick Up Girl, The Master Builder, Hot Summer Night, The Animal Kingdom, The Old Ladies; wrote TV Omnibus programs; gave R.S.A. theatre lectures. Devised-directed, Down With All Parties, Look, No Hands, My Brother, Willie, Lecturing, writing series of radio portraits; working on auto-biography. Publications: The Trial of Elvira Barney, Circus, The Man Called Mitch. 1978: Music Hall Tragedies, Charlie Chaplin Mervyn Peake (radio), The Diminutive One.; Pubs. 1982/83: Evelyn and John, Wilfred Lawson, The Barbirollis. Radio series The Old Stagers. Contributor to numerous periodicals.

COTTEN, JOSEPH: Actor. b. Petersburg, Va., 1905. In stock and on New York Stage, 1930–40, including Accent on Youth, Philadelphia Story; also Orson Welles' Federal Theatres productions and Mercury Theatre of the Air.
STAGE: Sabrina Fair, Once More With Feeling, Prescription: Murder, Calculated Risk.
TV: narrator, Hollywood and the Stars, own show.
PICTURES INCLUDE: Citizen Kane, Lydia, Magnificent Ambersons, Journey Into Fear, Shadow of a Doubt, Hers to Hold, Temptation, The Last Sunset, Two Flags West, September Affair, Walk Softly, Stranger, Half Angel, Peking Express, Man With a Cloak, The Untamed Frontier, The Steel Trap, Niagara, Blueprint for Murder, Special Delivery, Bottom of the Bottle, Killer Is Loose, Halliday Brand, From the Earth to the Moon, The Angel Wore Red, The Great Sioux Massacre, The Oscar, The Hellbenders, The Tramplers, The Money Trap, They Also Killed, The White Comanche, Petulia, The Grasshopper, The Abominable Dr. Phibes, Soylent Green, A Delicate Balance, Twilight's Last Gleaming, Airport '77, Caravans, Heaven's Gate.

COTY, HENRI ROLAND: Executive. b. Neuilly-sur-Seine, France, Feb. 13, 1922. e. Lycee Descartes, Tours, France. Baccalaureat, 1939–40, St. Jean DePassy, WWII Buchmaster Underground network; arrested 1942, deported to Dachau, Dora, Manthauson, Bergen-Belsen concentration camps; liberated, 1945. Sales mgr., Coty Perfume Co., 1946–55; found own company, s.a. Coty & Co., promotion, publicity, public relations, printing, now TV program prod.

COULOURIS, GEORGE: Actor. b. Manchester, England, Oct. 1, 1903. Stage debut, 1926, Outward Bound. Began screen career in 1933.
PICTURES INCLUDE: Citizen Kane, Watch on the Rhine, Hotel Berlin, Doctor in the House, King of Kings, Arabesque, Papillon, Murder on the Orient Express, It's Not the Size That Counts.

COURTENAY, TOM: Actor. b. Hull, England, Feb. 25, 1937 e. University Coll., London, Royal Academy of Dramatic Art, 1960–61; Old Vic. Ent. TV 1961 in Private Potter and The Lads; I Heard the Owl Call My Name (U.S.).
STAGE: Billy Liar, Andorra, Hamlet, She Stoops to Conquer, Otherwise Engaged (N.Y. debut).
PICTURES INCLUDE: Loneliness of the Long Distance Runner, Private Potter, Billy Liar, King and Country, Operation Crossbow, King Rat, Dr. Zhivago, Night of the Generals, The Day the Fish Came Out, A Dandy in Aspic, Otley, One Day in the Life of Ivan Denisovich, The Dresser, Happy New Year.

COURTLAND, JEROME: Actor-Producer-Director. Began career in 40s as actor, then turned to directing and producing.
PICTURES INCLUDE: Actor: Kiss and Tell, Man from Colorado, Battleground, The Barefoot Mailman, The Bamboo Prison, Tonka, Black Spurs. Director: Run, Cougar, Run, Diamond on Wheels. Producer: Escape to Witch Mountain, Ride a Wild Pony, Return from Witch Mountain.
TV: Actor: The Saga of Andy Burnett, Tonka. Director: Hog Wild (also co-prod.), Harness Fever.

COUSTEAU, JACQUES-YVES: Producer. b. France, 1910. Won Oscar for short, The Golden Fish, 1959.
PICTURES INCLUDE: The Silent World, World Without Sun, Voyage to the Edge of the World.
TELEVISION INCLUDES: Blind Prophets of Easter Island, Time Bomb at 50 Fathoms, The Nile, The Undersea World of Jacques Cousteau.

COWAN, THEODORE: Executive. b. Letchworth, Eng. e. Parmiters School. Entered m.p. ind., J. Arthur Rank Productions, pub. div., asst. dir. pub. & adv., 1960. Formed own pr. & publ. Co., 1962.

COWAN, WARREN J.: Publicist. b. New York, Mar. 13. e. Townsend Harris H.S., U.C.L.A., graduated 1941. Entered public relations, 1941, with Alan Gordon & Associates; three yrs. Air Force; joined Henry C. Rogers office in 1945; became partner, 1949, and changed name to Rogers & Cowan, Public Relations Advisor, Rogers & Cowan, Inc., 1960; pres., Rogers & Cowan, Inc., 1964–present. Active in various entertainment industry, civic and philanthropic organizations, including current post as national communications chm. for the United Way of America. On advisory board of the National Association of Film Commissioners; serves on the Second Decade Council of the American Film Institute.

COX, RONNY: Actor. b. Cloudcroft, NM, Aug. 23, 1938. e. Eastern New Mexico Univ.
PICTURES: The Happiness Cage, Delverance, Hugo the Hippo, Gray Lady Down, Harper Valley PTA, The Onion Field, Taps, Beverly Hills Cop, Vision Quest.
TELEVISION: Movies: Transplant, When Hell was in Session, Fugitive Family, Alcatraz—The Whole Shocking Story, The Jesse Owens Story, etc.

COYOTE, PETER: Actor. Studied with San Francisco Actors Workshop, Theatre includes The Minstrel Show (dir.), Olive Pits (also co-writer), The Red Snake, True West, etc.
PICTURES: Die Laughing, Tell Me a Riddle, The Pursuit of D.B. Cooper, Southern Comfort, E.T.: The Extra Terrestrial, Endangered Species, Timerider, Cross Creek, Stranger's Kiss, Slayground, Heartbreakers, Jagged Edge, Outrageous Fortune.
TELEVISION: Movies: The People Vs. Jean Harris, In the Child's Best Interest, Up and Coming, Golden Gate, Scorned and Swindled, Child's Cry, Time Flyer, etc.

CRAIG, MICHAEL: Actor. b. India, 1929. At 16 joined Merchant Navy. 1949 returned to England and made stage debut in repertory. M.P. debut as crowd artist 1950.
PICTURES INCLUDE: Malta Story, The Love Lottery, Passage Home, The Black Tent, Yield to the Night, Eye-Witness, House of Secrets, High Tide At Noon, Sea of Sand, Sapphire, Upstairs and Downstairs, The Angry Silence, Cone of Silence, Doctor In Love, The Mysterious Island, Payroll, No My Darling Daughter, A Pair of Briefs. Under contract Rank Organisation. A Life for Ruth, The Iron Maiden, Captive City, Summer Flight, Of a Thousand Delights, Life at the Top, Modesty Blaise, Star, a Town Called Hell, Ride a Wild Pony, The Irishman, Turkey Shoot, The Timeless Land.

CRAIN, JEANNE: Actress. b. Barstow, Calif., May 25, 1925. Model; crowned Miss Long Beach of 1941: Camera Girl of 1942.
PICTURES INCLUDE: Home in Indiana, In the Meantime Darling, Winged Victory, State Fair, Leave Her to Heaven, Margie, Centennial Summer, You Were Meant for Me, Apartment for Peggy, Letter to Three Wives, Pinky, Cheaper by the Dozen, Take Care of My Little Girl, People Will Talk, Model and the Marriage Broker, Belles on Their Toes, O. Henry's Full House, City of Bad Men, Dangerous Crossing, Vicki, Duel in the Jungle, Man Without a Star, Second Greatest Sex, Gentlemen Marry Brunettes, Fastest Gun Alive, Tattered Dress, The Joker, Guns of the Timberland, Skyjacked.

CRAMER, WM. DOUGLAS: Executive. b. Aug. 22, 1931. e. Northwestern U., Sorbonne, Cincinnati U., B.A.; Columbia U.M.F.A., M. Joyce Haber, columnist. Taught at Carnegie Inst. of Tech., 1954–55; Production asst. Radio City Music Hall 1950–51; MGM Script Dept. 1952; Manag. Dir. Cincinnati Summer Playhouse 1953–54. TV supvr. Procter and Gamble 1956–59; Broadcast supvr. Ogilvy, Benson and Mather, Adv. 1959–62; V-P Program Dev. ABC-TV 1962–66; V-P Program Dev. 20 Cent.-Fox TV 1966; Exec. v.p. in chg. of production, Paramount Television, 1968.
PLAYS: Love is a Smoke, Whose Baby Are You, Call of Duty.

CRAWFORD, MICHAEL: Actor. b. Salisbury, England, 1942. Early career as boy actor in children's films and sound radio.
TV: Still Life, Destiny, Byron, Move After Checkmate, Three Barrelled Shotgun, Home Sweet Honeycomb, Some Mothers Do 'ave 'em, Chalk and Cheese, BBC Play for Today, Private View.
PICTURES INCLUDE: Two Left Feet, The War Lover, Two Living, One Dead, The Knack, A Funny Thing Happened On The Way To The Forum, The Jokers, How I Won the War, Hello, Dolly!, The Games, Hello and Goodbye, The Adventures of Alice in Wonderland, Condorman.
STAGE: Come Blow Your Horn, Traveling Light, The Anniversary, Black Comedy (N.Y.), No Sex Please We're British, Billy, Same Time Next Year, Flowers for Algernon, Barnum.

CRENNA, RICHARD: Actor. b. L.A., Calif., Nov. 30, 1927. e. Belmont H.S., U. of Southern Calif.
RADIO: Boy Scout Jamboree, A Date With Judy, The Great Gildersleeve, Johnny Dollar, Our Miss Brooks.
TV: Our Miss Brooks, The Real McCoys, Slattery's People, All's Fair. Movies: Passions, A Case of Deadly Force, Doubletake. Mini-Series: On Wings of Eagles.
PICTURES INCLUDE: Pride of St. Louis, It Grows on Trees, Red Skies Over Montana, John Goldfarb, Please Come Home, Pendick Enterprises, The Sand Pebbles, Star, Marooned, The Deserter, Doctor's Wives, Red Sky at Morning, A Man Called Noon, Catlow, Dirty Money, Death Ship, First Blood, Table for Five, The Flamingo Kid, Rambo: First Blood Part II, Summer Rental.

CRICHTON, CHARLES: Director. b. Wallasey, Aug. 6, 1910; e. Oundle & Oxford. Collab. dir. Dead of Night.
PICTURES INCLUDE: Painted Boats, Hue and Cry, Against the Wind, Another Shore, Dance Hall, Lavender Hill Mob, Hunted (Stranger in Between), Titfield Thunderbolt, The Love Lottery, Divided Heart, Man in the Sky, Floods of Fear, Battle of the Sexes, The Third Secret, He Who Rides a Tiger.
TV: The Wild Duck, Danger Man, The Avengers, Man in a Suitcase, The Strange Report, Shirley's World, Black Beauty, The Protectors, Space 1999, Return of the Saint, Dick Tuirpin 1 & 2 Series, Smuggler, Video Arts Shorts.

CRICHTON, MICHAEL: Writer-Director. Entered Harvard Medical School in 1965; while there completed first novel, Easy God, under pseudonym, John Lange. Has written 15 books under four different names, including A Case of Need (filmed as The Carey Treatment) and The Andromeda Strain (first book to appear under his own name). Did post-graduate work at Salk Institute in La Jolla. Also wrote novels Dealing and The Terminal Man, both filmed.
PICTURES INCLUDE: Westworld (s.p., dir.), Coma (s.p., dir.), The Great Train Robbery (s.p., dir.), Looker (s.p., dir.)., Runaway (s.p., dir.).
TELEVISION: Pursuit (Movie of Week), dir.; script by Robert Dozier based on Chrichton's book, Binary.

CRIST, JUDITH: Journalist-Critic. b. N.Y.C., May 22, 1922. e. Hunter College, Columbia Univ. (School of Journalism). Joined New York Herald Tribune, serving as reporter, arts editor, assoc. drama critic, film critic. Continued as film critic for New York World Journal Tribune, NBC-TV Today Show, New York, New York Post. Now regular film critic for TV Guide, WOR-TV, Coming Attractions. Teaches at Col. Grad. School of Journ.
AUTHOR: The Private Eye, The Cowboy and the Very Naked Girl; Judith Crist's TV Guide to the Movies; Take 22: Movie Makers on Movie Making.

CRISTALDI, FRANCO: Producer. b. Turin, Italy, Oct. 3, 1924. Owner, prod. Vides Cinematografica; President of Italian Producer's Union.
PICTURES INCLUDE: White Nights, The Strawman, The Challenge, Big Deal On Madonna Street, Kapo, The Dauphins, Salvatore Giuliano, The Assassin, Divorce Italian Style, The Organizer, Bebo's Girl, Seduced and Abandoned, Time of Indifference, Sandra, A Rose for Every-One, China Is Near, A Quiet Couple, The Red Tent.

CRITCHFIELD, EDWARD: Producer. B. Cleveland, Ohio, Jan. 9, 1919. e. Glenville H.S., 1937. Gen. insurance broker; real estate mortgage financing; motion picture financier, Delta Diamond Productions; then joined Bernfield Publications Inc., as vice-pres.; assoc. prod. Terrified.

CRON, JOHN B.: Executive. b. Mt. Vernon, New York, June 11, 1923. e. Princeton U.: Exec. vice-pres., Robert Lawrence Productions; managing dir., Screen Gems (Europe); sales dir., N.B.C. Film Division; vice-pres., sales dir. SIB Productions.

CRONENBERG, DAVID: Writer-Director. b. Toronto, May 15, 1943. e. Univ. of Toronto. In college produced two short movies on 16mm. 1971, to Europe on a Canadian Council grant where shot in 1975 his first commercial, Shivers.
PICTURES: Rabid, Fast Company (both dir. only), The Brood, Scanners, Videodrome, The Dead Zone.

CRONKITE, WALTER: Correspondent. b. St. Joseph, Mo., Nov. 4, 1916; e. Univ. of Texas. Reporter: radio reporter; U.P. Correspondent. Joined CBS as Washington news correspondent, 1950; anchorman and mng. editor, CBS Evening News, 1962–81; special correspondent, CBS News, 1981–present. Many TV shows including You Are There, Twentieth Century, Eyewitness to History: CBS Reports: 21st Century, Walter Cronkite's Universe. Past nat'l pres. & mem. bd. Trustees, Acad. TV Arts & Sciences. Managing Editor of CBS Evening News since 1963.

CRONYN, HUME: Actor, writer, director. b. London, Ontario, Canada, July 18, 1911; e. Ridley Coll.; U. of McGill; Amer. Acad. of Dramatic Art; m. Jessica Tandy, actress. m.p. acting debut in Shadow of a Doubt.
STAGE: (Actor N.Y. plays) High Tor, Escape This Night, Three Men on a Horse, Boy Meets Girl, Three Sisters, Mr. Big, The Survivors; dir. plays Now I Lay Me Down to Sleep, Hilda Crane, Madam Will You Walk. N.Y. stage, The Fourposter, 1951–53; Madam Will You Walk, 1953–54; The Honeys, A Day by the Sea, 1955; The Man in The Dog Suit, 1957; Directed The Egghead, 1957; Directed and toured with his wife, Miss Tandy, in Triple Play, 1958–59; Big Fish, Little Fish, 1961; also in London, 1962; The Miser, 1963; The Three Sisters, 1963; Hamlet, 1964; The Physicists, 1964; Produced Slow Dance on The Killing Ground, 1964; Appeared at the White House; Hear America Speaking 1965; Richard III, 1965; Revival The Miser, 1965; A Delicate Balance, 1966 and tour, 1967; The Miser, 1968; Hadrian VII tour, 1969–70; Caine Mutiny Court Martial, 1971; Promenade All 1972–73; Krapp's Last Tape, Happy Days, Act Without Words I, 1972; Coward In Two Keys, 1974, Concert recital Many Faces Of Love 1974; National tour, Noel Coward in Two Keys, 1975, Merchant of Venice and A Midsummer Night's Dream, at Stratford Festival Theatre, Canada 1976. 1976; Many Faces of Love limited tour 1975–76 and at Theatre London, Ontario, Canada '76 as well as for CBC, Canada, 1977; Appeared in The Gin Game, Long Wharf Thea., New Haven, Conn. June, 1977. Co-produced with Mike Nichols and also appeared in The Gin Game, The Golden Theatre, N.Y.C. 1977–78. Toured U.S., Toronto, London, U.S.S.R., 1978–79. Co-authored and acted in Foxfire at Stratford, Ont., 1980, and Minneapolis, 1981 and N.Y.C. 1982–83.
TV: The Marriage, and other network dramatic shows, 1957.
PICTURES INCLUDE: Cross of Lorraine, Lifeboat, Seventh Cross, Main Street, After Dark, The Sailor Takes a Wife, A Letter for Evie, The Green Years, Brute Force, Bride Goes Wild, Postman Always Rings Twice, Top O' the Morning, People Will Talk, Crowded Paradise, Sunrise at Campobello, Cleopatra, Gaily, Gaily, The Arrangement, There Was A Crooked Man, Conrack, Parallax View, Honky Tonk Freeway, Roll-over, Garp, Impulse, Brewester's Millions.

CROSBY, BOB: Band leader, actor; r.n. George Robert C.; b. Spokane, Wash., Aug. 23, 1913; e. Gonzaga U. Began as singer; later featured vocalist Jimmie & Tommy Dorsey band. Org. own band (Bobcats); appeared with orch. on screen in Let's Make Music, 1940.
PICTURES INCLUDE: Sis Hopkins, Reveille with Beverly, Thousands Cheer, Presenting Lily Mars, See Here Private Hargrove; Meet Miss Bobby Socks, Kansas City Kitty, My Gal Loves Music, Pardon My Rhythm, Singing Sheriff, Two Tickets to Broadway.
TV: Bob Crosby Show.

CROSBY, CATHY LEE: Actress. b. Los Angeles, Dec. 2. e. Univ. of So. California. Studied with Lee Strasberg. Theatrical film debut in The Laughing Policeman (1973).
PICTURES: Call Me by My Rightful Name, Trackdown, The Dark, Coach.
TELEVISION: Movies: Wonder Woman, Keefer, Kingston Confidential, Roughnecks, Intimate Strangers. Series: Marcus Welby, Shaft, Cannon, Emergency. Specials: Battle of the Network Stars, The American Sportsman, Circus of the Stars, etc. Mini-Series: World War III.

CROSBY, KATHRYN: Actress. r.n. Kathryn Grandstaff. b. Houston, Tex., Nov. 25, 1933. e.. University of Texas, U.C.L.A. m. Bing Crosby.
CREDITS: Forever Female, Rear Window, Living It Up, Arrrowhead, Cassanova's Big Night, Unchained, Cell 2455 Death Row, Tight Spot, Five Against the House, Reprisal, Guns of Fort Petticoat, Phoenix City Story, Wild Party, Mister Cory, Night the World Exploded, Brothers Rico, Operation Mad Ball, The Big Circus, Bob Hope Chrysler Theatre (TV), Bing Crosby Christmas Specials (TV), Suspense Theatre (TV), Ben Casey (TV), The Kathryn Crosby Show KPIX-TV-San Francisco.

CROSS, PERRY: Performer. b. Brooklyn, N.Y., Feb. 26. e. R.I. State Coll. At various clubs; to NBC, 1947. Guest relations staff, then TV production supervisor, coordinator, unit mgr.
TV: Ernie Kovacs Show, Henie Ice Spectacular, Ruggles of Red Gap, Tonight, Jack Paar Show, Today, TV network programs, night time.

CROUSE, LINDSAY: Actress. b. New York City. Daughter of playwright Russel Crouse. e. Radcliffe. Began career as modern and jazz dancer; is also flutist and pianist. Has worked in films, theatre and TV.
PICTURES INCLUDE: All the President's Men, Slap Shot, Between the Lines, The Verdict, Daniel, Iceman, Places in the Heart.
TV: Eleanor and Franklin, The Tenth Level.

CRUEA, EDMOND D.: Executive. b. Jersey City, N.J., June 3. Joined Grand National Pictures, Los Angeles, 1935; Monogram Pictures, 1938–41 (L.A. & Seattle); U.S. Army Signal Corp., 1942–46; Monogram Pictures, Seattle, 1946–48; branch mgr., 1948–49; branch mgr. Allied Artists, 1950–65 (Seattle, Portland, San Francisco); v.p., gen. sls. mgr., 1965–71; dir. distribution, Abkco Films div. of Abkco Industries, Inc., 1971–73; pres. of Royal Dist. Corp., 1974; pres., Esco Film Corp., 1975; joined Film Ventures Intl. in 1976 as exec. v.p., succeeding to pres. and chief operating officer in August, 1976. Resigned Sept. 1977 to form Fil-Mark Inc. Co-founded New Image Releasing, Inc., 1982, as pres. & CEO 1985, v.p. theatrical, Cinetel Films.

CRYER, JON: Actor. On Bdwy. stage in Brighton Beach Memoirs. Feature film debut: No Small Affair (1984).
PICTURES INCLUDE: Pretty in Pink.

CRUISE, TOM: Actor. b. Syracuse, NY, 1962. Acted in high school plays; secured role in dinner theatre version of Godspell. First film role in Endless Love (1981).
PICTURES: Taps, The Outsiders, Risky Business, All the Right Moves, Legend, Top Gun, The Color of Money.

CRYSTAL, BILLY: Actor. b. Long Island, NY, Mar. 14, 1947. Father, Jack, produced jazz concerts; family owned Commodore jazz record label. e. Marshall Univ., New York Univ. Worked with Alumni Theatre Group at Nassau Community College. Later teamed with two friends (billed as 3's Company) and toured coffee houses and colleges. Became stand-up comedian on own, appearing on TV.
PICTURES INCLUDE: Rabbit Test, Spinal Tap, Running Scared.
TELEVISION: Tonight Show, Dinah, Mike Douglas Show, That Was the Year That Was, All in the Family, Love Boat, Soap. Movies: Death Flight, Breaking Up Is Hard To Do.

CULBERG, PAUL S.: Executive. b. Chicago, June 14, 1942. Began career in record industry, holding positions with Elektra Records & Wherehouse Record; 1977–80; v.p. sls. mktg., Cream Records.; 1980–82, dir. sls. Paramount Home Video; 1982, v.p. sls. mktg., Media Home Entertainment; 1986, pres., New World Video.

CULLEN, BILL: Performer. b. Pittsburgh, Pa., Feb. 18, 1920; U. of Pittsburgh, B.A. Asst. disc jockey; announcer, KDKA, Pittsburgh; sportscaster; staff announcer. CBS radio, 1943; then m.c., panel member; shows include; m.c. Three on a Match, To Tell the Truth, Winning Streak, 25,000 Pyramid; Love Experts.

CULLEN, JAMES V.: Executive. b. San Francisco, Dec. 29, 1938; e. City College of S.F. Sales mgr., M.P.I. Toys, Los Angeles, 1963–65; entered film industry 1965 with 20th-Fox in S.F. exchange as ass't. field man; Named Southwest ad-pub. mgr. for Fox 1966 and Western Division ad-pub mgr. 1968. Appointed Fox director of exploitation 1971; then nat'l. dir. field adv. & pro.; Joined Sandy Howard Prods., v.p. creative affairs, 1974. Produced The Devils' Rain, 1975.

CULP, ROBERT: Actor, Writer, Director. b. Berkeley, Cal., Aug. 16, 1930. e. Stockton, College of the Pacfic, Washington U., San Francisco State; to N.Y. to study with Herbert Berghof; starred in off B'way prod. He Who Gets Slapped. Best Actor of the Year in an off B'way Play; motion picture debut, 1962; P.T. 109; television guest appearances in Rawhide, Wagon Train, Bob Hope Presents the Chrysler Theatre; wrote and acted in Rifleman, Cain's Hundred, The Dick Powell Show.
PLAYS: The Prescott Proposls, He Who Gets Slapped, A Clearing in the Woods.
TELEVISION: Trackdown, I Spy. Movies: The Calendar Girl Murders, Brothers-in-Law, The Blue Lightning, The Gladiator.
PICTURES INCLUDE: PT 109, Sammy, The Way Out Seal, The Raiders, Sunday in New York, Rhino, The Hanged Man, Bob & Carol & Ted & Alice, The Grove, Hannie Caulder, Hickey and Boggs, Sky Riders, Great Scout and Cathouse, Thursday, Turk 182.

CUMMINGS, BOB: Godson of Orville Wright. Actor, dir. b. Joplin, Mo., June 9, 1910; e. Drury Coll., Carnegie Inst. Tech.; American Academy of Dramatic Arts: on dram. & musical stage, also radio.
TV: Bob Cummings Show; My Hero, Twelve Angry Men (Emmy, 1954).
PICTURES INCLUDE: Three Smart Girls Grow Up, Spring Parade, Saboteur, Heaven Only Knows, So Red the Rose, Kings Row, Flesh and Fantasy, Princess O'Rourke, You Came Along, Reign of Terror, The Accused, Free for All, Tell It to the Judge, Paid in Full, Petty Girl, For Heaven's Sake, Barefoot Mailman, The Lost Moment, Free and Easy, First Time, Marry Me Again, Lucky Me, Dial M for Murder, How to Be Very Very Popular, My Geisha, Beach Party, The Carpetbaggers, What A Way to Go, Stage Coach, Promise Her Anything, Gidget Grows Up, The Great American Beauty Contest, (TV). Has toured Dinner Theater Circuit since '73 and established new attendance records in 16 theaters playing Never Too Late, Marriage Go Round, No Hard Feelings, Harvey, Fun and Games.

CUMMINGS, CONSTANCE: Actress. b. Seattle, Wash., May 15, 1910; p. D.V. Halverstadt, attorney, and Kate Cummings, concert soprano; m. Benn Levy, English playwright. Was chorus girl in The Little Show and also appeared in June Moon.
PICTURES INCLUDE: Behind the Mask, Washington Merry-Go-Round, Broadway; Through a Keyhole, Channel Crossing, Glamour, Doomed Cargo, Busman's Honeymoon, This England, The Outsider, The Foreman Went to France, Somewhere in France, Blithe Spirit, Into the Blue, The Scream, John and Julie, The Intimate Stranger, Battle of the Sexes, A Boy 10 Feet Tall.
TV: Touch of the Sun, Clutterbuck, The Last Tycoon, Ruth, Late Summer.

CUMMINGS, JACK: Producer. b. New Brunswick, Canada. Started at MGM as office boy. Later worked as script boy, assistant director, director, producer of short subjects. Became producer of feature pictures. In 1934 produced The Winning Ticket.
PICTURES INCLUDE: Bathing Beauty, I Dood It, Broadway Melody, Girl from Rectors, Romance of Rosy Ridge, Neptunes Daughter, Two Weeks with Love, Three Little Words, Excuse My Dust, Texas Carnival, Lovely to Look At, Fiesta, Stratton Story, Sombrero, Give a Girl a Break, Kiss Me Kate, Seven Brides for Seven Brothers, Last Time I Saw Paris, Many Rivers to Cross, Interrupted Melody, Teahouse of the August Moon, Can Can, Bachelor Flat, Viva, Las Vegas.

CUMMINGS, SANDY: Executive. r.n. Sanford Cummings. b. Oct. 31, 1913. e. University of Southern Calif. Child actor; Broadway. Summer stock, 1935; asst. prod., Paramount; assist. to Walter Wanger, 1936; started Hollywood office of Benton & Bowles, 1937; major, army, 1939–46; Head American Forces Network, Germany; prod. Columbia, 1946; ABC Coordinator, Walt Disney Studios, 1954; manager, TV Net Programs, Western Div. ABC, 1957; dir. TV Net Prog., 1958; V.P. & Dir. of pgms., Western Div., 1958–62; prod. specials, STV, 1964; prod., 20th Fox Television, 1965–66; NBC Broadcast Standards; 1969 mgr., live nighttime and special programs, NBC.

CUMMINS, DWIGHT W.: Writer. b. San Francisco, Cal., Feb. 20, 1901; e. U. Calif., L.A., B.A. '26. m. Dorothy Yost, writer. Tech. dir. & prod. asst. Film Booking Office studio, 1926–27. Began writing scripts 1927. Ed. & story asst. various major producers 1932–38. Instructor in Cinematog., U. So. Calif., 1938–42. Member Phi Gamma Delta.
PICTURES INCLUDE: Naughty but Nice, None but the Brave, The River, Thunderhead, Smoky, The Strawberry Roan, The Saginaw Trail.
TV: Gene Autry, Range Rider; TV writer for Roy Rogers, 1955–60; TV free lance.

CUMMINS, PEGGY: Actress. b. Prestatyn, North Wales. e. Alexandra School, Dublin, Gate Theatre, Dublin. Starred in Let's Pretend on London Stage 1938. Made Dr. O'Dowd WB, Eng., 1939. In 1942; Salute John Citizen; Welcome Mr. Washington; On London Stage in Junior Miss, Alice in Wonderland, Peter Pan. From 1946 Hollywood, starred in Late George Apley.
PICTURES INCLUDE: Moss Rose, Green Grass of Wyoming, Escape, That Dangerous Age, Gun Crazy, My Daughter Joy, Returned to Eng. 1950. Who Goes There (Passionate Sentry), Street Corner (Both Sides of the Law), Meet Mr. Lucifer, Always a Bride, Love Lottery, To Dorothy a Son, Cash on Delivery, March Hare, Carry on Admiral, Night of the Demon, Hell Drivers, The Captain's Table, Your Money or Your Wife, Dentist in the Chair, In the Doghouse.
TV: The Human Jungle, Looks Familiar.

CUNNINGHAM, SEAN S.: Producer-Director. b. New York City, 1941. e. B.A. Franklin & Marshall, MFA Stanford Univ. Worked briefly as actor, moving into stage-managing. Became producer of Mineola Theatre (Long Island, NY) and took several productions to Broadway. Formed Sean S. Cunningham Films, Ltd., 1971. Produced commercials, industrial film, documetaries, features.
PICTURES: Together (prod.-dir.), Last House on the Left (prod.); The Case of the Full Moon Murders (prod.); Here Come the Tigers (prod.-dir.); Kick (prod.-dir.); Friday the 13th (prod.-dir.); A Stranger Is Watching (prod.-dir.); Spring Break (prod.-dir.); The New Kids (prod., dir.); House (prod.); House II (prod.).

CURTIN, JANE: Actress. b. Cambridge, MA, Sept. 6, 1947. e. Northeastern Univ. On stage in Proposition, Last of the Red Hot Lovers, Candida, etc.
PICTURES: Mr. Mike's Mondo Video, How to Beat the High Cost of Living.
TELEVISION: Series: Saturday Night Live, Kate & Allie. Movies: Divorce Wars—A Love Story, Candida, etc.

CURTIS, DAN: Producer-Director. b. Bridgeport, Conn., Aug. 12. e. Univ. of Bridgeport; Syracuse Univ. (BA, 1950). Was sales exec. for NBC and MCA before forming own company, Dan Curtis Productions, which he now heads. Producer/owner of CBS Golf Classic (1963–73).
PICTURES INCLUDE: House of Dark Shadows, Night of Dark Shadows (features for MGM, prod.-dir.), Burnt Offerings (prod., dir., co-s.p.).
TV: Producer; Dark Shadows (ABC serial, 1966–71), and following movies: The Night Stalker, Frankenstein, The Picture of Dorian Gray. Producer-Director of movies: The Night Strangler, The Norliss Tapes, The Turn of the Screw, Dracula, The Scream of the Wolf, Purvis.

CURTIS, JAMIE LEE: Actress. b. Los Angeles, Nov. 22, 1958. Daughter of Janet Leigh and Tony Curtis.

PICTURES: Halloween, The Fog, Terror Train, Halloween II, Road Games, Prom Night, Love Letters, Grandview, USA, Perfect.

CURTIS, KEN: Actor. b. Lamar, Colo., July 2, 1916. e. Colorado Coll. Success as songwriter for college prod. steered him to musical career in Hollywood. Sang with several groups, including Sons of the Pioneers, Tommy Dorsey Orchestra, Shep Fields band. In infantry and anti-aircraft unit in World War II. Signed by Columbia Pictures for series of westerns with "Big Boy" Williams in 1945.
PICTURES INCLUDE: The Searchers, The Alamo, The Quiet Man, Cheyenne Autumn, How the West Was Won, The Killer Shrews, The Giant Gila Monster, My Dog, Buddy.
TV: Ripcord, Perry Mason, Rawhide, Have Gun, Will Travel, Gunsmoke (joined later series as Festus Haggin in 1963).

CURTIS, TONY: Actor. r.n. Bernard Schwartz. b. New York, N.Y., June 3, 1925; e. Seward Park H. Sch. In U.S. Navy, amateur dramatics, NYC, started Empire Players Theatre, Newark, N.J., with Dramatic Workshop, Cherry Lane Theatre, Jr. Drama Workshop of Walt Whitman School; first prod. work with Stanley Woolf Players; m.p. debut in Criss-Cross; signed with U-I Star of Tomorrow, 1953.
PICTURES INCLUDE: City Across the River, Johnny Stool Pigeon, Francis, Sierra, I Was a Shoplifter, Winchester 73, Kansas Raiders, Prince Who Was a Thief, Flesh and Fury, Son of Ali Baba, No Room for the Groom, Houdini, All American, Forbidden, Beachhead, Johnny Dark, Black Shield of Falworth, 6 Bridges to Cross, So This is Paris, Purple Mask, Square Jungle, Rawhide Years, Trapeze, Mister Cory, Midnight Story, Sweet Smell of Success, Some Like It Hot, Spartacus, Operation Petticoat, Who Was That Lady?, The Rat Race, The Defiant Ones, Perfect Furlough, The Great Impostor, The Outsider, Taras Bulba, 40 Pounds of Trouble, Paris When It Sizzles, The List of Adrian Messenger, Captain Newman, M.D., Wild and Wonderful, Sex and the Single Girl, Goodbye, Charlie, The Great Race, Boeing-Boeing, Arrivederci, Baby!, Not With My Wife, You Don't!, Don't Make Waves, On My Way to The Crusades I Met a Girl Who—; The Boston Strangler; Those Daring Young Men in Their Jaunty Jalopies, Suppose They Gave a War and Nobody Came; You Can't Win 'Em All, Lepke, The Last Tycoon, The Manitou, Bad News Bears Go To Japan, The Mirror Crack'd, Insignificance.
TV: The Persuaders, Vegas, Movies: The Second Girl on the Right, Mafia Princess.

CUSACK, CYRIL: Actor. b. Durban, S. Africa, Nov. 26, 1910. e. Newbridge, Co. Kildare; University College, Dublin, Eire. LL.D (Honoris Causa-National University of Ireland). Stage debut: Candida, Abbey Theatre, 1932. Screen debut: Odd Man Out, 1945.
PICTURES INCLUDE: Esther Waters, Escape, The Blue Lagoon, Once a Jolly Swagman, All Over the Town, Small Back Room, The Elusive Pimpernel, Soldiers Three, Blue Veil, Secret of Convict Lake, Gone to Earth (Wild Heart), Saadia, Passage Home, Man in the Road, Man Who Never Was, March Hare, Jacqueline, Spanish Gardner, Ill Met By Moonlight, Rising of the Moon, Miracle in Soho, Shake Hands with the Devil, Floods of Fear, Gideon's Day, A Terrible Beauty, Johnny Nobody, The Waltz of the Toreadors, I Thank a Fool, 80,000 Suspects, Passport to Oblivion, The Spy Who Came In from The Cold, Fahrenheit 451, Taming of the Shrew, I Was Happy Here, Oedipus Rex, Galileo, King Lear, Country Dance, David Copperfield, Harold and Maude, Sacco Vanzetti, La La Polizia Ringrazia, The Day of the Jackal, Juggernaut, Homecoming, Gallileo, Tristan and Iseult, True Confessions.
TV: The Dummy, The Moon and Sixpence, What Every Woman Knows, The Enchanted, The Power and The Glory, The Chairs, Don Juan in Hell, The Lotus Eater, Krapp's Last Tape, Murder in the Cathedral, Six Characters in Search of An Author, The Big Toe, Workhouse Ward, In the Train, Purgatory, The Moon in the Yellow River, Passage to India, Deirdre, The Tower, Dial M for Murder, St. Francis, The Physicists, Trial of Marshal Petain, In the Bosom of the Country, Uncle Vanya, A Time of Wolves and Tigers, Them, Clochemerle, The Golden Bowl, The Reunion, I Stand Well With All Parties, Catholics, Crystal & Fox, Jesus of Nazareth, The Plough and The Stars, You Never Can Tell, The Hitchhiker.

CUSHING, PETER: Actor. b. Kenley, Surrey, Eng., May 26, 1913. e. Purley Secondary Sch. Stage debut with Worthington Repertory Co.
TV: Asmodee, Anastasia, 1984, Gaslight, Home at Seven, Tovarich, Beau Brummell, Epitaph for a Spy, Pride and Prejudice, The Moment of Truth, Uncle Harry, Eden End, Rookery Nook, The Creature, The Browning Version, Winslow Boy, Peace With Terror, Julius Caesar (Cassius), Monica. Daily Mail TV award actor, 1953–54; Guild of TV award, 1955; News Chronicle T.V. Top Ten award, 1956, The Plan, Caves of Steel, Sherlock Holmes series, 1968, Morecambe & Wise Show, Wild-life Spectacular, The Zoo Gang, Orson Welles Great Mysteries, Space 1999, The New Avengers, The Great Houdini, A Land Looking West, A Tale of Two Cities (1981); The Vordal Blade, Tales of the Unexpected (1982); Helen and Teacher (1983).
PICTURES INCLUDE: Vigil in the Night, Moulin Rouge, Hamlet, Black Knight, End of the Affair, Alexander the Great, Magic Fire, Time Without Pity, Curse of Frankenstein, Abominable Snowman, Dracula, John Paul Jones, The Hound of the Baskervilles, Violent Playground, The Mummy, Suspect, The Flesh and the Friends, The Revenge of Frankenstein, Cone of Silence, Brides of Dracula, Sword of Sherwood Forest, The Naked Edge, Cash on Demand, The Devil's Agent, Captain Clegg, Fury at Smuggler's Bay, Hell-Fire Club, The Man Who Finally Died, The Evil of Frankenstein, The Gorgon, Dr. Terror's House of Horrors, She, The Skull, Dr. Who and Daleks, The Frighten Bed Island, Daleks Invade Earth, Frankenstein Created Woman, Torture Garden, Some May Live, The Night of the Big Heat, Corruption, Death's Head Moth, Frankenstein Must Be Destroyed, Doctors Wear Scarlet, The Vampire Lovers, Scream and Scream Again, House That Dripped Blood, I Monster, Twins of Evil, Tales from the Crypt, Dracula Today, Fear in the Night, Horror Express, The Creeping Flesh, Asylum, Nothing But the Night, Bride of Fengriffen, Frankenstein and the Monster from Hell, The Satanic Rites of Dracula, The Revenge of Dr. Death, From Beyond the Grave, The Beast Must Die, Dracula and the Legend of the Seven Golden Vampires, Shatter, Tender Dracula, The Ghoul, Legend of the Werewolf, The Devil's People, Death Corps, Trial by Combat, At The Earth's Core, Star Wars, Battleflag, The Uncanny, Hitler's Son, Touch of the Sun, Arabian Adventure, Black Jack, House of the Long Shadows, Sword of the Valiant, Top Secret!, Biggles.

D

DA COSTA, MORTON: Director-Actor. b. Philadelphia, PA, March 7, 1914. e. Temple Univ. Director of many Bdwy. musicals and plays, including Man and Superman, The Wild Duck, Plain and Fancy, No Time for Sergeants, Auntie Mame, The Music Man, Hot Spot, Maggie Flynn, etc.
PICTURES: Auntie Mame, The Music Man, Island of Love.

DAFF, ALFRED EDWARD: Executive. b. Melbourne, Australia, Aug. 18, 1902. e. McDonald's Private Coll., Melbourne. Office boy Progressive Films, night asst. projectionist Moonee Ponds Theatre 6 mos., then in chg. of dispatch, adv. & accessory depts., booker & in chg. of shipping, repairing, adv. & accessory depts. Cooperative Films; joined Universal Mar., 1920 booker & suburban salesman 2 yrs., asst. mgr., then mgr. of Victoria & Tasmania; apptd. managing dir. of Japanese subsidiaries, 1935; Far Eastern supvr., 1938; also of Far and Middle East, 1940; to N.Y.C., 1942; apptd. foreign supvr. 1943; vice-pres. Universal Internatl Films, Inc., 1944; pres. same co., 1950; v.p. dir. world sales, Universal Pictures Co., since 1951. Named dir. Universal, May, 1952; exec. v.p., July, 1952; res. 1958; consultant motion pictures, TV.

DAHL, ARLENE: b. Aug. 11, 1928, Mpls., Minn., USA Actress-writer; Designer. e. Mpls. Bus. Coll.; Univ. of Minn., summers 1941–44; Mpls. Coll. of Music. m. (1) Fernando Lamas, 1954, 1 s, Lorenzo Lamas b. 1958, (2) Christian R. Holmes III, 1960, 1 d, Carole Christine b. 1961 (3) Rounsevelle W. Schaum, 1969, 1 s. Sonny b. 1970. Acting career begun at age 8, playing heroine of children's adventure serials on radio, Broadway stage debut in Mr. Strauss Goes to Boston, 1946; other Broadway starring roles include: Cyrano de Bergerac; Applause; other starring roles onstage in major US cities include: The King and I, One Touch of Venus, Pal Joey, Bell Book and Candle, The Camel Bell, Lilliom, Marriage Go Round, Blythe Spirit; 28 film appearances include: debut in My Wild Irish Rose (Warner Bros., 1947), Three Little Words, Desert Legion, Here Come the Girls, Sangaree, Woman's World, Journey to the Center of the Earth, Kisses for My President. Num. TV appearances include: Series of 65 films for ABC-TV—Arlene Dahl's Beauty Spot, 1965; Hostess, CBS Model of the Year Show, 1969, Arlene Dahl's Starscope, 1980. Appts: Internationally syndicated beauty columnist, Chgo. Tribune-N.Y. News Syndicate, 1951–71; Sleepwear Designer, A.N. Saab & Co., 1952–57; Nat. Beauty Advisor, Sears Roebuck & Co., 1970–75; v.p. Kenyon & Eckhart, pres., Women's World Div., Kenyon-Eckhart, 1967–72, Fashion Consultant, O.M.A. 1975–78, Int'l. Director of S.M.E.I., 1973–76, Pres., Dahlia Parfums Inc., 1975, pres., Dahlia Prods., 1978–Publs: Always Ask a Man, 1965 (6th ed.), Your Beautyscope (series of 12), 1969, Secrets of Hair Care, 1971, Your Beautyscope (series of 12) 1977–78. Profl. Assns. include: Screen Actors Guild, Actors Equity, Am. Fedn. of TV & Radio Artists, International Platform, Inc., Acad. of Motion Picture Arts and Sciences. Honrs.

include: 8 Motion Picture Laurel Awards, 1948–63; Hds. of Fame Award, 1971, Woman of Year, N.Y. Adv. Council, 1969.

DALE, JIM: Actor. b. Rothwell, Northants, England, Aug. 15, 1935. Debut as solo comedian at the Savoy, 1951. Joined National Theatre Co. at Old Vic. Toured Europe in plays and in New York in Taming of the Shrew, Scapino, Barnum.
PICTURES: Raising the Wind, Carry on Spying, Carry On Cleo, The Big Job, Carry On Cowboy, Carry on Screaming, Lock Up Your Daughters, The National Health, Digby, Joseph Andrews, Pete's Dragon, The Unidentified Flying Oddball, Scandalous.

DALEY, ROBERT: Producer. Began career in TV; later joined Clint Eastwood's Maplasco Co.
PICTURES INCLUDE: Dirty Harry, Magnum Force (both exec. prod.), Thunderbolt and Lightfoot (prod.), The Enforcer (prod.), The Gauntlet (prod.), Every Which Way But Loose (prod.), Escape from Alcatraz (exec. prod.)., Any Which Way You Can (exec. prod.); Stick (exec. prod.).
TV: The Untouchables, Ben Casey, The FBI, 12 O'Clock High, The Invaders, etc.

DALTON, TIMOTHY: Actor. b. Colwyn Bay, Wales, March 21, 1946.
PICTURES: The Lion in Winter, Cromwell, The Voyeur, Wuthering Heights, Mary Queen of Scots, Lady Caroline Lamb, Permission to Kill, Sextette, Agatha, Flash Gordon, Chanel Solitaire, The Doctor and the Devils.
TELEVISION: Movies: Mistral's Daughter, The Master of Sins, Ballantrae, Florence Nightingale. Mini-Series: Jane Eyre.

DALTREY, ROGER: Singer-Actor. b. London, England, March 1, 1944. Lead vocalist with The Who.
PICTURES: Woodstock, Tommy, Lisztomania, The Legacy, The Kids are Alright, McVicar (also prod.), The Beggar's Opera.

DALY, JOHN: Chm., Hemdale Group Ltd. b. London, England, 1937. After working in journalism joined Royal Navy. On leaving Service after three years, trained as underwriter with an Assurance Company. In 1966 became David Hemmings manager and in 1967 formed the Hemdale Company. Subsequently, in 1968, Hemdale obtained public status and produced features including The Passage, Sunburn, Cattle Annie and Little Britches, High Risk, Going Ape, Carbon Copy, Yellowbeard, Falcon and the Snowman, Terminator, Salvador, At Close Range, Hoosiers.

DALY, ROBERT A.: Executive. b. New York City, Dec. 8, 1936. e. Brooklyn Coll. Joined CBS-TV in 1955; dir. of program acct.; dir. of research and cost planning; dir. of business affairs. Later named v.p., business affairs, NY; exec. v.p. of network on April, 1976. Named producer, CBS Entertainment, Oct. 1977. In Nov., 1980, appointed co-chmn. and co-chief exec. officer of Warner Bros. Now sole title holder.

DALY, TYNE: Actress. b. Madison, WI, Feb. 21, 1947. Daughter of late actor James Daly. Wife of Georg Stanford Brown.
PICTURES: John and Mary, Angel Unchained, Play It As It Lays, The Entertainer, The Enforcer, Telefon, Speedtrap, Zoot Suit, The Aviator, Movers & Shakers.
TELEVISION: Series: Cagney and Lacey. Movies: Larry, Better Late Than Never, The Women's Room, A Matter of Life or Death, etc.

DAMON, MARK: Executive. b. Chicago, April 22, 1933. e. University of California at Los Angeles, B.A. Literature, M.A. Business Administration. Actor: 1958 under contract to 20th Century Fox, 1960 winner Golden Globe Award—Newcomer of the Year; early career includes The Fall of The House of Usher, The Longest Day; 1961 moved to Italy, stayed 16 years appearing in leading roles in 50 films; 1973 co-producer of The Arena with Roger Corman; 1974 head of foreign department for PAC, a leading film distributor in Italy; 1976 returned to the U.S.A. as executive producer of The Choirboys and in charge of its foreign distribution; 1977 founder and pres. of Producers Sales Organization, international distribution organization.

DAMONE, VIC: Singer, actor. r.n. Vito Farinola. b. Brooklyn, N.Y., June 12, 1928. e. Lafayette H. Sch., B'klyn. Winner Arthur Godfrey talent show, 1945; then night clubs, radio, theatres, hotels. m.p. debut in Rich, Young and Pretty; U.S. Army, 1951–53.
PICTURES INCLUDE: The Strip, Athena, Deep in My Heart, Hit the Deck, Kismet, Hell to Eternity.
TV: Vic Damone Show, 1958. Lively Ones, 1962.

DAMSKI, MEL: Director. b. New York City, July 21, 1946. e. Colgate; AFI. Worked as reporter, journalism professor.
PICTURES: Yellowbeard, Mischief.
TELEVISION: MASH, Lou Grant, Long Journey Back, The Child Stealer, Word of Honor, The Legend of Walks Far Woman, For Ladies Only, Making the Grade, An Invasion of Privacy, Attack on Fear, etc.

DANA, BILL: Actor-Writer. b. Quincy, MA, 1924. In night clubs and on TV.
PICTURES: The Barefoot Executive (actor only), The Nude Bomb.

D'ANGELO, BEVERLY: Actress. b. Columbia, Ohio. Studied visual arts and was exchange student in Italy before working as cartoonist for Hanna-Barbera Studios in Hollywood. Toured Canada's coffeehouse circuit as singer and appeared with rock band called Elephant. Joined Charlotte Town Festival Company. Bdwy. debut in rock musical, Rockabye Hamlet. Film debut in The Sentinel.
PICTURES: Annie Hall, First Love, Every Which Way But Loose, Hair, Coal Miner's Daughter, National Lampoon's Vacation, Finders Keepers, National Lampoon's European Vacation, Big Trouble.
TELEVISION: A Streetcar Named Desire, Doubletake.

DANGERFIELD, RODNEY: Actor-Comedian. b. Babylon, NY, 1921.
PICTURES: The Projectionist, Caddyshack, Easy Money (also co. s.p.), Back to School.

DANHEISER, MELVIN B.: Executive. Held positions at RKO Radio Pictures and National Telefilm Associates before joining United Artists in 1961 in intl. div.'s sls. dept. Since served in various capacities—asst. intl. sls. mgr. for Europe, Middle East, and English-speaking mkts. overseas. 1978 promoted to exec. asst. to foreign mgr. Appt. v.p. of UA in 1979; 1981, named exec. asst. to Norbert T. Auerbach, pres. & chief operating officer for UA 1982, named v.p., MGM/UA int. m.p. div.

DANIEL, SEAN: Executive. b. 1952. e. California Inst. of Arts film school. Was journalist for Village Voice before starting m.p. career as documentary filmmaker and asst. dir. for New World Pictures. In 1976 joined Universal Pictures as prod. exec.; 1979, named v.p. Now pres., production.

DANIELEWSKI, TAD: Director-Writer. b. Poland. Studied Royal Academy of Dramatic Art, London; Ohio University; State Univ. of Iowa. At Johns Hopkins Univ. won national award for research in prod. and dir. methods for TV. Produced and directed a series of dramatic shows on WAAM-TV in cooperation with NBC-TV, 1953–54.
PICTURES INCLUDE: Imperial Woman (co-writer), No Exit (dir.), The Guide (writer-dir.), Spain (writer-dir.), Copernicus (writer-dir. of English version).
TELEVISION: Omnibus, Wide Wide World, Eddie Fisher Show, Matinee Theatre, Robert Montgomery Presents, etc.
STAGE: Artistic director New York Repertory Theatre; directed Man with a Load of Mischief (London), A Desert Incident (Bdwy.), Brouhaha (off-Bdwy.), etc.

DANIELS, HAROLD: Director, producer, writer, b. Buffalo, N.Y. e. Carnegie Tech Drama Dept. B.A., U. of Pittsburgh, PHG.
STAGE: Director in Pittsburgh for Prof. Stage Guild Co., N.Y., Rhode Island and Boston Repertoire. Directed over 50 plays.
PICTURES INCLUDE: Joined MGM in 1940, directed shorts and won award from M.P. Council; joined David Selznick as director f1943–45; produced, directed and wrote Prince of Peace, won spec. award for dir., directed Woman from Tangier, Sword of Venus, Port Sinister, Roadblock, Daughter of the West Classics, Terror in the Haunted House, Date With Death, My World Dies Screaming, Bayou, Poor White Trash, Ten Girls Ago; directed, Night of the Beast, House of Black Death, Annabelle Lee, 1968–69, Moonfire, 1969–70. Pigmy, 1971.
TV: directed over 200 half-hour and hour films including My Hero, Readers Digest, Fury, Colt 45, Ellery Queen, Jim Backus Theatre, G.E. Theatre, etc. Wrote many original screenplays for both films and TV. The Phantom, On Guard, Death Valley Days, Hannibal Cobb.

DANIELS, JEFF: Actor. b. Georgia. 1955. e. Central Michigan Univ. Apprentice with Circle Repertory Theatre, New York.
THEATRE: Brontosaurus, Short-Changed Review, The Farm, Fifth of July, etc.
PICTURES: Ragtime (debut), Terms of Endearment, The Purple Rose of Cairo, Marie, Something Wild, Heartburn.
TELEVISION: Movies: A Rumor of War, Invasion of Privacy, Fifth of July. Series: Breaking Away (pilot), Hawaii 5-0, etc.

DANIELS, WILLIAM: Actor. b. Brooklyn, NY, Mar 31, 1927. e. Northwestern University. Stage debut in Life with Father. Brought to national attention by role in A Thousand Clowns in original Bdwy. play and film version.
PICTURES: Marlowe, The Parallax View, Two for the Road, Black Sunday, Oh God, Sunburn, The Blue Lagoon.
TELEVISION: The Adams Chronicle, A Case of Rape, Blind Ambition, The Nancy Walker Show, Captain Nice, Knight Rider, St. Elsewhere.
STAGE: On a Clear Day You Can See Forever, 1776, Dear Me, The Sky Is Falling, A Little Night Music, etc.

DANNER, BLYTHE: Actress. b. Philadelphia, 1944. e. Bard College. m. writer-producer Bruce Paltrow. Appeared in

repertory cos. in U.S. before Lincoln Center (N.Y.) productions of Cyrano de Bergerac, Summertree, and The Miser (Theatre World Award for last).
PICTURES INCLUDE: 1776, To Kill a Clown, Lovin' Molly, Hearts of the West, Futureworld, The Ace, Too Far To Go, Man, Woman and Child.
TV: Dr. Cook's Garden, To Confuse the Angel, George M, To Be Young, Gifted and Black, The Scarecrow, Adam's Rib (series), F. Scott Fitzgerald and The Last of the Belles, Eccentricities of a Nightingale, Guilty Conscience.

DANO, ROYAL: Actor. b. New York City, Nov. 16, 1922. On Broadway stage before entering films.
PICTURES: The Red Badge of Courage, Bend of the River, The Far Country, Moby Dick, Death of a Gunfighter, The Outlaw Josey Wales, In Search of the Historic Jesus, Take This Job and Shove It, Something Wicked This Way Comes, The Right Stuff.
TELEVISION: Death Valley Days, Planet of the Apes, Heroes of the Bible, From Here to Eternity.

DANSON, HAROLD L.: Executive. b. New York, N.Y., Nov. 15, 1905. e. Brooklyn Polytechnic Institute, 1926. Feature ed., Brooklyn Eagle, 1927; press rep., Shubert Theatrical Co., asst. city ed., Newark Star-Eagle, 1928; dir. of adv. pub., RCA Photophone, 1929–30; asst. nat'l adv. mgr., RKO, 1930–32; exploit. mgr., studio adv. dir., asst. nat'l adv. dir., head of trailer prod., Paramount, 1932–44; account exec., 20th Century-Fox, 1944–46; nat. adv. dir., Eagle Lion, 1946–49; v.p., gen. sales mgr., Adler Communications Labs., 1951–54; dir. of adv., pub., TV National Screen Service Corp., 1955; acct. exec. ZIV TV Programs, 1956; Nat'l Telefilm Assoc. program sales, 1959; nat'l sales mgr., syndication Independent Television Corp., 1961–68; consultant 1969.

DANSON, TED: Actor. b. Dec. 29, 1947. e. Kent School, Stanford Univ., Carnegie-Mellon Univ. Studied at Actors Institute with Dan Fauci. New York stage debut, The Real Inspector Hound, 1972. Film debut in The Onion Field, 1979. Television debut, The Doctors.
PICTURES: Body Heat, Creepshow, Little Treasure, A Fine Mess, Just Between Friends.
TELEVISION: Somerset, The Women's Room, The Good Witch at Laurel Canyon, Cowboy, Something about Amelia, Cheers.

DANTE, JOE: Director. b. Morristown, NJ. Managing editor for Film Bulletin before going to Hollywood to work in advertising, creating campaigns for many films. Became protege of Roger Corman, co-directing Hollywood Boulevard. Followed with Piranha, which directed and co-edited. At New World also co-wrote Rock 'n' Roll High School, edited Grand Theft Auto.
PICTURES: The Howling, Twilight Zone—The Movie (segment), Gremlins, Explorers.

DANTON, RAY: Actor. b. New York, N.Y., Sept. 19, 1931. e. Horace Mann School, Carnegie Tech. m. Julie Adams. Radio actor on many programs; summer stock; London prod. of Mr. Roberts; U.S. Army, 1951–53; then TV actor numerous programs. Became dir. in 1976 with Psychic Killer (also co-s.p.).
PICTURES INCLUDE: Chief Crazy Horse, The Looters, The Spoilers, I'll Cry Tomorrow, Outside the Law, The Night Runner, Onionhead, Too Much Too Soon, Ice Palace, Legs Diamond, Tarawa Beachhead, Majority of One, The George Raft Story, Fever In The Blood, Portrait of a Mobster, The Chapman Report, The Longest Day, Sandokan, FBI Code 98, New York Calling Superdrago.

D'ANTONI, PHILIP: Producer-Director. b. NYC, Feb. 19, 1929. e. Fordham Univ. Has degree in business admn. Joined CBS in mailroom, advanced into prod., sales development, prog. analysis, mkt. rsrch. Became indep. radio-TV repr. in 1954 for two years; then joined Mutual Broadcasting as sales manager; later, exec. v.p. Resigned in 1962 to form own prod. co. Made theatrical film debut with Bullitt as producer; directing debut with The Seven Ups. Heads Phil D'Antoni Prods.
PICTURES INCLUDE: Producer: Bullitt, The French Connection. Prod.-Dir.: The Seven Ups.
TELEVISION: Elizabeth Taylor in London, Sophia Loren in Rome, Melina Mercouri in Greece, Jack Jones Special, This Proud Land, and two movies: Mr. Inside/Mr. Outside, The Connection.

DANZ, FREDRIC A.: Executive. b. Seattle, Wash., Feb. 28, 1918. Is chairman of Sterling Recreation Organization Co., Seattle; member, Foundation of M.P. Pioneers; v.p., Variety Club Intl.

DANZA, TONY: Actor. b. Brooklyn, NY, Apr. 21. e. Univ. of Dubuque. Professional boxer before tested for role in TV pilot (Fast Lane Blues) which he won. Back to New York and fighting until called to coast to appear as Tony Banta in Taxi series.
PICTURES: Hollywood Knights, Going Ape.
TELEVISION: Taxi, Who's the Boss.

DARBY, KIM: Actress. r.n. Derby Zerby. b. July 8, 1948, Hollywood, Calif. e. Swanson's Ranch School, Van Nuys High School. Studied at the Desilu Workshop in Hollywood. Professional debut on the Mr. Novak TV series.
TV: Eleventh Hour, Gunsmoke, Flesh and Blood (special).
PICTURES INCLUDE: Bus Riley's Back in Town, True Grit, Generation, Norwood, The Strawberry Statement, The Grissom Gang, The One and Only, Better Off Dead.

DARK, JOHN: Producer. Films include, as associate: Light Up the Sky, Lost Innocence, The 7th Dawn, Casino Royale. Production exec., Paramount Pictures, exec. producer: Half a Sixpence, There's a Girl in My Soup. Produced: Wind of Change, Bachelor of Arts, Land That Time Forgot, At the Earth's Core, People That Time Forgot, Warlords of Atlantis, Arabian Adventure, Slayground.

DARLEY, DICK: Director, Producer network TV series and specials. Over 180 TV film shows; over 1,370 TV live/tape shows. Numerous pilots and commercials. Credits in U.S.A. and 27 foreign countries include drama, musical-variety, comedy, sports and documentary.

DARNBOROUGH, ANTONY: Producer, director. b. London, Eng., ent. m.p. ind. 1944.
PICTURES INCLUDE: Seventh Veil, Years Between, Daybreak, Girl in a Million, Upturned Glass, When the Bough Breaks, Dear Murderer, The Calendar, My Brother's Keeper, The Girl in the Painting, Helter Skelter, Once Upon a Dream, Traveller's Joy, Boys in Brown, The Astonished Heart, So Long at the Fair, Quartet, Trio, Highly Dangerous, Encore, The Net (Project M. 7), Personal Affair, To Paris With Love, Baby and the Battleship.
TV: Also made many TV and documentary films for own co. and in assoc. with NSS.

DARREN, JAMES: Actor. b. Philadelphia, Pa., June 8, 1936. Studied with Stella Adler group. Hollywood debut: Rumble on the Docks.
PICTURES INCLUDE: The Brothers Rico, Guns of Navarone, Gidget Goes Hawaiian, The Lively Set, 633 Squadron, Venus in Furs.
TELEVISION: T.J. Hooker.

DARRIEUX, DANIELLE: Actress. b. Bordeaux, France, May 1, 1917. e. Lycee LaTour; Conservatoire de Musique.
PICTURES INCLUDE: La Crise Est Finis, Mayerling, Club des Femmes, Abus de Confiance, Counsel for Romance, Mademoiselle Ma Mere, Katia, Orders from Tokyo, Oh Amelia, Rage of Paris, Rich Young and Pretty, 5 Fingers, La Ronde, Le Plaisir, Earrings of Madame De, Alexander the Great, Adorable Creatures, A Friend of the Family, Loss of Innocence.
THEATRE: Coco.

DARTIGUE, JOHN: Executive. b. Port-au-Prince,Haiti, Sept. 12, 1940. e. Brandeis Univ. (B.A., 1961), Columbia Univ. (M.A., 1965). United Artists: named director of worldwide pub. in 1975; appointed executive assistant to the senior vice president for advertising and publicity in 1977; named v.p. adv.-pub., 1978. Joined Warner Bros. in 1978 as project executive. Named sr. exec. asst. to the exec. v.p. of worldwide adv./pub., Jan., 1980, v.p., publicity, July 1980.

DARTNALL, GARY: Exec. b. Whitchurch, Eng., May 9, 1937. e. Kings Coll., Taunton. Overseas Div., Associated British Pathe; Eur. rep., 1958–60; Middle & Far East rep., Lion International Films; Amer. rep., 1962; pres., Lion International Inc., 1963; Amer. rep., Alliance International Films Distributors, Ltd., and London Independent Producers, Ltd.; pres., Alliance International Films Corp. & Dartnall Films Ltd., 1966; managing dir., Overseas Division, Walter Reade Organization, 1969. pres., EMI Film Distributors, Inc., 1971; vice chairman, EMI Television Programs, Inc., 1976; pres., EMI Videograms, Inc., 1979; pres., VHD Programs, Inc. & VHD Disc Mfg. Co., 1980; chm. & chief exec. officer, Thorn EMI Films, Ltd., & Thorn EMI Video, 1983. Also pres. & CEO, Thorn EMI Films, Inc.; chm., Thorn EMI Cinemas; CEO, Thorm EMI Screen Entertainment Ltd.

da SILVA, RAUL: Creative consultant, writer, director, producer, b. New York City. June 12. e. Adelphi U., B.A. 1958, elected to Academy of Distinction Adelphi Alumni Assoc. 1978. Specializes in script evaluation, analysis and rework, production design, graphics for promotion. Exp. Corporate AV dir., exec. prod. adv. agencies; indep. writer, producer, dir., univ. lecturer (business aspects of film prod. writing).
PUBLICATIONS: Making Money in Film & Video (Simon & Schuster, (1986); The World of Animation (Kodak, 1979); The Business of Filmmaking (Kodak, 1978); SOUND, Magnetic Recording for Motion Pictures (Kodak, 1977). Wrote articles for Millimeter, American Cinematographer, Back Stage and many other trades.
PICTURES: Fear No Evil (creative consultant).
TV: Nat Hurst, M.D.; The Strangest Voyage (dir., prod.),

Standing Tall (script consultant). On video cassette: The Ancient Mariner.
AWARDS: 1984 Writer's Digest screenwriting award and numerous as dir.-prod. for films; six in 1975–76 for Coleridge and his masterpiece, The Ancient Mariner with Sir Michael Redgrave.

DA SILVA, RAY: Director and designer of animated films, animator, illustrator, character designer. b. New York City, July 13, 1934. e. School of Visual Arts, NYC, also instructor there. Specializes in animation direction, character design. Numerous national and international TV spots for the advertising industry.
PICTURES: Raggedy Ann & Andy; Heavy Metal.
TELEVISION: The Strangest Voyage, Noah's Animals, The Little Brown Burro, Ichabod Crane.

DASSIN, JULES: Director. b. Middletown, Conn. Dec. 18, 1911. Actor on dramatic stage several years; radio writer. Joined MGM, 1940, as dir. short subjects; later dir. features.
PICTURES INCLUDE: Canterville Ghost, Brute Force, Naked City, Thieves' Highway, Night and the City, Rififi, He Who Must Die, Never On Sunday, Phaedra, 10:30 p.m. Summer, Promise At Dawn, Uptight, A Dream of Passion.
PLAYS: Ilya, Darling, 1967.

DAVEE, LAWRENCE W.: Engineer. b. Foxcroft, Me., March 28, 1900; e. U. Me., B.S. (elec. eng.). Research eng. Bell Telephone Lab.; Fox Case Corp.; studio mgr. Fox Hearst Corp.; Bronx Studio. Elec. Research Prods., Inc.; Century Projector Corp., N.Y.; engineer & sales mgr.; pres. 1959. Member: 25–30 Club (Honorary). Lifemember, N.Y. State Projectionists.

DAVENPORT, NIGEL: Actor. b. Cambridge, England, May 23, 1928. e. Trinity Coll., Oxford. Began acting after stint in British military at 18 years. First 10 years of professional career in theatre. Majority of screen work in British films in 1950s and 60s.
PICTURES INCLUDE: Peeping Tom, A High Wind in Jamaica, A Man for All Seasons, Royal Hunt of the Sun, No Blade of Grass, Villain, Mary, Queen of Scots, Island of Dr. Moreau, Zulu Dawn, Nighthawks, Chariots of Fire, Greystoke.

DAVID, SAUL: Producer. b. Springfield, Mass., June 27, 1921. e. Classical High School, Springfield, Mass., Rhode Island School of Design. Started in radio, newspaper work and as editorial director for Bantam Books. Worked for Columbia Pictures, 1960–62; Warner Bros., 1962–63; 20th Century-Fox, 1963–67, and Universal, 1968–69; Executive story editor at MGM, 1972.
PICTURES INCLUDE: Produced Von Ryan's Express, Our Man Flint, Fantastic Voyage, In Like Flint, Skullduggery, Logan's Run.

DAVIDSON, JOHN: Actor-Singer. b. Pittsburgh, Penna., Dec. 13, 1941. e. Denison Univ. In numerous school stage prods. before coming to N.Y. where won co-star role with Bert Lahr in Bdwy. show, Foxy. Signed as regular on The Entertainers with Carol Burnett.
PICTURES INCLUDE: The Happest Millionaire, The Concorde—Airport '79.
TELEVISION: The Fantasticks, USA, The FBI, The Interns, Owen Marshall, Kraft Summer Music Hall (own variety series), The Tonight Show, The Girl with Something Extra, The John Davidson Talk Show (1980), That's Incredible.

DAVIDSON, MARTIN: Director. b., New York City, Nov. 7, 1939. Acted in and directed off-Bdwy. plays, wrote material for Sid Caesar, worked as agent with N.Y. offices of Int'l. Famous Artists.
PICTURES: The Lords of Flatbush, Almost Summer, Hero at Large, Eddie and the Cruisers (also s.p.).

DAVIES, PAUL: Executive. b. Toronto, Canada, M.A. Columbia Univ. Service with RCAF. Prod. Your Man Everywhere, many documentaries; Isle of Rainbow, Kansanshe, African Heritage, etc. Originator and pilot prod. Jazz in Europe, Man About the House. Manager of Malachite Films, NBC reporter and cameraman, bureau chief for Visnews, Israel 1980; since 1983 M.D. Media High Technology.

DAVIES, WILLIAM C.: Director. b. Auburn, N.Y., June 17, 1932. e. Auburn Community Coll., School of Radio Technique. Radio & T.V. announcer & narrator, then cameraman & editor. Formed Virgo Productions, 1965.
PICTURES INCLUDE: Legend of Horror, Orgy of the Dead, The Seekers, Day the Adults Died, Pink Garter Gang, Night at the Feast, Laughter in Hell, The Crimson Cult, Submarine X-1.

DAVIS, ALFRED: Exhibitor. b. Brighton, England, Aug. 19, 1899. e. University College Sch., London. In Brit. Army 1914 before entering m.p. ind. as dir. & booking mgr. Davis Pavillion circuit; later same position Gaumont British, New Era Pictures. Chr. London & Home Counties Branch, C.E.A., 1937, 1953, 1955. Dep. asst. dir., War Office Army Kinematograph, World War II; v.p. CEA; 1959–60; pres. CEA, 1960–61.

DAVIS, ARTHUR: Executive. b. New York, N.Y., Dec. 28, 1927. e. N.Y. Univ. Began as exhibitor in U.S.; founded Arthur Davis Organization in Tokyo, Japan, in 1963, representing European and American films for sales to Japanese TV and motion picture industry. 1979, released two documentaries, Brutes and Savages, The Art of Killing.

DAVIS, BETTE: Actress. b. Lowell, Mass., April 5, 1908; e. Cushing Academy; Mariarden School of Dancing; John Murray Anderson Dram. School. Stage debut in "Broadway" (Rochester, N.Y.); with Provincetown & Cape Players; on Broadway in: Broken Dishes, Solid South; m.p. debut in "Man Who Played God" 1932; won Academy Award twice: best actress 1935, in Dangerous and 1938, in Jezebel; voted one of the 10 best Money-Making Stars in Motion Picture Herald-Fame Poll 1939, 40, 41, 44; founder & pres. Hollywood Canteen 1942; pres. AMPAS 1940. Received American Film Institute Life Achievement Award, 1977; 1979, Emmy for performance in Strangers; 1982, Film Advisory Board's Life Achievement Award; Amer. Acad. of Arts, 1983; Dept. of Defense Medal for Distinguished Public Service, 1983; Women in Films Crystal Award, 1983.
PICTURES INCLUDE: Of Human Bondage, Fog Over Frisco, Sisters, Dark Victory, Juarez, Old Maid, Private Lives of Elizabeth and Essex, All This and Heaven Too, Letter, Now Voyager, Corn Is Green, Little Foxes, Deception, Winter Meeting, N.Y. stage, Night of the Iguana, Sandburg, June Bride, Beyond the Forest, All About Eve, Payment on Demand, Another Man's Poison, Phone Call From a Stranger, The Star, Virgin Queen, Catered Affair, Storm Center, John Paul Jones, The Scapegoat, A Pocketful of Miracles, What Ever Happened to Baby Jane, Dead Ringer, Empty Canvas, Where Love Has Gone, Hush . . . Hush Sweet Charlotte, The Nanny, The Anniversary, Connecting Rooms, Bunny O'Hare, Madame Sin (TV in U.S.), Scientific Card Game, Burnt Offerings, Return from Witch Mountain, Death on the Nile, Watcher in the Woods.
TV: The Disappearance of Aimee, Laugh-In, The Dark Secret of Harvest Home, Strangers, The Story of a Mother and Daughter, White Mama, Skyward, Family Reunion, A Piano for Mrs. Cimino, Little Gloria—Happy at Last, Right of Way, Hotel, Murder with Mirrors, As Summers Die.

DAVIS, BRAD: Actor. b. Florida, Nov. 6, 1949. Won music talent contest at 17; moved to Atlanta and acted in theatres before settling in New York, N.Y. stage debut in Crystal and Fox; did several off-Bdwy. plays including The Normal Heart in 1985. Appeared in TV soap opera, How to Survive a Marriage, for 10 months.
PICTURES: Midnight Express, A Small Circle of Friends, Chariots of Fire, Querelle.
TELEVISION: Walt Whitman, Sybil, Roots, A Rumor of War, The Greatest Man in the World, Chiefs, Robert Kennedy and His Times.

DAVIS, FRANK I.: Executive. b. Poolesville, Md. Feb. 18, 1919. e. U. of Md., AB, 1941; Harvard Law School, LL.B., 1948; law firm, Donovan, Leisure, Newton, Lombard and Irvine, 1948–50; v.p., gen. counsel, Vanguard Films, 1951; v.p., gen. counsel, Selznick Releasing Org., 1951–53; pres., The Selznick Company, 1953–55; v.p., Famous Artists Corp., 1956–62; v.p. George Stevens Productions Inc., 1962–65; exec. prod., The Greatest Story Ever Told; v.p. in charge of m.p. affairs, Seven Arts, 1966; exec. in chg. talent and exec. asst. to v.p. in chg. prod., MGM, 1967; dir. m.p. business affairs, MGM, 1970; v.p., business affairs, MGM, 1972; sr. v.p., motion picture business affairs, MGM/UA, 1983.

DAVIS, GEENA: Actress. b. Wareham, MA, 1959. e. Boston Univ. Model before debut in Tootsie (1982).
PICTURES: Fletch, Transylvania 6-5000, The Fly.
TELEVISION: Series: Buffalo Bill, Sara.

DAVIS, GEORGE W.: Art director, b. Kokomo, Ind., Apr. 17, 1914. e. U. Southern California.
PICTURES INCLUDE: The Robe, The Diary of Anne Frank, Love Is A Many Splendored Thing, All About Eve, David and Bathsheba, Americanization of Emily, Unsinkable Molly Brown, Funny Face, Cimarron, Period of Adjustment, Mutiny on the Bounty, Twilight of Honor, How The West Was Won, Patch of Blue, The Wonderful World of the Bros. Grimm, Mr. Buddwing, The Shoes of the Fisherman, etc. Including 200 feature films and 2000 TV segments.

DAVIS, JORDAN P.: Executive. b. N.Y., N.Y., October 29, 1933. e. Lehigh University, 1954; Columbia University Law School, 1958. Attorney for five years. Director of Business Affairs, ABC TV Network, 1963–67. NBC TV Network 1967–69. Director of Talent and Program Admin. v.p. Warner Bros. Television, 1969–72. Executive, The Sy Fischer Company, 1972–73. Executive in charge of production, Four D. Productions, Inc.; The Mimus Corp., The

Triseme Corporation, 1973–82. Pres., Jorlee Ltd., 1982–present.

DAVIS, JUDY: Actress. b. Australia. Left convent school as teenager to become a singer in a rock band. Studied at West Australia Institute of Technology and National Institute of Dramatic Art. Worked with theatre companies in Adelaide and Sydney. Theatrical film debut in My Brilliant Career (1979).
PICTURES: Hoodwink, Heatwave, Winter of Our Dreams, The Final Option, A Passage to India.
TELEVISION: A Woman Called Golda.

DAVIS, LUTHER.: Writer, producer. b. N.Y., Aug. 29. Solo s.p., The Hucksters, B.F.'s Daughter, Black Hand, A Lion Is in the Streets, The Gift of Love, Holiday for Lovers, The Wonders of Aladdin; Across 110th St.; collab. book B'way musical Kismet, collab. s.p.; author, prod., Lady In A Cage; s.p. Across 110th St. Prod. and wrote book for Bdwy musical, Timbuktu!, 1978–79. Co-prod., Eden Court and Not About Heroes (off-Bdwy. plays, 1985).
TV: Wrote, prod., Kraft Suspense Theatre and several pilots for series (Run for Your Life, The Silent Force, etc.). Wrote, prod. Arsenic and Old Lace (TV special). Wrote teleplays for MOW's Daughter of the Mind, The Old Man Who Cried Wolf, Colombo.

DAVIS, MAC: Singer-Songwriter-Actor. b. Lubbock, TX, Jan 21, 1942. e. Emory Univ., Ga. State Coll. Employed as ditch digger, service station attendant, laborer, probation officer and record company salesman before gaining fame as entertainer-singer in 1969. Recording artist and composer of many popular songs.
PICTURES: North Dallas Forty, Cheaper To Keep Her, The Sting II.

DAVIS, MARTIN S.: Executive. b. New York City. e. City Coll., N.Y.: New York Univ. U.S. Army, 1943–46; joined Saml. Goldwyn Prod., Inc., 1944; Allied Artists, 1955; Paramount Pictures, 1958. Dir. adv., pub. expl. 1960; vice-pres., 1963; exec. v.p., 1966; exec. comm. & bd. of dir. Member of Bd., Gulf + Western, 1967. Exec. v.p. Gulf + Western, member exec. comm. 1983, elected G + W chm., CEO, & Chm. of exec. comm.

DAVIS, MARVIN: Executive. General partner, Davis Oil Co., Denver; co-owner, 20th Century Fox, 1981–.

DAVIS, SIR JOHN: Executive. b. London, Eng., 1906; e. City of London Sch.; fellow Inst. of Chartered Secretaries and Administrators. Secy. to various ind. gps.; entered m.p. ind. as acct.-secy. to Odeon Theatres, Ltd., 1938; joint man. dir., 1941; man. dir., 1948; deputy chmn. 1951–62; chmn. and chief exec. The Rank Organisation Plc. 1962–74; chmn. 1974–77; pres. 1977–1983. Retired July 5, 1982. Jt.-Pres. Rank Xerox Ltd., National Centre of Films for Children, Trustee, Westminster Abbey Trust and Chairman, fund raising committee, Westminster Abbey Appeal 1973–85. Knighted June, 1971; Hon. D. Tech. (Loughborough) 1975; Knight Commander of the Order of St. John. Commandeur de l'Ordre de la Couronne (Belgium) 1974; C.V.O. 1985.

DAVIS, OSSIE: Actor-Writer-Director. b. Cogdell, Ga., Dec. 18, 1917. e. Howard Univ., Washington, D.C. m. actress Ruby Dee. Studied acting in N.Y. with Rose McLendon Players, leading to Broadway debut in 1946 in Jeb. For 11 years thereafter was one of most well-known blacks on Broadway stage (Anna Lucasta, Jamaica, A Raisin in the Sun, etc.) Wrote and starred in Purlie Victorious, repeating role for film version.
PICTURES INCLUDE: Actor: The Joe Louis Story, Fourteen Hours, Shock Treatment, No Way Out, The Cardinal, The Hill, Man Called Adam, The Scalphunters, Sam Whiskey, Let's Do It Again. Director: Cotton Comes to Harlem, Black Girl, Gordon's War, Countdown at Kusini (also star), Harry and Son, Avenging Angel.
TELEVISION: Author: East Side/West Side, The Eleventh Hour. Acted in many top dramatic series.

DAVIS, ROGER H.: Attorney. b. June 19, 1923, Chicago. e. U. Calif.-Berkeley, 1951, A.B., LL.B. Private law practice, partner, Loeb and Loeb, Los Angeles, 1951–61; atty., William Morris Agency, head of west coast legal, literary and M.P. depts., exec./admin., asst. sec. WMA, Inc., 1969–present, made v.p., 1974. exec. v.p. & bd. member, 1980.

DAVIS, SAMMY, JR.: Entertainer. b. New York City, Dec. 8, 1925. Father: Sammy Davis, Sr., entertainer. Professional debut at age 2, Gibson Theatre, in act with father and uncle, Will Mastin; singer, dancer, comedian, vocal and acting impressions; song writer; recording artist; starred in Mr. Wonderful, & Golden Boy on B'way; in many major TV shows.
PICTURES INCLUDE: Anna Lucasta, Porgy & Bess, Ocean's 11, Robin and the Seven Hoods, Salt and Pepper, A Man Called Adam, Sweet Charity, One More Time, The Cannonball Run, Cannonball Run II.

DAVISON, BRUCE: Actor. b. Philadelphia. e. Penn State, New York University. debut, Lincoln Center Repertory.
PICTURES INCLUDE: Last Summer, The Strawberry Statement, Willard, Been Down So Long It Looks Like Up To Me, The Jerusalem File, Ulzana's Raid, Mame, Mother, Jugs, and Speed, Short Eyes, Brass Target, Crimes of Passion, Spies Like Us, The Ladies Club.

DAVISON, JON: Producer. b. Haddonfield, NJ, July 21, 1949. e. NY Univ. Film School. Taught film history there one summer and ran NYU Cinema two years. 1972, joined New World Pictures as natl. dir. of publ./adv.; 1977, named in charge of prod.; 1980, became indep. prod.
PICTURES: Hollywood Boulevard, Grand Theft Auto, Piranha, Airplane!, White Dog, Twilight Zone—The Movie (episode), Top Secret! (co-prod.).

DAWBER, PAM: Actress-Singer. b. Detroit, Mich., Oct. 18, 1954. e. Farmington High School, Oakland Community College. Travelled nationally to trade shows to introduce new auto model; also began working in commercials. In 1971 came to N.Y.C.; hired as model, also doing commercials. First professional performance as singer in Sweet Adeleine at Goodspeed Opera House, East Haddam, Conn. Signed by Robert Altman to appear in theatrical film, A Wedding. On TV in comedy special, Sister Terri. Played Mindy in Mork and Mindy.
TELEVISION: Last of the Great Survivors (movie).

DAY, DORIS: Singer, actress. r.n. Doris Kappelhoff. b. Cincinnati, Ohio, Apr. 3, 1924. e. dancing, singing. Toured as dancer; radio and band singer; screen debut in Romance on the High Seas, 1948. Voted one of Top Ten Money-Making Stars in Motion Picture Herald-Fame poll, 1951–52. Best female vocalist. M. P. Daily radio poll, 1952.
PICTURES INCLUDE: Young Man With a Horn, Tea for Two, Storm Warning, West Point Story, Lullaby of Broadway, On Moonlight Bay, I'll See You in My Dreams, Starlift, Winning Team, April in Paris, By The Light of the Silvery Moon, Calamity Jane, Lucky Me, Young at Heart, Love Me or Leave Me, Man Who Knew Too Much, Julie, Pajama Game, Teacher's Pet, Pillow Talk, Please Don't Eat the Daisies, Midnight Lace, Lover, Come Back, That Touch of Mink, Jumbo, Thrill of It All, Move Over, Darling, Do Not Disturb, Send Me No Flowers, Glass Bottom Boat, Caprice, The Ballad of Josie, Where Were You When the Lights Went Out, With Six You Get Eggrolls.
TV: The Doris Day Show 1968–73.

DAY, LARAINE: Actress. r.n. Laraine Johnson. b. Roosevelt, Utah, Oct. 13, 1920. In school dramatics; with Players Guild, Long Beach, Calif.; toured in church prod. Conflict; Professionally on stage in Lost Horizon, The Women, Time of the Cukoo, Angel Street; m.p. debut in Border G-Men 1938.
PICTURES INCLUDE: Story of Dr. Wassell, Those Endearing Young Charms, Locket, Tycoon, My Son, My Son, Foreign Correspondent, Woman on Pier 13, Without Honor, High and the Mighty, Mr. Lucky, Toy Tiger, Three for Jamie Dawn, The Third Voice, Yank on The Burma Road, The Bad Man, Fingers at the Window, Bride By Mistake, My Dear Secretary.
TV: Climax, Playhouse 90, Alfred Hitchcock, Wagon Train, Let Freedom Ring, Name of the Game, FBI, Sixth Sense, Medical Center, Murder on Flight #504 (ABC Movie), Fantasy Island, Love Boat, Lou Grant, Airwolf, Hotel.

DAYTON, LYMAN D.: Producer. b. Salt Lake City, Aug. 17, 1941. m. Elizabeth Doty Dayton. e. Brigham Young Univ. After college worked in film lab at MGM, 1967–68; joined Screen Gems and General DeLuxe, 1968–69; became indep. prod. 1969. Heads Doty-Dayton Productions.
PICTURES INCLUDE: Where the Red Fern Grows, Seven Alone, Against A Crooked Sky, Pony Express Rider, Baker's Hawk, Young Rivals, Powder Keg.

DEAN, EDDIE: Actor. r.n. Edgar D. Glosup. b. Posey, Texas; married. From 1930–33 in radio throughout middle west; 1934 National Barn Dance, Station WLS; 1935 on CBS & NBC with same program. Featured male singer on TV KTLA Western Varieties 1944–55. Came to Hollywood in 1936; since then has starred in many westerns. Featured performer in western series for PRC in 1945. Voted one of the ten best money making Western Stars in Motion Picture Herald-Fame Poll 1936–47; recording artists, personal appearances, rodeos, fairs, etc.; 1966 V.P. Academy of Country & Western Music; 1967–68 on Bd. of Dir. of Academy of Western Music, Calif. Winner, Pioneer Award of Academy of Country Music, 1978. In 1983 named ACM v.p.; also v.p. in 1985. Recorded video cassette 1986, A Tribute to Eddie Dean.

DEAN, JIMMY: Performer. b. Plainview, Tex., Aug. 10, 1928. Joined armed forces, 1946–49; first appeared in various clubs in Wash., 1949; then app. on Town and Country Jamboree; toured Caribbean and Europe with his troupe.
SONGS: Comp. of following songs; Bummin' Around,

Freight Train Blues, Glad Rags, Hello, Mr. Blues, I Found Out, Big Bad John, PT-109, Little Black Book, This Ole House.
TV: Sunday Night at the Palladium (London), The Jimmy Dean Show.

DEAN, MERRILL C.: Executive. b. May 24, 1941. e. UCLA, MBA (bus. admin.). 1967–68, involved with Walt Disney Productions, 11 yrs. starting in m.p. distribution internationally with Buena Vista Intl., concentrating on Latin America. Later involved with world-wide publications and gen. mgr. of direct mktg. Was v.p., & gen. mgr. Walt Disney Records Music Division, four years. 1978–82, pres. of Televisa Intl. Distribution Corp., whose activities are principally involved with dist. of films to the Hispanic mkt. in U.S. & Puerto Rico. Now pres. InterFilm, Inc., Los Angeles, and Azimuth Communications Corp.

DEAN, MORTON: Television Newsman. b. Fall River, MA., Aug. 22, 1935. e. Emerson Coll. News dir., NY Herald Tribune Net, 1957; corr. WBZ, 1960, corr. WCBS-TV, 1964; anchor, WCBW-TV News, 1967; corr., CBS News, 1967; anchor, CBS Sunday Night News, 1975; anchor, Sunday edition CBS Evening News, 1976; co-anchor, Independent Network News, 1985.

DE BELDER, GUIDO: Actor-Author-Screenwriter. b. Tienen, Belgium, Mar. 14, 1939.
PICTURES INCLUDE: Mirliton, Obsessie, Spielgelvan Het Geluk, Mireille Dans La Vie Des Autres, Exit Seven, Ten Years After, Chock, Slachtvee, Deterugtocht, Mama Dracula, Traverses Traversees, Une Femme en Fuite, The Afterman.
TELEVISION: De Machinist (serial in 3 parts), Portrait of Guido De Belder (documentary).

DE BROCA, PHILIPPE: Director. b. 1933. French director.
PICTURES INCLUDE: Les Jeux de l'Amour, L'Amant, de Cinq Jours, Cartouche, That Man from Rio, Un Monsieur de Compagnie, Tribulations, Chinoise en Chine, King of Hearts, Devil By the Tail, Give Her the Moon, Louise.

DECAE, HENRI: Cinematographer b. France, 1915. Career spans 30 years and 60 films.
PICTURES INCLUDE: Le Silence de la Mer, Les Enfants Terribles, Creve-Coeur, Bob le Flambeur, Lift to the Scaffold, Le Beau Serge, A Double Tour, Les Quatre Cents Coup, Les Cousins, Plein Soleil, Les Bonnes Femmes, Leon Morin, Priest, Sundays and Cybele, Dragees au Poivre, Viva Maria, Weekend at Dunkirk, Night of the Generals, La Voleur, The Comedians, Castle Keep, The Sicilian Clan, The Light at the Edge of the World, Bobby Deerfield, The Island, Exposed.

DE CAESAR, GABRIEL: Producer. b. New York, Nov. 15, 1928. e. L.A. City College, 1952. Dir.-mgr. Little Theatre, L.A. Group, 3 yrs.; actor, 6 years; acting member Catholic Coll. Thea., Santa Monica Thea. Group, Pilgrimage Play Thea. Group, 3 yrs., producer: Three Wishes for Jamie, Bullfight; assoc. prod., asst. prod., Viscount Films, Inc. 1957–59; dir., N.A.B.E.T.; acted: Unexpected, TV series; ABC-TV series; producer, TV pilots, 1958; asst. prod., pictures; Tank Battalian, Speed Crazy; pres., exec. prod. Marqhis Productions, Inc., 1959; assoc. prod., Why Must I Die?

DE CAMP, ROSEMARY: Actress. b. Prescott Ariz., 1913.
TV: Robert Cummings Show, That Girl, Life of Riley (with Jackie Gleason); Death Valley Days; Partridge Family; Love American Style, Police Story, Rockford Files, Days of Our Lives, Misadventures of Sheriff Lobo, Love Boat, Blind Ambition, B.J. & the Bear.
PICTURES INCLUDE: Cheers for Miss Bishop, Hold Back the Dawn, Jungle Book, Yankee Doodle Dandy, Eyes in the Night, Pride of the Marines, Look for the Silver Lining, Story of Seabiscuit, Big Hangover, Scandal Sheet, On Moonlight Bay, Treasure of Los Canyon, By the Light of the Silvery Moon, Main Street to Broadway, So This Is Love, Many Rivers to Cross, Strategic Air Command, Saturday the 14th.

DE CAPRIO, AL: Producer-director. e. Brooklyn Tech., NYU. Started as radio engineer, cameraman, tech. dir., prod. & dir. CBS; dir. Sgt. Bilko, Car 54 Where Are You?, Musical specials for ABC, CBS, NBC; v.p. exec. prod. dir., MPO Videotronics, Pres. World Wide Videotape.

DE CARLO, YVONNE: Actress. b. Vancouver, B.C., Sept. 1, 1924; e. Vancouver School of Drama, Fauchon & Marco, Hollywood; specialty dancing at Florentine Gardens, Earl Carroll's; m.p. debut in This Gun for Hire 1942.
PICTURES INCLUDE: Harvard Here I Come, Youth on Parade, Road to Morocco, Story of Dr. Wassell, Salome, Where She Danced; Frontier Gal, Brute Force, Song of Scheherazade, Black Bart, Casbah, River Lady, Criss Cross, Gal Who Took the West, Calamity Jane and Sam Bass, Buccaneer's Girl, Tomahawk, Hotel Sahara, Silver City, Scarlet Angel, San Francisco Story, Hurricane Smith, Sombrero, Sea Devils, Fort Algiers, Border River, Captain's Paradise, Passion, Tonight's the Night, Shotgun, Magic Fire, Flame of the Islands, Ten Commandments, Raw Edge, Death of a Scoundrel, Band of Angels, Timbuktu, Law of the Lawless, Hostile Guns, The Power, McClintock.
BROADWAY STAGE: Follies.

DE CORDOVA, FREDERICK: Director. b. New York City, Oct. 27, 1910; e. Northwestern U., B.S. '31. Gen. stage dir. Shubert enterprises, N.Y., 1938–41; same for Alfred Bloomingdale Prods., N.Y., and prod. Louisville (Ky.) Amphitheatre 1942–43; m.p. dir.
PICTURES INCLUDE: (dial. dir.) San Antonio, Janie, Between Two Worlds; (dir.) Too Young to Know, Her Kind of Man, That Way with Women, Always Together, Wallflower, For the Love of Mary, Countess of Monte Cristo, Illegal Entry, Girl Who Took the West, Buccaneer's Girl, Peggy, Desert Hawk, Bedtime for Bonzo, Katie Did It, Little Egypt, Finders Keepers, Here Come the Nelsons, Yankee Buccaneer, Bonzo Goes to College, Column South.
Under contract CBS-TV, prod., dir. Burns and Allen, 1955–56; prod., December Bride, 1954–55; prod. and dir., Mr. Adams and Eve, prod. dir. December Bride; prod. dir. George Gobel Show; prod. dir., Jack Benny Program, 1960–63; dir., program planning, Screen Gems, 1964; prod. dir., Smothers Bros. Show, 1965–66; 1965 dir. I'll Take Sweden and Frankie & Johnny; 1966–70 dir. My Three Sons; 1971–86, prod., Tonight Show.

DECUIR, JOHN: Art Director-Production Designer. b. San Francisco. Universal 1938–49; Mark Hellinger Prods., 1946. 20th Fox 1949. Nominated for Acad. Award 11 times.
PICTURES INCLUDE: The Naked City, Snows of Kilimanjaro, My Cousin Rachel, Call Me Madam, Three Coins in the Fountain, There's No Business Like Show Business, Daddy Long Legs, The King and I (A.A., Art Dir.), Island in the Sun, South Pacific, The Big Fisherman, A Certain Smile, Cleopatra (A.,A.: Prod. Des.), The Agony and the Ecstasy, The Honey Pot, Zefferelli's Taming of The Shrew, Dr. Faustus, Hello, Dolly! (A.A.: Prod. Des.), On A Clear Day You Can See Forever, The Great White Hope, Once Is Not Enough, That's Entertainment, Too!, The Other Side of Midnight, Ziegfeld: The Man and his Women, Love and Bullets, Charlie, Raise the Titanic, Monsignor, Ghostbusters, Jo Jo Dancer, Legal Eagles.

DE CUIR, JR., JOHN F.: Art Director-Production Designer. b. Burbank, CA, Aug. 4, 1941. Son of John F. De Cuir, Sr. e. Univ. of So. Calif. (bach. of architecture, 1965). 1966–68, U.S. Coast Guard (holds commission with rank of Lt. Commander, USCGR). 1968–72, project designer, Walt Disney World, Walt Disney Prods. 1972–74, dir. of design, Six Flags Corp. 1974–9, project designer, EPCOT, Walt Disney Prods. 1980–85, pres., John F. De Cuir, Jr. Design Consultants, Inc.
PICTURES: Illustrator: Cleopatra, The Honey Pot. Design Concepts: The Agony and the Ecstasy. Art Director: Raise the Titanic, Monsignor (also special effects consultant), Ghostbusters. Producer: The Building Puzzle. Production Designer: Fright Night.
TELEVISION: Art Director: Frank Sinatra Special—Old Blue Eyes Is Back, Annual Academy Awards Presentation 1971.

DEE, RUBY: Actress. b. Cleveland, Oct. 27, 1924. m., Ossie Davis. e. Hunter Coll. Stage appearances include Jeb, Raisin in the Sun, Purlie Victorious, Wedding Band, etc.
PICTURES: Jackie Robinson Story, Take a Giant Step, St. Louis Blues, Raisin in the Sun, Purlie Victorious, Buck and the Preacher.
TELEVISION: The Atlanta Child Murders.

DEE, SANDRA: Actress. b. Bayonne, N.J., April 23, 1942. Modeled, Harry Conover and Huntington Hartford Agencies, N.Y., 1954–56; signed long term exclusive contract, U-I, 1957.
PICTURES INCLUDE: Until They Sail, The Restless Years, Stranger in My Arms, The Reluctant Debutante, Gidget, The Wild and the Innocent, Imitation of Life, Summer Place, Portrait in Black, Romanoff and Juliet, Come September, Tammy Tell Me True, If a Man Answers, Tammy and the Doctor, Take Her, She Is Mine, I'd Rather Be Rich, That Funny Feeling, Doctor You've Got to Be Kidding!, Rosie, The Dunwich Horror.

DEELEY, MICHAEL: Producer. b. London, England, 1932. Ent. m.p. ind. 1951 and TV, 1967, as alt. dir. Harlech Television Ltd. Film editor, 1951–58. MCA-TV 1958–61, later with Woodfall as prod. and assoc. prod. Proc. One Way Pendulum. Assoc. prod. The Knack, The White Bus, Ride of the Valkyrie, Prod. Robbery, The Italian Job. Executive prod. Long Days Dying, Where's Jack, Sleep Is Lovely, Murphy's War, Convoy, The Deer Hunter (AA), Blade Runner. Great Western Investments Ltd.; 1972; Great Western Festivals Ltd.; 1973, man. dir. British Lion Films Ltd. 1975, purchased BLF, Ltd. Appt. Jnt. man. dir. EMI Films Ltd., 1977; pres., EMI Films, 1978, Member Film Industry Interim Action Committee, 1977–82.

DE GRUNWALD, DIMITRI: Producer. Managing director Script Development Ltd. de Grunwald Films Ltd. and Films include: That Lucky Touch, The Millionairess, Shalako, Stranger in the House, The McMasters, Murphy's War, The Virgin and the Gypsy, Time for Loving, Perfect Friday.

DE HAVILLAND, OLIVIA: Actress b. Tokyo, Japan, July 1, 1916. e. California schools and Notre Dame Convent, Belmont. Acting debut, Max Reinhardt's stage prod., Midsummer Night's Dream; film debut in m.p. version, 1935; won Academy Award twice, best actress performance in To Each His Own, 1946, and The Heiress, 1949; N.Y. Film Critics award twice, 1948-49; Women's Natl. Press Club Award, 1949; Look award, best perf. 3 times, 1941-48-49.

PICTURES INCLUDE: Anthony Adverse, Gone With the Wind, Strawberry Blonde, Hold Back the Dawn, Princess O'Rourke, Dark Mirror, Snake Pit, My Cousin Rachel, Not as a Stranger, Ambassador's Daughter, Proud Rebel, Libel, Light in the Piazza, The Adventurers, Pope Joan, Airport '77, The Swarm.

STAGE: Romeo and Juliet, 1951; U.S. tour Candida, 1951-52, N.Y., 1952; A Gift of Time, Bdwy. 1962.

TV: Noon Wine for Stage 67. Mini-Series: North & South Book II.

DEIN, EDWARD: Director-Writer. b. Chicago, Ill.

PICTURES INCLUDE: Dir., s.p. Shack Out on 101, Seven Guns to Sin, Curse of the Undead, Calypso Joe, I Trust My Wife, Hard Yellow, Come Die My Love (Spain), The Naked Sword (Mexico), Gaby (Brazil); story s.p. The Fighting Guardsman, Calling Dr. Death, The Gallant Blade, Leopard Man, All this and More, 13 French Street, Hang Me High; dir., prod., wrote, Capito, in Italy.

TV: Lawless Years, Hawaiian Eye, Bronco, Philip Marlowe, Not for Hire, Wild, Wild West series.

DE LANE LEA, JACQUES: Executive. b. Nice, France, 1931. Early career as prod. shorts, second features; later prod. sup. features. Ent. m.p. ind. 1952, prod. own films. Became man. dir. De Lane Lea Ltd., after death his father 1964. Also dir. Delmore Film Productions Ltd., Mole-Richardson (England) Ltd., Humphries Holdings, Ltd., Int'l Library Service Ltd., CTS Ltd. Pres., dir. gen., SIS (1982).

DELANNOY, JEAN: Director. b. Noisy-le-Dec, France, Jan. 12, 1908; e. Universite de Paris, Lycee Montaigne, Lycee Louis le Grand, La Sorbonne; actor, 1927-29; film edit., 1929-37; dir., 1937-52.

PICTURES INCLUDE: Black Diamond, The Eternal Return, Symphonie Pastorale, The Chips Are Down, Souvenir, The Secret of Mayerling, Savage Triangle, Moment of Truth, Daughter of Destiny, The Bed.

DE LAURENTIIS, DINO: Producer. b. Torre Annunziata, Italy, Aug. 8, 1919. Took part in Rome Experimental Film Center; dir., prod. Chairman of the Board and CEO, De Laurentiis Entertainment Group Inc.; founded in 1984 the DEG Film Studios in Wilmington, NC.

PICTURES INCLUDE: L'amore Canta, Il Bandito, La Figlia del Capitano, Riso Amaro, La Lupa, Anna, Ulysses, Mambo, La Strada, Gold of Naples, War and Peace, Nights of Cabiria, The Tempest, LaGrande Guerra, Five Branded Women, Barabbas, The Bible, Operation Paradise, The Witches, The Stranger, Diabolik, Anzio, Barbarella, Waterloo, Valachi Papers, Stone Killers, Serpico, Death Wish, Casanova, Mandingo, Three Days of the Condor, Drum, Face to Face, Buffalo Bill and the Indians, King Kong, The Shootist, Orca, White Buffalo, Serpent's Egg, King of the Gypsies, The Brink's Job, Hurricane, Flash Gordon, Halloween II, Ragtime, Conan the Barbarian, Fighting Back, Amityville II: The Possession, Halloween III, The Dead Zone, Amityville 3-D, Firestarter, The Bounty, Conan the Destroyer, Stephen King's Cat's Eye, Red Sonja, Year of the Dragon, Marie, Silver Bullett, Raw Deal, Maximum Overdrive, Tai-Pan, Blue Velvet, the Bedroom Window, Crimes of the Heart, King Kong Lives.

DE LA VARRE, ANDRE, JR.: Producer-Director. b. Vienna, Austria, Oct. 26, 1934. Prod. "Grand Tour" Travelogues; producer of promotion films for KLM, Swissair, tourist offices, recent productions: Bicentennial films for State of Virginia, City of Charleston, NY State; winner, Atlanta Film Festival, Sunset Travel Film Festival; Burton Holmes Travelogue subjects; V-P-R Educational Films; producer, director, lecturer, narrator.

del VALLE, JOHN: Publicist. b. San Francisco, Calif., Mar. 23, 1904; e. U. California. Adv., edit. staff various newspapers including asst. drama ed. S.F. Call-Bulletin, L.A. Mirror; adv.-publicity dir. San Francisco Fox Theatre 1933-36; publicist, Paramount Studio, 1936g, Orca, The Serpent's Egg, The Brinks Job, King of the Gypsies, Hurricane, Flash Gordon, Ragtime, Conan the Barbarian, Fighting Back, The Dead Zone, The Bounty, Firestarter, Conan the Destroyer, Dune, Cat's Eye, Red Sonja, Year of the Dragon, Marie.

DE LA VARRE, ANDRE, JR.: Producer-Director. b. Vienna, Austria, Oct. 26, 1934. Prod. "Grand Tour" Travelogues; producer of promotion films for KLM, Swissair, tourist offices, recent productions: Bicentennial films for State of Virginia, City of Charleston, NY State; winner, Atlanta Film Festival, Sunset Travel Film Festival; Burton Holmes Travelogue subjects; V-P-R Educational Films; producer, director, lecturer, narrator.

del VALLE, JOHN: Publicist. b. San Francisco, Calif., Mar. 23, 1904; e. U. California. Adv., edit. staff various newspapers including asst. drama ed. S.F. Call-Bulletin, L.A. Mirror; adv.-publicity dir. San Francisco Fox Theatre 1933-36; publicist, Paramount Studio, 1936-42; dir. pub., adv. Arnold Prod. 1946; Chaplin Studios, 1947; Nat Holt Prod., 1948-52; Editor, TV Family mag., N.Y., 1952-53; adv. pub. dir. Century Films, 1954; pub. rel. Academy M.P. Arts & Sciences, 1965; publicist, various U.A. indep. film prod., 1955-56; unit publicist, Para., 1956; TC-F 1957-62, Para., 1962-63; Universal 1964-65; Mirisch Corp.—UA Filming, "Hawaii," 1965; pub. re. and editor, Atomics Int'l div. North American Rockwell, 1966-71; present, free-lance writer residing Westlake Village, CA.

DEL BELSO, RICHARD: Executive. e. New York Univ. (1965). Began career in adv./research dept. at Benton & Bowles. Served as research dept. group head for Kenyon and Eckhart; group head for Gruden/Appell/Haley Research Co. (now known as A/H/F/ Marketing Research, Inc.). Two years as assoc. dir. of mktg., research for Grey Advertising (N.Y.). Joined MCA/Universal in 1977 as assoc. dir., mktg. research. In 1980 named v.p. & dir. of mktg. research for Warner Bros.

DELERUE, GEORGES: Composer-Conductor. b. Roubaix, France, 1924. Studied with Busser and Milhaud at Paris Cons. Was conductor for RTF (Radio-TV Francais).

PICTURES INCLUDE: Hiroshima Mon Amour, King of Hearts, Shoot the Pianist, Jules and Jim, Silken Skin, The Pumpkin Eater, Viva Maria, The 25th Hour, Interlude, The Day of the Jackal, The Day of the Dolphin, A Little Romance, True Confessions, Rich and Famous, A Little Sex, Partners, The Escape Artist, Man, Woman and Child, The Black Stallion Returns, Exposed, Silkwood, Maxie, Salvador.

TELEVISION: Aurora, Arch of Triumph.

DELFONT, BERNARD LORD: Chairman, Chief Executive First Leisure Corporation PLC. b. Tokmak, Russia, September 5, 1909. e. London, England. Dir. more than 30 companies incl. Delfont Productions. Ent. theatrical management 1941. Since presented over 250 shows in London; pantomimes in provinces and seaside shows; presented annual Royal Variety Performance. Controls Prince of Wales Theatre in London's West End. 1969: Chief Barker (Pres.) Variety Club of Great Britain; Companion of the Grand Order of Water Rats, President of Entertainment. Artistes' Benevolent Fund, member of Saints and Sinners organisation.

DELMAINE, BARRY: Writer, director. b. London. Began motion picture career as extra. Later roles in comedies; then asst. dir. for Gloria Swanson prod. in England. From 1936-39 wrote sketches, lyrics London stage musicals; radio scripts. In 1939 apptd. chief scenarist Gaumont-British Instructional. In 1941 dir. films for Brit. Ministry of Information; 1942-43 scenarist, Brit. War Office mi. training films. In 1944 author & dir. Here We Come Gathering, J. Arthur Rank experimental film for child audiences. In 1946 joined Film Producers Guild, writer, dir.; 1949-50, dir. Concord Productions, Ltd., freelance writer films, radio, TV; s.p. Heir Conditioned; dir. ind. films, Concord Prod. Ltd., ass't dir. Advance Films; The Great Game, Les Parent Terrible (Eng. version), Is Your Honeymoon Really Necessary? Unit dir. Don't Blame the Stork; Unit dir., loc. mgr. Douglas Fairbanks Ltd.; prod. mgr. 1955; prod. mgr. Chase a Crooked Shadow, Ice Cold in Alex, Jetstream; prod. sup. The Night We Dropped a Clanger. Prod. Sup., Nothing Barred; prod. mgr., The Hellions; prod. The Golden Rabbit; prog. sup., Man of The World, Sentimental Agent, assoc. prod., Danger Man (secret agent) series. Assoc. prod., Man in the Suitcase series; Assoc. prod., Strange Report series; assoc. prod. Mr. Jerico feature. TV series: assoc. prod. The Firechasers; prod. Shirley's World; assoc. prod. The Adventurers. Assoc. prod., Three For All. Currently: Freelance Writer and Prod. Consultant.

DELON, ALAIN: Actor. b. Sceaux, France, Nov. 8, 1935. Discovered by Yves Allgret. Served in French Navy as a Marine. Worked as cafe waiter, heavy-load carrier.

PICTURES INCLUDE: When a Woman Gets Involved, Be Beautiful, and Keep Quiet, Plein Soleil and Quelle Joie de Vivre, Rocco and His Brothers, L'Eclipse, The Leopard, The Big Crab, The Black Tulip, The Felines, The Yellow Rolls Royce, The Killers of San Francisco, The Centurions, Is Paris Burning?, Texas, Here We Come, The Adventurers, Extraordinary Stories, Le Samourai, Diaboliquement Votre, The Motorcycle, Goodbye Friend, The Swimming Pool, Jeff, The Sicilian Clan, Borsalino, Red Sun, Assassination of Trotsky, Scorpio, Dirty Money, Mr. Klein, The Concord-Airport '79, Swann in Love.

Del ROSSI, PAUL R.: Executive. b. Winchester, MA Oct. 19, 1942. e. Harvard Coll. (1964); Harvard Business School (1967). Sr. v.p., The Boston Co., 1977–1980; sr. consultant, Arthur D. Little, Inc.; presently pres., General Cinema Theatres.

DeLUISE, DOM: Comedian-Actor. b. Brooklyn, Aug. 1, 1933. e. Tufts Coll. Spent two seasons with Cleveland Playhouse. Launched TV career on The Garry Moore Show with character, Dominick the Great, a bumbling magician.
PICTURES INCLUDE: Fail Safe, The Busybody, The Glass Bottom Boat, 12 Chairs, Who Is Harry Kellerman?, Every Little Crook and Nanny, The Adventures of Sherlock Holmes' Smarter Brother, Silent Movie, The World's Greatest Lover, The End, The Cheap Detective, The Last Married Couple in America, Fatso, Wholly Moses, Smokey and the Bandit II, History of the World—Part I, The Cannonball Run, The Best Little Whorehouse in Texas, Cannonball Run II, Johnny Dangerously, Haunted Honeymoon.
TELEVISION: The Entertainers, The Dean Martin Summer Show, Dom DeLuise Variety Show, The Barrum-Bump Show, The Dean Martin Show, The Tonight Show, Lotsa Luck. Movie: Happy (also exec. prod.).
STAGE: The Student Gypsy, Last of the Red Hot Lovers, Here's Love.

DEMBY, EMANUEL H.: Producer, writer. b. New York, N.Y., Dec. 12, 1919. e. C.C.N.Y., New School. Chung Ang University (Ph.D.). Pioneered new programs for radio, 1936–47; story dept., Universal Pictures, 1937; writer, Gangbusters, Crime of the Week, Thrill of the Week (NBC, CBS); TV shows; What's Playing, 1950–52; Hollywood to Broadway, currently in TV syndication, How To Be a Cowboy; The Shadow; prod., theatrical features, filmed commercials; pub. rel. consultant. Author: My Forty Year Fight for Korea; Indonesia; King of The Hill; Hot Tip on Wall St.; prod. Cavalcade of Music (TV); The World in Space (TV, theatrical); The Edge of Violence (stage); Man Into Space; Year III-Space Age (TV); The Communications Gap, The Creative Consumer, (P.R. films). Book: Who's Alienated, Youth or Society? Research Consultant, NBC TV News; consultant, Radio Advertising Bureau, Smash, Crash, Pow! (feature).

DEMME, JONATHAN: Director-Writer. b. Rockville Center, N.Y., 1944. e. Univ. of Florida. First job in industry as usher; was film critic for college paper, The Florida Alligator. Did publicity work for United Artists, Avco Embassy, Pathe Contemporary Films; wrote for trade publication, Film Daily, 1966–68. Moved to England in 1969; served as musical co-ordinator on Irving Allen's EyeWitness in 1970. In 1972 produced and co-wrote first film, Angels, Hard As they Come.
PICTURES: Hot Box (prod., co-writer); Caged Heat (writer-dir.); Crazy Mama (writer-dir.); Fighting Mad (writer-dir.), Citizen's Band (dir.), Last Embrace (dir.), Melvin and Howard (dir.), Swing Shift (dir.), Stop Making Sense (dir.), Something Wild (co-prod., dir.).

De MORNAY, REBECCA: Actress. b. California, 1963, but spent childhood in Europe, graduating at high school in Austria. Returned to America, enrolling at Lee Strasberg's Los Angeles Institute; apprenticed at Zoetrope Studios. Motion picture theatrical debut in Risky Business (1983).
PICTURES: Testament, The Slugger's Wife, Runaway Train, The Trip to Bountiful.

DEMOSS, LYLE: Executive. b. Anthony Kansas, Sept. 14, 1907; e. York Coll. and U. of Nebraska School of Music; 1925. KGBZ in York, Nebr.; 1928. KFAB in Lincoln, Nebr.; in 1932 became Prog. Mgr. of KFAB-KFOR; held same position for WOW from 1936 to 1946; asst. gen. mgr. Meredith WOW, 1946–59. Allen & Reynolds v.p. radio-TV dept. Omaha Advertising Club, Variety Club Canvasman, past pres. Omaha Ad. Club. Radio KLNG, 1965–67; freelance TV; Elected to Nebr. Broadcasters Hall of Fame—1972; KYNN-community relations director.

DENBAUM, DREW: Director-Screenwriter. b. New York, Dec. 12, 1949. e. The Lawrenceville School, 1967; Yale Univ., 1971; NYU grad. Institute of Film & TV, 1973–75, assistant to visiting directors Frank Perry and Gilbert Cates. Represented by William Morris Agency.
PICTURES INCLUDE (Writer-Director): Nickel Mountain (based on novel by John Gardner); Lovesick (dramatic short); The Last Straw (dramatic short based on play by Charles Dizenzo).
AWARDS INCLUDE: First Prize, 20th Century Fox Screenwriting Competition (Caught In the Act); Silver Medal, Chicago Film Festival (Lovesick); Academy Award Finalist (Lovesick); Leo Jaffe Producer's Award (NYU Grad. Inst. of Film & TV); Saybrook Fellows Prize (Yale Univ.); American Legion Award (1964). Lovesick and The Last Straw featured in Cineprobe Series, New York Museum of Modern Art.

DENCH, JUDI: O.B.E. Actress. b. York, England, 1934. Studied for stage at Central School of Speech and Drama. Theatre debut Old Vic, 1961. Recent Theatre: Cymbeline, Juno and the Paycock, A Kind of Alaska, Importance of Being Earnest, Pack of Lies.
TELEVISION: Major Barbara, Pink String and Sealing Wax, Talking to a Stranger, The Funambulists, Age of Kings, Jackanory, Hilda Lessways, Luther, Neighbours, Parade's End, Marching Song, On Approval, Days to Come, Emilie, The Comedy of Errors, Macbeth (both RSC productions), Langrishe Go Down, On Giant's Shoulders, Love in a Cold Climate, Village Wooing, A Fine Romance (series), The Cherry Orchard, Going Gently, Saigon, Year of the Cat, Ghosts..
PICTURES: He Who Rides a Tiger, Study in Terror, Four in the Morning, A Midsummer Night's Dream (RSC Production), The Third Secret, Dead Cert, Wetherby, A Room with a View.

DENEAU, SIDNEY, G.: Sales executive. Head film buyer Fabian Theatres; U.S. Army 1942–46; gen. mgr. Schine Theatres 1947; v.p., gen. sales mgr., Selznick Releasing Orgn., 1949; 1956; v.p. asst. gen. sls. mgr., Para. Film Dist., 1958; exec. v.p., Rugoff Theatres, 1964. Resigned, September, 1969 to engage in own theatre consultant business.

DENEUVE, CATHERINE: Actress. b. 1945. r.n. Catherine Dorleac. Sister was the late Francoise Dorleac.
PICTURES INCLUDE: The Doors Slam, Vice and Virtue, Satan Leads the Dance, Umbrellas of Cherbourg, (received the French Film Academy's best actress award); Repulsion, Le Chant du Monde, La Vie de Chateau, Les Creatures, The Young Girls of Rochefort, Belle de Jour, Benjamin, Manon 70, Mayerling, La Chamade, April Fools, Mississippi Mermaid, Tristana, It Only Happens to Others, Dirty Money, Hustle, March or Die, The Last Metro, The Hunger, Fort Saganne.

DENHAM, MAURICE: Actor. b. Beckenham, Kent, Eng., Dec. 23, 1909. e. Tonbridge School. Started theatrical career with repertory com. 1934. Served in World War II and since demobilization played in numerous plays, films & radio shows.
PICTURES INCLUDE: Blanche Fury, London Belongs To Me, It's Not Cricket, Traveller's Joy, Landfall, Spider and the Fly, No Highway in the Sky, The Net, Time Bomb, Street Corner (Both Sides of the Law), Million Pound Note (Man With a Million), Eight O'Clock Walk, Purple Plain, Simon and Laura, 23 Paces to Baker Street, Checkpoint, Carrington V.C. (Court Martial), Doctor at Sea, Night of the Demon, Man With a Dog, Barnacle Bill, The Captain's Table, Our Man in Havana, Sink the Bismark, Two-Way Stretch, Greengage Summer, Invasion, Quartette, The Mark, HMS Defiant.
TV: appearances include: Uncle Harry, Day of the Monkey, Miss Mabel, Angel Pavement, The Paraguayan Harp, The Wild Bird, Soldier Soldier, Changing Values, Maigret, The Assassins, Saturday Spectacular, Vanishing Act, A Chance in Life, Virtue, Somerset Maugham, Three of A Kind, Sapper, Pig In The Middle, Their Obedient Servants, Long Past Glory, Devil in The Wind, Any Other Business, The Retired Colourman, Sherlock Holmes (series), Blackmail, Knock on Any Door, Danger Man, Dr. Finley's Casebook, How To Get Rid of Your Husband, Talking To a Stranger, A Slight Ache, From Chekhov With Love, Home Sweet Honeycomb, St. Joan, Julius Caesar, Golden Days, Marshall Petain, The Lotus Eaters, Fall of Eagles, Carnforth Practice. The Unofficial Rose, Omnibus, Balzac, Loves Labour Lost, Angels, Huggy Bear, The Portrait, The Crumbles Murder, A Chink In The Wall, Porridge, For God's Sake, Bosch, Marie Curie, Upchat Line, Secret Army, My Son, My Son, Edward and Mrs. Simpson, Gate of Eden, Potting Shed, Double Dealer, Minder, Agatha Christie Hour, Chinese Detective, The Old Men at the Zoo, The Hope and the Glory, Luther, Love Song, Mr. Palfrey, The Black Tower, Boon.
OTHER PICTURES: The Very Edge, Paranoiac, The Set Up, Penang, The Kings Breakfast, Downfall, Hysteria, The Uncle, Operation Crossbow, Legend of Dick Turpin, The Alphabet Murders, The Night Callers, The Nanny, Those Magnificent Men in Their Flying Machines, Heroes of Telemark, After the Fox, The Torture Garden, The Long Duel, The Eliminator, Danger Route, Attack on the Iron Coast, The Best House in London, Negatives, The Midas Run, Some Girls Do, The Touch of Love, The Virgin and the Gypsy, Bloody Sunday, Countess Dracula, Nicholas and Alexandra, The Day of the Jackal, Luther, Shout at the Devil, Julia, The Recluse, From a Far Country, Mr. Love, The Chain, Monsignor Quixote, Murder on the Orient Express, 84 Charing Cross Road.

De NIRO, ROBERT: Actor. b. New York City, Aug. 17, 1943. Studied acting with Stella Adler and Lee Strasberg. In off-Broadway productions and touring shows.
PICTURES INCLUDE: The Wedding Party, Jennifer on My Mind, Bloody Mama, Born To Win, The Gang That Couldn't Shoot Straight, Bang the Drum Slowly, Mean Streets, Godfather II, Taxi Driver, 1900, The Last Tycoon, New York, New York, The Deer Hunter, Raging Bull, True

Confessions, The King of Comedy, Once Upon a Time in America, Falling in Love, Brazil, The Mission, Angel Heart.

DENISON, MICHAEL: Actor. b. Doncaster, York, Eng., Nov. 1, 1915; e. Harrow & Magdalen Coll., Oxford and Webber Douglas Sch.; m. Dulcie Gray, prof. Served overseas, Capt. Intelligence Corps, 1940–46. On stage first, 1938, Charlie's Aunt. Screen debut 1940, Tilly of Bloomsbury.
THEATRE: 47 London plays including Ever Since Paradise, Rain on the Just, Queen Elizabeth Slept Here, Fourposter, Dragon's Mouth, Bad Samaritan; Shakespeare Season Stratford-on-Avon; Edinburgh Festival. Meet Me By Moonlight, Let Them Eat Cake, Candida, Heartbreak House, My Fair Lady (Australia), Where Angels Fear to Tread, Hostile Witness, An Ideal Husband, On Approval, Happy Family, No. 10, Out of the Question, Trio, The Wild Duck, The Clandestine Marriage, The Dragon Variation, At the End of the Day, The Sack Race, Peter Pan, The Black Mikado, The First Mrs. Fraser, The Earl and the Pussycat, Robert and Elizabeth, The Cabinet Minister, Old Vic Season: Twelfth Night, Lady's Not for Burning, Ivanov, Bedroom Farce, The Kingfisher, Relatively Speaking, Coat of Varnish, Capt. Brassbound's Conversion, School for Scandal, Song at Twlight, See How They Run, The Tempest, Ring Round the Moon, The Apple Cart.
PICTURES INCLUDE: Hungry Hill, My Brother Jonathan, The Blind Goddess, The Glass Mountain, Landfall, The Franchise Affair, Angels One Five, Tall Headlines, Importance of Being Earnest, There Was a Young Lady, Contraband Spain, The Truth About Women, Faces in the Dark.
TV: Boyd QC Series, Funeral Games, Unexpectedly Vacant, Tale of Piccadilly. 1973: The Twelve Pound Look, The Provincial Lady, Subject: This Is Your Life, 1977, Bedroom Farce, Private Schultz, Blood Money, The Critic, Scorpion, Cold Warrior, Good Behavior.

DENNEHY, BRIAN: Actor. b. Bridgeport, CT. e. Columbia Univ. In Marine Corps five years, including Vietnam. After discharge in 1965 studied with acting coaches in N.Y., while working at part time jobs. Cast by Michael Ritchie in Semi-Tough, 1977.
PICTURES: 10, Split Image, First Blood, Never Cry Wolf, Gorky Park, River Rat, Cocoon, Silverado, The Check Is in the Mail, F/X, Twice in a Lifetime, Legal Eagles.
TELEVISION: Films: The Jericho Mile, Dummy, The Seduction of Miss Leona, Acceptable Risks, etc. Series: Big Shamus, Little Shamus, Star of the Family.

DENNIS, SANDY: Actress. b. Hastings, Nebraska, April 27, 1937. m. Gerry Mulligan. Joined the Lincoln Community Theatre group. Made her professional acting debut in summer stock at London, N.H. Studied with Herbert Berghof, N.Y. Understudy for N.Y. prod. Dark at the Top of the Stairs. Broadway debut in Any Wednesday (Antoinette Perry Award), then A Thousand Clowns (Tony Award for best supporting actress).
PICTURES INCLUDE: Who's Afraid of Virginia Wolf? (won an Academy Award as best supporting actress), Up the Down Staircase, Sweet November, The Fox, Thank You All Very Much, That Cold Day in the Park, The Out-of-Towners, Nasty Habits, The Four Seasons.

DE NORMAND, GEORGE: Actor, director. b. New York, N.Y., Sept. 22. Actor many westerns & TV series; dir., TV series, Man of Tomorrow. Member: SAG, SEG, NSTP.

DENVER, BOB: Actor. b. New Rochelle, NY, 1935.
PICTURES INCLUDE: Take Her She's Mine, For Those Who Think Young, Who's Minding the Mint? The Sweet Ride, Do You Know the One About the Travelling Saleslady?
TELEVISION: Dobie Gillis, Gilligan's Island, Dusty's Trail, The Castaways on Gilligan's Island.

DE PALMA, BRIAN: Director. b. Newark, N.J., 1940. e. Columbia Univ. (B.A.) and Sarah Lawrence (M.A.). While in college made series of shorts, including Wotan's Wake, winner of Rosenthal Foundation Award for best film made by American under 25. Also judged most popular film of Midwest Film Festival (1963); later shown at San Francisco Film Festival.
PICTURES INCLUDE: The Wedding Party, Murder a La Mod, Greetings, Hi Mom, Dionysus in '69, Get To Know Your Rabbit, Sisters, Phantom of the Paradise, Obsession, Carrie, The Fury, Home Movies, Dressed to Kill, Blow Out, Scarface, Body Double (prod.-dir., s.p.), Wiseguys (dir.).

DEPARDIEU, GERARD: Actor. b. Chateuaroux, France, Dec. 27, 1948. Studied acting at Theatre National Populaire in Paris. Made film debut at 16 in short by Roger Leenhardt (Le Beatnik et Le Minet). Acted in feature film by Agnes Varda which was never finished.
PICTURES INCLUDE: Going Places, Stavisky, 1900, Get Your Handkerchiefs, LouLou, The Last Metro, Mon Oncle d'Amerique, The Moon in the Gutter, Fort Saganne, Police, A Woman or Two, Tenue de Soiree (Evening Dress).

DEPEW, RICHARD H.: Executive. b. New York, N.Y., Jan. 16, 1925. e. Princeton U. U.S. Navy; American Broadcasting Co., 1947; television director, 1950; assistant, Eastern TV network program director, 1953; mgr. of TV network program oper., 1954–57; Cunningham & Walsh; Radio & TV acct. supv. & programming coordinator, 1961–65 v.p. & dir. of TV programming; 1965 Broadcast supr., Ogilvy and Mather; 1967, v.p. dir. TV programing Fuller & Smith & Ross. V.P. Media and Programming 1969, FS&R.; 1973, Director of Corporate Underwriting Department WNET/13, Educational Broadcasting Corp. 1977 Management Supervisor, J. Walter Thompson, N.Y.C.; 1978, v.p., Account Director, 1980, Marsteller, Inc., mgt. supvr., v.p., corporate adv., Doremus & Co., 1983; exec. v.p., Knox Minisk & Harwood, Stowe, VT.

DEREK, BO: Actress. b. Torrance, CA., Nov. 20, 1956. r.n. Cathleen Collins. Discovered by John Derek, actor turned film producer, who changed her first name to Bo, now married to him. Film debut in "10" in 1979.
PICTURES INCLUDE: Change of Seasons, Tarzan, the Ape Man, Bolero.

DEREK, JOHN: Actor-Producer-Director. b. Hollywood, CA, August 12, 1926. Acting debut in 1945 in I'll Be Seeing You; appeared in numerous films throughought 1950s. In 1963 produced and directed first film, Nightmare in the Sun, followed by Once Before I Die in 1965.
PICTURES: Actor: Knock on Any Door, All the King's Men, Mask of the Avenger, Scandal Sheet, Mission Over Korea, The Adventures of Hajji Baba, Prince of Players, Run for Cover, The Leather Saint, The Ten Commandments, Omar Khayyam, Prisoner of the Volga, Exodus, etc. Producer-Director: A Boy . . . a Girl (also s.p. & cinematographer); Childish Things, Once Upon a Time, Tarzan, The Ape Man (1981; dir. only).

DERN, BRUCE: Actor. b. Chicago, Ill., 1937. e. University of Pennsylvania. Studied acting with Gordon Phillips, member, Actor's Studio, 1959 after N.Y. debut in Shadow of a Gunman.
PICTURES: The Trip, The Wild Angels, Hush, Hush, Sweet Charlotte, Support Your Local Sheriff, Thumb-tripping, Drive, He Said; They Shoot Horses, Don't They?; The Cowboys, Silent Running, Sweet Bird of Youth (Stage), Orpheus Descending (Stage), The King of Marvin Gardens, The Laughing Policeman, The Great Gatsby, Smile, Posse, Family Plot, Won Ton Ton, Black Sunday, Coming Home, The Driver, Middle Age Crazy, Tattoo, That Championship Season, On the Edge.
TELEVISION: Space, Toughlove.

DERN, LAURA: Actress. b. 1968. Daughter of Diane Ladd & Bruce Dern. Film debut at age 11 in Foxes (1980).
PICTURES: Mask, Smooth Talk, Blue Velvet.

DE SANTIS, GIUSEPPE: Director. b. Italy, 1917. Film publicists; asst. dir.
PICTURES INCLUDE: Tragic Hunt, Bitter Rice, Under the Olive Tree, Rome 11 O'Clock, A Husband for Anna Zaccheo, Days of Love.

DE SCHAAP, PHILIP: Dutch correspondent, Quigley Publications, N.Y. b. Amsterdam, Holland, May 26, 1911. Entered m.p. ind. 1934 as publicity mgr., MGM br. office, Amsterdam; in 1936 corresp. for Quigley Publications. Also in 1937 exploitation mgr., RKO Radio Pictures, Amsterdam; to Paris 1938 as spec. publicity repr. in Paris and Brussels, RKO: in 1939 org. own co. for exploitation and publicity; non-active 1940–45; on Oct. 1, 1945 estab. Phidesa Publiciteitsbureau voor de Filmbranche.

DESCHANEL, CALEB: Director-Cinematographer. b. Philadelphia, Sept. 21, 1941. e. Johns Hopkins Univ.; South Calif. Film School.
PICTURES: Cinematographer: More American Graffiti, Being There, The Black Stallion, The Right Stuff, The Natural, The Slugger's Wife. Director: The Escape Artist

DE TITTA ARTHUR A.: Newsreel editor. b. North Bergen, N.J., July 9, 1904. Began work 1916 in employ newspaper in Union City, N.J.; joined Fox Film Corp., N.Y. office & lab. staff; later became asst. & second cameraman, performing in that capacity numerous pictures Fox and other produs. (The Mountain Woman, When Knighthood Was in Flower, The Royale Girl, East Side, West Side, Untamed, etc.). In 1928 joined Movietonnews, Inc.; Wash. (D.C.) suprv. to 1938; asst. Europ. supvr. to 1940; Pacific Coast supvr. to 1943. Commis. Lt. USNR, assigned to M.P. Sect., 1943; ret. 1944. Appt. news ed. Movietonews; west coast superv., 1951–63; pub. rel., prod., documentaries; West Coast Bureau mgr. for foreign editions of Movietone News, now retired.

DE TOTH, ANDRE: Writer-Director-Producer. b. Hungary. Dr.-writer European films, 1931–39; U.S. assoc. Alexander Korda prod., 1940; dir. Columbia, 1943; assoc. David Selznick, 1943; assoc. Hunt Stromberg-UA, 1944–45; staff dir., Enterprise 1946–47; dir., 20th-Fox, 1948–49; collab. story, The Gunfighter; dir., Columbia & Warner Bros., 1951; contract dir., Warner Bros., 1952; U.A. Columbia, W.B., 1953–55; Palladiums U.A., Denmark, 1956; Col. U.A. 1957;

Columbia, 1960; assoc., Sam Spiegel, Horizon Pictures, Columbia, 1962; Harry Saltzman, Lowndes Prod., U.A. 1966–68; National General, 1969–70.
PICTURES INCLUDE: Passport to Suez, None Shall Escape, Since You Went Away, Pitfall, Springfield Rifle, Thunder Over the Plains, House of Wax, Bounty Hunter, Tanganyika, Indian Fighter, Monkey on My Back, Two Headed Spy, Man on a String, Morgan, The Pirate, The Mongols, Gold for the Caesars, Billion Dollar Brain, Play Dirty, El Condor.

DEUTCHMAN, IRA J.: Executive. b. Cherry Point, NC Mar. 24, 1953. e. Northwestern Univ. (BS, majoring in film). Began career with Cinema 5, Ltd. serving, 1975–79, as non-theatrical sls. mgr.; dir. theatrical adv./pub./dir. acquisitions. Joined United Artists Classics, 1981 as dir. of adv./pub. 1982, left to become one of the founding partners in Cinecom Intl. Films, where headed mktg./dist. div. from inception. On bd. of advisors for Independent Feature Project-West, the Sundance Institute and the U.S. Film Festival.

DEUTSCH, ARMAND S.: Producer. b. Chicago, Ill., Jan. 25, 1913. e. U. of Chicago, 1935; B.A. Producer, MGM.
PICTURES INCLUDE: Ambush, Right Cross, Magnificent Yankee, Three Guys Named Mike, Kind Lady, Girl in White, Carbine Williams, Girl Who Had Everything, Green Fire, Slander.

DEUTSCH, DAVID: Producer-Writer. b. Birmingham, England, January 10, 1926. e. in Birmingham and Queen Mary College, London Univ. Ent. m.p. ind. apprentice at Gainsborough Pictures, Ltd., 1949; asst. Sydney Box, 1954; J. Arthur Rank asst. to prod. 1955 Lost; assoc. prod. High Tide at Noon, The One That Got Away, Floods of Fear; prod. Blind Date; Anglo Amalgamated Film Dist. Ltd., as exec. in chrg. prod., 1960. Prod., Play It Cool, 1962, Nothing But the Best. 1963: Domino Prods. Ltd., Catch Us If You Can, 1965; Interlude, 1967; Lock Up Your Daughter, 1968. A Day in the Death of Joe Egg, 1970. Co-prod. The Day of the Jackal, 1972; s.p., The Blue Train, The Jacaranda Tree; 1982: Prod. Shakespeare, The Round House Workshops for Channel 4 TV.

DEUTSCH, HELEN: Writer. b. New York, N.Y. e. Barnard Coll., B.A. Author: The Provincetown.
PICTURES INCLUDE: Seventh Cross, National Velvet, King Solomon's Mines, Golden Earrings, Kim, Plymouth Adventure, Lili, The Glass Slipper, I'll Cry Tomorrow, Forever Darling.
TV: Jack and the Beanstalk, NBC Gen. Motors 50th Anniv. Show, 1957; book of Broadway musical, Carnival, 1961.

DEVANE, WILLIAM: Actor. b. New York City, Sept. 5, 1937. Appeared in some 15 productions with N.Y. Shakespeare Festival and off-Bdwy. shows before heading for California and films and TV. Has own theatre, Actors for Themselves, in Los Angeles. Has also directed plays.
PICTURES: Rolling Thunder, Marathon Man, Yanks, Honky Tonk Freeway, Testament.
TELEVISION: The Missiles of October, Fear on Trial, From Here to Eternity (series), Knot's Landing.

DE VITO, DANNY: Actor. b. Asbury Park, NJ, Nov. 17, 1944. e. Oratory Prep School. Married actress Rhea Perlman. Studied at American Academy of Dramatic Arts. On stage in Down the Morning Line, The Line of Least Existence, The Shrinking Bride, Call Me Charlie, Comedy of Errors, etc. Played role also in One Flew Over the Cuckoo's Nest which led to casting in the film version.
PICTURES : Goin' South, Lady Liberty, Scalawag, Hurry Up or I'll be 30, Terms of Endearment, Romancing the Stone, Johnny Dangerously, Head Office, Jewel of the Nile, Wiseguys, Ruthless People.
TELEVISION: Series: Taxi.

DEWHURST, COLLEEN: Actress. b. Montreal, Canada, June 3, 1926. Gained fame as stage actress, appearing in, among others, Mourning Becomes Electra, All Over, A Moon for the Misbegotten, More Stately Mansions, All the Way Home, The Ballad of the Sad Cafe, etc.
PICTURES: The Nun's Story, A Fine Madness, McQ, The Cowboys, The Last Run, Annie Hall, Ice Castles, When a Stranger Calls, Tribute, The Dead Zone, The Boy Who Could Fly.
TELEVISION: The Price, The Crucible, The Hands of Cormac Joyce, Jacob and Joseph, Studs Lonigan, The Kitty O'Neill Story, And Baby Makes Six, The Blue and the Gray, The Glitter Dome, A. D., Between Two Women, Johnny Bull.

DEWITT, JOYCE: Actress. b. Wheeling, W. Va., April 23, 1949. e. Ball State Univ. (B.A.), theatre. Performed in summer stock musical comedies (Damn Yankee, Li'l Abner, etc.). Worked at Indianapolis dinner theatres, directing, staging and starring in musical revues.
TELEVISION: Baretta, The Tony Randall Show, Most Wanted, Risko, Three's Company. Movie: With This Ring.

DEY, SUSAN: Actress. b. Pekin, IL, Dec. 10, 1952. Signed as magazine teen model at age 15. Made professional TV debut at 17, appearing in The Partridge Family, 1970–74.
TELEVISION: Series: Barnaby Jones, Hawaii Five-O, Switch, Loves Me, Loves Me Not, etc. Movies: Cage Without a Key, Terror on the Beach, Mary Jane Harper Cried Last Night, Little Women, The Comeback Kid, The Gift of Life, Sunset Limousine, Echo Park.
PICTURES: Skyjacked, First Love, Looker.

DE YOUNG, CLIFF: Actor. b. Inglewood, CA., Feb. 12, 1946. e. CA State Coll.; Illinois State Univ. On stage in Hair.
PICTURES: Sunshine, A Perfect Couple, Shock Treatment, Independence Day, The Hunger, Reckless, Protocol, Secret Admirer, F/X, Flight of the Navigator.
TELEVISION: Sticks and Bones, Centennial, Hunter's Mong, Scared Straight, Invasion of Privacy, Master of the Game, Deadly Intentions, etc.

DEZEL, ALBERT: Exhibitor. b. Russia, May 21, 1900; e. Chicago Acad. Fine Arts; also Art Inst. & Crane Coll., Chicago. Art work, theatre publicity, exploitation & Middle West. Org. Albert Dezel Roadshows, exploitation films, 1926; in 1945 owner, operator, Film Classics Franchise, Detroit, Cleveland, Cincinnati; in 1946 acquired rights in same territory for Screen Guild Products; operator, operator, Avon Art Theatre, South Bend; Cinema, Hamilton Theatre, Indianapolis; Guild Theatres, Detroit.

DIAMANT, LINCOLN: Executive. b. New York City, Jan. 25, 1923. e. Columbia College, AB cum Laude 1943; cofounder, Columbia University Radio Station. Advertising mgr., World Publ. Co.; writer-prod. CBS; prod.-dir., Blue Network (NBC); prom. dir., Book Find Club; creative dir., Ben Sackheim; group hd., McCann-Erickson; copy chief, DKG; Sr. TV prod., Ogilvy & Mather; TV prod. super., Grey Adv; founder, pres., Spots Alive, Inc., broadcast advertising consultants, 1969; author, The Broadcast Communications Dictionary, Anatomy of a Television Commercial, Television's Classic Commercials, contrib., to Effective Advertising, to Messages and Meaning; member, Broadcast Pioneers, Acad. TV Arts & Sciences; v.p. Broadcast Advertising Producer's Society of America. Adjunct faculty member, Pace College, Hofstra University. Fellow, Royal Society of Arts. President, Teatown Lake Reservation of Brooklyn Botanic Garden.

DIAMOND, BERNARD: Theatre Executive. b. Chicago, Jan. 24, 1918. e. Univ. of Indiana, Univ. of Minnesota. Except for military service was with Schine Theatre chain from 1940 to 1963, working up from ass't. mg., booker, buyer, dir. of personnel to gen. mgr. Then joined Loews Theatres; last position, exec. v.p. Retired, 1985.

DIAMOND, I.A.L.: Writer. b. Unghani, Roumania, June 27, 1920. r.n. Isidore Diamond. e. Col Univ. Came to US when 9 yrs. old. Hired as Junior writer by Paramount in 1941. Usually collaborates on scripts with other writers, particularly in recent years with Billy Wilder.
PICTURES INCLUDE: (All co-written except where indicated by (s) for solo) Murder in the Blue Room, Never Say Goodbye, Two Guys from Milwaukee, Two Guys from Texas, Always Together, The Girl from Jones Beach (s), It's a Great Feeling (s), Love Nest (s), Let's Make It Legal, Monkey Business, Something for the Birds, That Certain Feeling, Love in the Afternoon, Merry Andrew, Some Like It Hot, The Apartment, One, Two, Three, Irma La Douce, Kiss Me, Stupid, The Fortune Cookie, Cactus Flower (s), The Private Life of Sherlock Holmes, Forty Carats (s), Avantil, The Front Page, Fedora.

DIAMOND, NEIL: Singer-Songwriter. b. Brooklyn, NY, Jan. 24, 1941. Many concert tours and Bdwy. appearance in Dancin'.
PICTURES: Jonathan Livingston Seagull (music), Every Which Way But Loose (music), The Last Waltz (actor), The Jazz Singer (actor, music).

DICKINSON, ANGIE: Actress. b. Kulm, N.D. Sept. 30, 1931. Parochial Schools, Heart Coll., Glendale Coll., secretarial course. m. Burt Bacharach. Won a beauty contest.
PICTURES INCLUDE: Sins of Rachel Cade, Rio Bravo, Bramble Bush, Ocean's 11, Jessica, Capt. Newman, M.D., The Killers, The Art of Love, The Chase, The Last Challenge, Point Blank, Sam Whiskey, Young Billy Young, Pretty Maids All in a Row, The Outside Man, Dressed to Kill, Charlie Chan and the Curse of the Dragon Queen, Death Hunt.
TELEVISION: Movies: Jealousy, Hollywood Wives, A Touch of Scandal.

DICKINSON, ROBERT: Actor-Engineer, Chemical-Electrical; prof. Writer; Teacher, Drama; Producer. b. Newhall, W. Va. e. Va. Polytechnic Institute & State Univ.; (grad. upper 4.31% of Class); N.Y. Univ.; U. Calif., at L.A.; Pasadena Playhouse; Private drama schools, five; U.S. Army Signal Corps, W.W. II; U.S. chemical-aerospace firms: 10 yrs.;

Approx. 819 total performances in 58 show biz shows, incl. nigh clubs & circus, across USA. Chemical engr.-prof. "gag" writer; legit. Stage plays include: Murder in the Red Barn; Career; The Ponder Heart; & 25 Other plays. Motion pictures include: The Brain Eaters; Her Conversion. Elected member Int'l. Platform Ass'n; Assoc. Member: American Inst. of Chemical Engineers; AFTRA; SAG; AEA; DAV; Amer. Legion; Tau Beta Pi; Phi Lambda Upsilon; Phi Kappa Phi; First United Methodist Church; Boy Scouts.
TELEVISION: The Rank & File (Playhouse 90 series, CBS), (1962–1959); Weather Channel 9 (Puaski, Va.).

DIEHL, WALTER F.: Executive. International President, I.A.T.S.E. b. Revere, Mass., April 13, 1907. e. Northeastern Univ., Boston Catholic Labor Guild School. Became projectionist in Boston in 1927 and member of Boston Moving Picture Machine Operators Local 182 in 1933. After several years of service on the executive board became business agent in 1946 and held that post until 1953, when he resigned to accept an appointment as an International Representative, handling assignments throughout New England until 1957, when was appointed assistant international president. In 1952 made a member of the Minimum Wage Commission for the amusement industry in the state of Massachusetts. Also served several years on the executive board of the Boston Central Labor Union and as Labor Representative on the Suffolk County March of Dimes. IATSE pres. since March, 1974.

DIETRICH, MARLENE: Actress. r.n. Maria Magdalene von Losch. b. Berlin, Germany, Dec. 27, 1904; e. pvt. sch., Weimar; Musical Acad., Berlin; m. Rudolph Sieber; d. Maria Riva, actress. Stage training, Max Reinhardt's Sch. of Drama; debut in Viennese version of play, Broadway; then mus. com.
PICTURES INCLUDE: In German film, Blue Angel; in Hollywood: Morocco, Dishonored, Blonde Venus, Shanghai Express, Scarlet Empress, Song of Songs, Desire, Angel, Garden of Allah, Knight Without Armour, Destry Rides Again, Seven Sinners, Flame of New Orleans, Manpower, Pittsburgh, The Spoilers; with Army overseas (USO), 1942–45. Golden Earrings, Martin Roumagnac (French), Foreign Affair, Stage Fright, No Highway in the Sky, Rancho Notorious, Witness for the Prosecution, Judgment at Nuremberg.

DIFFRING, ANTON: Actor. b. Koblenz, Germany. Early career Academy of Drama, Berlin. Acted in Canada and U.S. before ent. m.p. ind. in Britain, 1951. Since 1970 in Rome, Munich, and Canneos.
PICTURES INCLUDE: I Am a Camera, Seven Thunders, House of Secrets, Albert RN, Circus of Horrors, The Man Who Could Cheat Death, A Question of Adultery, Lady of Vengeance, The Traitor, The Crooked Sky, The Sea Shall Not Have Them, The Colditz Story, The Black Tent, Enter Inspector Duval, Incident at Midnight. 1963/65 working in Germany, The Heroes of Telemark, The Blue Max, Farenheit 451, The Double Man, Counterpoint, Where Eagles Dare, Michael Kohlhaas, Horse Dealer, Uccidete Rommel, Piggies, Zeppelin, L'Iguana della lingua del Fuoco, Sutjeska, Corringa, Assassination of Little Sister, Dead Pigeon on Beethoven St., Der Stoff aus dem die Traume sind, The Day the Clown Cried, Das Schicksal ist der Jager, Tony Arzenta, The Beast Must Die, Shatter, Swiss Conspiracy, Vanessa, Operation Daybreak, Potato Fritz, Valentino, Les Indiens sont encore loin, L'Imprecateur, Waldrausch, Anna Ferroli, Das Einhorn, Return to Munich, Arsene Lupen, Escape to Victory, Jer Schnüffler S.A.S. Malko The Perfume of Old Memories, Operation Dead End.
TV: The Last Hours, A Small Revoltion, Wedding Day, The One Who Came Back, The Man in Half Moon Street, The Queen and the Rebels, The Cold Light, The Magnificent Egoist, The One Who Got Away, Autumn Crocus, The Fourposter, Dear Charles, Cross of Iron, One Step Beyond, Ghost Squad, Dr. Korczak and His Children, Dixon of Dock Green, The Joel Brandt Story, Firebrand, Scobie in September, The Trouble Shooters, The Million Pound Note, Strange Report, Kommissar, A Place in the Sun, Die Krise, Assignment Vienna, Liebe 74, Yoster, Kiss Me and Die, Die Himmlischen Tochter, Car along the Pass, MM Le Mutant, Flambards, Plutoniumaler Alte. Der Gast (Durbridge), The Winds of War, Tanzschule Kaiser Les Voleurs Des Moutons Weltunter Gang, End of the World, The Masks of Death, The Gentle Art of Murder.

DILLER, BARRY: Executive b. Fed. 2, 1942. Joined ABC in April, 1966, as asst. to v.p. in chg. programming. In March, 1968, made exec. asst. to v.p. in chg. programming and dir. of feature films. In May, 1969, named v.p., feature films and program development, east coast. In Feb., 1971, made v.p., Feature Films and Circle Entertainment, a unit of ABC Entertainment, responsible for selecting, producing and scheduling The Tuesday Movie of the Week, The Wednesday Movie of the Week, and Circle Film original features for airing on ABC-TV, as well as for acquisition and scheduling of theatrical features for telecasting on ABC Sunday Night Movie and ABC Monday Night Movie. On May 30, 1973, named v.p. in chg. of prime time TV for ABC Entertainment. In 1974 joined Paramount Pictures as bd. chm. and chief exec. officer. 1983, named pres. of Gulf & Western Entertainment and Communications Group, while retaining Paramount titles. Resigned from Paramount in 1984 to join 20th Century-Fox as bd. chm. and chief. exec. officer.

DILLER, PHYLLIS: Comedienne. b. Lima, O., July 17, 1917. e. Sherwood Music School, 1935–37; Bluffton College, O., 1938–39.
PICTURES INCLUDE: Boy, Did I Get A Wrong Number! 1966; Mad Monster Party, 1967; Eight on the Lam, 1967; Did You Hear the One About the Traveling Saleslady, 1967; The Private Navy of Serg. O'Farrell, 1967; The Adding Machine, Motel: The Great American Tradition (1981).
TV: Series, The Phyllis Diller Show, ABC 1966–67; The Beautiful Phyllis Diller Show (NBC) 1968. Guest spots on major shows here and abroad.
BOOKS: Phyllis Diller's Housekeeping Hints, 1968, Phyllis Diller's Marriage Manual, Phyllis Diller's The Complete Mother, The Joys of Aging and How to Avoid Them.
RECORDS: Verve and Columbia
BROADWAY: Hello, Dolly!
CONCERTS: A dozen annual piano concerts with symphony orchestras.

DILLMAN, BRADFORD: Actor. b. San Francisco, Calif., April 14, 1930. e. Yale, 1951.
PICTURES INCLUDE: A Certain Smile, In Love and War, Compulsion, Crack in the Mirror, Circle of Deception, Sanctuary, Francis of Assisi, A Rage to Live, Sergeant Ryker, Bridge at Remagen, Jigsaw, Suppose They Gave a War and Nobody Came, Mastermind, Brother John, The Mephisto Waltz, Escape from the Planet of the Apes, The Way We Were, The Iceman Cometh, Chosen Survivors, 99 and 44/100 ½ Dead, Gold, Bug, A Black Ribbon for Deborah, One Away, The Enforcer, Amsterdam Kill, The Lincoln Conspiracy, The Swarm, Love and Bullets, Piranha, Guyana-Crime of the Century, Running Scared, Sudden Impact, Treasure of the Amazon, Man Outside.

DILLON, MATT: Actor. b. New Rochelle, NY, Feb. 18, 1964. Casting director found him at age 14 in junior high school and put him in Over the Edge (1978).
PICTURES: Little Darlings, My Bodyguard, Tex, The Outsiders, Rumble Fish, The Flamingo Kid, Target, Rebel, Native Son.

DILLON, MELINDA: Actress. Launched career an Broadway in original company of Who's Afraid of Virginia Woolf? Screen debut with bit in The April Fools (1969).
PICTURES INCLUDE: Bound for Glory, Slap Shot, Close Encounters of the Third Kind, F.I.S.T., Absence of Malice, A Christmas Story, Songwriter.
TELEVISION: Space, The Shadow Box, Fallen Angel.

DILLOW, JEAN CARMEN: Producer, writer, actress, director. Began as baby star at age 5 on stage, screen. Last of the Wampas Baby Stars. Film work in England, Germany, Switzerland, Mexico, Italy. Play writing with George S. Kaufman; screenplay-writing with Andrew Solt. Wrote and produced with John Croydon, London producer. Wrote produced, directed and starred in The Pawn, filmed in Italy, Vienna, Warner Bros. TV feature. Latest play to music for London, in which she stars, There is No Other Prince But Aly. Also on stage in Stage Door, The Man Who Came to Dinner, What a Life. Completed scripts Spirit-Doll. The Resurrection, for Pinewood Studios, London. Star & leading lady in series of westerns for Republic, Monogram First National, Universal. Sang and danced in musicals and nightclubs. See Carmen Productions under Corporations. 1979, non-fiction books on phenomena: Do You Hear the Voices? and The Kidnapping of Aldo Moro. 1983 book Western Bullets are Blank, Mommy Angel; screenplay The Shoe Of The Ghost, India-Rome locale; teleplays: Jikoku-ten, The Ghost Of Palazzo Palladio, Give The Highest Award To Mommy Angel; The House in Athens. 1986, produced, directed and co-starred in film with Rossano Brazzi. Resides in Greenwich, CT and Rome working with son Grey.

DIMMOCK, PETER: CVO, OBE. Vice President-managing Director ABC Sports Worldwide Enterprises Ltd. & ABC Sports Intl., Inc., Director Screensport. b. Dec. 6, 1920. e. Dulwich Coll. & in France, R.A.F. pilot & Staff Officer during war. TV as prod. & commentator BBC Outside Broadcasts Dept., 1946. Prod. more than 500 TV relays including telecast from Windsor Castle of King George VI's funeral, 1952. Coronation telecast Westminster Abbey; State Opening Parliament. Commentator, introduced BBC-TV weekly Sportsview, 1954–64. Head of BBC-TV Outside Broadcasts 1954–72. Head of BBC Enterprises 1973, v.p. ABC Cos., Inc., 1977. Fellow Royal TV Society.

DIPIETRA, ROSEMARY: Executive. Joined Paramount Pictures in 1976, rising through ranks to become director-corporate administration. 1985, promoted to exec. dir.-corporate administration.

DISNEY, ROY E.: Prod.-dir.-writer, cameraman, film editor. b. January 10, 1930, Los Angeles; e. Pomona College, Calif. 1951 started as page, NBC-TV. Asst. film eidtor "Dragnet" TV series. 1952–78, Walt Disney Prods., Burbank, Calif., various capacities; now pres. Roy E. Disney Prods.; bd. chm., Shamrock Broadcasting Co., bd. dir., Walt Disney.
PICTURES INCLUDE: Perri, Mysteries of the Deep, Pacific High.
TV: Walt Disney's Wonderful World of Color; The Hound That Thought He Was A Raccoon, Sancho, The Homing Steer, The Silver Fox and Sam Davenport, Wonders of the Water World, Legend of Two Gypsy Dogs, Adventure in Wildwood Heart. Also, The Postponed Wedding, (Zorro series), (Wonder World of Color); An Otter in the Family, My Family Is A Menagerie, Legend of El Blanco, Pancho, The Fastest Paw In The West, The Owl That Didn't Give A Hoot, Varda the Peregrine Falcon, Cristobalito, The Calypso Colt, Three Without Fear, Hamade and the Pirates, Chango, Guardian of the Mayan Treasure, Nosey, the Sweetest Skunk in the World, Mustang!, Call It Courage, Ringo, the Refugee Raccoon, Shokee, the Everglades Panther, Deacon, the High-Noon Dog, Wise One, Whale's Tooth, Track of African Bongo, Dorsey, the Mail-Carrying Dog.

DIXON, BARBARA: Executive. b. Pasadena CA. e. Univ. of So. Calif. Served as staff member of Senate Judiciary Committee and was deputy dir. of legislation for Sen. Birch Bayh, 1974–79. Left to become dir. of Office of Government & Public Affairs of Natl. Transportation Safety Board. Named v.p., Fratelli Group, p.r. firm in Washington; took leave of absence in 1984 to serve as deputy press secty. to Democratic V.P. candidate, Geraldine Ferraro. In 1985 joined Motion Picture Assn. of America as v.p. for public affairs.

DIXON, WHEELER: Educator-Writer-Filmmaker. b. New Brunswick, NJ, March 12, 1950. e. Rutgers Univ. In 1969s asst. writer for Time/Life publications; during same period worked as editor for Interview magazine. 1976, directed TV commercials in New York. Two years with TVTV, Los Angeles, as post-prod. suprv.; produced programming for Theta Cable there. 1978, formed Deliniator Films, Inc., serving as exec. prod./dir. 1982, consultant to Vestron Industries, acquiring classic feature films. Since 1984 has directed film prod. program at Univ. of Nebraska, where holds rank of asst. prof. Author of book, The 'B' Directors, 1985; The Cinematic Vision of F. Scott Fitzgerald, 1986; PRC: A History of Producer's Releasing Corp., 1986.

DMYTRYK, EDWARD: Director. b. Grand Forks, B.C., Canada, Sept. 4, 1908. Entered employ Paramount 1923, working after school. Film editor 1930–1939; dir. from 1939.
PICTURES INCLUDE: Murder My Sweet, Back to Bataan, Cornered Crossfire, So Well Remembered, Till the End of Time, Give Us This Day, Mutiny, The Sniper, Eight Iron Men, The Juggler, Caine Mutiny, Broken Lance, End of the Affair, Left Hand of God, Soldier of Fortune, The Young Lions, Where Love Has Gone, Mirage, Alvarez Kelly, Anzio, Bluebeard.

DODD, WILFRID E.: Executive, b. Hamburg, Germany, March 19, 1923. e. Institut Fisher, Montreux (Switzerland), Downside College, Bath (England), Royal Military College, Sandhurst (England). In the '50s formed the Canadian Investing Banking firm: Oswald Drinkwater & Graham Ltd., Vice Pres. and partner. Pres. Allied Artists International Corp., 1964. President of Allied Artists Productions, Inc., 1969. Formed Cinepix Inc., Canadian dist. firm, 1963.

DOLGEN, JONATHAN L.: Executive. e. Cornell Univ., NYU School of Law. Began career with Wall Street law firm, Fried, Frank, Harris, Shriver & Jacobson. In 1976 joined Columbia Pictures Industries as asst. gen. counsel and deputy gen. counsel. 1979, named sr. v.p. in chg. of worldwide business affairs; 1980, named exec. v.p. Joined Columbia m.p. div., 1981; named pres. of Columbia Pay-Cable & Home Entertainment Group. Also pres. Columbia Pictures domestic operations, overseeing Music Group. 1985, joined 20th-Fox in newly created position of sr. exec. v.p. for telecommunications.

DOLLINGER, IRVING: Exhibitor. Columbia Amusement Co. b. N.Y.C., Sept. 20, 1905; e. U. of Pennsylvania. Stanley-Fabian mgr., 1926. Then with Warner Theatres in New Jersey. Owner and operator of theatre since 1929. Past pres. Allied Theat. Owners of N.J. Pres., Assoc. Theats. of N.J., booking org. 1938–44; v.p. & buyer, Independent Theatre Service Eastern regional v.p. Allied States Assoc., 1949–54; treas., Nat'l Allied, 1955–56; partner, Triangle Theatre Service, 1957; chief barker, N.Y. Tent 35, Variety Club, 1966.

DONAHUE, PHIL: Television Personality. b. Cleveland, Dec. 21, 1935. Started daytime talk show in Dayton, Ohio, 1967. Originally called The Phil Donahue Show. Syndicated show, Host, Donahue, now in 165 outlets in U.S. Home base: WGN—TV, Chicago, an independent station. In 1979 a mini-version of show became 3-times-a-week segment on NBC's Today Show. Winner of 2 Emmys.

DONAHUE, TROY: Actor. r.n. Merle Johnson, Jr. b. New York City, Jan. 17, 1937. e. Bayport H.S., N.Y. Military Acad. Directed, wrote, acted in school plays. Journalism, Columbia Univ.; Summer stock, Bucks County Playhouse, Sayville Playhouse; contract, Warner Brothers, 1959.
PICTURES INCLUDE: A Summer Place, The Crowded Sky, Parrish, Susan Slade, Palm Springs Weekend, Rome Adventure, A Distant Trumpet, My Blood Runs Cold, Come Spy With Me, Sweet Savior, Godfather, Part II, Grandview, U.S.A., Low Blow.
TV: Surfside 6, Hawaiian Eye.

DONALDSON, ROGER: Director. b. Australia. Emigrated to New Zealand at 19. Established still photography business; then began making documentaries. Directed Winners and Losers, a series of short dramas for NZ-TV. First theatrical feature, Sleeping Dogs.
PICTURES: Smash Palace (also s.p.), The Bounty, Marie.

DONCASTER, CARYL: TV writer, prod. b. Liverpool, Eng., Sept. 28, 1923. e. London U. (B.A. Honors). Educational film & film strip prod.; TV as BBC Talks producer in 1948; docum. writer & prod., 1950.
PRODUCTIONS: Made by Hand series, Report on Gambling, Report on Women, Born with the Century, The Rising Twenties, The Declining Years, Make Me an Offer, Pattern of Marriage, Children in Trust, Return to Living, New Canadians, Those Who Dare. Writer, dir., Canadian Venture, 1955; joined Associated Rediffusion, prod., Big City, This Week, People Are Talking, Secret Mission, Mantrap, Boyd Q.C., Outlook, Look In on London, Northern Journey, Members Mail, The Unwanted; head, Assoc. Rediffusion features; free lance TV writer-prod., writ., dir., School at Sea, Supermarket; Lecturer in prod., Thomson TV; Four Men of India. Prod. BBC TV, Report on Immigrant School Children, on Nurses, 1966; TV experiments in Sierra Leone, 1966. 1968 Nigerian TV; 1969 Documentaries in Mexico, Peru, Java, Zambia, Baffin Island, India.

DONEN, STANLEY: prod dir. b. Columbia, S.C., April 13; p. Mortie and Helen Donen; e. local public, high schools, U. of South Carolina.
PICTURES INCLUDE: Royal Wedding; Singin' in the Rain; It's Always Fair Weather, Deep in My Heart, Seven Brides for Seven Brothers, On the Town, Funny Face, Pajama Game, Kiss Them for Me, Indiscreet, Damn Yankees, Once More With Feeling, The Grass is Greener, Charade, Arabesque, Two for the Road, Bedazzled, Staircase, The Little Prince, Lucky Lady, Movie, Movie, Blame It on Rio.

DONIGER, WALTER: Writer-Director-Producer. b. New York City. e. Valley Forge Military Academy, Duke University, Harvard Graduate Business School. Entered m.p. business as writer later writer-prod-dir. Wrote documentaries in Army Air Forces M.P. Unit in World War II.
PICTURES INCLUDE: Rope of Sand; Desperate Search, Cease Fire, Safe At Home, House of Women, Duffy of San Quentin, Along the Great Divide, Tokyo Joe, Alaska Seas, Steel Cage, Steel Jungle, Hold Back the Night, Guns of Fort Petticoat, (dir., prod., s.p.).
TELEVISION: Delvecchio, Mad Bull, Switch, Moving On, Baa, Baa, Blacksheep, McCloud, The Man and the City, Sarge, Owen Marshall, Peyton Place (200 episodes), Mr. Novak, The Greatest Show On Earth, Travels of Jaimie McPheeters, Outlaws, Hong Kong, Checkmate, Bat Masterson, The Web, Bold Venture, Tombstone Territory, Maverick, Rough Riders, Captain Grief, Lockup, Dick Powell, The Survivors, Bracken's World, Bold Ones, Kung Fu, Barnaby Jones, Marcus Welby, Lucas Tanner, Movies of Week: Kentucky Woman, Mad Bull, The Outlaws and nine network-sold pilots.

DONLAN, YOLANDE: Actress, b. Jersey City, June 2; e. Immaculate Heart Convent, Hollywood, Calif. English stage debut in Born Yesterday at the Garrick Theatre (London) 1947; screen debut in Miss Pilgrim's Progress 1950.
PICTURES INCLUDE: To Dorothy a Son, The Body Said No, Traveller's Joy, Mr. Drake's Duck, Penny Princess, They Can't Hang Me, Expresso Bongo, Jigsaw, 80,000 Suspects, The Adventurers, Seven Nights in Japan.
TELEVISION: I Thought They Died Years Ago.

DONNELL, JEFF: Actress. b. South Windham, Me., July 10, 1921. r.n. Jean Donnell, e. Leland Powers Sch. of Theat., Yale Sch. Dram. On stage Farragut Playhouse, Rye Beach, N.H., before screen debut 1942. Summer stock, N.Y., Fla., Ohio, Wash., Calif.
PICTURES INCLUDE: Sweet Smell of Success, My Man Godfrey, Gidget Goes Hawaiian. Gidget Goes to Rome,

Fran Maidin, Stand Up and Be Counted.
TV: George Gobel Show, U.S. Steel Hour, Play of the Week, June Allyson, Ann Southern Shows.

DONNELLY, RALPH E.: Executive. b. Lynbrook, New York, Jan. 20, 1932. e. Bellmore (L.I.) Public School; W. C. Mepham High School (1949). Worked for Variety (publication) as writer, 1950; Long Island Press as daily columnist, 1951; joined Associated Independent Theatres, 1953, as gen. mgr.; later film buyer; in 1973 left to become independent buyer and booker for Creative Films; film buyer and v.p., RKO/Stanley Warner Theatres, 1976–79; now v.p. & gen. mgr. for Cinema 5 Ltd. circuit in New York.

DONNENFELD, BERNARD: Exec. b. New York, N.Y. Oct. 28, 1926. e. New York U., LL.B. Admitted to New York, Cal. Bar. Spvsr., corp. affrs., legal dept., Paramount Pictures Corp., New York, 1957–61; exec. asst., asst. secy. corp., Hollywood Studio, 1961–64; asst. to pres., asst. secy. corp., New York, 1964–65; assoc. hd. stud. activities, asst. secy. corp., Hollywood Studio, 1965, v.p. in charge of World Wide Production, Administration, Paramount, 1965–69. Pres. The Filmakers Group, 1970.

DONNER, CLIVE: Director. b. London, Eng. Ent. m.p. ind. 1942.
PICTURES INCLUDE: The Card, Meet Me Tonight, Genevieve, Million Pound Note, Purple Plain, I Am a Camera, The Secret Place, Heart of a Child, Marriage of Convenience, Some People, The Caretaker, Nothing But the Best, What's New Pussy Cat, Luv, Here We Go Round The Mulberry Bush, Alfred the Great, Vampira, Spectre, Rogue Male, Three Hostages, She Fell Among Thieves, The Thief of Baghdad, The Nude Bomb, Charlie Chan and the Curse of the Dragon Queen.
TV: Danger Man, Sir Francis Drake, Mighty and Mystical, British Institutions, Tempo, Oliver Twist, The Scarlet Pimpernel, Arthur The King, To Catch a King, A Christmas Carol, Arthur the King, Dead Man's Folly.

DONNER, RICHARD: Director. b. New York City. Began career as actor off-Bdwy. Worked with director Martin Ritt on TV production of Maugham's Of Human Bondage. Moved to California 1958, directing commercials, industrial films and documentaries. First TV drama: Wanted: Dead or Alive (Steve McQueen series).
TELEVISION: Many Movies of the Week; episodes of Kojak, Bronk, etc.; Portrait of a Teen-Age Alcoholic.
PICTURES: The Omen, Superman, The Final Conflict, The Toy (exec. prod.), Ladyhawke (prod.-dir.), Goonies (co-prod., dir.).

DONOVAN, ARLENE: Producer. Worked in publishing before entering industry as asst. to late dir. Robert Rosen on Cocoa Beach, uncompleted at his death. Worked as story editor, Columbia Pictures. 1969–82, literary head of m.p. dept. for ICM; involved in book publishing as well as stage and screen projects. Debut as film producer, Still of the Night (1982).

DONOVAN, HENRY B.: Executive. producer. b. Boston, Mass. Entered m.p. ind. for RKO Pathe Studios 1932; asst. cameraman, head of property dept., special effects dept., unit mgr., asst. dir., prod. mgr.; worked on over 300 pictures for many studios; dept. head Sherman Prod. 10 yrs., U.S. Army Signal Corps, as head of dept. of California studios prod. training m.p.; pres. Telemount Pictures, Inc. Prod., dir., writer Cowboy G Men (TV series). Wrote novel, Corkscrewed.
PICTURES INCLUDE: Hopalong Cassidy Features, Gone with the Wind, Becky Sharp, dir. Our Flag; Magic Lady (live-action TV show); Magic Lady (13 one-reel features), others. Prod. writer, Cowboy G Men (39 films), TV, 1952–54.
TV: programming, financing, distribution. Global Scope; International TV; Dist., Financing, programming; sls. consultant, Internat'l TV & motion pictures. Cable TV & distribution & program development, collector of movie memorabilia; DBS TV programming & financing: production software, etc.

DOOHAN, JAMES: Actor. b. Vancouver, B.C., Mar. 3. World War II capt. in Royal Canadian Artillery. 1946 won scholarship to Neighborhood Playhouse in NY and taught there later. 1953, returned to Canada to live in Toronto, becoming engaged in acting career on radio, TV and in film. Then to Hollywood and chief fame as Chief Engineer Scott in TV series, Star Trek.
PICTURES: The Wheeler Dealer, The Satan Bug, Bus Riley's Back in Town, Fellowship;, Star Trek—The Motion Picture, Star Trek II: The Wrath of Khan, Star Trek III: The Search for Spock.
TELEVISION: Hazel, Bonanza, The Virginia, Gunsmoke, Peyton Place, The Fugitive, Marcus Welby MD, Ben Casey, Bewitched, Fantasy Island, etc.

DOOLEY, PAUL: Actor. Began career on N.Y. stage in Threepenny Opera. Later member of Second City. Bdwy. credits include The Odd Couple, Adaptation/Next, The White House Murder Case, Hold Me, etc. Co-creator and writer for The Electric Company on PBS. Owns co. called All Over Creation, which produces original industrial films and shows and has created over 1,000 radio commercials.
PICTURES INCLUDE: What's So Bad About Feeling Good?, Slap Shot, Gravy Train, Death Wish, The Out-of-Towners, A Wedding, A Perfect Couple, Rich Kids, Breaking Away, Popeye, Paternity, Endangered Species, Kiss Me Goodbye, 16 Candles, Big Trouble.

DORAN, LINDSAY: Executive. b. Los Angeles. e. Univ. of Calif. at Santa Cruz. Moved to London where was contributing author to The Oxford Companion to Film and the World Encyclopedia of Film. Returned to U.S. to write and produce documentaries and children's programs for Pennsylvania public affairs station WPSX-TV. Career in m.p. industry began in story dept. at Embassy Pictures which she joined in 1979; 1982 promoted to dir. of development; then v.p., creative affairs. 1985, joined Paramount Pictures as v.p., production, for M.P. Group.

DORFMAN, IRVIN S.: Executive. b. New York, Sept. 3, 1924. e. Yale University, 1945 B.A. Following three years in U.S. Navy, joined Dorfman Associates, press rep. organ. handling film, and TV personalities. Handled pub. and promotion for more than 100 B'way shows and worked for 20th Cen.-Fox and U.A. Also produced off-B'way "The Lion In Love." Top ranking amateur tennis star, 1950; pres., Surrogate Releasing and Dandrea Releasing.

DORTORT, DAVID: Executive Producer. b. New York, Oct. 23, 1916. e. City Coll. of N.Y. Served U.S. Army, 1943–46. Novelist and short story writer, 1943–49. Also TV writer. Now pres. of Xanadu Prods. and Aurora Enterprises, Inc., Pres. TV branch, WGA, West, 1954–55; TV-radio branch, 1955–57; v.p. PGA, 1967; pres. 1968. Chairman of The Caucus for Producers, Writers and Directors, 1973–75. Pres., PGA, 1980–81; campaign director, Permanent Charities Comm., 1980–81; chm., Interguild Council 1980–81.
AUTHOR: Novels include Burial of the Fruit and The Post of Honor.
PICTURES INCLUDE: The Lusty Men, Reprisal, The Big Land, Cry in the Night, Clash by Night.
TV: Creator and exec. prod., Bonanza TV series; High Chaparral, The Chisholms. Producer: The Restless Gun, The Cowboys.

DOUGHERTY, MARION: Executive. Gained fame as casting director. Acted as co-executive producer on Smile (1975). In 1977 named v.p. in chg. talent for Paramount Pictures. In 1979 joined Warner Bros. v.p. in chg. talent to work with production dept. and producers and directors.

DOUGLAS, GORDON: Director, b. New York, New York. Actor. Hal Roach stock company; writer; callab. Topper series, Housekeeper's Daughter; dir., 30 Our Gang shorts.
PICTURES INCLUDE: Saps at Sea, Broadway Limited, Devil with Hitler, First Yank into Tokyo, San Quentin, If You Knew Suzie, Black Arrow, Walk a Crooked Mile, Doolins of Oklahoma, Mr. Soft Touch, The Nevadan, Between Midnight and Dawn, Kiss Tomorrow Goodbye, Great Missouri Raid, Only the Valient, I Was a Communist for the FBI, Come Fill the Cup, Mara Maru, Iron Mistress, She's Back on Broadway, So This Is Love, The Charge at Feather River, Them, Young at Heart, McConnell Story, Sincerely Yours, Santiago, The Big Land, Bombers B-52, Fort Dobbs, Yellowstone Kelly, Rachel Cade, Gold of 7 Saints, Follow That Dream, Call Me Bwana, Rio Conchos, Robin and the Seven Hoods, Sylvia, Harlow, Stagecoach, Way Way Out, In Like Flint, Chuka, Tony Rome, The Detective, Lady in Cement, Barquero, They Call Me Mr. Tibbs, Slaughter's Big Rip Off, Nevada Smith (MOW).

DOUGLAS, KIRK: Actor, Producer, Director. b. Amsterdam, N.Y. Dec. 9, 1918; e. St. Lawrence U; B.A. Stage debut in New York: Spring Again; others: Three Sisters, Kiss and Tell; U.S. Navy during World War II; resumed stage work in Kiss and Tell, then in Trio; did radio soap operas. Signed by Hal B. Wallis from The Wind is Ninety, B'way show, 1945. Screen debut: The Strange Love of Martha Ivers. Recipient of U.S. Freedom Medal, 1981. Three Academy Award nominations: Champion, The Bad and the Beautiful, Lust for Life. N.Y. Critics Award for Lust for Life. Cecile B. DeMille Award–1968 Cited in Congressional Record three times: on discrimination, on good will ambassador work, testimony on abuse of elderly. Received Jefferson Award in 1983 for public service by a private citizen. Made Goodwill Ambassador to U.N., 1983. Chevalier de la Legion d'Honneur, 1985.
TV: Mousey, 1974; The Money Changers, Draw! (HBO), Remembrance of Love, Amos.
PICTURES INCLUDE: Out of the Past, I Walk Alone, Mourning Becomes Electra, The Walls of Jericho, Letter to Three Wives, Champion, Young Man With a Horn, The Glass Menagerie, Big Carnival, Along the Great Divide, Detective Story, Big Trees, Big Sky, Bad and the Beautiful, Story of Three Loves, The Juggler, Art of Love, Ulysses, Man Without a Star, 20,000 Leagues Under the Sea, The

Racers, Indian Fighter, Lust for Life, Top Secret Affair, Gunfight at the OK Corral, Paths of Glory, The Vikings, Last Train from Gun Hill, The Devil's Disciple, Strangers When We Meet, Spartacus, The Last Sunset, Town Without Pity, Lonely Are the Brave, Two Weeks in Another Town, The Hook, List of Adrian Messenger, For Love or Money, Seven Days in May, In Harm's Way, Cast a Giant Shadow, Is Paris Burning?, The Way West, The War Wagon, Heroes of Telemark, A Lovely Way to Die, The Brotherhood, The Arrangement, There Was a Crooked Man, A Gunfight, Light at the Edge of the World, Catch Me a Spy,A Man to Respect. Producer: Indian Fighter, The Vikings, Spartacus, Lonely Are The Brave, List of Adrian Messenger, Seven Days in May, The Brotherhood, Summertree, (prod.) Scalawag; (prod., dir., act.) Once Is Not Enough, Posse (prod., dir., act.) The Chosen, The Fury, Home Movies, The Villian, Saturn III, The Final Countdown, The Man from Snowy River, Eddie Macon's Run, Tough Guys.

DOUGLAS, MICHAEL: Actor. b. N. Brunswick, N.J., Sept 25, 1945. f. Kirk Douglas. e. Black Fox Military Academy, Choate, U. of Cal. Worked as asst. director on Lonely Are The Brave, Heroes of Telemark, Cast A Giant Shadow; after TV debut in The Experiment, appeared off-Broadway in City Scene, Pinkville; m.p. debut in Hail Hero, followed by Adam at 6 A.M., Summertree, Napoleon and Samantha, Coma, China Syndrome (also prod.). Co-prod., One Flew Over the Cuckoo's Nest; Running (actor). It's My Turn (actor). Star Chamber (actor). Romancing the Stone (p., actor), A Chorus Line (actor); Jewel of the Nile (prod., actor).
TV: The FBI, Medical Center, When Michael Calls, Streets of San Francisco (series).

DOUGLAS, MIKE: TV host, commentator. r.n. Michael Delaney Dowd, Jr. b. Chicago, 1925. Started career singing with bands in and around Chicago. In 1950 became featured singer with Kay Kyser's band, staying four years. In 1953 became host of WGN-TV's Hi Ladies in Chicago; also featured on WMAQ-TV, Chicago, as singer and host. Moved to Hollywood in late '50s, working as piano bar singer. In 1961 hired as host for new show on station KYW-TV in Cleveland, owned by Westinghouse Bdg. Co., featuring celebrity guests. This became the Mike Douglas Show which was later nationally syndicated and moved base of operations to Philadelphia.

DOUGLAS, VALERIE: Executive. b. Hollywood, CA, Dec. 3. e. UCLA (Journalism). Uncle was actor Elmo Lincoln (first Tarzan). 1945–46, publicist, Vic Shapiro Public Relations; 1946–49, sub-agent, Manning O'Conner Agency; 1949–51, TV coordinator, Bing Crosby Enterprises, Fireside Theatre Series; 1951–52, publicist, RKO Studios; 1952–59, personal mgr., Richard Burton, v.p. & dir. Denham Films, Ltd., London; 1959–61, pub. coordinator, Hecht-Lancaster-Hill; 1961–64, dir. of pub. relations, IPAR Productions, France; 1964–67, v.p., Illustra Films, West Coast branch; 1967–75, asst. dir. pub., United Artists Corp., West Coast; 1975–78, exec. v.p., Guttman & Pam Public Relations; 1978, formed Suvarie, Inc., m.p. representation, of which is pres., Personal manager, Richard Burton.

DOURIF, BRAD: Actor. b. Huntington, WV. Stage actor before films and TV.
PICTURES INCLUDE: Split, W. W. and the Dixie Dancekings, One Flew Over the Cuckoo's Nest, Group Portrait with Lady, Eyes of Laura Mars, Wise Blood, Heaven's Gate, Ragtime, Dune.
TELEVISION: Mound Builders, The Gardeners's Son, Studs Lonigan, Guyana Tragedy—The Story of Jim Jones.

DOWN, LESLEY-ANN: Actress. b. London, England, March 17, 1954. At age of 10 modeled for TV and film commercials, leading to roles in features. At 14 appeared in All the Right Noises (debut).
PICTURES INCLUDE: Pope Joan, Scalawag, Brannigan, The Pink Panther Strikes Again, The Betsy, A Little Night Music, The Great Train Robbery, Hanover Street, Sphinx, Rough Cut, Nomads.
TELEVISION: Series: Upstairs, Downstairs; Heartbreak House, North & South Book II. Movies: The One and Only Phyllis Dixey, The Last Days of Pompeii, Arch of Triumph.
STAGE: Great Expectations, Hamlet, etc.

DOWNS, HUGH: Broadcaster. b. Akron, Ohio, Feb. 14, 1921. e. Bluffton Coll., 1938. Wayne Univ., 1941. Col. Univ., NYC, 1955; Supervisor of Science Programming, NBC's Science Dept. one yr.; science consultant for Westinghouse Labs., Ford Foundation, etc.; chm. of bd., Raylin Prods., Inc. Today, Chairman, U.S. Committee for UNICEF. Chm., National Space Institute.
TV: Hawkins Falls, Kukla Fran & Ollie, Short Story Playhouse, American Inventory, Home, Sid Caesar Show, Tonight (Jack Paar Show), Concentration, Today. Host: ABC-TV 20/20 Program, Host: Over-Easy-PBS Network.
RADIO: NBC's Monitor.

DOWSON, GRAHAM R.: Chairman, Erskine House Investments, 1975–1983. b. 1923. e. Alleyn Court School; City of London School; Ecole Alpina, Switzerland. Served RAF, 1941–46 (Pilot, sqdn-ldr.). Sales, U.S. Steel Corporation (Columbia Steel), Los Angeles, 1946–49; Sales & Senior Commentator, Mid-South Network (MBS), Radio, U.S., 1949–52; dir., Rank Organisation Ltd., 1960–75, Chief exec. 1974–75; Chm., Mooloya Investments, 1975–78; Pincus Vidler Arthur Fitzgerald, 1979–84; Marinex Petroleum, 1981–83; Deputy chm., Nimslo European Holdings; Nimslo Intl. Ltd.; Nimslo Limited 1979- (dir., 1978); dir.,: A.C. Nielsen Co., Oxford, 1953–58; Carron Co. (holdings) Ltd., 1976–82; Carron Investments Ltd., 1976–82; ROC Holdings PLC (formerly Barrowmill Ltd.) 1979 Nimslo Corp., dep. chm., 1979–. Chm., European League for Economic Cooperation (British section), 1972–1983; 1983- Joint Pres. V.p., N.P.F.A., 1974. Liveryman, Distillers' Co. 1985: Chairman & Chief Exec., Teltecit, Ltd. Dir., Film Bond.

DOYLE, KEVIN: Executive. b. Sydney, Aust., June 21, 1933. e. N. Sydney Tech. HS. Aust. Jr. exec., asst. adv. & pub. div., 20th Century-Fox, Aust., 1947–59; adv. & pub. dir., Columbia Pictures Aust., 1960–66; international ad/pub. mgr.; Columbia Pictures Int'l, N.Y. 1966; intl. pub./promo. mgr., 1980.

DRAGOTI, STAN: Director. b. New York City, Oct. 4, 1932. Worked in ad agency and did TV commercials (including I Love New York campaign). Theatrical director debut with Dirty Little Billy (1972).
PICTURES: Love at First Bite, Mr. Mom, The Man with One Red Shoe.

DRAI, VICTOR: Producer. b. Casablanca, Morocco, July 25, 1947. e. Lycee De Port Lyautey, 1957–63. In real estate in Los Angeles 1976–82; clothing designer/mfg. in Paris, France, 1969–76. Began producing features in 1984, The Woman in Red.
PICTURES: The Man with One Red Shoe, The Bride.

DRAKE, CHARLES: Actor. r.n. Charles Ruppert; b. New York City, Oct. 2, 1914; e. Nicholas Coll. 1937. With Electric Boat Co., Groton, Conn.; adv. salesman; in little theatres; in m.p. as an actor.
PICTURES INCLUDE: I Wanted Wings, Man Who Came to Dinner, Now, Voyager, Air Force, Mr. Skefflington, Whistle Stop, Pretender, You Came Along, Tender Years, Bowie Knife, Comanche Territory, Air Cadet, Winchester '73, Harvey, Little Egypt, You Never Can Tell, Treasure of Lost Canyon, Red Ball Express, Bonzo Goes to College, Gunsmoke, Lone Hand, It Came from Outer Space, War Arrow, Glenn Miller Story, Tobor the Great, Four Guns to the Border, Female on the Beach, All That Heaven Allows, Price of Fear, The Arrangement.

DRAKE, DONA: Actress. r.n. Rita Nevella; b. Mexico City, 1920.
PICTURES INCLUDE: Louisiana Purchase, Road to Morocco, Star Spangled Rhythm, So This is New York, Another Part of the Forest, Beyond the Forest, Valentino, Bandits of Corsica, Kansas City Confidential, Son of Belle Starr, Princess of the Nile.

DRAZEN, LORI: Executive. Began career as asst. to dir. of adv. for Orion Pictures; gen. mgr., Seiniger Advertising; creative dept. mgr., Kenyon & Eckhardt. Joined Warner Bros. 1985 as dir., world-wide adv. & pub. services.

DREIFUSS, ARTHUR: Producer-director-writer. b. Frankfurt on Main. e. Univ. of Frankfurt on Main, Germany, Conservatory of Music, Columbia University; choreographer, producer; many U. lectures; legit. producer: Allure, Baby Pompadour; producer many night club shows; associate producer Fanchon & Marco, Hollywood; dir. over 50 features, many musical shorts for Columbia, RKO, Universal, Allied Artists, Ind. to 1952; director Paul Muni debut Screen Gems-Ford Theatre, TV 1953; prod-director Secret File, U.S.A. Official Films; TV 1954–54; prod-dir: features Secret File and Assignment Abroad, Anglo-Amalgamated, London, 1956; dir: The Last Blitzkrieg; Life Begins at Seventeen; Juke Box Rythm, Columbia 1958–59; writer-director Brendan Behan's The Quare Fello British-Lion-Bryanston, London, 1961–62; director: Riot on Sunset Strip, AIP; The Love-Ins, For Singles Only, Columbia; The Young Runaways, A Time to Sing, MGM, 1963 to 1968; assoc. producer Angel, Angel, Down We Go, AIP, 1969; executive producer New Age Productions, 1970 to 1972; executive producer The Peter Hurkos Show, CBS; writer Owl Hill; Dolls behind Walls, 1973, director, Wildlife in Crisis, Viacom TV series 1975. Assoc. prod. Chennault China Tiger (Genson Prods.), 1978; assoc. video editor Creative Editing, Inc., 1979–80; dir. literary dept, George Michaud Agency, 1981; dir., literary dept., Schoeman Agency.

DREW, ELLEN: Actress. Previously known as Terry Ray. b. Kansas City, Mo. Nov. 23, 1915. Played on stage. Appeared in many pictures for major companies. In 1940: Women Without Names, Buck Benny Rides Again, Christmas in July, Texas Rangers Ride Again, Par. Many Others.

DREXLER, ELIAS J.: Executive. b. New York City, Dec. 24, 1911. e. Columbia University, Columbia Law School, LL.B.,

1936. Special agent. Div. of Investigations, U.S. Dept. of Interior, 1937–40; dir., Preclusive operations, 1940–45; dir., Surplus Property Div., Foreign Economic Admin; exec., National Screen Service, 1945–56; general counsel and nat. sales mgr. AGFA-Gavaert; 1956–65; nat. sales mgr. and exclusive U.S. and Mexican dist. of motion picture products manufactured by Fuji Photo Film Co., Ltd., Tokyo, Japan, 1965–present.

DREYFUSS, RICHARD: Actor. b. Brooklyn, N.Y., Oct. 29, 1947. e. Beverly Hills High. Prof. career began at Gallery Theatre (L.A.) in In Mama's House. Has also acted off-Bdwy. and on Bdwy.

PICTURES INCLUDE: Hello Down There, The Young Runaways, American Graffiti, The Apprenticeship of Duddy Kravitz, Jaws, Inserts, Close Encounters of the Third Kind, The Goodbye Girl, The Big Fix (also co-prod.) The Competition, Whose Life Is It Anyway?, The Buddy System, Down and Out in Beverly Hills, Stand by Me.

TV: The Big Valley, Room 222, Judd For the Defense, Mod Squad, The Bold Ones.

STAGE: Journey to the Day, Incident at Vichy, People Need People, Enemy, Enemy, Line, Whose Little Boy Are You, But Seriously, Major Barbara, The Time of Your Life.

DRU, JOANNE: Actress. r.n. Joanne La Cock; b. Logan, W. Virginia, Jan. 31, 1923. John Robert Powers model: on stage as showgirl in Hold on to Your Hats; a Samba Siren at Ritz Carlton & Paramount; with theatrical group under Batami Schneider. Hollywood: m.p. debut in Abie's Irish Rose, 1946.

PICTURES INCLUDE: Red River, She Wore a Yellow Ribbon, All the King's Men, Wagonmaster, Vengeance Valley, 711 Ocean Drive, Mr. Belvedere Rings the Bell, Siege at Red River, Outlaw Territory, Southwest Passage, Three Ring Circus, Day of Triumph, Hell on Frisco Bay, Sincerely Yours, The Warriors.

DRURY, JAMES: Actor. N.Y.C., 1934. ed. N.Y. Univ. Acting debut at age 8 in Biblical play for children at Greenwich Settlement Playhouse. Performed on stage while youngster. Signed by MGM in 1955, working one day in each of seven movies that year, including Blackboard Jungle. Then got two-year contract at 20th-Fox. Gained fame as hero of TV series, The Virginian, which had nine-year run.

PICTURES INCLUDE: Love Me Tender, Bernardine.

TELEVISION: The Virginian, The Devil and Miss Sarah (movie of the week), Firehouse (series).

DRURY, WESTON, JR.: Freelance casting director. b. Leeds, England, April 1916. Ent. m.p. ind. 1933. Rank Organization 1946–71, I.T.C. Ltd. 74–76. TV series include 1977: Return of the Saint; 1978: Danger UXB; 1979: Minder I; 1979: Masada; 1980: Minder II; 1980; The Acts of Peter & Paul; 1980: Flame Trees of Thika; 1981: Minder III. Dwain Glyndur, Strange But True, Minder IV, Minder V, Minder on the Orient Express.

DRUXMAN, MICHAEL B.: Publicist, producer. b. Seattle, Wash., Feb. 23, 1941. e. Univ. of Washington. exec. v.p., Seattle Civic Playhouse, 1962–63; founder, exec. dir., Actor's Theatre, Seattle; formed public relations firm, Michael B. Druxman and Associates.

CREDITS: Genesis (wrote, prod., dir.); produced and directed plays in the Los Angeles area—A Shot in the Dark, A Thousand Clowns.

DUBAND, WAYNE: Executive. Joined Warner Bros. 1969 as mgr. trainee in Australia. 1973, transferred to South Africa as mgr. dir.; 1977 gen. mgr. of CIC/Warner Bros. joint venture, also managing the CIC theatre operation there. 1980, named exec. asst. to Myron D. Karlin, pres. WB Intl., in Burbank. 1981, mgr. dir. of Warner/Columbia joint venture in France. 1985, appt. v.p. of sls. for WB Intl. division.

DUBBINS, DON: Actor. b. Brooklyn, N.Y., June 28, 1929. Appeared in stock company of Mr. Roberts, also Tea and Sympathy. Many television shows including Ed Sullivan show.

PICTURES INCLUDE: From Here to Eternity, Caine Mutiny, Tribute to a Bad Man, These Wilder Years, The D.I., Gunfight in Abilene, The Illustrated Man.

DUBENS, STANLEY: Writer-Producer. b. London, England, 1920. e. St. Paul's School, s. of Harry Dubens, Royal Corps Signals 1939–1945. From 1946, agent and theatrical productions. Ent. film production 1963. Currently making commercials, Doc., Film and video.

THEATRE: prod. incl. Sweet and Low, And No Birds Sing, The Train for Venice, The Man Who Let it Rain, The Hands of Eurydice, I Want to See Mioussov, Sign Here Please.

PICTURES INCLUDE: Operation Snatch, Live Now Pay Later, The World Ten Times Over, Modesty Blaise, Marble Heroes, Matchgirls, Archie's Caper. 1975 formed with Roger Moss, The Original Electric Picture Company, making commercials, doc., video, AV presentations.

DUBIN, JOSEPH S.: Attorney, Los Angeles, Calif.: Chief Studio Counsel, Universal Pictures, Calif., 1950–1970; Member, U.S. State Department International Copyright Panel, Panel of Consultants on General Revision of Copyright Law, Panel of Neighboring Rights; Chairman, Copyright Subsection, ABA (1956); Member of Council, Patent Trademark and Copyright Section, ABA (1957–61); Past Chairman, Committee on Related Rights, ABA; Past Chairman, Committee on Program for Revision of Copyright Law, ABA (1961–1969); Past Chairman, Committee on International Copyrights, AIPPI; Past Chairman, Committee on Copyright Law, APLA (1964–1969); Member, Board of Managers, APLA (1969–1972); President, Los Angels Copyright Society (1964–65).

AUTHOR: Copyright Relations Between Nations; Copyright—Duration of Protection; Copyright—Formalities; Moral Rights and Protection for U.S. Works; Copyright Aspects of Sound Recordings; Universal Copyright Convention; Motion Picture Recordings; Universal Copyright Convention; Motion Picture Rights—U.S. and International; An Exclusive Federal System for All Works; Neighboring Rights; The New French Copyright Law of 1957; Wartime Extensions of Copyright in Europe; International Developments in Copyrights; Copyright Relations with the Soviet Bloc and Less Industrialized Nations; The New German Copyright Law of 1965; Copyright Duration. Waiver of the exercise of the Droit Moral.

DUDELHEIM, HANS R.: Producer—Director—Editor. Began film career in Germany after World War II. Hired by U.S. Army Signal Corps as photographer, being sent to Far East Command. Came to New York, where joined ABC-TV as film editor. Beginning with hard news, moved to documentaries, editing many films. In 1981 estalished Cinema Arts Associates, Inc. as film society; 1966 expanded into indep. m.p. prod. co., of which he is pres.

DUDELSON, STANLEY E.: Executive. b. Cleveland, O., July 12, 1924. Regnl. sales mgr., Hygo-Unity; natl. sales mgr. Screen Gems; producer's rep., Selma Ent., Italian Intl. Uni-Export Films of Rome, AIP; first vice pres., American Intl. Television, Inc. Joined New Line Dist. Corp., pres., New Line Intl. Releasing. Left 1985 to be pres. & chief exec., Inter-pictures Releasing Corp.

DUFF, HOWARD: Actor. Bremerton, Wash. Nov. 24, 1917: e. Reportory Playhouse, Seattle. With KOMO radio station 1935; served with U.S. Army 1941–5; entered m.p. 1947. Radio's original Sam Spade.

PICTURES INCLUDE: Brute Force, Naked City, All My Sons, Calamity Jane and Sam Bass, Illegal Entry, Johnny Stoolpigeon, Woman in Hiding, Shakedown, Lady From Texas, Models Inc., Spaceways, Roar of the Crowd, Jennifer, Tanganyika, Private Hell 36, Women's Prison, Yellow Mountain, Flame of the Islands, Broken Star, Sierra Stranger, Blackjack Ketchum Desperado, While the City Sleeps, Boy's Night Out, Syria Against Babylon, Panic in the City, The Late Show, A Wedding, Kramer vs. Kramer, Oh, God! Book II.

TV: Mr. Adams and Eve, Dante, Felony Squad; Movies of the Week: The D.A., The Heist, This Girl for Hire.

DUFFY, JAMES E.: Executive. b. Decatur, Ill. e. Beloit College. Radio announcer, then reporter; joined publicity dept., ABC in 1949; named director of adv. & Promo., then account exec. for Central division of ABC Radio Network; director of sales ABC Radio, 1957; central division account exec., ABC Television Network, 1955; natl. director of Sales, ABC Radio central division, 1960; vice president, ABC Radio Network, 1961; exec. v.p. & natl. director of sales, 1962; vice president in charge of sales, ABC Television Network, 1963; president, ABC Television Network, 1970–85; pres., communications, 1985–86; v.p. Capital Cities/ABC, Inc.; pres., communications, ABC Network & Bdgst. Divisions.

DUFFY, PATRICK: Actor. b. Townsend, Mont., March 17, 1949. e. Univ. of Washington. Became actor-in-residence in state of Washington, where performed with various statefunded groups. Acted off-Bdwy. Taught mime and movement classes in summer camp in Seattle. Moved to L.A. and began TV acting career.

TELEVISION: Movies: The Stranger Who Looks Like Me, Hurricane. Series: Man from Atlantis (star), Switch (guest), Dallas (star).

DUIGAN, JOHN: Writer-Director. b. Australian. e. Melbourne Univ. (Philosophy, M.A.). taught for several years at Melbourne and Latrobe Universities before entering films. Made experimental short, The Firm Man (1974).

PICTURES: The Trespassers, Mouth to Mouth, Dimboola (d., only), Winter of Our Dreams, Far East.

DUKE, PATTY: Actress. b. New York, N.Y., Dec. 14, 1947. e. Quintano School for Young Professionals.

THEATRE: The Miracle Worker, Isle of Children.

PICTURES INCLUDE: The Miracle Worker, Valley of the Dolls, Billie, My Sweet Charlie, Me, Natalie, The Swarm.

TV: Armstrong Circle Theatre, The Prince and the Pauper,

Wuthering Heights, United States Steel Hour, Meet Me in St. Louis, Swiss Family Robinson, The Power and the Glory, The Patty Duke Show, George Washington, A Time to Triumph.

DUKES, DAVID: Actor. b. San Francisco. On Bdwy. in Don Juan, The Visit, Holiday, Dracula, Bent, Amadeus, etc.
PICTURES: The Whild Part, A Little Romance, The First Deadly Sin, Only When I Laugh, Without a Trace, The Men's Club.
TELEVISION: Beacon Hill, 79 Park Avenue, Family, Some Kind of Miracle, The Triangle Factory Fire Scandal, Mayflower—the Pilgrim Adventure, Portrait of a Rebel—Margaret Sanger, George Washington, Sentimental Journey, Space, Kane & Abel.

DULLEA, KEIR: Actor. b. Cleveland, Ohio, May 30, 1936. e. San Francisco State College, Sanford Meisner's Neighborhood Playhouse. Worked as ice cream vendor, carpenter with a construction co. Acted as resident juvenile at the Totem Pole Playhouse in Pa. N.Y. theatre debut in the revue Sticks and Stones, 1956; appeared in stock co. prods. at the Berkshire Playhouse and Philadelphia's Hedgerow Theatre, 1959, off-Broadway debut in Season of Choice, 1969, Butterflies Are Free.
TV: All Summer Long.
PICTURES INCLUDE: The Hoodlum Priest, David and Lisa (Best Actor Award, San Francisco Intern'l Film Festival), The Thin Red Line, Mail Order Bride, The Naked Hours, Madame X, Bunny Lake Is Missing, The Fox, 2001: A Space Odyssey, de Sade, Pope Joan, Paul and Michelle, The Paperback Hero, Silent Night, Evil Night, Leopard in the Snow, Brainwave, 2010.

DUNAWAY, FAYE: Actress. b. Bascom, Fla., Jan. 14, 1941. e. Texas, Arkansas, Utah, Germany, University of Fla., Awarded a Fulbright scholarship in Theatre. Boston U. of Fine Applied Arts. Appeared on N.Y. stage in: A Man For All Seasons, After the Fall (with Lincoln Center Repertory Co., three years), Hogan's Goat.
PICTURES INCLUDE: The Happening, Bonnie and Clyde, Hurry Sundown, The Thomas Crown Affair, The Extraordinary Seaman, A Place for Lovers, The Arrangement, Puzzle of a Downfall Child, Little Big Man, Doc, Oklahoma Crude, The Three Musketeers, Chinatown, The Towering Inferno, The Four Musketeers, Three Days of the Condor, Network, Voyage of the Damned, Eyes of Laura Mars, The Champ, The First Deadly Sin, Mommie Dearest, The Wicked Lady, Ordeal by Innocence, Supergirl.
TV: The Disappearance of Aimee, Evita, Ellis Island, 13 at Dinner, Beverly Hills Madam.

DUNCAN, SANDY: Actress. b. Henderson, Tex., Feb. 20, 1946, e. Len Morris Col.
STAGE: Ceremony of Innocence, Your Own Thing, Canterbury Tales, etc.
PICTURES INCLUDE: $1,000,000 Duck, Star Spangled Girl, The Cat From Outer Space.
TV: The Sandy Duncan Show, Roots.

DUNING, GEORGE: Composer, Conductor, Arranger. b. Richmond, Ind., Feb. 25; e. Cincinnati Conservatory of Music; University of Cincinnati. Musical director; music scores for many m.p. including: Jolson Sings Again, Eddy Duchin Story, From Here to Eternity, Picnic, World of Susie Wong, Devil at 4 O'Clock, Toys in the Attic, Any Wednesday, The Man with Bogart's Face. TV: No Time for Sergeants, Wendy and Me, The Farmer's Daughter, Big Valley, The Long Hot Summer, The Second Hundred Years, Star Trek, Mannix, Then Came Bronson; music dir. Aaron Spelling Prods., 1970–71, Bobby Sherman Show, "Movies" of the Week—NBC, CBS, ABC. OPT. Board of Directors, ASCAP.

DUNLAP, RICHARD D.: Producer, director. b. Pomona, Calif., Jan. 30, 1923; e. Yale U., B.A., 1944; M.F.A., 1948. U.S. Navy 1943–46; Instructor, English dept., Yale U., 1947–48; Prod.-dir., Kraft TV Theatre, 3 years; Dir, Assoc. Prod., Omnibus, 3 seasons; Dir., 25 half-hr. Dramatic Film Shows. Frank Sinatra Specials, Prod.-Dir., 10 Academy Award Shows, 4 Emmy Award Shows.

DUNNE, DOMINICK: Producer. Began career as stage manager at NBC-TV; then produced shows for CBS Studio One. Later exec. prod. at 20th-Fox TV, v.p. at Four Star.
PICTURES INCLUDE: Boys in the Band (exec. prod.), The Panic in Needle Park, Play It As It Lays, Ash Wednesday.

DUNNE, IRENE: Actress. b. Louisville, Ky., Dec. 20, 1904. e. Loretta Academy in St. Louis, Mo.; Chicago Coll. of Music (D.M., 1945), N.Y.; one child, Mary Frances. Screen debut 1931.
THEATRE: Stage prods. include Sweetheart Time, The City Chap, Show Boat.
PICTURES INCLUDE: Cimarron, Consolation Marriage, Back Street, Silver Cord, Ann Vickers, The Age of Innocence, Sweet Adeline, Roberta, The Magnificent Obsession, Showboat, The Awful Truth, Invitation to Happiness, My Favorite Wife, Penny Serenade, Lady in a Jam, A Guy Named Joe, The White Cliffs, Together Again, Over 21, Anna and the King of Siam, Life With Father, I Remember Mama, Never A Dull Moment, The Mudlark, It Grows on Trees, Love Affair, Theodora Goes Wild.

DUNNE, PHILIP: Writer-prod. dir. b. N.Y.C., Feb. 11, 1908; p. Finley P. and Margaret Abbott Dunne; e. Harvard Univ.; m. Amanda Duff.
PICTURES INCLUDE: How Green Was My Valley, Stanley and Livingstone, The Rains Came, Johnnie Apollo, Son of Fury, Suez, Lancer Spy, The Last of the Mohicans, The Count of Monte Cristo, The Late George Apley, Forever Amber, The Ghost and Mrs. Muir, Escape, Luck of the Irish, Pinky, David and Bathsheba, Anne of the Indies, Lydia Bailey, Way of a Gaucho, Demetrius and the Gladiators, The Egyptian, Prince of Players, View from Pompey's Head, Hilda Crane, Three Brave Men, Ten North Frederick, In Love and War, Blue Denim, Wild In The Country, Lisa, Blindfold, The Agony and the Ecstasy.
PUBLICATIONS: Mr. Dooley Remembers, Atlantic-Little Brown. Take Two (McGraw Hill, 1980).

DUNNING, JOHN: Film editor. b. Los Angeles, Calif., May 5, 1916; e. U.C.L.A., A.B., 1939. With MGM since 1935; U.S. Armed Forces, 1942–45.
PICTURES INCLUDE: Cass Timberlane, Homecoming, Julia Misbehaves, Battleground, Show Boat, Julius Caesar, Take the High Ground, Rhapsody, Last Time I Saw Paris, Tender Trap, Interrupted Melody, The Swan, Brothers Karamozov, Raintree County, Cimarron, Ben-Hur (Academy Award).
Post prod. supervisor, MGM, Inc.

DUNNOCK, MILDRED: Actress. b. Baltimore, Md., Jan. 25, 1906. e. Goucher Co., Baltimore, Teacher, Brearly Sch., N.Y.; acted in summer stock.
THEATRE: Prof. B'way debut, Corn Is Green; since in Richard III, Vicki, Lute Song, Another Part of the Forest, Cat on a Hot Tin Roof, The Chinese, Colette.
PICTURES INCLUDE: Corn Is Green, Kiss of Death, I Want You, Death of a Salesman, Viva Zapata, Girl in White, The Jazz Singer, Bad for Each Other, Hansel & Gretel (voice), Trouble with Harry, Love Me Tender, Sweet Bird of Youth, Whatever Happened to Aunt Alice?, Dragonfly.
TV: Death of a Salesman.

DUPONT, ADLEY: Actress. r.n. Adley Stoltz, b. New York City, Aug. 7, 1946. e. Geller School of Theatre, Film Industry Workshop, Desilu School.
PICTURES INCLUDE: Movie Star, The Golden Poodle.

DURBRIDGE, FRANCIS: Writer. b. Hull, England, Nov. 25, 1912. e. Birmingham University. Early career, radio playwright and novelist; entered TV 1946.
TV PLAYS AND SERIALS INCLUDE: Broken Horseshoe, Operation Diplomat, Teckman Biography, Protrait of Alison, My Friend Charles, A Time of Day, The Scarf, The Other Man, The Desperate People, Bat Out of Hell, The Passenger, The Doll, Breakaway.
TV: The World of Tim Frazier, Melissa.
PICTURES INCLUDE: The Teckman Mystery, The Vicious Circle.
THEATRE: London stage play: Suddenly At Home, The Gentle Hook, Murder With Love, House Guest, Nightcap.
RADIO PLAYS: Paul Temple plays, La Boutique.

DURNING, CHARLES: Actor. b. Highland Falls, N.Y. Many stage credits on Broadway (That Championship Season, The Happiness Cage, etc.).
PICTURES INCLUDE: Harry and Walter Go to New York, Twilight's Last Gleaming, The Choirboys, Breakheart Pass, The Hindenburg, Enemy of the People, The Sting, Dog Day Afternoon, The Fury, The Greek Tycoon, Tilt, The Muppet Movie, North Dallas Forty, Starting Over, When a Stranger Calls, The Final Countdown, True Confessions, Sharky's Machine, Tootsie, The Best Little Whorehouse in Texas, To Be Or Not To Be, Two of a Kind, Stick, Mass Appeal, The Man with One Red Shoe, Big Trouble, Stand Alone, Happy New Year, Tough Guys.
TELEVISION: Captains and the Kings, The Rivalry, The Dancing Bear, The Copy and the Kid (1975 series), Queen of the Stardust Ballroom, Studs Lonigan, Death of a Salesman.

DURSTON, DAVID E.: Writer-Director. b. Newcastle, Pa., Sept. 10, 1925. e. Evanston Township H.S. Served as TV-Radio director, Lynn Baker Adv. Agency, 1952–57; assoc. producer, Your Hit Parade, 1957–58. Acting credits include Winged Victory (B'way, film), Young Man's Fancy (B'way); TV writing credits include Tales of Tomorrow, Navy Log.
PICTURES INCLUDE: Felicia, Love Statue, Reflections, Blue Sextet (also edited), I Drink Your Blood, Stigma.

DURWOOD, RICHARD M.: Executive. b. Kansas City, MO., Aug. 18, 1929. e. Brown Univ. (A.B.). Pres. Crown Cinema Corp. Member: Motion Picture Assn. of Kansas City (pres.); United Motion Pictures Assn. (pres. 1972–73); Young

NATO (chm., 1968–69); National NATO bd., Past Chief Barker, Tent #8; exec. comm., National NATO.

DURWOOD, STANLEY H.: Chairman of the Board, American Multi-Cinema, Inc.; b. 1921. BS Harvard College (Football, Wrestling); Air Force navigator 3 years; six children. Member: Harvard Club of Kansas City; Harvard Club of New York; Chamber of Commerce (board of directors); Downtown, Inc. (board of directors), United Motion Picture Assoc. of America, Variety Club International. On board of United Missouri Bankshares.

DUSSAULT, NANCY: Actress. b. Pensacola, FL, Jun. 30, 1936. e. Northwestern Univ. On Bdwy. in Street Scene, The Mikado, The Cradle Will Rock, Do Re Mi, Sound of Music, Carousel, Fiorello, The Gershwin Years, etc.
PICTURE: The In-Laws.
TELEVISION: The Beggars Opera, Good Morning America (hostess), Too Close for Comfort.

DUTFIELD, RAY: Executive. Early career as chief accountant in Hawker Siddeley Group. Ent. m.p. ind. 1957, as exec. accountant with Rank Film Laboratories, gen. man., 1967; Appt. to board of dir., 1969; Appt. man. dir., 1970. Appt. man. dir., Rank Leisure Services, 1976 and vice-chm., Rank Film Labortories. 1979 January appt. chmn. and chief executive officer, Technicolor Limited, Fellow Member of Inst. Chartered Accounts, SMPTE, BKSTS, Member Institute of Directors, Institute of Marketing.

DUVALL, ROBERT: Actor. b. San Diego, Calif., Jan. 5, 1931.
PICTURES INCLUDE: To Kill a Mockingbird, Captain Newman, M.D., The Chase, Countdown, The Detective, Bullitt, True Grit, The Rain People, M*A*S*H*, The Revolutionary, THX-1138, The Godfather, Tomorrow, The Great Northfield, Minn. Raid, Joe Kidd, Lady Ice, Badge 373, The Outfit, The Conversation, Godfather, Part II, Breakout, The Killer Elite, 7% Solution, Network, The Eagle Has Landed, The Greatest, The Betsy, True Confessions, The Pursuit of D.B. Cooper, Tender Mercies, The Stone Boy, The Natural, The Lightship. Writer-Director: Angelo, My Love.

DUVALL, SHELLEY: Actress. b. Houston, TX, 1949.
PICTURES INCLUDE: Brewster McCloud, McCabe and Mrs. Miller, Thieves Like Us, Nashville, Three Women, Annie Hall, The Shining, Popeye, Time Bandits.
TELEVISION: Producer, Faerie Time Theatre.

DYER, TONY: Actor. b. Feb. 8, 1919; e. University of Missouri, Alvine School of Theatre. Acting debut: Cotton Blossom Showboat and Arthur Casey-Mary Hart Repertoire.
PICTURES INCLUDE: To Please A Lady, Children of An Loc, Apocalypse Now, Up From the Lower Depths, Bushido Blade.
TELEVISION: Shogun.

E

EASTWOOD, CLINT: Actor-Producer-Director. b. San Francisco, Calif., May 31, 1930. e. Oakland Technical High School, Los Angeles City College. Worked as a lumberjack in Oregon before being drafted into the Army. Starred in TV series Rawhide, for seven and a half years. Formed Malpaso Productions, 1969.
PICTURES INCLUDE: A Fistful of Dollars, For a Few Dollars More, The Witches, The Good The Bad and The Ugly, Paint Your Wagon, Hang 'Em High, Coogan's Bluff, Where Eagles Dare, Kelly's Heroes, Two Mules For Sister Sara, Beguiled, Play Misty For Me (dir. and star); Magnum Force; Breezy (dir.); Thunderbolt & Lightfoot; The Eiger Sanction, The Outlaw Josey Wales, The Enforcer, The Gauntlet (dir., star), Every Which Way But Loose, Escape from Alcatraz, Bronco Billy (dir., star), Any Which Way You Can, Firefox (prod., dir., star), Honky Tonk Man (prod., dir., star), Sudden Impact (prod., dir., star), Tightrope, City Heat, Pale Rider (dir., star).

EBERSON, DREW: Architect. Stamford, Conn; b. Hamilton, Ohio, Feb. 29, 1904; e. Northwestern Military and Naval Academy; University of Pennsylvania, Architect U.S.A. and England. WB production, Burbank. In 1931–38: Director, Coronet Pictures. Then theatre architect practicing throughout U.S.A. in 1942: Colonel, Corps of Engineers.

EBSEN, BUDDY: Actor. b. Belleville, Ill., April 2, 1908. r.n. Christian Ebsen, Jr. e. Univ. of Fla., Rollins College. Won first Broadway role as dancer in Ziegfeld's Whoopee in 1928. Sister, Vilma, became dancing partner and they played nighclubs and did road tours. Went to Hollywood and appeared in many musicals as single. Later became dramatic actor and appeared on TV.
PICTURES INCLUDE: Broadway Melody of 1936, Captain January, Banjo on My Knee, Four Girls in White, My Lucky Star, Thunder in God's Country, Red Garters, Davy Crockett, Attack, Breakfast at Tiffany's, Mail Order Bride, The Family Band.
TELEVISION: Hawaii Five-O, Gunsmoke, The Beverly Hillbillies, Davy Crockett, Barnaby Jones.
STAGE: Take Her, She's Mine, Our Town.

EBY, GEORGE W.: Executive. b. Pittsburgh, Pa., Jan. 2, 1914. e. Carnegie Tech.: Penna. State U., BA 1934. pres., Ice Capades, Inc., 1963–78, chm., Jan. 1, 1979; Int. Chief Barker Variety Clubs, 1958–60. Retired, 1983.

ECCLES, TED: Executive. Began career with Modern Film Effects developing special effects & title sequences for feature films. At Paramount Pictures for year as admin., west coast audio visual services. Joined Walt Disney Pictures 1985 as dir. of creative film svcs.

ECKERT, JOHN M.: Co-Producer, Assoc. Producer. b. Chatham, Ontario, Canada, 1948.
PICTURES INCLUDE: Middle Age Crazy, 1979 (co-prod.), Running 1978 (co-prod.), Power Play, 1977 (assoc. prod.), The Clown Murders, 1975 (Associate Prod.) As Prod. Man/Assit. Dir.; Second Wind, 1975, Sudden Fury, 1974. First assist. dir. Rituals, Find the Lady, It Seemed Like a Good Idea at the Time, Lions for Breakfast. Second unit asst. dir., Silver Streak. Second asst. dir., Equus, Black Christmas. Various TV dramas and series.

EDELE, DURAND (BUD) J.: Executive e. St. Louis U., Washington U. Reportorial staff, St. Louis Globe Democrat, 1934–35; booking dept., Paramount, 1935; booker & salesman, Warner Bros., 1936–41; branch & dist. mgr., Film Classics, 1946; branch mgr., United Artists, 1952–60; managed various divisions, United Artists, 1960–63; gen. sales mgr., v.p., Avco Embassy Pictures Corp., 1964, gen. sales mgr., Venture Dist. Inc., 1976; Consultant, RCMC 1976–78.

EDEN, BARBARA: Actress. b. Tucson, AZ, Aug. 23, 1934.
PICTURES: Back from Eternity, Twelve Hours to Kill, Flaming Star, Voyage to the Bottom of the Sea, Five Weeks in a Ballon, The Wonderful World of the Brothers Grimm, The Brass Bottle, Seven Faces of Dr. Lao, Harper Valley PTA.
TELEVISION: How to Marry a Millionaire, I Dream of Jeannie, etc. Movie: I Dream of Jeannie: 15 Years Later.

EDWARDS, BLAKE: Writer-director-producer. b. Tulsa, Okla., July 26, 1922. e. Beverly Hills High. Coast Guard during war.
RADIO: Johnny Dollar. Line-up; writer-creator: Richard Diamond.
TV: creator: Dante's Inferno, Peter Gunn, Mr. Lucky.
PICTURES INCLUDE: Panhandle, Stampede, Sound Off, Bring Your Smile Along, All Ashore, Crusin' Down the River, Rainbow Round My Shoulder, He Laughed Last, Drive a Crooked Road, My Sister Eileen, Mr. Cory, This Happy Feeling, The Perfect Furlough, Operation Mad Ball, Notorious Landlady, Operation Petticoat, High Time, Breakfast at Tiffany's, Experiment in Terror, Days of Wine and Roses, Soldier in the Rain, The Pink Panther, Shot in the Dark, The Great Race, What Did You Do in the War, Daddy, Gunn, Darling Lili, The Party, The Wild Rovers, Carey Treatment, The Tamarind Seed (dir. s.p.) The Return of the Pink Panther (prod., dir., co-s.p.), The Pink Panther Strikes Again (prod., dir., co-s.p.), Revenge of the Pink Panther (prod., dir., co-s.p.); "10" (co-prod., dir., s.p.). "S.O.B." (co-prod., dir., Victor/Victoria (co-prod., dir., s.p.); Trail of the Pink Panther (co-prod., dir., co-s.p.); The Man Who Loved Women (prod., dir., co-s.p.); Micki and Maude (dir.); A Fine Mess (dir., s.p.), That's Life (dir., co-s.p.).

EDWARDS, DOUGLAS: News Correspondent. b. Ada, Okla, July 14, 1917. Became radio reporter in Troy, Ala., at 15 yrs. e. Univ. of Ala., Emory Univ., Univ. of Ga. News reporter for WAGF, Dothan, Ala.; ass't. news editor for Atlanta Journal and its station, WSB. Transferred to WXYZ, Detroit, returning to WSB as ass't. news editor 2 yrs. later. Joined CBS Radio News staff, 1942, appearing on Report to the Nation, and The World Today. Chief of CBS News Paris Bureau. First major newsman to make transition to TV, 1947. Anchorman on CBS Afternoon News and Douglas Edwards with the News for 15 years on CBS-TV. Presently on CBS Mid-Day News with Douglas Edwards.

EDWARDS, JAMES H.: Executive. President, Storey Theatres, Inc. b. Cedartown, GA, Aug. 14, 1927. e. Georgia State. U.S. Navy, 1948–50. With Ga. Theatre Co., 1950–1952; Storey Theatres, 1952–present. Formerly pres. & chm., NATO of Ga; formerly pres., Variety Club of Atlanta. Former dir. at large, Nat'l. NATO. Director, numerous theatre cos.

EDWARDS, RALPH: Producer-Emcee. b. Merino, CO, June 13, 1913. e. Univ. of CA, Berkeley. Began career in radio in 1929 as writer-actor-producer-announcer at station KROW, Oakland. Later joined CBS & NBC Radio in New York as announcer. 1940, originated, produced and emceed Truth or Consequences for both radio & TV. Also has produced and hosted This Is Your Life, The Ralph Edwards Show, Name That Tune, Cross Wits, etc.

EDWARDS, VINCE: Actor. b. New York City, July 9, 1928. e. Ohio State U., Univ. of Hawaii, Amer. Acad. of Dram. Arts. N.Y. stage. High Button Shoes.
TV APPEARANCES INCLUDE: Studio One, Philco, Kraft, Ben Casey, The Untouchables, General Electric Theatre, Hitchcock, The Deputy, Firehouse (movie), The Rhinemann Exchange.
PICTURES INCLUDE: Sailor Beware, Hiawatha, Rogue Cop, Night Holds Terror, Serenade, The Killing, Hit and Run, The Scavengers, The Three Faces of Eve, City of Fear, Murder by Contract, The Victors, Devil's Brigade, The Desperados, Las Vegas, Los Angeles, The Seduction, Space Raiders, Deal of the Century.

EGAN, RICHARD: Actor. b. San Francisco, Calif., July 29, 1923. e. U. of San Francisco, B.A.; Stanford U., M.A.; U.S. Army, 1942–46; then taught public speaking; several TV appearances. Currently in Capitol (series).
PICTURES INCLUDE: Damned Don't Cry, Undercover Girl, Bright Victory, One Minute to Zero, Devil Makes Three, Blackbeard the Pirate, Split Second, Demetrius and the Gladiators, Wicked Woman, Gog, Khyber Pass, Underwater, Untamed, Violent Saturday, View from Pompey's Head, Seven Cities of Gold, Revolt of Mamie Stover, Love Me Tender, Tension At Table Rock, These Thousand Hills, A Summer Place, Pollyanna, Esther and the King, The Lion of Sparta, Valley of Mystery, The Big Cube.

EGGAR, SAMANTHA: Actress. b. London, Eng., March 5, 1939.
PICTURES INCLUDE: The Wild and the Willing, Dr. Crippen, Doctor in Distress, Psyche 59, The Collector, Walk Don't Run, Return From the Ashes, Doctor Dolittle, Molly Maguires, The Lady in the Car, Walking Stick, The Grove, Light at the Edge of the World, 7% Solution, Why Shoot the Teacher, Blood City, The Uncanny, Curtains.
TV INCLUDES: Anna and the King (CBS), Man of Destiny, Double Indemnity, The Hope Diamond, Columbo, Baretta, The Hemingway Play, Love Story, Kojak, McMillan & Wife, Streets of San Francisco, Starsky and Hutch.

EHRLICH, ROSEANNE: Executive. e. Sarah Lawrence Coll. (BA, English literature). Entered m.p. industry as freelance reader for Warner Bros., Avco Embassy and Robert Stigwood Organization. 1977–80, East Coast story editor for Lorimar Productions. 1981, joined Paramount Pictures as dir. of literary affairs. 1985, promoted to v.p., production, East Coast for M.P. Group.

EICHHORN, LISA: Actress. b. Reading, Pa. Went to England for literature studies at Oxford. Studied at RADA. Made film debut in Yanks (1979).
PICTURES: The Europeans, Why Would I Lie?, Cutter and Bone.

EIKENBERRY, JILL: Actress. b. New Haven, CT, Jan. 21, 1947. e. Yale Drama School. On Bdwy. in All Over Town, Watch on the Rhine, Onward Victoria, etc.
PICTURES: Between the Lines, the End of the World in Our Usual Bed in a Night Full of Rain, An Unmarried Woman, Butch and Sundance, The Early Days, Orphan Train, Rich Kids, Hide in Plain Sight, Arthur, Grace Quigley, The Manhattan Project.
TELEVISION: Sessions, Kane & Abel.

EILBACHER, LISA: Actress. b. May 5, Aravia. Moved to Calif. at age 7; acted on TV as child.
PICTURES: An Officer and a Gentleman, Ten to Midnight, Beverly Hills Cop.
TELEVISION: Series: Wagon Train, Laredo, My Three Sons, Gunsmoke, Combat, Ryan's Four. Movies: The War Between Men and Women, The Patty Hearst Story, Love for Rent, To Race the Wind, This House Possessed. Mini-Series: The Winds of War.

EISNER, MICHAEL D.: Executive. b. New York City, 1942. e. Denison Univ., (B.A.). Started career with programming dept. of CBS TV network. Joined ABC in 1966 as asst. to v.p. & natl. program director. Two years later named manager of specials and talent. Dec., 1968 became dir. of program development—east coast. In March, 1971 named v.p., daytime programming, ABC-TV. In June, 1975 made v.p., program planning and development. In May, 1976 named sr. v.p., prime time production and development, ABC Entertainment. In Nov., 1976, left ABC to join Paramount Pictures as pres. & chief operating officer. 1984, joined Walt Disney Prods. as chm.

EKBERG, ANITA: Actress. b. Malmoe, Sweden, Sept. 29, 1931. Started career as a model.
PICTURES INCLUDE: Man in the Vault, Blood Alley, Artists and Models, War and Peace, Back from Eternity, Zarak, Pickup Alley, Sheba and the Gladiator, Sign of the Gladiator, La Dolce Vita, Boccaccio '70, The Alphabet Murder, The Cobra, Fellini's Clowns.

EKLAND, BRITT: Actress. b. Stockholm, Sweden, 1942.
TV: England: A Cold Peace. U.S.A.: Trials of O'Brien, McCloud, Six Million Dollar Man.
PICTURES INCLUDE: After the Fox, Double Man, Bobo, Night They Raided Minsky's, At Any Price, Stiletto, Cannibals, Tintomara, Percy, Carter, Night Hair Child, Endless Night, Baxter, Asylum, Wickerman, Ultimate Thrill, Man With Golden Gun, Royal Flash, Cassanova and Company, Slaves, King Soloman's Treasures.

ELAM, JACK: Actor. b. Miami, AZ, Nov. 13, 1916. e. Santa Monica Jr. College, Modesto Jr. College. Worked in Los Angeles as bookkeeper and theatre mgr.; served in Navy in World War II. Introduction to show business was as bookkeeper for Sam Goldwyn. Later worked as controller for other film producers. Given first acting job by producer George Templeton in 1948; has since appeared in over 100 films.
PICTURES: Rawhide, Kansas City Confidential, The Moonlighter, Vera Cruz, Moonfleet, Kiss Me Deadly, Gunfight at OK Corral, Baby Face Nelson, Edge of Eternity, The Comancheros, The Rare Breed, The Way West, Firecreek, Once Upon a Time in the West, Support Your Local Sheriff, Rio Lobo, Support Your Local Gunfighter, Dirty Dingus Magee, The Cannonball Run, Cannonball Run II.
TELEVISION: The Texas Wheelers, The Dakotas, Temple Huston, Gunsmoke, Struck by Lightning, etc.

ELFAND, MARTIN: Executive b. Los Angeles, 1937. Was talent agent for ten years with top agencies; joined Artists Entertainment Complex in 1972. First film project as producer: Kansas City Bomber, first venture of AEC, of which he was snr. v.p. In 1977 joined Warner Bros. as production chief. 1980, produced It's My Turn. 1982, An Officer and a Gentleman; 1985, King David.

ELG, TAINA: Actress, dancer. b. Helsinki, Finland, March 9. e. Helsinki. Sadler's Wells Ballet. Toured with Marquis de Cuevas Ballet; m.p. debut in The Prodigal.
PICTURES INCLUDE: Diane, Gaby, Les Girls, Imitation General, The 39 Steps.

ELIAS, HAL: Executive. b. Bklyn,. N.Y., Dec. 23. Publicity dir., State Theatre, Denver; western exploitation mgr., MGM; adv. dept., pub. dept., MGM, Culver City studios; Head, MGM cartoon studio (Tom and Jerry); UPA Pictures, Inc., vice-pres. studio mgr.: Hollywood Museum; bd. dir., Academy of Motion Picture Arts & Sciences, 30 years; treasurer, AMPAS 1976–1979. Special Academy Award, 1979, for service to AMPAS.

ELIZONDO, HECTOR: Actor. b. N.Y.C. m. actress Carolee Campbell. Studied with Ballet Arts Co. of Carnegie Hall and Actors Studio. Many stage credits in N.Y. and Boston.
PICTURES INCLUDE: Pocket Money, Born to Win, Deadhead Miles, Stand Up and Be Counted, One Across, Two Down, The Taking of Pelham One Two Three, Report to the Commissioner, American Gigolo, The Flamingo Kid.
STAGE: Mr. Roberts, Island in Infinity, Madonna of the Orchard, Drums in the Night, The Prisoner of Second Avenue, Dance of Death, Steambath, The Great White Hope.
TV: The Impatient Heart (tf), Kojack, the Jackie Gleason Show, All in the Family.

ELKINS, SAUL: Producer. b. New York City, June 22, 1907; e. C.C.N.Y., B.S. 1927. Radio writer, dir., prod. 1930–2; dir., prod. stock co. touring Latin America 1932–4; writer Fox Films, 20th Century-Fox; writer RKO, Columbia 1937–42; writer, dial-dir., dir. Warner Bros. 1943–7; prod. Warner Bros. since 1947. Member: AMPAS, Screen Writer's Guild. Exec. prod., Comprenetics, Inc. Dir., Pioneer Prods., 1982.
PICTURES INCLUDE: Younger Brothers, One Last Fling, Homicide, House Across the Street, Flaxy Martin, Barricade, Return of the Frontiersmen, This Side of the Law, Colt 45, Sugarfoot, Raton Pass, The Big Punch, Smart Girls Don't Talk, Embraceable You.

ELLIOTT, DENHOLM: Actor. b. London, Eng., May 31, 1922; e. Malvern College. Screen debut in Dear Mr. Proback, 1948; films include: The Sound Barrier, The Holly and the Ivy, The Ringer, The Cruel Sea, Heart of the Matter, They Who Dare, Man Who Loved Redheads, Lease of Life, Night My Number Came Up, Pacific Destiny, Scent of Mystery; TV appearances; Stage: Write Me A Murder, N.Y., Seagull, N.Y., 1964.
PICTURES INCLUDE: Nothing But the Best, Station Six Sahara, King Rat, You Must Be Joking, The High Bright Sun, Alfie, Here We Go Round The Mulberry Bush, The Night They Raided Minskys, The Seagull, Too Late the Hero, The Rise and Rise of Michael Rimmer, A Doll's House, The Apprenticeship of Duddy Kravitz, Robin & Marion, To The Devil A Daughter, Russian Roulette, Voyage of the Damned, The Boys from Brazil, St. Jacques, Zulu Dawn, A Game for Vultures, Cuba, Illusions, Saint Jack, Bad Timing, Sunday Lovers, Marco Polo, Brimstone and Treacle, The Missionary, The Wicked Lady, Trading Places, The Razors Edge, A Room with a View, Defense of the Realm, Whoopee Boys.
TELEVISION: Mrs. Delafield Wants To Marry.

ELLIOTT, LANG: Producer-Director. b. Los Angeles, CA, Oct. 18, 1949. Given first job in films by his uncle, the late actor William Elliott (known as Wild Bill Elliott). Worked as actor from early years; employed by, among others the McGowan Brothers. Turned to film production; co-founded distribution co., The International Picture Show Company, serving as exec. v.p. in chg. of financing, production & distribution. Under banner of TriStar Pictures, Inc. also finances productions. 1982, formed Lang Elliott Productions, Inc.
PICTURES: Produced Ride the Hot Wind, Where Time Began, The Farmer, The Billion Dollar Hobo, They Went That-a-Way & That-a-Way, The Prize Fighter. Produced and directed the Private Eyes.
TELEVISION: Produced Experiment in Love (special).

ELLIOTT, RICHARD B.: Executive. b. San Francisco, Oct. 20, 1952. e. Stanford Univ. (MBA, 1983); Univ. of Calif. (BS, 1974). Worked for Price Waterhouse & Co. in Brussels, Belgium, as sr. tax acct., 1976–78; Touche Ross & Co. in Brussels, tax spvr., 1978–81; mgr. planning & special projects, Pay Cable and Home Entertainment Group of Columbia Pictures, 1983; dir. opns., Pay Cable & Home Entertainment Group, 1984; v.p., sls. planning, Marketing and Distribution Group, 1985.

ELLIOTT, SAM: Actor. b. Sacramento, CA, Aug.9, 1944. e. Univ. of Oregon.
PICTURES: The Games, Frogs, Molly and Lawless John, The Legacy, Mask.
TELEVISION: Movies: The Challenge, Assault on the Wayne, The Blue Knight, I Will Fight No More Forever, Once an Eagle, Aspen, The Sacketts, A Death in California. Series: Yellow Rose, The Blue Lightning.

ELLSWORTH, JAMES: Producer. b. Deltaville, Virginia, March 12, 1927. e. U.C.L.A., 1949. Pro. baseball player.
TV SERIES: Champions of Sports.
PICTURES INCLUDE: Naked Fury, Marine, Life Story of Lt. General Lewis B. (Chesty) Fuller, Door to Door Maniac (Five Minutes to Live).

ELMES, GUY: Writer. b. London, Eng., July 22, 1920; e. Aberdeen U. Painter and writer for radio after War Service (1939–45) in Royal Navy.
PICTURES INCLUDE: The Planter's Wife, The Flanagan Boy, Counterspy, Bang! You're Dead, Across the Bridge, Nor the Moon by Night, Wheel of Fate, Stranger's Hand, Serious Charge, Hello London, The Lady Takes a Gun, Joseph and His Brothers, Hannibal, The Blue Countess, Pontius Pilate, A Face in the Rain, The Captive City, Stranglehold, Flames Over India, El Greco, Submarine X, The Heroes, The Night Visitor, s.p.

ELSON, NORMAN: Executive. b. New York City, July 5, 1907; e. U. of Maryland. Contact clerk for Columbia; accessory mgr. N.Y. Columbia Exchange; district mgr. film buyer & gen. mgr. Brandt Theatres; gen. mgr. Trans-Lux Theatre Circuit, then apptd. vice-pres. 1950. Guild Enterprises, Inc., circuit pres. operating nine theatres in New York City.

ELWES, CARY: b. London, England, Oct. 26, 1962. e. Harrow. Studied for stage with Julie Bovasso at Sarah Lawrence, Bronxville, NY. Theatrical film debut, Another Country (1984).
PICTURES: Oxford Blues, The Bride, Lady Jane.

ENDERS, ROBERT: Producer, Writer. Began in television, being responsible for 64 hrs. of live programming weekly for industry and govt. as pres. of Robert J. Enders, Inc. In 1961 turned to theatrical prod. and writing.
PICTURES INCLUDE: A Thunder of Drums (prod.), The Maltese Bippy (prod.), How Do I Love Thee (prod.), Zig Zag (story), Voices (prod., s.p.), The Maids, (s.p.), Winter Rates (exec. prod.), Conduct Unbecoming (s.p.), Hedda (prod.), Nasty Habits (prod., s.p.), Stevie (prod., dir.).
TV: The Best of the Post (prod. of series), Ben Franklin, High Noon (prod., special). Co-prod. of Acad. Award Show, 1968.

ENDFIELD, CY: Producer, director, writer. b. Nov. 1914. Ent. m.p. ind. 1942; credits include: Joe Palooka series. Argyle Secrets, Underworld Story, Sound of Fury, Limping Man, Impulse, The Secret Child in the House, shorts for MGM; dir., Hell Drivers, Sea Fury.
PICTURES INCLUDE: dir., Jet Storm, Mysterious Island, Hide and Seek; dir., co-prod., co-scripted, Zulu, Sands of the Kalahari. Dir. De Sade.

ENGEL, CHARLES F.: Executive. b. Los Angeles, CA, Aug. 30, 1937. e. Mich. State Univ.; UCLA. Son of Samuel G. Engel. Pgm. devel., ABC-TV, 1964–68; v.p. Univ.-TV, 1972; sr. v.p., 1977; exec. v.p., 1980; pres., MCA Pay-TV New Programming, 1981.

ENGELBERG, MORT: Producer. b. Memphis, TN. e. Univ. of Illinois; Univ. of Missouri. Taught journalism; worked as reporter for UPI, AP. Worked for US government, including USIA, Peace Corps., Office of Economic Opportunity; President's Task Force on War on Poverty. Left government service in 1967 to become film unit publicist, working on three films in Europe: Dirty Dozen, Far From the Madding Crowd, The Comedians. Returned to US; appt. pub. mgr. for United Artists. Sent to Hollywood as asst. to Herb Jaffe, UA head of west coast production, which post he assumed when Jaffe left. Left to join with independent producer, Ray Stark.
PICTURES: Smokey and the Bandit, Hot Stuff, The Villian, The Hunter.

ENGLANDER, MORRIS: Executive. e. Wharton School, Univ. of PA. With General Cinema Corp. circuit before joining RKO Century Warner Theatres 1984 as exec. v.p., develp.; now co-vice chm. of circuit.

ENGLUND, GEORGE H.: Producer-Director. b. Washington, D.C., June 22, 1926. Producer, Paramount, Pennebaker Prods.; prod., MGM; prod.-dir., Universal.
PICTURES INCLUDE: The World the Flesh and the Devil, The Ugly American, Signpost to Murder, Snow Job.
TELEVISION: The Vegas Strip War (exec. prod., dir., s.p.)

ENGLUND, KEN: Writer. b. Chicago, Ill., May 6, 1914. e. Lane Tech., Chicago. Started career as magazine writer; then vaudeville routines, comedy radio shows. B'way revues and musicals. Twice elec. pres. screen branch Writers Guild of America, West, then pres. of WGAW. Member national council.
TV SHOWS INCLUDE: Jackie Gleason Show, Dear Phoebe, Ray Milland Show, Loretta Young Show, several spectaculars. Prod.-writer CBS-TV staff 1957; Sonja Henie Spect. London, 1958; 20th Fox and Warner Bros. TV Films, My Three Sons; sev. teleplays, Bewitched, 1965, That Girl!, Dr. Joyce Brothers (head writer for series).
PICTURES INCLUDE: Big Broadcast of 1938, Artists and Models Abroad, Good Girls Go to Paris, Slightly Honorable, Doctor Takes a Wife, No No Nanette, This Thing Called Love, There's That Woman Again, Nothing But the Truth, Springtime in the Rockies, Sweet Rosie O'Grady, Here Comes the Waves, Secret Life of Walter Mitty, Androcles and the Lion, Good Sam, A Millionaire for Christy, The Caddy, Never Wave at a Wac, Vagabond King, The Wicked Dreams of Paula Schultz, Surviving the Savage Sea.
AUTHOR: Tour D'Amour, Larks in a Casserole; B'way musical in work, and literary projects. Co-author (with George Marshall) The Ghost in Emily's Trunk.

EPSTEIN, JULIUS J: Screenwriter. b. New York City, Aug. 22, 1909. e. Penn State. Worked as publicist before going to Hollywood where began writing. Had long collaboration with twin brother, Philip G. Epstein. Under contract with Warner Bros. over 17 years.
PICTURES INCLUDE: Casablance (AA), Arsenic and Old Lace, The Man Who Came to Dinner, Four Daughters, Saturday's Children, Mr. Skeffington, My Foolish Heart, Pete 'n' Tillie, Reuben, Reuben, etc.

EPSTEIN, MEL: Producing. b. Dayton, O., Mar. 25, 1910, e. Ohio State U. Adv. & edit. depts. on newspapers; entered m.p. ind. as player in 1931; then asst. dir., unit prod. mgr., second unit & shorts dir.; U.S. Army Signal Corps (1st Lt.); apptd Para. prod., 1946. Now retired.
PICTURES INCLUDE: Whispering Smith, Hazard, Copper Canyon, Dear Brat, Branded, The Savage, Alaska Seas, Secret of the Incas.
TV: Broken Arrow, Men into Space, The Islanders, Asphalt Jungle, Rawhide, Long Hot Summer, The Monroes, Custer TV, Lancer TV Pilot, unit mgr. Lancer TV series, Medical Center, TV series.

ERDMAN, RICHARD: Actor-director. b. Enid, Okla., June 1, 1925, e. Hollywood High Sch.
PICTURES INCLUDE: Janie, Objective Burma, Time of Your Life, Four Days Leave, The Men, Cry Danger, Jumping Jacks, Happy Time, The Stooge, Stalag 17, The Power and the Prize, Saddle the Wind, Namu, The Killer Whale. Features directed: Bleep, The Brothers O'Toole.
TV: Ray Bolger Show, Perry Mason, Police Story, Tab Hunter Show, Alice, Bionic Woman, One Day at a Time, Playhouse of Stars, Twilight Zone, The Lucy Show, Lou Grant.
DIRECTED: The Dick Van Dyke Show, Mooch (special).

ERICSON, JOHN: Actor. b. Dusseldorf, Germany, Sept. 25, 1926. e. American Acad. of Dramatic Arts. Appeared in summer stock; m.p. debut, Teresa, 1951, then Stalag 17 on Broadway.
PICTURES INCLUDE: Rhapsody, Student Prince, Green Fire, Bad Day at Black Rock, Return of Jack Slade, Pretty Boy Floyd, Bedknobs and Broomsticks.
TV: Honey West.

ERIKSON, LAUNCELOT: Actor-singer. b. New York, Sept. 6, 1949. Industrial films, Stanley Neal Prod., Faith for Today, Gifts, Take My Name, Odds Against Tomorrow, dubbing for Carosello Napolitano; Commercials; Transcriptions, Radio comm. & dramas. Model.

TV LIVE: Studio One, Omnibus, U.S. Steel, Du Pont Show of the Month.

ERLICHT, LEWIS H.: Executive. b. New York City. e. Long Island Univ. Began career with ABC in 1962 with Television Spot Sales. Promoted to mgr. of research for spot sales in 1965 became sls. mgr., gen. sls. mgr. of WABC-TV, New York, from 1969 to 1974. Named v.p., gen. mgr. of WLS-TV, Chicago, in 1975. Moved to ABC Entertainment in 1977; named v.p., gen. mgr., in 1978; v.p., asst. to pres. in 1979. In 1980 made snr. v.p. & asst. to pres.; 1981, sr. v.p., prime time. Promoted to pres. of ABC Entertainment in June, 1983.

ERMAN, JOHN: Director. b. Chicago, Aug. 3, 1935. e. Univ. of California. Debut as TV director, Stoney Burke, 1962.
TELEVISION: Green Eyes, Alexander the Other Side of Dawn, Child of Glass, Just Me and You, My Old Man, Roots: The Next Generation, Family, Moviola, The Letter, Eleanor First Lady of the World, Who Will Love My Children?, A Streetcar Named Desire.
PICTURES: Making It, Ace Eli and Rodger of the Skies.

ESBIN, JERRY: Executive. Joined Paramount Pictures in 1975 as mgr. of branch operations; later named v.p., asst. sls. mgr. In 1980 named v.p., gen. sls. mgr. 1981, snr. v.p., domestic sls. & mktg. 1981, joined United Artists as snr. v.p., mktg. & dist.; 1982, named pres., MGM/UA m.p. dist. & mktg. div; 1983, sr. v.p., domestic dist., Tri-Star Pictures; 1985, promoted to exec. v.p.

ESMOND, CARL: Actor. b. Vienna, Austria, June 14, 1906; e. U. Vienna. On stage Vienna, Berlin, London, etc. (Shakespeare, Shaw, German modern classicals. On screen in Brit. prod. including Blossom Time, Even Song, Invitation to the Waltz. To U.S. in 1938.
PICTURES INCLUDE: The Catman of Paris, Smash-up, Story of a Woman, Slave Girl, Walk a Crooked Mile, Mystery Submarine, World In His Arms, Agent for H.A.R.M., Morituri.

ESSENFELD, BARRY: Executive. b. Bronx, N.Y., Feb. 16, 1936. e. De Witt Clinton, N.Y.U. Acct., American Broadcasting Company, 1957–62; division controller, International Paper Co., 1962–67; group controller & division exec., New England Industries, 1968–70; Controller & asst. secty., Allied Artists Pictures Corp., 1970–73; named asst. treas. & dir. admin., Sept. 1973; gen. sis. mgr. 1979. Allied Artists Industries, v.p., finance, 1980–.

ESSERT, GARY: Executive. b. Oakland, Calif., Oct. 15, 1938. e. UCLA. Entered entertainment field through m.p. exhibition; managed theatres in San Franciso and Los Angeles; has created advertising art campaigns for major studios and main titles for feature films. Technical consultant for professional motion picture presentation installations; coordinated and supervised design and planning of UCLA Motion Picture Center—Melnitz Hall (1964–67). Technical coordinator for the American Film Institute's Center for Advanced Film Studies (1968–1970) designing and outfitting complete facilities. Co-owned and operated a multi-media dance/concert hall in Hollywood known as The Kaleidoscope. Produced The Movies, a two-part, four-hour compilation documentary on the history of American motion pictures, telecast nationally on ABC-TV in March, 1975. Founder (1971) and CEO for 13 years of the Los Angeles International Film Exposition (Filmex). Founder (1983) and current artistic director of the American Cinematheque in Hollywood.

ESSEX, DAVID: Actor-singer. b. Plaistow, London, Eng. July 23, 1947. e. Shipman Sch., Custom House. Started as a singer-drummer in East London band. 1967: Joined touring Repertory Co. in "The Fantasticks," "Oh, Kay," etc. 1970: West End debut in "Ten Years Hard," 1972: Jesus Christ in Godspell, 1978: Che in Evita; 1981: Lord Byron in "Childe Byron" 1983/4: Fletcher Christian in own musical "Mutiny!", on album and stage. Phonogram recording artist. Variety Club of Great Britain show business personality of 1978. Many gold & silver disc intl. awards.
TV: appearances include: Top of the Pops, Own Specials, BBC series. Appearances on TV: France, Japan, Germany, Spain, Denmark, Australia.
PICTURES INCLUDE: Assault, All Coppers Are . . . , Recent pictures: That'll Be the Day, Stardust, Silver Dream Racer.
U.S. TV: Merv Griffin, Johnny Carson, Dinah Shore, American Bandstand, Midnight Special, Grammy Awards, Salute To The Beatles, Don Kirshners Rock Concert, A.M. America, Phil Everly in Session, Paul Ryan Show.

ESSEX, HARRY J.: Writer. b. New York City, N.Y. e. St. John's Univ., Brooklyn, B.A. With Dept. Welfare, author play Something for Nothing, on New York stage, followed by Stronger than Brass. Wrote orig. story, Man Made Monster, for Universal. During World War II in U.S. Army Signal Corps; scenarist, training films on combat methods, censorship. Since release has written orig. s.p. Boston Blackie and the Law, Dangerous Business, (s.p.) Desperate Bodygaurd, He Walked by Night, Dragnet, Killer That Stalked New York, Wyoming Mail, The Fat Man, Undercover Girl, Las Vegas Story, Models, Inc., Kansas City Confidential, The 49th Man, It Came From Outer Space; s.p., dir., I the Jury; s.p. Creature from the Black Lagoon; collab. s.p., story, Southwest Passage; adapt., Devil's Canyon; s.p., dir., Mad at the World; collab. s.p., Teen-age Crime Wave, Raw Edge; story, s.p. Lonely Man; play. One for the Dame; collab., Sons of Katie Elder, Man and Boy, s.p. & dir. Octman, s.p., dir., prod. The Cremators, The Amigos, story and SP Metro, release 1973. Collaboration with Oscar Saul; Chrysalis, in collaboration with Ray Bradbury.
TV: Untouchables (various series). The Racers, Alcoa Hour, Westinghouse, Desilu; story consultant and head writer: Target, The Corruptors, The Dick Powell Show, Bewitched, I Dream of Jeannie, Kraft Suspense Theatres, Terror in the Sky (NBC, 1986).
NOVELIST: I Put My Right Foot In, Little Brown. Stage prod., Fatty, B'way, Sept., 1976; Man and Boy, (Dell), 1971, Marina, Playboy Press, 1981.
PLAYS: Something for Nothing; Neighborhood Affair; One for the Dame; Fatty; Twilight, When the Bough Breaks, Dark Passion, Casa D'Amor.

ESTEVEZ, EMILIO: Actor. b. 1963. Oldest son of actor Martin Sheen.
PICTURES: Tex, The Outsiders, Repo Man, The Breakfast Club, That Was Then This is Now, (also s.p.), St. Elmo's Fire.
TELEVISION: In the Custody of Strangers (movie).

ESTRADA, ERIK: Actor. b. New York City, Mar. 16, 1949. Began professional career in Mayor John Lindsay's Cultural Program, performing in public parks. Joined American Musical Dramatic Academy for training. Feature film debut in The Cross and the Switchblade (1970).
PICTURES: The New Centurions, Airport '75, Midway, Trackdown.
TELEVISION: CHIPS, guest roles on Hawaii Five-O, Six Million Dollar Man, Police Woman, Kojak, Medical Center, etc.

ETKES, RAPHAEL: Executive. Joined MCA in 1961; named v.p. of Universal Pictures n 1973. Appt. v.p. of MCA, Inc. in 1978; named sr. v.p., Universal Pictures, 1979; 1980, named prs. chief exec. off., AIP; 1981, joined United Artists as snr. v.p.—Worldwide Prod; 1983–85, pres., production, Embassy Pictures.

ETTINGER, EDWIN D.: Publicist. b. New York City. 1921. Entered m.p. ind. as office boy, MGM; pub. rel. and publ. for industrial, comm. clients, 1946–52; joined Ettinger Co., pub. rel., 1952; pub. rel. dir., Disneyland Inc., 1955; marketing dir., Disneyland, 1955–65; v.p., M.C.A. Enterprises, Inc., 1955.

ETTLINGER, JOHN A.: Prod.-dir., distributor. b. Chicago, Ill., Oct. 14, 1924. e. Peddie Inst., Cheshire Acad., Signal Corps Photog. Center, 1942–45; with Paramount Theatres Corp., 1945–47; dir., KTLA, Paramount TV Prod., Inc., Los Angeles, 1948–50; radio-TV dir., Nat. C. Goldstone Agency, 1950–53; pres. Medallion TV Enterprises, Inc.; TV prod., View the Clue, Greenwich Village, High Road to Danger, Sur Demande, Star Route, Las Vegas Fights, Celebrity Billiards; Pres., KUDO-FM, Las Vegas.

EVANS, ANDREW C.: Executive. Joined Paramount Pictures 1987 as dir. of financial reporting. Named v.p., corporate controller, 1980; sr. v.p., 1984. Same year named exec. v.p., finance, for Motion Picture Group of co. 1985, promoted to sr. v.p., finance.

EVANS, BARRY: Actor-Director. b. Guildford, England, 1943. Trained Central School. Repertory: Barrow, Nottingham, Chester, Royal Court, Nat. Theatre, Hampstead Th. Club, Chips with Everything, London and B'way. Young Vic. Theatre Clwyd Mold.
TV: Redcap, Undermined, The Baron, The Class, Armchair Theatre, Love Story, Doctor at Large, Short Story, Crossroads, Mind Your Language, Dick Emery Show.
PICTURES INCLUDE: The White Bus, Here We Go 'Round the Mulberry Bush, Alfred the Great, Die Screaming, Marriane, The Adventures of a Taxi-Driver, Under the Doctor.

EVANS, GENE: Actor. b. Holbrook, Ariz., July 11, 1924; e. Colton H.S. Started career in summer stock, Penthouse Theatre, Altadena, Calif. Screen debut: Under Colorado Skies, 1947.
PICTURES INCLUDE: Crisscross, Larceny, Berlin Express, Assigned to Danger, Mother Was a Freshman, Sugarfoot, Armored Car Robbery, Steel Helmet, I was an American Spy, Force of Arms, Jet Pilot, Fixed Bayonets, Mutiny, Park Row, Thunderbirds, Donovan's Brain, Golden Blade, Hell & High Water, Long Wait, Cattle Queen of Montana, Wyoming Renegades, Crashout, Helen Morgan Story, Bravados, Sad Sack, The Hangman, Operation Petticoat, Support Your Local Sheriff, War Wagon, Nevada Smith, Young and Wild, Ballad of Cable Hogue, There

Was a Crooked Man, Support Your Local Gunfighter, Camper John, Walking Tall, People Toys, Pat Garrett & Billy The Kid, Magic of Lassie, Blame It on the Night.
TELEVISION: Matt Helm (series), Spencer's Pilots (series); Kate Bliss & Ticker Tape Kid Fire, the Sacketts, Shadow Riders, Travis McGee.

EVANS, LINDA: Actress. b. Hartford, CT, Nov. 18, 1942. e. Hollywood High School, Los Angeles. TV commercials led to contract with MGM and film debut in Twilight of Honor (1963). Formerly married to John Derek.
PICTURES: The Klansman, Avalanche Express, Tom Horn, etc.
TELEVISION: Series: The Big Valley, The Hunter, The Love Boat, Dynasty. Movies: Nowhere to Run, Standing Tall, Gambler II, etc. Mini-Series: Bare Essence, North & South Book II.

EVANS, MAURICE: Actor. b. Dorchester, Eng., June 3, 1901. On the stage since 1926.
THEATRE: London theatrical, career included Justice, Loyalties, Diversion, Journey's End, The Man I Killed, The Queen Bee. The Swan, See Ourselves, The Heart Line and starred for one season at the Old Vic; to U.S. 1935 and appeared in Romeo and Juliet, St. Helena, Richard II, Hamlet (Entirety), Henry IV (Part I), Twelfth Night, Macbeth, 1942; after War returned to Broadway, 1945 and appeared in G.I., Hamlet, Man and Superman, The Devil's Disiciple, The Wild Duck, Dial 'M' For Murder, The Apple Cart, Heartbreak House, Tenderloin, The Aspern Papers, Shakespeare Revisited, A Program for Two Players.
PICTURES INCLUDE: Kind Lady, Androcles and the Lion, Gilbert and Sullivan, Macbeth, Warlord, Planet of The Apes, Rosemary's Baby, The Body Stealers.
Prod. Teahouse of the August Moon. No Time for Sergeants, N.Y. stage.
TV SHOWS: Hamlet, Richard II, Macbeth, Devil's Disciple, Taming of the Shrew, Man and Superman, The Tempest, St. John, series of 7 plays for Hallmark, NBC; G.E. Theatre (Caesar & Cleopatra), Theatre Guild, etc. Gen. Motors Motorama, Bewitched.

EVANS, RAY: Songwriter. b. Salamanca, N.Y., Feb. 4, 1915. e. Wharton School of Pa. U. Musician on cruise ships, radio writer spec. material. Hellzapoppin', Sons o' Fun.
SONGS INCLUDE: To Each His Own, Golden Earrings, Buttons and Bows (Academy Award, 1948), Mona Lisa (Academy Award, 1950), Whatever Will Be Will Be (Academy Award, 1956), A Thousand Violins, I'll Always Love You, Dreamsville, Love Song From Houseboat, Tammy, Silver Bells, Dear Heart, Angel, Never Let Me To, Almost In Your Arms, As I Love You, In the Arms of Love, Wish Me a Rainbow.
PICTURES INCLUDE: Paleface, Sorrowful Jones, Fancy Pants, My Friend Irma, Capt. Carey U.S.A., Off LImits, Here Come the Girls, Red Garters, Man Who Knew Too Much, Stars Are Singing, Tammy, Houseboat, Blue Angel, A Private's Affair, All Hands on Deck, Dear Heart, The Third Day, What Did You Do In The War Daddy?, This Property Is Condemned.
BROADWAY MUSICAL: Oh Captain! Let It Ride!, Sugar Babies.
TV THEMES: Bonanza, Mr. Ed, Mr. Lucky, To Rome With Love.

EVANS, ROBERT: Producer. b. N.Y.C., June 29, 1930. Made appearance on radio as actor at age 11; went on to appear in more than 300 radio programs on major networks. Also appeared on TV in its early days. At 20 joined brother, Charles, and Joseph Picone, as partner in firm of Evans-Picone, Inc. In 1957 signed by Universal to play Irving Thalberg in The Man of a Thousand Faces after recommendation by Norma Shearer, Thalberg's widow. (See credits below for other acting assignments.) Turned to production and signed as independent by 20th Century-Fox. In August, 1966, joined Paramount Pictures as head of prod., a post he held ten years. Resigned to become indep. prod. again; has exclusive contract with Para.
PICTURES INCLUDE: Actor: The Sun Also rises, The Fiend Who Walked the West, The Best of Everything. Independent Producer: Chinatown, Marathon Man, Black Sunday, Players, Urban Cowboy, Popeye, The Cotton Club.

EVERETT, CHAD: Actor. b. South Bend, Ind., June 11, 1936. r.n. Ray Canton. e. Wayne State Univ., Detroit. Signed by William T. Orr, head of TV prod. for Warner Bros. to 3-year contract. Appeared in many TV series as well as films. Next became contract player at MGM.
PICTURES INCLUDE: Claudelle Inglish, The Chapman Report, The Singing Nun, The Last Challenge, Made in Paris, Johnny Tiger, Return of the Gunfighter, The Impossible Years, Airplane II; The Sequel, Fever Pitch.
TELEVISION: Hawaiian Eye, 77 Sunset Strip, Surfside Six, Lawman, Bronco, The Dakotas, The Lieutenant, Redigo, Route 66, Ironside, Medical Center, The Rousters.

EVERETT, RUPERT: Actor. b. Norfolk, England, 1961. e. Ampleforth Central School for Speech & Drama. Apprenticed with Glasgow's Citizen's Theatre. Originated role of Guy Bennett in Another Country on London stage in 1982 and made feature film debut in screen version in 1984.
PICTURES: Real Life, Dance with a Stranger.
TELEVISION: Arthur, the King.

EVERSON, WILLIAM K.: Writer. b. Yeovil, Eng., April 8, 1929. Pub. dir., Renown Pictures Corp., Ltd., London, 1944; film critic; m.p. journalist; in armed forces, 1947–49; thea. mgr., pub. & booking consultant, Monseigneur News Theatres, London, 1949; pub. dir., Allied Artists Inc. Corp., 1951; prod., writer Paul Killiam Dorg., 1956. Writer-editor-researcher on TV series "Movie Museum" and "Silents Please," also on TV specials and theatrical features "Hollywood the Golden Years," "The Valentino Legend," "The Love Goddesses" and "The Great Director."
AUTHOR: Several books on movie history, including "The Western," "The Bad Guys," "The American Movie," "The Films of Laurel & Hardy," "The Art of W. C. Fields," "Hal Roach." "The Detective in Film," "Classics of the Horror Film," "Claudette Colbert."
Lecturer, archival consultant, American Film Institute representative. Film History instructor at New York University, The New School and The School of Visual Arts, all in New York. Also, Harvard Univ.

EWELL, TOM: Actor. r.n. Yewell Tompkins. b. Owensboro, Ky., April 29. e. U. of Wisconsin. Active in coll. dramatics; salesman at Macy's. Stage debut, New York: They Shall Not Die, 1934; thereafter many unsuccessful plays. U.S. Navy 1942–46.
THEATRE: Returned to stage in John Loves Mary; Small Wonder; on road in Stage Door, Tobacco Road, Roberta, Key Largo; on Broadway in Seven-Year Itch, Tunnel of Love.
RADIO: Many programs.
PICTURES INCLUDE: Adam's Rib, Mr. Music, A Life of Her Own, American Guerilla in the Philippines, Up Front, Finders Keepers, Lost in Alaska, Willie & Joe Back at the Front, Seven-Year Itch, Lieutenant Wore Skirts, Girl Can't Help It, Tender Is the Night, State Fair, Suppose They Gave A War and Nobody Came?, To Find a Man, They Only Kill Their Masters, The Great Gatsby.

F

FABRAY, NANETTE: Actress. b. San Diego, Calif., Oct. 27, 1920. d. Raoul Fabares and Lillian (McGovern) Fabares; student Los Angeles City College. m. David Tebet 1947 (div. July, 1951); m. 2d Ranald MacDougall 1957, deceased Dec. 11, 1973. One son, Jamie. First prof. stage appearance at age of three and a half in vaudeville as Baby Nan. Leading lady in Charlie Chan radio series. Member of the cast, radio, Showboat. 1938, won two-year scholarship to Max Reinhardt school in Hollywood, and starred in his Calif. productions of The Miracle, Six Characters in Search of an Author, and Servant With Two Masters.
PICTURES INCLUDE: Elizabeth and Essex, A Child is Born, The Happy Ending, Cockeyed Cowboys, The Bandwagon.
TV: Own TV Series, Yes, Yes Nanette 1961–62. Also starred on shows with every major TV star. Two years on Caesar's Hour. Series: One Day at a Time.
BROADWAY SHOWS: Meet the People, By Jupiter, Jackpot, May Dear Public, Let's Face It, Bloomer Girl, Arms and the Girl, High Button Shoes, Make A Wish, Love Life, Mr. President, No Hard Feelings.
AWARDS: High Button Shoes 1948, two Donaldson Awards for best performance in a musical and best supporting performance; Love Life 1947, the Tony Awards best musical actress of the year; Three Emmy Awards for Caesar's Hour as best comedienne, 1955, 1956, best supporting actress 1955; Woman of the Year, 1955, Radio and TV Editors of America; Hollywood Women's Press Club, 1960; Honorary Mayor of Pacific Palisades 1967–68; One of Ten Best Dressed Women in America, Fashion Academy Award, 1950.

FABRIZI, ALDO: Actor. b. Rome, Italy. Stage actor to 1942.
PICTURES INCLUDE: Go Ahead, Passengers, Square of Rome, Open City, My Son, the Professor, To Live in Peace, Christmas at Camp 119, Emigrants, Welcome, Reverend, First Communion (Father's Dilemma), Flowers of St. Francis, Mishappy Family, Thieves and Cops, Times Gone By, Lucky Five, Too Young For Love, Voice of Silence.

FADIMAN, CLIFTON: Writer-Performer. b. Brooklyn, N.Y., May 15, 1904. e. Columbia Univ. Contributor to magazines since 1924. Asst. ed. Simon & Schuster, 1927–29, ed. 1929–35. Book ed. The New Yorker, 1933–43. Mc. on Information Please radio program 1938–48; TV, 1952; Judge, Book of the Month Club, since 1944; Mc. This Is Show Business, TV; author, Party of One; Any Number

Can Play; Enter Conversing; The Lifetime Reading Plan; editor, American Treasury, 50 years; m.c., Conversation, 1954; m.c., Quiz Kids, 1956; Metropolitan Opera Roving Reporter, 1955–60; m.c., Alumni Fun, 1964; bd. of editors, Encyclopaedia Britannica; Advisory Board, CRICKET: The Magazine for Children, Co-author, The Joys of Wine, 1975. Co-author, The Wine Buyers Guide, 1977; Co-author, Empty Pages: A Search for Writing Competence in School and Society, 1979; editor, World Treasury of Children's Literature, 1984–85; commentator, First Edition, 1983–84; Little Brown Book of Anecdotes, 1985; The Word of the Short Story, 1986.

FAICHNEY, JAMES B.: Producer-Director-Writer-Consultant. b. Yonkers, N.Y. Pathe News; RKO Pathe, film editor, writer, director; U.S. Army WW II, chief motion picture security censorship; Soundmasters; James B. Faichney Prod.; U.S. Dept. of State—USIA; Freelance producer, director, writer for CBS Films, ABC-CBS-NBC News, U.S. Army, National Foundation, Communications Four, Cul-Crieff Associates. Consultant to the U.S. Atomic Energy Commission, U.S. Air Force, Committee for Free Asia, Chm., Directors Guild of America Government Audio-Visual Committee; Coordinator, Joint Management-Labor Committee on Government Audio-Visual Policy. Currently engaged in cable-TV program production.

PICTURES INCLUDE: The Most Rewarding Law, The Third Pillar, Air Power, Dead Man's Voice, Dawn of a New Day, Kampong Sentesa.

TV: Air Power, Twentieth Century, 21st Century, David Brinkley's Journal, NBC White Paper, ABC Close-up, The Great Conventions (the Republicans, the Democrats), Viet Cong, The Green Scene, The Revolutionaries, The Will for Peace, A Better World, 1945, The Diplomat, The General.

AWARDS: George Foster Peabody, Sylvania. Billboard and United States Air Force exceptional service awards; two ATVAS nominations for best documentary program and series.

FAIN, SAMMY: Composer. b. New York City, June 17, 1892. e. Public and high schools. Self taught on piano. Commenced career in Tin Pan Alley as teenage staff pianist-composer for leading music publishers, then in vaudeville. Recording contract at Harmony Records (Columbia); featured solo performer on many New York radio stations. Joined ASCAP, 1926. Wrote first song hit, "Let A Smile Be Your Umbrella." Lyrics by Irving Kahal, 1927.

STAGE: Scores for Hellzapoppin, Son's of Fun, George White's Scandals, Ed Wynn's Boys & Girls Together, Flahooley, Christine & others.

PICTURES INCLUDE: Scores & Songs—Big Pond, Young Man of Manhattan, Footlight Parade, Sweet Music, Harold Teen, New Faces of '37, Geo. White's Scandals, Call Me Mister, Alice in Wonderland, Peter Pan, Jazz Singer, Weekend at the Waldorf, Anchors Aweigh, Imitation of Life, Mardi Gras, Calamity Jane, April Love, Marjorie Morningstar, Certain Smile, Love is a Many Splendored Thing, Tender is the Night, Made in Paris, The Stepmother and many others.

SONGS: Let a Smile Be Your Umbrella, Wedding Bells Are Breaking Up That Old Gang of Mine, When I Take My Sugar to Tea, You Brought a New Kind of Love to Me, Was That the Human Thing to Do, By A Waterfall, Are You Having Any Fun, I'm Late, I Can Dream Can't I, That Old Feeling, I'll Be Seeing You, Dear Hearts and Gentle People, April Love, A Certain Smile, A Very Precious Love, Tender Is the Night, Secret Love, Love Is a Many Splendored Thing, many others. Elected to Songwriters' Hall of Fame.

CITATIONS: Oscar awards for Secret Love and Love is a Many Splendored Thing, plus eight Acad. Oscar nominations: Internatinal awards—Diploma Di Benemerenza most coveted honor by the Hall of Artists in Nice, France, and Augasto Messinesse Gold Award from Messina, Italy. Also two Laurel Awards.

FAIRBANKS, DOUGLAS, JR.: Actor, prod. Bus. exec. b. N.Y. Dec. 9, 1909; son of late Douglas Fairbanks. e. Pasadena (Calif.) Polytech. Sch.; Harvard Mil. Acad., Los Angeles; Bovee and Collegiate Sch., N.Y.; also Paris, London. Began as screen actor 1923 in Stephen Steps Out; thereafter in more than 75 pictures. Stage from 1927 in U.S., U.K. (Young Woodley, Saturday's Children, etc.); 1934 in Manchester, England (The Winding Journey), London (Moonlight in Silver), 1968–77 My Fair Lady, The Secretary Bird, Pres ent Laughter (U.S.), The Pleasure of His Company (U.S., U.K., Ireland, Australia and Hong Kong), Out on a Limb, Sleuth (U.S.). Since sound in both British & U.S. prods.; formed own co. 1935, prod. & starring, The Amateur Gentleman, etc.; U.S. Navy, 1941; Silver Star Combat Legion of Merit; K.B.E., D.S.C., Legion of Honor, Croix de Guerre, etc. 1949. Entered TV film prod., 1952.

PICTURES INCLUDE: (since sound): Dawn Patrol, Little Caesar, Outward Bound, Union Depot, Captured, Catherine the Great, Accused, The Prisoner of Zenda, Having Wonderful Time, Gunga Din, Morning Glory, Angels Over Broadway, The Corsican Brothers, The Exile, Sinbad the Sailor, That Lady in Ermine, Joy of Living, Fighting O'Flynn, State Secret; prod. Another Man's Poison; Chase Crooked Shadow, Ghost Story.

TV: prod. Douglas Fairbanks Presents, The Rheingold Theatre, etc.

FAIRBANKS, JERRY: Executive Producer. b. San Francisco, Calif.; cameraman, 1924–29; prod., shorts, Universal, 1929–34; prod., Popular Science, Unusual Occupations, Speaking of Animals Series, Para., 1935–49; Winner two Acad. Awards; set up film div., NBC, 1948; formed, NBC Newsreel, 1949; devel. Zoomar Lens and Multicam System; formed Jerry Fairbanks Prods., 1950.

TV: Public Prosecutor (first film series for TV); other series: Silver Theatre, Front Page Detective, Jackson and Jill, Hollywood Theatre, Crusader Rabbit.

PICTURES INCLUDE: The Last Wilderness, Down Liberty Road, With This Ring, Counterattack, Collision Course, Land of the Sea, Brink of Disaster, The Legend of Amaluk, North of The Yukon, Damage Report, The Boundless Seas.

FAIRCHILD, MORGAN: Actress. b. Dallas, TX, Feb. 3, 1950. e. SMU.

PICTURES: Bullet for Pretty Boy, The Seduction.

TELEVISION: Search for Tomorrow, Murder in Music City, The Memory of Eva Ryker, Flamingo Road, The Dream Merchants, The Zany Adventures of Robin Hood, Time Bomb, North & South Book II.

FAIRCHILD, WILLIAM: Director, screenwriter, playwright. b. Cornwall, England. e. Royal Naval College, Dartmouth. Early career Royal Navy.

PICTURES INCLUDE: Screenplays: Morning Departure, Outcast of the Islands, The Gift Horse, The Net, Newspaper Story, Malta Story, The Seekers, Passage Home, Value For Money, Star!, Embassy, The Darwin Adventure, Invitation to the Wedding, Dir.: John and Julie, The Extra Day, the Horsemasters, The Silent Enemy.

SCREENPLAYS AND TV PLAYS INCLUDE: The Man With the Gun, No Man's Land, The Signal, Four Just Men, Some Other Love, Cunningham 5101, The Break, The Zoo Gang, Lady with a Past.

STAGE: Sound of Murder, Breaking Point, Poor Horace, The Pay-Off, The Flight of the Bumble B, The Paternal Optimist, Shooting Script.

BOOKS: A Matter of Duty, The Swiss Arrangement, Astrology for Dogs, Astrology Cats, Catsigns (U.S.A.).

FALK, PETER: Actor. b. New York City, Sept. 16, 1927. e. Syracuse Univ.

THEATRE: Off-Broadway: The Iceman Cometh, Comic Strip, Purple Dust, Bonds of Interest, The Lady's Not For Burning, Saint Joan, Diary of a Scoundrel. On Broadway: Saint Joan, The Passion of Josef D., The Prisoner of Second Avenue.

TV: Studio One, Kraft Theatre, Alcoa Theatre, N.T.A. Play of the Week, Armstrong Circle Theatre, Omnibus, Robert Montgomery Presents, Brenner, Deadline, Kraft Mystery Theatre, Rendezvous, Sunday Showcase, The Untouchables, N.B.C.'s Sacco—Vanzetti Story, Dick Powell Show—The Price of Tomatoes, Danny Kay Show, Edie Adams Show, Bob Hope Chrysler Hour, Columbo (1971).

PICTURES INCLUDE: Murder, Pocketful of Miracles, The Balcony, Robin and the Seven Hoods, Mad, Mad, Mad World, Italiano Brava Gente, Luv, Castle Keep, Anzio, Husbands, Machine Gun McCann, Mikey and Nicky, Murder by Death, The Cheap Detective, Brinks' Job, The In-Laws, All the Marbles, Big Trouble, Happy New Year.

FANTOZZI TONY: Theatrical Agent. b. May 1, 1933. New Britain, Conn. William Morris Agency.

FARBER, BART: Executive. Joined United Artists corp. in early 1960s when UA acquired ZIV TV Programs. Served as v.p. United Artists Television and United Artists Broadcasting. In 1971 named v.p. in charge of legal affairs of the cos. In January 1978, named snr. v.p.—TV, video and special markets; indep. consultant, TV, Pay TV, home video. 1981, joined Cable Health Network as v.p., legal & business affairs; 1982, v.p., business & legal affairs, Lifetime Network; 1986, independent communications consultant.

FARENTINO, JAMES: b. Brooklyn, N.Y., Feb. 24, 1938. m. Michele Lee, actress, singer. e. American Academy of Dramatic Arts.

THEATRE: Appeared in Broadway prod. of Night of the Iguana. A Streetcar Named Desire (revival, 1973).

TV INCLUDES: Naked City, daytime soap operas, Laredo, Route 66, The Alfred Hitchcock Hour, Ben Casey, Twelve O'Clock High, Death of a Salesman, Sins.

PICTURES INCLUDE: The Pad (And How to Use It) (Golden Globe Award, 1966), The Ride of Hangman's Tree, Banning Rosie!, The Story of A Woman, The Final Countdown, Dead & Buried.

FARNSWORTH, RICHARD: Actor. b. Los Angeles. Active as stuntman for 40 years before turning to acting.

PICTURES: Comes a Horseman, Tom Horn, Resurrection, Ruckus, The Legend of the Lone Ranger, The Grey Fox, The Natural, Into the Night, Sylvester.

FARR, FELICIA: Actress. b. Westchester, N.Y., Oct. 4. e. Penn State College. m. Jack Lemmon. Stage debut: Picnic (Players Ring Theatre).
PICTURES INCLUDE: Timetable, Jubal, Reprisal, First Texan, Last Wagon, 3:10 to Yuma, Hell Bent For Leather, Kiss Me Stupid, Kotch, Charley Varrick, That's Life.

FARR, JAMIE: Actor. r.n. Jameel Joseph Farah. b. Toledo, OH, July 1. e. Columbia Coll. Trained for stage at Pasadena Playhouse. Film debut in Blackboard Jungle, 1955. Gained fame as Klinger in TV series, MASH.
PICTURES: Cannonball Run, Murder Can Hurt You, Return of the Rebels, Cannonball Run II.
TELEVISION: Dear Phoebe, The Red Skelton Show, The Danny Kaye Show, Chicago Teddy Bears, MASH, After MASH (also dir. of both MASH series).

FARRAR, DAVID: Actor. b. Forest Gate, Essex, England, 1908.
PICTURES INCLUDE: Black Narcissus, Frieda, Mr. Perrin & Mr. Traill, Small Back Room, Diamond City, Gone to Earth. One of top ten British money makers Motion Picture Herald-Fame poll, Cage of Gold, Night Without Stars, The Golden Horde, Obsessed, Wild Heart, Duel in the Jungle, Black Shield of Falworth, Lilacs in the Spring, Escape to Burma, Sea Chase, Pearl of the South Pacific, Lost, Woman and the Hunter, I Accuse, Son of Robin Hood, John Paul Jones, Watusi, Solomon and Sheba, Best Girl, Middle of Nowhere, The 300 Spartans, Beat Girl.
TV: Dick Powell Show.

FARRELL, CHARLES: Actor. b. Onset Bay, Mass., Aug. 9, 1901; e. Boston U. Entered m.p. ind. in silent films.
PICTURES INCLUDE: Seventh Heaven, Street Angel, Lucky Star, Sunny Side Up, Wild Girl, Big Shakedown, Moonlight Sonata, Just Around the Corner, Tailspin.
U.S. Navy, 1942–45; mayor of Palm Springs since 1947.
TV: My Little Margie; The Charles Farrell Show.

FARRELL, HENRY: Author of novels and screenplays
SCREENPLAYS INCLUDE: Whatever Happened to Baby Jane? Hush . . . Hush, Sweet Charlotte, and What's the Matter with Helen?
TV: How Awful About Allan, The House That Would Not Die.

FARREN, JACK: Prod.-Writer. b. New York City; e. B.A., NYU. Theatre: prod., Take a Giant Step, Lorenzo 1967, Robert Anderson's You Know I Can't Hear You When the Water's Running; 1968, The Education of Hyman Kaplan.
PICTURES INCLUDE: Silent Night, Lonely Night; Fuzz.
TV: Goodson-Todman Productions; NBC, CBS.

FARROW, MIA: Actress. b. Los Angeles, Feb. 9. 1945. e. Marymount, Los Angeles, Cygnet House, London. Bway. debut. The Importance of Being Earnest, 1963. Screen debut: Guns at Batasi.
PICTURES INCLUDE: Guns at Batasi, A Dandy in Aspic, Rosemary's Baby, John and Mary, Secret Ceremony, See No Evil, The Public Eye. The Great Gatsby, Full Circle, A Wedding, Death on the Nile, Hurricane, A Midsummer Night's Sex Comedy, Zelig, Broadway Danny Rose, Supergirl, The Purple Rose of Cairo, Hannah and Her Sisters.
TV: Peyton Place, Johnny Belinda.
THEATRE: Mary Rose (London).

FASS, M. MONROE: Theatre Broker. b. New York City, Feb. 26, 1901. e. City College of N.Y. (M.E. degree, engineering). Firm: Fass & Wolper. Entered real estate business in 1925, making first deal with Marcus Loew for land on which Paradise Theatre, Bronx, N.Y., was built. Thereafter made theatre deals (sale or lease of land or building) in most major cities in the U.S. and in major shopping centers. Member: Real Estate Board of N.Y.: Natl. Institute of Real Estate Brokers, Natl. Assoc. of Real Estate Board; Amer. Society of Real Estate Appraisers, Natl. Assoc. of Theatre Owners.

FAWCETT, FARRAH: Actress. b. Corpus Christi, Texas, Feb. 2, 1947. e. Univ. of Texas. Picked as one of the Ten Most Beautiful Girls while a freshman; went to Hollywood and signed by Screen Gems. Did films, TV shows, and made over 100 TV commercials.
PICTURES INCLUDE: Love Is a Funny Thing, Myra Breckenridge, Logan's Run, Somebody Killed Her Husband, Sunburn, Saturn III, Cannonball Run, Extremities.
TV: Owen Marshall, Counselor at Law, The Six Million Dollar Man, Charlie's Angels (regular). Movies: The Feminist and the Fuzz, The Burning Bed, Between Two Women.

FAY, PATRICK J.: Director, producer. b. June 7. e. Carnegie Tech; Dumont TV Network, 10 years. Director of over 100 Army training films.
TV: Bishop Sheen, Broadway to Hollywood, Manhattan Spotlight, Life is Worth Living, Front Row Center, Ilona Massey Show, Alec Templeton Show, Maggi McNellis Show, Key to Missing Persons, Kids and Company; co-prod., dir., Confession; dir., TV film series, Confession; dir. IBM Industrials, IBM World Trade, Europe Industrial, The Big Picture.
AUTHOR: Melba, The Toast of Pithole, The Last Family Portrait in Oil, Coal Oil Johnny, French Kate, The Water's Fine, No Pardon in Heaven.
FILMS: Director for RCA, General Electric H.G. Peters Company, Bransby Films.

FEHR, RUDI: Executive. b. Berlin, Germany; m. Maris Wrixon actress. Started career with Tobis-Klangfilm, Berlin. Joined Warner Bros. editorial department, 1936. Became producer, 1952; promoted to executive, 1956; Post Production Exec. Warner Bros.; WB title changed to dir. of editorial & post-prod. operations. Now retired; is consultant to industry. Nominated for Oscar as co-editor of Prizzi's Honor.

FEINBERG, MILTON: Executive. b. Milwaukee, Wis. e. Univ. of Minn., school of Bus. Admin. Salesman, 20th Century-Fox, Des Moines, 1942–44; branch mgr., National Screen Service, Des Moines, 1945–57; branch mgr., in Chicago, superv. Chicago, Milwaukee, Des Moines exchange territories, National Screen Service, 1958–65; gen. sales mgr., NSS, 1966; v.p. & gen. sls. mgr. 1967; May, 1974, sr. v.p., N.S.S.

FEITSHANS, BUZZ: Executive. Worked for 10 years at American-International as supvr. of prod., jobs including film editing and supervision of editing and dubbing. Bowed as producer on Dillinger (1973). In 1975 formed A-Team Productions with John Milius.
PICTURES: Big Wednesday (prod.), Hardcore (prod.), 1941 (prod.), Extreme Prejudice (exec. prod.). Conan the Barbarian, First Blood, Uncommon Valor, Rambo II.

FELD, FRITZ: Actor. b. Berlin, Germany, Oct. 15, 1900. e. U. Berlin; Max Reinhardt Sch. of Drama, Berlin. Actor, prod. asst. dir. for Reinhardt in Berlin 7 yrs.; on screen 1918 in The Golem, Ufa. Since found variously assoc. U.S. m.p. prod., as writer, director, actor: has appeared in more than 410 pictures. 1971; nat'l bd. dir., Screen Actors Guild. 1968 chairman of the "American National Committee," Southern California Chapter. 1976 chairman Hollywood Museum Project committee—Screen Actors Guild, 20th Century-Fox Film corp. staged A Tribute To Fritz Feld-60 Years In The Movies and the Los Angeles City named a theater in Brentwood The Fritz Feld Community Theatre. In April 1979 Feld was elected honorary Mayor of Brentwood by the Chamber of Commerce.
TV: Dangerous Assignment, Racket Squad, Mr. & Mrs. North, Jimmy Durante Show, Jack Paar, Thin Man, Chevy Show, Red Skelton, Milton Berle, Colonel Flack, Accused, Peter Gunn, General Electric Thea., Kraft Music Hall, Danny Thomas, Bachelor Father, Commercials. Adventures in Paradise, Follow the Sun, The Donna Reed Show, Valentine Day, No Time for Sergeants, The Farmer's Daughter, The Bing Crosby Show, Batman, Lost in Space, The Man From U.N.C.L.E., Laredo, Please Don't Eat the Daisies, Girl From U.N.C.L.E., The Smothers Bros., The Wild, Wild, West, Bewitched, Donald O'Connor Show, The Beverly Hillbillies, Land of the Giants, Arnie, Love, American Style, The Merv Griffin Show, Movie of the Week, The New Bill Cosby Show, The Julie Andrews Hour, Fire House, The Odd Couple, The Night Couple, The Night Stalker, Only With Married Men, The Mike Douglas Show, The Tonight Show, Tabitha, The Hardy Boys, Flying High, Over Easy, Hizzonner, NBC's Sunday Show, General Hospital, Heidi, Supertrain, Love, Sidney, No Soap, Radio, Magnum P.I., Simon & Simon, Amazing Stories.
STAGE: The Miracle, Once More With Feeling, Would Be Gentleman, Midsummer Night's Dream, Arsenic and Old Lace, You Can't Take It With You.
PICTURES INCLUDE: Wives and Lovers, Promises, Promises, Who's Minding the Store?, Four for Texas, The Patsy, Harlow, Made in Paris, Three on a Couch, Way . . . Way Out, The Comic, Hello, Dolly!, The Computer Wore Tennis Shoes, The Phynx, Which Way to the Front? Herbie Rides Again, The Strongest Man in the World, Only With Married Men, Hoyd Axton's Country Western Rock 'Roll Show, The Sunshine Boys, Won Ton Ton, The Dog Who Saved Hollywood, Broadway Rose, Mel Brooks' Silent Movie, Pennsylvania Lynch, Freaky Friday, The World's Greatest Lover, Herbie Goes Bananas, Mel Brooks' History of the World, All the Marbles, The Last of the Great Survivors, A Fine Mess, Shell Game.

FELDMAN, EDWARD S.: Producer. b. New York, Sept. 5, 1929. e. Michigan State Univ. Trade press contact, newspaper and mag. contact, 20th Century Fox, 1950; dir. info. services, Dover Air Force Base. 1954–56; publicity coordinator, The World of Suzie Wong, Para., 1959; joined Embassy, dir. of publicity, 1969; vice pres. in chg., adv. & pub, Seven Arts Prods., 1962; v.p. exec. asst. to head prod. Warner-7 Arts Prods., 1967, pres., m.p. dept., Filmways, 1970; exec. prod., What's the Matter With Helen?,

1971, exec. prod. Fuzz, 1972, Save the Tiger, 1972; prod. The Other Side of the Mountain, 1974; prod. Two-Minute Warning, 1976; exec. prod. 21 Hours At Munich, 1976; prod., King, 1977. Formed Edward S. Feldman Co., 1978. Co-prod. The Last Married Couple in America; Exec. Prod.: Valentine, 300 Miles for Stephanie, Charles and Diana: A Royal Love Story, The Hitcher. Prod.: The Sender, Hot Dog...The Movie!, Witness, Explorers, The Golden Child, Wired.

FELDMAN, PHIL: Producer. b. Boston, Mass. Jan. 22, 1922. e. Harvard, 1943; Georgetown U., 1946; Harvard Law School, 1949, Harvard Business School, 1947. First Lieutenant, U.S. Army, 1943–46. Owner, Wholesale and retail dry goods firm, 1946–49. Law practice, 1950–51. Legal counsel Famous Artists Corp. 1951–53. Assoc. Dir. of Business Affairs CBS, 1953; Dir. of Business Affairs CBS, 1954–57. V.P. Talent & Contract Properties CBS, 1957–60. Exec. v.p. Broadcast Management, 1960–62. Head Business Relations 20th-Century Fox, 1962. V.P. 7 Arts Assoc. Corp. 1962–66 Pres., Phil Feldman Prods., Inc., 1967. Pres., First Artists, 1969; 1980, joined Rastar Films as exec. v.p.
PICTURES INCLUDE: You're a Big Boy Now, The Wild Bunch, The Ballad of Cable Hogue, Blue Thunder (exec. p.).

FELL, NORMAN: Actor. b. Philadelphia, March 24, 1924. e. Temple Univ. Studied acting with Stella Adler. Member, Actors Studio. Professional debut at Circle-in-the-Square Theatre in N.Y. in Bonds of Interest.
Summer Stock; appearances on TV; moved to Hollywood in 1958 to begin theatrical film career.
PICTURES: The Graduate, Pork Chop Hill, Oceans 11, Rat Race, Inherit the Wind, Bullitt, If It's Tuesday, This Must Be Belgium, Catch 22, The End.
TELEVISION: Over 150 live plays from New York and some 200 shows filmed in Hollywood. Series: Dan August, 87th Precinct, Joe and Mable, Tom Ewell Show, Needles and Pins, Three's Company, The Ropers. Mini-Series: Rich Man, Poor Man, Roots: The Next Generation.

FELLINI, FEDERICO: Director. b. Rimini, Italy. Jan. 8, 1920. Cartoonist, caricaturist; then m.p. dir., writer, actor; s.p., actor.
PICTURES INCLUDE: The Miracle, Open City, Paisa, Variety Lights, White Sheik, I Vitelloni, The Matrimonial Agency (Love in the City), Il Bidone, The Wastrels, La Strada, The Swindlers, La Dolce Vita, Boccaccio '70, "8½", The Nights of Cabiria, Juliet of the Spirits, Spirits of the Dead, Fellini Satyricon, The Clowns, Fellini's Rome, Amarcord, Casanova, City of Women, And The Ship Sails On, Ginger and Fred.

FELLMAN, DANIEL R.: Executive. b. Cleveland, Ohio, March 14, 1943. e. Rider College (BS, 1964). Joined Paramount N.Y. 1964; later sales mgr. Washington DC, Dallas. Next branch mgr. Cleveland; then Chicago. In 1969 joined Loews Theatres as film buyer. In 1971 joined Cinema National Theatres, division of Carrols Development Corp., as v.p./ chief film buyer. In 1973 named v.p./dir., Cinema National Theatres. 1977, pres., American Theatre Mgt. Joined Warner Bros. in 1978 as eastern sales mgr. 1979 named v.p./ass't. gen. sales mgr. 1982, v.p., sls. mgr., WB. 1985, named v.p. & gen. sls. mgr. Elected to: board directors NATO, 1975–76. Assistant Chief Barker Variety Club, Tent 35 NY 1976. President Variety Club Tent 35, 1977–78. 1980 Chairman Will Rogers Raffle Committee. v.p., bd. member, Variety Club Tent 25. 1986, chm., Will Rogers Fund raising; bd. member. Motion Picture Pioneers.

FELLMAN, NAT D.: Executive. b. New York, N.Y., Feb. 19, 1910. 1928. Started as office boy, Warner Bros. Pictures, 1928; transferred to Warner Bros. Theatres, asst. to chief booker; handled pool, partnership operations; head buyer, booker for Ohio zone, 1941; asst. to chief film buyer in New York, 1943; apptd. chief film buyer, 1952; exec. asst. to v.p. and gen. mgr., Stanley Warner Theatres, 1955; asst. gen. mgr., Stanley Warner Theatres, 1962; acting gen. mgr., Stanley Warner Theatres, July, 1964; Stanley Warner Theatres, v.p. and gen. mgr., 1965; v.p., NGC Theatre Corp. and division mgr. Fox Eastern Theatres, 1968; v.p. National General Corp., and pres., National General Theatres, 1969; 1974, formed Exhibitor Relations Co., operations consultant; sold it and retired in 1982. Served as vice pres., Variety Clubs International and NATO, Chrm., presidents' advisory comm.

FELTNER, JR., C. E.: Executive. b. Krypton, KY, Aug. 20, 1932. e. Lees Coll., Morehead Univ; degrees in radio & mgt. and bus. admin. Was news cameraman and station manager in West Virginia before managing station, WHIS-TV, Bluefield. 1963–74, founder and major stockholder, Trans America Film Corp. 1968–80, chm., American Diversified Industries. Producer of motion picture and TV shows for over 20 yrs. Now chm., Krypton Corp., Vanguard Films, Palm Beach Home Video. owns WSUL-FM, Monticello, N.Y.

FENADY, ANDREW J.: Producer-writer. b. Toledo, Ohio, Oct. 4, 1928. e. Univ. of Toledo, 1946–50. Radio-prod.-actor-writer, WTOD; Actor, Summer Stock, 1948–51; National Classic Theatre, 1950–51; writer-prod., confidential File, TV, 1954–56; joined Screen Gems as indep. prod. with own company, Fenady Associates, 1962.
PICTURES INCLUDE: Stakeout on Dope Street, The Young Captives, Ride Beyond Vengeance, Chisum, Terror in the Wax Museum, Arnold, The Man with Bogart's Face.
TV: The Rebel, Branded series, Hondo, Mission: Impossible.

FENNELLY, VINCENT M.: Producer. b. Brooklyn, July 6, 1920. e. Holy Cross, 1938–42. U.S. Navy, 1942–46; salesman, Monogram, Des Moines, 1947; entered prod. field, 1949; indep. prod. for Monogram, 1950; Ent. TV field, 1957; prod. Transwestern Films, Inc., Frontier Pictures, Silvermine Productions Co., Allied Artists; Malcolm Enterprises, Hilgarde Enter.
PICTURES INCLUDE: Kansas Territory, Wagons West, Fargo, Marksman, Star of Texas, Topeka, Texas Bad Man, Bitter Creek, The Desperado, Seven Angry Men, Dial Red O, Bobby Ware Is Missing, At Gunpoint, Crime in the Streets, Last of the Badmen.
TV: Four Star Films, Alcoa-Goodyear, Trackdown, Wanted Dead or Alive, David Niven Show, Richard Diamond, Stagecoach West, The Dick Powell Theatre, Target, The Corruptors, Rawhide; A Man Called Shenandoah, MGM.

FENNEMAN, GEORGE: M.C., Announcer. b. Peking, China, Nov. 10.; e. San Francisco State Univ.
CREDITS INCLUDE: Groucho Marx Show, You Bet Your Life, M.C. Host: Surprise Package, Funny Funny Films, Talk About Pictures, On Campus, Donny & Marie, Spokesman for Home Savings of America/Savings of America.

FERGUSON, HELEN: Public rel., career counsel. b. Decatur, Ill., July 23. e. Chicago Academy of Fine Arts. Film debut at 13, Essanay Studio, with Vitagraph, Lasky, Goldwyn, etc.; stage debut in Alias the Deacon, 1927.
THEATRE: New Brooms, Lomardi Ltd., This Thing Called Love, Intimate Strangers.
Freelance film work for many companies; retired from acting, 1930; entered pub. & pub. rel., 1933.
TV Panelist, RSVP, 1949–50.
Author: Loretta Young's The Things I Had to Learn, 1961. Bobbs-Merrill, other professional biographies.

FERGUSON, ROBERT S.: Executive. b. New York, N.Y., May 8, 1915. e. N.Y.U., BS, 1936. Started in newspaper field, Scripps Howard, 1936–37; m.p. ind., 1938 with Warner Bros. Pictures; Columbia Pictures, 1940; asst. dir. of adv. & pub., 1950; dir. adv., exploitation & pub., 1957; pres. Screen Publicists Guild, 1946; V.P. World-Wide Adv. & Pub. Columbia, 1963; v.p. Corporate Relations, Columbia Pictures Industries, 1974; v.p., world mktg., American Film Theatre, 1974–75; v.p. and mgr., Entertainment Division—Rosenfeld, Sirowitz and Lawson Advertising, 1975; Director Marketing—Horizon Pictures, 1976; pres. Cinema Think Tank 1977–; instructor, Adelphi University, 1978. Rejoined Columbia Pictures Industries as consultant to pres., 1979–83. Presently consultant to CPI board chm. Named to board, NATCO Industries, Inc., 1980–85.

FERRAZZA, CARL J.: Executive. b. Cleveland, OH, Aug. 29, 1920. e. Catholic Univ. of America (Washington, D.C.). Started career as asst. mgr. & mgr. for Loews Theatres. 1952, joined Cincinnati Theatre Co., first as mgr. for Keith's Theatre, Cincinnati, and after prom. dir. for circuit. 1963, field rep. for United Artists, covering midwest. 1968, UA prom. mgr., N.Y. 1975–83, dir. of field activities, MGM/UA; 1984, joined Orion Pictures Distributing Corp. as v.p. promotional and field activities.

FERRER, JOSE: Producer, director, actor. b. Santurce, Puerto Rico, Jan. 8, 1912; e. Princeton U.; Director and actor, New York stage, prior to screen career; dir. stage play, Strange Fruit; New York stage; Twentieth Century, 1951; dir., prod. Stalag 17, N.Y. stage, 1951; prod. and dir., The Chase; prod. dir., act., The Shrike, N.Y. stage, 1952; dir. My Three Angels.
PICTURES INCLUDE: Joan of Arc, Whirlpool, Crisis, Cyrano de Bergerac, Anything Can Happen, Moulin Rouge, Miss Sadie Thompson, Caine Mutiny, Deep in My Heart, The Shrike, Cockleshell Heroes, Great Man, I Accuse, State Fair; Lawrence of Arabia, Stop Train 349 From Berlin, Enter Laughing, Voyage of the Damned, The Sentinel, The Swarm, Fedora, A Midsummer Night's Sex Comedy, To Be Or Not To Be, The Evil That Men Do, Dune.
TELEVISION: This Girl for Hire, Hitler's SS: Portrait in Evil, Samson and Delilah, Blood & Orchids.

FERRER, MEL: Producer, director, actor. b. Elberon, N.J., Aug. 25, 1917; e. Princeton U. During Coll. and early career spent summers at Cape Cod Playhouse, Dennis, Mass.; then writer in Mexico, authored juvenile book, Tito's Hats; later ed. Stephen Daye Press, Vt. Left publishing upon reaching leading-man status at Dennis; first two Broadway appearances, dancing roles, You'll Never Know, Everywhere I Roam; others. Kind Lady, Cue For Passion; then to radio, serving apprenticeship in small towns; prod.-dir., NBC: dir. Land of the Free, The Hit Parade, and Hildegarde program. Entered m.p. ind., 1945, when signed by Columbia, dial. dir.: The Girl of the Limberlost; later, returned to Broadway, leading role, Strange Fruit; signed by David Selznick as producer-actor, on loan to John Ford as prod. asst. on The Fugitive; then to RKO for Vendetta. Acted in Lost Boundaries, Born to be Bad, Ondine on Bway., 1954.

PICTURES INCLUDE: The Secret Fury, The Brave Bulls, Rancho Notorious, Scaramouche, Lili, Knights of the Round Table, Saada, War and Peace, Paris Does Strange Things, The Vintage, The World, The Flesh, and the Devil, Blood and Roses, El Greco; prod., Wait Until Dark, "W."

TELEVISION: Falcon Crest. Movies: Seduced, Outrages, Dream West, Peter the Great.

FETZER, JOHN E.: Executive. b. Decatur, Ind., March 25, 1901. e. Purdue Univ., U. of Mich. A.B., Andrews U. Hon LL.D., West. Mich. Univ. 1958; chairman, owner Fetzer Broadcasting Co., Kalamazoo, Mich.; chmn., Detroit Baseball Club; pres., owner Fetzer Communications, Inc., Kalamazoo; chairman, dir., Cornhusker TV Corp.; Mem., former bd. dir., Amer. Nat'l Bank and Trust Co., former mem. Bd. of Trustees, Kalamazoo College. Radio research Europe, 1925; asst. dir., U.S. Censorship in charge of radio. 1944–46; served as war corr. in ETO, 1945; spl. assignment radio, TV, newspaper mission to Europe and Middle East, 1952. chmn., TV code review bd., NARTB, 1952–55. Pres., Pro Am Sports System, 1983; Member, bd., Domino's Pizzo, 1983.Fellow, Royal Society of Arts, London; mem., Acad. of Polit. Science. Clubs: Park, Kalamazoo Country, (Kalamazoo); Radio and Television Execs. Soc. (Assoc.); Broadcast Pioneers, N.Y.C.

FIEDLER, JOHN: Executive. Launched m.p. career with Technicolor as exec. in prod. svcs. in mktg. Joined Rastar as v.p., prod. devel. and asst. to Guy McElwaine, pres. & CEO. Joined Paramount as v.p. in prod.; then to Tri-Star Pictures in same post. Resigned to become exec. v.p., world-wide prod., at Columbia Pictures.

FIELD, DAVID M.: Executive. b. Kansas City, MO. e. Princeton University. Worked as reporter on city desk at Hartford (Conn.) Courant. In 1968 with NBC News in N.Y.C. and Washington, D.C. Entered film school at U.S.C. (L.A.) after which joined Columbia Pictures as west coast story editor. In 1973 went to ABC-TV Network as mgr., movies of the week. 1975, moved to 20th-Fox as v.p., creative affairs. Joined United Artists in 1978; named snr. v.p.—west coast production. Left in 1980 to become 20th-Fox exec. v.p. in chg. of worldwide production 1983, resigned to enter independent production deal with 20th-Fox, Consultant, Tri-Star Pictures.

FIELD, SALLY: Actress. b. Pasadena, Calif., 1946. Gained stardom lead of TV series, Gidget, 1965, followed by The Flying Nun, 1967–68. Theatrical film debut in The Way West (1967).

PICTURES INCLUDE: Stay Hungry, Smokey and the Bandit, Heroes, The End, Hooper, Norma Rae (Oscar), Beyond the Poseidon Adventure, Smokey and the Bandit II, Back Roads, Absence of Malice, Kiss Me Goodbye, Places in the Heart (Oscar), Murphy's Romance (also exec. prod.).

TV: Home for the Holidays, The Girl with Something Extra, Sybil.

FIELD, SHIRLEY ANNE: Actress. b. London. Ent. films after repertory experience 1955. Under contract to Ealing-M.G.M. 1958.

THEATRE: The Lily White boys, Kennedys Children, Fire Wait Unitl Dark, The Life and Death of Marilyn Monroe, How the Other Half Loves.

PICTURES INCLUDE: Saturday Night and Sunday Morning, The Man in the Moon, War Lover, Lunch Hour, Kings of the Sun, Doctor in Clover, Alfie, Hell is Empty, The Entertainer, The Damned, My Beautiful Laundrette.

TV: Risking It, Buccaneer.

FIELD, VIRGINIA: Actress. r.n. Margaret Cynthia Field. b. London; e. England, Paris, Vienna. On N.Y. stage in Victoria Regina & others. On screen from 1934.

PICTURES INCLUDE: The Lady is Willing, Little Lord Fauntleroy, Ladies in Love, Lloyds of London, Singapore Woman, Atlantic Convoy, The Crystal Ball, Christmas Eve, Repeat Performance, Ladies Man, Dial 1119, Weekend With Father, Veils of Bagdad.

THEATRE: The Doughgirls.

FIELDS, ALAN: Executive. Spent five years with Madison Square Garden before joining Paramount Pictures. Career there included various positions: v.p. for pay-TV and Home Video TV. Spent two years at studio lot in L.A. as part of network TV organization. 1981, named bd. director for Paramount Pictures (UK) in London, serving as liaison to United Intl. Pictures and Cinema Intl. Corp., serving on operating committees of both. 1985, appt. v.p., Entertainment & Communications Group of Gulf & Western Industries, Inc., parent co. of Paramount.

FIELDS, FREDDIE: Executive. b. Ferndale, N.Y. July 12, 1923. Vice-pres., member of bd. of directors, MCA-TV, MCA Canada Ltd., MCA Corp.; mem., Pres. Club, Wash., D.C.; pres., Freddie Fields Associates Ltd., 1961 Pres., Kam Ent., Ltd.; v.p. F/B Prod., Inc., pres., chief exec. officer Creative Management Assoc. Ltd. Agency, Chicago, Las Vegas, Miami, Paris, Los Angeles, N.Y., London, Rome, 1962. Exclusive agent of Henry Fonda, Phil Silvers, Joanne Woodward, Paul Newman, Peter Sellers, Barbara Streisand, Steve McQueen, Ali MacGraw, Woody Allen, Robert Redford, Ryan O'Neal, Liza Minnelli and others. Dir. Chelsea Nat'l Bank, N.Y., Polly Bergen Co., First Consolidated Corp. In 1975 resigned post with CMA (now International Creative Mgt.) but continued as consultant. Produced for Paramount Pictures. 1977: Looking for Mr. Goodbar. 1980: Wholly Moses. 1981: Victory. In 1983 named pres. and COO, MGM Film Co. Resigned 1984 to become independent producer for MGM/UA. 1985: Fever Pitch. 1986: Poltergeist, II.

FINBERG, JACK GERALD: Writer technician. b. London, England. Asst. to exec. prod., story dept., British National Studios; Offic. shorthand writer, Royal Courts of Justice and Central Criminal court; hon. sec., Film Studios Club; personal asst. to Sam Spiegel; verbatim report., nuclear weapons, testing and disarmament conferences, UN; asst. prod., ABC TV; two feature writing credits; six major, 18 second feature film adaptations; Film/TV prod., Australia.

FINCH, JON: Actor. b. England, 1941. Came to acting via backstage activities, working for five years as stage manager in repertory theatres all over Britain.

PICTURES: MacBeth, Sunday, Bloody Sunday, Frenzy, Lady Caroline Lamb, The Final Program, Une Femme Fidele, The Man of the Green Cross, Battleflag, Death on the Nile.

FINE, HARRY: Producer. e. St. Andrew's College and Dublin Univ.

FILMS INCLUDE: Up The Junction, The Liquidator, The Penthouse, Long Days Dying, Vampire Lovers, Fright, Twins of Evil, Too Far To Go, Quadrophenia, McVicar, Journey to a Safe Place.

TV FILM SERIES: Sir Francis Drake, Man of The World, The Sentimental Agent.

FINESHRIBER, WILLIAM H., JR.: Executive. b. Davenport, Ia. Nov. 4, 1909; e. Princeton U., B.A., 1931. Pub., CBS, 1931–34; mgr. Carnegie Hall, N.Y., 1934–37; script writer, dir., music comm., dir. of music dept., CBS, 1937–40; dir. of short wave programs, CBS, 1940–43; gen. mgr. CBS program dept. 1943–49; v.p. in charge of programs MBS, 1949–51; exec. v.p. & dir., MBS, 1951–53; v.p. & gen. mgr. of networks, NBC, 1953–54; v.p. in charge of Radio Network, NBC, 1955; v.p. Television Programs of America, 1956; director International operations, Screen Gems, 1957; v.p., Motion Picture Assoc. of America and Motion Picture Export Assoc. of America, 1960; bd. of dir., NARTB: exec. comm., bd. of dir., R.A.B; v.p. Radio Pioneers.

FINKELSTEIN, HERMAN: Attorney, b. Torrington, Conn., Jan. 9, 1903; e. Clark U., A.B.: Yale Law School, LL.B., member of Conn., Pa. & N.Y., U.S. Sup. Ct. bar; honorary L.L.D., New England Coll. of Law; director, ASCAP Nathan Burkan Memorial Competition; Mem.; American Law Institute; State Dept. Panel on intl. Copyright; U.S. National Commission for UNESCO 1957–62; Consultant to U.S. Delegation, Inter-Amer. Conf. of Copyright Exports, Wash., D.C., 1946; Mem. U.S. Delegation, Intergovernmental Conference on Universal Copyright Convention Geneva (1952), Berne Convention-Stockholm Revision Conf. 1967, Paris Revision Conf. 1971, Communication Satellite Conf. 1973, past pres., Copyright Soc. U.S.A., past pres., Exec. Bureau, CISAC: past pres., SCRIBES.

AUTHOR: Numerous articles on copyright.

FINNEY, ALBERT: Actor. b. Salford, England, May 9, 1936. Studied for stage at R.A.D.A. making his West End debut 1958 in The Party. Appeared at Stratford-on-Avon 1959 season playing title role in Coriolanus, etc. 1960; On West End stage in The Lily White Boys and Billy Liar, Luther; New York, 1963, Luther. National Theatre 1965; Much Ado About Nothing, Armstrong's Last Goodnight, Love for Love, Miss Julie, Black Comedy, A Flea in Her Ear; broadway, Joe Egg; London Stage, Alpha Beta, Krapp's Last Tape, Cromwell, Chez Nous, Hamlet, Tamburlaine, Uncle Vanya, Present Laughter. National Theatre: The Country Wife, The Cherry Orchard, Macbeth 1978, The Biko Inquest, Sergeant Musgrave, Musgrave's Dances.

PICTURES INCLUDE: The Entertainer, Saturday Night and Sunday Morning, Tom Jones, Night Must Fall, Two for the Road, Charlie Bubbles, Scrooge, Gumshoe, Alpha Beta, Murder on the Orient Express, Wolfen, Loophole,

Looker, Shoot the Moon, Annie, The Life of Pope John Paul II, The Dresser, Under the Volcano, Orphans.

FINNEY, EDWARD: Producer. b. New York City; e. C.C.N.Y. Began as engineer, Western Electric. Then property man, Johnny Hines, C.C. Burr comedies. To MGM as press sheet ed.; sales promotion mgr., Pathe; asst. adv. dir. UA; story ed. and adv. dir., Mon-Rep., prod. & adv. dir., Grand Natl.; then prod. Monogram, many westerns. In 1941 org. Edward Finney Prod. Discovered Tex Ritter and made his first 40 features. Prod. & dir. Silver Stallion, Code of the Redman, Queen of the Amazons, etc. Clubs: Masquers. ex. pres. Catholic Press Council, Board Member Permanent Charities, M.P. Acad. of Arts and Sciences Dramatic Guild; pres., Indep. M.P. Prod. Assn. Film chrm. Catholic Press Council.
PICTURES INCLUDE: Corregidor, Golden Stallion, Call of the Forest, Hi Diddle Diddle, Primitive Passion, Mormon Battalion, This Is Pippin (TV); Seven Wonders, Baron Munchausen, Enchanted Years, Buffalo Bill in Tomahawk Territory, Slash of the Knife, Gun Girls, Journey to Freedom, London After Dark, Dark Road, Halfway to Hell, The Prairie, Secret Tower, Barrels Away, Things That Make America Great, (TV); Spring Affair, Dragons Across Asia, The Madcaps, The Happy Clown, The Great Dogtown Robbery.
TV: Pilots for Law and the People and the Circle Kids. Now preparing Small Crossing, Dog House Blues and The Italian.

FIRTH, PETER: Actor. b. Bradford, Yorkshire, Oct. 27, 1953. Selected to appear in local TV children's show where casting director spotted him and got him role in series, The Flaxton Boys, Moved to London and worked in TV, first in children's show, later on dramas for BBC. Big break came in 1973 when signed for Equus at National Theatre, London, which role repeated for film.
PICTURES: Joseph Andrews, Aces High, Equus, When You Comin Back Red Ryder, Letter to Brezhnev.
STAGE: Equus, Romeo and Juliet, Spring Awakening.

FISHER, AL: Executive. b. Brooklyn, N.Y. Entered m.p. industry as office boy, Fox Metropolitan Theatres; U.S. Army Provost Marshal General's Office, 1942–46; Universal Pictures, mgr., Park Avenue Theatre, N.Y. & Copley Plaza Theatre, Boston, 1946; Eagle Lion Film Co., mgr., Red Shoe's Bijou Theatre, N.Y., 1947; Stanley Kramer Prods., exploitation, Cyrano de Bergerac, 1951; press agent, 1951; prod., Bway show, Daphine, 1952; joined United Artists Corporation, 1952, named dir. of exploitation; now freelancing as producer's repr.

FISHER, CARRIE: b. Beverly Hills, CA, Oct. 21, 1956. e. London Central School of Speech & Drama. Daughter of Debbie Reynolds and Eddie Fisher. On Broadway in revival of Irene and Censored Scenes from King Kong.
PICTURES: Shampoo, Star Wars, Mr. Mike's Mondo Video, The Empire Strikes Back, The Blues Brothers, Under the Rainbow, Return of the Jedi, Garbo Talks, The Man with One Red Shoe, Hannah and Her Sisters.

FISHER, EDDIE: Singer. b. Philadelphia, Pa., Aug. 10, 1928. Band, nightclub, hotel singer; discovered by Eddie Cantor, 1949; U.S. Army, 1951–53; many hit records include; Wish You Were Here, Lady of Spain; radio & TV shows, NBC.
PICTURES INCLUDE: Butterfield 8, Nothing Lasts Forever.

FISHER, LUCY: Executive. b. Oct. 2, 1949. e. Harvard U (BA). Story ed., Samuel Goldwyn Jr. Prods.; exec. story ed., MGM; exec. chg. creative affairs, MGM; v.p., creative affairs, 20th Century Fox; v.p., prod., Fox. 1980, prod. v.p., Zoetrope Studios; 1984, v.p., sr. prod. exec., Warner Bros.; 1983, sr. v.p. prod., WB.

FISK, JACK: Director. b. Ipava, IL, Dec. 19, 1934. E. Cooper Union. Married Sissy Spacek. Career in films as designer turning to direction with Heart Beat (1980).
PICTURES: Director: Raggedy Man, Violets Are Blue.

FISZ, BENJAMIN: Producer. b. Warsaw, Poland, Nov. 4, 1922. Formed in assoc. Golden Era Films, 1954. Later Aqua Films Ltd., 1957 as ind. prod. for Rank Org. and formed S. Benjamin Fisz Prod. Ltd., 1963 formed Benton Film Prod. Ltd. in assoc. with Anthony Mann. 1967 Spitfire Prods. with Harry Saltzman. 1969 Benmar Prods. Incorporated into Scotia Investments Ltd. Formed Scotia Intl. under name group for dist. Dir., Scotia-Barber. 1970: Created studios complex, Spain Esterdios, Madrid. 1972: Formed Scotia Int. (Film Sales.) Jointly formed Scotia Deutschland and International Film Theatre Ltd. For Intl. Films Theatre Ltd. with Kenneth Rive. Formed Sintel Intl. Ltd. for worldwide dist., 1976. Formed London Leisure Centre and acquired Wembley Stadium Complex, 1983.
PICTURES INCLUDE: Capri, The Secret, Child in the House, Hell Drivers, Sea Fury, On the Fiddle, The Heroes of Telemark, The Battle of Britain, A Town Called Bastard, Aces High, A Nightingale Sang in Berkeley Square, Jigsaw Man. Exec. in chg. prod.: Captain Apache, Bad Man's River, Pancho Villa, Royal Hunt of the Sun, Horror Express, Psychomania.

FITELSON, H. WILLIAM: Attorney, counsel to Fitelson, Lasky and Aslan, law firm, New York City, specializing in the field of communications (publishing, motion pictures, theatre, television, radio); born New York City Jan. 21, 1905; educated Columbia University (extension), New York Law School; newspaper and editorial work, librarian and tutor New York Law School, Story Department Tiffany-Stahl Productions 1929, counsel Tiffany-Stahl Productions 1929–32, United States counsel to British and foreign motion picture and theatrical producers, counsel to The Theatre Guild and numerous members motion picture industry, theatre industry, newspaper and publishing, television and radio interests, managing director Theatre Guild Television and radio divisions, including U.S. Steel Hour. Non-legal consultant on communications projects to Allen & Co., and Columbia Pictures Industries.

FITZGERALD, GERALDINE: Actress. b. Dublin, Eire, Nov. 24, 1914; e. Dublin Art Sch. On stage Gate theat., Dublin; then in number of Brit. screen prod. including Turn of the Tide, Mill on the Floss. On N.Y. stage in Heartbreak House. In U.S. screen prod. from 1939 Wuthering Heights. Pictures (U.S.) include Dark Victory, Till We Meet Again, Flight from Destiny, Gay Sisters, Ladies Courageous, Watch on the Rhine, Wilson, The Strange Affair of Uncle Harry, Three Strangers, Nobody Lives Forever, So Evil My Love, Obsessed, Ten North Frederick, The Pawnbroker, Rachel, Rachel, Believe in Me, The Last American Hero, Harry and Tonto, Echoes of a Summer, Arthur, Easy Money, Poltergeist II.
STAGE: A Long Day's Journey Into Night (1971).
TV: The Best of Everything, Do You Remember Love.

FITZGERALD, PEGEEN: Commentator, executive. b. Norcatur, Kans., Nov. 24, 1910. e. Coll. of St. Theresa, Winona, Minn.; LL.D. (hon.) Seton Hall U. m. Ed Fitzgerald. Sales prom. adv. in retail field; magazine editor; originator (with husband) of husband and wife radio-TV conversation; radio-TV commentator, WOR, N.Y.; pres. Vivisection Investigation League; founder, Mercy Animal Clinic Special Fund, president Millennium Guild; co-author of Cast of Characters, author of Meatless Cooking pub. by Prentice-Hall.

FLAKS, STEPHEN: Executive. b. Jan. 1, 1941, New York. e. City College of New York, B.B.A. Early career as an investment banker & stock broker for various companies, including First Hanover, First Devonshire, 1962–69. Founded Flaks-Zaslow in 1969. Entered motion picture industry in 1974 in capacity of production financing. Established VideoVision, Inc., in 1978.

FLATTERY, THOMAS L.: Executive-Lawyer b. Detroit, Mich., Nov. 14, 1922. e. U.S.M.A., West Point, B.S., 1944–47; U.C.L.A., J.D., 1952–55; U.S.C., LL.M. 1955–65. Gen'l counsel and asst. sec'y, McCulloch Corp., Calif., 1957–64; sec'y and corporate counsel, Technicolor, Inc., 1964–70; Vice President, Secretary & General Counsel, Amcord, Inc. (formerly American Cement Corporation) 1970–72; Vice President, Secretary & General Counsel, Schick Incorporated, 1972–75; counsel asst. secretary, C.F. Braun & Co., 1975–76; sr. vice pres., secretary & general counsel PCC Technical Industries, Inc. since 1976 to present.

FLAXMAN, JOHN P.: Producer. b. New York City, March 3, 1934. e. Dartmouth Univ. B.A. 1956; 1st Lt. U.S. Army, 1956–58. Ent. m.p. industry in executive training program, Columbia Pictures Corp., 1958–63; exec. story consultant, Profiles in Courage, 1964–65; head of Eastern Literary Dept., Universal Pictures, 1965; writer's agent, William Morris Agency, 1966; partner with Harold Prince in Media Productions, Inc. 1967; pro. m.p. Something for Everyone. Founded Flaxman Film Corp., 1975 Prod. Jacob Two-Two Meets the Hooded Fang, 1976. Prresident-Tricorn Productions 1977; pres. Filmworks Capital Corp., 1979–83; Becker/Flaxman & Associates, 1979–83; pres., Cine Communications, 1983–.

FLEISCHER, RICHARD O.: Director. b. Brooklyn, N.Y., Dec. 8, 1916; e. Brown U., B.A.; Yale U., M.F.A. Stage dir.; joined RKO Pathe 1942.
PICTURES INCLUDE: Flicker Flashbacks, This is America, Design for Death, Child of Divorce, Banjo, So This Is New York, Bodyguard, Follow Me Quietly, The Clay Pigeon, Narrow Margin, The Happy Time, Arena, 20,000 Leagues Under the Sea, Violent Saturday, Girl in the Red Velvet Swing, Bandido, Between Heaven and Hell, The Vikings, These Thousand Hills, Compulsion, Crack in the Mirror, The Big Gamble, Barabbas, Fantastic Voyage, Doctor Dolittle, Boston Strangler, Tora! Tora! Tora!, Ten Rillington Place, The Last Run, See No Evil, The New Centurions, Soylent Green, The Don is Dead, The Spikes Gang, Mister Majestyk, Mandingo, The Incredible Sarah, Crossed Swords, Ashante, The Jazz Singer, Tough Enough, Amityville 3-D, Conan the Destroyer, Red Sonja.

FLEMING, JANET BLAIR: Executive. b. Ottawa, Canada, November 29, 1944. e. Bachelor Arts Degree, Carlton University, Ottawa, Canada; Secretary to Canada's Federal Minister of Transport 1967–72; 1973–77, asst. to Sandy Howard—business affairs; 1977, co-founder and v.p./sales & admin. of Producers Sales organization; 1981, named sr. v.p., admin.; 1982, sr. v.p., acquisitions; 1983, exec. v.p., Skouras Pictures; 1985 promoted to pres., intl. div.

FLEMING, RHONDA: Actress. r.n. Marilyn Lewis. b. Los Angeles, Aug. 10, 1923. p. Harold and Effie Graham Lewis, prof.; e. Beverly Hills High School. Calif. Screen debut: Spellbound. L.A. Civic Light Opera in Kismet revival; 1976. Broadway debut in 1973: Revival of The Women.

PICTURES INCLUDE: Spiral Staircase, Adventure Island, Out of the Past; singing debut: A Connecticut Yankee in King Arthur's Court, The Last Outpost, Cry Danger, The Redhead and the Cowboy, The Great Lover, Crosswinds, Little Egypt, Hong Kong, Golden Hawk, Tropic Zone, Pony Express, Serpent of the Nile, Inferno, Those Redheads from Seattle, Jivaro, Yankee Pasha, Tennessee's Partner, While the City Sleeps, Killer Is Loose, Slightly Scarlet, Odongo, Queen of Babylon, Gunfight at the OK Corral, Buster Keaton Story, Gun Glory, Home Before Dark, Alias Jesse James, The Big Circus, The Crowded Sky, Instant Love, The American Wife, Won Ton Ton, The Dog Who Saved Hollywood, The Nude Bomb.

FLEMYNG, ROBERT: Actor. b. Jan. 3, 1912, Liverpool, Eng. e. Halleybury Coll. Stage debut: Rope 1931. Screen debut; Head Over Heels 1937.

PICTURES INCLUDE: Bond Street, The Guinea Pig, The Conspirators, The Blue Lamp, Blackmailed, The Magic Box, The Holly and the Ivy, Cast a Dark Shadow, Man Who Never Was, Funny Face, Let's Be Happy, Windom's Way, Blind Date, A Touch of Larceny, Radtus (Italian), The King's Breakfast, The Deadly Affair, The Spy with the Cold Nose, The Quiller Memorandum, Deathhead Avenger, Oh! What a Lovely War, Battle of Britain, Cause for Alarm, Young Winston, The Darwin Adventure, Travels with My Aunt, Golden Rendezvous, The Medosa Touch, The Four Feathers, The Thirtynine Steps.

TV: appearances in England, U.S. inc.: Rainy Day, Playhouse 90, Wuthering Heights, Browning Version, After the Party, Boyd Q.C., They Made History, Somerset Maugham Show, Woman in White, The Datchet Diamonds, Probation Officer, Family Solicitor (series), Man of the World, Zero One, Compact, (serial), Day By the Sea, The Living Room, Hawks and Doves, Vanity Fair, The Inside Man, The Doctor's Dilemma, The Persuaders, Major Lavender, Public Eye, Florence Nightingale, Edward VIII, Spy Trap, The Venturers' Loyalties, The Avengers, Crown Court, Enemy at the Door, Rebecca, Edward and Mrs. Simpson, The Ladykiller, Professionals, Fame Is the Spur, Crown Court, Spider's Webb.

FLETCHER, LOUISE: Actress. b. Birmingham, AL, 1935. Came to Hollywood at age 21; studied with Jeff Corey. Worked on TV shows (including Playhouse 90). Gave up career to be housewife for 10 yrs.; returned to work in 1973.

PICTURES INCLUDE: Thieves Like Us, One Flew Over the Cuckoo's Nest, Exorcist II: The Heretic, The Cheap Detective, Natural Enemies, Brainstorm, Firestarter, Invaders from Mars, The Boy Who Could Fly.

FLEXER, DAVID: Executive. b. Mt. Plasant, Tenn., June 29, 1909; e. Wallace U. School, 1926; Vanderbilt U., 1930; m. Eleanor Handmacher, concert pianist. Was adv. rep. on national magazines, 1930–32; joined United Artists 1932–33; entered exhib. 1933, head of Flexer Theatres, operating in Tenn. and Miss.; The Albany Corp.; Theatre Real Estate Corp.; v.p. Impossible pictures, Inc., producers of cartoons currently distrib. by Republic; constructed first drive-in theatres in Minneapolis, and St. Louis, 1947; pres., Flexer Theatres of Tenn., Inc., Flexer Theatres of Miss., Inc., The Albany Corp. Pres., Inflight Motion Pictures.

FLINN, JOHN C.: Publicist. b. Yonkers, N.Y. May 4, 1917; p. late John C. Flinn, pioneer m.p. executive; e. U. of Calif. In pub. dept. David O. Selznick, 1936–39; unit publicist, then head planner, Warner, 1936–46; joined Monogram as asst. to nat'l adv. & pub. head & pub. mgr. Aug. 5, 1946; apptd. nat'l dir. of pub. & adv. of Allied Artists Pictures Corp., March, 1951, appt'd studio dir. adv. & pub., Columbia, March, 1959; v.p., Jim Mahoney & Associates (pub. rel. firm) in 1971. Joined MGM West Coast publicity department as publicity coordinator, January, 1973; Rejoined Columbia Pictures in Feb., 1974 as studio pub. dir.; 1979, promoted to dir. industry relations.

FLOREA, JOHN: Producer-Director. b. Alliance, O., May 28, 1916. Served as photo journalist with Life magazine, 1940–50; assoc. editor Colliers magazine, 1950–53. Prod.-dir.

TV: Sea Hunt TV series, 1957–60; also dir. TV shows Bonanza, The Virginian, Honey West, Daktari, Gentle Ben, Cowboy in Africa. Prod.-dir. of film Islands of the Lost. With Ivon Tors Films. Nominated as one of the Top 10 directors in America by DGA for 1968 Mission Impossible episode. Dir. several Ironside episodes.

PICTURES INCLUDE: A Time to Every Purpose.

FLYNN, JOHN: Director-Writer. Began career as trainee script supvr. for dir. Robert Wise. Soon working as ass't. dir. on MGM-TV shows. Made dir. debut with The Sergeant, 1969.

PICTURES INCLUDE: The Jerusalem File (dir.), The Outfit (s.p., dir.), Rolling Thunder (dir.), Defiance (dir.), Touched (dir.).

FOCH, NINA: Actress. b. Leyden, Holland, April 20, 1924; daughter of Consuelo Flowerton, actress, & Dirk Foch, symphony orch. conductor. Many stage, radio, television appearances. Prof. Univ. South. Calif, 1966–67; 1978–80, senior faculty, American Film Institute, 1974–77; Board of Governors, Hollywood Acad. Television Arts & Sciences, 1976–77; Exec. Comm. Foreign Film Award, Acad. Motion Picture Arts & Sciences, 1970–. Co-chmn., exec. comm. foreign language film award.

PICTURES INCLUDE: Nine Girls, Song to Remember, My name is Julia Ross, An American in Paris, Scaramouche, Young Man in Hurry, Undercover Man, Sombrero, Fast Company, Executive Suite, Four Guns to the Border, Ten Commandments, Illegal, You're Never Too Young, Cry of the Werewolf, Escape in the Fog, I Love A Mystery, Johnny Allegro, Johnny O'Clock, Prison Ship, Return of the Vampire, Shadows In The Night, The Dark Past, The Guilt of Janet Ames, Three Brave Men, Spartacus, Cash McCall, Such Good Friends, Salty, Mahogany, Jennifer.

FOGARTY, JACK V.: Executive Producer-Writer. b. Los Angeles, Calif. e. UCLA. hd. travel dept., MGM, 1960–62; exec. prod. mgr., Cinerama, Inc., 1962–64; assoc. prod., The Best of Cinerama, 1963; est. own p.r. firm, 1965; pres., AstroScope, Inc., 1969–74. Partner, Sowards/Fogarty Prods.

TV: (writer) The Rookies, SWAT, Charlie's Angels, Most Wanted, Barnaby Jones, A Man Called Sloane, Trapper John, T.J. Hooker, Crazy Like a Fox, The Equalizer. Story Editor, Charlie's Angels; exec. story consultant: Most Wanted, A Man Called Sloane, Sheriff Lobo, T.J. Hooker. Producer: T.J. Hooker. Co-prod.: Jessie.

FOGELSON, ANDREW: Executive. b. New Rochelle, N.Y., August 5, 1942. e. Union College (1960–64). First entered m.p. industry in 1968 with Warner Bros., starting as copywriter and soon made exec. asst. to v.p. of adv.-pub. In 1973 appt. v.p., marketing services. Joined Columbia Pictures in Dec. 1973, as v.p. in chg. world-wide adv.-pub. In 1977 went to Warner Bros. as exec. v.p. in chg. worldwide adv.-pub. 1979 left to become pres. of Rastar Prods. Resigned 1981 to become indep. producer. 1981: Wrong Is Right (exec. prod.). 1983: Blue Thunder (exec. prod.). 1982: Spring Break. 1985: Just One of the Guys.

FOLSEY, GEORGE: Cameraman.

PICTURES INCLUDE: Reunion in Vienna, Storm at Daybreak, Stage Mother, Going Hollywood, MGM, Men in White, Operator 13, MGM. In 1935, Reckless, I Live My Life, The Great Ziegfeld. The Gorgeous Hussy, MGM; Hearts Divided, Meet Me in St. Louis, Mr. Imperium, Law and Lady, Lovely to Look At, Million Dollar Mermaid, All The Brothers Were Valiant, Executive Suite, Seven Brides for Seven Brothers, Deep in My Heart, The Cobweb, Fastest Gun Alive, House of Numbers, Imitation General, Cash McCall, Glass Houses.

FONDA, JANE: Actress. b. New York City, Dec. 21, 1937. p. Henry Fonda. e. Emma Willard School, Troy, N.Y. active in dramatics. Vassar. Appeared with father. Summer stock production. The Country Girl, Omaha, Neb. Studied painting, languages, Paris. Art Students League, N.Y. Appeared in The Male Animal, Dennis, Mass. Modeled, appeared on covers, Esquire, Vogue, The Ladies Home Journal, Glamour, and McCall's, 1959.

PICTURES INCLUDE: Tall Story (debut), Walk on the Wild Side, The Chapman Report, Period of Adjustment, In the Cool of The Day, Sunday in New York, The Love Cage, La Ronde, Cat Ballou, The Chase, La Curee, Any Wednesday, The Game Is Over, Hurry Sundown, Barefoot in the Park, Barbarella, Spirits of The Dead, They Shoot Horses, Don't They? (Acad. Award nom.), Klute, Steelyard Blues, F.T.A., A Doll's House, The Bluebird, Fun with Dick and Jane, Julia, Coming Home, Comes a Horseman, California Suite, The China Syndrome, The Electric Horseman, Nine To Five, Roll-Over, On Golden Pond, Agnes of God, The Morning After.

STAGE: There Was A Little Girl, Invitation to a March, The Fun Couple, Strange Interlude.

TELEVISION: The Doll Maker.

FONDA, PETER: Actor. b. 1939. Son of Henry Fonda. Brother of Jane Fonda.

PICTURES INCLUDE: Tammy and the Doctor, The Victors, Lilith, The Wild Angels, Easy Rider, The Last Movie, The Hired Hand (also dir.), Two People, Dirty Mary Crazy Larry, Open Season, Race with the Devil, 91 In the Shade,

Killer Force, Futureworld, Outlaw Blues, High Ballin!, Wanda Nevada (also dir.), Split Image, Certain Fury.
TELEVISION: A Reason to Live, The Hostage Tower.

FONTAINE, JOAN: Actress. b. Tokyo, Oct. 22, 1917; e. art, privately; sister of Olivia de Haviland, actress; on B'way in Tea and Sympathy; m.p. debut in "Quality Street" 1937; won Academy Award best performance, 1941, for "Suspicion."
PICTURES INCLUDE: Women, Rebecca, Man Who Found Himself, You Can't Beat Love, Music for Madame, Blond Cheat, Gunga Din, This Above All, Jane Eyre, Frenchman's Creek, Affairs of Susan, Emperor Waltz, Kiss the Blood Off My Hands, You Gotta Stay Happy, Letter from an Unknown Woman, Duke of West Point, Ivy, Born to Be Bad, Something to Live For, September Affair, Darling How Could You?, Ivanhoe, Decameron Nights, Flight to Tangier, The Bigamist, Casanova's Big Night, Island in the Sun, Until We Sail, A Certain Smile, Tender Is the Night, The Devil's Own.
TELEVISION: Crossings.

FOOTE, HORTON: Writer. b. Wharton, TX, March 14. Actor before becoming playwright. Plays include Out of My House, Only the Heart, Celebration, The Chase, Trip to Bountiful, Traveling Lady, etc.
PICTURES: To Kill a Mockingbird (Oscar, 1962); Tender Mercies (Oscar, 1983); 1918; The Trip to Bountiful, On Valentine's Day, etc.
TELEVISION: Trip to Bountiful, Young Lady of Property, Death of the Old Man, Flight, The Night of the Storm, etc.

FORBES, BRYAN: Actor, writer, producer, director. Former head of prod., man. dir., Associated British Prods. (EMI). b. Stratford (London) July 22, 1926. Stage debut, The Corn is Green (London), 1942; screen debut, The Small Back Room 1948.
PICTURES INCLUDE: All Over the Town, The Wooden Horse, Dear Mr. Prohack, Appointment in London, Sea Devils, Wheel of Fate, Million Pound Note (Man with a Million), An Inspector Calls, Colditz Story, Passage Home, Extra Day, It's Great to be Young, Satellite in the Sky, Quartermass 11, Cockleshell Heroes, Black Tent, House of Secrets, Baby and the Battleship, I was Monty's Double, A Piece of Cake, Man in the Moon, Whistle Down The Wind, League of Gentlemen, Only Two Can Play, The L-Shaped Room, Of Human Bondage, Station Six Sahara, Seance on a Wet Afternoon, King Rat, The Wrong Box, The Whisperers, Deadfall, The Madwoman of Chaillot, The Go-Between (executive producer), The Railway Children (exec. prod.) Tales of Beatrix Potter (exec. prod.) The Raging Moon (US title: Long Ago Tomorrow). Also: I Caught Acting Like the Measles (produced/directed for television), Goodbye Norma Jean and Other Things, The Stepford Wives (dir.), The Slipper & The Rose, International Velvet, Sunday Lovers, Jessie, Hopscotch (s.p.), Better Late Than Never (s.p./dir.) The Naked Face (s.p./dir.), Life of Henry Ford (s.p.).
TV: The Breadwinner, French Without Tears, Johnnie was a Hero, The Gift, The Road, The Heiress. Theatre: Flarepath, Fighters Calling, Gathering Storm, September Tide, The Holly and the Ivy, Tobias and the Angel, A Touch of Fear, Three Way Switch, December Flower, First Among Equals.
PUBLICATIONS: Truth Lies Sleeping (short stories) 1951; Distant Laughter (novel) 1972; Notes For a Life (Autobiog.) 1973/4. The Slipper & The Rose (Book of Film) 1975/6. Ned's Girl, 1977, International Velvet 1978 (novel); Familiar Strangers (novel), 1979 (US Title "Stranger"), That Despicable Race, 1980. the Rewrite Man 1983 (novel), The Endless Game (novel) 1986.

FORBES, DAVID: Executive. b. Omaha, Nov. 9, 1945. e. Univ. of Nebraska. Began career with MGM in 1968 as field man in Detroit; later named asst. natl. field coordinator at studio. director, Metrovision, 1973. Director special projects for 20th-Fox, 1974; made natl. dir. marketing services, 1976. In 1977 left to join Rastar Prods. as marketing dir. Named v.p. & asst. to pres., Columbia Pictures, 1980; 1982, joined Almi Distributing Corp. as vice chm.

FORBES, GORDON B.: Executive. b. New York, New York. e. Yale University Drama Dept. Republic Studio-1945 Budget and Cost Control Dept.; 1950 asst. to production mgr.; 1952 head of production operations; 1954–58 UPM Batjack Productions, production manager RKO-El Dorado Pictures (Cuba); 1959–76 v.p. Universal TV, studio operations mgr.; 1977 executive assistant to the pres. of The Burbank Studios and member of the executive committee. In 1979 named v.p. of studio operations for Paramount Pictures. 1985, dir. opns., Hollywood Center Studios and Hollywood Center TV Studios.

FORD, GLENN: Actor. r.n. Gwylin Ford; b. Quebec, Canada, May 1, 1916. On stage in western co. "Children's Hour" 1935; on Broadway in: Broom for a Bride, Soliloquy; served in U.S. Marine Corps 1942–45; m.p. debut in Heaven With a Barbed Wire Fence 1940.
PICTURES INCLUDE: Men Without Souls, Lady in Question, So Ends Our Night, Desperadoes, Stolen Life, Gilda, Framed, Mating of Millie, Return of October, Loves of Carmen, Mr. Soft Touch, Man from Colorado, Undercover Man, Lust for Gold, Doctor and the Girl, Flying Missile, The Redhead and the Cowboy, Follow the Sun, The Secret of Convict Lake, Green Glove, Young Man With Ideas, Affair in Trinidad, Man from the Alamo, Terror on a Train, Plunder of the Sun, Big Heat, Appointment in Honduras, Human Desire, The Americano, Violent Men, Blackboard Jungle, Interrupted Melody, Trial, Ransom, Fastest Gun Alive, Jubal, Teahouse of the August Moon, Don't Go Near the Water, Cowboy, The Sheepman, Imitation General, Torpedo Run, It Started with a Kiss, The Gazebo, Cimarron, Cry for Happy, The Four Horsemen of The Apocalypse, Experiment in Terror, Love Is a Ball, The Courtship of Eddie's Father, The Rounders, The Money Trap, Fate Is the Hunter, Dear Heart, The Last Challenge, Heaven With a Gun, Smith!, The Day of the Evil Gun, A Time for Killing, Midway, Superman, Happy Birthday To Me.
TV: The Brotherhood of Ty Bell (movie); Cade's County (series); Jarret; The Holvak Family.

FORD, HARRISON: Actor. b. Chicago, July 13, 1942. e. Ripon Coll.
PICTURES: Dead Heat on a Merry-Go-Round, Luv, Getting Straight, The Long Ride Home, Journey to Shiloh, Zabriskie Point, The Conversation, American Graffiti, Star Wars, Heroes, Force 10 from Navarone, Hanover Street, Apocalypse Now, The Frisco Kid, The Empire Strikes Back, Raiders of the Lost Ark, Blade Runner, Return of the Jedi, Indiana Jones and the Temple of Doom, Witness, Mosquito Coast.
TELEVISION: Dynasty, Trial of Lt. Calley, The Possessed.

FORD, TENNESSEE ERNIE: Singer. r.n. Ernest J. Ford, b. Bristol, Tenn., Feb. 13, 1919. e. Cincinnati Conserv. of Music. Radio anncr., 1939–41; U.S. Air Force, 1942–45; radio anncr., San Bernardino, Calif.; hillbilly disc jockey, Pasadena; Capital Recording Star.
TV: own TV shows, NBC; guest appearances on I Love Lucy, Red Skelton Show, Perry Como Show, George Gobel Show; own show, Tennessee Ford Show, ABC.
RECORDS INCLUDE: 16 Tons, etc.

FORD, TONY: Executive. b. August 6, 1925, New York City. e. St. Johns Univ. In U.S. Navy World War II; in life insurance business, 1946–48. Agent with MCA 1949–53. TV indep. prod., specials for Timex, Ringling Bros. Circus, Pontiac Victor Borge. Re-entered agency business, General Artists Corp., v.p., TV dept. Headed own agency, Tony Ford Mgt., Inc., which was acquired by William Morris Agency. Headed creative services division WMA representing producers, directors, writers specializing in the packaging of TV series and specials, left Morris Agency Jan. 1, 1977; now pres. of Tony Ford Productions, affiliated with Universal Studios.

FOREMAN, JOHN: Producer. b. Idaho Falls, Idaho. Cofounder of CMA Agency. Resigned Jan., 1968, to form production co. with Paul Newman: Newman-Foreman Company.
PICTURES INCLUDE: Winning, Butch Cassidy and the Sundance Kid, WUSA (co-prod.), Puzzle of a Downfall Child, They Might Be Giants, Sometimes a Great Notion, Pocket Money, The Effect of Gamma Rays on Man-in-the-Moon Marigolds (exec. prod.), The Mackintosh Man, The Man Who Would Be King, Bobby Deerfield, The Great Train Robbery, Prizzi's Honor.

FORMAN, SIR DENIS, O.B.E., M.A.: Executive. b. Moffat, Dumfriesshire, Scot., Oct. 13, 1917. e. Loretto School, Musselburgh, Pembroke College, Cambridge. Served in Argyll & Sutherland Highlanders, World War II. Entered film business May, 1946, production staff Central Office of Information, 1947; Chief Production Officer C.O.I. 1948; appointed dir. of the British Film Institute, 1949; joined Granada Television Ltd., 1955. Jnt. Mng. Dir., 1965 chm., British Film Institute, Bd. of Gov., 1971–73. Chmn. Granada T.V. 1975. Chmn. Novello & Co. 1972. Fellow, British Acad. Film & TV Arts, 1976.

FORMAN, MILOS: Director. b. Czechoslovakia, Feb. 18, 1932. Trained as writer at Czech Film School and as director at Laterna Magika. Won Int'l. attention with first film Black Peter, 1963. Emigrated to U.S. after collapse of Dubcek Govt. in Czech.
PICTURES INCLUDE: The Loves of a Blonde, Fireman's Ball, Taking Off, Visions of Eight (segment), One Flew Over the Cuckoo's Nest, Hair, Ragtime, Amadeus.

FORREST, FREDERIC: Actor. Began career off-Broadway in Futz, Massachusetts Trust and Tom Paine, all with La Mama Troupe under direction of Tom O'Horgan. Moved to Hollywood in 1970. Made film debut in When The Legends Die in 1972.

PICTURES INCLUDE: The Don is Dead, The Conversation, The Gravy Train, Permission to Kill, The Missouri Breaks, It Lives Again, Apocalypse Now, The Rose, One from the Heart, Hammet, Valley Girl, The Stone Boy.
TELEVISION: Movies: Best Kept Secrets, Calamity Jane, Right to Kill?, The Deliberate Stranger.

FORREST, STEVE: Actor. b. Huntsville, Texas, Sept. 29, 1925. e. UCLA, 1950 Acted at La Jolla Playhouse; appeared on radio, TV; m.p. debut in Geisha Girl.
PICTURES INCLUDE: Bad and the Beautiful, Battle Circus, The Clown, Band Wagon, Dream Wife, So Big, Take the High Ground, Phantom of the Rue Morgue, Prisoner of War, Rogue Cop, Bedeviled, It Happened to Jane, Heller in Pink Tights, Five Branded Women, Flaming Star, The Second Time Around, Rascal, The Wild Country, The Late Liz, North Dallas Forty, Mommie Dearest, Sahara, Spies Like Us.
TELEVISION: Hollywood Wives.

FORRESTER, LARRY: Writer. b. Glasgow, Scotland, 1924. Ent. TV industry with his wife Pauline as Special investigators on audience participation shows. Later scripting for TV.
SERIES INCLUDE: Ivanhoe, William Tell, Flying Doctor, International Detective, Interpol Calling, Knight Errant, No Hiding Place, The Golden Girl, Sir Francis Drake, Top Secret, Ghost Squad, This Man Craig, Danger Man, Espionage, The Saint.
PICTURES INCLUDE: Hercules and the Princess of Troy; Tora! Tora! Tora!
BOOKS INCLUDE: Battle of the April Storm, A Girl Called Fathom, Fly for Your Life, Skymen, Diamond Beach.

FORSTATER, MARK: Producer. b. Philadelphia, 1943. e. City College of New York, Temple Univ. In 1967 moved to England; studied at University of Manchester and London Intl. Film School. First job in industry with Anglia TV on program, Survival. Began producing in 1970 with British Film Institute. Set up Chippenham Films to make documentaries. Moved into features in 1974 with Monty Python and the Holy Grail.
PICTURES: The Odd Job, Marigolds in August, The Grass Is Singing, Xtro, etc. Shorts: The Glitterball, Wish You Were Here.
TELEVISION: The Cold Room.

FORSTER, ROBERT: Actor. b. Rochester, N.Y., July 13, 1941. e. Heidelberg College, Alfred University, Rochester U., B.S.
THEATRE: Plays, Mrs. Dally, 1965. Summer tour, A Streetcar Named Desire, 1967.
PICTURES INCLUDE: Reflections in a Golden Eye, Medium Cool, Justine, Journey Through Rosebud, The Don is Dead, the Black Hole, Alligator, Vigilante, Walking the Edge.

FORSYTHE, JOHN: Actor. b. Penn's Grove, N.J., Jan. 29, 1918.
STAGE CREDITS: Mr. Roberts, All My Sons, Yellow Jack, Teahouse of the August Moon, and others.
TV: Started in 1947; appeared on Studio One, Kraft Theatre, Robert Montgomery Presents, and others. Bachelor Father series; To Rome with Love series; Dynasty.
PICTURES INCLUDE: Captive City, It Happens Every Thursday, The Glass Web, Escape from Fort Bravo, Trouble With Harry, Ambassador's Daughter, Everything But the Truth, Kitten With a Whip, Madame X, In Cold Blood, The Happy Ending, Topaz, And Justice For All.

FORTE, FABIAN: Singer, Actor. b. Philadelphia, Feb. 6, 1940. e. South Philadelphia high sch. At 14, discovered by Marcucci and DeAngelis, voice teacher. Chancellor Records; signed contract. Studied with Carlo Menotti.
RECORDS INCLUDE: Turn Me Loose, This Friendly World, The Fabulous Fabian (Gold album), Foggy Foggy Dew (High Time).
PICTURES INCLUDE: Hound Dog Man, High Time, North To Alaska, Love in a Goldfish Bowl, Mr. Hobbs Takes a Vaction, Ride the Wild Surf, Dear Brigette, Longest Day, 10 Little Indians, Fireball 500, Thunder Alley, Five Weeks in a Balloon, Devil's Eight, The Longest Day, A Bullet for Pretty Boy, Little Laura and Big John.

FOSSE, BOB: Director, Choreographer, Actor. b. Chicago, June 23, 1927. Began dancing at age of 9 and made first professional appearance at 13. After service with U.S. Navy in World War II toured with Mary Ann Niles in Call Me Mister. Signed by MGM in 1953 and acted in three films. First big Broadway success as choreographer of Pajama Game in 1955.
PICTURES INCLUDE: Actor: Give a Girl a Break, My Sister Eileen, The Affairs of Dobie Gillis, Kiss Me Kate, Thieves, The Little Prince. Choreographer: My Sister Eileen. Director-Choreographer: Sweet Charity, Cabaret. Director: Lenny. All That Jazz (also co. s.p.). Star '80 (also s.p.).
BROADWAY: Choreographer: Pajama Game, Damn Yankees, Redhead, Little Me, New Girl in Town, How To Succeed in Business Without Really Trying, Sweet Charity, Pippin, Chicago. Director: Redhead, Little Me, Sweet Charity, Pippin, Chicago, Dancin! Director/choreographer/ Book: Big Deal.

FOSTER, DAVID: Producer. b. New York City, Nov. 25, 1929. e. Dorsey H.S., U. of Southern California (School of Journalism). U.S. Army, 1952–54; entered public relations field in 1952 with Rogers, Cowan & Brenner; Jim Mahoney, 1956; Allen, Foster, Ingersoll & Weber, 1958; left field in 1968 to enter independent m.p. production.
PICTURES INCLUDE: Co-produced (with Mitchell Brower) McCabe and Mrs. Miller, The Getaway, The Nickel Ride (exec. prod.), The Drowning Pool (co-prod.), The Legacy, Tribute (exec. prod.), Caveman (co-prod.), The Thing (co-prod.), Second Thoughts (co-prod.), Mass Appeal (co-prod.), The Mean Season (co-prod.), Short Circuit (co-prod.); Running Scared (co-prod.).

FOSTER, JODIE: Actress. b. Los Angeles, 1962.Acting debut on Mayberry, R.F.D. TV series. Followed with many TV appearances, from series to Movies-of-the-Week.
PICTURES INCLUDE: Napoleon and Samantha, Menace of the Mountain, One Little Indian, Tom Sawyer, Kansas City Bomber, Taxi Driver, Echoes of a Summer, Bugsy Malone, Freaky Friday, The Little Girl Who Lives Down the Lane, Candleshoe, Foxes, Carny, The Hotel New Hampshire.
TV: The Courtship of Eddie's Father (regular), My Three Sons (regular), Paper Moon (regular). Movies: Smile, Jenny, You're Dead, Rookie of the Year, The Blood of Others.

FOSTER, JULIA: Actress. b. 1944, in Lewes, Sussex, England. First acted with the Brighton Repertory Company, then two years with the Worthing, Harrogate and Richmond companies. 1956, TV debut as Ann Carson in Emergency Ward 10.
PICTURES INCLUDE: Term of Trial, The Loneliness of the Long Distance Runner, The Small World of Sammy Lee, The System, The Bargee, One Way Pendulum, Alfie, Half A Sixpence.
TV: A Cosy Little Arrangement, The Planemakers, Love Story, Taxi, Consequences, They Throw It At You, Crime and Punishment, The Image.
STAGE: No. 1 tour of The Country Wife; 1969, What the Butler Saw.

FOSTER KEMP, CECIL R.: (M.B.E.) Assoc. prod. and prod. supervisor. b. Shanghai. e. Brighton College.
PICTURES INCLUDE: Paris Holiday, Interpol, Tarzan and the Lost Safari, Around the World in Eighty Days, Front Page Story, Appointment in London, South of Algiers, Under Capricorn, Scott of the Antarctic, Untamed, John Paul Jones, King of Kings, Offbeat, El Cid, Fifty Five Days at Peking, The Fall of the Roman Empire, William The Conqueror, Girl on the Motorcycle, Arthur! Arthur!, I Saw Him Die, Ferdinand and Isabella, Wild Violets.

FOSTER, MAURICE DAVID: Prod.-Wrt. e. St. Paul's Ent. m.p. ind. 1943 as asst. to gen. man. and prod. sup. Easling Studios. From 1950–61, prod. sup. and dir. Film Finances, 1961–63, dir. and gen. man. MGM British Studios.
PICTURES INCLUDE: The Jokers (Universal), Assignment K (Columbia), The Osterman Weekend (Fox).

FOSTER, MEG: Actress. b. May 10, 1948. e. N.Y. Neighborhood Playhouse.
PICTURES: Adam at 6 A.M., Promise Her Anything, A Different Story, Once in Paris, Carny, Ticket to Heaven, The Emerald Forest.
TELEVISION: Movies: The Death of Me Yet, Sunshine, Things In This Season, James Dean, Washington: Behind Closed Doors, Sunshine Christmas.

FOWLER, HARRY: Actor. b. Lambeth Walk (London). Stage debut, Nothing Up My Sleeve (London) 1950; Screen debut, 1941.
PICTURES INCLUDE: Demi-Paradise, Don't Take It to Heart, Champagne Charlie, Painted Boats, Hue and Cry, Now Barabbas, The Dark Man, She Shall Have Murder, The Scarlet Thread, High Treason, The Last Page, I Believe in You, Pickwick Papers, Top of the Form, Angels One Five, Conflict of Wings (Fuss Over Feathers), A Day To Remember, Blue Peter, Home and Away, Booby Trap, Town on Trial, Lucky Jim, Birthday Present, Idle on Parade, Don't Panic Chaps, Heart of a Man, Crooks Anonymous, The Longest Day, Lawrence of Arabia, Flight From Singapore, The Golliwog, Ladies Who Do, Clash By Night, The Nanny, Life At the Top, Start the Revolution Without Me, The Prince & The Pauper, Fanny Hill.
TV: Stalingrad, I Remember the Battle, Gideon's Way, That's For Me, Our Man At St. Mark's, Dixon of Dock Green, Dr. Finlay's Case Book, I Was There, Cruffs Dog Show, The Londoners, Jackanory, Get This, Movie Quiz, Get This series, Going a Bundle, Ask a Silly Answer, London Scene, Flockton Flyer, Sun Trap, The Little World of Don Camillo, World's End, Minder, Dead Ernest, Morecambe Wise Show, Gossip, Entertainment Express, Fresh Fields.

FOWLEY, DOUGLAS: Actor. b. New York City, May 30, 1911; e. St. Francis Xavier's Mil. Acad., N.Y. In stock; operated dramatic sch. N.Y.; on screen in bit parts. From 1934 in regular roles. Has appeared in many pictures.
PICTURES INCLUDE: Battleground, Just This Once, This Woman Is Dangerous, Singin' in the Rain, Man Behind the Gun, Slight Case of Larceny, Naked Jungle, Casanova's Big Night, Lone Gun, High & Mighty, Three Ring Circus, Texas Lady, Broken Star, Girl Rush, Bandido, Nightmare in the Sun.

FOX, EDWARD: Actor. b. England, 1937. Comes from theatrical family; father was agent for leading London actors; brother is actor James Fox.
PICTURES INCLUDE: The Mind Benders, The Long Duel, Morgan, The Naked Runner, The Jokers, I'll Never Forget What's 'Is Name, The Battle of Britain, Oh! What a Lovely War, Skullduggery, The Breaking of Bumbo, The Day of The Jackal, A Doll's House, Galileo, The Squeeze, A Bridge Too Far, The Duellists, The Big Sleep, Force 10 from Navarone, The Mirror Crack'd, Gandhi, The Dresser, The Bounty, Wild Geese II.

FOX, JAMES: Actor. b. London, England, 1939. Ent. films as child actor in 1950 in The Magnet and Mrs. Minniver.
TV APPEARANCES INCLUDE: The Door, Espionage, Love Is Old, Love Is New, Nancy Astor, Country, New World.
PICTURES INCLUDE: The Loneliness of the Long-Distance Runner, Tamahine, The Servant, Those Magnificent Men in Their Flying Machines, King Rat, The Chase, Thoroughly Modern Millie, Arabella, Duffy, Loves of Isadora, Performance, Anna Pavola, Runners, A Passage to India, Absolute Beginners, The Whistler Blower, Comrades.

FOX, MICHAEL J.: Actor. b. Edmonton, Canada, June 9, 1961.
PICTURES: Midnight Madness, The Class of 1984, Back to the Future, Teen Wolf, Light of Day.
TELEVISION: Leo and Me, Letters from Frank, Palmerstown, Family Ties, High School USA, Poison Ivy, etc.

FOX, RICHARD: Executive. Joined Warner Bros. Intl. as mgt. trainee in October 1975, working in Australia and Japan. 1977, named gen. mgr. of Columbia-Warner Dist., New Zealand. Served as gen. mgr. of WB in Tokyo, 1978–1981. Joined WB in L.A. as exec. asst. to Myron D. Karlin, pres. of WB Intl., 1981; appt. v.p., sls. 1982; 1983, promoted to exec. v.p. of intl. arm; 1985, named pres. of WB Intl., assuming post vacated by Karlin.

FOX, RICHARD A.: Executive. b. Buffalo, NY, Jan 5, 1929. e. Univ. of Buffalo (1950). Owns theatre chain, Fox Theatres Management Corp. Pres., Nat'l. NATO (1984) & pres. Theatre Owners of PA.

FOXWELL, IVAN: Producer. b. Feb. 22, 1914, London, Eng. Entered m.p. ind. 1933 as technician with British & Dominions Film Corp., subsequently with Paramount British & London Films; Assoc. with Curtis Bernhardt in Paris 1937 becoming producer & collaborating on story, s.p. of Carefour, Le Train pur Venise, Sarajevo, others. In World War II with BEF and AEF 1939–46. Returned to British films 1947 as producer, co-author screen adapt., No Room at the Inn; prod., collab. s.p., Guilt Is My Shadow; prod., Twenty-Four Hours of a Woman's Life; co-author s.p. and prod. The Intruder, The Colditz Story (TV series adapt. 1972), Manuela, A Touch of Larceny, Tiara Tahiti, The Quiller Memorandum; s.p. and prod. Decline and Fall. Director, Foxwell Film Prods. Ltd.

FOXWORTH, ROBERT: Actor. b. Houston, TX, Nov. 1, 1941. e. Mellon Univ. Began acting at age 10 at Houston Alley Theatre and stayed with stage part-time while completing formal education. Returned to theatre on full-time basis after graduation from Mellon. Made TV debut in Sadbird, 1969.
TELEVISION: The Storefront Lawyers (series), Mrs. Sundance, Hogan's Goat, Falcon Crest.
PICTURES: Treasure of Matecumbe (debut), The Astral Factor, Airport '77, Damien-Omen II, The Black Marble, Invisible Strangler.
STAGE: P.S., Your Cat Is Dead.

FOXX, REDD: Actor, Performer. b. St. Louis, Mo., Dec. 9, 1922. Began career by running away from home to join a washboard band at age 13; first nightclub appearances as a single, then with Slappy White from 1951 to 1956; 50 record albums in last 17 years.
TV: Sanford and Son.
PICTURE: Norman, Is That You?

FRAKER, WILLIAM A.: Cinematographer—Director. b. Los Angeles, 1923. Graduate USC Film School. Worked as operator with Conrad Hall; moved to TV before feature films.
PICTURES: Cinematographer: Games, The Fox, President's Analyst, Fade In, Rosemary's Baby, Bullitt, Paint Your Wagon, Dusty and Sweets McGee, Day of the Dolphin, Rancho Deluxe, The Killer Inside Me, Aloha, Bobby and Rose, Gator, Close Encounters of the Third Kind, Looking for Mr. Goodbar, Heaven Can Wait, Odd Boyfriends, 1941. Director: Monte Walsh, Reflection of Fear, Bette Midler's Divine Madness, The Legend of the Lone Ranger, Sharky's Machine, the Best Little Whorehouse in Texas, WarGames, Irreconcilable Differences, Murphy's Romance, Fever Pitch, Murphy's Romance, SpaceCamp.
TELEVISION: Stony Burke, Outer Limits, Ozzie and Harriet, Daktari.

FRAMER, WALT: TV Producer. b. Pittsburgh, Pa., Apr. 7, 1908; e. Univ. of Pittsburgh. Former theatre magr.; news commentator, KDKA, Pitts.; sidewalk interviewer of Radio Swaps; creator-prod. Strike It Rich, The Big Payoff, Million Dollar Family, Futures Unlimited, Penny-a-Mile, Lady Luck, For Love or Money, Man on the Beat, It's in the Cards, Meet the People, Make It Big, The Fashion News Reel, Make Your Move, Holiday for Two, Take A Letter. Your Great Escape, Fun For the Money, Heartline U.S.A., Look For Tomorrow, What's It Worth?, Futures Unlimited.

FRANCIOSA, ANTHONY: Actor. b. New York City, Oct. 25, 1928. e. High School there. First stage part in Y.W.C.A. play; joined Off-Broadway stage group; stock at Lake Tahoe, Calif., Chicago and Boston.
THEATRE: N.Y. stage in End As a Man, The Wedding Breakfast; lead in A Hatful of Rain.
PICTURES INCLUDE: A Face in the Crowd, This Could Be The Night, A Hatful of Rain, Wild Is The Wind, The Long Hot Summer, The Naked Maja, Career Story, On Page One, Go Naked in the World, Period of Adjustment, The Swinger, Fathom, A Man Called Gannon, The Sweet Ride, Rio Conchos, In Enemy Country, Across 110th Street, The Drowning Pool, Firepower, Death Wish II.
TV: Valentine's Day, The Name of the Game, Search, Matt Helm, Stagecoach.

FRANCIS, ANNE: Actress b. Ossining, N.Y., Sept. 16, 1932. Child model; radio TV shows as child & adult; on B'way in Lady in the Dark.
PICTURES INCLUDE: Summer Holiday, So Young So Bad, Whistle at Eaton Falls, Lydia Bailey, Elopement, Dream Boat, Lion is in the Streets, Rocket Man, Susan Slept Here, Rogue Cop, Bad Day at Black Rock, Battle Cry, Blackboard Jungle, Scarlet Coat, Forbidden Planet, The Rack, Great American Pastime, Don't Go Near the Water, Crowded Sky, Girl of the Night, Satan Bug, Brainstorm, Hook, Line, and Sinker, More Dead Than Alive, The Impasse, The Love God, Funny Girl, Born Again.

FRANCIS, ARLENE: Actress. r.n. Arlene Kazanjian; b. Boston, Mass. e. Convent of Mount St. Vincent Academy, Riverdale, N.Y.; Finch Finishing School, Theatre Guild School, N.Y.; m. Martin Gabel, actor.
STAGE: All That Glitters, Doughgirls, The Overtons, Once More With Feeling, Tchin-Tchin, Beekman Place, Mrs. Dally, Dinner at Eight, Kind Sin, Lion in Winter, Pal Joey, Who Killed Santa Claus?, Gigi.
TV: Regular panelist What's My Line, WCBS-TV; Home, Arlene Francis Show, NBC-TV: Talent Patrol, etc.
RADIO: Arlene Francis Show, Emphasis, Monitor.
PICTURES INCLUDE: All My Sons, One, Two, Three, The Thrill of It All.

FRANCIS, CONNIE: Singer. r.n. Constance Franconero. b. Newark, N.J., Dec. 12, 1938. Appeared, Star Time since 12 years old; won Arthur Godfrey's Talent Scout Show, 12 years old.
GOLD RECORDS: Who's Sorry Now, My Happiness. Numerous vocalist awards: All Major TV shows.
PICTURES INCLUDE: Where the Boys Are, Follow the Boys, Looking For Love.

FRANCIS, FREDDIE: Producer-Director-Cameraman. b. London, 1917. Joined Gaumont British Studios as apprentice to stills photographer; then clapper boy at B.I.P. Studios, Elstree; camera asst. at British Dominion. After World War II returned to Shepperton Studios to work for Korda and with Powell and Pressburger as cameraman.
PICTURES INCLUDE: Director: Paranoiac, Vengeance, Evil of Frankenstein, Nightmare, Hysteria, Dr. Terror's House of Horrors, The Skull, Traitor's Gate, The Psychopath, The Deadly Bees, They Came from Beyond Space, Torture Garden, Dracula Has Risen from the Grave, Girly, Trog, Tales from the Crypt, The Creeping Flesh, Tales That Witness Madness, The Ghoul, Legend of The Werewolf, The Doctor and the Devils. Cameraman: Moby Dick (second unit photo., special effects), Room at the Top, Saturday Night and Sunday Morning, Sons and Lovers (Oscar), The Innocents, The Elephant Man, The French Lieutenant's Woman, Dune, Code Name: Emerald.

FRANCIS, KEVIN: Producer-Executive. b. London, England, 1948. 1967–70, production mgr., assoc. producer. 1970–72, produced It's Life, Passport, Trouble with Canada. 1972 founder, Tyburn Productions Limited; 1973, produced Persecution; 1974, produced The Ghoul & Legend of the Werewolf; 1975, founder, Tyburn Productions Inc.; 1976, prod. Film Techniques Educ. Course for BFI. Since 1977 exec. prod., Master of the Shell, The Masks of Death, Courier, Murder Elite, The Abbot's Cry, etc.

FRANCISCUS, JAMES: Actor. b. Clayton, Mo. 1934; e. Taft Prep, Yale U.
PICTURES INCLUDE: Four Boys And A Gun, I Passed For White, The Outsiders, The Miracle of the White Stallions, Youngblood Hawke, The Valley of Gwangi, Marooned, Beneath the Planet of the Apes, The Cat O' Nine Tails, The Greek Tycoon, City on Fire, When Time Ran Out, Butterfly.
TV: Naked City, Mr. Novak, Longstreet (TV film feature), The 500 Pound Jerk (TV feature).

FRANK, EDMOND: Executive. b. New York, N.Y., Feb. 11, 1945. e. American University (B.A.) Washington College of Law (J.D.) Admitted to Fla. Bar 1971. Vice-pres. and gen. counsel, World Film. pres., South Florida Entertainment Counsel Guild.

FRANK, MELVIN: Writer, producer, director. In 1942: collaborated on story, My Favorite Blonde, Par. In June, 1942: appointed consultant in the radio branch of the War Department, working under Lt. Col. E. M. Kirby. In 1942 collab. s.p. Happy-Go-Lucky, Thank Your Lucky Stars; collab. Star Spangled Rhythm, (collab. s.p.) And the Angels Sing, Monsieur Beaucaire, Road to Utopia, Duffy's Tavern, The Return of October, It Had To Be You.
PICTURES INCLUDE: Mr. Blandings Builds His Dream House, Southern Yankee, The Redhead and the Reformer, Strictly Dishonorable, Callaway Went Thataway, Above and Beyond, Knock on Wood, White Christmas, Court Jester, That Certain Feeling, Li'l Abner, A Funny Thing Happened on the Way to the Forum, The Facts of Life, The Road to Hong Kong, Strange Bedfellows, Buona Sera, Mrs. Campbell, A Touch of Class, The Prisoner of Second Avenue, The Duchess and the Dirtwater Fox, Lost and Found.

FRANKEL, DANIEL: Executive. b. New York City, Aug. 21, 1903; e. U. Mich., U. Berlin (Germany). Gen. mgr., Films Erka, Paris, 1925–30. Ran Theatre des Champs Elysees, 1928–29. Produced two French pictures. Returned to New York and joined Pathe 1930; dir. foreign dept., later of all sales to 1941; resigned to engage in prod. unit org. Vice-pres. & exec. dir., Four Continents Films, 1945; with U.A. in Europe 1953–56; ret. U.S. & org., pres., Zenith Int'l Film Corp., 1956, distr., Lovers, 400 Blows, Hiroshima, Mon Amour, etc. Governor IFIDA.

FRANKENHEIMER, JOHN: Director. b. Malba, N.Y. Feb. 19, 1930. e. Williams College. Actor, dir., summer stock; radio-TV actor, dir., Washington, D.C.; then joined CBS network.
TV: Mama, You Are There, Danger, Climax, Studio One, Playhouse 90, Du Pont Show of the Month; Ford Startime, Sunday Showcase.
PICTURES INCLUDE: The Young Stranger, The Young Savages, Birdman of Alcatraz, All Fall Down, The Manchurian Candidate, Seven Days in May, The Train, Seconds, Grand Prix, The Extraordinary Seaman, The Fixer, The Gypsy Moths, I Walk the Line, Horsemen, The Impossible Object, The Iceman Cometh, 99 and 44/100½ Dead, French Connection II, Black Sunday, Prophecy, The Challenge, The Holcroft Covenant, 52 Pick-Up.

FRANKLIN, MICHAEL HAROLD: Executive. b. Los Angeles, Dec. 25, 1923. e. Univ. of Cal. (A.B.), Univ. So. Cal. (LL.B.). Admitted to Cal. bar, 1951; pvt. practice in L.A. 1951–52; atty. CBS, 1952–54; atty. Paramount Pictures, 1954–58; exec. dir. Writers Guild Am. West, Inc. 1958–78; national exec. dir., Directors Guild of America 1978–. Mem. Am. Civil Liberties Union, Los Angeles Copyright Soc., Order of Coif.

FRANKLIN, PAMELA: Actress. b. Tokyo, Japan. Feb. 4, 1950. Attended, Elmshurst Ballet School, Camberley, Surrey.
PICTURES INCLUDE: The Innocents, The Lion, Flipper's New Adventure, The Prime of Miss Jean Brodie, The Night of the Following Day, And Soon the Darkness, The Legend of Hell House, Food of the Gods.

FRANKLIN, ROBERT A.: Executive. b. New York City April 15. e. Univ. of Miami (BBA, 1958); Columbia Pacific (MBA, 1979; PHD, 1980) majoring in marketing. Before entering film industry worked with House of Seagram (1959–64); Canada Dry Corp. (1964–66); J. M. Mathes Adv. (1966–67). In 1967 joined 20th Century-Fox as dir. of mkt. planning. Formed RP Marketing Intl. (entertainment consulting firm) in 1976 and World Research Systems (computer software marketer). In 1981 joined MPAA; 1983, named v.p., administration and information services. Chm., MPAA research comm.; member, AMA and ESOMAR.

FRANKLYN, ARTHUR R.: b. N.Y.C. July 19, 1928. Child actor with Life With Father, Farewell Tour and Just Because. New York stage 1941–44. Featured skater, Ice Frolic Latin American tour, 1948–49; star and prod. ice revues at Havana Coliseum, 1949–50; served with U.S. Marines, Korea 1950–51; prod. dir., Los Angeles Ice Palace, 1951–56; exploitation and special events, Fox West Coast Theatres, 1956–59; Lippert Theatres, 1960; purchased Amador Chain of Central California Theatres. Pres. U.S. Bowling Photographers, Inc.; 1960–65 Dist. Mgr. Theatre Amuse Co., Tarzana, Calif.; Mgr. Florida State Theas., Dist. mgr. Arlo Enterprises.

FRANKOVICH M. J.: Executive. b. Bisbee, Arizona, Sept. 29, 1910. e. U.C.L.A., B.A. Ent. Radio 1934 as producer, commentator; began writing screenplays for Universal, 1938; Republic Pictures, 1940–49 (except for period war service U.S. Army); to Europe 1949 to make Fugitive Lady, Lucky Nick Kane, Thief of Venice etc.; England 1952. prod., Decameron Nights, Malaga, Footsteps in the Fog, Joe Macbeth; apptd. man. dir. Columbia Pictures Corp. Ltd., in U.K. and Eire Aug. 1955; elected vice-pres., Columbia Pictures International Corp., Dec. 1955; head Col. Pictures Int. Prod., 1958; vice-pres., Col. Pics. Corp., 1959. Appt. Chrmn., Columbia Pics. Corp. Ltd., 1959. Variety Club Crew Member; chief barker, Tent 36 Variety Club, 1957. dir., BLC Films; chmn., Screen Gems Ltd.; first v.p. chge. world prod., Columbia; resigned July, 1967 to return to independent production. Long Term Deal, 1969, rel. through Columbia.
PICTURES INCLUDE: Bob & Carol & Ted & Alice, Marooned, Cactus Flower, The Looking Glass War, Doctors' Wives, There's A Girl in My Soup, The Love Machine, Dollars, Butterflies Are Free, Stand Up and Be Counted, 40 Carats, A Report to the Commissioner, From Noon Till Three, The Shootist.

FRANZ, ARTHUR: Actor. b. Perth Amboy, N.J. Feb. 29, 1920; e. Blue Ridge Coll., Md. U.S. Air Force. Radio, TV shows.
THEATRE: Streetcar Named Desire, Second Threshold.
PICTURES INCLUDE: Jungle Patrol, Roseanna McCoy, Red Light, Doctor and the Girl, Sands of Iwo Jima, Strictly Dishonorable, Submarine Command, Member of the Wedding, Flight Nurse, Bad for Each Other, Eddie Cantor Story, Caine Mutiny, Steel Cage, Battle Taxi, New Orleans Uncensored, Bobby Ware Is Missing, Atomic Submarine, The Human Factor, That Championship Season.

FRAWLEY, JAMES: Director. b. Houston, Texas. Studied drama at Carnegie Tech and Actors Studio, where later taught and ran the directors unit. Was charter member of comedy group, The Premise; has acted in plays on and off Bdwy. Won Emmy Award for Monkees series, where staged two musical numbers a week for two seasons.
PICTURES: Kid Blue, The Big Bus, The Muppet Movie.
TELEVISION: Columbo, Delancy Street, Capra, etc.

FRAZER, AUSTIN: Prod. consultant. b. London, England. Early career, designer and writer. Fellow SIAD. Writer's Guild Award 1967, Dante's Inferno.

FRAZIER, CLIFF: Director, actor. b. Detroit, Mich., Aug. 27, 1934; e. Wayne State U., Harold Clurman. Exec. dir., The Community Film Workshop Council; was co-founder & artistic dir.: Stable Theatre, Detroit, 1960–63; Concept East Theatre, Detroit, 1962–64; co-produced and acted in Study in Color, 1964–65; assoc. dir., Theatre of Latin America, Inc., N.Y.C., 1968; dir. of drama, Mobilization for Youth, N.Y.C., 1966–68; East Coast dir. of rsch., Brooks Foundation, Sta. Barbara, 1966–68.
TV ACTING INCLUDES: Today, Tell It Like It Is, NYPD. The Nurses, The Negro Experimental Theatre, Othello.
THEATRE: Stage repertories: Washington Theatre Club, Irish Hills Rep., Will-O-Way Playhouse.
Co-author, Discovery in Drama and book critic, Catholic Reporter, 1969.

FRAZIER, SHEILA E.: Actress. b. Bronx, N.Y., Nov. 13, 1948. e. Englewood, N.J. Was exec. sect'y. and high-fashion model. Steered to acting career by friend Richard Roundtree. Studied drama with N.Y. Negro Ensemble Co. and New Federal Theatre, N.Y.
PICTURES INCLUDE: Super Fly (debut), Superfly T.N.T., The Super Cops, California Suite.

FREDERIC, MARC: Producer. b. New York, Apr. 25, 1916. e. Washington & Lee Univ. Capt. U.S. Air Force. Prod., dist. "Little Theatre" 1948, 104 episodes. First to make deal through AFTRA for kinescope release of live shows for dist. Tales of Tomorrow series. Org., Marc Frederic Prods., Inc.
PICTURES INCLUDE: Giant of the Unknown, She Demon, Missile to the Moon, Frankenstein's Daughter, Girl in Room 13, Career Girl, Festival Girl.

FREDERICKSON, H. GRAY, JR.: Producer. b. Oklahoma City, Okla., July 31, 1937. e. U. of Lausanne, Switzerland, 1958–59; U. of Okla. B.A., 1960. m. Victoria Schmidlapp. Worked one yr. with Panero, Weidlinger & Salvatori Engineering Co., Rome Italy. In 1979 named v.p. of feature films, Lorimar Films.

PICTURES INCLUDE: Candy, Inspector Sterling, Gospel 70, An Italian in America, The Man Who Wouldn't Die, The Good, Bad & Ugly, Intrigue in Suez, How to Learn to Love Women, God's Own Country, Wedding March, An American Wife, Natika, Echo in the Village, Little Fauss & Big Halsey, Making It, The Godfather, The Godfather, Part II, Hit (exec. prod.), Apocalypse Now (co.-prod.), One From the Heart, The Outsiders.

TELEVISION: Producer: The Return of Mickey Spillane's Mike Hammer, Houston Nights.

FREEMAN, EVERRETT: Writer. b. New York City. Contrib. Sat. Eve. Post. From 1942 writer for screen.

PICTURES INCLUDE: George Washington Slept Here, Princess and the Pirate, It Happened on Fifth Ave., Secret Life of Walter Mitty, Too Youing to Kiss, Lady Takes a Sailor, Jim Thorpe—All American, Pretty Baby, Million Dollar Mermaid, Destination Gobi, Kelly and Me, My Man Godfrey, Marjorie Morningstar, Sunday In New York, The Glass Bottom Boat, Where Were You When the Lights Went out, The Maltese Bippy, How Do I Love Thee, ZigZag.

TV: Prod. Bachelor Father series.

FREEMAN, JOEL: Producer. b. Newark, N.J., June 12, 1922. e. Upsala Coll. Began career at MGM studios in 1941. In Air Force Mot. Pic. Unit 1942–46. Became assist. dir. at RKO in 1946. In 1948 returned to MGM as asst. dir.; later assoc. prod. In 1956 entered indep. field as prod. supv. on various features and TV series. In 1960 to Warner Bros., assoc. producing Sunrise at Campobello, The Music Man and Act One. After such films as Camelot and Finian's Rainbow, became studio exec. at Warners.

PICTURES: Producer: The Heart Is a Lonely Hunter, Shaft, Trouble Man, Love At First Bite, Octagon. Exec. Producer: The Kindred, Wired.

FREEMAN, SIR N. BERNARD: (C.B.E.) Executive. b. Sydney, Sept. 1, 1896; e. public schools, Xavier College, Melbourne; established MGM throughout Australia, New Zealand, man. dir., chmn., retired 1967. European War, 1914–18.

Member: Admin. Comm. of Brit. Centre, 1944–46. Chairman: Anzac House Appeal 1945, Anzac House Trust 1946, Miss Australia Quest, 1948–49. N.S.W. Comm. for World Refugee Year, 1960. Nat'l. Chmn., UNICEF, 1953; pres. Rotary Club of Sydney, 1960–61; Created C.B.E. (Civil) 1946; chmn., Motion Picture Distributors' Association of Australia, 1939–41, '63 Deputy Chairman, Council of International House, University of Sydney.

FREGONESE, HUGO: Director. b. Argentina. e. Buenos Aires College, Buenos Aires U. Prior to entering m.p. ind., newspaperman, Buenos Aires; ed. All Sports, in cattle ind., Azul; arrived New York City, for study at Columbia U.; to Los Angeles, as tech. adv.; back to Buenos Aires, 1938; made shorts in Argentina, cutter; asst. dir.; co-dir., Pampa Barbara; dir. Where Words Fail; signed by Hollywood, when MGM bought releasing rights; dir. Hardly A Criminal, Argentina; to Universal-International, 1949. Stanley Kramer Prod., 1951.

PICTURES INCLUDE: One Way Street, Saddle Tramp, Apache Drums, Mark of the Renegade, My Six Convicts, Untamed Frontier, Blowing Wild, Decameron Nights, Man in the Attic, The Raid, Black Tuesday, Thunders, Harry Black and the Tiger, I Girovaghi, Marco Polo, Moneta, Sperzzata (Italy), Shatterhand (Germany), The Tramps, Broken Coin, Savage Pampas (Spain).

FRELENG, FRIZ: Writer-Producer. b. Kansas City, MO, Aug. 21, 1906. Animator, Walt Disney Studio, 1928–29; Charles Mintz Studio, 1929–30, prod.-dir., Warner Bros., 1930–63. Formed partnership with David DePatie in 1963.

CARTOON FILMS INCLUDE: Tweetie Pie, Speedy Gonzales, Halloween Is Grinch Night, Pink Panther in Olympinks, Dr. Deuss' Pontoffel Pock. Recent compilations: The Looney, Looney Bugs Bunny Movie, Bugs Bunny's 3rd Movie: 1001 Rabbit Tales.

FRENCH, HAROLD: Film and stage director. b. London, England, April 23, 1900. Popular London player in revue musical comedy, etc., 1930–35. Started directing 1936. Cavalier of the Streets, at Pinewood. Since: The House of the Arrow, Dead Men Are Dangerous, Jeannie, Unpublished Story, The Day Will Dawn. Directed stage plays: Youth at the Helm, Design for Living, No Time for Comedy, French Without Tears. In 1942: Secret Mission, Helm-General Film: The Avengers, Par. In 1944 dir. Mr. Emmanuel.

PICTURES INCLUDE: English Without Tears, Quiet Weekend, My Brother Jonathan, The Blind Goddess, Quartet, Adam & Evelyn, The Dancing Years, Trio, Hour of Thirteen, Encore, Isn't Life Wonderful, Rob Roy, Man Who Watched Trains Go By (Paris Express), Man Who Loved Redheads.

FRENKE, EUGENE: Producer. b. Russia, Jan. 1, 1907. m. Anna Sten.

PICTURES INCLUDE: Life Returns, Two Who Dared, Three Russians Girls, Let's Live a Little, Lady in Iron Mask, Miss Robin Crusoe, Heaven Knows, Mr. Allison, Barbarian and the Geisha, The Last Sunset, Royal Hunt of the Sun.

FRESCO, ROBERT M.: Writer. b. Burbank, Calif., Oct. 18, 1928. e. Los Angeles City Coll. Newspaperman. Los Angeles, 1946–47; U.S. Army, 1948–49; staff writer, Hakim Prod., 1950–51; various screenplays, 1951–56.

PICTURES INCLUDE: Tarantula, They Came to Destroy the Earth, Monolith.

TV: Scripts for Science Fiction Theatre, Highway Patrol.

FRIEDBERG, A. ALAN: Executive. b. New York City, Apr. 13, 1932. e. Columbia Coll. (BA), Harvard Law School. President, Sack Theatres, Boston. NATO bd. mbr.

FRIEDKIN, JOHN: Executive. Entered industry in New York as publicist for Columbia Pictures; spent eight years at Young & Rubicam adv. agency. Formed Sumner & Friedkin with Gabe Sumner as partner; left to join Rogers & Cowan, where named v.p. In 1967 resigned to join 20th-Fox, moving to California in 1972 when home offices were transferred. Appointed Fox v.p. worldwide publ. & promo. In 1979 joined Warner Bros. as v.p.—adv. pub. for intl. div.

FRIEDKIN, WILLIAM: Director. b. Chicago, Ill., 1939. Joined NBC-TV, 1957, worked for National Education TV, did TV documentaries before feature films.

PICTURES INCLUDE: Good Times, The Night They Raided Minsky's, The Birthday Party, The Boys in the Band, The French Connection. (Academy Award, best picture, dir. 1971), The Exorcist, Sorcerer (prod.-dir.), Cruising (dir.-s.p.), Deal of the Century, To Live and Die in L.A. (dir., co-s.p.).

FRIEDMAN, ARNOLD J.: Executive b. New York, N.Y. Entered m.p. industry as exploiteer for Columbia Pictures Corp. 1957–60; advng dept. United Artists Corp. 1960–62; adv. mgr., Embassy Pictures Corp. and later director of adv., publ., prom. for Embassy Pictures Television, 1962–67; pres. Arnold Friedman's Company, 1967–70; dir. of ad./pub./promo for Metromedia Producers Corp., 1970–72; creative dir., ITC, 1973–76; vice pres. of theatrical adv. & TV pub./promo. for Cinema Shares International Television. Ltd., 1976–79; pres., Arcady Communications, 1980–present.

FRIEDMAN, DAVID F.: Executive. b. Birmingham, Ala., Dec. 24, 1923. e. Cornell Univ. With U.S. Army Signal Corps, 1944–46. With Paramount Pictures as booker office manager 1946–50; circus press agent, 1950–51; Para. publ. agent, 1952–55; partner, Modern Film Distributors, 1956–60; partner, Sonney Amusement, 1960–64. Formed Entertainment Ventures, Inc. in 1965, of which he is pres. Produced a total of 58 features between 1958 and 1984.

FRIEDMAN, JOSEPH: Executive. b. New York, N.Y. e. City Coll. of N.Y., 1940–42, N.Y. Univ., 1946–47. U.S. Navy 3 yrs. Asst. to nat'l. dir. field exploitation, Warner Bros. Pictures, 1946–58; nat'l. exploitation mgr., Paramount Pictures, 1958–60; exec. asst. to dir. of adv., publicity & exploitation, Para., 1961; dir. adv. & pub., Paramount 1964; a v.p., Para., 1966; v.p. in charge of Marketing, 1968; v.p., adv., and p.r., Avco Embassy Pictures, 1969; v.p., p.r. American Film theatre, 1973; v.p., adv. and p.r., ITC, motion picture div., 1976, pres., Joseph Friedman Marketing and Advertising, Inc., 1977. Exec. dir. New Jersey M.P. & T.V. Commission, 1978; v.p. worldwide adv./pub./promo., Edie & Ely Landau, Inc., 1980; exec. dir., New Jersey Motion Picture & Television Commission, 1981.

FRIEDMAN, MARTIN: Executive. b. New York City, Oct. 9. Warner 1928 sls. and contract dept.; booking sales, Cleveland 1939–42; U.S. Marine Corps, production unit; 1945 joined A.W. Schwalberg at Artists Producers, when company was dissolved in 1946 then joined Liberty Films as ass't. to E.K. (Ted) O'Shea. Liberty was taken over by Paramount Pictures; remained with Paramount in their sales division until 1957 at which time joined American Broadcasting-Paramount Theatres as their producers representative. Production was stopped, then Friedman assigned to the theatre division in 1960; v.p., gen. mgr., ABC Theas. of Penn. Inc., ABC Theas. of N.Y., Inc., New England Theas., Inc.; pres., Countrywide Theaters, 1970. In 1973 formed own corp., Martin Films, Inc., of which is pres. Co. buys and distributes indep. product.

FRIEDMAN, ROBERT L.: Executive. b. Bronx, N.Y., March 1, 1930. e. DeWitt Clinton High School. Started as radio announcer and disc jockey with Armed Forces Radio Service in Europe and U.S. v.p., marketing, United Artists Corp.; now pres. domestic distribution, Columbia Pictures. 1984, named pres., AMC Int'l., new subsidiary of AMC Entertainment.

MEMBER: M.P. Associated Foundation, Phila., pres. 2 yrs.; Variety Club (on board) M.P. Pioneers; (on board) area chm. and N.Y. participation in Will Rogers Hospital Foundation, American Film Institute, Academy of M.P. Arts & Sciences.

FRIEDMAN, SEYMOUR MARK: Director. b. Detroit, Mich., Aug. 17, 1917; e. Magdalene Coll., Cambridge, B.S. 1936; St. Mary's Hospital Medical School, London. Entered m.p. ind. as asst. film ed. 1937; 2nd asst. dir. 1938; 1st asst. dir. 1939, on budget pictures; entered U.S. Army 1942; returned to ind. 1946; dir. Columbia Pictures 1947. Member: Screen Directors Guild; Vice president & executive production for Columbia Pictures Television, division of Columbia Pictures Industries, since 1955.
PICTURES INCLUDE: To the Ends of the Earth, Rusty's Birthday, Prison Warden, Her First Romance, Rookie Fireman, Son of Dr. Jekyll, Loan Shark, Flame of Calcutta, I'll Get You, Saint's Girl Friday, Hyber Patrol, African Manhunt, Secret of Treasure Mountain.

FRIEDMAN, STEPHEN: Writer-Producer. e. Univ. of Penn., Harvard Law School. Worked as lawyer for Columbia Pictures and Ashley-Famous Agency. Formed and heads Kings Road Productions.
PICTURES INCLUDE: The Last Picture Show (prod.), Lovin' Molly (prod.-s.p.), Slap Shot (prod.), Bloodbrothers (prod.) Fast break (prod.), Hero at Large (prod.), Little Darlings (prod.), All of Me (prod.), Creator (prod.), Enemy Mine (prod.).

FRIEND, PHILIP: Actor. b. Horsham, Sussex, England, Feb. 20, 1915; e. Bradfield Coll.; m. Eileen Erskine, prof.
THEATRE: With musical comedy tour 1935; at Drury Lane Theatre 1936; Broadway debut in "French Without Tears" 1937; plays include: Pink Strings and Sealing Wax, First Gentlemen, Hide Out, 1969; Dictator's Slippers, The Ladder, 1970. Blindsight, Forgotten Factor, 1970.
Brit. m.p. debut in "Midas Touch" 1939; on Brit. radio; served in Brit. Army 3 yrs. World War II; made training m.p. for Brit. govt.
PICTURES INCLUDE: My Own True Love, In Which We Serve, Next of Kin, Great Day, Enchantment, Sword in the Desert, Buccaneer's Girl, The Highwayman, Thunder on the Hill, Desperate Moment, Background (Edge of Divorce), The Diamond, The Betrayal, Son of Robin Hood, Web of Suspicion, The Solitary Child, Stranglehold, The Fur Collar, Manutara.
TV: Rendezvous, Invisible Man series, The Third Man Series, Z Cars, Freewheelers, Short Story, Dial M for Murder, Moody & Peg, Suez.

FRIES, CHARLES W.: Executive. b. Cincinnati, Ohio. Ohio State U., B.S.; exec.-prod., Ziv Television; v.p., prod., Screen Gems; v.p., prod., Columbia Pictures; exec. v.p., prod. and exec. prod., Metromedia Prod. Corp., 1970–74; pres., exec. prod., Alpine Prods. and Charles Fries Prods. 1974–83; chm. & pres., Fries Entertainment, 1984. Nat'l. treas., TV Academy; pres., Alliance TV Film Producers; exec. comm., MPPA. Chm., Caucus of Producers, Writers and Directors, board of governors and exec. comm. of Academy of TV Arts and Sciences.

FRISCH, LARRY: Producer, Director, Writer. b. Indianapolis, Ind., Dec. 27, 1929; e. Univ. of So. California, 1947–49, Columbia Univ., 1951–54. Prof. child actor, Radio 1944–47; writer/dir. with Caravel Films, NYC, 1950; Assist. dir., Exodus, El Cid (Spain); Pro., Dir.; Writer, Tel Aviv Taxi, 1956 (Israel), Pillar of Fire 1962 (Israel), Casablan, 1963 (Greece).
TV: Dir., Story of a Teenage Drug Addict, Power of Pot Roast, Beyond Three Doors, Destination Vietnam, Bus to Sinai (NBC-TV), Biafra Eye-Witness (UPI-TV); Metromedia TV News, overseas correspondent 1969–71; prod., Miracle of Survival (TV special), An American Family In China, 1971.

FROBE, GERT: Actor. b. Zwickau, Germany, 1912. Began acting career in 1935 in German films and theatrical productions. In post-war period there became street comedian; later worked in more than 70 German and French films, usually as villain.
PICTURES: Those Magnificent Men in Their Flying Machines, Is Paris Burning?, The Three Penny Opera, He Who Must Die, Those Daring Young Men in Their Jaunty Jalopies, Chitty Chitty Bang-Bang, Goldfinger, Bloodline.

FRONTIERE, DOMINIC: Executive. b. New Haven, Conn., June 17, 1931. e. Yale School of Music. Studied composing, arranging and conducting; concert accordionist, World's Champion Accordionist, 1943; An Hour with Dominic Frontiere, WNHC-TV, New Haven, 3 years, 1947; exec. vice-pres., musical dir., Daystar Prods. Composer or arranger over 75 films.
PICTURES INCLUDE: Giant, Gentlemen Prefer Blondes, Let's Make Love, High Noon, Meet Me in Las Vegas, 10,000 Bedrooms, Hit the Deck; composer-conductor; Marriage-Go-Round, The Right Approach, One Foot in Hell, Hero's Island, Popi, Barquero, Chisum, A For Alpha, The Aviator.
TV: Composer-conductor: The New Breed, Stoney Burke, Bankamericard commercials (Venice Film Festival Award Best Use of Original Classical Music for filmed TV commercials), Outerlimits, Branded, Iron Horse, Rat Patrol, Flying Nun, The Invaders, Name of the Game, That Girl, Twelve O'Clock High, Zig Zag, The Young Rebel, The Immortal, Jean C. Killy, Fugitive, The Love War.

FRUCHTMAN, MILTON A.: Producer, director. b. New York, N.Y. e. Columbia U.
TV: High Adventure Series, CBS, Every Man's Dream, ABC, Verdict for Tomorrow, NBC Spectaculars, Assignment Southeast Asia, It Happened in Naples; Son of Sulan, worked for Columbia and independent producers in various production capacities, set up first worldwide TV network, Eichmann Trial, Capital Cities Broadcasting, The Makebelievers, Odyssey Prods.; received Peabody Emmy, and Gabriel awards.

FRYE, WILLIAM: Producer. Was agency exec. before beginning prod. career as associate prod. of Four Star Playhouse in assoc. with late Dick Powell, David Niven and Charles Boyer. Later joined Revue Prods., which became Universal TV; he produced General Electric Theatre and other series. Has produced many Movie of the Week entries for ABC-TV.
PICTURES INCLUDE: The Trouble with Angels, Where Angels Go, Trouble Follows, Airport 1975, Airport 1977, Raise the Titanic.

FUCHS, LEO L.: Indep. prod. b. Vienna, June 14, 1929; moved to U.S., 1939; ed. Vienna and New York; U.S. Army cameraman 1951–53; int'l. mag. photographer until entered motion pictures as producer with Universal in Hollywood in 1961.
PICTURES INCLUDE: Gambit, A Fine Pair; Jo (French version of The Gazebo).

FUCHS, MICHAEL: Executive. b. March 9, 1946, New York City. e. Union Coll., NYU. Show business lawyer before joining Home Box Office. HBO Entertainment Group pres. and HBO Licensing exec. v.p. of programming. 1984, HBO pres. & chief exec. off. Now chm.

FUEST, ROBERT: Director. Early career as painter, graphic designer. Ent. TV industry as designer with ABC-TV, 1958. 1962: directing doc., commercials. 1966: Wrote and dir. Just Like A Woman, 1967–68; dir. 7 episodes of The Avengers, 1969: wrote and directed 6 episodes of The Optimists.
PICTURES: And Soon the Darkness, Wuthering Heights, Doctor Phibes, Doctor Phibes Rides Again (also .p.); The Final Programme (also s.p., design), The Devil's Rain, The Geller Effect (s.p. only), The New Avengers, The Gold Bug, Revenge of the Stepford Wives, The Big Stuffed Dog, Mystery on Fire Island, Aphrodite, Worlds Beyond, Cat's Eyes.

FULLER, JACK DUBOSE: Exhib. b. Columbia, S.C. March 7, 1921. U. of So. Carolina, B. S. Palmetto Theatre Co. 1936–42; U.S. Navy, 1942–45; theatre mgr. Wilby-Kincey Service Corp., 1945–47; booker, 1947–51; partner Irvin-Fuller Theatres, operate 24 theatres No. & So. Carolina, since 1951; Pres., Theatre Owners of N.C. and S.C. 1957; dir. NATO since 1956.

FULLER, SAMUEL: Director, writer, producer. Copy boy, N.Y. Journal; reporter, rewrite man, N.Y. Graphic, N.Y Journal, San Diego Sun; journeyman reported many papers. Author of novel The Dark Page; many orig. s.p.; in U.S. Army, 16th Inf. 1st U.S. Inf. Div. 1942–45; s.p., dir., I Shot Jesse James, Baron of Arizona; prod., dir., also screen play author of The Steel Helmet; dir., Fixed Bayonets; s.p., dir., prod., Park Row; s.p., dir., Pickup On South Street; s.p., dir., Hell and High Water, House of Bamboo; prod. dir., s.p. Run of the Arrow, China Gate, Forty Guns, Verboten, The Crimson Kimono, Underworld U.S.A., Merril's Marauders, (collab. s.p., dir.), s.p., dir., prod. Shock Corridor, s.p. prod., dir., The Naked Kiss; s.p. dir., Dead Pigeon on Beethoven Street; s.p. dir., The Big Red One; co-s.p., dir., White Dog, Thieves After Dark.
AUTHOR: Novel, Crown of India. Novel; 144 Piccadilly Street; Dead Pigeon on Beethoven Street; The Rifle; The Big Red One, The Dark Page, La Grande Melee (Battle Royal), Pecos Bill and the Soho Kid.

FUNT, ALLEN: Producer—Performer. b. New York City, Sept. 16, 1914. Best known as producer and creator of Candid Camera series which originated on radio in 1947 as Candid Microphone which inspired theatrical film shorts. TV version began in 1948 as Candid Mike, changed in 1949 to Candid Camera which played off and on until 1960 when became regular series on CBS, lasting until 1967. Revived briefly in early '70s in new format; then syndicated as The New Candid Camera. Funt produced and starred in film, What Do You Say to a Naked Lady?

FURBER, PERCIVAL E.: b. Paris, France, May 16, 1906; e. Hotchkiss School, Princeton '27; chm. emeritus div., Trans-Lux Corp.; dir., Tampax, Inc., Fedders Corp. & Fedders Fin. Corp.

FURIE, SIDNEY J.: Director, writer, producer. b. Toronto,

Canada, 1933. Ent. TV and films 1954. Canadian features include: Dangerous Age, A Cool Sound from Hell. Also dir. many Hudson Bay TV series. To England 1960. Films since include Dr. Blood's Coffin, During One Night, Brewster's Millions, The Young Ones, The Boys. 1961 appt. exec. dir. Galaworldfilm Productions, Ltd.

PICTURES INCLUDE: The Leather Boys, Wonderful Life, The Incress File, The Appaloosa, The Naked Runner, The Lawyer, Little Fauss and Big Halsy, Lady Sings the Blues, Hit!, Sheila Levine, Gable and Lombard, The Boys in Company C, The Entity, Purple Hearts, Iron Eagle.

FURNESS, BETTY: Actress—TV Correspondent. b. New York City, Jan. 3, 1916. Stage and screen actress in the '40s; TV commercial spokeswoman in '50s' leading consumer advocate in '70s. Host on both local TV and radio shows in New York (At Your Beck and Call, Ask Betty Furness, etc.). Named President Johnson's asst. for consumer affairs in 1967. 1970, head of New York state's consumer protection board. Joined WNBC-TV in 1970 as consumer reporter and occasional contributor to network news specials and Today Shows.

FURSE, RUSSELL L.: Executive. b. Humansville, Mo., Jan. 27, 1908. e. Colorado Teachers College, Greely, Colo. Film. dir., prod. Warner Bros., Hal Roach: Prod. vice pres. Televisions Programs, Inc. Executive prod., ABC Television, Hollywood, Gen. mgr. network prog. dept., CBS Television: dir; prog. oper.; KEY T Santa Barbara. Gen. mgr. CHEK TV Victoria, B.C. Santa Barbara; exec. v.p. Santa Maria Telecasting Corp. Co-founder Academy of Televisions Arts & Sciences. Chmn. of board, Communications Foundation, pres. Tri-County Public Service Corporation, pres. KBBY-KBBQ Radio Oxnard, member Affiliated Producers Work Shop, Board of Directors Affiliates University of California Santa Barbara, Founder, Riviera Park Research & Communications Center; pres. & chief exec. off., California Video Communications.

G

GABOR, ZSA ZSA: Actress. r.n. Sari Gabor; b. Hungary, Feb. 6, 1919. e. Budapest, Lausanne, Switzerland; Stage debut in Europe.

PICTURES INCLUDE: Lovely to Look At, We're Not Married, The Story of Three Loves, Lili, Moulin Rouge, Three Ring Circus, Death of a Scoundrel, Girl in the Kremlin, For The First Time, Boys' Night Out, Picture Mommy Dead, Jack of Diamonds.

GAFFNEY, ROBERT: Prod.-dir. b. New York, Oct. 8, 1931. e. Iona College, 1949–51. Staff, Louis de Rochemont mer; prod., Rooftops of New York, in assoc. with Robert Associates, prod. staff, Cinerama Holiday, Man on a String; camera technical consultant, Cinemiracle prod., Windjam-McCarty, 1960; prod. industrial films, Seneca Prods., Prod., Light Fantastic; prod., Troublemaker; assoc. prod., Harvey Middleman Fireman; dir., Frankenstein Meets the Space Monster.

GALANTE, M. CHRISTINA: Executive. b. Tucson, AZ, Aug. 30, 1942. e. U. of Arizona, New School for Social Research (NYC). Started career as child model in 1948. Entered film career as stunt double in 1955 working in dozens of major films made in Arizona, 1962–66, feature vocalist with big bands for USO tours and major night clubs. 1967–70, spokeswoman and actress in TV commercials and feature films. 1970–74, television commercials producer. 1974–77, film coordinator for mayor's office, City of New York, coordinating and supervising all m.p. and television filming in City. 1977 named special consultant to California Motion Picture Council. 1980, named to Council by Governor Edmund G. Brown and elected it's Chairman. 1980, named to Los Angeles Film Commission by Mayor Tom Bradley, currently on executive board. 1981–82, special consultant for m.p. & TV development for City of Los angeles. Currently creative services director, Rogers and Cowan (public relations).

GALE, BOB: Writer-Producer. b. St. Louis, 1952. e. USC School of Cinema. Joined with friend Robert Zemeckis to write screenplays, starting with episode for TV series, McCloud. Also co-wrote s.p. for The Nightstalker series. Turned to feature films, co-writing with Zemeckis script for I Wanna Hold Your Hand, on which Gale also acted as associate producer.

PICTURES: 1941 (s.p.); Back to the Future (co. prod., s.p.).

GALE, GEORGE: Executive, e. Sorbonne U., Paris, France. Feature editor, Budapest Ed., U.S. Army Pictorial Service, Astoria, N.Y., 1944–45; feature and TV editor 1945–65, including MGM, Hal Roach, Disney Studios Assoc. prod. and prod. exec. with Ivan Tors, 1965–70; 1971–76, American National Enterprises, Inc., vice-president in charge of production. Producer and director. Supervised the production of approximately 30 features for television syndication. Producer-director of: UFO: Fact or Fiction, Animals Are the Craziest People, Mysteries From Beyond Earth (theatrical feature). Formed George Gale Productions, Inc. in 1976. Wrote story and produced feature, Escape from Angola, in South Africa; prod. for American National Ent., Mysteries from Beyond; The Force on Thunder Mountain, Mysteries of the Mind, Anne of the Seven Seas, Lure of the Blue Planet, Quest of Courage. Produced for own co.: Neptune's Squad (TV pilot). 1982: prod. exec., American Diary. 1983: Bimini Code (TV feature).

GALLOP, RICHARD C.: Executive. e. Harvard Law School. Now pres. & chief operating officer, Columbia Pictures Industries (appt. 1983); also chm. of m.p. div., Columbia Pictures. Previously exec. v.p-finance, law and admin. of Columbia (since 1982); also served as gen. counsel, 1981–83. Joined Columbia as sr. v.p. & gen. counsel, 1981. Began career in 1963 as associate of law firm, Milbank Tweed Hadley & McCloy, New York; named partner, 1970. 1979, partner of Washington D.C. law firm, Caplin & Drysdale, specializing in corporate and financial matters. In that capacity served as outside corporate legal counsel to Columbia two yrs. Member: finance committee, Williams College; board of trustees, Marymount College.

GANIS, SIDNEY M.: Publicist. b. New York, Jan. 8, 1940. e. Brooklyn College. Staff writer, newspaper and wire service contact, 20th Century-Fox 1961–62; radio, TV contact and special projects, Columbia Pictures 1963–64. Joined Seven Arts Prod. 1965 as publicity mgr.; 1967, appt. prod. publicity mgr. Warner-7 Arts, Ass't prod., There Was a Crooked Man, 1969. Studio Publicity dir., Cinema Center Films, 1970. Director of Ad-Pub for "Mame", Warner Bros., 1973; Director of Advertising, Warner Bros., 1974; named WB v.p., worldwide adv. & pub., 1977; 1979, snr. v.p., Lucasfilm, Ltd. 1982: Emmy winner, exec. prod., best documentary, The Making of 'Radiers of the Lost Ark'. 1986, joined Paramount Pictures as pres., world-wide mktg.

GARBO, GRETA: Actress. r.n. Greta Gustafson. b. Stockholm, Sept. 18, 1906; e. Stockholm. Stage career as a dancer in Sweden. Hollywood screen career started 1926 with Torrent. Voted one of the Ten best Money-Making Stars in Motion Picture Herald-Fame Poll 1932. Spec. Academy Award, 1954.

PICTURES INCLUDE: Temptress, Flesh and the Devil, Love, Divine Woman, Mysterious Lady, Single Standard, Wild Orchids, Woman of Affairs, Kiss, Anna Christie, Susan Lennox, Her Fall and Rise, Romance, Mata Hari, Grand Hotel, Queen Christina, Anna Karenina, Camille, Conquest, Ninotchka, Two-Faced Woman.

GARDENIA, VINCENT: Actor. b. Naples, Italy, Jan. 7, 1923. f. was actor and singer who brought Vincent to U.S. at age 2, formed theatrical co. in which Vincent took part. Vincent served in U.S. Army, World War II, and after landed first English-speaking role in summer stock prod. of Burlesque. Made off-Bdwy. debut in The Man with the Golden Arm; first Bdwy. role in The Visit (1958) with the Lunts.

PICTURES INCLUDE: Cop Haters, Cold Turkey, Little Murders, Hickey and Boggs, Bang the Drum Slowly, Luciano, The Manchu Eagle, Death Wish, The Front Page, Heaven Can Wait, Firepower, Home Movies, The Last Flight of Noah's Ark, Movers and Shakers.

TV: All in the Family.

STAGE: Machinal, Passing Through from Exotic Places, The Prisoner of Second Avenue.

GARDNER, ARTHUR: Producer, b. Marinette, Wis., Entered m.p.ind. as actor, in orig. cast All Quiet on the Western Front, Juvenile leads in: Waterfront, Heart of the North, Warner Bros., Assassin of Youth, Ind., Religious Racketeer, Ind. Into production asst. dir. King Bros. 1941, then asst. prod. U.S. Air Force 1st Motion Picture Unit, 1943–45.

PICTURES INCLUDE: (Asst. dir.) Paper Bullets, I Killed That Man, Rubber Racketeers, Klondike Fury, I Escaped From the Gestapo, Suspense; (Asst. prod.) Gangster, Dude Goes West, Badmen of Tombstone, Gun Crazy, Mutiny, Southside 1–1000; Formed Levy-Gardner-Laven Prods. with Jules Levy, Arnold Laven, 1951. Prod.: Without Warning, Vice Squad, Down Three Dark Streets, Return of Dracula, The Flame Barrier, The Vampire, The Monster That Challenged the World, Geronimo, The Glory Guys, Clambake, Scalphunters, Sam Whiskey, Underground, McKenzie Break, The Honkers, Hunting Party, Kansas City Bomber, White Lightning, McQ, Brannigan, Gator, Safari 3000.

TELEVISION: Rifleman, Robert Taylor's Detectives, Law of The Plainsman, The Big Valley.

MEMBER: Producers Guild of America, Directors Guild of America, Screen Actors Guild, Actors Equity.

GARDNER, AVA: Actress. b. Smithfield, N.C., Dec. 24, 1922. e. Atlantic Christian Coll.

PICTURES INCLUDE: We Were Dancing, Joe Smith,

American, Lost Angel, Three Men in White, Maisie Goes to Reno, Whistle Stop, The Killers, The Hucksters, Singapore, One Touch of Venus, The Bribe, Great Sinner, East Side, West Side, Show Boat, Pandora and the Flying Dutchman, Lone Star, Snows of Kilimanjaro, Ride Vaquero, Mogambo, Knights of the Round Table, Barefoot Contessa, Bhowani Junction, Little Hut, The Naked Maja, On The Beach, The Fair Bride, 55 Days at Peking, Night of the Iguana, The Bible, Mayerling, Life and Times of Judge Roy Bean, The Devil's Widow, Earthquake, The Bluebird, Permission to Kill, The Cassandra Crossing, The Sentinel, City on Fire, Priest of Love.
TELEVISION: Harem, The Long Hot Summer, etc.

GARFIELD, WARREN: Writer, publicist, b. Nov. 18, 1936. e. UCLA, Loyola Of Los Angeles School of Law. Story analyst, assistant to dir., Hecht-Hill-Lancaster, 1948–58; casting dir. Assist., assist. film editor, Columbia Pictures, films, featurettes, trailers, TV spots, Paramount Pictures, 1966–68; creative film services, Walt Disney Productions, 1968–present. Member: Academy of Motion Picture, Arts & Sciences.
CREDITS: A Stranger in Town (wrote s.p.), Cat Ballou, Wild and Wonderful, Flight From Ashiya, Taras Bulba (as assist. to Harold Hecht); The High Chaparral (wrote, TV).

GARFINKLE, LOUIS: Writer-Director-Producer. b. Seattle, Wash., February 11, 1928. e. U. of Calif., U. of Washington, U. of So. Calif. Writer KOMO, Seattle, 1945; Executive Research, Inc., 1948; Writer, educ. doc. screenplays, Emerson Films, EBF. 1948–50; s.p. You Can Beat the A-Bomb (RKO), 1950; Writer-dir. training films, info. films, Signal Photo, 1950–53; Copy, Weinberg Adv., 1953; Head of Doc. Reserch in TV, U. of Calif., Berkeley, 1954–55; staff, Sheilah Graham Show, 1955; story and s.p. The Young Guns (AA), formed Maxim Prod. Inc. with Albert Band, 1956; story, s.p. and co-producer I Bury the Living (UA), 1957 (Killer on the Wall); s.p. and co-producer Face of Fire (AA), 1958; Writer, 712 teleplays for Day in Court, Morning Court, Accused for Selmur—ABC-TV, 1959–66; Co-writer-creator Direct Line pilot, Selmur, 1960; Story and t.p. June Allyson Show, Threat of Evil, 1960; s.p. in collab. The Hellbenders (Embassy) 1967; story and t.p. Death Valley Days, Crullers At Sundown, 1967; story, Death Valley Days, Captain Dick Mine, 1967; s.p. in collab. A Minute to Pray A Second to Die (ABC-Cinerama) 1968; story, s.p. and co-producer The Love Doctors (Sigma III) 1969; story, s.p. and director Beautiful People, (I.P.C.) 1970; s.p. (collab.) The Models, 1971; head writer, No. 3 Peanut Place (pilot), 1972; story & s.p. (collab.) The Doberman Gang, (Dimension) 1971; story & s.p. (collab.) Little Cigars (AIP) 1973; The Deer Hunter (U-EMI) 1978, (story collab.)

GARFUNKEL, ART: Actor-Singer-Composer. b. New York City, Oct. 13, 1942. e. Columbia Univ. Began singing at age 4. Long partnership with Paul Simon began in grade school at 13 (Queens); first big success in 1965 with hit sigle, Sound of Silence. Partnership dissolved in 1970. Film debut in Catch 22 (1969).
PICTURES: Carnal Knowledge, Bad Timing/A Sensual Obsession.

GARLAND, BEVERLY: Actress. b. Santa Cruz, Calif., Oct. 17, 1930. e. Glendale College, 1945–47.
TV: starred, Decoy, Bing Crosby; Twilight Zone, Dr. Kildare, Medic, Emmy Nomination, 1954; My Three Sons; Scarecrow and Mrs. King. Movies: This Gun for Hire.
PICTURES INCLUDE: The Mad Room, Where the Red Fern Grows, Airport, 1975, Roller Boogie, It's My Turn.

GARNER, JAMES: Actor. b. Norman, Okla., April 7, 1928; e. High School there, then joined Merchant Marine, U.S. Army ser. in Korean War. Prod. Paul Gregory suggested acting career. Studied drama at N.Y. Berghof School. Toured with road companies; Warner Bros. studio contract followed with screen debut in Toward the Unknown.
PICTURES INCLUDE: Shoot-out at Medicine Bend, Darby's Rangers, Sayonara, Up Periscope, Cash McCall, The Children's Hour, The Great Escape. Thrill of It All, Move Over Darling, The Americanization of Emily, 36 Hours, The Art of Love, Mister Buddwing, Duel at Diablo, Grand Prix, Hour of the Gun, Support Your Local Sheriff, Marlowe, Support Your Local Gunfighter, Skin Game, They Only Kill Their Masters, One Little Indian, Hawaiian Cowboy, Health, The Fan, Victor/Victoria, Tank, Murphy's Romance.
TV: Cheyenne, Maverick, Rockford Files. Movies: The Glitter Dome, Heartsounds. Mini-Series: Space.

GARR, TERI: Actress. b. Hollywood. Began career as dancer, performing S.F. Ballet at 13. Later appeared with L.S. Ballet and in original road show co. of West Side Story. Did commercials; appeared in film written by a fellow acting student, Jack Nicholson, Head. Career boosted by appearance on TV as semi-regular on The Sonny and Cher Show.
PICTURES: The Conversation, Young Frankenstein, Oh, God!, Close Encounters of the Third Kind, The Black Stallion, One From the Heart, The Sting II, Tootsie, The Black Stallion Returns, Mr. Mom, Firstborn, Lies, Miracles, After Hours.
TELEVISION: Movies: Law and Order, Winter of Our Discontent, To Catch a King, Intimate Strangers.

GARRETT, BETTY: Singer, actress. b. St. Joseph, Mo., May 23, 1919. e. scholarships; Annie Wright Seminary, Tacoma, Wash., Neighborhood Playhouse, N.Y.C. Sang in night clubs, hotels, Broadway shows (1942–46); won Donaldson award for best musical comedy performance of 1946, Spoon River Anthology.
PICTURES INCLUDE: (Screen debut) The Big City, 1947, Star of Tomorrow, '49; Words and Music, Neptune's Daughter, On The Town, My Sister Eileen, Shadow on the Window.
TV: Laverne and Shirley.

GARRETT, LAWRENCE G. JR.: Executive. b. San Francisco, Nov. 5, 1942. e. Univ. of Calif.; Thunderbird Graduate Sch. 1967, joined Columbia Pictures Intl., Panama, Mexico; 1969, Paramount Pictures, mgr., Venezuela; 1973, asst. mgr., Mexico; 1973–76, Shearson Hayden Stone Institutional investment; 1977, United Artists, Argentina, Austral-Axis mgr. dir.; 1980, Avco Embassy, sls. supvr. Latin American-Far East; 1981, head intl. sls., Shapiro Entertainment; 1982, head intl. sls., Goldfarb Distributors; 1983–present, dir./intl. sls. & acquisitions, Arista Films.

GARRISON, PAUL: Writer, producer, director. Adv. photog, in N.Y., Hollywood; production of TV films since 1948; dir. first series of half hour TV pictures made, Cases of Eddie Drake; dir., writer for more than 100 TV film shows; currently in chge. of TV Workshop, Hollywood.

GARSON, GREER: Actress. b. County Down, Northern Ireland, 1908. e. London U., B.A. cum laude; Grenoble U.
THEATRE: Stage debut Birmingham (England) Rep. theat. 1932 in Street Scene; London debut 1935 in Golden Arrow; continued London stage to 1938 (Vintage Wine, Mademoiselle, Accent on Youth, Page From a Diary, Old Music, etc.).
Screen debut 1939 in Goodbye, Mr. Chips. Academy Award best performance by actress, 1942 (Mrs. Miniver, MGM). Voted one of the ten best Money-Making Stars in Motion Picture Herald-Fame Poll 1942–46 inclusive. Photoplay Mag. Gold Medal 1944–45.
PICTURES INCLUDE: Pride and Prejudice, Blossoms in the Dust, When Ladies Meet, Mrs. Miniver, Random Harvest, Mme. Curie, Mrs. Parkington, Valley of Decision, Adventure, Desire Me, Julia Misbehaves, That Forsythe Woman, The Miniver Story, The Law and the Lady, Scandal at Scourie, Julius Caesar, Her Twelve Men, Strange Lady in Town, Sunrise at Campobella, The Singing Nun, The Happiest Millionaire.

GASSMAN, VITTORIO: Actor. b. Genoa, Italy, Sept. 1, 1922; e. Academy of Dramatic Art, Rome. Stage actor, 1943; m.p. debut, 1946.
PICTURES INCLUDE: Daniele Cortis, Mysterious Rider, Bitter Rice, Lure of Sila, The Outlaws, Anna, Streets of Sorrow; to U.S., Cry of the Hunted, Sombrero, The Glass Wall, Rhapsody, Girls Marked Danger, Mambo, War and Peace, World's Most Beautiful Woman, Tempest, The Love Specialist, The Great War, Let's Talk About Women, Il Successo, The Tiger, Woman Times Seven, Ghosts—Italian Style, Scent of a Woman, Viva Italia!, A Wedding, Quintet, Immortal Bachelor, The Nude Bomb, Sharky's Machine, Tempest.

GAVIN, JOHN: Actor. b. Los Angeles, Calif., April 8, 1932. e. St. John's Military Acad., Villanova Prep at Ojai, Stanford Univ., Naval service: air intelligence officer. Married to actress Constance Towers, 1974. Four children. pres. Screen Actors Guild. Broadway Stage debut: Seesaw, 1973. Named U.S. Ambassador to Mexico, 1981.
PICTURES INCLUDE: A Time to Love and a Time to Die, Imitation of Life, Spartacus, A Breath of Scandal, Romanoff and Juliet, Tammy, Tell Me True, Back Street, Thoroughly Modern Millie, Mad Woman of Chaillot, Psycho, Midnight Lace.

GAYLARD, JAMES W., III: Exhibitor b. Knoxville, Tenn., Sept. 18, 1943. e. Henderson H.S., Troy, Ala., 1961. Troy State Univ. 1965 BS Mathematics Ent. industry, managed theatres, Troy Drive-In Theatres, Inc. 1966.

GAYLE, PETER: Producer, writer, actor. b. New York City. Attended American Academy of Dramatic Arts; New York School of Theatre Arts. Columbia Pictures Talent School.
TV: (Specials) Producer, writer, The World of Brigette Bardot, The Goldie Hawn Special, The Rolling Stones in Concert, The Janis Joplin Special, Hollywood: The Magic Kingdom, On Location With ABBA; Boy George Live from the London Paladium, John Belushi Remembered.
TV: (Series) The Young Rebels (ABC-TV), The Protectors (ABC-TV), Spindletop (Universal Studios), The Legends of Rock and Roll.
PICTURES INCLUDE: Without Each Other (winner of

Cannes Film Festival), The Gang; Never Too Young To Rock; Black Cobra; Shoot; The Boy Who Owned A Melephant (winner of the Venice Film Festival); Intercept, Scenes from a Murder.

GAYNOR, MITZI: Actress. b. Chicago, Ill. Sept. 4, 1931. e. Powers Professional H.S., Hollywood. Studied ballet since age four; was in L.A. Light Opera prod. Roberta.
OPERA: Fortune Teller, Song of Norway, Louisiana Purchase, Naughty Marietta, Great Waltz.
PICTURES INCLUDE: My Blue Heaven, Take Care of My Little Girl, Golden Girl, The I Don't Care Girl, We're Not Married, Bloodhounds of Broadway, There's No Business Like Show Business, Anything Goes, Birds and the Bees, The Joker, Les Girls, South Pacific, Surprise Package, Happy Anniversary, For Love or Money.

GAZZARA, BEN: Actor. b. N.Y.C., 1930. Won scholarship to study with Erwin Piscator; joined Actor's Studio, where students improvised a play, End As a Man, which then was performed on Broadway with him in lead. Screen debut (1957) in film version of that play retitled The Strange One.
PICTURES INCLUDE: Anatomy of a Murder, The Passionate Thief, The Young Doctors, Convicts Four, Conquered City, A Rage To Live, The Bridge at Remagen, Husbands, Capone, Killing of a Chinese Bookie, Voyage of the Damned, Bloodline, They All Laughed, Inchon.
TV: Arrest and Trial, Run for Your Life, Movies: An Early Frost, A Letter to Three Wives, etc.
STAGE: Cat on a Hot Tin Roof, A Hatful of Rain, Hughie, etc.

GEARY, ANTHONY: Actor. b. Coalville, UT, May 29, 1947. e. Univ. of Vermont. On screen in Johnny Got His Gun.
TELEVISION: Bright Promise, The Young and the Restless, Osmond Family Holiday Special, General Hospital, Intimate Agony, Sins of the Past, The Imposter, Kicks.

GEBHARDT, FRED: Prod.-writer, exhibitor. b. Vienna, Austria, Mar. 16, 1925. e. Schotten Gymnasium, Vienna. U.C.L.A., 1939. Usher Boyd Theatre, Bethlehem, Pa.; Mgr., Rivoli Thea. L.A., 1944; 18 yrs. mgr. many theatres. Fox West Coast, then Fine Arts Theatre. Writer, prod.: 12 To the Moon, The Phantom Planet; prod., Assignment Outer Space, Operation M; s.p., All But Glory, The Starmaker, Shed No Blood, Fortress in Heaven, Eternal Woman.
BOOKS: Mental Disarmament, All But Glory, Starmaker, Shed No Blood, The Last of the Templars.
Pres., Four Crown Prods., Inc.; recipient of Medal of Americanism, D.A.R., 1963; Honorary Lifetime Member, P.T.A., Young Man of The Year Award, 1956, 24 Showmanship Awards; Mem. Acad. M.P. Arts and Sciences, Ind. M.P. Prod. Assoc.

GEESON, JUDY: Actress. b. Arundel, Sussex, England, Sept. 10, 1948. e. Corona Stage School. Began professional career on British TV, 1960.
PICTURES INCLUDE: To Sir With Love, Circus of Blood, Here We Go Round the Mulberry Bush, Hammerhead, Three into Two Won't Go; Two Gentlemen Sharing, The Executioner, 10 Rillington Place, Brannigan, The Eagle Has Landed.
TV: Dance of Death, Lady Windermere's Fan, Room with a View, The Skin Game, Star Maidens, Poldark, She.
THEATRE: Othello, Titus Andronicus, Two Gentlemen of Verona, Section Nine, An Ideal Husband.

GEFFEN, DAVID: Executive. b. New York City, Feb. 21, 1943. Career began in 1964 in mail room of William Morris Agency. In 1968 left with co-worker Elliot Roberts to form Geffen-Roberts Management, clients eventually including Joni Mitchell, Crosby, Stills and Nash, Neil Young, Jackson Browne. Funded Asylum Records, later merging it with Elektra; roster including Joni Mitchell, Linda Ronstadt, Queen, Carly Simon, Bob Dylan, etc. In 1975 named vice chm. of Warner Bros. Pictures. Produced first film Personal Best (1981). Theatrical productions include Dreamgirls, Cats, Little Shop of Horrors, Master Harold...and the Boys, Good, etc.
PICTURES INCLUDE: Risky Business, Lost in America.

GELBART, LARRY: Writer. b. Chicago, Feb. 25, 1925. Began writing at 16; frist break job doing material for Danny Thomas on Fanny Brice Show. Followed by Duffy's Tavern, shaping routines for Eddie Cantor, Bob Hope, Jack Paar. Was one of Sid Caesar's stable of comedy writers on Show of Shows. Wrote A Funny Thing Happened on the Way to the Forum for Bdwy, with Bert Shevlove.
PICTURES INCLUDE: The Notorious Landlady, The Wrong Box, Oh, God!, Movie, Neighbors, Tootsie, Blame It on Rio (exec. prod., co.-s.p.).
TELEVISION: MASH (Emmy, 1974), United States, etc.

GELFAN, GREG: Executive. Was entertainment atty. with two firms before joining Paramount Pictures in 1983 as dir. of business affairs. 1985, named v.p., business affairs, for M.P. Group of Paramount.

GELLER, BRIAN L.: Executive. b. New York City, Feb. 3, 1948. e. Queens Coll. Entered industry with Columbia Pictures as sls. trainee in 1966, leaving in 1968 to go with American Intl. Pictures as asst. branch mgr. In 1969 joined Cinemation Industries as eastern div. sls. mgr.; 1978, left to become gen. sls. mr. of NMD Film Distributing Co. 1982, named dir. of dist., Mature Pictures Corp. 1983, gen. sls. mgr., Export Pix. Now with Concorde Cinema Group as east. sls. mgr.
Member: Motion Picture Bookers Club of N.Y.; Variety Tent 35.

GENDECE, BRIAN K.: Executive. b. St. Louis, Mo. e. Drury College, Springfield, Mo. 1981–85, Director of Business Affairs, Weinstein/Skyfield Productions and Skyfield Management. Currently pres., Clayton Prods.
PICTURES INCLUDE: Runaway Train, Queens.
STAGE: Lyndon.
VIDEO: Bad Habits, Shape, Up with Arnold.
MANAGEMENT: Jenny Burton (1981–85).

GENOCK, TED: Newsreel Editor. r.n. Edouard Paul Genock, b. Paris, France, Mar. 7, 1907; e. Chelsea Polytechnic London U. (BS), Columbia (MA). Initiated prod. and pictorial news, Egypt. From 1930–39 covered Ethiopia, Iraq, Iran, India, Malaya, Netherlands Indies, Australia as newsreel war correspondent. British Paramount News. Apptd. assignment editor, Paramount News (N.Y.C.), 1942. Tech. dir., Neighbor to North (1948), Cassino to Korea (1950) for Parat.; dev. 22-second high-speed processing machine for TV film recording, now inc. in Parat. theatre TV system. Ed. in chief, Telenews Prod., Inc., 1952; Television, Eastman Kodak adv. dept., 1954. Fellow: Soc. M.P. & TV Engineers. Member, Dir. American TV Commercials Festival, 1962; dir. TV adv. Eastman-Kodak; chmn. Assn. Nat'l Advertisers Television Committee, 1969; Director Media Development Film & TV, Mercer County College, N.J., 1972.

GEORGE, GEORGE LOUIS: Director. b. Moscow, Russia, July 31, 1907. e. U. Paris (law). Began as cutter, later asst. dir., French prods. To Hollywood 1935 as corresp. French pubs. Re-entered prod. 1939 as asst. dir. & prod. French version of The Four Hundred Million; in similar capacity numerous French versions of Hollywood prods. thereafter. In 1942 asst. prod. Our Russian Front. Became assoc. Natl. Film Board of Canada in prod. war information films; also dir. The Labor Front for World in Action series. In 1944 dir. University Town for Co-ord. Inter-Amer. Affairs; 1946–49 dir. 16 films for Signal Corps Photo. Center, Astoria, L.I., incl. Acad. Award winner Toward Independence. In 1949 dir. in TV, also Women of Tomorrow, WB. 1950, dir. in Israel for Palestine Films; dir., prod., TV & documentary films, 1950–55; exec. secr., Screen Directors International Guild, 1956–63; admin., SDIG Trust Fund, 1963–67; member, Natl. Bd. Directors Guild of America 1966–69; since 1966, member Eastern Directors Council, DGA; pres. Film & TV Book Club, Inc. 1967–69. Currently free-lancing.

GEORGE, GEORGE W.: Writer/Producer. b. New York, N.Y., Feb. 8, 1920. e. Williams College; U.S. Navy, 1941–44; screen writer since 1948. President, The Saga Group, Inc. N.Y.C. based, Industrial Video/film company.
PICTURES INCLUDE: Bodyguard, The Nevadan, Woman on Pier 13, Peggy Mystery Submarine, Red Mountain Experiment, Alcatraz, Fight Town, Smoke Signal, Desert Sands, Uranium Boom, Halliday Brand, Doc, The James Dean Story, The Two Little Bears.
PRODUCER STAGE: Dylan, Any Wednesday, Ben Franklin in Paris, The Great Indoors, Happily Never After, Night Watch, Via Galaetica, Bedroom Farce.
PRODUCER PICTURES: A Matter of Innocence, Twisted Nerve, Hello-Goodbye, Night Watch, Rich Kids, My Dinner with Andre.
TV: Climax, Screen Gems, Loretta Young Show, The Rifleman, Peter Gunn, The Real McCoys, Adventures in Paradise, Hong Kong, Follow The Sun.

GEORGE, LOUIS: Executive. Pres. & chief operating officer, Arista Films, Inc. b. Karavas, Kyrenia, Cyprus, June 7, 1935. e. Kyrenia Business Academy, Cyprus (honored 1951). Emigrated to U.S. in 1952. After brief stint in Foreign Exchange Dept. of City National Bank New York, served in U.S. Army, 1953–55. Entered industry in 1956 as theatre manager with Loew's Theatres in N.Y. metro area, managing Metropolitan, Triboro, New Rochelle, between 1958–66. In 1966 joined MGM as dir. of intl. theatre dept. In 1969 promoted to dir. of world-wide non-theatrical sales. From 1972 to 1974 served as regional dir. of MGM Far East operations. In 1974 left MGM to establish Arista Films, Inc., handling foreign sales of independently produced U.S. films.

GEORGE, SUSAN: Actress. b. Surrey, England, 1950. e. Corona Academy. m.p. debut Million Dollar Brain, 1965.
PICTURES: The Sorcerers, Up The Junction, The Strange Affair, The Looking Glass War, All Neat in Black Stockings, Twinky, Spring and Port Wine, Eye Witness, Die Screaming

Marianne, Fright, Straw Dogs, Sonny and I, Dr. Jekyll and Mr. Hyde, Dirty Mary Crazy Larry, Mandingo, Out of Season, A Small Town in Texas, Tiger Shark, Tomorrow Never Comes, Venom, A Texas Legend, House Where Evil Dwells, Jigsaw Man, The White Stallion.

TELEVISION: Swallows and Amazons, Adam's Apple, Weaver's Green, Compensation Alice, The Right Attitude, Dracula, Lamb to the Slaughter, Royal Jelly, Masquerade, Czechmate, Hotel, Blackie's Magic.

GERAGHTY, MAURICE: Writer, director, producer. b. Rushville, Ind., Sept. 29, 1908; e. Princeton. Western story suprv. Republic 3 yrs; prod Falcon series, China Sky, Action In Arabia at RKO; Flash Gordon (feature and serial).

PICTURES INCLUDE: Red Canyon, Dakota Lil, Calamity Jane and Sam Bass, Tomahawk, Sword of Monte Cristo, Rose of Cimarron, Mohawk, Love Me Tender (Elvis Presley), Tall In The Saddle (John Wayne), Gene Autry and Roy Rogers series, Hopalong Cassidy series, Mesquiteers series (John Wayne) Darby O'Gill And The Little People.

TV: Created Cheyenne series, Warner Bros. Director: Virginian, Bonanza, Daniel Boone, 87th Precinct, Thriller, 21 Beacon Street, Cavalcade of America, Panic, Whiplash (Australia). Writer: The Addams Family, Annie Oakley, Gene Autry series, Champion series. Director: No Warning, Flight, Jane Wyman Theater, Laramie, Lassie (Emmy and Peabody Awards).

GERALD, HELEN: Actress. b. New York City, Aug. 13. e. U. of Southern Calif. 1948. Stage: Italian Teatro D'Arte, Les Miserables, The Civil Death, Feudalism.

PICTURES INCLUDE: The Gay Cavalier, The Trap, Tarzan and the Leopard Woman, Cigarette Girl, Meet Miss Bobby Socks, G.I. War Brides, Gentleman's Agreement, A Bell For Adano, Tomorrow is Forever, Janie, Grand Prix, The Sandpiper, Make Mine Mink, Best of Everything.

TV: Robert Montgomery Presents, Frontiers of Faith, Valiant Lady, Kraft Theatre, Gangbusters, Adventures of The Falcon, Schlitz Playhouse of Stars, This Is the Answer, Man from UNCLE, Run for Your Life, Perry Mason.

GERARD, GIL: Actor. b. Little Rock, AZ, Jan. 23, 1940. On stage in I Do! I Do!.

PICTURES: Airport '77, Buck Rogers in the 25th Century.

TELEVISION: The Doctors, Killing Stone, Buck Rogers in the 25th Century. Movies: For Love or Money, Stormin' Home, International Airport.

GERARD, LILLIAN: Publicist-Writer, Publicity, Rialto Theatre, 1936; publicity-adv. Filmarte Theatre, 1938, Gerard Associates, 1938–47; V.P. and managing dir. of Paris Theatre, 1948–62; publicity-adv. dir., Rugoff Theatres, 1962. Film consultant to Times Films, Lopert Films, Landau Co., 1962–65. Exec. secy. to the National Soc. of Film Critics, 1966–68. Adjunct Professor, Film, 1968–70, Columbia Univ., School of the Arts, Special Projects Co-Ordinator, Museum of Modern Art, 1968–80. Contributor to American Film. Published by American Film Institute. Now associated with Philip Gerard in Gerard Associates.

GERARD, PHILIP R.: Executive. b. New York City, Aug. 23, 1913. e. C.C.N.Y., B.B.A. 1935; Columbia U.; Publicity dir. Mayer-Burstyn 1936–39; Gerard Associates, 1939–41; in public relations U.S. War Dept. 1942–44; with MGM 1944–48; with Universal Pictures since 1948; Eastern pub. mgr., 1950–59; Eastern ad. and pub. dir., Dec. 1959; N.Y. Production Exec., 1968–76. As of Jan. 1, 1977 formed Gerard Associates, film consultants on marketing, production and acquisitions. N.Y.C. Advisory Council of CSS/RSVP (retired seniors volunteer program); volunteer asst. to dir. of RSVP. Member: Visitor's Day Comm., New York Hospital.

GERBER, DAVID: Executive. b. Brooklyn, N.Y. e. Univ. of Pacific. m actress Laraine Stephens. Joined Batten, Barton, Durstine and Osborn ad agency in N.Y. as TV supvr. Left to become senior v.p. of TV at General Artists Corp. In Jan., 1956, named v.p. in chg. sales at 20th-Fox TV where sold and packaged over 50 prime-time series and specials. Entered indep. prod. with The Ghost and Mrs. Muir, followed by Nanny and the Professor. In 1970 was exec. prod. of The Double Deckers, children's series made in England. In 1971 was exec. prod. of Cade's County (CBS). In 1972 he joined Columbia Pictures Television as an independent producer and in 1974 was named executive vice president worldwide production for CPT. In 1976 he returned to independent production and has been the executive producer on such progrms as Police Story, Police Woman, The Lindbergh Kidnapping Case, Joe Forrester, The Quest and Gibbsville. For Police Story he received an Emmy award for best dramatic series. 1985, joined MGM/UA TV bdgst. group in chg. world-wide production.

GERBER, MICHAEL H.: Executive. b. New York City, Feb. 6, 1944. e. St. Johns Univ. (BA, '69); St. Johns Univ. School of Law (Juris Doctor, '69). Atty, for Screen Gems, 1969–71; asst. secy. & asst. to gen. counsel, Columbia Pictures Industries, 1971–74; corporate counsel and secretary, Allied Artists Pictures, 1974, v.p. Corporate affairs, Allied Artists, 1978; v.p., business affairs, Viacom Intl.

GERE, RICHARD: Actor. b. Philadelphia, 1950. e. Univ. of Massachusetts. Started acting in college; later joined Provincetown Playhouse and Seattle Repertory Theatre. Composed music for productions of these groups. Appeared on Broadway in Grease, Soon, Habeas Corpus, and Bent and in London in Taming of the Shrew with Young Vic.

PICTURES INCLUDE: Report to the Commissioner, Baby Blue Marine, Looking for Mr. Goodbar, Days of Heaven, Bloodbrothers, Yanks, American Gigolo, An Officer and a Gentleman, Breathless, Beyond the Limits, The Cotton Club, King David, Power, No Mercy.

TV: Kojak, Strike (movie).

GERETY, T. MICHAEL: Executive. b. Rockville Center, N.Y., Oct. 30, 1942. U.S., Navy, 1961–64. Started industry career in Chicago with MGM as regional adv/pub. repr.; transferred to Atlanta in same capacity, 1966 and then to Dallas, 1967–70. Joined Durwood Theatres in Dallas in 1971 as div. operations mgr. In 1972 returned to MGM as south west div. dir. adv./pub. in Dallas. Moved to MGM Studios in 1973 as asst. natl. adv. coordinator. In 1974 joined American International as dir. of cooperative adv./exploit. In 1976 named exec. dir. of adv./pub. for AIP. In 1980 joined the Milton I. Moritz Co., film marketing firm, as v.p. In 1981, named v.p., Market Relay Systems, a mktg./communications co. 1982–83, pres., The Newslink Corp. (videotext news service). Joined Hanson & Schwam p.r., 1985. Member: Academy of MP. Arts & Sciences.

GERSHENSON, JOSEPH: Musician, b. Russia, Jan. 12, 1904; e. N.Y. public sch.; Pace Inst., N.Y.; studied music priv. Conductor orch. B.F. Keith Theats. 1920–28; asst. genl. music dir. RKO Theats., 1928–33. Joined Universal Pictures 1939; exec. prod. & music dir. of shorts in 1939; exec. prod. (under name of Joseph G. Sanford) of features from 1940–49; in 1950 apptd. exec. prod.; head of music dept. Universal International. Retired 1969.

PICTURES INCLUDE: Glenn Miller Story, Magnificent Obsession, So This Is Paris, Man Without a Star, Foxfire, Benny Goodman Story, All That Heaven Allows. There's Always Tomorrow, Spoilers, Never Say Goodbye, Battle Hymn, Away All Boats, Written on the Wind, My Man Godfrey, Man of a Thousand Faces, Never Steal Anything Small, Imitation of Life, This Earth Is Mine, Pillow Talk, Operation Petticoat, Back Street, Come September, Lover Come Back, Spiral Road, Freud, Captain Newman, Father Goose, Send Me No Flowers, I'd Rather Be Rich, Warlord, Madame X, Shenandoah, Blindfold, Thoroughly Modern Millie, Sweet Charity.

GERTNER, RICHARD: Editor. b. Tampa, Florida, Nov. 1; e. Rollins College, B.A., 1949, Columbia U., M.A., 1950; editor, Hoffman Publications, 1950–52; editorial asst., Better Theatres, 1952; news editor, Motion Picture Daily, 1956; managing editor, Motion Picture Daily, 1962; managing editor, Motion Picture Herald, 1963; editor, Better Theatres, 1963; executive editor, Motion Picture Herald, 1964; editor, Motion Picture Herald, 1966; editor, Motion Picture Almanac and TV Almanac, 1970. Managing editor Motion Picture Daily, Oct. 1970; Editor, Motion Picture Daily, 1971; Editor-in-chief, Quigley Publications, Nov., 1971.

GERTZ, IRVING: Composer, musical director. b. Providence, R.I., May 19, 1915; e. Providence Coll. of Music, 1934–37. Assoc. with Providence Symph. Orch., comp. choral works for Catholic Choral Soc.; music dept., Columbia, 1939–41; U.S. Army, 1941–46; then comp. arranger, mus. dir. for many cos. incl. Columbia, U-I, NBC.

PICTURES INCLUDE: Bandits of Corsica, Gun Belt, Long Wait, The Fiercest Heart, First Travelling Saleslady, Fluffy, Nobody's Perfect, Marines, Let's Go! It Came From Outer Space, The Man From Bitter Ridge, Posse From Hell, The Creature Walks Among Us, The Incredible Shrinking Man, Hell Bent For Leather, Seven Ways From Sundown, Francis Joins the WACS, Raw Edge, East of Sumatra, A Day of Fury, To Hell and Back, Cult of the Cobra, Plunder Road, Top Gun, Tombstone Express, The Alligator People, Khyber Patrol, The Wizard of Baghdad.

Record album (Dot Records) Leaves of Grass; published works for mixed voices; Fluffy, feature, Universal. Marines, Let's Go! feature, 20th Century Fox Serenata for String Quartet, Divertimento for String Orchestra, Tableau for Orchestra.

TV: Orig. theme & scores for TV: America, The Golden Voyage, Across the Seven Seas, The Legend of Jesse James, Daniel Boone, Voyage to the Bottom of the Sea, Peyton Place, Land of the Giants, Lancer, Medical Center, Boutade for Wood-Wind Quartet, Salute to All Nations, A Village Fair.

GETTY, J. RONALD: Producer. b. -Berlin, Germany, Dec. 19, 1929. e. Zurich U., Heidelberg U., U. of Southern California. Prior to entering m.p. industry was oil executive, Tidewater Oil Co., mgn. dir. Veedol GmbH, 1955; Getty Oil, Hamburg,

1954–61; pres. & chm. of bd., Veedol Petroleum Int'l, Switzerland, 1961–69; dir., Huiles Veedol France, 1961–69. President & Chm. of bd., Getty Picture Corp.; pres. & chm., Getty Labs, Inc.; dir., Home Theatre Network.
PICTURES: Flare Up, Zeppelin, Shelia.

GIANNINI, GIANCARLO: Actor. b. Spezia, Italy, Aug. 1, 1942. Acquired degree in electronics but immediately after school enrolled at Academy for Drama in Rome. Cast by Franco Zeffirelli as Romeo at age of 20. Subsequently appeared in a play also directed by Zeffirelli, Two Plus Two No Longer Make Four, written by Lina Wertmuller.
PICTURES INCLUDE: Love and Anarchy, The Seduction of Mimi, Swept Away by an Unusual Destiny in the Blue Sea of August, Seven Beauties . . . That's What They Call Him, How Funny Can Sex Be?, A Night Full of Rain, The Innocent, Immortal Bachelor, American Dreamer, Fever Pitch, Saving Grace.
TELEVISION: Sins.

GIBSON, HENRY: Actor. b. Germantown, PA, Sept. 21, 1935. e. Catholic Univ. Amer. Appeared as child actor with stock companies, 1943–57; Bdwy. debut in My Mother, My Father and Me, 1962. Many appearances on stage since and in films and TV.
PICTURES: The Long Goodbye, Charlotte's Web, Nashville, The Last Remake of Beau Geste.
TELEVISION: Laugh-In co-star.

GIBSON, MEL: Actor. b. New York City, 1956. Emigrated in 1968 to Australia with family. Attended Natl. Institute of Dramatic Art in Sydney; in 2nd yr. was cast in his first film, Summer City. Graduated from NIDA, 1977. Joined South Australian Theatre Co. In 1978, appearing in Oedipus, Henry IV, Cedoona, etc. Also on TV in The Sullivans and The Oracle series.
PICTURES: Summer City, Mad Max, Tim, Attack Force Z, Gallipoli, The Road Warrior (Mad Max II), The Year of Living Dangerously, The Bounty, The River, Mrs. Soffel, Mad Max Beyond Thunderdome.

GIELGUD, SIR JOHN: Actor. b. London, England, Apr. 14, 1904; e. Westminster Sch., Lady Benson's Sch. (dram.), London; Royal Acad. Dram. Art. Knighted, 1953.
THEATRE: Began stage career in Shakespearean roles; on London stage also in the Constant Nymph, The Good Companions, Dear Octopus, The Importance of Being Earnest, Dear Brutus, etc., various Shakespearean seasons, London & N.Y.
PICTURES INCLUDE: On screen 1932 in Brit. prod. Insult; later (Brit.) films The Good Companions, Secret Agent (Warner-Brit.); The Prime Minister, Other films: Julius Caesar, Richard III. Around the World in 80 Days, Barretts of Wimpole Street, Becket. The Loved One, Chimes At Night, St. Joan, Sebastian, The Assignment, Charge of the Light Brigade, The Shoes of the Fisherman, Oh, What a Lovely War, Eagle in a Cage, Lost Horizon, 11 Harrowhouse, Gold, Murder on the Orient Express, Providence, Portrait of the Artists as a Young Man, Joseph Andrews, Murder by Decree, The Human Factor, The Elephant Man, The Formula, Sphinx, Lion of the Desert, Arthur, Chariots of Fire, Priest of Love, Gandhi, The Wicked Lady, Seandalous, Wagner.
TV: A Day by the Sea, The Browning Version (U.S.A.), The Rehearsal, Great Acting, Ages of Man, Mayfly and the Frog, Cherry Orchard, Ivanov, From Chekhov With Love, St. Joan, Good King Charles' Golden Days, Conversation at Night, Hassan, Deliver Us From Evil, Heartbreak House, Brideshead Revisited.

GIL, DAVID: Producer. b. Tel Aviv, Israel, Jan. 24, 1930; e. U. of Jerusalem; m. Joan Andre. After commission in Israeli Army worked for Israeli Embassy, Paris, 1950–52; Israeli Film ind., 1953–55; prod. educational films, 1955–61; headed Gilart Productions, 1962–68; foreign sales dir., Commonwealth United, 1968; prod. Guess What We Learned in School Today, Joe, A Journey Through Rosebud, A Change in the Wind.

GILBERT, ARTHUR N.: Producer. b. Oct. 17, 1920, Detroit; Lt., U.S.M.C., 1941–45; ed. Univ. of Chicago, 1946; Special Agent, FBI, 1946–53; world sales dir., Gen. Motors, Cadillac Div., 1953–59; investments in mot. pictures and hotel chains, 1959–64; exec. prod., Mondo Hollywood, 1965; exec. prod. Jeannie-Wife Child, 1966; assoc. prod., The Golden Breed, 1967; commissioned rank of Colonel U.S.M.C., 1968.
PICTURES INCLUDE: The Glory Stompers, Fire Grass, Cycle Savages, Bigfoot, Incredible Transplant.

GILBERT, BRUCE: Producer. e. University of Calif. Pursued film interests at Berkeley's Pacific Film Archive; in summer involved in production in film dept. of San Francisco State Univ. Founded progressive pre-school in Bay Area. Became story editor in feature film division of Cine-Artists; involved in several projects, including Aloha, Bobby and Rose. Partnered with Jane Fonda and IPC Films, Inc.
PICTURES: Coming Home (assoc. prod.); The China Syndrome (exec. prod.); Nine to Five (prod.); On Golden Pond (prod.); Rollover (prod.).

GILBERT, LEWIS: Producer, writer, director, actor. b. London, England, Mar. 6, 1920. In RAF, World War II. Screen debut, 1932; asst. dir. (1930–39) with London Films, Assoc. British, Mayflower, RKO-Radio; from 1939–44 attached U.S. Air Corps Film Unit (asst. dir., "Target for Today"). In 1944 joined G.B.I. as writer and dir. In 1948, Gainsborough Pictures as writer, dir., 1949; Argyle Prod. 1950; under contract Nettlefold Films, Ltd. as dir.
PICTURES INCLUDE: Under One Roof, I Want to Get Married, Haunting Melody, Once a Sinner, Scarlet Thread, There Is Another Sun, Time Gentlemen Please, Emergency Call, Cosh Boy, Johnny on the Run, Albert R.N., The Good Die Young, The Sea Shall Not Have Them, Reach for the Sky, Cast a Dark Shadow, The Admirable Crichton, Carve Her Name with Pride, A Cry from the Street, Ferry to Hong Kong, Sink the Bismarck, Light Up the Sky, The Greengage Summer, H.M.S. Defiant, The Patriots, Spare the Rod, Alfie, The Seventh Dawn, You Only Live Twice, The Adventurers, Friends, Paul & Michelle, Operation Daybreak, Seven Nights in Japan, The Spy Who Loved Me. 1978–79: Dir. Moonraker, Educating Rita, Not Quite Paradise.

GILBERT, MELISSA: Actress. b. Los Angeles, May 8, 1964. Made debut at age of 3 in TV commercial. Comes from show business family: father, late comedian Paul Gilbert; mother, former dancer-actress Barbara Crane.
TELEVISION: Gunsmoke, Emergency, Tenafly, The Hanna-Barbara Happy Hour, Christmas Miracle in Caufield U.S.A., Love Boat, Little House on the Prairie (regular). Movies: Choices of the Heart, Choices.
PICTURE: Sylvester (debut).

GILER, DAVID: Producer-Writer-Director. b. New York City. Son of Bernie Giler, screen and TV writer. Began writing in teens; first work an episode for ABC series, The Gallant Men. Feature film career began as writer on Myra Breckenridge (1970).
PICTURES: Writer: The Parallax View, Fun with Dick and Jane, The Blackbird (also dir.), Southern Comfort (also prod.), Alien (prod. only), Rustlers' Rhapsody (prod. only), etc.
TELEVISION: Writer: The Kraft Theatre, Burke's Law, The Man from UNCLE, The Girl from UNCLE, etc.

GILFORD, JACK: Actor. b. New York City, 1907. Made first stage appearances in amateur night performances as stand-up comic. Wrote own material, specializing in imitations. First theatrical role in 1952 in The World of Sholem Aleichem, which he repeated in TV special based on play.
PICTURES INCLUDE: They Might Be Giants, Catch-22, Save the Tiger, Harry and Walter Go to New York, Wholly Moses, Cocoon.
STAGE: The Diary of Anne Frank, Romanoff and Juliet, Once Upon a Mattress, Cabaret, No, No, Nanette.

GILLASPY, RICHARD M.: Producer, director. b. St. Louis, Mo., Dec. 10, 1927; joined NBC in New York as exec. trainee, 1947; headed Marine Corps Radio, 1952–54; rejoined NBC-TV as stage mgr., became prod. dir.; won Emmy Award, 1960, for Nixon-Khrushchev debate; pres., Seven League Productions, 1961–63, owner, Radio Station WIII, Homestead, Fla., 1963–67; freelance prod.-dir., 1967–70; v.p. of Ivan Tors Studios, N. Miami, 1970–72; pres. RMG Productions, 1972.

GILLIAM, TERRY: Writer-Director-Actor. b. Minneapolis, MN. Nov. 22, 1940. e. Occidental College. Freelance writer and illustrator for various magazines and ad agencies before moving to London. Member, Monty Python's Flying Circus.
PICTURES: Monty Python and the Holy Grail (co-dir.), Jabberwocky (dir.); Life of Brian (also s.p.), Time Bandits, Monthy Python's The Meaning of Life (s.p., act.), Brazil (s.p., dir.).

GILLIAT, LESLIE: Producer. b. New Malden, England, 1917. e. Epsom College. Ent. m.p. ind. 1935.
PICTURES INCLUDE: Only Two Can Play, The Amorous Prawn, Joey Boy, The Great St. Trinians Train Robbery, A Dandy in Aspic, The Virgin Soldiers, The Buttercup Chain, Endless Night, Priest of Love (prod. supvr.).

GILLIGAN, ZACH: Actor. b. NYC. e. Manhattan Collegiate School. On TV before theatrical debut in Nothing Lasts Forever.
PICTURES: Nothing Lasts Forever, Gremlins.
TELEVISION: It's a Fact of Life (ABC after-school special), Prisoner without a Name, Cell without a Number (movie).

GILLIN, DONALD T.: Executive. b. Council Bluffs, Iowa, June 17, 1914. e. Univ. of Minn., bus. adm., 1929–32; sls., Warner Bros., 1932–39; World War II; home office sup., Warner Bros., 1946–48; sls. exec., Universal, 1948–50; v.p., gen. sls. mgr., mgr., Sol Lesser, 1950–59; establ., Donald T. Gillin Inc., producers' rep., 1960. Muchnic-Gillin Internat'l, Inc., 1961; Producers' Representatives, Inc., 1967.

GILLIS, ANNE: Actress. r.n. Alma Mable O'Connor. b. Little Rock, Arkansas, Feb. 12, 1927. Screen debut 1936 in The Garden of Allah; thereafter in number child roles.
PICTURES INCLUDE: King of Hockey, Off to the Races, The Californian, The Adventures of Tom Sawyer, Peck's Bad Boy with the Circus, Little Orphan Annie, Edison the Man, All This and Heaven Too, Janie; A Wave, a Wac, a Marine; The Cheaters, Gay Blades, Big Town After Dark.

GILMORE, WILLIAM S.: Producer. Started career as film cutter before becoming asst. dir. and prod. mgr. at Universal Studios, where worked on 20 feature films. Headed prod. for Mirisch Co. in Europe; then to Zanuck/Brown Co. as exec. in chg. prod. Produced several TV movies for EMI-TV. Sr. v.p./prod. of Filmways Pictures, supervising literary development, prod. and post-prod.
PICTURES: Swashbuckler (assoc. prod.), The Last Remake of Beau Geste, Rock 'n' Roll Hotel, Another Woman's Child, Tough Enough, Deadly Blessing, Defiance, Against All Odds.
TELEVISION: Just You and Me, One in a Million—The Ron Lefore Story, The Legend of Walks Far Woman, S.O.S. Titanic, etc.

GIMBEL, ROGER: Producer. Began television production career as copy and creative chief of RCA Victor TV, then became assoc. prod. of the Tonight Show for NBC. Subsequently named head of program development of NBC daytime programming; later became producer of the 90-minute NBC Tonight Specials, including The Jack Paar Show and the Ernie Kovacs Show. Became prod. and co-packager of the Glen Campbell Goodtime Hour for CBS, 1969; vice pres. in charge of production for Tomorrow Entertainment, 1971. Produced 15 major movies for television including The Autobiography of Miss Jane Pittman, Born Innocent, Birds of Prey, Brand New Life, Gargoyles, Glass House, In This House of Brede (General Electric Theatre), I Heard the Owl Call My Name (G.E. Theatre), I Love You, Good-Bye, Larry (G.E. Theatre), Miles to Go (G.E. Theatre), Queen of the Stardust Ballroom, Tell Me Where It Hurts (G.E. Theatre), Things in Their Season (G.E. Theatre), War of the Children (Emmy award, Outstanding Single Program, Drama or Comedy). Formed his own production company, Roger Gimbel's Tomorrow Enterprises, Inc., 1975; produced two-hour CBS special, Minstrel Man. Became U.S. pres. of EMI-TV, 1976. Received special personal Emmy as exec. prod. of War of the Children, 1975. Produced 33 movies for TV under the EMI banner. In January, 1984, EMI-TV became The Peregrine Producers Group, Inc., of which he is pres. & COO.

GINGOLD, DAN: Freelance Executive Producer, Producer, Director. Credits include all types live and film prod. Specialist in Special Events and Documentary. Awards include Emmy, Ohio State, Northwestern, Ed Murrow, Assoc. Press, San Francisco State.

GINGOLD, HERMIONE: Actress. b. London, England, Dec. 9, 1897. Appeared with Old Vic and at Shakespeare at Stratford on Avon and in Paris before coming to America and Bdwy.
PICTURES: Gigi, Naked Edge, Music Man, Gay Paree, Harvey Middleman—Fireman, I'd Rather Be Rich, Promise Her Anything, Rocket to the Moon, Garbo Talks.
TELEVISION: Ed Sullivan Show, Omnibus, Matinee Theatre, Jack Paar, Alfred Hitchcock Presents, Merv Griffin Show, Mike Douglas Show, etc.

GINNA, ROBERT EMMETT, JR.: Producer-Writer. b. New York City, Dec. 3, 1925. e. U. of Rochester, Harvard (MA). In U.S. Navy, WWII. Journalist for Life, Scientific American, Horizon, 1950–55; 1958–61, contributor to many magazines. Staff writer, producer, director NBC-TV, 1955–58; v.p., Sextant, Inc., dir., Sextant Films Ltd., 1961–64; Founded Windward Productions, Inc., Windward Film Productions, Ltd., 1965. Active in publishing 1974–82; sr. ed. People; ed. in chief, Little Brown; asst. mgr., Life. Resumed pres., Windward Prods, Inc., 1982; publishing consultant.
PICTURES: Young Cassidy (co-prod.); The Last Challenge (co-s.p.); Before Winter Comes (prod.); Brotherly Love (prod.).

GINSBERG, SIDNEY: Executive. b. New York City, Oct. 26, 1920; e. City Coll., 1938; entered m.p. ind., as asst. mgr., Loew's Theatres; joined Trans-Lux 1943, as thea. mgr.; film booker; helped form Trans-Lux Distributing Corp., 1956; asst. to pres., Trans-Lux Dist. Corp.; asst. vice-pres., Trans-Lux Picture, Distributing and TV Corp., 1961, V.P. Trans-Lux Dist. Corp., 1967, V.P. in charge of world wide sales, 1969. Haven International Pictures, Inc., Haven Intern'l 1970; IFIDA gov., 1970, v.p. sales, Scotia International Films, Inc., 1971; exec. v.p., Scotia American Prods; 1977, pres., Rob-Rich Films Inc.; 1979, exec. v.p., A Major Studio, Inc.; 1980, exec. v.p., The Health and Entertainment Corp. of America; 1982, sr. acct. rep., 3M-Photogard; 1984, pres., Rob-Rich Films.

GINSBURG, LEWIS S.: Distrib., Import., prob. b. New York, May 16, 1914 e. City Coll., N.Y., 1931–32. Columbia Univ., 1932–33. Ent. film industry, tabulating dept., United Artists, Sept. 1932; sls. contract dept. 1933; asst. to eastern district mgr., 1938; slsmn., New Haven exch., 1939. Army, 1943. Ret. to U.S., then formed first buying & booking service in Connecticut, 1945–55; in chg., New England Screen Guild Exchanges, 1955; TV film distr., 1955; Formed & org. International Film Assoc., Vid-EX Film Distr. Corp., 1961. Prod., TV half-hour series; vice-pres. in chg., dist., Desilu Film Dist. C., 1962; organized Carl Releasing Co., 1963; Walter Reade-Sterling Inc., 1964–65; formed L.G. Films Corp.; contract and playdate mgr., 20th Fox, 1965–68. Cinerama Releasing Corp. Adm. Ass't to sales mgr., 1968–69; 20th Cent.-Fox. Nat'l sales coordinator, 1969–present. 1970, 20th Century-Fox, Asst. to the Sales Mgr. 1971, Transnational Pictures Corp., v.p. in chg. of dist., pres., Stellar IV Film Corp., 1972.

GIRARDOT, ANNIE: Actress. b. France, Oct. 25, 1931. Studied nursing. Studied acting at the Paris Conservatory, made her acting debut with the Comedie Francaise. Has acted on the French stage and in reviews in the Latin Quarter.
PICTURES INCLUDE: Rocco and His Brothers, The Organizer, Les Galoise Bleues, Live For Life, Trois Chambres A Manhattan (Best Actress Award at the Venice Film Festival), Story of A Woman, Love Is A Funny Thing, The Slap, No Time for Breakfast.

GISH, LILLIAN: Actress. b. Springfield, Ohio, Oct. 14, 1899; sister of Dorothy G., actress. At 5 appeared in In Convict's Stripes, at Rising Sun, Ohio; following year danced in Sarah Bernhardt prod. in N.Y. In 1913 appeared with Mary Pickford in A Good Little Devil, N.Y. Began screen career 1912 with Biograph, beginning there assn. with D. W. Griffith, dir., which culminated in such films as The Birth of a Nation, Intolerance, Hearts of the World, The Great Love, Broken Blossoms, Way Down East and Orphans of the Storm. Continued in films: White Sister, Romola, The Wind, La Boheme, Scarlet Letter. From 1930 on N.Y. stage in number orig. prods. & classics Uncle Vanya, Camille, 9 Pine Street, Within the Gates, Hamlet, Star Wagon, Old Maid, Dear Octopus, Life With Father, Mr.Sycamore, The Marquise, Legend of Leonora, Crime and Punishment, Miss Mable, Curious Savage, A Passage to India, Too True to be Good; Romeo and Juliet, Stratford Shakespeare Theatre, 1965. 1969–71, One woman int'l. concert tour, Lillian Gish and the Movies. Received honorary Oscar, 1971. International touring with illustrated lecture on the art of film and TV, 1974. Lecture tour on Queen Elizabeth 2, 1975.
PICTURES INCLUDE: One Romantic Night, His Double Life, Commandos Strike at Dawn, Duel in the Sun, Miss Susie Slagle's, Portrait of Jenny, Follow Me Boys!, Night of the Hunter, 1954; The Cobweb, 1955; The Unforgiven, Orders to Kill; Warning Shot, The Comedians, A Wedding (her 100th film), Hambone and Hillie, Sweet Liberty.
PLAYS: Theatre Guild play The Trip to Bountiful, 1954; Chalk Garden, 1956; Phoenix Theatre, N.Y., The Family Reunion; in Berlin, Ger., Portrait of a Madonna, Wreck of the 5:25, Uncle Vanya, 1973. All The Way Home, 1960; Anya, 1965; I Never Sang For My Father, 1968; A Musical Jubilee, 1976.
TV: I Mrs. Bibbs, Sound and the Fury, Day Lincoln Was Shot, Mornings at Seven, The Grass Harp, Grandma T.N.T., Mr. Novak, Alfred Hitchcock Hour, Breaking Point, The Defenders, The Silent Years (hostess). Twin Detectives—(ABC Movie-of-the-Week), 1976; Thin Ice; Hobson's Choice.
AUTHOR: The Movies, Mr. Griffith and Me, published by Prentice-Hall, 1969; Dorothy and Lillian Gish published by Charles Scribner, October, 1973.

GITHENS, W. FRENCH: Executive. b. New York City, April 30, 1906; e. Columbia U. in 1928 secy. Amer. embassy Madrid. Entered m.p. ind. 1929 as member ed. staff Movietonews, editing program Embassy Newsreel theat., N.Y.; asst. ed. Pathe News 1933. On 1934 org. Newsreel Theats. (Embassy theat., Broadway, N.Y. & others), becoming pres. & dir. Org. Sound Masters 1937 to prod. industrial & educational films. Lt. Comdr., U.S.N.R. Bureau Aeronautics World War II; com. U.S.N.R.; pres. National Educational Films, Inc.; on bd. of Viterama & Cinerama Corps. developers of 3-dimensional projection system, 1950. Mayor of Bernardsville, N.J., 2 terms; prod., Movietime Digest; prod., V.P. and dir. Steel Properties, N.Y.C.

GLASER, PAUL MICHAEL: Actor. b. Cambridge, Mass., March 25. e. Tulane Univ., Boston Univ. (M.A.). Did five seasons in summer stock before starting career in New York City, making stage debut in rock version of Hamlet in 1968. Appeared in numerous off-Bdwy. plays and got early TV training as regular in daytime series, Love of Life and Love Is a Many Splendored Thing.
PICTURES INCLUDE: Fiddler on the Roof, Butterflies Are Free. Director: Band of the Hand.
TV: Kojak, Toma, The Streets of San Francisco, The Rockford Files, The Sixth Sense, The Waltons. Movies: Trapped Beneath the Sea, The Great Houdini, Princess

Daisy, Jealousy, Attack on Fear, Single Bars Single Women. Series: Starsky & Hutch.

GLASER, SIDNEY: Exec. adv., prod. b. New York, N.Y., July 12, 1912. e. CCNY, b. Eng., 1936; NYU, m. Eng., 1942; office boy, adv. dept., Metro-Goldwyn-Mayer, 1929; prod. asst. 1934; prod. mgr., 1957; adv. prod. mgr., 1972; gen. adv. exec.

GLAZER, WILLIAM: Executive b. Cambridge, Mass.; e. State University of New York, Entered m.p. ind. with Ralph Snider Theatres 1967–69; General Cinema Corp. 1969–71; Loews Theatres 1971–73; Joined Sack Theatres 1973 as Dist. mgr.; 1974 Exec. Asst. to Pres.; 1976 Gen. Mgr.; 1980 V.P. Gen. Mgr.; 1982 Exec. V.P. Member of SMPTE; NATO (Bd of Dir); Theatre Owners of New England (Bd of Dir); President Theatre Owners of New England 1982–1985.

GLAZIER, SIDNEY: Producer. b. Philadelphia, May 29, 1918. Managed movie and legitimate theatres in Pennsylvania and Ohio. Air Force captain during World War II. Became v.p. of Washington Federal Savings and Loan Bank in Miami. Org. and became exec. dir. of Eleanor Roosevelt Cancer Foundation. Prod. network TV public service programs. First m.p. The Eleanor Roosevelt Story won Academy Award, 1966. Pres. of U-M Film Distributors, 1969.
PICTURES INCLUDE: The Producers, Take the Money and Run, The Gamblers, Quackser Fortune Has a Cousin in the Bronx, The 12 Chairs, Glen and Panda, The Night Visitor, The Only Way.

GLEASON, JACKIE: Performer. b. Brooklyn, N.Y., Feb. 26, 1916. Started as amateur entertainer, clubs, WB pact, appeared in Navy Blues, All Through the Night, Larceny, Inc., Orchestra Wives, Springtime in the Rockies; returned to Broadway appearing on the stage and summer stock.
BWY. STAGE: Take Me Along, 1959–60 (Tony Award).
TV: Started as lead in The Life of Riley; then star and m.c. Cavalcade of Stars on the Du Mont network; The Honeymooners; Jackie Gleason Show, CBS-TV network. Best comedian, Fame poll, 1953; best comedy show, 1954. Movie: Izzy and Moe.
PICTURES INCLUDE: The Hustler, Requiem For a Heavyweight, Gigot, Papa's Delicate Condition, Soldier in the Rain, Ski-doo; How to Commit a Marriage, Don't Drink the Water, How Do I Love Thee, The Late Show, Smokey and the Bandit, Smokey and the Bandit II, The Sting II, The Toy; Smokey and the Bandit, Part III, Nothing in Common.

GLEASON, LARRY: Executive. b. Boston, MA Apr. 30, 1938. e. Boston Coll. (MA, 1960). Held various positions, western div., mgr., General Cinema Corp.; 1968–84; gen. mgr., Gulf States Theatres, New Orleans, 1984–85; pres., Mann Theatres, 1985; joined DeLaurentiis Entertainment Group as pres., mktg./dist., Dec., 1985.

GLENN, CHARLES OWEN: Executive. b. Binghamton, N.Y., March 27, 1938; e. Syracuse U., (BA), U. of Pa. Capt., U.S. Army, 1961–63. Asst. to dir. of adv., 20th Cent. Fox, 1966–67; asst. adv. mgr., Paramount, 1967–68; acct. spvsr. & exec., MGM record & m.p. div., 1968–69; nat'l adv. mgr., Paramount, 1969–70; nat'l. dir. of adv., Paramount, 1970–71; v.p. adv.-pub.-prom., 1971–73; v.p. marketing, 1974; v.p. prod. mktg., 1975; joined American Intl. Pictures as v.p. in chg. of adv./creative affairs, 1979. 1980, when Filmways took AIP over he was named their v.p. in chg. worldwide adv./pub./promo.; joined MCA/Universal in 1982 as exec. v.p., adv.-promo.; 1984, appt. Orion Pictures adv.-pub.-promo. exec. v.p.
MEMBER: Exec. comm. public relations branch, Academy of M.P. Arts & Sciences. Holder of NATO mktg. exec. of year (1983) award. Variety Club. Motion Picture Pioneers.

GLENN, SCOTT: Actor. b. Pittsburgh. Worked as newspaper reporter before going to New York to study drama. Off-Bdwy. productions included Fortune in Men's Eyes, Long Day's Journey into Night. Member of Actors Studio. Film debut in The Baby Maker, 1970.
PICTURES: Apocalypse Now, Urban Cowboy, Personal Best, The Challenge, The Right Stuff, The Keep, The River, Wild Geese II, Silverado.
TELEVISION: Countdown to Looking Glass.

GLICK, HYMAN J.: Executive. b. Russia, Dec. 15, 1904; e. N.Y.U., B.C.S., '26, C.P.A. (N.Y.); with public accounting firm, N.Y., 1923–29; own public accounting Business, 1929–32. Became assoc. m.p. ind. as member comptrollers' com., repr. Republic; 1932–36, tax & financial counsel Mascot Pictures Corp. Joined Republic 1936 as comptroller; apptd. asst. secy.-asst. treas. Jan., 1945. Retired, 1985.
Member: B'nai Brith Lodge 1325; State Soc. of Certified Public Accountants, Am. Inst. of Accountants. Resigned Republic, 1959; CPA (Calif.), member, Calif. Soc. of CPA; Own Accounting and Tax Practice.

GLICK, PHYLLIS: Executive. b. New York City. e. Queens College of C.C.N.Y. Began career with Otto-Windsor Associates, as casting director; left to be independent. 1979, joined ABC-TV as mgr. of comedy series development; promoted 1980 to director, involved with all comedy series developed for network. 1985, joined Paramount Pictures as exec. dir., production, for M.P. Group.

GLICKMAN, JOEL: Producer. b. Los Angeles, July 29, 1930. e. UCLA (film dep't.). Was actor and director for LA little theatre groups and writer-director for industrial films. Early TV work on series, documentaries and commercials. Directed videotaping of off-Broadway shows. Was production assoc. on film, Wedding and Babies, 1958. Was assoc. prod. and prod. mgr. on films (Terror in the City, The Balcony, All the Way Home, For Love of Ivy, Hamlet (Richard Burton, assoc. director), Dion Brothers, Last Summer and TV (East Side, West Side, Mr. Broadway), N.Y.P.D., Love Song of Barney Kempinski, Among the Paths To Eden. Member Motion Picture Academy & D.G.A. Has own co.: Selznick/Glickman Productions.
PICTURES INCLUDE: Brother John, Buck and the Preacher, Trial of the Catonsville Nine (exec. prod.), Night Terror (NBC-TV movie), Angel on Horseback (CBS-TV movie), Kennedy-Hoffa War (NBC-TV miniseries).

GLOVER, JOHN: Actor. b. Sailsbury, MD, Aug. 7, 1944. e. Towson State coll., Baltimore. On regional theatre circuit; in plays off-Bdwy. Drama Desk award for The Great God Brown.
PICTURES: Julia, She Killed Her Husband, Last Embrace, The American Success Company, Melvin & Howard, The Mountain Men, The Incredible Shrinking Woman, A Little Sex, The Evil That Men Do, White Nights, 52 Pick-Up.
TELEVISION: An Early Frost, Apology (cable).

GOATMAN, ALAN H.: Consultant, Entered m.p. industry 1934. Officer of the Venerable Order of St. John of Jerusalem. Fellow Society of Company and Commercial Accountants. Memb. Brit. Computer Soc. Fellow Brit. Inst. Management; member Inst. Data Processing; Management Dir. British Film & TV Producers Assoc.; Exec. mem., intl. treas., AGICDA, Geneva.

GODARD, JEAN-LUC: Writer-Director. b. Paris, France, Dec. 3, 1930.
PICTURES INCLUDE: A Bout de Souffle, Une Femme Est Une Femme, Vivre Sa Vie, Le Petie Soldat, Les Carabiniera, Bande a Part, Une Femme Marlee, A Little Godard; Pierrot Le Fou, Made in USA, Weekend, Tout va Bien, First Name Carmen, Hail Mary.

GODBOLD, GEOFF: Executive. b. London, England, 1935. Ent. ind. 1959. Specialized in supply of location requirements for film and TV prods. Formed Prop Workshops Ltd., co-promoted Television Recordings Ltd. Man. dir. Facilities (Screen & Television) Ltd. Dir. TV Recordings, Investments, Ltd.; Centrepoint Screen Prod. Ltd.; Tape Commercials, Ltd. Council Mem. Film and TV Contractors Assoc. Dir. Lancair Export Services Ltd.; 1968 Freelance production buyer, Screen Gems and Tigon. 1969. Feature Prod. Rep. Film Div. N.A.T.T.K.E. Man. Dir. Setpieces Ltd. Film & TV Prop. Hire. 1984: Carlton Communication. 1985: mng. dir., Set Pieces Ltd.
PICTURES INCLUDE: Dubious Patriot, Every Home Should Have One, Melody, Up Pompeii. Morocco location, Young Winston. The Asphyx, Our Miss Fred, Death of a Snow Queen, Man in the Iron Mask. TV: The Professionals.

GODDARD, PAULETTE: Actress. b. Great Neck, N.Y., June 3, 1911. On N.Y. stage in Rio Rita; then member of Hal Roach Studios stock co. In 1936 opposite Charles Chaplin in Modern Times.
PICTURES INCLUDE: The Young in Heart, The Women, North West Mounted Police, The Great Dictator, Hold Back the Dawn, Reap the Wild Wind, Star Spangled Rhythm, I Love a Soldier, So Proudly We Hail, Standing Room Only, Duffy's Tavern, Kitty, Unconquered, An Ideal Husband, Hazard, On Our Merry Way, Bride of Vengeance, Anna Lucasta, Babes in Bagdad, Vice Squad, Paris Model, Sins of Jezebel, Charge of the Lancers, Unholy Four, Time of Indifference.

GODWIN, FRANK: Producer, writer, director.
PICTURES INCLUDE: Woman in a Dressing Gown, No Trees in the Street, Operation Bullshine, Don't Bother to Knock, The Small World of Sammy Lee, Danny the Dragon, Headline Hunters, Demons of the Mind, The Boy With Two Heads, The Firefighters, Sky Pirates, Sammy's Super T-Shirt, Electric Eskimo, The Boy Who Never Was, Break Out, Terry on the Fence.

GOLAN, MENAHEM: Producer-Director-Writer. b. Israel, 1931.
PICTURES INCLUDE: Director: Sallah, Teyve and His Seven Daughters, What's Good for the goose? Lepke, Diamonds, The Magician of Lublin, The goodsend, Happy Hooker Goes to Hollywood, Enter the Ninja. Producer-Writer-Director: The Apple. Producer-Director: It's a Funny, Funny World, The Uranium Conspiracy, Over the Brooklyn Bridge.

Producer: New Year's Evil, Body and Soul, The Wicked Lady, Cobra.

GOLD, MELVIN: Executive. b. Chicago, Ill., Sept. 3, 1909. In 1930 joined MGM, Chicago, as ssistant office manager. To Reinheimer Circuit 1932 to operate theatres Hammond, Indiana; in 1940 organized own advertising agency, Sales, Inc., mgr.; mgr. Vogue Theatre, Hollywood, Calif., 1943. Joined National Screen Service 1943 as editor Mister Showman; Feb., 1945 named director of advtsng. and publicity; assumed east coast film prod. and TV, Sept., 1948 to May, 1954. Formed Mel Gold Productions, Inc., June 1954.

Member Publicity Club of N.Y.; Associated Motion Picture Advertisers; founded National Television Film Council in 1948, elected Honorary Lifetime President, 1955. Partner Melmon Productions; Melvin L. Gold Enterprises, 1958; pres., Mesal Prods., Inc., 1961; wrote s.p., Not For Love, 1961; pres., Associated Motion Picture Advertisers, 1963–64–65–66; gen. sls. mgr., National Screen Service, 1963. Pres., Melvin L. Gold Enterprises, Inc. 1966. Pres. Manhatten Sound Studios 1967, v.p. in chg. m.p. div., National Showmanship Services, 1968; 1971, Pres. East Side Productions; Pres. Melvin L. Gold Enterprises. Motion picture consultant, Philip Morris, Inc., 1976–present. Operations director, Benson & Hedges 100, Film classics, 1976–79. Wrote s.p., The Sheriff is a Lady, 1979.

GOLDBERG, BERNARD: Executive. b. Bronx, N.Y., Aug. 25, 1932. e. Queens College (B.A.). Co-owner, Golden Theatre Mgt. Corp.; named vice pres. 1973.

GOLDBERG, FRED: Publicist. b. N.Y.C., Aug. 26, 1921. e. Pace College, School of Marketing and Advertising expl., Paramount, 1946; asst. expl. mgr., trade paper contact, syndicate contact, N.Y. newspaper contact promotion mgr., 1946–52; ass't publ. mgr., RKO, 1952,; national publ. mgr.; IFE, 1953; v.p. Norton and Condon, pub., 1953; returned to IFE Sept., 1954, as nat'l pub. mgr.; head of N.Y. office, Arthur Jacobs, then Blowitz-Maskel, 1956; exec. asst. to dir. pub., adv., United Artists Corp., 1958; exec. dir., adv., pub., exploitation, United Artists Corp., 1961; named vice pres., 1962, senior vice president, 1972, Senior Vice President, Director of Marketing, 1977. Left in 1978 to be consultant with Piener, Hauser & Bates Agency. In 1979 joined Columbia Pictures as snr. v.p. in chg. adv./pub. Left in 1981 to form new company.

GOLDBERG, LEONARD: Executive. b. Brooklyn, Nov. 24, 1934. . e. Wharton School, Univ. of PA. Began career in ABC-TV research dept.; moved to NBC-TV research div.; 1961 joined Batten, Barton, Durstine & Osborn ad agency in chg. of daytime TV shows and overall bdcst. coordinator. In 1963 rejoined ABC-TV as mgr. of program devel. In 1966 named VP in chg of network TV programming. Resigned in 1969 to join Screen Gems as VP in chg. of prod. Left for partnership with Aaron Spelling in Spelling/Goldberg Prods. Goldberg is now producing TV and theatrical films under own banner, Mandy Prods. 1981: co-prod. All Night Long. 1983: WarGames.

GOLDBLUM, JEFF: Actor. b. Pittsburgh, PA, Oct. 22, 1952. Studied at Sanford Meisner's Neighborhood Playhouse in New York. On Bdwy. in Two Gentleman of Verona, The Moony Shapiro Songbook.

PICTURES: Death Wish (debut), Nashville, Next Stop, Greenwich Village, Annie Hall, Between the Lines, Thank God, It's Friday, Invasion of the Body Snatchers, Threshold, The Big Chill, The Right Stuff, Buckaroo Banzai, Into the Night, Silverado, Transylvania 6-5000, The Fly.

TELEVISION: Movies: The Legend of Sleepy Hollow, Rehearsal for Murder, Ernie Kovacs: Between the Laughter. Series: Tenspeed and Brownshoe.

GOLDEN, HERBERT L.: b. Philadelphia, Feb. 12. e. Temple U., 1936, B.S. Reporter, rewrite man. asst. city ed., Philadelphia Record, 1933–38; joined Variety, 1938; on leave of absence, 1942–43, when asst. to John Hay Whitney and Francis Alstock, directors, M.P. Division, Coordinator of Inter-American Affairs (U.S.); commissioned in U.S. Navy, 1943, served on destroyer to 1946; then returned to Variety. M.p. ed. Consultant on motion pictures, Good Housekeeping magazine,, McGraw-Hill Publications, American Yearbook. Ent. Ind. Div. Bankers Trust Co., N.Y.C., 1952; named v.p. 1954–56; treas., Children's Asthma Research Institute, 1956; v.p. & mem. of bd. United Artists Corp., 1958; member of board, MPAA, 1959; pres., Lexington Int., Inc. investments, 1962; mem. bd., chmn. exec. com., Perfect Photo Inc., 1962; 1965 sect. & mem. bd. Century Broadcasting Group; chmn. G & G Thea. Corp.; pres. Diversifax Corp., 1966; consult. Pathe Lab, 1967; Mem. bd. Childhood Prod. Inc., 1967. Member bd. Music Makers Group, Inc., 1962. Mem. bd. Cinecom Corp., 1968; pres., Vere/Swiss Corp., 1977; mem. bd., Coral Reef Publications, Inc., 1977. Returned to Bankers Trust, 1979, to head its Media Group (service to film and TV industries).

GOLDEN, JEROME B.: Executive-Attorney. b. New York, N.Y., Nov. 26, 1917. e. St. Lawrence Univ., LL.B., 1942. Member legal dept., Paramount Pictures, Inc., 1942–50; United Paramount Theatres, Inc., 1950–53; American Broadcasting Companies, Inc., 1953; secy., ABC, 1958; vice-pres., ABC, 1959.

GOLDENSON, LEONARD H.: Executive. b. Scottsdale, Pennsylvania, December 7, 1905; e. Harvard College, B.A., Harvard Law School, LL.B. Practiced law, New York; counsel in reorg. Paramount theats. in New England, 1933–37; in 1937 apptd. asst. to vice-pres. Paramount in charge theat. operations; became head of theat. operations, 1938; elected pres. Paramount Theat. Service Corp., vice-pres. Paramount Pictures, Inc., 1938; dir. Paramount Pictures, 1942 (also pres. various Paramount theat. subsids., see Paramount circuits in Theatre Circuits section). Pres., chief exec. off. and director United Paramount Theatres, Inc., 1950, and of American Broadcasting-Paramount Theatres, Inc., 1953, result of merger of ABC and United Paramount Theatres, Inc.; name changed to American Broadcasting Companies, Inc. 1965; Chairman of the Board and Chief Executive Officer; of American Broadcasting Companies, Inc. since January 17, 1972; mem., board chm. of United Cerebral Palsy Assns.; trustee, John F. Kennedy Center for the Performing Arts; dir., Daughters of Jacob Geriatric Center; mem., International Radio and Television Society; Founder Member of Hollywood Museum; Trustee of Children's Cancer Research Foundation of the Children's Medical Center, Boston, Mass.; Director of Allied Stores Corporation; Trustee of Highway Users Federation for Safety and Mobility; Member of National Academy of Television Arts and Sciences; Member of Uptown Advisory Committee of Bankers Trust Company; Graduate Director of The Advertising Council, Inc.; Associate Trustee and Member of Advisory Council for the Performing Arts of University of Pennsylvania; Member of Broadcast Pioneers; Member of Inter Lochen Arts Academy-National Advisory Board; Member of Motion Picture Pioneers; Member of National Citizens' Advisory Committee on Vocational Rehabilitation; Member of United Negro College Fund-National Corporations Committee; Director of World Rehabilitation Fund, Inc.

GOLDFARB, HOWARD: Executive. b. New York City, Sept. 19, 1941. e. Wharton School of Business. Joined Columbia Pictures as exec. trainee; 1964–69 mgn. dir., U.A., central America; 1969–70, supervisor of sales, Buena Vista Intl.; 1972–75, pres. H.G. Entertainment Ltd.; 1975–76, dir. of dist., CIC London; v.p., intl. operations, NTA; 1978–79, v.p., intl. sls., Dino de Laurentiis pres., Goldfarb Distributors, since 1979.

GOLDFARB, HOWARD GERALD: Executive. b. New York, City, Sept. 19, 1941. Exec. trainee, Columbia Pictures, 1962–64; mgr. dir., United Artists Corp., in Panama/Central America, 1964–69; v.p. & foreign mgr., Cannon Releasing Corp., 1970–72; pres., H.G. Entertainment Ltd. & Salt Water Releasing Co., Inc., 1972–75; dir. dist., C.I.C. (cassettes co.), 1976; v.p., dir. intl. opns., National Telefilm Associates, 1976–78; dir. intl. sls., Dino de Laurentiis Corp., 1978–79; pres., Goldfarb Distributors, 1979–1980, distributing films for independent producers worldwide. Now represents Leisure Investment Co., Astral Films, National American, Hall Bartlett Films, Sewanee Prods., Western Pictures, Haruki Kadokawa Films, Highpoint Prods., Lawrence Schiller Prods., Market Prods.

PICTURES: Producer: The Unseen, Venus in 3-D, Mission Kills, Car Trouble, On the Fringe.

GOLDIN, BERNARD: Executive. Began career with Universal Pictures as branch mgr. in number of territories. Named Philadelphia mgr. for United Artists; 1977–81, Midwestern div. mgr. for Columbia Pictures. Returned to UA, 1981, as v.p. & asst. gen. sls. mgr.

GOLDING, DAVID: Executive. b. New York City, U. of Wisc., B.A. Now operating public relations consultancy in London, David Golding and Associates Ltd. Formerly Universal advertising and publicity representative in UK. During war, mg. ed. Mediterranean edition, The Stars and Stripes. Also pub. dir. Samuel Goldwyn, 20th-Fox, Hecht-Hill-Lancaster, Otto Preminger.

GOLDMAN, EDMUND: Executive-Producer. b. Shanghai, China, Nov. 12, 1906. e. in Shanghai and San Francisco. Entered ind. as assst. mgr., for Universal in Shanghai, 1935–36; named mgr. Columbia Pictures' Philippine office, 1937. In 1951 named Far East. supvr. for Columbia, headquartering in Tokyo. From 1953 to present indep. m.p. dist., specializing in foreign marketing, representing indep. producers and distributors. Now chm. of bd. for Manson International.

PICTURES: Surrender Hell (prod.), The Quick and the Dead (exec. prod.).

GOLDMAN, JANE: Executive. e. Barnard College; NY Univ. School of Law. Represented Warner Bros. in special assignments while in general law practice; joined Warner Communications Inc. in N.Y. as full-time attorney, counselling dist. div. in copyright and anti-trust matters. 1985, named v.p., gen. counsel for WB Dist. Corp., at Warner Studio.

GOLDMAN, MARVIN: Executive. b. New York City. e. Fordham & Univ. of Miami. Served in U.S. Navy in WW II, leaving with rank of Lt. commander. In 1947 went to Washington, D.C. to work for K-B Theatres; purchased the chain of five theatres. Circuit now operates 52 theatres in the D.C., Maryland, Virginia area. (Partnership now includes Goldman's son, Ronald.) Goldman also involved with son in indep. film prod. co., which has completed 6 features and planning more. Active in theatre organizations for many years; named pres. of National NATO in 1976. Former pres. of Metropolitan, Washington, D.C. area chapter of NATO and now bd. chmn. Past chief barker of Variety Club of Washingtron. Named exhibitor of year by IFIDA in 1966. With son operates European Classics, distributing imported films in U.S. & Canada.

GOLDMAN, MICHAEL F.: Executive. b. Manila, Philippines, Sept. 28, 1939. e. UCLA (B.S. in acct., 1962). C.P.A. certificate issued June, 1972. In 1962 incorporated Manson International, succeeding company to Manson Distributing Corp. Currently sole owner Manson International. Also owner and sole proprietor Taurus Film co. of Hollywood, founded 1964. Co-founder and first chief financial officer of American Film Marketing Association, sponsor of First American Film Market in Los Angeles in 1981; v.p. of AFMA 1982 and 1983 and President AFMA 1984–85. AFMA bd. mbr., 1986–87. Produced feature, Jessi's Girls in 1975.

GOLDMAN, WILLIAM: Writer. b. Chicago, 1931. e. Oberlin College (B.A.), Columbia Univ. (M.A.). Novels include The Temple of Gold, Soldier in the Rain (filmed), No Way to Treat a Lady (filmed), Father's Day, The Princess Bride, Marathon Man (filmed), Magic (filmed), Tinsel, control, etc.
PICTURES INCLUDE: Harper, Butch Cassidy and the Sundance Kid, The Great Waldo Pepper, Marathon Man (based on own book), All the President's Men, A Bridge Too Far, Magic (based on own book), Heart (based on own book).

GOLDSMITH, JERRY: Composer. b. Los Angeles, 1930. e. L.A. City College. Studied piano with Jacob Gimpel and music composition, harmony, theory with Mario Casteinuovo Tedesco. Taught music; went with CBS radio first with own show (Romance) and then moved on to others (Suspense). Began scoring for TV, including Climax, Playhouse 90, Studio One, Gunsmoke, etc.
PICTURES INCLUDE: Black Patch (debut), Freud, Lilies of the Field, The Stripper, The Prize, Seven Days in May, In Harm's Way, Von Ryan's Express, A Patch of Blue, Our Man Flint, Stagecoach, The Blue Max, Seconds, Sand Pebbles, In Like Flint, Patton, Papillon, The Reincarnation of Peter Proud, The Cassandra Crossing, Islands in the Stream, MacArthur, Coma, Damien-Omen II, The Boys from Brazil, The Great Train Robbery, Alien, Players, Star Trek, The Final Conflict, Outland, Raggedy Man, Poltergeist, The Challenge, Inchon, First Blood, Under Fire, The Lonely Guy, Gremlins, Supergirl, Runaway, Baby, Rambo: First Blood Part II, King Solomon's Mines, Legend, Poltergeist II.

GOLDSMITH, MARTIN M.: Writer. b. New York, N.Y., Nov. 6, 1913. Bush pilot.
AUTHOR: Novels include: Double Jeopardy, Detour, Shadows at Noon, Miraculous Fish of Domingo Gonzales.
PICTURES INCLUDE: Detour, Blind Spot, Narrow Margin, Mission Over Korea, Overland Pacific, Hell's Island.

GOLDSTEIN, MILTON: Executive. b. N.Y.C., Aug. 1, 1926. e. N.Y.U., 1949. In exec. capac., Paramount; foreign sales coord., "The Ten Commandments," "Psycho"; v.p. foreign sales, Samuel Bronston org.; asst. to Pres., Paramount Int'l., special prods., 1964; Foreign sales mgr., 1966; v.p., world wide sales, 1967, Cinerama; Sr. v.p. Cinema Center Films, 1969; pres., Cinema Center Films, 1971; v.p. Theatrical Mktg. & Sales, Metromedia Producers Corp., 1973; in March, 1974, formed Boasberg-Goldstein, Inc., consultants in prod. and dist. of m.p.; 1975, named exec. vice pres., Avco Embassy Pictures; 1978, named exec. v.p. & chief operating officer, Melvin Simon Prods. 1980, named pres.; 1985, pres. Milt Goldstein Enterprises, Inc.

GOLDSTONE, JAMES: Director. b. Los Angeles, Calif. June 8, 1931. e. Dartmouth College, BA, Bennington College, MA. Film Editor from 1950. Writer, story editor from 1957.
TELEVISION: From 1958, including pilots of Star Trek, Ironside, The Senator, etc., A Clear and Present Danger (Emmy nomination); Eric (Virgin Islands Int'l. Film Festival Gold Medal); Journey From Darkness (Christopher Award); Studs Lonigan, 6 hr. miniseries, 1978, Kent State, (Emmy, best direction, special), Things in Their Season, Calamity Jane; The Sun Also Rises; Dreams of Gold.
PICTURES INCLUDE: Jigsaw, Man Called Gannon, Winning, Brother John, Red Sky at Morning, The Gang That Couldn't Shoot Straight, They Only Kill Their Masters, Swashbuckler, Rollercoaster, When Time Ran Out.

GOLDSTONE, RICHARD: Producer. b. New York City, July 14, 1912. e. University of Cal., Los Angeles, B.A., '33. Capt., Army Air Forces, office of Motion Picture Services, World War II. Adv. exec. Entered m.p. ind. 1934 as writer, MGM; in 1935 asst. head short subjects dept.; in 1939 assoc. prod. short subjects; apptd. prod. mgr., MGM short subjects dept., co-holder 3 Academy Awards short subjects, 1942. Prod. The Set-Up, (RKO), 1948, won Int'l Critics Grand Prix, Cannes, 1949. v.p. Dudley Pict. Corp.; v.p., Goldcoast Productions, Inc.
PICTURES INCLUDE: The Outriders, Yellow Cab Man, Dial 1119, Inside Straight, The Tall Target, Talk About a Stranger, Devil Makes Three, Terror on the Train, Tabor the Great, The Big Search, East of Kilimanjaro, South Seas Adventures; No Man Is An Island, Rage, The Sergeant, The Babymaker.
TV: Prod. Adventures in Paradise, Combat, Peyton Place, We Ask, Why Not? (doc.)

GOLDWURM, JEAN: Executive. b. Bucharest, Rumania, Feb. 21, 1893. e. Univ. of Vienna. pres. Times Film Corp. officer French Legion of Honor; commander Italian Order of Merit, Commander French Order of Arts and Letters.

GOLDWYN, SAMUEL, JR.: Producer, director. b. Los Angeles, Calif., Sept. 7, 1926; e. U. of Va. U.S. Army, 1944; following war writer, assoc. prod., J. Arthur Rank Org.; prod. Gathering Storm on London stage; returned to U.S., 1948; assoc. prod., Universal; recalled to Army service, 1951; prod., dir., Army documentary films including Alliance for Peace (Edinburgh Film Festival prize); prod. TV shows, Adventure series for CBS, 1952–53; prod. TV series, The Unexpected, 1954; pres., The Samuel Goldwyn Company.
PICTURES INCLUDE: Man With the Gun, The Sharkfighters, The Proud Rebel, The Adventures of Huckleberry Finn, The Young Lovers, Cotton Comes to Harlem, Come Back Charleston Blue, The Golden Seal.

GOLIGER, NANCY: Executive. Began career in entertainment industry at Bill Gold Adv. & B.G. Charles. Joined Warner Bros. as natl. adv. mgr.; promoted to dir., creative adv. With Universal as dir. adv.; PolyGram Pictures, v.p., domestic & foreign adv./pub.; Seiniger Advertising, exec. v.p. & gen. mgr. 1985, joined Paramount Pictures as sr. v.p., prod./mktg. for M.P. Group.

GOLLINGS, FRANKLIN: Producer, writer, director. Llandudno, Wales. Ent. m.p. ind. 1936. Film prod. adviser to the Admiralty, 1945–8. Shorts pro. Rayant Pictures, 1948–52. Unit man. Mogambo. First asst. The Maggie. S.p. The Sitting Duck. Prod. man. Bhowani Junction. Exec. prod. Associated-Rediffusion. Writ. 2nd unit dir. assoc. prod. Yangtse Incident, 1960, Writ. Tempt Not the Stars, The Stirling Moss Story, 1961; Writ. Force 136 and The Stone; writer, dir., The Changing Face, 1963; dir., Woman; res., writer, The Story of Yang-Kwei-Fei; writer, prod., Jason and the Argonauts, 1964; writer, dir., Mystery Horse, A Price for Dorothy, The Big Design, 1965; Writer Dictionary of 1001 Famous People, Great Moments in Amer. History. S.P. dir. prod. Connecting rooms. Formed Four Cities Int. Corp., 1968; program of Internat'l co-prods., 1969. Research and Script High Risk (based on The Junkie Priest), 1970. Prod., dir. High Risk. Dir. The Todd Dossier.

GONZALEZ-GONZALEZ, PEDRO: Actor. b. Aguilares, Tex., Dec. 21, 1926. Comedian in San Antonio Mexican theatres.
PICTURES INCLUDE: Wing of the Hawk, Ring of Fear, Ricochet Romance, High and the Mighty, Strange Lady in Town, Bengazi, I Died a Thousand Times, Bottom of the Bottle, Gun the Man Down, Wetbacks, The Love Bug, Hellfighters, Support Your Local Gunfighter.
TV: O'Henry Stories, Felix, the Fourth, Hostile Guns.

GOOD, CHARLES E.: Executive. b. 1922. Joined Buena Vista in 1957 in Chicago office; progressed from salesman to branch manager and then district manager. Later moved to Burbank as domestic sales manager in 1975; 1978, named v.p. & general sales manager; 1980, appointed pres., BV Distribution Co. Resigned 1984; now BV consultant.

GOODMAN, DAVID Z.: Writer. e. Queens College, Yale School of Drama.
PICTURES: Straw Dogs, Lovers and Other Strangers, Farewell, My Lovely, Logan's Run, The Eyes of Laura Mars, Man, Woman and Child (co.-s.p.).

GOODMAN, GENE: Executive. Joined United Artists as salesman in 1954; promoted to branch mgr., Atlanta (1958–61). Served successively as branch mgr., New Orleans (1961–68); southern regional mgr. (1968–70); and southern div. mgr., (1970–78), New Orleans. Moved to N.Y. in 1978 to become asst. gen. sls. mgr. Promoted to v.p. & gen. sls. mgr. in 1980. Later in year named snr. v.p. for domestic sls.

GOODMAN, JULIAN: Executive. b. Glasgow, Ky., May 1, 1922. e. B.A. Western Kentucky Univ; B.A. Geo. Washington Univ; Office mgr., Comb. Prod. & Resources, 1943–45.

History at NBC: news writer, WRC, NBC owned station in Washington, D.C., 1945; Washington ed., News of the World, NBC Radio network; mgr. of news and special events, NBC-TV, 1951; dir. of news and public affairs, NBC News Div., 1959; v.p., NBC News, 1961; exec. v.p., 1965; sr. exec. v.p., Operations, Jan. 1, 1966; pres., NBC, April 1, 1966. Mem. bd. of dirs., NBC, 1966; chief executive officer, Jan. 1, 1970; elected director or RCA Corporation, Jan. 1, 1972; chmn., chief exec. off., NBC, April, 1, 1974; chmn., Jan. 5, 1977.

GOODMAN, MORT: Advertising-public relations executive. b. Cleveland, O., Oct. 17, 1910. e. Western Reserve U. With sports dept. Cleveland News 1928–29 joined pub. dept. Warner Bros. theatres (Ohio), 1930; transferred to Hollywood as pub. dir. for Pacific Coast zone, 1937; pub. dir. Republic Studios, 1946; res. 1952, apptd. v.-p. Stodel Adv. Agcy., formed Mort Goodman Adv., 1953; formed Goodman Org., advertising agency, pub. rel., 1955. Currently pres., Goodman Nemoy and Partners, adv.-p.r. firm started 1977. In 1980 became adv. & p.r. consultant for m.p. industry.

GOODRICH, ROBERT EMMETT: Executive. b. Grand Rapids, MI, June 27, 1940. e. Univ. of Mich. (BA, 1962; JD, 1964); New York Univ. LLM, 1966). Pres. & Secty., Goodrich Theaters, Inc. 1967–present, developed circuit from father's one theater to 39 screens at 11 locations in seven Mich. communities. Owns and operates 2FM and 2AM Mich. radio stations.
MEMBER: NATO; Will Rogers Institute advisory comm; bd., Mich. Millers Mutual Insurance Co.; State of Mich. Bar Assn.

GOODSON, MARK: TV producer; b. Sacramento, Jan. 24, 1918; s. Abraham Ellis and Fannie (Gross) G.; A.B., U. Cal., 1937. Announcer, newscaster, dir. Radio Sta. KFRC, San Francisco, 1938–41; radio announcer, dir., N.Y.C. 1941–43; producer—Appointment with Life, ABC, 1943; dir. Portia Faces Life, Young & Rubicam, advt. agy., 1944; radio dir. U.S. Treasury War Bond Drive, 1944–45; formed Goodson-Todman Prodns., 1946, originated radio shows Winner Take All, 1946, Stop the Music, 1947, Hit the Jackpot, 1947–49. Creator of TV game programs What's My Line, It's News To Me, The Name's the Same, I've Got a Secret, Two For The Money, To Tell the Truth, The Price Is Right, Password, Match Game, Family Feud, and others; TV film series, The Web, The Rebel, Richard Boone Theater, Branded. 1st v.p. Capitol City Pub. Co.; v.p. New Eng. Newspapers, Inc.; dir. City Center Music and Drama, Board American Film Institute. Recipient nat. television award Great Britain, 1951; Emmy award Acad. TV Arts and Scis., 1951, 52; Sylvania award. Pres. N.Y. Acad. TV Arts and Sci. 1957–58. Phi Beta Kappa.

GOODWIN, RICHARD: Producer. b. Bombay, India, Sept. 13, 1934. e. Rugby. Entered film world by chance: while waiting to go to Cambridge Univ. took temporary job as tea boy at studio which led to 20-year-long association with producer Lord Brabourne. First worked as asst. on Seven Thunders, of which Brabourne was assoc. prod. Named location manager for Brabourne's company, Mershal Productions; pro moted to prod. mgr. Named assoc. prod. for Brabourne's British Home Entertainment Productions in 1960 (now defunct.)
PICTURES: Prod. Mgr.: The Sheriff of Fractured Jaw, Carve Her Name with Pride, The Grass Is Greener, Sink the Bismarck, HMS Defiant. Prod.: The Tales of Beatrix Potter. Co-Prod.: Murder on the Orient Express, Death on the Nile, The Mirror Crack'd, Evil Under the Sun, A Passage to India.

GOODWIN, RONALD: Composer, arranger, conductor. b. Plymouth, England. Early career: arranger for BBC dance orchestra; mus. dir., Parlophone Records; orchestra leader for radio, TV and records. Fut. m.p. ind., 1958. Many major film scores. Guest cond. R.P.O., B.S.O., Toronto Symph. Orch. New Zealand Symphony Orch., Sydney Symphony Orch. Scottish National Orch., BBC Scottish Symphony Orch., BBC Welsh Symphony Orch., BBC Radio Orch., BBC Concert Orch., BBC Concert Orch., London Philharmonic Orch., Gothenberg Symphony Orch., Norwegian Opera Orch. & Chorus.
PICTURES INCLUDE: The Trials of Oscar Wilde, 633 Squadron, Those Magnificent Men in Their Flying Machines, The Trap, Where Eagles Dare, Monte Carlo or Bust, Battle of Britain, The Executioner, The Selfish Giant, Frenzy (1972), Diamonds on Wheels, The Little Mermaid, The Happy Prince, One of Our Dinosaurs Is Missing, Escape From the Dark, Born to Run, Beauty and the Beast, Candleshoe, Force Ten from Navarone, Spaceman and King Arthur, Clash of Loyalties, Valhalla.

GORDON, ALEX: Producer. b. London, Eng., Sept. 8, 1922; ed. Canford Coll., Dorset, 1939. Writer, m.p. fan magazines, 1939–41; British Army, 1942–45; pub. dir. Renown Pictures Corp., 1946–47; P.R. and pub. rep. for Gene Autry, 1948–53; v.p. and prod. Golden State Productions, 1954–58; prod. Alex Gordon Prods., 1958–66; producer Twentieth Century-Fox Television, 1967–76; film archivist/preservationist, 1976–84; v.p., Gene Autry's Flying A Pictures, 1985.
PICTURES INCLUDE: Lawless Rider, Bride of the Monster, Apache Woman, Day the World Ended, Oklahoma Woman, Girls in Prison, The She-Creature, Runaway Daughters, Shake Rattle and Rock, Flesh and the Spur, Voodoo Woman, Dragstrip Girl, Motorcycle Gang, Jet Attack, Submarine Seahawk, Atomic Submarine, The Underwater City, The Bounty Killer, Requiem for a Gunfighter.
TV: Movie of the Year, Golden Century, Great Moments in Motion Pictures.

GORDON, BERT I.: Producer-director-writer. b. Kenosha, Wis., U. of Wisconsin, grad.
PICTURES INCLUDE: Beginning of the End, The Amazing Colossal Man, The Fantastic Puppet People, The Cyclops, The Spider, Tormented, Boy and The Pirates, The Magic Sword, Village of the Giants, Picture Mommy Dead, How to Succeed With the Opposite Sex, Necromancy, Geronimo, The Mad Bomber, The Police Connection, The Food of the Gods, The Coming, The Big Bet.

GORDON, BRUCE: Executive. b. Sidney, Australia, Feb. 4, 1929. Began career in Australian entertainment industry 1952 with Tivoli Circuit, live theatre chain; acted as advance man, front-of-house mgr., adv. dir.; promoted to busn. mgr., 1958. Named Tivoli membr. bd. of management, 1960–62. Joined Desilu Studios in 1962, developing Far East territories; promoted 1968 when Paramount acquired Desilu to mng. dir. Para. Far East opns. Named to bd. of TV Corp., 1969, operator of Channel 9 TV stns. & co.'s theatres in Sydney, Melbourne. Dir. on bd. of Academy Investments, operator of Perth theatre chain; responsible for building Perth Entertainment Centre. Named pres., Paramount TV Intl. Services, Ltd., 1974, in New York office.

GORDON, GALE: Actor. r.n. Charles T. Aldrich, Jr. b. New York City, Feb. 2, 1906. Stage debut in the Dancers; m.p. debut in The Pilgrimage Play, 1929.
PICTURES INCLUDE: Rally Round the Flag Boys, All in a Night's Work, Don't Give Up the Ship, Visit to a Small Planet, All Hands on Deck, Speedway.
TV: My Favorite Husband, Our Miss Brooks, The Brothers, Dennis The Menace, The Lucy Show, Here's Lucy.

GORDON, JACK: Executive. b. Brooklyn, N.Y., Mar. 13, 1929. e. UCLA. Father is Mack Gordon, songwriter. Started in industry as TV production asst. in 1949. Served in U.S. Infantry, Korea, 1951–52. Joined MGM in 1953; named dir. of non-theatrical div., 1956; v.p., MGM Intl., 1972. Appointed exec. v.p., MGM, Intl. 1979; sr. v.p., MGM/UA International Motion Pictures Distribution, 1981; pres., 1983.
Member: ASCAP, Motion Picture Pioneers, Academy of Motion Picture Arts & Sciences.

GORDON, LAWRENCE: Producer. b. Yazoo, Miss., March 25, 1936. e. Tulane Univ. First show business venture with TV producer Aaron Spelling on Burke's Law series, 1964. Joined ABC-TV as head of west coast talent development 1965, left to become v.p. of Screen Gems (now Columbia Pictures TV) where worked on developing new projects. Joined American Intl. Pictures as v.p. in chg. of world-wide production. Resigned to form his own company, Lawrence Gordon Productions, Inc. 1984, named pres., 20th Century-Fox m.p. prod. group.
PICTURES: Hard Times, Rolling Thunder, The Driver, The End, Hooper, Warriors, Xanadu, Paternity, 48 Hrs., Streets of Fire, Brewster's Millions.

GORDON, MICHAEL: Director. b. Baltimore, Md., Sept., 1909; e. Johns Hopkins Univ., B.A.; Yale, M.F.A. Stage experience as technician, stage mgr., actor, stage dir. (Stevedore, Home of the Brave, Anna Christie, One Bright Day; m.p. debut: dial. dir. Columbia on over 20 films; dir. in 1942. Professor of Theater Arts, UCLA.
PICTURES INCLUDE: Boston Blackie Goes Hollywood, Underground Agent, One Dangerous Night, The Crime Doctor, The Web, Another Part of the Forest, An Act of Murder, The Lady Gambles, Woman in Hiding, Cyrano de Bergerac, I Can Get It for You Wholesale, The Secret of Convict Lake, Any Way the Wind Blows, Pillow Talk, Portrait in Black, Boy's Night Out, For Love or Money, Move Over Darling, Texas Across the River, A Very Special Favor, The Impossible years, How Do I Love Thee?
OTHER PLAYS: Deadfall, The Lovers, Tender Trap, Male Animal, His & Hers, Champagne Complex, Home of the Brave, etc.

GORDON, RICHARD: Producer. b. London, Eng., Dec. 31, 1925; e. U. of London, 1943. Served in Brit. Royal Navy, 1944–46; ed. & writer on fan magazines & repr. independent American cos. 1946, with publicity dept. Assoc. Brit. Pathe 1947; org. export-import business for independent, British and American product; formed Gordon Films, Inc., 1949; formed Amalgamated prod., 1956; formed Grenadier Films, Ltd. 1971.

PICTURES INCLUDE: The Counterfeit Plan, The Haunted Strangler, Fiend Without a Face, The Secret Man, First Man into Space, Corridors of Blood, Devil Doll, Curse of Simba, The Projected Man, Naked Evil, Island of Terror; Tales of the Bizarre, Tower of Evil, Horror Hospital, The Cat and the Canary, Inseminoid.

GORDY, BERRY: Executive. Was working on auto assembly line in Detroit when decided to launch record co., Motown. In 1961 wrote song, Shop Around; recording by Smokey Robinson made it his first million dollar record. Expanded into music publishing, personal mgt., recording studios, film and TV, also backing stage shows. Now bd. chm., Motown Industries.
PICTURES INCLUDE: Lady Sings the Blues (prod.), Mahogany (dir.), Almost Summer, The Last Dragon (exec. prod.).

GORING, MARIUS: Actor. b. Newport, Isle of Wight. e. Cambridge & Universities of Frankfurt-on-Main, Munich, Vienna, Paris. Early career with Old Vic; stage debut 1927, Jean Sterling Rackinlay's Children's Matinees.
PICTURES INCLUDE: Rembrandt, UA-London Films. Dead Men Tell No Tales, Flying 55 Admiral Films, Consider Your Verdict, Spy in Black, Pastor Hall, The Case of the Fightened Lady, Br. Lion. 1940–46 serving with H. M. Forces & Foreign Office. In 1942, The Big Blockade, The Night Raider. In 1944, Lilli Marlene. Others: Stairway to Heaven, Night Boat to Dublin, Take My Life, Red Shoes, Mr. Perrin and Mr. Traill, Odette, Pandora and the Flying Dutchman, Circle of Danger, Highly Dangerous, So Little Time, The Man Who Watched Trains Go By, Rough Shoot, The Barefoot Contessa, Break in the Circle, Quentin Durward, Ill Met By Moonlight, The Moonraker, Family Doctor, Angry Hills, Whirlpool, Treasure of St. Teresa, Monty's Double, Beyond the Curtain, Desert Mice, The Inspector, Girl On a Motorcycle, Subterfuge.
TV: Numerous appearances, Sleeping Dog, Man In a Suitcase, Scarlet Pimpernel, The Expert.

GOROG, LASZLO: Writer. b. Hungary, Sept. 30, 1903. e. U. of Sciences, Budapest. Playwright, short story writer, asst. editor, Budapest, 1928–39.
PICTURES INCLUDE: Tales of Manhattan, The Affairs of Susan, She Wouldn't Say Yes, The Land Unknown, for U-I.
TV: 4 Star, Dupont, The Roaring Twenties, 77 Sunset Strip, Maverick, etc.

GORTNER, MARJOE: Actor—Producer. b. Long Beach, CA, Jan. 14, 1944. Was child evangelist, whose career as such was basis for documentary film, Marjoe (AA). Acted in films and TV; turned producer in 1978 for When You Comin' Back, Red Ryder.
PICTURES: Bobbie Joe and the Outlaw, The Food of the Gods, Viva Knievel, Sidewinder One, Earthquake, When You Comin' Back, Red Ryder, Mausoleum, Hellhole.
TELEVISION: Films: The Marcus-Nelson Murders, The Gun and the Pulpit, Pray for the Wildcats. Guest appearances on Police Story, Mayday: 40,900 Feet, etc.

GOSSET, LOUIS, JR.: Actor. b. brooklyn, NY, May 27, 1936. e. NYU (BS). On stage in Take a Giant Step, Lost in the Stars, Raisin in the Sun, Golden Boy, The Blacks, Blood Knot, etc.
PICTURES: The Landlord, River Niger, choirboys, The Deep, It Rained All Night the Day I Left, An Officer and a Gentleman (Oscar), Jaws 3-D, Finders Keepers, Enemy Mine, Iron Eagle.
TELEVISION: Movies: Campions in Nightmare, It's Good to Be Alive, Sidekicks, Delancey Street, Roots, Little Ladies of the Night, to Kill a Cop, The Critical List, Backstairs at the White House, This Man Stands Alone, Sadat, The Guardian.

GOTTLIEB, ALEX: Producer, writer. b. Dec. 21, 1906; e. U. of Wisconsin. Pub. Dir. Paramount theatre, New York; adv. mgr. United Artists, Columbia 1930–37; prod., W.B., Universal, RKO, 1941–50; then ind. prod. Member, ASCAP, WGA, Dramatists Guild, Academy of Motion Picture Arts and Sciences, Sigma Delta Chi, Pi Lambda Phi.
RADIO: Writer for Al Jolson, Eddie Cantor, Edgar Bergen, George Jessel.
TV: writer, prod., Dear Phoebe, The Gale Storm Show, The Tab Hunter Show, Bob Hope Chrysler Theatre, Donna Reed Show, The Smothers Brothers Show, ABC Movie of the Week.
PICTURES INCLUDE: I'll Take Sweden, Frankie and Johnny, Arizona Ranger, Blue Gardenia, Hellzapoppin, Macao, Susan Slept Here, Hollywood Canteen, Buck Privates.
AUTHOR OF B'WAY PLAYS: Wake Up Darling, Separate Rooms, Susan Slept Here, Stud, Your Place or Mine?, Divorce Me, Darling; Two for the Money, One Big Happy Family.
ONE-ACT PLAYS: Published in Best Short Plays of 1969, Best Short Plays of 1976, Best Short Plays of 1985.

GOTTLIEB, STAN: Actor, Film Distributor. b. N.Y.C. April 22, 1917. e. N.Y.U., Col. Univ. Has acted in films, theatrical, stage and TV since 1970. Gen. mgr. for Impact Films, Inc. 1966–72. Gen. Mgr., Mammoth Films (1973–76).
PICTURES INCLUDE: Actor: Putney Swope, You Gotta Walk It Like You Talk It, The Owl and the Pussycat, Pound, The Anderson Tapes, Cold Turkey, Slaughterhouse Five, Black Fantasy, Greaser's Place, Compliments to the World.
TV: Actor: Sticks & Bones, Hot L Baltimore, The Jeffersons.
STAGE: Steambath.

GOUGH, MICHAEL: Actor. b. Malaya, Nov. 23, 1917. e. Rose Hill School in Kent, England, and at Durham School. Studied at Old Vic School in London; first stage appearance in 1936 at Old Vic Theatre. N.Y. stage debut 1937 in Love of Women. London debut in 1938 in The Zeal of They House. M.P. debut in 1948 in Blanche Fury; since in over 50 films.
PICTURES INCLUDE: Anna Karenina, The Man in the White Suit, Rob Roy, The Sword and the Rose, Richard III, Reach for the Sky, Horror of Dracula, The Horse's Mouth, Konga, Mr. Topaze, The Phantom of the Opera, The Skull, Women in Love, Julius Caesar, Trog, The Go-Between, Henry VIII and His Six Wives, Savage Messiah, The Legend of Hell House, The Boys from Brazil, The Dresser, Top Secret!
TELEVISION INCLUDES: Smiley's People, To the Lighthouse, The Citadel, etc.

GOULD, ELLIOTT: Actor. b. Brooklyn, N.Y., August 29, 1938. Broadway debut in Rumple.
STAGE: Say Darling, Irma La Douce, I Can Get It For You Wholesale, On the Town (London), Fantasticks (tour), Drat the Cat, Little Murders, Luv (tour), A Way of Life.
TV: Once Upon A Mattress. Movie: Vanishing Act.
PICTURES INCLUDE: The Night They Raided Minsky's, Bob & Carol & Ted & Alice, M*A*S*H, Getting Straight, Move, Little Murders, The Touch, I Love My Wife, The Long Goodbye, Busting, S*P*Y*S!*, California Split, Who?, Nashville, (guest), Whiffs, I Will . . . I Will . . . For Now, Harry and Walter Go to New York, A Bridge Too Far, Capricorn One, Matilda, Escape to Athena, The Last Flight of Noah's Ark, The Devil and Max Devlin, Dirty Tricks, The Naked Face.

GOULD, JON J.: Executive. e. New England College, Harvard Graduate Program in Publishing. In 1977 joined Straight Arrow Publishers as east coast sales mgr. for publications, Rolling Stone and Outside. In 1978 left for post at Paramount Pictures in m.p. div. as dir. of mktg. admin. for mktg. group. 1979, appt. exec. asst. to Frank G. Mancuso, then exec. v.p., dist. & mktg. In 1980 named v.p., corporate communications, for Paramount.

GOULD, JOSEPH: Executive. b. New York, N.Y. Jan. 30, 1915. e. B.A., New York U., 1935; M.S., Pulitzer School of Journ., Columbia U., 1936. Adv. dept., United Artists, 1939–46; Universal, 1947–48; asst. adv. mgr. 20th Century-Fox. 1949–52; adv. consultant, Joseph Burstyn. Louis De Rochemont Assoc., I.F.E. Releasing Corp. 1953–55; adv. mgr. United Artists, 1955–60; adv. mgr. Paramount Pictures, 1960–62; David Singer Associates, 1962–64; partner, Konheim Gould & Ackerman, 1968–74; principal, Joseph Gould Associates, 1974–77; creative services director, WIXT-TV, Syracuse, 1978–82; Joseph Gould Associates, Falls Church, Va., 1982–84; Center for Defense Information, Public Affairs, Washington, D.C., 1984–.

GOULET, ROBERT: Singer, actor. b. Lawrence, Mass., Nov. 26, 1933. e. attended school, Edmonton; scholarship, Royal Conservatory of Music. Sang in choirs, appeared with numerous orchestras; disk jockey, CKUA, Edmonton; pub. rel., The Merrick Co.
STAGE: Camelot, The Happy Time.
TV: The Ed Sullivan Show, Garry Moore, The Enchanted Nutcracker, Omnibus, The Broadway of Lerner and Loewe, Rainbow of Stars, Judy Garland Show, Bob Hope Show, The Bell Telephone Hour; England: Granada—TV special, Jack Benny; Dean Martin; Andy Williams; Jack Paar; Red Skelton; Hollywood Palace; Patty Duke Show, Star of Robert Goulet Show, Blue Light series for ABC-TV, Brigadoon & Carousel for ABC-TV. Kiss Me Kate.
PICTURES INCLUDE: Honeymoon Hotel, I'd Rather Be Rich, I Deal in Danger, Underground.
RECORDS: Always You, Two of Us, Sincerely Yours, The Wonderful World of Love, Robert Goulet in Person, This Christmas I Spend With You, Manhattan Tower, Without You, My Love Forgive Me, Travelling On, Robert Goulet on Tour, Robert Goulet on Broadway, Robert Goulet on Broadway II, Camelot, Happy Time.

GOWDY, CURT: Sportscaster. b. Green River, Wyoming, 1919. Basketball star at U. of Wyoming. All-Conference member; graduated U. of Wyoming. 1942; officer in U.S. Air Force WWII, then became sportscaster. Voted Sportscaster of the Year, 1967, Nat'l Assn. of Sportwriters Broadcasters. Best Sportscaster, FAME, 1967. Sports staff at NBC; American Sportsman, ABC. Won Peabody Award 1975. Host of The Way It Was on PSS.

GRADE, LORD: Chmn. & Chief exec., Embassy Communication Intl. Ltd.

GRADUS, BEN: Producer-Director-Writer. b. N.Y.C. e. Brooklyn Coll. Is principal in Directors Group Motion Pictures, Inc. Positions held include v.p. Filmways, Inc.; prod.-dir. for Screen Gems. Specialist in educational and doc. films; also has done feature, children's comedy TV shows and series, Decision: The Conflicts of Harry S. Truman. Author, Directing the Television Commercial. Nominee for Emmy, Grammy.
CREDITS INCLUDE: Dawn over Ecuador, Gentlemen of the Jury, To Save Your Life, Lifewatch Six, Ford Around the World, Art Heritage, A Girl from Puerto Rico, Span of Life, Crowded Paradise.

GRAF, BILLY: Executive. b. 1945. Entered industry 1965. Was asst. dir.; unit/location mgr./production mgr. for American, British and European companies.
PICTURES: Alfie, A Man for All Seasons, Billion Dollar Brain, Scrooge, Run Wild Run Free, The Best House in London, Chitty Chitty Bang Bang, Galaxina, Khartoum, You Only Live Twice, Women in Love, Song of Norway, Prudence and the Pill, Hammerhead, Underground Aces.
TELEVISION: Secret Agent, The Saint, "Q" Branch, Private Eye Public Ear, The Avengers, Department "S", The Dave Cash Radio Show.

GRAF, WILLIAM N.: Executive. b. New York City. Entered industry in 1934. 1937–42, exec. secty./asst. to Mark Hellinger at Warner Bros. & 20th-Fox. 1942–45, writer of armed forces training films. 1946–50, exec. secty./asst. to Harry Cohn, pres., Columbia Pictures; 1951, prod. asst. to Jack Fier, prod. head, Columbia. 1952–65, Amer. repr. for British productions, Columbia Pictures; 1965–66, exec. asst. to J. J. Frankovich, Columbia Pictures, London; 1965–66, v.p., Columbia Pictures Intl., London; 1969–70, indep. prod., Cinema Center Films; 1980, v.p. in chg. of prod., Legion Films, Inc., Beverly Hills; 1984, pres., Billy Graf Prods.
PICTURES: (Producer): The Red Beret, A Man for All Seasons, Sinful Davey, The African Elephant.

GRAFF, RICHARD B.: Executive. b. Milwaukee, WI, Nov. 9; e. U. of Illinois; served U.S. Air Force; Universal Pictures 1956 to 1964 in Chicago, Detroit, Chicago and New York home office as Asst. to genl. sales manager; 1964 went to National General in Los Angeles. In 1967 became v.p. and general sales mgr. of National General Pictures and formed and operated company. 1968, exec. v.p. in charge of world-wide sales and marketing. 1968 v.p. of parent company; v.p. general sales mgr. AIP in 1971; 1975, pres. Cine Artists Pictures; pres. The Richard Graff Company Inc 1977; pres., Domestic distribution, MGM/UA June 1983.

GRAFF, ROBERT D.: Producer. b. New York City 1919. Early career 1951–60 with National Broadcasting Co. and consultant to m.p. and t.v. orgs. in Iran, Venezuela, U.S.A. Formed Sextant Inc., 1960. Sextant Films Ltd., 1963.
PICTURES INCLUDE: Young Cassidy.

GRANET, BERT: Producer, writer. b. New York City, July 10, 1910; e. Yale U., Sch. Fine Arts (47 Workshop). From 1936 author s.p. orig. & adapt. numerous pictures. Exec. prod.: Universal, 1967–69, CBS, Desilu Studios.
PICTURES INCLUDE: Quick Money, The Affairs of Annabel, Mr. Doodle Kicks Off, Laddie, A Girl a Guy and a Gob, My Favorite Wife, Bride by Mistake, Sing Your Way Home, Those Endearing Young Charms, The Locket, Do You Love Me?, The Marrying Kind, Berlin Express, The Torch, Scarface, Mob.
TV: Desilu (1957–61), Twilight Zone, The Mob, The Untouchables Pilot, Scarface Mob; Loretta Young Show (1955–56), Walter Winchell File 1956–57, Lucille Ball-Desi Arnaz Show 1957–60, Westinghouse Desilu Playhouse, The Great Adventure.

GRANGER, FARLEY: Actor. b. San Jose, Calif., July 1, 1925; e. Hollywood. School prior to m.p. career; screen debut in North Star 1943; in U.S. Armed Forces 1944–46.
PICTURES INCLUDE: They Live by Night, Rope, Enchantment, Roseanna McCoy, Side Street, Our Very Own, Edge of Doom, Strangers on a Train, Behave Yourself, I Want You, O. Henry's Full House, Hans Christian Andersen, Story of Three Loves, Small Town Girl, Summer Hurricane, Brass Ring, Naked Street, Girl in the Red Velvet Swing, Arrow Smith, The Heiress, The Prisoner of Zenda, Senso, The Serpent, A Man Called Noon, Those Days in the Sun, The Chief of Homicide, The Painter and the Red Head, Call Me Trinity, The Syndicate, Arnold, A Crime for a Crime, The Imagemaker.
TV: Playhouse of Stars, U.S. Steel Hour, Producer's Showcase, Climax, Ford Theatre, Playhouse 90, 20th Century Fox Hour, Robert Montgomery Presents, Arthur Murray Dance Party, Wagon Train, Masquerade Party, Kojak, 6 Million Dollar Man, Ellery Queen, 9 Lives of Jenny Dolan, Widow, National Repertory Co., One Life To Live, As the World Turns.

GRANGER, STEWART: Actor. r.n. James Stewart. b. May 6, 1913; e. medicine; Webber-Douglas Sch. of Acting, London. m. Jean Simmons, actress. In Brit. Army, World War II. On stage from 1935, Hull Repertory theat.; Birmingham Repertory; Malvery Festivals (1936–37); Old Vic Co. Screen debut 1940 in So This Is Voted one of Brit. top ten money-making stars in M.P. Herald-Fame Poll, 1945, 1946, 1947, 1949.
PICTURES INCLUDE: Convoy, Secret Mission, Thursday's Child, Man in Grey, The Lamp Still Burns, Fanny by Gaslight, Love Story, Waterloo-Road, Madonna of the Seven Moons, Caesar and Cleopatra, Caravan, Magic Bow, Captain Boycott, Blanche Fury, Saraband for Dead Lovers, Woman Hater, Adam and Evalyn, King Solomon's Mines, Soldiers Three, Light Touch, Wild North, Scaramouche, Prisoner of Zenda, Salome, Young Bess, All the Brothers Were Valiant, Beau Brummell, Green Fire, Moonfleet, Deadlock, Bhowani Junction, Last Hunt, Footsteps in the Fog, The Little Hut, Gun Glory, The Secret Invasion, Flaming Frontier, The Trygon Factor, The Last Safari, The Wild Geese.

GRANT, CARY: Actor. r.n. Archibald Alexander Leach. b. Briston, England, Jan. 18, 1904. On dram. stage in England, then to U.S. and appeared with St. Louis (Mo.) Municipal Opera Co. a season. Screen debut 1932 in Paramount prod. This is the Night. Voted one of the ten best Money-Making Stars in M.P. Herald-Fame Poll 1944, 1949.
PICTURES INCLUDE: Gambling Ship, Alice in Wonderland, Sylvia Scarlett, Suzy, Holiday, Gunga Din, The Philadelphia Story, The Howards of Virginia, Penny Serenade, Suspicion, Once Upon a Honeymoon, Mr. Lucky, Destination Tokyo, Once Upon a Time, None But the Lonely Heart, Arsenic and Old Lace, Bachelor and the Bobby Soxer, The Bishop's Wife, Every Girl Should Be Married, Mr. Blandings Builds His Dream House, I Was a Male War Bride, Crisis, People Will Talk, Room for One More, Monkey Business, Dream Wife, To Catch A Thief, The Pride and the Passion, An Affair to Remember, Kiss Them for Me, Houseboat, North by Northwest, Operation Petticoat, The Grass is Greener, That Touch of Mink, Charade, Father Goose, Walk Don't Run.

GRANT, LEE: Actress. b. New York City, Oct. 31, 1931. At 4 was member of Metropolitan Opera Company; played princess in L'Orocolo. Member of the American Ballet at 11. e. Juilliard School of Music, studied voice, violin and dance. At 18 with road co. Oklahoma as understudy. Acting debut: Joy To The World.
THEATRE: acted in a series of one-acters at ANTA with Henry Fonda. 1949, played shoplifter in The Detective Story (won Critics Circle Award); Lo and Behold, A Hole in the Head, Wedding Breakfast; road co. Two for the Seesaw, The Captains and the Kings; toured with Electra, Silk Stockings, St. Joan, Arms and the Man, The Maids (Obie Award), Prisoner of Second Avenue.
TV: Studio One, The Kraft Theatre, Slattery's People, The Fugitive, Ben Casey, The Nurses, The Defenders, East Side/West Side, Peyton Place (Emmy Award, Best Supporting Player, 1966), Bob Hope Show (Emmy nom.), The Love Song of Bernard Kempenski, BBC's The Respectful Prostitute, The Neon Ceilings (Emmy Award), Fay (series), The Spell (movie). Mussolini - The Untold Story (mini-series) Director: Nobody's Child (movie).
PICTURES INCLUDE: The Detective Story, Terror in the Streets, Affair of the Skin, The Balcony, Divorce American Style, Valley of the Dolls, In the Heat of the Night, Buona Sera, Mrs. Campbell, The Big Bounce, Marooned, The Landlord, There Was a Crooked Man, Plaza Suite, Portnoy's Complaint, Shampoo, Voyage of the Damned, Airport '77, When You Comin' Back, Red Ryder, Charlie Chan and the Curse of the Dragon Queen, Teachers.

GRANVILLE, BONITA: Actress-Producer. b. New York City, Feb. 2, 1923. Child actress of the '30s before turning producer in the '50s with Lassie series on TV. Produced two features on Lassie: Greatest Adventure (1963) and The Magic of Lassie (1980).
PICTURES INCLUDE: Cradle Song, These Three, Maid of Salem, Call It a Day, Nancy Drew Detective, Escape, Glass Key, Now, Voyager, Hitler's Children, Youth Runs Wild, Love Laughs at Andy Hardy, Treason, The Lone Ranger, etc.

GRASGREEN, MARTIN: Executive. b. New York City, July 1, 1925. Entered m.p. ind. Jan., 1944, Columbia Pictures h.o. in contract dept. Promoted to travelling auditor April, 1946. Appt. office mgr. Omaha branch Dec., 1948; salesman Omaha, Dec., 1950. Transferred to Indianapolis, 1952, as city salesman; transferred to Cleveland as sales mgr., 1953. Left Columbia in 1960 to become 20th-Fox branch mgr. in Cleveland. Transferred to Philadelphia in 1965 as branch mgr.; transferred to N.Y. in 1967 as Eastern dist. mgr. Resigned in 1970 to form Paragon Pictures, prod.-dist. co. In Jan., 1975, formed Lanira Releasing Corp., representing producers for U.S. and Latin American sales and dist. of films in U.S., Canada.

GRASSHOFF, ALEX: Writer, producer, director. b. Boston, Mass. e. Tufts Coll., and U. of Southern Calif., 3 Academy Award nominations for feature documentaries; 1974, Journey to the Outer Limits; 1966, Really Big Family; 1968, Young Americans won Oscar; Future Shock: 1973 Cannes Film Festival. T.V. Series (Dir.): The Rockford Files, Chips, Night Stalker. 1982, The Wave (Emmy).

GRAVES, PETER: Actor. b. London, Oct. 21, 1911: e. Harrow. With Knight, Frank & Rutley, then Lloyds prior to theat. career. First stage appearance 1934 in Charles B. Cochran's Streamline.

THEATRE: Novello musicals at Drury Lane; repertory at Windsor, Old Chelsea, The Merry Widow, The Sound of Music, Private Lives. Recent: The Reluctant Peer, The Last of Mrs. Cheyney, Dear Charles, An Ideal Husband (S. Africa), A Boston Story (tour), His, Hers, and Theirs, The Great Waltz, No Sex Please We're British.

PICTURES INCLUDE: Mrs. Fitzherbert, Spring in Park Lane, Maytime in Mayfair, Lady With a Lamp, Encore, Derby Day (Four Against Fate), Lilacs in the Spring (Let's Make Up), Admirable Crichton, Alfie, The Wrong Box, The Jokers, I'll Never Forget What's Is Name, How I Won the War, Assassination Bureau,The Adventurers, The Slipper and the Rose.

TV: Those Wonderful Snows, Chelsea at 9, One O'Clock Show, Lunch Box, 2 Cars, Dickie Henderson Show, Ivor Novello Series, East Lynne, Ninety Years On, The Sleeping Doe, The Frobisher Game, The Jazz Age series, Kate series, Crown Court, Softly, Softly, 10 from the 20s. Quiller, Duchess of Duke Street, Looks Familiar.

GRAVES, PETER: Actor, b. Minneapolis, Minn., March 18, 1926. brother, James Arness, e. U. of Minn. Played with bands, radio announcer, while at school; U.S. Air Force 2 yrs.; summer stock appearances; m.p. debut in Rogue River.

PICTURES INCLUDE: Fort Defiance, Stalag 17, East of Sumatra, Beneath the 12-Mile Reef, The Raid, Black Tuesday, Wichita, Long Gray Line, Night of the Hunter, Naked Street, Fort Yuma, Court Martial of Billy Mitchell, The Ballad of Josie, Sergeant Ryker, The Five Man Army, Sidecar Racers, Airplane!, Airplane II: The Sequel.

TV: Fury, 1955–58, Mission Impossible, 1967–73.

GRAY, COLEEN: Actress. r.n. Doris Jensen. b. Staplehurst, Neb., Oct. 23, 1922; e. Hamline U., B.A. summa cum laude, 1943, Actor's Lab.: m. Fritz Zeiser. Member: Nat'l Collegiate Players, Kappa Phi, a Capella choir, little theatres, 1943–44; screen debut State Fair, 1945.

PICTURES INCLUDE: Kiss of Death, Nightmare Alley, Fury at Furnace Creek, Red River, Sleeping City, Riding High, Father Is a Bachelor, Models Inc., Kansas City Confidential, Sabre Jet, Arrow in the Dust, The Fake, The Vanquished, Las Vegas Shakedown, Twinkle in God's Eye, Tennessee's Partner, The Killing, Wild Dakotas, Death of a Scoundrel, Frontier Gambler, Black Whip, Star in the Dust, The Vampires, Hell's Five Hours, Copper Sky, Johnny Rocco, The Leech Woman, The Phantom Planet, Town Tamer, P.J., The Late Liz, Cry from the Mountain.

TV: Days of Our Lives, NBC-TV, 1966–67. Family Affair, Ironside, Bonanza, Judd for the Defense, Name of the Game, Bright Promise, The FBI, The Bold Ones, World Premiere, Mannix, Sixth Sense, McCloud, The Best Place To Be, Tales from the Dark Side.

GRAY, DULCIE: C.B.E. Actress b. Malaya, Nov. 20; e. Webber Douglas Sch., London Stage debut 1939, Aberdeen, Hay Fever, Author: Love Affair (play), 18 detective novels, book of short stories. 8 radio plays; co-author with husband Michael Denison, An Actor and His World; Butterflies on My Mind, The Glanville Women, Anna Starr.

STAGE: 40 West End plays including Little Foxes, Brighton Rock, Dear Ruth, Rain on the Just, Candida, An Ideal Husband, Where Angels Fear to Tread, Heartbreak House, On Approval, Happy Family, No. 10, Out of the Question, Village Wooing, Wild Duck, At The End of the Day, The Pay Off, A Murder Has Been Announced, Bedroom Farce, A Coat of Varnish, School for Scandal.

PICTURES INCLUDE: Two Thousand Women, A Man About the House, Mine Own Executioner, My Brother Jonathan, The Glass Mountain, They Were Sisters Wanted for Murder, The Franchise Affair, Angels One Five, There Was a Young Lady, A Man Could Get Killed, The Trail of the Pink Panther, The Curse of the Pink Panther.

TV: Milestones, The Will, Crime Passionel, Art and Opportunity, Fish in the Family, The Governess, What the Public Wants, Lesson in Love, The Happy McBaines, Winter Cruise, The Letter, Tribute to Maugham, Virtue, Beautiful Forever, East Lynne, Unexpectedly Vacant, The Importance of Being Earnest, This Is Your Life, Crown Court, Making Faces, Read All About It, The Voysey Inheritance, Life After Death, The Pink Pearl, Britain in the Thirties, Rumpole (The Old Boy Net.), Cold Warrior, Hook Line & Sinker, Howard's Way, 1985–86.

GRAY, GORDON: Broadcast Management Consultant. b. Albert Lea, Minn., Nov. 16, 1905; e. U. of Missouri. Entered broadcasting ind. 1932, v.p., gen. mgr., WOR, WOR TV; pres. WKTV, Utica, N.Y., KAUZ, Wichita Falls, Tex. Founded Central N.Y. Cable, Utica, N.Y. Chm., Board of Governors, WFTV, Orlando, Fla. and management consultant, presently.

GRAY, VERNON: Actor b. Saskatoon, Canada, e. Elk Point. Early career engineering plant; repertory Canada and America; studied Irving School of the Theatre; in Britain for more repertory; London stage, Stalag 17; screen debut: A Day to Remember.

PICTURES INCLUDE: To Paris With Love, Now and Forever, Barretts of Wimpole Street.

GRAYSON, KATHRYN: Actress. r.n. Zelma Hedrick; b. Winston-Salem, N.C. Feb. 9, 1923. e. St. Louis schools. Singer. Screen debut; Andy Hardy's Private Secretary, 1940; The Vanishing Virginian, Rio Rita, Seven Sweethearts,Thousands Cheer; achieved stardom in Anchors Aweigh, 1945.

PICTURES INCLUDE: Ziegfeld Follies of 1946, Two Sisters from Boston, Showboat, That Midnight Kiss, Grounds For Marriage, The Toast of New Orleans, The Kissing Bandit, Lovely To Look At, Desert Song, So This Is Love, Kiss Me Kate, Vagabond King.

TV: GE Theatre, Emmy Nomination, 1960; Die Fledermaus, ABC, '66.

STAGE: Debut in N.Y. and tour, Camelot, 1963; Rosalinda, Merry Widow, Kiss Me Kate, Showboat, (N.Y. and U.S. tour).

GREEN, ADOLPH: Writer. b. New York City, Dec. 2, 1915. Wrote book, sketches & lyrics for many Broadway shows including: On the Town, Billion Dollar Baby, Two on the Aisle, Wonderful Town, Peter Pan (Mary Martin), Bells Are Ringing, Applause (Tony Award).

PICTURES INCLUDE: Good News, On the Town, Barkleys of Broadway, Take Me Out to the Ball Game, Singin' in the Rain, Band Wagon, It's Always Fair Weather, Auntie Mame; all in collab. with Betty Comden.

GREEN, GUY: Director. b. Somerset, Eng. 1913. Joined Film Advertising Co. as projectionist & camera asst. 1933; camera asst., Elstree Studios (BIP) 1935; started as camera operator on films including One of Our Aircraft Is Missing, In Which We Serve, This Happy Breed. 1944: Director of Photography; Dir of Allied Film Makers Ltd.

PICTURES INCLUDE: The Way Ahead, Great Expectations, Oliver Twist, Captain Horatio Hornblower, I Am A Camera, River Beat, Tears For Simon, House of Secrets, Sea of Sand, The Angry Silence, The Mark, Light In The Piazza, Diamond Head, A Patch of Blue, Pretty Polly, A Matter of Innocence, The Magus, A Walk in the Spring Rain, Luther, Once Is Not Enough, The Devil's Advocate.

GREEN, JANET: Actress, screen writer. b. Hertfordshire, England, 1914. Early career as actress; Wrote first play, 1945; Ent. m.p. ind. 1947, wrote orig. s.p., The Clouded Yellow; further orig. s.p. incl. The Good Beginning, Lost Eye Witness, The Long Arm (in coll.), The Fever Tree, Sapphire, Cast a Dark Shadow, Midnight Lace, Gathering of Eagles, Ashenden, Victim, Life for Ruth, Christobel; Show Me A Murderer, Walk in the Shadow, Seven Women, The Golden Keel, It Happened in Havana, My Turn Now, Gutsy, The Sweetest Voice in the World (USA), The Fox is Female, Little Individual.

GREEN, JOHN, (JOHNNY): Composer-Music Director-Conductor Arranger-Pianist. b. New York City, Oct. 10, 1908; e. Horace Mann School, Harvard U., 1928, A.B. Entered m.p. industry as rehearsal pianist. Paramount Astoria, N.Y.; composer-conductor 1930–32. Conductor, Paramount-Publix Theatres, 1930–33. Name band leader, 1933–40. Made numerous shorts, appeared on many TC commercial radio programs. Composer of songs: Coquette, I'm Yours, Out of Nowhere, I Cover the Waterfront, Song of Raintree County, Body and Soul, Easy Come, Easy Go, I Wanna Be Loved etc.; also symphonic works performed by major orchestra U.S. and abroad; Symphony, Mine Eyes Have Seen, 1978 Joined MGM, composer-conductor, 1942–46; Univ. Internat'l. 1947; returned to MGM for Easter Parade (Acad. Award, scoring of musical); Warner 1948–49. Inspector General (Golden Globe Award 1949, best score of year). Apptd. gen. music dir. and exec-in-chg-of-music MGM 1949; produced shorts series MGM Concert Hall (Acad. Award, best one reel short 1953); Acad. Award, best scoring of musical, American in Paris 1951; composed score Raintree County (Acad. Nom. 1957): left MGM to freelance 1958. Prod. Desilu 1958–59. Comp. many original scores. V.p., Academy M.P. Arts and Sciences, 1953–55; chmn. Music Br. several terms: Acad. Life Member; prod. Acad.'s first Award Show TV, 1953. Acad. Award, best scoring of musical, West Side Story, 1961, nominated for Acad. Award, 14 times. Other films incl. High Society, Bye Bye Birdie, The Great Caruso, etc. Music dir. film, Oliver, won Acad. Award, 1968. Assoc. prod. They Shoot Horses, Don't They? (Acad. Award nomination, best music score). Pres. Screen Comp. Assoc., U.S.A. 1966–72; Member Bd of Governors Performing Arts Council L.A. Music Center, 1965–71; Chmn. bd. Emeritus, Young Musicians Foundation since 1965. Pres., Young Musicians Foundation 1973–77; Since 1949, guest conductor, many U.S. orchestras; 1983–31st. season Hollywood Bowl; co-chairman, music branch and v.p., Academy of Motion Picture Arts and Sciences, 1973–77; Music Branch Exec. Committee, 1980; 1981, ASCAP board; 1985, asst. secty.

GREEN, JOSEPH: Executive. b. Warsaw, Poland, Apr. 23, 1905. e. high school, prep school. Industry, legitimate theatre prod. Foreign film dist. since 1933; headed Green Film Co., Warsaw, Poland; head of Sphinx Film Dist. Co., N.Y., until 1940. co-owner, Art Theatre Circuit, N.Y., 1940–52; pres., Globe Dist. Co. of Foreign Films; formed President Films, Inc., 1954, now Globe Pictures, Inc. Beginning in 1979 a renaissance of Josoeph Green's Yiddish film Classics produced in Pland in pre-World War II days, including Yiddle with He's Fiddle, Abriele der Mamen, Der Purinspieler, Mamele.

GREEN, MALCOLM C.: theatre Executive. b. Boston, Mar. 1, 1925. e. Harvard Coll. Began career as asst. mgr., Translux Theatre, Boston & Revere Theatre, Revere, MA. Treas., Interstate Theatres, 1959-64. Film Buyer, Interstate, 1959–72. Formed Theatre Management Services in 1972 with H. Rifkin and P. Lowe and Cinema Centers Corp. with Rifkin and Lowe families in 1973. Currently operating 116 theatres in six northeast states. Now treas., Cinema Center, & pres., Theatre Mgmt. Services.
Pres., Theatre Owners of New England, 1964–65; chmn bd., 1955–69; treas., 1970–84. Dir., Natl. Assoc. Theatre Owners. Chm., NATO of New York State. Chmn., Vision Foundation.

GREEN, MICHAEL L.: Executive-chm. Entertainment Film Distributors Ltd., chm. Entertainment in Video Ltd., chm. Michael Green Enterprises Ltd., mng. dir., Blackwater Film Productions Ltd.

GREEN, NATHANIEL CHARLES: Executive (Retired) b. Spokane, Wash. Feb. 16, 1903. e. Pleasant Prairie School until 14 yrs. of age; ent. banking bus., Spokane & Eastern Trust Co., until 1921; came to Calif., became associated Bank of America. Br. bank mgr., 26 yrs. of age, youngset in the U.S. at the time; became vice-pres., 1941; Jan. 1960 became v.p., and senior pub rel. officer between bank and m.p. and TV industry.

GREENE, CLARENCE: Producer, writer. b. New York City. e. St. John's Univ. (L.L.B.); author of play Need a Lawyer. Formed Greene-Rouse prods. with Russell Rouse; Acad. Oscar co-orig. story Pillow Talk. Acad. award nom. co-orig. s.p. The Well. Two Writers Guild nominations. Writers Guild award outstanding teleplay, One Day in the Life of Ivan Deni sovitch.
PICTURES INCLUDE: Prod., collab. s.p. The Town Went Wild, D.O.A., The Well, The Thief, Wicked Woman, New York Confidential, A House Is Not a Home, The Oscar. Prod. Unidentified Flying Objects, The Gun Runners, Fastest Gun Alive, Thunder in the Sun, The Caper of the Golden Bulls. collab. prod., writer TV series Tightrope.

GREENE, DAVID: Director, Writer. Early career as actor. To U.S. with Shakespeare company early 1950's; remained direct TV in Canada, New York and Hollywood.
TV: The Defenders. Emmy Awds. The People Next Door, Rich Man, Poor Man, Roots, Friendly Fire, The Guardian, Fatal Vision, Guilty Conscience.
PICTURES INCLUDE: The Shuttered Room, Sebastian, The Strange Affair, I Start Counting, Madame Sin, Godspell, Count of Monte Cristo, Gray Lady Down, Hard Country.

GREENE, LORNE: Actor. b. Ottawa, Can., Feb. 12, 1915. e. Queene's University, where began acting and directing plays. Entered radio and became chief announcer for Canadian Broadcasting Corp. and chief news broadcaster. Following World War II service returned to Canadian radio. Came to N.Y. and appeared in TV production and Broadway plays. Went to Hollywood for films and gained biggest fame as Ben Cartwright in Bonanza series started in Sept., 1959.
PICTURES INCLUDE: The Silver Chalice, Autumn Leaves, The Gift of Love, The Buccaneer, etc. 1974: Earthquake. 1975: Tidal Wave.
TV: Destiny of a Spy, The Harness (films), Lorne Greene's American West, Christmas Special with UNs Children's Chorus, Lewis and Clark Expedition, Big Cats, Little Cats, Wonderful World of Horses, Swing Out Sweet Land, Andy Williams Show, Johnny Cash Show, Sonny and Cher Show, Clebration, The Barnum & Bailey NBC-TV Special, Roots, Battlestar Galactica, The Bastard.

GREENFIELD, IRVING H.: b. Nov. 15, 1902; e. Brooklyn Law School. Formerly president, Cinema Lodge, B'nai B'rith. Former sec'y, attorney, Metro-Goldwyn-Mayer, Inc. and Key chairman M.P. Amusement Div. of U.J.A. Federation. Engaged in law practice: Greenfield, Lipsky, and Bress.

GREENFIELD, LEO: Executive, b. N. Y. C., Education: St. John's Univ, college Arts & Sciences; v.p., gen. sales mgr. Buena Vista, 1962; Columbia road show sales mgr. 1966; v.p.-gen. sales mgr., Cinerama Rel. Corp. 1966; pres.-gen. sales mgr., Warners, 1969; sr. v.p. worldwide distribution, MGM 1975; v.p. distribution & marketing, Marble Arch Productions, 1978; exec. v.p. Associated Film Distribution, 1979; pres., Greenlee Assoc., Inc., 1985.

GREENWALD, ROBERT: Director-Producer-Teacher. b. New York City, Aug. 8, 1945. e. Antioch Coll., New School for Social Research. Teaches Film and theatre at New York Univ., New Lincoln, New School.
TELEVISION: Director: In the Custody of Strangers, Burning Bed, Mistress.
STAGE: A Sense of Humor, I Have a Dream, Me and Bessie.

GREENWOOD, JACK: Producer. b. 1919.
PICTURES INCLUDE: Horrors of the Black Museum, Concrete Jungle, Invasion, Act of Murder, We Shall See, Face of A Stranger. Also prod. Scotland Yard, The Scales of Justice and the Edgar Wallace series, Avengers series, 1967–68.
TV: From a Bird's Eye View, TV series with Sheldon Leonard 1969 for NBC. Prod. exec. with ATV Network (ITC) since 1970.

GREENWOOD, JOAN: Actress. b. Chelsea, London, Eng. Mar. 4, 1921. e. St. Catherines, Bramley, Surrey, Royal Academy Dramatic Art. Stage debut: Le Malade Imaginaire, London; in other London plays & repertory.
PICTURES INCLUDE: The Gentle Sex, They Knew Mr. Knight, Latin Quarter, Girl In a Million, The Man Within, The October Man, The White Unicorn, Saraband for Dead Lovers, Bad Lord Byron, Whiskey Galore, Kind Hearts & Coronets, Train of Events, Flesh & Blood, Young Wives' Tale, Mr. Peek-A-Boo, Man in the White Suit, Importance of Being Earnest, Father Brown (The Detective), Knave of Hearts (Lovers, Happy Lovers), Moonfleet, Stage Struck, Mysterious Island Pawn, The Amorous Pawn, Tom Jones, The Moonshiners, Boy Stroke Girl, Water Babies, The Uneasy, Hound of the Baskervilles.
THEATRE: N.Y. Stage, Confidential Clerk 1954, Those That Play the Clowns. London Stage, Moon & the Chimney, Bell Book and Candle, Doll's House, Grass is Greener, Hedda Gabler, Irregular Verb to Love, Au Pair, Chalk Garden, Eden End, In Praise of Love, The Understanding.
TV: Doll's House, Confidential Clerk, King and Mrs. Candle, Man and Superman, Fat of the Land, Good King Charles, Golden Days, Love is the Flame, Love Among the Artists, Wainwright's Law, Bognor, The Best of Friends, Country, Triangle, Wagner, Strangers and Brothers, One by One, Girls on Top, Caring, Little Dorrit.

GREER, JANE: Actress. b. Washington, D.C., Sept. 9, 1924. Orchestra singer; photograph as WAC on Life Magazine cover won screen debut in Pan-Americana 1945.
PICTURES INCLUDE: They Won't Believe Me, Out of the Past, Station West, Big Steal, You're in the Navy Now, The Company She Keeps, You For Me, Prisoner of Zenda, Desperate Search, The Clown, Down Among the Sheltering Palms, Run for the Sun, Man of a Thousand Faces, Where Love Has Gone, Billie, The Outfit, Against All Odds, Just Between Friends.

GREGORY, JOHN R.: Executive, producer, writer. b. Bklyn, N.Y., Nov. 19, 1918. e. Grover Cleveland H.S., 1935, New Institute of M.P. & Telev; Sls., adv. dept. Fotoshop, Inc., N.Y., 1938–42; Spec. Serv., Photo. instructor, chief projecionist, supv., war dept. theatres, U.S. Army, 1942–46; sls. mgr., J. L. Galef & Son, N.Y.; 1948–49, gen. mgr., Camera Corner Co.; 1949–58, pres.; City Film Center, Inc., 1957; exec. v.p., Talent Guild of New York, 1958; pres., Teleview Prods., Inc., 1961; executive producer, City Film Productions, 1970. Executive post-production supervisor, Jerry Liotta Films, 1977.
AUTHOR: many articles in nat'l publications dealing with m.p. practices and techniques; tech. editor, "Better Movie-Making" Magazine, 1962; editor, pub., National Directory of Movie-Making Information, 1963; assoc. ed., Photographic Product News, 1964; contrib. editor, U.S. Camera. M.P. columnist, contributing ed. Travel and Camera magazine, 1969; Advisory panelist, Photo-methods (NY), 1975. Consultant, Photographic Guidance Council, 1957, assoc. Society of M.P. & Television-Engineers, 1952.

GRESHLER, ABNER J.: Producer. b. New York City. e. Fordham U., St. John's School of Law. Prior to entering m.p. ind., prod. shows for resort hotels; mgd., booked artists for vaudeville, hotels, cafes. Now pres., York Pictures Corp.; Abner J. Greshler Prod., Inc. Executive prod. At War with the Army, 1951; Hundred Hour Hunt, Yesterday and Today, 1953; Johnny and the Gaucho, 1955; prog. consultant, NBC; coord. of prog. development dept., NTA; pres., R.G. Prod., Ltd. Pres. Damond Artists Ltd.; dir. Yesterday and Today, The Fugitive, Odd Couple; v.p., Astron Prod Ltd.

GREY, JOEL: Actor-Singer. b. Cleveland, 1932. e. Alexander Hamilton High, L.A. Acting debut at 10 years in On Borrowed Time at Cleveland Playhouse. Extensive nightclub appearances before returning to theatres and TV.
PICTURES INCLUDE: About Face, Calypso Heat Wave, Come September, Cabaret, Man on a Swing, Buffalo Bill and the Indians, 7 percent Solution, Remo Williams.
TV: Maverick, December Bride, Jack and the Beanstalk (special), Ironside, Night Gallery, The Burt Bacharach Show, The Tom Jones Show, The Englebert Humperdinck Show, George M! (special), The Carol Burnett Show, The Julie Andrews Hour.
STAGE: Come Blow Your Horn, Stop the World—I Want to Get Off, Half a Sixpence, Harry, Noon and Night, West Side Story, Finian's Rainbow, Tom Sawyer, Mardi Gras, Littlest Revue, Cabaret, George M!.

GREY, VIRGINIA: Actress. b. Los Angeles, Calif., March 22, 1923. Screen career started 1935 with She Gets Her Man.
PICTURES INCLUDE: Who Killed Doc Robbin, Bullfighter and the Lady, Highway 301, Slaughter Trail, Desert Pursuit, Perilous Journey, Forty-Niners, Target Earth, Eternal Sea, Last Command, Rose Tattoo, All That Heaven Allows, Tammy Tell Me True, Bachelor In Paradise, Back Street, Madame X, Rosie, Airport.

GRIEM, HELMUT: Actor. b. Hamburg, Germany, 1940. e. Hamburg Univ.
PICTURES: The Damned, The Mackenzie Break, Cabaret, Ludwig, Voyage of the Damned, Sergeant Steiner, Breakthrough, The Glass Cell, Berlin Alexanderplatz, La Passante.
TELEVISION: Peter the Great.

GRIFFIN, MERV: Singer, M.C. b. San Mateo, Calif., July 6, 1925. e. Univ. of San Francisco and Stanford. w. Julann Wright. The Merv Griffin Show, KFRC-Radio, 1945–48; vocalist, Freddy Martin's orch., 1948–52; Contract Warner Bros., 1952–54. co-starred, So This Is Love, The Boy From Oklahoma; CBS-TV, toured Niteclubs, 1954–55; Prod. Finians Rainbow, City Center, N.Y.C., 1955; Vocalist, CBS-TV, Morning Show, and Robt. Q. Lewis Show, 1956; M.C., Look Up and Live, CBS-TV, Going Places, ABC-TV, 1957, Merv. Griffin Show, 1958, Play Your Hunch, 1960; M.C., Keep Talking, ABC-TV, 1960; Merv. Griffin Show, NBC-TV, 1962; Word for Word, NBC-TV, 1963; Merv. Griffin Show, Westinghouse Broadcasting, 1965; pres., Griffin Prods.

GRIFFITH, ANDY: Actor. b. Mount Airy, N.C., June 1, 1926. e. U. of North Carolina.
THEATRE: Broadway stage: No Time for Sergeants, Destry Rides Again.
TV: The Andy Griffith Show, Andy of Mayberry, No Time for Sergeants, The Headmaster (series). Movies: Go Ask Alice, Salvage I, Crime of Innocence, Diary of a Perfect Murder, Return to Mayberry.
PICTURES INCLUDE: A Face in the Crowd, No Time for Sergeants, Onionhead, The Second Time Around, Angel in My Pocket, Hearts of the West, Rustler's Rhapsody.

GRIFFITH, MELANIE: Actress. b. New York City, Aug. 9, 1957. Dauther of Tippi Hedren. Wife of actor Steven Bauer.
PICTURES: Night Moves, The Drowning Pool, Smile, Roar, One on One, Joyride, Fear City, Body Double.
TELEVISION: Steel Cowboy, She's in the Army Now, Golden Gate, Alfred Hitchcock Presents, etc.

GRILLO, BASIL F.: Executive. b. Angel's Camp, Calif., Oct. 8, 1910, e. A.B., Univ. of Calif., Berkeley. Certified public accountant, exec. vice-pres., dir., Bing Crosby Ent., Inc., 1948–57; bus. mgr., Bing Crosby, 1945; co-organizer, dir., 3rd pres., & treas., Alliance of T.V. Film Producers, 1950–54; exec. prod., BCE, Inc., shows incl. Fireside Thea., Rebound, Royal Playhouse, The Chimps; dir., KCOP, Inc., 1957–60; dir. KFOX, Inc., 1958–62; pres., dir., Bing Crosby Prods., 1955–69; dir., Seven Leagues Ent., Inc., 1958; dir. Electrovision Prods., 1970, chief exec. off., Bing Crosby Enterprises.

GRIMALDI, ALBERTO: Producer. b. Naples, 1927. Studied law, serving as counsel to Italian film companies, before turning to production with Italian westerns starring Clint Eastwood and Lee Van Cleef. Is pres. of P.E.A. (Produzioni Europee Associate, S.A.S.).
PICTURES INCLUDE: For a Few Dollars More, The Good, the Bad and the Ugly, Three Steps in Delerium, Satyricon, Burn!, The Decameron, The Canterbury Tales, 1001 Nights, Salo, or the 100 Days of Sodom, Bawdy Tales, Man of La Mancha, Last Tango in Paris, Avanti, Fellini's Casanova, 1900, The True Story of General Custer.

GRIMES, GARY: Actor. b. San Francisco, 1955. Family moved to L.A. when he was nine. Made film debut at 15 yrs. in Summer of '42, 1971. Voted Star of Tomorrow in QP poll, 1971.
PICTURES INCLUDE: The Culpepper Cattle Company, Cahill, United States Marshall, Class of '44, The Spikes Gang, Gus.

GRIMES, TAMMY: Actress. b. Lynn, MA, Jan. 30, 1934. e. Stephens Coll. On Bdwy. in Bus Stop, Amazing Adele, The Lark, Unsinkable Molly Brown, High Spirits, Finian's Rainbow, Only Game in Town, Private Lives, California Suite, 42nd Street, etc.
PICTURES: Three Bites of an Apple, Play It As It Lays, Somebody Killed Her Husband, The Runner Stumbles, Can't Stop the Music.
TELEVISION: Movies: The Other Man, The Horror at 37,000 Feet, The Borrowers, You Can't Go Home Again.

GRIPPO, JAN: Producer. b. Beacon, N.Y., Dec. 15, 1906; e. Eastman Coll., 1925; N.Y. Sch. of Design; m. Flo Browne. From 1926–28 cartoonist New York Herald-Tribune Syndicate; com. artist, caricaturist for Shubert shows, cartoonist national magazines; agent in Hollywood, 1940–49; prod. since 1945. Produced 23 Bowery Boys features for Mono gram; assoc. producer Edward Small on Valentino for Columbia, 1950 prod. Bowery Battalion, Ghost Chasers, Let's Go Navy for Monogram, 1951.
MEMBER: Soc. American Magicians.

GRISSMER, JOHN: Executive. b. Houston, TX, Aug. 28, 1933. e. Xavier Univ. (BS, 1955); Catholic Univ. (MFA in dramatic writing, 1959). Taught drama courses, directed student productions at Univ. of Connecticut & American Univ., Washington, D.C. Produced and co-wrote House That Cried Murder (1973); co-produced, wrote and directed Scalpel (1978); directed Slasher (1986). Partner in P.J. Productions Co. & Stillman Grissmer, Inc. (film & TV dist. co.).

GRIZZARD, GEORGE: Actor. b. Roanoke Rapids, N.C., 1928. Debut on Broadway in The Desperate Hours. Has been member of APA repertory company and Tyrone Guthrie resident company in Minneapolis. Broadway plays include The Disenchanted, The Country Girl, The Royal Family, Who's Afraid of Virginia Woolf, California Suite, etc.
PICTURES: From the Terrace, Advise and Consent, Warning Shot, Happy Birthday, Wanda June, Comes a Horseman, Wrong Is Right.
TELEVISION: Robert Kennedy and His Times, International Airport, The Deliberate Stranger, Under Siege.

GRODIN, CHARLES: Actor-Director. b. Pittsburgh, PA, April 21, 1935. e. Univ. of Miami. Studied acting with Uta Hagen and Lee Strasberg; began directing career in New York 1965 in New York as asst. to Gene Saks. Has appeared in some 75 plays all over country and has been guest of major network TV shows. Has also written scripts produced plays.
PICTURES INCLUDE: Actor: Rosemary's Baby, Catch-22, The Heartbreak Kid, 11 Harrowhouse, Thieves, King Kong, Heaven Can Wait, Real Life, Sunburn, It's My Turn, Seems Like Old Times, The Incredible Shrinking Woman, Great Muppet Caper, The Lonely Guy, The Woman in Red, Movers and Shakers (also co-prod.-s.p.).
TV: Candid Camera (writer, dir.); Simon and Garfunkel Special (writer, dir.); Acts of Love and Other Comedies (dir.); Paradise (prod., dir.).

GROSS, JERRY: Executive, producer, writer, director. e. N.Y. pub. schools, night sch.
PICTURES INCLUDE: Girl on a Chain Gang, Teen Age Mother and Female Animal.
Pres., Jerry Gross Productions, 1962; Pres., Cinemation Industries, Inc., 1964–75. Pres., Jerry Gross Org., 1979.

GROSS, KENNETH H.: Executive. e. New School for Social Research, Univ. of London. Conducted film seminars at New School and active in several indep. film projects. Published film criticism in various journals and magazines. Joined ABC Entertainment Oct. 1971. Named supvr. of feature films for ABC-TV. Appt. mgr. of feature films, Jan. 1974. Promoted in Nov, 1975 to program executive, ABC Entertainment Prime Time/West Coast. Moved to L.A. offices, Nov. 1976, pro moted to exec. producer, movies for TV, ABC Ent.; 1978, with literary agency F.C.A. as partner in Los Angeles; 1979 producer for Lorimar; then with Intl. Creative Mgt; 1982, formed own literary talent agency, The Literary Group; 1985, merged agency with Robinson-Weintraub & Assoc. to become Robinson-Weintraub-Gross & Assoc.

GROSSBERG, JACK: Producer/Executive. b. Brooklyn, N.Y., June 5, 1927. Member: Academy of Motion Picture Arts & Sciences, New York Friars Club, Producers Guild of America, Directors Guild of America.
PICTURES: Requiem for a Heavyweight, Leadbelly, Pretty

Poison, The Betsy, King Kong, Sleeper, Don't Drink the Water, Everything You Always Wanted to Know About Sex, Bananas, Take the Money and Run, The Producers, Fast Break, A Stranger Is Watching, Brainstorm, Strange Brew, Touch and Go, Made in Heaven. Exec. prod. superv. for American Film Theatre on: The Iceman Cometh, Rhinoceros, A Delicate Balance, Luther.

GROSSMAN, ERNIE: Exec. b. N.Y.C., Sept. 19, 1924. Still dept., pressbook edit., asst. field mgr., Warner Bros., 1940–58; Studio publicist, 1958–60; exploitation, promo. mgr. field dept., 1960–64; nat'l mgr., pub., exploit., promo.; 1964–67 exec. co-ord. advt., pub. & promo., Warner-7 Arts, 1967; WB nat'l supv. ad.-pub., 1970. exec. assist. to Richard Lederer, 1971–72; 1973 nat'l dir. of Pub. & Promotion, Warner Bros. Inc.; 1977, natl. dir. of adv.-pub.; 1980–85, natl. dir. promo.

GROSZ, PAUL: Art Director. b. New York, N.Y. e. Cooper Union, 1928–30; Pratt, 1930–32; National Academy. Ent. m.p. ind. as artist-apprentice, Universal Pictures, 1929; art, adv., Warner Bros., Paramount, Buchanan Ad Agency, Monroe Greenthal Agency, Roxy Theatre; 20th Century-Fox, 1948–62; art dir. United Artists, 1962–82, art director; now consultant.

GRUEN, ROBERT: Executive. b. New York, N.Y., Apr. 2, 1913. e. Carnegie Mellon University. B.A. Stage designer, 1934–35; designer, 20th-Fox, 1936; prod. exec., National Screen Service Corp., 1936; head, Robert Gruen Associates, ind. design org., 1940; nat. pres. Industrial Designers Institute, 1954–55; dir. and v.p., National Screen Service Corp. since 1951; senior v.p. 1975–78; dir., NSS Corp., Contintental Lithograph and NSS, Ltd., 1978–85.

GRUENBERG, JERRY: Executive. b. Minneapolis, Minn., June 7, 1927. e. U. of Minn. United Artists, Minneapolis, 1952; m.p. exhibitor 1952–67; v.p. Sigma III Corp. 1965–67. division mgr., 20th Century-Fox, 1967–71; Senior V.P., general sales mgr., Allied Artists Pictures, 1971–79. Now pres., Blossom Pictures, Inc. Member of Variety Club, Friars Club. Director of Will Rogers Memorial Fund.

GRUENBERG, LEONARD S.: Executive. b. Minneapolis, Minn., Sept. 10, 1913. e. Minnesota U. Began as salesman Republic pictures (Minneapolis), 1935; with RKO in same capacity, 1936; promoted to city sales mgr., (St. Louis), 1937, then branch mgr. (Salt Lake City), 1941; later that year apptd. Rocky Mt. Dist. Mgr. (hqts., Denver, Colo.); 1946 Metropolitan, div. mgr., v.p. NTA, v.p. Cinemiracle Prods.; Pres., Chmn. of bd., Sigma III Corp., 1962. Chmn. of bd., Filmways, 1967. Chmn. of bd. Gamma III Dist. Co. & Chmn of bd. and Pres. Great Owl Corp., 1976. Member variety Club, Sigma Alpha Mu Fraternity; Lieut. Civil Air Patrol, Lieut. Comdr., U.S.N.R.

GRUSIN, DAVID: Composer-Conductor-Performer. Directed music for the Andy Williams Show on TV for 7 yrs in the 1960s, where met Norman Lear and Bud Yorkin, producers of the series. They signed him to score their first feature film, Divorce, American Style.

PICTURES INCLUDE: Winning, The Heart Is a Lonely Hunter, Tell Them Willie Boy Is Here, The Front, Murder by Death, The Yakuza, Three Days of the Condor, Bobby Deerfield, And Justice for All, My Bodyguard, Absence of Malice, On Golden Pond, Reds, Author! Author!, Scandalous, Racing with the Moon, The Pope of Greenwich Village, The Little Drummer Girl, Falling in Love, Goonies.

GUARDINO, HARRY: Actor. b. Brooklyn, N.Y., Dec. 23, 1925. e. Haaren H.S.

THEATRE: B'way: End As A Man, A Hatful of Rain, Anyone Can Whistle, One More River, Natural Affection, The Rose Tatoo (revival), Seven Descents of Myrtle, Woman of the Year.

TV: Studio One, Playhouse 90, The Alcoa Theatre, Naked City, Dr. Kildare, The Untouchables, The Dick Powell Show, The Reporter, The New Perry Mason.

PICTURES INCLUDE: Pork Chop Hill, The Five Pennies, Houseboat, The Pigeon That Took Rome, Treasure of San Grennaro, Madigan, Lovers and Other Strangers, Red Sky at Morning, Dirty Harry, They Only Kill Their Masters, St. Ives, The Enforcer, Rollercoaster, Matilda, Any Which Way You Can.

GUBER, PETER: Producer. e. Syracuse Univ. (B.A.); Univ. at Florence (Italy), (S.S.P.); N.Y.U. School of Law (Juris Doctor, L.L.M.). Recruited by Columbia Pictures as exec. asst. in 1968 while pursuing MBA degree at N.Y.U. Graduate School of Business Adm. With Col. seven yrs. in key prod. exec. capacities, serving last three as exec. v.p. in chg. of worldwide prod. Formed own company, Peter Guber's Filmworks, which in 1976 was merged with Casablanca Records to become Casablanca Record and Filmworks. He was chm of bd. of co. called PolyGram, and co.-mgr. dir.

PICTURES INCLUDE: The Deep (first under own banner), Midnight Express (6 Golden Globes, 2 Oscars). Six Weeks (co-prod.), Visionquest (co-prod.), Clue (exec. prod.), The Color Purple (exec. prod.).

GUEST, LANCE: Actor. b. Saratoga, CA, July 21, 1960. e. UCLA.

PICTURES: I Ought To Be in Pictures, Halloween II, The Last Starfighter.

TELEVISION: Lou Grant, St. Elsewhere. Movies: Between Two Loves, Why Us?, Please Don't Hit Me Mom, Confessions of a Married Man, One Too Many, My Father My Rival.

GUEST, VAL: Writer, dir., prod. b. London, England, e. England and America. Journalist with Hollywood Reporter, Zit's Los Angeles Examiner and Walter Winchell.

PICTURES INCLUDE: Murder at the Windmill, Miss Pilgrim's Progress, The Body Said No, Mr. Drake's Duck, Happy Go Lovely, Another Man's Poison, Penny Princess, The Runaway Bus, Life With the Lyons, Dance Little Lady, Men of Sherwood Forest, Lyons in Paris, Break in the Circle, It's A Great Life, Quatermass Experiment, They Can't Hang Me, The Weapon, The Abominable Snowman, Carry on Admiral, It's a Wonderful World, Camp on Blood Island, Up the Creek, Further Up the Creek, Life is a Circus, Yesterday's Enemy, Expresso Bongo, Hell Is a City, Full Treatment, The Day the Earth Caught Fire, Jigsaw, 80,000 Suspects, The Beauty Jungle, Where the Spies Are, Casino Royale, Assignment K, When Dinosaurs Ruled the Earth, Tomorrow, The Persuaders, Au Pair, Girls, The Adventurers, Confessions of a Window Cleaner, Killer Force, Diamond Mercenaries. TV. Space 1999, The Shillingbury Blowers, The Band Played On, Sherlock Holmes & Dr. Watson, Shillingbury Tales, Dangerous Davies, The Last Detective. 1983: the Boys in Blue. 1984–85: In Possession, Mark of the Devil, Child's Play.

GUILLAUME, ROBERT: Actor. b. St. Louis, Nov. 30. e. St. Louis Univ., Washington, Univ. Studied voice; acting career debut in Carousel. Has appeared in many Bdwy. plays and musicals.

TELEVISION: Dinah, Mel and Susan Together, Rich Little's Washington Follies, Jim Nabors, All in the Family, Sanford and Son, The Jeffersons, Marcus Welby, M.D., Soap, Benson.

PICTURE: Seems Like Old Times.

GUILLERMIN, JOHN: Director. b. London, England, Nov. 11, 1925. e. City of London School, Cambridge Univ. RAF pilot prior to entering film industry.

PICTURES INCLUDE: The Blue Max, The Towering Inferno, King Kong, Death on the Nile, Sheena, King Kong Lives.

GUINNESS, SIR ALEC: Actor. b. London, Eng., April 2, 1914. e. Pembroke Lodge, Southbourne & Roborough School, Eastbourne. created C.B.E. 1955; Knighted 1959. Stage debut: London, 1934. Theatre appearances in London, New York & Continent. Special AA (1979) for services to film.

PICTURES INCLUDE: Great Expectations, Oliver Twist, Kind Hearts & Coronets, Run For Your Money, Last Holiday, The Mudlark, Lavender Hill Mob (Academy Nomination), The Man in the White Suit, The Card (The Promoter), Malta Story, Captain's Paradise, Father Brown (The Detective), To Paris With Love, The Prisoner, The Ladykillers, The Swan, The Bridge On the River Kwai (Academy Award 1957, best actor); The Horse's Mouth (Academy Nomination for s.p.), The Scapegoat, Our Man in Havana, Tunes of Glory, A Majority of One, H.M.S. Defiant, Lawrence of Arabia, Dr. Zhivago, The Comedians, Cromwell, Scrooge, Brother Sun and Sister Moon, Hitler: The Last Ten Days, Murder by Death, Star Wars (Academy Nomination), The Empire Strikes Back, Little Lord Fauntleroy, Return of the Jedi, Lovesick, A Passage to India, Little Dorrit.

TV: The Wicked Scheme of Jehel Deeks (National Academy Nomination), Twelfth Night, Conversation at Night, Solo, E.E. Cummings, Little Gidding, The Gift of Friendship, Caesar & Cleopatra, Tinker, Tailor, Soldier, Spy (7-part series), Smiley's People (series), Edwin.

GULAGER, CLU: Actor. Father, John Gulager, cowboy entertainer. e. Baylor Univ. Starred at school in original play, A Different Drummer, where spotted by prod. of TV's Omnibus; invited to New York to recreate role on TV.

PICTURES INCLUDE: The Last Picture Show, Winning, The Other Side of Midnight, Touched by Love, The Return of the Living Dead, etc.

TELEVISION: The Virginian, San Francisco International, Glass House, Ski Lift to Death, Space, etc.

GUMBEL, BRYANT: Announcer—News Show Host. b. Chicago, e. Bates Coll. Started as sports dir., KNBC, Los Angeles. Now co-host on Today Show, New York.

TELEVISION: Super Bowl games, Games People Play, Different as Night and Day.

GUMPERT, JON: Executive. e. Cornell Univ. Law School. Sr. v.p., business affairs, MGM/UA Entertainment; pres., World Film Services, Inc., indep. prod. co. in N.Y. 1985, named v.p., business affairs, Warner Bros.

GUNN, MOSES: Actor. b. St. Louis, Oct. 2, 1929. e. Tenn. State Univ. Taught speech and drama at Grambling College. Came to N.Y. and first cast in off-Bdwy. prod. of Genet's The Blacks. Later joined Negro Ensemble Company.
PICTURES INCLUDE: WUSA, The Great White Hope, The Wild Rovers, Shaft, Shaft's Big Score, Eagle in a Cake, Hot Rock, Amazing Grace, The Iceman Cometh, Rollerball, Aaron Loves Angela, Ragtime, Amityville II: The Possession, Firestarter.
STAGE: In White America, Day of Absence, Song of the Lusitanian Bogey, Summer of the 17th Doll, Daddy Goodness, Harvest, Titus Andronicus, Measure for Measure, Romeo and Juliet, The Tempest, As You Like It, Macbeth, Othello, A Hand Is on the Gate.
TELEVISION: Mr. Carter's Army, The Borgia Stick, Of Mice and Men, Haunts of the Very Rich, Hawaii Five-O, The FBI, Kung Fu, If You Give a Dance, You Gotta Pay the Band, The Cowboys, Roots.

GUNSBERG, SHELDON: Executive. b. Jersey City, N.J., Aug. 10, 1920; e. St. Peters Coll., N.J. State Normal, N.Y. Univ. With Night of Stars, Madison Sq. Garden, 1942; for. pub., 20th-Fox 1942; United Artists, 1945–47; Universal, roadshows. Rank product, asst. adv., pub. dir., 1947–54; v. pres., Walter Reade Theatres; exec. v.p. & dir., Walter Reade Org. 1962; Made chief operating officer, 1971; president, and Chief Executive Officer, 1973; chm. & CEO, 1984.

GUNZBURG, M.L.: President, Natural Vision Corporation. b. Denver, Colo. e. UCLA: Columbia U. Newspaper man, columnist, Los Angeles Times, New York Times; radio writer, screen writer many m.p. cos.
Developed 3-D process, Natural Vision; contract Polaroid Corp. for 3-D, 1953.

GURIAN, PAUL R.: Executive. b. New Haven, CT., Oct. 18, 1946. e. Lake Forest Coll., Univ. of Vienna, N.Y. Univ. Started producing films in 1971 with Cats and Dogs, a dramatic short which won prizes at Chicago Int. Film Fest and Edinburgh Fest. In 1977 formed Gurian Entertainment Corp., to acquire film properties for production.
PICTURES INCLUDE: The Garden Party (PBS program), Profile Ricardo Alegria (short), Bernice Bobs Her Hair (shown at 1977 N.Y. Film Festival); Cutter and Bone (United Artists, distributor).

GUTTENBERG, STEVE: Actor. b. Brooklyn, NY, Aug. 24, 1958. e. School of Performing Arts, NY. In off- Bdwy. in The Lion in Winter; studied under John Houseman at Julliard; classes with Lee Strassberg and Uta Hagen. Moved to West Coast in 1976; landed first TV role in movie, Something for Joey. Theatrical film debut in The Chicken Chronicles (1977).
PICTURES: The Boys from Brazil, Players, Can't Stop the Music, Diner, The Man Who Wasn't There, Police Academy, Police Academy 2, Cocoon, Bad Medicine, Police Academy 3, Short Circuit, The Bedroom Window.
TELEVISION: Series: Billy, No Soap, Radio, Police Story, Doc, etc. Movies: To Race the Wind, Miracle on Ice, The Day After.

GWYNNE ANNE: Actress. r.n. Marguerite Gwynne Trice. b. Waco, Tex., Dec. 10, 1918. e. San Antonio High School, Stephens Coll.
THEATRE: Stage Door, Inside Story, The Colonel's Lady.
PICTURES INCLUDE: Charlie McCarthy, Detective; Framed, Unexpected Father, Honeymoon Deferred, Fear, Ghost Goes Wild, Glass Alibi, Dick Tracy Meets Gruesome, Panhandle, Enchanted Valley, Blazing Sun, Call of Klondike, Breakdown, Teenage Monster.

GWYNNE, FRED: Actor. b. New York City, Jul. 10, 1926. e. Harvard Univ. On stage in Mrs. McThing, Irma La Douce, Cat on a Hot Tin Roof, Winter's Tale, etc.
PICTURES: Luna, Simon, So Fine, The Cotton Club, Off Beat, Water, The Boy Who Could Fly.
TELEVISION: Movies: Captains Courageous, Vanishing Act. Series: The Munsters. Mini-Series: Kane & Abel.

H

HABEEB, TONY G.: Executive. b. San Francisco, Calif., Oct. 26, 1927. e. San Francisco City College, 1945–47, Univ. of Calif., 1947–49, Lincoln Univ. Law School, LLB, 1949–53. TV Editor, San Francisco Chronicle, 1949–54; Information Specialist, U.S. Army, 1954–56; managing editor; Torrance Press, 1956–57; CBS-TV Network Press information Division, 1957–61; ass't. dir. promo. and pub., Screen Gems, 1961–63; dir. promo. and pub., Screen Gems, 1963–67; world-wide dir. advertising, pub. and promo., Paramount Television; 1967–70. v.p., adv. and publicity, Metromedia Producers Corp. 1970–74. v.p. adv. and publicity, Irwin Allen Productions, 1974–81, pres., Publicist Guild of America; now dir., adv., Warner Bros.-TV.

HABER, JOYCE: Writer, syndicated Hollywood columnist. r.n. Mrs. Joyce Haber Cramer. b. Dec. 28, 1932, New York, N.Y. e. Brearley School, N.Y.C., class of '48; Bryn Mawr College, 1949–50, Cum Laude List; Barnard College, B.A., 1953.
Researcher, Time magazine, 1953–63; Hollywood Reporter, L.A. Bureau Time, 1963–66; Columnist, Los Angeles Times, 1966–75; contributing editor, Los Angeles Magazine, 1977–80.
Published "Caroline's Doll Book," illus. by R. Taylor, 1962. freelance writing: Esquire, Herald Tribune's New York Magazine, Harper's Bazaar, New York Magazine, Town and Country. Published "The Users," a novel, 1976.

HACK, SHELLEY: Actress. b. Connecticut, July 6. e. Smith College. Made modeling debut at 14 on cover of Glamour Magazine. Gained fame as Revlon's Charlie Girl on TV commercials.
PICTURES: Annie Hall, If Ever I See You Again, The King of Comedy, Troll.
TELEVISION: Death Car, Charlie's Angels. Movies: Trackdown, Found Money, Single Bars Single Women.

HACKER, CHARLES R.: Executive. b. Milwaukee, Oct. 8. e. Univ. Wisconsin. Thea. mgr., Fox Wisc. Amuse. Corp., 1940; served in U.S.A.F., 1943–45; rejoined Fox Wisconsin Amusement Corp.; joined Standard Theatres Management Corp. 1947, on special assignments; apptd. district mgr. of Milwaukee & Waukesha theatres 1948; joined Radio City Music Hall Corp. as administrative asst. July, 1948; mgr. of oper., 1952; asst. to the pres., Feb. 1957; v.p., Radio City Music Hall Corp., 1964; appointed executive vice president and chief operating officer, February 1, 1973. Pres., Landmark Pictures, May, 1979. Elected treas. Will Rogers Memorial Fund, 1978. Award: Quigley Silver Grand Award for Showmanship, 1947.

HACKETT, BUDDY: Actor, comedian. b. Brooklyn, Aug. 31, 1924. Prof. debut, Borscht Circuit.
TV: Stanley series, Bud and Lou (movie).
THEATRE: B'way, Lunatics and Lovers, I Had A Ball.
PICTURES INCLUDE: God's Little Acre, All Hands on Deck, The Music Man, Everything's Ducky, It's a Mad, Mad, Mad, Mad World, Muscle Beach Party.

HACKFORD, TAYLOR: Director. b. 1945. Bagan career with KCET in Los Angeles as prod.-dir. Won Oscar for short, Teenage Father, 1978. Theatrical film debut as director with The Idolmaker (1980).
PICTURES: An Officer and a Gentleman, Against All Odds (also co.-prod.), White Nights (also co-prod.).

HACKMAN, GENE: Actor. b. San Bernardino, Calif., Jan. 30, 1930. First major broadway role in Any Wednesday. Other stage productions include: Poor Richard, Children from their Games, A Rainy Day in Newark, The Natural Look. Formed own production co., Chelly Ltd.
TV: CBS Playhouse's My Father, My Mother, The F.B.I., The Invaders, The Iron Horse, etc.
PICTURES INCLUDE: Lilith, Bonnie and Clyde (Acad. Award nom. for Best Supporting Actor), First to Fight, Out by the Country Club, Hawaii, Riot, The Split, The Gypsy Moths, Downhill Racer, Marooned, I Never Sang for My Father, Doctor's Wives, Cisco Pike, The French Connection (Acad. Award best actor, 1971), Prime Cut, The Poseidon Adventure, Scarecrow, The Conversation, Zandy's Bride, Young Frankenstein, Night Moves, Bite the Bullet, French Connection II, Lucky Lady, The Domino Principle, A Bridge Too Far, March or Die, Superman, All Night Long, Superman II., Eureka, Under Fire, Uncommon Valor, Misunderstood, Power, Target, Twice in a Lifetime.

HADLOCK, CHANNING M.: Mktg. TV exec. b. Mason City, Iowa e. Duke Univ., Univ. of North Carolina. Newspaperman, Durham, N.C. Herald, war corr., Yank; NBC, Hollywood; television prod.-writer, Cunningham & Walsh Adv.; v.p. account supr. Chirug & Cairns Adv.; v.p. Marketing Innovations; dir. mktg. Paramount Pictures; mktg. svcs, Ogilvy & Mather; mktg, Time Life Books.

HAGERTY, JULIE: Actress. b. Cincinnati. Studied drama for six years before leaving for New York. Made acting debut in her brother Michael's theatre group in Greenwich Village called the Production Company. Film debut in Airplane! (1980).
PICTURES: A Midsummer Night's Sex Comedy, Airplane II: The Sequel, Lost in America, Bad Medicine.

HAGGAR, PAUL: Executive. Veteran of over 30 yrs. with Paramount Pictures, working way up from studio mail room to become apprentice editor in 1953; promoted to asst. editor 1955; music editor, 1957. In 1968 named head of post-prod. for all films made by Paramount. 1985, named sr. v.p., post-prod. for Studio Group.

HAGGARD, PIERS: Director. b. Scotland, 1939. Son of actor Stephen Haggard and great grandnephew of author Rider Haggard. e. Univ. of Edinburgh. Began career in theatre in 1960 as asst. to artistic dir. at London's Royal Court. Named director at Glasgow Citizens' Theatre. 1963–65 worked with the National Theatre, where co-directed Hobson's Choice and The Dutch Courtesan. Has directed many plays and series for TV.
PICTURE: Venom, The Fiendish Plot of Dr. Fu Manchu.
TELEVISION: Pennies from Heaven, Quatermass.

HAGMAN, LARRY: Actor. b. Fort Worth, TX, Sept. 21, 1931. Son of actress Mary Martin. e. Bard College. First stage experience with Marg Jones Theatre in the Round in Dallas. Appeared in N.Y. in Taming of the Shrew; two years with London production of South Pacific. 1952–56 was in London with US Air Force where produced and directed show for servicemen. Returned to N.Y. for plays on and off Bdwy. Starred in daytime serial, Edge of Night, for over 2 years.
PICTURES: Fail Safe, Ensign Pulver and the Captain, The Cavern, Stardust, 3 in the Cellar, Mother, Jugs and Speed, Harry and Tonto, The Eagle Has Landed, Superman, etc.
TELEVISION: Series: I Dream of Jeannie, The Good Life, Here We Go Again, Dallas. Movies: The President's Mistress, Last of the Good Guys, Battered.

HAHN, HELENE: Executive. b. New York City. e. Loyola Univ. Instructor of entertainment law at Loyola. Attorney for ABC before joining Paramount in 1977 in studio legal dept. 1979, moved to business affairs; promoted to dir. 1980, v.p., 1981; sr. v.p., 1983. Left in 1985 to join Walt Disney Pictures as sr. v.p., business & legal affairs for m.p. division.

HAIM, COREY: Actor. b. Toronto, Canada, 1972. Performed in tv commercials; signed as regular on children's show, The Edison Twins. Theatrical m.p. debut, Firstborn (1984).
PICTURES: Secret Admirer, Silver Bullet, Lucas.

HALAS, JOHN: Director. b. Budapest, Apr. 16, 1912; e. Hungary & Paris. Entered m.p. ind. 1928; prod. over 500 documentary, educational shorts & cartoons.
PICTURES INCLUDE: Animal Farm, The Owl and the Pussycat (3-D), History of the Cinema, Animal Vegetable and Mineral, The Candlemaker; anim. seq., The First 99, The Energy Picture, Habatales, A Christmas Visitor, Hamilton Cartoon series, Automania 2000, Is There Intelligent Life On Earth, Midsummer Nightmare, Hoffnung Cartoon Series, Dodo, The Kid From Outer Space (series), Ruddigore, The Question, Children and Cars, Parkinson's Law, Tomfoolery Show, Max and Moritz series, Ten for Survival, Autobahn, Dilemma, Players, Botticelli—A New Vision, Toulouse-Lautrec, Leonardo da Vinci.

HALE, ALAN, JR.: Actor. b. Los Angeles, 1918. Son late Alan Hale, actor.
PICTURES INCLUDE: Short Grass, The Gunfighter, West Point Story, At Sword's Point, Wait Till the Sun Shines Nellie, Big Trees, Lady in the Iron Mask, Springfield Rifle, Man Behind the Gun, Capt. John Smith & Pocahontas, Iron Glove, Silver Lode, Rogue Cop, Young at Heart, Many Rivers to Cross, Destry, A Man Alone, Sea Chase, Indian Fighter, Killer Is Loose, Up Periscope, Advance to the Rear, Hang 'Em High, The True Story of Jesse James, Hambone & Hillie.
TV: The Lucy Show, Hazel, Wagon Train, Cheyenne, Maverick, Route 66, Jack Benny Show, Biff Baker, U.S.A. (series), Casey Jones (series), Gilligan's Island (series).

HALE, BARBARA: Actress. b. DeKalb, Ill., April 18, 1922; e. Chicago Acad. Fine Arts. Beauty contest winner, Little Theatre actress. Screen debut, 1943: Higher and Higher. On TV in Perry Mason series.
PICTURES INCLUDE: Belle of the Yukon, Goin' to Town, Boy with Green Hair, Window, Jolson Sings Again, And Baby Makes Three, Emergency Wedding, Jackpot, Lorna Doone, First Time, Last of the Comanches, Seminole, Lone Hand, Lion Is in the Streets, Unchained, Far Horizons, Houston Story, Buckskin.
TELEVISION: Perry Mason Returns (movie).

HALE, MONTE: Actor, b. San Angelo, Texas, June 8, 1919. Night clubs and theatres, radio singer. Under contract to Republic Pictures, 1942–50.
PICTURES INCLUDE: Home on the Range, Timber Trail, Prince of the Plains, Bandits of the Badlands, Pioneer Marshal, The Old Frontier, Giant, The Chase.
TV: Gunsmoke, Honey West, Circus Boy, Wild Bill Hickok.

HALEY, JR., JACK: Executive. b. Los Angeles, Oct. 25. Son of late film star. e. Loyola Univ. Sr. v.p. at Wolper Productions before joining MGM. Named dir. of creative affairs. Produced, wrote and directed That's Entertainment! (1974). Left Nov., 1974, to join 20th Century-Fox as pres. of TV Div. and v.p., TV for 20th-Fox Film Corp. Winner of 2 Peabody Awards, best prod. at Int'l. TV Festival at Monte Carlo and 3 Silver Lion Awards at Venice Film Festival. Won Emmy for best dir. in music or variety shows for Movin' On with Nancy. Directed M.P. Academy Awards Show in 1970; prod. it in 1974 and 1979. Left Fox 1976 to be indep. prod. 1985: That's Dancing.

HALL, CONRAD: Cinematographer. b. Tahiti, 1926. Worked as camera operator with Robert Surtees, Ted McCord, Ernest Haller; moved to TV as director of photography before feature films.
PICTURES INCLUDE: Wild Seed, The Sabateur—Code Name Morituri, Harper, The Professionals, Rogue's Gallery, Incubus, Divorce, American Style, In Cold Blood, Cool Hand Luke, Hell in the Pacific, Butch Cassidy and the Sundance Kid, Tell Them Willie Boy Is Here, The Happy Ending, Fat City, Electra-Glide in Blue, The Day of the Locust, Smile, Marathon Man.

HALL, HUNTZ: Actor. b. Boston, MA, 1920. In 1937 appeared in stage and screen production Dead End.
PICTURES INCLUDE: Crime School, Angels with Dirty Faces, They Made Me a Criminal, Hell's Kitchen, Muggs Rides Again, Live Wires, A Walk in the Sun, Jinx Money, Smuggler's Cove, Fighting Fools, Blues Busters, Bowery Battalion, Ghost Chasers, Crazy Over Horses, Let's Go Navy, Here Come the Marines, Hold That Line, Feudin' Fools, No Holds Barred, Private Eyes, Paris Playboys, Bowery Boys Meet the Monsters, Clipped Wings, Jungle Gents, Bowery to Bagdad, High Society, Spy Chasers, Jail Busters, Dig That Uranium, Up in Smoke, Second Fiddle to a Steel Guitar, Gentle Giant.
TV: The Teddy Bears (series).

HALL, KEN G.: Producer, director. b. Sydney, Australia, Feb. 22, 1901. Reporter. Joined pub. dept., Union Theats., Sydney; adv. mgr. 1920. In 1922 adv. mgr. FN (Asia) Ltd. Became adv. mgr. & pub. dir., State theat., Sydney, 1928; then asst. to managing dir., Union Theats. In 1931 gen. mgr. & dir., Cinesound Prods., Ltd.
PICTURES INCLUDE: (dir.) On Our Selection, Squatter's Daughter, Tall Timbers, Lovers and Luggers, Mr. Chedworth Steps Out, Vengeance of the Deep, Pacific Adventure.

HALPERN, NATHAN L.: Executive. b. Sioux City, Ia., Oct. 22, 1914; e. U. of South. Calif. 1936, B.A.; Harvard Law School 1939, L.L.B. With general counsel's office, U.S. Securities & Exchange commission, 1939–41; exec. asst. to dir., Civilian Supply, U.S. War Prod. Board, 1941–43; naval officer, Psychological Warfare Div., Supreme Headquarters, Allied Expeditionary Force, 1943–45; exec. asst. to dir., U.S. Information Service, Paris, 1945; asst. to pres., Columbia Broadcasting System, 1945–49; 1949–present; pres., TNT Communications, Inc.

HAMADY, RON: Producer. b. Flint, MI, June 16, 1947. e. Univ. of Calif. (BA). 1971, co-founder of The Crystal Jukebox, record productions, music management and music publishing co. Produced 12 hit albums for Decca Records of England and London Records, USA. Entered m.p. industry in 1975-76, producing Train Ride to Hollywood for Taylor-Laughlin dist. Co. 1979-80, produced Fade to Black for American Cinema Corp. Now producer for Solar Survival Film Corp. 1983; Co-produced Surf II for Arista Films.

HAMEL, VERONICA: Actress. b. Philadelphia, PA, Nov. 20, 1943. e. Temple Univ.
PICTURES: Cannonball, Beyond the Poseidon Adventure, When Time Ran Out.
TELEVISION: Ski Lift, 79 Park Avenue, The Gathering, The Gathering II, Valley of the Dolls, Sessions.

HAMILL, MARK: Actor. b. Oakland, CA, Sept. 25, 1952. Started in TV, including General Hospital (serial) and the Texas Wheelers (series). Film debut in Star Wars.
PICTURES INCLUDE: Star Wars, Corvette Summer, The Empire Strikes Back, The Night the Lights Went Out in Georgia, Return of the Jedi.
TV: Sarah T: Portrait of A Teenage Alcoholic, The F.B.I., Owen Marshall, Room 222, The Partridge Family.

HAMILL, PETE: Journalist-Writer. b. Brooklyn. Worked as ad designer, NBC page boy and sheetmetal worker before joining staff of New York Post. In 1962 won Mike Berger Award of Col. Univ. Graduate School of Journalism for N.Y.'s worst slum. Received citation from Newspaper Reporters' Assn. for series on NY Police Dept. Made s.p. writing debut with Doc, 1971.
PICTURES INCLUDE: Doc, Death at an Early Age, Badge 373, Report from Engine Co. 82.
BOOKS: A Killing for Christ (novel), Irrational Ravings (collection of N.Y. Post columns), The Seventeenth Christmas (novel).

HAMILTON, GEORGE: Actor. b. Memphis, Tenn. Aug. 12, 1939. e. grammar, Hawthorne, Calf.; military sch., Gulfport, Miss., N.Y. Hackley Prep Sch., Florida, Palm Beach H.S. Won Best Actor Award for the State of Florida, high sch. contest.

TV: Rin Tin Tin, The Donna Reed Show, The Veil, Roots, Two Fathers' Justice.
PICTURES INCLUDE: Crime and Punishment, USA (debut), Home from the Hill, All The Fine Young Cannibals, Angel Baby, Where the Boys Are, By Love Possessed, A Thunder of Drums, Light in the Piazza, Two Weeks in Another Town, The Victors, Your Cheatin' Heart, Viva Maria, That Man George, Doctor, You've Got to Be Kidding!, The Long Ride Home, Jack of Diamonds, A Time for Killing, The Power, Evel Knievel, The Man Who Loved Cat Dancing, Once is Not Enough, Love at First Bite (also exec. prod.), Zorro, the Gay Blade (also co-prod.)

HAMILTON, GUY: Director. b. Paris, Sept. 1922. Ent. m.p. industry 1939 as apprentice at Victorine Studio, Nice; Royal Navy, 1940–45, in England asst. dir., Fallen Idol, Third Man, Outcast of the Islands, African Queen.
PICTURES INCLUDE: The Ringer, The Intruder, An Inspector Calls, Colditz Story, Manuela, The Devil's Disciple, A Touch of Larceny, The Best of Enemies, The Party's Over, Man In the Middle, Goldfinger, Funeral in Berlin, Battle of Britain, Diamonds Are Forever, Live and Let Die, The Man with the Golden Gun, Force Ten From Navarone, The Mirror Crack'd, Evil Under the Sun, Remo Williams.

HAMLIN, HARRY: Actor. b. California, 1952. e. Univ. of Calif., Yale (graduate 1974 in theatre, psychology). Joined American Conservatory Theatre (San Francisco) for two years' study before joining as professional actor. Screen debut in Movie, Movie (1979).
PICTURES: King of the Mountain, Clash of the Titans, Making Love, Blue Skies Again.
TELEVISION: Mini-Series: Studs Lonigan, Master of the Game, Space.
STAGE: Hamlet, Awake and Sing.

HAMLISCH, MARVIN: Composer. b. New York City. Winner of Tony Award for score of Broadway show, A Chorus Line.
PICTURES INCLUDE: The Way We Were (Oscars for original score and song), The Sting (Oscar for adaptation), The Spy Who Loved Me, Starting Over, Ordinary People, The Fan, Sophies' Choice, Romantic Comedy, D.A.R.Y.L.

HAMMOND, PETER: Actor, writer, dir. b. London, Eng., Nov. 15, 1923. e. Harrow School of Art. Stage debut: Landslide, Westminster Theatre. Screen debut: Holiday Camp.
PICTURES INCLUDE: The Huggetts, Helter Skelter, Fools Rush In, The Reluctant Widow, Fly Away Peter, The Adventurers, Operation Disaster; Come Back, Peter; Little Lambs Eat Ivy, Its Never Too Late, The Unknown, Morning Departure, Confession, dir.: Spring and Port Wine.
TV: William Tell, Robin Hood, The Buccaneers series. 1959–61. writ., dir. TV plays. TV dir. credits: Avengers, 4 Armchair Theatres, Theatre 625, BBC classic serials Count of Monte Cristo, Three Musketeers, Hereward the Wake, Treasure Island, Lord Raingo, Cold Comfort Farm, The White Rabbit, Out of the Unknown, Follyfoot; Lukes Kingdom, Time to Think, Franklin's Farm, Sea Song, Shades of Greene, Our Mutual Friend, The House that Jack Built, The King of the Castle, The Black Knight, Kilvert's Diary, Turgenev's Liza, Wuthering Heights, Funnyman, Little World of Don Camillo, Rumpole of the Bailey, Bring on the Girls, Hallelujah Mary Plum, Aubrey Beardsley, The Happy Autumn Fields, The Combination, Tales of the Unexpected, The Glory Hole, The Hard Word, Shades of Darkness—The Maze, The Blue Dress.

HAMNER, EARL: Producer-Writer. b. Schuyler, VA, July 10, 1923. With WLW, Cincinnati, as radio-writer-producer; joined NBC 1949 as writer; 1960, freelance.
PICTURES: Spencer's Mountain, You Can't Get There from Here, The Homecoming.
TELEVISION: The Waltons (creator, co-prod.); Joshua's World, Falcon Crest (exec. prod.); A Wedding on Walton's Mountain (exec. prod.); A Day of Thanks on Walton's Mountain (exec. prod. actor), The Gift of Love—A Christmas Story (exec. prod., s.p.).

HAMPSHIRE, SUSAN: Actress. b. London, Eng., May 12, 1941.
STAGE: Expresso Bongo, Follow That Girl, Fairy Tales of New York, Ginger Man, Past Imperfect, She Stoops to Conquer, On Approval, The Sleeping Prince, A Doll's House, Taming of the Shrew, Peter Pan, Romeo & Jeanette, As You Like It, Miss Julie, The Circle, Arms and the Man, Man and Superman, Tribades, An Audience Called Edward, The Crucifer of Blood, Night and Day, The Revolt, House Guest.
TV: Andromeda, The Forsyte Saga, Vanity Fair, Katy, The First Churchills; An Ideal Husband, The Lady is a Liar, The Improbable Mr. Clayville, musical version of Dr. Jekyll and Mr. Hyde, The Pallisers, Barchester Chronicles, Leaving, Leaving II, Going to Pot I and II..
PICTURES INCLUDE: The Three Lives of Thomasina, Night Must Fall, Wonderful Life, Paris Au Mois d'Aout, The Fighting Prince of Donegal, The Trygon Factor, Monte Carlo or Bust, Rogan, David Copperfield, A Room in Paris, Living Free, Time for Loving, Malpertius, Baffled, Neither the Sea nor the Sand, Roses and Green Peppers, David the King, Bang.

HANCOCK, JOHN: Director. b. Kansas City, Mo., Feb. 12, 1939. e. Harvard. Was musician and theatre director before turning to films. Nominated for AA for short, Sticky My Fingers, Fleet My Feet.
PICTURES INCLUDE: Let's Scare Jessica to Death, Bang the Drum Slowly, Baby Blue Marine, California Dreaming, The In-Laws.

HAND, BETHLYN J.: Executive. b. Alton, Illinois. e. University of Texas. Entered motion picture industry in 1966 as administrative assistant to president of Motion Picture Association of America, Inc. In 1975 became associate director of Code for advertising of MPAA. In 1976 became director of Code for advertising; v.p.—west coast activities, board of directors, Los Angeles. S.P.C.A. 1981, appointed by Governor to Calif. Motion Picture Council 1983, elected vice chm., California Motion Picture Council.

HANDEL, LEO A.: Producer. Dir. audience research, MGM, 1942–51; organized Meteor Prod., 1951; organized Leo A. Handel Prod., for TV films, 1953; author, Hollywood Looks at Its Audience, also TV plays; pres., Handel Film Corp; prod. TV series including Everyday Adventures, Magic of the Atom. Exec. prod. & v.p., Four Crown Prods., Inc., exec. prod., Phantom Planet, 1961; prod.-writer-dir., feature film, The Case of Patty Smith, 1961; Americana Series, 1963; book, A Dog Named Duke, 1965. TV specials, Age of the Atom, 1966; Sweden-Vikings Now Style, 1968, Benjamin Franklin, 1969; The Mexican American Heritage and Destiny, 1970, The American Indian, 1971, Police Dog (TV special), 1972; Art in America, 10 half-hour films, 1981; Stress-Distress (special), 1982; Computer and You, 1983–84; Thailand, 1983; The Philippines, 1984; Germ Wars, 1985.

HANKS, TOM: Actor. b. Oakland, CA, July 9, 1956. e. CA State Univ. Began career with Great Lakes Shakespeare Festival, Cleveland.
PICTURES: He Knows You're Alone, Splash, Bachelor Party, The Man with One Red Show, Volunteers, The Money Pit, Nothing in Common, Love Is Ever Young.

HANNA, WILLIAM: Executive. b. Melrose, N.M. Studied engineering and journalism. Joined firm in Calif. as structural engineer; turned to cartooning with Leon Schlessinger's company in Hollywood. In 1937 hired by MGM as director and story man in cartoon dept. There met Joseph R. Barbera and created famous cartoon series Tom & Jerry, continuing to produce it from 1938 to 1957. Left MGM in 1957 to form Hanna-Barbera Productions to make cartoons for TV. Series have included Yogi Bear, Huckleberry Hound, The Flintstones. Hanna-Barbera became a subsidiary of Taft Bdg. Co. in 1968 with both men operating studio under long-term agreements with Taft. Hanna is senior v.p. of Hanna-Barbera Productions. Company entered theatrical production with Charlotte's Web in 1973. 1983: Heidi's Song.

HANNAH, DARYL: Actress. b. 1961.
PICTURES: Blade Runner, Summer Lovers, Splash, The Pope of Greenwich Village, Reckless, Clan of the Cave Bear, Legal Eagles.

HANNEMANN, WALTER A.: Film editor. b. Atlanta, G., May 2; U.S.C., the Class of 1935. Editorial training, RKO 1936–40; edit. supvr., Universal, 1941–42; consultant 1970–75 national educational media.
PICTURES INCLUDE: Interval, The Revengers, Dream of Kings, Guns of the Magnificent Seven, East of Java, Pay or Die, Al Capone, Hell's Five Hours, Armoured Command, Only the Valiant, Time of Your Life, Kiss Tomorrow Goodbye, Blood on the Sun, Guest in the House, Texas Masquerade, Cannon for Cardoba, El Condor, Maurie, Lost in the Stars, Mad Mad Movie Making, Big Mo, Two Minute Warning, (Oscar nominee) The Peter Hill Puzzle, Smokey and the Bandit, Other Side of the Mountain—Part II, The Visitor, The Villain, Return of Maxwell Smart.
TV: Death Valley Days, Reader's Digest, Rosemary Clooney Show, The New Breed, The Fugitive, Twelve O'Clock High, The Invaders, Hawaii Five-O, Streets of San Francisco, Cannon, Barnaby Jones, Caribe.

HANSON, PETER: Actor. b. Oakland, Calif.; p. Sydney and Lee Hansen; e. Cranbrook Acad. of Arts, Mich.; U. of Mich., 1940–41. Studied acting at Pasadena Playhouse, Calif., 1946, following war service as marine fighter pilot. Campagne, Arsenic and Old Lace, This Happy Breed; m.p. debut in Branded.
PICTURES INCLUDE: Molly, Something to Live For, When Worlds Collide, Passage West, Darling How Could You, The Savage, Violent Men, Proud and Profane, Harlow.

HARBACH, WILLIAM O.: Producer. b. Yonkers, N.Y., Oct. 12, 1919; p. Otto Harbach, lyricist, author; e. Brown U. U.S. Coast Guard, 1940–45; actor, MGM, 1945–47; broadcast co-ordinator. NBC, 1947–49; stage mgr., 1949–50; dir.,

NBC, 1950–53; prod., Tonight, 1954; prod. Steve Allen Show, 1960–61 prod., dir., Bing Crosby shows; prod., Milton Berle Special, 1962; prod., Hollywood Palace Shows, 1963–69.; co-produced Julie Andrews Show, 1972–73. Emmy for Shirley MacLaine's Gypsy In My Soul, 1976; Bob Hope Special, 1981 and 1982.

HARDIMAN, JAMES W.: Publicist. b. Brighton, England 1926. Director Advtg. & Pub., Rank Organization of Canada & Odeon Canada, 1947–56. Asst. dir. ad & pub, National Theatres, 1956–58. Dir. radio & TV promotion, Walt Disney, 1959–60. Dir. pub, Screen Gems Hollywood, 1960–64. Dir. press infmtn, CBS TV Network, Hollywood, 1964–67. Studio dir. promtn. & pub, Screen Gems, Hollywood, 1967–70. VP Yuni public rels, Tokyo and v.p. and resident director, Sijohn o Enterprises, Japan, 1970–75. Dir. pub, (entertainment) Rogers & Cowan, Beverly Hills, 1975–77. President, Suhosky & Hardiman Public Rels, 1977 to date. 1968 named Hollywood Showman of the Year by the Publicists Guild.

HAREWOOD, DORIAN: Actor. b. Dayton, OH, Aug. 6. 3. Univ. Cincinnati. On stage in Jesus Christ Superstar, Two Gentlemen of Verona, Miss Moffat, Streamers, etc.
PICTURES: Foster & Laurie, Gray Lady Down, Looker, Tank, Against All Odds, The Falcon and the Snowman.
TELEVISION: Roots—The Next Generation, An American Christmas Carol, High Ice, Strike Force, Trauma Center, The Jesse Owens Story, Dirty Work, etc.

HARGREAVES, JOHN: Executive. Joined Gainsborough Pictures 1945. Transferred to Denham Studios 1946 and later Pinewood Studios. Joined Allied Film Makers 1960, then Salamander Film Productions as Bryan Forbes' financial controller and Asst. Prod. 1965. Joined EMI Film Prods. Ltd. as Asst. Man. Dir. and prod. controller May 1969–May 1972. Produced Don Quixote (with Rudolf Nureyer, in Australia), 1973. Asst. Prod. The Slipper & The Rose 1975, Man. Dir; Cinderella Promotions Ltd, 1978: assoc. prod., International Velvet. Orion repr., 1979, The Awakening; post prod. exec., Fiendish Plot of Dr. Fu Manchu, 1980; Orion rep. for Excalibur, 1981; MGM rep., Year of Living Dangerously, Australia, 1982. 1983, U.K. consultant for Completion Bond Company, Inc.

HARINGTON, JOY: Producer. b. London, Eng., Feb. 22, 1914. e. private school, Kate Rorke Dram. School. 6 years in English theatre; New York theatre and radio; Hollywood Studios. Since 1971, freelance writer, producer and actress.
PICTURES INCLUDE: Our Hearts Were Young and Gay, Gaslight, National Velvet, Salome Where She Danced, Tony Draws A Horse.
TV: Treasure Island, Holly and the Ivy, Bridesman Danger, Midsummer Night's Dream, Beauty and The Beast, Billy Bunter of Greyfriars, Heidi, Heidi Grows Up, Clementine, Vice Versa, Robin Hood, Kidnapped, Jesus of Nazareth, Little Women, Jo's Boys, Paul of Tarsus, Hurricane, The Chen-Lab. Mystery serials. Prod. Fothergale Co. Ltd., Law and Life, Make the Best of Yourself.
AUTHOR: Jesus of Nazareth, Paul of Tarsus, TV Script Pollyanna, Radio Play, Play It By Ear.

HARMON, MARK: Actor. b. Burbank, CA, Sept. 2. Son of actress Elyse Knox and football star Tom Harmon.
PICTURES: Beyond the Poseidon Adventure; Comes a Horseman.
TELEVISION: Series: Sam, Laverne & Shirley, Nancy Drew, Police Story, Adam-12, 240-Robert, St. Elsewhere. Movies: Eleanor and Franklin: The White House Years, Little Moe, Getting Married, The Deliberate Stranger, Prince of Bel Air.

HARMON, TOM: Performer. b. Rensselaer, Ind., Sept. 28, 1919; e. U. of Mich., B.S., 1941; m. Elyse Knox, actress. All American football player, 1939–40; U.S. Air Corps, 1941–46; sports dir., WJR, Detroit, 1941; KFI, Los Angeles, 1947; broadcaster, many football, baseball games; sports dir., Columbia Pacific Radio Network, 1948–61; Tom Harmon Sports Show (ABC) 1961–70; Golden West Braodcasters (Channel 5, Hollywood), 1970; 1974—Hughes Television Network—sports dir.; 1976—Editor-Publisher—Tom Harmon's Football Today. (weekly national football paper).

HARNELL, STEWART D.: Executive. b. New York City, Aug. 18, 1938. e. Univ. of Miami, UCLA, New School of Social Research, Entertainer with Youth on Parade in Coral Gables, 1948–55, performing for handicapped children, Variety Club, etc. Singer, dancer, musician. Had own bands, Teen Aces & Rhythm Rascals, 1950–56; performed on Cactus Jim TV show and Wood & Ivory, 1959–61, WTVJ. Miami. Catskills, Sand Lake, N.Y., 1954–55. Joined National Screen Service as exec. trainee in 1960 in Chicago; worked as booker & salesman. Transferred to N.Y. home office, 1963; worked in special trailer production. Promoted to asst. gen. sls. mgr., 1964–66; New Orleans branch mgr., 1966–67; Atlanta division mgr., 1967–70. Formed own independent distribution co., 1970–Harnell Independent Productions. Resumed post as gen. sls. mgr. of NSS, New York, 1977–78; resigned to become pres. of Cinema Concerts Theatre Service, Atlanta, in 1978 to present. Pres. of Variety Club of Atlanta, Tent 21, 1972, 1976, 1979. In 1986 formed Cinema Concepts Communications, film-video animation studio in Altanta.

HARPER, JESSICA: Actress. b. Chicago, 1949. e. Sarah Lawrence Coll. Understudied on Broadway for Hair for one year. Appeared in summer stock and off-Bdwy shows. Theatrical film debut in Phantom of the Paradise (1974).
PICTURES: Inserts, Taking Off, Love and Death, Stardust Memories, Suspiria, Shock Treatment, Pennies from Heaven, My Favorite Year, The Imagemaker.
TELEVISION: Series: Little Women. Min-series: Aspen, Studs Lonigan.

HARPER, JOE: Theatre Executive. b. Dallas, Texas, Aug. 11, 1941. e. El Centro Coll., Dallas; Ga. State Univ. Was in public relations, N.Y.C., 1961–65 when joined Academy Theatres, Dallas. In 1968–69, with American Multi-Cinema, Dallas. In 1969 joined R. C. Cobb Theatre, Atlanta. Now v.p. in chg. booking, buying, Member: Democratic Executive Committee, Officer Ruritan International Active in Scouting and Little League sports.

HARPER, RICHARD A.: TV Executive, b. Johnstown, Pa. e. Univ. of So. Calif. 1939; Columbia Univ. 1943 (MA); Harvard Grad. School of Bus. Admin. 1945; National City Bank of New York in Japan, China, Malaya, India and Burma 1939–42; Lt. Cmd. USNR 1942–45; MGM-New York, ass't to gen. sales mgr., circuit sales mgr. 1945–56; director world-wide syndication MGM-TV 1956–63; gen. sales mgr. Samuel Goldwyn Prod's. 1963–64; Warner Bros.-Seven Arts v.p.-administration 1964–71; Twentieth Century-Fox Television, v.p. World-Wide syndication 1971; sr. v.p., 20th-Fox Intl. TV, 1980.

HARPER, VALERIE: Actress. b. Aug. 22, 1940. Suffern, N.Y. m. actor-writer Dick Schaal. Started as dancer in stage shows at Radio City Music Hall. First professional acting in summer stock in Conn. Appeared on Bdwy. in Take Me Along, Wildcat, Subways Are for Sleeping. Won 3 Emmys for best performance in supporting role in comedy for portrayal of Rhoda on The Mary Tyler Moore Show.
PICTURES INCLUDE: Freebie and the Bean, Chapter Two, The Last Married Couple in America, Blame It on Rio.
TV: The Mary Tyler Show, Rhoda. Movie: The Execution.

HARPER, WILLIAM A.: Producer, b. Port Jervis, N.Y., Sept. 3, 1915; e. Univ. So. Calif. (BS), 1936. Founder member Delta Kappa Alpha frat (cinematography), U.S.C.; started in m.p. ind. in pub.; later asst. dir., prod. mgr., director; In WW II Major, USMC. Organized Marine Corps Photo Service, then in chg. Marine Corps Photo activities Pacific Ocean Areas. End of war organized Reliance Film Co., Inc., eng. in prod., dist., early TV prod. Recalled active duty for Korean War, headed USMC Photo Service. Co-prod. with Navy (Adm. John Ford) feat. documentary, This is Korea; govt. liaison with March of Time, Crusade in Pacific and with NBC US Navy Victory at Sea; prod. dir., writer, Loucks & Norling Studios, 1952; free lance writer-director 1953–55; with Fred Feldkamp Prods. 1955–56; in Europe 1956–58. Assoc. prod. The Silken Affair (RKO) 1956; Producer, The Stranding in Holland 1957; prod. advisor The Last Blitzkreig (Col.), Europe, (1958); producer, The Stone, 1962; Managing Director, St. James Productions Ltd., (England) and Pres. American-European Entertainments, Inc. (Paris).

HARRINGTON, CURTIS: Director, writer. b. Los Angeles, Calif., Sept. 17; e. U. Southern Calif., B.A. Exec. assts. to Jerry Wald, 1955–61 Associate Producer at 20th Cent. Fox.
PICTURES INCLUDE: Hound Dog Man, Return to Peyton Place, The Stripper, Night Tide and Queen of Blood, released by A.I.P. For Universal, What's the Matter with Helen? (UA) 1971, Gingerbread House, The Killing Kind.

HARRINGTON, PAT (JR.): Actor. b. New York City, Aug. 13, 1929. e. Fordham U. Served USAF as 1st Lt., 1952–54. Time salesman for NBC, 1954–58. Some 150 TV appearances on Jack Paar, Steve Allen and Danny Thomas TV shows, 1958–61; nightclub appearances, 1960–63. TV and films, 1963 to present. Television Series include: Mr. Deeds Goes to Town, Owen Marshall, and One Day at a Time.
PICTURES INCLUDE: The Wheeler Dealers, Move Over Darling, Easy Come, Easy Go, The President's Analyst, 2000 Years Later, The Candidate.

HARRIS, BARBARA: Actress. b. Evanston, Ill., 1935. e. Wright Junior College (Chicago), Goodman School of the Theatre and U. of Chicago. Joined acting troop, The Compass, and came to N.Y. where first role was in Oh, Dad, Poor Dad, Mamma's Hung You in the Closet and I'm Feeling So Sad, repeating in m.p.
PLAYS: On a Clear Day You Can See Forever,The Apple Tree.
PICTURES INCLUDE: Thousand Clowns, Who Is Harry Kellerman?, The War Between Men and Women, Mixed

Company, Nashville, Family Plot, Movie Movie, The North Avenue Irregulars, The Seduction of Joe Tynan.

HARRIS, BURTT: Producer. Began career as actor; later worked with Elia Kazan as prod. asst. and asst. dir. on America America, Splendor in the Grass, and The Arrangement. Worked as second unit dir. and asst. dir. on many films as well as producer and actor.
PICTURES: Associate Producer: Little Murders, The Wiz, Cruising, Gilda Live. Executive Producer: The Verdict, Just Tell Me What You Want. Producer: Prince of the City, Daniel, Deathtrap, Garbo Talks. Co-Producer: D.A.R.Y.L. Actor: Splendor in the Grass, Fail Safe, The Taking of Pelham 1-2-3, The Wanderers, The Verdict, Daniel, Garbo Talks, D.A.R.Y.L., etc.

HARRIS, ED: Actor. b. Tenafly, NJ, 1950.
PICTURES: Borderline, Knightriders, Creepshow, The Right Stuff, Under Fire, Swing Shift, Places in the Heart, Alamo Bay, A Flash of Green, Sweet Dreams, Code Name: Emerald.

HARRIS, EDWARD M.: Exhibitor. b. Holdenville, Okla., Aug. 21, 1916. e. Tulsa U. Theatre mgr. in Neosho, Mo., since 1933; now mgr., co-owner, Gardner Theatres there. Member: Kans.-Mo. Theatre Assn. (pres. 1954-56).

HARRIS, JAMES B.: Prod. Dir. b. New York City, Aug. 3, 1928; e. Julliard School. U.S. film export, 1947; Realart Pictures, 1948; formed Flamingo Films, 1949; formed Harris-Kubrick Productions, 1954. Producer of The Killing, Paths of Glory, Lolita; formed James B. Harris Prods., Inc., 1963; prod., dir., The Bedford Incident, 1965; produced, directed & wrote screenplay, Some Call It Loving, 1973; prod., Telefon, 1977; Fast-Walking, 1981 (prod., dir., s.p.).

HARRIS, JULIE: Designer. b. London, England. e. Chelsea Arts School. Entered industry in 1945 designing for Gainsborough Studios. First film, Holiday Camp.
PICTURES INCLUDE: Greengage Summer, Naked Edge, The War Lover, Fast Lady, Chalk Garden, Psyche 59, A Hard Day's Night, Darling, Help, The Wrong Box, Casino Royale, Deadfall, Prudence and the Pill, Decline and Fall, Goodbye Mr. Chips, Sherlock Holmes, Follow Me!, Live and Let Die, Rollerball, Slipper and The Rose, Dracula.
TV: Laura (with Lee Radziwill), Candleshoe, The Sailor's Return, Lost and Found, The Kingfisher, Arch of Trumiph, Sign of Four, Hound of the Baskervilles.

HARRIS, JULIE: Actress. b. Grosse Pointe, Mich., Dec. 2, 1925; e. Yale Drama Sch. m.p. debut in Member of the Wedding.
PICTURES INCLUDE: East of Eden, I Am a Camera, The Trouble with Women, The Haunting, Harper, Reflection in a Golden Eye, The Poacher's Daughter, You're a Big Boy Now, The Split, The People Next Door, The Hiding Place, Voyage of the Damned, The Bell Jar.
B'WAY PLAYS: Sundown Beach, Playboy of the Western World, Macbeth, Young and the Fair, Magnolia Alley, Monserrat, Member of the Wedding, I Am a Camera, Colombe, The Lark, And Miss Reardon Drinks a Little, The Last of Mrs. Lincoln (Tony Award).
TV: Little Moon of Alban, Johnny Belinda, A Doll's House, Ethan Frome, The Good Fairy, The Lark, He Who Gets Slapped, The Heiress, Victoria Regina, Pygmalion, Anastasia, The Holy Terror, The Power and The Glory. Series: Knot's Landing.

HARRIS, PHIL: Orchestra leader. b. Linton, Ind., June 24, 1906; husband of Alice Faye, actress. In 1933: with orchestra in Melody Cruise. In 1936: Vitaphone short prod. In 1937: Turn Off the Moon. In 1939: Man About Town. IN 1940: Buck Benny Rides Again, Dreaming Out Loud.
PICTURES INCLUDE: I Love a Bandleader, Wabash Avenue, Wild Blue Yonder, Starlift, High and the Mighty, Anything Goes, Good-Bye My Lady. Co-starred with Alice Faye in weekly radio show; many TV appearances.

HARRIS, RICHARD: Actor. b. Limerick, Ireland, Oct. 1, 1930.
PICTURES INCLUDE: Alive and Kicking, Shake Hands With the Devil, The Long, The Short and The Tall, Guns of Navarone, Mutiny on the Bounty, This Sporting Life, The Red Desert (Italy), Major Dundee, The Heroes of Telemark, The Bible, Hawaii, Camelot, The Molly Maguires, A Man Called Horse, Cromwell, Bloomfield (actor & dir.), Man in the Wilderness, The Snow Goose, The Deadly Trackers, Gulliver, 99 and 44/100% Dead, Juggernaut, Echoes of a Summer, Robin and Marian, Return of the Man Called Horse, The Cassandra Crossing, Orca, Golden Rendezvous, The Wild Geese, The Ravagers, The Number, Game for Vultures, High Point, Your Ticket is No Longer Valid, Martin's Day.

HARRIS, ROBERT: Executive. Senior v.p., Universal TV, with responsibility of supervising Universal programming on CBS network. In 1981 named pres. of Universal TV.

HARRIS, ROSEMARY: Actress. b. Ashby, Suffolk, 1930; e. India and England. Early career, nursing; studied Royal Acad. of Dramatic Art, 1951-52.
PLAYS INCLUDE: Climate of Eden (New York), Seven Year Itch, Confidential Clerk (Paris Festival), and with Bristol Old Vic, The Crucible, Much Ado About Nothing, Merchant of Venice.
Screen debut in Beau Brummell, The Shiralee, TV, Cradle of Willow, Othello, The Prince and the Pauper, The Tale of Two Cities, Dial M for Murder, etc. On stage, at Old Vic, 1955-56; U.S. tour, 1956-57; U.S. stage, 1958-63.
TV: Profiles in Courage, A Dickens Chronicle, Athens Where the Theatre Began; Blithe Spirit.
Chichester Festivals 1962 and 63; Nat'l Theatre 1963-64; You Can't Take It With You, 1965; The Lion in Winter, 1966, (U.S. Stage); 1967, APA Repertory Co., A Lion in Winter.
PICTURES INCLUDE: Camelot, The Boys from Brazil, The Ploughman's Lunch.

HARRISON, GREGORY: Actor. b. Avalon, Catalina Island, off coast of California, May 31, 1950. Started acting in school plays; then joined Army. Studied at Estelle Harman Actors Workshop; later with Lee Strasberg and Stella Adler. Film debut in Jim, the World's Greatest (1976). Also in Fraternity Row and Razorback.
TELEVISION: Series: Logan's Run, MASH, Barnaby Jones, Trapper John. Movies: The Gathering, Enola Gay, Trilogy in Terror, the Best Place To Be, The Women's Room, For Ladies Only, The Fighter, Seduced. Mini-series: Centennial.

HARRISON, JOAN: Writer, producer. b. Guildford, Surrey, England; e. U. Sorbonne; Oxford U., B. A. Began screen career in England as asst. & writer with Alfred Hitchcock, dir. To U.S. 1939 to write s.p. Rebecca.
PICTURES INCLUDE: Foreign Correspondent, Suspicion, Saboteur, Phantom Lady, Dark Waters, The Strange Affair of Uncle Harry, Ride A Pink Horse, Circle of Danger, Eye Witness.
Prod. Alfred Hitchcock Presents, TV.

HARRISON, KATHLEEN: Actress. b. Lancashire, Eng., Trained at R.A.D.A.
PLAYS: Night Must Fall, Corn Is Green, Flare Path, Winslow Boy, Flowers for the Living, The Silver Box, Waters of the Moon, All for Mary, Nude With Violin, How Say You, Watch It Sailor, The Chances, Norman, Collapse of Stout Party, Mrs. Puffin, Harvey, She Stoops to Conquer (1972).
PICTURES INCLUDE: Bank Holiday, A Girl Must Live, Night Must Fall, In Which We Serve, Major Barbara, Holiday Camp, Bond Street, Oliver Twist, Winslow Boy, Trio, Magic Box, Waterfront, Here Comes the Huggetts, Vote for Huggett, Huggetts Abroad, Scrooge, The Happy Family, Pickwick Papers, Turn the Key Softly, Lilacs in the Spring, Where There's a Will, Cast a Dark Shadow, All for Mary, It's a Great Life, Big Money, Home and Away, Seven Thunders, A Cry From the Streets, Alive and Kicking, Mrs. Gibbons Boys, Fast Lady, West Eleven, Lock Up Your Daughters, Our Mutual Friend.
TV: Mrs. Thursday, series, Waters of the Moon, High Finance, Dixon of Dock Green, Spring & Autumn, VXB.

HARRISON, REX: Actor. b. Derry House, Huyton, Lancashire, England, Mar. 5, 1908; m. Rachel Roberts. In the RAF, World War II. Stage debut 1924 in "Thirty Minutes in a Street," Liverpool Repertory theatre, England; later on British tour ("Charley's Aunt," "Alibi," etc.) London debut 1930 in "Getting George Married." To New York, 1936, in "Sweet Aloes."
PLAYS INCLUDE: London, repertory, tour. New York stage: Anne of a Thousand Days, Henry VIII, 1948; Cocktail Party, London, 1950; Bell, Book & Candle, New York, 1951; Venus Observed, Love of 4 Colonels, N.Y.: Bell, Book & Candle, London.
PICTURES INCLUDE: Began screen career, 1929. Films include Men Are Not Gods, Storm in a Teacup, School for Husbands, Over the Moon, The Citadel, Ten Days in Paris, Sidewalks of London, Night Train, Major Barbara, Blithe Spirit. Voted one of top ten British money-making stars in Motion Picture Herald-Fame Poll, 1945-46. To Hollywood, 1946. I Live in Grosvenor Square, The Rake's Progress, Anna and the King of Siam, The Ghost and Mrs. Muir, Foxes of Harrow, Escape, Unfaithfully Yours, The Long Dark Hall, The Four Poster, King Richard & the Crusaders, Constant Husband, The Reluctant Debutante, Midnight Lace, Once a Thief, Cleopatra, My Fair Lady, The Yellow Rolls-Royce, The Agony and the Ecstasy, The Honey Pot, Dr. Doolittle, A Flea In Her Ear, Staircase, The Prince and the Pauper, A Time To Die.
BROADWAY STAGE: in My Fair Lady, 1956-57; B'way stage in The Fighting Cock, 1959-60; London, My Fair Lady, 1958-59; Platinov, London, 1960; 1961, August for The People. Both Seasons at Royal Court Theatre, London. nom. best actor for Cleopatra; acad. award, 1965, My Fair Lady; New York Film Critics Award, 1965; Golden Globe, 1965; David di Donatello award, 1965; Top ten world box office star, 1966.

HARROLD, KATHRYN: Actress. b. Tazewell, VA. e. Mills College. Studied acting at Neighborhood Playhouse in N.Y.: also with Uta Hagen. Appeared in off-off-Bdwy. plays for year; then joined experimental theatre group, Section Ten, touring East, performing and teaching at Connecticut College and New York univ. Cast in TV daytime serial, The Doctors.
PICTURES: Nightwing (debut), The Hunter, Modern Romance, The Pursuit of D.B. Cooper, Yes, Gorgio, The Sender, Into the Night, Raw Deal.
TELEVISION: Movies: Son-Rise, a Miracle of Love, Vampire, Bogie, An Uncommon Love. Series: Starsky and Hutch, Women in White.

HARRYHAUSEN, RAY: Producer, Writer, Special Effects Expert. b. L.A. e. L.A. City Coll. While at coll. made 16mm animated film, Evolution, which got him job as model animator for George Pal's Puppetoons in early '40s. Served in U.S. Signal Corps; then made series of filmed fairy tales with animated puppets for schools and churches. In 1946 worked on Mighty Joe Young as ass't. to Willis O'Brien. Designed and created special visual effects for The Beast from 20,000 Fathoms; then began evolving own model animation system called Dynarama. In 1952 joined forces with prod. Charles H. Schneer, using new process for first time in It Came from Beneath the Sea. Subsequently made many films with Schneer in Dynarama.
PICTURES INCLUDE: Twenty Million Miles to Earth, The Three Worlds of Gulliver, Jason and the Argonauts, the First Men in the Moon, One Million Years B.C., The Valley of Gwangi, The Golden Voyage of Sinbad, Sinbad and the Eye of the Tiger, Clash of the Titans (co. prod., special effects).

HART, HARVEY: Director. b. Canada, Mar. 19, 1928. Began career on TV in native country then went to Hollywood.
PICTURES INCLUDE: Bus Riley's Back in Town, Sullivan's Empire, The Sweet Ride, Fortune and Men's Eyes, The Pyx, Aliens Are Coming, Utilities.
TELEVISION: East of Eden, Master of the Game, Beverly Hills Madam.

HARTFORD, K.: Executive, b. New York, July 5, 1922. Graduate Univ. Cincinnati, Los Angeles City college. Active in Film Financing, co-production, packaging. Executive of Hartford Industries, Latin Ameican Developmnet & Investment Co., Western International. Has offices in 8 countries.

HARTLEY, MARIETTE: Actress. b. New York City, June 21, 1940.
PICTURES: Ride the High Country, Marooned, Skyjacked, Marnie, Improper Channels.
TELEVISION: Peyton Place, Stone, the Incredible Hulk, Second Time Around, Good Night Beantown. Movies: Earth II, Sandcastles, Genesis II, Killer Who Wouldn't Die, Last Hurrah, Silence of the Heart, My Two Loves.

HARTMAN, DAVID: Actor. b. Pawtucket, R.I., May 19, 1935. e. Duke Univ. Was 2nd Lt. in Air Force; entered Amer. Acad. of Dramatic Arts in N.Y. Appeared in off-Bdwy. musicals and summer stock; Bdwy. debut in Hello, Dolly!
PICTURES INCLUDE: The Island at the Top of the World.
TV: World Premiere: I Love a Mystery, Nobody's Perfect, Ballad of Josie. Series: The Virginian, The Bold Ones, Lucas Tanner, Good Morning, America.

HARTMAN, ELIZABETH: Actress. b. Youngstown, O., December, 1943. e. Carnegie Tech.
PICTURES INCLUDE: Patch of Blue, The Group, You're a Big Boy Now, The Fixer, The Beguiled, Walking Tall, Full Moon High.

HARTMAN, PAUL: Actor, dancer, comedian. e. U. of Calif.; pr. Ferris Hartman. In show business since a child; toured West Coast with own vaude. act; toured Asia & Europe; worked in supper clubs.
BROADWAY: Red Hot & Blue, You Never Know, Of Thee I Sing, Angel in the Wings, Tickets Please, Ballyhoo, Topnotchers, Keep 'Em Laughing, All for Love, Showboat, The Pajama Game, Drink to Me Only, What A Killing, A Funny Thing Happened on the Way to the Forum.
PICTURES INCLUDE: 45 Fathers, Sunny, Higher & Higher, Man on a Tightrope, Inherit the Wind, The Thrill of It All, Soldiers in the Rain, Those Calloways, How To Succeed in Business Without Really Trying, The Reluctant Astronaut, Luv.
TV: Our Town, Petrified Forest, 12 Angry Men, Good Old Charlie Faye, Alfred Hitchcock, Ben Casey, The Defenders, Have Gun, Will Travel, Mary Martin Easter Show, Hazel, Ozzie & Harriet, Chrysler Thea., Pride of the Family, Andy Griffith Show, Petticoat Junction, Mayberry RFD, The Hartmans At Home.
AWARDS: Tony Award, Comedian of the Year; Donaldson Award, Best Comdeian on Broadway; Newspaper Guild Page One Award, Best Night Club Act; Lambs Club Award, contribution to Amer. Theatre; Daily MIrror Night Club Award; Critics Award for Best Comedian in Musical; Variety Poll Award, 1947–48.

HARTZ, JIM: TV Newsman and Panelist. b. Feb. 3, 1940, Tulsa, Okla. Pre-med student at University of Tulsa, where worked in spare time as reporter for radio station KRMG. In 1963 left studies for career as newsman and joined KOTV in Tulsa. In 1964 moved to NBC News in New York, acting as reporter and anchorman. In 1974 became co-host of Today Show, joined Barbara Walters.

HARVEY, ANTHONY: Director. b. London, Eng., June 3, 1931. Royal Academy of Dramatic Arts; two yrs. as actor. Ent. m.p. ind. 1949 with Crown Film Unit.
PICTURES INCLUDE: Private's Progress, Brothers-in-Law, Man in the Cocked Hat, Carlton Brown of the F.O., I'm Alright Jack, The Angry Silence, The Millionairess, Lolita, The L-Shaped Room, Dr. Strangelove, Spy Who Came In From the Cold, The Whisperers, Directed Dutchman; Dir. The Lion in Winter, They Might Be Giants, Eagles' Wing, Players, The Abdication, The Glass Menagerie, Richard's Things, The Ultimate Solution of Grace Quigley.
TV: The Disappearance of Aimee, Svengali, The Pat Neal Story, Glass Menagerie.

HARWOOD, RONALD: Writer. b. Cape Town, South Africa, 1934. To England to study acting at RADA, 1951.
TV: The Barber of Stamford Hill, Private Potter, Take a Fellow Like Me, The Lads, Convalescence, Guests of Honor, The Paris Trip, New Assistant, The Guests. Adapted several of the Tales of the Unexpected.
PICTURES INCLUDE: Barber of Stamford Hill, Private Potter (written with Casper Wrede), subsequently High Wind in Jamaica, Eye Witness, One Day in the Life of Ivan Denisovich, Operation Daybreak, The Dresser.

HASSANEIN, RICHARD C.: Executive. b. New York City, Aug. 13, 1951. e. Staunton Military Academy (1966–70); Amer. Univ. (1970–74). booker/real estate dept. opns., United Artists Theater Circuit, 1974–77; joined United Film Distribution Co., 1977; named pres. 1978.

HASSANEIN, SALAH M.: Executive. b. Suez, Egypt, e. British School, Alexandria, Egypt, Nat'l Bank of Egypt, Cairo, 1939–42. Asst. division mgr. Middle East, 20th-Fox, Cairo, Egypt, 1942–44: U.S. armed forces, 1945–47; usher, asst. mgr., Rivoli Theatre, N.Y., 1947–48. Film buyer, booker, oper. v.p. U.A. Eastern Theas., 1948–59; pres. 1960; exec. v.p. U.A. Communications, Inc. 1960; v.p. United Artists Cable News Corp.; pres. Todd-AO Corp., 1963.

HASSELHOFF, DAVID: Actor. b. Baltimore, MD, July 17, 1952.
PICTURE: Starcrash.
TELEVISION: The Young and the Restless, Knight Rider. Movies: Griffin and Phoenix, Semi Tough, After Hours—Getting to Know Us, The Cartier Affair, Bridge Across Time, etc.

HASTINGS, DON: Performer; b. Apr. 1, 1934, Bklyn., N.Y., e. Professional Children's Sch.; on B'way in Life With Father, I Remember Mama, Summer and Smoke, etc.; on various radio shows, video ranger on Capt. Video since 1949, also occasional TV guest appearances.

HATFIELD, BOBBY: Performer. b. Beaver Dam, Wis., Aug. 10, 1940. e. Long Beach State Coll. Mem., Righteous Bros. recording team.
TV: Shindig, The Danny Kaye Show, Ed Sullivan Show.
PICTURES INCLUDE: Beach Ball, Swingin' Summer.

HATFIELD, HURD: Actor. b. New York City, 1918. e. Morristown prep, Horace Mann; Riverdale Acad., Columbia U., Chekhov Drama School, Devonshire, Eng., on dramatic stage, Lower Depths, Twelfth Night, Cricket on the Hearth, King Lear, then Screen debut Dragon Seed, The Picture of Dorian Gray, 1943–44.
PICTURES INCLUDE: The Unsuspected, Joan of Arc, Destination Murder, Tarzan & Slave Girl, Left-Handed Gun, Mickey One, Harlow, Von Richtofen and Brown, King David.
N.Y. stage 1952, Venus Observed. TV appearances.

HATFIELD, TED: Executive. b. Wilton Junction, Iowa, Aug. 26, 1936. e. Hot Springs, Ark., U.S. Army-NCO Academy (1954). Entered industry as usher, ABC Paramount Theatre, Hot Springs, Ark (1949) continuously employed by ABC Theatres as doorman, ass't manager, manager, city manager (1949–1967). Joined MGM Studios as assistant exploitation director (1967) assistant national advertising coordinator (1970) national advertising coordinator (1971). Now v.p., field operations, MGM/UA.
MEMBER: Variety Club; Motion Picture Pioneers; past v.p., Louisiana Jr. Chamber of Commerce; Past pres. Ark.-La.-Miss. Advertising Club; Great Western Boy Scout Council of L.A.; v.p., Culver City Chamber of Commerce.

HAUER, RUTGER: Actor. b. Breukelen, Netherlands, Jan. 23, 1944. Stage actor in Amsterdam for six years. Motion picture debut in Turkish Delight, 1975.
PICTURES INCLUDE: The Wilby Conspiracy, Keetje Tippl'e, Max Havelaar, Soldier of Orange, Pastorale 1943, Femme Entre Chien et Loup, Mysteries, Nighthawks, The Blade Runner, Chanel Solitaire, Eureka, The Osterman

Weekend, A Breed Apart, Ladyhawke, Flesh and Blood, The Hitcher.

HAVELOCK-ALLAN, SIR ANTHONY: Baronet; film producer, born Durham County, England; e. Charterhouse, Switzerland; 1924–1929 Artists and Recording Manager, Brunswick Grammophone Co. London & Vox AG. Berlin; 1930 Advertising Dept. "Evening Standard"; 1930–1933 presented Cabaret-Ciro's Club, London; 1933 entered Films asst Casting Director and Producer's Assistant; 1935–1937 produced 23 Quota Films for Paramount; 1938–1940 produced for Pinebrook Ltd. and Two Cities Films; 1941 Associate producer to Noel Coward; 1942 with David Lean and Ronald Neame formed Cineguild; 1942–1947 Producer, associate producer or in charge of production for Cineguild; 1949 formed constellation Films, independent company producing for Rank Org. and British Lion; from 1948–1951 Member of the Cinematographic Films Council and the National Film Production Council; also Member of Home Department's Committee on Employment of Children in Entertainment; 1952 Chairman of the British Film Academy; 1958 formed with John Brabourne and Daniel Angel British Home Entertainment; 1962 and 1963 Chairman of the Council of the Society of Film and Television Arts (B.A.F.T.A.); Member of National Film Archive Committee; from 1958–1965 a Governor of the British Film Institute and Member of the Institute's Production Committee; 1970 Member of the U.S. Academy of Motion Pictures Arts & Sciences.

PICTURES INCLUDE: This Man Is News, This Man in Paris, Lambeth Walk, Unpublished Story, From the Four Corners (documentary produced and directed), Brief Encounter (shared Academy script nomination), Great Expectations (shared Academy script nomination), Take My Life, Blanche Fury, Shadow of the Eagle, Never Take No for an Answer, Young Lovers, (director Anthony Asquith), Orders to Kill, (director Anthony Asquith), Brendon Behan's The Quare Fellow, An Evening with The Royal Ballet (directed two ballets); (for Television only): National Theatre's "Uncle Vanya"; Olivier's "Othello," Zeffirelli's "Romeo and Juliet," David Lean's "Ryan's Daughter."

HAVOC, JUNE: Actress. r.n. Hovick. b. Seattle, Wash., 1916. Sister of Gypsy Rose Lee, actress. Made film bow when two in Hal Roach prod. Danced with Anna Pavlova troupe, then entered vaudeville in own act. Later, joined Municipal Opera Company, St. Louis, and appeared in Shubert shows. To Hollywood, 1942.

PICTURES INCLUDE: Hello Frisco, Hello, No Time for Love, Sweet and Low Down, Brewster's Millions, Intrigue, Gentleman's Agreement; Red, Hot and Blue; Chicago Deadline, Once a Thief, Follow the Sun, Lady Possessed, Can't Stop the Music.

PLAYS: Pal Joey, Sadie Thompson, Mexican Hayride, Dunnigan's Daughter, Dream Girl, Affairs of State, The Ryan Girl, The Infernal Machine, The Beaux Strategem.

American Shakespeare Festival, Stratford, 1958; The Skin of Our Teeth, Tour for U.S. Dept. of St., 1961; wrote Marathon 33.

TV: Anna Christie, The Bear, Cakes and Ale, Daisy Mayme, The Untouchables; co-owner, Willy.

HAWN, GOLDIE: Actress. b. Washington, D.C., November 21, 1945; was a professional dancer and made TV debut dancing on an Andy Griffith Special; TV acting debut, "Good Morning World" followed by "Laugh-In." Screen debut: Cactus Flower.

PICTURES INCLUDE: There's A Girl In My Soup, Dollars, Butterflies Are Free, The Sugarland Express, The Girl from Petrovaka, Shampoo, The Duchess and the Dirtwater Fox, Foul Play, Private Benjamin (also prod.), Seems Like Old Times, Best Friends, Swing Shift, Protocol (also exec. prod.); Wildcats.

HAYDEN, STERLING: Actor. b. Montclair, N.J.; e. Browne and Nichols School, Cambridge, Mass. In 1937: cruised around world as mate. In 1939: captain of the "Aries" owned by Warner Buxton.

PICTURES INCLUDE: Virginia, Bahama Passage, Blaze of Noon, El Paso, Manhandled, The Asphalt Jungle, Flaming Feather, Journey Into Light, Denver and Rio Grande, Golden Hawk, Hellgate, Flat Top, The Star, Take Me to Town, So Big, Crime Wave, Arrow in the Dust, Prince Valiant, Johnny Guitar, Naked Alibi, Suddenly, Battle Taxi, Timberjack, Eternal Sea, Last Command, Shotgun, Top Gun, The Killing, Hard Contract, The Godfather, The Long Goodbye, King of the Gypsies, Winter Kills, Nine to Five, Gas, Venom.

TELEVISION: The Blue and the Gray.

HAYES, HELEN: Actress, r.n. Helen H. Brown. b. Wash., D.C., Oct. 10, 1901; e. Sacred Heart Convent, Wash.; wife of Charles MacArthur, writer. Started film career in 1931.

PLAYS INCLUDE: What Every Woman Knows, Coquette, Petticoat Influence, The Good Fairy, Mary of Scotland, Victoria Regina, Harriet, Happy Birthday, Wisteria Trees, Mrs. McThing, Skin of Our Teeth, Glass Menagerie, The Show Off, Front Page (revivals).

PICTURES INCLUDE: Arrowsmith, The White Sister, Another Language, Night Flight, A Farewell to Arms, Academy Award 1931–32 (The Sin of Madelon Claudet), My Son, John, Main Street to Broadway, Anastasia, Airport (AA, 1970), Herbie Rides Again, One of Our Dinosaurs Is Missing, Candleshoe.

TV: Twelve Pound Look, Mary of Scotland, Dear Brutus, Skin of Our Teeth, Christmas Tie, Drugstore on a Sunday Afternoon, Omnibus, A Caribbean Mystery, Murder with Mirrors.

HAYES, JOHN MICHAEL: Writer. b. Worcester, Mass., May 11, 1919; e. University of Massachusetts, 1941.

PICTURES INCLUDE: Red Ball Express, Thunder Bay, Torch Song, War Arrow, Rear Window, To Catch a Thief, Trouble with Harry, It's A Dog's Life, Man Who Knew Too Much, The Matchmaker, Peyton Place, But Not For Me, Butterfield 8, The Children's Hour, Where Love Has Gone, The Chalk Garden, Judith, Nevada Smith.

HAYES, PETER LIND: Actor: m. b. San Francisco, June 25, 1915. m. Mary Healy, prof.

PICTURES INCLUDE: Million Dollar Legs, All Women Have Secrets, These Glamour Girls, Seventeen, Dancing on a Dime, Playmates, Seven Days Leave.

Was radio singer, actor, vaudeville, night clubs. Producer, Grace Hayes Lodge Review: on TV show with Mary Healy; 5000 Fingers of Dr. T. Recent films: Once You Kiss A Stranger.

HAYS, ROBERT: Actor. b. Bethesda, MD, July 24, 1947. e. Grossmont College, San Diego State. Left school to join Old Globe Theatre for five years. Cast in ABC series, Harry O.

PICTURES: Airplane, Take This Job and Shove It!, Some Summer Day, Airplane II: The Sequel, Utilities, Trenchcoat, Touched, Scandalous, Cat's Eye.

TELEVISION: Series: Love Boat, Laverne & Shirley, Most Wanted, Wonder Woman, Angie. Movie: California Gold Rush. Mini-series: Will Rogers: Champion of the People, The Girl, The Gold Watch, and Everthing.

HAYWORTH, RITA: Actress. r.n. Margarita Cansino; b. New York City, Oct. 17, 1919; e. private schools. Danced at Foreign Club in Tiajuana, Mexico, then at Agua Caliente. Started screen career 1935 with Dante's Inferno. Formed prod. co. with Dick Haymes, Crystal Bay Prods., 1955.

PICTURES INCLUDE: Meet Nero Wolfe, Who Killed Gail Preston?, There's Always a Woman, Convicted, The Lone Wolf, Spy Hunt, Gilda, Cover Girl, Tonight and Every Night, Down to Earth, Lady from Shanghai, Loves of Carmen, Affair in Trinidad, Salome, Miss Sadie Thompson, Fire Down Below, Pal Joey, Separate Tables, They Came to Cordura, Story on Page One, The Happy Thieves, Circus World, Money Trap, The Poppy Is Also a Flower, The Naked Zoo, Road to Salina, The Wrath of God.

HAZEN, JOSEPH H.: Attorney b. Kingston, N.Y., May 23, 1898; e. George Washington U. & Law School. Formerly assoc. as member of firm, Thomas and Friedman. In 1939 member ind. com. in discussions with Commerce Dept. Member com. which negotiated consent decree. Member ind. Committee of Six, lawyers to study and reorganize ind. activities. Mem. War Activities Committee. In 1944 resigned as v.p. and dir., Warner Bros. to join Hal Wallis Prods. as pres., 1944–48; pres. Wallis-Hazen, Inc., Tillco. dissolved, June 1953; photoplay prod., Hal B. Wallis, Paramount Pictures Corp., since 1953. Dir. USO Camps, Inc., M.P.A.A.

HEALEY, MYRON: Actor, writer, dialogue director. b. Petaluma, Calif., e. East Central State Teachers Coll., Okla.; bombardier, navigator, World War II.

PICTURES INCLUDE: Monsoon, Son of Belle Starr, The Longhorn, African Manhunt, Gang Busters, Man from Bitter Ridge, Cattle Queen of Montana, Rage at Dawn, Shoot Out at Medicine Bend.

Writer on several s.p.; TV shows. Stars in numerous live and filmed TV shows.

HEALY, JOHN T.: Executive. e. Brooklyn Coll. Taught economics and was associated with Lehigh Valley Industries and General Food Corp. before joining ABC, Inc. in 1970 as assoc. dir. of corp. planning. Named dir. of planning and develop. June, 1972. Elected v.p., planning and admin. of ABC Leisure Group, March, 1974; elected vice pres. of corporate planning, Feb., 1976.

HEARD, JOHN: Actor. b. 1947. Married, actress Margot Kidder. Career began at Organic Theatre, starring in Chicago & N.Y. productions of Warp. Other stage roles include Streamers, G.R. Point, Othello.

PICTURES: Between the Lines, On the Yard, Head Over Heels, Heartbeat, Cutter and Bone, Cat People, Heaven Help Us, Lies, After Hours, The Trip to Bountiful.

TELEVISION: The Scarlet Letter, Tender Is the Night.

HEATHERTON, JOEY: Actress. b. Rockville, Centre, NY, Sept. 14, 1944.
PICTURES: Twilight of Honor, Where Love Has Gone, My Blood Runs Cold, Bluebeard, The Happy Hooker Goes to Washington.

HECKART, EILEEN: Actress. b. Columbia, Ohio, Mar. 29, 1919. e. Ohio State U., American Theatre Wing. m. Jack Yankee.
BROADWAY: Bad Seed, View from the Bridge.
TV: Kraft, Suspense, Philco Playhouse, The Web (CBS Playhouse). m.p. debut in Miracle in the Rain.
AWARDS: Daniel Blum and Outer Circle (Picnic), Foreign Press, and Donaldson, Oscar nom. and Film Daily Citation, (Bad Seed), TV Sylvania for the Haven, Variety Poll of N.Y. and Drama Critics (Dark at The Top of the Stairs); Emmy, (Save Me a Place at Forest Lawn).
PICTURES INCLUDE: Somebody Up There Likes Me, Bus Stop, Hot Spell, Heller in Pink Tights, My Six Loves, Up the Down Staircase, No Way to Treat a Lady, Butterflies Are Free, Zandy's Bride, The Hiding Place, Burnt Offerings.
STAGE: Bad Seed, Family Affair, Pal Joey, Invitation to a March, Everybody Loves Opal, Dark at the Top of the Stairs, And Things That Go Bump in the Night, You Know I Can't Hear You When the Water's Running, Too True to Be Good, Butterflies Are Free.

HECKERLING, AMY: Director. b. New York City, May 7, 1954. e. Art & Design High School; NYU; AFI. Made shorts (Modern Times, High Finance, etc.) before turning to features.
PICTURES: Fast Times at Ridgemont High, Johnny Dangerously.

HEDWIG, GORDON W.: President, Nu-Art Films, Inc. b. Jersey City, N.J., April 27, 1913; p. William K. and Elsa Hedwig; e. Newtown high school, Rensselaer Polytechnic Inst., Lt., Signal Corp. World War II. Part-time work film lab., 1927–33; salesman, 1933–35. Started 16 mm. distribution in 1935 as Nu-Art Film co., an individual enterprise and incorporated as Nu-Art Films, Inc., 1937. President NuArt Films, Inc., org. Telecast Films, Inc., org. in 1947 for TV film distribution. Sec. Theatre-on-films, Inc. Now active in all corporations, in TV & non theatrical.

HEFFNER, RICHARD.: Executive. b. Aug. 5, 1925. e. Columbia Univ. Instrumental in acquisition of Channel 13 (WNET) as New York's educational tv station; served as its first general manager. Previously had produced and moderated Man of the Year, The Open Mind, etc. for commercial TV. Served as dir. of public affairs programs for WNBC-TV in N.Y. Was also dir. of special projects for CBS TV Network and editorial consultant to CBS, Inc. Editorial Board. Was radio newsman for ABC. Taught history at Univ. of Calif. at Berkeley, Sarah Lawrence College, Columbia Univ. and New School for Social Research, N.Y. Served as American specialist in communications for U.S. Dept. of State in Japan, Soviet Union, Germany, Yugoslavia, Israel, etc. Now produces and moderates The Open Mind on Channel 11 (WPIX) in New York and is exec. editor of From The Editor's Desk. Is Univ. Prof. of Communications and Public Policy at Rutgers University. In July, 1974 appt. chmn. of classification and rating admin. rating board.

HEFFRON, RICHARD T.: Director. b. Chicago, Oct. 6, 1930.
PICTURES INCLUDE: Fillmore, Newman's Law, Trackdown, Futureworld, Outlaw Blues, I, the Jury.
TV: The Morning After, Dick Van Dyke Special, I Will Fight No More Forever, Toma (pilot), Rockford Files (pilot). Movies: The Mystic Warrior, V: The Final Battle, Anatomy of an Illness.

HEIDER, FREDERICK: Producer. b. Milwaukee, Wis., April 9, 1917. e. Notre Dame U., Goodman Theatre, Chicago. Actor in Globe Theatre, Orson Welles' Mercury Theatre.
TELEVISION & RADIO: Chesterfield Supper Club, Sammy Kaye's So You Want to Lead a Band, Frankie Carle Show, Jo Stafford Show, prod., writer, Paul Whiteman Goodyear Revue, Billy Daniels Show, Martha Wright Show, Earl Wrightson Show, Club Seven, Mindy Carson Show; prod., ABC, Ted Mack Family Hour, Dr. I.Q., Miss America Pageant, Bishop Sheen's Life Is Worth Living, Voice of Firestone, Music for a Summer Night. Music for a Spring Night, The Bell Telephone Hour. (Warner Bros. TV) publisher, Television Quarterly, National Academy of Television Arts and Sciences. Presently columnist, The Desert Sun, Palm Springs, CA.

HELD, DAVID: Executive. Entered industry as atty. in United Artists' legal dept. 1976, joined Paramount as sr. atty. in legal dept.; transferred to business affairs 1977; promoted to v.p., business affairs, 1979. Left for sabbatical 1983; re-entered industry with Sameuel Goldwyn Co. as v.p., business affairs. 1984, returned to Paramount as sr. v.p. in chg. business affairs.

HELLER, FRANKLIN: Producer-director. b. Dover, N.J.; e. Carnegie Inst. of Tech., B.A., 1934. Actor, 1934–36; stage mgr., Sam Harris-Max Gordon Prods., 1936–44; exec. prod., USO shows N.Y., 1944–45; prod. & dir., Paramount, 1945–47; dir., summer stock, 1947–48; prod. & dir., CBS TV, 1949–54; exec., prod. and dir. Goodson-Todman Prods., 1954–69; exec. prod. Protocol Prods., 1969–72 Literary Representative 1972. Dirs. Guild of America, Nat'l bd. 1965–77; Treas. 1965–69; Sec. 1970–73; Chr. Publications 1966–76.
TV SHOWS: What's My Line?, Beat the Clock, The Front Page, The Web, Danger, To Tell the Truth, I've Got a Secret.

HELLER, LUKAS: Writer. b. Germany, 1930. Started as reader at Pinewood Studios, England; later working in various production capacities. Writing career began when Robert Aldrich assigned him to script for What Ever Happened to Baby Jane? (1962). Long collaboration with Aldrich followed.
PICTURES: The Killing of Sister George, The Flight of the Phoenix, Too Late the Hero, The Dirty Dozen, Hush Hush Sweet Charlotte, Monty Walsh, The Deadly Trackers, Damnation Alley, Blue City, etc.
TELEVISION: Hitler's SS—Portrait in Evil.

HELLER, PAUL M.: Producer. b. N.Y.C. Sept. 25, 1927. e. Hunter Coll., Drexel Inst. of Technology. President, Intrepid Productions. Studied engineering until entry into U.S. Army as member of security agency, special branch of signal corps. Left Army and went into fine arts and theatre. Worked as set designer (Westport, East Hampton, Palm Beach) and in live TV and then on theatrical films. Debut as film producer, David and Lisa (1963). From 1964 to 1969 was president of MPO Pictures Inc. Joined Warner Bros. as prod. exec., 1970. In 1972 founded Sequoia Pictures, Inc. with Fred Weintraub. Now pres. of Paul Heller Prods. Inc.
PICTURES INCLUDE: David & Lisa, The Eavesdropper, Secret Ceremony, Enter the Dragon, Truck Turner, Golden Needles, Dirty Knight's Work, Outlaw Blues, The Pack, The Promise, First Monday in October.

HELLMAN, JEROME: Producer. b. New York City. e. N.Y.U. Joined ad dept. of New York Times then went to William Morris Agency as apprentice. Made Asst. in TV dept. Worked as agent for Jaffe Agency. After hiatus in Europe joined Ashley-Steiner Agency (later IFA) where clients included Franklin Schaffner, Sidney Lumet, George Roy Hill, John Frankenheimer. Functioned as TV prod., including Kaiser Aluminum Hour. Left to form own agency, Ziegler, Hellman and Ross. Switched to feature prod. with The World of Henry Orient in 1964.
PICTURES INCLUDE: A Fine Madness, Midnight Cowboy (AA), The Day of the Locust, Coming Home, Promises in the Dark (also dir.).

HELLPMANN, ROBERT SIR: CBE., Actor-dancer, producer, choreographer. b. Mount Gambier, Australia, April 9, 1909; e. Prince Alfred's Coll., Adelaide, Aus.; studied dancing under Laurent Novikoff. Solo dancer, 1923, Theatre Royal, Adlaide. London debut, 1931, at Sadler's Wells. Appeared on screen, 1942 in One of Our Aircraft Is Missing.
PICTURES INCLUDE: Henry V, Caravan, The Red Shoes, Tales of Hoffmann, Iron Petticoat, Big Money, The Quiller Memorandum, 55 Days at Peking, Chitty Chitty Bang Bang, Alice's Adventures in Wonderland, Don Quixote, The Mango Tree, Patrick.
London & N.Y. stage in Caesar and Cleopatra, Anthony and Cleopatra, The Millionaires, TV, U.S. and England; Old Vic Australian tour, 1955; Old Vic London, 1956–57, Nude with Violin, Royal Ballet, 1958–59; Australian tour. Prod.: The Sleeping Beauty, Paris 1960; The Ghost Sonata, BBC TV play, 1962; awarded CBE 1965; Australian of the Year, 1966; co-artistic dir. of Australian Ballet, 1965–76. Knighted, 1968.

HEMINGWAY, MARGAUX: Actress. b. Portland, OR, Feb. 1955. Granddaughter of the late Ernest Hemingway. Model.
PICTURES: Lipstick, Killer Fish, A Fistful of Chopsticks, Over the Brooklyn Bridge.

HEMINGWAY, MARIEL: Actress. b. November, 1961. Granddaughter of novelist Ernest Hemingway. Sister of Margaux Hemingway, model and actress.
PICTURES: Lipstick (debut, 1976), Manhattan, Personal Best, Star 80, The Mean Season, Creator.
TELEVISION: I Want to Keep My Baby.

HEMMINGS, DAVID: Actor, director. b. Guildford, England, 1941. Early career in opera. Ent. m.p. ind. 1956.
THEATRE: Dylan Thomas in Adventures in the Skin Trade.
TV: Auto Stop, The Big Toe, Out of the Unknown, Beverly Hills Cowgirl Blues.
PICTURES INCLUDE: Some People, Two Left Feet, The System, The Eye of the Devil, Blow Up, Camelot, Charge of the Light Brigade, Only When I Larf, Barbarella, The Best House in London, Alfred The Great, The Walking Stick, Fragment of Fear, Unman Wittering and Zigo, Voices,

Juggernaut, Crossed Swords. Directed: Running Scared, The 14, Quilp, Profundo Rosso, Islands In The Stream, The Squeeze, Murder by Decree, Man, Woman, and Child, Prisoners (also exec. prod.).

HENDERSON, MARCIA: Actress. b. Seattle, Wash., Dec. 11, 1934. e. Univ. of Arizona. Appeared in stock in west; m.p. debut in Delicate Delinquent, 1957.
PICTURES INCLUDE: Short Cut to Hell, I Married a Monster from Outer Space, G.I. Blues, Guns of Wyoming, Town Tamers, Dear Phoebe.
Many TV appearances.

HENDERSON, SKITCH: Mus. dir. r.n. Lyle Henderson, b. Birmingham, England, Dec. 7, 1918. e. U. of Calif.
TV: Steve Allen Show, Tonight Show.

HENDRICKS, BILL L.: Owner/Director Bill Hendricks Films; writer, prod. dir. of documentaries & shorts and TV commercials. b. Grand Prairie, Texas, May 3; e. St. John's College. Formerly Warner Bros. Studio Publicity Director; special asst. to Jack Warner; and Director WB Cartoon Studios. Winner first Quigley Grand Award; mgr., Friendship Train & Merci Train. Author "Encyclopedia of Exploitation" with Howard Waugh, "Showmanship in Advertising" with Montgomery Orr; writer, prod., A Force in Readiness, (Academy Award). The John Glenn Story (Oscar nomination), The FBI, Seapower, The Land We Love, A Free People, Top Story, A World of Pleasure, Red Nightmare, Star Spangled Revue, This is Eucom, An American Legend, Scenes to Remember, Freedom and You, Jobs, Wonderful World of Warner, Global Marine; Football Safety; An American Partnership, Free Enterprise, Today's Demand, Tomorrow's Challenge, That's Us in the USA, A Special Day. As ASCAP lyricist, songs include Wintersong; Vaya Con Dios, Amigo; March of the Americans; Paris Je T'aime; Hollywood!; Toys For Tots Parade; Merry Christmas!; Happy Song; On With the Show; Ho! To the West; Wait For Me. Colonel, USMCR (Ret); Founder Marine Corps Toys For Tots program.

HENKIN, HOWARD, H.: Executive writer, producer, director. b. New York, Sept. 13, 1926. e. U. of Delaware, 1944. U.S. Army, 1944–46, TV dept., Newell Emmett Agency, 1947–48; gen. mgr., TelePrompter, 1950–54; eastern sales mgr., Shamus Culhane Prod. 1955–57; Academy Pictures 1957–58; pres. HFH Productions, 1958; pres., Henkin Prods. Inc. & Henkin-Faillace Prods. Inc., 1962–68; ch. of bd., Trio Prods., Inc., 1968–80; author of "The Dot System".

HENNER, MARILU: Actress. b. Chicago, Apr. 6, 1952. e. Univ. of Chicago. Studied singing and dancing, appearing in musicals in Chicago and on Broadway in Over Here and Pal Joey. Gained fame as Elaine in TV series, Taxi.
PICTURES: Between the Lines, Blood Brothers, Hammett, The Man Who Loved Women, Cannonball Run II, Johnny Dangerously, Rustler's Rhapsody.
TELEVISION: Movie: Stark.

HENNING, LINDA KAY: Actress, singer. b. Toluca Lake, Calif. Sept. 16, 1944. e. San Fernando Valley State College.
STAGE: Gypsy, Applause, Damn Yankees, I Do, I Do, Pajama Game, Sugar, Wonderful Town, Fiddler on the Roof, Sound of Music, Vanities, Born Yesterday, Mary, Mary, Bus Stop, etc.
PICTURES INCLUDE: Bye Bye Birdie.
TELEVISION: Series: Petticoat Junction, Happy Days, Mork & Mindy, Double Trouble, Barnaby Jones, Love American Style, Adam 12. Pilots: Kudzu, The Circle, Family. Movies: The Dog Days of Arthur Kane, The Return of the Beverly Hillbillies, Gift of Terror.

HENNING, PAUL: TV producer-writer. b. Independence, Mo., Sept. 16, 1911. e. Kansas City School of Law. grad. 1932. Radio singer and disc jockey. Also acted, ran sound effects, sang, wrote scripts. To Chicago 1937–38, to write Fibber McGee and Molly. w. Don Quinn. To Hollywood as writer for Rudy Vallee, 1939. Wrote scripts for Burns and Allen 10 years, including transition radio to TV. In 1953 wrote, produced live and film shows for Dennis Day. Created, wrote, produced Bob Cummings Show, 1954–59. Wrote Beverly Hillbillies, 1962 to date. Created, prod. wrote Petticoat Junction. Exec. prod. Green Acres series. Wrote motion pictures, Lover Come Back, Bedtime Story.

HENREID, PAUL: Actor, director. b. Trieste, Italy, 1907; son of Carl Alphons Hernried Knight of Wasel-Waldingon. Baron Carl von Henreid. e. Maria Theresianishe Academy Inst. Graphic Arts, Vienna. With book pub. taking night courses at Konservatorium, dramatic arts school in Vienna. In Max Reinhardt's Vienna Theat., then in Austrian films. On dramatic stage and in films among them Jersey Lily and Victoria Regina, London. Arrived in N.Y. 1940 for stage play Flight to the West. In Brit. film Night Train. In 1980 awarded Austrian Cross of Honor, 1st Class, for Science and Arts. 1980: Received The American Classic Screen Award from National Film Society. 1983: Texas Film Society Award for Artistic Achievement. 1984: Legend Silver Screen Award.
PICTURES INCLUDE: Joan of Paris, Now Voyager, Casablanca, Of Human Bondage, Song of Love, In Our Time, Devotion, Deception, Between Two Worlds, The Spanish Main, Conspirators, Rope of Sand, Last of the Buccaneers, Pardon My French, So Young—So Bad, Stolen Face, Man in Hiding, Pirates of Tripoli; actor, dir., prod. For Men Only. Actor, dir., Acapulco; Actor, prod.: Hollow Truimph, Ten Thousand Bedrooms, etc. Dir. of TV films for Revue Productions, Warner, Desilu, 4-Star, CBS, Screen Gems, Universal, 20th Century-Fox Studios, Actor; Holiday for Lovers, Never So Few, The Four Horsemen of The Apocalypse, The Great Spy Mission; dir., Live Fast Die Young, Take Five From Five, Deadringer, Blues For Lovers, actor. The Madwoman of Chaillot, Colors of Love, Exorcist II: The Heretic; dir., Bracken's World, dir., The Man and the City, 1972–73, "Don Juan in Hell" on major theatrical tour in the U.S. and Canada for 6 months.
TV: Film: Any Number Can Kill and many other films and series.

HENRY, BUCK: Actor, writer. b. New York City. e. Dartmouth College. Acted in Life with Father, tour, 1948; Fortress of Glass, Circle in the Square; Bernardine, Bwy; 1952–54, U.S. Army; No Time for Sergeants, Nat'l. Co.; The Premise, improvis. theatre, off-Bwy; TV's The Steve Allen Show, writer, performer; That Was the Week That Was, writer, performer.
TV: Garry Moore Show; Steve Allen Show; Get Smart, co-creator with Mel Brooks, story editor; producer of Captain Nice series, pilot for NBC-TV.
PICTURES INCLUDE: The Troublemaker; The Graduate, 1966 for Laurance Turman, (producer); Catch 22 (author & actor); Taking Off, Candy, The Owl and the Pussycat, What's Up, Doc?, The Day of the Dolphin (s.p.), The Man Who Fell to Earth, Heaven Can Wait (actor, co-s.p.), Gloria, First Family (s.p., dir., act.), Protocol (s.p.).

HENRY, FRED: Producer. b. L.A., Calif., May 30, USC Journalism and business administration; CBS-LA radio station KNX newscaster, writer; news, spec. events dir., KMPC-LA. Co-News commentator, CBS, Let's Talk Over the News; Served, U.S.N. Office of Naval Intelligence, Radio Relations Officer on Staff of Supreme Allied Commander, C-B-I Theatre, Admiral Lord Louis Mountbatten; officer, chg. short-wave broadcasting, AFRS, S.F., 1945; appointed news, spec. events dir., KLAC, Don Fedderson; prg. dir. asst. gen. mgr., prg. dir. combined radio-tv operations, KLAC; res. KLAC, Jan. 1954, as vice-pres., exec. prod., Don Fedderson Prod.; supv. prod.: The Millionaire, Do You Trust Your Wife, Betty White Show, Date With Angels, Liberace, Life with Elizabeth, Who Do You Trust; My Three Sons, 1960; Family Affair, 1966; To Rome With Love, 1969; Henry Fonda Show, 1970.

HENRY, JUSTIN: Actor. b. Ryne, NY, May 25, 1971. Debut in Kramer Vs. Kramer (1979) at age 8.
PICTURES: Sixteen Candles, Martin's Day.
TELEVISION: Tiger Town.

HENSLEY, PAMELA: Actress. b. Los Angeles, Oct. 3, 1950. Game show model on The New Treasure Hunt at age 18. Under contract to Universal Studios for seven years, appearing in TV series and movies.
PICTURES: Buck Rogers, Rollerball, Doc Savage, Double Exposure.
TELEVISION: Movies: Any Member Can Kill, Mrs. R., Kingston, Confidential. Series: Toma, Banacek, The Six Million Dollar Man, Switch, Marcus Welby, Buck Rogers, 240 Robert, Matt Houston.

HENSON, JIM: Producer-Director-Writer. b. Greenville, MIss., Sept. 24, 1936. e. Univ. of Maryland. Early TV work with Washington station, appearing with puppets he built called The Muppets. Did commercials in Washington area, followed by bookings on Today, Tonight shows and Ed Sullivan Show. Followed with Sesame Street, The Muppet Show, and series of TV specials he produced and/or directed. Heads own production company, Henson Associates. First theatrical feature: The Muppet Movie, 1979.
PICTURES: The Great Muppet Caper, The Dark Crystal, The Muppets Take Manhattan, Labyrinth.

HENSON, LISA: Executive. e. Harvard Univ. Joined Warner Bros., 1983, as exec. asst. to heads of prod. 1985, named dir. of creative affairs. 1985, promoted to v.p., prod.

HEPBURN, AUDREY: Actress. b. Brussels, May 4, 1929. Appeared in London plays; screen debut in Laughter in Paradise; on B'way in Gigi, Ondine; Star of Tomorrow, 1954.
PICTURES INCLUDE: One Wild Oat, Young Wives' Tales, Lavender Hill Mob, Secret People, Roman Holiday (Academy Award, best actress, 1953), Sabrina, War and Peace, Funny Face, Love in the Afternoon, Green Mansions, The Nun's Story, The Unforgiven, Breakfast at Tiffanys, Paris When it Sizzles, Charade, My Fair Lady, Two for

the Road, Wait Until Dark, Robin and Marian, Bloodline, They All Laughed.
TV: Producers Showcase, Mayerling, 1957.

HEPBURN, KATHARINE: Actress. b. Hartford, Conn., Nov. 8, 1909. On stage in Death Takes a Holiday, Warrior's Husband, The Lake, Philadelphia Story, (film version 1940), As You Like It, Millionairess. Started screen career 1933 with A Bill of Divorcement; then Christopher Strong and won Academy Award same year for Morning Glory. On stage in Merchant of Venice, Taming of the Shrew, Measure for Measure, Coco, West Side Waltz, etc.
PICTURES INCLUDE: Little Women, Spitfire, The Little Minister, Alice Adams, Sylvia Scarlett, Mary of Scotland, A Woman Rebels, Quality Street, Stage Door, Bringing Up Baby, Holiday, Woman of the Year, Keeper of the Flame, Dragon Seed, Without Love, Song of Love, State of the Union, Adam's Rib, Sea of Grass, African Queen, Pat and Mike, Summertime, Iron Petticoat, The Rainmaker, Desk Set, Suddenly Last Summer, Long Day's Journey Into Night, Guess Who's Coming to Dinner, Lion in Winter, The Madwoman of Chaillot, The Trojan Women, A Delicate Balance, Rooster Cogburn, Olly, Olly, Oxen Free, On Golden Pond, Grace Quigley.
TV: The Glass Menagerie, Love Among the Ruins, The Corn Is Green, Mrs. Delafield Wants To Marry.

HEPPEL, ALAN: Executive. e. Harvard Univ. (BA), Yale Univ., Stanford Law School. With Haldeman and Peckerman as associate, practicing entertainment law. 1985, joined Paramount Pictures as atty. for M.P. Group. Mbr., California Bar Assn.

HERALD, PETER: Executive. e. UCLA, BA.
PICTURES INCLUDE: assoc. prod. Almost Angels, Magnificent Rebel, Miracle of the White Stallions, Waltz King, Emil and the Detectives, The Young Loner, prod. supr. There Was a Crooked Man, Soldier Blue; co-prod., Outrageous Fortune, Ballerina, National Lampoon's Class Reunion, Doctor Detroit, D. C. Cab; assoc. prod. The Great Waltz, Assignment: Vienna, Crazy World of Julius Vrooder, Foul Play, Nightwing. Also: W. W. and the Dixie Dancekings, Mandingo, W. C. Fields and Me, Alex and the Gypsy, Silver Streak, Fire Sale, Star Wars.

HERB, THOMAS: Executive. Joined Warner Bros. Intl. 1981 as trainee; 1981–83 in Australia, also as trainee, before moving to Brazil as asst. gen. mgr., 1982–84. Returned to Burbank 1984 as asst. dir. of sls. 1985, named dir. of sls. for WBI.

HERBERT, HOLMES: Actor. b. Mansfield, Nottinghamshire, England, July 3, 1882; e. Rugby, England. First appearance on stage 1890, London; later with John Sanger circus, Robys Minstrels. F. R. Benson Co., in English provinces; also in many London prods.; on Amer. stage with Charles Frohman Co. Began m.p. career in The Terror 1928.
PICTURES INCLUDE: Gentlemen Prefer Blondes, Sporting Age, Madame X, The Kiss, Untamed, Dr. Jekyll and Mr. Hyde (1931), The House of Rothschild, Captain Blood, Lloyds of London, Lancer Spy, British Intelligence, This Above All, Sherlock Holmes in Washington, The Verdict, The Swordsman, Singapore, The Brigand.

HERDER, W. ED: Producer. b. New York City. Univ. of Miami (BBA). Pres. and chm. of bd., Worldfilm Corp. Financial investor in many m.p. and t.v. prods.
PICTURES: Without Each Other, Force of Impulse, Black Cobra, Shoot, Never Too Young to Rock, The Siberian Move, The Gang, Intercept, Scenes From A Murder.
TELEVISION: The World of Brigette Bardot, The Goldie Hawn Special, The Rolling Stones in Concert, The Janis Joplin Special, The Young Rebels, Hollywood: The Magic Kingdom.

HERMAN, NORMAN: Producer-Director. b. Newark, N.J. e. Rutgers Univ., N.Y. Univ. Was accountant in California; in 1955 switched to film ind., joining American Int'l Pictures. Headed AIP prod. dept. 4 years, incl. prod., post-prod., labor negotiations, supervising story dept., etc. Now pres. of Zide-Herman Co., Inc.
PICTURES INCLUDE: All producer in some capacity except where noted as also directing and/or writing: Sierra Stranger, Tokyo After Dark (dir.), Hot Rod Girl, Hot Rod Rumble, Crime Beneath Seas, Look in any Window, Mondy Teeno (dir., co-s.p.), Glory Stompers, Three in the Attic, Bloody Mama, Pretty Boy Floyd, Dunwich, Three in the Cellar, Angle Unchained, Bunny O'Hare, Psych-Out, Killers Three, Frogs, Blacula, Legend of Hell House, Dirty Mary Crazy Larry.
TELEVISION: Writer: Robert Taylor Detectives, Iron Horse, Invaders, Adam 12, Lancer. Director-Producer: Hannibal Cobb, You Are the Judge.

HERMAN, PINKY: Journalist, songwriter. b. N.Y.C., Dec. 23, 1905; e. N.Y.U. Song writer; member, ASCAP. Counsel member, S.P.A.; writer, M.P. News, 1930; 1934; charter member, Songwriters Protective Assoc.; writer, M.P. Daily, 1935–43; columnist, Radio Daily, 1943–50; TV columnist for M.P. Daily. Retired, 1973.
SONGS INCLUDE: (collab.) Face the Sun, All Around the Town, Boom Ta Ra Ra, It Must Be LUV, Piano Teacher Song, Manhattan Merry Go Round, Lucky, I'm Still in Love With You, Havin' A Wonderful Time, Where Can You Be, Seven Days a Week, Texas Lullaby, Lighthouse in the Harbor, I'm Cuckoo Over Your, It's a Coincidence, If I Had a Million Dollars, Masquerade of Love, Mademoiselle Hortensia, Come Back to Me My Love, Someday When Shadows Fall, Myrtle the Turtle & Flip the Frog, Cowboy Isn't Speaking to His Horse, Gotta Horse That Loves to Rhumba, Girl on My Grandfather's Shaving Mug, Definition Song, Got a Gal in a Town Way Out West, Sing Something Irish, Little Sweetheart of the Mountains, Make a Million, Music Sets Me Free, She's the Daughter of the Sweetheart of Sigma Chi, Who Wants Love, Good-Lookin' It's Good Lookin' at You, Carib Gold, What Makes the Rainbow, Right Across de Ribber, Shadows in the Moonlight, Bible My Mother Left to Me, Poor Little Doll, Little Bit O'Ryhthmn in the Best of Us, Lovely Lady, When a Girl's In Love, Never Leave A Lady When She Loves You, Without You, That's The Way to Live, It's Time to Sing, Acapulco (By The Sea), Councilman; The Lambs.

HERRMANN, EDWARD: Actor. b. Washington, DC, July 31, 1943. e. Bucknell Univ. On stage in Mrs. Warren's Profession, The Philadelphia Story, Plenty, Tom and Viv, etc.
PICTURES: The Paper Chase, The Day of the Dolphin, The Great Gatsby, The Great Waldo Pepper, The Betsy, The North Avenue Irregulars, Brass Target, Take Down, Harry's War, Reds, Death Valley, A Little Sex, Annie, Mrs. Soffel, The Purple Rose of Cairo.
TELEVISION: Beacon Hills, Eleanor and Franklin, Eleanor and Franklin: The White House Years, The Lou Gehrig Story, Portrait of a Stripper, Dear Liar, The Gift of Life, Concealed Enemies, etc.

HERSHEY, BARBARA: Actress. b. Los Angeles, Feb. 5, 1948. e. Hollywood H.S.; Screen debut in With Six You Get Eggroll.
PICTURES INCLUDE: Last Summer, The Liberation of Lord Byron Jones, The Baby Maker, The Pursuit of Happiness, Boxcar Bertha, Vrooder's Hooch, Diamonds, The Last Hard Men, The Stunt Man, Take This Job and Shove It, The Entity, The Right Stuff, The Natural, Hannah and Her Sisters..
TV: Gidget, The Monroes, The Farmer's Daughter, Run For Your Life, The Invaders, Daniel Boone, CBS Playhouse, Chrysler Theatre. Movies: My Wicked, Wicked Ways, Passion Flower.

HERSKOVITZ, ARTHUR M.: Executive. b. Mukden, China. Nov. 28, 1920. e. CCNY, 1939. Joined RKO, scenario dept., 1939. U.S. Army, 1942–46; appt. mgr., RKO Radio Pictures of Peru, 1955; RKO Pict. Peru, 1958; Warner Bros., Peru, 1958–64; MGM, Panama, 1965–67; MGM rep. in Japan, 1968; Far East supvr., 1970; Joined National General Pictures, 1973 as foreign sls. mgr. In 1974 appt. dir. of sls., JAD Films Int'l.; named v.p., 1978; pres., 1979.

HERZOG, WERNER: Producer-Director. b. Germany, 1942.
PICTURES: Signs of Life, Even Dwarfs Started Small, Fata Morgana, The Land of Silence and Darkness; Aguirre—Wrath of God, Foufriere, Heart of Glass, Stroszek, Kaspar Hauster, Nosferatu, Woyzeck (also s.p.), Fitzcarraldo, Where the Green Ants Dream.

HERTZ, WILLIAM: Executive. Began theatre career in 1939; 1946 joined Fox West Coast Theatres; theatre mgr., booking dept.; 1965 appointed Los Angeles first-run district mgr.; promoted to Pacific Coast Division Mgr., National General Corp., 1967; v.p. Southern Pacific Div. Mgr., National General Theatres, Inc. 1971. Now with Mann Theatres as dir. of marketing, public relations, and labor relations.

HESSLER, GORDON: Producer, director. b. Berlin, Germany. e. Reading U., England; dir., vice pres., Fordel Films, Inc., 1950–58; dir., St. John's Story (Edinborough Film Festival), March of Medicine Series, Dr. Albert Lasker Award; story edit., Alfred Hitchcock Presents 1960–62; assoc. prod., dir., Alfred Hitchcock Hour, 1962; prod., Alfred Hitchcock Hour; prod., dir., Universal TV 1964–66.
PICTURES INCLUDE: The Woman Who Wouldn't Die, The Last Shot You Hear, The Oblong Box, Scream and Scream Again, Cry of the Banshee, Murders of the Rue Morgue, Sinbad's Golden Voyage, Medusa, Next Week Rio, Puzzle, Starlock, Pray for Death.
TV: Alfred Hitchcock Presents, 1960–62; Alfred Hitchcock Hour, 1962–65; Run For Your Life, Convoy, Bob Hope Chrysler Show, 1964–66; ABC Suspense Movies of the Week, ABC Movies of the Week, 1973. Lucas Tanner, Night Stalker, Amy Prentis, Switch, 1974; Kung Fu, Sara, Hawaii Five O, 1975–76; Blue Knight; Wonder Woman.
Pilots: Tender Warriors, Chips, Master, Thief, Tales of the Unexpected.

HESTON, CHARLTON: Actor. b. Evanston, Ill., Oct. 4, 1924; e. Northwestern U. School of Speech, Radio, stage, TV experience. Following coll. served 8 yrs. 11th Air Force, Aleutians. After war, co-acted (leads) and dir. with wife, Thomas Wolfe Memorial Theatre, Asheville, N.C. in State of the Union, Glass Menagerie; member, Katharine Cornell's Co., during first year on Broadway; Anthony and Cleopatra, other Bway. plays, Leaf and Bogh, Cockadoodle Doo; Studio One (TV): Macbeth, Taming of the Shrew, Of Human Bondage, Julius Caesar, etc.

PICTURES INCLUDE: Dark City, Greatest Show on Earth, The Savage, Ruby Gentry, President's Lady, Pony Express, Arrowhead, Bad for Each Other, Naked Jungle, Secret of the Incas, Far Horizons, Lucy Gallant, Private War of Major Benson, Ten Commandments, The Maverick, Ben Hur, Wreck of the Mary Deare, El Cid, The Pigeon That Took Rome, 55 Days at Peking, Major Dundee, The Agony & The Ecstasy, The War Lord, The Greatest Story Ever Told, Khartoum, The Battle Horns, Planet of the Apes, Beneath the Planet of the Apes, The Omega Man, Anthony and Cleopatra, (star & dir.), Skyjacked, Soylent Green, The Three Musketeers, Airport 1975, Earthquake, The Four Musketeers, The Last Hard Men, Midway, Two Minute Warning, The Prince and the Pauper (Crossed Swords), Gray Lady Down, The Awakening, Mother Lode (also dir.).

TELEVISION: Chiefs, The Narobi Affair.

HETZEL, RALPH D.: Executive. b. Corvallis, Ore., August 18, 1912; e. Penn. State Univ. (A.B.), 1933; University of London, 1935–36; Private secy. to Gov. Pinchot of Pa. 1933–35; did research & study, 1936–39; exec. secty. natl. hdqts., CIO, 1937–40; economic dir., 1938–40; in service, 1942–45. Consultant on labor, Natl. Selective Service hdqts., 1942; manpower consultant War Prod. Bd., 1942–43; dept. vice chmn., manpower requirements, W.P.B., 1943–45; acting vice-chmn., 1945; dir. Office of Labor Requirements, Civilian Prod. Admin., 1945–46; asst. to Secy. of Commerce, U.S. Dept. of Comm., 1946–48; asst. to secty. & dir. Office of Program Planning, 1948–51; asst. admin., Economic Stabilization Agency, 1951; exec. v.p. Motion Picture Association, MP Export Assn., 1951–71, Past president, International Federation of Film Producers Assns.; member of Board of Trustees, California Institute of the Arts and of Penn State University; member of Film Advisory Committee of Museum of Modern Art, and of Advisory Council of Edward R. Murrow Center of Public Diplomacy at Tufts University. Dean, College of Fine and Professional Arts, Professor of Art, Kent State University, 1971–76; provost and vice president, academic affairs, California Institute of the Arts 1976–80; faculty member, 1976–.

HEYMAN, JOHN: Producer. b. England, 1933. e. Oxford Univ. Started with British TV, creating writing and producing entertainment and documentary programs; expanded into field of personal management, forming International Artists, largest independent p.r. agency in Europe. 1963, formed World Film Services, Ltd. to produce, package and finance films. 1973, formed Genesis Project, educational film co. whose first venture was to translate the Bible onto film.

PICTURES: Privilege, Boom!, Secret Ceremony, Twinky, Bloomfield, The Go-Between, Daniel, Beyond the Limit, The Dresser, A Passage to India (co-prod.), Martin's Day, Steaming, D.A.R.Y.L., etc.

HEYWOOD, ANNE: Actress. b. England, 1931. m. Raymond Stross.

PICTURES INCLUDE: Checkpoint, Doctor at Large, Dangerous Exile, The Depraved, Violent Playground, Floods of Fear, Heart of a Man, Upstairs and Downstairs, A Terrible Beauty, Carthage in Flames, Petticoat Pirates, Stork Talk, Over My Dead Body, The Very Edge, 90 Degrees In The Shade, The Fox, A Run On Gold, The Most Dangerous Man in the World, The Nun of Monza, I Want What I Want, and Presumed Dead.

HICKMAN, DARRYL: Actor. b. Hollywood, July 28, 1933. Started screen career 1938 with The Starmaker. Was with CBS as exec. prod., daytime programming. Returned to acting with Network in 1977.

PICTURES INCLUDE: Grapes of Wrath, Young People, Jackass Mail, Northwest Rangers, Keeper of the Flame, And Now Tomorrow, Salty O'Rourke, Captain Eddie, Kiss and Tell, Leave Her to Heaven, Black Gold, Happy Years, Submarine Command, Destination Gobi, Island in the Sky, Sea of Lost Ships, Southwest Passage, The Human Comedy, Men of Boystown, Fighting Father Dunn, Tea and Sympathy, Looker, Sharky's Machine.

HIFT, FRED: Executive. b. Vienna, 1924. e. Vienna, London and Chicago. Early career reporter Chicago Sun and radio work with CBS News, New York. 1946 joined Boxoffice magazine; 1947 Quigley Publications; 1950 Variety. 1960 began career as publicist on Exodus. 1961 dir. pub., The Longest Day for Darryl Zanuck. 1962 joined Fox in Paris as ad-pub. dir. for Europe. 1964 became dir. European prod. pub. with headquarters London. Formed own pub., p.r. Co., Fred Hift Associates, 1970. 1979, joined Columbia Pictures as dir. of eastern ad-pub operations in N.Y.; 1980, to United Artists as intl. adv./pub. v.p. Left to establish Fred Hift Associates, intl. mktg. consultant in New York. 1983, joined Almi Pictures as v.p., mktg. 1985, reactivated F.H.A.

HIGGINS, COLIN: Writer-Director. b. New Caledonia, July 28, 1941. e. Sanford Univ., Sorbonne, UCLA (masters in film). Co-wrote The Ik for Peter Brook's International Center of Theatrical Research; brought to U.S. in 1977 where toured college campuses. Wrote s.p. for Harold and Maude and Silver Streak before turning to directing with Foul Play (also s.p.).

PICTURES: Nine to Five (co. s.p., dir.), The Best Little Whorehouse in Texas (s.p., dir.).

HILL, ARTHUR: Actor. b. Saskatchewan, Canada, 1922. e. U. of British Columbia. Moved to England in 1948, spending ten years in varied stage & screen pursuits; starred on Broadway in Who's Afraid of Virginia Woolf? (Tony Award), later in More Stately Mansions; film debut in Miss Pilgrim's Progress; other British work includes The Body Said No, Raising A Riot, The Deep Blue Sea.

PICTURES INCLUDE: The Young Doctors, The Ugly American, In the Cool of the Day, Moment to Moment, Harper, Petulia, Don't Let the Angels Fall, The Chairman, The Pursuit of Happiness, Rabbit Run, The Andromeda Strain, The Killer Elite, Future World, A Bridge Too Far, A Little Romance, The Champ, Dirty Tricks, Making Love, The Amateur, One Magic Christmas.

TV: Owen Marshall, Counselor-At-Law. Movies: Death Be Not Proud, Churchill and the Generals, The Guardian.

HILL, BENJAMIN (BENNY): TV performer. b. Southampton, England, Jan. 21, 1925. TV debut 1952; since many TV appearances including Showcase, Benny Hill Show; Midsummer Night's Dream, 1964; winner Daily Mail Award TV personality of the year 1954; m.p. debut, Who Done It, 1955; Light Up the Sky, 1960; Those Magnificent Men in Their Flying Machines, 1965; Chitty Chitty Bang Bang.

HILL, DEBRA: Producer. b. Haddonfield, NJ. Started in film business with Adventure Films helping make documentaries in Africa, the Caribbean, etc. Career on feature films started with work as script supvr., asst. dir. and 2nd unit dir. of 13 pictures. Producer's debut with Halloween (1980), for which also co-wrote script with director John Carpenter.

PICTURES: The Fog, Escape from New York, Halloween II, Halloween III: Season of the Witch, The Dead Zone, Head Office.

HILL, GEORGE ROY: Director. b. Minneapolis, Dec. 20, 1921. e. Yale and Trinity College in Dublin. Started as actor, Irish theatres and U.S. Shakespeare repertory company, also off-Broadway. Served as Marine pilot in World War II and again in Korean War. Wrote TV play, My Brother's Keeper, for Kraft Theatre, later rose to director with show. TV assignments included A Night to Remember, The Helen Morgan Story, Judgment at Nuremberg. Directed first Broadway play in 1957, Look Homeward Angel, followed by The Gang's All Here, Greenwillow. First film, Period of Adjustment, 1962.

PICTURES INCLUDE: Toys in the Attic, The World of Henry Orient, Hawaii, Thoroughly Modern Millie, Butch Cassidy and the Sundance Kid, Slaughterhouse Five, The Sting, The Great Waldo Pepper, Slap Shot, A Little Romance, The World According to Garp, The Little Drummer Girl.

HILL, TERENCE: Actor. b. Venice, March, 1941. r.n. Mario Girotti. First attracted attention as actor in Visconti's The Leopard (1963). Gained fame in European-made westerns.

PICTURES INCLUDE: God Forgives, I Don't, Boot Hill, Ace High, Barbagia, Anger of the Wind, They Call Me Trinity, Trinity Is Still My Name, My Name Is Nobody, Mr. Billion, March or Die.

HILL, WALTER: Writer-Director-Producer. b. Long Beach, Calif. Jan. 10, 1942. e. Michigan State Univ.

PICTURES INCLUDE: Writer: Hickey & Boggs, The Getaway, The Thief Who Came to Dinner, The Mackintosh Man, The Drowning Pool. Writer-Director: Hard Times, The Driver, The Warriors, The Long Riders, Southern Comfort, 48 Hrs., Streets of Fire. Co-Producer: Alien. Writer-Producer: Blue City. Director: Brewster's Millions, Crossroads, Blue City (co-prod., co-s.p.), Extreme Prejudice (dir.), Aliens (co-prod.).

HILLER, ARTHUR: Director. b. Edmonton, Alberta, Can., Nov. 22, 1923. e. Univs. of Alberta, Toronto, Brit. Columbia.

TV: Matinee Theatre, Playhouse 90, Climax, Alfred Hitchcock Presents, Gunsmoke, Ben Casey, Rte. 66, Naked City, The Dick Powell Show.

PICTURES INCLUDE: The Careless Years, Bryne Prods., Americanization of Emily, Tobruk, The Tiger Makes Out, Popi, The Out-of-Towners, Love Story, Plaza Suite, The Hospital, Man of La Mancha, The Man in the Glass Booth, W. C. Fields and Me, Silver Streak, Nightwing, Making

Love, Romantic Comedy, Lonely Guy (also prod.), Teachers, Outrageous Fortune.

HILLER, WENDY: (DBE, 1975, OBE, 1971), Hon. LLD (Manchester) 1984. Actress. b. Bramhall, Cheshire, England, Aug. 15, 1912. e. Winceby House Sch., Bexhill. On stage 1930, Manchester Repertory Theatre, England; then on British tour. London debut 1935 in "Love On the Dole"; to N.Y., same role 1936. m.p. debut in "Lancashire Luck," 1937.
PLAYS: First Gentleman, Cradle Song, Tess of the D'Urbervilles, Heiress, Ann Veronica, Waters of the Moon, Night of the Ball, Old Vic Theatre, Wings of the Dove, Sacred Flame, Battle of Shrivings, Crown Matrimonial, John Gabriel Borkman, Waters of the Moon (revival), Aspern Papers (revival).
PICTURES INCLUDE: Pygmalion, Major Barbara, I Know Where I'm Going, Outcast of the Islands, Single Handed (Sailor of the King), Something of Value, Uncle George, Separate Tables, Sons and Lovers, Toys in the Attic, Man For All Seasons, David Copperfield, Murder on the Orient Express, Voyage of The Damned, The Elephant Man, Making Love.

HILLMAN, WILLIAM BRYON: Writer-Director-Producer. b. Chicago, Feb. 3. e. Oklahoma Military Academy–U.C.L.A. Head of production at Intro-Media Productions; Fairchild Spectro Productions; Double Eagle Entertainment Corp; Excellent Films. Creative consultant for The Hit 'Em Corp. Presently head of SpectroMedia Entertainment.
PICTURES INCLUDE: Fast & Furious (dir., s.p.), Lovelines (s.p.), the Master (Dir., s.p.), The Passage (dir. s.p.), Double Exposure (dir., s.p., co-prod.), Campus (dir., s.p.), The Photographer (dir., prod., s.p.), The Man From Clover Grove (dir., s.p., co-prod.), Thetus (dir., s.p.), The Trail Ride (dir., s.p., co-prod.), Betta Betta (dir., s.p., prod.).
TELEVISION: Working Together (pilot s.p.), Disco-Theque Pilot (dir., s.p.), Everything Will Be Alright (s.p.), Money (dir., s.p.).
NOVELS: Silent Changes, The Combination, The Liar, Additives The Perfect Crime, Why Me, The Loner.

HILLERMAN, JOHN: Actor. b. Denison, TX, Dec. 20, 1932. e. Univ. of Texas. While in US Air Force joined community theatre group and went to New York after completing military service. Studied at American Theatre Wing, leading to summer stock and off-Bdwy.
PICTURES: Paper Moon, The Day of the Locust, Chinatown, Up the Creek, etc.
TELEVISION: Series: Ellery Queen, The Betty White Show, Magnum P.I. Movies: The Law, Kill Me If You Can, Betrayal, Marathon, Battles, Little Gloria . . . Happy at Last, etc.

HINES, GREGORY: Actor-Dancer. b. Feb. 14, 1946. Early career as junior member of family dancing act starting at age 2. Later landed role in The Last Minstrel Show in New York, going on the Eubie, Comin- Uptown, Sophisticated Ladies, etc. Motion picture debut in Wolfen (1981).
PICTURES: History of the World—Part I, Deal of the Century, The Cotton Club, White Nights, Running Scared.

HINGLE, PAT: Actor. b. Denver, CO, July 19, 1923.
THEATRE: Man for All Seasons (Oherbein College, Ohio); The Price, Macbeth (American Shakespeare Festival).
RADIO: Voice of America.
PICTURES INCLUDE: On the Waterfront, The Strange One, No Down Payment, Splendor in the Grass, The Ugly American, Sol Madrid, Hang Em High, Jigsaw, Norwood, Bloody Mama, WUSA, Corporal Crocker, The Carey Treatment, One Little Indian, The Super Cops, The Gauntlet, When You Comin' Back, Red Ryder, Norma Rae, Sudden Impact, Running Brave, Going Berserk, The Falcon and the Snowman, Brewster's Millions.
TELEVISION: The Lady from Yesterday.

HINKLE, ROBERT: Actor-Prod.-Dir. b. Brownfield, Texas, July 25, 1930; e. Brownfield High School. Joined Rodeo Cowboys Association, 1950 and rodeoed professionally until 1953 when began acting career in Outlaw Treasure.
PICTURES INCLUDE: Giant, All the Fine Young Cannibals, Hud, The First Texan, Dakota Incident, Gun the Man Down, The Oklahoman, First Traveling Saleslady, No Place to Land, Under Fire, Speed Crazy, The Gunfight at Dodge City, Broken Land, Law in Silver City, Ole Rex (award for Family Entertainment), Born Hunter, Trauma, Something Can Be Done, Mr. Chat, Stuntman, Hud, Jumping Frog Jubilee, Mr. Chat-Mexico Safari, Trail Ride, Virginia City Cent., Texas Today, Texas Long Horns, Kentucky Thoroughbred Racing, Produced & Directed country Music, Guns of a Stranger, Old Rex.
TV: Test Pilot, Dial 111, Juvenile Squad, X13 Vertijet, Cellist Extraordinary, Sunday Challange.
Pres. Hinkle Pictures, Inc.

HIRD, THORA: Actress. b. Morecambe (Lancs), Eng., May 28, 1914. e. The Nelson School, Morecambe.
PICTURES INCLUDE: (Screen debut, 1940) The Black Sheep of Whitehall; Street Corner, Turn the Key Softly, Personal Affair, The Great Game, Storks Don't Talk, Shop Soiled, For Better or Worse; Love Match, One Good Turn, Quatermass Experiment, Simon and Laura, Lost, Sailor Beware, Home and Away, Good Companions, The Entertainer, A Kind of Loving, Term of Trial, Bitter Harvest, Rattle of A Simple Man, Some Will, Some Won't, The Nightcomers.
TV: The Winslow Boy, The Bachelor, What Happens to Love, The Witching Hour, So Many Children, The Queen Came By, Albert Hope, All Things Bright and Beautiful, Say Nothing, Meet the Wife, Who's A Good Boy Then? I AM! Dixon of Dock Green, Romeo & Juliet, The First Lady, Ours Is a Nice House, The Foxtrot, Seasons, She Stoops to Conquer, Villa Maroc, When We Are Married, In Loving Memory, Flesh and Blood, Your Songs of Praise Choice, Hallelujah, Happiness, Thats the Main Thing, Intensive Care, In Loving Memory, Hallelujah, Praise Be.

HIRSCH, JUDD: Actor. b. New York City, March 15, 1935. e. City College of N.Y. Studied physics but turned to acting; first job in 1962 when performed with stock co. in Colorado. Returned to N.Y. to work on stage and since has also done films and TV.
PICTURES INCLUDE: Serpico, Ordinary People, Without a Trace, The Goodbye People, Teachers.
TV: Medical Story, Delvecchio. Movies: Fear on Trial, Valentino, The Law, The Keegans, Taxi.

HIRSCHFIELD, ALAN J.: Executive. e., University of Oklahoma (BA); Harvard Business School (MBA). Current: Investments. 1980–84, chm. and chief exec. officer, 20th Century-Fox. Film Corp. V.P., Allen & Co., 1959–66; Financial v.p. & dir. Warner/7 Arts, 1967–68; v.p. & dir., American Diversified Enterprises, 1969–73; pres. & chief exec. officer, Columbia Pictures Industries, 1973–78; consultant, Warner Communications, 1979.
Vice Chairman and trustee: Cancer Research Institute. Director: American Film Institute, Billboard Publications, Chappell Music Publishers, Charvo 2 Carsen Corp., Jackson Hole Land Trust.

HIRSHAN, LEONARD: Theatrical Agent. b. Dec. 27, 1927, New York City. e. NYU. Joined William Morris Agency as agent trainee, New York, 1951. Agent legit theatre & TV dept. 1952–54. Sr. exec. agent M.P. dept., California office, 1955; sr. v.p., 1983.

HIRT, AL: Musician. b. New Orleans, La., Nov. 7, 1922. e. Cincinnati Conservatory of Music. Military service four years. Played with Tommy and Jimmy Dorsey bands, Ray McKinley and Horace Heidt; appeared, Dunes Hotel, Harrah's Club, Basin Street East, Cloisters, Palmer House, Eden Roc Hotel, Greek Theatre. European tour concerts. Inaugural Ball, President John F. Kennedy, Jan., 1961.
TV: Dinah Shore Show, Jack Paar Show, Ed Sullivan, NBC Special Home For the Holidays, Bell Telephone Hour Rainbow of Stars, Andy Williams Show, Tonight Show, Today Show, Perry Como Show, Lively Ones, Jerry Lewis Show.
PICTURES INCLUDE: World By Night, Rome Adventure.
RECORDINGS: RCA: The Greatest Horn in the World, Al—He's the King—Hirt, Horn-A-Plenty, Al Hirt at the Mardi Gras, Trumpet & Strings, Our Man in New Orleans, Honey In The Horn, Beauty And The Beard, Pop Goes the Trumpet, Boston Pops.

HITT, J. T.: Executive. b. Spearman, Texas, Dec. 16, 1922. e. Grad., Gentry, Ark. H.S., 1940. Farming and ranching. Ent. motion picture industry 1947; Pres., Independent Theatre Owners of Arkansas, 1961–63; chmn. bd., 1964; sec.-treas., Tri-States Theatre Owners, mem. bd., Theatre Owners of America; pres. Tri-State T.O. Ark., Tenn. & Miss., 1965–66. Retired.

HOARE, VICTOR J.: Executive. Entered m.p. ind. with United Artists 1931; Dir., British Lion Films, 1961; man. dir., BLC Films, 1962; dep. chmn., BLC Films, 1965; man. dir. British Lion Films, 1965; v.p. in chg. of Continental Europe, Columbia International, in Paris, 1966; v.p., theatres, C.I.C., 1974 Exec. dir. CIC NV; Pres. Theatre Div. 1982. Pres., CIC Developments, 1985.

HOBERMAN, DAVID: Executive. Started career as prod. exec. with TAT Communications for five years. 1982–85, worked as m.p. agent with Writers and Artists Agency and later at Ziegler Associates and ICM. 1985, named v.p. of prod. for Walt Disney Pictures based at studio.

HOBIN, BILL: TV prod. dir.; r.n. Charles W. Hobin; b. Nov. 12, 1923, Evanston, Ill.; e. U. of So. Calif.; prod. mgr., Coronet Instructional Films, Glenview, Ill.; dir., Garroway at Large, Wayne King Show from Chic., 1949–51; dir., Assignment Manhunt, 1952; Nothing But the Best, 1953; Les Paul and Mary Ford, 1953; Your Show of Shows, 1951–54; assoc. prod.-dir., Max Liebman Presents (Spectaculars), prod. dir. Fred Waring Show, Andy Williams Show, Pat Boone, Timex All-Star Jazz Show. dir. Your Hit

Parade. Prod.-dir. The Golden Circle, 1959; The Bell Telephone Hour, 1959–60; The American Cowboy, 1960; Sing Along with Mitch, 1960–63; dir., Judy Garland Show, 1963; prod., dir., Victor Borge at Carnegie Hall, 1964; dir., m.p. Chrysler Show-Go-Round, N.Y. World's Fair. 1964. Dir.: Meredith Wilson Special, 1964; Jack Jones on the Move Special, 1966; Red Skelton Hour, 1964–68; prod.; Red Skelton Hour, 1968–70; prod. and dir. The Bill Cosby Special I, 1968; prod., dir., The Tim Conway Comedy Hour, 1970–71; prod., dir. The CBS Newcomers series, 1972; dir. An Evening With My Three Sons special, prod., dir. Michel Legrand Special; prod., dir. Fred Astaire special; director, Maude, 1972; director, A Touch of Grace, 1972–73; 1974, prod.-dir. credits: Dinah, Won't You Please Come Home! (NBC Special); Bobby Goldsboro Show (syn); Your Hit Parade (CBS), prod.-dir. Flip Wilson Special, Dionne Warwick Special, Wayne Newton Special, all 1975; 1976—dir., Welcome (Back), Kotter, Prod.-dir., Monty Hall's Variety Special. Dir., Bert Convy Show; 1976 Director, George Burns Special; McLean Stevenson Show, 1976–78, Director, Three's Company. Producer-director Bob Hope Specials, (1978–79) (NBC); director Celebrity Challenge of the Sexes, 1979 (CBS); director, Steve Allen Special (PBS), 1981; director, No Soap Radio (ABC-TV), 1982.

HOBLEY, McDONALD: b. Port Stanley, Falkland Islands; e. South America; Brighton Coll. Early career in repertory cos. tours, etc.; entered TV in 1946 as TV announcer; won Nat'l TV Award for Personality of the Year, 1953–54; resigned from BBC, 1956; now free-lance.
PICTURES INCLUDE: Checkpoint, The Entertainer.
TV: Holiday Town Parade, The Dave King Show, Tell the Truth, The Tommy Steele Show, Close-up.

HOCK, MORT: Executive. b. New York, N.Y., June 24, 1929. Blaine-Thompson Agency; A. E. Warner Bros., 1945; David Merrick B'way Prod., 1958; asst. adv. mgr., Paramount Pictures Corp., 1960; adv. mgr., United Artists Corp., 1962; dir. adv., United Artists Corp., July 1964; adv. dir., Para., 1965; v.p. advertising and public relations, Paramount Pict. Corp., 1968–71; pres., Atina Enterprises, Inc. 1971; v.p., marketing, Rastar Prods., 1973; exec. v.p., Charles Schlaifer & Co., 1974; sr. v.p. entertainment div., Doyle Dane Bernbach, 1983.

HODGE, PATRICIA: Actress. b. Lincolnshire, England, 1946.
PICTURES: The Elephant Man, Betrayal.

HOFFMAN, DUSTIN: b. Los Angeles, Calif., Aug. 8, 1937. m. Lisa Hoffman. e. Los Angeles Conservatory of Music, Santa Monica College, Pasadena Playhouse, 1958. Worked as an attendant at a psychiatric institution, a demonstrator in Macy's toy dept., and a waiter. First stage role in Yes Is For A Very Young Man, at Sarah Lawrence College. Acted in summer stock, television and dir. at community theatre. Broadway and Off Broadway plays include: 1964, Harry, Noon and Night (American Place Theatre); 1966, Journey of the Fifth Horse (APT, won Obie Award); Eh? (won Vernon Rice & Theatre World Award); Jimmy Shine. Asst. Dir.: A View From The Bridge. Dir. (1974): All Over Town; 1984, Death of a Salesman (Drama Desk Award).
TV: Journey of the Fifth Horse, The Star Wagons, Death of a Salesman.
PICTURES INCLUDE: Madigan's Millions, The Graduate (Acad. Award nom.); Midnight Cowboy (Acad. Award nom.); John and Mary, Little Big Man, Who Is Harry Kellerman?, Straw Dogs, Alfredo, Papillon, Lenny (Acad. Award nom), All the President's Men, Marathon Man, Straight Time, Agatha, Kramer vs. Kramer (AA), Tootsie, Ishtar.

HOFFMAN, HERMAN: Wrt. Dir. b. Montgomery, Ala., e. Baltimore City Coll., U.S. Navy.
FEATURE DIRECTING: The Bar Sinister, Great American Pastime, The Invisible Boy, The Battle of Gettysburg.
FEATURE WRITING: Attack on the Iron Coast, Guns of the Magnificent Seven, Escapeline, Reluctant Heroes (Movie-of-Week), The Icemen.
TV DIRECTING: Alcoa Premiere, Untouchables, Bonanza, Virginians, M-Squad, The Nurses, Room 222, Run Joe Run, Monster Squad, The Phantom Rebel, (NBC special).

HOFFMAN, JOSEPH: Writer. b. New York City, Newspaperman, radio writer, magazine writer. TV prod. Now TV and screen free lance writer.
PICTURES INCLUDE: China Sky, Don't Trust Your Husband, Gung-Ho, And Baby Makes Three, Weekend with Father, Duel at Silver Creek, At Sword's Point, Has Anybody Seen My Gal?, Against All Flags, No Room For the Groom, Lone Hand, Yankee Pasha, Rails into Laramie, Tall Man Riding, Chicago Syndicate, Live A Little, How to Make Love and Like It, Sex and the Single Girl.
TELEVISION: Producer: Ford Theatre, Colt 45. Writer: Leave It To Beaver, My Three Sons, The Virginian, Love American Style, etc.

HOGARTH, JOHN M.: Executive. b. Hampstead, London, England, 1931. Man. Dir. Enterprise Pictures Ltd. 1977.

HOLBROOK, HAL: Actor. b. Cleveland, O., Feb. 17, 1925. Gained fame as impersonator of Mark Twain on stage.
PICTURES INCLUDE: The Group, Wild in the Streets, They Only Kill Their Masters, Magnum Force, The Girl from Petrovka. All the President's Men, Midway, Julia, Capricorn One, Natural Enemies, The Fog, Creepshow, Star Chamber.
TELEVISION: Mark Twain Tonight, Celebrity, George Washington, Undersiege, Behind Enemy Lines, Dress Gray, North & South Book II.

HOLDEN, GLORIA: Actress. b. London, Eng. Sept. 5, 1911. e. Amer. Acad. of Dramatic Arts. Church soloist and singer, artists' & clothes model; mgr. Elizabeth Arden salon, Southhampton, L.I.; stage and radio roles, lead in As Husbands Go, Theatre Guild road tour. Began screen career 1937.
PICTURES INCLUDE: Life of Emile Zola, The Girl of Limberlost, Dracula's Daughter, Test Pilot, Girls' School, Behind the Rising Sun, The Hucksters, Kiss for Corliss, Dream Wife, Music by Duchin.
TV: Lux Theatre, Hallmark Theatre.

HOLLENDER, ALFRED L.: Advertising executive. b. Chicago, Ill.; e. U. of Illinois. Was associated with Radio Stations WIND-WJJD, Chicago as continuity ed., program dir. & asst. to pres.; entered military service in 1943; exec. v.p. & partner of Louis G. Cowan, Inc., exec. v.p. and dir. radio-TV dept., Grey Adv. Agency; pres., Grey Int'l.

HOLLIMAN, EARL: Actor. b. Tennasas Swamp, Delhi, La., Sept. 11, 1928. e. Louisiana State U., U.C.L.A.
PICTURES INCLUDE: Girls of Pleasure Island, Destination Gobi, East of Sumatra, Devil's Canyon, Tennessee Champ, Bridge at Toko-Ri, Broken Lance, Big Combo, I Died a Thousand Times, Forbidden Planet, Giant, Burning Hills, Gunfight at the OK Corral, The Rainmaker, Hot Spell, Visit to a Small Planet, The Power, Sharky's Machine.

HOLLOWAY, STERLING: Actor. b. Cedartown, Ga., 1905. e. Ga. Military Acad., Atlanta, Amer. Acad. of Dramatic Art.
THEATRE: N.Y. Plays include: Shepherd of the Hills, The Failures, Garrick Gaieties (4 editions), Donna Magana; vaude.; night clubs; radio; U.S. armed forces, 1943.
PICTURES INCLUDE: Walk in the Sun, Death Valley, Beautiful Blonde from Bashful Bend, Her Wonderful Lie, Alice in Wonderland, Live a Little, Love a Little, The Jungle Book (voice).

HOLM, CELESTE: Actress. b. New York City, Apr. 29, 1919. p. Theodor Holm and Jean Parke Holm. Ed. Univ. School for Girls, Chicago, Francis W. Parker, Chicago, Lyceé Victor Durui (Paris), Chicago U & UCLA.
THEATRE: On Bdwy incl. Time of Your Life, Return of the Vagabond, Papa Is All, Oklahoma, Bloomer Girl, Affairs of State, Anna Christie, The King and I, Third Best Sport, Invitation to a March, A Month in the Country; Theatre-in-Concert for the US State Department in 8 countries May–July 1966. Appeared on B'way 1975–76, Habeas Corpus.
PICTURES INCLUDE: The Little Girls in Blue, won Academy Award 1947, Gentlemen's Agreement, Come to the Stable, All About Eve, Snake Pit, Road House, Chicken Every Sunday, Everybody Does It, Champagne for Caesar, Tender Trap, High Society, Bachelor Flat, Doctor, You've Got To Be Kidding, Tom Sawyer, Bittersweet Love.
TV: A Clearing House in the Wood, Play of the Week, Cinderella, This Girl for Hire.
RADIO: People at the U.N.

HOLM, IAN: Actor. b. Ilford, Essex, England, Sept. 12, 1931. e. RADA. On British stage—Love Affair, Titus Andronicus, Ondine, Becket, The Homecoming, The Seat, etc.—before entering films.
PICTURES: The Bofois Gun, A Midsummer Night's Dream, The Fixer, A Severed Head, Nicholas and Alexandra, Mary Queen of Scots, Young Winston, The Homecoming, Juggernaut, Shout at the Devil, Alien, Chariots of Fire, Time Bandits, Brazil, Dreamchild.
TELEVISION: Les Miserables, S.O.S. Titanic, Napoleon, We, the Accused.

HOMEIER, SKIP: Actor. r.n. George Vincent Homeier. b. Chicago, Oct. 5, 1930. e. U.C.L.A. Started in radio, 1936–43; on B'way stage, Tomorrow the World, 1943–44.
PICTURES INCLUDE: Tomorrow the World, Boy's Ranch, Mickey, Arthur Takes Over, The Big Cat, The Gunfighter, Halls of Montezuma, The Black Widow, Cry Vengeance, Dakota Incident, The Captives, No Road Back, Decision at Durango, Showdown.
TV: Playhouse 90, Alcoa Hour, Kraft Theatre, Studio 1, Armstrong Circle Theatre, Alfred Hitchcock, etc.

HONG, WILSON S.: Cinematographer. b. Butte, Mont., Dec. 18, 1934; ed. Montana State University, Brooks Institute of Photography; 1965 Free lance photographer for national magazine and world-wide newspaper syndication; 1966, Photographic Director of U.S Forest Service Fire & Research Division; 1967, first cameraman on various documentaries, industrials, commercials, sports specials.

PICTURES INCLUDE: Bigfoot, Operation North Slope, John Wayne's 'No Substitute for Victory', The Hellcats, Dear Dead Delilah, Zodiac Killer, Velvet Vampire, Mrs. McGrudy, The Day The Adults Died, Sundown in Watts, Parallax View, 1776, Don't Go West, Drum, White Buffalo, MacArthur, An Enemy of the People, Sergeant Pepper's Lonely Hearts Club Band, Mulefeathers, Winterkills, Mission to Glory, The Unfinished, They Only Kill Their Masters, The Fearless Five.

TELEVISION: Snowmobile Grand Prix (ABC), Indianapolis International Drag Races (ABC), The Great Outdoors (23 episodes, ABC), Thank you America (spec.), The Unser Story (ABC), Gun Hawks (pilot), Keep it Up (pilot), Where are they Now? (pilot), Hunting and Fishing the North American Continent (spec.), The Blue Knight, A Dream for Christmas, The Toy Game, Moose (pilot), The Jerry Show, Apple's Way, The Moneychangers, Young Maverick, Rudi Gernreich/Future, Ours, Max Factor and Pepsi-Cola Commercials, The Groovy Seven (pilot).

HOOPER, TOBE: Director. b. Texas. Began film career making documentary and industrial films and commmercials in Texas. Was asst. dir. of Univ. of Texas film program, continuing filmmaking while working with students. First feature film: Eggshells.

PICTURES: Eaten Alive, The Texas Chainsaw Massacre, Funhouse, Poltergeist, Lifeforce, Invaders from Mars, The Texas Chainsaw Massacre Part 2.

HOPE, BOB: Actor. b. Eltham, England., May 29, 1903. Started in vaude.; plays include: Roberta, Ziegfeld Follies, Red, Hot & Blue; author, They Got Me Covered, I Never Left Home, So This Is Peace. Voted one of ten best Money-Making Stars in M.P. Herald-Fame Poll, 1941–47, 49–53. On radio and TV.

PICTURES INCLUDE: Big Broadcast of 1938, College Swing, Give Me a Sailor, Thanks for the Memory, Never Say Die, Some Like It Hot, Cat and Canary, Road to Singapore, Ghost Breakers, Road to Zanzibar, Caught in the Draft, Louisiana Purchase, My Favorite Blonde, Road to Morocco, Nothing But the Truth, They Got Me Covered, Star Spangled Rhythm, Let's Face It, Road to Utopia, Princess and Pirate, Monsieur Beaucaire, My Favorite Brunette, Where There's Life, Road to Rio, Paleface, Sorrowful Jones, Great Lover, Fancy Pants, Lemon Drop Kid, My Favorite Spy, Son of Paleface, Road to Bali, Off Limits, Here Come the Girls, Casanova's Big Night, Seven Little Foys, That Certain Feeling, Iron Petticoat, Beau James, Paris Holiday, Alias Jesse James, Facts of Life, Bachelor In Paradise, Road to Hong Kong, Call Me Bwana, A Global Affair, I'll Take Sweden, Boy Did I Get a Wrong Number, Eight on the Lam, The Private Navy of Sgt. O'Farrell, How to Commit Marriage, Cancel My Reservation.

HOPE, HARRY: Producer, director, writer. e. UCLA, Etudes Universitaires Internationales, Ph.D. Entered m.p. industry as special effects man, Republic Studios, 1944; associate producer Star Productions; formed Blue Bird Film Co. Has since produced, directed and written 33 feature films, including Like the Gull, 1967, which won creative classical film award as Asian Film Festival. Founded Western International and directed First Leisure Corp. as exec. v.p. until 1972. From then until present, pres. of Harry Hope Production. Among recent film credits: Smokey and The Judge, Sunset Cove, Doomsday Machine, Death Dimension, Thunderfist, Tarzana, The Mad Butcher, Death Blow.

HOPKINS, ANTHONY: Actor. b. Port Talbot, Dec. 31, 1937. Trained at Royal Academy of Dramatic Arts. Joined National Theatre, gaining fame on stage in England, then TV and films.

PICTURES INCLUDE: White Bus, Lion in Winter, Hamlet, The Looking Glass War, When Eight Bells Toll, Young Winston, The Girl from Petrovka, Audrey Rose, A Bridge Too Far, International Velvet, Magic, Change of Seasons, The Elephant Man, The Bounty, 84 Charing Cross Road.

TV: QB VII, All Creatures Great and Small, The Bunker, Peter and Paul, A Married Man, Hollywood Wives, Guilty Conscience, Arch of Triumph.

HOPKINS, BO: Actor. B. Greenwood, S.C. Studied with Uta Hagen in N.Y. then went to Calif. with Desilu Playhouse training school in Hollywood. Parts in several prods. for that group won him an agent, an audition with director Sam Peckinpah and his first role in latter's The Wild Bunch.

PICTURES INCLUDE: Monte Walsh, The Culpepper Cattle Co., The Moonshine War, White Lightning, The Getaway, The Man Who Loved Cat Dancing, American Graffiti, The Nickel Ride, The Day of the Locust, Posse, The Killer Elite, A Small Town in Texas, More American Graffiti, The Fifth Floor, Sweet Sixteen, Night Shadows.

TV: Doc Elliott (series).

HOPPER, DENNIS: Actor. b. Dodge City, Kans., May 17, 1936. e. San Diego, Calif., public schools.

TV: Medic, Loretta Young Show.

PICTURES INCLUDE: Jagged Edge, Rebel Without a Cause, Giant, Wrote, dir. starred in Easy Rider, The Last Movie, Hex, The American Friend, King of the Mountain, Rumble Fish, The Osterman Weekend, The Texas Chainsaw Massacre Part 2, Blue Velvet.

HOPPER, JERRY: Director. b. Guthrie, Okla., July 29, 1907. Wrote radio scripts; asst. dir. & actor. Universal, MGM; casting office, Paramount; Combat/photog—U.S. Army, m.p. div.; asst. edit. dept. head, Paramount; dir., Paramount.

PICTURES INCLUDE: The Atomic City, Hurricane Smith, Pony Express, Alaska Seas, Secret of the Incas, Everything But the Truth, Something to Live For, Naked Alibi, Smoke Signal, Private War of Major Benson, One Desire, Square Jungle, Never Say Goodbye, Toy Tiger, Shark Fighters, Missouri Traveler, Blueprint for Robbery, Maharlica, Madrone.

TV: pilots—Bachelor Father, Leave it to Beaver, Naked City, Wagon Train, Witchita Town. Many television productions, including The Fugitive, Addams Family, Gilligan's Island, Perry Mason, Get Smart, Voyage to the Bottom of the Sea, The Rifleman, etc. Specials: Bob Hope Shows, Nanette Fabray Shows.

HORDERN, MICHAEL, SIR: Actor. Berkhampstead, England, 1911. e. Brighton College. early career in business before stage appearance, 1937. M.P. debut 1939. TV debut 1946. 1939–45 Naval Service. Knighted 1983.

PICTURES INCLUDE: Passport to Pimlico, The Constant Husband, Alexander the Great, The Black Prince, Storm Over The Nile, Pacific Destiny, The Baby and the Battleship, The Spanish Gardener, No Time for Tears, Windom's Way, Monty's Double, Girls at Sea, Moment of Danger, Sink the Bismarck, Man in the Moon, El Cid, Cleopatra, V.I.P.s, Dr. Syn, The Yellow Rolls Royce, Ghengis Khan, The Spy Who Came in From the Cold, Khartoum, Cast a Giant Shadow, A Funny Thing Happened on the Way to the Forum, Taming of the Shrew, The Jokers, How I Won the War, I'll Never Forget What's 'Is Name, Prudence and the Pill, The Bed-sitting Room, Where Eagles Dare, Anne of the Thousand Days, Futtocks End, Some Will, Some Won't, Up Pompeii, The Possession of Joel Delaney (USA), Pied Piper, Blood Will Have Blood, England Made Me, Girl Stroke Boy, Alice's Adventures in Wonderland, Theatre of Blood, The Mackintosh Man, Quilp, Barry Lyndon (narrator), The Slipper and the Rose, Joseph Andrews, The Medusa Touch, Wildcats of St. Trinians, Gandhi, Ivano, Oliver Twist, The Missionary, Yellowbeard, Robin Hood, Trouble at the Royal Rose, Lady Jane, Comrades.

TV: Doctor's Dilemma, The Great Adventure, The Witness, The Indifferent Shepherd, Dock Brief, Mr. Kettle & Mrs. Moon, Guinea Pig, The Gathering Dusk, Farewell My City, Flowering Cherry, I Have Been Here Before, Without the Grail, The Outstation, The Square, Any Other Business, The Stone Dance, The Quails, A Waltz on the Water, August for the People, Land of My Dreams, Condemned to Acquittal, Nelson, The Browning Version, Whistle and I'll Come to You, The Man Who Murdered in Public, A Crack in the Ice, Sir Jocelyn the Minister Would Like A Word, Six Dates With Barker, Don Juan in Hell, Tartoffe, Tall Stories, The Magistrate, Edward VII, King Lear, Cakes and Ale, Chester Mystery Cycle, Paddington Bear (story teller), The Saints Go Marching In, Mrs. Bixby and the Colonel's Coat, Romeo and Juliet, The Tempest, All's Well That Ends Well, You're Alright: How Am I?, King Lear, Rod and Line, Cymbeline, Trelawney of the Wells, Paradise Postponed.

HORN, ALAN: Executive. b. New York City, Feb. 28, 1943. e. Union Coll.; Harvard Business School. 1972, joined Tandem Prods., 1972; named v.p., business affairs, and of sister co., T.A.T. Communications, 1973; 1977, exec. v.p. & COO; pres., 1978. In 1983 named pres. Embassy Communications. 1986 joined 20th Century Fox as pres. B COO.

HORNE, DAVID: Actor. b. Balcome, Sussex, July 14, 1898; e. Eton & Sandhurst. Began screen career 1931.

PICTURES INCLUDE: Doomed Cargo, The Mill on the Floss, The Wrecker, Four Dark Hours, The First and the Last, Inspector Hornleigh Goes To It, Chamber of Horrors, Spitfire, Adventure in Blackmail, Rake's Progress, Seventh Veil, Men of Two Worlds, Gaiety George, The Magic Bow, Saraband for Dead Lovers, Easy Money, Martin Luther, Spaceways, Five Pound Note, Policewoman, Wedding Gift, The Intruder, 3 Cases of Murder, Beau Brummell.

HORNE, LENA: Vocalist, actress. b. Brooklyn, N.Y. June 30, 1917.

THEATRE: Blackbirds, Dance With Your Gods.

Radio with Noble Sissle, Charlie Barnet, other brands. Floor shows at Cotton Club, Cafe Society, Little Troc, etc. Started screen career 1942.

PICTURES INCLUDE: Panama Hattie, Cabin in the Sky, Stormy Weather, I Dood It, Thousands Cheer, Broadway Rhythm, Swing Fever, Two Girls and a Sailor, Ziegfeld Follies, Till the Clouds Roll By, Words and Music, Meet Me in Las Vegas, Death of a Gunfighter, The Wiz.

HORNER, HARRY: Director. b. Holic, Czechoslovakia, July 24, 1910; e. U. of Vienna, Dept. of Architecture, 1928–33; Acad. of the Theatre, Vienna, 1930–32, Max Reinhardt's Seminary. Joined Max Reinhardt Thea. Co., Vienna and Salzburg Festivals; to U.S. as asst. to Reinhardt on pageant, The Eternal Road. Stage designer, N.Y. theatre 10 yrs. (Lady in The Dark, Family Portrait, others). First m.p. as prod. designer, 1938, Our Town (co-credit, Wm. Cameron Menzies). later Little Foxes, Stage Door Canteen. Army service, 1942–45; designed Winged Victory for Air Force. In 1949, won Acad. award black and white art dir., The Heiress. Other films designed: Born Yesterday, Separate Tables, They Shoot Horses; Acad. nomination, The Hustler; (Acad. award). Since 1959 prod., dir., TV series, The Royal Canadian Mounted Police; exec. prod., dir., Enterprise Films of Can., Anglo Ent. Films, London; co-prod., Fahrenheit 451, 1966, They Shoot Horses, Don't They? (Acad. nom.), Who Is Harry Kellerman?, Up the Sandbox (Streisand).

FURTHER PICTURES INCLUDE: Born Yesterday, He Ran All the Way, Androcles and the Lion, Outrage. Films Directed: Beware My Lovely, Red Planet Mars, Vicki, New Faces, Life in the Balance, Step Down to Terror, Lonesome Gun, Wild Party Man From Del Rio, Winner of 2 acad. awards, 6 acad. nominations for Art Dir. 1975: The Black Bird, Harry and Walter Go To New York, Audrey Rose, The Driver, Moment by Moment, The Jazz Singer.

TV: Omnibus, Cavalcade, Reader's Digest, Author's Playhouse, Four Star Theatre, Gunsmoke, Revue Productions, Dupont Theatre.

OPERA: designer & director at San Francisco Opera, Metrop. Opera N.Y. Vancouver Festivals Hollywood Bowl Operas designed & directed: David, Joan at the Seake, Magic Flute. Amer. Premiere of New Opera, Midsummers Night Dream. Designed Idiots Delight, Ahmanson Theatre, 1970, winner, L.A. Drama Critics Award, best stage design. Designed Time of the Cuckoo, Ahmanson Theatre 1974.

HORSLEY, LEE: Actor. b. Muleshow, TX, May 15. e. Univ. of No. Colorado. Appeared in stage productions locally of Oklahoma, Fiddler on the Roof, Lion in Winter, etc. Did stage work in New York. Starred in theatrical film, The Sword and the Sorcerer.

TELEVISION: Series: Nero Wolfe, Matt Houston.

HORTON, ROBERT: Actor. b. Los Angeles, July 29, 1924. e. Miami Univ., U.C.L.A. U.S. Coast Guard; many legit. plays; many radio & TV appearances; co-star, Wagon Train; screen debut in The Tanks Are Coming.

PICTURES INCLUDE: Return of the Texan, Pony Soldier, Apache War Smoke, Bright Road, The Story of Three Loves, Code Two, Arena, Prisoner of War, Men of the Fighting Lady, The Green Slime.

TELEVISION: Wagon Train, As the World Turns.

HORWITZ, SOL: Executive. b. Chicago, April 2, 1920. e. Univ. of Chicago. U.S. Navy, 1942–45. Film booker and buyer for Balaban and Katz and Allied Theatres of Illinois, in Chicago before moving to New York where served in same capacity for Walter Read Org., Cinema 5, Loews, Inc. In sls. divisions of EDP Films, Screenvision, and Castle Hill Prods. Now project administrator for Short Film Showcase.

HOSKINS, BOB: Actor. b. England, Oct. 26, 1942. Porter and steeplejack before becoming actor at 25. Veteran of Royal Shakespeare Co. Appeared with Britain's National Theatres (Man Is Man, King Lear, Guys and Dolls, etc.)

PICTURES: Royal Flash, Zulu Dawn, The Wall, The Long Good Friday, Beyond the Limit, Lassiter, The Cotton Club, Brazil, Sweet Liberty.

TELEVISION: Flickers, Pennies from Heaven.

HOUGH, JOHN: Director, Worked in British film prod. in various capacities; impressed execs. at EMI-MGM Studios, Elstree, London, so was given chance to direct The Avengers series for TV. Began theatrical films with Sudden Terror for prod. Irving Allen, 1971.

PICTURES INCLUDE: Twins of Evil, Treasure Island, The Legend of Hell House, Dirty Mary Crazy Larry, Escape to Witch Mountain, Return to Witch Mountain, Brass Target, Watcher in the Woods.

HOUSEMAN, JOHN: Producer, director, writer. r.n. J. Haussmann. b. Rumania, Sept. 22, 1902. e. Clifton Coll., Eng. Moved to Argentina 1923 to conduct wheat export business. To U.S., Canada, 1925; contrib. to magazines; adapt. plays from German, French. In 1932 prod. Four Saints in Three Acts; later dir. Valley Force, Panic, for Theatre Guild. Assoc. with Orson Welles in founding Mercury Theat., 1937; apptd. assoc. prof. English at Vassar same yr. Prod. Julius Caesar, Native Son for stage. Co-author Woodrow Wilson (prod. on stage as In Time to Come), bought by 20th Century-Fox. Wrote radio scripts for Helen Hayes. Exec. Selznick Prod., 1941–42. Chief of overseas radio div. OWI, 1942–43. In 1943–44 (joint s.p.) Jane Eyre; New York stage; dir. Lute Song, 1948; King Lear, 1950; Coriolanis, 1953.

PICTURES INCLUDE: Miss Susie Slagle's, The Unseen, Blue Dahlia, Letter from an Unknown Woman, They Live By Night, The Company She Keeps; prod. On Dangerous Ground, Holiday For Sinners, The Bad and The Beautiful, Julius Caesar, Executive Suite, Her Twelve Men, Moonfleet, The Cobweb, Lust For Life, All Fall Down, Two Weeks in Another Town, In The Cool of the Day. Actor: The Paper Chase, 1973, Rollerball, 1975, Three Days of the Condor, St. Ives, The Cheap Detective, The Fog, Wholly Moses, Ghost Story, Murder by Phone.

TV: Paper Chase (series), The Winds of War, A.D..

HOVEY, TIM: Actor. b. Los Angeles, Calif., June 19, 1945. Child model; on TV in Lassie.

PICTURES INCLUDE: Queen Bee, Private War of Major Benson, Toy Tiger, Everything But the Truth, Man Afraid, Slim Carter, Money Women and Guns.

TV: Playhouse 90, Lux Theatre, Kraft Theatre, Matinee Playhouse, Schlitz Playhouse, G.E. Theatre, Cimarron City.

HOWARD, CY: Producer, director. b. Milwaukee,Wis., Sept. 27, 1915. e. U. of Minnesota, U. of Wisconsin, Entered radio Station KTRH, Houston, Tex. as writer, prod., actor; served 1 yr. Army Air Corps; to WBBM, Chicago, as writer, prod., actor, 1942; to Jack Benny's radio writing staff; actor, Storm Operation (stage), 1943; to ABC as writer, comedian on What's New program; to NBC where orig. wrote Palmolive Party; radio writer for Milton Berle, Danny Thomas, Bert Lahr, Jerry Lewis; orig. My Friend Irma, Life with Luigi, radio and TV shows; to Hall B. Wallis Prod. as writer and assoc. prod. My Friend Irma; exec. prod., Desilu Studios, created and produced Harrigan & Son, Westward Ho, Fair Exchange, My Friend Irma Goes West (films), That's My Boy; writer, Marriage on the Rocks; co-writer: Won Tonton, The Dog Who Saved Hollywood; director, Lovers & Other Strangers and Every Little Crook and Nanny.

HOWARD, CYRIL: Managing Director of Rank's Pinewood Studios, England. Formerly Secretary and general manager of the studios. Joined Rank Organization 1942.

HOWARD, KEN: Actor. b. El Centro, CA, March 28, 1944. e. Yale Drama School. Left studies to do walk-on in Bdwy. musical, Promises, Promises. Starred at Thomas Jefferson in 1776 on Bdwy. (Theatre World Award).

PICTURES: Tell Me That You Love Me, Junie Moon (debut), Such Good Friends, 1776, Second Thoughts.

TELEVISION: Series: Manhunter, Bonanza, Medical Center, Adam's Rib, The White Shadow. Movies: The Trial of George Armstrong Custer, He's Not Your Son.

STAGE: Child's Play, Seesaw, 1600 Pennsylvania Avenue, The Norman Conquests, Equus.

HOWARD, ROBERT T.: Executive. b. Red Bank, N.J. e. Univ. of Virginia, Columbia Univ. (N.Y.). Began prof. career as NBC page, joining guest relations staff in N.Y., 1947. Moved up to NBC TV research dept., where worked in program testing and audience measurement. Became head of research for NBC Radio Spot Sales in 1953; 1955, promoted to acct. exec. in same dept. Joined TV Spot Sales in 1959 and named natl. sales mgr. of WNBC-TV, New York in 1963 named gen. mgr. of KNBC, Los Angeles. Elected v.p. of NBC a month later. Returned to N.Y and named pres. of NBC TV Network April 1, 1974. Elected to NBC bd. and named exec. v.p.; 1977, v.p. & gen. mgr. WNBC TV, New York; 1980, pres. & chm., Citicom Communications Co.

HOWARD, RON: Actor. b. Duncan, Okla., March 1, 1954. e. Univ. of South Calif. Acting debut at age of two with parents, Rance and Jean Howard, in The Seven Year Itch at Baltimore's Hilltop Theatre. Two years later travelled to Vienna for his first film, The Journey. Many TV appearances over years. Is brother of Clint Howard, also actor from childhood.

PICTURES INCLUDE: Actor: The Journey, Wild Country, The Music Man, Courtship of Eddie's Father, Happy Mother's Day . . . Love, George, American Graffiti, The Spikes Gang, The Shootist, More American Graffiti. Director: Night Shift, Splash, Cocoon, Gung Ho (also exec. prod.).

TELEVISION: Red Skelton Hour, Playhouse 90, Dennis, the Menace, Many Loves of Dobie Gillis, Five Fingers, Twilight Zone, Dinah Shore Show, Andy Griffith Show (regular), The Fugitive, Dr. Kildare, Big Valley, I Spy, Danny Kaye Show, Gomer Pyle, USMC, The Monroes, The FBI, Judd for the Defense, Daniel Boone, Lancer, Land of the Giants, Gentle Ben, Gunsmoke, Disney TV films (A Boy Called Nuthin', Smoke), Happy Days (regular), Movie: Return to Mayberry.

HOWARD, SANDY: Producer. b. Aug. 1, 1927. Ent. m.p. ind. 1946.

PICTURES INCLUDE: Perils of the Deep, One Step to Hell, Jack of Diamonds, Tarzan and the Trappers, A Man Called Horse, Man in the Wilderness, Together Brothers, Neptune Factor, The Devil's Rain, Sky Riders, The Last Castle, Embryo, Magna I—Beyond the Barrier Reef, The

Battle, Island of Dr. Moreau, City on Fire, Death Ship (exec. prod.), Avenging Angel, The Boys Next Door.
TV: Over 50 TV series.

HOWARD, TREVOR: Actor. b. Kent, England, Sept. 29, 1916; e. Clifton Coll., Bristol, Royal Acad. of Dramatic Art. Stage debut: Revolt in a Reformatory, 1933; played Petruchio in Old Vic production of The Taming of the Shrew and in James Bridie's The Anatomist. Screen debut: The Way Ahead, 1943. In H. M. Forces in World War II.
PICTURES INCLUDE: Brief Encounter, Way to the Stars, Green for Danger, So Well Remembered, Passionate Friends, Third Man, Golden Salamander, Odette, Outcast of the Islands, Lovers of Lisbon (French), The Clouded Yellow, The Gift Horse, Heart of the Matter, Stranger's Hand, Cockelshell Heroes, Run for the Sun, Around the World in 80 Days, Interpol, Manuela, The Key, Roots of Heaven, Moment of Danger, Sons and Lovers, Mutiny On the Bounty, Father Goose, The Great Spy Mission, Von Ryan's Express, The Sabateur Code Name-Morituri, The Lion, Man in the Middle, Pretty Polly, A Matter of Innocence, The Battle of Britain, Ryan's Daughter, Pope Joan, Ludwig, 11 Harrowhouse, Who?, Hennessy, Conduct Unbecoming, The Bawdy Adventures of Tom Jones, The Last Remake of Beau Geste, Superman, Hurricane, Meteor, The Sea Wolves, Gandhi, The Missionary.
TELEVISION: Hedda Gabler, Mr. Disraeli, Napoleon, Catholics, Night Flight, George Washington, Peter the Great.

HOWELL, C. THOMAS: Actor. b. 1967. Former junior rodeo circuit champ.
PICTURES: E.T.: The Extra Terrestrial, The Outsiders, Tank, Grandview U.S.A., Red Dawn, Secret Admirer, The Hitcher.
TELEVISION: Series: Little People (only 4 yrs. old), Two Marriages.

HOWELLS, URSULA: Actress. b. Sept. 17, 1922. e. St. Paul's Sch., London. Stage debut, 1939, at Dundee Repertory with Bird in Hand followed by several plays inc. Springtime for Henry in N.Y., 1951; m.p. debut in Flesh and Blood, 1950; TV debut in Case of the Frightened Lady for BBC, 1948.
TV: Many appearances including The Small Back Room, A Woman Comes Home, For Services Rendered, Mine Own Executioner, The Cocktail Party.
PICTURES INCLUDE: The Oracle (Horse's Mouth), Track the Man Down, They Can't Hang Me, Keep It Clean, Long Arm (Third Key), Death and The Sky Above, Mumsy, Nanny, Sonny, and Girly.

HOWERD, FRANKIE: Performer. b. York, Eng., e. Shooters Hill, London, Sch. Stage debut, Sheffield Empire, 1946. Film: Runaway Bus; BBC radio & TV appearances include Tons of Money, Frankie Howerd Show, Howerd Crowd.
PICTURES INCLUDE: Jumping for Joy, An Alligator Names Daisy, The Lady Killers, A Touch of the Sun, Further Up the Creek, Cool Mikado, Fast Lady, The Great St. Trinian's Train Robbery, Carry On Doctor, Up Pompei, Up the Chastity Belt, Up The Front, The House in Nightmare Park, Sgt. Pepper's Lonely Hearts Club Band.
TV: BBC series. Comedy Playhouse, Frankie Howerd Show, Up The Convicts—Series (4) (Australia 1975), The Frankie Howerd Show—Series (13) (Canada 1976), Up Pompeii. TV-Viedo: HMS Pinafore, Trial by Jury.
STAGE: Old Vic Midsummers Night's Dream, A Funny Thing Happened on the Way to the Forum, Way Out in Piccadilly, Wind in the Sassafras Trees, Die Fledermaus.

HUDGINS, TORRENCE B.: Film Buyer. b. Merkel, Tex. e. SMU. Interstate Theatres, Inc. 1923–52; Trans-Texas Theatres, 1951–54, advertising; Cinema Art Theatres Inc., 1954–74, film buyer and advertising. 1974–78 Torrence Hudgins Buying and Booking Service.

HUDDLESTON, DAVID: Actor-Producer. b. Vinton, VA, Sept. 17, 1930. e. AADA. On stage in A Man for All Seasons, Front Page, Ten Little Indians, Silk Stockings, Fanny, Guys and Dollas, Mame, etc.
PICTURES: All the Way Home, A Lovely Way to Die, Slaves, Norwood, Rio Lobo, Fools Parade, Country Blue, Bad Company, Blazing Saddles, McQ, Capricorn I, World's Greatest Lover, Gorp, Smokey and the Bandit II.
TELEVISION: Movies: The Priest Killer, The Homecoming, Tenafly, Heatwave, The Oregon Trail, Sherlock Holmes in New York, Kate Bliss and the Ticket Tape Kid, Finnegan Begin Again, etc.

HUDSON, HUGH: Producer-Director. b. England; e. Eton. Began career with ad agency in London; left for Paris to work as editor for small film co. Returned to London to form Cammell-Hudson Film Co., production house., turning out documentaries. 1970, joined with Ridley Scott to make TV commercials. 1975, formed Hudson Films to produce. Debut as director of theatrical features with Chariots of Fire (1982).
PICTURES: Greystoke: The Legend of Tarzan, Lord of the Apes (prod./dir.), Revolution (dir.).

HUGGINS, ROY: Writer, director. b. Litelle, Wash., July 18, 1914; e. U. of Calif 1935–39; U. of Calif. Grad. Sch., 1939–41; m. Adele Mara, actress. Spec. rep., U.S. Civil Service Comm., 1941–43; industrial eng., 1943–46; writer 3 novels and many stories for Sat. Eve. Post; pres., Public Arts, Inc., 1968. V.P., 20th Century-Fox TV, 1961.
PICTURES INCLUDE: I Love Trouble, Too Late for Tears, Lady Gambles; story, Fuller Brush Man, Good Humor Man; adap., Woman in Hiding; collab., s.p., Sealed Cargo; Sp., dir., Hangman's Knot; collab. s.p., Gun Fury, Three Hours to Kill; s.p., Pushover; Prod. motion picture A Fever in the Blood for Warner Bros.
TV: Prod. Warner Bros. Presents Cheyenne series, anthologies, 1955–56; Conflict (series); Produced Pilots of Colt .45, 77 Sunset Strip, Maverick, Prod. Maverick, 1957–58; won Emmy Award 1958. Created, The Fugitive, 1962; v.p., MCA Revue, 1963; exec.-prod. Run For Your Life, 1965; exec. prod., The Outsiders, The Bold Ones, Alias Smith and Jones, Toma, 1968–74. ABC Movie of Week, Pretty Boy Floyd. 1974: Co-creator of The Rockford Files pilot and series for NBC; 1975: Co-creator of City of Angels for NBC; 1976: executive producer of Captains and the Kings, a segment of Best Sellers for NBC. 1977: exec. prod. of Aspen, a segment of best sellers for NBC: 1978: exec. prod. of Wheels, a segment of The Big Event for NBC.

HUGHES, BARNARD: Actor. b. Bedford Hills, N.Y., July 16, 1915. Winner of Emmy for role as Judge in Lou Grant series (1978) and Tony for Da (1978). Acted for over 47 years.
PICTURES INCLUDE: Midnight Cowboy, Oh, God!, Where's Poppa, The Hospital, Rage, Sisters, Cold Turkey, Pursuit of Happiness, Deadhead Miles, Tron, Best Friends, Maxie, Where Are the Children?.
TELEVISION: Doc, See How She Runs, The Caryl Chessman Story, Tell Me My Name, Look Homeward, Angel, Father Brown: Detective, Nova, Homeward Bound, The Sky's No Limit, A Caribbean Mystery.

HUGHES, JOHN: Writer-Director-Producer. Editor of National Lampoon before writing film scripts of National Lampoon's Vacation and Mr. Mom (both in 1983). Made directorial debut with Sixteen Candles in 1984 which also wrote. In 1985 entered into deal with Paramount Pictures to write, direct and produce films with his own production unit, The John Hughes Co.
PICTURES: The Breakfast Club (s.p., dir.); Weird Science (s.p., dir.); Pretty in Pink (s.p., dir., prod.).

HUGHES, KATHLEEN: Actress. r.n. Betty von Gerkan; b. Hollywood, Calif., Nov. 14, 1928; e. L.A. City Coll., UCLA. m. Stanley Rubin, producer, mother of 4, Michael played Baby Matthew on Peyton Place. Studied drama; under contract, 20th-Fox, 1948–51; starred in 7 Year Itch 1954, La Jolla Playhouse; parts m.p.; signed by UI, 1952.
PICTURES INCLUDE: For Men Only, Sally and Saint Anne, Golden Blade, It Came From Outer Space, Thy Neighbor's Wife, Glass Web, Dawn at Socorro, Cult of the Cobra, Three Bad Sisters, Promise Her Anything, The President's Analyst, The Late Liz, The Take.
TV: Bob Cummings Show, Hitchock, 77 Sunset Strip, G.E. Theatre, Bachelor Father, The Tall Man, Dante, Tightrope, Markham, I Dream of Jeannie, Peyton Place, Gomer Pyle, Kismet, Ghost and Mrs. Muir, Bracken's World, The Survivors, Julia, Here's Lucy, To Rome with Love, The Interns, The Man and the City, Mission Impossible, The Bold Ones, Lucas Tanner, Marcus Welby, Barnaby Jones, Medical Center, Babe (mov.).

HUGHES, KEN: Writer, dir. b. Liverpool, Eng. Ent. ind. as sound engineer, BBC, 1940; dir., doc. films. Novels: High Wray, The Long Echo.
TV: Script of serials Solo for Canary, An Enemy of the State; Sammy (Eddie in USA); The Haunting, Lenin in 1917 (Fall of Eagles); The Voice (Dial M For Murder).
PICTURES INCLUDE: Joe Macbeth, Confession, The Trials of Oscar Wilde, The Small World of Sammy Lee, Arrivederci Baby, Casino Royale, Chitty Chitty Bang, Bang, Cromwell, The Internecine Project, Sextette.
AWARDS INCLUDE: Golden Globe, Emmy, Script Writer of Year, W.G. Merit Award.

HUKE, BOB, B.S.C.: Cinematographer. Ent. m.p. ind. 1937, Asst. cameraman Pygmalion, French Without Tears, etc.; 1939–44 Royal Navy. 1945–9 camera operator Great Expectations, Uncle Silas, Seven Days To Noon and others. 1950–56 Brazil. Contract dir. of photo. for Cia Cinematographica Vera Cruz, 1957–59 dir. own company, Zenith, 1960. dir. photo, 3 Dinah Shore Shows, Spain, Paris, Copenhagen. NBC 1961. Dir. photo. Reach For Glory, The War Lover, The Very Edge, 1962; The Brain, 8 Danny Thomas Shows in Europe. 1963 Sandres of the River. 1964, Ballad in Blue, License to Share. TV & Cinema Commercials, 1955. 1966, 2nd Unit You Only Live Twice; 1968, 2nd Unit, Battle of Britain, 1969; dir. photo, Virgin and Gypsy. 1971; Under Milk Wood.

HUNNICUT, GAYLE: Actress. b. Fort Worth, Texas, February 6, 1943. e. BA (with honors) University of California, Los Angeles, (UCLA) Theater Arts & English major. Early career, community theatres in Los Angeles. Ent. m.p. ind. 1967.

PICTURES INCLUDE: PJ (New Face in Hell), Eye of the Cat, Marlowe, Fragment of Fear, The Freelance, Voices, Running Scared, New Face in Hell, Scorpio, L'Homme Sans Visage, The Spiral Staircase, The Sell Out, Tony Siatta, Once in Paris, One Take Two, Fantomas, Return of the Man from UNCLE, Privilege, Sherlock Holmes, Target, Dream Lover.

TV: Man and Boy, The Golden Bowl, The Ripening Seed, Fall of Eagles, The Switch, Humboldts Gift, The Life and Death of Dylan Thomas, Return of the Saint, Martian Chronicles, A Man Called Intrepid, Kiss Inc., Love Boat—The Mallory Quest, The Lady Killers, Marlowe, The Quest, Fantasy Island, Taxi, Savage in the Orient, The First Modern Olympics, Dream West, Strong Medicine.

THEATRE: The Ride Across Lake Constance, Twelfth Night, The Tempest, Dog Days, The Admirable Crichton, A Woman of No Importance, Hedda Gabler, Peter Pan, Macbeth, Uncle Vanya, The Philadelphia Story, Miss Firecraker Contest, Exit The King-Ionsco, The Doctor's Dilemma.

HUNT, LINDA: Actress. b. Morristown, N.J., 1945. e. Interlochen Arts Academy (Michigan) and Chicago's Goodman Theatre & School of Drama.

PICTURES: The Year of Living Dangerously, Dune, The Bostonians, Silverado, Eleni.

THEATRE: Mother Courage, End of the World, etc.

HUNT, MARSHA: Actress. b. Chicago, Ill., Oct. 17, 1917. Started screen 1935.

B'WAY PLAYS INCLUDE: Devils Disciple, Joy to the World, Legend of Sarah, Born in Texas, Tunnel of Love, The Paisley Convertible.

PICTURES INCLUDE: Virginia Judge, College Holiday, Easy to Take, Blossoms in the Dust, Panama Hattie, Joe Smith American, These Glamour Girls, Winter Carnival, Irene, Pride and Prejudice, Flight Command, Cheers for Miss Bishop, Trial of Mary Dugan, Thousands Cheer, None Shall Escape, Lost Angel, Cry Havoc, Bride by Mistake, Music for Millions, Valley of Decision, A Letter for Evie, Smash-Up, Carnegie Hall, Raw Deal, Take One False Step, Actors and Sin, Happy Time, No Place To Hide, Bombers B-52, Blue Denim, Johnny Got His Gun.

TV: Philco, Studio One, Ford Theatre, Show of Shows, G.E. Theatre, Climax, Hitchcock, Peck's Bad Girl Series, The Defenders, Twilight Zone, Cains Hundred, Gunsmoke, The Breaking Point, Outer Limits, Profiles in Courage, Ben Casey, Accidental Family, Run For Your Life, My Three Sons, The Outsiders, Name of the Game, Univ.'s 120, Ironside, Marcus Welby, M.D., Police Story, The Young Lawyers.

HUNT, PETER: Director—Editor. b. London, England. 1928. e. Romford England—Rome, Italy. London School of Music. Actor English Rep. Entered film as camera asst. Documentary, later asst editor documentary, then asst editor features. London Films then editor—credits incl. Hill in Korea, Admirable Crichton, Scripting films. Editor: Cry From the Streets, Greengage Summer (Loss of Innocence in USA), Ferry To Hong Kong, H.MS Defiant (Damn the Defiant in USA), Supervising editor/2nd Unit Director, Dr. No, Call Me Bwana, From Russia With Love, Goldfinger, Ibcress File, Thunderball, You Only Live Twice, . . . associate producer, Chitty Chitty Bang Bang . . . Director, On Her Majesty's Secret Service, Gullivers Travels (Live & Animation) Gold, Shout At The Devil, Death Hunt, Chandle Town; Wild Geese II.

HUNT, PETER H.: Director. b. Pasadena, Calif., Dec. 16, 1938. e. Hotchkiss, Yale, Yale Drama School. m. actress Barbette Tweed. Director for Williamston Theatre since 1957. Lighting designer on Bdwy. (1963–69)

PICTURES INCLUDE: 1776; Give 'Em Hell, Harry; Bully, Adventures of Huckleberry Finn.

TELEVISION: Huckleberry Finn (mini-series), It Came Upon the Midnight Clear, The Parade, Life on the Mississippi, A Private History of a Compaign That Failed, A New Start, Sheezer, Mysterious Stranger. Pilots: Adams Rib, Hello Mother Goodbye, Ivan the Terrible, Quark, Mixed Nuts, Flying High, Wilder and Wilder, Rendezvous Hotel, The Main Event, Nuts and Bolts, The Good Witch of Laurel Canyon, Masquerade, Stir Crazy, Charley Hannah, The Wizard of Elm Street.

CABLE: Sherlock Holmes, Bus Stop.

STAGE: 1776 (London & Bdwy.), Georgy (Bdwy.), Scratch (Bdwy.), Goodtime Charley (Bdwy.), Give 'Em Hell Harry (Tour), Magnificent Yankee (Kennedy Center), Bully, Three Penny Opera, Sherlock Holmes, Bus Stop (last four all tours).

AWARDS: Tony, Ace, Peabody, N.Y. Drama Critics, London Drama Critics, Edgar Allan Poe, Christopher.

HUNT, WILLIE: Executive Producer. b. Van Nuys, Ca., Oct. 1, 1941. e. Utah State Univ. (BA, 1963). Married to actor Tim Considine. Started in industry as secretary at Warner Bros., 1965; named exec. secty. to Ted Ashley, WB, 1969; story analyst, WB, 1974; story editor, WB, 1975; named West Coast story editor for WB, 1978; joined MGM in 1979 as v.p., motion picture development. Moved to United Artists as v.p.-prod., 1982. In 1983 sr., v.p. of prod. at Rastar Prods.; 1984, indep. prod., Tri-Star Pictures; 1986, sr. v.p., Freddie Fields Prods.

HUNTER, KIM: Actress. r.n. Janet Cole; b. Detroit, Nov. 12, 1922. d. Donald and Grace Mabel (Lind) Cole; ed. pub. schs.; student acting with Carmine Lantaff Camine, 1938–40, Actors Studio; m. William A. Baldwin, Feb. 11, 1944 (div. 1946); 1 dau., Kathryn Emmett; m. 2nd, Robert Emmett, Dec. 20, 1951; 1 son, Sean Emmett; First stage appearance, 1939; played in stock, 1940–42; Broadway debut in A Streetcar Named Desire, 1947.

STAGE: Two Blind Mice (tour), 1950; Darkness at Noon (N.Y.C.), 1951; The Chase (N.Y.C.), 1952; They Knew What They Wanted (tour), 1952; The Children's Hour (revival) (N.Y.C.), 1952; The Tender Trap (N.Y.C.), 1954; Write Me a Murder (N.Y.C.), 1961; Weekend (N.Y.C.), 1968; The Penny Wars (N.Y.C.), 1969; And Miss Reardon Drinks a Little (tour), 1972–72; The Glass Menagerie (Atlanta), The Women (N.Y.C.), 1973; In Praise of Love (tour), 1975; The Lion in Winter (N.J.), 1975; The Cherry Orchard (N.Y.C.), 1976; The Chalk Garden (Pa.), 1977; Elizabeth the Queen (Buffalo), 1977; Semmelweiss (Buffalo), 1977; The Belle of Amherst (N.J.), 1978; The Little Foxes (Mass.), 1980; To Grandmother's House We Go (N.Y.C.), 1981; Another Part of the Forest (Seattle), 1981; When We Dead Awaken (N.Y.C.), 1982; Ghosts (Garden City and Tarrytown, N.Y.), 1982; Territorial Rites (N.Y.C.), 1983; Death of a Salesman (Stratford, Ont.), 1983; Cat on a Hot Tin Roof, 1984; Life With Father (Coconut Grove, Fla.), 1984; Sabrina Fair (BTF, Mass.), 1984; Faulkner's Bicycle (Yale Repertory and Joyce Theatre, N.Y.C.), 1985; Antique Pink (U. of Mich. Theatre), 1985; The Belle of Amherst (N.H.), 1986; Painting Churches (Stamford, Conn.), 1986; A Delicate Balance (BTF, Mass.), 1986; frequent appearances summer stock and repertory theater, 1940–; appeared Am. Shakespeare Festival, Stratford, Conn., 1961.

PICTURES: Film debut in The Seventh Victim, 1943; other motion pictures include: Tender Comrade, 1943; When Strangers Marry (re-released as Betrayed), 1944; You Came Along, 1945; A Canterbury Tale, 1949; Stairway to Heaven, 1946; A Streetcare Named Desire, 1951; Anything Can Happen, 1952; Bermuda Affair, 1957; The Young Stranger, 1957; Money, Women and Guns, 1958; Lilith, 1964; Planet of the Apes, 1968; The Swimmer, 1968; Beneath the Planet of the Apes, 1970; Escape from the Planet of the Apes, 1971; Dark August, 1975; The Kindred, 1986.

TELEVISION: Made TV debut on Actors Studio Program, 1948; numerous TV appearances include: Requiem for a Heavyweight, 1956; The Comedian, 1957 (both on Playhouse 90); Give Us Barabbas on Hallmark Hall of Fame, 1961; Love, American Style; Columbo; Cannon; Night Gallery; Mission Impossible; The Magician, 1972–73; Marcus Welby; Hec Ramsey; Griff; Police Story; Ironside; Medical Center; Bad Ronald; Born Innocent; Once an Eagle; Baretta; Gibbsville; Hunter, 1976; The Oregon Trail, 1977; Project: U.F.O.; Stubby Pringle's Christmas, 1978; Backstairs at the White House, 1979; Specter on the Bridge, 1979; Edge of Night, 1979–80; F.D.R.'s Last Year; 1980; Skokie, 1981; Scene of the Crime, 1984; Private Sessions, 1985; Three Sovereigns for Sarah, 1985; Hot Pursuit, 1985; Martin Luther King, Jr.: The Dream and the Drum, 1986.

RECORDED: From Morning 'Til Night (and a Bag Full of Poems), RCA Victor, 1961; Come, Woo Me—Unified Audio Classic, 1964.

AWARDS: Recipient Donaldson Award for best supporting actress in A Streetcar Named Desire, 1948, also on Variety N.Y. Critics Poll, 1948, for film version, 1952; winner Acad. award, LOOK award, Hollywood Fgn. Corrs. Golden Globe award; Emmy nominations for Baretta, 1977, Edge of Night, 1980; Carbonnell award for Big Mama in Cat on a Hot Tin Roof, So. Fla., 1984.

HUNTER, ROSS: Producer. r.n. Martin Fuss. b. Cleveland, Ohio, May 6, 1926. e. Western Reserve U., M.A. School teacher, 1938–43; actor, Columbia Pictures, 1944–46; returned to school teaching; stage prod. & dir.; m.p. dialogue dir.; assoc. prod. U-I, 1950–51; prod., U-I, 1951. Moved production Co. from Universal to Columbia, April 1, 1971. Moved to Paramount, Oct.1, 1974.

PICTURES INCLUDE: Louisiana Hayride, Ever Since Venus, Bandit of Sherwood Forest, Groom Wore Spurs, Take Me to Town, All I Desire, Tumbleweed, Taza Son of Cochise, Magnificent Obsession, Naked Alibi, Yellow Mountain, Captain Lightfoot, One Desire, The Spoilers, All That Heaven Allows, There's Always Tomorrow, Battle Hymn, Tammy and the Bachelor, Interlude, My Man Godfrey, The Wonderful Years, Stranger in My Arms, Imitation of

Life, Pillow Talk, Portrait in Black, Midnight Lace, Back Street, Flower Drum Song, Tammy and the Doctor, The Thrill of It All, The Chalk Garden, I'd Rather Be Rich, The Art of Love, Madame X, The Pad, Thoroughly Modern Millie, Rosie, Airport, Lost Horizon.

HUNTER, TAB: Actor. b. New York, N.Y., July 11, 1931. U.S. Coast Guard; odd jobs. discovered in 1948.
PICTURES INCLUDE: The Lawless, Island of Desire, Gun Belt, Steel Lady, Return to Treasure Island, Track of the Cat, Battle Cry, Sea Chase, Burning Hills, Girl He Left Behind, Lafayette Escadrille, Gunman's Walk, Damn Yankees, That Kind of Woman, Pleasure of His Company, The Golden Arrow, War Gods of the Deep, Ride the Wild Surf, Hostile Guns, Life and Times of Judge Roy Bean, Grease 2, Lust in the Dust (also prod.).

HUNTLEY, RAYMOND: Actor. b. Birmingham, England, Apr. 23, 1904. On stage from 1922 repertory, tour; London debut in "Back to Methuselah" 1924; N.Y. debut in "Venetian Glass Nephew" 1931; m.p. debut 1934; many TV appearances.
PICTURES INCLUDE: Rembrandt, Knight Without Armour, Night Train to Munich, They Came to a City, Pimpernel Smith, Freedom Radio, Way Ahead, I See a Dark Stranger, School for Secrets, Broken Journey, So Evil My Love, Mr. Perrin and Mr. Traill, It's Hard to Be Good, Passport to Pimlico, Trio, I'll Never Forget You, The Last Page, Laxdale Hall, Meet Mr. Lucifer, Mr. Denning Drives North, Hobson's Choice, Orders Are Orders, Constant Husband, Geordie, The Prisoner, Doctor at Sea, Dam Busters, Teckman Mystery, Green Man, Brothers in Law, Room at the Top, Carlton-Browne of the F.O., Suspect, A French Mistress, Pure Hell of St. Trinians, Only Two Can Play, Waltz of The Toreadors, Crooks Anonymous, On the Beat, Carry On Nurse, The Great St. Trinian's Train Robbery, Hostile Witness, The Gaunt Woman, Arthur! Arthur!, Young Winston, That's Your Funeral, Symptoms.

HURLOCK, ROGER W.: Pres. Hurlock Cine-World. b. Cambridge, Md., May 30, 1912. e. Baltimore City College; ent. m.p. ind. as publicist, Hippodrome Theatre, Balt.; asst. mgr., Lessor-operator Imperial and Majestic Theatres, Balt., 1931–35; real estate, bldg., farming, Md. and Alaska, 1936–58; elected bd. mem., Allied Artists, 1958; asst. to pres., 1961–63; chmn. budget comm., 1963; chmn. policy comm., 1964; c.p. exec. comm. member, 1964; v.p., chf. operating officer 1965; chmn. exec. comm., 1966; pres., 1967. pres., Hurlock Cine-World, 1969.

HURT, JOHN: Actor. b. Shirebrook, Derbyshire, Jan. 22, 1940. e. St. Martin's School for Art, London. Professional debut in 1962 in British film, The Wild and the Willing.
PICTURES: A Man for All Seasons, Before Winter Comes, Sinful Davey, In Search of Gregory, 10 Rillington Place, Forbush and the Penguins, East of Elephant Rock, Disappearance, Spectre, Pied Piper of Hamelin, The Ghoul, Little Malcolm, The Shout, Midnight Express, Alien, Heaven's Gate, The Elephant Man, Partners, Night Crossing, The Osterman Weekend, Champions, The Hit.
TELEVISION: Playboy of the Western World, A Tragedy of Two Ambitions, Green Julia, Nijinsky, Shades of Green, Ten from the Twenties, The Pedlar, The Naked Civil Servant, I, Claudius, Crime and Punishment.
STAGE: The Dwarfs, Little Malcolm and His Struggle Against the Eunuchs, Man and Superman, Belcher's Luck, Ride a Cock Horse, The Caretaker, Romeo and Juliet, Ruffian on the Streets, The Dumb Waiter, Travesties, The Arrest.

HURT, MARY BETH: Actress. b. Marshalltown, IA, Sept. 26. e. NYU School of Arts. Stage debut in 1973 in N.Y. Shakespeare Festival prod., More Than You Deserve. Other stage work includes Trelawny of the Wells, Father's Day.
PICTURES: Interiors, Head Over Heels, Change of Seasons, The World According to Garp, D.A.R.Y.L.
TELEVISION: Secret Service (NET Theatre), Kojak, etc.

HURT, R. N.: Circuit executive. b. Veedersburg, Ind., Jan. 30, 1902; e. Brown's Business Coll., Danville, Ill.; m. Entered m.p. ind. as operator at Veedersburg for H.C. Whisler, 1918–22; owned, oper. Lyric Edinburgh, Ind., 1920; for six months, operator and later booker Lincoln Paris, Ill., for Mrs. L. Jarodsky. To Crown Point, Ind., Palace Theatre, manager four years; State, Princeton, in 1930 as mgr., later owner. Sold out to E. E. Alger, 1932 and became mgr. Apollo, Princeton. Transferred to main office, Alger Circuit as booker in 1934, then gen. mgr. oper. in 10 towns controlling 14 theatres. Left 1945; Dixon Theatre Co., 1945–46; Isis Theatre, Toluca, Ill., 1946–48; returned to Alger Sept. 1948–58; booker, Kerasotes Theatres, hdq. Springfield, Ill., 1958–71. Mgr., Times, Danville, Ill., Oct. 1, 1971. Retired.

HURT, WILLIAM: Actor. b. Washington, D.C., Mar. 20, 1950. e. Tufts, Julliard. Leading actor with New York's Circle Repertory Company since 1976, appearing in among other plays, The Fifth of July, My Life, Ulysses in Traction, The Runner Stumbles, Hamlet, Childe Byron. Also appeared with the New York Shakespeare Festival and in Hurly Burly off-Bdwy and on Bdwy.
PICTURES: Altered States (debut), Eyewitness, Body Heat, The Big Chill, Gorky Park, Kiss of the Spiderwoman (Academy Award), Children of a Lesser God.
TELEVISION: Verna: USO Girl, Best of Families, All The Way Home.

HUSSEIN, WARIS: Director. b. India, 1938. TV incl: Sleeping Dog, Death of a Teddy Bear, Toggle, Spoiled, Days In the Trees, A Passage to India, Girls in Uniform, St. Joan, A Casual Affair, Divorce His, Divorce Hers, Shoulder To Shoulder, Gorges Sand, Chips With Everything, The Glittering Prizes, Love Letters on Blue Paper, Sarah Bernhardt, Blind Love, Romance, Daphne Laureola, Waiting for Sheila, Armchair Thriller, Edward and Mrs. Simpson, Death Penalty, And Baby Makes Six, The Henderson Monster.
PICTURES INCLUDE: A Touch of Love, Quackser Fortune, Melody, The Possession of Joel Delaney, Henry VIII and His Six Wives, Coming Out of the Ice.
TV Film: Baby Comes Home, Callie and Son, Little Gloria: Happy at Last, Princess Daisy. Winter of Our Discontent, Arch of Triumph, Copacabana.

HOUSTON, ANJELICA: Actress. b. 1952. daughter of John Huston.
PICTURES: Sinful Davey, A Walk with Love and Death, The Last Tycoon, The Postman Always Rings Twice, The Ice Pirates, Prizzi's Honor (Oscar).

HUSTON, JOHN: Director, writer. b. Aug. 5, 1906, Nevada. Mo. p. Walter Huston. In 1938: collab. s.p., Amazing Dr. Clitterhouse, WB. In 1939: Juarez, In 1940: Dr. Ehrlich's Magic Bullet, WB. In 1941: High Sierra, Sergeant York, WB.; dir., s.p., The Maltese Falcon, WB, in 1942: dir. In This Our Life, Across the Pacific, WB. U.S. documentaries (dir.).
PICTURES INCLUDE: Three Strangers, Treasure of the Sierra Madre, Key Largo, WB. 1949 founded Horizon Films with S.P. Eagle, Were Strangers, The Asphalt Jungle, The Red Badge of Courage, The African Queen, Moulin Rouge, Beat the Devil, Moby Dick, The Misfits, Freud, List of Adrian Messenger, The Night of the Iguana, The Bible, Reflections in a Golden Eye, Candy, acted in De Sade, Walk with Life and Death, The Kremlin Letter, The Deserter, acted in Man in the Wilderness, Fat City, The Life and Times of Judge Roy Bean (dir. & acted), Battle for the Planet of the Apes (actor), The McIntosh Man, Chinatown (actor), The Wind and The Lion (actor), The Man Who Would Be King (dir.), Winter Kills (actor), Wise Blood (dir.), Victory (dir.), Annie (dir)., Lovesick (actor), Under the Volcano (dir.), Prizzi's Honor (dir.).
TV: The Rheinmann Exchange.

HUSTON, VIRGINIA: Actress. b. Omaha, Neb., Apr. 24, 1925. Did radio and stage work while in school; acted at Omaha Community playhouse; started in m.p. with RKO 1945.
PICTURES INCLUDE: Nocturne, Out of the Past, Tarzan's Peril, The Highwayman, Racket, Flight to Mars, Night Stage to Galveston, Sudden Fear, Knock on Wood.

HUTTON, BETTY: Actress. b. Battle Creek, Mich., Feb. 26, 1921. Made screen debut in 1942.
PICTURES INCLUDE: The Fleet's In, Star Spangled Rhythm, Happy Go Lucky, Miracle of Morgan's Creek, Incendiary Blonde, And the Angels Sing, Here Come the Waves, Duffys Tavern, The Stork Club, Perils of Pauline, Annie Get Your Gun, Let's Dance, The Greatest Show on Earth, Somebody Loves Me, Spring Reunion.
TV: Goldie.

HUTTON, BRIAN, G.: Director. b. N.Y. City, 1935.
PICTURES INCLUDE: The Wild Seed (Universal); The Pad (Universal); Sol Madrid (MGM); Where Eagles Dare (MGM); Kelly's Heroes (MGM); X, Y, and Zee, Night Watch, The First Deadly Sin, High Road to China.

HUTTON, LAUREN: Actress. b. Charleston, S.C., 1944. e. Univ. of So. Florida, Sophie Newcombe College. As model featured on more covers than any other American.
PICTURES: Paper Lion (debut, 1968), Little Fauss and Big Halsey, The Gambler, Gator, Welcome to L.A., A Wedding, American Gigolo, Zorro, the Gay Blade, Paternity, Starflight One, Lassiter, Once Bitten.
TELEVISION: The Cradle Will Fall, The Rhinemann Exchange, Someone Is Watching Me, Scandal Sheet, Sins.

HUTTON, ROBERT: Actor. r.n. R. Winne. b. Kingston, N.Y., June 11, 1920. e. Blair Acad., N.J. In summer stock prior to screen career, 1943.
PICTURES INCLUDE: Destination Tokyo, Janie, Roughly Speaking, Hollywood Canteen, Too Young to Know, Love and Learn, Always Together, Steel Helmet, New Mexico, Racket, Slaughter Trail, Casanova's Big Night, Cinderella; co-prod., dir., star, The Slime People; asso. prod., Now It Can Be Told. The Vulture, You Only Live Twice, They Came From Beyond Space, Torture Garden, Tales From the Crypt.

HUTTON, TIMOTHY: Actor. b. Malibu, CA, Aug. 16, 1960. Father, late actor Jim Hutton. In plays in high school; toured with father in Harvey during vacation. Theatrical film debut in Ordinary People (1980).
TELEVISION: Movies: Zuma Beach, Best Place To Be, Baby Makes Six, Sultan and the Rock Star, Young Love, First Love, Friendly Fire.
PICTURES: Ordinary People, Taps, Daniel, Iceman, The Falcon and The Snowman, Turk 182, Made in Heaven.

HUYCK, WILLARD: Writer-Director. e. USC. Went to work as reader for Larry Gordon, executive at American-International Pictures; named Gordon's asst., working on scene rewrites for AIP films. First screen credit on The Devil's Eight as co-writer with John Milius, also USC graduate. Left AIP to write original scripts, joining with Gloria Katz. Both signed by Francis Ford Coppola to write and direct films for his America Zoetrope but projects never materialized. Co-wrote American Graffiti with Katz (1973) and Lucky Lady (1975). Huyck made directorial debut in 1979 with French Postcards, co-written with Katz, who also produced.
PICTURES: Indiana Jones and the Temple of Doom (dir., co.-s.p.); The Best Defense (co.-s.p.); Howard the Duck (dir., co.-s.p.).

HYAMS, JOSEPH: Adv. & pub. exec. b. N.Y., Sept. 21, 1926. e. N.Y. Univ.; ent. industry, 1947. Various publicity posts, 20th Century-Fox, Columbia Pictures, 1947–55; eastern pub. mgr., Figaro Prods., 1955–56; West Coast pub. mgr., Hecht-Hill-Lancaster, 1955–58; pub. adv. dir., Batjac Prods. 1959–60 national adv. & pub. dir., Warner Bros., Seven Arts, 1960. v.p., world-wide pub., Warner Bros., Inc., 1970–present.

HYAMS, PETER: Director-Writer. b. N.Y.C., July 26, 1943. e. Hunter College, Syracuse Univ. Joined CBS news staff N.Y. and made anchor man. Filmed documentary on Vietnam in 1966. Left CBS in 1970 and joined Paramount in Hollywood as writer. Hired by ABC to direct TV features.
PICTURES INCLUDE: Busting (s.p., dir.), Our Time (dir.), Peeper, Telefon (co-s.p.), Carpicorn One (s.p., dir.), The Hunter (co-s.p.), Outland (dir., s.p.), Star Chamber (s.p., dir.), 2010 (prod., dir., s.p.), Running Scared (exec. prod., dir.).
TELEVISION: The Rolling Man, Goodnight My Love (both s.p., dir.).

HYDE, JOHN W.: Executive. b. Jackson, MI. e. New York University, B.A. 1963. Joined ABC upon graduation from N.Y.U. 1963 hired by MCA-Universal as executive assistant to then v.p. Ned Tanen. As Tanen's assistant, became assoc. prod. on several MCA features. Also wrote, produced and directed musical shorts for MCA Records. 1969 joined Filmways, Inc. as v.p. and exec. asst. to then-pres. Richard R. St. Johns. 1972 formed own company, Acmelab, Ltd., multi-faceted special effects, commercial and post-production facility, which included Cinefex, Videoconversion and Acme Film Laboratories. 1976 Hyde sold Acmelab to produce The Ravagers for Columbia Pictures. During production of that film, Hyde rejoined Richard St. Johns as v.p. of the Morison Film Group, a Guinness co. 1977 Hyde became vice president in charge of production for all Morison films; 1981, named pres. of MFG.
TELEVISION: The Andy Williams Show, The Lloyd Thaxton Show.
PICTURES INCLUDE: Games, Midnight Patient, Skulduggery, The Ravagers, Death Hunt, Rituals, The Uncanny, Silent Flute (Circle of Iron), Matilda, The Wanders, Nightwing, The Mountain Men, The Final Countdown, A Change of Seasons, Dead & Buried, American Pop, Venom, Fire and Ice.

HYDE, TOMMY: Executive. r.n. Thomas L. b. Meridian, Miss., June 29, 1916. e. Lakeland H.S., grad., 1935. Worked E.J. Sparks Theatres, 1932–41. Florida State Theatres, 1941–42. U.S. Navy, 1942–46. Florida State Theatres, 1946–47; city mgr. (Tallahassee). Talgar Theatres, 1947–58; v.p. and gen. mgr. Kent Theatres, 1958–86; vice-pres. Motion Picture Films, Inc.; pres., NATO of Florida, 1961–62; chmn. bd. 1963–70.

HYDE-WHITE, WILFRID: Actor. b. Gloucestershire, Eng.; e. Marlborough Coll. Stage debut, 1925; screen debut in Rembrandt, 1936. TV appearances.
PICTURES INCLUDE: The Winslow Boy, Britannia Mews, Adam and Evelyn, The Third Man, Golden Salamander, Trio, Mr. Drake's Duck, The Browning Version, Outcast of the Islands, Mr. Denning Drives North, Gilbert & Sullivan, Million Pound Note (Man With a Million), Betrayed, Duel in the Jungle, Rainbow Jacket, To Dorothy, A Son, Quentin Durward, March Hare, The Silken Affair, Libel, North West Frontier, Two-Way Stretch, Let's Make Love, On the Double, Ada, The Castaways, Crooks Anonymous, My Fair Lady (Hollywood), 1964; You Must Be Joking, Ten Little Indians, The Sandwich Man, Marrakesh.

HYER, MARTHA: Actress. b. Fort Worth, Tex., Aug. 10, 1924. e. Northwestern Univ., Pasadena Playhouse.
PICTURES INCLUDE: Thunder Mountain, Indian Summer, Roughshod, Velvet Touch, The Lawless, Outcast of Black Mesa, Salt Lake Raiders, Frisco Tornado, Abbott and Costello Go to Mars, Scarlet Spear, So Big, Sabrina, Kiss of Fire, Paris Follies of 1956, Francis in the Navy, Red Sundown, Showdown at Abilene, Kelly and Me, Battle Hymn, Mister Cory, My Man Godfrey, Paris Holiday, Once Upon a Horse, Houseboat, Some Came Running, Big Fisherman, Best of Everything, Ice Palace, Desire In the Dust, The Right Approach, The Last Time I Saw Archie, Girl Names Tamiko, Man From the Diner's Club, Wives and Lovers, Pyro, The Carpetbaggers, First Man in the Moon, Blood On the Arrow, Bikini Beach, Sones of Katie Elder, The Chase, Night of the Grizzly, Picture Mommy Dead, The Happening, Some May Live, House of a Thousand Dolls, Once You Kiss A Stranger, Crossplot.

I

IANNUCCI, SALVATORE J.: Executive. b. Brooklyn, N.Y., Sept. 24, 1927. e. NYU 1949 B.A., Harvard Law School 1952 J.D. 2 yrs. legal departments RCA and American Broadcasting Company, Inc.; 14 yrs. with CBS Television Network: asst. dir. of bus. affairs, dir. of bus. affairs, v.p. of bus. affairs; 2 yrs. v.p. admin. National General Corp.; 2½ yrs. pres. of Capital Records; 4½ yrs. Corpor. Vice pres. and dir. of Entertainment Div. of Playboy Enterprises, Inc.; 4 yrs. partner with Jones, Day, Reavis & Pogue in Los Angeles office, handling entertainment legal work; Pres., Filmways Entertainment, and sr. v.p., Filmways, Inc.; exec. v.p., Embassy Communications; now COO, Aaron Spelling Prods.

IBBETSON, ARTHUR: Cinematographer. b. England, 1922.
PICTURES INCLUDE: The Horse's Mouth, Tunes of Glory, Whistle Down the Wind, Nine Hours to Rama, I Could Go On Singing, The Chalk Garden, A Countess from Hong Kong, Where Eagles Dare, Anne of the Thousand Days, A Doll's House, A Little Night Music, Hopscotch, The Bounty, Santa Claus, etc.
TELEVISION: Frankenstein: the True Story, Little Lord Fauntleroy (Emmy).

IBERT, LLOYD: Executive. Began career as mgng. editor, Independent Film Journal. 1973, joined Paramount Pictures pub. dept.; named sr. publicist. 1985, appointed dir., natl. pub. for M.P. Group.

IMAMURA, SHOHEI: Director, Producer. b. Tokyo, Japan, Sept. 15, 1926. e. Waseda U. Joined Shochiku Ofuna Studio 1951 asst. dir., transferred Nikkatsu in 1954 as asst. dir., director Stolen Desire 1958 then 4 more films before refusing to work on any film distasteful to him; and wrote play later made into film directed by him in 1968; later turned to documentaries and from 1976 onward as independent; Ballad of Narayamá awarded Golden Palm Prize, Cannes Festival, 1983.
PICTURES: Stolen Carnal Desire, Big Brother, Hogs and Warships, Insect Woman, God's Profound Desire, Human Evaporation, Postwar Japan, Vengeance is Mine, Swing Along.

IMI, TONY: Cinematographer. Has worked primarily in England and Germany.
PICTURES: The Slipper and the Rose, International Velvet, Brass Target, Night Crossing, Enemy Mine.
TELEVISION: Inside the Third Reich, Not Quite Jerusalem, A Christmas Carol.

IMMERMAN, WILLIAM J.: Producer. b. Dec. 29, 1937. Joined 20th Century-Fox in 1972 as v.p., business affairs. Promoted 1975 to senior vice pres., administration and worldwide business affairs of the Feature Film Division. Previously was with American International Pictures for 6 yrs. as v.p. business affairs & assoc. counsel. From 1963–65 was deputy dist. atty. for Los Angeles County. Presently bd. chm. of Cinema Group, Inc. Exec. prod., Highpoint, Southern Comfort.

INGALLS, DON: Producer, writer. b. Humboldt, Nebr. e. George Washington U. Columnist, Washington Post; producer-writer, ATV England and Australia; writer-producer, Have Gun Will Travel, CBS, also produced for TV: The Travels of Jamie McPheeters, The Virginian, Honey West, Serpico, Kingston: Confidential. Exec. story consultant The Sixth Sense, ABC; producer, Fantasy Island, T.J. Hooker.
WRITER: Gunsmoke, Have Gun Will Travel, The Bold Ones, Marcus Welby M.D., Mod Squad, Star Trek, Honey West, Bonanza, The Sixth Sense, Then Came Bronson, Police Story, World Premier Movie, Shamus, Flood, Capt. America, The Initiation of Sarah, Blood Sport, and others.
FEATURE FILMS: Airport-1975, Who's Got the Body?

INGELS, MARTY: Actor. b. Brooklyn, N.Y., Mar. 9, 1936. U.S. Infantry 1954–58. Ent. show business representing Army, Name That Tune. Stage: Sketchbook revue, Las Vegas.

TV: Phil Silvers Show, Steve Allen, Jack Paar, Playboy Penthouse, Bell Telephone Hour, Manhunt, Ann Southern Show, Peter Loves Mary, The Detectives, Joey Bishop Show, Hennessey, Dick Van Dyke Show, I'm Dickens... He's Fenster, Burke's Law, Hollywood Palace.
PICTURES INCLUDE: Ladies Man, Armored Command, Horizontal Lieutenant, Wild & Wonderful.

INGIS, ROBERT L.: Executive. b. Brooklyn, N.Y., Feb. 19, 1935. e. N.Y.U. Accounting staff, S. D. Leidesdorf & Co., 1956–61; officer of Kalvex, Inc., 1961 to present.

INGSTER, BORIS: Writer, director. In 1935; collaborated on adaptation, The Last Days of Pompeii, RKO. In 1936: Dancing Pirate, RKO. In 1937: collaborated on screen play Thin Ice, 20th-Fox. In 1938: Happy Landing.
PICTURES INCLUDE: Judge Steps Out, Southside 1-1000; Something for the Birds, Abdullah's Harem, California-story, Cloak & Dagger, The Amazing Mrs. Holliday.
TV: Wagon Train, The Alaskans, The Roaring 20's, Travel of Jaimie McFeathers, The Man From U.N.C.L.E.

IRELAND, JILL: Actress. b. London, England, 1936. Began career in music halls of England at age of 12; went on to sing, dance and entertain at London's Palladium, in cabarets and a tour of the continent in ballet. Began acting in West End repertory; then signed to major film studio contract at 16 by J. Arthur Rank. Screen debut as ballet dancer in Oh, Rosalinda, first of 16 feature films for Rank.
PICTURES INCLUDE: Three Men in a Boat, Hell Drivers, Robbery Under Arms, Carry On, Nurse, Raising the Wind, Twice Round the Daffodils, Villa Rides, Rider on the Rain, Cold Sweat, The Family, Someone Behind the Door, The Mechanic, The Valdez Horses, The Valachi Papers, Breakout, Hard Times, Breakheart Pass, From Noon Till Three, Death Wish II.
TV: Shane (series), The Man from U.N.C.L.E., Ben Casey, Night Gallery, Daniel Boone, Mannix, Star Trek (series).

IRELAND, JOHN: Actor. b. Vancouver, B.C., Jan. 30, 1915; m. Stock 5 yrs. To Hollywood, 1945.
THEATRE: On N.Y. stage: Macbeth, Moon Is Down, Native Son, Counter Attack, etc.
PICTURES INCLUDE: A Walk in the Sun, Wake Up and Dream, Red River, The Gangsters, Roughshod, All The King's Men, Return of Jesse James, Vengeance Valley, Red Mountain, Basketball Fix, Bushwackers, Hurricane Smith, 49th Man, Combat Squad, Southwest Passage, Security Risk, Steel Cage, Outlaw Territory, Fast and Furious, Good Die Young, Queen Bee, Hell's Horizon, Faces in the Dark, I Saw What You Did, Fort Utah, Once Upon a Time in the West, The Adventurers, The Dirty Heroes, Escape to the Sun, Farewell, My Lovely, Martin's Day.

IRETON, KIKUKO MONICA: Managing Editor. Movie/TV Marketing; Tokyo, Japan. b. May 22, 1929. e. Seijo Gaguen, Tokyo. Daughter of late Shoichiro Kobayashi, manager of Bank of Japan in New York (1937–41) and later director. Co-founder with husband (Glenn F. Ireton) of Far East Film News in 1953, renamed Movie Marketing in 1961, Movie/TV Marketing in 1966.

IRONS, JEREMY: Actor. b. Isle of Wight, 1949. e. Sherbourne School, Dorset. Stage career began at Marlowe Theatre, Canterbury, where he was student asst. stage manager. Accepted at Bristol Old Vic Theatre School for two-yr. course; then joined Bristol Old Vic Co. In London played in Godspell, Much Ado About Nothing, The Caretaker, Taming of the Shrew, Wild Oats, Rear Column, An Audience Called Edouard, etc. N.Y. stage debut, The Real Thing, 1984.
PICTURES: The French Lieutenant's Woman, Moonlighting, Betrayal, The Wild Duck, Swann in Love, The Mission.
TELEVISION: The Pallisers, Notorious Woman, Love for Lydia, Langrishe Go Down, Brideshead Revisited.

IRVINE, RICHARD H: Executive. b. 1942. e. Univ. of So. Calif. Early career in marketing positions with Time-Life & Campbell Soup Co.; dir. of mktg., Disneyland; suprv. worldwide non-theatrical dist. for Walt Disney Prods. Pres. & CEO of Straight Arrow Publishing; v.p.-mktg. for Trans American Video, Inc. Served as exec. v.p. & COO of Talent Payments, Inc., Production Payments, Inc. & Central Casting Corp., all subsidiaries of IDC Services, Inc., of which he was also corp. sr. v.p.–west coast, 1976–78. In 1978 joined in formation of Aurora Pictures, of which is pres. & CEO.
PICTURES: Exec. Prod.: Why Would I Lie?, The Secret of NIMH, Eddie and the Cruisers, Heart Like a Wheel, East of the Sun, West of the Moon.

IRVIN, JOHN: Director. b. England, May 7, 1940. In cutting rooms at Rank Organization before making first film—documentary Gala Day (on grant from British Film Institute). Other documentaries before turning to features.
PICTURES: Dogs of War, Ghost Story, Champions, Turtle Diary, Raw Deal.
TELEVISION: Hard Times, Tinker Tailor Soldier Spy.

IRVING, AMY: Actress. b. Palo Alto, CA, Sept. 10, 1953. e. American Conservatory Theatre, London Academy of Dramatic Art. Daughter of late Jules Irving.
PICTURES: Carrie, The Fury, Honeysuckle Rose, The Competition, Voices, Yentl, Micki and Maude, Rumpelstiltskin.
TELEVISION: Movies: James Dean, Dynasty, Panache, Once an Eagle.

IRWIN, CHRISTOPHER: Producer-Executive, b. England 1948. e. University of Sussex, Eng., from where he holds a B.A. degree in social studies. From 1967 to 1969 worked as freelance producer-presenter for BBC Radio Brighton. Was with the Federal Trust (the institute concerned with European affairs) 1969 to 1975, during which time worked for the Secretariat of the North Atlantic Assembly. Joined the BBC's External Services as talks producer in 1975, moving in 1977 to the BBC's central Secretariat. From 1977 to 1978 was seconded to the International Institute for Strategic Studies. In 1978 went to Scotland as Secretary, BBC Scotland, and was closely associated with early stages of Radio Scotland. Is a member of BBC's Future Policy Group, the "think tank" of the Corporation. Appointed Head of Radio Scotland May 1980.

ISAACS, CHERYL BOONE: Executive. Entered m.p. industry 1977 as staff publicist for Columbia Pictures. Worked five years after that for Mel Simon Prods.,; named v.p. Left to become dir. of adv./pub. for The Ladd Co. 1984, named dir., pub. & promo., West Coast, for Paramount Pictures.

ISAACS, PHIL: Executive. b. N.Y.C. e. City College of N.Y. In U.S. Navy, 1943–46. Joined Paramount Pictures in 1946 as bookers asst., N.Y. exch. Branch mgr. in Washington; then mgr. Rocky Mt. div. In 1966 was Eastern-Southern sls. mgr.; 1967 joined Cinema Center Films as v.p. domestic dist. In 1972 named v.p., marketing, for Tomorrow Entertainment; Joined Avco-Embassy 1975 as v.p., gen. sls. mgr., named exec. v.p., 1977. 1978 joined General Cinema Corp. as v.p. 1980 v.p., gen. sls. mgr., Orion Pictures. 1983, formed Phil Isaacs Co.

IVANEK, ZELJKO: Actor. b. Yugoslavia, 1957. Came to U.S. with family in 1960 and returned to homeland before settling in Palo Alto, CA, in 1967. Studied at Yale, majoring in theatre studies: graduated in 1978. Also graduate of London Academy of Music and Dramatic Arts. Regular member of Williamstown Theatre Festival, appearing in Hay Fever, Charley's Aunt, Front Page, etc. Bdwy. debut in The Survivor; also in Master Harold . . . and the Boys.
PICTURES: Tex, The Sender, Mass Appeal.
TELEVISION: The Sun Also Rises.

IVERS, IRVING N.: Executive. Worked for 10 years in radio and TV in variety of executive capacities in station management before entering film business. Joined Columbia Pictures in 1973, serving as director of mktg. and dir. of adv. 1973–77; named Canadian sls. mgr. 1977–78; v.p. of adv./pub. 1978–80. In 1980 joined 20th Century-Fox as snr. v.p. of adv./pub./promo.; exec. v.p., worldwide adv., pub., promo. 1980–83; pres., worldwide mkt., MGM/UA/Entertainment Co., 1983–86. In 1986 to Warner Bros. as v.p., intl. adv./pub.

IVES, BURL: Ballad singer. b. Hunt Township, Ill., June 14, 1909. e. Teacher's College, Charleston, Ill. Professional football player, itinerant worker, radio singer, specializing ballads.
STAGE: On B'way in Cat on a Hot Tin Roof.
PICTURES INCLUDE: Smoky, Green Grass of Wyoming, Station West, So Dear to My Heart, Sierra, East of Eden, The Big Country, Cat on a Hot Tin Roof, Day of the Outlaw, Our Man in Havana, Robin and the Seven Hoods, Just You and Me, Kid.

IVEY, JUDITH: Actress. b. El Paso, TX, Sept. 4, 1951. e. Illinois State Univ. Stage debut in The Sea in Chicago, 1974. Film debut in Harry and Son, 1984. Television debut in The Sandy Hill Kidnapping.
PICTURES: The Lonely Guy, The Woman in Red.
TELEVISION: Dixie: Changing Habits.
STAGE: The Goodbye People, Oh, Coward!, Design for Living, Piaf, The Rimers of Eldritch, Pastorale, Two Small Bodies, Steaming, etc.

IVORY, JAMES: Director. b. June 7, 1928. e. Univ. of Oregon, USC. American director who gained his reputation making films in India.
PICTURES: the Householder, Shakespeare Wallah, The Guru, Bombay Talkie, Savages, The Wild Party, Autobiography of a Princess, Roseland, The Europeans (also prod.), Jane Austen in Manhattan, Quartet, Heat and Dust, The Bostonians, A Room with a View.

J

JACKS, ROBERT L.: Producer. b. Oxnard, Calif., June 14; e. Santa Monica City Coll.; U.S.C. U.S. Navy; expl. dept., 20th-Fox, 1949; then story dept.; admin. asst. to prod. Julian Blaustein & Samuel G. Engel; prod., 1952.
PICTURES INCLUDE: Lure of the Wilderness, Man on a Tightrope, Desert Rats, Prince Valiant. Prod (with late Leonard Goldstein) as Panoramic Prod. for 20th-Fox: The Gorilla, Gambler from Natchez, Man in the Attic, Princess of the Nile; The Raid, Siege at Red River, Three Young Texans, White Feather, A Life in the Balance, Robt. Jacks Prods.: Killer Is Loose, A Kiss Before Dying, Proud Ones, Bandido, Man from Del Rio, Roots of Heaven, Darryl Zanuck Prods.; prod. rep. 20th Century-Fox, 1963; Man in the Middle, The Third Secret, Guns at Batasi, Zorba the Greek; prod. exec. 20th Century-Fox TV, 1964. Prod.; Victor Borge Show (pilot), 1964; Three Coins in the Fountain (pilot), 1964; The Man Who Never Was, 1965; Custer (pilot), 1967; Honeymoon With a Stranger (ABC Movie of Week), 1969; Arnie (pilot), 1970; Bandolero (film), The Undefeated (film).
TELEVISION: Eight Is Enough (series), 1977–78; State Fair (1 hour pilot); Crunch (2 hour pilot); The Waltons (series), 1972–76; Lovejoy (pilot); Pomroy's People (pilot/co-creator); The Girls of Huntington House (MOW); Binary (MOW); The Homecoming (CBS 2 hour special), Do Not Fold, Spindle or Mutilate (MOW); A Girl and a Boy (MOW); Wild, Wild West Revisited (special), Mr. Horn (mini-series); Young Pioneers (mini-series); Young Love, First Love (MOW); Murder Can Hurt You (MOW); More Wild Wild West (MOW); A Matter of Death & Life (MOW); The Day the Loving Stopped (MOW), A Few Days in Weasle Creek (MOW), The Dukes of Hazzard (series), Flag (pilot).

JACKSON, ANNE: Actress. b. Allegheney, PA, Sept. 3, 1926. e. Neighborhood Playhouse, Actors Studio. Married to actor Eli Wallach. Stage debut in The Cherry Orchard, 1944. Film debut in So Young So Bad, 1950.
PICTURES: The Secret Life of an American Wife, Zig Zag, Lovers and Other Strangers, Dirty Dingus Magee, etc.

JACKSON, BRIAN: Actor—Film/Stage Producer. b. Bolton, England, 1931. Early career in photography then numerous stage performances incl. Old Vic, Royal Shakespeare. Ent. film/TV industry 1958. Formed Quintus Plays, 1965; formed Brian Jackson Productions 1966; formed Hampden Gurney Studios Ltd. 1970. Co-produced The Others 1967; presented The Button, 1969; co-produced the documentary film Village in Mayfair, 1970; 1971: Formed Brian Jackson Films Ltd.; produced Yesterday, The Red Deer; 1972: produced The Story of Tutankhamen.
TV INCLUDES: Moon Fleet, Private Investigator, Life of Lord Lister, Z Cars, Vendetta, Sherlock Holmes, Mr. Rose, Hardy Heating International, Nearest & Dearest, The Persuaders, The Paradise Makers, The New Avengers, Smugglers Bay, The Tomorrow People, Secret Army, Last Visitor for Hugh Peters, Six Men of Dorset.
PICTURES INCLUDE: Incident in Karandi, Carry On Sergeant, Gorgo, Jack the Ripper, Taste of Fear, Heroes of Telemark, Only the Lonely, The Deadly Females, The Revenge of the Pink Panther, Deceptions.
STAGE INCLUDES: Mame, Drury Lane, Fallen Angels, Seasons with Old Vic and Royal Shakespeare Co., In Praise of Love.
RADIO INCLUDES: Westward Ho., Jude the Obscure.

JACKSON, FREDA: Actress. b. Nottingham, Eng., Dec. 29, 1909; e. U. Coll., Nottingham. Stage debut 1933, Northampton Repertory Theatre; London debut 1936, Old Vic; screen debut in Canterbury Tale, 1942.
PICTURES INCLUDE: Henry V, Beware of Pity, Great Expectations, No Room at the Inn, Flesh and Blood, Women of Twilight, The Good Die Young, The Crowded Day, The Enchanted Doll, Bhowani Junction, Last Man to Hang, The Flesh Is Weak, Brides of Dracula, Greyfriar's Bobbie, Shadow of the Cat, Attempt to Kill, West Eleven, Monster of Terror, The Third Secret, Gwangi, Tom Jones, Clash of the Titans.
TV: Macadam and Eve, Sorry Wrong Number, Trial of Marie Lafarge, Release, Colombe, Maigret in Montmartre, Sergeant Musgrave's Dance, Dr. Finlay's Casebook, Sunset, Knock On Any Door, The Spies, Adam Adamant, Midland Profile, Owen Md., The Kilvert Diaries, She Fell Among Thieves, Randall and Hopkirk, The Old Curiosity Shop.

JACKSON, GLENDA: Actress. b. Birkenhead, England, May 9, 1936. Ent. m.p. ind. 1955.
PICTURES INCLUDE: Marat-Sade, Negatives, Women In Love, The Music Lovers, Sunday, Bloody Sunday, Mary Queen of Scots, Triple Echo, The Nelson Affair, A Touch of Class, The Maids, The Tempter, The Romantic Englishwoman, Hedda, Sarah, Nasty Habits, House Calls, Stevie, The Class of Miss McMichael, Lost and Found, Hopscotch, The Patricia Neal Story, Giro City, The Return of the Soldier, Turtle Diary.
TV: Queen Elizabeth, Sakharov.

JACKSON, GORDON: Actor. b. Glasgow, Scotland, Dec. 19, 1923; e. Glasgow. On radio since 1939; screen debut in "Foreman Went to France" 1940.
PICTURES INCLUDE: Nine Men, San Demetrio, Millions Like Us, Pink String & Sealing Wax, Captive Heart, Against the Wind, Eureka Stockade, Whiskey Galore, Floodtide, Stop Press Girl, Bitter Springs, Happy Go Lovely, The Lady with the Lamp, Meet Mr. Lucifer, Malta Story, Castle in the Air, Quartermass Experiment, Pacific Destiny, Baby and the Battleship, Sailor Beware, Seven Waves Away (Abandon Ship), As Long As You're Happy, Hell Drivers, Rockets Galore, Bridal Path, Yesterday's Enemy, Blind Date, Cone of Silence, Tunes of Glory, Greyfriar's Bobbie, Mutiny on the Bounty, The Great Escape, The Long Ships, Those Magnificent Men in Their Flying Machines, The Great Spy Mission, The Ipcress File, Cast A Giant Shadow, Fighting Prince of Donegal, Night of the Generals, Triple Cross, The Eliminator, Prime of Miss Jean Brodie, Run Wild, Run Free, Hamlet, Scrooge, Kidnapped, Madame Sin, Russian Roulette, Spectre, Golden Rendezvous, Medusa Touch, Last Giraffe, Shooting Party, The Masks of Death.
TV: Numerous TV appearances incl: Upstairs, Downstairs, The Professionals, A Town Like Alice, Hart to Hart.

JACKSON, JOHN HENRY: Executive. b. New York, April 27, 1916. e. Holy Cross Academy, 1930; Professional Children's School, 1934; Georgia Tech, 1936. Performed as vaudeville artist touring Europe, 1928–29; Fair dates and indoor circus, 1929–35; Texas Centennial, 1936; George Abbott's Too Many Girls, 1938. Joined Radio City Music Hall, 1943 with Glee Club; stage manager, 1944–51; director of stage operations, 1958; v.p., 1970; prod., 1971; pres., Tri-Marquee Productions, Ltd., 1979.

JACKSON, KATE: Actress. b. Birmingham, Ala., Oct. 29, 1949. e. Univ. of Mississippi, Birmingham Southern Univ. Did summer stock before going to N.Y. to enter American Academy of Dramatic Arts, appearing in Night Must Fall, Constant Wife, Lttle Moon of Alban, etc. Worked as model and became tour guide at NBC. First role on TV in Dark Shadows (series).
PICTURES INCLUDE: Thunder and Lightning, Dirty Tricks, Making Love.
TV: The Jimmy Stewart Show (pilot). Movies: Killer Bees, The Shrine of Lorna Love, The Jenny Storm Homicide. Series: Charlie's Angels, Scarecrow and Mrs. King.

JACKSON, MICHAEL: Singer-Composer. b. Aug. 29, 1958. Musical recording artist with family group known as The Jacksons: all brothers, Jackie, Tito, Marlon, Randy and Michael.
PICTURE: The Wiz.

JACOBI, DEREK: Actor. b. London, England, Oct. 22, 1938. e. Cambridge. On stage in Pericles, The Hollow Crown, Hobson's Choice, The Suicide.
PICTURES: Day of the Jackal, Blue Blood, The Odessa File, The Medusa Touch, The Human Factor, Enigma.
TELEVISION: She Stoops to Conquer, Man of Straw, The Pallisers, I, Claudius, Philby, Burgess and MacLean, Hamlet.

JACOBS, BARRY: Executive. b. London, England, 1924. Ent. m.p. ind. 1938. Served in RAF 1943–46. Circuit rep. Warner Bros. 1938–59. Overseas sales rep. independent producers 1960–62. Formed Eagle Films Ltd. dist. organization UK 1962. Entered prod. 1969. Exec. prod. The Wife Swappers, Groupie Girl, Bread, Naughty, The Love Box, Sex and The Other Woman, On the Game, Eskimo Nell. Formed Elephant Entertainment Ltd. & Elephant Video Ltd., 1986.

JACOBS, JOHN: Executive. b. New York City. e. Syracuse Univ.'s Newhouse Communications School. Full-service agency background, including 13 years with Grey Advertising agency, where handled Warner Bros. & Warner Home Video accts. Supvr. media on RCA, ABC-TV, Murdoch Publishing, Radio City Musical Hall, etc. Named v.p. & group media dir. for Grey. 1986, left to join Warner Bros. as v.p., media.

JACOBY, FRANK DAVID: Director/Producer. b. New York, N.Y., July 15, 1925. Hunter College, Brooklyn College. m. Doris Storm, producer/director educational films, actress. 1949–52: NBC network TV director; 1952–56: B.B.D.O., Biow Co., TV producer/director; 1956–58 Metropolitan Educational TV Association, Director of Production; 1958–65: United Nation, film producer/director; 1965 to present: President, Jacoby/Storm Productions, Inc., Westport, Conn., documentary, industrial, educational films and filmstrips. Clients include Xerox Corp., Random House, Publ., Lippincott Co., IBM, Heublein, G.E., and Pitney Bowes. Winner, Sherwood Award, Peabody Award. Member, Director's Guild of America; winner, Int'l TV & Film Festival, National Educational Film Festival, American Film Festival.

JACOBY, JOSEPH: Producer-Director-Writer. b. Brooklyn, N.Y., 1942. e. N.Y. Univ. School of Arts and Sciences, majoring in m.p. As undergraduate worked part-time as prod. asst. on daytime network TV shows and as puppeteer for Bunin Puppets. In 1963 joined Bill Baird Marionettes as full-time puppeteer, working also on Baird film commercials. Made feature m.p. debut as prod.-dir of Shame, Shame, 1968.
PICTURES INCLUDE: Hurry Up, or I'll Be 30, The Great Georgia Bank Hoax (co.-prod., dir., s.p.).

JACOBY, SCOTT: Actor. b. Chicago, Nov. 19, 1956.
PICTURES: The Little Girl Who Lives Down the Lane, Midnight Auto Supply, Our Winning Season.
TELEVISION: Movies: No Place to Run, That Certain Summer, The Man Who Could Talk to Kids, Bad Ronald, Smash-Up on Interstate 5, 79 Park Avenue, No Other Love, The Diary of Anne Frank.

JACON, BERNARD: Executive. b. Louisiana. Manager, promotion, Small & Strausberg Theatres, New York; buyer & gen. mgr., Mantell Theatres N.Y., gen. mgr. & assoc., Rockaway Beach Theatres, Universal Pictures, home office & field, br. operations & sales. Mgr., sales & dist. (Continental Films) Superfilms Distribution Corp., New York 1946–49; vice-pres. in chg. of sales & dist., Lux Film Distributing Corp., N.Y., 1949–52; v.p. sales, dist. IFE Releasing, 1952–55; org. nat'l distrib. co., Jacon Film Distributors, Inc., as pres., 1956; nat'l consultant to independent distributors, producers & exhibitors, member of the Pioneers & Variety; 1979, formed Bernie Jacon, Inc., natl. co-ordinator for producers and distributors.

JACQUEMIN, ROBERT: Executive. Began career as media buyer; later in station representation as v.p. of regional sls. for Telerep, Inc. Entered syndication as pres. of Television Marketing Services, St. Louis. Joined Paramount Domestic Television and Video Programming as midwest div. mgr. in St. Louis; later sr. v.p., sls. in N.Y. 1981, named exec. v.p., sls. & mktg. 1985, joined Walt Disney Pictures as sr. v.p., domestic TV dist., a new syndication div. formed by the co.

JACQUES, ROBERT C.: Film editor. b. Cincinnati, Ohio, Feb. 24, 1919. e. U. of Mich., U.S.C. Asst. film ed., RKO Radio 1939–42; film ed., Pathe News, 1942–44; chief film ed., NBC Television, 1944–48; prod. chief, Ziv TV film dept. 1948–51; free lance m.p. film ed., 1951–52; supervising film ed., prod. mgr., American Film Prod., 1952–53; prod. supvr., ed., Telenews and Screen Gems 1953; film ed., RKO Radio, 1953–55; supervising film ed., George Blake Enterprises, 1955–57; v.p. Peter Elgar Productions 1957–60; supv. film editor, Transfilm-Caravel Inc. 1960–62; v.p. in chg. of completion, Filmex, Inc., 1962. V.P. in charge of completion, Filmex Inc. 1962–69. Free lance film editor, May–Nov. 1969. V.P. of own co., Double Image Inc., film and videotape editorial service, Nov. 1969–1983. Free lance post-prod. consultant, 1983–present.

JAECKEL, RICHARD HANLEY: Actor. b. Long Beach, N.Y., Oct. 10, 1926; e. Hollywood High School, 1943. Performed odd jobs upon graduation, with plans toward entering Navy when of age; worked as delivery boy in mail room, 20th Century-Fox; signed for role of Baby Marine, in Guadalcanal Diary.
PICTURES INCLUDE: The Gunfighter, Sea Hornet, Hoodlum Empire, My Son John, Come Back Little Sheba, Big Leaguer, Sea of Lost Ships, Shanghai Story, Violent Men, Apache Ambush, Sands of Iwo Jima, Fragile Fox, The Dirty Dozen, Sometimes a Great Notion, Ulzanas Raid, Pat Garrett and Billy the Kid, The Outfit, Chosen Survivors, The Drowning Pool, Part II—Walking Tall, Twilights Last Gleaming, All the Marbles, Starman.
TV: U.S. Steel Hour, Elgin Hour, Goodyear Playhouse, Kraft, Firehouse (movie).

JAFFE, HERB: Executive-Producer. b. New York, N.Y. e. Brooklyn Coll., Columbia U. Press agent; then talent agent, MCA personal appearance div.; sales exec., MCA-TV, Ltd., syndic. film div.; eastern sales mgr., Motion Pictures for Television; joined Official Films as v.p., sales mgr.; Herb Jaffe Assoc. 1957; sold Herb Jaffe Assoc. to Ashley-Steiner-Famous Artists, Inc.; v.p. in prod., United Artists, 1965; v.p. of West Coast Operations, 1966. 1970, v.p. charge of World-Wide prod, 1973 entered field of independent motion picture production. Now pres., TVO Productions, Inc.
PICTURES: The Wind and the Lion, Demon Seed, Who'll Stop the Rain, Time After Time, Those Lips, Those Eyes, Motel Hell, Jinxed, The Lords of Discipline, Little Treasure, Fright Night.

JAFFE, LEO: Executive. b. April 23, 1909. e. New York U. Columbia, 1930; v.p., Columbia Pictures, January, 1954; 1st v.p., treas., member of board, 1956; v.p. & treas., 1958; exec. v.p., Columbia Pictures, 1962; Pres. Columbia Pictures, 1968; pres., Columbia Pictures Industries, Inc, 1970, president & chief executive officer Columbia Pictures Industries, Inc., 1973; chm., August, 1973, Chairman of Board of directors since Aug., 1973. Currently chm. emeritus.

JAFFE, STANLEY R.: Producer. b. New Rochelle, N.Y., July, 1940. Graduate of University of Pennsylvania's Wharton School of Finance. Joined Seven Arts Associates, 1962; named exec. ass't to president, 1964; later, head of East Coast TV programming. Produced Goodbye, Columbus, in 1968 for Paramount; then joined that company as exec. v.p., 1969. Produced A New Leaf, 1970. Named pres. of Paramount in 1970; resigned June 10, 1971 to form own prod. unit. First film: Bad Company (1972); Man on the Swing, Bad News Bears. Joined Columbia as v.p. of global prod. in 1976, but resigned to be independent producer. 1979: Kramer vs. Kramer; 1981: Taps (co. prod.); 1983: Without a Trace (prod.-dir.). 1984: Racing with the Moon, Firstborn.

JAFFE, STEVEN-CHARLES: Producer. b. 1954. e. Univ. of So. Calif. (cinema). Worked on production in Holland and Switzerland; served as prod. asst. on The Wind and the Lion in Spain. Assoc. prod. on Demon Seed (written by brother Robert); served as location mgr. on Who'll Stop the Rain; assoc. prod. on Time After Time. Full producer on Those Lips, Those Eyes.

JAFFE, WILLIAM B.: Attorney. b. New York City, Mar. 11, 1904; e. Union Coll. 1926, A.B.; Columbia U. Law School 1929, LL.B.; m. Evelyn Annenberg. Assoc. Nathan Burkan 1929–35; gen. counsel Allied Artists; 1933–69 spcl. counsel to interests financing independent prod.; to leading personalities m.p. ind.; dir. MPPDA rep. Columbia; gen. counsel & dir. Allied Artists Internat'l 1933–69; chmn. Manning Plan, State of N.Y.; counsel, War Manpower Commission, N.Y. Region Spec. counsel to Revlon, Inc., in TV field; s.p. counsel Triangle Pub.; chmn., Art Advisory Committee Dartmouth College; trustee, Union Coll., Schenectady, N.Y. Vice Chr. & Bd. of Gov. Jewish Museum, N.Y.C.: Benefactor Metropolitan Museum of Art; Patron, Museum of Modern Art, Group Chairm. United Hospital Fund 1964–69; Trustee, Phi Epsilon Pi Foundation. Recipient Phi Epsilon Pi Achievement Award, 1964; Doctor Humane Letters, Dartmouth College 1964; Trustee Mt. Sinai Hospital, N.Y., N.Y. Eye & Ear Infirmary. Partner, law firm, Shea, Gallop, Climenko & Gould.

JAFFEY, HERBERT: Executive. b. Somerville, N.J., Cap't. U.S. Army, pressbook writer, 20th Century-Fox; theatre management, Loew's; field exploitation, United Artists, Ad. pub. dir. 20th Century-Fox Int and Inter-Amer. Corp.; dir., adv. & publicity, Rugoff Theatres; Independent Film Prod.; Paramount Foreign Advertising & Publicity Manager, screenplay writer.

JAGGER, DEAN: Actor. b. Lima, Ohio, Nov. 7, 1903; e. Wabash Coll. (Crawfordsville, Ind.). On N.Y. stage, stock, vaudeville. Screen debut 1929 in Woman from Hell. Academy Award sup. role 1949 for 12 O'Clock High.
PICTURES INCLUDE: College Rhythm, Home on the Range, Car 99, Woman Trap, 13 Hours By Air, Woman in Distress, Escape by Night, Brigham Young, Western Union, Valley of the Sun, I Escaped from the Gestapo, North Star, Alaska, When Strangers Marry, Pursued, Driftwood, Dark City, Rawhide, Warpath, Denver and Rio Grande, My Son John, It Grows on Trees, The Robe, Executive Suite, Private Hell 36, White Christmas, Bad Day at Black Rock, The Eternal Sea, On the Threshold of Space, It's a Dog's Life, Red Sundown, Great Man, Three Brave Men, The Nun's Story, Cash McCall, Elmer Gantry, Parrish, Jumbo, Stay way Joe, Firecreek, Smith, The Kremlin Letter, Vanishing Point, Tiger by the Tail.
TV: Glass House, Mr. Novak (series), Brotherhood of the Bell, The Lie.

JAGGER, MICK: Singer-Composer-Actor. b. Dartford, Kent, England, July 26, 1943. Lead singer with Rolling Stones.
PICTURES: Performance, Ned Kelly, Gimme Shelter, Sympathy for the Devil, Ladies and Gentlemen, The Rolling Stones, The Lond Rock 'n' Roll Show, Let's Spend the Night Together.

JAGLOM, HENRY: Director-Writer-Editor. b. New York City, Jan. 26, 1943. Studied acting, writing and directing at Univ. of Pennsylvania and with Actors Studio. Did off-Bdwy. shows; went to West Coast where appeared in TV series (Gidget, The Flying Nun, etc.). Started shooting documentary film in Israel during Six Day War; turned it into 3-hr. silent film. Hired to edit Easy Rider by producer Bert Schneider. Acted in Drive, He Said and Last Movie. Directed first feature, A Safe Place, in 1971.
PICTURES: Tracks (1977); Sitting Ducks (1980); Can She Bake a Cherry Pie? (1983); A Lovely Ride (1984); Always (1986).

JALBERT, JOE JAY: Executive. e. Univ. of Washington. Was ski captain in school and began film career as technical director on Downhill Racer, 1969, also cinematographer and double for Robert Redford. 1970, produced Impressions of Utah, documentary, with Redford. Won Emmy for cinematography on TV's Peggy Fleming Special. In 1970 formed Jalbert Productions, Inc., to make feature films, TV sports, specials, commercials, etc. Co. has produced official films at Innsbruck Winter Olympics (1976), Lake Placid (1980), Sarajevo (1984).

JAMES, CLIFTON: Actor. b. N.Y.C., May 29, 1923. e. Oregon Univ. Studied at Actors Studio. Made numerous appearances on stage and TV, as well as theatrical films.
PICTURES INCLUDE: On The Waterfront, The New Centurions, Live and Let Die, The Last Detail, Bank Shot, Juggernaut, The Man with the Golden Gun, Rancho DeLuxe.

JAMES, DENNIS: Performer. b. Jersey City, N.J. Aug. 24, 1917. e. St. Peter's Coll., Jersey City. TV personality for over 30 years. Formerly M.C., actor, sports commentator in Radio; award winning sports commentator for wrestling, 25 TV first to credit; currently pres., Dennis James Prod.
TV: Chance of A Lifetime, High Finance, First Impressions, What's My Line, PDQ, Your All-American College Show; host new Price Is Right, Nightime; Host, "Name That Tune," Daytime.

JAMES, LAURA: Actress. b. Hazelton, Penn., 1933. e. The Theatre Wing, The American Academy of Dramatic Arts, 1948–50; worked Off-Broadway, Summer Stock, TV; starred in West Coast premieres of The Second Man, Champagne Complex.
PICTURES INCLUDE: Four Girls in Town, St. Francis of Assisi.
TV: Matinees Theatre, The Big Story, Day in Court, Divorce Court, Official Detective, Congressional Investigator, Sheriff of Cochise; now working overseas.

JAMES, POLLY: Writer. b. Ancon, Canal Zone; e. Smith Coll. Newspaper work, Panama; with trade mag., N.Y.; screen writer since 1942.
PICTURES INCLUDE: Mrs. Parkington, The Raiders, Redhead from Wyoming, Quantrill's Raiders.
TV: Several shows.

JAMESON, JERRY: Director. b. Hollywood. Started as editorial asset; then editor and supv. editor for Danny Thomas Prods. Turned to directing.
PICTURES: Dirt Gang, The Bat People, Brute Core, Airport '77, Raise the Titanic.
TELEVISION: Movies: Heatwave!, The Elevator, Hurricane, Terror on the 40th Floor, The Secret Night Caller, The Deadly Tower, The Lives of Jenny Dolan, The Call of the Wild, The Invasion of Johnson County, Superdome, A Fire in the Sky, High Noon—Part II, The Return of Will Kane.

JANKOWSKI, GENE F.: Executive. b. Buffalo, NY, May 21, 1934. e. Canisius (BS), Michigan State Univ. (MA). Joined CBS radio network sls, 1969 as acct. exec.; eastern sls. mgr., 1966; moved to CBS-TV as acct. exec. 1969; gen. sls. mgr. WCBS-TV, 1970; dir. sls, 1970; v.p. sls., CSB-TV, 1973, v.p., finance & planning, 1974; v.p., controller, 1976; v.p. adm., 1977; exec. v.p. CBS Broadcast Group, 1977; pres., 1977.

JANNI, JOSEPH: Producer. b. Milan, Italy, May 21, 1916. e. Milan University; Rome Film School. Entered m.p. industry 1941. Assistant producer. Founded Vic Films Ltd.
PICTURES INCLUDE: Own productions: The Glass Mountain, White Corridors, Something Money Can't Buy, Romeo and Juliet (co-prod.), A Town Like Alice (prod.); The Captain's Table, Savage Innocents, A Kind of Loving, Billy Liar, Darling, Modesty Blaise, Far From The Madding Crowd, Poor Cow, In Search of Gregory, Sunday, Bloody Sunday, Made, Yanks (co-prod.).

JARMAN, CLAUDE, JR.: Actor. b. Nashville, Tenn., Sept. 27, 1934; e. MGM School. Film debut in "Yearling," 1946.
PICTURES INCLUDE: High Barbaree, Sun Comes Up, Intruder in the Dust, Roughshod, Outriders, Inside Straight, Rio Grande, Hangman's Knot, Fair Wind to Java, Great Locomotive Chase.

JARRE, MAURICE: Composer. b. Lyon, France, 1924. Studied at Paris Cons. Was orchestra conductor for Jean Louis Barrault's theatre company four years. In 1951 joined Jean Vilar's nat'l theatre co., composing for plays by Shakespeare, Moliere, O'Neill, Eliot, and Victor Hugo. Started writing music for films in 1952.
PICTURES INCLUDE: Hotel des Invalides, La Tete contre les Murs, Eyes without a Face, Crack in the Mirror, Sundays and Cybele, The Longest Day, Lawrence of Arabia (AA, 1962), The Collector, Is Paris Burning?, Weekend at Dunkirk, Dr. Zhivago (AA, 1965), Night of the Generals, The Professionals, Grand Prix, Five Card Stud, Isadora, The Damned, Ash Wednesday, The Life and Times of Judge Roy Bean, The Mackintosh Man, The Effect of Gamma Rays on Man-in-the-Moon Marigolds, Island at the Top of the World, Mandingo, Posse, Winter Kills, The Black Marble, Taps, Firefox, Young Doctors in Love, The Year of Living Dangerously, Dreamscape, A Passage to India, Witness, Mad Max Beyond Thunderdome.

JARRICO, PAUL. Writer, Producer. b. Los Angeles, Jan. 12, 1915.
PICTURES INCLUDE: Salt of the Earth, Tom, Dick & Harry (Academy nomination), Thousands Cheer, The Search (Academy Award), The White Tower, Not Wanted, The Girl Most Likely.

JARROTT, CHARLES: Director. b. London, England June 16, 1927. Son of British businessman and former singer-dancer at Gaiety Theatre. Joined British Navy; wartime service in Far East. After military service turned to theatre as asst. stage mgr. with Arts Council touring co. In 1949 joined Nottingham Repertory Theatre as stage dir. and juvenile acting lead. In 1953 joined new company formed to tour Canada; was leading man and became resident leading actor for Ottawa Theatre. In 1955 moved to Toronto and made TV acting debut opposite Katharine Blake whom he later wed. In 1957 made directing debut in TV for Canadian Bdcstg. Co. Became CBC resident dir. Moved to London to direct for Armchair Theatre for ABC-TV. Then became free-lance dir., doing stage work, films, TV.
PICTURES INCLUDE: Anne of the Thousand Days, Mary, Queen of Scots, Lost Horizon, The Dove, The Littlest Horse Thieves, The Other Side of Midnight, The Last Flight of Noah's Ark, The Amateur, The Boy in Blue.
TELEVISION: The Hot Potato Boys, Roll On, Bloomin' Death, Girl in a Birdcage, The Picture of Dorian Gray, Rain, The Rose Affair, Roman Gesture, Silent Song, The Male of the Species, The Young Elizabeth, A Case of Libel, Dr. Jekyll and Mr. Hyde, A Married Man.
STAGE: The Duel, Galileo, The Basement, Tea Party, The Dutchman, etc.

JASON, RICK: Actor. b. New York City, May 21, 1926. e. American Academy of Dramatic Arts.
THEATRE: Broadway debut: Now I Lay Me Down To Sleep (Theatre World award).
PICTURES INCLUDE: Sombrero, Saracen Blade, This Is My Love, Lieutenant Wore Skirts, Wayward Bus.
TV: The Case of the Dangerous Robin, Combat.

JAY, LESLIE: Executive. b. New York City, May 12. e. Fordham Univ. (BA, 1977). Entered industry in 1969 as publicist with Bob Perilla Associates. 1970, pub. asst. on Such Good Friends, 1976–present, with Penthouse Films Intl., Ltd., asst. to producers on Caligula; then world-wide project coordinator on Caligula. Director of pub. & promo. for Omni: The New Frontier for Omni Productions Intl., Ltd. Director of p.r. for Penthouse Int'l., Ltd; 1984, v.p. & dir. public relations, Penthouse.

JAYSTON, MICHAEL: Actor. b. Nortingham, England, Oct. 28, 1935. Member of Old Vic theatre Co. & Bristol Old Vic.
PICUTRES: Cromwell, The Nelson Affair, Nicholas and Alexandra, A Midsummer Night's Dream, The Public Eye.
TELEVISION: She Fell Among Thieves, Tinker, Tailor, Soldier, Spy.

JEFFEE, SAUL: Executive. b. Elizabeth, N.J., March 30, 1918. Established Movielab, Inc., 1936, pres., bd. chmn., & chief exec. officer. Also chm. & CEO, Movielab Video, Inc.; chm. & pres. 619 West 54th St. Corp.; chm. & pres., MLH Realty Corp.; chm. & pres., Film Recoupment Corp. Fellow, SMPTE, Treas.; Pres. & chm., Movielab Theatre Service; Pres. Assoc. of Cinema Labs, 1963; American Tech. Rep. & Deleg. in the U.S.-U.S.S.R. Cult. Exch. 1965; Ch. Enter. & Commu. Div., U.J.A., 1967–68; Life member, Motion Picture Pioneers, Friars, City Athletic Club; Author of Narcotics—An American Plan, chmn. Bd. of Trustees, Lorge School, 1968–81; Pres. & Chm., Movielab-Hollywood, Inc., vice chrm., Film Society of Lincoln Center, Patron, Lincoln Center for The Performing Arts, Mem. Bd. of Gov. U.J.A., life member, chm., Life Patron Program, Variety Clubs International, holder of 16 patents, Professional Motion Picture Equipment, Trustee, Federation of Jewish Philanthropies; Trustee, Will Rogers Hospital & Research Center; Mason (Shriner, 32 deg); Life Member, The Jewish Chautagui Society. Member, Boy Scouts Advisory Committee on Scouting For The Handicapped; Advisory Board, Cinema Lodge No. 6000 B'nai B'rith. Academy of Motion Picture Arts & Sciences; Mayor of N.Y.C. Advisory Council on Motion Pictures. Member, Natl. Academy of TV Arts & Sciences, Film Acquisition Comm., U.S.I.A.

JEFFREYS, ANNE: Actress. b. Goldsboro, N.C.
PICTURES INCLUDE: I Married an Angel, Step Lively, Dillinger, Sing Your Way Home, Trail Street, Riffraff, Return of the Bad Men, Boys' Night Out.
THEATRE: On Bway. in Street Scene, Kiss Me Kate, Romance, Three Wishes for Jamie, Kismet.
TELEVISION: Topper, Love That Jill, many guest appearances, Delphi Bureau, Falcon Crest, General Hospital, Finder of Lost Loves.
STOCK: Camelot, King & I, Kismet, Song of Norway, Bells Are Ringing, Marriage Go Round, No Sex Please, We're British, Take Me Along, Carousel, Anniversary Waltz, Do I Hear a Waltz, Ninotchka, Pal Joey, Name of the

Game, Destry Rides Again, The Merry Widow, Bitter Sweet, Desert Song, High Button Shoes, Sound of Music.

JEFFRIES, LIONEL: Actor. b. Forest Hill, London, England, 1926. Ent. m.p. ind. 1952.
PICTURES INCLUDE: The Nun's Story, Two-Way Stretch, The Trials of Oscar Wilde, Fanny, The Notorious Landlady, The Wrong Arm of the Law, First Men in the Moon, Call Me Bwana, The Truth About Spring, You Must Be Joking, The Crimson Blade, Arrividerci Baby, Spy with the Cold Nose, Journey to the Moon, Camelot, Chitty Chitty Bang Bang, Eye Witness, The Prisoner of Zenda. Dir. s.p., Railway Children, 1970. Gingerbread House, Dir. Baxter, Dir. s.p., The Amazing Mr. Blunden, The Water Babies, Cream in My Coffee.
TELEVISION: Father Charlie, Tom, Dick, and Harriet.

JENKINS, CHARLES: Animation producer. b. Yorkshire, England, 1941. Ent. m.p. ind. 1957. Joined T.V.C. as gen. ass't 1958. Animated and prod. various prods. Joined Dick Williams, pioneered use of Oxberry Camera for animation, 1966. Esta. Trickfilm Ltd., prod. optical effects for Yellow Submarine, 1967.

JENKINS, DAN: Public Relations Executive. b. Montclair, N.J., Dec. 5, 1916. e. Univ. of Va., 1938. U.S. Army, 1940–45; major, infantry. P.R. officer, Hq. Eighth Army. Mng. ed., Motion Picture Magazine, 1946–48; editor, Tele-Views Magazine, 1949–50; TV editor, columnist, Hollywood Reporter, 1950–53; Hollywood bureau chief, TV Guide, 1953–63; v.p., exec. dir. TV dept., Rogers, Cowan & Brenner, Inc., 1963–71. Formed Dan Jenkins Public Relations, Inc. 1971. Joined Charles A. Pomerantz Public Relations, Ltd. as v.p., 1975, while retaining own firm. Sr. associate, Porter, Novelli, Assocs., 1981.Mem. bd. trustees, Natl. Academy of TV Arts & Sciences; bd. gov., Hollywood chapter, Natl. Academy of TV Arts & Sciences, 1967–71. Rejoined Rogers & Cowan, 1983, v.p., TV dept.

JENKINS, GEORGE: Art dir. b. Baltimore, Md.; e. Univ. of Pennsylvania. Holly-N.Y. art dir. since 1946; TV pictures for Four Star Playhouse and revue productions; NBC-TV opera, Carmen; color dir., CBS-TV, 1954; NBC color spec. Annie Get Your Gun, 1957; TV music with Mary Martin, 1959. Professor, Motion Picture Design, UCLA, 1985.
STAGE: Mexican Hayride, I Remember Mama, Dark of the Moon, Lost in the Stars, Bell, Book & Candle, Bad Seed, Happiest Millionaire, Two for the Seawaw, Icecapades. Jones Beach spec., Song of Norway, Paradise Island, Around the World in 80 Days, Mardi Gras, Miracle Worker, Critics Choice, A Thousand Clowns, Jennie, Generation, Wait Until Dark, Only Game in Town, Night Watch, Sly Fox.
PICTURES INCLUDE: Best Years of Our Life, Secret Life of Walter Mitty, Miracle Worker, Mickey One, Up The Down Staircase, Wait Until Dark, Subject Was Roses Klute, 1776, Paper Chase, Parallax View, Night Moves, Funny Lady. Won Oscar 1977 for All the President's Men, Comes A Horseman, China Syndrome, Starting Over, The Postman Always Rings Twice, Rollover, Sophies' Choice, The Dollmaker, Orphans.

JENNINGS, PETER. TV Newsman. b. Toronto, Canada, July 29, 1938. e. Carleton Univ; Rider Coll. Started career as newsman CFJR (radio), Ottawa; then with CJOH-TV and CBS before becoming co-anchor of first national news program on Canadian commercial network, CTV. Joined ABC in 1964 as NY corr.; 1965, anchor, Peter Jennings with the News; 1968, natl. corr., ABC News; 1969, overseas assignments; 1975, Washington corr. and anchor for AM America; 1977, chief foreign corr.; 1978, foreign desk anchor; 1978, foreign desk anchor, World News Tonight; 1983, anchor, sr. editor, World News Tonight.

JENS, SALOME: Actress. b. Milwaukee, May 8, 1935. e. Northwestern Univ. On stage in The Disenchanted, USA, Night Life, Winter's Tale, Mary Stuart, Antony and Cleopatra, etc.
PICTURES: Angel Baby, The Fool Killer, Seconds, Me, Natalie, Cloud Dancer, Harry's War, Just Between Friends.
TELEVISION: Movies: In the Glitter Palace, Sharon: Portrait of a Mistress, From Here to Eternity, The Golden Moment: an Olympic Love Story, A Killer in the Family, Playing with Fire.

JEPHCOTT, SAMUEL C.: Executive. b. 1944, Southampton, England. e. Arts Educational School, London. Entered industry as child actor The Grove Family BBC TV, 1956. Eight years in advertising producing TV Commercials. Emigrated to Toronto, Canada in 1968. Exec. Secty., Directors Guild of Canada, 1969–72. Film production management, 1972–75. Joined Compass Film Sales Ltd., a division of Quadrant Film Ltd. 1975–77. Joined Nielsen-Ferns Intl. Ltd. in chg. of distribution and production, 1977–81. Mgr. distribution, CBC Enterprises, 1982–84. Currently exec. dir., Canadian Film & TV Assn., & pres., Cyclops Communications Corp. Is director of the Canadian Association of Motion Picture Producers.
PICTURES INCLUDE: The Hard Part Begins 1973. Odyssey Films (prod. Manager); Sunday In The Country, 1973, Quadrant (2nd A.D.); Me, 1974, Muddy York Prods. (prod. Manager); Lions For Breakfast, 1974, Burg Prod. (prod. Manager), It Seemed Like A Good Idea At The Time, 1975, Quadrant (2nd A.D.); Love at First Sight, 1976 (prod. accountant) Quadrant; Find The Lady, 1976 (stills) Quadrant; The New Avengers, TV, 1977 (prod. manager) Neilson-Ferns Inc.; The Wars (prod. supvr.) 1981; The Last Frontier (prod.), 1985–86.

JERGENS, ADELE: Actress. b. Brooklyn, N.Y., Nov. 28, 1922. Began career in musical shows during summer vacation at 15; won contest, New York's World Fair, as model; appeared on New York stage; night clubs, U.S. and abroad.
PICTURES INCLUDE: Edge of Doom, Side Street, A&C Meet the Invisible Man, Sugarfoot, Try and Get Me, Show Boat, Somebody Loves Me, Aaron Slick From Punkin' Crick, Overland Pacific, Miami Story, Fireman Save My Child, Big Chase, Strange Lady in Town, The Cobweb.

JESSEL, IAN: Executive. b. London, England, 1939. e. Oxford. Joined Rank Organization in 1962 as graduate trainee and became responsible for acquisition of indep. product. Formed Target International Pictures in 1968. In 1970 joined World Film Sales becoming man. dir. 1972. World Film Sales merged with ITC in 1974. Elected to board 1975. Appointed dir. Classic Cinemas and ITC Film Distributors (UK), 1979. Appt. man. dir. ITC Films Int., 1980. Joined CBS Theatrical Films, Sept. 1981, as vice-pres. int. distribution, now based in Los Angeles.

JEWISON, NORMAN P.: Producer-director. b. Toronto, Canada, July 21, 1926. e. Malvern Collegiate Institute, Toronto, 1940–44; Victoria College, Univ. of Toronto, Canada, 1946–50 (BA).
TV: Exec. prod. of 8 Judy Garland shows; prod.-dir., Judy Garland specials.
PICTURES INCLUDE: 40 Pounds of Trouble, The Thrill of It All, Send Me No Flowers, Art of Love, The Cincinnati Kid, The Russians Are Coming, The Russians Are Coming, Dir. In The Heat of the Night. Prod.-dir. Gaily, Gaily, Prod.: The Landlord, Fiddler on the Roof, Prod./dir.: Jesus Christ Superstar; Prod.: Billy Two Hats; Prod.-dir.: Rollerball. Prod.-dir.: F.I.S.T.; co-prod.-dir.: And Justice For All; co.-prod.-dir.: Best Friends; co-prod.: Iceman; co-prod., dir.: A Soldier's Story; co-prod., dir.: Agnes of God.

JILLIAN, ANN: Actress. b. Cambridge, MA. Jan. 29, 1951. Began career at age 10 in Disney's Babes in Toyland; in film version of Gypsy at age 12. On stage in musical, Sugar Babies. Has own company: 9-J Productions, developing TV movies.
TELEVISION: Series: It's a Living, Jennifer Slept Here. Movies: Mae West, Death Ride to Osaka, Girls of the White Orchid. Many appearances on series (Love Boat, Fantasy Island, etc.) and numerous talk shows. Mini-series: Ellis Island. Movies: Mae West, Killer in the Mirror.
PICTURES: Gypsy, Mr. Mom.

JOELS, MERRILL E.: Performer. b. Hartford, Conn.; began career, Hartford, 1930; organ. Mark Twain Masquers Thea.; radio, New York since 1945; TV since 1946; actor, announcer, narrator; over 500 TV shows; feature, Army, Navy and industrial films; narr., children's records, dir., AFTRA; member, The Players; Credits also Off-Broadway, Summer Stock, Daytime TV Drama. Announcer and Co-host WEVD Home Show 29 years. Announcer-engineer, WEVD.
AUTHOR: Acting is a Business, How to Get Into Show Business, Touring in Theatre of Peretz and Three by Chayefsky; Talking Books for Library of Congress.

JOFFE, CHARLES H.: Executive. b. Brooklyn, N.Y. e. Syracuse Univ. Joined with Jack Rollins to set up management-production org., clients including Woody Allen, Ted Bessell, Billy Crystal, David Letterman, Tom Poston, Robin Williams.
PICTURES INCLUDE: Produced: Don't Drink the Water, Take the Money and Run, Everything You Always Wanted to Know About Sex but Were Afraid To Ask, Love and Death, Annie Hall, House of God, Arthur. Exec. prod.: Play It Again Sam, Bananas, Sleeper, Arthur, Mahattan, Interiors, Stardust Memories, A Midsummer Nights' Sex Comedy, Zelig, Broadway Danny Rose, The Purple Rose of Cairo, Hannah and Her Sisters.
TV: Woody Allen specials. Star of the Family, Good Time Harry.

JOFFE, EDWARD: producer, director, writer. Worked in m.p., theatre, commercial radio and as Journalist before ent. TV ind. in Britain 1957 as writer/prod with ATV. Has prod. & dir. over 4000 progs. 1959–61 staff prod. Granada TV, 1962, dir., Traitor's Gate & Traveling Light for Robt Stigwood, prod. dir., numerous series for Grampian TV; 1967, dir. film The Price of a Record—Emmy finalist, Special Mention Salerno Film Fest shown in over 70 countries; 1967—8 films, Columba's Folk & So Many Partings ITV entries in Golden Harp Fest.; 1968, prod. dir., Tony Hancock's last film in Australia, prod. dir. Up At The Cross for ATN 7;

prod. dir. ind. film, Will Ye No' Come Back Again for ITV; 1969–70, dir., This Is . . . Tom Jones; prod. dir., The Golden Shot; 1971, senior production lecturer, Thomson TV College; dir., films for USA for London Television Service; Evening Standard Commercials for Thames TV. Co. prod. dir.,ind. film Sound Scene, 1972–8, Contract prod. dir. Thames TV various series: Magpie, Today, Opportunity Knocks. The David Nixon Show, Seven Ages of Man, Problems, Finding Out; 1980; production consultant, CBC-tv, 1978–82, prod. dir. series Writers' Workshop, About Books; 1978, film, Places & Things (British Academy Award nomination), 1979, film, Who Do You Think You Are? (British Academy Award nomination, ITV's Japan Prize entry, Special Jury Award San Francisco Int Film Fest), 1981, Film Images, British Academy Award nomination; Gold Plaque Chicago Int Film Fest.) 1982: The Protectors (medal winner Intl. Film & TV Festival, N.Y.). 1982–86: Film Rainbow Coloured Disco Dancer. Various Series: Taste of China, Jobs Ltd. Spin-offs.

JOFFE, ROLAND: Director. e. Manchester Univ., England. Worked in British theatre; 1973 became youngest director at National Theatre. 1978, moved into directing TV as preparation for career in films making debut in 1984 with The Killing Fields.
TELEVISION: Documentaries: Rope, Anne. Plays: The Spongers, Tis Pity She's a Whore, United Kingdom (also co-wrote). Series: The Stars Look Down.

JOHNS, GLYNIS: Actress. b. Durban, So. Africa, Oct. 5, 1923; daughter of Mervyn Johns, actor, and Alys Steele, pianist; e. In England. On London stage from 1935 (Buckie's Bears, The Children's Hour, A Kiss for Cinderalla, Quiet Week-End; Gertie, N.Y. stage, 1952; Major Barbara, N.Y., 1956–57.) On screen 1936: South Riding. Voted one of top ten British Money-making stars in Motion Picture Herald-Pathe poll, 1951–54.
STAGE: N.Y. 1964, Too Good to Be True, London, 1967: The King's Mare; 1970, Come As You Are. 1971–2 Tour of Britain, Canada and USA in The Marquise, A Little Night Music, NY 1973 (Tony Award); Cause Celebre (London, 1977); Harold and Maude (Canada, 1977); Hayfever (UK tour, 1978); The Boy Friend (Toronto, 1984).
PICTURES INCLUDE: Murder in Family, Prison Without Bars, Mr. Brigg's Family, 49th Parallel, Adventures of Tartu, Half-Way House, Perfect Strangers, This Man Is Mine, Frieda, An Ideal Husband, Miranda, Third Time, Lucky Mr. Proback, The Great Manhunt, Flesh and Blood, No Highway in the Sky, Appointment With Venus (Island Rescue), Encore, The Card (The Promoter), The Sword and the Rose, Rob Roy, Personal Affair, The Weak and the Wicked, The Seekers (Land of Fury), The Beachcomber, Mad About Men, Court Jester, Josephine and Men, Loser Takes All, Day They Gave Babies Away, Another Time Another Place, Shake Hands With the Devil, The Sundowners, The Spider's Web, The Chapman Report, Mary Poppins, Dear Brigette, Don't Just Stand There, Lock Up Your Daughters.
TV: Own series (US): Glynis. Guest star TV includes: Dr. Kildare, Roaring Twenties, Naked City, The Defenders, Danny Kaye Show, Noel Coward's Star Quality, Mrs. Amworth, All You Need Is Love, Across A Crowded Room, Little Gloria, Skagg, various series.

JOHNSON, ARTE: Actor. b. Chicago, Jan. 20, 1934. Gained fame on TV's Laugh-In.
PICTURES: Miracle in the Rain, The Subterraneans, The Third Day, The President's Analyst, Love at First Bite.

JOHNSON, BEN: Actor. b. Pawhuska, Okla., 1918, Stunt rider & performer in rodeos, touring country; did stunt work in War Party; m.p. debut in Mighty Joe Young.
PICTURES INCLUDE: Three Godfathers, She Wore a Yellow Ribbon, Wagonmaster, Rio Grande, Wild Stallion, Fort Defiance, Shane, Rebel in Town, The Wild Bunch, The Undefeated, Chisum, The Last Picture Show, (Academy Award, Best Supporting Actor, 1971), Junior Bonner, The Getaway, Dillinger, The Train Robbers, Kid Blue, The Sugarland Express, Bite The Bullet, Hustle, The Town That Dreaded Sundown, The Greatest, Grayeagle, The Swarm, The Hunter, Terror Train, Tex, Champions.

JOHNSON, DON: Actor. b. Flatt Creek, MO, Dec. 15, 1950. Worked at ATC, San Francisco.
PICTURES: The Magic Garden of Stanley Sweetheart, The Harrad Experiment, A Boy and His Dog, Zaachariah, Return to Macon County, Soggy Bottom, USA, Cease Fire.
TELEVISION: The Rebels, Miami Vice. Movies: From Here to Eternity—The War Years, Beulah Land, Revenge of the Stepford Wives, Elvis and the Beauty Queen, The Long Hot Summer, etc.

JOHNSON, G. GRIFFITH: Executive. b. New York, Aug. 15, 1912; e. Harvard U., 1934. (AM). 1936, (Ph.D), 1938; U.S. Treasury Dept. 1936–39; Dept. of Comm., 1939–40; O.P.A. & predecessor agencies, 1940–46; consulting economist, 1946–47; dir., Econ. Stab. Div., Nat'l. Security Resources Bd., 1948–49; chief econ., U.S. Bur. of Budget, 1949–50; econ. advisor to Econ. Stab. Admin. 1950–52; Exec. v.p. MPEAA, 1965, MPAA, 1971; Asst. Sec'y of State for Economic Affairs, 1962–65; v.p. MPAA, 1953–62; Author of several books & articles.

JOHNSON, J. BOND: Producer, Exec. b. Fort Worth, Texas, June 18, 1926. e. Texas Wesleyan Coll., B.S., 1947; Texas Christian Univ. M. Ed., 1948; Southern Methodist Univ., B.D., 1952; Ph.D., Univ. of Southern Calif., 1967. Army Air Forces, WW II; public information officer, captain, U.S. Marine Corps. Korean War. Formerly member Marine Corps Reserve, Motion Picture Production Unit, Hollywood. Now Colonel, U.S. Army Reserve. Newspaper reporter, Fort Worth Star-Telegram, 1942–48; pres., West Coast News Service, 1960; pres., exec. prod., Bonjo Prods., Inc., 1960, President, chief executive officer, Cine-Media International, 1975 managing partner, Capra-Johnson Productions, Ltd., 1978.
PICTURES INCLUDE: Sands of Iwo Jima, Retreat Hell, Flying Leathernecks; photographed aerial portions, Jamboree 53, Norfleet, Devil at My Heels, Kingdom of the Spiders, Ordeal at Donner Pass, Place of the Dawn, Lies I Told Myself, Backstretch, Airs Above The Ground, The Jerusalem Concert, The Berkshire Terror, The Seventh Gate.
TV: Creator, story consultant, tech. advisor, Whirlpool, 1962, one hour dramatic series for Screen Gems/CBS-TV, Executive Producer, Creator, On The Go. (½ hour TV News-Sports series), 1977, Coasties (1 hour TV series), 1978, Desert Rangers (1 hour series) 1979. Producer, Fandango (series), 1981.

JOHNSON, LAMONT: Director, producer, actor. b. Stockton, Calif.; e. UCLA.
TV: The Defenders, Profiles in Courage, Twilight Zone, That Certain Summer, My Sweet Charlie, The Execution of Pvt. Slovik, Fear On Trial, Ernie Kovacs: Between the Laughter, Wallenberg: A Hero's Story (co-prod., dir.).
PLAYS: The Egg, Yes is For a Very Young Man; dir., two operas, L.A. Philharmonic, 1964; founder, dir., UCLA Professional Theatre Group.
THEATRICAL PICTURES INCLUDE: McKenzie Break, A Gunfight, The Groundstar Conspiracy, You'll Like My Mother, The Last American Hero, Lipstick, One on One, Somebody Killed Her Husband, Cattle Annie and Little Britches, Spacehunter.

JOHNSON, LAURIE: Composer, mus.; dir. b. 1927. Studied Royal College of Music.
STAGE: Lock Up Your Daughters, Pieces of Eight, The Four Musketeers.
PICTURES INCLUDE: Good Companions, Moonraker, Girls at Sea, Operation Bullshine, Tiger Bay, I Aim at the Stars, Spare The Road, What a Whopper, Bitter Harvest, Seige of the Saxons, Dr. Strangelove, The First Men in The Moon, Beauty Jungle, East of Sudan, Hot Millions, And Soon the Darkness, Mister Jerico, Cause for Alarm, The Beltstone Fox, Hedda, It Lives Again, All Things Bright and Beautiful.

JOHNSON, RICHARD: Actor. b. Essex, England, July 30, 1927. Studied at RADA. First stage appearance Opera House, Manchester, then played in John Gielgud's repertory season, 1944. Served in Royal Navy 1945–48. Subsequent stage appearances incld. The Mad Woman of Chaillot, The Lark. Visited Moscow with Peter Brook's production of Hamlet. Royal Shakespeare Thea.: Stratford & London, 1957–62. Royal Shakespeare Company 1972–73. National Theatre, 1976–77.
PICTURES INCLUDE: The Haunting, 80,000 Suspects, Moll Flanders, Operation Crossbow, Khartoum, La Strega in Amore, Deadlier than the Male, The Rover, Danger Route, Twist of Sand, Oedipus The King, Trajan's Column, Lady Hamilton, Some Girls Do, Julius Caesar, The Deserters, The Beloved, Hennessy, Aces High, The Four Feathers, Turtle Diary.

JOHNSON, RUSSELL: Actor. b. Ashley, Pa. e. Girard College, Actors Laboratory, L.A.: W.W. II, Army Air Corps.
PICTURES INCLUDE: For Men Only, The Greatest Story Ever Told.
TV: Black Saddle, Climax, You Are There, Rawhide, Twilight Zone, Gilligan's Island.

JOHNSON, VAN: Actor. b. Newport, R.I., Aug. 28, 1916. Began in vaudeville; then on N.Y. stage New Faces of 1937, Eight Men of Manhattan, Too Many Girls, Pal Joey. On screen 1941 in Murder in Big House. Voted one of the top ten Money Making Stars in Motion Picture Herald-Fame Poll 1945–46.
PICTURES INCLUDE: War Against Mrs. Hadley, Dr. Gillespie's New Assistant, Pilot No. 5, Dr. Gillespies's Criminal Case, Guy Named Joe, Three Men in White, Two Girls and a Sailor, Thirty Seconds Over Tokyo, Ziegfeld Follies, Between Two Women, Thrill of Romance, Week-End at the Waldorf, Romance of Rosy Ridge, Bride Goes Wild, State of the Union, Command Decision, In the Good Old Summertime, Scene of the Crime, Battleground, Big Hang-

over, Three Guys Named Mike, Grounds for Marriage, Go For Broke, Too Young To Kiss, It's A Big Country, Invitation, When In Rome, Washington Story, Plymouth Adventure, Confidentially Connie, Remains to Be Seen, Easy to Love, Caine Mutiny, Siege at Red River, Men of the Fighting Lady, Brigadoon, Last Time I Saw Paris, End of the Affair, Bottom of the Bottle, Miracle in the Rain, 23 Paces to Baker Street, Slander, Kelly and Me, The Lost Blitzkreig, Beyond This Place, Subway in the Sky, Web of Evidence, Enemy General, Wives and Lovers, Where Angels Go . . . Trouble Follows, Eagles Over London, The Purple Rose of Cairo.

JOHNSTON, MARGARET: Actress. e. Sydney Univ., Australia. London stage debut: Murder Without Crime. Screen debut: Rake's Progress, 1945.
TV: Always Juliet, Taming of the Shrew, Man With a Load of Mischief, Light of Heart, Autumn Crocus, Androcles and the Lion, Sulky Five, Windmill Near a Frontier, The Shrike, The Out of Towners, Looking for Garrow, The Typewriter, The Glass Menagerie, That's Where The Town's Going, The Vortex.
PICTURES INCLUDE: A Man About the House, Portrait of Clare, The Magic Box, Knave of Hearts, Touch and Go, Night of the Eagle, The Nose on My Face, Life at the Top, Schizo, Mr. Sebastian.
THEATRE: Ring of Truth, The Masterpiece, Lady Macbeth, Merchant of Venice, Measure for Measure, Othello.

JOHNSTONE, DAVID: b. Kilmarnock, Scotland, July 4, 1926. e. Ayr Academy. Journalist: Ayrshire Post; Glasgow Herald. Night News Editor Scottish Daily Mail; Scottish Correspondent News Chronicle. Joined Scottish Television May, 1958 as News Editor. Later producer, director. Originated daily magazine, Here and Now. Producer ITV World Cup (part) 1976. Head of News, Current Affairs, Documentaries and Sport. Assistant controller of programmes; controller (now director) of programmes 1977.

JOLLEY, STAN: Producer-Director-Production Designer-Art Director. b. New York City, May 17, 1926. e. Univ. of S. Calif., col. of architecture, son of actor I. Stanford Jolley. In Navy in World War II. Has acted in capacities listed for many feature films and TV series.
PICTURES INCLUDE: Producer and Production Designer: Knife For the Ladies. Assoc. Producer and Prod. Designer, The Good Guys & The Bad Guys,; Director: Today's FBI, Macgyver; 2nd Unit director, Superman. Production Designer: Witness, Taps, Caddyshack, Cattle Annie and Little Britches, Americathon (also second unit director), Swarm, Drum, Framed, Dion Brothers, Mixed Company, Walking Tall, Terror In The Wax Museum, Night of The Lepus (also second unit director), War Between Men & Women, Law Man, The Phynx. Art Director: Young Billy Young, Ride Beyond Vengeance, Broken Saber, The Restless Ones, Mail Order Bride, Toby Tyler, Nine Lives of Elfego Baca. Assoc. producer & prod. designer & 2nd unit director, Happily Ever After.
TV FEATURES: 2nd Unit Director and Production Designer: Swiss Family Robinson, Adventures of The Queen, Woman Hunter, Production Designer: No Man's Land, Last of the Great Survivors, Like Normal People, Howard Hughes, Flood, Voyage of The Yes, The Stranger, Punch & Jody, City Beneath the Sea, Women of San Quentin.
TV SERIES: Art Director: Walt Disney Presents, Pete & Gladys, Gunsmoke, Mr. Ed., Branded, Voyage to The Bottom of The Sea, Land of The Giants, O'Hara, etc. Production Designer: Walking Tall, Today's F.B.I., For Love and Honor, Macgyver. Pilots: 8, including Get Smart.

JONES, BARRY: Actor. b. Guernsey (Channel Islands) March 6, 1893. Stage debut in 1921 acting extensively in London and United States. Film debut in Arms and the Man, 1931. During World War II, in Royal Navy.
PICTURES INCLUDE: Dancing with Crime, Frieda, Uneasy Terms, Seven Days to Noon, Clouded Yellow, White Corridors, Plymouth Adventure, Return to Paradise, Prince Valiant, Brigadoon, Demetrius and the Gladiators, Glass Slipper, Alexander the Great.
THEATRE: Starred B'way in Mis-Alliance.

JONES, CHUCK: Producer, Director, Writer. b. Spokane, Wash., Sept. 21, 1912. e. Chouinard Art Institute. Dir., Warner Bros. Animation until 1962 where he created and directed Roadrunner & Coyote, Pepe le Pew; directed and helped create Bugs Bunny, Porky Pig, Daffy Duck etc. Created Snafu character, U.S. Armed Service. Co-prod., wrote, dir., Bugs Bunny Show, ABC-TV. Headed MGM Animation Dept. dir. How the Grinch Stole Christmas, Horton Hears a Who, The Dot and the Line, Pogo, The Phantom Tollbooth. Lecturer and teacher at many universities. Currently independent, Chuck Jones Enterprises, Producer, Director, Writer (for ABC-TV) The Cricket in Times Square; A Very Merry Cricket; Yankee Doodle Cricket and (for CBS-TV) Rudyard Kipling's Rikki-Tikki-Tavi; The White Seal; Mowgli's Brothers, Saint-Saens' The Carnival of the Animals, Ogden Nash lyrics, with Daffy Duck & Bugs Bunny; A Connecticut Rabbit in King Arthur's Court, based on Mark Twain's original story, with Bugs Bunny, Daffy Duck, Porky Pig, Elmer Fudd, etc., two specials featuring Raggedy Ann and Andy in The Great Santa Claus Caper and The Pumpkin Who Couldn't Smile; plus a feature compilation of past work: Chuck Jones' Bugs Bunny Road Runner Movie. Most recently: Daffy Duck's Thanks-for-Giving Special and Bugs Bunny's Bustin' Out All Over. Recipient Academy Award for best animated cartoons for Scenti-Mental Reasons-1950, The Dot and The Line-1965; best documentary short subject for So Much for So Little, 1950. Honored with retrospectives at Deauville Film Fest (1978), British Film Institute (1979). N.Y. Film Festival (1982); Tellwide Film Festival (1976). N.Y. Museum of Modern Art (1985), 25 gallery exhibition of cartoon art and unique art (1983–84–85). Cartoon and other art displayed in gallery exhibitions throughout U.S., 1983–84. Honored at Cambridge Film Festival, 1985; received Great Director Award, USA Film Festival, 1986; received best animation award from National Society of Cartoonists, 1986; appeared for Children's Hospital Telethon New Orleans, 1985, 1986; Children's Hospital Benefit St. Louis, 1985; Lecturer Emeritus Univ of Calif San Diego, 1986; Children's book "William the Backwards Skunk" 1986 by Crown Publ.

JONES, CHUCK: Public Relations Executive. b. Detroit, Mich., Dec. 6. e. Michigan State University (B.A. Advertising) U.S. Marine Corps 1964–66. Staff writer, Pacific Stars & Stripes, Tokyo, Japan and DaNang, Vietnam. Contributing editor, Leatherneck Magazine, Naval Aviation News, Navy Times. Entered motion picture industry 1969. Critic/writer Motion Picture Daily, 1969. Publicist, Harold Rand & Co., Public Relations, 1970–71. Publicist, American International Pictures, 1971. Radio/TV, newspaper, magazine & syndicate contact, United Artists Corp., 1972–73. Established Chuck Jones Public Relations in 1973 and has been pres. since then. Had stint as eastern adv./pub. dir., Embassy Pictures, 1981–82.

JONES, CLARK R.: Prod. dir. b. Clearfield, Pa., April 10, 1920. e. Northwestern U.
TV SHOWS INCLUDE: The Tony Awards, Peter Pan, Sleeping Beauty Ballet, Ford 50th Anniversary Show, Caesar's Hour, Your Hit Parade, Jack & the Beanstalk; Romeo & Juliet, Perry Como, Bell Telephone Hour, Carol Burnett series; Carol Channing and Pearl Bailey on Broadway, Tony Awards, 6 Rms Riv Vu, Twigs, CBS 50th Anniversary, Emmies, Miss USA, Miss Universe.

JONES, DAVID: CBE until retirement, publicity director, EMI Films Ltd. and also of EMI Cinemas. b. London, Eng., 1913. Entered industry through the CEA Organ, "Cinematograph Times"; editorial assistant RKO-Radio, 1930–36; served in advertising and editorial sections, London "Hollywood Reporter"; rejoined RKO-Radio as exploiteer, appointed press representative, 1938; became director of publicity, 1942 until 1958, chairman, FIPC, 1951–52, 1955–62; president FIPC, 1952–54, 1960–63; Press Guy, Variety Club of Gt. Britain, 1949–50, 1953–63, Chief Barker, Variety Club, 1964, International Press Guy Variety Club of Great Britain, 1965–86.

JONES, DEAN: Actor. b. Morgan County, Ala., Jan. 25, 1936; e. Asbury College, Wilmore, Ky.; prof. debut as blues singer, New Orleans; U.S. Navy, 1953.
TV: Ensign O'Toole, The Teddy Bears.
STAGE: There Was a Little Girl, Company.
PICTURES INCLUDE: Handle With Care, Never So Few, Under the Yum-Yum Tree, The New Interns, That Darn Cat, Two On A Guillotine, The Ugly Daschshund, Monkeys, Go Home, Blackbeard's Ghost, The Love Bug, The $1,000,000 Duck, Snowball Express, Mr. Super Invisible, The Shaggy D.A., Herbie Goes to Monte Carlo, Born Again.

JONES, GRACE: Singer-Actress. b. Spanishtown, Jamaica, May 19, 1952. e. Syracuse Univ. Modelled and appeared in several Italian pictures before career as singer.
PICTURES: Conan the Destroyer, A View to a Kill.

JONES, GRIFFITH: Actor. b. London, England. e. University College, London; Royal Academy Dramatic Art (gold medal 1932). In H.M. Forces, World War II. Stage debut, London, 1930, in Carpet Slippers; N.Y. debut 1935 in Escape Me Never. Many stage successes. In many Brit. pictures from 1932.
PICTURES INCLUDE: Escape Me Never, Four Just Men, Atlantic Ferry, This Was Paris, The Day Will Dawn, Uncensored, Henry V. Rake's Progress, Wicked Lady, They Made Me a Fugitive, Good Time Girl, Miranda, Look Before You Love, Once Upon a Dream, Honeymoon Deferred, Star of My Night, Scarlet Web, The Sea Shall Not Have Them, Face in the Night, Wanted on Voyage, The High Wall, Hidden Homicide, Strangler's Web, Decline and Fall.
PLAYS: The Moonraker, Quadrille, Alice Thro' the Looking Glass, Love Machine, Dead on Nine, The Entertainer, Expresso, The Sound of Murder, Treasure Island, Two Accounts Rendered, The Cavern, The Doctor's Dilemma,

Jockey Club Stakes. 1973, Nottingham P'House, 1974 Crucible, Sheffield. Member of Royal S'Peare Co. 1975–80,1981–86.

TV: The Breaking Point, The Ware Case, When in Rome, A Moment in the Sun, Hell Hath no Fury, Margret, No Hiding Place, The Collection, By Invitation Only, A Woman of No Importance, Freedom in September, Blythe Spirit, Treasure Island, The Three Sisters, Emergency Ward, Vendetta, The Cabinet Papers, Man in a Suitcase, Boy Meets Girl, Troubleshooters, Strange Report, Avengers, Inside Man, A Matter of Principle, Doom Watch, Warm Feet, Warm Heart, Paul Temple, The Persuaders, The Lotus Eaters, The Black Arrow, Arrow, Spy Trap, Crown Court, Fallen Eagles, The Apple Cart, Comedy of Errors, Macbeth, The Three Sisters, Nicholas Nickleby.

JONES, HENRY: Actor. b. Philadelphia, Aug. 1, 1912. e. St. Joseph's Coll. On stage in Time of Your Life, My Sister Eileen, Bad Seed, Sunrise at Campobello, Advise and Consent, etc.

PICTURES: Never Too Late, Stay Away Joe, Support Your Local Sheriff, Rascal, Angel iln My Pocket, Butch Cassidy and the Sundance Kid, Rabbit Run, Dirty Dingus Magee, Skin Game, Tom Sawyer, Pete 'n' Tillie The Outfit, Nine to Five, etc.

JONES, JAMES EARL: Actor. b. Arkabutla, MS, Jan. 17, 1931. e. Univ. of Mich. Son of Robert Earl Jones. On stage in The Cool World, The Great White Hope (Tony, 1969), The Iceman Cometh, Of Mice and Men, A Lesson from Aloes, Master Charley and the Boys.

PICTURES: Dr. Strangelove, The Comedians, The End of the Road, the Great White Hope, The Man, Claudine, The Swashbuckler, The Bingo Long Travelling All-Stars and Motor Kings, The Greatest, The Last Remake of Beau Geste, A Piece of the Action, The Bushido Blade, Soul Man.

TELEVISION: Movies: The UFO Incident, Jesus of Nazareth, The Greatest Thing That Almost Happened, Roots: The Next Generation, Guyana Tragedy—The Story of Jim Jones, Golden Moment: An Olympic Love Story, Philby, Burgess and MacLean, The Atlanta Child Murders, The Vegas Strip War.

JONES, JENNIFER: Actress. r.n. Phyllis Isley. b. Tulsa, Okla., Mar. 21, 1919. e. Northwestern U., Amer. Acad. Dram. Arts; daughter of Phil R., Flora Mae (Suber) Isley, exhib.; m. David O. Selznick prod. Toured with parents stock company as child; in summer stock in East; little theat. East & West. Began screen career (as Phyllis Isley) in several Republic Westerns, first major role 1943 as Marie Soubirous in The Song of Bernadette, Winning Academy Award 1943 (best performance by an actress).

PICTURES INCLUDE: Since You Went Away, Love Letters, Duel In the Sun, Cluny Brown, Portrait of Jennie, We Were Strangers, Madame Bovary, Carrie, Wild Heart, Ruby Gentry, Indiscretion of an American Wife, Beat the Devil, Love Is a Many-Splendored Thing, Good Morning Miss Dove, Man in the Gray Flannel Suit, Barretts of Wimpole Street, Farewell to Arms, Tender Is the Night, The Idol, Angel, Down We Go, The Towering Inferno.

JONES, KATHY: Executive. Joined Paramount Pictures in 1977 as exec. dir., field mktg. Left to join Time-Life Films as v.p., domestic mktg., for m.p. div. Returned to Paramount 1981 as v.p., domestic pub. & promo. 1984, appt. sr. v.p., domestic pub. & promo. for Motion Picture Group, Paramount.

JONES, QUINCY: Composer. b. 1935. Formerly in trumpet section of Lionel Hampton's band; has played with Dizzy Gillespie, Count Basie before scoring films.

PICTURES INCLUDE: In the Heat of the Night, In Cold Blood, (Acad. Award nom.), The Pawnbroker, Mirage, The Slender Thread, Made In Paris, Walk, Don't Run, Banning, The Deadly Affair, Enter Laughing, A Dandy in Aspic, The Counterfeit Killer, For Love of Ivy, The Split, Bob & Carol & Ted & Alice, The Lost Man, Cactus Flower, John and Mary, The Last of the Mobile Hotshots, The Out-of-Towners, They Call Me Mister Tibbs, Brother John, Dollars, The Anderson Tapes, The Hot Rock, The New Centurions, The Getaway, The Color Purple (also co-prod.).

JONES, SAM J.: Actor. b. Chicago, IL, Aug. 12, 1954.

PICTURES: 10, Flash Gordon, My Chauffeur.

TELEVISION: Stunts Unlimited, Code Red, No Man's Land.

JONES, SHIRLEY: Actress. b. Smithon, Pa., March 31, 1934.

THEATRE: Appeared with Pittsburgh Civic Light Opera in Lady in The Dark, Call Me Madam. Broadway: South Pacific, Me and Juliet, Maggie Flynn.

PICTURES INCLUDE: Oklahoma, Carousel, Bobbikins, Elmer Gantry, Pepe, A Ticklish Affair, The Secret of My Success, Fluffy, The Happy Ending, Beyond the Posiedon Adventure.

TV: Silent Night, Lonely Night, The Partridge Family (series).

JONES, TOMMY LEE: Actor. b. San Saba, Texas, Sept. 15, 1946. Worked in oil fields; studied acting at Harvard, where earned a degree in English. Broadway debut in A Patriot for Me; appeared in Four in a Garden, Ulysses in Nighttown, Fortune and Men's Eyes. Film debut in Love Story (1970).

PICTURES INCLUDE: Jackson County Jail, Rolling Thunder, The Betsy, Eyes of Laura Mars, Coal Miner's Daughter, Back Roads, Nate and Hayes, River Rat, Block Moon Rising.

TELEVISION: The Amazing Howard Hughes, The Executioner's Song, Cat on a Hot Tin Roof (Showtime).

JORDAN, HENRIETTA: Exec. b. New York, N.Y., Feb. 26. Ent. m.p. ind. as ass't to exec. v.p., UPA Pictures, 1950; v.p. in charge of sales, Format Prods, Inc. v.p. and assoc. prod., 1962–71. Assoc. prod. Levitow-Hanson Films, Inc., 1972–74; Producer, Image West, Ltd., 1975–84; dir. sls., Cause & EFX, 1984–85; dir. sls., Modern Videofilm Graphics, 1986.

JORDAN, RICHARD: Actor. b. New York City, July 19, 1938. e. Harvard.

PICTURES: The Yakuza, Rooster Cogburn, Old Boyfriends, Interiors, Raise the Titanic, A Flash of Green (also prod.), Dune, The Mean Season, The Men's Club.

TELEVISION: Captains and the Kings, Les Miserables, The French Atlantic Affair, The Bunker, Washington Mistress, etc.

JOSEPH, KENNETH. Executive. b. New York City, July 15, 1922. e. Syracuse U. Entered industry as announcer and program director of various NY radio stations, including WNYC, 1946–53; exec. in various capacities of United Artists Television and predecessor companies, 1953–68; exec. v.p., syndication, Four Star Entertainment Corp., 1968–70; exec. v.p., world-wide syndication, Metromedia Producers Corp., 1970 to present.

JOSEPHSON, MARVIN: Executive. b. New York City, June 5, 1935. e. Long Island Univ. Started with Liebling-Wood Agency as agent; later with Music Corp. of America, General Artists Corp., Agency for the Performing Arts. Now chm. bd., Marvin Josephson Associates, parent co. of International Creative Management.

JOSIAH, JR., WALTER J.: Executive. b. New York City. e. Fordham college BS:SS (1955–58): Harvard Law School (LLB, 1962). United States Air Force, 1955–58, First Lt. and Pilot. Associate, Simpson Thacher & Bartlett, 1962–67. Legal staff, Paramount Pictures, 1967–69. Asst. resident counsel, 1969; chief resident counsel, 1970 and v.p. & chief resident counsel, 1971–82. v.p. & general counsel, Motion Picture Association of America, Inc., 1983.

Professional Associations: Chairman, Committee 307, Authors Rights, 1981–82, Patent, Trademark & Copyright Law Section of the American Bar Assn.; Association of the Bar of the City of New York (Committee on Copyright and Literary Property, 1976–79, 1982–85): Copyright Society of the U.S.A.—Member of the Board of Trustees commencing June, 1981; member, Motion Picture Academy of Arts and Sciences; Copyright Office Advisory Committee, 1981–82; National Sculpture Society—advisor to the president; Advisory Board, Publication: Communications and the Law; Member, President's Club Executive Committee and Annual Fund Council, Fordham University.

JOURDAN, LOUIS: Actor, b. Marseille, France, June 19, 1921. Stage actor, prior to m.p.

PICTURES INCLUDE: Her First Affair, La Boheme L'Arlesienne, La Belle, Adventure, Felicie Nanteuil, The Paradine Case, Letter from an Unkown Woman, Madame Bovary, Bird of Paradise, Anne of the Indies, The Happy Time, Three Coins in the Fountain, No Minor Voices, Decameron Nights, The Swan, Julie, Gigi, Streets of Montmartre, Story of the Count of Monte Cristo, VIP's, Made in Paris, A Flea in Her Ear, To Commit a Murder, Silver Bears, Octopussy.

TELEVISION: Beverly Hills Madam.

JUDD, EDWARD: Actor. b. Shanghai, 1934. e. Far East. Stage; The Long and the Short and the Tall, The Tinker. Numerous TV appearances.

PICTURES INCLUDE: The Day the Earth Caught Fire, Stolen Hours, The World Ten Times Over, Mystery Submarine, The Long Ships, First Men On the Moon, Strange Bedfellows, Invasion, Island of Terror, The Vengeance of Shee, Shakedown.

JULIA, RAUL: Actor. b. San Juan, PR, Mar. 9, 1940. e. Univ. of Puerto Rico; studied for theatre with Wynn Handman. New York stage debut in La Vida Es Sueno, 1964. Film debut in Panic in Needle Park, 1971.

PICTURES: The Organization Man, Been Down So Long It Looks Like Up to Me, Gumball Rally, The Eyes of Laura Mars, Tempest, The Escape Artist, One from the Heart, Kiss of the Spider Woman, The Morning After.

TELEVISION: Sesame Street (running role), King Lear, The National Health, McCloud, Love of Life, Aces Up, Death Scream, etc.

JUNKIN, RAYMOND: Executive. b. New York, N.Y., Nov. 4, 1918. e. Univ. of Alabama, Univ. of Penn. Air Force, World War II. Eastern sls. mgr., Robert H. Clark Co., southwestern sls. mgr., then ass't to president; v.p., director of sales, Official Films, Inc., 1951–58; self-employed as a film and program consultant, 1959–60; pres. Program Sales Inc.; gen. sls. mgr., Programs For Television, Inc., since 1961; v.p. & gen. mgr., Screen Gems (Canada), Ltd.; v.p. Domestic Sales Mgr. Screen Gems Internat'l; 1967 gen. sls. mgr., Trans-Lux TV Corp., v.p. & gen. sls. mgr., 1968 to date. CTV Television Network Ltd.

JURADO, KATY: Actress. r.n. Maria Christina Jurado Garcia. b. Guadalajara, Mexico, 1927. Numerous Mexican films m.p. columist for Mexican publications; American m.p. debut in Bullfighter and the Lady.
PICTURES INCLUDE: High Noon, San Antone, Arrowhead, Broken Lance, The Racers, Trial, Trapeze, Man from Del Rio, The Badlanders, One Eyed Jacks, Barabbas, A Convenant with Death, Pat Garrett and Billy the Kid, Under the Volcano.
TELEVISION: Lady Blues.

JUROW, MARTIN: Producer. b. New York, N.Y. e. William and Mary, Harvard Law School. Associated with MCA, William Morris, pres., Famous Artists; prod., G & E Productions; co-prod. with Richard Shepherd Jurow-Shepherd Productions.
PICTURES INCLUDE: The Hanging Tree, The Fugitive Kind, Love In a Goldfish Bowl, Breakfast At Tiffany's, The Great Race, A Shot in the Dark, Solider in the Rain, Terms of Endearment, Sylvester.

JUSTIN, GEORGE: Executive. Major credits include producer on Middle of the Night and The Tiger Makes Out; assoc. prod. for Marathon Man and On the Waterfront; prod. exec. on The Goddess and Twelve Angry Men. V.p. & exec. prod. mgr. at Paramount Pictures; four years; left to join Columbia as prod. exec, where was assoc. prod. for The Deep and Prod. exec. on The Eyes of Laura Mars. In April, 1979 joined Orion Pictures; named exec. prod. mgr. Promoted to v.p./exec. prod. mgr. in April, 1980.

JUSTIN, JOHN: Actor. b. London, Nov. 23, 1917; e. Bryanston (Dorset). Stage debut, repertory at Plymouth 1933; entered m.p. ind. in 1939. Many TV appearances.
PICTURES INCLUDE: Thief of Bagdad, Journey Together, The Sound Barrier, The Village, Melba, Crest of the Wave, King of the Khyber Rifles, The Man Who Loved Redheads, The Teckman Mystery, Untamed, Safari, Crime Passionelle, Guilty?, Island in the Sun, Spider's Web, Les Hommes Veulent, Vivre, The Savage Messiah, Barcelona Kill, Lisztomania, Valentino, The Big Sleep, Trenchcoat.

K

KAEL, PAULINE: Critic. b. June 19, 1919, Sonoma County, CA. e. Univer of Calif. at Berkeley (1936–40), majoring in philosophy. Managed two art theaters in Calif. for which she wrote program notes. Broadcast weekly about films on Pacifica network. Made experimental shorts. Has written on films for many magazines. Since 1968 movie critic for The New Yorker.
AUTHOR: I Lost it at the Movies, Kiss Kiss Bang Bang, Going Steady, The Citizen Kane Book, Deeper into Movies, Reeling, When the Lights Go Down, 5001 Nights at the Movies, Taking It All In, State of the Art.
AWARDS: Guggenheim Fellow, 1964; George Polk Memorial Award for Criticism, 1970; The National Book Award, 1974, for Deeper into Movies; Front Page Award for best magazine column in 1974 from Newswomen's Club of N.Y and for distinguished journalism, 1983.

KAGAN, JEREMY PAUL: Director-Writer. b. Mt. Vernon, NY, Dec. 14, 1945. e. Harvard; NYU.
PICTURES: Heroes, The Big Fix, The Chosen, The Sting II, The Journey of Natty Gann.
TELEVISION: Columbo, The Bold Ones, Unwed Father, Judge Dee, Katherine (also s.p.), Scott Joplin, etc.

KAHN, JUDITH: Executive. Background in mktg., including graphic design, adv./promo. Creative dir. at Intralink Film Graphic Design; art dir. for Seiniger & Associates. 1983, returned to New York as consultant to corporate clients, including cable, TV, and m.p. accts. 1985, joined Paramount Pictures as v.p., creative svcs. of M.P. Group.

KAHN, MADELINE: Actress-Singer. b. Boston, MA., Sept. 29, 1942. Broadway bow in New Faces of '68. Featured in off-Broadway musical Promenade. Trained as opera singer and appeared in La Boheme, Showboat, Two by Two, Candide.
PICTURES INCLUDE: What's Up Doc? (debut), Paper Moon, From the Mixed-Up Files of Mrs. Basil E. Frankweiler, Blazing Saddles, At Long Last Love, Young Frankenstein, The Adventures of Sherlock Holmes' Smarter Brother, Won Ton Ton, High Anxiety, The Cheap Detective, Simon, Happy Birthday, Gemini, Wholly Moses, First Family, History of the World—Part I, Yellowbeard, City Heat, Clue.
RECENT THEATRE: In the Boom Boom Room, On the Twentieth Century.
TELEVISION: Oh Madeline!

KAHN, RICHARD: Executive. b. New Rochelle. N.Y., Aug. 29, 1929; e. Wharton School, U. of Penn., B.S., 1951; U.S. Navy, 3 yrs.; joined Buchanan & Co., 1954; ent. m.p. ind., pressbook writer, Columbia Pictures, 1955; exploitation mgr., 1958; natl. coord. adv. and pub., 1963; natl. dir. of adv., pub. and exploitation, 1968; v.p., 1969; 1974 v.p. in chg. of special marketing projects; 1975; moved to MGM as v.p. in chg. of worldwide advertising, publicity and exploitation; 1978, named sr. v.p. in chg. worldwide mktg. & pres., MGM Intl. 1980, elected bd. of governors, m.p. Academy of Arts & Sciences. 1982, named exec. v.p. of adv., pub., promo. for MGM/UA; 1983, formed the Richard Kahn Co., dist. & mktg. consultancy. Elected v.p., M.P. Academy of Arts & Sciences.

KALB, MARVIN: TV news reporter. e. CCNY: Harvard, M.A., 1953, Russian Language School, Middlebury College. Worked for US State Dept., American Embassy, Moscow; CBS News, 1957; writer, reporter-researcher. Where We Stand: reporter-assignment editor; Moscow Bureau Chief, 1960–63; first dip. corres., Washington Bureau, 1963.
BOOKS: Eastern Exposure, Dragon in the Kremlin, A Day in the Life of Ivan Denisovich, Roots of Involvement, The U.S. in Asia, 1784–1971.

KALISH, EDDIE: Executive. Reporter/reviewer, Variety, 1959–64; sr. publicist, Paramount Pictures, 1964–65; adv./pub./promo dir., Ken Greengras Personal Management, 1965–66; pub. dir., Harold Rand & Co., 1966–67; independent publicist overseas, 1967–75; rejoined Paramount Pictures in 1975 as dir. of intl. mktg.; later named v.p.; 1978, named v.p., worldwide pub. & promo. In 1980 appt. senior v.p., mktg. United Artists v.p.—domestic mktg.; sr. v.p., adv., pub., promo, for MGM/UA 1981–82; now sr. v.p., worldwide mkt., PSO, 1982–present.

KALSER, KONSTANTIN: Executive, b. Munich, Germany, Sept. 4, 1920; e. Switzerland, and UCLA in United States. Color photographer, newsreel cameraman, founded Marathon International Prods., Inc., pres., executive producer; Crashing the Water Barrier, 1956 (Acad. Award); Give and Take (Venice Award), The Carmakers, Chris Award. Director, The One for the Road, 1973 Gold Award, Internatl. Film & Festival of N.Y. Director, We Did It! 1978 Gold Medal Intl. Film & TV Festival of N.Y.; Production Executive, The Unknown War 1978 Grand Award, Intl. Film & TV Festival of N.Y. 1984, For Years To Come! (dir., s.p.), winner of CINE Golden Eagle.

KAMBER, BERNARD M.: Executive. e. U. of Pa. New England exploitation rep. U.A. 1940; Army service 1941–43; dir. special events dept. U.A., 1943; asst. to Gradwell L. Sears, nat'l distrib. chmn. 6th War Loan Drive; dir. pub. 7th War Loan Drive, 1943–47; dir. pub. & prom. Eagle Lion Classics, 1951; org. Kamber Org., pub. rel. rep. for ind. prod. v.p. sales, adv. pub. Ivan Tors Prod. Greene-Rouse Prods.; June 1953; exec. asst. Hecht-Hill-Lancaster, chg. of N.Y. off., 1957; v.p. Hecht-Hill-Lancaster Companies, 1958; formed Cinex Distr. Corp., 1962; Pres. Cinex and Posfilm, Inc.; 1967 v.p. in chg. sls. Du Art Film Lab. Inc; 1975 joined Technicolor, Inc.

KAMEY, PAUL: Executive. b. New York, N.Y., Aug. 25, 1912. Worked on newspapers including NY Journal American. Ent. m.p. industry 1938; worked for MGM and 20th Century Fox; during war, writer, Office of War information; joined Universal, 1949; eastern pub. mgr., Universal Pictures. 1968, Freelance publicist.

KAMINS, BERNIE: Publicist. b. Cambridge, Mass., Jan. 2, 1915; e. Harvard U., B.A. Harvard U. corresp. various newspapers and press services while in coll.; joined Russell Birdwell & Assoc., publicists unit man. Paramount studios. Author screen story Forty Thieves; co-author Sky Princess. Dir. adv. & publ. Harry Sherman Prod., then Charles R. Rogers Prod.; apptd. same Principal Artists Prods., April, 1944; later same yr. joined Chas. R. Rogers Prods.; identical posts Cagney Prod. Inter-American Prod., Jesse L. Lasky Prod. Author, The Copy Rider; pub. relations, Hollywood Actors Council; 1951, book, Basic Propaganda; 1953. instructor, propaganda, UCLA; 1953–54 pub. Peter Goelet Ent. Nat'l Bd. of Review of M.P., Inc.; 1954–57. p.r. and exec. v.p. national Audience Board, Inc.; p.d. Clarion Enterprises, 1956; p.d. Romson Productions, 1957; p.r. Guy Madison Prod., 1958; Julian Lesser Prod., Principal Securities, 1959. Pacific Title and Art Studio p.r., Counsel, 1960; elected pres. Opinion Builders, Inc., 1961. Exec. hd. of United Republican Finance Committee of Los Angeles

County, 1962; Buddy Ebsen Enterprises (Turquoise Prods.), 1963; finance pub. rel. counsel. Herts-Lion International Corp., 1963–64; acting P.R. chmn., Republican State finance committee; P.R. chmn., Western US Amer. Jewish Comm., 1964; Publicists Assoc. Awards Comm. 1966–67; V.P. Commu. Rel. South. Calif. Industry-Educ. Council, 1966–68; Co-ord. Harvard Med. School Alumni Assoc. 1967; Exec. Sect. Insurance Research Foundation, 1968. Statewide education comm. of Calif. State Chamber of Commerce. National advisory comm. for UCLA Allied Health Projects Div.; staff, UCLA Alumni & Development; board member, Foundation for California Community Colleges; Advisory board, L.A. City Board-of-Education on Unified School District Proposal for Utilization of UHF-TV Channel 58; Exec. Secty., American Consumers Council, 1966–; Member, general advisory board, Santa Monica College; 1972–; Exec. Secty., Foundation of Oral and Maxillofacial Surgery Inc., 1976–, 1977 appointed to Los Angeles County Youth Commission; 1977—UCLA Chancellor's Associates member. 1978—lecturer on P.R. for Community Organizations, West Los Angeles College. 1979—lecturer, same, Santa Monica College. 1979—Appointed to Board of Directors of International Students Center, UCLA, 1979—Coordinator and public relations consultant, Foundation for Effective Government Inc.

KANANACK, ARTHUR: Executive. e. Cornell Univ.; Cornell Law School. Started in industry in business affairs dept., ABC-TV, New York. Moved to London 1966 with Creative Management Associates (now ICM); returned to N.Y. 1969 to join business affairs dept. of 20th Century Fox. 1971–79, v.p., Warner Bros of business affairs intl., London. 1979–82, V.P., business affairs, WB-TV Distribution. 1982, joined ITC Productions as exec. v.p. 1985, named pres., ITC Entertainment.

KANE, CAROL: Actress. b. Cleveland, Ohio, June 18, 1952. Began professional acting career at age 14, touring in The Prime of Miss Jean Brodie. Other stage credits include, Arturo UI, The Enchanted, The Tempest, Macbeth, Tales of the Vienna Woods, etc.
PICTURES INCLUDE: Wedding in White, The Last Detail, Carnal Knowledge, Hester Street, Dog Day Afternoon, Annie Hall, The World's Greatest Lover, The Muppet Movie, When a Stranger Calls, Over the Brooklyn Bridge, Racing with the Moon, The Secret Diary of Sigmund Freud, Transylvania 6-5000.

KANE, STANLEY D.: Judge. b. Minneapolis, Minn., Dec. 21, 1907; e. U. of Minn., B.A. (magna cum laude, 1930), M.A., 1931; Minn. Coll. of Law, LL.B., 1940. Instructor, U. of Minn., 1930–33; exec. sec. Allied Theatre Owners of the Northwest, 1933–37; city attorney, Golden Valley, Minn., 1940–63; City Atty., Champlin, Minn., 1955–60; on faculty, Minn. Coll. of Law, 1940–44; trial attorney & trial examiner, NLRB, Minneapolis, New Orleans, N.Y., 1943–46; special, gen. counsel, Puerto Rico Labor Relations Bd., 1946; exec. vice-pres. & gen. counsel, North Central Allied Independent Theatre Owners, 1946–63; recording sec. Allied States Assn., 1947 to 1956; Dist. Court Judge, Hennepin County, 1963; elected to 6-yr. term, 1964; re-elected, 1970.

KANIN, FAY: Writer. b. New York, N.Y. e. Elmira Coll., U.S.C., m. Michael Kanin, writer. Contrib. fiction to mags.; mem. and officer of WGA., AMPAS. also bd. mem. of latter.
PICTURES INCLUDE: Blondie for Victory, Sunday Punch, My Pal Gus, Rhapsody, The Opposite Sex, Teacher's Pet, Swordsman of Siena, The Right Approach.
BROADWAY: Goodbye My Fancy, His and Hers, Rashomon, The Gay Life.
TELEVISION: Heat of Anger, CBS Friday Night Movie 1972; Tell Me Where It Hurts, CBS General Electric Theater, 1974.

KANIN, GARSON: Director, writer. b. Rochester, N.Y., Nov. 24, 1912; e. American Acad. Dram. Arts; m. Ruth Gordon, actress. Musician actor, appearing in Spring Song, Little Ol' Boy, and others. Prod. assist. George Abbott on Three Men on a Horse, Brother Rat, Room Service; dir. Hitch Your Wagon, Too Many Heroes, Broadway plays; In June, 1937, Samuel Goldwyn's prod. staff, 1938, joined RKO, prod.-dir. contract. In 1942: prod. for U.S. Office of Emergency Management. Joined armed forces, World War II; co-dir. True Glory.
PICTURES INCLUDE: A Double Life, Adam's Rib, Born Yesterday, Marrying Kind, Pat and Mike, It Should Happen to You, Next Time I Marry, Man to Remember, Great Man Votes, Bachelor Mother, My Favorite Wife, They Knew What They Wanted, Tom, Dick and Harry, From This Day Forward, The Girl Can't Help It, The Rat Race, High Time, The Right Approach, Where It's At, Some Kind of a Nut, Woman of the Year, The More the Merrier.
THEATRE: Born Yesterday, The Smile of the World, The Rat Race, The Live Wire, A Gift of Time, Do Re Mi, Come on Strong, The Amazing Adele, The Good Soup, Dreyfus in Rehearsal. (Writer &/or Dir.) Dir.: The Rugged Path; Years Ago; How I Wonder; The Leading Lady; The Diary of Anne Frank; Into Thin Air; Small War on Murray Hill; Hole in the Head; Sunday in New York; Funny Girl; I Was Dancing; A Very Rich Woman; We Have Always Lived in a Castle; Idiot's Delight; Ho! Ho! Ho!
BOOKS: Remembering Mr. Maugham, Cast of Characters, Tracy and Hepburn; Hollywood; Blow Up A Storm; The Rat Race; A Thousand Summers; One Hell of an Actor; It Takes a Long Time to Become Young; Moviola, Smash, Together Again!, Cordelia.
TELEVISION: Hardhat and Legs (movie); Mr. Broadway (series, 1964).

KANIN, MICHAEL: Writer. b. Rochester, N.Y., Feb. 1, 1910; m. Fay Mitchell. Member SWG, officer; WGA, AMPAS. Commercial artist, musician, N.Y. prior to m.p. career; contrib. fiction mags.; s.p. Panama Lady, They Made Her a Spy, 1939.
PICTURES INCLUDE: Anne of Windy Poplars, Woman of the Year, Sunday Punch, The Cross of Lorraine, Centennial Summer Honeymoon, A Double Life, My Pal Gus, When I Grow Up, Rhapsody, The Opposite Sex, Teacher's Pet, The Right Approach, The Swordsman of Siena, The Outrage, How to Commit Marriage.
BROADWAY: Goodbye My Fancy, Seidman and Son, His and Hers, Rashomon, The Gay Life.

KANTER, HAL: Writer, director, producer. b. Savannah, Ga., Dec. 18, 1918. Writer, Danny Kaye Show, Amos 'n Andy, Bing Crosby Show, Ed Wynn TV Show, 1949; creator, writer, prod., stager, George Gobel Show; writer, Paramount, 1951–54; dir., RKO Radio, 1956; Prod., dir., writer, Kraft Music Hall, 1958–59; exec. prod., TCF-TV; Valentine's Day; writer, prod. dir. Chrysler Theatre 1966–67. Creator W.D.P., Julia, NBC, 1968–71; creator W.D.P., Jimmy Stewart (NBC), 1971. W.P. Many TV specials. 1975–76 exec. prod. All In The Family (CBS). Sup. Prod. Chico & The Man (NBC), 1976–77; exec. prod., WB-TV; 1978; prod./writer, Lucille Ball Prod., 1979–80; dir./writer, ABC TV Movies, 1980; Walt Disney Prods., 1981; Savannah Prods., 1982–86. Writer, AFI Life Achievement Awards: Henry Fonda, Alfred Hitchcock; writer, 21 Annual Academy Awards.
PICTURES INCLUDE: My Favorite Spy, Off Limits, Road to Bali, Casanova's Big Night, About Mrs. Leslie, Money from Home, Artists and Models, Mardi Gras, Rose Tattoo, I Married a Woman, Loving You, Once Upon a Horse, Blue Hawaii, Pocketful of Miracles, Bachelor in Paradise, Move Over, Darling, Dear Brigitte, etc.

KANTER, JAY: Executive. b. 1927. Entered industry with MCA, Inc., where was v.p. Left after more than 20 yrs. to become pres. of First Artists Production Co., Ltd. In 1975 joined 20th-Fox as v.p. prod.; 1976, named sr. v.p., worldwide prod. Named v.p., The Ladd Co., 1979. Joined MGM/UA Entertainment Co. as pres., worldwide prod., Motion Picture Division, 1984. In 1985, named pres., world-wide prod., UA Corp.; now pres., MGM Film Co.

KANTOR, IGO: Producer, Film Editor. b. Vienna Austria, Aug. 18, 1930. e. UCLA, AA. 1950. BS, 1952. MS, 1954. Foreign corres., Portugal magazine, FLAMA, 1949–57, music supvr., Screen Gems, Columbia 1954–63; post-prod. supvr., film ed., features, TV; assoc. prod., 1963–64; prod., exec., International Entertainment Corp., 1965. pres., Synchrofilm, Inc., post-production co. and Duque Films, Inc., production co. 1968–74. 1975—present, produced and edited films. 1982, pres., Laurelwood Prods.
PICTURES INCLUDE: Bye Bye Birdie, Under the Yum Yum Tree, Gidget Goes to Rome, A House Is Not a Home, Pattern for Murder, Willy. Co.-prod., editor: Assault on Agathon (1975); assoc., prod., editor, Dixie Dynamite (1976); prod., editor, music supvr., Kingdom of the Spiders; assoc. prod., The Dark (1977); prod. supvr., Good Luck Miss Wyckoff, (1978); prod., Hardly Working,: (1980); Kill and Kill Again (1981); Mutant (1983), Shaker Run (1985).
TELEVISION: From Hawaii with Love (1984); The Grand Tour (1985); It's a Wonderful World (prod.-dir., 1986; Nasotros Golden Eagle Award (prod., 1986).

KAPLAN, BORIS: Executive. b. New York City, Sept. 23, 1897; m.; e. Coll. of City of New York. General mgr. of Selwyn Theatrical Enterprises, 1925–32. Prod. Plays for legitimate stage, Broadway; joined Paramount Pictures Corp., 1933; head of eastern casting and talent dept., Paramount 1936–62; independent casting dir.; m.p. consultant.

KAPLAN, GABRIEL: Actor/Comedian. b. Brooklyn, N.Y., March 31, 1945. After high school worked as bellboy at Lakewood, N.J. hotel, spending free time studying comedians doing routines. Put together a comedy act, landing engagements in small clubs and coffee houses all over U.S. Made several appearances on Tonight Show, Merv Griffin Show, Mike Douglas Show, etc. Has played Las Vegas clubs.
TV: Welcome Back, Kotter.
PICTURES INCLUDE: Fast Break, Tulips, Nobody's Perfect.

KAPLAN, MURRAY M.: Executive. In motion picture distribution since 1936. Distributor for Warner Bros., Paramount, Monogram, Eagle-Lion, United Artists, Allied Artists, Cinemation Industries. Became independent distributor in 1950, independent producer in 1966. Co-founder of PRO-International Films, 1975; 1978, formed M & M Films, to produce and distribute worldwide. Member: Motion Picture Pioneers of America.

KARLIN, FRED: Composer. Won Academy Award for Best Song for For All We Know (from Lovers and Other Strangers) and Emmy for original music in The Autobiography of Jane Pittman on TV. Adapted Huddie Ledbetter melodies for film Leadbelly.
PICTURES INCLUDE: Up the Down Staircase, Yours, Mine and Ours, The Sterile Cuckoo, Westworld, Gravy Train, Mixed Company, Leadbelly, Loving Couples.

KARLIN, MYRON D.: Executive. b. Revere, Mass., Sept. 21, 1918, e. UCLA. Joined m.p. business in 1946 as gen. mgr. for MGM in Ecuador. Two yrs. later assigned same spot for MGM in Venezuela. In 1952–53 was gen. sales mgr. for MGM in Germany, after which held same post in Argentina, returning to Germany as mgr. dir. in 1956. Named mgn. dir. for United Artists in Italy. 1960–68 was pres. of Brunswick Int'l., while also serving as advisor to World Health Organization and UNESCO. In 1969 was European mgr. for MGM and mgn. dir. in Italy. Joined Warner Bros. Int'l. in May, 1970 as v.p. of European dist. In March, 1972 appt. v.p. in chg. of int'l. operations for WB; 1977, appt. pres., WB Intl. & exec. v.p., Warner Bros., Inc; 1985, named exec. v.p., intl. affairs, WB, Inc.

KARRAS, ALEX: Actor. b. Gary, IN, July 15, 1935. e. Iowa Univ. Former professional football player.
PICTURES: Blazing Saddles, Another Day at the Races, Jacob Two-Two Meets the Hooded Fang, When Time Ran Out, Nobody's Perfekt, Victor, Victoria.
TELEVISION: Movies: Hardcase, The 500-Pound Jerk, Babe, Mulligan's Stew, Mad Bull, Centennial. Series: Webster.

KASDAN, LAWRENCE: Writer-Director. b. West Virginia. e. Univ. of Michigan. In advertising before becoming screen writer. Became director with Body Heat (1981).
PICTURES INCLUDE: The Empire Strikes Back (co-s.p.); Raiders of the Lost Ark (s.p.); Continental Divide (s.p.); Return of the Jedi (co-s.p.); Body Heat (dir., s.p.); The Big Chill (co-exec. prod., dir., co-s.p.); Silverado (prod., dir., co-s.p.).

KASLOFF, STEVE: Executive. b. New York City, Nov. 13, 1952. e. Pratt Institute (1974, cum laude). Writer/supvr., Young & Rubicam, 1974–76; writer/sprv., Ally & Gargano, 1976; writer/supvr., Marsteller Inc., 1976–79; writer/creative supvr., Scali, McCabe, Sloves, 1979–82. hired as youngest v.p., Columbia Pictures, 1982; promoted to sr. v.p., creative dir., Columbia, 1983.
AWARDS: Winner of numerous Clio Awards when at ad agencies and over 100 other awards & medals for creative work (trailers, TV commercials, radio commercials, posters, etc.) on such films as Body Double, Tootsie, Karate Kid, Ghostbusters, Soldier's Story, Agnes of God, etc. Has directed stage production (Wait Until Dark), and commercials & special teaser trailers. Now working on screenplay.

KASTNER, ELLIOTT: Executive. b. N.Y.C. Was agent before becoming indep. prod., financing and personally producing 23 feature films in 9 yrs. Based in London.
PICTURES INCLUDE: Harper, Kaleidoscope, Sweet November, Laughter in the Dark, Where Eagles Dare, When Eight Bells Toll, X, Y, Zee, The Nightcomers, Fear Is The Key, The Long Goodbye, Cops and Robbers, Jeremy, 11 Harrowhouse, Rancho Deluxe, 92 in the Shade (exec. prod.,) The Missouri Breaks (co-prod.), Equus (co-prod.), The Big Sleep (co-prod.); ffolkes (prod.); Death Valley (prod.); Man, Woman, and Child (prod.); Garbo Talks (co-prod.).

KATLEMAN, HARRIS L.: Executive. b. Omaha, Neb., Aug. 19, 1928. e. U.C.L.A. (B.A. in Admin., 1949). Joined MCA in 1949; in 1952 transferred to N.Y. as head of TV Packaging Dept. Left to join Goodson-Todman Prods. in 1955, where named v.p., 1956; exec. v.p., 1958; sr. exec. v.p., 1968. Was directly responsible for all film prod. in L.A., including such shows as The Rebel, Branded, The Richard Boone Show (Emmy nominations, Fame Award of Year), and Don Rickles Show, on which was exec. prod. Joined Metro-Goldwyn-Mayer in 1972 as v.p. of MGM-TV; promoted following year to pres., MGM-TV and sr. v.p. of MGM, Inc. Resigned as pres., MGM-TV September, 1977. Formed Bennett/Katleman Productions under contract to Columbia Pictures. Exec. prod.: From Here to Eternity, Salvage 1; 1980, named bd. chm. 20th-Fox Television.

KATSELAS, MILTON: Director. b. Pittsburgh. e. drama dept. Carnegie Tech (now Carnegie Mellon Univ.). Has directed more than 30 stage prods., including in New York, The Rose Tattoo and Camino Real (both revivals), The Zoo Story, Butterflies Are Free, etc.
PICTURES INCLUDE: Butterflies Are Free (debut), 40 Carats, Report to the Commissioner, When You Comin' Back, Red-Ryder.

KATT, WILLIAM: Actor. Son of Barbara Hale and Bill Williams. e. Orange Coast College. Majored in music, playing piano and guitar. Acted with South Coast Repertory Theatre, later working in production at the Abmanson and Mark Taper Theatres in L.A. Made theatrical film debut in Carrie.
PICTURES INCLUDE: Carrie, First Love, Big Wednesday, Butch and Sundance: The Early Days, Baby, House.
TELEVISION: Perry Mason Returns.

KATZ, GLORIA: Producer-Writer. e. UCLA Film School. Joined Universal Pictures as editor, cutting educational films. Later joined forces with Willard Huyck, whom she had met at UCLA. Pair signed by Francis Ford Coppola to write and direct for his newly created company, American Zoetrope. Projects didn't materialize but Katz and Huyck teamed to write script for America Graffiti for director Paul Lucas. Wrote Lucky Lady (1975) together. Katz made debut as producer with French Postcards in 1979 which co-wrote with Huyck, who directed.
PICTURES: Indiana Jones and the Temple of Doom (co.-s.p.); The Best Defense (prod., co.-s.p.); Howard the Duck (prod., co.-s.p.).

KATZ, MARTY: Executive. b. Landsburg, West Germany, Sept. 2, 1947. e. UCLA, Univ. of Maryland. Served in Vietnam War as U.A. Army first lt.; awarded Bronze Star as combat pictorial unit director. 1971, dir. of film prod., ABC Circle Films; 1976, exec. v.p., prod., Quinn Martin Prods.; 1978–80, prod. consultant, prod., Paramount Pictures' 1981–85, independent producer (Lost in America, Heart Like a Wheel, etc.). 1985, joined Walt Disney Prods. as sr. v.p., m.p. & tv prod.

KATZ, NORMAN B.: Executive. b. Scranton, Penna., Aug. 23, 1919. e. Columbia Univ. In U.S. Army 1941–46 as intelligence officer, airborne foices. Entered m.p. industry in 1947 with Discina Films, Paris, France, as prod. asst. Named exec. asst. to head of prod. in 1948. In 1950 named v.p. Discina Int'l. Films and in 1952 exec. v.p. In 1954 joined Associated Artists Prods. as foreign mgr.; named dir. of foreign operation in 1958. In 1959 became dir. of foreign operations for United Artists Associated. 1961 joined Seven Arts Associated Corp. of v.p. in chg. of foreign operations; named exec. v.p., Seven Arts Prods. Int'l. in 1964. Named exec. v.p. Warner Bros.—Seven Arts Int'l. in 1967. In 1969 appt. exec. v.p. and chief exec. off. Warner Bros. International and bd. mem. of Warner Bros. Inc. In 1974 named snr. v.p. int'l. div. of American Film Theatre. Pres. of Cinema Arts Associated Corp. 1979, exec. v.p. and bd. member, American Communications Industries and pres., chief exec. off. of ACI subsidiary, American Cinema; 1983, pres., The NORKAT Co., Also, bd. chm., CEO, American Film Mktg. Assoc., 1985–87.

KATZENBERG, JEFF: Executive. b. 1951. Pres., production, for the motion picture division of Paramount Pictures. Joined co. in 1975 in New York as asst. to chm., Barry Diller. 1977, became exec. dir. of mktg.; later same year moved to west coast as v.p. of programming for Paramount TV. May, 1978, promoted to v.p., feature production, for Paramount Pictures. July, 1980, promoted to sr. v.p. prod. of m.p. div. in 1982. Left in 1984 to join Walt Disney Prods. as pres., motion pictures & TV.

KAUFMAN, HAL: Creative director, TV writer-producer. b. New York, N.Y., Dec. 16, 1924; e. U. of Texas. 1943–44; U. of Michigan. 1944–47. Started career as petroleum geologist, Western Geophysical Co., 1947–48; TV writer-prod-dir., KDYL-TV, Salt Lake City, 1948–49; prog. dir., WLAV-TV, Grand Rapids, 1949–51; prod. mgr., WOOD-TV, Grand Rapids, 1951–54; Radio-TV dir., Webber Advertising Agency, Grand Rapids, 1951–54; TV writer-prod., Leo Burnett Company, Chicago, 1954–56; TV writer-prod., Gordon Best Company, Chicago, 1956–59; senior writer, TV/Radio creative dept., Needham, Louis & Brorby, Inc., 1959; vice-pres., asst. copy dir., Needham, Louis & Brorby, Inc., 1962; dir., TV, Radio prod., Needham, Louis & Brorby, Inc., 1963; dir., broadcast design, production, Needham, Louis & Brorby, Inc., 1964; assoc. creat. dir., asst. Exec. v.p., Needham, Harper & Steers, Inc., 1965; Creat. dir. L.A., 1966; Sr. v.p. and Member Bd. of Dir., 1966. Aug. 1969, creative & marketing consultant in Beverly Hills. Aug., 1970 v.p., principle, Kaufman, Vinson, Lansky Inc., Beverly Hills and San Diego; Aug. '72, Exec. V.P., principle, Kaufman, Lansky Advertising, Inc., Los Angeles and San Diego, Member, Directors Guild of America, SAG, AFTRA. 1979, program dir., Z Channel, Theta Cable TV. 1979 named snr. v.p./adv. & p.r. & asst. to pres. & bd. chmn., World Airways, Inc.; 1981–pres. Hal Kaufman Inc., mktg. & adv. consultant; 1982–v.p., Creative director, Admarketing, Inc., Los Angeles; 1985, mktg. & adv. consultant; copy dir., Teleflora, Inc.

KAUFMAN, J. L. (Les): Publicist. b. Chicago, Ill., June 3: e. Morgan Park (Ill.) Military Acad. Police reporter, City News Bureau, Chicago. In 1926 adv. dept., Balaban & Katz Theats. In 1929 pub. Paramount Public Theats. To Columbia, 1933 asst. exploit, dir. In 1938 adv. & pub. dir., Fanchon & Marco Serv. Corp., St. Louis. Adv.-pub. dir., Republic Studios, 1944–46; Nat'l. adv. pub. dir., International Pictures Corp. In 1947 named studio pub. dir., Universal-International; sales prom. counsel, Kaiser-Frazer Corp., 1950; v.p. in chge. West Coast, Ettinger Co., 1950; v.p. Grant Adv. Inc., Hollywood, Detroit, 1952–55; v.p., adv. dir., UPA Pictures, Inc., 1956; P.R. dir., Fedderson Productions & Lawrence Welk, 1957–83; My Three Sons, Hollywood Palladium, 1961, Family Affair, To Rome with Love. The Smith Family; pres., Hollywood Press Club, 1964–65, 1967–68. Bd. governors—NATVAS, Hollywood chapter. Director/promotion, Nederlander Companies, 1983.

KAUFMAN, LEONARD B.: Producer, writer, director. b. Newark, N.J., Aug. 31. e. N.Y.U. In World War II served with Army Special Services writing and directing camp shows. Nat'l magazine writer, 1945–48; radio writer, including Errol Flynn Show, 1948–50; radio and TV writer, 1950–52. Headed own public relations firm: Kaufman, Schwartz, and Associates, 1952–64. Joined Ivan Tors Films as writer-prod., 1964. Films Corp., 1958.
PICTURES INCLUDE: Clarence, the Cross-eyed Lion, Birds Do It, Story.
TV: Daktari, Ivan Tors' Jambo, O'Hara, U.S. Treasury (CBS) pilot feature and series for Mark VII Prods.

KAUFMAN, PHILIP: Writer-Director. b. Chicago, Oct. 23, 1936. e. Univ. of Chicago, Harvard Law School. Was teacher in Europe before turning to film medium.
PICTURES INCLUDE: Goldstein, Fearless Frank, The Great Northfield, Minnesota Raid, The White Dawn, Invasion of the Body Snatchers, The Wanderers, The Right Stuff.

KAUFMANN, CHRISTINE: Actress. b. Lansdorf, Graz, Austria, Jan. 11, 1945. e. attended school in Munich, Germany. Film debut as a dancer. Salto Mortale at 7 yrs of age.
PICTURES INCLUDE: Rosenrosli (Little Rosie), Schweigende Engel (Silent Angel), Maedchen in Uniform, Winter Vacation, The Last Days of Pompeii, Red Lips, Town Without Pity, Taras Bulba (first American-made film), Murder in the Rue Morgue.

KAVANAGH, DECLAN M.: Executive. b. Hollywood, CA Oct. 29, 1956. e. Calif State Univ. (BA, acct. & mktg.); Univ. of So. Calif. (MBA). Co-producer of original Jane Fonda Workout, 1981; founded Video Associates (formerly Video Odyssey), 1981; co-producer home video, Everyday with Richard Simmons, 1982; organized first home video dist. deal with V.C.I. and Media Home Entertainment, 1983; founded Active Home Video, 1984; produced Bruce Jenner Winning Workout, 1984; sold Active Home Video, 1985. Now v.p. mktg. & sls., Video Associates, Inc.

KAY, EDWARD: Musical director, composer. b. New York City, Nov. 27, 1898; e. U. of Pennsylvania; later musical study. Became musical director, vaudeville, New York stage productions; similar work in radio. Musical director, Gaumont-British, 1932–33. To Hollywood, 1933, as musical director, Paramount, Allied Artists.
PICTURES INCLUDE: Highway Dragnet, Thunder Pass, Treasure of Ruby Hills, Big Tip Off, Las Vegas Shakedown, Betrayed Women, Night Freight, Toughest Man Alive.

KAY, GILBERT LEE: Director-Writer. b. Chicago, Ill., June 28. e. Los Angeles City Coll. Was asst. dir. at various studios from 1942–53; started directing on own in 1954. Formed Pearly Gate Productions, London.
PICTURES INCLUDE: Three Bad Sisters, The Tower, Ocean's 11 (s.p.), Comeback, (s.p.), Take Five (s.p.), Fame! (s.p.), Anything for Money (s.p.), The Wrong Mrs. Wright, Now It Can Be Told (s.p.), It Happened in Lisbon (s.p.), The Secret Door, A Harvest of Evil (s.p., dir.), Sometimes I Love You (s.p.), White Comanche, Ragan, Devil May Care, Maybe September (s.p.), Recent screenplays: The Oedipus Vendetta, The Lotus Affair, Candle in the Wind, Royal Flush.
TV: Directed: Treasury Men in Action, Man Behind the Badge, Reader's Digest, Passport To Danger, Hollywood Profile, Highway Patrol, Arabian Nights, Telephone Time, Silent Service, The Grey Ghost, Man with a Camera, Adventures in Paradise, Shotgun Slade, Perry Mason, Follow the Sun, Frontier Circus. Wrote: The Uncivil Engineer, 8:46 to Southampton.
PLAYS: Directed: Two Faced Coin, Some Call It Love, French without Tears, Burlesque, London by Night, The Man from Madrid, Paris, With Love. Wrote and Directed: West End, Please Omit Flowers, The Girl From Soho.

KAY, GORDON: Producer. b. Montreal, Canada, Sept. 6, 1916; e. Williams Coll. (Mass.); married. Asst. prod. Republic 1946, assoc. prod., 1947. apptd. secy.-treas.; exec. asst. to head of prod. at Republic, Feb., 1951; prod., Univ. 1955; pres. Gordon Kay & Assoc., 1958.
PICTURES INCLUDE: Wild Frontier, Bandits of Dark Canyon, Oklahoma Badlands, Bold Frontiersman, He Rides Tall, Fluffy, Taggart, Gunpoint, Beardless Warriors.

KAYAMA, YUZO: Actor. b. April 11, 1937. e. law school Keio Univ. Debut Toho Studio 1959 in Man Against Man.
PICTURES INCLUDE: Westward desperado, Man from the East, Blood in the Sea, Three Dolls series, Bull of Ginza, Tsubaki Sanjuro.

KAYE, DANNY: Actor. b. Brooklyn, N.Y., Jan. 18, 1913. On stage summer theatres; toured U.S. in act La Vie Paree; in night clubs; toured Orient, 1934; m.p. debut in Up in Arms, 1944; formed prod. co. Nov., 1952; Ambassador-at-Large UNICEF-U.N. Children's Fund. Recipient of Scopus Laureate for 1977; first award for International Distinguished Service from the United Nations Children's Fund; Honorary Degree from Colgate University, Doctor of Humane Letters.
TV: The Secret Life of Danny Kaye, numerous Danny Kaye Specials, Danny Kaye Show. Danny Kaye's "Look In" at Metropolitan Opera since 1973; televised, 1975; Pinocchio, 1976; Skokie, 1981; Live from Lincoln Center, 1981.
BROADWAY: Straw Hat Revue, Play's The Thing, Death Takes a Holiday, Lady in the Dark, Let's Face It, Two by Two, 1970–71.
PICTURES INCLUDE: Wonder Man, Kid from Brooklyn, Secret Life of Walter Mitty, Song Is Born, Inspector General, On the Riviera, Han Christian Anderson, Knock on Wood, White Christmas, Court Jester, Merry Andrew, The Five Pennies, On the Double, Man for the Diner's Club, The Madwoman of Chaillot.

KAZAN, ELIA: Director. b. Constantinople, Turkey, Sept. 7, 1909; e. Williams Coll., Yale Dramatic School. With Group Theatre as apprentice & stage mgr.; on stage, 1934–41; plays include: Waiting for Lefty, Golden Boy, Gentle People, Five-Alarm Lilliom; m.p. acting debut in Blues in the Night, 1941; stage dir.; won Critics Award best direction of Skin of Our Teeth. All My Sons, Streetcar Named Desire, Death of a Salesman, Cat on a Hot Tin Roof; also dir.: One Touch of Venus, Harriet, Jocobowsky and the Colonel, Tea and Sympathy, Dark at the Top of the Stairs, J.B., Sweet Bird of Youth; co-dir., prod., Lincoln Center Repertory Theatre; dir., After The Fall, But For Whom Charlie; m.p. dir., 1944; Academy Award best direction, 1947, for Gentleman's Agreement; author novel, The Arrangement. 1967–68, novel, The Assassins; 1974 novel, The Understudy.
PICTURES INCLUDE: City of Conquest, Tree Grows in Brooklyn, Boomerang, Sea of Grass, Panic in the Streets, Pinky, Streetcar Named Desire, Viva Zapata, Man on a Tightrope, On the Waterfront (Acad. Award, best dir., 1954), East of Eden, Baby Doll, Face in the Crowd, Wild River, Splendor In the Grass, America, America, The Arrangement, The Visitors, The Last Tycoon.

KAZAN, LAINIE: Singer-Actress. b. New York City, May 15, 1943. e. Hofstra Univ. On stage and performed in niteries.
PICTURES: Romance of a Horse Thief, Lady in Cement, Dayton's Devils, One from the Heart, May Favorite Year, Lust in the Dust, The Delta Force.
TELEVISION: A Cry for Love, Sunset Limousine, The Jerk Too, Obsessive Love.

KEACH, STACY: Actor-Director-Producer. b. Savannah, GA. 1942. Began professional acting career as Marcellus, Player King in Joseph Papp's 1964 production of Hamlet in Central Park. Performances since have won three Obie Awards, Vernon Rice Drama Desk Award for Macbird, Drama Desk Award, Tony Nomination for Indians and include Peer Gynt, Hamlet, Cyrano de Bergerac, Barnum and Hughie, Deathtrap.
PICTURES: The Heart Is a Lonely Hunter, End of the Road, The Traveling Executioner, Brewster McCloud, Doc, Judge Roy Bean, The New Centurions, Fat City, The Killer Inside Me, Conduct Unbecoming, Luther, Street People, The Squeeze, Gray Lady Down, The Ninth Configuration, Longriders, (also exec. prod.), Road Games, Butterfly, Up in Smoke, Nice Dreams, That Championship Season.
TELEVISION: Caribe, The Blue and the Gray, Princess Daisy, Murder Me, Murder You, More Than Murder, Wait Until Dark, Mistral's Daughter, Mickey Spillane's Mike Hammer. Director: Incident at Vichy, Six Characters in Search of an Author.
STAGE: Long Day's Journey into Night, Macbird, Indians, Hamlet, Deathtrap, Hughie, Barnum, Cyrano de Bergerac, Peer Gynt, Henry IV Parts I & II, Idiot's Delight.

KEACH, SR., STACY: Executive. b. Chicago, May 29, 1914. Father of actors, Stacy and James. e. Northwestern Univ. (MA). Was instructor in theatre arts at Northwestern and Armstrong College and dir. at Pasadena Playhouse before entering industry. For 4½ yrs. was under contract at Universal Pictures; 3 yrs. at RKO; had own productions on NBC, CBS. In 1946 began producing and directing industrial stage presentations for Union Oil Co. and from then on became full-time prod. of m.p. and stage industrial shows. In 1946 formed Stacy Keach Productions, of which he is pres. In addition to directing, producing and writing he occasionally appears as actor in films. Plays Clarence Birds Eye on TV commercials.

KEATON, DIANE: Actress. b. Santa Ana, CA, 1949. e. Santa Ana College. Appeared in summer stock and studied at Neighborhood Playhouse in N.Y. Made prof. debut in Bdwy. prod. of Hair (1968); then co-starred with Woody Allen in Play It Again, Sam, repeating role for film version.
PICTURES INCLUDE: Lovers and Other Strangers, The Godfather, Play It Again, Sam, Sleeper, The Godfather, Part II, Love and Death, I Will . . . I Will . . . for Now, Harry and Walter Go to New York, Annie Hall, Looking for Mr. Goodbar, Interiors, Manhattan, Reds, Shoot the Moon, The Little Drummer Girl, Mrs. Soffel, Crimes of the Heart.

KEATON, MICHAEL: Actor. b. Pittsburgh, PA, Sept. 9, 1951. Started career as stand-up comic.
PICTURES: Night Shift, Mr. Mom, Johnny Dangerously, Touch and Go, Gung Ho.

KEEL, HOWARD: Actor. r.n. Harold Keel. b. Gillespie, Ill., April 13, 1917. e. high school, Fallbrook, Calif.; m. Helen Anderson, dancer; d. Kaiye Liana. Stage and screen. Began career following George Walker scholarship award for singing, L.A.; appeared in plays, Pasadena Auditorium, concerts; won awards, Mississippi Valley and Chicago Musical Festivals. Stage debut: Carousel, 1945; principal role (Oklahoma). Screen debut, The Small Voice, London, 1948.
PICTURES INCLUDE: Annie Get Your Gun, Pagan Love Song, Three Guys Named Mike, Show Boat, Texas Carnival, Callaway Went Thataway, Lovely to Look At, Desperate Search, Ride Vaquero, Fast Company, Kiss Me Kate, Calamity Jane, Rose Marie, Seven Brides for Seven Brothers, Deep in My Heart, Jupiter's Darling, Kismet, Floods of Fear, Big Fisherman, Armored Command, Arizona Bushwackers.
PLAYS: Saratoga, No Strings.
TELEVISION: Dallas.

KEESHAN, BOB: Performer. b. Lynbrook, N.Y., June 27, 1927. e. Fordham U. As network page boy became assistant to Howdy Doody's Bob Smith and originated role of Clarabelle the Clown; created children's programs Time for Fun (1953), Tinker's Workshop (1954), Captain Kangaroo (1955), Mister Mayor, 1965.

KEITEL, HARVEY: Actor. b. Brooklyn, N.Y., 1941 Served in U.S. Marine Corps. Over 10 yrs. experience in summer stock repertory and little theatre after study at Actors Studio with Lee Strasberg and Frank Corsaro. Read for male lead in collegiate film prod. of Who's That Knocking at My Door?; Martin Scorsese, director, gave him the role. Has since become repertory member of Scorsese films.
PICTURES INCLUDE: Who's That Knocking at My Door?, Street Scenes, Mean Streets, Alice Doesn't Live Here Anymore, Taxi Driver, Mother, Jugs and Speed, Welcome to L.A., The Duellists, Fingers, Blue Collar, Bad Timing, The Border, Exposed, Falling in Love, Off Beat, Wise Guys, The Men's Club.

KEITH, BRIAN: Actor. b. Bayonne, N.J., Nov. 14, 1921; p. Robert Keith, actor. U.S. Marines, 1942–45; worked in stock co., radio shows, comm. films for TV; on B'way in Mr. Roberts, Darkness at Noon; dramatic TV shows including: Studio One, Suspense, Philco Playhouse, star of Crusader; m.p. debut in Arrowhead. Recent TV: Hardcastle and McCormick.
PICTURES INCLUDE: Jivaro, Alaska Seas, Bamboo Prison, Violent Men, Tight Spot, Five Against the House, Storm Center, Run of the Arrow, Nightfall, Sierra Baron, Those Calloways, The Raiders, The Young Philadelphians, Dino, A Tiger Walks, The Parent Trap, The Hallelujah Trail, Rare Breed, Nevada Smith, Reflections in a Golden Eye, Krakatoa, East of Java, Gaily, Gaily, Suppose They Gave a War and Nobody Came, McKenzie Break, Scandalous John, Something Big, The Yakuza, The Wind and the Lion, Nickelodeon, Hooper, Meteor, Charlie Chan and the Curse of the Dragon Queen, Sharkey's Machine.

KEITH, DAVID: Actor. b. Knoxville, TN, 1955. e. Univ. of Tenn., where majored in drama. Appearance at Goodspeed Opera House in musical led to role in CBS sitcom pilot, Co-Ed Fever. Followed by first film role in The Rose with Bette Midler.
PICTURES: The Great Santini, Brubaker, Back Roads, Take This Job and Shove It, An Officer and a Gentleman, Lords of Discipline, Independence Day, Firestarter.
TELEVISION: Friendly Fire, Gulag. Mini-Series: Golden Moment, If Tomorrow Comes.

KELLER, HARRY: Prod.-dir. b. Los Angeles, Calif., Feb. 22, 1913. Film ed., Nat'l Screen Service, Universal, Republic, 1936–50; dir., Republic 1950–53; TV dir., Loretta Young show, 1954–55; dir., Univ. Int., 1956–57; dir. Walt Disney, 1958–59; dir., Universal, 1960–62; for Univ. Prod-Dir. 1963–69; prod., WB, 1970–71.
PICTURES INCLUDE: The Unguarded Moment, Brass Bottle, Send Me No Flowers, That Funny Feeling, Voice in the Mirror, Tammy Tell Me True, Mirage, Texas Across the River, In Enemy Country, Skin Game.

KELLER, MARTHE: Actress. b. Switzerland, 1946. Started acting in France and attracted attention of U.S. directors after appearing in Claude Lelouch's And Now My Love.
PICTURES INCLUDE: The Devil by the Tail (debut), And Now my Love, Marathon Man, Black Sunday, Bobby Deerfield, Fedora, The Formula, The Amateur, Wagner, Femmes de Personne.

KELLERMAN, SALLY: Actress. b. Long Beach, Calif., June 2, 1936. e. Hollywood High. Studied acting in N.Y. at the Actors Studio and in Hollywood with Jeff Corey.
TV: Mannix, It Takes a Thief, Chrysler Theatre.
PICTURES INCLUDE: The Boston Strangler, The April Fools, M*A*S*H*, Brewster McCloud, Last of the Red Hot Lovers, Lost Horizon, Slither, Rafferty and the Gold Dust Twins, The Big Bus, Welcome to L.A., A Little Romance, Foxes, Loving Couples, Moving Violations, Back to School, That's Life.

KELLEY, DeFOREST: Actor. b. Atlanta, GA, Jan. 20, 1920.
PICTURES: Fear in the Night, Canon City, The Men, House of Bamboo, Man in the Gray Flannel Suit, Tension at Table Rock, Gunfight at the O.K. Corral, Raintree County, The Law and Jake Wade, Warlock, Where Love Has Gone, Marriage on the Rocks, Star Trek—The Motion Picture, Star Trek II—The Wrath of Khan, Star Trek III: The Search for Spock, Star Trek IV: The Voyage Home.
TELEVISION: Star Trek.

KELLEY PATRICK: Executive. Joined MCA in 1950 as agent; with them for 20 years; named v.p. in chg. of talent for Universal's theatrical and TV project in 1964. Left MCA in 1970 to form First Artists with star partners Barbra Streisand, Sidney Poitier, Paul Newman (later joined by Steve McQueen and Dustin Hoffman). Resigned 1975 as F.A. bd. chmn. to head Pan Arts Corp., prod. co. of which George Roy Hill is bd. chmn.
PICTURES INCLUDE: A Little Romance (exec. prod.), The Little Drummer Girl (exec. prod.).

KELLOGG, PHILIP M.: executive. b. March 17, 1912, Provo, Wash. e. UCLA. Special feature writer for Hearst papers and magazines, 1933–34; MGM story dept., production dept., Irving Thalberg unit, 1934–35; Warner Bros. Film editor, 1935–41; Berg-Allenberg Agency, 1941–50; U.S. Naval Reserve officer, 1941–46; William Morris Agency, 1950–present, co-head of m.p. dept., dir. WMA, Ltd., London.

KELLY, GABRIELLE: Producer. b. Ireland. e. Univ. of Sussex. Moved to U.S. in 1975, working at the New York Review of Books before going into independent film production. Has worked with producers Jay Presson Allen, Burtt Harris and director Sidney Lumet, optioning, developing and producing projects. Co-producer of D.A.R.Y.L.

KELLY, GENE: Actor. b. Pittsburgh, Pa., Aug. 23, 1912. e. Penn State U., U. Pittsburgh. Bricklayer, concrete mixer, soda clerk, dance instructor before going on stage, in N.Y. prods. (Leave It to Me, One for the Money, The Time of Your Life, Pal Joey). On screen 1942 in For Me and My Gal; Summer Stock.
PICTURES INCLUDE: Pilot No. 5, Du Barry Was a Lady, Thousands Cheer, The Cross of Lorraine, Christmas Holiday, Anchors Aweigh, Cover Girl, Ziegfeld Follies, Pirate, Three Musketeers, Words and Music, Take Me Out to the Ball Game, Black Hand, On the Town, An American in Paris, Singin' in the Rain, It's A Big Country, Devil Makes Three, Brigadoon, Crest of the Wave, Deep in My Heart, Invitation to the Dance, It's Always Fair Weather, The Happy Road, Les Girls, Special Academy Award for advancing dance films, Gigot, A Guide for the Married Man, The Young Girls of Rochefort, Hello, Dolly!, The Cheyenne Social Club, 40 Carats, That's Entertainment, That's Entertainment, Part Two, Viva, Knievel!, Xanadu, That's Dancing.
TELEVISION: Sins.

KELLY, JIM: Actor. b. Paris, Ky. e. Univ. of Louisville. Studied karate at univ., winning trophies and int'l. middleweight championship. Opened school for karate in L.A. Did modelling and TV commercials. Was technical advisor for fight scenes on Melinda and played role in it.
PICTURES INCLUDE: Enter the Dragon (debut), Black Belt Jones, Three the Hard Way.

KELLY, NANCY: Actress. b. Lowell, Mass., March 25, 1921. e. Immaculate Conception Acad., N.Y.; St. Lawrence Acad., L.I.; Bentley Sch. for Girls. In number of pictures as child, and on stage in Susan and God (N.Y. prod. 1937). In 1938 on screen.

PICTURES INCLUDE: Torando, Women in Bondage, Gamblers Choice, Show Business, Double Exposure, Song of the Sarong, Woman Who Came Back, Murder in the Music Hall, Crowded Paradise, Bad Seed.
STAGE: Season in the Sun, 1950–51; Bad Seed, 1954–55.

KEMENY, JOHN: Producer. b. Budapest, Hungary. Producer for National Film Board of Canada, 1957–69. Formed International Cinemedia Center, Ltd. in 1969 in Montreal, as partner.
PICTURES INCLUDE: The Apprenticeship of Duddy Kravits, White Line Fever, Shadow of the Hawk, La Castles, Bay Boy.

KEMP, JEREMY: Actor. b. Chesterfield, England, Feb. 3, 1935. e. Abbottsholme School, Central School of Speech and Drama. Service with Gordon Highlanders. Early career on stage incl. Old Vic Theatre Company, 1959–61. Recent theatre: Celebration, Incident at Vichy, Spoiled, The Caretaker. National Theatre, 1979–80.
TV: Z Cars, The Lovers of Florence, The Last Reunion, Colditz, Brassneck, Rhinemann Exchange, Lisa, Goodbye, Henry VIII, St. Joan, The Winter's Tale, Unity, The Contract, Winds of War, Sadat, King Lear, Sherlock Holmes, George Washington, Peter the Great.
PICTURES INCLUDE: Cast a Giant Shadow, Operation Crossbow, The Blue Max, Assignment K, Twist of Sand, Strange Affair, Darling Lilli, The Games, The Saltzburg Connection, The Blockhouse, The Bellstone Fox, 7% Solution, A Bridge Too Far, East of Elephant Rock, Caravans, The Prisoner of Zenda, The Return of the Soldier, Top Secret!

KEMPER, VICTOR: Cinematographer.
PICTURES: Oh, God!, Hospital, The Candidate, The Jerk, Mr. Mom, Eyes of Laura Mars, National Lampoon's Vacation, The Friends of Eddie Coyle, The Four Seasons, Dog Day Afternoon, Husbands, Pee Wee's Big Adventure, Clue, etc.

KEMP-WELCH, JOAN: Free lance, TV director-producer, actress. First appearance on stage 1927. Subsequently many stage parts and stage directorial assignments. First appeared in films 1938. Films included 60 Glorious Years, They Flew Alone, The Citadel, Busman's Honeymoon. Over 200 repertory and touring productions. West End theatre prods. include: Dead on Nine, Vicious Circle, Our Town, Desire Under the Elms. Since 1954 TV dir. Received TV Oscar for Light Entert., 1958. Desmond Davis Award for services to TV 1963. Silver Dove Monte Carlo Award, 1961 for Electra. The Lover, awarded Prix Italia 1963 (drama). Many other productions, incl. musicals, ballet, dramas, series, outside broadcasts. Dear Octupus, The Birthday Party, The Collection, View from the Bridge, Electra, 3 Sisters, A Midsummer Nights Dream, Dangerous Corner. Upstairs, Downstairs; prod. Armchair Theatre, 1973–74. 1974–75. French Without Tears, Wait Till Dark, The Price, Cranford Musical. 1976: The Other Side of the Swamp, TV. Romeo & Juliet. 1977 in S. Africa. Deep Blue Sea, The Kingfisher, The Monkey Walk in Vienna, The Circle 1978 Hay Fever. TV Hay Fever, London, It Happened in Harrods 1979. A Man & His Wife, You Can't Take it With You, In South Africa, Home. Cause Celebre your Place or Mine, TV. The Piano 1980 Shades of Brown, Winter Journey, I Am Who I Am, TV Lady Killers. In S. Africa The Elocution of Benjamin Franklyn, The Unvarnished Truth 1981. Pitlochry. Gaslight & The Unvarnished Truth. S. Africa Happy Birthday in Vienna, Murder at the Viccarage, Revival. Other Side of the Swamp, 1982. Vienna. Dangerous Corner. Arsnic & Old Lace, The Killing of Sister George. 1983 in Australia On the Razzle, Romeo & Juliet. Tales from Chekov in New York. Shades of Brown. 1984: On Golden Pond, The Voices in S. Africa; Sleuth in Vienna; An Inspector Calls in Cincinnati, USA; West Side Waltz, The Amorous Prawn, Outside Edge.

KENNEDY, ARTHUR: Actor. b. Worcester, Mass., February 17, 1914; p. Dr. and Mrs. J. T. Kennedy; e. Carnegie Institute of Technology; m. Mary Cheffey, prof. Has worked for George M. Cohan; Guthrie McClintic, Marc Connelly and others well known to theatregoers. Film debut: City for Conquest.
PICTURES INCLUDE: Champion, They Died With Their Boots On, High Sierra, Strange Alibi, Knockout, Highway West, Air Force, Devotion, Boomerang, The Window, Chicago Deadline, The Glass Menagerie, Red Mountain, Bright Victory, Bend of the River, Rancho Notorious, Girl in White, Lusty Men, Man from Laramie, Trial, Naked Dawn, Desperate Hours, Crashout, Rawhide Years, Peyton Place, Some Came Running, Claudelle Inglish, Adventures of a Young Man, Barabbas, Laurence of Arabia, Italiano Brava Gentle, Stay Away Joe, A Minute to Pray, a Second to Die, Hail Hero, Shark, My Old Man's Place, The Sentinel.

KENNEDY BURT: Director. b. Muskegon, Mich. Began as writer of TV and film scripts, and most recently was writer, producer and director of Combat series.
PICTURES INCLUDE: Mail Order Bride. The Rounders, The Money Trap, Return of the Seven, The War Wagon, Support Your Local Sheriff, Young Billy Young, The Devil's Backbone, Dirty Dingus Magee, Support Your Local Gunfighter, Hannie Caulder, The Train Robbers (also s.p.).

KENNEDY, GEORGE: Actor. b. N.Y., N.Y., Feb. 18, 1925. f. orchestra leader at N.Y. Proctor Theatre, m. dancer with Le Ballet Classique in vaudeville. At 2 acted in touring co. of Bringing Up Father. At 7, disc jockey with his own radio show for children. Joined W.W. II Army at 17, earned two Bronze Stars and combat and service ribbons. In Army 16 years, became Capt. and Armed Forces Radio and TV officer. 1957, opened first Army Information Office, N.Y. Served as technical advisor to Phil Silvers's Sergeant Bilko TV series. Began acting in 1959 when discharged from Army.
TV: Sugarfoot, Cheyenne. Movie: International Airport.
PICTURES INCLUDE: Lonely Are the Brave, Strait Jacket, The Silent Witness, Island of the Blue Dolphins, The Man From the Diners Club, Little Shepherd of Kingdom Come, Mirage, See How They Run, McHale's Navy, Charade, In Harm's Way, The Sons of Katie Elder, Shenandoah, Hush . . . Hush Sweet Charlotte, The Dirty Dozen, Hurry Sundown, Cool Hand Luke (Acad. Award Best Supporting Actor), The Ballad of Josie, Jolly Pink Jungle, Bandolero!, The Boston Strangler, Guns of the Magnificent Seven, Gaily, Gaily, The Good Guys and the Bad Guys, Airport, . . . tick . . . tick . . . tick, Zigzag, Dirty Dingus Magee, Fool's Parade, Lost Horizon, Cahill, Thunderbolt and Lightfoot, Airport 1975, Earthquake, The Human Factor, Airport '77, Death on the Nile, Brass Target, The Concorde—Airport 79, Death Ship, The Delta Force.

KENNEDY, KATHLEEN: Producer. e. San Diego State Univ. Early TV experience on KCST, San Diego, working as camera operator, video editor, floor director and news production coordinator. Produced talk show, You're On. Left to enter m.p. industry as prod. asst. on Steven Spielberg's 1941.
PICTURES: Raiders of the Lost Ark (prod. assoc.); Poltergeist (assoc. prod.); E.T.: The Extra-Terrestrial (co-prod.); Indiana Jones and the Temple of Doom (assoc. prod.); Gremlins (exec. prod.); Goonies (exec. prod.); Back to the Future (exec. prod.); The Color Purple (co-prod.); Young Sherlock Holmes (co-prod.).

KENNEY, H. WESLEY: Producer-Director, stage, TV, film. b. Dayton, O., grad. Carnegie Tech. Six-time Emmy winner; 1974–75 dir., All in the Family; exec. prod. Days of Our Lives; 1979–81, dir., Ladies Man, Filthy Rich, 1981. Now exec. prod. Young and Restless.

KENT, JEAN: Actress. b. London, Eng., June 29, 1921. e. Marist Coll., Peekham, London; p. prof. Fields & Norrie. First stage appearance at 3 and at 10 played in parents' act; chorus girl at Windmill Theatre, London, 1935; 2 yrs. repertory; Screen debut: It's That Man Again, 1941.
PICTURES INCLUDE: Trottle True, Her Favorite Husband, The Reluctant Widow, The Woman in Question, The Browning Version, Big Frame, Before I Wake, Shadow of Fear, Prince and the Showgirl, Bon Jour Tristesse, Grip of the Strangler, Beyond This Place, Please Turn Over, Bluebeard's Ten Honeymoons, Shout At the Devil.
TV: A Call on the Widow, The Lovebird, The Morning Star, November Voyage, Love Her to Death, The Lion and the Mouse, The Web, Sir Francis Drake series, Yvette, Emergency Ward 10, County Policy, Coach 7, Smile On the Face of the Tiger, No Hiding Place, Kipling, This Man Craig, The Killers, Vanity Fair, A Night with Mrs. Da Tanka, United serial. The Family of Fred, After Dark, Thicker than Water series, The Young Doctors, Brother and Sister, Up Pompei, Steptoe and Son, Doctor at Large, Family at War, K is for Killing, Night School, Tycoon series, Crossroads (series), Lyttons Diary.

KENT, JOHN B.: Theatre executive and attorney. b. Jacksonville, Fla., Sept. 5, 1939. e. Yale Univ., Univ. of Fla., Law School, N.Y. Univ. grad. school of law (LLM in taxation, 1964). Partner in Kent, Watts & Durden, (1967 to present); Pres. & dir, Kent Investments, Inc. (1977 to present); dir. and off. Kent Theatres, Inc. and affiliated corps (1961 to present); v.p. and gen. counsel, (1970 to present). Was pres. 1967–70 when resigned to devote full time to law practice. NATO dir. (1972) and Presidents' Advisory Cabinet, 1979 to present) v.p. NATO of Fla., 1968–72, dir; 1973 to present. Member of Rotary Club of Jacksonville, Fla. Bar Ass'n., American Bar Ass'n., American Judicature Society.

KENYON, CURTIS: Writer.
TV PLAYS: Cavalcade of America, Fireside Theatre, Schlitz Playhouse, U.S. Steel Hour, 20th Century-Fox Hour.
PICTURES INCLUDE: Woman Who Dared, Lloyds of London, Wake Up and Live, Love and Hisses, She Knew All the Answers, Twin Beds, Seven Days' Leave, Thanks

for Everything, Princess and the Pirate, Bathing Beauty, Fabulous Dorseys, Tulsa, Two Flags West.

KERASOTES, GEORGE G.: Exhibitor. Springfield, IL, e. U of IL, 1929–33; Lincoln Coll. of Law 1935–37. Past pres. Theatre Owners of Illinois. Past pres. Kerasotes Theatres, 1935–85. Past pres., Theatre Owners of America, 1959–60. Chmn. of board of TOA 1960–62; chmn. ACE Toll TV com.; bd. mem. Code Appeal Board; mem. exec comm. NATO, bd of dir. NATO. Chm. insurance committee. Chm. GKC Theatres and Kerasotes Michigan Theatres. Director St. Anthony's Hellenic Church—Hellenic Golf Classic. Director, Will Rogers Hospitals; Director, Pioneers.

KERASOTES, LOUIS G., Exhibitor. b. Springfield, IL, Dec 22, 1920. e. Univ of IL, 1943, BA, business admins. 1st Lt., U.S. Army Infantry (WWII: 1943–46, Korea: 1951–53). Head film buyer, head of purchasing dept., v.p./treas. Kerasotes Theatres, 1953–85. Pres., Kerasotes Theatres, 1985.

KERKORIAN, KIRK: Executive. b. Fresno, CA, June 6, 1917. e. Los Angeles public schools. Served as capt., transport command, RAF, 1942–44. Commercial air line pilot from 1940; founder Los Angeles Air Service (later Trans Intl. Airlines Corp.), 1948; Intl. Leisure Corp., 1968; controlling stockholder, Western Airlines, 1970; chief exec. officer, MGM, Inc., 1973–74; chm. exec. com., vice-chm. bd., 1974—

KERR, DEBORAH: Actress. b. Helensburgh, Scotland, Sept. 30, 1921; e. Phyllis Smale Ballet Sch.; m. Anthony Bartley. On stage 1939 in repertory. Began Brit. screen career 1940 in Major Barbara; voted "Star of Tomorrow" Motion Picture Herald-Fame Poll, 1942. Voted one of top ten British money-making stars in Motion Picture Herald-Fame Poll, 1947. B'way debut in Tea & Sympathy, 1953.

PICTURES INCLUDE: Major Barbara, Love on the Dole, Hatler's Castle, The Day Will Dawn, The Avengers, Perfect Strangers, Colonel Blimp, Black Narcissus, The Hucksters, If Winter Comes, Edward My Son, Please Believe Me, King Solomon's Mines, Quo Vadis, Thunder in the East, Prisoner of Zenda, Dream Wife, Julius Caesar, Young Bess, From Here to Eternity, End of the Affair, King and I, Proud and Profane, Tea and Sympathy, Heaven Knows Mr. Alison, Affair to Remember, Count Your Blessings, Beloved Infidel, Sundowners, The Grass Is Greener, The Innocents, The Naked Edge, The Chalk Garden, Night of the Iguana, Marriage On the Rocks, Casino Royale, Eye of the Devil, The Gypsy Moths, The Arrangement, The Assam Garden.

TELEVISION: A Woman of Substance, Reunion at Fairborough.

KERR, FRASER: Actor. b. Glasgow, Scotland, 1931. Early career in repertory. Tours of Canada and America. Ent. TV 1956. Series incl. Emergency Ward 10, Dixon of Deck Green, Murder Bag. Many Shakespeare plays. Radio: BBC Drama Rep. Co., 39 Steps, The Ringer, The Bible, What Every Woman Knows.

STAGE & TV: Night Must Fall, Never a Cross Word, The Inside Man, On the Buses, Dr. Finlay's Casebook, Wicked Woman, Madelaine July, Doctor in the House, Counterstrike, Waggoner's Walk, Juno and the Paycock, Aquarius, Ev, Upstairs and Downstairs, Cover to Cover, Janine, Robert the Bruce, Caliph of Bagdad, Watch it, Sailor!, The Fosters, Weekend World, Doctor at Sea, Dads Army, Algernon Blackwood, Waiting for Sheila, Weekend Show, Mind Your Language, Yes, Minister, Dick Emery Show, Bottle Boys, The Hard Man.

PICTURES INCLUDE: What a Whopper, Carry on Regardless, Way of McEagle, Thomasina, Theatre of Death, Tom, Dick and Harriet, Granny Gets the Point, Nothing But The Night, The Lord of the Rings, Kidnapped, The Derelict, Bloomfield, Ace of Diamonds, Andy Robson, It's a Deal!

RECORD PRODUCER: Tales of Shakespeare Series, The Casket Letters of Mary Queen of Scots.

KERR, JOHN: Actor. b. New York, N.Y., Nov. 15, 1931. p. Geoffrey Kerr, actor, and June Walker, actress. e. Harvard U., B.A., Columbia U., M.A. Actor in summer stock, TV; on Broadway in Bernardine, Tea and Sympathy, All Summer Long.

PICTURES INCLUDE: The Cobweb, Gaby, Tea and Sympathy, The Vintage, South Pacific, Girl of the Night, Pit and the Pendulum, Seven Women from Hell.

TV: Peyton Place.

KERSHNER, IRVIN: Director. b. Phila., Pa., April 29, 1923. e. Tyler School Fine Arts of Temple Univ., 1946, Art Center School, Univ. of Southern Calif. Designer, photography, adv., documentary, architectural; doc. film maker, U.S.I.S., Middle East, 1950–52; dir., cameraman, TV doc., Confidential File, 1953–55; dir.-prod.-writer, Ophite Prod.

PICTURES INCLUDE: Stakeout on Dope Street, Young Captives, Hoodlum Priest, The Luck of Ginger Coffey, A Fine Madness, The Flim Flam Man, Loving, Up the Sandbox, S*P*Y*s, Return of a Man Called Horse, Raid on Entebbe. (TV in U.S.): Eyes of Laura Mars, The Empire Strikes Back, Never Say Never Again.

TV: The Rebel, Naked City, numerous pilots and other nat'l. shows.

KEYES, EVELYN: Actress. b. Port Arthur, Texas, 1925. e. high school; began career as a dancer in night clubs; m. Artie Shaw.

PICTURES INCLUDE: The Buccaneer, Union Pacific, Gone with the Wind, A Thousand and One Nights, The Jolson Story, Mating of Millie, Johnny O'Clock, Enchantment, Mr. Soft Touch, The Prowler, The Killer That Stalked New York, Smuggler's Island, The Iron Man, One Big Affair, Shoot First, 99 River Street, Hell's Half Acre, Top of the World, Seven-Year Itch, Around the World in 80 Days.

KEYLOUN, MARK: Actor. b. Dec. 20, 1960. e. Georgetown Univ. Worked in New York theatre.

PICTURES: Those Lips, Those Eyes, Sudden Impact, Forty-Deuce, Mike's Murder.

TELEVISION: Evergreen.

KIDDER, MARGOT: Actress. b. Yellowknife, Canada, Oct. 17, 1948.

PICTURES: Gaily, Gaily, Quackser Fortune Has a Cousin in the Bronx, Sisters, The Great Waldo Pepper, Superman, Mr. Mike's Mondo Video, The Amityville Horror, Willy and Phil, Superman II, Some Kind of Hero, Little Treasure.

TELEVISION: Louisiana, The Glitter Dome, Bus Stop, Vanishing Act.

KIEL, RICHARD: Actor. b. Detroit, Sept. 13, 1939.

PICTURES: The Human Duplicators, Skidoo, The Longest Yard, The Spy Who Love Me, Force 10 from Navarone, They Went Thataway and Thataway, Flash and the Firecat, Moonraker, So Fine, Cannonball Run II, Pale Rider.

KILEY, RICHARD: Actor. b. Chicago, Ill., Mar. 31, 1922; e. Loyola U. Started prof. career radio, Jack Armstrong, All American Boy.

STAGE: Streetcar Named Desire, Misalliance, Kismet, Time Limit, No Strings, Man of LaMancha, Her First Roman.

PICTURES INCLUDE: The Mob, The Sniper, Eight Iron Men, Pick-Up on South Street, Blackboard Jungle, Phoenix City Story, Spanish Affair, Pendulum, The Little Prince, Looking for Mr. Goodbar.

TELEVISION: The Thorn Birds, George Washington, The Bad Seed, A.D., Do You Remember Love, If Tomorrow Comes.

KILLIAM, PAUL: Producer-performer. b. Mass., Sept. 12, 1916. e. Harvard. News supervisor, WOR-Mutual; prod.-performer TV Hometown. Matinee in NY units for CBS-TV Morning Show, NBC-TV Home Show; ind. prod. cartoons, shorts, comedies: prod. film series, Paul Killiam Show, Movie Museum, Silents Please.

KIMBLEY, DENNIS: Sales Manager, Motion Picture Sales, Kodak Limited., in U.K. Early career in Kodak Testing Dept. responsible for quality control motion picture films. Joined Marketing Division 1966. Chairman BKSTS FILM 75 and FILM 79 Conference Committee. President BKSTS 1976–78. Governor, London International Film School, 1983.

KIMMINS, ANTHONY: Director, writer. b. Harrow Middlesex, England, Nov. 10, 1901; e. R.N. Coll., Dartmouth. Capt. in Royal Navy, World War II. Playwright (While Parents Sleep, Night Club Queen, Chase the Ace, Winter Sport, The Amorous Prawn.) Began screen career 1934 in How's Chances?; since author variously orig., s.p., collab., dial, many Brit. features (Talk of the Devil, Come On George, Laburnum Grove, etc.); in 1936 dir. & s.p. All at Sea; pictures dir. since include I See Ice, It's in the Air, Trouble Brewing. In 1946 returned to m.p. to write, produce and direct.

PICTURES INCLUDE: Mine Own Executioner, Bonnie Prince Charlie, Flesh and Blood, Mr. Denning Drives North, Who Goes There (Passionate Sentry), Captain's Paradise, Smiley, Smiley Gets a Gun, The Amorous Prawn.

KING, ALAN: Actor-Producer. b. New York City, Dec. 26, 1927. Author, Anybody Who Owns His Own Home Deserves It, Help I'm a Prisoner in a Chinese Bakery.

TV: The Tonight Show, Kraft Music Hall, Comedy is King. Prod-star NBC-TV specials. Hosts and guest star, Tonight Show. Stars semi-annually at Sands Hotel, Las Vegas, Seventh Avenue (mini-series).

STAGE: The Impossible Years, The Investigation, Dinner At Eight, A Lion in Winter, Something Different.

PICTURES INCLUDE: Bye Bye Braverman, Anderson Tapes, Just Tell Me What You Want, Author! Author! Producer: Happy Birthday, Gemini, Lovesick, Cat's Eye.

KING, ANDREA: Actress, r.n. Georgette Barry; b. Paris, France; e. Edgewood High School, Greenwich, Conn.; m. N.H. Willis, attorney. Started career on N.Y. stage, following high school; in Growing Pains & Fly Away Home, Boy

Meets Girl, Angel Street (Boston); Life with Father (Chicago); signed by Warner, 1943. Screen debut: The Very Thought of You. TV actress, CBS.
PICTURES INCLUDE: My Wild Irish Rose, Ride the Pink Horse, Mr. Peabody and the Mermaid, Song of Surrender, Southside 1-10001, Dial 1119, Lemon Drop Kid, Mark of the Renegade, World In his Arms, Red Planet Mars, Daddy's Gone A-Hunting.

KING, HERMAN: Producer. b. Chicago, Ill. Was engaged in vending machine business; mfr. Hollywood Talkitone Soundie Projectors; org. prod. co., King Bros. Prod. (with bros. Maurice and Franklin), 1941.
PICTURES INCLUDE: When Strangers Marry, Dillinger, Suspense, The Gangster, The Dude Goes West, Badman of Tombstone, Gun Crazy, Southside 1-1000, Drums in the Deep South, Mutiny, The Ring, Carnival Story, The Brave One, Gorgo, Captain Sinbad, Maya, Return of The Gunfighter, Heaven with a Gun.
TV: Maya series, King International Corp.

KING, PERRY: Actor. b. Alliance, Ohio, e. Yale. Studied with John Houseman at Julliard.
PICTURES INCLUDE: The Possession of Joel Delaney (debut), Slaughterhouse-Five, Big Truck, Poor Clare, The Lords of Flatbush, Mandingo, The Wild Party, Lipstick, Andy Warhol's Bad, The Choirboys, A Different Story, The Clarivoyant.
TV: Medical Center, Hawaii Five-O, Apple's Way, Cannon.

KING, PETER: Executive. b. London, Eng., 1928. e. Marlborough College, Oxford U.; bd., Shipman & King Cinemas Ltd., 1956; borough councillor, 1959–61; chmn., London & Home counties branch, CEA, 1962–63; pres., CEA, 1964; dir. film ind. Defense Organization dir., Grade Org. 1966–68; man. dir. Shipman & King Cinemas Ltd., 1959–68. Ch. man. dir. Paramount Pictures (U.K.) Ltd. Britain, 1968–70. Man., dir., EMI Cinemas and Leisure Ltd., 1970–74. Chairman: King Publications Ltd.; Publisher: Screen International.

KING, STEPHEN: Writer. Best-selling novelist specializing in thrillers many of which have been adapted to film by others (Carrie, Salem's Lot, The Shining, The Dead Zone, Christine, Cujo, Firestarter, Cat's Eye, etc.).
PICTURES: Creepshow (s.p., actor), Silver Bullet (s.p.).

KINGMAN, DONG: Fine Artist. b. Oakland, Calif., Mar. 31, 1911. e. Hong Kong 1916–1920; 1928, mem. motion picture co., Hong Kong branch; 1935; began to exhibit as fine artist in San Francisco; promotional, advertising or main title artwork for following films: World of Suzie Wong, Flower Drum Song, 55 Days of Peking, Circus World, King Rat, The Desperados, The Sand Pebbles, Lost Horizon-1973. 1966–7, created 12 paintings for Universal Studio Tour for posters and promotion; 1968, cover painting for souvenir program for Ringling Bros.-Barnum and Bailey Circus; treasurer for Living Artist Production since 1954; Exec. V.P. 22nd-Century Films, Inc. since 1968, Prod. & dir. short, Hongkong Dong. Also short subject film Dong Kingman, filmed and directed by James Wong Howe.

KINGSLEY, BEN: Actor. b. Yorkshire, England, Dec. 31, 1943. Started career with Salford Players, amateur co. in Manchester. Turned pro in 1966 and appeared on London stage at a Chichester Festival Theatre. 1967, joined Royal Shakespeare Co., where has been lead player in A Midsummer Night's Dream, Tempest, Measure for Measure, Merry Wives of Windsor, volpone, Cherry Orchard, etc. Played Squeers in Nicholas Nickleby in 1980 in London. Film debut in Gandhi, 1982. 1983: Betrayal. 1985: Turtle Diary.

KINGSLEY, DOROTHY: Writer. (Mrs. William W. Durney): b. New York City, Oct. 14. e. Detroit Arts and Crafts Acad. Radio writer for Bob Hope, 1938; Edgar Bergen, 1939–43.
PICTURES INCLUDE: Date With Judy, Neptune's Daughter, Two Weeks With Love, Angels in the Outfield, Texas Carnival, It's a Big Country, When In Rome, Small Town Girl, Dangerous When Wet, Kiss Me Kate, Seven Brides for Seven Brothers, Jupiter's Darling, Don't Go Near the Water, Pal Joey, Green Mansions, Can-Can, Pepe, Half a Sixpence, Valley of the Dolls.
TV: Created series, Bracken's World.

KINGSLEY, WALTER: Executive. b New York, Oct. 20, 1923. e. Phillips Academy, Andover; Amherst Coll., B.A., 1947. Charter member Big Brothers of Los Angeles. WCOP, Boston, 1947–50; Ziv Television Programs, Inc., 1950–58; President, Independent Television Corp., 1958–61. Member bd. dir Big Brothers of Amer.; pres. Kingsley Co., 1962–66; exec. v.p. Wolper Prods. Metromedia Prods. Corp., 1966–72; faculty, Inter-Racial Council of Business Opportunity, N.Y.C.; 1972–82, pres., Kingsley Company, Commercial Real Estate; 1982–present, special consultant, American Film Institute; Board Member: Big Brothers/Big Sisters of America; Big Brothers of Greater Los Angeles.

KINOSHITA, KEISUKE: Director. b. Japan, 1912. Entered Shochiku studio as film processor and progressed to director.
PICTURES INCLUDE: Twenty-four Eyes, Sun and Rose, Wild Chrysanthemum, A Japanese Tragedy, Times of Joy and Sorrow, Snow Flurry, Candle in the Wind, Carmen's Pure Love.

KINOY, ERNEST: Writer. Started career in radio writing sci. fic. programs (X Minus One, Dimension X). Created and wrote religious radio show, The Eternal Light. Moved in to TV and wrote for nearly all dramatic shows, including Studio One, Philco Playhouse, Playhouse 90.
PICTURES INCLUDE: Brother John, Buck and the Preacher, Leadbelly.
TV: The Defenders, Naked City, Dr. Kildare, Jacob and Joseph (special), David, the King (special).

KINSKI, KLAUS: Actor. b. Poland, 1928. r.n. Nicolaus Naksznski. Drafted into German army at 16; became British prisoner. After release began acting career in postwar German theatre. Since early 1950s has made nearly 170 films throughout Europe.
PICTURES INCLUDE: Cold Blooded Beast, Pleasure Girls, The Bloody Hands of the Law, Doctor Zhivago, For a Few Dollars More, Aguirre: The Wrath of God, Woyzeck, Nosferatu, the Vampyre, Love and Money (American debut), The Soldier, The Little Drummer Girl.

KINSKI, NASTASSJA: Actress. b. Berlin, Germany, Jan. 24, 1960. Daughter of actor Klaus Kinski.
PICTURE: To the Devil a Daughter, Passion Flower Hotel, Stay As You Are, Tess, Cat People, Exposed, The Moon in the Gutter, Unfaithfully Yours, The Hotel New Hampshire, Maria's Lovers, Paris, Texas, Revolution.

KIRK, PHYLLIS: Actress. b. Syracuse, N.Y., Sept. 18, 1930. Perfume repr. model, Conover Agcy.; B'way play debut in My Name Is Aquilon; actress, summer stock; screen debut in Our Very Own; B'way production of Point of No Return.
TV: The Thin Man.
PICTURES INCLUDE: A Life of Her Own, Two Weeks With Love, Mrs. O'Malley and Mr. Malone, Three Guys Named Mike, About Face, Iron Mistress, Thunder Over The Plains, House of Wax, Crime Wave, River Beat, Canyon Crossroads, City After Midnight.

KIRKPATRICK, DAVID: Executive. e. Calif. Institute of Arts. Wrote screenplay, The Great Texas Dynamite Chase, produced by New World Pictures. Joined Paramount Pictures 1979 as analyst in story dept; left to head Sidney Beckerman's production co. at United Artists. Returned to Paramount 1982 as exec. dir. of production. 1984, promoted to v.p., prod., Paramount. 1985, named exec. v.p., prod.

KITT, EARTHA: Actress, singer. b. Columbia, S.C., Jan. 26, 1928. Professional career started as dancer in Katherine Dunham group; toured U.S., Mexico & Europe with group, then opened night club in Paris; in Orson Welles stage prod. of Faust for European tour; N.Y. night clubs; stage in U.S., New Faces; at Macambo Hollywood, 1953; author, Thursday's Child; on screen, 1954, New Faces; 1958, The Mark of the Hawk, St. Louis Blues, Anna Lucasta.

KLEES, ROBERT E.: Executive. b. New York, N.Y., Feb. 21, 1927. e. Duke Univ. (1947–51); Univ. of Calif. Graduate School of Management (1973–75). U.S. Navy, 1944–46; Union Carbide Corp., 1951–57; director of communications, Beckman Instruments, Inc., 1957–69; co-founder and v.p. mktg., International Biophysics Corp., 1969–73; sr. v.p., mktg., Deluxe Laboratories, Inc., 1975–83; Int'l. Exec. Service Corps & Senior Corps of Retired Executives, 1983–present.

KLEIN, ALLEN: Producer. b. Dec. 18, 1931. Pres. ABKCO industries, Inc.
PICTURES INCLUDE: Force of Impulse, Pity Me Not, Mrs. Brown, You've Got A Lovely Daughter, Stranger in Town, The Stranger Returns, Samuri on a Horse, The Silent Stranger, Pete, Pearl & The Pole, The Grand Bouffe, Come together, Let It Be, The Holy Mountain, El Topo, The Concert for Bangladesh, The Greek Tycoon.

KLEIN, HAROLD J.: Executive. b. New York, N.Y., e. U. of West Virginia, N.Y. Law School; reviewer, sales staff. Showman's Trade Review; booker, Brandt Theatres; booker, later vice-pres., gen. mgr., J&J Theatres, 1941–59; account executive; Exec. vice-pres., dir. of world-wide sales, ABC Films, Inc., N.Y., Pres., Klein Film Assn.; Exec. Vice President, Plitt Theatres, Inc.

KLEIN, MALCOLM C.: Executive. b. L.A., Calif., Nov. 22, 1927. e. UCLA, grad., 1948, U. of Denver; Prod. dir. managment, KLAC-TV (KCOP), L.A., 1948–52; acct. exec., KABC-TV, 1952–56; asst. gen. sales mgr., KABC-TV, 1956–59; exec. vice-pres. gen. mgr., NTA Broadcasting, N.Y., 1959; v.p., gen. mgr., RKO-General-KHJ-TV, 1960; joined National General Corp. 1968, vice-pres. Creative Services and Marketing. Pres. National General Television Productions, Inc., Pres. NGC Broadcasting Corp.; 1971, pres. Filmways TV Presentations; 1972, pres. Malcolm C. Klein & Assoc. mgmt. & mktng. consultants; 1973 gen'l. exec. Sterling

Recreation Organization & Gen'l Mgr. Broadcast Division; pres., American Song Festival. Exec. v.p., Telease Inc. & American Subscription Television; and mgt. & mktng. consultant; 1981, sr. v.p., mng. dir., STAR-TV (subscription TV); 1982, sr. v.p., InterAmerican Satellite TV Network.

KLEIN, PAUL L.: Television Executive. e. Brooklyn Coll. Veteran of U.S. Army Air Corps. Research analyst with Biow Co., ad agency, 1953–54; research manager for Doyle Dane Bernbach ad agency, 1955–60. Started with NBC in 1961 as supervisor, ratings, and rose to position of v.p., audience measurement in October, 1965. In August, 1970, left NBC to found Computer Television Inc., first independent pay-per-view TV co. in world. Time, Inc. bought his interest in CTI. Returned to NBC in March, 1976. as v.p., network mktg. & planning; then named v.p., programs. Appointed exec. v.p., programs, NBC-TV, November, 1977. Became independent 1978.

KLEINER, HARRY: Writer, producer. b. Phila., Penna. e. Temple University (B.S.); Yale University (M.F.A.).
TV: Writer: The Virginian, Bus Stop, musical Robin Hood, Rosenberg Trial.
PICTURES INCLUDE: Screenplay: Carmen Jones, Street With No Name, Miss Sadie Thompson, Salome, Garment Jungle (also prod.), Fantastic Voyage, Bullitt (co-s.p.), Le Mans.

KLEISER, RANDALL: Director. b. July 20, 1946. e. USC.
PICTURES: Grease, Street People, The Blue Lagoon, Grandview, U.S.A., Flight of the Navigator.
TELEVISION: Movies: All Together Now, Dawn: Portrait of a Teenage Runaway, The Boy in the Plastic Bubble, The Gathering. Series: Marcus Welby, M.D., The Rookies, Starsky and Hutch, Family.

KLINE, FRED W.: Publicist. b. Oakland, CA May 17, 1918. e. U. Calif. Berkeley; M.P. pub. rel. since 1934; pres. The Fred Kline Agency; pres. Kline Communications Corporation; Owner, Fred Kline Agency, Inc.; Kline Communications Corp.; Fred W. Kline Prod., Inc.; Capitol News Service, Sacramento; L.A. News Bureau; Capitol Radio News Service, Inc.; Commissioner, Motion Picture Council, State of California; Commissioner, Los Angeles County Fire Commission.

KLINE, KEVIN: Actor. b. St. Louis, MO, Oct. 24, 1947. e. Indiana Univ. Studied at Julliard and became founding member of John Houseman's The Acting Company, with whom performed in classics, including The School for Scandal, She Stoops to Conquer, The Three Sisters, etc. Bdwy. debut in musical, On the Twentieth Century.
PICTURES: Sophie's Choice (debut), The Pirates of Penzance, The Big Chill, Silverado, Violets Are Blue.

KLINGER, HENRY: Eastern story editor, 20th Century-Fox Film Corp. b. New York, N.Y., Mar. 15, 1908. e. CCNY, BA: NYU, BBA. Assoc. ed., Chatterbox, nat'l mag., 1931–33; pres. Booklovers' Guild, 1930–33; freelance story dept. work, RKO, Cosmopolitan & Fox Films, 1931–33; story dept., pub. contract, Fox, 1934; asst. story ed., 20th-Fox, 1936; acting story ed., 1941; assoc. story ed., 1942; story ed., 1956; exec. story ed., 1964; exec. aide, 1971–73. Lecturer, Author.

KLINGER, MICHAEL: Producer. Managing Dir. Klinger Films, Ltd., Avril Films Ltd., Avton Film Productions, Peregrine Entertainments Ltd.
PICTURES INCLUDE: Cul-de-Sac, Repulsion, Saturday Night Out, The Projected Man, Yellow Teddy Bears, Black Torment, Study in Terror, The Penthouse, Baby Love, Something to Hide, Get Carter, Pulp, Rachel's Man, Tomorrow Never Comes, Gold, Shout at the Devil, Riding High. Exec. Prod. Confessions series, Blood Relatives, A Certain Fury, War Story, Judgement in Stone.

KLUGMAN, JACK: Actor. b. Philadelphia, Pa., April 27, 1922. e. Carnegie Tech. m. Brett Somers. After several menial jobs appeared on Broadway in Saint John, Stevedore; later understudied in Mister Roberts, taking over the doctor role; recent stage work includes Gypsy.
PICTURES INCLUDE: Timetable, Twelve Angry Men, Cry Terror, The Scarface Mob, Days of Wine and Roses, I Could Go On Singing, The Yellow Canary, Act One, Hail Mafia, The Detective, The Split, Goodbye Columbus, Who Says I Can't Ride a Rainbow?, Two Minute Warning.
TV: The Defenders (Emmy Award for role in 'Blacklist' segment), The FBI, Ben Casey, 90 Bristol Court, etc.; The Odd Couple (Emmy, 1971 and 1973), Quincy.

KNIGHT, ARTHUR: Critic, educator. b. Phila., Pa., Sept. 3, 1916. e. CCNY. BA 1940. Asst. curator Museum of Modern Art Film Library, 1939–49; film consultant CBS-color television, Omnibus, Odyssey, Seven Lively Arts, etc; film courses at CCNY, New School for Social Research, Hunter College; contributor to Encyclopedia Britannica, Collier's Encyclopedia, etc.; author: "The Liveliest Art," The Hollywood Style; film critic, Hollywood Reporter; formerly Saturday Review; prof. USC School of Cinema/TV.

KNIGHT, DAVID: Actor. b. Niagara Falls, N.Y., Jan. 16, 1928. e. Whittier College, Calif.; 1944–52 teacher Putney School, Vermont; 1952–53 student Royal Academy of Dramatic Art.
LONDON STAGE: Trial of Mary Dugan, The Tenth Man, How to Succeed in Business Without Really Trying, Caine Mutiny Court Martial.
PICTURES INCLUDE: Young Lovers (Chance Meeting), Out of the Clouds, Lost, Eyewitness, Across the Bridge, V.I., The Story of David, Nightmare, Bedtime Story.
TV: Lincoln in Illinois, Berkeley Square, The Philadelphia Story, The Unquiet Spirit, A Question of Pride, Trial and Error.

KNIGHT, SHIRLEY: Actress. b. Goessell, Kansas, 1937. e. University of Wichita, University of California. Joined the Pasadena Community Playhouse.
PICTURES INCLUDE: Five Gates to Hell (debut), Ice Palace, The Dark At the Top of the Stairs, (Acad. Award nom.) The Couch, Sweet Bird of Youth, House of Women, Flight from Ashiya, The Group, Dutchman, Petulia, The Counterfeit Killer, The Rain People, Juggernaut, Beyond the Poseidon Adventure, Endless Love, The Sender, Prisoners.

KNOPF, DAVID A. Producers Representative. b. Boston, MA, Feb. 9, 1942. e. University of Wisconsin. m. Jane Gibbons. vice-pres., Knopf/Polier Representation. 1964 started in Universal Studios mailroom, moved up to publicity department. Began career in exhibition 1968 as film buyer, National General Theatres. Head film buyer for S. Cal, UA Theatres and General Cinema before joining Warner Bros. as sales exec. in Boston. Returned to Los Angeles as S. Cal. film buyer for Mann theatres. Started Knopf/Polier, 1979.

KNOTTS, DON: Actor. b. Morgantown, W.VA, July 21, 1924. e. West Virginia Univ., Univ. of Arizona. Drafted into US Army where became part of show called Stars and Grapes, teamed with comedian Mickey Shaughnessy. After schooling resumed, was offered teaching fellowship but went to New York to try acting instead. Appeared on radio and TV, leading to role in No Time for Sergeants on Bdwy.; appeared in film version.
PICTURES: It's a Mad, Mad, Mad, Mad World, The Incredible Mr. Limpet, The Shakiest Gun in the West, The Apple Dumpling Gang, Herbie Goes to Monte Carlo, The Apple Dumpling Gang Rides Again, Cannonball Run II.
TELEVISION: Garry Moore Show, Steve Allen Show, Andy Griffith Show (played Barney Fife), The Don Knotts Show, Three's Company, Return to Mayberry.

KNOWLES, PATRIC: Actor. r.n. Reginald Lawrence Knowles; b. Horsforth, Yorkshire, England, Nov. 11, 1911. Joined Abby Repertory Theatre, 1930; m.p. debut (Ireland) in Irish Hearts, 1934; on London stage in By Appointment; U.S. m.p. debut in Charge of the Light Brigade, 1936; served in Canadian RAF & as civilian instructor USAF, World War II.
PICTURES INCLUDE: Honours Easy, Mister Hobo, Two's Company, Give Me Your Heart, It's Love I'm After, Expensive Husbands, Adventures of Robin Hood, How Green Was My Valley, Forever and a Day, Of Human Bondage, Bride Wore Boots, Ivy, Kitty, Monsieur Beaucaire, Dream Girl, Big Steal, Quebec, Three Came Home, Mutiny, Tarzan's Savage Fury, Jamaica Run, Flame of Calcutta, World Ransom, Khyber Patrol, No Man's Woman, Band of Angels, Auntie Mame, The Way West, In Enemy Country, The Devil's Brigade, Chisum, The Man, Terror in the Wax Museum, Arnold.

KNOX, ALEXANDER: Actor. b. Strathroy, Ont., Jan. 16, 1907. e. Western Ontario U. Author, novels: Bride of Quietness, Night of the White Bear, The Enemy I Kill, Raider's Moon, The Kidnapped Surgeon; plays, Old Master, The Closing Door, Red On White.
TELEVISION: Potsdam, Tinker Tailor Soldier Spy, Suez, Churchill And The Generals, Helen and Teacher, Empire, Darwin, Oppenheimer, The Last Place on Earth, Lovejoy.
STAGE: (NY) Romeo and Juliet, The Three Sister, Jupiter Laughs, Jason, The Closing Door; (London) King of Nowhere, Geneva, In Good King Charles' Golden Days, The Jealous God, Winter Journey, Henry VIII, Geneva, King of Nowhere, Return to Tyassi, Burnt Flower Bed, When We Dead Awaken.
PICTURES INCLUDE: The Sea Wolf, This Above All, Commandos Strike at Dawn, None Shall Escape, Over 21, Wilson, Sign of the Ram, Judge Steps Out, Sister Kenny, I'd Climb the Highest Mountain, Saturday's Hero, Sleeping Tiger, Divided Heart, Crack in the Mirror, The Viking, The Night My Number Came Up, Reach for the Sky, High Tide at Noon, Davy, Operation Amsterdam, The Longest Day, Wreck of the Mary Deare, Man in the Middle, Woman of Straw, Mr. Moses, Accident, Villa Rides, Shalako, Skullduggery, Pupper on a Chain, Khartoum, Nicholas and Alexandra, Gorky Park, Joshua Then and Now.

KNOX, GORDON: Producer. b. Greenville, TX. e. Univ. of Missouri; married. In addition to making documentary films for several years has been employed by Warner Bros., and Walter Wanger Prods. Joined Princeton Film Center in 1940; Pres. SKS Prod. Inc., Santa Fe, N.M. Pres., PAC Productions, Inc., Princeton, N.J.

KOBAYASHI, MASAKI: Director. b. Japan, Feb. 4, 1916. e. Waseda Univ. Joined Shochiku 1941 as asst. Director. Army. Rejoined Shochiku 1946.
PICTURES INCLUDE: No Greater Love, Road to Eternity, A Soldier's Prayer, Black River, Room with Thick Walls, Somewhere Beneath Wide Sky, Fountainhead, I'll Buy You, The Human Condition, The Inheritance.

KOCH, HOWARD: Writer. b. New York City, Dec. 12, 1902. e. St. Stephen's Coll., '22. B.A.; Columbia Law School, '25. LL.B. Hon. degree Doctor of Human Letters, Bard. Coll., 1972. Playwright (Give Us This Day, In Time To Come, Straitjacket). Began screen career collab. s.p. The Sea Hawk. Radio: wrote War of the Worlds play for Orson Welles' broadcast. book: The Panic Broadcast (Little, Brown & Co.); Academy Award best s.p. (Casablanca). As Time Goes By, Memoirs of a Writer in Hollywood, New York and Europe published by Harcourt, Brace and Jovanovich.
PICTURES INCLUDE: The Letter, Shining Victory, In This Our Life, Casablanca, Mission to Moscow, Letter From an Unknown Woman, The Thirteenth Letter, The War Lover, The Fox, Loss of Innocence, No Sad Songs for Me, Sergeant York, Three Strangers.

KOCH, HOWARD W.: Prod., dir. b. New York, N.Y., Apr. 11, 1916. Runner on Wall St., asst. cutter, 20th-Fox; asst. dir., 20th-Fox, Eagle Lion, MGM; 2nd unit dir., freelance; prod. Aubrey Schenck Prod.; 1961–64, exec. prod. Frank Sinatra Enterprises; v.p., chg. prod., Paramount Pictures Corp., 1964–66, Past pres. of the Academy of Motion Picture Arts and Sciences, 1977–79. On June 11, 1977, elected to the National Board of Directors Guild of America for two year term. Produced eight Academy Award shows, 1972 thru 1983.
TV: Director, Miami Undercover, The Untouchables, Maverick, Cheyenne, Hawaiian Eye, Hollywood Wives (1985 mini-series), Crossings (1986 mini-series).
PICTURES INCLUDE: War Paint, Beachhead, Yellow Tomahawk, Shield for Murder, Big House USA, Crime Against Joe, Emergency Hospital, Ghost Town, Broken Star, Rebel in Town, Pharaoh's Curse, Three Bad Sisters, Fort Yuma, Desert Sands, Quincannon Frontier Scout, Black Sheep, Hot Cars, "X-1," Sergeants 3, The Manchurian Candidate, Come Blow Your Horn, Four For Texas, Robin and the Seven Hoods, None But the Brave, The Odd Couple, On A Clear Day You Can See Forever, Plaza Suite, Star Spangled Girl, (Prod.), Last of the Red Hot Lovers, (Prod.), Badge 373 (Prod.-Dir.) 1973, (Prod.) Once Is Not Enough; MATI (prod.), 1977; Airplane! (prod.) 1980; Dragonslayer (exec. prod.), 1981; Some Kind of Hero (prod.), 1982; Airplane II: The Sequel (prod.) 1982.

KOCH, HOWARD W., JR.: Producer. b. Los Angeles, Dec. 14, 1945. Was asst. dir. and in other industry posts before turning to production. Currently pres. & chief exec. off., Rastar.
PICTURES: Heaven Can Wait, The Other Side of Midnight, The Frisco Kid, The Idolmaker, Gorky Park, The Keep, A Night in Heaven, The Pope of Greenwich Village.

KOENEKAMP, FRED J.: Cinematographer. Member of American Society of Cinematographer. Winner of Oscar for Towering Inferno.
PICTURES: Beyond the Valley of the Dolls, Billy Jack, Embryo, The Other Side of Midnight, The Champ, Amityville Horror, The Domino Principle, Towering Inferno, The Hunter, Yes, Giorgio, Two of a Kind.

KOENIG, WALTER: Actor-Writer-Director-Producer. b. Chicago, Sept. 14. e. Grinnell College (Iowa), Univ. of Calif. Performed in summer stock; after college enrolled at Neighborhood Playhouse, NY; first acting job in TV's Day in Court.
PICTURES: The Deadly Honeymoon, Star Trek—The Motion Picture, Star Trek II: The Wrath of Khan, Star Trek III: The Search for Spock, etc.
TELEVISION: Actor: Colombo, Medical Center, Ironside, Mannix, Alfred Hitchcock Presents, Mr. Novak, Ben Casey, The Untouchables, Combat. Films: The Questor Tapes, Goodbye Raggedy Ann. Writer: Family, The Class of '65, The Powers of Matthew Starr.

KOHLER, FRED, JR.: Actor.
PICTURES INCLUDE: The Prisoner of Shark Island, Sins of Man, Pigskin Parade, Hold That Coed, Young Mr. Lincoln, Big Bonanza, Why Girls Leave Home, Feudin', Fussin', and A-Fightin', Spoilers of the Plains, Baron of Arizona, Hollywood Thrill-Makers, Racing Blood.

KOHN, HOWARD E., II: Executive. b. McKeesport, Pa. National dir. of adv., publicity, roadshow dept., United Artists; indep. prod., Hidden Fear, 1957; pres. Lioni-Warren-Kohn, Inc., 1958; national roadshow dir., Columbia Pictures, Porgy & Bess, 1959; World wide co-ordinator, national co-ordinator adv. & pub. for El Cid, June 1961; named world wide co-ordinator adv., pub. all Samuel Bronston Productions, April 1962; pres., Starpower Inc., 1968; exec. v.p., Avanti Films, 1970; v.p. Avariac Prods., 1971; Pres., Blossom Films, 1973. Elected member of ASCAP, 1975. Pres., Avanti Associates, 1976. Pres. Channel Television Prods., Inc., 1985. Assoc. prod.: Lois M. O'Brien.

KOHNER, SUSAN: Actress, b. L.A., Calif., Nov. 11, 1936. e. Univ. of Calif., 1954–55.
TV: Alcoa Hour, Schlitz Playhouse, Four Star Theatre, Matinee Theatre, Climax, Suspicion, Playhouse 90, Route 66, Dick Powell Theatre.
STAGE: Love Me Little, He Who Gets Slapped, A Quiet Place, Rose Tatoo, Bus Stop, St. Joan, Sunday in New York, Take Her She's Mine, Pullman Car, Hiawatha.
PICTURES INCLUDE: To Hell and Back, The Last Wagon, Dino, Imitation of Life, The Big Fisherman, The Gene Krupa Story, All the Fine Young Cannibals, By Love Possessed, Freud.

KONIGSBERG, FRANK: Executive. b. Kew Gardens, NY. e. Yale and Yale Law School. Worked as lawyer at CBS for six years; moved to NBC for seven years in legal dept. Left to package TV special for Artists Agency Rep. (later AFA) in Los Angeles. being sr. v.p. of West Coast office seven years. Executive producer of many TV series, pilots, variety specials and made-for-TV movies. Formed own Konigsberg Company. Theatrical film debut as prod., Joy of Sex (1984).
TELEVISION: Movies (all exec. prod.): Pearl, Dummy, Before and After, Guyana Tragedy, A Christmas Without Snow, The Pride of Jesse Hallam, Divorce Wars, Coming Out of the Ice, etc. Series (all exec. prod.): It's Not Easy, Breaking Away, Dorothy.

KONTOS, SPERO L.: Thea. Equip. Dealer. b. Chicago, Ill., Dec. 17, 1922. e. Illinois Inst. of Technology, B.S. BM., eng.; ECLA Ent. Ind. as Chicago exhib., 1937; thea. mgmt. until 1942. U.S. Army, 1942–46; sis. eng., Abbott Theatre Equip. Co., 1946–48; sis. mgr., 1948–51; gen. mgr. 1951–54; sis. mgr. John P. Filbert Co. Inc., 1954–59; hd. Century 70/35 mm. projector program, 1959–60; Filbert Co., v.p. chg. sis. & eng., 1960–64; pres., 1964; pres. Theatre Equipment Dealers Assoc., 1965–67; bd. chm., TEDA, 1967–69; chief barker, L.A. Variety, 1971–72; pres., Megaron Corp., 1973, Academy of Motion Picture Arts & Sciences, 1975.

KOPELSON, ARNOLD: Producer-Packager-Financier-Distributor. b. New York City, Feb. 14, 1935. e. NY Law School (JD, 1959); N.Y. Univ. (BS). Has executive-produced, produced, packaged, developed or distributed over 100 films. Handled intl. dist. of Twice in a Lifetime. 1986, prod. The Platoon. Chm., Film Packages Intl. Co-chm. Inter-Ocean Film Sales, Ltd.

KORBAN, BERNARD: Executive. b. New York City, Nov. 28, 1923; e. RCA Inst. of Tech., NYU. U.S. Army 1942–46; 1951–58, Public Relations and Promotions for Davega Stores; 1959–62, exploitation fieldman for Universal Pictures; 1962–66, supvr. of fieldmen and exploitation activities; 1966–68, exec. in chrg. field activities; exec. assist. to v.p., adv. pub. and promotion; 1972 dir. of exploitation, National General Pictures; 1973, dir. of Marketing, promotion and worldwide distribution for Brut Prods; 1974, dir. of mkt., Avco Embassy Pictures, 1975, vice pres. of advertising/publicity/promotion, Cine Artists Pictures Corp.; advertising/publicity, United Artists Corp. West Coast ad. mgr.; then UA v.p., West Coast adv.; v.p. West Coast adv./promo., MGM/UA; 1983, v.p., gen. mgr., Diener/Hauser/Bates, San Diego.

KORMAN, HARVEY: Actor-Director. b. Chicago, Feb. 15, 1927. e. Wright Junior College. Began dramatic studies at Chicago's Goodman School of Drama at the Arts Institute. Acted in small roles in Broadway plays and did TV commercials until break came as comedian for Danny Kaye Show on TV. Staged comedy sketches for Steve Allen variety series in 1967. Became Carol Burnett's leading man on her show in 1967 and continued as regular to present. Has directed two episodes of The New Dick Van Dyke Show.
PICTURES INCLUDE: Actor: Three Bites of an Apple, Lord Love a Duck, Last of the Secret Agents, The April Fools, Blazing Saddles, Huckleberry Finn, High Anxiety, Americathon, First Family, History of the World–Part I, Trail of the Pink Panther, Curse of the Pink Panther, The Longshot.
TV: The Danny Kaye Show, Carol Burnett Show.

KORTY, JOHN: Director, Producer, Writer, Cameraman, Animator. b. Lafayette, IN, 1936; B.A. Antioch College 1959; President, Korty Films, Inc., Mill Valley, CA.
THEATRICAL FEATURES: Alex & the Gypsy (Fox 1976);

Oliver's Story (Paramount 1978); Twice Upon a Time (Ladd/WB 1982).
TELEVISION FEATURES: The Autobiography of Miss Jane Pittman (CBS 1974), Emmy, DGA Award; Farewell to Manzanar (NBC 1976), Humanitas, Christopher Awards; Forever (CBS 1977); A Christmas Without Snow (CBS 1980), A Deadly Business (CBS; 1986); Resting Place (CBS; 1986). INDEPENDENT FEATURES: Crazy Quilt (1964); Funnyman (1967); Riverrun (1969). DOCUMENTARIES: Who Are the DeBolts? (ABC 1978), Oscar, Emmy, DGA Award; Can't It Be Anyone Else? (ABC 1980); Stepping Out: the DeBolts Grow Up, (HBO 1980), The Ewok Adventure (ABC 1984).
SHORT FILMS: The Language of Faces (AFSC 1961); Imogen Cunningham, Photographer (AFI grant 1970); The Music School (PBS 1975). ANIMATION: Breaking the Habit (1964), Oscar Nominee; Various children's films; Segments for Sesame Street and The Electric Company.

KORVIN, CHARLES: Actor. r.n. Geza Korvin Karpathi: b. Czechoslovakia, Nov. 21; e. U. of Paris, Sorbonne, 1933–36. Cameraman, dir., documentary films in Europe; to U.S.A. in 1937; Barter Theatre, 1940–42; on B'way, Dark Eyes, 1943; m.p. debut in Enter Arsene Lupin, 1945.
PICTURES INCLUDE: This Love of Ours, Temptation, Berlin Express, Killer That Stalked N.Y., Lydia Bailey, Tarzan's Savage Fury, Sangaree, Ship of Fools, The Man Who Had Power Over Women.

KOSCINA, SYLVA: Actress. b. Yugoslavia, Aug. 22, 1933. Grew up in Italy; as model placed under contract for films by Carlo Ponti.
PICTURES INCLUDE: The Railroad Man (debut), Juliet of the Spirits, Deadlier Than the Male, The Hornet's Nest, Casanova & Co., Sunday Lovers.

KOSINER, HARRY: Executive. b. New York City, Jan. 29. e. City Coll. N.Y. Stenographer, Fox Films, 1923; asst. to pres., Deluxe Lab., N.Y. 1930–36; eastern rep. Walter Wanger Prod., 1937–40; assistant to western div. mgr. United Artists, 1941–42; on staff m.p. bur., OWI, 1943; apptd. same yr. east. rep. Edward Small Prods., hdqts. N.Y.; home office staff, Columbia Pictures, 1951; v.p. National Screen Service, 1965.

KOSLECK, MARTIN: Actor. b. Barkotse. Pommern Mar. 24, 1907. Six years with Max Reinhardt's dramatic school and theatre in Berlin.
PICTURES INCLUDE: Espionage Agent, Calling Philo Vance, Nurse Edith Cavell, Bomber's Moon, North Star, Secrets of Scotland Yard, Hitler Gang, Gangs of the Waterfront, The Spider, The Wife of Monte Cristo, Pursuit to Algiers, The Frozen Ghost, The Mummy's Curse, Crime of the Century, Assigned to Danger, Smuggler's Cove, Something Wild, 36 Hours, Morituri, The Flesh Eaters.

KOSTER, HENRY: Director. b. Berlin, May 1, 1905. Comm. artist, cartoonist, newspaperman, critic; scenarist, Ufa, Terra, Aafa, Berlin; dir. Berlin, Vienna, Budapest, to Hollywood, 1936.
PICTURES INCLUDE: 100 Men and a Girl, Rage of Paris, It Started With Eve, Spring Parade, Music for Millions, Two Sisters from Boston, The Bishop's Wife, Come to the Stable, Inspector General, My Blue Heaven, Harvey, No Highway in the Sky,, Mr. Belvedere Rings the Bell, Elopement, seq. O. Henry's Full House, Stars & Stripes Forever, My Cousin Rachel, The Robe, Desiree, A Man Called Peter, Good Morning Miss Dove, Power and the Prize, My Man Godfrey, Flower Drum Song, Mr. Hobbs Takes a Vacation, Take Her, She's Mine, Dear Brigitte, The Singing Nun.

KOTCHEFF, WILLIAM THEODORE (Ted): Director. b. Toronto, Canada, 1931. Ent. TV ind. 1952. After five years with Canadian Broadcasting Corp. joined ABC-TV in London, 1957.
PLAYS INCLUDE: Of Mice and Men, Desperate Hours, The Human Voice, Edna the Inebriate Woman, Signalman's Apprentice, Lights Out, Rx for the Defence.
STAGE: Progress The Park, Play With A Tiger, Luv, Maggie May, The Au Pair Man, Have You Any Dirty Washing, Mother Dear?
PICTURES INCLUDE: Life At The Top, Two Gentlemen Sharing, Outback, Billy Two Hats, The Apprenticeship of Duddy Kravitz, Fun with Dick and Jane, Who Is Killing The Great Chefs of Europe?, North Dallas Forty (also co-s.p.), Captured, First Blood, Split Image, Uncommon Valor (also exec. prod.), Joshua Then and Now.

KOTTO, YAPHET: Actor. Has many stage credits, including starring roles on Broadway in The Great White Hope and The Zulu and the Zayda. Off-Bdwy.: Blood Knot, Black Monday, In White America, A Good Place To Raise a Boy.
PICTURES INCLUDE: The Limit (star, prod.), Nothing But a Man, The Liberation of L. B. Jones, Live and Let Die, Across 110th Street, Truck Turner, Bone, Report to the Commissioner, Sharks' Treasure, Hey Good Lookin', Friday Foster, Drum, Blue Collar, Brubaker, Fighting Back, Star Chamber.
TELEVISION: Movies: Badge of the Assassin, Harem.

KOVAKS, LASZLO: Cinematographer.
PICTURES INCLUDE: Hell's Angels On Wheels, The Savage Seven, Targets, Easy Rider, That Cold Day In the Park, Getting Straight, Alex In Wonderland, The Last Movie, Marriage of a Young Stockbroker, The King of Marvin Gardens, Pocket Money, What's Up, Doc?, Paper Moon, Huckleberry Finn, For Pete's Sake, Freebie and the Bean, Shampoo, Baby Blue Marie, Harry and Walter Go to New York, New York, New York, F.I.S.T., The Last Waltz, Paradise Alley, Butch and Sundance: The Early Days, The Runner Stumbles, Heart Beat, Frances, The Toy, Crackers, Mask, Legal Eagles.

KRAMER, JEROME: Executive-Producer-Director. b. Los Angeles, 1945. Graduated USC Law School 1971. Joined Braverman Productions, Inc. 1971; named exec. v.p. Co-producer with Charles Braverman of network specials (21 Years of A.I.P., Horror Hall of Fame), show titles (Rhoda, Cher) corporate and promotional films for Xerox, Petersen Publishing, etc. Producer and director of various television commercials (for Chevrolet, United Artists Records, Gulf Oil), educational films for United States Information Agency, special films and montages.

KRAMER, LARRY: Writer, producer. b. Bridgeport, Conn. U.S.A., 1935. e. Yale Univ. B.A. 1957. Ent. m.p. ind. 1958. Story edit. Columbia Pictures, N.Y. London 1960–65. Asst. to David Picker and Herb Jaffe, UA, 1965. Assoc. prod. and additional dialogue Here We Go Round The Mulberry Bush, 1968. Writ. prod. Women in Love, 1969. Writer: Lost Horizon, 1971; A Sea Change, 1972.

KRAMER, SIDNEY: Sales executive. b. New York City. e. LL.B., New York Law School and C.C.N.Y., married. Gen. sales mgr., RKO Pathe, June 1953; dir. and v.p. Cellofilm Corp. 1941–56; foreign sales mgr., RKO Radio, 1954–59; v.p. Cinemiracle Intl. 1960–61; v.p. T.P.E.A., 1960–61; foreign sls. mgr., Cinerama, Inc., 1962–65; Exec. Commonwealth Theatres, Puerto Rico, Inc., 1965–68; Exec. v.p. Cobian Jr. Enterprises Inc. 1968. M.P. consultant-exhibition, dist., foreign and Caribbean area, Oct., 1968–70. Pres. Coqui Internat'l. Inc.; 1970–80; vice. pres. of UAPR, Inc., Puerto Rico, U.A. Eastern Theatres, Inc. 1981–present, consultant in Florida, UA Theatres.

KRAMER, STANLEY E.: Executive producer, director. b. New York City, Sept. 29, 1913; e. N.Y.U., B.Sc. 1933. Entered m.p. ind. via back lot jobs; with MGM research dept.; film cutter 3 yrs.; film ed.; m.p. & radio writer; served in U.S Signal Corps, 1st Lt.
PICTURES INCLUDE: Champion, Home of the Brave, The Men, Cyrano de Bergerac, Death of a Salesman, High Noon, My Six Convicts, The Sniper, The Four Poster, The Happy Time, Eight Iron Men, 5,000 Fingers of Dr. T, Wild One, The Juggler, Caine Mutiny, Not As a Stranger, Pride and the Passion; prod. dir., s.p., The Defiant Ones, On the Beach, Inherit the Wind, Judgment at Nuremberg; prod., dir., It's a Mad, Mad, Mad, Mad World, Invitation To A Gunfighter, prod., Ship of Fools, Prod. Dir. Guess Who's Coming to Dinner, The Secret of Santa Vittoria, R.P.N.*, Bless the Beasts and Children, Oklahoma Crude, The Domino Principle, The Runner Stumbles.

KRANTZ, STEVE: Exec. b. New York, N.Y., May 20, 1923. e. Columbia U., B.A. Dir. progs., NBC, New York, 1953; dir. prog. dev., Screen Gems, N.Y., 1955; v.p., gen. mgr. Screen Gems, Canada, 1958; dir. int. sls., 1960; formed Krantz Films, Inc. 1964.
TV: Steve Allen Show, Kate Smith Show, Hazel, Dennis the Menace, Winston Churchill—The Valiant Years, Telefilms, Marvel Super Heroes, Rocket Robin Hood, Animated Films.
PICTURES INCLUDE: Fritz the Cat, Heavy Traffic (prod.).

KREIMAN, ROBERT T.: Executive. b. Kenosha, Wis., Sept. 16, 1924. Served W. W. II Capt Army Corps of Engineers-ETO. e. Stanford, 1943; Univ. of Wis., 1942—1946–49. Dir., sales training, mgr., audio visual sales, Bell & Howell Co., 1949–58; V.P., Argus Cameras, Inc., 1958–61; V.P., gen. mgr., Commercial & Educ. Div., Technicolor 1961–69, v.p. gen. mgr., The Suburban Companies; 1969–71: pres. and chief exec. officer, Deluxe General, Inc. Pres. and Director of Movietonews, Inc. Bd. chm. Keith Cole Photograph, Inc. 1972–78. bd. chm., pres. and chief exec. officer, Pace International Corp., 1969 to present. past pres. of UCLA Executive Program Ass'n. Fellow SMPTE, Member M.P. Academy; TV Academy; assoc. mem., American Society of Cinematographers.

KRESS, HAROLD F.: Director, film editor. b. Pittsburgh, Pa., June 26, 1913. e. U. of Calif., L.A. Film ed., Command Decision, Madame Curie, Mrs. Miniver, The Yearling; crime shorts; 5-reel Army documentary short, Ward Care for Psychotic Patients. Member: Acad. of M.P. Arts and Sci-

ences, Screen Directors Guild, Film Editors Guild.
PICTURES INCLUDE: Painted Hills, No Questions Asked, Apache War Smoke, Ride Vaquero, Saadia, Rose Marie, Valley of the Kings, The Cobweb, The Prodigal, I'll Cry Tomorrow, Teahouse of the August Moon, Silk Stockings, Until They Sail, Merry Andrew, Imitation General, The World, The Flesh and The Devil, Count Your Blessings, Home from the Hills, The Greatest Story Ever Told, Walk Don't Run, Alvarez Kelly, Academy Award for Film Editing on How the West Was Won.
FILM EDITOR: Poseidon Adventure, The Iceman Cometh, 99-44/100ths % Dead, The Towering Inferno.

KREUGER, KURT: Actor. b. St. Moritz Switzerland, July 23, 1917; e. U. Lausanne, U. London. Came to U.S. 1937, partner in travel bureau: acted in Wharf Theat. group. Cape Cod, 1939; Broadway debut in Candle in the Wind with Helen Hayes, 1941.
PICTURES INCLUDE: Mademoiselle Fifi, Hotel Berlin, Paris Underground, Dark Corner, Unfaithfully Yours, Fear, The St. Valentine's Day Massacre, What Did You Do in the War Daddy?

KRIER, JOHN N.: Executive. b. Rock Island, Ill. e. Augustana Coll. Joined A. H. Blank Theatres, Grad. Publix Theatres Manager Training School, 1930: managed theatres in Illinois, Iowa, Nebraska; joined Intermountain Theatres, Salt Lake City, 1937: appointed Purchasing Head, 1946: buyer-booker, 1952: v.p., gen. mgr., 1955: appt. v.p. gen mgr. ABC Theas., Arizona, 1968: appt. v.p. director Film Buying ABC Theatres of California & ABC Intermountain Theatres, Feb. 1972. Became consultant ABC Southern Theatres, 1974. Joined Exhibitors Relations Inc. as partner, 1978. Elected pres., 1982.

KRIM, ARTHUR B.: Attorney. b. New York City, 1910. e. Columbia U., B.A., '32, 1932 became member law firm Philips, Nizer, Benjamin, Krim & Ballon, N.Y. elected pres. United Artists Feb. 20, 1951; chairman of bd., 1969 to January 1978; Ch. of Board, Orion Pictures Company, March, 1978.

KRISTOFFERSON, KRIS: Actor-singer. b. Brownsville, Texas, 1936. e. Pomona College, Oxford Univ. (Rhodes Scholar). Joined U.S. Army briefly and taught English Literature at West Point. Started writing songs (country music) and hits have included Me and Bobby McGee, Why Me, Lord, Sunday Mornin' Comin' Down, etc. Film debut in Cisco Pike, 1971. Continues to make records, do concert tours and appear in films.
PICTURES: Cisco Pike, Pat Garrett and Billy the Kid, Blume in Love, Bring Me the Head of Alfredo Garcia, Alice Doesn't Live Here Anymore, Vigilante Force, The Sailor Who Fell from Grace with the Sea, A Star Is Born, Semi-Tough, Convoy, Heaven's Gate, Roll-Over, Songwriter, Flashpoint, Trouble in Mind.
TELEVISION: The Lost Honor of Kathryn Beck, Blood & Orchids, Stagecoach, The Last Days of Frank and Jesse James.

KRONICK, WILLIAM: Writer-director. b. Amsterdam, N.Y. e. Columbia College, A.B.; U.S. Navy photography; wrote, dir. featurette, A Bowl of Cherries.
TV DOCS: Wrote, dir., prod.: To the Ends of the Earth, Mysteries of the Great Pyramid; George Plimpton Specials; National Geographic, Ripley's Believe It or Not, et. al. Wrote: Raiders of the Lost Ark, Great Movie Stunts. Prod.: In Search of . . . series.
FEATURE FILMS: Horowitz in Dublin (dir., s.p.); Flash Gordon and King Kong (2nd unit dir.); The 500 Pound Jerk (dir., TV movie).

KROST, BARRY: Producer. Partner with Doug Chapin and Mel Simon in The Movie Company, a film, TV, and theatrical production co. Also pres., BKM Management, involved in managing stars. Credits are as exec. prod.
PICTURES: When a Stranger Calls, Uforia, Pandemonium, American Dreamer.
TELEVISION: Movies: Second Sight, Missing Pieces, The Rules of Marriage, When the Circus Comes to Town, Belle Starr.

KRUEGER, RONALD P.: Executive. b. St. Louis, MO, Oct. 19, 1940. e. Westminister Coll. (1961). Began working in theatres as a teenager when father headed Wehrenberg Theatres. Assumed presidency when father died, 1962.
MEMBER: NATO and regional v.p.; American Film Institute; advisory bd. mbr., Salvation Army.

KRUGER, HARDY: Actor. b. Berlin, Germany, April 12, 1928; ent. m.p. ind. 1943; on stage since 1945.
PICTURES INCLUDE: The One That Got Away, Bachelor of Hearts (Rank). German version of The Moon is Blue (U.A.). 1959: The Rest is Silence (German film of Hamlet), Blind Date (Britain). He has also starred in twenty-four German films. 1960: Filming in France and Germany. 1961–62: Films include: Taxi Pour Tobrouk (France), Hatari (Paramount, Hollywood). 1962: Les Dimanches de Ville d'Avray (France), etc. 1963: Le Gros Coup (France). 1964: Les Pianos Mecaniques (France), Le Chant Du Monde (France). 1965: Flight of the Phoenix (Hollywood) 1966: The Defector (U.S.A.), La Grande Sauterelle (France). 1967: Le Franciscain de Bourge (France). 1968–9: The Battle of the Neretva, The Red Tent, The Nun of Monza, The Secret of Santa Vittoria. 1971: Night Hair Child. 1972: Death Of A Stranger (Israel). 1973–74: Le Solitaire (France), Barry Lyndon (England). 1974–75: Paper Tiger (England/Germany), Potato Fritz (Germany). 1976: A Bridge Too Far (England/U.S.A.), L'Autopsie d'un Monstre (France). 1977: The Wild Geese (England); Wrong Is Right (U.S.A.).

KRUGER, JEFFREY S.: Producer, concert impresario, record and music publisher, film distribution exective. Born 19th April, 1931, London. Chairman of the Kruger Organisation (Concert Promotions) Ltd., Bulldog Records Ltd., Kruger Leisure Organisation Ltd., Visual and Audio Leisure Co. Ltd. Produced feature films Rock You Sinners; Sweet Beat; The Amorous Sex. Distributor of Jack Nicolson's the Shooting, Love Child (Dyan Cannon), Dial Rat For Terror (Yaphet Kotto), Starcrash, (Christopher Plummer: David Hasselhoff: Caroline Monro); Kill the Shogun; Red Light In The Whitehouse; Enforcer From Death Row; A Whale Of A Tale, Vengeance Of The Barbarians, From Nashville With Music, togetherness, Forbidden Love, Search For The Evil One, Gallery Of Horrors, Grave Of The Vampire, Tomb Of The Undead, Sex And the Lonely Woman, House Of Terror, Smoke In The Wind, Ten Fingers Of Steel, Psychopath, Choppers, Deadwood 76, Good Time Outlaws, Ground Zero, Journey To The Centre Of Time, and others. Produced (in association with B.B.C.-TV): 20 musical specials including six one-hour musicals starring Glen Campbell as well as shows starring Marvin Gaye, Jacksons, Charley Pride, George Burns, Charlie Rich, Anne Murray, Helen Reddy, Dionne Warwick, Blood, Sweat & Tears, War, David Soul, Frankie Laine, Jerry Lee Lewis and many others. Concert presentations include Glen Campbell, HElen Reddy, Anne Murray, Jack Benny, George Burns, Charlie Rich, Charley Pride, Stylistics, Trini Lopez, Jerry Lewis, Dionne Warwicke, Sara Vaughan, Wayne Newton, Billie Holiday, Abbe Lane, Marvin Gaye, Supremes, Lena Horne, Tony Bennett, Marty Allen, Barry White, Isaac Hayes, Chi-Lites, Vic Damone, Bill Anderson, Faron Young, Vera Lynn, Edwin Starr, Ray Stevens, Temptations, Bill Haley And The Comets, Jerry Lee Lewis, The Jacksons, Frankie Valli And The Four Seasons, David Soul, Don Williams, Commodores, Frankie Laine, Gloria Gaynor, etc. Music publ. through Songs For Today. Own record production and distribution via Bulldog Records and Visual and Audio Leisure Co. Ltd. Director The Kruger Organisation (Concerts) Ltd. Songs For Today Ltd. Ember Enterprises Inc. Visual and Audio Leisure Co. Ltd. Hillbrow Productions Ltd. Recipient, certificate of merits from City of Beverly Hills & commendation from City of Los Angeles.

KUBRICK, STANLEY: Producer, director, writer. b. New York, N.Y., July 26, 1928; e. Taft H.S. Staff photog., Look magazine; writer, prod., dir., documentaries including Day of the Fight, Flying Padre; prod., dir., s.p., Fear and Desire, Killer's Kiss; dir., s.p., The Killing; writer-dir., Paths of Glory; dir. Spartacus; prod. dir., Lolita; prod. dir., writer, Dr. Strangelove; prod. dir., writer, 2001; A Space Odyssey; A Clockwork Orange; Barry Lyndon; The Shining; Full Metal Jacket (dir., co-prod., co-s.p.).

KUHN, THOMAS G.: Executive. b. Chicago, Ill., Nov. 10, 1935. e. Northwestern Univ., 1957; Univ. of So. Calif. (MBA), 1966. Singer on Roulette Records, 1958–59. KNBC-TV sales 1960–62; NBC business affairs, 1962–64; NBC mgr. live night time progs., 1965–67; dir. live night time progs., 1968–69. Warner Bros. TV, v.p. program dev. 1970; v.p. TV prod., 1971; exec. prod., Alice (WB-CBS), 1976; exec. prod., The Awakening Land (WB-NBC), 1977; exec. v.p. for Alan Landsburg Prods., 1977; exec. prod., Torn Between Two Lovers, 1978; exec. prod., The Jayne Mansfield Story, 1980; Long Way Home, 1982. Staff, v.p., west coast, for RCA Selectavision Video Discs, 1980; division v.p., 1981. Pres., RCA Video Prods., 1984.

KULIK, SEYMOUR (BUZZ): Producer-dir. b. N.Y.C., TV: Lux Video, Kraft; joined CBS-TV as prod.-dir., 1956; dir., You Are There, Climax, Playhouse 90, Defenders, Dr. Kildare, Twilight Zone, Dick Powell Playhouse; exec. prod., Kentucky Jones. 1964: v.p. chg. West Coast Prods., Bob Banner Associates Inc., 1965; 1967 Prod-Dir. with Paramount Studios, Brian's Song (TV); Shamus.
PICTURES: Warning Shot, The Riot, Villa Rides, The Hunter, Pursuit.
TELEVISION: Kane & Abel.

KUNO, MOTOJI: Sr. Managing Director. Tokyo Shibaure Electric Co., Ltd. (Toshiba), Tokyo, Japan. Graduated Law Dept., Tokyo Imperial Univ. Mar., 1923. Became Toshiba auditor June, 1941; dir. June, 1942; sr. managing dir. Nov., 1948, perm. auditor Apr. 1949; dir. Fem., 1950; exec. dir. May, 1952; sr. managing dir. May, 1958.

KUPPER, W. J.: Executive. b. New York, N.Y., Oct. 17, 1896. World Film Corp. 2 yrs.; h.o. 20th-Fox, Aug., 1919; asst. mgr. Dallas, 1920; br. mgr., Washington, Oct. 1921; later, br. mgr., Albany, Charlotte, Pittsburgh, Chicago; asst. gen. sales mgr., h.o., Jan., 1924; spcl. rep., 1928; west div. mgr., Aug., 1932; gen. sales mgr., U.S., Canada, 1942; mag. dir., 20th-Fox Films of Gt. Brit., 1947–54; v.p., gen. sales mgr. Chromart Colour Org., England; 1954. Member: M.P. Pioneers; Variety Club of Gt. Brit.

KURALT, CHARLES: TV News Correspondent. b. Wilmington, NC. e. Univ. of North Carolina. Reporter-columnist for Charlotte News until joining CBS News as writer in 1956. Promoted to news assignment desk in 1958. Became first host of CBS News series, Eyewitness, in 1960. Named CBS News chief Latin American correspondent (based in Rio de Janeiro) in 1961 Appt. CBS News chief west coast correspondent in 1963; transferred to New York, 1964. Has worked on CBS Reports, CBS News Specials, and On the Road series for CBS Evening News with Walter Cronkite (latter 11 years). Now anchor man for CBS News Sunday Morning.

KURI, EMILE: Set decorator. b. Mexico City, Mex., June 11, 1907; e. Chaminade Coll., 1924–27. Interior decorator Be Hennesey Art Studio, 1929–32; then set decorator property dept. dir.
PICTURES INCLUDE: I'll Be Seeing You, Silver Queen, Spellbound, Duel in the Sun, Paradine Case, The Heiress (Academy Award, 1949), A Place in the Sun, Carrie, Shane, The Actress, Executive Suite, 20,000 Leagues Under the Sea (Academy Award, 1954); in charge of interior exterior decorations Disneyland. Several Golden Chair Awards (L.A. Furniture Mart). Mem.: Nat'l Acad. of TV Arts and Sciences, American Institute of Interior Designers, Bd. of Gov. Acad. of M.P. Arts and Sciences (1959–69). Honorary Sir Knights of Royal Rosarians, State of Oregon (1970), Decorating Consultant, Disney World, Fla.

KURODA, TOYOJI: Executive. b. Tokyo. April 29, 1920. e. Waseda Univ. Joined Motion Picture Producers Association 1945; appointed inspectorate Board of Trade in export film division 1948. On occasion of founding of Association for Diffusion Japanese Films Abroad (UniJapan Film) became manager.

KUROSAWA, AKIRA: Director. b. Japan. March 23, 1910. Entered PCL Studio 1936 and made director 1943.
PICTURES INCLUDE: Sanshiro Sugata, The Most Beautiful, Those Who Tread on The Tiger's Tail, No Regrets For Our Youth, The Quiet Duel, Scandal, Stray Dog, Rashomon, The Seven Samurai, The Drunken Angel, The Lower Depths, The Idiot, Ikiru, I Live in Fear, The Hidden Fortress, Throne of Blood, Yojimbo, High and Low, Red Beard, The Bad Sleep Well, Sanjourno, Kagemusha, Ran.

KURTIS, BILL: News Correspondent-Anchor. b. Pensacola, FL, Sept. 21, 1940. e. Univ. of Kansas and Washington Univ. School of Law, Topeka. Member of American Bar Assn. Career in broadcast jounalism began at WIBW Radio in Topeka. Joined CBS News as reporter-producer at Los Angeles bureau in 1970; named CBS news correspondent in 1971. Joined WBBM-TV, Chicago, in 1973 as co-anchor of news broadcasts. In 1982 returned to CBS News as correspondent and co-anchor of CBS Morning News. Left in 1985.

KURTZ, GARY: Producer-Director. b. Los Angeles, 1941. e. Univ. of So. Calif., Cinema School. Began prof. career during college. Has worked as cameraman, soundman, editor for Roger Corman, other prods. Also worked on documentaries. Was asst. dir. for two Monte Hellman westerns, Ride in the Whirlwind, The Shooting. Was prod. supvr. for The Hostage before being drafted into Marines. Spent 2 yrs. in Photo Field as cameraman, editor and still photo.
PICTURES INCLUDE: Two-Lane Blacktop (asst. prod.), Chandler (asst. prod.), American Graffiti (co.-prod.); Star Wars (prod.), The Empire Strikes Back (prod.); Return to Oz (exec. prod.).

KURTZ, SWOOZIE: Actress. b. Omaha, Sept. 6. On Broadway in Enter a Free Man, Fifth of July, etc.
PICTURES: Slap Shot, First Love, Oliver's Story, The World According to Garp, Against All Odds, Wildcats.
TELEVISION: Uncommon Women, Marriage Is Alive and Well, Mating Season, Love Sidney, The Fifth of July, A Caribbean Mystery, Guilty Conscience, A Time To Live.

KUTNER, MARTIN: Executive. Joined Paramount Pictures in 1971 as eastern div. mgr.; has held various positions in sls. dept. Named v.p., gen. sls. mgr.; in 1980 appt. senior v.p., domestic distribution; 1983, exec. v.p., distribution; 1984, exec. v.p., intl. mkt. & dist.

KWIT, NATHANIEL TROY, JR.: Executive. b. N.Y.C., 1941. B.A. Cornell Univ.; M.B.A. New York Univ. 1964–68, American Broadcasting Co., Inc., exec. asst. to pres. of ABC Films. 1968–71, National Screen Service Corp., New York branch mgr., asst. genl. sls. mgr. 1971, founder, CEO Audience Marketing, Inc., later acquired by Viacom International as operating subsidiary. 1974 named v.p. marketing services, Warner Bros., Inc. 1979, named v.p. in charge video and special markets division, United Artists Corp.; 1981, named sr. v.p. in chg. UA television, video, special market div. Following acquisition of UA Corp. by MGM in 1981 promoted to pres., dist. & mktd. for MGM/UA Entertainment Co. 1983, pres. & CEO, United Satellite Communicationa, direct broadcast TV co. formed with Prudential Insurance Co. backing.

KYO, MACHIKO: Actress. b. Osaka, Japan. e. Osaka, Japan. Dancer in Osaka and Tokyo music halls; entered films 1948 with Daiei Studio; has appeared in numerous Japanese films.
PICTURES INCLUDE: Rashomon, Gate of Hell, Golden Demon, Story of Shunkin, Tales of Genji, Street of Shame, Teahouse of the August Moon, Ugetsu.

L

LADD, JR., ALAN: Executive. b. Los Angeles, Oct. 22, 1937. Motion picture agent, Creative Management Associates, 1963–69. M.p. producer, 1969–73; produced 9 films in 4 yrs. Joined 20th Century-Fox in 1973 in chg. of creative affairs in feature div. Promoted to v.p., production, 1974. In 1975 named sr. v.p. for worldwide prod.; 1976, promoted to pres. of 20th Century-Fox Pictures. Resigned & formed The Ladd Co., 1979. In 1985 appt. pres. & COO, MGM/UA Entertainment Film Corp.

LADD, CHERYL: Actress. b. Huron, S.D., July 2, 1951. r.n. Cheryl Stoppelmoore. M. film actor David Ladd. Joined professional Music Shop Band while in elementary school; left with it on tour, ending up in Los Angeles. Cast as voice of Melody character in animated Josie and the Pussycats. Studied acting with Milton Katselas. Did TV commercials, small parts in TV, made film Jamaica Reef (unreleased).
TELEVISION: Series: Charlie's Angels. Guest star on Ben Vereen . . . His Roots, General Electric's All-Star Anniversary, John Denver and the Ladies, Police Woman, Happy Days, Switch, etc. Had own special, Cheryl Ladd. Movies: A New Start, Romance on the Orient Express, A Death in California, Crossings.
PICTURE: Purple Hearts.

LADD, DAVID ALAN: Actor. b. Los Angeles, Feb. 5, 1947. Son of late Alan Ladd. On stage in the Glass Menagerie and Alpha Beta.
PICTURES: The Lone Ranger, The Big Land, Raymie, Misty, R.P.M., Catlow, Deathline, Jamaica Reef, Day of the Locusts, Kansan, Wild Geese.
TELEVISION: Zane Gray Theatre, Wagon Train, Playhouse 90, Pursuit, Ben Casey, Gunsmoke, Love American Style, Kojak.

LADD, DIANE: Actress. b. Meridian, MS, Nov. 29, 1939. e. St. Aloysius Academy; trained for stage with Frank Corsaro in NY. New York stage debut in Texas Trilogy. Film debut in Wild Angels, 1966.
PICTURES: Wild Angels, The Reivers, Macho Calahan, W.U.S.A., White Lightning, Alice Doesn't Live Here Anymore, Chinatown, Embryo, All Night Long, Something Wicked This Way Comes.
TELEVISION: Alice, Rose and Eddie, Addie and the King of Hearts, Willa, Black Beauty, The Secret Storm, Love Boat, Crime of Innocence.

LAFFERTY, PERRY: Executive. b. Oct. 3, 1920. With CBS-TV as v.p., programs, Hollywood, 1965–76. Joined Filmways as exec. prod. In 1979 named sr. v.p., programs and talent, west coast, for NBC Entertainment. 1985, resigned. Now indep. producer.

LAHTI, CHRISTINE: Actress. b. Detroit, MI, April 4, 1950. e. Univ. of Mich. Trained for stage at Herbert Berghof Studios with Uta Hagen. NY stage debut in The Woods, 1978. Film debut in And Justice for All, 1980.
PICTURES: Whose Life Is It, Anyway?, Swing Shift, Just Between Friends.
TELEVISION: The Last Tenant, The Executioner's Song.

LAI, FRANCIS: Composer. b. France, 1933.
PICTURES INCLUDE: A Man and a Woman, Mayerling, House of Cards, Rider on the Rain, Love Story (Oscar), Le Petit Matin, Another Man, Another Chance, Bilitis, The Good and the Bad, Widow's Nest, Cat and Mouse, International Velvet, Oliver's Story (Oscar), Beyond the Reef, A Second Chance.

LAKE, ARTHUR: Actor. r.n. Arthur Silverlake; b. Corbin, Ky. Stage debut at 3 yrs. of age; m.p. debut in silent Western 1924; sound m.p. debut Air Circus 1928; in vaudeville; on radio in "Blondie and Dagwood" series; owner of plastics

household products co.; org. Arthur Lake Productions.
PICTURES INCLUDE: Sweet Sixteen comedies, Cradle Snatchers, Dance Hall, Annapolis Salute, Everybody's Doing It, There Goes My Heart, Blondie series, Sixteen Fathoms Deep.

LAMARR, HEDY: Actress. b. Vienna, 1915. At 15 starred in Ecstasy (awarded top Italian film-prize).
PICTURES INCLUDE: Algiers, I Take This Woman, Lady of the Tropics, Boom Town, Comrade X, Come Live With Me, Ziegfeld Girl; H. M. Pulham, Esq.; Tortilla Flat, Crossroads, White Cargo, Heavenly Body, Conspirators, Strange Woman, Samson and Delilah, A Lady Without a Passport, Dishonored Lady, Experiment Perilous, Let's Live a Little, Copper Canyon, My Favorite Spy, Story of Mankind, The Female Animal.

LAMAS, LORENZO: Actor. b. Los Angeles, Jan. 20, 1958. e. Santa Monica City College. Son of the late Fernando Lamas and Arlene Dahl. Studied at Tony Barr's Film Actors Workshop (Burbank Studios).
PICTURES: Grease, Tilt, Take Down, Body Rock.
TELEVISION: Series: The Love Boat, Switch, Sword of Justice, California Fever, Secrets of Midland Heights, Falcon Crest. Movie: Detour.

LAMB, GIL: Actor. b. Minneapolis, Minn., June 14, 1906; e. U. Minn. On stage before screen debut 1939 in The Fleet's In, Lambs Clubs (N.Y.) On screen 1943.
PICTURES INCLUDE: Riding High, Rainbow Island, Practically Yours, Hit Parade of 1947, Make Mine Laughs, Humphrey Takes a Chance, Bye Bye Birdie, The Gnome-Mobile, Blackbeard's Ghost, The Love Bug.

LAMBERT, CHRISTOPHER: Actor. b. New York City; reared in Geneva. Parents French. Studied at French Conservatorie. Won role in small French film, Le Bar du Telephone.
PICTURES: La Dame de Coeur, Legitime Violence, Greystoke: The Legend of Tarzan, Lord of the Apes, Subway, Highlander.

LAMBERT, VERITY: Producer. b. London, England. Ent. TV 1954, prod. Dr. Who, Adam Adamant Lives, Detective, Somerset Maugham (all BBC series). Since 1971: Shoulder to Shoulder (series), Budgie, Between The Wars. 1974: Appt. controller of Drama, Thames Television. 1979: Chief exec. Euston Films. 1983: Director of Production Thorn EMI Films Ltd. Relinquished her position as controller of Drama Thames and retaining pos. as chief exec., Euston Films.

LAMOUR, DOROTHY: Actress. b. Dec. 10, 1914, New Orleans, La.; e. Spence's Business Sch. Miss New Orleans 1931; sang on radio programs; screen debut in Jungle Princess 1938.
PICTURES INCLUDE: Spawn of the North, St. Louis Blues, Man About Town, Disputed Passage, Johnny Apollo, Typhoon, Road to Singapore, Caught in the Draft, Star Spangled Rhythm, Road to Utopia, Practically Yours, Medal for Benny, Duffy's Tavern, My Favorite Brunette, Road to Rio, Wild Harvest, Miracle Can Happen, Lulu Belle, Girl from Manhattan, Lucky Stiff, Slightly French, Manhandled, The Greatest Show on Earth, Road to Bali, Road to Hong Kong, Donovan's Reef, The Phynx.

LANCASTER, BURT: Actor. b. New York City, Nov. 2, 1913; e. N.Y.U. Was circus acrobat, in vaudeville; served in U.S. Army Special Service in Italy & N. Africa, World War II; screen debut in The Killers, 1946. Formed Hecht-Lancaster Orgn. in partnership with Harold Hecht.
PICTURES INCLUDE: Desert Fury, I Walk Alone, Brute Force, Sorry Wrong Number, Kiss the Blood Off My Hands, Criss Cross, All My Sons, Rope of Sand, Mister 880, Flame and the Arrow, Vengeance Valley, Ten Tall Men, Jim Thorpe—All American, Crimson Pirate, Come Back Little Sheba, South Sea Woman, From Here to Eternity, His Majesty O'Keefe, Apache, Vera Cruz, The Kentuckian, Rose Tattoo, Trapeze, The Rainmaker, Gunfight at the OK Corral, Sweet Smell of Success, Separate Tables, The Devil's Disciple, Elmer Gantry, The Young Savages, Birdman of Alcatraz, The Leopard, Seven Days in May, Hallelujah Trail, The Swimmer, The Gypsy Moths, Castlekeep, Airport, Valdez Is Coming, Lawman, Ulzana's Raid, Scorpio, Executive Action, The Midnight Man (prod., dir. & star), Conversation Piece, Buffalo Bill and the Indians, The Cassandra Crossing, Twilight's Last Gleaming, The Island of Dr. Moreau, 1900, Go Tell the Spartans, Cattle Annie and Little Britches, Atlantic City, Local Hero, The Osterman Weekend, Little Treasure, Tough Guys.
TELEVISION: Scandal Sheet, On Wings of Eagles.

LANCHESTER, ELSA: Actress and authoress. b. London, England, Oct. 28, 1902. m. Charles Laughton. Acted in London, New York. At 16, started the Children's Theatre in London. Acted in London and New York with her husband. First British film was The Constant Nymph, silent version; The Private Life of Henry VIII, 1933, London Films. In 1935: David Copperfield, Naughty Marietta, MGM, and The Bride of Frankenstein, U. In 1936: The Ghost Goes West, Rembrandt, UA-London Films. In 1938: the Beachcomber, Mayflower-Par. In 1938: authoress of Charles Laughton and I. In 1939–40: Hollywood and on stage. In 1941: on screen, Ladies in Retirement, Col. In 1942: Son of Fury, Tales of Manhattan, 20th-Fox. In 1943: Forever and a Day, Lassie Come Home, Passport to Adventure, Witness for the Prosecution, Bell, Book and Candle.
PICTURES INCLUDE: The Spiral Staircase, The Razor's Edge, Northwest Outpost, Bishop's Wife, Come to the Stable, Secret Garden, Inspector General, Buccaneer's Girl, Mystery Street, Frenchie, Petty Girl, Androcles and the Lion, Dreamboat, Les Miserables, The Girls of Pleasure Island, Hell's Half Acre, Three Ring Circus, Glass Slipper, Mary Poppins, That Darn Cat, Blackbeard's Ghost, Easy Come Easy Go, Rascal, Me, Natalie, My Dog, The Thief, Willard, Arnold, Murder by Death.
TV: Studio One, Omnibus, Schlitz Playhouse, John Forsythe Show, Dick Cavett, Johnny Carson, Merv Griffin, David Frost Shows. Guest appearances on Mannix, Bill Cosby, To Catch a Thief, Then Came Bronson, Lucy Show.
BOOKS: Charles Laughton and I (1939); Elsa Lanchester, Herself (1983).

LANDAU, ELY A.: Executive. b. New York, N.Y., Jan. 20, 1920; formed National Telefilm Associates, Inc., 1954; org. NTA Film Network, 1956; pres., chmn. of bd., National Telefilm Associates, Inc., 1957; resigned, 1961; formed Ely Landau Company, Inc., 1963; dist. The Servant, King and Country, Umbrellas of Cherbourg; prod. Long Day's Journey Into Night, The Fool Killer, The Pawnbroker, A Face of War, The Madwoman of Chaillot. Prod. King—A Filmed Record—Montgomery to Memphis, 1968; organized, directed one-night simultaneous charity showing 633 theatres U.S., 1970; 1972 Formed American Film Theatre, and the Ely Landau Organization, Inc. 1972–74 produced Iceman Cometh, Rhinoceros, The Homecoming, A Delicate Balance, Luther, Lost In The Stars, Burley Galileo, In Celebration, The Man in the Glass Booth, 1978: The Greek Tycoon. 1980: 1981; Hopscotch; 1982: The Chosen; Beatlemanie—The Movie, 1981; The Deadly Game, 1982; Separate Tables, 1983; Mr. Halpern and Mr. Johnson. 1984: The Holcroft Covenant.

LANDAU, MARTIN: Actor. b. N.Y.C., June 20, 1934. Cartoon and staff artist on N.Y. Daily News; studied 3 yrs. at Actors Studio.
PICTURES INCLUDE: Pork Chop Hill, North by Northwest, Gazebo, Stagecoach to Dancer's Rock, Cleopatra, The Hallelujah Trail, The Greatest Story Ever Told, Nevada Smith, A Town Called Hell, Black Gunn, Strange Shadows in an Empty Room, Meteor, The Last Word.
TV: Mission Impossible (1966–68), etc.
STAGE: Middle of the Night, Uncle Vanya, Stalag 17, Wedding Breakfast, First Love, The Goat Song.

LANDAU, RICHARD H.: Writer. b. New York City, Feb. 21, 1914; e. U. Arizona, Yale U. With Small-Landau agency handling writers and stories; shorts dept. writer MGM 1939; writer for RKO Radio since 1942; wrote documentaries and raining films for U.S. Army.
PICTURES INCLUDE: Gun in His Hand, Strange Confession, Challenge in the Night, Back to Bataan, Little Iodine, Christmas Eve, Crooked Way, Johnny One Eye, Roadblock, Lost Continent, F.B.I. Girl, Stolen Face, Bad Blonde, Spaceways, Sins of Jezebel, Blackout, Deadly Game, A Race for Life, Pearl of the South Pacific, Creeping Unknown.

LANDIS, JOHN: Director. b. Chicago, Aug. 30, 1950.
PICTURES: Schlock, Kentucky Fried Movie, National Lampoon's Animal House, The Blues Brother (also s.p.), American Werewolf in London, Trading Places, Twilight Zone—The Movie (prod., s.p. also), Into the Night, Spies Like Us, Three Amigos (dir.).

LANDON, MICHAEL: Actor-Writer-Director. b. Forest Hills, N.Y., Oct. 31. e. U.S.C. Was athlete before signed by Warner Bros. to attend acting school. Roles in films and TV followed; big break came with Bonanza.
TV: Actor: Restless Gun, Bonanza, Little House on the Prairie. Guest appearances on Variety Shows. Writer-Director: Love Came Laughing (Love Story series). Director: Roy Campanella Story. Producer: Little House on the Prairie.

LANDRES, PAUL: Director. b. New York, N.Y., Aug. 21, 1912. e. U.C.L.A. Started as asst. Film Editor at Universal 1931. Editor 1937 to 1949 of many feature films. Director of feature films and TV since 1949. Under Directorial contract to Warner Bros. 1961–62. Director of 22 feature films for theatrical release.
PICTURES INCLUDE: Oregon Passage, A Modern Marriage, Mark of the Vampire, Navy Bound, The Curse of Dracula, Miracle of the Hills, 54 Washington Street and Son of a Gunfighter made in Spain for MGM release.
TELEVISION: 91 hour films and over 300 half hour shows including among many others, multiple episodes of Bonanza, Daktari, The Rifleman, 77 Sunset Strip, Maverick

Hawaiian Eye, The Plainsman, Readers Digest, Topper, Wyatt Earp, Blondie, etc.

LANDSBURG, ALAN: Executive, producer. b. New York City, May 10, 1933. e. New York University, Producer for NBC News Dept., 1951–59; producer-writer, CBS, 1959–60; exec. prod., Wolper Productions/Metromedia Producers Corp., 1961–70; pres., Alan Landsburg Productions, 1970–present.

LANE, DIANE: Actress. b. New York City, Jan., 1963. Debut in A Little Romance (1979).
PICTURES: Touched by Love, Six Pack, Ladies and Gentlemen: The Fabulous Stains, The Outsiders, Rumble Fish, The Cotton Club.
STAGE: The Cherry Orchard, Agamemmon, Runaway, etc.

LANG, CHARLES: Cinematographer. b. Bluff, Utah, March 27, 1902. e. Lincoln H.S., Los Angeles, U.S.C. Entered m.p. ind. with Paramount Film Laboratory, then asst. cameraman; dir. of photography, Paramount, 1929–52; then freelance.
PICTURES INCLUDE: A Farewell to Arms (Academy Award for best photography, 1933); Ghost and Mrs. Muir, A Foreign Affair, September Affair, Ace in the Hole, Sudden Fear, Sabrina, Queen Bee, Man from Laramie, The Rainmaker, Some Like It Hot, The Magnificent Seven, Facts of Life, One-Eyed Jacks, Summer and Smoke, Charade, Father Goose, Wait Until Dark, Inside Daisy Clover, Hotel, Flim Flam Man, The Stalking Moon, Cactus Flower, Bob & Carol & Ted & Alice, The Love Machine, Doctors' Wives, Butterflies Are Free.

LANG, DAVID: Writer. b. New York City, Nov. 30, 1913. Was in Merchant Marine three years. Joined Charles Mintz Studio (Columbia) as cartoonist. Moved to MGM cartoon dept. 1938–40. Radio writer, Calling All Cars, KNX, Los Angeles, 1941. Contract writer at MGM, 1941–43. Yank on the Burma Road, Gambler's Choice, Hired Gun, North West Mounted Police. For Par. Midnight Manhunt, People Are Funny, Caged Fury, One Exciting Night. For Warner Bros. Flaxy Martin, Smart Money. For Columbia, Chain of Circumstance, Ambush at Tomahawk, The Nebraskan, Black Horse Canyon for U.I. Also Screaming Eagles, Hellcats of the Navy, Buckskin Lady. For PRC, Queen of Burlesque.
TELEVISION: Cheyenne, 87th Precinct, Ford Theatre, Gallant Men, Westinghouse Theatre, Adventures in Paradise, Bonanza, Trackdown, Wanted Dead or Alive, Rifleman, Rawhide, Have Gun Will Travel. At least two hundred credits in above series. Novelist. Oedipus Burning. Publisher, Stein and Day.

LANG, JENNINGS: Executive. b. New York City, May 28, 1915. e. St. John's Univ. & Law School. m. actress-singer Monica Lewis. Went into law practice in 1937 with Seligsburg and Lewis, m.p. law specialists. In 1938 went to Hollywood and became 2nd asst. dir. at Grand National Studios. Opened own office as actor's agent; first client, comedian Hugh Herbert. In 1940 joined Jaffe Agency; made partner and v.p. in 1942. Was pres. from 1948 to May, 1950, when resigned to join MCA. Worked in all phases of MCA operations; in 1952 made v.p. of MCA TV Ltd., and bd. mem. Involved with prod. and sales of TV prods. from inception of Revue (now Universal City Studios) in 1950. Organized Revue's New Projects Dept., creator and exec. in chg. of prog. dev. Involved with creation and sales of such series as Wagon Train, The Robert Cummings Show, Bachelor Father, Wells Fargo, Mike Hammer, etc. Most recently has been supvr. of Universal's World Premiere films, airing on Tuesday Night at the Movies and Saturday Night at the Movies (NBC).
Made Executive Producer at MCA (Universal) for motion pictures. Executive Producer on following films: Winning, They Might Be Giants, Puzzle of a Downfall Child, Coogan's Bluff, The Beguiled, Act of the Heart, Tell Them Willie Boy is Here, Play Misty for Me, Pete 'N Tillie, High Plains Drifter, Slaughterhouse Five, Charley Varrick, Breezy, The Great Waldo Pepper, Airport '75, Earthquake, Joe Kidd, The Great Northfield Minnesota Raid, The Eiger Sanction, Airport 1977, The Front Page, The Hindenburg. Producer: Swashbuckler, Roller Coaster, House Calls, Nunzio, Airport '79—The Concorde, Little Miss Marker, The Nude Bomb, The Sting II, Stick.

LANG, OTTO: Producer-Director, Four Academy Award nominations for Cinemascope Specials, Twentieth Century-Fox Film Corp. Saga of Western Man; ABC-TV Specials—The Legend of Cortez; Beethoven: Ordeal and Triumph.
TV: Man from U.N.C.L.E.; Daktari; Iron Horse; Cheyenne; Dick Powell Show; Zane Gray Theatre; Ann Sothern Show; Rifleman; Bat Masterson; Seahunt; The Deputy; Surfside 6; Hawaiian Eye. Prod. Twentieth Century Fox Hour. Dir. Man and the Challenge; Aquanauts; World of Giants. Dir. feature for Cinerama: Search for Paradise, Lancer, Felony Squad.
PICTURES: Prod., Call Northside 777; Five Fingers; White Witch Doctor. Specialist for foreign locations. Many segments for This World of Ours; Wide, Wide World. 1969. Assoc. prod: Tora! Tora! Tora!, 20th Century-Fox.

LANGAN, GLENN: Actor. b. Denver, Colo., July 8, 1917; e. Wheatridge H.S. Started career as asst. mgr. Elitch Gardens, Denver; traveled to N.Y., worked at odd jobs, until walk-on part in play, Swing Your Lady; signed by Hollywood after appearance in A Kiss for Cinderella, oppos. Luise Rainer.
PICTURES INCLUDE: Riding High, Four Jills in a Jeep, Something For The Boys, Margie, Homestretch, Forever Amber, Iroquois Trail, Treasure of Monte Cristo, Rapture, Hangman's Knot, One Girl's Confession, 99 River Street, Big Chase, Mutiny in Outer Space.

LANGE, HOPE: Actress. r.n. Hope Elise Ross Lange; b. Redding Ridge, Conn., Nov. 28, 1933. e. Reed Coll., Portland, Ore. & Barmore Jr. Coll., N.Y. Parents: John Lange, musician (Arr. music for stage shows, including Show Boat); Minnette Buddecke Lange, actress. Prof. stage debut at age 12 in The Patriots on Broadway; then in The Hot Corner; seen on TV by 20th-Fox prod. Buddy Adler and signed for Bus Stop, her screen debut.
PICTURES INCLUDE: Jesse James, Peyton Place, The Young Lions, In Love and War, The Best of Everything, A Pocketful of Miracles, How the West Was Won, Love is a Ball, Jigsaw, Death Wish, A Nightmare on Elm Street: Part 2.
TV: The Ghost and Mrs. Muir, The New Dick Van Dyke Show, That Certain Summer, I Love You—Goodbye.

LANGE, JESSICA: Actress. b. Minnesota, Apr. 20, 1949. e. Univ. of Minn. Studied mime 2 years under Etienne Decroux in Paris. Worked in experimental theatre in New York. Theatrical film debut in King Kong (1976).
PICTURES: All That Jazz, How To Beat the High Cost of Living, The Postman Always Rings Twice, Frances, Tootsie, Country (also co-prod.), Sweet Dreams, Crimes of the Heart.
TELEVISION: Cat on a Hot Tin Roof.

LANGELLA, FRANK: Actor. b. Bayonne, NJ, Jan. 1, 1940. Studied acting at Syracuse Univ.; later in regional repertory, summer stock, and on and off Bdwy. Film debut in The Twelve Chairs (1970).
PICTURES: Diary of a Mad Housewife, Dracula, Those Lips, Those Eyes, Sphinx, The Men's Club.

LANGFORD, FRANCES: Singer-actress. b. Lakeland, Fla., April 4, 1913. e. Southern Coll. Stage experience in vaudeville, nightclubs, national radio programs. In 1935: collab. on lyrics and appeared in Every Night at Eight, Collegiate Broadway Melody of 1936, Palm Springs, Born to Dance, The Hit Parade, Hollywood Hotel, Dreaming Out Loud, Too Many Girls, The Hit Parade of 1941, All-American Coed, Swing It Soldier, Mississippi Gambler, Yankee Doodle Dandy, This Is the Army, Career Girl, The Girl Rush, Dixie Jamboree, Radio Stars on Parade, People Are Funny, Deputy Marshall, Purple Heart Diary, Glenn Miller Story; TV appearances with Don Ameche.

LANGNER, PHILIP: Producer, b. New York, N.Y., Aug. 24, 1926. e. Yale U. President of The Theatre Guild and Theatre Guild Films, Inc. Producer the Westport Country Playhouse 1947–53. Joined The Theatre Guild 1954. Produced 28 plays on Broadway for the Theatre Guild including the Matchmaker, Bells Are Ringing, The Tunnel of Love, Sunrise At Campobello, A Majority of One, The Unsinkable Molly Brown, A Passage To India, Seidman and Son, The Royal Hunt of the Sun, The Homecoming, Absurd Person Singular and Golda.
FILMS: Producer of The Pawnbroker, Slaves and Born To Win. Associate Prod., Judgment At Nuremberg, and A Child Is Waiting.

LANSBURY, ANGELA: Actress. b. London, England, Oct. 16, 1925; e. South Hampstead School for Girls, England; Academy of Music, London; Feagin Dramatic School, N.Y.; p. Moyna Macgill, actress; also rel. to Robert B. Mantell, actor, & Rt. Hon. George Lansbury, gov't. official. Screen debut in "Gaslight," 1943, which won Hollywood Foreign Correspondents' Assoc. award.
PICTURES INCLUDE: National Velvet, Picture of Dorian Gray, Harvey Girls, Hoodlum Saint, Till the Clouds Roll By, Tenth Avenue Angel, If Winter Comes, State of the Union, Three Musketeers, Red Danube, Samson and Delilah, Kind Lady, Mutiny, Remains to be Seen, Purple Mask, A Lawless Street, A Life at Stake, Court Jester, Please Murder Me, A Breath of Scandal, All Fall Down, In the Cool of the Day, The Manchurian Candidate, Mr. Buddwing, Dear Heart, Something for Everyone, Bedknobs and Broomsticks, Death on the Nile, The Mirror Crack'd, The Pirates of Penzance.
BROADWAY: Mame, Dear World, Gypsy, Sweeney Todd.
TELEVISION: Sweeney Todd, Lace, The First Olympic Race, The Gift of Love. Series: Murder She Wrote.

LANSBURY, BRUCE: Executive. b. London, England, Jan. 12, 1930. e. UCLA. m. actress Moyna Macgill. writer, prod.

KABC-TV, Los Angeles, 1957–59; joined CBS-TV, 1959, was ass't. dir., program dev., Hollywood, director for daytime and nighttime programs, producer of Great Adventure series; and v.p., programs, New York; 1964–66, indep. prod., Broadway stage; 1966–69 producer, Wild Wild West, CBS series; 1969–72, prod. Mission: Impossible, Paramount Movies of Week; now v.p., creative affairs, Paramount TV.

LANSBURY, EDGAR: Producer-Designer. b. London, England, Jan. 12, 1930. e. UCLA. Brother of Angela and Bruce Lansbury. Started career as scenic designer and art director. 1955–60, art dir., CBS; 1962–63, exec. art dir. prod. for WNDT-TV, educational sta.; On Bdwy. produced such shows as The Subject Was Roses, Promenade, Waiting for Godot, Long Day's Journey into Night, Gypsy, The Night That Made America Famous, American Buffalo, etc.
PICTURES: Producer: The Subject Was Roses, Godspell, The Wild Party, Squirm, Blue Sunshine, He Knows You're Alone.
TELEVISION: The Defenders (art. dir.); Summer Girl (exec. prod.), etc.

LANSING, SHERRY: Executive. b. Chicago, July 31, 1944. e. Northwestern Univ. Taught math, English and drama in L.A. city high schools, 1966–69. Acted in films (Loving, Rio Lobo) and numerous TV shows. Story editor for Wagner Intl. Prod. Co., 1972–74. Talent Associates, in chg. West Coast development (all projects), 1974–75. Appt. MGM story editor, 1975. In 1977 named MGM v.p. of creative affairs, Nov., 1977, appointed vice pres., production, at Columbia Pictures. January, 1980, appointed pres., Twentieth Century-Fox Productions. Resigned 1982 to form new production co. with Stanley R. Jaffee: Jaffee—Lansing Prods.
PICTURES: Racing with the Moon, Firstborn.

LANTZ, WALTER: Animated cartoon producer. b. New Rochelle N.Y., April 27, 1900. Producer and creator of Woody Woodpecker, Andy Panda, Chilly Willy. Started with Gregory La Cava, 1916 with Katzenjammer Kids, Happy Hooligan and Krazy Kat. Joined J. R. Bray in 1922, producing Col. Heeza Liar, Dinky Doodle. Started with Universal Pictures in 1928. Produced first Technicolor cartoon for Paul Whiteman's King of Jazz. Produced Oswald Rabbit. Created Woody Woodpecker in 1941. Produced the first Woody Woodpecker TV show in 1957. Toured the Pacific War Zone on a handshake tour for the USO, with wife Gracie, the voice of Woody Woodpecker. Has been awarded the Golden Globe Award, the ASIFA Award, and in 1979 the OSCAR for achievement in the field of animation. Now producing the Woody Woodpecker TV show. 1986, award a star on Hollywood Walk of Fame.

LARDNER, RING W., JR.: Writer. b. Chicago, Aug. 19, 1915; married; p. Ring W. and Ellis A.; e. Phillips Acad. and Princeton U. Was reporter on New York Daily Mirror. Publ. writer, Selznick International. Shared Academy Award with Michael Kanin. Orig. Screenplay, Woman of the Year, 1942.
PICTURES INCLUDE: The Cross of Lorraine, Tomorrow the World, Forever Amber, Forbidden Street, Four Days Leave, Cloak and Dagger, The Cincinnati Kid, M*A*S*H, The Greatest.

LARKIN, JAMES J.: Executive. B. Brooklyn, N.Y., Nov. 2, 1925; e. Columbia U., 1947–52. U.S. Air Force, 1943–46; BOAC rep. to entertainment ind., 1948–60; pres., Transportation Counselors Inc., 1960–62; pres., Larkin Associates, Inc., 1962–65; exec. Radio N.Y. Worldwide, 1965–68, V.P. Grolier Educational Corp., 1968–69; V.P. Visual Informational Systems, 1969–73. Pres., Business Television Services, Inc., 1973; exec. prod., Madhouse Brigade, 1977–79; prod.-writer, All Those Beautiful Girls, 1979–80.

LARSEN, KEITH: Actor. e. Univ. of Utah. Little theatre work.
TV: Series: The Hunter, Brave Eagle.
PICTURES INCLUDE: Green Glove, Son of Belle Star, Chief Crazy Horse, Desert Sands, Night Freight, Arrow in the Dust, Dial Red O, Security Risk, Wichita, Women of the Prehistoric Planet.

LARSON, G. BENNETT: Executive. Joined KDYL, Salt Lake City as announcer, prog. mgr., 1926. Prod., dir., NBC, New York, 1929–34. Shows included Ed Wynn Texaco Show, Fleischmann House and Chase & Sanborn Hour. Radio exec. with Joseph Katz Co., Ruthrauff & Ryan, and Young & Rubicam, 1934–42. Gen. mgr. and part owner of WWDC, Washington, 1942–45. Mgr. of WPEN, Phila., 1945–47. v.p. of TV, WCAU-TV 1947–50, App'd v.p. and gen. mgr., WPIX, New York, 1950; pres., Intermountain Broadcasting Corporation, KDYL AM-FM & TV, Salt Lake City, Utah, Exec. v.p. and gen. mgr. of Flower City Television Corporation, WOKR-TV, Rochester, New York, 1979–80, pres. Larson/Walker & Co., media brokers, Los Angeles; pres., G. Bennett Larson & Associates (broadcast consultants), 1981.

LASKY, JESSE JR.: Writer. b. New York City, Sept. 19, 1910; p. Jessie and Bessie Gains Lasky; e. Blair Academy, Hun School of Princeton, Grand Central School of Art, U. Of Dijon; entered m.p. industry, foreign dept., Paramount, Spain, 1930. Was censorship editor for Paramount on story board. Assistant to Sol Wurtzel Fox.
NOVELS INCLUDE: Curtain of Life, No Angels in Heaven, Spendthrift, Naked in a Cactus Garden, The Offer (with Pat Silver); autobiography, Whatever Happened to Hollywood?
OTHER MATERIAL: Three books of verse. Short stories published in Cosmopolitan Magazine; The Gehenna of the Bone; (plays) Hope and Pray and Private Beach (in collab.); Ghost Town: (collab. s.p. or story) Secret Agent; The Red Head (s.p.); Back in the Saddle; The Singing Hill (collab. s.p.); Steel Against the Sky (film script); Union Pacific; Northwest Mounted Police; Reap the Wild Wind; (collab. narr.); Land of Liberty, dir. orig. story, s.p. Omaha Trail; U.S. Army, 1942–46; (collab. s.p.) Unconquered. Samson and Delilah; (orig. s.p.) Sickle or Cross Thief of Venice (Italy); (s.p.) Women Without Names, City of Violence (Italy); (s.p.) Lorna Doone, Mask of the Avenger, Never Trust a Gambler, The Brigand, The Silver Whip, (collab. s.p.) Mission Over Korea, (story) Salome, (collab. s.p.) Hell and High Water, Iron Glove, (s.p.) Pearl of the South Pacific, Hot Blood, (collab. s.p.) Ten Commandments, (collab. s.p.) The Buccaneer, John Paul Jones, (collab. with Pat Silver) Wizard of Bagdad, Pirates of Tortuga, River Gambler, 7 Women From Hell, The Land Grabbers (orig. story), One of Those Things (English version).
TV: Naked City, Rescue 8, Shannon, 7 of the New Breed (in collab. with Pat Silver), Avengers, Danger Man, The Saint, The World of Lowell Thomas, The Baron, The Protectors, and four musical specials for BBC; Ten Who Dared (serial with Pat Silver).

LASSER, LOUISE: Actress. b. New York City, 1941. Brandeis Univ., New Sch. for Social Research. Appeared on stage before theatrical film debut in 1965 with What's New, Pussycat?
PICTURES: What's Up, Tiger Lily?, Take the Money and Run, Bananas, Everything You Always Wanted to Know About Sex, Such Good Friends, Slither, Stardust Memories, Crimewave.
TELEVISION: Masquerade, Mary Hartman, Mary Hartman (series); The Lie, Isn't It Shocking? (movies).

LASZLO, ANDREW: Cinematographer. b. Hungary, 1926.
PICTURES: You're a Big Boy Now, The Night They Raided Minskys, Popi, Teacher, Teacher, The Out of Towners, Lovers and Other Strangers, The Owl and the Pussycat, Class of 44, the Warriors, The Funhouse, Southern Comfort, Streets of Fire, Thief of Hearts, Remo Williams, Poltergeist II.

LATHROP, PHILIP: Cinematographer. b. Jan. 12, 1916.
PICTURES INCLUDE: Experiment in Terror, Lonely Are the Brave, Days of Wine and Roses, The Pink Panther, The Americanization of Emily, Thirty Six Hours, The Cincinnati Kid, The Russians Are Coming, Point Blank, Finian's Rainbow, The Gypsy Moths, The Illustrated Man, They Shoot Horses Don't They?, Airport '77, Earthquake, A Different Story, The Concrode—Airport '79, Little Miss Marker, Foolin' Around, Loving Couples, A Change of Seasons.

LATSIS, PETER C.: Publicist. b. Chicago, Ill., Mar. 9, 1919. e. Wright Junior College, Chicago, Newspaper reporter, Chicago Herald-American, 1942–45; Army, 1943; joined Fox West Coast Theatres, Los Angeles, in theatre operations 1945; adv.-pub. dept. 1946; asst. dir. adv.-pub. 1955; press rep. National Theatres, 1958; press relations dir., National General Corp., 1963; home office special field pub. repr., American International Pictures, 1973; Filmways Pictures, 1980–82; Recipient of Publicists Guild's Robert Yeager Award, 1983.

LATTUADA, ALBERTO: Director. b. Milan, Italy, 1914. Son of Felice Lattuada, musician, opera composer, and writer of scores of many of son's films. Studied architecture; founded the periodical Cominare. Later founded Italian Film Library, of which he is still pres. Also, pres., Cinema D'Essay, First screen work as scriptwriter and asst. dir. of two films, 1940.
PICTURES INCLUDE: Mill on the Po, Anna, The Overcoat, La Lupa, Love in the City, White Sister, Flesh Will Surrender, Without Pity, The She Wolf, Tempest, The Unexpected, Mafioso, The Mandrake, Matchless, The Betrayal, The Steppe, Oh, Serafina, Stay As You Are.

LAUGHLIN, TOM: Actor-Producer-Director-Writer. b. Minneapolis, 1938. e. Univ. of Indiana, Univ. of Minn. where had athletic scholarships. m. actress Delores Taylor. Travelled around world, studying in Italy with Dr. Maria Montessori. Established, ran a Montessori school in Santa Monica for several yrs. Worked his way to Hollywood, where acted in bit parts until stardom came in Born Losers in 1967. Produced and starred in Billy Jack and The Trial of Billy Jack, also writing s.p. with wife under pseudonym Frank

Christina. Heads own prod. co., Billy Jack Enterprises.
PICTURES INCLUDE: South Pacific, Tea and Sympathy, Gidget, Born Losers, Billy Jack, The Trial of Billy Jack, The Master Gunfighter, Billy Jack Goes to Washington.

LAURENCE, DOUGLAS: Producer. b. Totowa, N.J., Dec. 16, 1922. U.S. Air Force. 1947–50; wrote, prod., dir., shows for NBC Radio. Exec. prod. talent buyer for Teleways Radio, TV Prod. 1958–59; ent. dir., Flamingo Hotel. Advisor to Brazilian govt. on building film industry.
PICTURES INCLUDE: Quick Before It Melts, Mister Buddwing, Doctor You've Got to Be Kidding, Speedway, Stay Away Joe, Live a Little Love a Little, The Outside Man, Rio Man.
STAGE: General Motors Motorama, L.A. Home Show, Calif., Wisc., Texas State Fairs, Ford Motor Auto Shows, Stay Eastern Univ. Dance Troupe, Jazz America.
TV: Strange Wills, John Charles Thomas Show, Sons of the Pioneers, All Star Hit Parade, John Gunther's High Road.

LAURENTS, ARTHUR: Writer-Director. b. New York City, e., Cornell, B.A. 1937. First professional writing as radio script writer in 1939. In Army 1941–45.
STAGE PLAYS: Author: Home of the Brave, The Bird Cage, The Time of the Cuckoo, West Side Story, Gypsy, Hallelujah, Baby! Director: Invitation to a March, I Can Get It For You Wholesale. Author-Director: Anyone Can Whistle, Do I Hear a Waltz?
SCREENPLAYS: Rope, Caught, Anastasia, The Way We Were (from his own novel), The Turning Point.

LAURIE, PIPER: Actress. r.n. Rosetta Jacobs. b. Detroit, Mich. Jan. 22, 1932. e. Los Angeles H.S. Acted in school plays, signed by U.I. in 1949; m.p. debut in Louisa; Broadway, The Glass Menagerie (revival).
PICTURES INCLUDED: The Milkman, Francis Goes to the Races, Prince Who Was A Thief, Son of Ali Baba, Has Anybody Seen My Gal, No Room for the Groom, Mississippi Gambler, Golden Blade, Dangerous Mission, Johnny Dark, Dawn at Socorro, Smoke Signal, Ain't Misbehavin', Until They Sail, The Hustler, Carrie, Ruby, Return to Oz.
TELEVISION: The Days of Wine and Roses, Rainbow, Thorn Birds, Love Mary, Tender Is The Night, etc.

LAUTER, ED: Actor. b. Long Beach, NY, Oct. 30, 1940.
PICTURES: The Last American Hero, Executive Action, Lolly Madonna, The Longest Yard, The French Connection II, Breakheart Pass, Family Plot, King Kong, Magic, Death Hunt, Timerider, Lassiter, Cujo, Finders Keepers, Death Wish 3, Youngblood, Raw Deal.
TELEVISION: Movies: Class of '63, The Migrants, The Godchild, Satan's Triangle, A Shadow in the STreets, Last Hours Before Morning, The Clone Master, The Jericho Mile, Undercover with the KKK, The Boy Who Drank Too Much, Guyana Tragedy—The Story of Jim Jones, Alcatraz—The Whole Shocking Story.

LAVEN, ARNOLD: Director-Producer. b. Feb. 23, 1922. Chicago, Ill.
PICTURES INCLUDE: Without Warning, Vice Squad, Down Three Dark Streets, The Rack, Slaughter on 10th Ave., Anna Lucasta, The Glory Guys, Rough Night in Jericho, Sam Whiskey.
TELEVISION: Part creator and director TV pilots: The Rifleman, Robert Taylor's Detectives, The Plainsmen. Many TV films.

LAVIN, LINDA: Actress. b. Portland, Me. Oct. 15, 1937. e. College of William & Mary. First professional job in chorus of Camden County (N.J.) Music Circus. Worked in plays both off and on Broadway before turning to TV, where guest-starred on such series as Family, Rhoda, Phyllis and Harry O; had recurring role in Barney Miller—all before advent of her own series, Alice.

LAW, JOHN PHILIP: Actor. b. Hollywood, 1937. e. University of Hawaii. Trained at Repertory Theatre of Lincoln Center under Elia Kazan. Did numerous Italian films before discovery in U.S.
PICTURES INCLUDE: The Russians Are Coming, The Hawaiians, Barbarella, Von Richtofen and Brown, The Last Movie, The Sergeant, The Love Machine, The Golden Voyage of Sinbad, The Cassandra Crossing, Tarzan, the Ape Man, Night Train to Terror, American Commandos.

LAWRENCE, BARBARA: Actress. b. Carnegie, Okla., Feb. 24, 1930; e. UCLA: mother Berenice Lawrence. Child model; successful screen try-out, 1944; screen debut in Billy Rose Diamond Horse Shoe.
PICTURES INCLUDE: Margie, Captain from Castile, You Were Meant for Me, Give My Regards to Broadway, Street With No Name, Unfaithfully Yours, Letter to Three Wives, Mother is a Freshman, Thieves Highway, Two Tickets to Broadway, Here Come the Nelsons, The Star, Arena, Paris Model, Her 12 Men, Oklahoma, Man With a Gun, Pay The Devil, Joe Dakota.

LAWRENCE, JODY: Actress. r.n. Josephine Lawrence Goddard. b. Fort Worth, Tex., Oct. 19, 1930; e. Beverly Hills H.S.; Hollywood Professional Sch. Signed by Columbia; m.p. debut in Mask of Avenger.
PICTURES INCLUDE: Family Secret, Son of Dr. Jekyll, Ten Tall Men, The Brigand, All Ashore, Capt. John Smith & Pocahontas, Scarlet Hour, Leather Saint.

LAWRENCE, MARC: Actor. b. New York City; e. City Coll. N.Y. On stage in Sour Mountain, Waiting for Lefty.
PICTURES INCLUDE: White Woman, Lttle Big Shot, Dr. Socrates, Road Gang, San Quentin, I Am the Law, While New York Sleeps, Dillinger, Flame of Barbary Coast, Club Havana, Don't Fence Me In, The Virginian, Life with Blondie, Yankee Fakir, Captain from Castile, I Walk Alone, Calamity Jane and Sam Bass, The Asphalt Jungle, Hurricane Island, My Favorite Spy, Girls Marked Danger, Helen of Troy, Custer of the West, Nightmare in the Sun, Night Train to Terror.

LAWRENCE, STEVE: Actor. b. New York City, July 8, 1935. Singer in nightclubs and on TV.
PICTURES INCLUDE: Stand Up and Be Counted, The Blues Brothers, The Lonely Guy.
TELEVISION: Steve and Eydie Celebrate Irving Berlin.

LAWRENCE, VICKI: Actress. b. Inglewood, CA, March 26, 1949. Singer and recording artist appearing with Young Americans group for several years. Gained fame on The Carol Burnett Show as comedienne. 1982: TV series, Mama's Family.

LAWSON, SARAH: Actress. b. London, Eng., Aug. 6, 1928. e. Heron's Ghyll School (Sussex). stage debut in Everyman (Edinburgh Festival) 1947; screen debut in The Browning Version, 1949.
PICTURES INCLUDE: Street Corner, You Know What Sailors Are, Blue Peter, It's Never Too Late, Links of Justice, Three Crooked Men, Man with a Dog, Night Without Pity, The World Ten Times Over.
TV: Face to Face, River Line, Whole Truth, Lady From the Sea, Mrs. Moonlight, Silver Card, An Ideal Husband, Love and Money, Rendezvous, Invisible Man, Saber Buccaneers, White Hunter, Flying Doctor, On the Night of the Murder, Haven in Sunset, The Odd Man, Zero 1 series, The Innocent Ceremoney, Department S, The Marrying Kind, The Expert, The Persuaders, Trial, Starcast, The Midsummer of Colonel Blossum, Callen, Crimes of Passion, Full House, Father Brown, Within These Walls Series, The Standard, The Purple Twilight, The Professionals, Bergerac, Cuffy.

LAYE, EVELYN: Actress, singer. b. London, England, July 10, 1900. London stage debut 1918 The Beauty Spot. Subseq. in numerous musicals, dramas, London, including The Merry Widow, Madame Pompadour, Lilac Time, Blue Eyes, The New Moon, Paganini, Wedding in Paris, The Amorous Prawn, Strike a Light!, Let's All Go Down the Strand, Phil the Fluter, No Sex Please, We're British (1971–72). B'way stage debut, 1929, Bitter Sweet; m.p. debut 1927 silent production The Luck of the Navy.
PICTURES INCLUDE: One Heavenly Night, Waltz Time, Princess Charming, Evensong, The Night is Young, Make Mine a Million, Theatre of Death, Within and Without, Say Hello to Yesterday.
TV: Stars and Garters, Not Just An Act; 1969: Late Night Line Up, The Golden Shot, The Simon Dee Show, The David Niven Show, This Is Your Life, Omnibus.
PUBLICATION: Boo To My Friends (Autobiography).

LAZARUS, PAUL N.: Executive. b. Brooklyn, N.Y., March 31, 1913. e. Cornell U., B.A., '33. In U.S. Army, World War II. Entered m.p. ind. 1933 as gen. asst., press book dept., Warner Bros.; pres., AMPA, 1939–40. Joined Buchanan & Co., 1942 as m.p. account exec. To United Artists 1943 as dir. adv. & pub. Named asst. to pres., July 1948; joined Columbia exec. staff, New York, Aug. 1950; elected v.p. Columbia, Jan., 1954–62; exec. vice-pres. Samuel Bronston Prods., 1962–64; v.p., chg. Motion Pictures, Subscription Television Inc., 1964; exec. officer and partner, Landau Releasing Organization, 1964–65, exec. v.p., member bd. of dir., Nat'l Screen Serv. Corp., 1965–75. Lecturer and consultant, Film Studies Dept., Univ. of California at Santa Barbara. 1975 to present. Consultant to Kenya Film Corp., Nairobi, 1983. Director, Santa Barbara Intl. Film Festival, 1986–87.

LAZARUS, PAUL N. III: Motion Picture Executive. Third generation film exec. Began career with Palomar Pictures Int'l. as exec. v.p.; joined ABC Pictures Corp. as v.p. in chg. of creative affairs. Mng. dir., CRM Productions, maker of educational films; v.p. for motion pictures. Marble Arch Productions; 1983, v.p. in chg. of prod., Home Box Office.
PICTURES INCLUDE: Extreme Close-Up, Westworld, Futureworld, Capricorn One, Hanover Street, Barbarosa.

LAZARUS, THEODORE R.: Executive. b. Brooklyn, N.Y., Aug. 5, 1919. e. Yale U. B.A., 1940. Adv. mgr., Eagle Lion

Classics, 1951; adv., sales prom. mgr., WMGM, New York, 1951; then with Donahue and Coe adv. agency; secy., treas., George Blake Enterprises, TV film prod. firm, 1955; v.p. Gommi-TV, 1956; Charles Schlaifer and Co., Inc., 1957; adv. mgr., Paramount Pictures Corp., 1964; pres., Cinema Lodge, B'nai B'rith, 1968–71.

LEACHMAN, CLORIS: Actress. b. Des Moines, Iowa, June 30, 1930. e. Northwestern Univ. Broadway stage, television, motion pictures.
TV: Lassie, A Brand New Life, The Migrants, Phyllis (series). Movies: Twigs, Ernie Kovacs: Between the Laughter, Deadly Intentions, Love Is Never Silent.
PICTURES INCLUDE: Butch Cassidy and the Sundance Kid, The Steagle, The Last Picture Show, (Acad. award best supporting actress, 1971), Dillinger, Daisy Miller, Young Frankenstein, Crazy Mama, High Anxiety, The North Avenue Irregulars, Scavenger Hunt, History of the World—Part I.

LEACOCK, PHILIP: Producer-Director. b. London, England, Oct. 8, 1917. Moved from British film industry to American films and TV.
PICTURES: The Brave Don't Cry, Appointment in London, The Kidnappers, Escapade, The Spanish Gardener, High Tide at Noon, Innocent Sinners, The Rabbit Trap, Let No Man Write My Epitaph, Hand in Hand, Take a Giant Step, Reach for Glory, West Street, The War Lover, Tamahine, Adam's Woman.
TELEVISION: Movies: The Birdmen, When Michael Calls, The Daughters of Joshua Cabe, Baffled, The Great Man's Whiskers, Dying Room Only, Key West, Killer on Board, Wild and Wooly. Series: Gunsmoke, Cimarron Strip, Hawaii 5-O, Three Sovereigns for Sarah, etc.

LEADER, ANTON MORRIS: Director-producer. b. Boston, Mass., e. Hebrew Coll., New Eng. Conservatory of Music. Dir., announcer, actor, Boston radio stations; prod. mgr., WMCA, N.Y.; Army Air Corp.; prod. dir., NBC; winner, Variety Showmanship Award, Peabody Award for Words at War; winner Brotherhood Award, Peabody Award for Eternal Light; Western Heritage Award, dir. TV Film, The Horsefighter (The Virginian); inst., Fordham U., prod., dir., Suspense, CBS; prod., dir., writer Columbia Pictures; prod., U-1.
PICTURES INCLUDE: It Happens Every Thursday, Sally and St. Anne, Go Man Go!, Children of the Damned, Cockeyed Cowboys of Calico County.
TV: The Virginian, Rawhide, Tarzan, Daniel Boone, Playhouse 90, Father of the Bride, It Takes a Thief, Ironside, Star Trek, Lost in Space, I Spy, Get Smart, Hawaii Five-O, Firehouse, Movin' On, This Is The Life.

LEAN, SIR DAVID: Director. b. Croydon, England, Mar. 25, 1908; e. Leighton Park. Entered m.p. ind. 1928 as camera asst. Graumont Pictures; asst. dir. & ed.; co-dir. 1942; dir. Knighted in 1984.
PICTURES INCLUDE: Escape Me Never, Pygmalion, Invaders, In Which We Serve, This Happy Breed, Blithe Spirit, Brief Encounter, Great Expectations, Oliver Twist, Madeleine, One Woman's Story. The Sound Barrier, Hobson's Choice, Summertime, The Bridge on the River Kwai (Academy Award 1957, best direction), Lawrence of Arabia (Academy Award), Dr. Zhivago, Ryan's Daughter, A Passage to India (also s.p. and editor).

LEAR, NORMAN: Producer-Director-Writer. b. New Haven, Ct., July 27, 1922. Began in TV as co-writer of weekly one-hour variety show, The Ford Star Revue in 1950. Followed as writer for Dean Martin and Jerry Lewis on the Colgate Comedy Hour and for the Martha Raye and George Gobel TV shows. With partner, Bud Yorkin, created and produced such specials as Another Evening with Fred Astaire, Henry Fonda and the Family, An Evening with Carol Channing, and The Many Sides of Don Rickles. In 1965 their company also produced the original Andy Williams Show. Moved into motion pictures in 1963, writing and producing Come Blow Your Horn.
PICTURES: Never Too Late (prod.), Divorce-American Style (prod., s.p.), The Night They Raided Minsky's (co. prod., co-s.p.), Start the Revolution without Me (exec.-prod.), Cold Turkey, (s.p., prod., dir.).
TELEVISION: Exec. prod. of All in the Family, Maude, Good Times, The Jeffersons, Mary Hartman, Mary Hartman, One Day at a Time, The Baxters, Palmerstown, I Love Liberty, Heartsounds.

LEARNED, MICHAEL: Actress. b. Washington, D.C., Apr. 9, 1939. Studied ballet and dramatics in school. Many stage credits include Under Milkwood, The Three Sisters, A God Slept Here, etc.; resident performances with Shakespeare festivals in Canada, Stratford, CT, and San Diego, CA. Gained fame on hit TV series, The Waltons, as the mother, Olivia. Theatrical film debut in 1980, Touched by Love.
TELEVISION: Gunsmoke, Police Story, Widow, Little Mo, A Deadly Business, etc.

LE BORG, REGINALD: Director. b. Vienna, Austria Dec. 11; e. U. Vienna, B.A.; Sorbonne, Paris; Columbia U. Banker, playwright & stage dir., Europe; then staged musical and operatic sequences, Columbia, Paramount. To MGM as dir. short subjects. In 1941 joined Universal. Entered U.S. armed services, 1942; returned to Universal, 1944; Rec'd citation from OWL; free lance since 1946. Wrote Academy Award winning short Heavenly Music, 1945. directed two films in England, one in Mexico.
PICTURES INCLUDE: She's for Me, The Mummy's Ghost, Calling Dr. Death, Weird Woman, Dead Man's Eyes, Jungle Woman, Destiny, Honeymoon Ahead; San Diego, I Love You; (prod.), Philo Vance's Secret Mission; (dir.) Fighting Fools, Hold That Baby, The Squared Circle, Young Daniel Boone, Wyoming Mail, Triple Cross, G.I. Jane; Models, Inc., Bad Blonde, Great Jesse James Raid, Sins of Jezebel, Joe Palooka, Champ, Port Said, Fall Guy, Formed Cosmos Prod., prod., White Orchid (dir.), Black Sleep, Voodoo Island, War Drums, The Dalton Girls.
TV: for Sovereign, 4 Star Schlitz Playhouse, Wire Service, Navy Log, Maverick, Desilu Revue; Court of Last Resort, Warner Bros., Screen Gems, MGM, Ziv; recent features: The Flight That Disappeared, Deadly Duo, The Diary of A Madman, The Eyes of Annie Jones, So Evil, My Sister.

LEDER, HERBERT JAY: Writer-director, producer, b. New York City, Aug. 15, 1922. e. B.A., PHD. Play Doctor on Broadway; Director TV dept., Benton and Bowles Adv. chg. all T.V. & Film production, 13 yrs.; Features: writer, Fiend Without a Face; writer-director co-prod., Pretty Boy Floyd; writer-director, co-producer, Nine Miles to Noon; writer, Aquarius Mission, Love Keeps No Score of Wrongs; writer, prod-dir., The Frozen Dead, It; Mia, writer-dir., Candyman, writer-director; writer, The Winners, The Way It Is, The Cool Crazies. Sponsored Films: Child Molester, Bank Robber, Shoplifter, Untouchables.

LEDERER, RICHARD: Executive. b. New York, N.Y. Sept. 22, 1916; e. Univ. of Virginia. B.S., 1938; Free lance writer, 1939–41; U.S. Army. Cryptanalyst, Signal Intell. Serv 1941–45; Adv. copywriter, Columbia Pictures, 1946–50; Adv. copywriter, Warner Bros., 1950–53; copy chief, Warner Bros., 1950–53; copy chief, Warner Bros., 1953–57; Asst. Nat'l Adv. mgr., Warner Bros. studios, 1957–59; Prod., theatrical, TV. Warner Bros. studios, 1959–60; Dir. of adv., publicity, Warner Bros. Pictures, 1960; v.p. Warner Bros. Pictures, 1963. V.P. production, Warner Bros. Studio, 1969–70; indep. prod. to May, 1971, when returned to WB as adv.-pub., v.p. Independent producer. 1980: Hollywood Knights. Joined Orion Pictures as v.p., adv. Resigned, 1984.

LEE, ANNA: Actress. b. England; seen in First a Girl, The Camels Are Coming, You're in the Army Now, King Solomon's Mines.
PICTURES INCLUDE: Flesh and Fantasy, Summer Storm, Abroad with Two Yanks, High Conquest, Ghost and Mrs. Muir, Best Man Wins, Fort Apache, Prison Warden, This Earth is Mine.
Many TV shows.

LEE, BONNI: Executive. Prod. exec. at MGM/UA, 1982; joined Warner Bros. as v.p.—creative affairs, 1984; v.p., production, 1986.

LEE, CHRISTOPHER: Actor. b. London, England, May 27, 1922. e. Wellington College. Served RAF 1940–46. Ent. m.p. ind. 1947. Over 40 TV films.
PICTURES INCLUDE: Corridor of Mirrors, Hamlet, Moulin Rouge, Moby Dick, River Plate, Truth About Women, Tale of Two Cities, Curse of Frankenstein, Dracula, Man Who Could Cheat Death, The Mummy, Too Hot to Handle, Beat Girl, City of the Dead, Two Faces of Dr. Jekyll, The Terror of the Tongs, The Hands of Orlac, Taste of Fear, The Devil's Daffodil, Pirates of Blood River, Devil's Agent, Red Orchid, Valley of Fear, Katharsis, Faust '63, The Virgin of Nuremberg, The Whip and the Body, Carmilla, The Devil Ship Pirates, The Gorgon, The Sign of Satan, The House of Blood, The Dunwich Horror, Dr. Terror's House of Horrors, She, The Skull, The Mask of Fu Manchu, Dracula, Prince of Darkness, Rasputin, Theatre of Death, Circus of Fear, The Brides of Fu Manchu, Five Golden Dragons, Diabolica, Vengeance of Fu Manchu, Night of the Big Heat, The Pendulum, The Face of Eve, The Devil Rides Out, The Blood of Fu Manchu, The Crimson Altar, Dracula Has Risen from the Grave, The Oblong Box, De Sade 70, Scream and Scream Again, The Magic Christian, Julius Caesar, One More Time, Count Dracula, Bloody Judge, Taste the Blood of Dracula, Private Lives of Sherlock Holmes, El Umbragolo, Scars of Dracula, House That Dripped Blood, I Monster, Hannie Caulder, Dracula 72, Horror Express, Creeping Flesh, Death Line, Nothing but the Night, The Wicker Man, Poor Devil, Dark Places, Dracula Is Dead?, Eulalie Quitte les champs, The Three Musketeers, Earthbound, Man With The Golden Gun, The Four Musketeers, Killer Force, Diagnosis-Murder, Whispering Death, The Keeper, To The Devil a Daughter, Pere Et Fils, Airport 77, Alien Encounter, The End of the World, Return from Witch Mountain, Caravans, The Silent Flute, The Passage, The Pirates, Jaguar Lives, Arabian Adventure, An Eye for an Eye, House of Long Shadows, Howling II,

The Far Pavilions, The Return of Captain Invincible, Roadtrip, Mio My Mio, The Girl.
TELEVISION: The Disputation, Metier du Seigneur.

LEE, JOHN: Actor. b. Launceston, Tasmania, March 31, 1928. Early career on Australian stage and radio. Ent. m.p. ind. in England 1957.
PICTURES INCLUDE: Dunkirk, Cat Girl, Silent Enemy, Flying Scot, Gypsy and The Gentleman, Under Ten Flags, The Liar, Seven Keys, The Secret Partner, Dr. Crippen, Stitch in Time, Go Kart Go, Space Flight.
TV: Adventures of the Sea Hawk, International Detective, Rendezvous, Flying Doctor, Danger Man, Shadow Squad, Man and Superman, A Man Involved, Aren't We All, Probation Officer, Ladies of the Corridor, Golden Girl, After the Crash, The Net, Emergency Ward 10, Zero One, Sapper Series, Dr. Fancy, The Shifting Heart, Sergeant Cork, Dr. Who, The Materialists, The July Plot.

LEE, MICHELE: Actress. b. Los Angeles, June 24, 1942. On Broadway in Seesaw.
PICTURES: How To Succeed in Business without Really Trying, The Love Bug, The Comic.
TELEVISION: Knots Landing, The Tim Conway Show.

LEE, PEGGY: Singer, actress. r.n. Norma Egstrom; b. Jamestown, N.D., May 26, 1920. Began career as night club vocalist in Fargo & radio singer, WDAY, then with Sev Olsen, bandleader, Minneapolis, Will Osborne; Benny Goodman; collab. (with Dave Barbour) popular songs, Manana, It's a Good Day, What More Can a Woman Do? Leading feminine vocalist. TV & records; screen debut in Mr. Music (Bing Crosby); singer on Bing Crosby program, CBS, TV appearances.
PICTURES INCLUDE: Jazz Singer, Pete Kelly's Blues, act., collab. songs, Lady and the Tramp.

LEEDS, MARTIN N.: Film-TV Executive. b. New York City, Apr. 6, 1916. e. NYU, BS, 1936; J.D., 1938. Admitted N.Y. Bar, 1938, Calif. Bar, 1948; dir. indsl. relations Wabash Appliance Corp., 1943–44 indsl. bus. relations cons. Davis & Gilbert. 1944–45; dir. indsl. relations Flying Tiger Lines, 1947; dir. bus. affairs CBS. TV div., 1947–53; exec. v.p. Desilu Productions, Inc., 1953–60; v.p. Motion Picture Center Studios, Inc.: mem. Industry comm. War Manpower Comm., 1943; chmn. Com. to form Television Code of Ethics: U.S. Army 1941. Mem. Los Angeles Bar Assn., Century City Bar Assn.; exec. v.p. in chg. of West Coast oper. & member of bd. of dir. Talent Associates—Paramount Ltd., Hollywood, 1962; TV production consultant; exec. v.p., Electronovision Prods. Inc., 1964; TV prod. & MP prod. consultant, 1965. Pres., chief exec. officer member of bd., Beverly Hills Studios, Inc., 1969, senior v.p., American Film Theatre, 1973; 1975, motion picture and TV attorney & consultant.

LEENHOUTS, LEWIS GRANT: Executive. b. Los Angeles, California; m. Edith Hargrave. From 1934–38 variously stunt man, unit manager, cutter & asst. dir., Collab. orig. story No More Women, wrote orig. Heroes at Leisure. In 1939 wrote training films, U.S. Officer of Education; 1940–41 assoc. prod., writer, dir., Caravel Films Inc.; 1942–45 head of planning and production U.S. Navy Training Film & Motion Picture branch, Navy Dept.; 1946–47 gen. mgr. in charge of prod., National Educational Films, Inc. Later coordinator-producer, Industry Film Project, Motion Picture Assoc.; prod. California's Golden Beginning, Paramount assoc. chief and head of prod., International M.P. Div., U.S. Dept. of State, 1950–51; exec. v.p., Cinerama, Inc., 1952–53; planning and prod. head, Ford Foundation Fund for Adult Education, 1954, v.p., prod. head Cinerama, Inc., 1955–60. Ind. producer; prod. consultant Macbeth, Compass Prods. and Grand Prize Films, London; pres., Leehouts Prods., Inc., 1961; prod., 20th Century Fox, Movietone Digest, Children's Digest, 1963; Prod. Consultant, Cascade Pics. of Calif., 1964–65; 1967, dir. prod., Breakfast At the Capitol; prod., New Sounds in Africa; prod. head, Eddie Albert, Inc., 1971.

LEEWOOD, JACK: Producer. b. New York City, N.Y., e. Upsala Coll., Newark U. and New York U. From 1926–31 with Gottesman-Stern circuit as usher, asst. and relief mgr.; 1931–43 Stanley-Warner mgr. of Ritz, Capitol and Hollywood theatres 1943–47. Joined Warner Bros. field forces in Denver-Salt Lake; Seattle-Portland, 1947–52. Dir. pub. & adv. Screen Guild Prod.; Lippert Productions; prod. exec. in chge. story dept.; 1953–56 Allied Artists; 1957–62 Prod. 20th Cent. Fox; 1965–68 prod., Universal; 1976–78. Affiliated Theatre Serrio; 1978–79. Aubrey/Hammer Prod.
PICTURES INCLUDE: Holiday Rhythm, Gunfire, Hi-Jacked; Roaring City, Danger Zone, Lost Continent, F.B.I. Girl, Pier 23, Train to Tombstone, I Shot Billy the Kid, Bandit Queen, Motor Patrol, Savage Drums, Three Desperate Men, Border Rangers, Western Pacific Agent, Thundering Jets, Lone Texan, Little Savage, Alligator, People, 13 Fighting Men, Young Jesse James, Swingin' Along, We'll Bury You, 20,000 Eyes, Thunder Island, The Plainsman, Longest 100 Miles, Escape to Mindanao, Dallas Cowboys Cheerleaders, When Hell Was in Session.

LEFFERTS, GEORGE: Producer, writer, director. b. Paterson, N.J., dir., numerous award-winning TV series, films, exec. prod.-Time-Life films 1977–78; prod./writer, Movie of the Week (NBC) 1977–78. Biog: Who's Who in America, Who's Who in the World. 1975 Emmy Award Benjamin Franklin Specials (CBS).
TV: 1969 Emmy Award, prod. Hallmark Hall of Fame "Teacher Teacher," 1963 Emmy Award, wrote, prod., directed Purex Specials for Women. 1965 Producer's Guild Award, exec. prod. "Breaking Point" series. Other shows: The Bill Cosby Show, Studio One, Kraft Theatre, Chrysler Theatre, Sinatra Show, Lights Out, Alcoa, The Harness (Movie of the Week), The Bold Ones, Exec. prod., Bing Crosby Productions, prod., NBC 10 yrs, Independent.
PICTURES INCLUDE: The Stake, Mean Dog Blues, 1977–78, The Living End, The Boat, The Teenager.
BROADWAY: The Boat, 1968, Hey Everybody, 1970.

LEFKO, MORRIS E.: b. March 30, 1907. Entered m.p. ind. as poster clerk; booker, salesman, br. mgr., Indianapolis, RKO, June 1941; br. mgr., Pittsburgh, July 1944; East Central dist. mgr., July, 1948; appt. sales exec. of Ten Commandments Unit. Para. Film Dist. Corp., N.Y.C. 1956; v.p. in chg. sls., Michael Todd Co., 1958. Joined MGM, Inc., July 1960 sls. mgr., of road shows, Ben-Hur, King of Kings, Mutiny on the Bounty; vice pres., gen. sales mgr., MGM, 1963. Exec. consultant to Pres., Cinema 5 Ltd., Jan. 1970. v.p., Network Cinema Corp., 1972; American Film Theatre, Ely Lando Co., Nov., 1972; v.p., sls. mgr. Brut Prods., 1976.

LE GALLIENNE, EVA: Actress—Producer. b. London, England, Jan. 11, 1899. Stage career began in 1914. Founded Civic Repertory Theatre in 1926, starring in and directing such classics as Hedda Gabler, Romeo and Juliet, Alice in Wonderland, Camille, The Cherry Orchard. Also co-founder of American Repertory Theatre; toured with National Repertory Theatre.
TELEVISION: Alice in Wonderland, The Corn Is Green, The Bridge of San Luis Rey, Mary Stuart, The Royal Family (Emmy award, 1977).
PICTURES: Prince of Players, The Devil's Disciple, Resurrection.

LEGG, STUART: Producer. b. London, England, August 31, 1910. m. e. Marlborough Coll., 1923–28; St. John's Coll., Cambridge, 1928–31. Began as dir. and ed., prod. of documentary and public information shorts. From 1931–32, with British Instructional Films; 1932–34, Empire Marketing Board film unit; 1934–37, G.P.O. Film Unit; 1937–38. Film Centre, London; 1938–39, Strand Films, London; 1939–42. National Film Board, Ottawa. In 1945, head N.Y. br., John Grierson's co.; editor, World in Action, shorts enterprises.

LEGRAND, MICHEL JEAN: Composer-Conductor. b. France, 1931. Son of well-known arranger, composer and pianist, Raymond Legrand. At 11 Michel, a child prodigy, entered Paris Cons. and graduated nine years later with top honors in composition and as solo pianist. In late Fifties turned to composing for films and has composed, orchestrated and conducted scores of more than 50 films.
PICTURES INCLUDE: Lola, Eva, Vivre Sa Vie, La Baie des Anges, The Umbrellas of Cherbourg, Banda a Part, Un Femme Mariee, Les Demoiselles de Rochefort, Ice Station Zebra, The Thomas Crown Affair, Pieces of Dreams, The Happy Ending, Wuthering Heights, The Go-Between, Summer of '42, Picasso Summer, The Nelson Affair, Breezy, The Three Musketeers, Sheila Levine, Gable and Lombard, The Hunter, Best Friends, Never Say Never Again, Yentl, Secret Places.
TV: Brian's Song, The Jesse Owens Story, A Woman Called Golda.

LEHMAN, ERNEST: Writer-Producer, Director. b. New York City. e. City College of New York. Began career as financial editor and free-lance short story and novelette writer. Recently published first novel, The French Atlantic Affair followed by second, Farewell Performance, and first non-fiction book, Screening Sickness. First screenplays were Executive Suite, Sabrina, Sweet Smell of Success, based on own novelette.
PICTURES INCLUDE: The King and I, Somebody Up There Likes Me, North by Northwest, From the Terrace, West Side Story, The Prize, The Sound of Music. Became a prod.-wr. for first time with Who's Afraid of Virginia Woolf? Prod.-wr. Hello Dolly; prod.-wr.-dir., Portnoy's Complaint; Family Plot (s.p.), Black Sunday (co.-s.p.).

LEHMAN, GLADYS: Writer, Scenarios identified with such Reginald Denny pictures as Out All Night, Clear the Deck, On Your Toes and Companionate Trouble; joined Columbia in 1929.
SCRIPTS INCLUDE: The Little Accident, A Lady Surrenders, The Cat Creeps, Many a Slip, Seed, Strictly Dishonorable, Back Street, Embarrassing Moments, Nice Women,

Good Girls Go to Paris, Blondie, Two Girls and a Sailor, Thrill of a Romance, Her Highness and the Bellboy, This Time for Keeps, collab. s.p. Luxury Liner, Golden Girl.

LEIBMAN, RON: Actor. b. New York City, Oct. 11, 1938. e. Ohio Wesleyan Univ. Joined Actor's Studio in N.Y.; first professional appearance in summer theatre production of A View from the Bridge.
STAGE: The Premise, We Bombed in New Haven, Cop Out, Room Service, I Oughta Be in Pictures.
PICTURES INCLUDE: Where's Poppa (debut), The Hot Rock, Slaughterhouse Five, Your Three Minutes Are Up, Super Cops, Won Ton Ton, Up the Academy, Zorro, the Gay Blade, Romantic Comedy, Rhinestone.
TV: A Question of Guilt (ff), Kaz (series).

LEIBOWITZ, SAM: Executive. b. New York City, Feb. 12, 1913. Service mgr., Reel Photos, 1931–34; svg. mgr., Consolidated Film Ind., 1935; Apco Photo Co., Inc., treas., 1936–62; Apco-Apeda Photo Co., Inc., 1962–present, pres. & chief operating officer.

LEIDER, GERALD J.: Producer-Executive. b. Camden, New Jersey, May 28, 1931. e. Syracuse Univ. 1953; Bristol Univ., Eng. 1954 Fulbright Fellowship in Drama. m. Susan Trustman, son Matthew Trustman, born April 14, 1972, son Kenneth Harold, born June 18, 1975. 1955 MCA, Inc., N.Y.; 1956–59 theatre producer in N.Y., London; Shinbone Alley, Garden District, and Sir John Gielgud's Ages of Man. 1960–61; director of special programs, CBS/TV; 1961–62, dir. of program sales, CBS-TV; 1962–69, vice pres., television operation, Ashley Famous Agency, Inc. Sept. 1969–Dec. 1974, pres. Warner Bros. Television, Burbank. Jan. 1975–Dec. 1976, exec. vice pres. foreign production Warner Bros. Pictures, Rome. Jan. 1977–1982, independent producer under Jerry Leider Productions; 1982–present, pres., ITC Prods., Inc.
PICTURES: Wild Horse Hank, The Jazz Singer (1980), Trenchcoat.
TELEVISION: And I Alone Survived, Willa, The Hostage Tower.

LEIGH, JANET: Actress, r.n. Jeanette Helen Morrison; b. Merced, Calif., July 6, 1927. e. College of Pacific (music). Screen debut in Romance of Rosy Ridge, 1947.
PICTURES INCLUDE: If Winter Comes, Hills of Home, Words and Music, Act of Violence, Little Women, That Forsyte Woman, Red Danube, Doctor and the Girl, Holiday Affair, It's a Big Country, Two Tickets to Broadway, Strictly Dishonorable, Angels in the Outfield, Just This Once, Naked Spur, Confidentially Connie, Houdini, Walking My Baby Back Home, Prince Valiant, Living It Up, Black Shield of Falworth, Rogue Cop, My Sister Eileen, Pete Kelly's Blues, Safari, The Vikings, The Perfect Furlough, Psycho, The Manchurian Candidate, Bye, Bye, Birdie, Wives and Lovers, Kid Rodello, Grand Slam, Hello Down There, One Is A Lonely Number, Night of the Lepus, Boardwalk, The Fog.

LEIGH, JENNIFER JASON: Actress. Theatrical film debut in Wrong Is Right (1982). Won L.A. Valley Colelge best actress award for The Shadow Box on stage (1979).
PICTURES: Fast Times at Ridgemont High, Eyes of a Stranger, The Hitcher.
TELEVISION: Movies: The Best Little Girl in the World, the Killing of Randy Webster, Angel City.

LEIGH, SUZANNA: Actress. b. England, 1945. Studies at the Arts Educational School and Webber Douglas School. Film debut 1961 in Oscar Wilde, followed by Bomb in the High Street. 1964: TV series made in France, Three Stars. 1965–66: Under contract to Hal Wallis and Paramount, Boeing Boeing, Paradise Hawaiian Style, 1966: The Deadly Bees, Deadlier Than The Male. 1967: The Lost Continent. 1968: Subterfuge. TV film series in West Indies, One On An Island. 1969: TV play, The Plastic People. 1970.
PICTURES INCLUDE: To Love a Vampire, Beware My Brethren, Son of Dracula.
TV: The Persuaders.

LELOUCH, CLAUDE: Director-Cinematographer. b. Paris, France, Oct. 30, 1937. Began m.p. career with short subjects, 1956; French military service, motion picture department, 1957–60; formed Films 13, 1960; publicity Films and Scopitones, 1961–62.
PICTURES INCLUDE: Le Propre de L'homme (Man's Own), L'amour avec des Si (Love With Ifs), Une fille et des Fusils (Guns and a Girl), To be A Crook, Un Homme et une Femme (A Man and A Woman), Vivre pour Vivre (Live for Life), Life, Love, and Death, Love Is a Funny Thing (dir., photog., s.p.); The Crook (dir., photog., s.p.) Adventure Is Adventure (prod., dir., s.p.). Smic, Smac, Smoc, La Bonne Anne, Another Man, Another Chance, Edith and Marcel (prod., s.p.); A Man and a Woman: 20 Years Later.

LeMAT, PAUL: Actor. b. New Jersey. Studied with Milton Katselas, Herbert Berghof.
PICTURES: American Graffiti, Citzen's Band, Melvin and Howard, Death Valley, Jimmy the Kid, Strange Invaders.
TELEVISION: Movies: Firehouse, The Night They Saved Christmas, The Burning Bed, Long Time Gone. Mini-Series: On Wings of Eagles.

LEMLEIN, NEAL C.: Executive. e. Tulane Univ.; New York Univ. Began career at Young & Rubicam in N.Y.; later joined Doyle Dane Bernbach, Inc., where named snr. acct. exec. assigned to 20th-Fox feature films account and CBS-TV Entertainment Division. In March, 1980, joined Universal Pictures as dir. of mktg. 1986, v.p., mktg., 20th Century Fox.

LEMMON, JACK: Actor. b. Boston, Mass. Feb. 8, 1925. e. Harvard U. Stage debut as a child; radio actor on soap operas; stock companies; U.S. Navy, WWII; many TV shows; B'way debut in Room Service 1953; other Broadway shows include: Face of a Hero (1960) and Tribute (1978). Other legitimate theatre appearances include: Idiot's Delight (1970, Los Angeles), Juno and the Paycock (1975, Los Angeles), Tribute (1979, Denver and Los Angeles), A Sense of Humor (Denver, L.A., S.F., 1983–84); Long Day's Journey into Night (Bdwy., Washington DC, London, Israel, L.A.). m.p. debut in It Should Happen to You.
PICTURES INCLUDE: Three for the Show, Phfft, My Sister Eileen, Mr. Roberts (Academy Award, best supporting actor, 1955), You Can't Run Away From It, Fire Down Below, Operation Mad Ball, Bell Book and Candle, It Happened to Jane, Some Like It Hot, The Apartment, The Wackiest Ship in the Army, Notorious Landlady, Days of Wine and Roses, Irma La Douce, Under the Yum Yum Tree, Good Neighbor Sam, How To Murder Your Wife, The Great Race, The Fortune Cookie, Luv, The Odd Couple, The April Fools, The Out of Towners. Debut as director: Kotch, 1971, The War Between Men and Women, 's Wonderful, 's Marvelous, 's Gershwin (TV Emmy Award 1972), Save the Tiger (Academy Award, Best Actor), Avanti, The Prisoner of Second Avenue, The Front Page, The Entertainer (TV in U.S.), Alex & The Gypsy, Airport '77, The China Syndrome (Cannes festival award for best actor, 1979), Tribute, Buddy, Buddy, Missing (Cannes award for best actor 1982), Mass Appeal, Macaroni, That's Life.

LEMONT, JOHN: Producer, director, screenwriter. e. Canada, U.S.A. and England. Ent. m.p. ind. as actor and writer/technician. Early career working on features and documentaries. Service with Army Kinematograph Service as writ./dir. A.B.P. Director of Trans-Oceanic Telefilm Productions, Zodiac Productions Ltd., Venture Productions Ltd. V. Chmn. Writers Guild of Gt. Britain. Awards: WGGB Laurel, Edgar Allen Poe, NY/USA Festival Gold Award.
PICTURES INCLUDE: Vacation Rhythm, The Patrol, The Green Buddha, Cross Channel, Missing Person, Harvest of the Seas, People's Playground, Port of London, Mirror and Markheim, And Women Shall Weep, The Shakedown, Konga, The Frightened City, Deep Waters, Horse Called Jester, Woman On the Stair.
TV: Fabian of the Yard, British Heritage, Frances Drake, Strange Study, Errol Flynn Theatre, Ivanhoe; prod., Sixpenny Corner, Dir. The Glorification of Al Toolum; dir, Witness in The Dark; TV Playhouse series.

LENZ, KAY: Actress. b. Los Angeles, March 4, 1953. Wife of David Cassidy.
PICTURES: American Graffiti, Breezy, White Line Fever, The Great Scout and Cathouse Thursday, The Passage, House.
TELEVISION: Movies: The Weekend Nun, Lisa, Bright and Dark, A Summer without Boys, Unwed Father, The Underground Man, The FBI Story: The FBI Versus Alvin Karpis, Journey from Darkness, Rich Man, Poor Man, The Initiation of Sarah, The Seeding of Sarah Burns, Sanctuary of Fear, The Hustler of Muscle Beach.

LEON, SOL: Executive. b. July 2, 1913, New York City. e. N.Y.U., CCNY, Brooklyn Law School, BBL, master of law. Sr. v.p., William Morris Agency, L.A.

LEONARD, SHELDON: Actor. r.n. Sheldon Leonard Bershad. b. New York, N.Y., Feb. 22, 1907; e. Syracuse U., B.A. Theatre mgr., Publix; N.Y. stage, 10 yrs.; sec., Directors Guild of America. 3 Emmy awards, Sylvania award, 4 TV Director of the Year nominations by D.G.A.
PICTURES INCLUDE: Another Thin Man, Tall, Dark and Handsome, Tortilla Flat, Rise and Shine, Lucky Jordan, Somewhere in the Night, Her Kind of Man, Its a Wonderful Life, The Gansters, If You Knew Susie, Sinbad the Sailor, My Dream Is Yours, Take One False Step, Iroquois Trail, Here Come the Nelsons, Young Man with Ideas, Stop You're Killing Me, Diamond Queen, Money from Home, Guys and Dolls; dir. Real McCoys, Pocketful of Miracles.
TV: 1953–56: dir. Make Room for Daddy, Damon Runyon, G.E. Theatre, Electric Theatre, Jewelers' Showcase, Jimmy Durante Show; prod.-dir. Danny Thomas Show; package & exec. prod., Andy Griffith Show, Dick Van Dyke Show; exec. prod., Gomer Pyle, U.S.M.C., I Spy, My World and

Welcome To It. In 1975 starred in Big Eddie (CBS), 1977, exec. prod. and co-star in Top Secret.

LEONE, ALFRED: Producer, b. Nov. 30, 1926. In entertainment industry since 1958. Assistant producer for Braken Productions and Hallmark Productions. In 1968 formed Europa-America in Rome, Italy. 1974, formed Leone Intl. SPA in Rome. In 1978 opened offices in Beverly Hills. Produced and distributed over 35 films, among them: Vengeance, Four Times That Night, Baron Blood, Lisa And The Devil, House of Exorcism, Love by Appointment, Gold of the Amazon Women, The Snake.

LEONE, SERGIO: Director-Writer. b. Rome Italy, 1921. Started career as asst. to dir. Robert Wise on Helen of Troy, followed by asst. to Fred Zinnemann on The Nun's Story, 1958. Served in same capacity for William Wyler on Ben Hur in 1959. Wrote screenplays for Italian films. Made debut as director in 1964 with A Fistful of Dollars (starring Clint Eastwood) under psuedonym Bob Robertson. Followed with several Italian "oaters" that gained him renown.
PICTURES: A Fistful of Dollars, For a Few Dollars More, The Good, the Bad and the Ugly, Once Upon a Time in the West, A Fistful of Dynamite, Duck, You Sucker! Once Upon a Time in America.

L'EPINE-SMITH, ERIC: Producer, director, writer. b. Thornton Heath Eng. m. Brenda Cameron. Stage as actor, prod. playwright, formed own co. Aldwitch Films; joined Wieland's Agency; apptd. dir. of co.; casting dir. Warner Bros. 1st Natl.; assoc. prod. Edward Dryhurst Productions, then prod. Now artists' mgr., L'Epine-Smith, Ltd.
PICTURES INCLUDE: Down on the Farm, Pitchfork and Powder-Puff, Making a Man of Him, House of Silence, Five Pound Man, Coming of Age, While I Live, Noose, Romantic Age, Come Die My Love.

LERNER, JOSEPH: Producer, director, writer. m. Geraldine Lerner, film ed. radio stage mgr. & actor on Broadway; with RKO, Columbia and Republic as dir., dial. dir., writer, 2nd unit dir., test dir., dir.-writer & head of special productions U.S. Army Signal Corps Photographic Center; writer of commercial and educational films 1946–47; vice-pres. in chg. of prod. Visual Arts Productions 1947; vice-pres. in chg. prod. Laurel Films 1949; prod.-dir., TV Gangbusters series, Grand Tour series; Girl on the Run, com. ind. films, Three Musketeers series TV, dir.-prod, 1961; Director, producer, writer, MPO Videotronics, Inc. 1967–73. President, The Place for Film Making, Inc.; pres., Astracor Associates Ltd. in production: The Ditch Digger's Daughter, The Little Hat, The Mapmakers. Also lecturer and instructor at New York University, Wm. Patterson College, Broward Community College (Florida).
CREDITS INCLUDE: (writer-dir.) Fight Never Ends; (prod.-writer) Kings of the Olympics, Olympics Cavalcade; (prod.-dir.-writer) United Nations Case Book (for CBS-TV), C-Man; (prod.-dir.) Guilty Bystander, Mr. Universe, writer, director co-producer, The Dark of Day, Polish and/or rewrite. Many others.

LEROY, MERVYN: Producer, director, b. San Francisco, Calif., Oct. 15, 1900. In vaudeville before entering m.p. ind. as contrib. comedy & other situations. From 1927 dir. many pictures, & from 1927 variously dir. & prod. In 1942 apptd. dir. supvr. Hollywood prod. for coordinator Inter-Amer. Affairs. In 1955 orig. own prod. co., Mervyn LeRoy Prods.; A "Champion Directors" in Fame ratings Special Acad. Award 1945 for dir. The House I Live In. In 1976 won the Irving Thalberg Award.
PICTURES INCLUDE: Wizard of Oz, King and the Chorus Girl, High Pressure, Thirty Seconds Over Tokyo, I Am a Fugitive from a Chain Gang, Hard to Handle, Gold Diggers of 1933, Five Star Final, Oil for the Lamps of China, Little Caesar, Tugboat Annie, Anthony Adverse, Three Men on a Horse, Escape, Johnny Eager, Random Harvest, Madame Curie, Without Reservations, Homecoming, Little Women, Any Number Can Play, East Side West Side, Quo Vadis, Lovely to Look At, Million Dollar Mermaid, Latin Lovers, Rose Marie, Mister Roberts, Strange Lady in Town, Bad Seed, Toward the Unknown, No Time for Sergeants, Home Before Dark, The FBI Story, Wake Me When It's Over, Majority of One, The Devil at 4 O'Clock.

LESLIE, ALEEN: Writer. b. Pittsburgh, Pa., Feb. 5, 1908; e. Ohio State U. Contributor to magazines; columnist Pittsburgh Press; orig. & wrote radio series A Date with Judy 1941–50. Bway play Slightly Married, 1943; wrote, prod. Date with Judy, TV series; author, The Scent of the Roses, The Windfall.
PICTURES INCLUDE: Doctor Takes a Wife, Affectionately Yours, Henry Aldrich Plays Cupid, Stork Pays Off, Henry Aldrich Gets Glamour, It Comes Up Love, Rosie the Riveter, Father Was a Fullback, Father Is a Bachelor.

LESLIE, JOAN: Actress. Star of Tomorrow, 1946. r.n. Joan Brodell; b. Detroit, Mich., January 26, 1925; p. Agnes and John Brodell; e. St. Benedicts, Detroit; Our Lady of Lourdes, Toronto; St. Mary's Montreal; Immaculate Heart. H.S., Los Angeles. Now on bd. of dir., St. Anne's Hospital, Damon Runyon Foundation.
PICTURES INCLUDE: The Sky's the Limit, This Is the Army, Yankee Doodle Dandy, Thank Your Lucky Stars, Rhapsody in Blue, Cinderella Jones, Hollywood Canteen, Where Do We Go From Here?, Too Young to Know, Repeat Performance, Northwest Stampede, Born To Be Bad, Skipper Surprised His Wife, Man in the Saddle, Hellgate, Flight Nurse, Jubilee Trail, Revolt of Mamie Stover.
TV: Ford Theatre, G.E. Theatre, Queen for a Day. Movies: Charley Hannah, The Keegans, Various commercials.

LESTER, MARK: Actor. b. Oxford, England, 1958. Ent. m.p. ind. 1963.
PICTURES INCLUDE: Allez France, Our Mother's House, 1967; Oliver, 1968; Run Wild, Run Free, 1969; The Boy Who Stole the Elephant, Eye Witness, SWALK (Melody), Black Beauty, Whoever Slew Auntie Roo?, Redneck, Crossed Swords.
TV: Special for Disney in Hollywood. 1970: American series for Krofft Television Productions, Scalawag, 1972; Graduation Trip, 1972; Danza Alla Porto Gli Olmi (Italian Entry Berlin '75), Seen Dimly Before Dawn '75.
STAGE: The Murder Game '76; The Prince & The Pauper '76.

LESTER, RICHARD: Director, composer. b. Philadelphia, Pa., 1932. Early career: dir. and mus. dir. TV, CBS, Phila., CBC-TV, Toronto. Ent. m.p. ind. 1957. TV: dir. TV Goon Shows. Composed (with Reg. Owen) Sea War Series. Films: Composed and dir., Running, Jumping and Standing Still Film.
PICTURES INCLUDE: It's Trad, Dad, Mouse On the Moon, Hard Day's Night, The Knack, Help! A Funny Thing Happened on the Way to the Forum, How I Won The War, Petulia, The Bedsitting Room, The Three Musketeers, Juggernaut, The Four Musketeers, Royal Flash, Robin & Marian, The Ritz, Butch and Sundance: The Early Days, Superman (prod. only), Cuba, Superman II, Superman III, Finders Keepers (also exec. prod.).

LESTZ, EARL: Executive. Affiliated for 18 years with Federal Department Stores, of which was sr. v.p. of operations for its Bullock's chain before joining Paramount Pictures in April, 1983, as sr. v.p. of studio operations. 1985, named pres., operations for Paramount Studio Group.

LETTER, LOUIS N.: Executive, b. New York City, August, 1937. e. Brooklyn College Business Administration, v.p. and dir. of operations, Century Theatres, New Hyde Park, N.Y. Exec. v.p., RKO Century Warner Theatres, New York City.

LEVEE, MICHAEL: Producer. e. Stanford Univ. Four years as U.S. Navy officer in World War II. After service went to work for father's company. M.C. Levee Agency. In 1947 formed Levee-Stark Agency with Ray Stark. Joined MCA in 1950; 1952, appt. v.p. in chg of TV division. When MCA phased out of agency business became exec. v.p. at CMA. Later joined Robert Radnitz as exec. v.p. of Radnitz/Mattel division of Mattel Toys, formed to finance family-oriented films. In 1975 rejoined Starr as exec. v.p. of Rastar Group. Left to produce independently.
PICTURES: The Black Bird (exec. prod.), Casey's Shadow (exec. prod.), Slow Dancing in the Big City (co.-prod.).

LEVEN, BORIS: Art director, production designer. b. Moscow, Russia. e. Certificate of Beaux Arts Inst. of Design, N.Y., U.S.C.—Bachelor of Architecture degree. Painter of water colors, many awards in architectural competitions; sketch artist, set designer, Paramount Studios, 1933–35; asst. art dir., Major Pictures Corp., 1936; art dir., 20th Century-Fox, 1937–38, 41–42, 45–46, Universal, 1947–48, freelance from 1948. Nominated for Acad. Award 8 times. Academy award in art direction for West Side Story. Member: Academy of M.P. Arts & Sciences, Soc. of M.P. & TV Art Dirs., United Scenic Artists, Delta Phi Delta, Tau Sigma Delta, Skull & Dagger. U.S. Army Air Force 1942–45.
PICTURES INCLUDE: Alexander's Ragtime Band, Tales of Manhattan, Shanghai Gesture, Hello Frisco Hello, I Wonder Who's Kissing Her Now, Criss-Cross, Mr. Peabody and The Mermaid, The Senator Was Indiscreet, The Prowler, Sudden Fear, The Star, The Invaders from Mars, Silver Chalice, Giant, Anatomy of Murder, West Side Story, Two For the Seesaw, The Sound of Music, The Sand Pebbles, Star! A Dream of Kings, The Andromeda Strain, The New Centurions, Jonathan Livingston Seagull, Mandingo, New York, New York, The Last Waltz, The King of Comedy, Fletch.

LE VIEN, JACK: Producer/Director. b. N.Y., N.Y., 1918; film ed., reporter, Pathe News; military service, 1941–46; news ed., gen. mgr., v.p., Pathe News; chmn, American Newsreel Assoc., 1956–59; dir. of prod., Hearst Metrotone News; prod. in assoc., ABC-TV, The Valiant Years; exec. prod., Black Fox; prod. The Finest Hours, A King's Story; chmn., exec. prod., Le Vien Films Ltd.; prod.; Other World of

Winston Churchill (NBC, BBC), The Gathering Storm, Walk With Destiny, The Amazing Voyage of Daffodil & Daisy, The Queens Drum Horse, Where The Lotus Fell, Churchill and the Generals, The Glittering Crowd, A Question of Choice.

LEVIN, ALAN M.: Executive. b. New York City, 1943. e. Brooklyn Coll., Brooklyn Law School. In law practice before joining CBS News Business Affairs dept. in 1969 as asst. dir.; 1970, talent and program negotiator for network business affairs; 1971, assoc. dir. business affairs; 1974, dir. talent and program contracts; 1975, dir., talent and program negotiations; 1976, v.p., business affairs, CBS, New York; 1977, v.p. business affairs CBS Entertainment. April 1978, v.p. and asst. to pres.; then v.p., business affairs. In 1980 named to business affairs and admin.; 1982, exec. v.p.; 1984, head of CBS Productions.

LEVIN, IRVING H.: Executive. b. Chicago, Ill., Sept. 8, 1921. e. grad., U. of Ill. U.S. Air Force, 1943–45; entered m.p. ind. as partner of Kranz-Levin Pictures and Realart Pictures of Calif. Inc.; indep. exch. in 1948; formed Mutual Prod, 1952; pres., Filmakers Releasing Org., 1953; secy., Filmakers Prod., Inc., 1952; pres. AB-PT Pictures Corp., 1956; pres., exec. prod., Oakhurst Television Prod., Inc., Sindee Prod., Inc.; pres., exec. prod. Atlas Enterprises, Inc.; pres., prod. Atlantic Pictures, 1959; exec. vice-pres., mem. of bd. of dir., National General Corp. (formerly NT&T) 1961 and Pres. National General Prod. Inc. 1966 & Pictures Corp. 1967. Pres. and chief operating officer, NGC. In 1975 formed Levin-Schulman Prods. 1983, pres., Royal Theatres, Hawaii.

LEVIN, ROBERT B.: Executive. b. Chicago. e. Univ. of Illinois. Operated own adv. firm for five years. 1982, named sr. v.p., Needham Harper World Wide Advertising Agency, Chicago. 1985, joined Walt Disney Pictures as sr. v.p., mktg.

LEVINE, JOSEPH E.: Executive. b. Boston, Massachusetts, Sept. 9, 1905. Entered motion picture industry as owner of theatre in New Haven, Connecticut. Entered national distribution in 1943. Named "Pioneer of the Year", Variety Club of N.Y.; "Showman of the Year", 1960. Named "Producer of the Year" by Allied States Assoc. of M.P. Exhibitions, 1962. Named "Master Showman of the World" by TOA, 1963; winner of Cecil B. DeMille Award for "Showman of the Year" from Hollywood Foreign Press, 1964; winner First Annual Award, Conference of Personal Mgrs., East, for outstanding contributions to World of Entertainment, 1965. President Avco Embassy Pictures. Resigned 1974 to form own co., Joseph E. Levine Presents.
PICTURES INCLUDE: Hercules, 1959; Two Women, 1962; Boccaccio '70, The Sky Above, The Mud Below, Long Day's Journey Into Night, Federico Fellini's 8½, The Easy Life, Yesterday, Today and Tomorrow, Marriage Italian Style, Divorce Italian Style, The Carpetbaggers, Zulu, Casanova '70, Darling, Woman Times Seven, The Graduate. The Producers, The Lion in Winter, Carnal Knowledge, Day of the Dolphin, A Bridge Too Far, Magic, Tattoo.

LEVINE, ROBERT J.: Executive. b. Brooklyn, N.Y. July 22, 1946. e. Brooklyn College (BA honors 1968); Cornell Law School, (JD 1971). Spec. in international affairs. 1971–73, staff attorney in securities and insurance field. 1973–present, sole practitioner in commercial field; 1977–present, in-house counsel to C. E. Feltner's enterprises in entertainment and tax field. Co-author and assoc. prod. of Carnival Magic. Adapter and assoc. prod. of Mars in the 8th House. Author and assoc. prod. of Nothing's As It Seems (tent. title) & play, The Black Widow Conspiracy.

LEVINSON, BARRY: Director. b. Baltimore, MD. e. American Univ. Wrote and acted in tv comedy show in L.A., leading to work on network tv. Wrote and performed on The Carol Burnett Show. Worked on film scripts with Mel Brooks and co-wrote scrips with Valerie Curtin: And Justice for All, Inside Moves, Best Friends, Unfaithfully Yours.
PICTURES: Diner, The Natural, Young Sherlock Holmes.

LEVINSON, NORM: Executive. b. New Haven, Conn., March 17, 1925. Started theatre business as usher for Loew's Theatres, 1940. U.S. Army, 1943–46. Returned Loew's Theatres managerial positions New Haven and Hartford, Connecticut. MGM press representative, Minneapolis, Jacksonville, Atlanta, Dallas. General Manager, Trans-Texas Theatres, Dallas. President, Academy Theatres, Inc., Dallas. Promoted Championship Boxing, Dallas and Johannesburg, South Africa. Executive Vice President, Cobb Theatres, Birmingham, Alabama; v.p., world-wide mktg., Artists Releasing Corp., Encino, CA.; head film buyer, Chakeres Theatres, Ohio & Kentucky.

LEVITT, RUBY REBECCA: Set decorator. b. Corinth, N.Y., Sept. 10, 1907; e. Pratt Inst., Brooklyn. Buyer, interior decorator, department stores; store mgr.; set decorator, Universal, since 1944.
PICTURES INCLUDE: Letter From an Unknown Woman, Magnificent Obsession, The Shrike, Six Bridges to Cross, Private War of Major Benson, This Earth Is Mine, Pillow Talk, 40 Pounds of Trouble, For the Love of Money, Sound of Music, Willie Boy, The Scavengers, Colossus, Change of Habit, Andromeda Strain, Vanished, Happy Birthday, Wanda June, The Other, Freebie and The Bean, The Manchn Eagle, Chinatown, Once Is Not Enough, Let's Do It Again, Harry and Walter Go To New York, A Star Is Born, New York-New York, Looking for Mr. Goodbar, The One The Only, Matilda, Promises in the Dark, The Jazz Singer.
TV: Mr. Ed, Addams Family, Double Life of Henry Phyffe, Movies of the Week, ABC, Banyon TV Series, Genesis II, Name of the Game, Love Story, Having Babies, Return Engagement.
Staff Decorator for television commercials, Filmways of California, Inc. Staff of Filmways of Calif., 1966. Universal Studios, 1968.

LEVY, BERNARD: Executive. b. Boca Raton, Florida. e. Brooklyn Law School, L.L.B. Legal staff of Superintendent of Insurance of the State of New York in the rehabilitation and liquidation of guaranteed title and mortgage companies, 1934–36; private practice of law, 1936–46; legal staff, Paramount Pictures, Inc., 1946–50; legal staff, United Paramount Theatres, 1950–51; exec. asst. to Edward L. Hyman, vice-pres., American Broadcasting Companies, Inc., in chg. of theatre administration, north, 1951–62; apptd. exec. liaison officer for southern motion picture theatres, ABC, Inc., 1962–64; exec. liaison officer, m.p. theas., ABC, Inc., 1965–72; vice pres., ABC Theatre Division, 1973. Retired, 1976.

LEVY, BUD: Executive. b. Jackson Heights, N.Y. April 3, 1928. e. New York Univ. Exec. v.p. Trans-Lux Corp., N.Y. Member: Variety Clubs Int'l., M.P. Pioneers, bd. of Indep. Theatres Owners Ass'n.; dir., Trans-Lux Corp.; New York area chm., Will Rogers Memorial Fund; Member, President's Advisory Board-NATO; director: NATO, TOP, CATO. Elected pres., Trans-Lux Corp., 1980.

LEVY, DAVID: Executive. b. Philadelphia, Pa., January 2, 1913; e. Wharton, U. of Pa.; exec. v.p., Four Star International, Inc. As v.p. & assoc. dir., Young & Rubicam. Inc., 1938–59, acquisitions for clients include: Father Knows Best, Goodyear Playhouse, Life of Riley, Gunsmoke. Was v.p. in charge of network TV programs & talent, NBC, 1959–61.
TV: Bonanza, Dr. Kildare, Dick Powell Show, Saturday Night at the Movies, Bat Masterson, Klondike, Americans, Outlaws, The Addams Family, Double Life of Henry Phyffe, The Chameleons, The Gods of Foxcroft Carbor House, as well as numerous TV plays.

LEVY, HERMAN M.: Attorney, Hamden, Conn. b. New Haven, Conn., Sept. 27, 1904; e. Yale, BA, '27, Yale Law School, LL.B., '29; Phi Beta Kappa, was in legal dept. RCA Photophone; newspaper reporter; admitted to Connecticut bar, 1929. In 1939 elected exec. secy. of MPTO of Connecticut. In 1943: Elected general counsel MPTOA. Elected gen. counsel, Theatre Owners of America, 1947–63. Pres., New Haven County Bar Assn., 1964; legislative agent, Conn. Assn. of Theatre Owners. Retired as legistative agent, 1981.
AUTHOR: More Sinned Against . . . Natl. Bd. of Review Magazine, 1941. Proving the Death of a Non-Resident Alien, Conn. Bar Journal, 1950; Need for a System of Arbitration M.P. Ind., Arbitration Journal, 1950; reprint of Industry Case Digest, 20th Century-Fox vs. Boehm in the Journal (Screen Producers Guild); Book Review of Antitrust in the Motion Picture Industry, by Michael Conant (Univ. of Calif. Law Review).

LEVY, JULES V.: Producer. b. Los Angeles, Calif., Feb. 12, 1923; e. U.S.C. Property dept., W.B., 1941; Army Air Force, 1942–45.
PICTURES INCLUDE: The Vampire, Return of Dracula, Vice Squad, Without Warning, Down Three Dark Streets, Geronimo, Glory Guys, Clambake, Scalphunters, Sam Whiskey, Underground, McKenzie Break, The Hunting Party, The Honkers', McQ, Brannigan, White Lightning, Gator, Kansas City Bomber, Safari 3000.
TV: Rifleman, Robert Taylor's Detectives, Law of the Plainsman, The Big Valley.

LEVY, MICHAEL: Executive. b. Brooklyn, NY. e. Brown Univ. Started in industry in editorial dept. of trade-paper Variety; held posts in New York with ABC Motion Pictures and with Diener/Hauser/Bates Advertising. Worked for Lawrence Gordon Productions as exec. asst. to Gordon and as story editor. Joined 20th Century Fox in January, 1985, as dir. of creative affairs for studio. 1986, named v.p., production, m.p. div., Fox.

LEVY, NORMAN: Executive. b. Bronx, New York, Jan. 3, 1935. e. City College. In 1957 joined Universal Pictures, holding various sales positions; 1967, went to National General Pictures, ultimately being named v.p. and exec. asst. to pres.; 1974, Columbia Pictures, v.p., gen. sls. mgr. In 1975 named Columbia exec. v.p. in chg. of domestic sls.; 1977, exec. v.p., mktg; 1978. pres., Columbia Pictures Domestic Distribution. In 1980 joined 20th-Fox as pres. of Entertainment Group; 1981, vice-chm., 20th Century-Fox Film Corp. Resigned 1984 to become mktg./dist. consultant. 1986, joined New Century Productions as head of domestic production.

LEWELLEN, A. WAYNE: Executive. b. Feb. 16, 1944. e. Univ. of Texas. Joined Paramount Pictures 1973 as brch. mgr., Dallas-Oklahoma City territory; named South. dist. mgr.; 1978, South. div. mgr. July, 1984, named v.p., domestic dist., South. div.; 1985, appt. exec. v.p., gen. sls. mgr. (New York). 1986, named pres., domestic dist.

LEWINE, ROBERT F.: Executive. b. New York, N.Y., Apr. 16, 1913; e. Swarthmore Coll. Worked for restaurant chain, in real estate; U.S. Navy, 1942; creative staff, Cine-Television Studios, Inc.; v.p. in charge of oper., 1946; formed own co., 1947, for prod. of TV comm., industrial m.p.; also eastern rep., Dudley Films; radio-TV dir., Hirshon-Garfield, Inc., 1953; eastern prog. dir., ABC, 1953; dir., ABC-TV network prog. dept., 1954; v.p. in charge of programming and talent ABC-TV network, 1956; v.p., NBC, prog. dept. chg. nighttime programming, 1957; v.p. network programs, 1958; v.p. Figaro, Inc., 1958; v.p. programs, CBS Films, 1959; v.p. programs, Hollywood CBS Television Network, Apr., 1962; officer Acad. TV Arts & Sciences from 1954, Exec. comm., dir., Acad. TV Arts & Sciences. Pres., N.Y. Chapter 1959; nat'l. pres., 1961; nat'l. trustee, 1961–63; National pres., Academy TV Arts & Sciences, 1961–63; first vice pres., dir., Academy TV Arts & Sciences Foundation; pres., 1964; exec. v.p., Creative Management Associates Ltd.; v.p., Warner Bros., TV Pres. Nat'l Acad. of Television Arts and Sciences; trustee, Columbia College, L.A., Calif.; trustee, American Women in Radio and Television Foundation. 1977-NBC Television Network, exec. prod. dir.; chairman, PAW Society (Preservation of Animal Wildlife); Member International Advisory Council, Population Institute; Chairman of the Board, Riverside Broadcasting Company. Since 1978 guest lecturer at UCLA and USC.

LEWIS, ARTHUR: Producer—Director—Writer. b. New York City. e. Univ. of So. Calif. and Yale. Began career as writer and assoc. prod. on the Jones Family TV series. Five years in U.S. Army; returned to screenwriting before producing Three Wishes for Jamie on Broadway and producing and directing Guys and Dolls in London's West End. In mid-60' produced plays with Bernard Delfont at Shaftesbury Theatre in London.
PICTURES: Producer: Loot, Baxter, The Killer Elite, Brass Target.
TELEVISION: Brenner, The Asphalt Jungle (prod. writer).

LEWIS, EDWARD: Producer. Began entertainment career as script writer, then co-produced The Admiral Was a Lady and teamed with Marion Parsonnet to bring the Faye Emerson Show to TV. Subsequently prod. first Schlitz Playhouse and China Smith series. Was v.p. of Kirk Douglas' indep. prod. co., where was assoc. prod. and writer-prod. Collaborated with John Frankenheimer on 8 films.
PICTURES INCLUDE: Lizzie (assoc. prod.), The Careless Years (prod., s.p.), Spartacus, The Last Sunset, Lonely Are the Brave, The List of Adrian Messenger, Seconds, Grand Prix, The Fixer (exec. prod.), The Gypsy Moths (exec.), I Walk the Line (exec.), The Horsemen, The Iceman Cometh (exec.), Crackers, The River.

LEWIS, EMMANUEL: Actor. b. Brooklyn, NY, March 9, 1971. Began in TV commercials and has done TV and radio voice-overs. Sings and dances and, following personal appearance tours in Japan, became recording star there. Theatrical debut in A Midsummer Night's Dream at N.Y. Shakespeare Festival (1982).
TELEVISION: Tonight Show, The Phil Donahue Show, Webster (star). Movie: Lost in London.

LEWIS, HAROLD G: Executive. b. New York City, Sept. 18, 1938. e. Union College; graduated 1960, electrical engineer. Joined ATA Trading Corp. in 1960 and has been pres. since 1977. Producer of feature animation. Importer and exporter for theatrical and TV features, documentaries, series, classics, etc.

LEWIS, JERRY: Actor. b. Newark, N.J., Mar. 16, 1926. e. Irvington H.S. m. Patti Palmer, vocalist, Jimmy Dorsey & Ted Florita bands; has six sons. Began his career in school theatricals, at 14, awarded plaque by American Red Cross for amateur show, Mosque Theatre. Formed comedy-team with Dean Martin (singer, straight man) at 500 Club, Atlantic City, N.J., 1946; appeared Latin Casino, Phila., then other nightclubs, on NBC television; played many m.p. theatres; signed by Hal Wallis; team m.p. debut in My Friend Irma (see biog. Dean Martin). Voted Most Promising Male Star in Television in m.p. Daily's 2nd annual TV poll, 1950. Voted (as team) one of top ten money making stars in m.p. Herald-Fame poll, 1951, 1953–54–57. Number 1, 1952; best comedy team in m.p. Daily's 16th annual radio poll, 1951, 1952, 1953; 1956 formed Jerry Lewis Prods. Inc., functions as prod., dir., writer & star.
PICTURES INCLUDE: My Friend Irma Goes West, At War With the Army, That's My Boy, The Stooge, Sailor Beware, Jumping Jacks, The Caddy, Scared Stiff, Money From Home, Living It Up, Three Ring Circus, You're Never Too Young, Artists and Models, Pardners, Hollywood or Bust, Delicate Delinquent, Sad Sack, Rock-A-Bye Baby, Geisha Boy, Don't Give Up the Ship, Visit to A Small Planet, Cinderfella, Bellboy, The Ladies Man, The Errand Boy, It's Only Money, The Nutty Professor, Who's Minding the Store?, The Patsy, The Disorderly Orderly, Boeing-Boeing, The Family Jewels, Three on a Couch, Way . . . Way Out, The Big Mouth, Don't Lower the Bridge Raise the River, Hook Line and Sinker, Which Way to the Front?, One More Time, Hardly Working (star, dir., co-s.p.), King of Comedy, Smorgasbord (also dir.).

LEWIS, JOSEPH H.: Director. b. New York, N.Y., Apr. 6. e. DeWitt Clinton H.S. Camera boy, MGM; then asst. film ed. in chge. film ed., Republic; dir. in chge. 2nd units; dir. Universal; U.S. Signal Corps., WW II; dir. RKO, Columbia, W.B.
PICTURES INCLUDE: My Name is Julia Ross, So Dark the Night, Jolson Story, The Swordsman, Return of October, Undercover Man, Gun Crazy, Lady Without Passport, Retreat Hell!, Desperate Search, Cry of the Hunted, Big Combo, A Lawless Street.
TV: Rifleman series, Barbara Stanwyck Show: The Big Valley.

LEWIS, LESTER: talent rep. b. New York, N.Y. Sept 23, 1912. e. H.S. of Commerce, N.Y. Pres. Lester Lewis Associates, Inc., talent agency.

LEWIS, MICHAEL J.: Composer. b. Wales, 1939. First film score 1968, The Mad Woman of Chaillot, won Ivor Novello Award for best film score. 1973: first Broadway musical, Cyrano, Grammy Nomination '74, Caesar & Cleopatra (T.V. '76); The Lion, the Witch, and the Wardrobe (Emmy, 1979).
PICTURES INCLUDE: The Man Who Haunted Himself, Julius Caesar. 1970: Upon This Rock, 1971: Unman, Wittering and Zigo, Running Scared, Baxter, Theatre of Blood, 11 Harrowhouse, 92 In The Shade, Russian Roulette, The Stick-Up, The Medusa Touch, The Legacy, The Passage, The Unseen, Sphinx, Yes, Giorgio, The Hound of Baskerville, On the Third Day, The Naked Face.

LEWIS, MONICA: Singer, actress. b. Chicago, Il., May 5, 1925. e. Hunter Coll., N.Y. p. Leon Lewis, concert pianist, former medical dir. CBS; Jessica Lewis, child star with Nazimova; member Ben Greet's Shakespearean players, sang leading roles. Chicago Opera Co.; now vocal teacher. Started career as radio singer, own show, WMCA, N.Y.; on Beat the Band, 1946; co-star Chesterfield program; sang leading role, Girl Crazy, Ford Sunday Evening Hour, Own program, Monica Makes Music; co-star Revere Camera show. Among first ten feminine singers in country on recording polls. Vocalist: Stork Club, Astor Roof, Copacabana, Persian Room.
PICTURES INCLUDE: Inside Straight, Excuse My Dust, The Strip, Everything I Have is Yours, Affair With a Stranger.

LIBERACE: Performer, pianist, r.n. Wladziu Valentino Liberace. b. Milwaukee, Wis., May 16, 1920. e. Wisconsin College of Music. Guest soloist with Chicago Symphony at 16, then hotel, night club entertainer, concert and recording artist. Own TV shows since 1952; m.p. debut in Sincerely Yours.

LIBERMAN, FRANK P.: Publicist, b. N.Y., N.Y., May 29, 1917. e. Cheshire Acad., Conn. 1934; Lafayette College, Easton, Pa., B.A. 1938. m. Patricia Harris, casting dir. Worked as copy boy, NY Daily News, 1938–39. Began career as publicist at Warner Bros., home office as messenger, 1939, promoted to pressbooks dept., transferred to Warner's Chicago office as field exploitation man. U.S. Signal Corps, 1941, public relations officer, Army Pictorial Service, on temporary duty with War Dept., Bureau of Public Relations in Pentagon. Discharged as Capt., 1946. Rejoined Warner Bros. on coast 2 years, 1947, est. own public relations office. Owner, Frank Liberman and Associates, Inc.

LICCARDI, VINCENT G.: Executive. b. Brooklyn, N.Y., Started as messenger at Universal Pictures, asst. adv. mgr. on Around the World in 80 Days, asst. to exec. coord. of States & Adv. on Spartacus; National Dir. of Adv. & Publ., Continental; Nat. Dir. Adv. & Publ., Braintree Prod., adv. pub. mgr. Allied Artists, ad. mgr. Paramount, National Dir. Adv.-Pub., UMC Pictures, Screenwriter, Playboy to Priest, The Rivals, The Rivals-Part II, The Greatest Disaster of All Time, The Lady on the 9:40, All That Heaven Allows, All Mine To Love.

LIDER, EDWARD W. Executive. b. New Bedford, Mass., March 13, 1922. e. Dartmouth, Harvard Law. Served as attorney-at-law, 1948–50. President & treasurer, Fall River Theatres Corp. & Nathan Yamins Enterprises, 1950 to present;

member of bd., Theatre Owners of New England; past pres., Theatre Owners of New England; past member of bd. & past treas., Allied States Assoc. of M.P. Exhibitors; general manager of Sonny & Eddy's Theatres in Boston: Exeter St., Academy, Harvard Square, Central Square, Allston C1nema-C2nema and Galeria Theatres.

LIEBER, PERRY W.: Publicist. b. Pleasant Prairie, Wis., June 1, 1905; e. U. of Illinois. Was in adv. dept. of J. P. Seaburg Co., Chicago, Ill. Pub. dept. RKO Radio Studio 1930; publ. dir. 1939; nat'l dir. pub., exploit. supv. N.Y. office, 1953–55. 20th Century-Fox pub. dept. 1956; in chg. studio adv. pub. dept., 20th Century Fox Studio, Aug. 1962. 1966 pub. dept. 20th Century-Fox. Mgr./P.R. Summa Corp. since 1970, Consultant, P.R., Summa Corp. since July, 1977.

LIEBERFARB, WARREN: Executive. e. Wharton School of Commerce and Finance, Univ. of Penna (BS, Economics); Univ. of Michigan (Master of Business Admin.). Started career in industry at Paramount Pictures as dir. of mktg. and exec. asst. to Stanley Jaffe, then pres. Later joined 20th-Fox as v.p.—special market dist. (cable, pay-TV, non-theatrical), also representing 20th in all MPAA matters on cable and pay/TV. Joined Warner Bros. as v.p., exec. asst. to Ted Ashley, bd. chm.; later named v.p., intl. adv.-pub. In 1979 joined Lorimar as v.p., of Lorimar Productions, Inc., the parent company, based in New York, Promoted to snr. v.p. 1982, named v.p. mktg., Warner Home Video; named pres., 1985.

LIEBERSON, SANFORD: Producer. b. 1936. 1979, named pres. of 20th-Fox Productions, which company he joined in 1977 as v.p.—European production. Previously an independent producer (Performance, Bugsy Malone, Jabberwocky, etc.). Prior to that exec. in chg. of European operations of Creative Management Associates. In 1980 named int'l. v.p. for Ladd Co., based in London. Now prod. chief, Goldcrest Film & TV.

LIGHTMAN, M. A.: Exhibitor. b. Nashville, Tenn., Apr. 21, 1915; e. Southwestern U., Vanderbilt U., 1936, B.A. bd. chmn. Malco Theatres, Inc., Memphis, Tenn.

LINDBLOM, GUNNEL: Actress-Director. b. Gothenburg, Sweden, 1931. Discovered by Ingmar Bergman while studying at drama school of Gothenburg Municipal Theatre (1950–53); she moved to Malmo, where he was director of the local Municipal Theatre. Under Bergman's direction she played in Easter, Peer Gynt, Faust, etc. between 1954–59. Later appeared in many Bergman films. Since 1968 has been on staff of Stockholm's Royal Dramatic Theatre, assisting Bergman and then beginning to direct on her own. Made film debut as director with Summer Paradise in 1977.
PICTURES INCLUDE: Actress: The Seventh Seal, Wild Strawberries, The Virgin Spring, Winter Light, The Silence, Rapture, Loving Couples. Director: Summer Paradise.

LINDEN, HAL: Actor. b. Bronx, N.Y., March 20, 1931. e. City College New York. Began career as saxophone player and singer, playing with bands of Sammy Kaye, Bobby Sherwood, etc. Drafted and performed in revues for Special Services. After discharge enrolled at N.Y.'s American Theatre Wing; appeared on Bdwy. in Bells Are Ringing, replacing Sydney Chaplin. On many TV talk and variety shows.
THEATRE: On a Clear Day, Wildcat, Something More, Subways Are for Sleeping, Ilya Darling, Apple Tree, Three Men on a Horse, Pajama Game, The Rothschilds.
TELEVISION: Host on ABC series, Animals Animals Animals; Barney Miller.
PICTURE: When You Comin' Back Red Ryder?

LINDFORS, VIVECA: Actress. b. Uppsala, Sweden, Dec. 29, 1920; e. Royal Dramatic School, Stockholm. Stage debut in Ann-Scofi Hedvig school prod. Screen debut in The Crazy Family, 1941; reached stardom in If I Should Marry the Minister. U.S. screen debut in Night Unto Night.
PICTURES INCLUDE: Adventures of Don Juan, Dark City, Flying Missile, Gypsy Fury, No Sad Songs For Me, Journey Into Light, Four In a Jeep, The Raiders, No Time for Flowers, Run for Cover, Captain Dreyfus, Coming Apart, Puzzle of a Downfall Child, The Way We Were, Welcome to L.A., Girl Friends, A Wedding, Voices, The Hand, Creepshow, The Sure Thing.
TELEVISION: A Doctor's Story, Passions, The Three Wishes of Billy Grier.

LINDNER, TERRELL M.: Executive. b. Dromana, Australia. Aug. 10, 1915. Entered m.p. ind. in pub. dep. Columbia Pictures, Melbourne, Australia, 1942. Columbia, mgr. Western Australia, Dec. 1946. gen. mgr. Columbia, New Zealand, 1948. United Artists home office rep. for India, Burma, Pakistan, Ceylon, 1952. apptd. United Artists dist. supvr. for Southeast Asia. hdqts. Bombay. Dec. 1953. Rank overseas. 1957. Opened West Indies offices. man. dir. Rank Filmes do Brasil, 1958. man. dir. Filmcenter Internacional Ltda., Brazil, (successors Rank) 1970.

LINKLETTER, ART: Emcee, prod. b. Moose Jaw, Saskatchewan, Canada, July 17, 1912. e. San Diego State Coll. Radio prg. mgr., San Diego Exposition, 1935; radio pgm. mgr. S.F. World's Fair, 1937–39; freelance radio ann. and m.c. 1939–42; m.c. People are Funny since 1942. Starred Inside Beverly Hills, NBC-TV, 1955; exec. prod. host, NBC-TV spec. Salute to Baseball, 1956; host, Art Linkletter's Secret World of Kids, NBC-TV's Ford Startime, 1959; 1969 House Party series became the Linkletter Show.
Author of: The Secret World of Kids, 1959, Kids Say the Darndest Things, 1957, Linkletter Down Under, 1969, Yes, You Can, 1979.

LINSON, ART: Producer-Director. b. Chicago. e. UCLA. Was rock music manager before turning to film production. Debuted as director also with Where the Buffalo Roam.
PICTURES: Rafferty and the Gold Dust Twins, (co.-prod.), Wash, American Hot Wax (also co-s.p.), Melvin and Howard, The Wild Life (dir.), Singles.

LIPPERT, ROBERT J., JR.: Producer. director, film editor. b. Alameda, Calif. Feb. 28, 1928. e. St Mary's College 1946; all conference Football 1947. Film Editor of 65 motion pictures. Produced and directed nine pictures for Lippert Pictures and 20th Century Fox. Present position is president, for Lippert Theatres headquartered in Pebble Beach, CA.

LIPSTONE, HOWARD H.; Executive, producer. b. Chicago, Ill., Apr. 28. e. UCLA, Univ. of So. Calif. Ass't to gen. mgr. at KLTA, 1950–55; program dir. at KABC-TV, 1955–65; exec. ass't to pres. at Selmur Prods., ABC subsidiary, 1965–69. Ivan Tors Films & Studios as exec. v.p., 1969–70; pres., The Landsburg Co., 1970 to present.

LIPTON, DAVID A.: Executive. b. Chicago, Nov. 6, 1906. U.S. Army, WW II. Entered m.p. ind. 1921 as office boy, Balaban & Katz, Chicago; in 1922 joined pub. dept.; in 1929 transf. Detroit; in 1930 joined Famous Players Canadian Corp., org. pub. dept.; ret'd to Chicago office 1931; res. 1933 to become publ. dir. for Sally Rand. In 1937 joined CBS, N.Y. as press relations counsel. Named publ. dir. Universal N.Y., 1938; later to West Coast as studio publ. dir. In 1941 to N.Y. as dir. adv. publ. & exploit., Columbia; returned to Universal as exec. coordinator of adv. & promotion, 1946; nat'l dir. adv. pub., Jan. 1949; elected v.p. in chge. adv. pub.; 1974, MCA Discovision, Inc., public relations director; 1979, consultant.

LISI, VIRNA: Actress. b. Ancona, Italy, Nov. 8, 1937.
PICTURES: How To Murder Your Wife, Casanova 70, Not with My Wife You Don't, Assault on a Queen, The Lady and the General, Arabella, Better a Widow, Ernesto.

LISTER, MOIRA: Actress. b. Capetown, So. Africa. e. Holy Family Convent, Johannesburg. Stage debut at 6 yrs. of age in Vikings of Heligoland; screen debut in Shipbuilders, 1943. Numerous TV appearances.
PICTURES INCLUDE: Love Story, Wanted for Murder, Don Chicago, Uneasy Terms, So Evil My Love, Another Shore, Once a Jolly Swagman, Run for Your Money, Pool of London, White Corridors, Something Money Can't Buy, Cruel Sea, Grand National Night, Limping Man, Trouble in Store, John and Julie, Deep Blue Sea, Seven Waves Away, The Yellow Rolls Royce, Joey Boy, Double Man, Stranger in the House.

LITHGOW, JOHN: Actor. b. Rochester, NY, Oct. 19, 1945. e. Harvard. Early career on Bdwy.; won Tony for The Changing Room. Acted and directed in London with Royal Shakespeare Co. and Royal Court Theatre. Also on Bdwy. in My Fat Friend, The Comedians, A Memory of Two Mondays, Anna Christie, Once in a Lifetime, etc.
PICTURES: Rich Kids, Obsession, Blow Out, All That Jazz, Twilight Zone—The Movie, Terms of Endearment, Footloose, 2010, Santa Claus, The Manhattan Project.
TELEVISION: Movies: The Day After, The Glitter Dome, Resting Place.

LITTLE, RICH: Actor. b. Ottawa, Canada, Nov. 26, 1938. Impersonator in night clubs. On screen in Dirty Tricks.
TELEVISION: Rich Little's Christmas Carol, Rich Little's Washington Follies, You Asked for It, Parade of Stars, The Christmas Raccoons, Rich Little and Friends in New Orleans, etc.

LITTO, GEORGE: Executive. b. Philadelphia, Dec. 9, 1930. e. Temple Univ. Joined William Morris Agency in New York and then became indep. literary agent. Opened own office in Hollywood, 1962. Packaged film and TV productions, including six films for Robert Altman. 1981, named chmn. bd. & CEO, Filmways.
PICTURES INCLUDE: That Cold Day in the Park, M*A*S*H, McCabe and Mrs. Miller, Images, Brewster McCloud, Thieves Like Us (debut as exec. prod.), Drive-In (exec. prod.), Dressed To Kill (prod.). Blow Out (prod.).
TV: Hawaii Five-O.

LITVINOFF, SI: Producer. b. New York City, April 5, 1929. e. Adelphi College (A.B.); NYU School of Law (LLB). Theatrical

lawyer, personal and business manager in New York until 1967 when left firm of Barovick, Konecky & Litvinoff to produce plays and films.
PICTURES: The Queen, All the Right Noises, Walkabout, A Clockwork Orange (exec. prod.), Glastonbury Fayre (exec. in chg. prod.); The Man Who Fell to Earth (exec. prod.)
STAGE: Leonard Bernstein's Theatre Songs, Cry of the Raindrop, Girl of the Golden West, Little Malcolm and His Struggle Against the Eunuchs, I and Albert (London).

LIVINGSTON, JAY: Comp. & Lyric. b. McDonald, Pa., March 28, 1915; e. U. Pa., 1937, UCLA, 1964–65. Army, World War II. Accompanist and arranger for various NBC singers and singing groups 1940–42, N.Y.; author music and special material for Olsen & Johnson, including various editions of Hellzapoppin, and Sons O'Fun: began composing picture songs, 1944. Under contract to Paramount, 1945–55; then free lance. Composed songs for over 100 films. Writer of songs and special material for Bob Hope, 1965–present.
SONG HITS INCLUDE: G'bye Now, Stuff Like That There, To Each His Own, Golden Earrings, Silver Bells, Buttons and Bows (Acad. Award, 1949), Mona Lisa (Acad. Award, 1951), Que Sera Sera (Acad. Award, 1957), Tammy (Acad. nom.), Almost In Your Arms (Acad. nom.), Bonanza (TV Theme), Mister Ed (TV Theme), Dear Heart, (Acad. nom.), Wish Me a Rainbow, In the Arms of Love, Never Let Me Go, As I Love You, All the Time, Maybe September, Collab. music and lyrics for B'way show Oh Captain! 1958; Let It Ride, 1961. Two songs for Sugar Babies, 1980.
PICTURES INCLUDE: The Paleface, Fancy Pants, The Lemon-Drop Kid, Houseboat, Tammy and the Bachelor, The Man Who Knew Too Much, Dear Heart, Here Come the Groom, My Friend Irma, The Night of the Grizzly, This Property is Condemned, The Oscar, Never Too Late, Harlow, What Did You Do In The War Daddy?, Wait Until Dark, Red Garters, Sorrowful Jones.

LIVINGSTONE, PERCY: Executive. b. Leeds, England, 1913. e. City of Leeds School, School of Accountancy. Entered m.p. industry Aug. 1931 in clerical capacity with old Fox Company. Joined sales force 3 years later; appointed Dublin Branch Manager, 1939; attached to Head Office, 1945 southern district mgr., 1948; assistant sales mgr., 1951; sales mgr., 1956; dir. of sales, 1957; bd. member; gen. sales mgr. Warner-Pathe Dist., 1959; man. dir. 20th Century-Fox, 1961; 20th Cent.-Fox Inter'l, N.Y., 1967; sr., v.p., 20th-Fox Intl. Corp., 1975; Chrm. 20th-Fox Film Co. Ltd. 1977; Chrm., 20th-Fox Productions Ltd.

LLOYD, CHRISTOPHER: Actor. b. Connecticut. Studied at Neighborhood Playhouse, NY. Starred off-Bdwy. in Kaspar, winning Drama Desk and Obie Awards, 1973. Feature film debut in One Flew Over the Cuckoo's Nest, 1975.
PICTURES: Butch and Sundance: The Early Days, The Onion Field, The Black Marble, The Legend of the Lone Ranger, Mr. Mom, To Be or Not To Be, Star Trek III: The Search for Spock, Adventures of Buckaroo Bonzai, Back to the Future, Clue.

LLOYD, EUAN: Producer. b. Rugby (Warwick), Dec. 6, 1923. e. Rugby. Entered m.p. ind. in 1939 as theatre manager, then pub. dir.; dir. of Publ. Rank, 1946; joined Associated British-Pathe, Ltd. in same capacity; 1952 asst. to prod., Warwick Film Prod. Ltd. v.p. Highroad Productions, 1962–64. Rep. Europe Goldwyn's Porgy & Bess 1959.
PICTURES INCLUDE: April in Portugal, Heart of Variety, Invitation to Monte Carlo, The Secret Ways, Genghis Khan, Poppy Is Also A Flower, Murderer's Row, Shalako, Catlow, The Man Called Noon, Paper Tiger, The Wild Geese, The Sea Wolves, Who Dares Wins, Wild Geese II.

LLOYD, NORMAN: Producer. b. Jersey City, N.J., Nov. 8, 1914. e. N.Y.U., 1932. Acted on B'wy in: Noah, Liberty Jones, Everywhere I Roam, 1935–44; in various stock companies.
PICTURES INCLUDE: (actor) Spellbound, The Southerner, Green Years, Limelight. Prod. asst. on Arch of Triumph and The Red Pony, 1946. Assoc. prod. on The Alfred Hitchcock Show, 1957 (TV) and exec. prod. 1963. Also prod. of Up Above the World, Universal feature film; prod. of TV package deal, 2 hr. film.
STAGE: The Cocktail Party, The Lady's Not for Burning, Madame Will You Walk, The Golden Apple.

LO BIANCO, TONY: Actor. b. New York City. Oct. 19. Has performed on N.Y. stage as well as in films and TV. Won Obie Award for performance in Yanks 3, Detroit 0, Top of the Seventh. Also acted on stage in The Office, The Rose Tattoo, The Royal Hunt of the Sun, etc.
PICTURES INCLUDE: The French Connection, The Honeymoon Killers, F.I.S.T., Bloodbrothers, City Heat.
TELEVISION: Lady Blue, Marco Polo, Welcome Home Bobby, etc.

LOCKE, SONDRA: Actress. Debut in The Heart Is a Lonely Hunter (1968).
PICTURES: The Second Coming of Suzanne, Willard, A Reflection of Fear, The Outlaw—Josey Wales, The Gauntlet, Every Which Way But Loose, Bronco Billy, Any Which Way You Can, Sudden Impact.

LOCKHART, JUNE: Actress. b. New York City, June 25, 1925. p. Gene and Kathleen Lockhart. On TV in Lassie series.
PICTURES INCLUDE: All This and Heaven Too (1940, Warner Bros.), Sergeant York, Miss Annie Rooney (1942, United Artists), Meet Me in St. Louis, Son of Lassie, White Cliffs of Dover, Keep Your Powder Dry, Bury Me Dead, T-Men, It's a Joke, Son, Time Limit, Troll.

LOCKWOOD, GARY: Actor. b. Van Nuys, Calif., 1937. Began in Hollywood as stuntman.
PICTURES INCLUDE: Tall Story, Splendor in the Grass, Wild in the Country, The Magic Sword, It Happened at the World's Fair, Firecreek, 2001: A Space Odyssey, They Came to Rob Las Vegas, Model Shop, The Body, R.P.M., Stand Up and be Counted.

LOCKWOOD, ROGER: Executive. b. Middletown, Conn., June 7, 1936. e. Ohio Wesleyan Univ. Sports writer for Akron Beacon Journal, 1960–62. On executive staff of Lockwood & Gordon Theatres; exec. v.p. SBC Theatres, 1969–73. In 1974 asst. to exec. v.p., General Cinema Corp. In 1975 formed Lockwood/Friedman Theatres, buying-booking and exhibition organization. Pres., Theatre Owners of New England, 1971–72; pres., Young NATO 1965–67; bd. of dir. NATO, 1962–present; pres., Jimmy Fund, present; 1979–80, Variety Club of New England, pres. Director, Dana-Farber Cancer Institute, 1983–present.

LOEWE, FREDERICK: Composer. b. Vienna June 10, 1904. Studied piano at Stern Conservatory; at 13 was youngest solo pianist to appear with Berlin Symphony Orchestra. Came to U.S. in 1924; played organ at Keith Albee's, Brooklyn. Became partner with Alan Jan Lerner for series of stage musicals, many of them filmed.
PICTURES INCLUDE: Brigadoon, Paint Your Wagon, My Fair Lady, Gigi, Camelot, The Little Prince.

LOGAN, JOSHUA: Director, writer, producer. b. Texarkana, Tex., Oct. 5, 1908; e. Princeton U., Moscow Art Theatre.
STAGE: Camille, On Borrowed Time, I Married an Angel, Knickerbocker Holiday, Star in Your Eyes, Morning's at Seven, Charley's Aunt, By Jupiter, Happy Birthday, John Loves Mary, South Pacific, Mister Roberts, Wish You Were Here, Picnic, Fanny.
PICTURES INCLUDE: Garden of Allah, History is Made at Night, I Met My Love Again, Mister Roberts (collab.), Picnic, Fanny, Camelot, Paint Your Wagon.

LOLLOBRIGIDA, GINA: Actress. b. Subiaco, Italy, July 14, 1927. e. Acad. of Fine Arts, Rome, m.p. debut (Italy) in Love of a Clown.
PICTURES INCLUDE: The City Defends Itself, The White Line, Fanfan the Tulip, Times Gone By, Beat the Devil, Crossed Swords, The Great Game, Beauties of the Night, Wayward Wife, Bread Love and Dreams, Bread Love and Jealousy, Young Caruso, World's Most Beautiful Woman, Trapeze, Hunchback of Notre Dame, Solomon and Sheba, Never So Few, Go Naked in the World, Come September, Imperial Venus, Woman of Straw, That Splendid November, Hotel Paradisio, Buona Sera, Mrs. Campbell, Bambole, Plucked.
TELEVISION: Deceptions, Falcon Crest.

LOM, HERBERT: Actor. b. Prague, 1917. e. Prague U. Stage training London Embassy, Old Vic—Sadlers Wells and Westminster Schools. First British Picture 1941 (Mein Kampf—My Crimes); on TV, The Human Jungle Series.
PICTURES INCLUDE: Tomorrow We Live, Secret Mission, Young Mr. Pitt, Dark Tower, Cage of Gold, Whispering Smith vs. Scotland Yard, Two on the Tiles, Mr. Denning Drives North, Hell is Sold Out, Gaunt Stranger, Rough Shoot, The Net, The Love Lottery, Star of India, Beautiful Stranger, The Ladykillers, War and Peace Action, Fire Down Below, Hell's Drives, Chase a Crooked Shadow, Passport to Shame, Roots of Heaven, The Big Fisherman, North-West Frontier, I Aim at the Stars, Spartacus, Mysterious Island, Mr. Topaz, The Frightened City, El Cid, Tiara Tahiti, The Phantom of the Opera, Horse Without a Head, A Shot in the Dark, Uncle Tom's Cabin, Return From the Ashes, Gambit, The Assignment, Three Faces of Eve, Villa Rides, Doppelganger, Mr. Jericho, Dorian, Mark of the Devil, Count Dracula, Murders in the Rue Morgue, Dark Places, Death in Persepolis, Return of the Pink Panther, The Pink Panther Strikes Again, Charleston, Revenge of the Pink Panther, The Man with Bogarts' Face, Hopscotch, The Acts of Peter and Paul, The Trail of the Pink Panther, The Curse of the Pink Panther, Memed, My Hawk, Dead Zone, King Solomon's Mines, Whoops Apocalypse.

LOMBARDO, GOFFREDO: Executive. b. Naples, Italy, May 13, 1920. President Titanus Films.
PICTURES INCLUDE: Rocco and His Brothers, Sodom and Gomorrah, The Leopard, Four Days of Naples.

LOMITA, SOLOMON: Executive. b. New York City, April 23, 1937. Entire industry career with United Artists Corp. as follows: adm., intl. dept., 1962; asst., intl. sales, same year. 1963, asst. intl. print mgr.; 1965, intl., print mgr. In 1973 appt. dir. of film services. 1981, v.p., film services. In 1985 named exec. v.p., post-prod., Orion Pictures.

LONDON, BARRY: Executive. Joined Paramount Pictures 1971 in L.A. branch office as booker; later salesman. 1973, sls. mgr., Kansas City-St. Louis; 1974, branch mgr. Transferred to San Francisco, first as branch mgr.; later as district mgr. 1977, eastern div. mgr. in Washington, D.C. 1978–81, western div. mgr. In March, 1981, named v.p., gen. sls. mgr. June, 1983, advanced to sr. v.p., domestic distribution. 1984, named pres., domestic div., for Motion Picture Group of Paramount.

LONDON, JULIE: Singer-Actress. b. Santa Rosa, Calif., Sept. 26, 1926. r.n. Julie Peck. Launched as actress by agent Sue Carol (wife of Alan Ladd) who arranged screen test, followed by contract for 6 films. As singer has appeared in nightclubs and recorded.
PICTURES INCLUDE: The Red House, The Fat Man, The Great Man, Saddle the Wind, Man of the West, The Third Voice.
TELEVISION: Perry Como Show, Steve Allen Show, Ed Sullivan Show, Emergency (series).

LONDON, MILTON H.: Executive. b. Detroit, Mich., Jan. 12, 1916. e. U. of Mich. BA, 1937. Wayne U. Law School, 1938. U.S. Army 1943–46. Invented Ticograph system of positive admissions control for theatres, 1950; pres. Theatre Control Corp., 1950–62; secy-treas. Co-op. Theas. of Michigan Inc., 1956–63; exec. comm., Council of M.P. Organizations, 1957–66; dir. M.P. Investors, 1960–67; exec. dir. Allied States Assoc. of M.P. Exhib., 1961–66; exec. dir. National Assoc. of Theatre Owners, 1966–69 pres., NATO of Michigan, 1954–74; Mich. State Fire Safety Bd., Chief Barker, Variety Club of Detroit, Tent No. 5. 1975–76; Life Patron and Lifeliner, Variety Clubs International; trustee, Variety Club Charity for Children; chm., Variety Club Electronic Limb Research Center; dir., Motion Picture Pioneers; advisory comm., Will Rogers Institute; trustee, Detroit Institute for Children; pres., Metropolitan Adv. Co.; Intl. ambassador, Variety Clubs Int'l.

LONERGAN, ARTHUR: Art director. b. New York City, Jan. 23, 1906. e. Columbia U. Instructor in history of architecture, NYU; architect with N.Y. School of Decoration and Design; joined MGM as illustrator in art dept., 1938; freelance art dir., 1945; pres. Soc. of M.P. Art Dir., 1952–54; Acad. Award nomination, art. dir., The Oscar. 1975-The Georges Melies Award for outstanding cinematic achievement for art direction in Science Fiction category. Design consultant on Disney Theme Park, Japan.
TV: Loretta Young show, The Falcon, Mr. and Mrs. North, Topper, Life of Riley, Adventures of Hiram Holiday, Hitchcock Presents, GE Theatre, M. Squad, Restless Gun. etc.
PICTURES INCLUDE: Song in My Heart, Intrigue, Tender Years, Maneaters of Kumaon, Pitfall, Outpost in Morocco, Ride Vaquero, The Actress, It's Always Fair Weather, Tender Trap, Ransom, Forbidden Planet, On the Double, My Geisha, Who's Got the Action, Papa's Delicate Condition, A New Kind of Love, Who's Sleeping in My Bed, Robinson Caruso On Mars, Tickle Me, Red Line 7000, The Caper of the Golden Bull, Yours Mine and Ours, How Sweet It Is, Che, M*A*S*H, Plaza Suite.

LONG, ROBERT A.: Executive. b. McLune, KS, Oct. 31, 1931. e. Univ. Kansas (1957). Mng. partner, K.C., Arthur Anderson & Co., 1970–80; now exec. v.p., Commonwealth Theatres, Inc.
MEMBER: Past. pres., Civic Council of Greater Kansas City; past pres., Chamber of Commerce Greater Kansas City; Heart of America Council of Boy Scouts; United Way; bd. mbr., Rockhurst Coll., Univ. of Kansas, city trustess; Advertising Council, Univ. of Kansas, school of business & medicine; bd. trustees, Endowment Assoc. of Univ. of Kansas. Named Mr. Kansas City, 1981.

LONG, SHELLEY: Actress. b. Ft. Wayne, IN, Aug. 23, 1949. e. Northwestern Univ.
PICTURES: A Small Circle of Friends, Caveman, Night Shift, Losin' It, Irreconcilable Differences, The Money Pit, Outrageous Fortune.

LONGSTREET, STEPHEN: Writer. b. New York City, April 18, 1907; e. Rutgers U.; Parsons Coll.; Rand Sch., London, B.A. Humorist, cartoonist (New Yorker, Collier's, etc.) 1930–37; ed. Free World Theat., radio plays; ed. film critic, Saturday Review of Literature, 1940, U.S. at War, Time 1942–43; writer for screen from 1942. On staff U.C.L.A. Elected pres. Los Angeles Art Assoc. 1970. 1974: appointed Prof. English Dep. Univ. of So. Calif. Modern Writing Course.
WRITINGS: Decade, The Golden Touch, The Gay Sisters, Last Man Around the World, Chico Goes to the Wars, Pedlocks, Lion at Morning, Promoters, Boy in the Model T, Sometimes I Wonder, Wind at My Back, The Young Men of Paris, The Wilder Shore, War Cries on Horseback, Yoshiwara, Geishas and Courtesans, Canvas Falcons, Men and Planes of World War I, We All Went to Paris. New publications in 1973: Chicago 1860–1919, (show business & society), Divorcing (a novel); The General (novel, 1974), All Star Cast, 1977; The Queen Bees (1979), Our Father's House (1985).
STAGE: High Button Shoes.
PICTURES INCLUDE: The Gay Sisters, Golden Touch, Stallion Road, Jolson Story, Silver River, Helen Morgan Story, First Traveling Saleslady, Untamed Youth, Duel in the Sun, Greatest Show on Earth, Streets of Montmarte, The Crime, Uncle Harry, Rider on a Dead Horse, The Imposter.
TV: Casey Jones (series), Clipper Ship, Agent of Scotland Yard, m.c. author of The Sea, NBC; m.c. Press & Clergy, 1960–63; Viewpoint, CBS, 1963–65; series Boy in the Model T, Young Man From Boston, 1967, Blue and the Grey, Donald O'Connor Show, John J. Anthony talk shows, L.A. Guest; Art Linkletter Show, CBS Boutique, Writers Guild, Comm. of Public Relations. Film and Book critic for Readers' Syndicate since 1970. Professor performing arts dept. Univ. So. Calif. since 1973, where in 1979, presented 12 great silent films, The Art & Entertainment of Silent Films in the cinema section of the college Rutgers Univ., lecturer, 1986.

LONSDALE, PAMELA: Freelance Producer/director. Devised and was first producer of Rainbow for Thames T.V. Other programmes include: Ace of Wands, The Squad (also devised) Cranford, S.W.A.L.K., Marmalade Atkins, Spooky, Chocky and Mr. Stabs. Recently produced Exploits at West Poley, a film for the C.F.T.F. In 1975 won the British Academy Award for the best children's programme.

LOOS, MARY: Writer. b. San Diego, Calif. May 6, 1914. e. Stanford U., 1933. Actress m.p.; in public relations field N.Y. 1938; jewelry designer for Paul Flato; author of novel Return in the Vineyard, 1945. secy. Voyager Films, Inc., literary exec. M. J. Frankovich Prod. Novel: The Beggars Are Coming, Bantam Books, 1974, Belinda, 1976; The Barstow Legend, 1978; A Pride of Lovers, 1981.
PICTURES INCLUDE: Rose Marie, Maytime, Crusades, Cleopatra, Mr. Belvedere Goes to College, Mother Was a Freshman, Ticket to Tomahawk, When Willie Comes Marching Home, Father Was a Fullback, I'll Get By, Meet Me After the Show, Let's Do It Again, The French Line, Gentlemen Marry Brunettes, Over-Exposed, Woman's World.

LORD, JACK: Actor-writer-artist-director-producer. b. N.Y.C., Dec. 30, 1930. e. N.Y.U. (Chancellor Chase scholarship), B.S. Artist, represented in various museums including Metropolitan Museum of Art, Museum of Modern Art, Brooklyn Museum, in New York. Bibliotheque National, Paris; British Museum; Fogg Museum, Harvard University. St. Gandens Plaque for Fine Arts; creator of Tramp Ship, McAdoo, Yankee Trader, The Hunter TV series. On Bway in Traveling Lady (Theatre World Award), Cat on a Hot Tin Roof. Fame Award, new male star, 1963, mem. of Directors Guild of America. Recent Awards: G. Washington Honor Medal from Freedom Foundation at Valley Forge, 1984; Veterans Administration, Administrator's Award, 1980; Salute to Hospitalized Veterans, Tripler Army Medical Center, 1985; East-West Center Distinguished Service Award, 1981.
PICTURES INCLUDE: Court Martial of Billy Mitchell, Williamsburg Story, Tip On a Dead Jockey, God's Little Acre, Man of the West, The Hangman, True Story of Lynn Stuart, Walk Like a Dragon, Doctor No, Doomsday Flight, Ride to Hangman's Tree, Counterfeit Killer.
TV: Leads on all networks, including Omnibus Constitution series, Playhouse 90, Goodyear Playhouse, Studio One, U.S. Steel, etc. (Film shows incl.) Have Gun Will Travel (pilot), Untouchables, Naked City, Rawhide, Bonanza, The Americans, Route 66, Gunsmoke, Stagecoach West, Dr. Kildare, Greatest Show on Earth, Combat, Chrysler Theatre, 12 O'Clock High, The Loner, Laredo, The FBI, The Invaders, The Fugitive, The Virginian, Man from UNCLE, High Chaparral, Ironside, Star of Stoney Burke and Hawaii Five-O series. Director of Death with Father, How to Steal a Masterpiece; Honor Is An Unmarked Grave, The Bells Toll At Noon, Top of the World, Why Won't Linda Die, Who Says Cops Don't Cry episodes of Hawaii Five-O. Creator, director, and exec. Producer of M Station: Hawaii (2-hr film for TV), 1979. Pres., Lord and Lady Enterprises, Inc.

LORD, ROSEMARY: Actress—Writer. b. May 16, Taunton, Somerset, England. Now living in Hollywood.
PICTURES INCLUDE: Actress: The Whisperers, Dr. Jekyll & Sister Hyde, The Watchers, Touch of Class, Duchess and the Dirtwater Fox, Return from Witch Mountain, Frances.

LOREN, SOPHIA: Actress. b. Rome, Italy, Sept. 20, 1934. e. Naples. m.p. debut, 1952.
TELEVISION: 30-Minute Theatre, Softly, Softly, Rivals of Sherlock Holmes, Fantasy Island, Aurora (movie).
PICTURES INCLUDE: Africa Beneath the Seas, Village

of the Bells, Good People's Sunday, Neapolitan Carousel, Day in the District Court, Pilgrim of Love, Aida, Two Nights with Cleopatra, Our Times, Attila, Scourge of God, Too Bad She's Bad, Pride and the Passion, Gold of Naples, Boy on a Dolphin, Scandal in Lorrinto, Miller's Beautiful Wife, Desire Under the Elms, Houseboat, The Black Ordeal, That Kind of Woman, Heller With a Gun, Anatomy of Love, Breath of Scandal, Heller in Pink Tights, Bay of Naples, Two Women, El Cid, Boccaccio 70, Il Coltello nello Piaga, French, The Fall of the Roman Empire, The Great Spy Mission, Lady L, Marriage Italian Style, Judith, Arabesque, The Countess from Hong Kong, Happily Ever After, More than a Miracle, Ghosts—Italian Style, Sunflower, The Priest's Wife, Lady LIberty, White Sister, Man of La Mancha, The Voyage, The Verdict, The Cassandra Crossing, A Special Day, Angela, Brass Target, Firepower.

LOUIS, JEAN: Designer. b. Paris, France, Oct. 5, 1907. Head designer, Hattie Carnegie, 7 yrs., before accepting post as Chief Designer Columbia Pictures. Later Universal Studios. Free lance in m.p. & TV. Pres. Jean-Louis, Inc.

LOUISE, TINA: Actress. b. New York City, 1934. e. Miami U., N.Y. Neighborhood Playhouse, Actors Studio, B'way.
STAGE: Two's Company, The Fifth Season, Almanac, Li'l Abner.
PICTURES INCLUDE: God's Little Acre, For Those Who Think Young, The Wrecking Crew, How to Commit Marriage, The Happy Ending, The Stepford Wives.
TV: Gilligan's Island, Mannix, Ironside, Kung Fu, Police Story, Kojak.

LOWE, PHILIP L.: Executive. b. Brookline, Mass. Apr. 17, 1917. e. Harvard. Army 1943–46. Checker, Loew's 1937–39; treasurer, Theatre Candy Co., 1941–58; Pres., ITT Sheraton Corp., 1969–70; pres., Philip L. Lowe and Assoc.

LOWE, PHILIP M.: Executive. b. 1944. e. Deerfield Academy, Harvard College (cum laude in psychology, 1966); Columbia Business School (1968). Work experience includes major marketing positions at General Foods, Gillette, Gray Advertising, and Estee Lauder Cosmetics before co-founding Cinema Centers Corp. and Theatre Management Services in Boston. Pres. of Lowe Group of Companies (cable television, broadcasting, hotels, real estate and management consulting). Past pres. and chm. of the bd; National Association of Concessionaires (NAC); past director, National Association of Theater Owners (NATO). Past professor of marketing, Bentley College, Waltham, MA.; Contributing Editor; The Movie Business Book, Prentice-Hall, Inc. 1983.

LOWE, ROB: Actor. b. Virginia, 1964.
PICTURES: The Outsiders, Class, The Hotel New Hampshire, Oxford Blues, St. Elmo's Fire, Youngblood, Square Dance.
TELEVISION: Schoolboy Father, A Matter of Time, Thursday's Child.

LOWRY, HUNT: Producer. b. Oklahoma City, Aug. 21, 1954. e. Rollins College, Wake Forest. Abandoned plans to study medicine to enter film-making industry; first job for New World Pictures where he met Jon Davison, with whom was later to co-produce. Next made TV commercials as prod. asst. and then producer. Left to go freelance as commercials producer. 1980, appt. assoc. prod. to Davison on Airplane!
PICTURES: Humanoids from the Deep, Top Secret!, Get Crazy.
TELEVISION: Rascals and Robbers: The Secret Adventures of Tom Sawyer and Huckleberry Finn.

LOY, MYRNA: Actress. r.n. Myrna Williams; b. Helena Mont., Aug. 2, 1905; e. Westlake Sch. for Girls. Appeared in stage presentations, Grauman's Chinese theatre, then Hollywood. On screen in What Price Beauty, 1925; thereafter in many pictures, variously starred, co-starred & featured. Voted one of the ten best Money Making Stars in Motion Picture Herald-Fame Poll, 1937, 38.
STAGE: Marriage-Go-Round, There Must Be A Pony, Good Housekeeping, Barefoot in the Park, Dear Love, The Women, Don Juan in Hell, Relatively Speaking.
PICTURES INCLUDE: Last of the Duanes, Transatlantic, Arrowsmith, Vanity Fair, Animal Kingdom, The Prizefighter and the Lady, The Thin Man, Evelyn Prentice, Wife Versus Secretary, After the Thin Man, Test Pilot, The Rains Came, Another Thin Man, Third Finger, Left Hand; Shadow of the Thin Man, The Thin Man Goes Home, Best Years of Our Lives, Mr. Blanding Builds His Dream House, Red Pony, If This Be Sin, Cheaper by the Dozen, Belles on Their Toes, Ambassador's Daughter, Lonely Hearts, From the Terrace, Midnight Lace, The April Fools, Airport 1975, The End, Just Tell Me What You Want.
TV: Meet Me in St. Louis, Minerva, George Gobel, Perry Como, Happy Birthday—June Allyson Show, Family Affair, The Virginians, Do Not Spindle or Mutilate, Death Takes a Holiday, The Couple Takes a Wife, Ironside, The Elevator, It Happened at Lakewood Manor, Summer Solstice.

LUBCKE, HARRY R.: Registered Patent Agent. b. Alameda, Calif., Aug. 25, 1905. e. U. of Calif. 1929. B.S. Holds numerous U.S. and foreign patents on television. In 1931: station W6XAO went on air on what is now television Channel No. 2 to become first station of kind in nation. New Mt. Lee studios built at cost of $250,000 in 1941, housing then largest TV stage 100x60x30 ft. Pioneered present television standard of 525 line (Aug., 1940). In 1942, television programs to promote war bonds sale. 1942–46 dir. war research for which certificates of commendation were received from Army & Navy.
MEMBER: Pres., Acad. TV Arts & Sciences, 1949. Dir. TV Don Lee Broadcasting System to Dec. 31, 1950; cons. TV engineer, 1951; registered patent agent, 1952. Life Fellow, 1951, IEEE, AAAS, SMPTE, 1967. Board of Governors, Patent Law Association of Los Angeles, 1974. Life Member National Academy of Television Arts & Sciences, member engineering Emmy Awards Committee. Member Blue Ribbon panel Emmy Awards Committee; 1978; Diamond Circle, of Pacific Pioneer Broadcasters, 1980; American Bar Assn., 1982.

LUBIN, ARTHUR: Director. b. Los Angeles, Calif. Since 1935 has directed numerous pictures, including John Wayne's first four films at Universal: Hell on Ice, California Straight Ahead, Adventure's End, I Covered the War.
PICTURES INCLUDE: Buck Privates in the Navy, Hold That Ghost, Keep 'Em Flying, Ride 'Em Cowboy, Eagle Squadron, Phantom of the Opera, White Savage, Ali Baba and the Forty Thieves, Delightfully Dangerous, Francis, Queen for a Day, Francis Goes to the Races, Rhubarb, Francis Covers the Big Town, Francis Goes to West Point, It Grows on Trees, South Sea Woman, Star of India, Lady Godiva, Francis in the Navy, Footsteps in the Fog, First Traveling Saleslady, Escapade in Japan, The Thief of Baghdad, The Incredible Mr. Limpett, Rain for a Dusty Summer, Night in Paradise, The Spider Woman Strikes Back, New Orleans, Impact, Queen for a Day, Star of India, Hold On!
TV: Maverick (Henry Fonda episodes), 77 Sunset Strip, Bonanza, the entire Mister Ed series (prod.-dir.).

LUCAS, GEORGE: Producer-Director-Writer. b. Modesto, CA, 1945. e. USC (cinema). Made short film called THX and won National Student Film Festival Grand Prize, 1967. Signed contract with WB. Ass't. to Francis Ford Coppola on The Rain People, during which Lucas made 2-hr. documentary on filming of that feature. Debut as director with THX 1138 for WB.
PICTURES INCLUDE: THX 1138 (dir., co-s.p.), American Graffiti (dir., co-s.p.), Star Wars (dir., s.p.); More American Graffiti (exec. prod.); The Empire Strikes Back (exec. prod.); Raiders of the Lost Ark (exec. prod.); Return of the Jedi (exec. prod.); Indiana Jones and the Temple of Doom (exec. prod.); Labyrinth (exec. prod.); Howard the Duck (exec. prod.).

LUCKINBILL, LAURENCE: Actor. b. Fort Smith, AZ, Nov. 21, 1934. e. Univ. of Arizona, Catholic Univ. of America. On Bdwy. in A Man for All Seasons, Arms and the Man, The Boys in the Band, Alpha Beta, The Shadow Box, etc.
PICTURES: The Boys in the Band, Such Good Friends, The Money, The Promise, Not for Publication.
TELEVISION: Movies: The Delphi Bureau, Death Sentence, Panic on the 5:22, Winner Take All, The Lindbergh Kidnapping Case, Ike.

LUDWIG, IRVING H.: Executive. b. Nov. 3. Rivoli Theatre, N.Y., mgr., theatre oper., Rugoff and Becker, 1938–39; opened first modern art type theatre, Greenwich Village, 1940. With Walt Disney Prod. in charge of theatre oper. on Fantasia, 1940–41; buyer-booker, Rugoff and Becker, 1942–45; film sales admin., Walt Disney Prod. home office, 1945–53; v.p. and domestic sales mgr., Buena Vista Dist. Co., 1953; pres. gen. sales mgr., 1959–80. Now exec. v.p., Exhibitor Relations Co.
MEMBER: Bd. of dir., Will Rogers Memorial Fund, Foundation of M.P. Pioneers; M.P. Bookers of NY; Academy of M.P. Arts & Sciences.

LUFKIN, DAN W.: Executive. Chairman of Exec. Comm., Columbia Pictures Industries (appt. July, 1978). Co-founder of Donaldson, Lufkin & Jenrette Securities Corp., investment banking and brokerage firm. Served as first commissioner of Dept. of Environmental Protection for State of Connecticut. Joined Columbia board in November, 1977.

LUKE, KEYE: Actor, artist. b. Canton, China, 1904. e. Franklin High Sch., Seattle; Formerly artist for Fox West Coast Theats. & RKO Studios; also technical advisor on Chinese films. Screen debut as actor in Painted Veil, 1935.
STAGE: Flower Drum Song (3 yr).
PICTURES INCLUDE: Charlie Chan series, Oil for the Lamps of China, King of Burlesque, The Good Earth, International Settlement, Sued for Libel, Disputed Passage, Dragon Seed, Three Men in White, Between Two Women, First Yank in Tokyo, Tokyo Rose, Sleep My Love, Hell's

Half Acre, World for Ransom, Bamboo Prison, Love is a Many Splendored Thing, 80 Days Around the World, Their Greatest Glory, Battle Hell, Fair Winds to Java, Nobody's Perfect, Project X, The Chairman, The Hawaiians, Noon Sunday, Won Ton Ton, Amsterdam Kill, Just You and Me, Kid, They Call Me Bruce, Gremlins, A Fine Mess.

TV: Gunsmoke, Danger, December Bride, Crusader, Wireservice, Crossroads, Soldiers of Fortune, My Little Margie, Annie Oakley, Ray Milland Show, Medic, Citizen Chang, Climax, Jerry Jewis, Trackdown, Perry Mason Show, The Littlest Hobo, This Is the Life, Smothers Bros., I Spy, FBI, Wackiest Ship in Army, Mickey Rooney Show, Johnny Quest, Kentucky Jones, Never Too Young, Bob Hope Chrysler Show, Family Affair, Big Valley, Dragnet, It Takes a Thief, Star-Trek, Adventures of Huck Finn, The Outsider, Scooby Doo, Paris 7000, Johnny Carson Show, Marcus Welby, M.D., Adam 12, Hawaii 5-O, Dinah Shore Show, The Lucy Show, Anna and the King of Siam, Kung Fu, Amazing Chan and Chan Clan, Follow The Sun, Target, The Corrupters, Fair Exchange, Cannon, Cat Creature, Love American Style, Judgment—trial of Yamashita, Judge Dee, Khan, Harry O, MASH, Quincy, How the West Was Won, Meeting of Minds, Vegas, Battle of the Planets, The Yee Family, Might Man and Yukk, Rickety Racket, Tang Face, Charlie's Angels, Reach for the Sun, Fly Away Home, Brothers, Adventures of Goldie Gold, Spider Man, Unit Four, Remington Steele, Magnum P.I., Falcon Crest, Voyagers, The A- Team, Mike Hammer, Cocaine and Blue Eyes, Miami Vice, Street Hawk, Trapper John, Blade in Hong Kong, Mr. T, Night Court, Mac Gyver, T. J. Hooker, Crazy Like a Fox, Kung Fu.

LUKE, PETER: Playwright director. Author of plays for TV: Small Fish Are Sweet, 1958; Pigs Ear with Flowers, 1960; Roll on Bloomin' Death, 1961; A Man on Her Back (with William Sansom), 1965; Devil a Monk Won't Be, 1966. wrote and directed films for BBC-TV: Anach 'Cuan (about the late Sean O Riada) 1967; Black Sound—Deep Song (About Federico Garcia Lorca) 1968; Author of Stage play, Hadrian VII, first produced at Birmingham rep in 1967 and at time of going to press has been playing in one part of the world or another ever since. Stage Play, Bloomsbury. Author of autobiography, Sisyphus & Reilly, publ., 1972, Prod. Phoenix Theatre 1974.

LUMET, SIDNEY: Director. b. Philadelphia, Pa., June 15, 1924. e. Professional Children's Sch.; Columbia U. Child actor in plays: Dead End, George Washington Slept Here, My Heart's in the Highlands. U.S. Armed Forces, WW II, 1942–46; dir. summer stock, 1947–49; taught acting, H.S. of Prof. Arts. Assoc. dir. CBS, 1950, dir. 1951.

TV: Mama, Danger, You Are There, Omnibus, Best of Broadway, Alcoa, Goodyear Playhouse.

PICTURES INCLUDE: 12 Angry Men, Stage Struck, That Kind of Woman, Fugitive Kind, A View From the Bridge, Long Day's Journey into Night, Fail Safe, The Pawnbroker, The Hill, The Group, The Deadly Affair, Bye Bye Braverman, The Sea Gull, The Appointment, Last of the Mobile Hot-Shots, The Anderson Tapes, Child's Play, The Offence, Lovin' Molly, Serpico, Murder on the Orient Express, Dog Day Afternoon, Network, Equus, The Wiz, Just Tell Me What You Want, Prince of the City, Deathtrap, The Verdict, Daniel, Garbo Talks, Power, The Morning After.

LUPINO, IDA: Actress-director. b. London, England, Feb. 4, 1918. e. Royal Academy of Dramatic Art, London. Daughter of Stanley Lupino, English stage and screen comedian. Brit. m.p. debut in "Her First Affair," 1932; in U.S. m.p. 1934; ent. independent prod., variously dir., prod. collab. s.p. and acting.

PICTURES INCLUDE: Money for Speed, High Finance, High Sierra, Ladies in Retirement, Moontide, Hard Way, Devotion, Man I Love, Escape Me Never, Deep Valley, Road House, Lust for Gold, Not Wanted, Never Fear, Outrage, Hard Fast & Beautiful, On Dangerous Ground, Beware My Lovely, The Hitch-Hiker, Jennifer, The Bigamist, Private Hell 36, Women's Prison, Big Knife, While the City Sleeps, Trouble With Angels, Junior Bonner, The Devil's Rain, The Food of the Gods.

TV: Mr. Adams and Eve. No. 5 Checked Out, The Trial of Mary Surrat, Honey West, Virginian, I Love a Mystery, Sam Benedict, Untouchables, G. E. Theater, Have Gun Will Travel, Thriller, Mr. Novac, Hong Kong, The Rogues, Chrysler Theatre, Kraft Theatre, Gilligan's Island, The Ghost and Mrs. Muir, The Bill Cosby Show, To Catch a Thief, Mod Squad, Family Affair.

LURASCHI, LUIGI G.: Exec. b. London, Jan 7, 1906. e. U. of Zurich. Long Island Studio, Paramount, 1929; home officer mgr. For. dept. hd, For. & dom. Censorship; Hollywood to 1960. Asst. Prod., Dino De Laurentiis Prod. 1960–65; asst. to pres. for prod. activities, Paramount, 1965. 1967 continental prod. exec. Paramount-Rome. Now v.p., intl.

LYDON, JAMES: Actor. b. Harrington Park, N.J., May 30, 1923; e. St. Johns Mil. Sch. On NY stage in Prologue to Glory, Sing Out the News. On screen 1939, Back Door to Heaven.

PICTURES INCLUDE: Thoroughbreds, Naval Academy, Henry Aldrich series, Twice Blessed, Life With Father, Out of the Storm, Joan of Arc, Miss Mink of 1949, Tucson, Gasoline Alley, Island in the Sky, The Desperado, Battle Stations, My Blood Runs Cold (assoc. prod.), Brainstorm, An American Dream, A Covenant With Death, First to Fight, The Cool Ones, Chubasco, Countdown, Assignment to Kill, The Learning Tree, Scandalous John.

TV: Frontier Circus (assoc. prod.), Wagon Train, Alfred Hitchcock hour, McHale's Navy, 77 Sunset Strip, Mr. Roberts.

LYLES, A. C.: Producer. b. Jacksonville, Florida. May 17. e. Andrew Jackson High School; Paramount Publix's Florida Theatre, 1928; interviewed Hollywood celebrities, Jacksonville Journal, 1932; mail boy, Paramount Studios, Hollywood, 1937; publicity dept., 1938; hd. of adv., publ. dept., Pine-Thomas unit at Paramount, 1940; assoc. prod., The Mountain; prod., Short Cut to Hell; assoc. prod., Rawhide. President, A. C. Lyles Productions, Inc. (Paramount Pictures).

PICTURES INCLUDE: Raymie, The Young and the Brave, Law of the Lawless, Stage to Thunder Rock, Young Fury, Black Spurs, Hostile Guns, Arizona Bushwackers, Town Tamer, Apache Uprising, Johnny Reno, Waco, Red Tomahawk, Fort Utah, Buckskin, Rogue's Gallery, Night of the Lepus, The Last Day.

LYNCH, DAVID: Director-Writer. b. Montana, 1947. e. Pa. Academy of Fine Arts, where received an independent filmmaker grant from America Film Institute. Made 16mm film, The Grandmother. Accepted by Center for Advanced Film Studies in Los Angeles, 1970. Wrote and directed Eraserhead (with partial AFI financing) which became cult movie. Co-wrote and directed The Elephant Man (1980). 1984: Dune. 1986: Blue Velvet (s.p., dir.).

LYNCH, RICHARD: Actor. b. Apr. 29, 1936. Made Bdwy. debut in The Devils, latter both on and off Bdwy in The Balcony, Lion in Winter, etc. Film debut in Scarecrow (1973).

PICTURES: The Premonition, Steel, The Formula, The Delta Fox, Savage Dawn, Cut and Run.

TELEVISION: Vampire.

LYNDON, VICTOR: Producer-writer. b. London. Ent. m.p. ind. as asst. dir., Gainsborough Pictures, 1946–56; prod. mgr., 26 feature pictures; since 1957 prod., assoc. prod., pictures for Columbia, United Artists, M-G-M, Paramount, British Lion. 1984: novel, Bermuda Blue.

PICTURES INCLUDE: as prod. mgr. The African Queen, Albert R.N., The Admirable Crichton, As assoc. prod., Dr. Strangelove, Darling, 2001 A Space Odyssey. As prod., Spare The Rod, Station Six—Sahara, The Optimists.

LYNLEY, CAROL: Actress. b. New York City, Feb. 13, 1942.

PICTURES: The Light in the Forest, Holiday for Lovers, Blue Denim, Return to Peyton Place, The Last Sunset, The STripper, The Cardinal, The Pleasure Seekers, Bunny Lake Is Missing, The Maltes Bippy, Norwood, The Poseidon Adventure, Harlow, The Cat and the Canary, The Shape of Things to Come.

TELEVISION: Movies: Shadow on the Land, The Smugglers, The Immortal, Weekend of Terror, The Cable Car Murder, The Night Stalker, The Elevator, Death Stalk, Flood, Fantasy Island, Having Babies II, Cops and Robin, The Beasts Are on the Streets.

LYNN, ANN: Actress. b. London, England. Ent. films and TV, 1958.

PICTURES INCLUDE: Naked Fury, Piccadilly Third Stop, The Wind of Change, TV film series: The Cheaters, The Other Side of the Underneath.

TV: After The Show, All Summer Long, Trump Card, Man at the Top, The Expert, Hine, The Intruders, Too Far, King Lear, The Zoo Gang. Recent films incl: The Uncle, Morning Tide, Shot In The Dark, Black Torment, Four In The Morning, Baby Love, Hitler—The Last Ten Days, Estuary, Who Pays The Ferryman, The Professionals, Zeticula, Westway. The Perfect House, Minder, To the Sound of Guns, Crown Court.

LYNN, JEFFREY: Actor. b. Auburn, Mass., 1909: e. Bates Coll. m.p. debut in 1938.

PICTURES INCLUDE: Four Daughters, Yes My Darling Daughter, Daughters Courageous, Espionage Agent, Roaring Twenties, Four Wives, Child Is Born, Fighting 69th, It all Came True, All This and Heaven, Too; My Love Came Back, Four Mothers, Million Dollar Baby, Law of the Tropics, Body Disappears, For the Love of Mary, Black Bart, Letter to Three Wives, Strange Bargain, Home Town Story, Up Front, Captain China, Lost Lagoon, Tony Rome.

BROADWAY: (Revival) Dinner at Eight.

LYNN, ROBERT: Director, producer. 100 TV films. Assoc. prod. for Mid-Atlantic Films. 1970 prod. The Railway Children.

TV: Space 1999.

PICTURES INCLUDE: Dr. Crippen, Postman's Knock,

Victim 5, Mozambique, Coast of Skeletons, Carnival of Killers, 2nd unit dir., Superman.

LYON, EARLE: Producer, Executive. b. Waterloo, Ia., April 9, 1923. e. UCLA. Entered m.p. industry 1947. Independent prod. 1954–55 and 1958–59; 20th Century-Fox prod., 1956–57; at Columbia, 1959–60; Universal, 1960–63; developed new TV projects with Bob Banner Assoc., 1963; v.p. and gen. mgr. United Pictures Corp.
PICTURES INCLUDE: Silent Raiders, The Lonesome Trail, The Silver Star, Stagecoach Fury, The Quiet Gun, The Rawhide Trail, The Rebel Set, The Destructors, Cyborg 2087, Dimension 5, Destination Inner Space, Haunting at Castle Montego, The Ten Billion Dollar Caper, Panic in the City. TV: Tales of Wells Fargo.

LYON, FRANCIS D. "PETE": Director. b. Bowbells, N.D., July 29. e. Hollywood H.S., Univ. of Calif. at L.A.; writer, prod., dir., OWI, W.W. II; assoc. with training, exploitation and information films. Maj. U.S. Army Signal Corps.
PICTURES INCLUDE: Shape of Things to Come, Knight Without Armour, Rembrandt, Intermezzo, Adam Had Four Sons, The Great Profile, Four Sons, Daytime Wife, Body and Soul, He Ran All the Way, Crazylegs, The Bob Mathias Story, Walt Disney's The Great Locomotive Chase, The Oklahoman, Gunsight Ridge, Bailout at 43,000, Escort West, Cinerama South Seas Adventure, The Young and The Brave, Destination Inner Space, The Destructors, The Money Jungle, The Girl Who Knew Too Much, Tiger By the Tail.
TV: Laramie, Perry Mason, Zane Grey Theatre, Bus Stop, M. Squad, Wells Fargo, Draft Suspense Theatre, etc.

LYON, SUE: Actress. b. Davenport, Iowa, July 10, 1946. e. Hollywood Prof. School.
PICTURES INCLUDE: Lolita, Seven Women, Night of the Iguana, The Flim Flam Man, Evel Knievel, Crash, End of the World, Astral Factor.

LYONS, RICHARD E.: Producer. b. Boston, Mass.; e. Titlon Jr. Coll. & Dartmouth College. Eastern sls. dept., MGM Pictures, 1933–41: Field Photographic Br., U.S. Navy, 1941–46; eastern artist, repertoire exec., MGM Records, 1946–55; story ed., Edward Small Prod., 1955–56; assoc. story ed., Univ., 1956–57; staff prod., MGM Studios, 1960.
PICTURES INCLUDE: Frontier Gun, The Sad Horse, The Miracle of the Hills, Ride The High Country, Mail Order Bride, The Rounders, The Plainsman, Winchester 73, Stranger on the Run, Something for a Lonely Man, Coogan's Bluff, Death of a Gunfighter, Dirty Dingus Magee.
TV: The Daughters of Joshua Cabe, The Jerico Mile (ABC-TV), Shootout in A One Dog Town (ABC-TV movie of the week, 1973). The Daughters of Joshua Cabe Return (ABC-TV M.O.W.); Welcome to Xanadu. (ABC-TV M.O.W.), Kate Bliss and the Ticker Tape Kid (ABC-TV M.O.W.); Roughnecks (4 hr. mini series), Metromedia Prod. I Married Wyatt Earp (NBC-TV M.O.W.).

LYONS, STUART: Producer. b. Manchester, England, 1928. e. Manchester University. Ent. m.p. ind. 1955. Asst. dir. TV series 1955–56. Casting dir. Associated British, 1956/60. Freelance cast. dir., 1960/63. Joined 20th Century-Fox Productions as cast. dir., 1963. Appt. director 20th Century-Fox Productions Ltd., 1967, man. dir. 1968. 1971: left Fox on closure Europe prod. Joined Hemdale Group as head of production, May, 1972. Left Hemdale Aug. 1973 to resume indep. prod.
PICTURES INCLUDE: As casting director: Over thirty films including Those Magnificent Men in Their Flying Machines, Cleopatra, The Long Ships, Guns at Batasi, High Wind in Jamaica, Rapture, The Blue Max. As indep. producer: The Slipper & The Rose, Meetings with Remarkable Men, Danses Sacrees, Turnaround. As prod. consultant, Eleni.

M

MAC ARTHUR JAMES: Actor. b. Los Angeles, Calif., Dec. 8, 1937; e. Harvard. p. Helen Hayes, Charles MacArthur. Stage debut, summer stock; The Corn Is Green, 1945; Life With Father, 1953.
PICTURES INCLUDE: The Young Stranger, The Light in the Forest, The Third Man on the Mountain, Kidnapped, Swiss Family Robinson, The Interns, Spencer's Mountain, The Love-Ins, Cry of Battle, Angry Breed.
TV: Strike a Blow, Hawaii Five-O.

MACCHIO, RALPH: Actor. b. Long Island, NY. Started with TV commercials; first theatrical film role in Up the Academy (1980).
TELEVISION: Eight is Enough (regular); Movies: Journey to Survival, Dangerous Company.
PICTURES: Up the Academy, The Karate Kid, Teachers, Crossroads, The Karate Kid: Part II.

MacCORKINDALE, SIMON: Actor. b. England, Feb. 2, 1953. Husband of actress Susan George. On stage in Dark Lady of the Sonnets, Pygmalion, French without Tears, etc.
PICTURES: Death on the Nile, Riddle of the Sands, Quatermass Conclusion, Caboblanco, The Sword and the Sorcerer, Jaws 3-D, etc.
TELEVISION: I Claudius, Romeo and Juliet, Jesus of Nazareth, Obsessive Love. Regular on Falcon Crest.

MAC DONALD, PHILIP: Writer. b. Scotland; e. St. Paul's School, London. Novelist, playwright. Began screen career 1933.
PICTURES INCLUDE: Sahara, Action in Arabia, The Body Snatcher, Strangers in the Night, Dangerous Intruder, Man Who Cheated Himself, Circle of Danger, Mask of the Avenger, Ring of Fear, Tobor the Great.

MAC GRAW, ALI: Actress. b. Pound Ridge, NY, 1938. Was top fashion model.
PICTURES INCLUDE: Goodbye Columbus, Love Story, The Getaway, Convoy Players, Just Tell Me What You Want.
TELEVISION: The Winds of War, China Rose.

MACKERRAS, SIR (ALAN) CHARLES (MACLAURIN): Kt 1979; CBE 1974; Chief Conductor, Sydney Symphony Orchestra, Australian Broadcasting Commission, from 1982–85; frequent Guest Conductor, Vienna State Opera, Geneva and Zurich Opera, Royal Opera House Covent Garden, English National Opera, San Francisco Opera; b. Nov. 17, 1925; s of late Alan Patrick and Catherine Mackerras, Sydney, Australia; m. 1947, Helena Judith (Née Wilkins); two d. Educ: Sydney Grammar Sch. Principal Oboist, Sydney Symphony Orchestra, 1943–46; Staff Conductor, Sadler's Wells Opera, 1949–53; Principal Conductor BBC Concert Orchestra, 1954–56; freelance Conductor with most British and many continental orchestras, concert tours USSR, S. Africa, N. America, 1957–66; Conductor, Hamburg State Opera, 1966–69; Musical Dir. Sadler's Wells Opera, later ENO, 1970–77; Chief Guest Conductor, BBC SO, 1976–79; frequent radio and TV broadcasts; many commercial recordings, notably Handel series for DGG and Janáček operas for Decca; appearances at many internat. festivals and opera houses. Evening Standard Award for Opera, 1977; Janáček Medal, 1978; Gramophone Record of the Year Award, 1978, 1980 and 1983. Grammy Award for best opera recording 1981 The House of the Dead by Janáček. Prix Fondation Jacques Ibert and the Stereo Review's Records of the Year Award 1983 and 1985 for Cunning Little Vixen by Janáček Publications: ballet arrangements of Pineapple Poll and of Lady and the Fool; articles in Opera Magazine, Music and Musicians and other musical jls. Recreations: languages, yachting. Musical dir., Welsh National Opera, from 1987.

MAC LAINE, SHIRLEY: Actress. b. Richmond, Va., April 24, 1934; e. Washington and Lee H.S., Arlington, Va. Dancer, singer; signed by Hal Wallis; m.p. debut in Trouble with Harry. Producer of film documentary on China, The Other Half of The Sky, Author of 2 best-selling books: Don't Fall off the Mountain and You Can Get There from Here.
PICTURES INCLUDE: Artists and Models, Around the World in 80 Days, The Matchmaker, Some Came Running, Ask Any Girl, Career, Can-Can, The Apartment, All in a Night's Work, Two Loves, My Geisha, The Children's Hour, Two for the Seesaw, Irma La Duce, What A Way To Go, John Goldfarb Please Come Home, The Yellow Rolls Royce, Gambit, Woman Times Seven, Sweet Charity, Two Mules for Sister Sara, Desperate Characters, The Possession of Joel Delaney, The Turning Point, Being There, Loving Couples, Change of Seasons, Terms of Endearment, Cannonball Run II.
TV: Shirley's World, Specials.
AUTHOR: Don't Fall off the Mountain, You Can Get There from Here, Out on a Limb, Dancing in the Light.

MACLEOD, GAVIN: Actor. b. Mt. Kiseo, NY, Feb. 28, 1931. e. Ithica Coll.
PICTURES: I Want to Live, Compulsion, Operation Petticoat, McHale's Navy, The Sand Pebbles, Deathwatch, The Party, Kelly's Heroes.
TELEVISION: Hogan's Heroes, Mary Tyler Moore Show, The Love Boat. Movies: The Intruders, Only with Married Men, Ransom for Alice, Murder Can Hurt You, Scruples.

MAC MAHON, ALINE: Actress. b. McKeesport, Pa., May 3, 1899; e. Erasmus Hall, Barnard College Stage experience; Once in a Lifetime, Candida, others. Screen debut 1931 in Five Star Final.
PICTURES INCLUDE: The Mouthpiece, One Way Passage, Gold Diggers of 1933, World Changes, Babbitt, Side Streets, Mighty McGurk, Search, Roseanna McCoy, Flame and the Arrow, Eddie Cantor Story, Man From Laramie, All the Way Home.

MAC MURRAY, FRED: Actor. b. Kankakee, Ill., Aug. 30, 1908; e. Carroll College, Wis. Sang and played in orchestra to earn tuition. To Hollywood with band; extra roles on screen;

to N.Y. with comedy stage band, then joined "Three's a Crowd" revue; vaudeville circuits, night clubs. Began screen career 1935.

PICTURES INCLUDE: Grand Old Girl, Beyond Suspicion, Murder He Says, Double Indemnity, Oregon Trail, The Absent Minded Professor, The Happiest Millionaire, Follow Me Boys, Charlie and the Angel, Car 99, Gilded Lily, Hands Across the Table, Bride Comes Home, Alice Adams, Trail of the Lonesome Pine, Maid of Salem, Exclusive, True Confession, Men with Wings, Coconut Grove, Sing You Sinners, Cafe Society, Invitation to Happiness, Honeymoon in Bali, Smoky, Pardon My Past, Suddenly It's Spring, Egg and I, Singapore, A Miracle Can Happen, Miracle of the Bells, Don't Trust Your Husband, Family Honeymoon, Never a Dull Moment, Callaway Went Thataway, Millionaire for Christy, Fair Wind to Java, The Moonlighter, Caine Mutiny, Pushover, Woman's World, Far Horizons, There's Always Tomorrow, At Gunpoint, Rains of Rachipur, Gun For a Coward, Quantez, Good Day for a Hanging, The Shaggy Dog, Face of a Fugitive, The Oregon Trail, Bon Voyage, Son of Flubber, Kisses For My President, The Swarm.

TV: My Three Sons (12 years).

MACNAUGHTON, ROBERT: Actor. b. New York City, Dec. 19, 1966. Entered entertainment industry in 1979. Member Circle Rep. Co., N.Y.

TELEVISION: Angel City, Big Bend Country, The Electric Grandmother.

PICTURE: E.T.: The Extra-Terrestrial, I Am the Cheese.

STAGE: Critic's Choice, Thousand Clowns, Camelot, The Diviners, The Adventures of Huckleberry Finn, Henry V, Tobacco Road, Master Harold . . . and the Boys, Tomorrow's Monday, Talley and Son.

MAC RAE, JEAN: Actress. b. Montreal, Quebec, Mar. 24, 1930. Worked for National Film Bd. of Canada, Canadian Bdcst. Corp., and repertory theatre in Canada; U.S. studios, including MGM, 20th-Fox, Columbia, and Paramount; as TV studios at Desilu and 20th-Fox.

MADDEN, BILL: Executive. b. New York City, March 1, 1915; e. Boston U. Joined Metro-Goldwyn-Mayer as office boy, 1930; student salesman, 1938; asst. Eastern div. mgr., 1939; U.S. Navy, 1942–46; Boston salesman, M.G.M., 1947–53; Philadelphia branch mgr., 1954–59; Midwest div. sales mgr., 1960–68; roadshow sales mgr., 1969; v.p., general sales mgr., M.G.M.; corp., v.p. & gen. sls. mgr., MGM, 1973; retired from MGM, 1975; 1976-present, exec. consultant to motion picture industry; lecturer and instructor at UCLA. Member: Academy M.P. Arts & Sciences.

MADDEN, DAVID: Executive. e. Harvard Univ. (1976), UCLA (MA, 1978). Joined 20th Century-Fox in Nov., 1978 as story analyst. Named story editor, 1980; exec. story editor, 1982. Appt. v.p., creative affairs for 20th-Fox Prods., 1983; v.p., prod., 20th Century-Fox Prods; 1980, v.p., production, Paramount Pictures.

MADIGAN, AMY: Actress. b. Chicago, 1957.

PICTURES: Love Child, Streets of Fire, Places in the Heart, Alamo Bay, Twice in a Lifetime.

TELEVISION: The Laundromat.

MADISON, GUY: Actor. r.n., Robert Moseley. b. Bakersfield, Calif., Jan. 19, 1922; e. Bakersfield Jr. Coll.; m. Sheila Connolly, U.S. Navy; m.p. debut in Since You Went Away, 1944; Wild Bill Hickok radio and TV shows, Star of Tomorrow, 1954.

PICTURES INCLUDE: Till the End of Time, Honeymoon, Texas, Brooklyn and Heaven, Massacre River, Drums in the Deep South, Red Snow, Charge at Feather River, The Command, Five Against the House, Beast of Hollow Mountain, Last Frontier, On the Threshold of Space, Hilda Crane, Bullwhip, Gunmen of The Rio Grande, Sandokan Fights Back, Sandokan Against the Leopard of Sarawak, Mystery of Thug Island, Shatterhand, Payment in Blood.

MAGILL, MORT: Sales executive. b. Philadelphia, Pa., Oct. 10, 1907; e. U. of Pennsylvania, B.S. 1927. Silk salesman in southern U.S. 9 yrs.; salesman United Artists, Harrisburg 1936; city salesman Philadelphia 1938; br. mgr. Pittsburgh 1941; br. mgr. Philadelphia; part-owner Principal Films 1949; district mgr. for M.P. Sales Corp., Philadelphia & Pittsburgh 1949; br. mgr., U.A. Philadelphia; dist. mgr. Buena Vista, (Phila., Pittsburgh, Washington) 1954; dist. mgr. Nat'l Gen. Pictures, 1971, independent distribution in partnership with John Turner-Firm called Turner-Magill, Inc., covering New York, Washington, Philadelphia and Pittsburgh. Firm now called Magill Films, Inc.

MAHARIS, GEORGE: Actor. b. Sept. 1, 1928.

PICTURES: Exodus, Sylvia, Quick Before It Melts, The Satan Bug, Covenant with Death, The Happening, The Desperadoes.

TELEVISION: Route 66. Movies: Escape to Mindanao, The Monk, The Victim, Murder on Flight 502, Rich Man, Poor Man, Look What's Happened to Rosemary's Baby, SST-Death Flight, Return to Fantasy Island, Crash.

MAHONEY, JOCK: Actor. r.n. Jacques O'Mahoney. b. Chicago, Ill., Feb. 7, 1919. e. U. of Iowa. Fighter pilot instructor, U.S.M.C.; enter m.p. ind. as stuntman; then started in westerns; TV show, Range Rider, many appearances on Loretta Young Show.

PICTURES INCLUDE: Away All Boats, Day of Fury, Showdown at Abilene, Battle Hymn, I've Lived Before, Land Unknown, Joe Dakota, Money, Women & Guns, Moro Witch Doctor, Walls of Hell, Tarzan Goes to India, Tarzan's Three Challenges.

MAIBAUM, RICHARD: Writer, Producer, b. New York City, May 26. educ. NYU, Univ. of Iowa, B.A., M.A., Ph. Beta Kappa. Plays on Broadway: The Tree, Birthright, Sweet Mystery of Life, See My Lawyer (1939), Member, Shakespearean Repertory Theatre in New York as player, 1933, From 1935 to 1942 worked on screenplays in Hollywood: MGM (They Gave Him a Gun, Stablemates, etc.); Columbia (Amazing Mr. Williams); Paramount (I Wanted Wings); 20th-Fox (Ten Gentlemen from West Point). Army, 1942–46, dir. Combat Film Div., final rank Lt. Col. To Para. prod.-writer, 1946, wrote-produced O.S.S., Song of Surrender; collab. & prod. The Great Gatsby. Prod. Sainted Sisters, The Big Clock, Bride of Vengeance, Dear Wife, No Man of Her Own, Capt. Carey, U.S.A.; free lance, 1953; collab. s.p., Paratrooper; adapt., Hell Below Zero; writer of Teleplays; exec. prod. MGM-TV, 1958–60.

PICTURES INCLUDE: Ransom, Cockleshell Heroes, Bigger Than Life, Zarak, Tank Force, Killers of Kilimanjaro, The Day They Robbed the Bank of England, Battle at Bloody Beach, Dr. No, From Russia With Love, Goldfinger, Thunderball, Chitty, Chitty, Bang Bang, On Her Majesty's Secret Service, Diamonds Are Forever, The Man With The Golden Gun, The Spy Who Loved Me, For Your Eyes Only, Octopussy, A View to a Kill.

MAIDMENT, GEORGE JOSEPH: Executive. Apptd. chief continental auditor, Fox Film Co., Ltd., 1924; was later comptroller of that co. and of British Movietonews, Ltd.; dir., Fox British Pictures, Ltd. 1933, treas. & secy., Columbia Pictures Corp., Ltd., Columbia Pictures Export Ltd., and Columbia British Productions, Ltd. In War Service as regional officer. Ministry Home Security, then on production planning for engineering and aircraft, finally on reorganization work. Ministry of Agriculture. 1944; gen. mgr., London Films Export, Ltd. 1947 gen. mgr., Omnia Films Ltd., Producers Re presentations Ltd., 1951 gen. mgr. Pendennis Pictures Corp. Ltd., Tower Films Ltd., Pax Films Ltd., Vicar Prod. Ltd., Orb. Prod. Ltd., Orb. Intl. Ltd. Fellow, Inst. of Chartered Accountants, Fellow Chartered Institute of Secretaries; Fellow, Institute of Linguists.

MAIN, DAVID: Writer, Producer. b. Essex, England, 1929. Extensive television experience in Britain producing and directing for A.T.V., Granada, A.B.C. and B.B.C. Emigrated to Canada in 1960. Directed Moment of Truth for N.B.C., and Quentin Durgens M.P. for C.B.C., Famous Jury Trials for 20th Century Fox. In 1977–78 directed King of Kensington, Le Club, A Gift to Last for CBC. President of Velvet Screen Plays Ltd. a subsidiary of Quadrant Films Ltd.

PICTURES INCLUDE: Sunday In The Country, 1973 (story & co-writer), and It Seemed Like A Good Idea At The Time, 1975 (co-writer); Find The Lady, 1976 (story, co-writer, co-producer); Double Negative, 1978 (co-prod.); Nothing Personal, 1979 (co-prod.).

MAJORS, LEE: Actor. b. Wyandotte, Mich., April 23, 1940. m. actress-model Farrah Fawcett-Majors. Star athlete in high school; turned down offer from St. Louis Cardinals in final year at Eastern Kentucky State College to pursue acting career. In L.A. got job as playground supervisor for park dept. while studying acting at MGM Studio.

PICTURES INCLUDE: Will Penny (debut), The Liberation of L. B. Jones.

TV: The Big Valley, The Man From Shiloh, The Six Million Dollar Man, The Fall Guy. Movies: The Ballad of Andy Crocker, Weekend of Terror, The Gary Francis Powers Story, The Cowboy and the Ballerina.

MALDEN, KARL: Actor. r.n. Malden Sekulovich. b. Gary, Ind., Mar. 22, 1914.

B'WAY PLAYS: Golden Boy, Key Largo, Flight to West, Missouri Legend, Uncle Harry, Counterattack, Truckline Cafe, All My Sons, Streetcar Named Desire, Desperate Hours, Desire Under the Elms.

PICTURES INCLUDE: Boomerang, The Gunfighter, Where the Sidewalk Ends, Hall of Montezuma, Streetcar Named Desire, (Acad. Award best supporting actor, 1951), The Sellout, Diplomatic Courier, Operation Secret, Ruby Gentry, I Confess, Take the High Ground, Phantom of the Rue Morgue, On the Waterfront, Bombers B-52, Desperate Hours, Fear Strikes Out, Egghead, The Hanging Tree, One Eyed Jacks, Parrish; dir., Time Limit, Billion Dollar Brain, Hot Millions, Blue Hotel, Patton, Cat O'Nine Tails, Wild

Rovers, Summertime Killer, Beyond the Poseidon Adventure, Meteor, The Sting II, Twilight Time.
TV: Streets of San Francisco, Captains Courageous, Word of Honor, With Intent to Kill, Fatal Vision.

MALICK, TERENCE: Producer-Writer-Director. b. Texas, Nov. 30, 1943. e. Harvard. Attended Oxford on Rhodes scholarship. Worked for Newsweek, Life and The New Yorker; lectured for year in philosophy at M.I.T. Studied at American Film Institute in Bev. Hills and made short funded by AFI.
PICTURES INCLUDE: Badlands (prod., dir., s.p.), Days of Heaven (s.p., dir.).

MALIN, AMIR JACOB: Executive. b. Tel-Aviv, Israel, Mar. 22, 1954. e. Brandeis Univ. (1972–76); Boston Univ. School of Law (1976–79). Staff atty., WOBH-TV, Boston, 1979–81; ABM Industries, chief exec. off., 1979; now pres. & CEO, Cinecon Intl. Films, Inc. Films acquired and distributed include Come Back to the 5 & Dime, Jimmy Dean; Angelo My Love; El Norte; Pumping Iron II; Metropolis; The Brother from Another Planet; Stop Making Sense; Coca-Cola Kid; A Room with a View.

MALKOVICH, JOHN: Actor. b. 1955. e. Illinois State Univ. Started Steppenwolf Ensemble in Chicago with group of college friends. Starred in True West which then was brought to New York. Stage work includes Death of Salesman on Bdwy. and TV with Dustin Hoffman.
PICTURES: The Killing Fields (debut), Places in the Heart, Eleni, Making Mr. Right.

MALLE, LOUIS: Director. b. Thumeries, France, 1932. Started in film industry as assistant to Robert Bresson. Began career somewhat ahead of most young French directors referred to as the Nouvelle Vague (New Wave). Became internationally known with Les Amants (The Lovers) in 1958. Has also acted in films.
PICTURES INCLUDE: The World of Silence (co-dir. with J. Y. Cousteau); A Man Escaped (asst. to Bresson); Elevator to the Gallows, The Lovers, Zazie in the Metro, Private Life, Vive Le Tour, The Fire Within, Bon Baisers de Bangkok, Viva Maria, The Thief, William Wilson, Phantom India, Murmur of the Heart, Humain, Trop Humain, Lacombe, Lucien, Black Moon, Pretty Baby, Atlantic City, My Dinner with Andre, Crackers, Alamo Bay (also prod.).

MALLERS, ANTHONY: Theatre Owner. b. Portland, Ind., Oct. 4, 1933. e. Indiana Univ. (B.S., business admin.). Entered industry in 1957. Now pres. of Mallers Theatres, headquartered in Muncie, Ind.

MALMUTH, BRUCE: Director. b. Brooklyn, N.Y., Feb. 4, 1937. e. City Coll., Brooklyn Coll. Acted in college productions. Moved to California and obtained job as page at TV center. In Army assigned to special services as director; reassigned to New York. Upon release began 10-year production stint in TV commercials. Debut as director of feature with Nighthawks, 1981.
PICTURES: Nighthawk, The Man Who Wasn't There, Where Are the Children?.

MALONE, DOROTHY: Actress. b. Chicago, Ill., Jan. 30, 1925. e. So. Methodist U. Screen debut in The Big Sleep, 1946.
PICTURES INCLUDE: Young at Heart, Battle Cry, Pillars of the Sky, Written on the Wind (Acad. Award, best supporting actress, 1956), Man of a Thousand Faces, The Last Voyage, The Last Sunset, Beach Party, Abduction, Golden Rendezvous, Winter Kills.
TV: Dick Powell Theatre, Dr. Kildare, Bob Hope Show, Jack Benny Show, The Untouchables, The Greatest Show On Earth, Peyton Place (series), Peyton Place: The Next Generation (movie).

MAMET, David: Writer. b. Chicago, IL. e. Goddard Coll. Husband of actress Lindsay Crouse. Co-founder Dinglefest Theatre; assoc. artistic dir., Goodman Theatre, Chicago. Plays include Lakefront, The Woods, American Buffalo, Sexual Perversions in Chicago, Duck Variations, The Long Canoe, Edmond, Glengarry Glen Ross, etc.
PICTURES: The Postman Always Rings Twice, The Verdict.

MAMOULIAN, ROUBEN: Director. b. Tiflis, Caucasus (Russia), Oct. 8, 1897; e. Lycee Montaigne, Paris, Moscow U., (law). Stage dir. since 1918; first English prod., Beating on the Door, London, 1922; came to U.S., 1923; prod. dir., Eastman Theatre, Rochester, N.Y., 1923–26; dir. operas, operetta, musicals; organizer, 1925, dir., 1925–26, Eastman Theatre School; dir. Oklahoma for Berlin Art Festival, 1951; dir. Oklahoma! for Paris, France (Salut a La France), 1955; Oklahoma! for Rome, Milan, Naples and Venice, Italy; author of short stories, verse, articles; pub. books: Abigayil, 1964; "Shakespeare's Hamlet, A New Version," 1966; 1966. prod. Hamlet; 1967. Tribute to R.M.'s 40th Anniv. on stage & screen at Mod. Art in N.Y.: 1968, Festival of R.M. Films at National Film Thea. in London, Washington, D.C., and Montreal. Tribute to Rouben Mamoulian: Retrospectives of all his films and personal appearances for discussion at: San Francisco International Film Festival, Science Center in Toronto, Canada, Museum of Science in Buffalo, New York, University of California at Los Angeles, University of South Florida, Yale University, New York (all in 1971). Seminar for USA Educators by Rouben Mamoulian at the American Film Institute, 1970. Guest of Honor of U.S.S.R. at the International Film Festival in Moscow, 1971. The Art of Survival—symposium at University of Southern California, 1972. Musical Mamoulian—Retrospective of R.M.'s musical films at the Academy of Motion Pictures Arts & Sciences, Hollywood, 1972. Publication: Foreword to the book Chevalier, 1973. Retrospective showing of Rouben Mamoulian's films at UCLA, 1973. Special showing of Blood and Sand and discussion at Filmex, Hollywood, 1973. President of the international jury at the International Film Festival of San Sebastian, Spain, 1973. Festival of Mamoulian's films in San Sebastian, 1973. Festival of Rouben Mamoulians films at the Cinematheque Francaise, Paris, France, 1973. Symposium on the Coming of Sound to the American Film 1925–1940—George Eastman House, Rochester, New York, 1973. Showing of Dr. Jekyll & Mr. Hyde and stage appearance Filmex 1974—Hollywood, 1974. Festival of Mamoulian's films in Sydney and Melbourne, Australia, 1974. Establishment of the "Rouben Mamoulian Award for the Best Australian Short Film" in perpetuity, June, 1974. Showing of Mamoulian musicals and appearance at the American Film Institute's "History of American Musicals" at Kennedy Center of Performing Arts, Washington, D.C., Sept., 1974. Guest of honor and member of international jury at International Film Festival, Tehran, Iran, 1974. Guest of Honor at festivities in Ispahan, Shiraz and Persipolis, December, 1974. Lecture on "The State of films and the state of the World" at Washington Club, Washington, D.C., December, 1974. Lectures, seminar and showing of Mamoulian films at University of California at Santa Barbara, February, 1975.
BROADWAY PLAYS: Porgy, Marco's Millions, Wings over Europe, Congai, A Month in the Country, Solid South, Farewell to Arms, Porgy and Bess, Oklahoma, Sadie Thompson, Carousel, St. Louis Woman, Lost in the Stars, Arms and the Girl.
PICTURES INCLUDE: Applause, City Streets, Dr. Jekyll and Mr. Hyde, Love Me Tonight, Song of Songs, Queen Christine, We Live Again, Becky Sharp, Gay Desperado, High, Wide and Handsome, Golden Boy, Mark of Zorro, Blood and Sand, Rings On Her Fingers, Summer Holiday, Silk Stockings, Never Steal Anything Small (co-author) 1959.

MANASSE, GEORGE: Producer. b. Florence, Italy, Jan. 1, 1938; e. U. of N.C. Producer, GSF Productions, Inc.; for Cannon was assoc. prod., Joe, Jump; prod. Who Killed Mary What's Her Name; for GSF was exec. prod., Journey Through Rosebud, Change in the Wind.

MANBY, C. R.: Executive. b. Battle Creek, Mich., Feb. 24, 1920; e. Hillsdale Coll., Mich., A.B., 1942; Harvard Grad. School of Bus. Admin., 1953; v.p., RKO General Inc., 1955–58; pres. Show Corp. of Amer., 1958–75; pres., RKO Pictures, 1978–84; chm., 1985–present.

MANCINI, HENRY: Composer. b., Cleveland, OH, April 16, 1924. Arranged music for the Glen Miller Story, The Benny Goodman Story, then began composing scores.
PICTURES INCLUDE: Touch of Evil, High Time, Breakfast at Tiffany's (AA, 1961), Bachelor in Paradise, Hatari, The Pink Panther, Charade, A Shot in the Dark, Dear Heart, What Did You Do in the War, Daddy?, Two for the Road, Visions of Eight, Oklahoma Crude, 99 44/100% Dead, The White Dawn, The Girl from Petrovka, The Great Waldo Pepper, W. C. Fields and Me, The Pink Panther Strikes Again, Silver Streak, Revenge of the Pink Panther, Who Is Killing the Great Chefs of Europe?, Prisoner of Zenda, Nightwing, "10," Little Miss Marker, Change of Seasons, Back Roads, "S.O.B.", Mommie Dearest, Whose Little Girl Are You?, Trail of the Pink Panther, Curse of the Pink Panther, The Man Who Loved Women, Harry and Son, Life Force, Santa Claus.

MANCUSO, FRANK G.: Executive. b. Buffalo, N.Y., July 25, 1933. e. State Univ. of New York. Film buyer and operations supvr. for Basil Enterprises, theatre circuit, from 1958 to 1962. Joined Paramount as booker in Buffalo branch, 1962. Named sls. repr. for branch in 1964 and branch mgr. in 1967. In 1970 appt. v.p./gen. sls. mgr., Paramount Pictures Canada, Ltd., becoming pres. in 1972. In 1976 relocated with Paramount in U.S. as western div. mgr. in L.A. In Jan., 1977, appt. gen. sls. mgr. of N.Y., office; two months later promoted to v.p.—domestic distribution; 1979, named exec. v.p., distribution & mktg. In 1983 made pres. of entire Paramount Motion Picture Division. 1984, appointed chm. and chief exec. officer, Paramount Pictures.

MANCUSO, FRANK, JR.: Producer. b. Buffalo, NY, Oct. 9, 1958. Son of Frank G. Mancuso, pres. m.p. div. of Paramount Pictures. e. Upsala College. Began with industry at age 14, booking short subjects in Canadian theatres. Worked in gross receipts dept. in Paramount corporate

offices in New York City and later with paralegal div. Initial prod. work as location asst. for Urban Cowboy in Houston, TX. Served as assoc. prod. of Friday the 13th Part II and prod. of Friday the 13th Part III in 3-D.
PICTURES: Off the Wall, The Man Who Wasn't There, April Fool's Day.

MANDEL, HARRY: Theatre executive. b. New York City, dir., adv. & publicity, RKO Theatres, 1938; added duties asst. to v.p. theatre operations, 1952; v.p. theatre operations, 1957; pres., 1961–66.

MANDEL, LORING: Writer. Long career writing scripts for TV, dating back to 1956 when penned A House of His Own for NBC.
PICTURES: Countdown, Promises in the Dark, The Little Drummer Girl, etc.
TELEVISION: Tom and Joann, Breaking Up, The Best of Family, etc.

MANDELL, ABE: Executive. e. U. of Cincinnati. Entered broadcasting as actor on Cincinnati radio station prior to WW II. Served U.S. Army in Southwest Pacific, 1942–45. Formed independent motion picture distribution company in the Far East. Company, which became the largest independent motion picture distributor in the Far East, also operated and owned motion picture theaters throughout the Phillipine Islands and Indonesia, 1946–56; network-regional sales exec., Ziv Television, 1956–58; dir. foreign operations, Independent Television Corporation, 1958; v.p.-foreign oper., 1960; v.p.-sales and adm., 1961; exec. v.p., 1962; pres. 1965. In 1976 ITC changed its corporate name from Independent Television Corp. to ITC Entertainment, Inc. President to 1983 of ITC Entertainment.

MANES, FRITZ: Producer. TV ad exec. and stuntman before becoming exec. prod. on films for Clint Eastwood.
PICTURES: Firefox, Honkytonk Man, Sudden Impact, Tightrope.

MANGANO, SILVANA: Actress. b. Rome, Italy. Apr. 23, 1930. e. Dance Academy of Jia Ruskaja. Model to 1949; m.p. debut in L'Elisir D'Amore.
PICTURES INCLUDE: Bitter Rice, Lure of Sila, Musolino, The Brigand; Anna, Ulysses, Mambo, Gold of Naples, This Angry Age, Tempest, Five Branded Women, Barabbas, Teorama, Death in Venice, Decameron, Ludwig, Conversation Piece, Dune.

MANKIEWICZ, DON M.: Writer. b. Berlin, Germany, Jan. 20, 1922. p. Herman J. Mankiewicz e. Columbia, B.A., 1942; Columbia Law School. Served in U.S. Army, 1942–46; reporter, New Yorker magazine, 1946–48; author of novels See How They Run, Trial, It Only Hurts a Minute; magazine articles, short stories.
TV: Studio One, On Trial, One Step Beyond, Playhouse 90, Profiles in Courage.
PICTURES INCLUDE: Trial, I Want to Live.
TV PILOTS: Ironside, Marcus Welby, M.D., Sarge; Lanigan's Rabbi (collaboration); Rosetti and Ryan (collab.)

MANKIEWICZ, JOSEPH L.: Writer, director. b. Wilkes-Barre, Pa., Feb. 11, 1909; e. Columbia U. Asst. corr. in Berlin, Chicago Tribune; Ufa studio, translating subtitles into Eng. for release in Eng. & U.S.; returned to U.S. 1929 to join brother, Herman, on Paramount writing staff; MGM, 1933; Fox, 1943–51; dir., La Boheme, Metropolitan Opera House, 1953. Academy Awards: 1949, Letter to Three Wives, best s.p., dir.; 1950, All About Eve, best s.p., dir.
PICTURES INCLUDE: Skippy, Million Dollar Legs, If I Had a Million, Alice in Wonderland, Fury, Gorgeous Hussy, Mannequin, Three Comrades, Shopworn Angel, Philadelphia Story, Woman of the Year, Keys of the Kingdom, Dragonwyck, Somewhere in the Night, No Way Out, Late George Apley, Ghost and Mrs. Muir, House of Strangers, Letter to Three Wives, All About Eve, 1950, People Will Talk, 5 Fingers, Julius Caesar, Barefoot Contessa, Guys and Dolls, Quiet American, Suddenly Last Summer, The Honey Pot, There was a Crooked Man, Sleuth.

MANKIEWITZ, TOM: b. Los Angeles, June 1, 1942. Writer. Specializes in adventure/suspense films.
PICTURES INCLUDE: The Sweet Ride (debut), Diamonds Are Forever, Live and Let Die, The Man with the Golden Gun, Mother, Jugs and Speed, The Cassandra Crossing, The Eagle Has Landed, Mother, Jugs and Speed.
TELEVISION: Hart to Hart (s.p., dir.).

MANKOWITZ, WOLF: Author, playwright, producer & impresario. B. London, 1924. Journalist. Ent. m.p. in 1952. Musical play based his story Expresso Bongo, 1958. Musical play, Make Me An Offer, 1959; Belle, 1961; Pickwick, 1963; Passion Flower Hotel.
PICTURES INCLUDE: Make Me An Offer, Kid For Two Farthings, The Bespoke Overcoat, Trapeze, Expresso Bongo, The Millionairess, The Long and Short and Tall, The Day The Earth Caught Fire, Where the Spies Are, Assassination Bureau 1969; Bloomfield, 1970: Black Beauty, Treasure Island. 1973: The Hireling.
TV: Make Me An Offer, The Baby, The Girl, It Should Happen To A Dog, Conflict, The Killing Stones, A Cure for Tin Ear, The Model Marriage, ABC of Show Business, The Battersea Miracle, Dickens of London, 1976–77.

MANN, ABBY: Writer. b. Philadelphia. e. N.Y.U. First gained fame on TV; adapted own teleplay Judgment at Nuremberg into theatrical film.
PICTURES INCLUDE: Judgment at Nuremberg, A Child Is Waiting, Ship of Fools, The Detective, Report to the Commissioner, War and Love.
TELEVISION: The Marcus-Nelson Murders, The Atlanta Child Murders.

MANN, DANIEL: Director. b. New York, N.Y., Aug. 8, 1912. e. Erasmus Hall, Brooklyn; Professional Children's School. Started as musician in resort hotels; then in Canada, on road; U.S. Army, World War II; then received scholarship to Neighborhood Playhouse, N.Y.; dir. teaching, TV dir.
BROADWAY: Come Back Little Sheba, Rose Tattoo, Streetcar Named Desire (City Center prod.), Paint Your Wagon.
PICTURES INCLUDE: Come Back Little Sheba, About Mrs. Leslie, Rose Tattoo, I'll Cry Tomorrow, Teahouse of the August Moon, Hot Spell, Last Angry Man, Mountain Road, Butterfield 8, Ada, Judith; A Dream of Kings, Who's Got the Action?, Who's Been Sleeping in my Bed?, For Love of Ivy, Willard, The Revengers, Maurie, Interval, Lost in the Stars, Matilda.

MANN, DELBERT: Director, Producer. b. Lawrence, Kans., Jan. 30, 1920; e. Vanderbilt Univ., Yale Univ., U.S. Air Force, 1942–45; stage mgr., summer stock, dir. Columbia, S.C. Town Theatre, 1947–49; asst. dir., NBC-TV, 1949; dir., NBC-TV, 1949–55. Past pres. Directors Guild of America.
PROGRAMS: Philco-Goodyear TV Playhouse, Producer's Showcase, Omnibus, Playwrights '56, Playhouse 90, Ford Star Jubilee, Lights Out, Mary Kay and Johnny, The Little Show, Masterpiece Theatre, Ford Startime.
STAGE: A Quiet Place, Speaking of Murder, Zelda, opera: Wuthering Heights; New York City Center.
PICTURES INCLUDE: Marty (Academy Award, best director, 1955), Bachelor Party, Desire Under the Elms, Separate Tables, Middle of the Night, The Dark at the Top of the Stairs, The Outsider, Lover Come Back, That Touch of Mink, A Gathering of Eagles, Dear Heart, Quick Before It Melts, Mister Buddwing, Fitzwilly, The Pink Jungle, Kidnapped, Birch Interval, Night Crossing.
TV: Heidi, David Copperfield, Jane Eyre. The Man Without A Country, A Girl Named Sooner, Breaking Up, Tell Me My Name, Home To Stay, All Quiet on the Western Front, To Find My Son, All the Way Home, The Member of the Wedding, Bronte, The Gift of Love, Love Leads the Way, A Death in California, The Last Days of Patton.

MANN, MICHAEL: Producer-Director-Writer. b. Chicago. e. Univ. of Wisc., London Film School. From 1965–72 directed commercials and documentaries in England, including Insurrection for NBC in Paris during the 1968 riots. Directed short film, Jaunpuri, winner of Juris Prize at Cannes Film Festival. Returned to U.S. in 1972 to direct documentary, 18 Days Down the Line. Wrote for prime-time TV (episodes of Starsky and Hutch, Police Story, Vegas).
PICTURES: Thief (exec. prod., s.p., dir.), The Keep (s.p. dir.).
TELEVISION: The Jericho Mile (s.p., dir.). (DGA, 1980 best director award). Miami Vice (exec. prod.).

MANNE, S. ANTHONY: Executive. b. New York, N.Y., July 19, 1940. e. Wharton School Univ. of Pa. (B.S., economics). Joined Columbia Pictures 1963; international dept. 1964; asst. mgr., Brazil, 1968; mgr., Brazil, 1972–76. Joined JAD Films, 1976; appointed v.p. 1978, exec. v.p., 1979.

MANNIX, DAVID K.: Executive. b. Brooklyn, N.Y., 1952; e. B.S., Fordham University, M.B.A., Pepperdine Univ. Joined Paramount Pictures in 1973 as supervisor, TV accounting; 1976, Mgr. financial analysis; 1978, asst. studio controller; 1979, director, production operations; 1981, executive director, studio operations; 1984, promoted to v.p. 1986, sr. v.p., theatrical distribution, Columbia Picture Industries.

MANSON, ARTHUR: Executive. b. Brooklyn, N.Y., Feb. 21, 1928; e. CCNY, grad. (Inst. Film Technique) '45; editor, American Traveler, U.S. Army, 1946; Advance agent, co. mgr., Henry V, U.S., 1948–50; producer's publ. rep., Stanley Kramer Distributing Corp., Samuel Goldwyn Productions, Lopert Films, dir. of adv. and publ., MGM Pictures of Canada, Ltd., 1952–53; publ. and adv. rep., Cinerama Corp., 1953–58; worldwide ad-pub Cinerama (wide screen process) 1958–60; adv. mgr., Columbia Pictures, 1961–62; nat'l dir. of adv., publ., Dino De Laurentiis, 1962–64; exec. asst. to v.p. chg. adv. & pub., 20th Century-Fox, 1964–67; v.p. chg, adv. & pub. Cinerama. Inc., and Cinerama Releasing Corp.; 1967–74; exec. v.p., sales & marketing, BCP, service of Cox Braodcasting Corp., 1974–75; v.p.

chg. worldwide adv.-pub. Warner Bros., 1976. In 1977 formed own company, Cinemax Mkt. & Dist. Corp. and is pres.

MANULIS, MARTIN: Prod.-dir. b. N.Y.C. May 30, 1915; e. Columbia Univ., B.A. 1935. Head of prod. John C. Wilson, 1941–49; mgr. dir., Westport Country Playhouse, 1945–50; dir. B'way plays; staff prod. & dir. CBS-TV, 1951–58; head prod. 20th-Fox Television. Now pres. Martin Manulis Prods. Ltd.
BROADWAY: Private Lives, Made in Heaven, The Philadelphia Story, Pride's Crossing, Laura, The Men We Marry, The Hasty Heart, The Show Off.
TV: Suspense, Studio One, Climax, Best of Broadway, Playhouse 90. Mini-Series: Chiefs, Space, The Day Christ Died.
PICTURES INCLUDE: Days of Wine and Roses, The Out-of-Towners, Luv, Duffy.

MARA, ADELLE: Actress. r.n. Adelaida Delgado; b. Dearborn, Michigan, April 28, 1923. m. Roy Huggins. Singer, dancer with Xavier Cugat orchestra; Col. contract.
PICTURES INCLUDE: Shut My Big Mouth, Blondie Goes to College, Alias Boston Blackie, You Were Never Lovelier, Riders of the Northwest Mounted, Magnificent Rogue, Passkey to Danger, Traffic in Crime, Exposed, The Trespasser, Blackmail, Campus Honeymoon, Sands of Iwo Jima, Sea Hornet, Count The Hours, Wake of the Red Witch, Back from Eternity.

MARAIS, JEAN: Actor. b. Cherbourg, France, Dec. 11, 1913; e. Coll. St. Germain, Lycee Janson de Sailly & Lycee Condorcet Painter; photog; stage actor; French Air Army; m.p. debut in Pavillon Brule.
PICTURES INCLUDE: Carmen, Eternal Return, Beauty and the Beast, Ruy Blas, Les Parents Terribles, Secret of Mayerling, Souvenir, Orpheus, Eagle with Two Heads, Inside a Girl's Dormitory, Royal Affairs in Versailles, Paris Does Strange Things, Le Capitan, Le Bossu La Princesse de Cleves, Le Capitaine Fracasse, Honorable Stanilleu, Agent Secret, Patute, Fantomas, Le Gentleman de Cocody.

MARANS, MARDI: Executive. ed. Univ. of Calif. Worked in L.A. office of Doyle Dane Bernbach ad agency. Joined Warner Bros. in March, 1975, as asst. to media director. In 1979 appt. v.p. and director of media for WB, responsible for planning and placement of all advertising for all films distributed by co. on world-wide basis. 1986, exec. v.p., worldwide mktg., Paramount Picture.

MARCH, DONALD: Production Executive. b. New York City, July 26, 1942. Held senior programming positions with ABC-TV network and Robert Stigwood Organization before joining CBS in 1977 as director, special projects, motion pictures for TV and mini-series. Later promoted to v.p., motion pictures for TV. Left CBS to serve as pres. of Filmways' theatrical division in early 1979; later that year rejoined CBS as v.p., theatrical films, with responsibility for selection, development and production of pictures for theatrical release. 1984, sr. v.p., HBO Premiere Films.

MARCHAND, NANCY: Actress. b. Buffalo, NY, June 19, 1928. On Bdwy. in Playboy of the Western World, On the Town, The Duel, Parents' Day, Morning's at Seven, Awake and Sing, etc.
PICTURES: The Rise and Rise of Michael Rimmer, Promise at Dawn, Goodbye Mr. Chips, Ladybug, Ladybug, Me, Natalie, Tell Me That You Love Me, Junie Moon.
TELEVISION: Lou Grant. Movies: Some Kind of Miracle, Willa, The Golden Moment—An Olympic Love Story, Sparkling Cyanide. Mini-Series: North & South Book II.

MARCUS, LOUIS: Producer, Director, Writer. b. Cork, Ireland, 1936. e. Natl. Univ. of Ireland (B.A., 1959). Based in Dublin since 1959, where has made nearly 30 theatrical documentary films. Produces and directs for Louis Marcus Documentary Film Production of Dublin and Louis Marcus Films Ltd. of London. In 1964 appt. by Irish govt. as bd. mem. of Dublin's Abbey Theatre. In 1972 appt. by govt. as mem. of Cultural Relations Comm. of Dept. of Foreign Affairs. Elected mem. of Academy of M.P. Arts & Sciences (short subject branch) 1974.
PICTURES INCLUDE: Fleadh Cheoil, Horse Laughs, Woes of Golf, Children at Work, Conquest of Light.
AUTHOR: The Irish Film Industry (1968).

MARDEN, MICHAEL: Executive. e. Princeton Univ. Joined CBS in N.Y. in 1957. Later was TV prog. exec. for Benton & Bowles, Inc. Returned to CBS in April, 1966 as gen. prog. exec. for the network in N.Y. Named director, feature films, and was responsible for the CBS Late Movie (premiere: 1972). In June, 1976 named director, motion pictures for TV and mini-series, Hollywood.

MARENSTEIN, HAROLD: exec. b. New York, N.Y., e. C.C.N.Y., 1937. Shipping, picture checking service, Warner Bros., 1935–45; Booking, Loew's Inc., 1945–48; Booking, contracts, Selznick Rel. Org., 1948–51; contracts, Paramount, 1951–52; asst. sls. gr., International Rel. Org., 1952; asst. sls. mgr., Janus Films, 1961–64; sls. exec., Rizzoli Films, 1965; 1967, nat'l. sales dir., Continental Dist.; gen. sales mgr., Cinemation Industries, 1968. v.p.-sales, dir., Cinemation Industries, 1971; 1976, gen. sls. mgr., General National Films; 1980, gen. sls. mgr., Lima Productions. Now retired.

MARGOLIN, JANET: Actress. b. New York City, 1943. e. N.Y. High School of Performing Arts. Discovered by Frank Perry while playing in Bdwy. show, Daughter of Silence, and hired by him for lead in David and Lisa.
PICTURES: The Greatest Story Ever Told, Bus Riley's Back in Town, Morituri, Nevada Smith, Enter Laughing, Buena Sera, Mrs. Campbell, Take the Money and Run, Annie Hall, Last Embrace.

MARGRAF, GUSTAV B.: Executive. b. Cape Giradeau, Mo., May 14, 1915; e. Southeast Missouri State Coll. and Duke Univ. Law Sch.; attorney with Cahill, Gordon, Zachry & Reindel 1939–48; v.p., gen. atty., NBC, 1948–53; v.p. for talent NBC, 1953–55; gen. counsel, dir. and v.p. Reynolds Metal Co.; mgng. dir., British Aluminum Co., Ltd.; pres., chmn. bd., Canadian British Aluminum Co., Ltd.; v. chmn., Manicouagan Power Co., chmn., Aluminum Wire & Cable Co. Ltd.; chr. dir., Reynolds Jamaica Mines, Metal Development Corp., Caribbean Steamship Co., Haitian Mines Inc.; chmn. Aluminum Foils Ltd.; pres. Aluminum Fed. of Gt. Britain.

MARGULIES, IRWIN: Attorney, executive. b. Austria. June 24, 1907; e. N.Y.U., BA, 1929; N.Y.U. Law Sch., LL.B., 1931. Assoc. with father in m.p. theatres, 1918; treas., counsel or Jayem Management Corp.; MGM legal dept., N.Y., 1930–42; asst. to v.p.; gen. counsel J. Robert Rubin, 1943–47; asst. secy, counsel, MGM Intern'l Films. Inc., 1945–47; in private practice since 1947. Member Calif. bar since 1948; counsel for many m.p. prod. & dist., cos., literary agencies, radio & TV prod., dist., & personalities; 1954–67 v.p. Horizon Pict. Inc.; 1967, v.p. in charge of bus. affairs, Warner-7 Arts; 1969, with Harry Saltzman; exec. prod., "Digby—The Biggest Dog in The World."

MARGULIES, STAN: Producer. b. New York, N.Y. Dec. 14, 1920. e. De Witt Clinton High School, New York Univ., B.S., June, 1940; Army Air Force, May, 1942; pub. rels. Air Force and the Infantry, wrote service magazines, newspapers including Yank; spec. feature writer & asst. Sunday editor, Salt Lake City Tribune; publicist, RKO Studios, Hollywood, March, 1947; continued publicity work at CBS-Radio, 20th Century-Fox, Walt Disney Productions. Bryna Films, 1955; became vice-pres., 1958; also served exec. prod., TV series, Tales of the Vikings; prod. aide. Spartacus. 1984, with ABC Circle Films.
PICTURES INCLUDE: 40 Pounds of Trouble, Those Magnificent Men In Their Flying Machines, Don't Just Stand There, The Pink Jungle, If It's Tuesday, This Must Be Belgium, I Love My Wife, Willy Wonka and the Chocolate Factory, One Is A Lonely Number, Visions of Eight.
TV: The Morning After, I Will Fight No More Forever, Collision Course, Roots, Roots: The Next Generation, Moviola, Murder Is Easy, The Thorn Birds, A Caribbean Mystery, Sparkling Cyanide, A Killer in the Family, The Mystic Warrior, A Bunny's Tale.

MARIN, RICHARD: Actor-Writer. b. Los Angeles, July 13, 1946. Teamed with Tommy Chong in improvisational group. Has made comedy recordings with him.
PICTURES: Cheech and Chong's Up in Smoke, Cheech and Chong's Next Movie, Cheech and Chong's Nice Dreams, Things Are Tough All Over, It Came from Hollywood, Still Smokin', Cheech and Chong's The Corsican Brothers, After Hours.

MARK, LAURENCE M.: Producer/Executive. b. New York City. e. Wesleyan Univ., New York Univ. Started career as trainee and publicist for United Artists; also asst. to producer on Lenny, Smile, etc. Joined Paramount Pictures as mktg./prod. liaison dir. and then exec. dir., pub. for m.p. division in New York. Named v.p., prod./mktg. at Paramount Studio; 1980, v.p., west coast mktg.; 1982 promoted to post as v.p., prod. 1984, joined 20th Century-Fox as exec. v.p., prod.; 1986, established Laurence Mark Productions at Fox while remaining senior prod. exec.
PICTURES: Black Widow (exec. prod.)

MARKHAM, MONTE: Actor. b. Monatee, Fla., June 21, 1938. e. Univ. of Ga. Military service in Coast Guard after which joined resident theatre co. at Stephens College, Missouri, where also taught acting. Joined ACT Theatre, San Francisco, for three years. Made TV debut in Mission: Impossible episode then starred in two series.
PICTURES INCLUDE: One Is a Lonely Number, Hour of the Gun, Guns of the Magnificent Seven, Midway, Airport '77, Ginger in the Morning, Jake Speed.
TELEVISION: The Second Hundred Years (series), Mr. Deeds Goes to Town (series), The New Perry Mason (series), Visions (movie), The Astronaut (movie), Death

Takes a Holiday (movie).
BROADWAY: Irene.

MARKLE, FLETCHER: Writer, director, producer. b. Canada, March 27, 1921. Writer, dir., prod. Canadian Broadcasting Co. & BBC, London, 1942–46; prod., dir. Studio One series, CBS, 1947–48; Ford Theatre, CBS, 1948–49; writer, ed. & narrator The Robot Bomb, prize-winning doc. short, 1941; first m.p. dir. Jigsaw, 1949; thereafter Night Into Morning, The Man With a Cloak; prod. Studio One series, CBS, 1952–53; prod., dir., Life with Father, CBS-TV, 1953–55; Front Row Center, 1955. Contributing dir. and/or prod. to various TV film series: Mystery Theatre, Panic, No Warning, Colgate Theatre, Lux Playhouse, M Squad, Buckskin, Rendezvous, Tales of the Vikings, Thriller, Hong Kong, 1956–61. Dir. Father of the Bride, 1961; dir. m.p., The Incredible Journey, 1962; Telescope series, CBC-TV, 1963–72. Head of TV Drama, Canadian Broadcasting Corp. 1970–73, Exec. prod., CBC-TV features and writer in residence. University of Toronto, 1974–75.

MARKOE, JERRY: Composer-Arranger-Conductor. b. New York, N.Y. March 22, 1941. e. Manhattan School of Music (BM, MM in composition, 1968); Julliard School of Music. Winner of ASCAP music for theatre awards.
MUSICALS: Macbird, Fair Play for Eve, Another Time.
MUSIC FOR FILM, THEATER and TV: Faust, The Chinese Wall, He Who Gets Slapped, Ethan Frome, The Lion in Winter, Indulgences in the Louisville Harem, The Cycle, The Ancient Art of Tai Chi.
CHILDREN'S MUSICALS FOR STAGE & TV: Alice in Wonderland, Punch & Judy, Alladin, Cinderella, The Black Princess, Forgotten Treasure, Androcles and the Lion.

MARKOWITZ, ROBERT: Director. Mostly on TV before theatrical debut with Voices, 1979.
TELEVISION: The Deadliest Season, Song of Myself, With All Deliberate Speed, The 34th Star, The Storyteller, Kojak: The Belarus File, Alex: The Life of a Child.

MARKS, ALFRED: Actor-Comedian. b. London, TV, own series, Alfred Marks Time with wife, comedienne Paddie O'Neil.
PICTURES INCLUDE: Desert Mice, There Was A Crooked Man, Weekend With Lulu, The Frightened City, She'll Have To Go.
TV: Blanding's Castle, Hobson's Choice, Paris 1900, The Memorandum.

MARKS, ARTHUR: Producer, Director, Writer, Film Executive. b. Los Angeles, Calif., Aug. 2, 1927. M. Has 4 children. At 19 began work at MGM Studios as Production Messenger. Became Asst. Dir. in 1951, youngest dir. member of Directors Guild of Amer., 1957. Prod. of Perry Mason TV Show from 1961–66. Dir. of over 100 Perry Mason episodes. Prod.-dir.-writer of feature film Togetherness. Writer-director of Class of '74, writer-director of Bonnie's Kids, writer-director of The Roommates, producer-director of Detroit 9000, producer-director of The Centerfold Girls, director of A Woman For All Men, executive producer of Wonder Woman, executive producer, The Candy Snatchers. President and board member of Arthur Prod., Inc. & Arm Service Co. Exec. head of prod., Henry Plitt Theatres. Writer-director of numerous TV shows: I Spy, Mannix, Starsky & Hutch, Dukes of Hazzard, etc.
RECENT CREDITS: Bucktown (dir.), Friday Foster (prod., dir.) J.D.'s Revenge (prod.-dir.), Monkey Hustle (prod., dir.).

MARKS, RICHARD E.: Executive. e. UCLA; UCLA School of Law. 1978–82, v.p., legal & business affairs for Ziegler/Diskant Literary Agency. Appt. pres., Major Business Brokers. Joined Paramount Pictures 1984 as sr. atty. for Network TV Div., as project atty. for Family Ties & Cheers. 1985, named sr. atty. for M.P. Group.

MARKSON, BEN: Writer. b. Creston, Ia., Aug. 6. Army Capt., W.W. II. Reporter, feature writer columnist, playwright (Is My Face Red?). Joined Warners, 1932 as writer; since author orig. s.p. dial., adapt., collab., many pictures. Writes many TV plays.
PICTURES INCLUDE: Here Comes the Navy, Woman-Wise, Danger, Love at Work, Is My Face Red?, Brides Are Like That, Half-Naked Truth, Lady Killer, That I May Live, White Cockatoo, Goodbye Again, Great Mr. Nobody, The Beautiful Cheat, A Close Call for Boston Blackie, Prison Ship, The Falcon in San Francisco, Mr. District Attorney, It Happened on Fifth Ave., Edge of Eternity, With My Face to The Enemy.

MARLEY, J. PEVERELL: Cameraman. b. San Jose, Calif., Aug. 14, 1901; Chief cameraman for C.B. DeMille for The Ten Commandments, The Volga Boatman, King of Kings.
PICTURES INCLUDE: Night and Day, Of Human Bondage, Two Mrs. Carrolls, Life with Father, Off Limits, House of Wax, Serenade.

MARLOW, LUCY: Actress. r.n. Lucy Ann McAleer; b. Los Angeles, Calif., Nov. 20, 1932; e. U. of Ariz.
PICTURES INCLUDE: A Star Is Born, Lucky Me, Tight Spot, My Sister Eileen, Queen Bee, Bring Your Smile Along.

MARLOWE, LOUIS J.: Producer, director. r.n. L. J. Goetten. b. St. Cloud, Minn., Jan. 4, e. Hollywood H.S., USC. Prop man, asst. dir., unit mgr., dr. special effects, shorts, second units Warner Bros., freelance dir. comedy series; Director features both theatrical and TV programs.
PICTURES INCLUDE: On the Air, Always Tomorrow, Handing It Back, Tradition, One Above All, Just a Boy.

MARLY, FLORENCE: Actress. b. Czechoslovakia, June 2; e. Sorbonne, Paris. Appeared in 9 films in France inc. L'Alibi, Cafe de Paris, Les Maudits; also films in Argentina, Czechoslovakia.
PICTURES INCLUDE: Sealed Verdict, Tokyo Joe, Tokyo File 212, Gobs and Gals, Queen of Blood, Games.

MARQUAND, RICHARD: Director. b. England. Did commercials and TV films before theatrical m.p. debut, The Legacy (1979).
PICTURES: Eye of the Needle, Return of the Jedi, Until September, Jagged Edge.
TELEVISION: The Search of the Nile, Birth of the Beatles.

MARRIOTT, PETER: Executive. b. Isle of Wright, England, 1921. Ent. ind. 1949. Assoc. prod. TV series Douglas Fairbanks Presents. Assoc. prod. Chase A Crooked Shadow, Moment of Danger, etc. Man. dir. Desilu Sales Inc. Dir. U.K. and Continental TV Sales 20th Century-Fox. Now man. dir. and dir. European operations NBC International (G.B.) Ltd.

MARSHALL, E. G.: Actor. b. Minnesota, June 18, 1910. Acting debut with Oxford Players, 1933. Numerous TV appearances on all networks; m.p. debut in House on 92nd St.
BROADWAY: Jason, Jacobowsky and the Colonel, Skin of Our Teeth, Iceman Cometh, Woman Bites Dog, The Survivors, The Gambler, The Crucible, The Little Foxes.
PICTURES INCLUDE: 13 Rue Madeleine, Call Northside 77, Caine Mutiny, Pushover, Bamboo Prison, Broken Lance, Silver Chalice, Left Hand of God, Scarlet Hour, 12 Angry Men, Bachelor Party, Town Without Pity, The Chase, Tora, Tora, Tora, The Bridge at Remagen, The Pursuit of Happiness, Interiors, Superman II, Creepshow, Power, My Chauffeur.
TV: The Defenders, The Bold Ones. Movies: The Winter of Our Discontent, Under Seige.

MARSHALL, FRANK: Producer. Worked on first feature film in 1967 while still a student at UCLA. Protege of Peter Bogdanovich, working on his production crew and serving as assoc. prod. on Paper Moon, Daisy Miller, Nickelodeon, etc. Line producer on Orson Welles' The Other Side of the Wind (unreleased) and Martin Scorsese's The Last Waltz. Worked with Walter Hill on The Driver (assoc. prod.) and The Warriors (exec. prod.). Began collaboration with Steven Spielberg as prod. for Raiders of the Lost Ark.
PICTURES: Poltergeist (exec. prod.); E.T.: The Extra-Terrestrial (prod. supvr.); Twilight Zone—The Movie (exec. prod.); Indiana Jones and the Temple of Doom (exec. prod.); Gremlins (exec. prod.); Goonies (exec. prod.); Back to the Future (exec. prod.); The Color Purple (co-prod.); Young Sherlock Holmes (co-prod.).

MARSHALL, GARRY: Producer-Director-Writer. b. New York City, Nov. 13, 1934. e. Northwestern Univ. Copy boy and reporter for NY Daily News while writing comedy material for Phil Foster, Joey Bishop. Partner with Jerry Belson many years.
PICTURES: Writer-Producer: How Sweet It Is, The Grasshopper. Director: Young Doctors in Love (also exec. prod.), The Flamingo Kid (also s.p.). Acted in Lost in America.
TELEVISION: Writer for Jack Paar Show, Joey Bishop Show, Danny Thomas Show, Lucy, Dick Van Dyke Show, I Spy, etc. Creator and exec. prod.: Happy Days, Laverne & Shirley, Mork and Mindy, etc.

MARSHALL, LARRY: Comedian, actor, writer, songwriter. b. Clarkston, Scotland. Trained Rutherglen repertory theatre. Own daily lunchtime television show for eight years. Appeared in many major television drama series; and light entertainment show; own evening shows; comedy and panel games. Since 1973 written, produced and starred in summer show, Jamie's Scottish Night Out currently running to 1987.

MARSHALL, PENNY: Actress. b. New York City, Oct. 15, 1944. m. actor Bob Reiner. Dropped out of Univ. of New Mexico to teach dancing. Acted in summer stock before going to Hollywood to make TV debut in The Danny Thomas Hour. Debut as theatrical director 1986: Jumpin' Jack Flash.
TV: The Bob Newhart Show, The Mary Tyler Moore Show, Chico and the Man, The Odd Couple (regular), Laverne & Shirley (regular). Movies: Let's Switch, Love Thy Neighbor, Challenge of a Lifetime.
PICTURES: 1941, Movers and Shakers.

MARSHALL, PETER: Actor-TV Show Host. b. Huntington, W. Va., March 30. r.n. Pierre La Cock. Began career as NBC page in N.Y.C. Did plays both on and off Bdwy., starring with Julie Harris in Skyscraper. Teamed with the late Tommy Noonan in comedy act for nightclubs, guesting on Ed Sullivan Show and other variety shows. In 1974 made Las Vegas stage debut and since has been headliner there and in Reno and Lake Tahoe.
PICTURES INCLUDE: Ensign Pulver, The Cavern, Americathon.
TV: Two of the Most (local N.Y. show), The Hollywood Squares (host).

MARSHALL, TRUDY: Actress. b. Brooklyn, N.Y. Commercial photographers' model before entering pictures, 1942.
PICTURES INCLUDE: Secret Agent of Japan, Girl Trouble, Sentimental Journey, Dragonwyck, Talk About a Lady, Boston Blackie and the Law, Alias Mr. Twilight, Too Many Winners, Joe Palooka in the Knockout, Key Witness, Fuller Brush Man, Disaster, Shamrock Hill, Mark of Gorilla, The President's Lady.

MARSHALL, WILLIAM: Actor. b. Chicago, Ill., Oct. 12, 1917. In 1936, vocalist with Fred Waring's Orchestra; from 1937 orch. leader; on stage 1943, Army Air show Winged Victory. Screen debut 1940 in Sante Fe Trail.
PICTURES INCLUDE: Flowing Gold, City for Conquest, Flying with Music, Murder in the Music Hall, Earl Carroll's Sketchbook, That Brennan Girl, Calendar Girl, Blackmail, Adventures of Captain Fabian, Seven Different Ways.

MARSHALL, ZENA: Actress. b. Kenya (East Africa). e. France and finishing school in Ascot (England). Made her stage debut in repertory. Many TV appearance U.S. and England including Bob Hope show, Harpers W.I., Ghost Squad.
PICTURES INCLUDE: Marry Me, Dark Interval, Blind Man's Bluff, Love's a Luxury, Deadly Nightshade, My Wife's Family, Bermuda Affair, Let's Be Happy, Dr. No, The Guilty Party, Those Magnificent Men In Their Flying Machines, The Terrornauts.
TV: International Detective, Invisible Man, Dial 999, Danger Man, Sir Francis Drake, Man of The World, Human Jungle, Sentimental Agent, Court Martial.

MARTA, JACK: Cameraman, Republic Studios. b. Butte, Montana, 1905; e. Los Angeles public schools. Began as laboratory worker for Fox. Then to Columbia. Later with Republic.
PICTURES INCLUDE: In Old Sacramento, Bells of San Angelo, Bill and Cool, Fair Wind to Java, Jubilee Trail, Timberjack, Last Command, Come Next Spring, Maverick Queen.

MARTEL, GENE: Producer, director. b. New York, N.Y., June 19, 1916. e. C.C.N.Y., University of Alabama, Sorbonne, Paris; newspaperman, New York and Birmingham, Ala.; dancer, actor, choreographer, director Broadway; prod. dir., many documentaries; films for State Department, others; dir. for Paramount Pictures. Joined Princess Pictures 1952 to make films in Europe; formed own company, Martel Productions Inc., 1954.
PICTURES INCLUDE: Check-mate, Double-barrelled Miracle, The Lie, Double Profile, Sergeant and the Spy, Black Forest, Eight Witnesses, Fire One, Phantom Caravan, Doorway to Suspicion, Diplomatic Passport, Immediate Disaster.

MARTENS, RALPH R.: Executive b. New York, N.Y. e. N.Y. Suny At Albany. USMC-USMCR 1962–Present, 1970–1973 Tampax Inc. 1973–1979 Pannell Kerr Forster and Co., CPA's 1979–84, asst. treas. Motion Picture Association of America, MPEAA, AMPECA, AFRAM FILMS, 1984 Treas., MPAA, MPEAA, AMPECA and AFRAM.

MARTIN, AL: Writer since 1932, including: (s.p.) The Last Alarm; (orig., s.p.) Flying Wild; (collab. orig., s.p.) Mississippi Gambler; (s.p.) Stagecoach Buckaroo, The Devil with Hitler; (joint orig. s.p.) Gang Busters, serial: s.p., Amazon Quest; orig. story, Standing Room Only, Adventures of Rusty; s.p., Nine Girls, Strange Mrs. Crane; collab. s.p. Racing Luck; s.p., Army Bound, In the Money.
TV: Trouble with Father, Mystery Theatre, Ramar of the Jungle, Joe Palooka, Hank McCune Show, Wild Bill Hickok, Craig Kennedy Series, Mayor of the Town, Ford Theatre, Frontier Doctor, Lone Ranger, Damon Runyon Theatre, Roy Rogers, Screen Gems, Dupont Theatre, Gray Ghost, Restless Gun, Whirlybird, Trouble Shooters, Huckleberry Finn (serial), Spark Tarzan, 77 Sunset Strip, Man Trap, Laramie, My Favorite Martian; co-creat., My Living Doll.

MARTIN, DEAN: Actor. b. Steubenville, Ohio, June 17, 1917. e. Steubenville High School. Was amateur prizefighter; worked at odd jobs, mill hand, gasoline attendant, prior to acting career. Joined Jerry Lewis, comedian at 500 Club, Atlantic City, N.J., as straight man-singer, 1946; played many theatres, night clubs (see biography: Jerry Lewis). Team m.p. debut: My Friend Irma. Voted (with Jerry Lewis) one of the top ten Money-Making Stars in Motion Picture Herald-Fame poll, 1951, 1953–55; Number One, 1952.
PICTURES INCLUDE: My Friend Irma Goes West, At War With the Army, That's My Boy, The Stooge, Sailor Beware, Jumping Jacks, The Caddy, Scared Stiff, Money from Home, Living It Up, Three Ring Circus, You're Never Too Young, Artists and Models, Pardners, Hollywod Or Bust, 10,000 Bedrooms, The Young Lions, Some Came Running, Rio Bravo, Career, Who Was That Lady?, Bells Are Ringing, Ocean's 11, Ada, Sergeants 3, Who's Got the Action?, Toys In the Attic, Who's That Sleeping in My Bed, Robin and the Seven Hoods, Kiss Me Stupid, Sons of Katie Elder, Rough Night in Jericho, How To Save a Marriage, Airport, The Ambushers, The Wrecking Crew, Something Big, Showdown, Mr. Ricco, The Cannonball Run, Cannonball Run II.
TV: Club Oasis, Dean Martin Show. Golden Globe Award.

MARTIN, DEWEY: Actor. b. Katemcy, Texas, Dec. 8: e. U. of Ga., Louisiana State Teachers Coll. U.S. Navy, W.W. II; actor, little theatres & stock; m.p. debut in Knock on Any Door.
PICTURES INCLUDE: The Thing, Big Sky, Tennessee Champ, Prisoner of War, Men of the Fighting Lady, Land of the Pharaohs, Desperate Hours, Proud and Profane, 10,000 Bedrooms.

MARTIN, EDWIN DENNIS: Executive. b. Columbus, Ga., Jan. 30, 1920, e. grad., Univ. of Georgia, B. S., 1940; Past pres., Martin Theatre Cos.; past pres. TOA, International. Retired.

MARTIN, HENRY H.: Executive. b. Holcomb, Miss., March 22, 1912. Joined Universal poster clerk, Oklahoma City, 1935; then booker, then salesman. Military service 1943–46. Rejoined Universal as salesman, Oklahoma City, then branch manager; to Dallas as branch manager, 1948, to district manager, 1951, to New York as southern division manager 1956; general sales manager, 1957. Elected v.p. Universal Pictures Co., Inc., Nov. 2, 1959. Named v.p. of MCA, Inc., Dec., 1972 and president of Universal, Jan. 1, 1973. Retired.

MARTIN, MARY: Actress. b. Wetherford, Texas, Dec. 1, 1914; e. Ward-Belmont Sch., Nashville, Tenn.; m.p. debut in 1939.
STAGE: Lute Song, Leave It to Me, One Touch of Venus, South Pacific, Annie Get Your Gun, Kind Sir, Peter Pan, Jennie, I Do I Do.
PICTURES INCLUDE: Great Victor Herbert, Rhythm on the River, Love Thy Neighbor, Kiss the Boys Goodbye, New York Town, Birth of the Blues, Happy Go Lucky, Night and Day.
TV: Ford anniversary show, Rodgers & Hammerstein Cavalcade show. Peter Pan, Together with Music (with Noel Coward).

MARTIN, MILLICENT: Actress, singer. Toured U.S. The Boy Friend, 1954–57.
STAGE: Expresso Bongo, The Crooked Mile, Our Man Crichton, Tonight at 8, The Beggars Opera, Puss 'n Boots, The Card, Absurd Person Singular, Aladdin, Side By Side By Sondheim, Move Over Mrs. Markham, Meet Mr. Stewart, 42nd Street (N.Y. & L.A.).
TV: International Detective Series, Millie, That Was the Week That Was, Harry Moorings; own series, Mainly Millicent, Kiss Me Kate; 1966 own series, Millicent TV; 1967: London Palladium Color Show, USA, Danny Kaye, Piccadilly London; From a Bird's Eye View (own series); Tom Jones show, Englebert Humperdinck show.
PICTURES INCLUDE: The Horsemaster, The Girl on the Boat, Nothing But the Best, Alfie, Stop the World I Want To Get Off.

MARTIN, PAMELA SUE: Actress. b. Westport, CT, Jan. 15, 1953. Did modelling and TV commercials before entering films.
PICTURES: To Find a Man, The Poseidon Adventure, Buster and Billie, Our Time, The Lady in Red, Torchlight (also assoc. prod. & s.p.).
TELEVISION: Series: Nancy Drew Mysteries, Dynasty. Movies: The Gun and the Pulpit, The Girls from Huntington House, Angel on My Shoulder, etc.

MARTIN, RICHARD: Producer-Director. b. New York City, Feb. 2, 1938. e. Harvard. Stage and TV actor in N.Y. from 1959 to 1969; writer from 1969–73.
PICTURES INCLUDE: The Bengal Tiger, The Chase Expedition, Jaws of Death (also s.p.).

MARTIN, STEVE: Actor. b. Waco, TX, 1945. e. Long Beach Coll., UCLA. Writer for various TV comedy shows (Smothers Brothers, Sonny & Cher, etc.). Acted on TV in Steve Martin—A Wild and Crazy Guy, Steve Allen Comedy Hours, Comedy Is Not Pretty, etc.
PICTURES: The Kids Are Alright, The Muppet Movie, The Jerk, Pennies from Heaven, Dead Men Don't Wear

Plaid (also co.-s.p.), The Man with Two Brains, Lonely Guy, All of Me, The Little Shop of Horrors, Three Amigos (also co-s.p.).

MARTIN, TONY: Singer, musician, actor. b. Oakland, Calif., Dec. 25, 1913; e. Oakland H.S., St. Mary's Coll.; m. Cyd Charisse, actress-dancer. Sang, played saxophone & clarinet in high school band, engaged by nearby theatres for vaudeville; with Five Red Peppers, jazz group at 14 yrs.; two yrs. later with band, Palace Hotel, San Francisco; radio debut Walter Winchell program, 1932; joined Tom Gerund's band, World's Fair Chicago, 1933; played night clubs. First starring radio show, Tune Up Time (singer & emcee); on Burns and Allen program; own show for Texaco, Carnation Contented Hour.

RECORDINGS INCLUDE: Begin the Beguine, Intermezzo, The Last Time I Saw Paris, I'll See You in My Dreams, Domino, September Song.

PICTURES INCLUDE: Sing Baby Sing, Follow The Fleet, You Can't Have Everything; Ali Baba Goes toTown, Music in My Heart, Ziegfield Girl, Till The Clouds Roll By, Cabash, Two Tickets to Broadway, Here Come the Girls, Easy to Love, Deep in My Heart, Hit the Deck, Quincannon Frontier Scout, Let's Be Happy, The Big Store.

MARTINI, ALLEN V.: Executive. b. San Francisco, Dec. 14, 1919. e. Stanford U. Since resigning from Air Force ent. m.p. ind., 1945. Executive capacity RKO Studios; partner Filmakers Prod., 1950; United Artists Television, 1953; associated with National General Corporation since 1963; man. dir., Carthay Center Productions Ltd., National General's subsidiary, London, 1966; vice-pres., National General Productions Inc.; formerly vice-president, National General Television Corporation..

MARTINS, ORLANDO: Actor, singer, b. Lagos, Nigeria; e. Eko High School, Lagos, Stage debut, Stevedore, 1937; screen debut; Men Of Two Worlds, 1946.

PICTURES INCLUDE: The Hasty Heart, Where No Vultures Fly, West Of Zanzibar, Simba, Safari, Seven Waves Away, Naked Earth, The Nun's Story, Sapphire, Frankie & Johnnie, Cry the Beloved Country, In Judea, This Book Is News, Killers of Kilimanjaro, Sammy Going South, Call Me Bwana, Mister Moses.

MARTON, ANDREW: Director. b. Budapest, Hungary, Jan. 26, 1904. Vita Film, Vienna, 1922; to Hollywood, with Ernst Lubitsch, 1923; started directing in Berlin, then in London, Wolf's Clothing, Secret of Stamboul, School for Husbands; in Hollywood, Little Bit of Heaven, Gentle Annie, Gallant Bess.

PICTURES INCLUDE: King Solomon's Mines, Wild North, Storm Over Tibet, Devil Makes Three, Gypsy Colt, Prisoner of War, Men of the Fighting Lady, Green Fire, Underwater Warrior, Cinerama Seven Wonders of the World, It Happened In Athens, The Longest Day, The Thin Red Line, Crack in the World, Clarence the Crosseyed Lion, Around the World Under The Sea, Birds Do It, Africa-Texas Style, Mohammed, Messenger of God.

TV: Man and The Challenge, Daktari, Cowboy in Africa, The Sea Hunt.

MARVIN, LEE: Actor. b. New York, N.Y., Feb. 19, 1924. Played in summer stock cos.; Bway, debut in Billy Budd; m.p. debut in You're in the Navy Now.

PICTURES INCLUDE: Diplomatic Courier, We're Not Married, Down Among the Sheltering Palms, Eight Iron Men, Stranger Wore a Gun, Big Heat, Gun Fury, Wild One, Caine Mutiny, Gorilla at Large, The Raid, Bad Day at Black Rock, Life in the Balance, Violent Saturday, Not As a Stranger, Pete Kelly's Blues, I Died a Thousand Times, The Rack, Shack Out on 101, Attack!, The Killers, Ship of Fools, Cat Ballou, The Professionals, The Dirty Dozen, Point Blank, Sergeant Ryker, Paint Your Wagon, Monte Walsh, Pocket Money, Prime Cut, Emperor of the North, The Spikes Gang, The Iceman Cometh, The Klansman, Great Scout, and Cathouse Thursday, Shout at the Devil, Death Hunt, Gorky Park, The Delta Force.

TELEVISION: The Dirty Dozen: The Next Mission.

MARX, SAMUEL: Writer-producer. b. New York City, Jan. 26, 1902.

PICTURES INCLUDE: Lassie Come Home, This Man's Navy, My Brother Talks to Horses, The Beginning or End, A Lady Without Passport, Grounds for Marriage, Kiss of Fire, Ain't Misbehavin', Waterloo, Rome, The Ravine.

MASEFIELD, JOSEPH R.: Executive, Producer, Director, Writer. b. N.Y., N.Y., June 20, 1933, 1950 American Academy of Dramatic Arts. Writer-performer, club work (as Steve Parker). Later, actor in stock; formed EEF Film Productions, 1956; prod. A Story Like Two (short), A City Eats (doc.). In m.p. as unit mgr., asst. dir. and prod. mgr. Later writer and film editor: Montage (Time-Life); Ages of Man (IBM); Festival of Two Worlds (Bell Telephone Hour) and special, The New Face of Israel. Asst. dir., prod. mgr., Mitgebracht Aus New York (German TV), The Devils Doubloon, (feature); Writer-director, Citizen Smith, feature documentary. Co-director and assoc. prod. Hear My Song, (Cavalier Films), 1969 producer The Spy. 1969, vice pres. in charge of prod. PCI, Inc. Public Relations director, The Max Steiner Music Society; pres., Joseph R. Masefield & Associates. In 1974, formed Majer Prods. with Steve Jerro.

PICTURES INCLUDE: A New Life, The Vanquished, Trio, Living Planet, The Burning Man.

MASLANSKY, PAUL: Producer—Director—Writer. Studied filmmaking at Cinemateque Francais where made a documentary (Letter from Paris) which won Cannes Festival award. Asst. dir. on Counterfeit Traitor; followed by prod. mgr. on several films in Europe, including The Running Man and Jason and the Argonauts. Wrote and produced Gothic horror films, including Castle of the Living Dead. Covered Israeli war in 1967 with CBS film group; spent year in Russia on The Red Tent, followed by The Blue Bird. Filmed Big Truck and Poor Claire in Israel; Miracles Still Happen in Brazil.

PICTURES: Damnation Alley (co-prod.), When You Comin' Back, Red Ryder (co-prod.), Hot Stuff, The Villain, Scavenger Hunt, Police Academy 2, Return to Oz, Police Academy 3.

MASON, JOHN DUDLEY: Executive. b. Ashland, KY, Oct 29, 1949. e. Amherst College (B.A., cum laude, 1971), Claremont Graduate School and University Center (M.A., 1973), Amos Tuck School of Business Administration , Dartmouth College (M.B.A., 1978). Program officer, National Endowment for the Humanities, 1972–1976; analyst1978–1979), asst. mgr. (1979–1980), mgr. (1980) strategic planning, Consolidated Rail Corp.; Consultant, Frito-Lay, Division, PepsiCo (1980–1982); mgr, corporate planning, The Dun & Bradstreet Corp (1982–1986); finance director, anti-piracy, Motion Picture Association of America, Inc. (1986–present).

MASON, KENNETH M.: Executive. b. Rochester, N.Y. Sept. 21, 1917. e. Washington and Jefferson College; Univ. of Rochester (graduate work). Began career with Eastman Kodak Co. in Kodak Park cine processing dept. in 1935; transferred following year to film developing dept. at Kodak Research Laboratories. Returned to college in 1938 to complete studies and returned to Kodak year later to same dept. Later joined film planning dept., remaining there until entering military service in 1943. Returned to Kodak in 1946 as staff engineer in Kodak Office motion picture film dept. In 1950 appt. mgr. of Midwest Division, of M.P. Film Dept.; became gen. mgr., Midwest Division, m.p. products sales dept. in 1963; named sls. mgr. of New York City region in 1965; appt. regional sls. mgr., Pacific Southern Region, Hollywood, in 1970. On Jan. 1, 1974 appt. mgr., product programs and research, Motion Picture and Audiovisual Markets Division, Kodak Office. On March 18, 1974 named gen. mgr. of that division. Elected asst. v.p. of co. on March 28, 1974, v.p., Dec. 11, 1978. Retired Oct. 1, 1982, now chm., Inter-Society Committee for the Enhancement of Theatrical Presentation.

MEMBER: Pres., Board of Trustees of Washington and Jefferson College; past pres. of Society of Motion Picture & Television Engineers and honorary member, honorary fellow of British Kinematograph Sound & Television Society; mbr. of University Film Assn., Motion Picture Academy, American Society of Cinematographers, Variety Club. Board of Directors: Will Rogers Institute, Institute of Allied Film & Video. Univ. Film & Video Foundation.

MASON, MARSHA: Actress. b. St. Louis. April 3, 1942. m. Neil Simon. Came to N.Y. to continue dramatic studies and embark on theatre career. Appeared off-Broadway (Happy Birthday, Wanda June, Deerpark) and on Broadway (Cactus Flower). Now member of American Conservatory Theatre, San Francisco.

PICTURES INCLUDE: Blume in Love (debut), Cinderella Liberty, Audrey Rose, The Goodbye Girl, The Cheap Detective, Promises in the Dark, Chapter Two, Only When I Laugh, Max Dugan Returns.

TV: Love of Life (series), Brewsie and Willie, Cyrano de Bergerac, Surviving, Trapped in Silence.

MASON, PAMELA: Actress, writer. b. Westgate. England. Mar. 10, 1918; Stage debut 1936, The Luck of the Devil, London; also playwright (in collab. James Mason, Flying Blind, Made in Heaven), Author novels This Little Hand, A Lady Possessed, The Blinds Are Down, Ignoramus, Began Brit. screen career 1938, I Met a Murderer (orig. story & s.p.; cast); also in They Were Sisters, 1944. In 1946 (s.p. & Cast) The Upturned Glass; (acted) Pandora and the Flying Dutchman; acted, collab. s.p. Lady Possessed, Syndicated TV, Pamela Mason Show, author Marriage Is the First Step Toward Divorce. syndicated TV The Weaker Sex?; author, The Female Pleasure Hunt; lectures at women's clubs countrywide.

MASSEN, OSA: Actress. b. Denmark, Copenhagen. Jan. 13, 1916.

PICTURES INCLUDE: Honeymoon in Bali, Honeymoon for Three, A Woman's Face, Accent on Love, You'll Never

Get Rich, The Devil Pays Off, Ireland, Strange Journey, Night Unto Night, Deadline at Dawn, Gentleman Misbehaves, Rocketship XM.

MASSEY, ANNA: Actress. b. Sussex, England, Aug. 11, 1937. Daughter of Raymond Massey. On London stage in Spoiled, Doctor's Delimma, School for Scandal, etc.
PICTURES: Peeping Tom, Bunny Lake Is Missing, The Looking Glass War, David Copperfield, Frenzy, A Little Romance, Sweet William.
TELEVISION: A Doll's House, Remember the Germans, Wicked Woman, The Corn Is Green, Sakharov, Hotel Du Loc.

MASSEY, DANIEL: Actor. b. London, Eng., Oct. 10, 1933. e. Eaton and King's Colleges f. Raymond Massey. Active on stage and TV.
PICTURES INCLUDE: Girls at Sea, Upstairs and Downstairs, The Queen's Guard, Go to Blazes, Moll Flanders, The Jokers, Star!, Fragment of Fear, Mary, Queen of Scots, Victory.

MASSIE, PAUL: Actor. b. Ontario, Canada. July 7, 1932. Early career on Canadian stage. Attended Central School, London, 1952, later jnd. Scottish National Children's Theatre. Entered m.p. ind. 1954 in Orders to Kill.
PICTURES INCLUDE: High Tide at Noon, Sapphire, Libel, The Two Faces of Dr. Jekyll, The Rebel, The Pot Carriers, Raising the Wind.
STAGE: Cat On a Hot Tin Roof.
TV: The Mark of the Warrior, The Last of the Brave, Ring Around the Moon, Secret Mission and Her Romeo.

MASTORAKIS, NICO: Writer-Director. b. Athens, Greece, 1941. Writer of novels and screenplays. Books include Fire Below Zero and The Ephesus Scrolls (co-author).
PICTURES: The Next One (s.p., dir.).

MASTROIANNI, MARCELLO: Actor. b. Fontane Liri, Italy, Sept. 28, 1923. e. U. of Rome theatrical company. Draftsman in Rome, 1940–43. Theatrical debut in Rome in Angelica, 1948.
PLAYS INCLUDE: Death of a Salesman, Streetcar Named Desire, Ciao Rudy.
PICTURES INCLUDE: Three Girls from Rome, The Miller's Beautiful Wife, Fever to Live, The Ladykillers of Rome, Love a La Carte, Days of Love, La Dolce Vita, White Nights, Divorce Italian Style, La Notte, A Very Private Affair, Bell Antonio, Where the Hot Wind Blows, The Organizer, 8½, Yesterday, Today and Tomorrow, Marriage Italian Style, Casanova '70, The 10th Victim, The Poppy Is Also a Flower, Shoot Loud, Louder . . . I Don't Understand, The Stranger, A Place for Lovers, Leo the Last, Diamonds for Breakfast, Sunflower, Jealousy Italian Style, The Priest's Wife. Formed indep. prod. co., Master Films, 1966; What?, The Grande Bouffe, Massacre in Rome, Down the Ancient Stairs, The Sunday Woman, A Special Day, Stay As You Are, Blood Feud, City of Women, Gabriella, Macaroni, Ginger and Fred.

MATALON, DAVID A.: Executive. Senior exec. v.p. and theatrical mgr. of Columbia Pictures International before joining Tri-Star Pictures in 1983 as exec. v.p. with responsibility for worldwide marketing and distribution. 1985, named Pres.

MATHESON, TIM: Actor. b. Los Angeles, Dec. 31, 1947. e. Calif. State Univ. Debut on tv at age 12 in My Three Sons. At 19 contract player for Universal regular on Bonanza. 1985, turned to direction: St. Elsewhere episode and music videos. Set up own productions co. at Burbank Studios 1985, acted off-Bdwy. in True West.
PICTURES: Divorce American Style, Yours, Mine and Ours, How to Commit Marriage, The Apple Dumpling Gang Rides Again, 1941, Magnum Force, Almost Summer, National Lampoon's Animal House, Dreamer, A Little Sex, To Be or Not To Be, Up the Creek, Impulse, Fletch.
TELEVISION: Movies: Owen Marshall, Counselor-at-Law, Lock, Stock and Barrel, Hitched, Remember When, The Last Day, The Runaway Barge, The Quest, Mary White, Obsessed with a Married Woman, Blind Justice.

MATHEWS, CAROLE: Actress. b. Montgomery, Ill., Sept. 13. e. Aurora, Ill. H.S. Started as night club, radio entertainer; to Hollywood, 1944.
PICTURES INCLUDE: Massacre River, Great Gatsby, Special Agent, Meet Me At the Fair, Swamp Woman, Port of Heil, Shark River, Treasure of Ruby Hills, Requirement for a Redhead, Look In Any Window, Thirteen Men, Female Fiend, Tender Is The Night, End of the Road.
TV: Steel Hour, Kraft Theatre, Lux Video, Hitchcock Presents, Studio One, Californians, Texan, 77 Sunset Strip, Perry Mason, Four Star Theatre, M-Squad, Death Valley Days, Guestward Ho, Two Faces West, Johnny Midnight, Pete & Gladys, 87th Precinct, Ben Casey.

MATLACK, JACK D.: Theatre executive, publicist. b. Manton, Calif., Feb. 22, 1914; e. Chico, Calif. State Teachers Coll. Entered m.p. ind. as doorman Criterion, Medford, Ore.; then mgr. dir.; joined J.J. Parker Theatres, Portland, Ore., 1943; as exec. asst. to pres. and adv. dir. eight theatres; now pres. Jack Matlack Promotions. Portland, Ore., N.W.P.R. for studios; well known showman, winner 20 exploit. awards including Grand (Silver) Quigley Award, 1943; Quigley War Showmanship Award, 1942–44; numerous Quigley Pub. citations; cited by U.S. Govt. for outstanding contrib. to World War II effort; active as civic worker; on bd. Portland, Ore. C. of C. Kiwanis, Portland City Planning Comm., Oregon Advertising Club; named First Citizen of Portland, 1944.

MATTHAU, WALTER: Actor. b. New York, Oct. 1, 1920. Served in Air Force WW II. Studied journalism at Columbia, then acted in summer stock. First Broadway role, 1948, in Anne of a Thousand Days.
THEATRE: Will Success Spoil Rock Hunter? and The Odd Couple.
PICTURES INCLUDE: A Face in the Crowd, The Kentuckian, Slaughter on Tenth Avenue, Indian Fighter, No Power on Earth, Middle of the Street, Onion Head, Voice in the Mirror, King Creole, Lonely Are the Brave, Strangers When We Meet, Who's Got the Action, The Gangster Story, Charade, Goodbye Charlie, Mirage, The Fortune Cookie, A Guide for the Married Man, The Odd Couple, Candy, Cactus Flower, Hello Dolly, A New Leaf, Plaza Suite, Pete 'n' Tillie, Charley Varrick, The Laughing Policeman, The Taking of Pelham One, Two, Three, The Front Page, The Sunshine Boys, The Bad News Bears, Casey's Shadow, House Calls, California Suite, Little Miss Marker, Hopscotch, First Monday in October, Buddy, Buddy, I Ought To Be in Pictures, The Survivors, Movers and Shakers, Pirates.

MATURE, VICTOR: Actor. b. Louisville, Ky., Jan. 29, 1916. TV retail store; trainee, Pasadena Theatre, Playbox Theatre; on B'way in Lady in the Dark; U.S. Coast Guard, WW II.
PICTURES INCLUDE: Housekeeper's Daughter, One Million B.C., Captain Caution, No No Nanette, I Wake Up Screaming, Shanghai Gesture, Song of the Islands, My Gal Sal, Footlight Serenade, Seven Days Leave, My Darling Clementine, Moss Rose, Kiss of Death, Cry of the City, Red Hot and Blue, Fury at Furnace Creek, Easy Living, Samson and Delilah, Wabash Avenue, Stella, Gambling House, Las Vegas Story, Androcles and the Lion, Million Dollar Mermaid, Something for the Birds, Glory Brigade, Affair with a Stranger, The Robe, Veils of Bagdad, Dangerous Mission, Betrayed, Demetrius & The Gladiators, The Egyptian, Chief Crazy Horse, Violent Saturday, Last Frontier, Safari, Zarak Pickup Alley, Tank Roce, The Bandit of Zhobe, Escort Wst., Big Circus, Timbuktu, Hannibal The Tartars, After the Fox, Every Little Crook and Nanny, Won Ton Ton, the Dog That Saved Hollywood, Firepower, The Screamer.
TELEVISION: Samson and Delilah.

MAUREY, NICOLE: Actress. b. France, 1925. Studied dancing; French films include Blondine, Pamela, Le Cavalier Noir; stage appearances in France; U.S. debut in Little Boy Lost.
PICTURES INCLUDE: Secret of the Incas, Bold and the Brave, House of The Seven Hawks, Day of the Triffids.

MAXWELL, RONALD F.: Writer-Director. b. Jan. 5, 1947. e. NY Univ. Coll. of Arts & Sciences; NY Univ. School of the Arts, Institute of Film & Television Graduate School (MFM, 1970). Producer-Director for PBS Theater-in-America.
PICTURES: Little Darlings (dir.); The Night the Lights Went Out in Georgia (dir.); Kidco (dir.); The Killer Angels (prod., dir., co-s.p.).
TELEVISION: Sea Marks (prod., dir.); Verna: USO Girl (prod., dir.).

MAY, ELAINE: Actress, Screenwriter. b. Philadelphia, Pa., April 21, 1932. Repertory theatre in Chicago, 1954; comedy team with Mike Nichols, 1955.
PICTURES INCLUDE: Luv, Enter Laughing. 1970: writer, dir., star, A New Leaf; dir., The Heartbreak Kid; dir., s.p., Mikey and Nicky. 1978; co-s.p. Heaven Can Wait; actress, California Suite; s.p., dir., Ishtar.

MAYEHOFF, EDDIE: Comedian. b. Baltimore, Md., July 7, 1914. e. Yale Sch. of Music. Adv. salesman, 1932; dance band leader, 6 yrs.; on radio with Norman Corwin; own show, Eddie Mayehoff on the Town; night clubs; B'way shows.
THEATRE: Let Freedom Sing, Early to Bed, Rhapsody, Billy Rose's Concert Varieties, Season in the Sun, Visit to a Small Planet.
TV: Adventures of Fenimore J. Mayehoff.
PICTURES INCLUDE: That's My Boy, The Stooge, Off Limits, Artists and Models, How to Murder Your Wife, Luv.

MAYER, BEN: Executive. b. Nov. 22, 1925. e. Manchester All Saints School of Art (England); Royal College of Art. President, Ben Mayer Design, Inc.

MAYER, GERALD: Producer, director. b. Montreal, Canada; p. both deceased: Jerry G., mgr. MGM studio, and Rheba

G Mayer (later Mrs. Hal Elias); e. Stanford (Journalism); corr. for San Francisco Examiner; pres. Sigma Delta Chi, prof. journalism soc. Navy lieut. amphibious forces, World War II. Entered m.p. ind. in prod. dept. MGM studios; first dir. job Dial 1119.

PICTURES INCLUDE: Dial 1119, Inside Straight, Sellout, Holiday for Sinners, Bright Road (Christopher Award for direction), The Marauders, African Drumbeat, and The Man Inside (Canadian).

TV: Canadian Broadcasting Corp. (prod./dir., TV Drama), prod. The Swiss Family Robinson (British-Canadian TV series). Director for U.S. TV: One Last Ride (mini-series), Airwolf, Lou Grant, Eight Is Enough, Quincy, Logan's Run, Mannix, Mission Impossible, Police Surgeon, Cimarron Strip, Peyton Place, Judd for the Defense, Bonanza, The Fugitive, Chrysler Thea., Ben Casey, Slattery's People, Profiles in Courage, The Defenders, Gunsmoke, etc.

MAYER, MICHAEL F.: Attorney-Executive b. White Plains, N.Y., Sept. 8, 1917; Harvard College B.S., 1939; Yale Law School L.L.B., 1942. Armed Forces 1942–46, Air Medal (1945); vice-pres. Kingsley International Pictures Corp., 1954–62. Executive Director and General Counsel, Independent Film Importers and Distributors of America Inc. (IFIDA), 1959–67. Special Counsel, French Society of Authors, Composers and Publishers, 1961–72; British Performing Rights Society, 1962–67. Author: Foreign Films on American Screens (1966); Divorce and Annulment (1967); What You Should Know About Libel and Slander (1968); Rights of Privacy (1972); The Film Industries (1973)—revised edition published in 1978). Lecturer on motion picture problems at N.Y.U., Stanford, Univ. of Pennsylvania, Dartmouth and New York State University (Albany). Teacher of courses on Business Problems in Film, New School (1971–1982). Secty. of Film Society of Lincoln Center, Inc.

MAYER, ROGER LAURANCE: Executive. b. New York City, Apr. 21, 1926. e. Yale Univ. (1948 graduate); Yale Law School (1951 graduate). In 1952 was practicing attorney; joined Columbia Pictures that year as atty. and named corp. exec., 1957. Left in 1961 to join MGM Studio as asst. gen. mgr. Since with MGM as follows: v.p., operations, 1964; v.p., administration, 1975–84. Also exec. v.p., MGM Laboratories, 1974–83. Now pres., MGM Laboratories and sr. v.p., studio admin.

MEMBER: Los Angeles County Bar Assn., Los Angeles Copyright Society, Academy of Motion Picture Arts & Sciences. Chm. & trustee for both Directors Guild Pension Plan and Producers Guild Pension Plan. Trustee, Motion Picture & TV Relief Fund and director, Permanent Charities.

MAYER, SEYMOUR R.: Executive. b. New York, N.Y., July 30, 1912; e. N.Y.C. schools. Div. mgr., Loew's in-town theatres, 1933; Armed Forces, WW II, as Major in charge of overseas m.p. service; with Loew's International: 1946, 1st v.p.; MGM Int'l.: 1963–69; pres., MGM Int'l.; worldwide sales, 1970; pres., MSD Int'l. worldwide sales.

MAYES, WENDELL: Writer. b. Hayti, Missouri e. Johns Hopkins, Columbia. Military service in Pacific, World War II. Began career as actor legit theatre, turned to writing for television. Gained television recognition before moving to Hollywood as motion picture writer.

PICTURES INCLUDE: Spirit of St. Louis, The Way to the Gold, Enemy Below, The Hunters, From Hell to Texas, The Hanging Tree, Anatomy of A Murder, Advise And Consent, In Harm's Way, Von Ryan's Express, Hotel, The Stalking Moon, The Poseidon Adventure, The Revengers, Bank Shot, Death Wish, Love & Bullets, Charlie, Go Tell The Spartans, Monsignor.

MAYO, VIRGINIA: Actress. r.n., Virginia Jones. b. St. Louis, Mo., Nov. 30, 1920. e. St. Louis dramatic school. With Billy Rose's Diamond Horseshoe; then N.Y. stage (Banjo Eyes).

PICTURES INCLUDE: Kid from Brooklyn, Best Years of Our Lives, Secret Life of Walter Mitty, Out of the Blue, Smart Girls Don't Talk, The Girl From Jones Beach, Flaxy Martin, Colorado Territory, Always Leave Them Laughing, Flame and the Arrow, West Point Story, Along the Great Divide, Captain Horatio Hornblower, Painting the Clouds with Sunshine, Starlift, She's Working Her Way Through College, Iron Mistress, She's Back on Broadway, South Sea Woman, Devil's Canyon, King Richard & the Crusaders, Silver Chalice, Pearl of the South Pacific, Great Day in the Morning, Proud Ones, Congo Crossing, Big Land, Young Fury, Fort Utah, Castle of Evil.

MAZURKI, MIKE: Actor. b. Ukrainian descent; Tarnopal, Austria, Dec. 25, 1909; e. Manhattan Coll., New York, B.A., 1930; married. Toured United States and Canada as heavyweight wrestler. Screen debut 1941 in Shanghai Gesture.

PICTURES INCLUDE: I Walk Alone, Unconquered, Nightmare Alley, Relentless, Neptune's Daughter, Come to the Stable, Rope of Sand, Samson & Delilah, Light Touch, Criminal Lawyer, Ten Tall Men, My Favorite Spy, The Egyptian, New Orleans Uncensored, New York Confidential, Blood Alley, Kismet, Davy Crockett, King of the Wild Frontier, Comanche, Around the World in 80 Days, Mad, Mad, Mad, Mad World, Four for Texas, Cheyenne Autumn, 7 Women, Bullwhip Griffin, Challenge to be Free, The Magic of Lassie, The Man with Bogart's Face, Doing Time.

MAZURSKY, PAUL: Producer-Director-Writer-Actor. b. Brooklyn, N.Y. April 25, 1930. Started acting in 1951 in the theatre, TV and films. Was nightclub comic 1954–1960 and directed plays. Began association with Larry Tucker by producing, directing, writing and performing in Second City, semi-improvisational revue. For four years they wrote the Danny Kaye TV show and created and wrote the Monkees series. First theatrical film I Love You, Alice B. Toklas (1969) which he wrote with Tucker and both men acted as exec. prod.

PICTURES INCLUDE: Bob and Carol and Ted and Alice, (dir., co-s.p.), Alex in Wonderland (dir., co-s.p., actor), Blume in Love (dir., s.p., prod., actor), Harry and Tonto (prod., dir., co-s.p.); Next Stop, Greenwich Village (prod., dir., s.p.); Unmarried Woman (prod., dir., s.p.); A Man, A Woman and A Bank (actor): Willie and Phil (prod., dir., s.p.); Tempest (prod., dir., s.p.); Moscow on the Hudson (prod., dir., co-s.p.); Down and Out in Beverly Hills (prod., dir., co-s.p.).

McBRIDE, JIM: Writer-Director. Began in underground film scene in New York. First film: David Holzman's Diary (1967), which won grand prize at Mannheim and Pesaro Film Festivals.

PICTURES: My Girlfriend's Wedding (actor, s.p., d.), Glen and Randa (s.p., d.), Pictures for Life's Other Sides (d.), Hot TImes (d.), Moviegoer (co. s.p.), Beathless (co. s.p., d.).

McCALL, JOAN: Actress-Writer. b. Grahn, Kentucky. e. Berea College, Starred on Broadway in Barefoot In The Park, The Star Spangled Girl, A Race of Hairy Men, and road companies of Barefoot In The Park, Star Spangled Girl, and Don't Drink The Water, Los Angeles Company of Jimmy Shine.

PICTURES INCLUDE: Grizzly, Act of Vengenance, The Devil Times Five. Screenwriter: The Predator, The Concision, Fly Away Home. 1980: Staff writer for The Days of Our Lives, Another World, As the World Turns, under the pen name Joan Pommer; Search for Tomorrow, Capitol, Santa Barbara.

McCALLUM, DAVID: Actor. b. Scotland, Sept. 19, 1933. Early career in rep. theatres and dir. plays for Army. Ent. m.p. Ind. 1953.

PICTURES INCLUDE: The Secret Place, Hell Drivers, Robbery Under Arms, Violent Playground, A Night to Remember, The Long and the Short and the Tall, Billy Budd, Freud, The Great Escape, The Greatest Story Ever Told, To Trap A Spy, Three Bits of the Apple, Sol Madrid, Mosquito Squadron, Watcher in the Woods.

TV: The Man From Uncle, The Invisible Man.

McCALLUM, JOHN: Actor, Producer, Director. b. Brisbane, Australia, CBE. Mar. 14, 1918; e. Royal Academy Dramatic Arts; served in Australian Imperial Forces. World War II. Appeared in repertory with Old Vic & Stratford-on-Avon seasons. On stage, 1937 in Judgment Day, Australian tour, 1955–56; on screen first 1944, Australia is Like This. Asst. man. dir. J. C. Williamson Theatres, Ltd., Australia, 1958; man. dir., 1960–66. Resigned chmn. Williamson-Powell Int. Films, 1965; chmn. Fauna Prod.; dir. Relatively Speaking on stage in Australia, 1968. Dir.; Plaza Suite, My Fair Lady, for Australian stage, 1969–70. Prod. TV Series, Skippy, Barrier Reef, Boney, Shannons Mob; London Stage 1973–74 Constant Wife. 1974 Comedy Theatre, Melbourne. 1976 Chichester Fest. 1976–77 The Circle. Exec. prod. Bailey's Bird, TV series.

PICTURES INCLUDE: A Son Is Born, Joe Goes Back, Root of All Evil, The Loves of Joanna Godden, It Always Rains on Sunday, Miranda, The Calendar, A Boy, a Girl and a Bike, Traveler's Joy, The Woman in Question, Valley of the Eagles, Lady Godiva Rides Again, Derby Day (Four Against Fate), Trent's Last Case, The Long Memory, Melba, Devil on Horseback, Trouble in the Glen, Smiley (in Australia), Safe Harbour, Nickel Queen (dir.); The Z Men (prod.); The Highest Honor (exec. prod.).

McCAMBRIDGE, MERCEDES: Actress. b. Joliet, Ill., March 17, 1918. e. Mundelein College Chicago, Ill., B.A. Did some radio work while in college; opposite Orson Welles two seasons, on Ford Theatre, other air shows; New York stage in: Hope for the Best, 1945; others: Place of Our Own, Twilight Bar, Woman Bites Dog, The Young and Fair; left latter play for Hollywood. Screen debut: All the King's Men (Academy Award for best supporting actress, 1950); own radio show, 1952.

PICTURES INCLUDE: Lightning Strikes Twice, Inside Straight, The Scarf, Johnny Guitar, Giant, A Farewell to Arms, Suddenly Last Summer, Cimarron, Angel Baby, Last

Generation, Jigsaw, 99 Women, Thieves, The Concord-Airport '79.
AUTHOR: The Two of Us.
TV: Numerous appearances.

McCARTHY, ANDREW: Actor. b. Westfield, NY. 1963. e. NYU. Studied acting at Circle-in-the-Square; on stage in Ah, Wilderness, A Midsummer Night's Dream, etc. Theatrical m.p. debut, Class (1984).
PICTURES: Heaven Help Us, St. Elmo's Fire, Pretty in Pink.

McCARTHY, FRANK: Producer. b. Richmond, Va., June 8, 1912. e. Virginia Military Institute and U. of Virginia, serving at VMI as instructor and tactical officer, and as police reporter for Richmond News-Leader, 1933–37. Press agent for producer George Abbott, 1937–39. During WW II was Asst. Secy. and later Secy. of War Dept. General Staff and military secy. to General George C. Marshall. Decorated with U.S. Distinguished Service, U.S. Legion of Merit, Order of the British Empire. Brigadier General in Army Reserve, Retired. In 1945, named Asst. Secy. of State for Administration; joined MPAA 1946 as asst. to v.p., later European mgr. Signed by 20th Century-Fox two years later as exec. and prod. Co-prod. Decision Before Dawn; prod., Sailor of the King, A Guide for the Married Man, Patton, Fireball Forward; at Universal, MacArthur.

McCARTHY, KEVIN: Actor. b. Seattle, Wash., Feb. 15, 1915. e. Minnesota U. Acted in sch. plays, stock; B'way debut in Abe Lincoln in Illinois. In U.S. Army; m.p. debut: Death of A Salesman.
PLAYS INCLUDE: Flight to West, Winged Victory, Truckline Cafe, Joan of Lorraine, Biography, Death of a Salesman, Anna Christie.
PICTURES INCLUDE: Drive a Crooked Road, Gambler from Natchez, Stranger on Horseback, Annapolis Story, Nightmare, Invasion of the Body Snatchers, A Big Hand for the Little Lady, Hotel, Kansas City Bomber, Buffalo Bill and the Indians, Hero at Large, Those Lips, Those Eyes.
TELEVISION: Movies: The Making of a Male Model, Deadly Intentions, The Midnight Hour, A Masterpiece of Murder.

McCARTNEY PAUL: Singer-Musician. b. Liverpool, England, Feb. 25, 1943. Member of The Beatles. Wrote songs for several films on own, including Live and Let Die (title), Oh Heavenly Dog. Formed group Wings for tours and recordings. Wrote script and music and acted in Give My Regards to Broad Street.

McCLORY, SEAN: Actor. b. Dublin, Ireland, March 8, 1924; e. Jesuit Coll., U. of Galway. With Gaelic Theatre, Galway; Abbey Theatre. Dublin. Brought to U.S., in 1946 under contract to RKO Pictures. Produced and directed numerous plays, member of the Directors Guild of America and is the author of the produced drama, Moment of Truth.
PLAYS INCLUDE: Shining Hour, Juno and the Paycock, Anna Christie, Escape to Autumn, King of Friday's Men, Lady's Not for Burning, Billy Budd, Dial M for Murder, The Winslow Boy, Shadow of A Gunman, Saint Joan.
PICTURES INCLUDE: Film debut: Dick Tracy vs. The Claw, Rough-Shod, Beyond Glory, Daughter of Rosie O'Grady, Storm Warning, Lorna Doone, What Price Glory, The Quiet Man, Diane, Island in the Sky, Ring of Fear, Them, Long Grey Line, Cheyenne Autumn, Plunder of the Sun Bay, Anne of the Indies, I CCover the Underworld, Botany Man in the Attic, Guns of Fort Petticoat, Kings Thief, Moonfleet, Bandolero, Day of the Wolves, Valley of the Dragons, Follow Me Boys, Rogues March, The Gnomobile, Well of the Saints, In Search of the Historical Jesus, Roller Boogie.
TV: Matinee Theatre, Climax, Lost in Space, My Three Sons, Suspense, The Untouchables, Hitchcock, Thriller, Bonanza, Gunsmoke, Mannix, Little House On The Prairie, S.W.A.T., The New Daughters of Joshua Cabe, The Captains And The Kings, One An Eagle, Fish, Columbo, How the West Was Won. Co-starred in two series: The Californians, also directing several episodes, and Kate McShane and General Hospital.

McCLURE, DOUG: Actor. b. Glendale, CA, May 11, 1935. e. UCLA.
PICTURES: Because They're Young, The Unforgiven, Shenandoah, Beau Geste, The King's Pirate, Nobody's Perfect, The Land That Time Forgot, At the Earth's Core, Warlords of Atlantis, Humanoids from the Deep, Cannonball Run II.
TELEVISION: Movies: The Longest Hundred Miles, Terror in the Sky, The Birdmen, The Death of Me Yet, Playmates, The Judge and Jake Wyler, Shirts/Skins, Death Race, Satan's Triangle, Roots, SST-Death Flight, Wild and Woolly, The Rebels. Series: Overland Trail, The Virginian.

McCLURE, WENDY: Actress, Dancer. b. Glasgow, Scotland, March 9, 1934. m. David Knight. e. Lowther College, North Wales. On London stage from 1955 in The Punch Revue, Alice Through the Looking Glass, Zuleika. M.P. debut in 1956 in Helen of Troy.
PICTURES INCLUDE: Helen of Troy, It's A Wonderful World, The Girl on the Boat, The Comedy Man, A King in New York.
TV: Knock on Any Door, Dr. Finlay's Casebook, The Newcomers, Over to Una, Z-Cars, The Borderers, Young Man in Trouble.

McCLURE, WILLIAM K.: Producer-Director. b. Knoxville, Tenn., Sept. 8, 1922; e. U. Tennessee & Catholic U., Washington, D.C. Contact man Washington staff, Pathe Newsreel, 1942; Los Angeles staff, 1943; asst. dir., "This Is America" series, 1943. Combat photographer, U.S. Army, 1944–46; Pub. mgr., RKO Pathe, Inc., 1947; Cameraman, corr., Warner Pathe Newsreel, 1948–51; Cameraman-corr., in Europe, Middle East for See It Now, CBS-TV, 1951–52, London, 1953; dir., cameraman, See It Now, 1952–54, Report on Africa. 1955–56, Burma, Buddhism. Neutralism, 1957, Watch on the Ruhr, 1958; dir. oper. Europe Small World. 1958–59. Prod., CBS Reports, co-prod.: CBS Reports, Iran Brittle Ally 1959, Berlin: End of the line 1960. Prod., CBS Reports: Britain, Blood Sweat and Tears, plus 20 1961 prod., Mr. Europe and the Common Market; prod., Germany Since Hitler; Adenauer Sums-up; prod., DeGaulle: The Challenge, DeGaulle: Roots of Power, East Europe, Satellites Out of Orbit; prod., CBS News, Henry Moore: Man of Form; Eur. prod., Town Meeting of the World, 1965–66. Prod. 1967 If you're appalled at my Texas I'm bewildered with your England. Prod. 1968 Don't Count the Candles.

McCOWEN, ALEC: Actor. b. Tunbridge Wells, England, May 26, 1925. e. RADA. On stage in London in Ivanhoe, The Mask and the Face, Hadrian the Seventh, etc. On Bdwy. in Antony and Cleopatra, No Laughing Matter, After the Rain, The Assam Garden, etc.
PICTURES: The Cruel Sea, Time Without Pity, A Midsummer Night's Dream, The Loneliness of the Long Distance Runner, The Agony and the Ecstasy, The Devil's Own, The Hawaiians, Frenzy, Travels with My Aunt, Stevie, Hanover Street.

McCREA, JOEL: Actor. b. Los Angeles, Calif., Nov. 5, 1905; e. Pomona College; husband of Frances Dee, actress. Stage experience: amateur dramatics and community plays taking male lead in "The Patsy" "Laff That Off" and "The Little Journey." In many pictures since 1932.
PICTURES INCLUDE: In 1940 He Married His Wife, Primrose Path, Foreign Correspondent. In 1941 Reaching for the Sun, Sullivan's Travels. In 1942 The Great Man's Lady, The Palm Beach Story. In 1943 The More the Merrier, Virginian, Ramrod, Four Faces West, South of St. Louis, Outriders, Colorado, Territory, Stars in My Crown, Saddle Tramp, Cattle Drive, San Francisco Story, Lone Hand, Shoot First, Border River, Black Horse Canyon, Stranger on Horseback, Wichita, First Texan, The Oklahoman, Trooper Hook, Fort Massacre, The Gunfight at Dodge City, Ride the High Country, Mustang Country.

McCULLOUGH, JIMMIE B.: Producer-Director. b. Mansfield, La., May 12, 1929. e. UCLA (1955). U.S. Marine Corps Reserve 1948–50; Ziv Studio, Hollywood, 1949–56: Acted on TV: Highway Patrol, CBS Playhouse 90, The Shadow, Teenage Monster, Crime File. Officer-director, American Metal Window Co., 1959–63. Owned and operated Macco Prod. Co., Inc., 1966–72. Now heads Jim McCullough Prods., Inc., Ry-Mac Intl. Film Dist., Inc., and Macco Prods., Inc.
PICTURES: Sheperd of the Hills (prod.-dir.), Where the Red Fern Grows (co-prod.), Creature from Black Lake (prod.-dir.), Charge of the Model Ts (prod.-dir.).

McDOWALL, BETTY: Actress. b. Sydney, Australia; e. Mt. Bernard Convent, N. Sydney. Early career radio, stage in Australia; ent. BBC TV, 1952; since in West End plays, many TV and radio plays and films.
STAGE: Age of Consent, Ghost Train, The Kidders, The Dark Halo, Period of Adjustment, Rule of Three, Signpost to Murder, Hippolytus, The Winslow Boy, Woman in a Dressing Gown, As Long As It's Warm, Caprice—In A Pink Palazzo, Sweet Bird of Youth, There was an Old Woman, What the Butler Saw, Two Dozen Red Roses, A Boston Story, The Man Most Likely To . . . , Sleeping Partner.
TV: Mid-Level and Glorification of Al Toolum, The Black Judge, Phone Call for Matthew Quade, Thunder on the Snowy, Shadow of Guilt, Traveling Lady, Torment, Biography, Notes for a Love Song, Esther's Altar, The Corridor People, The Braden Beat, The Douglas Fairbanks, Ivanhoe, The Foreign Legion, Fabian of the Yard, Four Just Men, Flying Doctor, No Hiding Place, 'Z' Cars, Days of Vengeance, Flower of Evil, Outbreak of Murder, Call Me Sam, The Prisoner, Public Eye, The Forgotten Door, All Out for Kangaroo Valley, Barry Humphries Scandals, Castle Haven, Albert and Victoria, Follyfoot, The Man Who Came to Dinner, Anne of Avoniea, Little Lord Fauntleroy, The Bass

Player and the Blond (4 plays), The Gingerbread Lady. Series: Boyd Q.C.

PICTURES INCLUDE: First lead in England, Timelock, She Didn't Say No, Jack the Ripper, The Shiralee, Jackpot, Dead Lucky, Spare the Rod, Golliwog, Echo of Diana, First Men in the Moon, Ballad in Blue, The Liquidators, Willy Wagtails by Moonlight, The Omen.

RADIO: Anna Christie, The Little Foxes, Another Part of the Forest, The Archers.

McDOWALL, RODDY: Actor (Star of Tomorrow, 1944.) b. London, England, Sept. 17, 1928; e. St. Joseph's London. First appeared in Murder in the Family at age of 8. Later, You Will Remember, The Outsider, Just William, Hey, Hey, U.S.A., This England, all made in England. In 1940 signed by 20th Century-Fox.

PICTURES INCLUDE: Man Hunt, How Green Was My Valley, Confirm or Deny, Son of Fury, On the Sunny Side, The Pied Piper, My Friend Flicka, Lassie Come Home, White Cliffs of Dover, Macbeth, Act, assoc. prod., Rocky, Kidnapped, Big Timber, Tuna Clipper, Black Midnight, Killer Shark, Steel Fist, The Subterraneans, Midnight Lace, Cleopatra, The Longest Day, The Greatest Story Ever Told, Shock Treatment, That Darn Cat, The Loved Ones, The Third Day, Daisy Clover, Bullwhip Griffin, Lord Love A Duck, The Defector, It, The Cool Ones, Planet of the Apes, Hello, Down There, Midas Run, Escape from the Planet of the Apes, Conquest of the Planet of the Apes. Directorial Debut, The Devil's Widow, 1971. Actor: The Legend of Hellhouse, The Poseidon Adventure, Arnold, Funny Lady, The Cat from Outer Space, Scavenger Hunt, Charlie Chan and the Curse of the Dragon Queen, Evil Under the Sun, Class of 1984, Fright Night.

THEATRE: On B'way in Misalliance, Escapade, Doctor's Dilemma, No Time for Sergeants, Good as Gold, Compulsion, Handful of Fire, Look After Lulu, The Fighting Cock, 1959–60, Camelot, 1960–61, The Astrakhan Coat, 1966.

RADIO & TV: Stratford Shakespearean festival, 1955. Movies: This Girl for Hire, The Zany Adventures of Robin Hood, Hollywood Wives.

McDOWELL, MALCOLM: Actor. b. Leeds, England, June 1943. Was spear-holder for the Royal Shakespeare Co. in season of 1965–66 when turned to TV and then to films. Made debut in small role in Poor Cow, 1967.

PICTURES INCLUDE: If . . . , Figures in a Landscape, The Raging Moon, A Clockwork Orange, O Lucky Man!, Royal Flash, Aces High, Voyage of the Damned, Caligula, The Passage, Time after Time, Cat People, Britannia Hospital, Blue Thunder, Cross Creek, Get Crazy.

TELEVISION: Arthur the King, Gulag.

McELWAINE, GUY: Executive. Started career in pub. dept. of MGM, 1955; 1959, joined m.p. div. of Rogers and Cowen. 1964, formed own public relations firm; then joined CMA. Left to become sr. exec. v.p. in chg. worldwide m.p. production, Warner Bros., 1975. In 1977 became sr. exec. v.p. in chg. worldwide m.p. activities and pres. of intl. film mktg. at Intl. Creative Management (ICM), formerly CMA. 1981, named pres. and chief exec. officer Rastar Films. Left in 1982 to become pres., Columbia Pictures; given additional title of chief exec. officer, 1983. In 1985 named chm. and on board of Columbia Pictures Industries. Resigned, 1986.

McEVEETY, BERNARD: Director. Comes from film family; father was pioneer as unit mgr. at New York's Edison Studios; brothers Vincent, also a dir., and Joseph, writer are at Disney Studios. Bernard's career began in 1953 at Paramount where was asst. dir. for 6 yrs. Earned full dir. responsibility on The Rebel, TV series.

PICTURES INCLUDE: Napoleon and Samantha, One Little Indian, The Bears and I.

TV: Episodes on Bonanza, Gunsmoke, Combat and Cimarron Strip (also prod.)

McEVEETY, VINCENT: Director. Joined Hal Roach Studios in 1954 as second asst. dir. Then to Republic for The Last Command. First Disney assignments: Davy Crockett shows and Mickey Mouse Club. Moved to Desilu as first asst. dir. on The Untouchables; made assoc. prod. with option to direct. Did segments of many series, including 34 Gunsmoke episodes. First theatrical film: Firecreek, 1968.

PICTURES INCLUDE: $1,000,000 Duck, The Biscuit Eater, Charley and the Angel, Superdad, The Strongest Man in the World, Gus, Treasure of Matecumbe, Herbie Goes to Monte Carlo.

TELEVISION: High Flying Spy.

McFADDEN, FRANK: Publicist. b. San Diego, Calif., June 3, 1914. e. Southwestern Bus. Coll. Pub. dept., Warner Bros. Studio, 1933–35; asst. pub. dir., Universal Studio, 1936–53; adv., pub. dir., Leonard Goldstein Prod., 1954; president pub. rel. agency, McFadden and Eddy, Inc., 1955; partner, McFadden, Strauss & Irwin, 1963. TV, 1956. Became partner in ICPR in 1975.

McGAVIN, DARREN: Actor. b. San Joaquin Valley, Calif., May 7, 1922. e. C. of the Pacific.

PLAYS INCLUDE: Death of a Salesman, My Three Angels, The Rainmaker, The Lovers, Dinner at Eight (revived).

PICTURES INCLUDE: Summertime, The Man with the Golden Arm, Court Martial of Billy Mitchell, Beau James, Delicate Delinquent, The Great Sioux Massacre, Bulley For a Badman, Mission Mars, Airport '77, A Christmas Story, The Natural, Turk 182. Directorial Debut: Happy Mother's Day . . . Love, George (1973).

TV: Mike Hammer, The Outsider, The Night Stalker, My Wicked Wicked Ways.

McGOOHAN, PATRICK: Actor. b. New York, Mar. 19, 1928. Early career in repertory in Britain. London stage 1954 in Serious Charge; 1955 Orson Wells' Moby Dick. Ent. films 1955.

PICTURES INCLUDE: Passage Home, High Tide at Noon, Hell Drivers, The Gypsy and the Gentleman, Nor the Moon by Night, Two Living, One Dead, All Night Long, The Quare Fellow, Thomasina, Dr. Syn, Ice Station Zebra, The Moonshine War, Brass Target, Scanners, Baby.

TV: Plays and star of ATV's Danger Man series; also directed some of these; Secret Agent, The Prisoner.

McGOVERN, ELIZABETH: Actress. b. Evanston, IL, July 18, 1961. Acted in high school in California; studied at American Conservatory Theatre, Julliard School of Dramactic Art. Film debut in Ordinary People (1980).

PICTURES: Ragtime, Lovesick, Racing with the Moon, Once Upon a Time in America, The Bedroom Window, Native Son.

McGOWAN, BROTHERS: Dorrell & Stuart. Writers, Directors, Producers. Independent producers since 1950. TV series: Death Valley Days, The Littlest Hobo. Features: Billion Dollar Hobo, Mister Too Little.

McGOWAN: ROBERT A.: Writer. b. Denver, Colo., May 22, 1901. Cartoonist; from 1923–29, writer of Hal Roach "Our Gang" comedies for his uncle, Robert Francis McGowan. Directed under the name of Anthony Mack, s.p., Babes in Toyland, collab. s.p., Too Many Parents, Boy Friend shorts for Warner-Vitagraph, N.Y. Prod. manager, four technicolor shorts. Wrote new series "Our Gang" comedies for MGM.

McGRATH, THOMAS J.: Producer. b. New York City. e. Washington Square Col. of N.Y.U. (B.A. 1956), N.Y.U. School of Law (LLB 1960). Has practiced law in N.Y.C. from 1960 to date. Became indep. prod. with Deadly Hero in 1976; Author, Carryover Basis Under The 1976 Tax Reform Act, published in 1977.

McGREGOR, CHARLES: Executive. b. Jersey City, N.J., April 1, 1927. e. N.Y.U. 1958–1969, Co-founder, pres. and chief exec. officer, Banner Films, Inc. (World Wide TV Distribution), 1955–58, salesman and div. mgr., Flamingo Films (domestic TV Dist.). 1953–55; Professional mgr. ABC Music Publishing. 1951–53: Prod. and partner Telco Prods. and G&M Productions (prods. of network and local shows). 1969–77: exec. v.p. in chg. of w-w dist., WB-TV; 1977: pres. WB-TV Distribution.

McGUIRE, DON: Writer, director. b. Chicago, Ill., Feb. 28, 1919. U.S. Army, 4 yrs.; press agent, Chicago and Hollywood; newsman, Hearst papers, Chicago; then actor, writer.

PICTURES INCLUDE: Double Deal, Dial 1119, Meet Danny Wilson, Willie and Joe in Back at the Front, Walking My Baby Back Home, Three Ring Circus, Bad Day at Black Rock, Artists and Models, Johnny Concho, Delicate Delinquent, Suppose They Gave a War and Nobody Came.

TV: Writer, dir. & co-prod., Hennessey series, creator, series Not for Hire; creator, writer, prod. series, Don't Call Me Charlie.

AUTHOR: Novels, The Day Television Died, 16000 Floogle Street.

McGUIRE, DOROTHY: Actress. b. Omaha, Neb., June 14, 1919; e. Ladywood convent, Indianapolis; Pine Manor, Wellesley, Mass.

STAGE: Bachelor Born, Our Town, My Dear Children, Swinging the Dream, Claudia, Legend of Lovers, Night of the Iguana (1976).

PICTURES INCLUDE: Claudia, Tree Grows in Brooklyn, Enchanted Cottage, Spiral Staircase, Claudia and David, Gentleman's Agreement, Mister 880, Callaway Went Thataway, I Want You, Make Haste to Live, Invitation, 3 Coins in the Fountain, Trial, Friendly Persuasion, Old Yeller, This Earth Is Mine, Remarkable Mr. Pennypacker, Dark at The Top of the Stairs, Summer Place, Susan Slade, Flight of the Doves.

TELEVISION: Rich Man, Poor Man.

McHUGH, JAMES: Agent/Manager. b. Boston, Mass., Oct. 21, 1915; e. Holy Cross Coll. Joined MCA 1939. U.S. Army Signal Corps, 1944–46. MCA-British and European, 1945–

50. Formed James McHugh, Talent Agency 1953. Pres., Artists Mgr. Corp., pres., Turquoise Prod., Inc., v.p.

McINTIRE, JOHN: Actor. b. Spokane, Wash., June 27, 1907; e. Local schools; m. Jeanette Nolan, actress; Radio announcer, actor teamed with wife.
PICTURES INCLUDE: Asphalt Jungle, Francis, Saddle Tramp, Winchester '73, Ambush, Scene of the Crime, You're in the Navy Now, Under the Gun, Raging Tide, Westward the Women, World in His Arms, Glory Alley, Sally & St. Anne, Horizons West, Lawless Breed, Mississippi Gambler, The President's Lady, Lion Is In the Street, War Arrow, Apache, Four Guns to the Border, Yellow Mountain, Far Country, Stranger on Horseback, Scarlet Coat, Phoenix City Story, Backlash, The Spoilers, The Kentuckian, World in My Corner, Away All Boats, The Tin Star, Who Was That Lady, Flaming Star, Two Rode Together, Summer & Smoke, Herbie Rides Again, Honkytonk Man, Cloak and Dagger.
TV: Wagon Train, Naked City, The Virginian.

McKEE, LONETTE: Actress. b. Detroit, MI, 1954. Started career as singer at age of 14 on dance show, Swingin' Time. Film debut in Sparkle, 1976. On stage in revival of Showboat on Bdwy.
PICTURES: Which Way Is Up?, Cuba, The Cotton Club, Brewster's Millions.

McKELLAR, KENNETH: Singer. b. Paisley, Scotland. singer, stage prods., radio & TV; appeared, concerts, Edinburgh International Festival; toured, Scots Concert groups; created role, Jamie in A Wish For Jamie, A Love for Jamie. Many BBC-TV and ITV appearances in V.K. Records regularly.

McKELLEN, IAN: Actor. b. Burnley, England, May 25, 1939. e. Cambridge. Many performances on London stage: A Scent of Flowers, Much Ado About Nothing, Trelawny of the Wells, A Lily in Little India, The Man of Destiny, Black Comedy, Dr. Faustus, King John, etc. On Bdwy. in The Promises, Amadeus (Tony; 1981), Ian McKellen Acting Shakespeare, etc.
PICTURES: Alfred the Great, The Promise, A Touch of Love, Priest of Love, The Keep, Plenty.
TELEVISION: Hamlet, David Copperfield, Hedda Gable, Ian McKellen Acting Shakespeare, etc.

McKENNA, SIOBHAN: Actress. b. Belfast, Ireland, May 24, 1923; e. St. Louis Convent, Monaghan; National Univ. of Ireland, B.A. Stage debut at Abbey Theatre, 1943; then London stage in The White Steed, 1947. Screen debut: Hungry Hill, 1946. London film and stage parts, also stage in Dublin; interested in development of Gaelic Theatre in Galway for which she has translated several plays including G. B. Shaw's Saint Joan.
PICTURES INCLUDE: Daughter of Darkness, The Lost People, The Adventurers, King of Kings, Of Human Bondage, Dr. Zhivago.
STAGE: (London) Saint Joan; (N.Y.) Chalk Garden.
TV: appearances in U.S include The Last Days of Pompeii (1984).

McKERN, LEO: Actor. b. Sydney, New South Wales, Mar. 16, 1920. On stage in She Stoops to Conquer, Hamlet, Merry Wives of Windsor, Cat on a Hot Tin Roof, A Man for All Seasons, etc.
PICTURES: A Man for All Seasons, Ryan's Daughter, Candleshow, The Blue Lagoon, The Frendh Lieutenant's Woman, Ladyhawke.

McKINNEY, BILL: Actor. b. Tennessee, Sept. 12.
PICTURES INCLUDE: Hollywood Secret File, She Freak, The Road Hustlers, Smack, Breakheart Pass, Josey Wales, Deliverance, Junior Bonner, Judge Roy Bean, Kansas City Bomber, The Outfit, Thunderbolt & Lightfoot; Parallax View, Every Which Way But Loose, The Gauntlet, For Pete's Sake.
THEATRE: No Time For Sergeants, A Cook For Mr. General, Time Limit, Bus Stop, Of Mice and Men, The Garbage Hustler, Roadside, As You Like It, Hassan Of Bagdad, No Place To Run, Career, Hat Full Of Rain, The Gamblers, The Devil's Disiciple, All My Sons, Deadwood Dick, Chanticleer, Hoot And Holler, War And Peace, Grapes Of Wrath, El Camino Real, The Little Prince.
TV: Showcase for Success, The Monkeys, Holvak, Baretta, Bronk, Sarah, Bold Ones, Smith & Jones, McCloud, Columbo, Ironside, Pvt. Slovak, The Healers.

McLAGLEN, ANDREW V.: Dir. b. London, Eng., July 28, 1920. e. U. of Virginia, 1939–40. prod. dept., Lockheed Aircraft Corp., 1940–44; asst. m.p. dir., 1944–54; dir., 1955–65; dir., CBS-TV. 1956–63.
PICTURES INCLUDE: Man in the Vault, Gun the Man Down, The Abductors, Freckles, The Little Shepherd of Kingdom Come, McLintock!, Shenandoah, The Rare Breed, Seven Men From Now, The Way West, The Ballad of Josie, Monkeys, Go Home, Devil's Brigade, Bandolero, The Undefeated, Fool's Parade, Something Big, One More Train To Rob, Cahill, U.S. Marshall, Mitchell, The Last Hard Men, The Wild Geese, ffolkes, The Sea Wolves, Sheena.
TV: Gunsmoke, Have Gun—Will Travel, Perry Mason, Rawhide, The Lineup, The Lieutenant, The Dirty Dozen: The Next Mission, On Wings of Eagles, etc.

McLERIE, ALLYN: Actress. b. Grand Mere, Quebec, Canada, Dec. 1, 1926; e. High School, N.Y. Dancer since 15 in many B'way shows.
SHOWS INCLUDE: One Touch of Venus, On the Town, Finian's Rainbow, Where's Charley, Miss Liberty, Time Limit.
PICTURES INCLUDE: Where's Charley, Desert Song, Calamity Jane, Phantom of the Rue Morgue, Battle Cry, They Shoot Horses, Don't They?, The Cowboys, Jeremiah Johnson, The Magnificent Seven Ride, Cinderella Liberty.

McMAHON, ED: Performer. b. Detroit, Mich., March 6, 1923. e. Boston Coll.; Catholic U. of America, B.A., 1949. U.S. Marines, 1942–53.
TV: Tonight Show, Monitor, Fortune Phone, Who Do You Trust, The Missing Links, commercials.
THEATRE: Stock Bdwy., Impossible Years.
PICTURES INCLUDE: The Incident, Fun with Dick and Jane.

McMAHON, JOHN J.: Executive. b. Chicago, Ill., 1932. e. Northwestern U. Served with U.S. Army in Korea, beginning career on WGN-TV, Chicago; associated with ZIV-United Artists TV Productions during 1950s; joined American Broadcasting Company in 1958; v.p. & gen. mgr., WXYTZ-TV, Detroit, then KABC-TV, Los Angeles, 1968; v.p., ABC, 1968–72; joined National Broadcasting Company in 1972 as v.p., programs, west coast, NBC-TV; president, Hollywood Radio & Television Society; board member, Permanent Charities Committee. June, 1980, named pres. of Carson Prods. (Johnny Carson's prod. co.).

McMILLAN, KENNETH: Actor. b. Brooklyn, NY, July 2, 1932. e. High School of the Performing Arts; trained for theatre with Uta Hagen and Irene Dailey at HB Studios, NY. Stage debut in Sweet Bird of Youth, touring co., 1962.
PICTURES: Serpico, The Taking of Pelham 1, 2, 3, The Stepford Wives, Oliver's Story, Blood Brothers, Hide in Plain Sight, Little Miss Marker, Carny, Borderline, Eyewitness, Whose Life Is It Anyway?, True Confessions, Ragtime, Heartbeeps, The Killing Hour, Blue Skies Again, Head Over Heels, Reckless, Dune, Pope of Greenwich Village, Runaway Train, Armed and Dangerous.
TELEVISION: King, Rhoda, The Hustler of Muscle Beach, Breaking Up, Joe Dancer, Salem's Lot, Lou Grant, The Rockford Files, Kojak, Maggie Briggs, etc.

McNALLY, STEPHEN: Actor r.n. Horace McNally; b. New York City, July 29; e. Fordham U., LL.B. In school dramatics; practiced law 2 yrs.; N.Y.; stage, films, 1942.
PICTURES INCLUDE: Winchester 73, Wyoming Mail, No Way Out, Air Cadet, Apache Drums, Raging Tide, Lady Pays Off, Devil's Canyon, Make Haste to Live, A Bullet Is Waiting, Man From Bitter Ridge, Tribute to a Bad Man, Once You Kiss a Stranger, Black Gunn.

McNEIL, ROBERT A.: Exhibitor. b. San Francisco, Cal., Jan. 14, 1889; e. public schools of San Francisco; m. Started show career when 17. Sang on stage, also operated projection machine and played in three shows a week in San Francisco. Worked on Pantages circuit for two years. Expanded theatre enterprises after San Francisco fire, owning five houses. Joined E. H. Emmick in forming Golden State Circuit in 1927. Associated with Mike Naify of T. and D. Jr. enterprises to form United California Theatres, Inc., sold interest to Naify, retired; maintains interest in small San Francisco chain.

McNICHOL, KRISTY: Actress. b. Los Angeles, Sept. 11, 1962. Made debut at age of 7 performing in commercials. Given regular role in Apple's Way; began appearing on such series as Love, American Style and The Bionic Woman. Attracted attention of Spelling-Goldberg Productions, who cast her as Buddy Lawrence in Family series.
PICTURES: The End, Little Darlings, The Night the Lights Went Out in Georgia, Only When I Laugh, White Dog, The Pirate Movie, Just the Way You Are, Dream Lover.
TELEVISION: Movies: Like Mom, Like Me, Summer of My German Soldier, My Old Man, Love Mary.

McQUEENEY, ROBERT: Actor. b. Bridgeport, Conn., March 5. e. Taft School, Watertown, Bard College; lieutenant, U.S. Army; prof. debut, summer theatre group, Jennerstown, Pa.
SHOWS INCLUDE: Billy Budd, Dial M for Murder, Affairs of State, Fragile Fox, Macbeth, Rain, The Second Man, The Tender Trap, Brainstorm, The Glory Guys.
TV: Robert Montgomery Presents, Philco, Kraft Theatre, Studio One, Omnibus Playwrights '56, Love of Life, The Guiding Light, The Gallant Men.

McRANEY, GERALD: Actor. b. Collis, Miss., Aug. 19. e. Univ. of Mississippi. Left school to become surveyor in oil fields after which joined acting company in New Orleans. Studied acting with Jeff Corey; landed guest role on TV series, Night Gallery.
TELEVISION: Series: The Incredible Hulk, The Rockford

Files, The Dukes of Hazzard, Eight Is Enough, How the West Was Won, Hawaii Five-O, Barnaby Jones, Gunsmoke, Simon & Simon, etc. Movies: Roots II, The Jordan Chance, Women in White, Trial of Chaplain Jenson, The Law, Love Story, The Haunting Passion, etc.
PICTURES: Night of Bloody Horror, Keep Off My Grass, etc.

McSHANE, IAN: Actor. b. Blackburn, England, Sept. 29, 1942. e. RADA. Stage work includes The House of Fred Ginger, The Easter Man, The Glass Menagerie in England and The Promise on Bdwy.
PICTURES: The Wild and the Willing, The Pleasure Girls, The Battle of Britain, If It's Tuesday This Must Be Belgium, Pussycat Pussycat I Love You, Villain, The Last of Sheila, Ordeal by Innocence, Too Scared to Scream, etc.
TELEVISION: Wuthering Heights, The Pirate, Disraeli, The Letter, Marco Polo, Bare Essence, Grace Kelly, Evergreen, A.D.

MEADES, KENNETH RICHARDSON: Communications Consultant. b. Montreal, Can., March 2, 1943; e. Cote des Neiges Comm. Coll., Geo. Williams U., Sta. Ana Coll., Western Tech. Inst. Obtained first class Radiotelephone lic. with FCC; eng. dept., CFCF Radio & TV, 1960–63; technician with Broadcast Engineering Services, Garden Grove, Calif.; presently priv. consultant.

MEANEY, DONALD V.: Executive. b. Newark, N.J. e. Rutgers Univ. School of Journ. Worked as reporter for Plainfield (N.J.) Courier-News, Newark Evening News. Became news director of radio station WCTC in New Brunswick N.J. and later for WNJR, Newark. Joined NBC in 1952 as news writer; two years later became nat'l. TV news editor. Promoted to mgr., national news, 1960 and mrg., special news programs, 1961. Appt. dir. of news programs 1962 and gen. mgr., NBC News, 1965; v.p., news programming, NBC, 1967; v.p. news, Washington, 1974; mrg. dir., affiliate & intl. liaison, 1979; sr. mng. editor, intl. liaison, 1984; retired from NBC, 1985. Now on faculty of American University's School of Communications.

MECHANIC, BILL: Executive. b. Detroit. e. Mich. State Univ.(BA); Univ. of So. Calif. (PhD in film). Entered industry 1978 as dir. of programming for SelecTV; promoted to v.p., 1980. Joined Paramount 1982; 1984, to Disney as v.p., pay TV sls. 1985, named sr. v.p., video, of new Walt Disney video div.

MEDAK, PETER: Director. b. Budapest, Hungary. Entered industry in 1956 in London with AB-Pathe as trainee. Worked sound, editing and camera depts. Later was asst. dir., second unit dir. on various action pictures. In 1963 under contract to Universal Pictures, where started directing TV films. In 1967 under contract to Paramount Pictures.
PICTURES INCLUDE: Kaleidoscope (assoc. prod., 2nd unit dir.), Funeral in Berlin (2nd unit dir.), Fathom (assoc. prod.; 2nd unit dir.) Negatives (dir.), Day in the Death of Joe Egg (dir.), Ruling Class (dir.), Ghosts in the Noonday Sun (dir.), Odd Job, The Changeling, Zorro, the Gay Blade, Men's Club.
TV: Third Girl from the Left, The Babysitter, The Dark Secret of Black Bayou, Mistress of Paradise, Cry for the Stranger, Fairy Tale Theatre, Twilight Zone, Nabokov.

MEDAVOY, MIKE: Executive. b. Shanghai, China, Jan. 21, 1941. Lived in China until 1947 when family moved to Chile. Came to U.S. in 1957. e. UCLA, graduating in 1963 with honors in history dept. Started working in mail room at Universal Studios and became a casting director, from which he went to work for Bill Robinson as an agent trainee. Two years later joined GAC and CMA where he was a v.p. in the motion picture department. In 1971 joined IFA as vice-president in charge of motion picture dept. Represented American and foreign creative talents, among whom were Jane Fonda, Donald Sutherland, Michelangelo Antonioni, Jean-Louis Trintignant, Karel Reisz, Steven Spielberg, Robert Aldrich, George Cukor, John Milius, Terry Malick, Raquel Welch, Gene Wilder and Jeanne Moreau. While at IFA was involved in packaging The Sting, Young Frankenstein, Jaws and others, before joining United Artists Corp. in May, 1974, as senior v.p. in chg. of West Coast prod. In 1978 named exec. v.p., Orion Pictures Co. (In 1982 Orion team took over Filmways, Inc.) While production head received four Oscars for best picture: One Flew Over the Cuckoo's Nest, Rocky, Annie Hall, Amadeus.
MEMBER: Filmex board; board of trustees, UCLA Foundation; advisory board, College for Intl. Strategic Affairs at UCLA; steering committee of Royce 270, UCLA; visiting committee, Boston Museum of Fine Arts; advisory board, Tel Aviv Univ.; board, Museum of Science & Industry; Co-Chmn.: Olympic Sports Federation, Music Center Unified Fund Campaign; board of governors Sundance Institute.

MEDFORD, DON: Director. b. Detroit, Mich.; e. Purdue U., U. of N.C., B.A., Yale U., M.F.A., actor, stage mgr., summer theatres; producer, B'way stage, Christopher Award.
TV: Kraft Theatre, General Electric Theatre, Alfred Hitchcock Presents, Climax, Twilight Zone, U.S. Steel Hour, Dick Powell, Eleventh Hour, Dr. Kildare, Fugitive, 12 O'clock High, The FBI, Man From UNCLE, Cimarron Strip, Baretta, Police Story, Kaz, Streets of San Francisco, Dynasty, Sizzle, Helltown.
FILMS: The Hunting Party, The Organization, The November Plan, Incident in San Francisco, The Coach.

MEDINA, PATRICIA: Actress. b. London, Eng. July 9, 1921. In many British films.
PICTURES INCLUDE: Secret Journey, Hotel Reserve, Don't Take It to Heart, Waltz Time. U.S. screen debut: Secret Heart, 1946; others: Moss Rose, Foxes of Harrow, Sangaree, Drums of Tahiti, Phantom of the Rue Morgue, Black Knight, Pirates of Tripoli, Duel on the Mississippi, Uranium Boom, Stranger At My Door, The Killing of Sister George.

MEDLEY, WM. THOMAS: Actor-singer. b. Hollywood, Calif., Sept. 19, 1940. Mem., Righteous Bros. rec. team.
TV: Shindig, The Danny Kaye Show, Ed Sullivan Show.
PICTURES INCLUDE: Beach Ball, Swingin' Summer.

MEDMAN, EDWARD A: Executive. b. Philadelphia, Pa. Nov. 11, 1937. e. University of Pennsylvania (Wharton School) 1955–58; University Pennsylvania Law School 1958–61, JDS; Joined General Counsel's Staff National Labor Relations Board, Washington, D.C., 1962–66; Trial Attorney NLRB, New York 1966–69; Joined Law firm of Poletti, Freidin, Prashker, Feldman & Gartner, 1969; Senior Labor Attorney, National Broadcasting Company 1970–72; Joined The Burbank Studios, Dec. 1972, v.p., legal/business affairs.

MEDWIN, MICHAEL: Actor, writer, producer. b. Eng., 1925; e. Institut Fischer. Switzerland. Stage debut 1940; m.p. acting debut in Root of All Evil, 1946.
PICTURES INCLUDE: My Sister and I, Mrs. Christopher, Gay One, Children of Chance, Operation Diamond, Black Memory, Just William's Luck, Ideal Husband, Picadilly Incident, Night Beat, Courtney's of Curzon Street, Call of the Blood, Anna Karenina, William Comes to Town, Woman Hater, Look Before You Love, Forbidden, For Them That Trespass, Queen of Spades, Trottie True, Boys in Brown, Trio, Long Dark Hall, Curtain Up, Street Corner (Both Sides of the Law). I Only Asked, Carry on Nurse, Wind Cannot Read, Heart of a Man, Crooks Anonymous, It's All Happening, Night Must Fall, I've Gotta Horse, 24 Hours To Kill. Prod: Charlie Bubbles, If . . . , Spring and Port Wine, O Lucky Man! Gumshoe, Law and Disorder, Memoirs of a Survivor.
TV: Granada's Army Game, The Love of Mike, Three Live Wires, Memorial Films Ltd.
THEATRE: Spring and Port Wine, Joe Egg, Forget-me-not Lane, Chez Nous, Alpha Beta, Another Country, Crystal Clear, Interpreters, Orpheus.

MEEKER, RALPH: Actor: b. Minneapolis, Minn., Nov. 21, 1920; e. Northwestern U. In school plays; served in U.S. Navy.
THEATRE: On B'way in Doughgirls, Strange Fruit, Cyrano de Bergerac, Mr. Roberts, Streetcar Named Desire (also road co.), Picnic, Mrs. Dally; off-B'way: House of Blue Leaves.
PICTURES INCLUDE: Teresa, Four in a Deep Shadow, Sky, Somebody Loves Me, Glory Alley, The Naked Spur, Jeopardy, Code Two, Big House U.S.A., Kiss Me Deadly, Desert Sands, Ada, Dirty Dozen, Gentle Giant, The Devil's Eight, I Walk the Line, Anderson Tapes, The Happiness Cage, Food of the Gods, Winter Kills.
TV: Lost Flight (Special).

MELAMED, DAVID J.: Executive. b. N.Y., Dec. 11, 1911; e. NYU; accountant, Columbia Pictures Corp., 1933–35; acct., RKO Radio Pictures, 1935–40; comptroller, Pathe Labs., Inc., 1941–43; U.S. Army, 1943–46; treas., Eagle Lion Films, 1947–51; exec. v.p., dir., Pathe Labs, Inc. 1952–58; dir. of adm., asst. to chmn. of bd., Nat'l General Corp., 1959–61; sr. exec. v.p., American International Pictures, 1961–80; v.p., SLM, Inc. 1981–84; presently director, Fries Entertainment.

MELCHIOR, IB: Director, writer. b. Copenhagen, Denmark, Sept. 17, 1917. p. Lauritz Melchior; e. Coll., Stenhus, Denmark, 1936; Univ. of Copenhagen, 1937. Actor. stage mgr., English Players, 1937–38; co-dir. 1938; actor in 21 stage prod. in Europe and U.S. on radio; set designer; stage man. dept., Radio City Music Hall, 1941–42; U.S. Military Intelligence, 1942–45; writer, dir., m.p. shorts for TV, 1947–48; TV actor, 1949–50; assoc. dir., CBS-TV, July, 1950; assoc. prod., G-L Enterprises, 1952–53; dir., Perry Como Show, 1951–54; dir. March of Medicine, 1955–56; writer, dir. of M.P. & TV films. 1957. Documentary writ. & dir. awarded Top Award by Nat'l. Comm. for Films for Safety, 1960. Golden Scroll Award, Academy of Science Fiction, Best Writing, 1976; Hamlet Award, Shakespeare Society of America, excellence in playwriting, Hour of Vengeance, 1982.

PICTURES INCLUDE: When Hell Broke Loose, Live Fast Die Young, The Angry Red Planet, Reptilicus, Journey to the Seventh Planet, The Case of Patty Smith, Robinson Crusoe on Mars, The Time Travellers, Ambush Bay, Planet of the Vampires, Death Race 2000.
AUTHOR: Novel, Order of Battle, 1972; Sleeper Agent, 1975; The Haigerloch Project, 1977; The Watchdogs of Abaddon, 1979; The Marcus Device, 1980; The Tombstone Cipher, 1982; Eva, 1984; V–3, 1985; Code Name: Grand Guignol.

MELFORD, AUSTIN: Actor, author, director. b. Alverstoke. England, Aug. 24, 1884; Actor & prod., Theatre Royal, Drury Lane, London, Gaiety Theatre, London, and others.
STAGE PLAYS: (Author) It's a Boy, Battling Butler, Night of the Garter, Nippy, Bob's Your Uncle, Blue for a Boy.
PICTURES INCLUDE: Oh, Daddy, Car of Dreams, Getting Married, We'll Smile Again, Heaven Round the Corner, Champagne Charlie, Sailors Three.

MELNICK, DANIEL: Executive. b. N.Y.C., April 21, 1934. e. N.Y. Univ. In 1954 was staff prod. for CBS-TV; then exec. prod., East Side West Side and N.Y.P.D. Joined ABC-TV as v.p. in chg. of programming. Partner in Talent Associates. Joined MGM as v.p. in chg. of prod.; in 1974 named sr. v.p. & worldwide head of prod.; 1977 in charge of worldwide production, Columbia Pictures; named pres., 1978. Resigned to be indep. prod.
PICTURES INCLUDE: Straw Dogs, That's Entertainment! (exec. prod.); That's Entertainment, Two! (co-prod.); All That Jazz (exec. prod.); Altered States (exec. prod.); First Family (prod.), Making Love (co-prod.), Footloose (exec. prod.), Quicksilver (co-prod.).

MELNIKER, BENJAMIN: Motion Picture Producer—Attorney; b. Bayonne, N.J., e. Brooklyn College; LL.B., Fordham Law School, Loew's Theatres usher, private law practice employed Legal Department Metro-Goldwyn-Mayer, vice president and general counsel, 1954–1969, executive vice president, 1968–1970, resigned from MGM December 1971; also member MGM bd. dir. and mem. MGM exec. com.; Adjunct associate professor, New York Law School, 1976–77; prod. & exec. prod. motion pictures, 1974–86; former motion picture chmn. Anti-Defamation League, B'nai B'rith; Mem. Am., N.Y. State bar assns., Bar Assn. City N.Y., Acad. Motion Picture Arts and Scis.
PICTURES: Mitchell, Shoot, Winter Kills, Swamp Thing.
TELEVISION: Three Sovereigns for Sarah, Television's Greatest Bets.

MELSON, JOHN: Writer-Lyricist. b. Anderson, Ind., Dec. 17, 1930. e. Univ. of Paris (La Sorbonne, 1952 B.A.) and Univ. of Madrid (P.G. studies, 1953–54). m. Maria Perschy, actress. Reporter, Detroit Labor News, 1951; taught French and Italian in various commercial schools in Paris, 1954–55; orchestra musician 1946–50. Script writer for films since 1962. Member: WGAW, BMI.
PICTURES INCLUDE: Battle of the Bulge (co-story, co-s.p.); Savage Pampas (co-s.p.); Cauldron of Blood (co-story, co-s.p.); Simon Bolivar (co-story, co-s.p.); Special Delivery (co-story, co-s.p.); Where Time Began (co-story, co-s.p.); Love and Bullets, Charlie (co-s.p.); The Animal (co-s.p.).
TV: Hawaii Five-O.
SONG LYRICS: Like a Dream (from the Summertime Killer); Cotton Candy Kingdom and The Familiar Stranger (both from Where Time Began).

MENGERS, SUE: Talent Agent. b. Bronx, N.Y. Started as receptionist, secretary with Music Corp. of America in New York. In 1963 became agent in small partnership. Two years later joined Creative Management Associates and sent to Hollywood. Now with Intl. Creative Mgt. (co. formed by merger of CMA and Marvin Josephson Associates). Clients include Barbra Streisand, Gene Hackman, Ryan O'Neal, Tatum O'Neal, Ali MacGraw, Cybill Shepherd, Peter Bogdanovich, Sidney Lumet, Arthur Penn, Nick Nolte, Robin Williams, Roman Polanski, Michael Caine.

MENGES, CHRIS: Cinematographer.
PICTURES: If.... The Empire Strikes Back (second unit), Local Hero, The Killing Fields, Marie, etc.
TELEVISION: World in Action, Opium Warlords, Opium Trail, East 103rd Street, etc.

MERCHANT, ISMAIL: Producer-Director. b. Bombay, India, 1936. e. St. Xavier's Coll., Bombay and NYU. Formed Merchant Ivory Prods., 1961.
PICTURES: The Householder, Shakespeare Wallah, The Guru, Bombay Talkie, Savages, Autobiography of a Princess, The Wild Party, Roseland, Hullabaloo Over Georgie and Bonnie's Pictures, The Europeans, Jane Austen in Manhattan, Quartet, Heat and Dust, The Bostonians, A Room with a View.

MERCHANT, LAWRENCE H., JR.: Producer. b. Cambridge, Mass. e. Boston Latin School, Hebron Academy, Maine, Columbia University, New York University. Pres., Educational Book Div., Prentice-Hall; pres., Pillsbury Productions; prod. exec., TV-Today, Home, Tonight, Milton Berle, Show of Shows, Hallmark Hall of Fame, Eye Witness, R. Montgomery Presents, Wide, Wide World, Walter Winchell; TV advisor, Gen. Dwight D. Eisenhower; prod. CBS films; pres., Kachina Productions.
PICTURES INCLUDE: Hands of Dr. Maniacal, Back Track, Present Tense of Love.

MERCOURI, MELINA: Actress, b. Athens, Oct. 18, 1925. schooling and training in Athens, fluent in French, German and English; Stage debut on Athens stage in avant-garde work; early stage career in Paris. Also made vocal recordings.
PLAYS INCLUDE: Morning Becomes Electra, La Nuit de Samaracande, Les Compagnons de la Marjolaine, Il Etait une Gare, Le Moulin de la Galette; to Greece 1954, in Stella. Also: A Streetcar Named Desire, Helen or the Joy of Living, The Queen of Clubs, The Seven Year Itch, Sweet Bird of Youth, Ilya Darling.
PICTURES INCLUDE: Stella, The Gypsy and the Gentleman, The Law, Never on Sunday, Phaedra, The Victors, Topkapi, He Who Must Die, 10:30 P.M. Summer, A Man Could Get Killed, Gaily, Gaily, Promise at Dawn, Earthquake, Once is Not Enough, Nasty Habits, A Dream of Passion.

MEREDITH, BURGESS: Actor. b. Cleveland, Ohio, Nov. 16, 1909; e. Amherst Coll., M.A. (hon.); m. Kaja Sundsten. Capt. U.S. Army Air Corps, World War II. On stage 1929 Civic Repertory Co., N.Y.
STAGE PLAYS: Little Ol' Boy, She Loves Me Not, The Star Wagon, Winterset, High Tor, Remarkable Mr. Pennypacker, etc.
PICTURES INCLUDE: Began screen career 1936 in Winterset. Idiot's Delight, Of Mice and Men, Second Chorus, That Uncertain Feeling, Tom, Dick and Harry, Street of Chance, Miracles Can Happen, Story of G.I. Joe, Diary of a Chambermaid, Magnificent Doll, Mine Own Executioner, Man on the Eiffel Tower, Gay Adventure, Joe Butterfly, Advise and Consent, Hurry Sundown, Fortune Garden, Stay Away Joe, McKenna's Gold, Hard Contract, There Was a Crooked Man, The Clay Pigeon, Such Good Friends, Golden Needles, The Day of the Locust, 92 in the Shade, The Hindenburg, Burnt Offerings, Rocky, The Sentinel, The Manitou, Foul Play, Magic, The Great Georgia Bank Hoax, Golden Rendezvous, Rocky II, When Time Ran Out, Clash of the Titans, True Confessions, Rocky III, Santa Claus.

MERRALL, MARY: Actress. b. Liverpool, England; e. convents in Belgium and London; m. Franklyn Dyall. First stage appearance in 1907. Managed Abbey Theatre, Dublin, in 1918 with Franklyn Dyall and produced several plays. Has toured Canada, U.S. and South Africa; many plays since. On screen in 1939–40; Dr. O'Dowd & since in many British films.
PICTURES INCLUDE: Squadron Leader X, Dead of Night, Pink String and Sealing Wax, This Man Is Mine, Nicholas Nickleby, They Made Me a Fugitive, Three Weird Sisters, Badgers Green, For Them That Trespass, Trio, The Late Edwina Black, Out of True, Tale of Five Cities, Encore, Meet Me Tonight, Pickwick Papers, Weak and the Wicked, Duel in the Jungle, Belles of St. Trinians, Pay-Roll Robbery, Green Buddha, Its Great To Be Young, Campbell's Kingdom, Family Doctor, Camp on Blood Island, Spare the Rod, Everything I Have, Moll Flanders, Futtocks End.
TV: The Guardians, Idle at Work, Cider with Rosie, I can See it All, His Lordship Entertains, Kate, Justice, Hunter's Walk, Willy.

MERRICK, DAVID: Producer. b. Hong Kong, Nov. 27, 1912. Famed Broadway stage impressario with long record of hits, including Fanny, The Matchmaker, Hello Dolly!, Look Back in Anger, The Entertainer, Jamaica, World of Suzie Wong, Gypsy, Take Me Along, Becket, Sunday in New York, Oliver!, I Do! I Do!, Private Lives, etc. Recent: 42nd Street.
PICTURES: Child's Play (debut), The Great Gatsby, Semi-Tough, Rough Cut.

MERRILL, DINA: Actress. r.n. Nedinia Hutton; b. N.Y.C. Dec. 9, 1925. e. George Washington Univ., 1940–41; American Academy of Dramatic Arts, 1942–44. Fashion model, 1941–42. Acting debut: Here Today, Mrs. January and Mr. X, Newport 1942.
PLAYS INCLUDE: My Sister Eileen, Major Barbara, Misalliance, On Your Toes.
PICTURES INCLUDE: Debut, Desk Set, Catch Me If You Can, Operation Petticoat, Butterfield 8, Young Savages, I'll Take Sweden, The Greatest, A Wedding, Just Tell Me What You Want.
TV: debut, Kate Smith Show 1956; Four Star Theatre, Playwrights '56, Climax!, Playhouse 90, Westinghouse Presents, The Investigators, Checkmate, The Rogues, Bob Hope Presents, To Tell the Truth.

MERRILL, GARY: Actor. b. Hartford, Conn., Aug. 2, 1915. e. Loomis Prep. School, Bowdoin Coll., Trinity Coll. Stage career started in 1937, minor role, stage play, The Eternal

Road; toured Brother Rat co.; then, Morning Star, See My Lawyer; on air in Young Dr. Malone, Helen Hayes Theatre, Theatre Guild, Gangbusters, Superman; army service 1941–45; upon disch. to stage in Born Yesterday, At War With the Army. Screen debut: Slattery's Hurricane, supporting role, then Twelve O'Clock High.
PICTURES INCLUDE: Where the Sidewalk Ends, All About Eve, The Frogmen, Decision Before Dawn, Another Man's Poison, Phone Call From a Stranger, Girl in White, Night Without Sleep, Blueprint for Murder, Black Dakotas, Human Jungle, Pleasure of His Company, The Woman Who Wouldn't Die, Clambake, The Incident, The Last Challenge, The Power, Huckleberry Finn, Thieves.
TV: The Mask, Justice, Dr. Kildare.

MERSON, MARC: Producer. b. New York City, Sept. 9, 1931. e. Swarthmore. Entered Navy in 1953; assigned as publicist to Admiral's Staff of Sixth Fleet Command in the Mediterranean. Upon discharge joined trade paper Show Business as feature editor. Joined CBS-TV as asst. to casting director. Left after 3 yrs. to work for Ely Landau as casting dir., packager and sometime producer of The Play of the Week on TV. Returned to CBS for 3-yr. stint doing specials and live programs. Left to organize Brownstone Productions as indep. prod. Now partner with Alan Alda in Helix Productions to package and produce TV shows.
PICTURES INCLUDE: The Heart Is a Lonely Hunter, People Soup (short), Leadbelly.
TV: Stage 67, Androcles and the Lion, Dummler & Son (pilot), The David Frost Revue (synd. series), We'll Get By.

MESMER, MARIE: Drama, film reviewer. b. Newark, N.J. Feb. 14, 1920; e. Syracuse Univ., Brooklyn (N.Y.) Inst. of Arts & Sciences; Radio adv. Crowell Pub. Co., 2 yrs.; danced with Ted Lewis and orchestra on tour; exhibiting artist in art galleries throughout U.S. for number years; currently drama reviewer Los Angeles (Calif.) Daily News, specializing in covering jazz music & personalities. Member: Los Angeles Press Club.

MESSENGER, GARY L.: Executive, b. Fresno, Calif., Jan. 14, 1941. e. University of Southern California-Cinema. 1967, joined MCA, Inc., asst. to exec. v.p.; 1970, independent motion picture & television producer; 1976, v.p. director production services, The Burbank Studios. Member of USC Cinema Circulus, Producers Guild of America.

MESSICK, DON: Actor. b. Buffalo, NY, Sept. 7, 1926. e. Ramsay Street, School of Acting; American Theatre Wing. Began performing as ventriloquist at age 13 in rural Maryland. Own radio show at 15 in Salisbury, MD (WBOC) for two years, writing and portraying all the characters in a one-man weekly comedy show. Worked in Hanna-Barbera cartoons since company began in 1958, voicing Ruff in their first series on NBC, 1959. Voiced Boo Boo Bear and Ranger Smith on Yogi Bear Show, Astro and The Jetsons. Voices Scooby Doo and Scrappy Doo on Scooby Doo series; Papa Smurf and Azrael on Smurfs. Has done numerous national commercials.

MESTRES, RICARDO: Executive. b. New York City, 1958. e. Harvard Univ. Gained filmmaking experience during summers as prod. asst. on TV features. Joined Paramount Pictures as creative exec. 1981. Promoted to exec. dir. of production, 1982 and to v.p., production, for Motion Picture Group, Paramount, 1984. Named v.p. of prod., Walt Disney Pictures, Promoted to sr. v.p., prod.,1986.

METZGER, RADLEY: Producer-Director-Writer.
PICTURES: Dark Odyssey (p.d., s.p.); Carmen, Baby (p.d,); Therese and Isabelle (p., d.); Camille 2000 (p.,d.); The Lickerish Quartet (p., d.); Score (p.d.); Little Mother (p., d.); Naked Came the Stranger (d.); The Image (d.).

METZLER, JIM: Actor. b. Oneonda, NY. e. Dartmouth Coll.
PICTURES: Four Friends, Tex.

METZLER, ROBERT: Writer. b. Buffalo, N.Y., Dec. 26, 1914; e. U. of S. California. Joined MGM writing staff 1939. In 1941: collaborated on screenplay Riders of the Purple Sage, 20th-Fox. In 1942: Sundown Jim, Dr. Renault's Secret; (s.p.) Circumstantial Evidence; (adapt.) The Undercover Woman.

MEYER, BARRY M: Executive. With ABC-TV in legal and business affairs depts. before joining Warner Bros. TV in 1971 as dir. of business affairs. 1972, named v.p. of business affairs for Warner TV arm; promoted to exec. v.p. of div. 1978. 1984, named exec. v.p. of Warner Bros., Inc.

MEYER, NICHOLAS: Director-Writer. b. Dec. 24, 1945. e. Univ. of Iowa. Was unit publicist for Love Story, 1969.
PICTURES: The Seven-Per-Cent Solution (s.p.), Time After Time (s.p., dir.), Star Trek II: The Wrath of Khan (dir.).
TELEVISION: Judge Dee (s.p.), The Night That Panicked America (s.p.); The Day After (dir.).

MEYER, RUSS: Producer, director. b. Oakland, Calif.; in 1942 joined Army Signal Corps, learned m.p. photography and shot combat newsreels.
PICTURES INCLUDE: The Immoral Mr. Teas, Eve and the Handyman, Finders Keepers, Lovers Weepers, Goodmorning and Goodbye, Vixen, Beyond the Valley of The Dolls, The Seven Minutes, and Sweet Suzy.

MEYERS, ROBERT: Executive. b. Mount Vernon, N.Y., Oct. 3, 1934. e. N.Y.U. Entered m.p. industry as exec. trainee in domestic div. of Columbia Pictures, 1956. Sales and adv. 1956–60; transferred to sales dep't. Columbia Pictures International, N.Y., posts there included supervisor of international roadshows and exec. ass't. to continental mgr. Joined National General Pictures as v.p.-foreign sales, 1969. Created JAD Films International Inc. in Feb. 1974 for independent selling and packaging of Motion Pictures around the world. September, 1977, joined Lorimar Productions Inc. as senior vice pres. of Lorimar Distribution International. Became pres. in April, 1978. Joined Filmways Pictures in 1980, named pres. & co-o. Pres. of American Film Mktg. Assn.; 1982, formed new co., R.M. Films International.

MICHAELI, JOHN EDWARD: Executive. b. Los Angeles, Calif., Nov. 20, 1938; e. Mt. Carmel H.S., Sta. Monica City Coll., S. California State University, B.A., 1965; M.A. 1977. Merch. buyer & dir. of Adv., Maymart div. of May Co.; police beat reporter, KGIL; pub. ed. Bunker-Ramo Corp.; Off. boy then publicist, MGM, 1965; v.p. communications, Hanna-Barbera Prods.

MICHAELS, RICHARD: Director. b. Brooklyn, NY, Feb. 15, 1936. e. Cornell Univ. Script supervisor 1955–64 and associate producer before starting directing career in 1968 with Bewitched (54 episodes), of which was also assoc. prod.
TELEVISION: Series: episodes of Love, American Style, Delvecchio, Ellery Queen, Room 222. Movies: Once an Eagle (mini-series), Charlie Cobb, Having Babies II, Leave Yesterday Behind, My Husband Is Missing, . . . And Your Name Is Jonah (winner, Christopher Award), Once Upon a Family, The Plutonium Incident, Scared Straight, Another Story (winner, Scott Newman Drug Abuse Prevention Award), Homeward Bound (winner, Banff Intl. TV Festival special & Christopher Award), Berlin Tunnel 21, The Children Nobody Wanted, One Cooks, The Other Doesn't, Sadat (mini-series), Jessie (pilot), Silence of the Heart, Heart of a Champion: The Ray Mancini Story, Rockabye, Kay O'Brien—Surgeon (pilot), I'll Take Manhattan (mini-series).
PICTURE: Blue Skies Again.

MICHAUD, HENRI: Executive. b. Ismailia, Egypt, Sept. 24, 1912. e. H.E.C. (Commercial Acdmy.), Paris, 1932. Warner Bros., Paris, 1934, 1944. Paramount Internat'l Films, 1944–68; pres. Para. Intern'l., 1968–70; co-chmn., Cinema Int'l Corp., July, 1970–77. Producer's rep., 1978.

MICHAUD, HENRY A.: Executive. b. Gastonia, N.C., Mar. 19, 1914. e. Loyola Coll., Tech. School (Science) 1932–37. Amateur photographer. Cameraman on animation and title stand, Associated Screen News, 1939; cameraman, Naval and Air Force training films, industrial and tourist films, 1940–47. Partner, founded, Phoenix Studios, 1947 which later was reorganized as Omega Prods., 1951; in chg. technical services, multiple camera shooting methods, rear-projection techniques, etc., using 16mm negative for TV shows, 1952; dir. on numerous industrial and government films. Pres., Assoc. of Motion Picture Producers and Labs. of Canada, 1961. v.p. Omega Prod. of Montreal.

MICHEL, WERNER: Executive. b. March 5, 1910. e. U. of Berlin, U. of Paris, Ph.D. Radio writer, dir., co-author two Broadway revues, 1938, 1940; dir. French feature films; dir. Broadcast Div., Voice of America, 1942–46; prod., dir., CBS, 1946–48; asst. prog. dir., CBS, 1948–50; dir. of Kenyon and Eckhart TV dept., 1950–52; prod., DuMont TV network, 1952–55; dir., Electronicam TV-Film Prod., 1955–56; prod., Benton and Bowles; Procter and Gamble, 1956–57; v.p. & dir. TV-radio dept., Reach, McClinton Advertising, Inc., 1957–62; consultant, TV Programming & Comm'l-Prod., N. W. Ayer & Son, Inc.; v.p., dir., TV dept., SSC&B Advertising, 1963, pgm. exec., ABC-TV Hollywood, 1975; director, dramatic programs, 1976; sr. v.p., creative affairs, MGM-TV, 1977; exec. v.p., Wrather Entertainment Intl., 1979; sr. v.p., creative affairs, MGM-TV, 1980–82; COO, Guber-Peters TV, 1982–84; sr. v.p., corporate TV dept., Kenyon & Eckhart, NY, 1984.

MICHELET, MICHEL: Composer. b. Kieff, Russia. Prof., Kieff & Vienna Conserv.; composed concert compositions, ballets, stage music; ent. m.p. industry, composed scores 105 films, France; to U.S. 1941; author many concert compositions.
PICTURES INCLUDE: Voice in the Wind (AA nom.), Hairy Ape (AA nom.), Music for Millions, The Chase, Lured, Siren of Atlantis, Man on the Eiffel Tower, Once a Thief, Tarzan's Peril, Fort Algiers, Un Missionaire, Le Secret de Soeur Angele, Petersburger, Nachte, Challenge (Tribute to Modern Art). Also did scores for many U.S. Information

Service documentaries; arr. of Russian music Anastasia; Afrodife (score); The January (orig. songs & arr. of Russian music). Member: French Soc. of Composers (SACEM).

MICHELL, KEITH: Actor. b. Adelaide, Australia. Early career as art teacher, radio actor; toured Australia with Stratford Shakespearean Co. 1952–53; Stratford Memorial Theatre 1954–55, Old Vic Theatre 1956–57. Irma la Douce, Chichester, Art of Seduction, The First 400 Years, Robert & Elizabeth, Kain, The King's Mare, 1969: Don Quijote in Man of La Mancha, London, N.Y. 1970: Abelard & Heloise, London; 1971, NY and LA, 1972, Hamlet, London, in October 1973–76. Artistic Director, Chichester Festival Theatre. Toured Australia with Chichester Festival Co., London 1979: Crucifer of Blood, London 1980: On the Twentieth Century, Melbourne Theatre Co. 1981: Pete McGynty (adaptation of Peer Gynt), London 1981–82: Captain Beaky Christmas Show. Chichester 1982: On the Rocks, Brisbane 1982: The Tempest, UK tour 1983: Amadeus San Francisco. 1984–85: La Cage Aux Folles (USA and Australia).
TV: Pygmalion, Act of Violence, Mayerling Affair, Tiger At The Gates, Traveller Without Luggage, Guardian Angel, Wuthering Heights, The Bergonzi Hands, Ring Round The Moon, Spread of the Eagle, The Shifting Heart, Loyalties, Soldier in Love, Hallmark Hall of Fame, series; Kain, The Ideal Husband, The Six Wives of Henry VIII (series). Keith Michell at various London theatres, Dear Love. Selections from Keith Michell in Concert at Chichester, Captain Beaky & his Band, Captain Beaky, Volume 2. 1983 TV Video: The Gondoliers, The Pirates of Penzance, Ruddigore.
PICTURES INCLUDE: True As A Turtle, Dangerous Exile, Gypsy and the Gentleman, The Hellfire Club, All Night Long, Seven Seas to Calais, Prudence and the Pill, House of Cards, Henry VIII and his Six Wives, Moments.

MIDLER, BETTE: Actress-Singer. b. Honolulu, Dec. 1, 1945. e. Univ. of Hawaii. Appeared on Bdwy. in Fiddler on the Roof; Salvation, 1970; Tommy, Seattle Opera Co., 1971. Gained fame as singer-comic in nightclubs and cabarets. Has toured extensively with own stage shows: Divine Miss M, Clams on the Half-Shell, etc.
PICTURES: The Rose, Divine Madness, Jinxed, Down and Out in Beverly Hills, Ruthless People, Outrageous Fortune.

MIFUNE, TOSHIRO: Actor. b. Tsingtao, China, April 1, 1920. e. Japanese schools. Served five years Japanese army. Joined Toho Studio 1946.
PICTURES INCLUDE: Snow Trail, Drunken Angel, Eagle of Pacific, Seven Samurai, I Live in Fear, Legend of Musashi, Throne of Blood, Rikisha Man, Three Treasures, Last Gunfight, I Bombed Pearl Harbor, Rose in Mud, Rashomon, Yojimbo, Animus Trujano (Mexican), Kiska, Red Beard, High and Low, Judo Sag, The Lost World of Sinbad, Hell in the Pacific, Paper Tiger, Midway, Winter Kills, 1941, Shogun, The Challenge, Inchon, The Bishudo Blade.

MIGDEN, CHESTER L.: Executive. b. New York, N.Y., May 21, 1921; e CCNY, B.A., 1941, Columbia U. LLB 1947; Member New York Bar. Attorney for National Labor Relations Board 1947–51. Currently exec. dir., Assn. of Talent Agents. Was exec of Screen Actors Guild 1952–81; nat'l. exec. secty., 1973–81.

MIKELL, GEORGE: Actor. b. Lithuania. In Australia 1950–56 acting with Old Vic Co. Ent. films 1955. TV 1957. To England 1957; since appeared in numerous film and TV prod.
TV: Counsel at Law, Six Eyes on a Stranger, The Mask of a Clown, Green Grows the Grass, Opportunity Taken, OSS Series, Espinage, The Danger Man, Strange Report, The Survivors, The Adventurer, Colditz, The Hanged Man, Quiller, Martin Hartwell, Flambards, Sweeney, The Secret Army, Sherlock Holmes, When the Boat Comes In, Brack Report, Bergerac, The Brief, Glass Babies (Australia).
PICTURES INCLUDE: The Guns of Navarone, The Password Is Courage, The Great Escape, Deadline for Diamonds, Where The Spies Are, The Spy Who Came in From the Cold, I Predoni Del Sahara, Sabina, The Double Man, Attack on the Iron Coast, Zeppelin, Young Winston, Scorpio, The Tamarind Seed, Sweeney Two, The Sea Wolves, Escape to Victory, Emerald.
STAGE: Five Finger Exercise, Altona, The Millionairess, Love from a Stranger, Portrait of A Queen, Farewell, Judas, Flare Path.

MILES, LORD: C.B.E. Actor, dir., writer. b. Hillingdon, Middlesex, Sept. 27, 1907; e. Pembroke Coll., Oxford. Brit. stage debut 1930 in Richard III, London. Brit. screen debut in Channel Crossing. Awarded C.B.E., 1953; founded Mermaid Theatre, 1959.
PICTURES INCLUDE: Pastor Hall, The Big Blockade, This Was Paris; (collab. s.p.) Thunder Rock; The Day Will Dawn, One of Our Aircraft Is Missing, In Which We Serve; (author, co-dir., actor) Tawney Pipit; Carnival, Great Expectations, Fame is the Spur, Nicholas Nickleby, Guinea Pig, Never Let Me Go, Moby Dick, Man Who Knew Too Much, Zarak, Tiger In the Smoke, Fortune Is a Woman, Smallest Show on Earth, St. Joan, Tom Thumb, Sapphire, Heavens Above, Run Wild, Run Free, The Specialist.
TV: Treasure Island, etc.

MILES, SARAH: Actress. b. 1941; e. R.A.D.A.; film debut, Term of Trial.
PICTURES INCLUDE: The Servant, The Ceremony, Six-Sided Triangle, Those Magnificent Men In Their Flying Machines, Blowup, Ryan's Daughter, Lady Caroline Lamb, The Man Who Loved Cat Dancing, The Sailor Who Fell from Grace with the Sea, The Big Sleep, Venom, Ordeal by Innocence, Steaming.
THEATRE: Vivat! Vivat Regina!
TELEVISION: Harem.

MILES, VERA: Actress. b. Boise City, Okla., Aug. 23, 1930. e. public schools, Pratt and Wichita, Kans.
TV: Climax, Pepsi Cola Playhouse, Schlitz Playhouse, Ford Theatre. Movie: International Airport.
PICTURES INCLUDE: For Men Only, Rose Bowl Story, Charge at Feather River, Pride of the Blue Grass, Wichita, The Searchers, 23 Paces to Baker Street, Autumn Leaves, Wrong Man, Beau James, Web of Evidence, FBI Story, Touch of Larceny, Five Branded Women, Psycho, The Spirit Is Willing, Gentle Giant, Sergeant Ryker, Kona Coast, It Takes All Kinds, Hellfighters, The Wild Country, One Little Indian, Psycho II, Brainwaves.

MILFORD, JOHN: Actor. b. Johnstown, MI, Sept. 7, 1929.
TV: Delvecchio; Code R; Little House On The Praire; ABC Circle Short Story Theatre; Hip; $6 Million Man; Bionic Woman; Police Story; Streets of San Francisco; Gemini Man; The Hunter; Faith for Today; Barnaby Jones; Blue Knight; Policewoman; Cannon; Joe Forrester; Medical Story; Men In Green; The Name Of The Game; Gold Ones; Mannix; The Magician; Twelve O'Clock High; The Invaders; Firehouse; The Sound Of Anger; The Sixth Sense; The Plainsman; Tombstone Territory; The Lieutenants; Columbo; The FBI; Petrocelli; Longstreet; Mod Squad; Dan August; King Of Diamonds; Men In Space; High Chaparral; Family Affair; Toma; Ironside; Rifleman; Jesse James; Wyatt Earp; Gunsmoke; The Virginian; Big Valley; Bonanza; Hawkins; Guns Of Will Sonnett; Robert Taylor Detectives.
PICTURES INCLUDE: Brannigan's Rebels; The Ten Commandments; For Pete's Sake; Heart Of The Rebel; Marty; Gunfight At Commanche Creek.
THEATRE: What Every Woman Knows; Pygmalion; The Prime Of Miss Jean Brodie; Happy Birthday, Wanda June; Silent Night, Lonely Night; Child's Play; Diary Of A Scoundrel; Miss Julie; Apollo Of Bellac; Do You Know The Milky Way; The Vigil; Portrait Of A Madonna; State Of The Union; Night Must Fall; The Long Voyage Home; Murder In The Cathedral; The Male Animal; The Admirable Crichton; Aria De Capo; Nothing But The Truth; The Happy Prince; The Purging of Simon Madden; Peterson House; Where Is Thy Victory; Harry; Noon And Night; Room Service; The American Nightmare.

MILGRAM, HENRY: Theatre Executive. b. Philadelphia, April 20, 1926. e. Univ. of Pa., Wharton School. In industry 40 years; now exec. v.p. Milgram Theatres. Variety Club Board Member for past 20 years, past president and chairman of the board of Variety Club of Phila.; presently Variety Club Intl. v.p. Board member. Hahnemann University, trustee.

MILIUS, JOHN: Writer-Director. b. 1945. e. L.A. City College, USC (cinema course). While at latter won National Student Film Festival Award. Started career as ass't. to Lawrence Gordon at AIP. Began writing screenplays, then became director with Dillinger.
PICTURES INCLUDE: Devil's 8, Evil Knievel, The Life and Times of Judge Roy Bean, Jeremiah Johnson (co-s.p.), Dillinger (s.p.-dir.), Magnum Force (o.-s.p.), The Wind and the Lion (s.pm., dir.), Big Wednesday (dir. co.-s.p.); Apocalypse Now (s.p.); 1941 (exec. prod.-co. s.p.); Conan the Barbarian (dir., co. s.p.); Red Dawn (dir., co-s.p.).

MILLAR, STUART: Producer-Director. b. New York, N.Y., 1929. e. Stanford; Sorbonne, Paris. Ent. industry working for Motion Picture Branch, State Dept., Germany. documentaries, Army Signal Corps, Long Island, Germany; journalist, International News Service, San Francisco; assoc. prod.-dir., The Desperate Hours; assoc. prod.-dir., Friendly Persuasion.
PICTURES INCLUDE: The Young Stranger; Stage Struck; Birdman of Alcatraz. I Could Go On Singing, The Young Doctors, Stolen Hours, The Best Man, Paper Lion, Little Big Man, When The Legends Die, Rooster Cogburn.
TELEVISION: Vital Signs.

MILLER, ANN: Actress. r.n. Lucille Ann Collier; b. Houston, Tex., Apr. 12, 1923; e. Albert Sidney Johson H.S., Houston; Lawler Prof., School, Hollywood. Studied dance as child; played West Coast vaudeville theatres, Screen debut: New Faces of 1937.
STAGE: George White's Scandals, 1940, Mame, 1969.
PICTURES INCLUDE: Life of the Party, Stage Door,

New Faces of 1937, Radio City Revels, Having a Wonderful Time, Room Service, You Can't Take It With You, Too Many Girls, Time Out for Rhythm, Priorities on Parade, Reveille With Beverly, Jam Session, Eve Knew Her Apples, Thrill of Brazil, Easter Parade, The Kissing Bandit, On the Town, Watch the Birdie, Texas Carnival, Two Tickets to Broadway, Lovely To Look At, Small Town Girl, Kiss Me Kate, Deep in My Heart, Hit the Deck, Opposite Sex, Great American Pastime.

MILLER, ARTHUR: Writer. b. New York City, Oct. 17, 1915. e. Univ. of Mich. Plays include All My Sons, Death of a Salesman, The Crucible, A View from the Bridge, After the Fall, Incident at Vichy, The Price, Up for Paradise, Situation Normal, The American Clock.
PICTURE: The Misfits.
TELEVISION: Death of a Salesman, Fame, Playing for Time.

MILLER, CHERYL: Actress. b. Sherman Oaks, Calif., Feb. 4, 1943. e. UCLA, Los Angeles Conservatory of Music.
PICTURES INCLUDE: First film, Casanova Brown, age 19 days. Appeared in over 100 films as child, more recently in the Monkey's Uncle, Clarence the Cross-Eyed Lion, The Initiation, The Man From Clover Grove, Doctor Death.
TV: Perry Mason, Bachelor Father, Flipper and as co-star in Daktari, Donna Reed, Leave it to Beaver, Farmers Daughter, Wonderful World of Color, Dobie Gillis, Bright Promise, Love American Style, Emergency, Cades County.

MILLER, DAVID: Director. b. Paterson, N.J., Nov. 28, 1909, U.S. Army, World War II. Film ed. 1930, Columbia; Walter Futter prods. In 1933 short subjects ed. MGM; then dir. short subjects. Dir. features 1941.
PICTURES INCLUDE: Billy the Kid, Sunday Punch, Flying Tigers, Love Happy, Top O The Morning, Our Very Own, Saturday's Hero, Sudden Fear, Twist of Fate, Diane, Opposite Sex, The Story of Esther Costello, Midnight Lace, Backstreet, Lonely are the Brave, Captain Newman, MD, Hammerhead, Hail Hero, Executive Action, Bittersweet Love.
TELEVISION: Best Place To Be, Goldie and The Boxer, Love for Rent.

MILLER, DICK (RICHARD): Actor/Writer. b. N.Y.C., Dec. 25, 1928. e. CCNY, Columbia Univ. Grd. NYU, Theater School of Dramatic Arts. Commercial artist, Psychologist; Bellevue Mental Hygiene Clinic, Queens General Hospital Psychiatric dept. U.S. Navy, WWII. Boxing champ, U.S. Navy. Semi-pro football. Broadway stage, radio; Disc jockey, The Dick Miller Show, WMCA, WOR-TV Over 500 live shows. Did first live night talk show, Midnight Set, CBS Wrote, produced and directed many early radio and TV shows. Wrote Screenplays; T.N.T. Jackson, Which Way To The Front, Four Rode Out and others.
PICTURES INCLUDE: Has appeared in over 65 features, including: Not of This Earth, Thunder Over Hawaii, Rock All Night, Sorority Girl, The Terror, Bucket of Blood, Little Shop Of Horrors, Targets, War Of The Satelittes, The Long Ride Home, St. Valentine Day Massacre, Capone, Executive Action, White Line Fever, Cannonball, Mr. Billion, N.Y., N.Y.

MILLER, GEORGE: Director. b. Chinchilla, Queensland, Australia. Practiced medicine in Sydney; quit to work on films with Byron Kennedy, who became longtime partner. First worldwide success with Mad Max.
PICTURES: The Road Warrior, Twilight Zone—The Movie (segment), Mad Max Beyond Thunderdome.

MILLER, JAMES R.: Executive. Began m.p./industry career in 1971 in legal dept. of United Artists (N.Y.). Left to go with Paramount Pictures in legal dept.; then moved to Columbia in 1977 as snr. counsel; later assoc. gen. counsel. In 1979 named Warner Bros. v.p.—studio business affairs; 1984, v.p. chg. world-wide business affairs.

MILLER, JP: Writer. b. San Antonio, Tex., Dec. 18, 1919. e. Rice Univ., 1937–41, Yale Drama School, 1946–47 U.S. Navy, Lieut., 1941–46; pub. poetry, short stories.
ORIGINAL DRAMAS INCLUDE: Philco TV Playhouse: Hide and Seek, Old Tasslefoot, The Rabbit Trap, The Pardon-me Boy; Playhouse 90, Days of Wine and Roses, CBS Playhouse, The People Next Door, The Unwanted, The Lindbergh Kidnapping Case, Gauguin The Savage.
PICTURES INCLUDE: The Rabbit Trap, (story, s.p.) Days of Wine and Roses (story s.p.) The Young Savages (co-author, s.p.) Behold A Pale Horse, (s.p.) The People Next Door (story, s.p.), Helter Skelter (s.p.)
NOVELS: The Race for Home, Liv, The Skook.

MILLER, JASON: Writer-Actor. b. Scranton, PA., April 22, 1940. Entered regional playwriting contest during high school in Scranton, Penna. and since has moved back and forth between acting and writing. Wrote That Championship Season, winner of N.Y. Drama Critics Best Play award, 1972, Tony Award, 1973, and Pulitzer Prize for Drama.
PICTURES INCLUDE: The Exorcist (actor), That Championship Season (s.p.), The Nickel Ride (actor), A Home of our Own (actor), Fitzgerald in Hollywood (actor), A Love Story (s.p.); Monsignor (actor).

MILLER, MAX B.: Executive. Father, Max Otto Miller, producer silent features and shorts. e. Los Angeles Valley Coll., UCLA, Sherwood Oaks Coll. Writer of articles on cinema for American Cinematographer and other publications. Owns and manages Fotos Intl., entertainment photo agency with offices in 46 countries. Recipient of Golden Globe Award in 1976 for Youthquake, documentary feature. Also director of Films International (currently producing Shoot Los Angeles) and pres. of MBM Prod., Inc. Active member of Hollywood Foreign Press Assn. (from 1974–82 bd member; twice chm.), Independent Feature Project, Acad. of TV Arts & Sciences, LA Int'l, Film Exhibition.

MILLER, ROBERT ELLIS: Director. b. New York City, July 18, 1932. Worked on Broadway and TV before feature film debut with Any Wednesday (1966).
PICTURES INCLUDE: Sweet November, The Heart Is a Lonely Hunter, The Buttercup Chain, Big Truck and Poor Claire, The Girl from Petrovka, The Baltimore Bullet, Reuben, Reuben.
TV: The Voice of Charlie Pont, And James Was a Very Small Snail, The Other Lover.

MILLER, RONALD W.: Producer. b. April 17, 1933, Los Angeles, e. U. of Southern Calif. Football player with Los Angeles Rams. Two years U.S. Army. 1957 joined Walt Disney Productions as 2nd asst. dir. Old Yeller. Assoc. prod. TV series Walt Disney Presents; assoc. or co-prod. additional 37 episodes Disney TV. Exec. prod. Walt Disney's Wonderful World of Color. 1980, named pres. & chief operating off.; 1983, pres. & chief executive off., Disney Productions. Resigned in 1984.
PICTURES INCLUDE: Bon Voyage, Summer Magic, Son of Flubber, Moon Pilot, The Misadventures of Merlin Jones, A Tiger Walks, The Monkey's Uncle, That Darn Cat, Robin Crusoe, U.S.N., Monkey's Go Home, Prod. of: Never A Dull Moment, The Boatniks, The Wild Country, No Deposit, No Return, Treasure of Matecumbe, Freaky Friday, The Littlest Horse Thieves, Herbie Goes to Monte Carlo, Pete's Dragon, Candleshoe, Return from Witch Mountain, Cat from Outer Space, The North Avenue Irregulars, The Black Hole, Midnight Madness, Watcher in the Woods, The Last Flight of Noah's Ark, Night Crossing, Tron.
Assisted Walt Disney, Pageant Direct 1960 U.S. Olympics. By 1968, v.p., exec. prod. mem. bd. of dir. Walt Disney Productions.

MILLER, WINSTON: Writer. b. St. Louis, Mo., June 22, 1910; e. Princeton U. In 1935 entered m.p. ind.
PICTURES INCLUDE: Good Morning, Judge, Song of Texas, Home in Indiana, One Body Too Many, They Made Me a Killer, Double Exposure, My Darling Clementine, Relentless, Station West, Last Outpost, Rocky Mountain, Hong Kong, Blazing Forest, Carson City, The Vanquished, Boy from Oklahoma, Jivaro, Bounty Hunter, Run for Cover, Far Horizons, Lucy Gallant, Tension at Table Rock, April Love, A Private's Affair, Hound Dog Man, Escapade In Japan, Mardi Gras.

MILLS, DONNA: Actress. b. Chicago, Dec. 11. e. Univ. of Illinois. Left school to pursue career in theatre, beginning as dancer with stage companies around Chicago. Toured and landed in New York City, breaking into TV as regular of soap opera, The Secret Storm. On Bdwy. in Don't Drink the Water; theatrical film debut in The Incident.
TELEVISION: Series: Love Is a Many Splendored Thing, Lancer, Dan August, The Good Life, Knots Landing. Movies: Waikiki, Doctor's Private Lives, Superdome, The Hunted Lady, Woman on the Run, Fire!, The Bait. Mini-Series: Hanging by a Thread, Bare Essence.
PICTURES: The Incident, Play Misty for Me, etc.

MILLS, HAYLEY: Actress. b. London, Eng., April 18, 1946. e. Elmhurst Boarding School, Surrey. m.p. debut Tiger Bay 1959; Pollyanna, 1960; signed Disney contract 1960.
PICTURES INCLUDE: The Parent Trap, Whistle Down the Wind, The Castaways, Summer Magic, The Chalk Garden, The Moonspinners, The Truth About Spring, Sky West and Crooked, Trouble With Angels, The Family Way, Pretty Polly, A Matter of Innocence, Twisted Nerve, Take a Girl Like You, Sillouettes, What Changed Charley Farthing, The Diamond Hunters, That Darn Cat, Forbush and the Penguins, Endless Night.
TELEVISION: The Flame Trees of Thika.

MILLS, JULIET: Actress. b. London, Nov. 21, 1941. Daughter of John Mills. Made stage debut at 14 in Alice Through the Looking Glass.
PICTURES: So Well Remembered, The History of Mr. Polly, No, My Darling Daughter, Twice Around the Daffodils, Nurse on Wheels, Carry on Jack, The Rare Breed, Wings of War, Oh, What a Lovely War!, The Challengers, Avanti!, Beyond the Door, The Second Power, The Last Melodrama.
TELEVISION: Movies: Wings of Fire, The Challengers,

Letters from Three Lovers, QB VII, Once an Eagle, Alexander: The Other Side of Dawn, The Cracker Factory, etc.

MILLS, SIR JOHN: Actor, Producer. b. Suffolk, England, February 22, 1908, m. Mary Hayley Bell. Previously clerk. Film actor since 1933. In 1942: "The Young Mr. Pitt." "In Which We Serve," One of top ten money-making Brit. stars in Motion Picture Herald-Fame Poll, 1945, 1947, 1949–50, 1954, 1956–58, Oscar for Ryans Daughter.
PICTURES INCLUDE: We Dive at Dawn, This Happy Breed, Blue for Waterloo, Cottage To Let, Way to the Stars, Waterloo Road, Great Expectations, So Well Remembered, October Man, Scott of the Antarctic, Operation Disaster, Mr. Denning Drives North, Gentle Gunman, Long Memory, Hobson's Choice, End of the Affair, Colditz Story, Above Us the Waves, Escapade, It's Great to be Young, Around the World in 80 Days, War and Peace, Baby and the Battleship, Town on Trial, Monty's Double, Dunkirk, Summer of the 17th Doll, Tiger Bay, Swiss Family Robinson, Tunes of Glory, The Singer Not The Song, Flame In the Streets, Tiara Tahiti, The Valiant, The Chalk Garden, The Truth About Spring, The Great Spy Mission, King Rat, The Wrong Box, 1965; dir., Sky West and Crooked; acted The Family Way, Cowboy in Africa, Chukka, A Black Veil For Lisa, Oh! What a Lovely War, Run Wild, Run Free, Ryan's Daughter, Adam's Woman, Dulcima, Oklahoma Crude, Young Winston, Lady Caroline, The Human Factor, Trial By Combat, Lamb, The Big Sleep, 39 Steps, Gandhi, Sahara.
STAGE: Good Companions, 1975; Great Expectations, 1976; Separate Tables, 1977; Goodbye, Mr. Chips, 1982; Little Lies, 1983; Little Wes (Toronto, 1984).
TELEVISION: Masks of Death, Murder with Mirrors, Woman of Substance, Edge of the Wind, When the Wind Blows.

MILNER, JACK: Exec. Prod. b. Jersey City, N.J., Nov. 2, 1910. e. Roosevelt H.S., L.A., Calif. M.P. industry 1927. Worked many phases from laboratory-camera-editorial dept. to financing and co-producing feature pictures; formed Milner Bros. Productions with brother Dan Milner, 1955; prod. Phantom from 10,000 Leagues, From Hell It Came, Jail Break, etc.
TV: prod. My Dog Sheppy, From Here to Now, Come As You Are.

MILNER, MARTIN: Actor. b. Detroit, Mich., Dec. 28, 1931. e. USC debut in Life with Father, 1947; U.S. Army 1952–54, directed 20 training films.
PICTURES INCLUDE: Sands of Iwo Jima, The Halls of Montezuma, Operation Pacific, The Captive City, Battle Zone, Mr. Roberts, Pete Kelly's Blues, On the Threshold of Space, Gunfight at the O.K. Corral, Sweet Smell o' Success, Marjorie Morningstar, Too Much, Too Soon, Compulsion, 13 Ghosts, Valley of the Dolls.
TV: Route 66 (4 yrs.), Adam-12 (6 yrs.), Swiss Family Robinson.

MILO, GEORGE: Set Decorator, r.n. George Milo Vescia. b. New York, N.Y., Dec. 19, 1909. e. High School, Art Schools; landscape, seascape, still life painter, portrait sculptor; set decorator since 1937.
TV: Republic Studios, Revue Studios; Dangerous Assignment, Stories of the Century, Thriller, Alfred Hitchcock, Checkmate, General Electric.
PICTURES INCLUDE: Wake of the Red Witch, Fair Wind to Java, Borderline, Jubilee Trail, Make Haste to Live, Eternal Sea, Last Command, Come Next Spring, Psycho, Judgement at Nuremberg, The Last Cowboy, That Touch of Mink, The Birds.

MIMIEUX, YVETTE: Actress. b. Los Angeles, Calif., Jan. 8, 1944. e. Vine Street School, Le Conte Junior High, Los Angeles, Los Ninos Heroes de Chapultepec, Mexico City, Hollywood High School, Calif. Appeared with a theatrical group, Theatre Events; Sympn. Concert: Persephone, Oakland Orchestra, 1965, N.Y. Philharmonic, Linc. Ctr., L.A. Philharmonic, Hollywood Bowl.
PICTURES INCLUDE: debut, Time Machine, Where the Boys Are, The Four Horsemen of the Apocalypse, Light in the Piazza, The Wonderful World of the Brothers Grimm, Diamond Head, Toys In the Attic, Joy In The Morning, Reward, Monkeys Go Home, Dark of the Sun, Caper of the Golden Bulls, Picasso Summer, Three in the Attic, Skyjacked, The Neptune Factor, Jackson County Jail, The Black Hole.
TV: Tyger Tyger, 1964. 1970: series, Most Deadly Game. Movies: Death Takes A Holiday, Black Noon, Obsessive Love.
STAGE: I Am A Camera, 1963; Owl and the Pussycat, 1966.
CONCERTS: Persephone—Houston Symphony, London Royal Philharmonic.

MINDLIN, MICHAEL, JR.: Executive. b. New York, N.Y. e. Columbia U., 1940–41; Duke U., 1941–43. U.S. Air Force; short subject pub., W.B., 1946–47; assoc., George & Dorothy Ross pub., 1947; pub., adv. dir., Ballet Russe de Monte Carlo, 1947–49; asst. to prod. Joseph Kaufman, 1950; with We the People, radio & TV show, 1950–51; Alfred Katz pub. & mgt., 1951–53; adv. & pub. dir., Lopert Films, 1953, pub., Hecht-Lancaster, 1955; adv., pub. dir., Figaro, Inc., 1956–58; assoc. prod. David Merrick Prod., 1958–59; formed prod. co. with Raoul Levy, 1959; v.p. chg. adv., publ., Filmways, Inc., 1963, v.p. prod., Filmways, Inc., 1968. Formed own prod. co. 1969, v.p., prod., Warren Bros., 1972–74; Paramount Pictures, Producer, 1974–75; Frank Yablans Enterprises, 1975.

MINNELLI, LIZA: Actress-singer. b. 1946; p. Judy Garland & Vincente Minnelli; After repertory work & off-broadway roles starred on Broadway in Flora, The Red Menace (Tony award), Chicago, The Rink.
PICTURES INCLUDE: Charlie Bubbles, The Sterile Cockoo, Tell Me That You Love Me Junie Moon, Cabaret, That's Entertainment!, Lucky Lady, Silent Movie, A Matter of Time, New York, New York, Arthur.
TELEVISION: Liza with a Z. Movie: A Time to Live.

MINSKY, HOWARD G.: Writer-Producer-Sales and Distribution Exec. Paramount-Twentieth Century-Fox. Agency Exec. Wm. Morris Pres. Cinema Consultants. Produced Love Story. 1970.

MIRISCH, DAVID: Executive. b. Gettysburg, Pa., July 24, 1935. e. Ripon College. United Artists Corp., 1960–63; former exec. with Braverman-Mirisch adv. public rel. firm.

MIRISCH, MARVIN E.: Executive. b. New York, N.Y., March 19, 1918. e. College of the City of New York, B.A., 1940. Print dept., contract dept., asst. booker, N.Y. exch.; head booker, Grand National Pictures, Inc., 1936–40; officer, gen. mgr. vending concession operation 800 theatres, Midwest, Theatres Candy Co., Inc., Milwaukee, Wisc., 1941–52; exec., corporate officer in chg., indep. producer negotiations, other management functions, Allied Artists Pictures, Inc., 1953–57; Chmn. of Bd., Chief Exec. Officer in chg. of all business affairs, admin. & financing, distr. liaison, The Mirisch Company, Inc., 1957 to present. Member of Board of Governors and currently vice-president of Academy of Motion Pictures Arts & Sciences. Member Motion Pictures Pioneers. Currently president of Academy of MPAA Foundation.

MIRISCH, WALTER: Producer. b. New York City, Nov. 8, 1921; e. U. Wisconsin, B.A., 1942; Harvard Grad. Sch. Business Admin., 1943. In m.p. indust. with Skouras Theatres Corp., 1938–40; Oriental Theatre Corp., 1940–42. 1945 with Monogram, A.A.: apptd. exec. prod. Allied Artists, July, 1951; pres. and exec. head of prod. The Mirisch Corporation 1969; 1960–61; pres. Screen Prod. Guild; 1962, mem. bd. dir., MPAA; bd. Gvnrs., Academy of Motion Pictures Arts and Sciences, 1964; 1967, pres., Center Thea. Group of L.A.; bd. dir., Wisconsin Alum. Assn.; bd. of dir. Cedars-Sinai Medical Center, Bd. of Advisors, California State University—Northridge, Board of Governors, Academy of Motion Picture Arts & Sciences—1972. President, Permanent Charities Committee 1962–63; President, Academy of Motion Picture Arts & Sciences—1973–77.
PICTURES INCLUDE: By Love Possessed, Two for the Seesaw, Toys in the Attic, Hawaii, Fitzwilly, In the Heat of the Night, They Call Me Mister Tibbs, The Organization, Mr. Majestyk, Midway, Gray Lady Down, Same Time, Next Year, Prisoner of Zenda, Dracula, Romantic Comedy.

MIRREN, HELEN: Actress. b. England, 1946. On stage in various Shakespearan roles as well as The Silver Tassle, Enemies, The Sea Gull, Faith Healer, etc.
PICTURES: Age of Consent, Savage Messiah, O! Lucky Man, Hamlet, Caligula, The Long Good Friday, The Fiendish Plot of Dr. Fu Manchu, Excalibur, Cal, 2010, White Nights.
TELEVISION: Miss Julie, The Applecart, The Little Minister, A Midsummer Night's Dream, etc.

MR. T: Actor. r.n. Lawrence Tureaud. b. Chicago, 1953. Professional bodyguard when hired by Sylvester Stallone in 1980 to play prizefighter in Rocky III.
TELEVISION: The A Team (series); The Toughest Man in the World (movie).
PICTURES: Rocky III, D.C. Cab.

MITCHELL, ANDREW: Producer. b. Giffnock, Scotland, 1925. e. Fettes College, Edinburgh; early career, banking; Associated British Picture Corporation, Elstree Studios; gen. mgr., Elstree Distributors, 1961; dir., Kenwood Films Ltd., 1963; assoc. prod., Hand in Hand, The Young Ones, Summer Holiday, French Dressing, Wonderful Life. 1965; Pro., Up Jumped a Swagman. Asst. to mgr. dir., Assoc. British Prods., Ltd. Prod. con. Associated British Productions Ltd. 1969–70: Film Finances, Mng. dir., Leslie Grade Film Ltd, 1973. Mng. Dir. Thorn E.M.I. Elstree Studios. 1977 Prod. Are You Being Served?

MITCHELL, CAMERON: Actor. b. Dallastown, Pa., Nov. 4, 1918; e. Theatre School (New York City); New York Theatre

Guild, 1938–40; on stage with Lunt & Fontanne, "Taming of the Shrew." Radio announcer, sportscaster before joining U.S. Army Air Forces 1942–44. Star of Tomorrow, 1954.
PICTURES INCLUDE: Mighty McGurk, High Barbaree, Cass Timberlane, Leather Gloves, The Sellout, Death of a Salesman, Japanese War Bride, Flight to Mars, Man in the Saddle, Outcasts of Poker Flat, Okinawa, Les Miserables, Pony Soldier, Powder River, Man on a Tightrope, How To Marry a Millionaire, Hell & High Water, Gorilla At Large, Garden of Evil, Desiree, Strange Lady in Town, Love Me Or Leave Me, House of Bamboo, Tall Men, View from Pompey's Head, Carousel, Monkey on My Back, Face of Fire, Inside The Mafia, The Unstoppable Man, The Last of the Vikings, Three Came to Kill, Blood and Black Lace, Ride in the Whirlwind, Hombre, Island of the Doomed, Nightmare in Wax, Buck and the Preacher, Slaughter, The Midnight Man, The Klansman, Viva, Knievel!, The Swarm, Night Train to Terror, Low Blow.
TV: High Chapparel, Andersonville Trial, Swiss Family Robinson.

MITCHELL, GUY: Singer. actor. b. Detroit, Mich., Feb. 22, 1927 e. High Sch., San Francisco. Studied singing; U.S. Navy, 1945–46; singer, radio stations; vocalist with Carmen Cavallaro orch.; sings with Columbia records; m.p. debut in Those Redheads from Seattle; also in: Red Garters.
TV: Guy Mitchell TV Show, Whispering Smith Series NBC.

MITCHELL, JOHN H.: Executive. b. Rochester, N.Y., Apr. 27, 1918; e. University of Michigan. radio dept., Erwin Wasey & Co., 1939; mgr. sales service dept., Mutual Broadcasting System, 1939; U.S. Navy; WVET and Honel Corp., 1946; dir. of television, United Artists, 1948; v.p. & gen. mgr. UA television dept., to 1952; Screen Gems, Inc., 1952; on bd. dirs., 1961, and first v.p. Columbia Pictures Ind., Inc. 1969 Pres. Screen Gems Div. of Columbia Pictures Industries; 1973, pres. Columbia Pictures Television, Division of Columbia Pictures Industries, and executive vice president of Columbia Pictures Industries Inc. 1975, elected to board of directors of Columbia Pictures Industries; 1975, elected pres. of Hollywood Radio and Television Society. Resigned all offices-Columbia Pictures Industries 1977. Formed John H. Mitchell Co., Inc. 1977. Located in Los Angeles, television program and distribution consultants. First v.p.-Academy of Television Arts & Sciences, 1978–79; chmn., Academy of TV Arts & Sciences, forum luncheons, 1979–82; pres., Academy of TV Arts & Sciences 1980–83; chm., TV Academy Hall of Fame, 1984–87.

MITCHELL, STEVE: Actor. b. New York, Dec. 15; e. Univ. of Wisconsin; grad. Feagin School of Drama, New York. U.S. Navy World War II and Korean War. Summer stock, Hilltop Md. Bway appearances Diamond Lil. Toured with Strike a Match. Screen debut in Walk East on Beacon St. 1952. M.P. and TV rep. State of Ark. (consultant).
PICTURES INCLUDE: Above and Beyond, Tender Hearts, Battle Circus, Fearless Feagin, Gypsy Colt, Gunsight Ridge, Big Combo, The Killing, Deep Six, Terror in a Texas Town, Seven Men From Now, China Doll, Submarine Sea Hawk, Girl in the Red Bikini, Most Dangerous Man Alive, Cause of Death, Once A Thief, Nevada Smith, Young Runaways.

MITCHUM, JIM: Actor. b. Los Angeles, May 8, 1941. m. actress Wendy Wagner. Son of Robert Mitchum. e. Univ. High School in L.A. Went directly from school to Hollywood Professional School. On-job prof. training at Barter Theatre in Virginia.
PICTURES INCLUDE: Thunder Road (debut), The Last Time I Saw Archie, The Victors, Ambush Bay, Tramplers, In Harm's Way, Invisible Six, Moonrunners, Beat Generation, Ride the Wild Surf, Trackdown.

MITCHUM, ROBERT: Actor. b. Bridgeport, Conn., Aug. 6, 1917. Odd jobs; to California; joined Long Beach Players Guild; appeared in Hopalong Cassidy series with William Boyd; in Westerns 8 yrs. RKO.
PICTURES INCLUDE: Story of G.I. Joe, Undercurrent, Pursued Locket, Til' the End of Time, Desire Me, Crossfire, Out of the Past, Rachel and the Stranger, Blood on the Moon, Red Pony, Big Steal, His Kind of Woman, Where Danger Lives, Her Forbidden Past, Macao, Racket, One Minute to Zero, Lost Men, Angel Face, White Witch Doctor, Second Chance, She Couldn't Say No, River of No Return, Track of the Cat, Night of the Hunter, Not as a Stranger, Man with the Gun, Foreign Intrigue, Bandido, Heaven Knows Mr. Allison, Fire Down Below, Wonderful Country, Home from the Hill, Sundowners, The Last Time I Saw Archie, Cape Fear, The Longest Day, List of Adrian Messenger, Two for the Seesaw, Rampage, Mr. Moses, El Dorado, Anzio, Villa Rides, Five Card Stud, Secret Ceremony, Young Billy Young, Good Guys and the Bad Guys, Ryan's Daughter, Going Home, Wrath of God, Friends of Eddie Coyle, The Yakuza, Farewell My Lovely, Midway, The Last Tycoon, Amsterdam Kill, The Big Sleep, Matilda, That Championship Season, Maria's Lovers, The Ambassador.
TELEVISION: The Winds of War, A Killer in the Family, The Hearst and Davies Affair, Reunion at Fairborough, Promises to Keep, Thompson's Lost Run.

MITOSKY, ALAN P.: Executive. b. Philadelphia, March 13, 1934. e. Univ. of Penna., School of Fine Arts (BFA, 1957). Was curator of museums in Phila. (1957–65) and later assoc. dir. of Philadelphia Civic Center, handling performing arts and film programs, promotion of trade shows, conventions, etc. In 1970–72 v.p., production, Madison Square Garden. In 1972 named pres. Leisure Presentations of America, packaging and producing film properties and rock and pop concerts. In 1974 named gen. mgr. Dragon Aire Ltd. and No Moss Films, handling distribution of theatrical properties. In 1975 pres. of Coliseum Films and Athena Films Ltd., natl. theatrical film dist., prod., foreign sales and prod. repr. in 1977–81 project administrator, National Endowment for the Arts Short Film Showcase—dist. of special films; 1981–83, v.p., sls., TVC Video; v.p. mktg., Video Works, Inc., 1984; pres. CEL Video Services, 1986.

MOBERLY, LUKE: Producer, director, writer. b. Richmond, Ky., Nov. 1, 1925. e. Univ. of Cincinnati, 1947, Univ. of Miami, 1951. Designed and built studio buildings; designer and set builder.
PICTURES INCLUDE: Country A-Go-Go, The Misfits, Gavilan, Devil's Sisters, Go-Go-A-Go-Go, etc. Wrote screenplay: Psychedelic, Rhinemans Seven, Ride Roxie Ride, In the Skin with Me, Easy Little Laura, Old Time Religion. Dir. and prod.: Moonlight Maniac, Assoc., prod.: That Nice Boy, writer, producer, director.: Sweet Talker, Skunk Aper, Moberly/Gordon Studios Inc. Production Company for feature films, 1975.

MOCIUK, YAR W.: Executive. b. Ukraine, Jan. 26, 1927. e. CCNY, World Univ., Peoples Univ. of Americas (Puerto Rico). Expert in field of m.p. care and repair; holds U.S. patent for method and apparatus for treating m.p. film. Has also been film producer and director. Founder and pres. of C&M Films Service, Inc. until 1973. Now chm. of bd. and pres. of Filmtreat International Corp. Member: M.P. & TV Engineers; Univ. Film Assn. Pres., Ukrainian Cinema Assn. of America.

MODINE, MATTHEW: Actor. Studied with Stella Adler.
PICTURES: Baby It's You, Private School, Streamers, Hotel New Hampshire, VisionQuest, Mrs. Soffel, Birdy, Full Metal Jacket.

MOGER, ART.: Publicity executive-Author. b. Boston, Mass., April 4. e. Boston U. Coll. of Journalism (BS) Cartoonist & caricaturist, stage & screen attractions; feature writer. nat. mag.; script writer, guest appearances with Fred Allen, and many radio, TV shows (Mike Douglas Show, Merv Griffin); creator cartoon strip Seymour Shoze, dealing with m.p. and comic strip, Groucho, based on Groucho Marx: orig., About Faces, puzzle series; in 1937 syndicated cartoon series; pressbook cartoonist; handled personal appearances of celebrities. Pub. exec., Warner Bros. & other m.p. cos. Holds record for "My Favorite Jokes" in Parade Magazine. (8 consecutive times) First honorary trustee of Nat'l. Broadcasters Hall of Fame; member Sigma Delta Chi, professional journalism society. Kentucky Colonel and Admiral.
AUTHOR: You'll Dial Laughing, Pros and Cons, Some of My Best Friends Are People, The Complete Pun Book, Hello! My Real Name Is. . ., Have You Played Your Numbers Today?, The Swindlers. Pres., Advertising Enterprises, Boston; exec., Amuse-A-Menu Co.; dorArt Enterprises; pres. and originator Tub Thumpers of Amer. Charter member, Nat'l. Hall of Humor.

MOGER, STANLEY H.: Executive. Pres., SFM Entertainment, Exec. Vice Pres., SFM Media Corp. b. Boston, Nov. 13, 1936. e. Colby Coll., Waterville, ME (BA, 1958). m. Marcia Fleishman, May 29, 1960, children—Robin 22, Wendy 20; announcer/TV personality/WVDA and WORL (Boston) 1953–54; WGHM (Skowhegan) 1955–56; WTWO-TV (Bangor) 1955; WMHB (Waterville) 1956–57; WTVL (Waterville) 1957–58; unit pub. dir., Jaguar Prods., 1958–59; US Army reserve, 1958–64, with calls to active duty in 1958–59 and 1961–62; account exec., NBC Films/California National Productions, Chicago; 1959–60, asst. sales manager, Midwest, RCA/NBC Medical Radio System; acct. exec. Hollingbery Co., Chicago, 1960–63; and New York 1963–66; account executive, Storer Television Sales, 1966–69; co-founded SFM, Sept. 29, 1969. In 1978, named pres., SFM Entertainment which is responsible for the revival of Walt Disney's "Mickey Mouse Club," "The Adventures of Rin-Tin-Tin"; Mobil Showcase Network; SFM Holiday Network. Executive producer-"Television-Annual 1978–79" ABC-TV Network; Executive Producer-"Your New Day" with Vidal Sassoon, The Origins Game; Believe You Can and You Can (from Disneyland, Walt Disney Presents Sport Goofy Series); exec. prod., The World of Tomorrow. Exec. prod., March of Time. . .on the March (channel 4, England).
PROPERTIES INCLUDE: SFM Holiday Network, SFM Documentary Network, Car Care Central, Your New Day

with Vidal Sassoon, March of Time series, Co-Packager Superstars-ABC-TV Adventures of the Wilderness Family-ABC-TV; Across the Great Divide-CBS-TV; Mysteries from Beyond Earth-NBC-TV; To the Ends of the Earth-PBS; Challenge To Be Free-ABC-TV, CBS-TV; Wonder of Lt. Allen ABC-TV; Great American Cowboy-ABC-TV; Dayan-ABC-TV and WTBS-TV; Sports Illustrated (a series for TV); General Foods Golden Showcase Network—Shock Trauma; 1983 official film of the America's Cup Challenge; Countdown to the Cup; Pinocchio in Outer Space; Rudyard Kipling's Jungle Book; The Heisman Trophy Annual Award Specials; Walt Disney World's Very Merry Xmas Parade (ABC); The Indomitable Teddy Roosevelt; (ABC); Crusade in the Pacific; Rosepetal Place; Hugga-Bunch; Jayce and the Wheeled Warriors (animated); Time Travel: Fact, Fiction and Fantasy; Zoobilee Zoo.

MOLINARO, EDOUARD: Director. b. Bordeaux. Made amateur films at university and launched professional career via award-winning technical shorts. First feature film, Le Dos au Mur (1957).
PICTURES INCLUDE: Girls for the Summer, A Ravishing Idiot, Gentle Art of Seduction, La Cage Aux Folles (also Part II), Sunday Lovers, Just the Way You Are.

MOLL, ELICK: Writer. b. New York City, Mar. 20, 1907; e. U. Illinois; U. Chicago. Short story writer, novelist, playwright; Seidman and Son, Memoir of Spring, Night Without Sleep, Image of Tallie, Seidman and the Geisha, Perilous Spring of Morris Seidman; worked with Samuel Goldwyn, MGM, Fox, Columbia stories appear in magazines, texts on short story; won 2nd prize O'Henry Memorial Award Prize Stories 1937.
PICTURES INCLUDE: You Were Meant for Me, Wake Up and Dream, House on Telegraph Hill, Night Without Sleep, Storm Center, Spring Reunion.
TV: Playhouse 90, Chrysler Theatre, others.
AWARDS: Academy of TV Arts & Sciences for best teleplay: Sizeman & Son; TV Writers award for best script: The Fabulous Irishman.

MONASH, PAUL: Producer-Writer. b. New York City. e. Univ. of Wisconsin, Columbia Univ. Was in U.S. Army Signal Corps and Merchant Marine; newspaper reporter; high school teacher; and civilian employee of U.S. gov't. in Europe. Wrote two novels: How Brave We Live, The Ambassadors. Entered industry writing TV scripts on such shows as Playhouse 90, Studio One, Theatre Guild of the Air, Climax, etc. Authored two-part teleplay which launched The Untouchables. In 1958 won Emmy award for The Lonely Wizard, dramatization of life of German-born electrical inventor Charles Steinmetz. Made m.p. debut as exec. prod. of Butch Cassidy and the Sundance Kid, 1969.
PICTURES INCLUDE: Slaughterhouse-Five (prod.), The Friends of Eddie Coyle (prod., s.p.), The Front Page (prod.), Carrie (prod.).

MONICELLI, MARIO: Director. b. Rome, Italy, May 15, 1915. Ent. m.p. industry in production; later co-authored, collab., comedies. Dir.: Big Deal on Madonna Street, The Great War, Tears of Joy, Boccaccio '70, The Organizer.

MONKHOUSE, BOB: TV-radio-cabaret comedian & comedy writer. b. Beckenham, Kent, June 1, 1928; e. Dulwich College. Debut 1948 while serving in RAF, own radio comedy series 1949–83 (winters), own TV series, BBC 1952–56, ITV 1956–83; BBC (ongoing). Several West End revues, Boys from Syracuse (Theatre Royal, Drury Lane); Come Blow Your Horn, (Prince of Wales) (2 yrs); The Gulls; others. Films include: Carry On, Sergeant; Weekend with Lulu; Dentist in the Chair; She'll Have to Go; Bliss of Mrs. Blossom; others. Major cabaret attraction U.K., Australia, Hong Kong. British star of numerous TV series including: What's My Line?; Who Do You Trust?; Mad Movies; Quick On The Draw; Bob Monkhouse Comedy Hour; The Golden Shot (8 years); Celebrity Squares (4 yrs); I'm Bob, He's Dickie! (1978–81); Family Fortunes (1979–83); Bob Monkhouse Tonight (1983–ongoing). Regular dramatic guest spots ITV & BBC-TV, now under exclusive contract to BBC till 1986 for Tonight Show and new game shows.

MONKS, JOHN, JR.: Writer, actor, prod., dir. b. Brooklyn, N.Y. e. Virginia Military Institute, A.B.; actor, stock, b'way, radio, m.p. U.S. Marines, 1942; commissioned Major, 1945. Playwright Co-author Brother Rat.
PICTURES INCLUDE: Brother Rat, Co-author Brother Rat And A Baby, Strike Up the Band, The House on 92nd Street, 13 Rue Madeleine, Wild Harvest, Dial 1119., The West Point Story, People Against O'Hara. Where's Charley. So This Is Love, Knock On Any Door, No Man Is An Island.
TV: Climax: The Gioconda Smile, A Box of Chocolates; 20th Century-Fox Hour: Miracle on 34th St.; Gen. Electric Theatre: Emily; CBS Special: High Tor; SWAT; Creator serial: Paradise Bay.

MONTAGNE, EDWARD J.: Producer-director. b. Brooklyn; e. Loyola University, of Notre Dame. RKO Pathe, 1942; U.S. Army, 1942–46; prod. many cos. after army.
PICTURES INCLUDE: Tattooed Stranger, The Man With My Face, McHale's Navy, McHale's Navy Joins The Air Force, P.J.
TV: Man Against Crime, Cavalier Theatre, The Vaughn Monroe Show, The Hunter, I Spy, Mchale's Navy; exec. prod. of film-CBS-N.Y., Phil Silvers Show. Prod. & head of programming, Wm. Esty Adv. Co., 1950; Program consultant, William Esty Co.; v.p. Universal TV prod. & dir.: 5 Don Knotts features; prod.: Andy Griffith, Angel in My Pocket, Ellery Queen, A Very Missing Person, Short Walk to Daylight, Hurricane, Terror on the 40th Floor, Francis Gary Powers, Million Dollar Ripoff, Crash of Flight 401, High Noon—Part 2, Harper Valley PTA.

MONTALBAN, RICARDO: Actor. b. Mexico City, Mex., Nov. 25, 1920. Appeared in Mexican pictures 1941–45; to U.S.
PICTURES INCLUDE: Fiesta, On an Island With You, Kissing Bandit, Neptune's Daughter, Battleground, Mystery Street, Right Cross, Two Weeks with Love, Across the Wide Missouri, Mark of Renegade, My Man and I, Sombrero, Border Incident, Latin Lovers, Saracen Blade, Life in The Balance, Sayonara, Hemingways Adventures of a Young Man, The Reluctant Saint, Love Is a Ball, Sol Madrid, Blue, Sweet Charity, Conquest of the Planet of the Apes, The Train Robbers, Star Trek II: The Wrath of Khan, Cannonball Run II.
TELEVISION: Series: Fantasy Island.

MONTAND, YVES: Actor, singer. r.n. Yvo Livi. b. Monsumano, Italy, Oct. 13, 1921. Worked as a truck loader, waiter in dock-side bar, and barber. Performed in Marseilles as singer in clubs and music halls. m. Simone Signoret, actress, 1951.
PICTURES INCLUDE: Etoile Sans Lumiere, Les Portes de La Nuit, L'Idole, Souvenir Perdus, Le Salaire de la Peur (Wages of Fear), Nostri Tempi, Mar, Napoleon, Les Heros Sont Fatigues, Marguerite de la Nuit, Uomini e Lupi, Les Sorcieres de Salem (The Crucible), La Lunga Strada, Un Denomme Squarcio, Le Pere et L'enfant, La Loi (Where the Hotwind Blows), Let's Make Love, Sanctuary, My Geisha, Goodbye Again, The Sleeping Car Murders, La Guerre est Finie, Is Paris Burning?, Grand Prix, Live for Life, Z, On A Clear Day You Can See Forever, The Vow, State of Siege.

MONTGOMERY, ELIZABETH: Actress. b. Los Angeles, April 15, 1933. e. AADA. Daughter of the late Robert Montgomery.
PICTURES: The Court Martial of Billy Mitchell, Johnny Cool, Who's Been Sleeping in My Bed?
TELEVISION: Series: Bewitched. Movies: The Victim, Mrs. Sundance, A Case of Rape, The Legend of Lizzie Borden, Dark Victory, A Killing Affair, The Awakening Land, Jennifer: A Woman's Story, Missing Pieces, Second Sight: A Love Story, Amos.

MONTGOMERY, GEORGE: Actor. r.n. George Montgomery Letz; b. Brady, Mont., Aug. 29, 1916; e. U. of Montana. Armed Services, World War II.
PICTURES INCLUDE: Cisco Kid and the Lady (1939), Star Dust, Young People, Charter Pilot, Jennie, Cowboy and the Blonde, Accent on Love, Riders of the Purple Sage, Last of the Duanes, Cadet Girl, Roxie Hart, Ten Gentlemen from West Point, Orchestra Wives, China Girl, Brasher Doubloon, Three Little Girls in Blue, Lulu Belle, Belle Starr's Daughter, Girl From Manhattan, Sword of Monte Cristo, Texas Rangers, Indian Uprising, Cripple Creek, Pathfinder, Jack McCall Desperado, Fort Ti, Gun Belt, Battle of Rogue River, Lone Gun, Masterson of Kansas, Seminole Uprising, Robbers' Roost, Too Many Crooks, Stallion Trail, The Steel Claw, Watusi, Samar, Hallucination Generation, Hostile Guns.

MONTY PYTHON: Group of six British comedians who performed for BBC-TV during the '60s and '70s. they include Eric Chapman, John Cleese, Terry Gilliam, Eric Idle, Terry Jomes, and Michael Palin.
PICTURES: And Now for Something Completely Different, Monty Python and the Holy Grail, The Life of Brian, Monty Python at the Hollywood Bowl, Monty Python's The Meaning of Life.

MOONJEAN, HANK: Producer-Director. Began as asst. dir. at MGM. Later turned to producing.
PICTURES INCLUDE: Assoc. Prod.: The Great Gatsby, WUSA. Exec. Prod.: The Fortune, The End. Producer; Hooper, Smokey and the Bandit II, The Incredible Shrinking Woman, Paternity, Sharky's Machine, Stroker's Ace (prod.).

MOORE, CONSTANCE: Actress. b. Sioux City, Iowa, Jan. 18, 1922. Sang on radio; Lockheed prog., 2 yrs; Jurgen's Show, 2 yrs. Screen debut 1938. TV shows, nightclubs. N.Y. Stage: The Boys From Syracuse, By Jupiter.
PICTURES INCLUDE: Prison Break, A Letter of Introduction, I Wanted Wings, Take A Letter Darling, Show Business, Delightfully Dangerous, Earl Carroll Sketchbook, In Old Sacramento, Hit Parade of 1947.

MOORE, DEMI: Actress. b. Roswell, NM, Nov. 11, 1962.
PICTURES: Choices, Young Doctors in Love, Blame It on Rio, No Small Affair, St. Elmo's Fire, One Crazy Summer.
TELEVISION: General Hospital, Bedrooms.

MOORE, DICKIE: Actor. b. Los Angeles, Cal., Sept. 12, 1925. Began picture career when only 11 months old, appearing with John Barrymore in The Beloved Rogue.
PICTURES INCLUDE: Oliver Twist, Peter Ibbetson, Dangerous Years, Out of the Past, Eight Iron Men, Member of the Wedding.

MOORE, DUDLEY: Actor-Writer-Musician. b. England, April 19, 1935. e. Oxford, graduating in 1958. Toured British Isles with jazz group before joining with three other Englishmen to put on revue, Beyond the Fringe, which was a hit in U.K. and N.Y. Appeared later with Peter Cook in N.Y. in Good Evening.
PICTURES: Monte Carlo or Bust, The Bed Sitting Room, Bedazzled, Foul Play, "10", Wholly Moses, Arthur, Six Weeks, Lovesick, Romantic Comedy, Unfaithfully Yours, The Best Defense, Micki and Maude, Santa Claus.

MOORE, ELLIS: Executive. b. New York, N.Y., May 12, 1924. e. Washington and Lee U., 1941–43. Newspaperman in Arkansas, Tenn., 1946–52; Joined NBC 1952; mgr. of bus. pub., 1953; dir., press dept., 1954; dir., press & publicity, Dec. 22, 1959; vice-pres., 1961; pub. rel. dept., Standard Oil Co. (N.J.), 1963–66; v.p. press relations, ABC-TV Network, 1966–68; v.p. public relations ABC-TV Network, 1968–70; v.p. public relations, ABC, 1970, v.p. public relations, ABC, Inc., 1972; v.p. corporate relations, ABC, Inc., 1979; v.p., public affairs, ABC, Inc., 1982–85. P.R. consultant, 1985.

MOORE, GARRY: Performer. r.n. Thomas Garrison Morfit; b. Baltimore, Md., Jan. 31, 1915. Continuity writer, WBAL; announcer, sports commentator, KWK, St. Louis; comedian, writer, Club Matinee show, Chicago; Everything Goes, N.Y.; teamed with Jimmy Durante on radio to 1947; m.c., Take It or Leave It, Breakfast in Hollywood.
TV: Star of Garry Moore Show, I've Got A Secret. Best TV daytime show: Fame Poll, 1958; To Tell The Truth.

MOORE, KIERON: Actor. b. Skibereen, Co. Cork, Eire, 1925; e. St. Mary's Coll. (Dublin). Stage debut, 1945 in Desert Rats; appeared in Red Roses For Me. Film debut 1947 in A Man About The House.
PICTURES INCLUDE: Anna Karenina, Mine Own Executioner, Ten Tall Men, David and Bathsheba, Saints and Sinners, Naked Heart, Honeymoon Deferred, Man Trap (Man in Hiding), Conflict of Wings (Fuss Over Feathers), Green Scarf, Blue Peter, Satellite in the Sky, Three Sundays to Live, The Key, The Angry Hills, The Day They Robbed the Bank of England, League of Gentlemen, The Seige of Sidney Street, Faces of Evil, Lion of Sparta, Steel Bayonet, I Thank a Fool, Double Twist, The Day of the Triffids, The Thin Red Line, The Main Attraction, Crack in the World, Son of a Gunfighter, Never Love a Savage, Run Like a Thief, Custer of the West, Ryan International, The Dolmetch Story, Zoo Gang, The Progress of Peoples, The Parched Land.

MOORE, KINGMAN T.: Director. b. Macon, Ga., Sept. 13, 1919; e. Wharton Sch. of Finance, U. of Pa., BS; Member: Lambs Club, Phi Delta Theta, Actor, 1939–41; U.S. Army, 1941–46; asst. cutter, RKO Radio Pictures, 1946–47; production asst., 1947–48; CBS-TV, N.Y., 1948–49; NBC-TV, N.Y., Hollywood, 1949–52; dir. CBS shows include: Places Please, Backstage with Barry Wood, Kobbs Korner, Adventures in Jazz.
TV: Candid Camera, Lights Out, Your Show of Shows, Colgate Comedy Hour.

MOORE, MARY TYLER: Actress. b. Brooklyn. N.Y., Dec. 29, 1936; Began as professional dancer.
TV: Steve Canyon, Richard Diamond, 77 Sunset Strip, Hawaiian Eye, Bachelor Father; feature role on The Dick Van Dyke Show (2 Emmy awards); star, The Mary Tyler Moore Show, Mary. Movies: Heartsounds, Finnegan Begin Again.
PICTURES INCLUDE: X-15, Thoroughly Modern Millie, Don't Just Stand There, What's So Bad About Feeling Good, Change of Habit, Ordinary People, Six Weeks, Just Between Friends.

MOORE, ROGER: Actor. Dir. b. London, England, Oct. 14, 1927. e. Art School, London; Royal Acad. of Dramatic Art.
PLAYS: Mr. Roberts, I Capture the Castle, Little Hut, others.
BROADWAY: A Pin to See the Peepshow.
TV: Maverick, The Alaskans, Ivanhoe, The Saint, The Persuaders.
PICTURES INCLUDE: Last Time I Saw Paris, Interrupted Melody, King's Thief, Diane, The Miracle, Gold of the Seven Saints, Rachel Cade, Rape of the Sabines, No Mans Land, Crossplot, The Man Who Haunted Himself, Live and Let Die, Gold, The Man with the Golden Gun, That Lucky Touch, Street People, Shout at the Devil, Sherlock Holmes in New York, The Spy Who Loved Me, The Wild Geese, Escape To Athena, Moonraker, ffolkes, The Sea Wolves, Sunday Lovers, For Your Eyes Only, The Cannonball Run, Octopussy, The Naked Face, A View to a Kill.

MOORE, TERRY: Actress. r.n. Helen Koford; b. Los Angeles, Cal., Jan. 1, 1932; mother Luella Bickmore, actress. Photographer's model as a child; on radio; with Pasadena Playhouse 1940; in m.p. 1933.
PICTURES INCLUDE: Gaslight, Son of Lassie, Sweet and Low Down, Shadowed, Devil on Wheels, Return of October, Mighty Joe Young, He's a Cockeyed Wonder, Gambling House, Two of a Kind, Sunny Side of the Street, Star of Tomorrow: 1958, Man on a Tightrope, Beneath the 12-mile Reef, King of the Khyber Rifles, Daddy Long Legs, Shack Out on 101, Postmark for Danger, Come Back Little Sheba, Bernardine, Why Must I Die?, Platinum High School, A Private's Affair, Cast a Long Shadow, City of Fear, Black Spurs, Town Tamer, Waco, A Man Called Dagger.

MOORE, THOMAS W.: Executive. e. U of Mo.; Naval aviator, USNR, 1940–45. Adv. dept., Star, Meridian, Miss.; v.p., adv. mgr., Forest Lawn Memorial Park; account exec., CBS-TV Film Sales, Los Angeles; gen. sales mgr., CBS-TV Film Sales, 1956; v.p. in chg. programming & talent, 1958; pres., ABC-TV Network, 1962; chmn. bd., Ticketron, 1968; pres., Tomorrow Entertainment, Inc. 1971; chm., 1981.

MOREAU, JEANNE: Actress. b. Paris, France, 1928. e. Nat'l Conservatory of Dramatic Art. Stage debut with Comedie Francaise, acting there until 1952 when she joined the Theatre Nationale Populaire, Director: Lumiere (film), 1976. L'Adolescente.
PLAYS: A Month in the Country, La Machine Infernale, Pygmalion, Cat on a Hot Tin Roof.
PICTURES INCLUDE: The She-wolves, Elevator to the Scaffold, The Lovers, Le Dialogue Des Carmelites, Les Liaisons Dangereuses, Moderato Cantabile, La Notte, Jules and Jim, A Woman is a Woman, Eva, The Trial, Bay of Angels, The Victors, Le Feu Follet, Diary of a Chambermaid, The Yellow Rolls-Royce, The Train, Mata Hari, Viva Maria, Mademoiselle, Chimes at Midnight, Sailor From Gibraltar, The Bride Wore Black, The Immortal Story, Great Catherine, Monte Walsh, Alex in Wonderland, The Little Theatre of Jean Renoir, The Last Tycoon, Mr. Klein, Querelle, The Trout.

MORENO, FRANK: Executive. Distribution executive for First Artists and v.p. of dist. & world-wide mktg. for New World Pictures, before setting up own company, The Frank Moreno Co. In January, 1984, joined Almi Pictures as pres. & CEO.

MORENO, RITA: Actress. b. Humacao, Puerto Rico, Dec. 11, 1931. Spanish dancer since childhood; night club entertainer; m.p. debut in 1950.
PICTURES INCLUDE: Pagan Love Song, Toast of New Orleans, Singin' in the Rain, The Ring, Cattle Town, Latin Lovers, Jivaro, Yellow Tomahawk, Garden of Evil, Untamed, Seven Cities of Gold, Lieutenant Wore Skirts, King and I, This Rebel Breed, Summer and Smoke, West Side Story, The Night of the Following Day, Marlowe, Popi, Carnal Knowledge, The Ritz, Happy Birthday, Gemini, The Four Seasons.
TELEVISION: Nine to Five, Eva Peron, Anatomy of a Seduction.

MORGAN, ANDRE: Producer. b. Morocco, 1953. e. Univ. of Kansas, majoring in Oriental languages-literature. Met Raymond Chow and joined his film production co. in Hong Kong. Produced Enter the Dragon, Bruce Lee kung-fu picture. Now acts as prod. on Golden Harvest's Chinese language films as well as new division established to produce English-language films.
PICTURES INCLUDE: Enter the Dragon, The Amsterdam Kill, The Boys in Company C, Cannonball Run II.

MORGAN, DENNIS: Actor. r.n. Stanley Morner; b. Prentice, Wisc., Dec. 10, 1910; e. Carroll Coll. Started with State Lake Theat., Chicago. Toured midwest in Faust, sang in Empire Room of Palmer House, Chicago, appeared on NBC programs and sang lead in Xerxes. Screen debut, 1936.
PICTURES INCLUDE: Susy, The Fighting 69th, Three Cheers for the Irish, My Wild Irish Rose, Two Guys from Milwaukee, Two Guys from Texas, Cheyenne, Perfect Strangers, To the Victor, One Sunday Afternoon, Raton Pass, Pretty Baby, Painting the Clouds with Sunshine, Star of Tomorrow (1941), This Woman is Dangerous, Cattle Town, Gun That Won the West, Pearl of the South Pacific, Uranium Boom.

MORGAN, HARRY: Actor. r.n. Harry Bratsburg; b. Detroit, Mich., Apr. 10, 1915; e. U. Chicago. Screen debut 1942.
TV: December Bride, Pete and Gladys, MASH, Dragnet, After MASH, etc.

PLAYS: Gentle People, My Heart's in the Highlands, Thunder Rock, Night Music, Night Before Christmas.

PICTURES INCLUDE: To the Shores of Tripoli, Loves of Edgar Allen Poe, Orchestra Wives, Dragonwyck, Appointment with Danger, The Highwayman, When I Grow Up, The Well, Blue Veil, Bend of the River, Scandal Sheet, My Six Convicts, Boots Malone, High Noon, What Price Glory, Stop You're Killing Me, Arena, Torch Song, Glenn Miller Story, About Mrs. Leslie, Forty-Niners, Far Country, Not As a Stranger, Backlash, Strategic Air Command, Support Your Local Sheriff, Charlie and the Angels, Snowball Express, The Apple Dumpling Gang, The Greatest, Cat from Outer Space.

MORGAN, LESLIE: Executive. b. Santa Ana, CA. e. Vice Pres., production, for 20th Century-Fox which co. she joined in Dec., 1984. Prior to that served as v.p. prod., Warner Bros.; story editor for British producer David Puttnam; story editor for Casablanca Records & Filmworks; same post with Charles Fries Prods.

MORGAN, MICHELE: Actress. r.n. Simone Roussel; b. Paris, France, Feb. 29, 1920; e. Dieppe, dramatic school, Paris. Decided on acting career at 15 yrs., won role at 17 opposite Charles Boyer in Gribouille (later filmed as The Lady in Question, Hollywood). Made several pictures abroad; to U.S. 1940. First Amer. film Joan of Paris, 1942.

PICTURES INCLUDE: The Chase, Symphonie Pastorale, Fallen Idol, Fabiola, 7 Deadly Sins, Moment of Truth, Daughters of Destiny, Naked Heart, Proud and the Beautiful, Grand Maneuver, Oasis, Lost Command, Benjamin.

MORGAN, TERENCE: Actor. b. London, Eng., Dec. 8, 1921; e. Ewell Castle, Surrey & R.A.D.A. Stage debut: There Shall Be No Night, London 1943; m.p. debut: Hamlet, 1948.

PICTURES INCLUDE: Capt. Horatio Hornblower, Encore, Mandy, It Started in Paradise, Steel Key, Street Corner, Turn the Key Softly, Always a Bride, Forbidden Cargo, Dance Little Lady, Femina, Svengali, They Can't Hang Me, March Hare, It's a Wonderful World, The Scamp, Tread Softly Stranger, The Shakedown, Picadilly Third Stop, The Curse of the Mummy's Tomb, The Penthouse, Hide and Seek, The Lifetaker.

TV: Perchance to Dream, More Than Robbery (serial), Now Barabbas, Women in Love, Sir Francis Drake (series of 26), The Persuaders, etc.

MORIARTY, MICHAEL: Actor. b. Detroit, April 5, 1941. e. Dartmouth. Studied at London Academy of Music and Dramatic Arts. Appeared with New York Shakespeare Festival, Charles Street Playhouse (Boston), Alley Theatre (Houston) and Tyrone Guthrie Theatre (Minneapolis). Broadway debut in The Trial of the Catonsville Nine.

PICTURES INCLUDE: Glory Boy (debut), Hickey & Boggs, Shoot It, Bang the Drum Slowly, The Last Detail, Report to the Commissioner, Who'll Stop the Rain, Too Far To Go, The Winged Serpent, Pale Rider, The Stuff, Troll.

TV: The Glass Menagerie, Girls of Summer, The Deadliest Season, Holocaust.

STAGE: Find Your Way Home, Richard III, The Caine Mutiny Courtmartial.

MORIN, ROBERT B.: Executive. b. New York, N.Y., Nov. 24. e. Harvard Coll., Merch, Mgr., ad agency. AAP sis., 1955; AAP mgr. program sls., 1956; eastern sis. mgr., MGM-TV, 1957; sls. mgr., Lopert-UA, 1959; v.p., Allied Artists TV; formed Scandia Films, pres., 1965; joined RKO, 1966, in chg. foreign operations; 1968, pres. Lin Medallion Pict. Corp.; 1970–73, Talent Associates; 1973–76, exec. v.p., Heritage Eng.; 1976–78, v.p., MGM TV; 1978–80, pres. Lorimar Syndication; 1980, exec. v.p., 20th Century Fox; 1985, pres., New Century Telecommunications.

MORITA, NORIYUKI "PAT": Entertainer-Actor. Began show business career as opening act in night clubs for such stars as Ella Fitzgerald, Johnny Mathis, Diana Ross and the Supremes, Glen Campbell, etc. Worked in saloons, coffee houses, and dinner theatres before becoming headliner in Las Vegas showrooms, Playboy Clubs, Carnegie Hall, etc. Guest on most TV talk and variety shows and regular on many series: MASH, Love Boat, Magnum, P.I., etc. Regular role on series, Happy Days.

PICTURES: Thoroughly Modern Millie, Midway, Savannah Smiles, Jimmy the Kid, The Karate Kid, The Karate Kid: Part II.

TELEVISION: The Vegas Strip War, Amos.

MORITZ, MILTON I: Executive. b. Pittsburgh, Pa., Apr. 27, 1933; e. Woodbury College, grad. 1955. Owned, operated theatres in L.A., 1953–55; U.S. Navy 1955–57; American International Pictures asst. gen. sls. mgr., 1957; nat'l. dir. of adv. and publ. 1958; v.p. and bd. mem. of American International Pictures, 1967; 1975, named Senior v.p.; in 1980 formed own co., The Milton I. Moritz Co., Inc., Inc., mktg. & dist. consultant. Pres. of Variety Club of Southern California Tent 25, 1975–76.

MORLEY, KAREN: Actress. r.n. Mabel Linton; b. Ottumwa, Iowa; e. Calif. U. Campus Baby Star, 1931; bit part in Scarface, 1932.

PICTURES INCLUDE: Arsene Lupin, Fast Life, Gabriel Over the White House, Dinner at Eight, Crime Doctor, Thunder in the Night, Devil's Squadron, Beloved Enemy, Outcast. Pride and Prejudice, Jealously, Unknown, 13th Hour, Framed, Six Gun Serendade, Code of the Saddle, M..

MORLEY, ROBERT: Actor, writer. b. Wiltshire, England, May 26, 1908; e. Royal Acad. Dram. Arts, London. U.S. Air Force, 1943; prod., assoc. prod., Captain Gallant, Arsen, Chicot, Forbidden Cargo; TV Series: Captain Gallant; Scene of the Crime; TV Advisor, Telepictures of Morroco, Telerama, Ltd., Eng., 1954–59; helped org., Alliance of TV Film Producers; prod., Telerama, Inc., Georgetown Films, Inc., 1960; prod., dir., TV film series closeup, Telefilm, Inc. Presently president, Creative Assoc., Inc. and co-prod. with Helen Ainsworth; exec. prod. with Leon Fromkess, The Long Corridor.

PLAYS: Brit. stage debut London 1929 in Treasure Island, also tour and repertory; N.Y. debut 1938 in Oscar Wilde; other appearances include Great Romancer, Pygmalion; 1948, Edward My Son, co-author, lead London and B'way stage; author several plays (Short Story, Goodness, How Sad, Staff Dance).

PICTURES INCLUDE: Marie Antoinette, You Will Remember, Major Barbara, Big Blockade, This Was Paris, Foreman Went to France, Young Mr. Pitt, I Live in Grosvenor Square, Outcast of the Islands, African Queen, Edward My Son, Curtain Up, The Final Test, Melba, Gilbert & Sullivan, Beat the Devil, Beau Brummell, Rainbow Jacket, Good Die Young, Quentin Durward, Loser Takes All, Six Months Grace, Full Treatment, Hippo Dancing, Around the World in 80 Days, Sheriff of Fractured Jaw, The Journey, The Doctor's Dilemma, Battle of the Sexes, Libel, Oscar Wilde, Go To Blazes, The Young Ones, Nine Hours to Rama, Murder at the Gallop, Topkapi, Amanda, Take Her She's Mine, Genghis Khan, Hot Enough for June, The Alphabet Murders, Sinful Davey, Hot Millions, Some Girls Do, The Trygon Factor, Song of Norway, The Blue Bird, Who Is Killing the Great Chefs of Europe?, Scavenger Hunt, The Human Factor, The Great Muppet Caper.

TV: Call My Bluff (series), Charge!

MORRICONE, ENNIO: Composer-Arranger. b. Rome. Studied with Goffredo Petrassi at the Academy of Santa Cecilia in Rome.

PICTURES INCLUDE: A Fistful of Dollars, El Greco, Fists in the Pocket, Matcheless, Theorem, Once Upon a Time in the West, Investigation of a Citizen, The Bird with the Crystal Plumage, Cat O'Nine Tails, The Red Tent, Four Flies in Grey Velvet, The Decameron, The Black Belly of the Tarantula, Battle of Algiers, Burn, Partner, Orca, The Heretic, Exorcist II, 1900, Days of Heaven, The Island, Tragedy of a Ridiculous Man, Butterfly, So Fine, Once Upon a Time in America.

MORRIS, HOWARD: Actor. b. New York, N.Y., Sept. 4, 1919; e. N.Y.U. U.S. Army, 4 yrs.; dir., Who's Minding the Mint, Don't Drink the Water.

BROADWAY: Hamlet, Call Me Mister, John Loves Mary, Gentlemen Prefer Blondes.

TV: Your Show of Shows, Caesar's Hour.

MORRIS, NELSON: Producer. b. Warsaw, Poland, July 25; e. Columbia Univ. Began in m.p. ind. as child actor, Paramount Studio, Astoria, L.I.; photographer, Life Mag.; WWII, training film div. Army Pictorial Service. After war continued career in advertising, industrial and mag. photography. Org., American Society of Magazine Photographers. Formed, Nelson Morris Prods., 1953; engaged in prod. of industrial and doc. film; prod. films for TV, theatrical feature films; producer, stage prod., Bicycle Ride to Nevada. Now pres., Astoria Pictures Corp.

MORRIS, OSWALD: Cinematographer. b. London. Left school at 16 to work for two years as camera dept. helper at studios. Was lensman for cameraman Ronald Neame who gave Morris first job as cameraman; in 1949 when Reame directed The Golden Salamander he made Morris dir. of photography.

PICTURES INCLUDE: The Golden Salamander, The Card, The Man Who Never Was, Mister Moses, Moulin Rouge, Beat the Devil, Moby Dick, Heaven Knows, Mr. Allison, The Roots of Heaven, Reflections in a Golden Eye, The Mackintosh Man, Oliver!, Scrooge, The Pumpkin Eater, The Hill, The Spy Who Came in from the Cold, A Farewell to Arms, The Key, The Guns of Navarone, Lolita, Term of Trial, Fiddler on the Roof, Sleuth, The Odessa File, The Man Who Would Be King, Seven Per Cent Solution, Just Tell Me What You Want, The Great Muppet Caper, The Dark Crystal.

MORRIS, R. A.: Executive. b. London, England, 1925; e. Imperial Services College, Windsor. Served Royal Navy 1942–46. Ent. m.p. ind. Animation Dept. Polytechnic Studios 1947; AB-Pathe, 16MM salesman, 1948; assist. to overseas sales mgr., 1951: Appt. overseas sales mgr. incl. from 1957 had responsibility for overseas sales of ABC-TV products. 1959 formed Programme Exchange Ltd., 1960; formed Anthony Morris (London) Ltd., 1968.

MORRIS, RICHARD: Director, writer. b. San Francisco, Cal., May 14, 1924; e. Burlingame High School, 1939–42, Chouinard Art Institute, 1946–47; Neighborhood Playhouse, 1947–48; U.S. Army special services, writing shows, Victory Bond; Universal-Int., talent dept., writing directing skits, writing music for acting class and Korean War entertainment troups; s.p. Take Me to Town, Finders Keepers.
AUTHOR, STAGE: The Unsinkable Molly Brown.
PICTURES INCLUDE: If a Man Answers, Thoroughly Modern Millie, Change of Habit.
TV: Wrote & dir. teleplays, Loretta Young Show, wrote & dir. The Pearl (Loretta Young Show), wrote teleplays, Private Secretary, Ford Theatre, Kraft Television Theatre, dir., The Wild Swans (Shirley Temple Show-Christopher Award).

MORRIS, SEYMOUR: Executive. b. Aug. 26, 1906. Started in show business with B.S. Moss, juvenile theatricals; entered m.p. ind. with C.B.C. Pictures on adv. accessories; exp. dept., U.A., Columbia. Ran own theatres, N.Y. State; mgr., upstate N.Y. theatres, Skouras Bros., until 1933; then mgr., dist. mgr., Schine; dir. of adv., pub., pub. rel., Schine Ent. Inc. including theatres, hotels, radio station etc. In 1961 opened own adv. & p.r. agency, Seymour Morris Associates Inc.; also pres. of Northeast Film Enterp. (1967); pres. PMK Prod. Inc.

MORRIS, WILLIAM, JR.: Consultant, retired president, William Morris Agency, Inc. b. New York, Oct. 22, 1899.

MORRISSEY, PAUL: Writer-Director. b. New York City, 1939. e. Fordham Univ. Service in Army; worked for insurance co. and Dept. of Public Welfare before becoming film-maker. Was involved in indep. film prod. for four years prior to joining Andy Warhol with whom he worked on such films as Chelsea Girls, Four Stars, Bike Boy, Nude Restaurant, Lonesome Cowboys, Blue Movie, L'Amour, Women in Revolt.
PICTURES INCLUDE: Flesh, Trash, Heat, Andy Warhol's Frankenstein, Dracula, Forty Deuce, Mixed Blood.

MORRISON, JR., HENRY T.: Executive. b. Mt. Pleasant, NY, Dec. 21, 1939. e. Univ. Minnesota (BA, 1963), IMEDE, Switzerland (PED, 1971); Yale Univ. Divinity School (MA, 1980). Has been ordained Episcopal priest 1983 to present. Positions in banking and marketing before entering m.p. industry 1972 in Minneapolis as assoc. prod., Dangerous Relations. 1976–85, independent financial consultant to industry. 1986, pres. & CEO, Mill City Entertainment, Minneapolis.
PICTURES: Mitchell (assoc. prod.); The Devil's Men (exec. prod.) Author: Intercept, s.p., based on his own novel.

MORRISON, BURTON J.: Executive. Joined 20th Century-Fox in 1963; named snr. financial officer for 20th Century-Fox Pictures. In 1980 named v.p., finance & administration, for The Ladd Company; 1985, v.p., Warner Bros. 1986, joined MGM Entertainment Co. as exec. v.p., finance & admin.

MORROW, JEFF: Actor. b. New York, N.Y., Jan. 13, 1917; e. Pratt Institute. Worked as commercial illustrator. Many radio and TV appearances including TV, Iron Horse.
BROADWAY: Romeo and Juliet, St. Joan, January Thaw, Billy Budd, Three Wishes for Jamie, Lace on Her Petticoat, The Suspects.
PICTURES INCLUDE: The Robe, Flight to Tangier, Siege at Red River, Tanganyika, Sign of the Pagan, Captain Lightfoot, This Island Earth, World in My Corner, Creature Walks Among Us, Giant Claw, Story of Ruth, Harbor Lights.

MORSE, ROBERT: Actor. b. Newton, Mass., May 18, 1931. Served U.S. Navy. Studied with American Theatre Wing, New York, where he had small role in film The Proud and the Profane, 1956. Following radio work, appeared on Broadway stage in The Matchmaker, 1956.
BROADWAY: Say, Darling, Take Me Along, How to Succeed in Business Without Really Trying, Sugar.
PICTURES INCLUDE: The Matchmaker, Honeymoon Hotel, Quick Before it Melts, The Loved One, Oh Dad Poor Dad, How to Succeed in Business Without Really Trying, Guide for the Married Man, The Boatniks.
TV: That's Life series.

MORTON, ARTHUR: Composer, arranger. b. Duluth, Minn., Aug. 8, 1908; e. U. of Minn., 1929. Composer for various film cos. including Universal, RKO, United Artists; with Columbia since 1948.
PICTURES INCLUDE: Night Life of the Gods, Princess O'Hara, Riding On Air, Fit for a King, Turnabout, Walking Hills, The Nevadan, Rogues of Sherwood Forest, Father is a Bachelor, Never Trust a Gambler, Harlem Globetrotters, Big Heat, Pushover, He Laughed Last.
ORCH. ARRANGEMENTS: Laura, Smokey, From Here to Eternity, Jolson Story, Salome, Phfft, No Sad Songs For Me, Born Yesterday, Long Gray Line, Man from Laramine, My Sister Eileen, Queen Bee, Picnic, Jubal, Autumn Leaves, Johnny Concho, Harder They Fall, 3:10 to Yuma, Full of Life, Garment Jungle, They Came to Cordura, Strangers When We Meet, Touch of Mink, Critics Choice, Diamond Head, Toys in the Attic, Man from the Diners' Club, Von Ryan's Express, The Saboteur, Code Name—Morituri, In Harm's Way, What a Way to Go, The New Interns, Rio Conchos, Dear Briggitte, Our Man Flint, Planet of the Apes, Flim Flam Man, Justine, Patton, Tora Tora Tora, Mephisto Waltz, Ballad of Cable Hogue, Traveling Executioner, Escape From the Planet of the Apes, Cold Turkey, Wild Rovers, The Other, Ace Eli, One Little Indian, The Don is Dead, Papillon, Chinatown, Breakout, The Wind and the Lion, Logan's Run, The Omen, Islands in the Stream, Passover Plot, Twilight's Last Gleaming, Damnation Alley, MacArthur, Capricorn One, Coma, The Swarm, Omen II (Damien), Boys from Brazil, Magic, Superman, Alien, Players, Meteor, Star Trek, Inchon, Masoda, The Final Conflict, Outland, Raggedy Man, Night Crossing, Poltergeist, The Secret of NIMH, First Blood, Psycho II, Twilight Zone, Under Fire, The Lonely Guy, Gremlins, Supergirl, Rambo: First Blood Part II, Explorers, King Solomon's Mines, Link, Poltergist II.
TV: Black Saddle, Laramie, Bus Stop, Follow the Sun, My Three Sons, Peyton Place, Medical Center, Daniel Boone, Lancers, National Geographic, Say Goodbye, How to Stay Alive, Hooray For Hollywood, The Waltons, Apple's Way, Medical Story.

MOSES, CHARLES ALEXANDER: Executive-Writer-Producer. b. Chicago, March 1; e. Aeronautical U., Northwestern U., Englewood Eve. Jr. Coll., Antioch U.; Pub. rel. dir., Goldblatt Bros. dept. store chain, Chicago; field adv-promo exec., United Artists, unit publicist for over 30 films, exec., Screen Gems; European adv-pub superv., Paris, United Artists; adv-pub dir., Bel Air Prod., V.P. adv-pub dir., Associates & Aldrich Co., adv-pub dir., Sinatra Enterprises, assoc. studio pub. dir., Universal Studios, adv-pub rep., Universal Studios from Paris for Europe, exec-in-chge New York domestic & foreign adv-pub dept., Universal, adv-pub superv., Orion Pictures Co. Own firm, Charles A. Moses Co., adv-marketing-pub. rel., acc'ts included United Artists, Columbia Picts., 20th Century-Fox, UA-TV, Brut Prod., Michael Klinger Ltd., ITT, Cinecom, Cinemation Industries, Hemdale Leisure Corp., Faberge, Stein & Day Publishers; Information, Inc., Automated Learning, Darrell Waters Ltd., Ebefilms, Phoenix Films, Valley Cable TV, Jensen Farley Picts., Taft Internat'l Picts, auto shows, TV shows, art galleries, events, guilds, Cinevent Prod., Dimitri Tiomkin, Dale Wasserman, American Internat'l Picts., Filmways. Orig. stories, Frankenstein 1970 (Allied Artists), Department Store (Brut Prod.); Prod., Radio Free Europe, Munich, Goldblatt radio, TV shows (WGN); Writer-prod-dir., documentaries, Carson Prod., Mason City; Screenplays, Abigail, The Callers; Musical book, Daddy. Past pres., The Publicists Guild of America (IATSE, Local 818).

MOSES, GILBERT: Director. b. Cleveland, Aug. 20, 1942. New York Stage director; m.p. debut Willie Dynamite, 1973; The Fish That Saved Pittsburgh, 1979.
STAGE: Ain't Supposed to Die a Natural Death, Slave Ship.
TV: Roots.

MOSLEY, ROGER E.: Actor. b. Los Angeles. Planned career in broadcasting but turned to acting, first appearing in small roles in TV series: Night Gallery, Baretta, Kojak, Cannon, Switch, etc. Theatrical film debut in The New Centurions (1972).
PICTURES: Stay Hungry, The Greatest, Semi-Tough, Leadbelly.
TELEVISION: Series: Swtch, Magnum P.I. Movies: I Know Why the Caged Bird Sings, The Jericho Mile, Attica, etc.

MOSS, ARNOLD: Actor-dir. b. New York, Jan. 28, 1910. e. CCNY, BA; Columbia U., MA; New York U., Ph.D.; Teacher, B'klyn Coll. 1932–39; visiting prof., U. of Conn. 1973; Pace U., 1975; College of William and Mary, 1976; Purdue U., 1977. Neighborhood Playhouse School of the Theatre, 1974–76; Univ. Wisconsin, 1985; Theatre, film & TV actor-director.
PICTURES INCLUDE: Temptation, Loves of Carmen, Reign of Terror, Border Incident, Kim, Mask of the Avenger, My Favorite Spy, Viva Zapata, Salome, Casanova's Big Night, Bengal Brigade, Hell's Island, Jump Into Hell, The 27th Day, The Fool Killer, Caper of the Golden Bulls, Gambit.

MOSS, CHARLES B., JR.: Theatre Executive and Producer. b. New York City, Aug. 29, 1944. e. Univ. of Penn. (B.A., 1966), Boston Univ. School of Law (LIB, 1969). Was asst. prof. of law at Boston Univ. 1969–70. Entered ind. as v.p. of B.S. Moss Enterprises, 1970; now pres. Has produced three films: Let's Scare Jessica to Death, Stigma, Diary of the Dead.

MOSS, FRANK L.: Writer-producer. b. New York, N.Y.: e. Duke & Columbia U: Reporter, drama & film critic, N.Y.: U.S. Army Air Force, 1942–46.
PLAYS: author: Glamour Girl, Call To Arms, (colab), So Goes The Nation, (colab), Some People's Children, American Pastoral, City On A Hill.
PICTURES INCLUDE: The Unvanquished, Whiphand, Carribean, Sangaree, Papago Wells, The Half Breed, Sweetheart of Sigma Chi. MILITARY: 22 Air Force Training Films; 17 documentaries.
TV PILOTS: Outer Limits, Grand Jury, The Texan.
TV SCRIPTS: Telephone Hour, Four Star Playhouse, Winston Churchill's Valiant Years, Route 66, Wagon Train, Laramie, Wild Wild West, The Texan, G.E. Theater, Wire Service, U.S. Marshall, M-Squad, Stoney Burke, Tales of The Texas Rangers, T.V. Reader's Digest, Sheriff of Cochise, Whirlybirds, Line-Up, Wyatt Earp, Rin Tin Tin, Walter Winchell File, Daniel Boone, Man Who Never Was, Felony Squad, Richard Diamond, Lassie, Like The Rich People, Hired Mother, Shenandoah, Counterspy, White Hunter.
PROD-STORY ED: Screen Televideo, Sovereign Prod., Wire Service, T.V. Reader's Digest, Wyatt Earp.

MOSS, IRWIN: Executive. e. Syracuse Univ., Harvard Law School, Member NY State Bar. Began industry career as director of package negotiations for CBS-TV; 1970–80, exec. v.p. & natl. head of business affairs for I.C.M.; 1978–80, snr. v.p., NBC Entertainment; 1980, pres., Marble Arch TV. 1982, joined Paramount Pictures as snr. v.p. for motion picture div. 1984, exec. v.p., L. Taffner Ltd.

MOUND, FRED: Executive. b. St. Louis, Mo., April 10, 1932. e. St. Louis Univ., Quincy Coll. 1946–52, assoc. with father, Charles Mound, at Park Theatre in Valley Park, Mo.; 1952–53, Universal Pictures (St. Louis); 1953, booker, UA, St. Louis; 1955 promoted to salesman in Kansas City; 1957, salesman, St. Louis; 1962, Indianapolis branch mgr. In 1967 named UA regional mgr., Dallas and in 1970 became S.W. Div. mgr; 1977–78, asst. gen. sls. mgr. for Southern, N.W. and S.W. Division operating out of Dallas. In June, 1978 appt. v.p., asst. gen. sls. mgr. of UA; 1984, sr. v.p., gen. sls. mgr., Universal Pictures.

MOYERS, BILL: TV Correspondent. b. Hugo, OK, June 5, 1934. e. Univ. Texas; Southwestern Baptist Theological Sem. Asst. to Lyndon B. Johnson, 1959–60, 1961–63; assoc. dir., Peace Corps, 1961–63; spec. asst. to Pres. Johnson, 1963–67 and press secty. 1965–67. Editor and chief corr., CBS Reports. Bill Moyers Journal on PBS.

MOYERS, BILL: TV Correspondent. b. Hugo, OK, June 5, 1934. e. Univ. Texas; Southwestern Baptist Theological Sem. Asst. to Lyndon B. Johnson, 1959–60, 1961–63; assoc. dir., Peace Corp, 1961–63; spec. asst. to Pres. Johnson, 1963–67 and press secty. 1965–67. Editor and chief corr., CBS Reports. Bill Moyers Journal on PBS.

MOYLAN, WILLIAM J: (M.B.K.S.) Producer-director, script editor and researcher, journalist. Entered m.p. ind. 1927; credits include 59 features and over 200 shorts; in charge prod. in various studios 1933–42; prod. and ed. Indian News Parade for Indian Govt. and war corr. with India and South East Asia Commands, 1943–46; prod. information films of India 1947; Indep. prod. documentaries in Ireland 1948; dir. eastern language versions De Lane Lea Process Ltd., 1949–51; films advisor to Pakistan Govt. apptd. by Commonwealth Relations Office under Tech. Co-op. Scheme of the Colombo Plan, 1952–58; overseas adv. De Lane Lea Process, 1959–60. Founded Munster House Prods. in Ireland, 1961.

MUDD, ROGER: Newscaster. b. Washington, D.C., Feb. 9, 1928. e. Washington Lee Univ., Univ. N.C. Reporter for Richmond-News-Leader, 1953; news. dr., WRNL, 1954; WTOP, Washington, 1956; joined CBS News 1961 as Congressional corr. 1977, Natl. Aff. corr.; 1978, corr., CBS Reports; 1980 joined ABC as chief Washington corr.

MUHL, EDWARD E.: Executive and Producer. b. Richmond, Ind. Feb. 17, 1907; gen. mgr., Universal 1948–53; v.p., chg. production 1953–68. Bd. member, Cinema Group, Inc., 1984. In 1985, co-author, s.p. & treatment, Audie Murphy, American Soldier. Retired.

MUIR, GRAEME: TV producer, actor. b. London, Feb., 1916; e. Oundle and St. John's, Oxford. Awarded Silver Medal Royal Academy of Dramatic Art 1938; first broadcast in Alcestis, 1940; many TV plays since; now freelance producer.
TV: Its Magic, The Dancing Years, Showtime, Perchance to Dream, Gilbert and Sullivan, Brothers In Law, Mr. Justice Duncannon, Christmas Night with the Stars, The Marriage Lines, Charley's Aunt, Comedy Playhouse, The Whitehall Worrier, Harry Worth, Not in Front of the Children, The Very Merry Widow, Bachelor Father, Birds on the Wing, My Wife Next Door, Oh Father!, Second Time Around, It Ain't Half Hot Mum, Oneupmanship, You're Only Young Twice, Life Begins at Forty, Hows' Your Father?, That's My Boy, Third Time Lucky.

MUIR, E. ROGER: Producer. b. Canada, Dec. 16, 1918. e. U. of Minn. Partner Minn Advertising Services Co., Photographer, Great Northern Railway; motion picture producer Army Signal corps; NBC TV producer, Howdy Doody, exec. producer, Concentration. Now pres. Nicholson-Muir Prods, TV program packager, U.S. Spin-Off, Pay Cards, Canada Pay Cards, Headline Hunters, Definition, Celebrity Dominoes; co-creator Newlywed Game, exec. prod. I Am Joe's Heart, I Am Joe's Lung, I Am Joe's Spine, I Am Joe's Stomach, The New Howdy Doody Show, Supermates, Second Honeymoon, Groaner, Generation Jury, Shopping Game, Guess What, I Am Joe's Kidney, I Am Joe's Liver, etc.

MULDAUR, DIANA: Actress. Began on New York stage the turned to films and TV, appearing on numerous major network shows.
PICTURES INCLUDE: The Swimmer, Number One, The Lawyer, One More Train To Rob, The Other, Chosen Survivors, Beyond Reason.

MULGREW, KATE: Actress. b. Dubuque, IA, April 29, 1955. e. NYU. Stage work includes stints with American Shakespeare Festival, O'Neill Festival and at Hartman Theatre, Stamford.
PICTURES: Jennifer, Tristan and Isolt, A Stranger Is Watching.
TELEVISION: Ryan's Hope, The Word, Jennifer, A Woman's Story, Mrs. Colombo, Kate Loves a Mystery, A Time for Miracles, The Manions of America.

MULHOLLAND, ROBERT E.: Executive. e. Northwestern Univ. Joined NBC News as newswriter in Chicago in 1962. In 1964 made midwestern field producer for Huntley-Brinkley Report. In 1964 moved to London as European producer for NBC News; 1967, named Washington producer of Huntley-Brinkley Report. Transferred to L.A. in 1967 to be director of news, west coast. Named exec. prod. of NBC Nightly News. In 1973 appt. v.p., NBC news.; 1974 exec. v.p. of NBC News. In 1977 appt. pres. of NBC Television Network; also elected to board of directors. Resigned.

MULL, MARTIN: Actor. b. Chicago, IL, Aug. 18, 1943. e. Rhode Island School of Design. Started as humorist, making recordings for Warner Bros., Capricorn, ABC Records, etc. Theatrical m.p. debut, FM (1978).
PICTURES: My Bodyguard, Serial, Take This Job and Shove It, Private School, Growing Pains, Flicks, Mr. Mom, Clue, O.C. and Stiggs.
TELEVISION: Mary Hartman Mary Hartman, Fernwood 2-Night, America 2-Night, Domestic Life, numerous talk shows, etc. Wrote produced and starred in The History of White People in America for HBO.

MULLIGAN, RICHARD: Actor. b. New York City, Nov. 13, 1932. On stage in All the Way Home, Never Too Late, Thieves, etc.
PICTURES: The Mixed Up Files of Mrs. Basil E. Frankweiler, Irish Whiskey Rebellion, One Potato, Two Potato, The Group, the Big Bus, Little Big Man, Scavenger Hunt, S.O.B., Teachers, Micki and Maude, A Fine Mess, Quicksilver.
TELEVISION: Having Babies, The Hero, Soap.

MULLIGAN, ROBERT: Director. b. Bronx, N.Y.; e. Fordham U., A.B. With CBS-TV, asst. supv. in radio oper.; prod. asst. on Supense, TV; then asst. dir. & dir.: TV Playhouse, NBC, Alcoa-Goodyear, Studio One, Playhouse 90, Hallmark Hall of Fame.
PICTURES INCLUDE: Fear Strikes Out (1957), The Rat Race, The Great Imposter, Come September, To Kill a Mockingbird, The Spiral Road, Love with the Proper Stranger, Baby the Rain Must Fall, Inside Daisy Clover, Up the Down Staircase, Pursuit of Happiness, Summer of '42, The Other, The Nickel Ride, Bloodbrothers, Same Time Next Year, Kiss me Goodbye (also prod.).

MURDOCH, RUPERT: Executive. b. Australia, March 11, 1931. Son of Sir Keith Murdoch, head of The Melbourne Herald and leading figure in Australian journalism. e. Oxford, Univ., England. Spent two years on Fleet St. before returning home to take over family paper, The Adelaide News. Acquired more Australian papers and in 1969 expanded to Britain, buying The News of the World. Moved to U.S. in 1973, buying San Antonio Express and News. Conglomerate in 1985 included New York Post, New York Magazine, The Star, The Times of London, The Boston Herald, The Chicago Sun-Times along with TV stations, book publishing companies, airline, oil and gas companies, etc. March, 1985, made deal to buy half of 20th Century-Fox Film Corp. from owner Martin Davis.

MURPHY, BEN: Actor. b. Jonesboro, AR, March 6, 1942. e. Univ. of Illinois. Degree in drama from Pasadena Playhouse. Acted in campus productions and toured in summer stock.

Film debut with small role in The Graduate (1967).
PICTURES: The Thousand Plane Raid, Yours, Mine and Ours, Sidecar Racer.
TELEVISION: Series: The Name of the Game, Alias Smith and Jones, Griff, Gemini Man, The Chisholms, Lottery! Movies: Wild Bill Hickock, Bridger, Heat Wave, Runaway, This Is the West That Was, Hospital Fire, The Cradle Will Fall. Mini-Series: The Winds of War.

MURPHY, EDDIE: b. Hempstead, NY, 1961. Wrote and performed own comedy routines at youth centers and local bars at age 15. Worked on comedy club circuit; at 19 joined TV's Saturday Night Live. 1982, became writer for SNL as well as staf. Theatrical film debut, 48 Hrs. (1982).
PICTURES: 48 Hrs., Trading Places, The Best Defense, Beverly Hills Cop, The Golden Child.

MURPHY, GEORGE: U.S. Senator. b. New Haven, Conn., July 4, 1902; e. Yale U. Toolmaker for Ford Co., miner, real estate agent, nightclub dancer, actor. On stage from 1927 (Good News, Of Thee I Sing, Roberta, etc.). Screen debut 1934 in Kid Millions. Member: Screen Actors Guild (pres.); Nat'l. Com. WAC. Spcl. Academy Award "for interpreting m.p. ind. correctly to country at large," 1940; chmn., Hollywood Coordinating Com.; bd. mem., USO Inc.; v.p., Acad. of M.P. Arts & Sciences; div. of pub. rel., MGM, 1954–58; bd. mem. & past pres., Screen Actors Guild; bd. mem., M.P. Relief Fund. Joined Desilu Productions as v.p. in chg. public affairs, 1959; v.p., bd. of dir., Technicolor Corp. Elected U.S. Senator, California.
PICTURES INCLUDE: I'll Love You Always, You're a Sweetheart, London by Night, Broadway Melody of 1938, Risky Business, Two Girls on Broadway, A Girl, a Guy and a Gob, Tom, Dick and Harry, Ringside Maisie, Mayor of 44th Street, For Me and My Gal, Powers Girl, This Is the Army, Up Goes Maisie, Arnelo Affair, Cynthia, Tenth Avenue Angel, Big City, Battleground, Border Incident, No Questions Asked, Talk About a Stranger, It's a Big Country, Walk East on Beacon, Jamboree (Boy Scout film), This is the Army, Broadway Melody.

MURPHY, JOHN F.: Theatre executive. b. Brooklyn, N.Y., Mar. 25, 1905; e. CCNY. Entire career with Loew's Theatres; started over 45 yrs. ago as asst. mgr. Hillside & Valencia Theatres, Jamaica, N.Y.; apptd. gen. mgr. in chg. of out-of-town Theatres, 1942–54; v.p., Loew's Theatres, Aug., 1954; dir., Loew's Theatres, Oct., 1956; exec. v.p., Loew's Theatre, 1959; ret. July 1963; continues on bd. as advisor and director emeritus.

MURPHY, MARY: Actress. b. Washington, D.C., Jan. 26; e. University High Sch., Santa Monica, 1949; m.p. debut in Lemon Drop Kid.
PICTURES INCLUDE: Carrie, When Worlds Collide, Atomic City, Turning Point, Come Back Little Sheba, Off Limits, Houdini, Main Street to Broadway, Wild One, Beachhead, Mad Magician, Make Haste to Live, Sitting Bull, Hell's Island, Desperate Hour, A Man Alone, Maverick Queen, Zex, Harlow, Junior Bonner.

MURPHY, MICHAEL: Actor. b. Los Angeles, May 5, 1938. e. Univ. of Arizona. Taught English and Drama in L.A. city school system, 1962–64. NY stage debut as director of Rat's Nest, 1978–79.
PICTURES: The Legend of Lylah Clare, The Arrangement, Brewster McCloud, MASH, McCabe and Mrs. Miller, What's Up Doc?, Nashville, An Unmarried Woman, The Front, Manhattan, The Year of Living Dangerously, Strange Behavior, Cloak and Dagger, Salvador.
TELEVISION: Saints and Sinners, Ben Casey, Dr. Kildare, Bonanza, Combat, Autobiography of Miss Jane Pittman, John Cheever's Oh Youth and Beauty, Two Marriages, etc.

MURPHY, RICHARD: Writer, director. b. Boston, Mass.; E. Williams Coll. Entered m.p. Ind. 1937 Capt. U.S. Army Sig. Corps. SWPA, 1942–45. Contract writer, 20th Century-Fox, 1945–54 Writer-Prod., 20th-Fox, 1964–72; pres. Cinecom World Ent. Ltd., 1974.
PICTURES INCLUDE: Boomerang, Deep Waters, Cry of the City, Panic in the Streets, You're in the Navy Now, Les Miserables, Desert Rats, Broken Lance, Three Strips in the Sun, Wackiest Ship in the Army, Compulsion, Last Angry Man.
TV: Our Man Higgins, Screen Gems, creator, TV series, The Felony Squad.

MURRAY, BARBARA: Actress. b. London, England, Sept. 27, 1929. Stage debut in Variety, 1946; screen debut in Badger's Green, 1948. Various TV appearances.
PICTURES INCLUDE: Passport to Pimlico, Don't Ever Leave Me, Boys in Brown, Poets Pub, Tony Draws a Horse, Dark Man, Frightened Man, Mystery Junction, Another Man's Poison, Hot Ice, Street Corner (Both Sides of the Law), Meet Mr. Lucifer, Doctor At Large, Campbell's Kingdom, A Cry from the Streets, Girls in Arms.

MURRAY, BILL: Actor. b. Chicago, Sept. 21, 1950. Was pre-med student; left to join brother, Brian, in Second City, the Chicago improvisational troupe. Appeared with brother on radio, National Lampoon Show, and in off-Bdwy. revue, of same name. Hired by ABC for Saturday Night Live; then by NBC.
PICTURES: Meatballs (debut), Where the Buffalo Roam, Caddyshack, Stripes, Tootsie, Ghostbusters, The Razor's Edge (also co-s.p.), Nothing Lasts Forever.

MURRAY, DON: Actor-director, writer. b. Hollywood, Calif., July 31, 1929.
PLAYS: Insect Comedy, Rose Tattoo, The Skin of Our Teeth, The Hot Corner, Smith (a musical), The Norman Conquests.
PICTURES INCLUDE: Bus Stop, Bachelor Party, Hatful of Rain, The Hoodlum Priest, Advise & Consent, Baby the Rain Must Fall, Sweet Love, Bitter, The Cross and the Switchblade, Conquest of the Planet of the Apes, One Man's Way, The Plainsman, Escape From East Berlin, Shake Hands with the Devil, From Hell to Texas, Confessions of Tom Harris, Call Me by My Rightful Name, The Borgia Stick, Deadly Hero, Damien, Endless Love.
TELEVISION: License to Kill, A Touch of Scandal.

MURRAY, JAN: Performer. b. New York City, N.Y., 1917. Performed in nightclubs, vaudeville, B'way, radio, TV, films. Was m.c., Songs for Sale, and Sing It Again, CBS-TV; TV guest star many programs; on Dollar a Second, ABC; Jan Murray Time, NBC; Treasure Hunt, ABC.
PLAYS: A Funny Thing Happened on the Way to the Forum.
PICTURES INCLUDE: Who Killed Teddy Bear?

MURRAY, KEN: Actor. r.n. Don't Court. b. New York City, July 14, 1903. On N.Y. stage as master of ceremonies; also Hollywood stage in Blackouts of 1942–49. Screen debut 1929 in Half Marriage. Since in numerous features and short subjects.
PICTURES INCLUDE: Leathernecking, You're a Sweetheart, Swing Sister Swing, A Night at Earl Carroll's, Swing It Soldier, Juke Box Jenny, Special Academy award 1947 (Bill and Coo)., Follow Me Boys, The Power, The Man Who Shot Liberty Valance, Sound of Flubber.
TV: Ken Murray Show TV; p. d., act.: Marshall's Daughter; prod.: Where Were You, El Coyote, Hollywood, My Home Town, Hollywood Without Makeup.
BROADWAY: Ken Murray's Hollywood.
LITERARY: The Golden Days of San Simeon—Doubleday, 1971, Now in 8th Edition.

MUSANTE, TONY: Actor. b. Bridgeport, Conn., June 30, 1936. e. Oberlin College. Taught High School, directed local theatre, then appeared off-Broadway and on Dupont Show of the Month (Ride With Terror).
PICTURES INCLUDE: Once A Thief, The Incident, The Detective, A Professional Gun, The Love Circle, The Bird With The Crystal Plumage, The Last Run, Anonymous Venetian, The Pope of Greenwich Village.
TV: Toma (series); Rearview Mirror (movie).

MUSTO, MICHAEL J.: Producer-writer. b. N.Y.C. Jan. 16, 1917; e. S. Niagara U. Apprentice for J. J. Shubert. Comedy Workshop, N.Y.C. W-Co.P Hellzapoppin, Wrote, Prod. Dir. Burlesque shows and stage revues. Prod. Industrial Films, Commercials, Operas, Fund Raising Shows. Prod. Films: The Glass House, Phenomena 7-7, Down Tin Pan Alley, Single Room Furnished, Educated Heart, Agnes, Spring Fancy, The Atheist, Man Who Cried Wolf, Several Robert Montgomery Presents, Hallmark Hall of Fame, TV Specials, The Bold Ones, Strange Is The Wind. Wrote: Due-Bill Marriage, Spring Fancy, Granada, Seppi and His Brothers, Amato and The Yenta, The Cliffdwellers, Other. Owner. Empire Films and Cinema City Studios. Manager, Ruth Burch.

MUTSU, IAN YONOSUKE: Producer-Distributor. b. London, England, Jan. 14, 1907. e. Univ. of Birmingham, England. Journalist 1931–48. Daily Express, UPI, etc.; Japan repr. MGM-Hearst Metrotone News, U.S. Newsreel Pool, later Telenews, UPI-Movietone News, ITN London; 1952 pres. International Motion Picture Co. for news coverage, documentaries, custom films for worldwide clients; 1966 agent BBC TV sales, Modern Talking Picture Service NYC; 1973 founded Mutsu Inc. (Canada). Productions include numerous documentaries on Japan, Japanese background films for overseas clients.

MYERS, JULIAN F.: Public relations. b. Detroit, Mich., Feb. 22, 1918; e. Wayne Univ., 1935–37, Univ. Southern Calif., 1937–39. Distribution, Loew's Detroit, 1941–42; asst. story editor, idea man, Columbia, 1942–46; publicist, 20th Century-Fox, 1948–62; public relations, Julian F. Myers, Inc., 1962; pres., Myers Studios, Inc., 1966; pres., New Horizons Broadcasting Corp., 1968–69; snr. publicist American Intl. Pictures, 1970–80. Executive Board Hollywood Press Club; member Variety Clubs; Academy of Motion Pictures Arts & Sciences; Board of Governors Film Industry Workshops, Inc. 1977, western vice-pres., The Publicists Guild; Recipient of Publicists Guild's Robert Yeager Award; 1979, re-elected western v.p., Publicists Guild. First male member Hollywood Women's Press Club. Co-founder HANDS (Hollywood Answering Needs of Disaster Survivors). Member, m.p. Pioneers. Winner, 1980 Publicists Guild Les Mason Award. Instructor in publicity, UCLA, 1979 to present. Filmways Pictures, pub. dept., 1980–81. Exec. v.p., worldwide m.p. and TV pub./mktg., Hanson & Schwam Public Relations 1981 to present.

MYERS, LAURENCE: Executive. Chairman, GTO Films & Video Intl. Handled Scum, The Wanderers, Breaking Glass and Caligula. Production credits incl. Never Too Young Too Rock, The Greek Tycoon (co-prod.), The Survivor (co-prod.), In the House of Death (exec. prod.), Bloodbath.

MYERS, PETER S.: Executive. b. Toronto, Ont., Canada, May 13, 1923; e. U. of Toronto, R.C.A.F. 1944–46. Toronto br. mgr., 20th Century-Fox, 1948; Canadian div. mgr., 1951; Canadian gen. mgr., 1955; man. dir. Canada, 1959; gen. sales mgr. in chg. of dom. distribution, 1968; v.p., 1969; named snr. v.p.; domestic dist., 1979; snr. v.p., 20th-Fox Entertainment, 1980; pres., 20th-Fox Classics, 1983; pres., PSM Entertainment, 1985.

MYERSON, BERNARD: Executive. b. New York, N.Y., March 25, 1918. Entered m.p. ind. with Fabian Theatres, 1938–63; last position as exec. v.p.; joined Loew's Theatres as v.p., 1963; exec. v.p. and board member, Loew's Corp.; pres. Loew's Theatres, 1971. Chm. & pres., Loews Theatre Management Corp., 1985. Vice chm. & mem. of Executive Committee Greater N.Y. Chapter, National Foundation of March of Dimes; Honorary chm. & bd. mem., Will Rogers Memorial Fund; Mem. exec. comm., bd., National Assn. Theatre Owners; chm., Motion Picture Pioneers. Vice pres., Variety International; mem., finance comm., Friars; Board of Directors Burke Rehabilitation Center; mem. NYS Governor's Council on M.P. & T.V. Development; mem. M.P. & T.V. Com. USIA.

N

NABORS, JIM: Actor. b. Bylacauga, AL, June 12, 1932.
PICTURES: The Best Little Whorehouse in Texas, Stroker Ace, Cannonball Run II, etc.
TELEVISION: Andy Griffith Show, Gomer Pyle USMC, The Jim Nabors Show, etc. Movie: Return to Mayberry.

NADEL, ARTHUR: Producer, director, writer. b. New York, N.Y. Film editor for Paramount, 20th Century-Fox, Walt Disney, U.S. Air Force m.p. div., United Artists; superv. editor, McCann-Erickson; prod., dir., writer, Universal; v.p., Levy-Gardner-Laven.
PICTURES INCLUDE: Clambake, Lola, Underground, No Trumpets, No Drum.
TV: The Rifleman, The Plainsman, Great Adventure, Arrest and Trial, Kraft Theatre, The Virginian, Big Valley, Daniel Boone, Cowboy in Africa, Bonanza, Delphi Bureau, Banyon, Streets of San Francisco; NBC Specials, Welcome Home (Emmy Winner); This Year in Jerusalem, Vortex in Oatmeal, Universal Studios, The Chase: NBC Special, Crime Without Punishment; executive consultant Filmation Studios, Shazam, The Secrets of Isis.

NADER, GEORGE: Actor. b. Pasadena, Calif.; e. Occidental College, B.A., Pasadena Playhouse. Served in U.S. Navy. Many TV appearances, m.p. debut in Monsoon. First novel, Chrome, recently published by Putnam's.
PICTURES INCLUDE: Carnival Story, Miss Robin Crusoe, Sins of Jezebel, Fours Guns to the Border, Six Bridges to Cross, Lady Godiva, Second Greatest Sex, Away All Boats, Congo Crossing, Unguarded Moment, Four Girls in Town, Man Afraid, Joe Butterfly, Nowhere to Go, The Secret Mark of D'artagnan, The Great Space Adventure, Zigzag, Walk by the Sea, The Human Duplicators, Sumuru, House of a Thousand Dolls, Alarm on 83rd Street, Murder at Midnight, Count-Down for Manhattan, Dynamite in Green Silk, The Check and Icy Smile, The Murder Club From Bklyn, Death in a Red Jaguar, End Station of the Damned, Bullets on Broadway, Beyond Atlantis.
TV: Letter to Loretta, Fireside Theatre, Chevron Theatre, Ellery Queen, Man and the Challenge, Shannon.

NAIFY, MARSHALL: Executive. b. Sacramento, Calif., March 23, 1920; e. U. So. Calif. U.S.A.F. Ch. exec. comm. & bd. chm., United Artists Communications, Inc.; pres., Magna Pictures Corp.

NAIFY, ROBERT: Pres., United Artists Communications Inc.; pres., Magna Pictures Corp.

NAKAMURA, MOTOHIKO: Executive. b. Tokyo, Japan, Aug. 10, 1929. e. U. of California at Berkeley, U. of Pennsylvania, Tokyo University. Joined Fuji Film Co., Ltd. in Tokyo, 1953; assigned to Japan Camera Center, New York City, 1956–67; North American rep. for Fuji Photo Film Co., Ltd., 1957–63; assistant export sales mgr., Fuji Photo Co., Ltd. in charge of international marketing of all products, 1964–71; exec. v.p., resident mgr., Fuji Photo Film U.S.A., Inc.

NALLE, BILLY: Theatre concert organist, popular field, ASCAP composer. b. Fort Myers, Fla.; graduate, The Julliard School. Over 5000 major TV shows from New York; now artist-in-residence, Wichita Theatre Organ, Inc. Reader's Digest, Telarc & WTO Records Artist. Public Relations: Billy Nalle Music, Wichita.

NAMATH, JOE: Actor. b. Beaver Falls, PA, May 31, 1943. e. univ. of Alabama. Former professional football star. Film debut in Norwood (1970).
PICTURES: C.C. & Co., The Last Rebel, Avalanche Express.
TELEVISION: The Waverly Wonders, Marriage Is Alive and Well, All American Pie.

NAPIER, ALAN: Actor. b. Jan. 1903, Caste, Nettleford; In a Monastery Garden, Hagen; Loyalties, AIP, 1933; Wings Over Africa, Premier Stafford, 1936; For Valour, Capitol, 1937; Wife of General Ling, Four Just Men, 1938.
PICTURES INCLUDE: The Uninvited, The Song of Bernadette, Action in Arabia, Ministry of Fear, The Hairy Ape, Mlle. Fifi, Dark Waters, Hanover Square, Isle of the Dead, Three Strangers, High Conquest, Driftwood, Forever Amber, Macbeth, Joan of Arc, Hills of Home, Tripoli, Highwayman, Strange Door, Blue Veil, Across the Wide Missouri, Big Jim McLain, Young Bess, Julius Caesar, Desiree, Moonfleet, Court Jester, Miami Expose, Mole People, Until They Sail, Journey to the Center of the Earth, Batman.
TV: Many TV dramatic shows and Batman series.

NARDINO, GARY: Executive. e. Seton Hall Univ. Awarded honorary degree of Doctor of Laws. Entered industry in 1949 as agent, representing Lorimar Prods. and Talent Associates, among others. Named sr. v.p. of ICM's New York TV dept; then v.p. of William Morris Agency, heading NY TV dept. Pres. of Paramount TV Production Division, 1977–1983. Served as exec. prod. of Star Trek III: The Search for Spock. Now pres., of Gary Nardino Prods., Inc., formed 1983, to develop and produce theatrical features and TV programming.
PICTURES: Star Trek III (exec. prod.); Fire with Fire (prod.).

NARIZZANO, SILVIO: Producer-Director. b. Montreal, Canada, 1927. e. Univ. of Bishop's, Lennoxville, Quebec (B.A.). Was active as actor-director in Canadian theatre before going to England for TV and theatrical film work.
PICTURES INCLUDE: Director: Under Ten Flags (co-dir.), Die! Die! My Darling!, Georgy Girl, Blue, The Man Who Had Power Over Women, Loot, Redneck, The Sky Is Falling. Producer: Negatives, Fadeout, Redneck.

NASH, N. RICHARD: Writer.
BROADWAY: author: Second Best Bed, The Young and Fair, See the Jaguar, The Rainmaker, Girls of Summer, Handful of Fire, Wildcat, 110 in the Shade, The Happy Time, Echoes.
PICTURES INCLUDE: Nora Prentiss, Vicious Years, The Rainmaker, Porgy and Bess, Sainted Sisters, Dear Wife, Welcome Stranger, Dragonfly.
dTV: Many TV plays for Television Playhouse, U.S. Steel, General Electric.
NOVEL: Cry Macho; East Wind, Rain; The Last Magic; Aphrodite's Cave; Radiance; Behold the Man.

NATHAN, WYNN: Executive. e. U. of So. Calif. Casting dept., Universal, 1941; then U.S. Air Force 4 yrs.; asst. oper. mgr., Universal, 1946; talent agent, Wm. Morris Agency; talent agent, Century Artists; then United TV Programs; v.p., MCA, 1954; v.p. chg. syndication & bd. of dir., MCA; pres., TV Marketeers, 1961; v.p. & gen. mgr., Metromedia Program Sales, 1966; vice president, Worldwide Syndication Time-Life Television 1970-May, 1981; pres. & chief exec. officer, Lionheart TV Intl., 1981–84; now v.p., mktg., worldwide TV & cable, RKO Pictures, Inc.

NATWICK, MILDRED: Actress. b. Baltimore, Md., June 19, 1908; e. Bryn Mawr Sch., Baltimore, Bennett Sch., Millbrook. Prof. stage debut in Carry Nation, 1932; London debut in Day I Forget.
PLAYS: Wind and the Rain, Distaff Side, End of Summer, Love From a Stranger, Candida, Missouri Legend, Stars in Your Eyes, Grass Harp, Blithe Spirit, (Barter Theatre award), Waltz of the Toreadors (nominated for Tony), The Firstborn, The Good Soup, Critic's Choice, Barefoot in the Park, Our Town, Landscape, 70, Girls 70, (nominated for Tony), Bedroom Farce.
PICTURES INCLUDE: Long Voyage Home, Enchanted Cottage, Yolanda and the Thief, Late George Apley, Woman's Vengeance, Three Godfathers, Kissing Bandit, She Wore a Yellow Ribbon, Cheaper by the Dozen, Quiet Man, Against All Flags, Trouble with Harry, Court Jester,

Teenage Rebel, Tammy and the Bachelor, Barefoot in the Park (nominated for Oscar), If It's Tuesday This Must be Belgium, Trilogy, The Maltese Bippy, Daisy Miller, At Long Last Love, Kiss Me Goodbye.
TELEVISION: Blithe Spirit (nominated for Emmy), House Without an Xmas Tree, Thanksgiving Treasure, Money to Burn, The Snoop Sisters (Emmy award), The Easter Promise, Little Women, McMillan & Wife, Hawaii Five-O, Love Boat, You Can't Take It With You, Alice-Made in America.

NAZARRO, CLIFF: Actor. b. New Haven, Conn., January 31, 1904. Stock, vaudeville, master of ceremonies in all leading theatres. Appeared with "Two Marjories" in Vitaphone No. 2116. In 1936: "Romance Rides the Range," Spectrum.
PICTURES INCLUDE: Outside of Paradise, a Desperate Adventure, King of the Turf, St. Louis Blues, Arise, My Love, In Old Colorado, Mr. Dynamite, Artists and Models Abroad, Dive Bomber, Night of January 16, World Premiere, Rookies on Parade, Sailors on Leave, Blondie Goes to College, Melody for Three, You'll Never Get Rich, Pardon My Stripes, Call of the Canyon, Hillbilly Biltzkrieg, Shantytown, I'm from Arkansas, Swing Hostess, Gentleman Joe Palooka.

NEAL, PATRICIA: Actress. b. Packard, Ky., Jan. 20, 1926; e. Northwestern U. Doctor's asst., cashier, hostess, model, jewelry store clerk. In summer stock; Broadway debut in "Another Part of the Forest" 1947, winning the Donaldson & Drama Critic Awards, also in Children's Hour. M.p. debut in John Loves Mary, 1948. Academy Award—Best Actress, 1963.
TV: The Bastard.
PICTURES INCLUDE: Fountainhead, Hasty Heart, Bright Leaf, Three Secrets, Breaking Point, Raton Pass, Operation Pacific, Day the Earth Stood Still, Weekend With Father, Diplomatic Courier, Washington Story, Something for the Birds, Face in the Crowd, Hud (Academy Award), Psych 59, In Harms Way, The Subject Was Roses, The Night Digger, Baxter!, Happy Mother's Day . . . Love, George, The Passage (1978), Ghost Story.

NEAME, RONALD: Cinematographer, producer, director. b. 1911; e. U. Coll. Sch., London; son, Elwin Neame, London photog. & Ivy Close, m.p. actress. Entered m.p. ind. 1928; asst. cameraman on first full-length Brit. sound "blackmail," dir. by Alfred Hitchcock, 1929; became chief cameraman & lighting expert, 1934; in 1945 joint assoc. prod., Noel Coward Prods.
PICTURES INCLUDE: Elizabeth of England, Invitation to the Waltz, Brief Ecstasy, It's in the Air, Gaunt Stranger, Four Just Men, Major Barbara, A Yank in the R.A.F. (Brit. flying sequence), One of Our Aircraft is Missing, In Which We Serve, This Happy Breed, Blithe Spirit, Brief Encounter, Great Expectations, Oliver Twist, Passionate Friends, Take My Life, Magic Box, Golden Salamander, The Card (The Promoter), Million Pound Note (Man With a Million), Man Who Never Was, Seventh Sin, Windom's Way, The Horse's Mouth, Tunes of Glory, Escape From Zahrain, I Could Go on Singing, The Chalk Garden, Mister Moses, Gambit, The Prime of Miss Jean Brodie, Scrooge, The Poseidon Adventure, The Odessa File, Meteor, Hopscotch, First Monday in October.

NEEDHAM, HAL: Director. In industry over 25 years. Was popular stuntman and second unit action director before full directorial debut with Smokey and the Bandit.
PICTURES INCLUDE: Hooper, The Villain, Smokey and the Bandit II, The Cannonball Run, Megaforce (also co-s.p.), Stroker Ace (also co-s.p.), Cannonball Run II (also co-s.p.).
TELEVISION: Hal Needham's Wild World of Stunts (syndicated series he wrote, directed and starred in): Directed Death Car on the Freeway (movie); Stunts Unlimited.

NEFF, HILDEGARDE: Actress, author. r.n. Hildegard Knef. b. Ulm, Germany, Dec. 28, 1925; e. Art Acad., Berlin. Film cartoonist for UFA, Berlin; on Berlin stage after war; appeared in German films: Murderers Are Among Us, Between Yesterday and Tomorrow, Film Without Title, The Sinner. On B'way in: Silk Stockings. U.S. m.p. debut in Decision Before Dawn. Author of best-selling autobiography, 1971.
PICTURES INCLUDE: Diplomatic Courier, Night Without Sleep, Snows of Kilimanjaro, Holiday for Henrietta, Man Between, Svengali, Subway in the Sky, Mozambique.

NEGULESCO, JEAN: Director. b. Rumania (Craiova), Feb. 29, 1900; e. Liceul Carol Univ., Rumania. Stage dir., artist, painter, Came to U.S. in 1927.
PICTURES INCLUDE: The Mask of Dimitrios, The Conspirators, Nobody Lives Forever, Three Strangers, Humoresque, Deep Valley, Johnny Belinda, Road House, Forbidden Street, Three Came Home, Under My Skin, Mudlark, Take Care of My Little Girl, The Full House, Phone Call From a Stranger, Lydia Bailey, Lure of the Wilderness, Titanic, Scandal at Scourie, How to Marry a Millionaire, The Rains of Ranchipur, Woman's World, Three Coins in The Fountain, Daddy Long Legs, Boy on a Dolphin, The Gift of Love, A Certain Smile, Count Your Blessings, The Best of Everything, Jessica, The Pleasure Seekers, Hello, Goodbye.

NEILL, SAM: Actor. b. New Zealand, 1948. e. Univ. of Canterbury. In repertory before joining N.Z. National Film Unit, acting and directing documentaries and shorts.
PICTURES: Landfall, Ashes, Sleeping Dogs, The Journalist, My Brilliant Career, Just Out of Reach, Attack Force Z, The Final Conflict, Possession, From a Far Country—Pope John Paul II, Enigma, The Country Girls, The Blood of Others, Robbery Under Arms, Plenty.
TELEVISION: The Sullivans, Young Ramsay, Lucinda Brayford, Ivanhoe, Reilly Ace of Spies, Kane & Abel.

NELLIGAN, KATE: Actress. b. London, England, March 16, 1951. On stage in Barefoot in the Park, A Streetcar Named Desire, Playboy of the Western World, Private Lives, Plenty, etc.
PICTURES: The Count of Monte Cristo, The Romantic Englishwoman, Dracula, Mr. Patman, Eye of the Needle, Without a Trace, Eleni.
TELEVISION: The Onedin Line, The Lady of the Camelias, etc.

NELSON, BARRY: Actor. r.n. Robert Neilson. b. Oakland, Calif., 1920. e. U. of Calif. London stage: No Time for Sergeants, 1957.
PICTURES INCLUDE: A Guy Named Joe, Winged Victory, Man with My Face, First Traveling Saleslady, Mary, Mary, The Borgia Stick, Airport, Pete 'n Tillie, The Shining.
BROADWAY: Light Up the Sky, Rat Race, Moon is Blue, Mary, Mary, Cactus Flower, Everything in the Garden, Seascape, The Norman Conquests, The Act.
TV: series: The Hunter, My Favorite Husband, Washington: Behind Closed Doors.

NELSON, CRAIG T.: Actor. Began career as writer/performer on Lohman and Barkley Show in Los Angeles. Wrote for Tim Conway Show, Alan King TV special; guest appearances on talk shows and Mary Tyler Moore Show. Produced series of 52 half-hour films on American artists, American Still. Returned to L.A. in 1978 and acting career. Theatrical film debut in And Justice for All, 1979.
PICTURES: The Formula, Where the Buffalo Roam, Private Benjamin, Poltergeist, The Osterman Weekend, Silkwood, All the Right Moves, The Killing Fields, Poltergeist II.
TELEVISION: Wonder Woman, Charlie's Angels, How the West Was Won, Diary of a Teenage Hitchhiker, Alex: The Life of a Child.

NELSON, DAVID: Actor. b. New York, N.Y., Oct. 24, 1936; e. Hollywood H.S., U. of Southern Calif.
PICTURES INCLUDE: Here Comes the Nelsons, Peyton Place, The Remarkable Mr. Pennypacker, Day of the Outlaw, The Big Circus, "30," The Big Show, No Drums, No Bugles, The Wheel, The Sinners.
TV: Adventures of Ozzie and Harriet; dir.: Easy To Be Free (special), OK Crackerby series.

NELSON, EDWARD, J.: Executive. b. July 15, 1911, St. Louis, Mo. e. Iowa State. Started as commercial m.p. & aerial photographer. With National Theatre Supply, 1934–42. AAFMPS, mgr., engineering E. To., 1942–52. Joined Ballantyne of Omaha in 1952; made pres. 1973, which post now holds. Member: T.E.A. pres., May 1974–76. and bd. mbr., 1970–74. SMPTE. Variety Club. Nominated for Academy Award 1973 for designing VIP, automated projection system.

NELSON, GENE: Dancer, actor. r.n. Gene Berb. b. Seattle, Wash., March 24, 1920; e. Santa Monica, Calif. H.S. Began dancing and ice skating in school; joined Sonja Henie ice show; played in This is the Army, World War II; after discharge, featured in It Happens on Ice, Center Theatre, New York. To Hollywood for I Wonder Who's Kissing Her Now; joined Hollywood group prod. stage musical, Lend an Ear; to Warner for Daughter of Rosie O'Grady.
PICTURES INCLUDE: Tea for Two, West Point Story, Lullaby of Broadway, Painting the Clouds With Sunshine, Starlift, She's Working Her Way Through College, She's Back on Broadway, Three Sailors and a Girl, Crime Wave, Oklahoma, Way Out, Atomic Man, So This Is Paris. Directed, The Hand of Death, Hootenany Hoot, The Cool Ones, Your Cheatin' Heart, Kissin' Cousins, Wake Me When the War is Over, The Letters, Harum Scarum.
TV: Directed Mod Squad, I Dream of Jeannie, Hawaii Five-O, Farmer's Daughter, Donna Reed Show, Burke's Law, Felony Squad, Laredo, The Rifleman, The Wackiest Ship, Iron Horse, FBI, The Rookies.
BROADWAY: Follies, 1970; Music, Music, 1974.

NELSON, GEORGE: Executive. Army veteran, World War II. Started with journalistic career, including service with NY newspaper PM and Newark Evening News; also positions with the US Office of War Information and U.S. State Dept. Held publicity posts with United Artists and Horizon Pictures before joining Warner Bros. in 1958. Served successively as pub. copy chief, dir. of press information, east. pub. dir., east. dir. of pub./adv. In 1985 named v.p.

NELSON, HARRIET: r.n. Harriet Hilliard. b. Des Moines, Iowa, July 18, 1914, e. High Sch., Kansas City, m. Ozzie Nelson. Appeared in dramatic & musical roles in shows; singer with Ozzie Nelson band; on radio shows: Believe It or Not, Seeing Stars, Red Skelton, Adventures of Ozzie & Harriet. Appeared in m.p.: Here Come the Nelsons.
TV: Adventures of Ozzie & Harriet, ABC-TV.
STAGE: Marriage-Go-Round; rec.: Ozzie & Harriet.
PLAYS: Impossible Years, State Fair.

NELSON, JUDD: Actor. b. Portland, ME, 1964. e. Haverford/Bryn Mawr Coll. Studied acting at Stella Adler Conservatory. Theatrical m.p. debut, Making the Grade (1984).
PICTURES: Fandango, The Breakfast Club, St. Elmo's Fire, Blue City.

NELSON, LORI: Actress. r.n. Dixie Kay Nelson; b. Santa Fe, N.M., Aug. 15, 1933; e. High Sch., L.A. Child actress; photographer's model; m.p. debut in Ma and Pa Kettle at the Fair.
PICTURES INCLUDE: Bend of the River, Francis Goes to West Point, All I Desire, All-American, Walking my Baby Back Home, Tumbleweed, Underwater, Destry, Revenge of the Creature, I Died a Thousand Times, Sincerely Yours, Mohawk, Day the World Ended, Pardners, Hot Rod Girl, Ma and Pa Kettle at Waikiki, Gambling Man, Untamed Youth.
TV: How to Marry a Millionaire, Wagon Train, Laramie, Bachelor Father, The Texan, Wanted Dead or Alive, Sam Spade, G.E. Theatre, Riverboat, Sugarfoot, The Young and the Restless, etc.

NELSON, RALPH: Producer, director, playwright, actor. b. New York City. Stage actor 1933–41; Wrote play, Angels Weep, for Cleveland Playhouse, 1943; also two Bdwy. plays: Mail Call (1944) and The Wind Is Ninety (1945). Directed plays: Here's Mama (1952); The Trouble-Makers (1953) and The Man in the Dog Suit (1957). From 1948 to 1960 directed over 1,000 dramatic shows on all TV networks. Has made film appearances in many pictures he produced and/or directed, now president Rainbow Productions. Honorary Doctor of Humane Letters, Columbia College, 1975.
PICTURES INCLUDE: Director: Requiem for a Heavyweight, Lilies of the Field, (also prod.) Soldier in the Rain, Fate Is the Hunter, Father Goose, Duel at Diablo, (also prod.) Charly, (also prod.) Counterpoint, Tic-Tic-Tic, Soldier Blue, Flight of the Doves, (also prod.) The Wrath of God, (also prod.) The Wilby Conspiracy, Embryo, A Hero Ain't Nothin' But a Sandwich, Because He's My Friend, You Can't Go Home Again. Screenplays: The Man in the Funny Suit, Flight of the Doves, The Wrath of God.
TV: Director: Playhouse 90, Studio One, Philco Playhouse, G.E. Theatre, Ford Startime, Omnibus, ABC Theatre, Elgin Hour, Dick Powell Theatre, Dupont Show of the Month, Front Row Center, Climax, Desilu Playhouse, and specials: Cinderella, Aladdin, This Happy Breed, Nutcracker Suite. Producer: Climax Series, Studio One, The Old Vic Hamlet, The Man in the Funny Suit, Doyle Against the House, Three Soldiers, John J. Digges, Farmer's Daughter (pilot). Christmas, Lilies of the Field.

NELSON, RAYMOND E.: Executive. b. Cleveland, O., Feb. 12, 1907; e. Baldwin-Wallace Univ. Eastern prod. mgr., NBC: supervisor of TV, Mutual; prod.-conductor, light operas; stock co. dir.; prod.-dir. TV shows on all networks: Television Follies, Fashions on Parade, Western Theatre, Boys from Boise, etc.; prod.-dir.-writer, Rod and Gun Club of the Air on Mutual, radio and TV; prod., dir., Story Time, ABC-TV. Pres., Keystone Ad Agency, Nelson Prod., Inc.; dir. of spot sales, TV Bureau of Adv.; v.p., gen. mgr., NTA Film Network.

NELSON, WILLIE: Composer-Singer-Actor. b. Abbott, TX, April 30, 1933. Started writing songs in the 60s; performing in the 70s. Film debut in Electric Horseman (1979).
PICTURES: Honeysuckle Rose, Thief, Barbarosa, Songwriter.
TELEVISION: Movies: The Last Days of Frank and Jesse James, Stagecoach.

NEPOMUNCENO, LUIS: Producer, director. b. Manila, Philippines, July 24, 1930; e. De La Salle College, Manila, Phil., New York Inst. of Photography, N.Y. Tech. Ass't. to pres., Nepomunceno Productions, 1946–54; gen. mgr., Mepro, Inc., 1954–59; pres., Film Advertising Media Exhibitions, Inc., 1959 to date; pres., Luis Nepomunceno & Sons, Inc., 1961 to date; pres., Filipino Theas. Ass'n., 1969. Awards include: Filipino Academy of Motion Pictures Arts & Sciences 3 Awards 1968, 8 Awards 1969. Grand Prix, 2nd & 3rd Manila Film Festivals; 6 Awards, 4th Manila Film Festival. Asian Film Festivals: 2 Awards 14th Festival, 4 Awards 15th Festival.
PICTURES INCLUDE: Tears in the Dark, Manila, Open City, Because of a Flower, Heaven on Earth, Mountain Maiden, The Beggar, A Time for Dying, The Hunted.

NETTER, DOUGLAS: Producer. Todd A.O., 1955–1957. Sam Goldwyn Productions, 1958–1960. Formed own company rep. producers, 1961–67. Jalem Prod., 1968–1969. Exec. v.p. MGM, 1969–1974. Producer, Mr. Ricco (MGM), 1975. American Co-producer, The Wild Geese, 1977. Producer, Louis L'Amour's The Sacketts, four hour mini-series (NBC), 1978. Executive Producer, The Buffalo Soldiers, NBC Pilot, 1979. Producer, Wild Times, four hour mini-series (Metromedia), 1980. Producer Roughnecks, four hour mini-series (Metromedia), 1981. Executive Producer Cherokee Trail (Walt Disney Productions and CBS), 1982. Executive Producer, Five Mile Creek, Austrialian based television series for Disney Channel and Austrialian Network Seven, 1983–85. Producer, Captain Power television series, syndication, 1986.

NETTLETON, LOIS: Actress. e. Studied at Goodman Theatre, Chicago. Replaced Kim Hunter in Darkness At Noon on Broadway.
PLAYS INCLUDE: Cat on a Hot Tin Roof, Silent Night, Lonely Night, God & Kato Murphy, The Wayward Stork, The Rainmaker, A Streetcar Named Desire.
PICTURES INCLUDE: Period of Adjustment, Come Fly With Me, Mail Order Bride, Valley of Mystery, Bamboo Saucer, The Good Guys and the Bad Guys, Dirty Dingus Magee, The Sidelong Glances of a Pigeon Kicker, The Honkers, Echoes of a Summer, Butterfly.
TELEVISION: Brass.

NEUMAN, ALAN: Producer, director. b. New York City. July 25, 1924; e. N.Y. Univ., B.A. American Theatre Wing. Dir., NBC-TV, 1947; prod., dir. of over 4000 TV shows; winner of 48 Nat'l Awards for excellence in TV. Now pres., Alan Neuman Prods.
TV: Exploring the Unknown (NBC Big Event), Person to Person, America Pause-Coke Special, Wide Wide World, General Motors Special Show, Inner Sanctum film series, Colgate Comedy Hour, Lights Out, Blind Date, Chevrolet Teletheatre, We the People, Kate Smith Show, Believe It or Not, Little Show, Dagmar's Canteen, Meet the Press, Ellery Queen; exec. prod.: College of the Air, Beat the Odds, Let. T, Laugh-In, This Is Your Life, You Asked For It.

NEWBERY, CHARLES BRUCE: Executive. b. Melbourne, Australia; e. All Saints Grammar School, Melbourne and Melbourne U. Entered m.p. ind. with Hoyt's Theatres, Ltd., Melbourne, 1929; publ. mgr., Fox Studios, Eng., 1934; controller, Fox Newsreel Theatres, 1935; managing dir., Fox Films, India, 1937; Supvr., India, China, Malaya, Fox Films, 1940; Film advisor, Government of India, 1941; estab. film studios & Newsreel for Government of India. suprv. Far East & Australia Republic, 1945; supvr. Middle, Near & Far East. Republic, 1947; supvr. Eng. & Europe, Republic, 1948; estab. Republic Productions Great Britain, 1952; v.p. bd. mem. dir. of sales, Republic, U.S.A., 1953; pres., Charles Newbery Assoc., Newbery-Warden Associates, London, 1960; mgr. dir., Santor Film Prods., Americon Prods, Inc., 1964; sen. v.p., bd. mem., administration, In-Flight Motion Pictures Inc., v.p., Intransit Motion Pictures, Inc., 1965. Senior v.p. Sales and Marketing 1967, President and Chief Operating Office, May 1973; vice chm. bd., Inflight, June, 1979; Dir. of Mktg., Life Services Co., of America June, 1979 chm. bd., Inflight and sls.—Europe, East and Africa, 1980. Bd. member/consultant to Inflight, 1985.
PICTURES INCLUDE: Deadlier Than the Male, Catch Me if You Can, Kiss Her Goodbye.

NEWBROOK, PETER: Producer and director of photography. Entered m.p. ind. Warner Bros. Studios, Teddington. Chmn. Titan Int'l. Productions, Ltd. Esquire Records Ltd. & Esquire Music Co. Pres., British Society of Cinematographers.
PICTURES INCLUDE: After working on such pictures as The Sound Barrier, The Captain's Paradise, Hobson's Choice, Summer Madness, The Deep Blue Sea, Anastasia, The Bridge on the River Kwai; became dir. photog.: Lawrence of Arabia (2nd unit), 1961; In The Cool of the Day, That Kind of Girl, 1962; The Yellow Teddybears, Saturday Night Out, 1963; The Black Torment, 1964. Prod. and photog; Gonks Go Beat, 1965; prod. and photog; The Sandwich Man, 1966; Press For Time, Corruption, The Smashing Bird I Used to Know, Bloodsuckers, She'll Follow You Anywhere, Crucible of Terror, The Asphyx, The Wonderful World of Greece, 1982: Bosom Friends, Where's Your Sense of Humor?, Last of the Midnight Gardeners.

NEWCOM, JAMES E.: Associate producer. b. Indianapolis, Ind., Aug. 29, 1907; e. U. California. Reader, MGM, 1926, then in stocks and bonds with E. F. Hutton; then actor and film editing dept., MGM, 1930; film ed. 1933; asst. prod., 1952. Now retired.
PICTURES INCLUDE: Gone With the Wind, Rebecca, Since You Went Away, Annie Get Your Gun, Trial, Somebody Up There Likes Me, Wings of Eagles, Until They Sail, Farewell to Arms, The Inn of the Sixth Happiness; Revue Television; Paramount Studios. Nine Hours to Rama, The Impossible Years, editor: Tora Tora Tora.

NEWGARD, ROBERT M.: Executive. b. Des Moines, Iowa, Jan. 14, 1925; e. U. of Notre Dame, 1948; Mirisch Bros., Theatres Candy Co., built and operated theas. in midwest, 1948–50; operated record dist. business 1949–53, Columbia and MGM records; prod. shows at KTTV Hollywood, 1952; Interstate Television Subsidiary Allied Artists, dist. and prod'n of TV films, 1953–56; midwestern and western sales mgr., Screen Gems, 1956–66; v.p. world syndication, Paramount Television, 1967–73; now v.p., intl. mkt., Film Services Corp.

NEWHART, BOB: Actor-Comedian. b. Chicago, Sept. 5, 1929. e. Loyola Univ. In Army 2 yrs.; then law school; left to become copywriter and accountant. Acted with theatrical stock co. in Oak Park; hired for TV man-in-street show in Chicago. Recorded comedy album for Warner Bros. Record Co., The Button Down Mind of Bob Newhart, which was big hit. Followed by two more successful albums. Did series of nightclub engagements and then acquired own TV variety series in 1961. Frequently appears in Las Vegas and headlines college concerts. Has guested on most major TV variety and comedy series.
PICTURES INCLUDE: Cool Millions, Catch 22, Cold Turkey, First Family.
TV: The Bob Newhart Show, Thursday's Game (movie), Newhart.

NEWLAND, JOHN: Director, actor. b. Cincinnati, Ohio. Musicals, many TV appearances. Actor, dir., Robert Montgomery Show, My Lover, My Son.

NEWLEY, ANTHONY: Actor, writer, composer, singer. b. Sept. 24, 1931.
PICTURES INCLUDE: Cockleshell Heroes, Battle of the River Plate, Port Afrique, Fire Down Below, Good Companions, X the Unknown, High Flight, No Time to Die, The Man Inside, The Bandit, The Lady is a Square, Idle on Parade, Killers of Kilimanjaro, Let's Get Married, Jazz Boat, In The Nick, The Small World of Sammy Lee, Dr. Dolittle, 1966; Can Hieronymus Merkin Ever Forget Mercy Humpee and Find True Happiness?, Sweet November, Quilp (star, music) Willie Wonka and the Chocolate Factory (score); Summer Tree (dir.).
TV: Sammy, Sunday Night Palladium, The Strange World of Gurney Slade (series), Saturday Spectaculars, The Johnny Darling Show, Hollywood Squares, Merv Griffin Show, The Tonight Show, Anthony Newley Special (London), Blade in Hong Kong (movie).
PLAYS: West End stage; Stop The World—I Want to Get Off. N.Y. stage: Roar of the Greasepaint (wrote, composed with Leslie Bricusse), Good Old Bad Old Days, Chaplin.

NEWMAN, ALFRED S.: Executive. b. Brooklyn, N.Y., Nov. 16, 1940. e. New York University. Public relations work for Equitable Life Insurance, Trans World Airlines prior to joining Columbia Pictures in 1968 as writer in publicity dept.; named New York publicity mgr., 1970; national publicity mgr., 1972; joined MGM as East adv't-pub. dir., 1972; named director of adv't, pub. and promotion, 1974; named v.p., worldwide adv., pub., promo., 1978; v.p., pub./promo., MGM/UA, 1981. With 20th Century-Fox as v.p. adv./pub./promo. for TV & corporate, 1984–85; joined Rogers & Cowan as sr. v.p. & head of corporate entertainment, 1985.

NEWMAN, DAVID: Writer. b. N.Y.C., Feb. 4, 1937. e. Univ. of Mich. (M.S., 1959). Was writer-editor at Esquire Magazine where he met Robert Benton, an art director, and formed writing partnership. All credits co-written with Benton.
PICTURES INCLUDE: Bonnie and Clyde, There Was a Crooked Man, Floreana, What's Up, Doc?, Money's Tight, Bad Company, Superman (co-s.p.), Superman II (co-s.p.), Jinxed (co-s.p.), Santa Claus.
STAGE: It's a Bird . . . It's a Plane . . . It's Superman (libretto), Oh! Calcutta (one sketch).

NEWMAN, EDWIN: News Correspondent. Joined NBC News in 1952, based in N.Y. since 1961. Reports news on NBC-TV and often assigned to anchor instant specials. Has been substitute host on Today, appeared on Meet the Press and has reported NBC News documentaries. Hosts interview series, Speaking Freely, on WNBC-TV, N.Y.C. station of NBC.

NEWMAN, JOSEPH M.: Producer, Director, writer. b. Logan, Utah. Aug. 7, 1909. Started as office boy MGM, 1925; jobs in production dept. to 1931; asst. to George Hill, Ernst Lubitsch, etc., 1931–37; asstd. in organization of MGM British studios 1937; dir. short subjects 1938; dir. "Crime Does Not Pay" series 1938–42; Major in U.S. Army Signal Corps 1942–46; dir. 32 Army Pictorial Service Pictures. Member: AMPAS, SDG Masons.
PICTURES INCLUDE: Northwest Rangers, Abandoned, Jungle Patrol, Great Dan Pitch, 711 Ocean Drive, Lucky Nick Cain, Guy Who Came Back, Love Nest, Red Skies of Montana, Outcasts of Poker Flat, Pony Soldier, Dangerous Crossing, Human Jungle, Kiss of Fire, This Island Earth, Flight to Hong Kong, Fort Massacre, Big Circus, Tarzan The Ape Man, King of the Roaring Twenties, Twenty Plus Two, The George Raft Story, Thunder of Drums.

NEWMAN, LIONEL: Composer-Conductor. b. Los Angeles. Began career at 16 as lead pianist with Earl Caroll's Vanities; wrote first song, Dust in Your Eyes, featured in Vanities. Joined brother, the late Alfred Newman, at 20th Century-Fox where Alfred was head of music dept. Lionel became head in 1970 when Alfred died. 1977, named v.p. of Fox; 1982, snr. v.p., 20th Century-Fox Feature Film and Television Divisions. Has composed or conducted for 250 films, earning 11 Academy Award nominations. Won Oscar, 1969, for Hello, Dolly.

NEWMAN, MARTIN H.: Executive. b. Brooklyn, N.Y. m. Nov. 16, 1913; e. N.Y.U., 1934, Certified Public Accountant (N.Y.); Century Theatres, 1936–1974, exec. v.p. 1966–1974; National Association of Theatre Owners, 1975–1977; exec. dir., Will Rogers Memorial Fund, 1977–present.

NEWMAN, NANETTE: Actress-writer. b. Northampton, England; m. to Bryan Forbes. Ent. films in 1946 and TV in 1951. Publications include God Bless Love, That Dog, Reflections, The Root Children, Amy Rainbow, Pigalev, Archie, Christmas Cookbook, etc.
TV: The Glorious Days, The Wedding Veil, Broken Honeymoon, At Home, Trial by Candlelight, Diary of Samuel Pepys, Faces in the Dark.
FILMS INCLUDE: The Personal Affair, The League of Gentlemen, The Rebel, Twice Around the Daffodils, The L-Shaped Room, Wrong Arm of the Law, Of Human Bondage, Seance on a Wet Afternoon, The Wrong Box, The Whisperers, Deadfall, The Madwoman of Chaillot, The Raging Moon, (U.S. title: Long Ago Tomorrow), The Stepford Wives, It's A 2′2″ Above the Ground World (The Love Ban), Man at the Top, International Velvet.
RECENT TV: Balzac (BBC), Fun Food Factory, TV series, Stay with Me Till Morning, Let There Be Love (series) West Country Tales, Jessie.

NEWMAN, PAUL: Actor. Director. b. Cleveland, Ohio, Jan. 26, 1925. e. Kenyon Coll., Yale School of Drama. Summer stock; on Broadway in Picnic, The Desperate Hours, Sweet Bird of Youth, Baby Want A Kiss.
TV: Philco, U.S. Steel, Playhouse 90.
PICTURES INCLUDE: The Silver Chalice, The Rack, Somebody Up There Likes Me, The Long, Hot Summer, Cat on a Hot Tin Roof, Rally Around the Flag Boys, The Young Philadelphians, Exodus, The Hustler, Sweet Bird of Youth, Adventures of a Young Man, Hud, A New Kind of Love, The Prize, The Outrage, What a Way to Go, Lady L., Harper, Hombre, Cool Hand Luke, The Secret War of Harry Frigg, Winning, Butch Cassidy and the Sundance Kid. Dir. Rachel, Rachel. Formed First Artists Prod. Co. Ltd. 1969 with Sidney Poitier, Steve McQueen and Barbra Streisand, 1971; actor, director, Sometimes A Great Notion; Pocket Money (actor), 1971; Life & Times of Judge Roy Bean, 1972, The Effect of Gamma Rays (dir., 1972), The Mackintosh Man, The Sting, The Towering Inferno, The Drowning Pool, Buffalo Bill and the Indians, Slap Shot, Quintet, When Time Ran Out, Fort Apache, The Bronx, Absence of Malice, The Verdict, Harry and Son (co-s.p., actor, dir.), The Color of Money.

NEWMAN, SAMUEL: Producer, writer, attorney. b. Jersey City, New Jersey, Dec. 14, 1919; e. N.Y.U., USFV College of Law, B.A., Juris Doctor; Captain, Armed Forces, WW II; writ. prod. Armed Forces Radio Service; freelance, contract writ. 30 m.p.; asst. exec. prod., Columbia Pictures; Pres., Samuel Newman Prods., Inc.; Head writer, story consultant, Perry Mason Show, CBS-TV 1960–64; head writer, story consultant, associate producer, Tarzan Series, NBC-TV, 1966–67; practicing licensed member, California and Federal Bar.

NEWMAN, SYDNEY.: O. C. (F.R.S.A.) Chief Creative Consultant for Canadian Film Development Corp. b. Toronto, Canada. Studied painting, drawing, commercial art at Central Techn. Schl. To Hollywood in 1938. Joined National Film Board of Canada under John Grierson. Prod. over 300 shorts. Later became exec. prod. all Canadian government cinema films, 1947–52; Canadian Broadcasting Corp., 1952, as dir. outside broadcasts, features and documentaries. Later became drama sup. and prod. Canadian Television Theatre. Joined ABC-TV in England, 1958. as sup. of drama and producer of Armchair Theatre: Head of Drama Group, TV, BBC, 1963. Commissioned and prod. first TV plays by Arthur Hailey, Harold Pinter, Alun Owen, Angus Wilson, Peter Lake. Fellow Society of Film & TV Arts, 1968; Prod. Associated British Pictures. SFTA award 1968; Zeta award, Writers Guild, Gt. Btn., 1970. 1970: Special advisor, ch. dir., Broadcast Programmes branch, Canadian Radio & TV Commission, Ottawa. Aug., 1970: Appt. Canadian Govt. Film Commissioner and chm., National Film Board of Canada; Trustee, National Arts Centre, Ottawa; board member, Canadian Broadcasting Corporation, Canadian

Film Development Corp., Canadian Picture Pioneers Special Award. Special Advisor on Film to the Secretary of State for Canada, 1975–77; pres., Sydney Newman Enterprises. 1981: Made Officer of the Order of Canada.

NEWMAN, WALTER BROWN: Writer.
PICTURES INCLUDE: Ace in the Hole (co-s.p.), Underwater, The Man with the Golden Arm (co-s.p.), The True Story of Jesse James, Crime and Punishment, USA, The Interns (co-s.p.), Cat Ballou (co-s.p.), Bloodbrothers, The Champ.

NEWTON-JOHN, OLIVIA: Actress-Singer. b. Sept. 26, 1948, Cambridge, England. Brought up in Melbourne, Australia, where won first talent contest at 15, with prize trip to England. Stayed there 2 yrs. performing as part of duo with Australian girl singer, Pat Carroll, in cabarets and on TV. Started recording; several hit records. Became a regular guest on TV series, It's Cliff Richard. Gained world-wide prominence as singer, winning several Grammys and other music awards.
PICTURES: Grease, Xanadu, Two of a Kind.

NEY, RICHARD: Actor, writer, prod., financier. b. N.Y. e. Columbia Univ., B.A. Acted in RCA TV demonstration, New York World's Fair; on stage in "Life with Father." On screen 1942 in Mrs. Miniver, War Against Mrs. Hadley, In armed services, World War II. Many TV shows. Financial advisor consultant, Richard Ney and Associates; financial advisor, lecturer; author, The Wall Street Jungle.
PICTURES INCLUDE: Late George Apley, Ivy, Joan of Arc, The Fan, Secret of St. Ives, Lovable Cheat, Babes in Bagdad, Miss Italia, Sergeant and The Spy.

NIBLEY, SLOAN: Writer. b. Ore.; e. U. of Utah, U.C.L.A., m. Linda Stirling, actress, Three yrs. U.S. Navy; employed as writer at major studios; contributor to mags.; wrote many western pictures incl.: Carson City, Springfield Rifle; prod., and writer many TV shows on film and live TV for Ralph Edwards.

NICHOLS, MIKE: Actor-Director. b. Berlin, Ger., Nov. 6, 1931. e. Chicago U. Compass Players, teamed with Elaine May; night clubs.
TV: Broadway, An Evening with Mike Nichols and Elaine May.
STAGE: Barefoot in the Park, The Knack, Luv, The Odd Couple, The Apple Tree, The Little Foxes, Plaza Suite, Uncle Vanya, The Prisoner of 2nd Avenue, Streamers, Comedians, The Gin Game. Produced Annie, 1976. 1984: Directed The Real Thing (Tony award), Hurlyburly, Social Security.
PICTURES INCLUDE: Who's Afraid of Virginia Woolf, The Graduate, Catch 22, Carnal Knowledge, The Day of the Dolphin, The Fortune, Silkwood (also co-prod.), Heartburn.

NICHOLSON, ELWOOD J.: Cinematographer, research engineer, physicist. b. Dewitt Co., Clinton, Ill., Mar. 8, 1908; e. Chicago Eng. Coll., D.E.E. 1925; Amer. Eng. Coll., N.Y.C., Ph.D., 1929, 1927 cameraman & technician U.S. Army Air Corps, Panama; 1928 photog. & tech. Chas. A. Lindbergh; 1929 aerial photog. skywriting, Curtiss Field, L.I.; 1930 pilot & photog., newsreels & Curtiss Flying Service; 1931 newsreel cameraman, prod. & ed., Bermuda; 1932, Natl. Theat. Supply; 1934 designed equip. for Billy Rose's Jumbo, N.Y.C.; 1935 newsreels; 1936 designed equip. sound & lighting Max Reinhardt's Eternal Road, N.Y.C.; 1937–40 eng., George Teegue Process, Hollywood; 1940–44 research eng., U.S. Army Wright Field, Dayton, Ohio; 1944–45 photo research developing color tem. meter; color photog. & design eng., Wolff Studios, Hollywood. In 1947 designed & built new type 16mm sound on film recorder; invented "Cinematic" sound; mag. tape; electro devices.
PICTURES INCLUDE: Pansy the Horse, Clyde Beatty series, Operation Airstrip, Drink Up series.
MEMBER: SMPTE, IATSE. Sec'y, treas., Magna-Sound Inc., 1954.

NICHOLSON, JACK: Producer, director, actor, writer. b. Neptune, N.J.; April 22, 1936. Began career in cartoon department of MGM. Made acting debut in Hollywood stage production of Tea and Sympathy.
PICTURES INCLUDE: (Acting credits) The Shooting, Psych Out, Hell's Angels on Wheels, Little Shop of Horrors, The Raven, Ride the Whirlwind, Flight to Fury, Ensign Pulver, Too Young To Live, Studs Lonigan, Cry Baby Killer, Easy Rider, Five Easy Pieces, Carnal Knowledge, A Safe Place, (Writing credits) The Trip, Head, Flight to Fury, Ride the Whirlwind, Drive, He Said. (Producing credits) Ride the Whirlwind, The Shooting, Head, Drive, He Said. Directing debut with Drive, He Said, 1971. Acting: The Last Detail, 1973, Chinatown, Tommy, The Passenger, The Fortune, One Flew Over the Cuckoo's Nest, The Missouri Breaks, The Last Tycoon, Goin' South (also dir.), The Shining, The Postman Always Rings Twice, The Border, Reds, Terms of Endearment, Prizzi's Honor, Heartburn.

NICHOLSON, ROBERT (NICK): Producer, actor, composer, arranger. b. Buffalo, N.Y. Musical dir., WBEN, WGR Buffalo, N.Y.; Musical dir., Howdy Doody, Ruff & Reddy, Top Dollar, Look To Win, How Do You Rate. Prod., Do, Re, Mi. VP., Nicholson-Muir Prod. Package Prod. creator Newlyweds Game, Matches 'n Mates, Big Spender, Pay Cards, Video Encyclopedia, Reader's Digest, "Joe" series, The Joy of Sewing, Headline Hunters, Family Challenge, Ladies 'n Gentlemen.

NICKELL, PAUL: Director. e. Morehead, Ky., State Teachers College, U. of No. Carolina English instructor, North Carolina State College; then cameraman, asst. dir., dir. WPTZ, Philadelphia; dir. CBS-TV 1948.
TV: Studio One, Best of Broadway, Climax, Playhouse 90.

NICKSAY, DAVID: Executive. e. Mass. Hampshire Coll. Entered industry thru Directors Guild of America's training program, apprenticing on Rich Man Poor Man and rising to second asst. dir. on Oh, God. Producer of many TV projects and theatrical films with Edgar Scherick prod. co. 1986, joined Paramount Pictures as v.p., prod., for M.P. Group.
PICTURES: Mr. Soffel (prod.), Lucas (prod.).
TELEVISION: Call to Glory (pilot), Little Gloria Happy at Last, etc.

NICOL, ALEX: Actor, Director. b. Ossining, N.Y., Jan. 20, 1919; e. Fagin Sch. of Dramatic Arts, Actor's Studio; U.S. Cavalry.
THEATRE: Forward the Heart, Sundown Beach, Hamlet, Richard II, South Pacific, Mr. Roberts, Cat on a Hot Tin Roof.
PICTURES INCLUDE: Sleeping City, Target Unknown, Air Cadet, Raging Tide, Meet Danny Wilson, Red Ball Express, Because of You, Tomahawk, Redhead From Wyoming, Lone Hand, Law and Order, Champ for a Day, Black Glove, Heat Wave, About Mrs. Leslie, Dawn at Socorro, Strategic Air Command, Man from Laramie, Great Day in the Morning, Sincerely Yours, Five Branded Women, Via Margutta, Under 10 Flags, Gunfighters at Casa Grande. Dir., Sleeping Skull, Then There Were Three. Acted in: The Brutal Land, Bloody Mama, Homer, The Gilded Cage. Director: Point of Terror. Actor: Hells Black Night: Director: Screaming Skull, Then There Were Three.

NIELSEN, LESLIE: Actor. b. Regina, Sask., Canada, Feb. 11, 1926. e. Victoria H.S., Edmonton. Disc jockey, announcer for Canadian radio station; studied at Neighborhood Playhouse; N.Y. radio actor summer stock.
TV APPEARANCES: Studio One, Kraft, Philco Playhouse, Robert Montgomery Presents, Putlizer Prize Playhouse, Suspense, Danger, Justice, Man Behind the Badge, Death of a Salesman, The New Breed, Swamp Fox, Peyton Place, Ben Casey, Wild Wild West, The Virginian, The Loner, Blade in Hong Kong.
PICTURES INCLUDE: Vagabond King, Forbidden Planet, Ransom!, Opposite Sex, Hot Summer Night, Tammy and the Bachelor, Night Train To Paris, Harlow, Dark Intruder, Beau Geste, Gunfight in Abilene, The Reluctant Astronaut, Counterpoint, Rosie, Dayton's Devils, How to Commit Marriage, Change of Mind, The Resurrection of Zachary Wheeler, The Poseidon Adventure, Viva, Knievel!, City on Fire, Airplane!, Wrong Is Right, Creepshow.

NIEMEYER, HARRY: Publicist. b. New York, N.Y., May 31, 1909. Drama ed. St. Louis Times; pub. depts., Warner Bros., RKO, Paramount and Columbia. In January, 1946 appointed asst. pub. dir., Benedict Bogeaus Prods. Hollywood correspondent St. Louis Post-Dispatch. Apptd. pub. dir. Samuel Bischoff Prod., 1948; Universal-International studio pub. dept., 1949; asst. pub. dir., 1958; Free lance pub., major studios, 1965–71. Retired.

NIGH, JANE: Actress. r.n. Bonnie Lenora Nigh. b. Hollywood, Calif., Feb. 25, 1926; e. Polytechnic H.S., Long Beach, Calif. Defense plant worker.
PICTURES INCLUDE: Something for the Boys; State Fair, Dragonwyck, Unconquered, Give My Regards to Broadway, Red, Hot and Blue, Blue Grass of Kentucky, County Fair, Captain Carey, U.S.A., Blue Blood, Disc Jockey, Fort Osage, Rodeo.

NILES, FRED A.: Executive. b. Milwaukee, Wisc., Sept. 12, 1918. e. Univ. of Wisc. Was radio news commentator and capt. of office of educ. and information of U.S. Army in World War II. Now heads own film studio, Fred A. Niles Communications Centers, Inc., Chicago.

NIMOY, LEONARD: Actor. b. Boston, Mass., Mar. 26, 1931. Along with active career in films, TV and stage, has been writer and photographer. Author of three books on photography and poetry, as well as autobiography, I Am Not Spock. Has also been speaker on college lecture circuit.
PICTURES: Queen for a Day, Rhubarb, The Balcony, Catlow, Invasion of the Body Snatchers, Star Trek—The Film, Star Trek II; The Wrath of Khan, Star Trek III: The

Search for Spock (also dir.), Star Trek IV: The Voyage Home (also. dir.).
TELEVISION: Star Trek, Mission: Impossible, etc. Movie: The Sun Also Rises.
STAGE: Equus, Sherlock Holmes, Vincent (one-man show).

NIVEN, DAVID, JR.: Executive. b. London, Dec. 15, 1942. Joined William Morris Agency in Beverly Hills in 1963. Transferred same yr. to New York; in next five yrs. worked for agency's European offices in Rome, Madrid and London. In 1968 joined Columbia Pictures' U.K. office as a prod. exec.; 1972, named mg. dir. of Paramount Pictures in U.K. In 1976 became indep. prod., forming partnership with Jack Wiener.
PICTURES INCLUDE: The Eagle Has Landed, Escape to Athena, Monsignor, That's Dancing!

NIX, WILLIAM PATTERSON: Executive. b. Philadelphia, April 10, 1948. e. Georgetown Univ. (A.B., 1970), Antioch Graduate School (M.A., 1971), Hofstra Univ. School of Law (J.D., 1976). New York University School of Law (LL.M., 1979). In 1976 joined the legal staff of the Motion Picture Association of America. Chairman of MPAA committee on copyright and literary property matters, and worldwide director of film industry's anti-piracy programs.

NIZER, LOUIS: Author-Attorney. b. London, Eng., Feb. 6, 1902. e. Columbia Coll., B.A., 1922; Columbia Univ. Law School, LLB, 1924. Recipient of Columbia Univ. Curtis Oratorical Prize two times. Sr. partner of law firm, Phillips, Nizer, Benjamin, Krim & Ballon & special counsel to the Motion Picture Assn. of America. Writer of numerous books and articles in leading periodicals and newspapers; lecturer on legal subjects at many universities and bar associations. Also painter and writer of musical compositions.
BOOKS: Reflections without Mirrors, The Implosion Conspiracy, The Jury Returns, My Life in Court, What to Do With Germany, Thinking on Your Feet, Between You and Me, New Courts of Industry, Legal Essays. Excerpt from My Life in Court adapted to Bdwy. play, A Case of Libel, and also for TV movie. Chapter of The Jury Returns adapted for TV movie.

NOBLE, PETER: Writer, producer, actor, TV personality. b. London, Eng., June 18; e. Hugh Myddelton Sch.; Latymer Sch. Author several books on m.p. ind.; writer & conducts movie radio prog. for B.B.C. & Luxembourg (Film Time, Movie-Go-Round, Peter Noble's Picture Parade). Formed Peter Noble Productions, 1953; Acted in many pictures; Ed. Screen International since 1975. Editor Screen International Film & TV Yearbook since 1974.
PICTURES INCLUDE: Production assoc., Runaway Bus; asst. prod., to Dorothy a Son; co-prod., s.p. Fun at St. Fanny's; s.p.; Three Girls in Paris; assoc. prod., Lost; s.p., Captain Banner; prod., Strange Inheritance; London Columnist; Hollywood Reporter etc. 1967–75.
AUTHOR: Editor, British Film Year Book; author of biographies of Bette Davis, Erich Von Stroheim, Ivor Novello, Orson Welles. Author book, I Know That Face. Wrote screen plays, the King of Soho, Love in the Limelight, The Story of Ivor Novello, The Negro in Films.
TV: Find the Link, Other Screen, Film Fanfare, Movie Memories, Yakity Yak, Startime, Thank Your Lucky Stars, Juke Box, Jury, Simon Dee Show, Star Parade, Who's Whose, Movie Magazine, The Big Noise, The Name Game, Line Up, Tea Break, Today. Prod. consult. On The Braden Beat, The Frost Program, Dee Time. 1969–70 Prod. Cons. Simon Dee Show. Appeared on Anything You Can Do Looks Familiar, Password, Etc. 1971–1975. Wrote scripts and prod. consultant Movie Quiz (series). Appears frequently on Today TV series. 1976, Two's Company, Looks Familiar. Prod. con. Musical Time Machine BBC2 series, Talking about films on radio, including BBC Star Sound, Radio Luxembourg, Film Focus, Newsnight, Looks Familiar Nationwide, Hotel TV Network, 1981–3. Recent TV: The Time of Your Life, Channel 4 News, Nationwide. Numerous radio shows. TV series: Show Business, This Is Britain. TV appearances: Looks Familiar, Electric Picture Show, Gossip, Entertainment Tonight (USA). 1984–85: This Is Britain (TV cable series; Cannes Film Festival (Premiere TV Cable).

NOIRET, PHILIPPE: Actor. b. France, 1931. Has played character roles in numerous international films.
PICTURES INCLUDE: Zazie dans le Metro, Les Copains, The Night of the Generals, Topaz, Murphy's War, A Time for Loving, The Serpent, Let Joy Reign Supreme.

NOLTE, C. ELMER, JR.: Executive v.p., b. Baltimore, Md., Oct. 19, 1905. Managing dir., F. H. Durkee Enterprises, Baltimore. Pres., NATO of Md., 1955–56; treas., 1957–59; pres., 1952–66, 67–69. Now v.p. & gen. mgr.

NOLTE, NICK: Actor. b. Omaha, Nebr., 1942. Attended 5 colleges in 4 yrs. on football scholarships, including Pasadena City College and Phoenix City College. Joined Actors Inner Circle at Phoenix and appeared in several plays. Did stock in Colorado. In 1968 joined Old Log Theatre in Minneapolis and after 3 yrs. left for New York, appearing at Cafe La Mama. Went to L.A. and did several TV series before big break in mini-series Rich Man, Poor Man as Tom Jordache.
PICTURES INCLUDE: Return to Macon County Line, The Deep, Who'll Stop the Rain, North Dallas Forty, Heart Beat, Cannery Row, 48 Hrs., Under Fire, Teachers, Grace Quigley, Down and Out in Beverly Hills, Extreme Prejudice.
TV: Guested on Medical Center, Gunsmoke, etc. Starred in Rich Man, Poor Man, Book I. Movies: Feather Farm.

NORDEN CHRISTINE: Actress, singer. r.n. Mary Lydia Thornton. b. Sunderland, England, Dec. 28, 1924. m. Jack Clayton, director (q.v.). On British stage in Tell the World, 1942; Take It Easy, 1944; Cinderella, 1951–52; The Marriage-Go-Round, 1979–80. On Broadway in Tenderloin, 1960–61; The Butler and Egg Man, 1966; Marat de Sade, 1967; Scuba Duba, 1968 etc. Signed by Sir Alexander Korda 1945 to seven year contract with London Films and Metro Goldwyn Mayer.
PICTURES INCLUDE: Night Beat, Mine Own Executioner, An Ideal Husband, Idol of Paris, A Yank Comes Back (in U.S.: A G.I. Returns), Saints and Sinners, The Interrupted Journey, Black Widow, A Case for PC 49, Reluctant Heroes.
TELEVISION: Angel's Ransom, The Virginia Graham Show, Playhouse 90, Give My Regards to Broadway, Time to Spare, Love and Marriage.

NORMAN, STANLEY: Producer-Director. b. Dec. 22, 1921. e. Filmacademy Berlin.
PICTURES INCLUDE: The Hot Country, Dangerous Journey, Land without Grace, The Devil from Cape Town, Nobodies Land, Operation Yellow Viper, The Man Who Came To Kill, El Cisco, Tests to Kill, The Spy Pit, Taste of Savage, The Manipulator, The Big Game, In a Colts Shadow.

NORRIS, CHARLES GLENN: Executive. b. Taylorsville, N.C., Nov. 24, 1906; e. Nat'l U. Law Sch., Wash., D.C. Asst. poster clerk, Fox Film Co., 1928; booker, Wash., D.C., 1934; ad-sales mgr., Aug., 1935; salesman, Phila.; Wash., July, 1937; Baltimore, July, 1944; br. mgr., Wash., Jan. 1946; dist. mgr., July, 1946; br. mgr., Wash., Apr., 1948; Atlantic div. mgr., Wash., Jan., 1952; eastern sales mgr., April, 1954; central Canadian sales mgr., April, 1956; asst. gen. sales mgr., April, 1959; gen. sls. mgr., 1960–69; exec. capacity in distribution, 20th Century-Fox, The Glenoris Corp.
MEMBER: Variety Club, English Speaking Union, M.P. Pioneers.

NORRIS, CHUCK: Actor. b. California, 1939. Gained renown as karate expert. Film debut in Return of the Dragon (1973).
PICTURES: Breaker! Breaker!, Good Guys Wear Black, A Force of One, The Octagon, An Eye for an Eye, Slaughter in San Francisco, Silent Rage, Forced Vengeance, Lone Wolf McQuade, Missing in Action, Missing in Action 2, Code of Silence, Invasion U.S.A. (also s.p.), Delta Force.

NORRIS, EDWARD: Actor. b. Philadelphia, Pa.; e. Culver Mil. Acad. Ran away to sea; later reporter on Phildelaphia Ledger, Philadelphia Bulletin & Morning Record. Joined Philadelphia Professionals, then to Theatre Union Group, N.Y. On stage (Doomsday Circus). Screen debut Queen Christina, 1934.
PICTURES INCLUDE: Boys' Town, Dr. Ehrlich's Magic Bullet, Mystery of Marie Roget, Great Impersonation, Decoy, Heartaches, Trapped by Boston Blackie, Forgotten Women, Breakthrough, Killer Shark, Highway 301, Murder Without Tears, The Kentuckian.

NORRIS, KATHI: Performer. b. Newark, Ohio. e. Univ. of Chicago; banker; acct. exec., Grant Advertising, Inc., 1940–45; columnist and writer, 1944–46; star, TV, Kathi Norris Show, WABD, WNBC, 1949–54; Today Show, NBC, 1954; spokeswoman, General Electric television shows, NBC, CBS, ABC, 1954–57; hostess-narrator, True Story, NBC TV, 1957–61; panelist, Leave It to the Girls, 1962–63; radio-TV spokeswoman, Ralston Purina, 1962–64; syndication and commercials, 1964–66.

NORTH, ALEX: Composer. b. Chester, Pa., Dec. 4, 1910; e. Curtis Inst., 1928–29; Julliard Sch. of Music, 1932–34. Composer for ballet, radio, TV, theatre; U.S. Army, 1942–46; Guggenheim Fellowship, 1947–48; comp., 40 documentary films, 1937–50; comp. Revue for Clarinet & Orch. for Benny Goodman, 1947. Member ASCAP; Dramatists Guild.
PICTURES INCLUDE: Streetcar Named Desire, Death of a Salesman, Viva Zapata, Les Miserables, Pony Soldier, Member of the Wedding, Go Man Go, Desiree, Unchained, The Racers, Man with the Gun, Rose Tatoo, I'll Cry Tomorrow, Cleopatra (Composers and Lyricists Award, best film score, 1964), Shoes of the Fisherman Golden Globe Award; best film score 1968), The Children's Hour, The Misfits, Cheyenne Autumn, Spartacus, The Rainmaker, The Agony an the Ecstacy, Who's Afraid of Virginia Woolf?, A Dream of Kings, Willard, Pocketmoney, Rebel Jesus, Once Upon a Scoundrel, Lost in the Stars, (musical director)

Journey Into Fear, Shanks, Bite the Bullet, Somebody Killed Her Husband, Wise Blood, Carny, Dragonslayer, Under the Volcano, Prizzi's Honor. 15 Acad. Awards nominations.
AWARDS: Honorary Oscar, 1986; ASCAP Golden Soundtrack Award, 1986; Society for Preservation of Film Music Award, 1986; American Society of Music Arrangers & Composers Golden Score Award, 1986.

NORTH, EDMUND H.: Writer. b. New York City, e. Stanford Univ., U.S. Army Signal Corps, five yrs., World War II, sep. as major.
PICTURES INCLUDE: One Night of Love, I Dream Too Much, Dishonored Lady, Flamingo Road, Young Man with a Horn, In a Lonely Place. collab. Only the Valiant; s.p. Day the Earth Stood Still, Outcasts of Poker Flat; collab. s.p., Destry, Far Horizons, Proud Ones; s.p. Cowboy; screen story and s.p., Sink the Bismarck!; collab. s.p., H.M.S. Defiant; collab. story and s.p. Patton; story and collab. s.p. Meteor.

NORTH, SHEREE: Actress. r.n. Dawn Bethel. b. Los Angeles, Calif., Jan. 17, 1933. e. Hollywood H.S. Amateur dancer with USO at 11; prof. debut at 13; many TV appearances; on Broadway in Hazel Flagg.
PICTURES INCLUDE: Excuse My Dust, Living It Up, How To Be Very Very Popular, Lieutentant Wore Skirts, Best Things in Life Are Free, Way to the Gold, Destination Inner Space, The Gypsy Moths, Charley Varick, The Outfit, Breakout, The Shootist, Telefon.
TV: Eddie, Scorned and Swindled.

NOSSECK, MAX (Alexander M. Norris): Director. b. Nakel, Poland, Sept. 19, 1902. e. U. of Berlin; studied art in Vienna; stage actor four years Poland and Germany. In 1919: Actor, assist. dir., film ed., dir. (DLS Berlin, Biograph, U.F.A.). In 1931: dir. The Unhappy Man, DLS Berlin. In 1938: first picture in Portuguese; also dir. in Spain, France, Holland; dir. Gado Bravo, Overture to Glory, Girls Under 21. In U.S., 1939–40.
PICTURES INCLUDE: The Brighton Strangler, Dillinger, Black Beauty, Return of Rin-Tin-Tin, Kill or Be Killed, the Hoodlum.

NOURI, MICHAEL: Actor. b. Washington, DC, Dec. 9, 1945. e. Avon Old Farms, Rollins College, Emerson College. Studied for theatre with Larry Moss and Lee Strasberg. New York stage debut in Forty Carats, 1969. Film debut in Goodbye Columbus, 1969.
PICTURE: Flashdance, The Imagemaker.
TELEVISION: Beacon Hill, The Gangster Chronicles, Contract on Cherry Street, Between Two Women.

NOVAK, KIM: Actress. r.n. Marilyn Novak. b. Feb, 13, 1933. e. Wright Junior Coll., Los Angeles City Coll. Started as model, named World's Favorite Actress, Brussels World Fair; m.p. debut in Pushover.
PICTURES INCLUDE: Phfft, Five Against the House, Picnic, Man with the Golden Arm, Eddy Duchin Story, Jeanne Eagles, Pal Joey, Middle of the Night, Bell, Book and Candle, Vertigo, Pepe, Strangers When We Meet, The Notorious Landlady, Boys' Night Out, Of Human Bondage, Kiss Me, Stupid, The Amorous Adventures of Moll Flanders, The Legend of Lylah Clare, The Great Bank Robbery, Tales That Witness Madness, The White Buffalo, The Mirror Crack'd.

NUREYEV, RUDOLF: Dancer—Actor. b. Russia, Mar. 17, 1938. e. Leningrad Ballet School. Joined Kirov Ballet Co. as soloist. Asked for and granted political asylum in 1961 in Paris while performing. Joined Marquis de Cuevan Ballet Co.
PICTURES: An Evening with the Royal Ballet, Swan Lake, Romeo and Juliet, The Sleeping Beauty, Don Quixote, Valentino, Exposed.
TELEVISION: Julie Andrews Invitation to the Dance with Rudolf Nureyev.

NYKVIST, SVEN: Cinematographer. b. 1922, Sweden. Became internationally known through photographing most of Ingmar Bergman's pictures.
PICTURES INCLUDE: Sawdust and Tinsel, Karin Mansdotter, The Silence, Loving Couples, Persona, Hour of the Wolf, Cries and Whispers (AA), The Dove, Black Moon, Scenes from a Marriage, The Magic Flute, Face to Face, The Tenant, The Serpents' Egg, Pretty Baby, Autumn Sonata, King of the Gypsies, Hurricane, Starting Over, Willie and Phil, The Postman Always Rings Twice, Fanny and Alexander, Agnes of God.

NYREN, DAVID O.: Prod. b. Des Moines, Iowa, Nov. 9, 1924. e. Columbia U., 1945–47. U.S. Marine Corps, 1943–45; radio & TV prod. supervision, W. Wallace Orr Adv. Agency, 1947–49; radio & TV dir., Ruthrauff & Ryan, Baltimore, 1949; TV supervisor & commercial prod. TV shows, Ruthrauff & Ryan, N.Y., 1950; also dir. of new program development & talent, 1951–52; radio-TV acct. exec., Dancer-Fitzgerald-Sample, 1952–55; vice-pres. in chge. of TV programming, 1955. Sr. V.P. in chg. TV Programs, 1966; David Nyren Prods., 1971.

O

OBOLER, ARCH: Writer. b. Chicago, Ill.; e. U. Chicago. Began writing for radio 1936 as author Lights Out, "Arch Oboler's Plays," Plays for Americans; 5 vols. radio scripts published; collab. s.p. Escape.
PICTURES INCLUDE: Bewitched, Arnelo Affair, Five, The Twonky. Org. Arch Oboler Prod., August, 1952. Prod. Bwana Devil, 1952, first 3-D feature, winner Peabody Award. Writer, dir., exec. Prod., 1 & 1, 1961. prod., writer, dir. The Bubble, (in space-vision).

O'BRIAN, HUGH: Actor. b. Rochester, N.Y., Apr. 19, 1930; r.n. Hugh J. Krampe; Univ. of Cincinnati; U.S. Marine Corps; actor, stock cos.; actor with many m.p. cos.
PICTURES INCLUDE: Young Lovers, Never Fear, Vengeance Valley, Little Big Horn, On the Loose, The Cimarron Kid, Red Ball Express, Sally and Saint Anne, The Raiders, The Lawless Breed, Meet Me at the Fair, Seminole, Man from the Alamo, Back to God's Country, Saskatchewan, Fireman Save My Child, Drums Across the River, Broken Lance, There's No Business Like Show Business, White Feather, The Fiend Who Won the West, Twinkle in God's Eye, Brass Legend, Rope Law, Come Fly With Me, Love Has Many Faces, In Harm's Way, Ten Little Indians, Ambush Bay, Cowboy in Africa, Harpy, Killer Force, The Shootist, Game of Death.
TV: Wyatt Earp, ABC; Special Dial M for Murder; Hallmark Hall of Fame, A Punt, A Pass and A Prayer; It's a Man's World. TV movie: Wild Women, ABC, Probe, NBC series, Tomorrow is Now, Space in the Age of Aquarius, Search (NBC series) Murder on Flight 502 (ABC Movie), Fantasy Island (ABC Movie), Cruise Into Terror (ABC Movie).
THEATRE: B'way Plays: Destry Rides Again, First Love, Guys and Dolls. National co. of Cactus Flower.
Pres. H.O.B. Inc. Bev. Hills, 1956. Chm., Flounder: Hugh O'Brian Youth Foundation; Nat'l Chmn., Cystic Fibrosis Research Foundation 1969–74, Pres. Thalians 1956–57; Founder Hugh O'Brian Annual Acting Awards at UCLA.

O'BRIAN, PETER: Producer. b. Toronto, 1947. e. University of Toronto, Emerson College, Boston. Assistant dir. in feature films, television series, and commercials. Prod. for Quadrant Films Ltd., 1975. Also pres. of Muddy York Motion Pictures Ltd.
PICTURES INCLUDE: Me (prod.) 1974; The Mourning Suit (Line Producer) 1974; Clown Murders (principal) 1975; Love At First Sight (prod.) 1975; Blood and Guts, 1977; Fast Company, 1978.

O'BRIEN, LIAM: Writer. b. New York, N.Y., March, 1913; e. Fordham U., Manhattan Coll., A.B., 1935. Author B'way play Remarkable Mr. Pennypacker, 1953.
PICTURES INCLUDE: Chain Lightning, Redhead and the Cowboy, Of Men and Music, Diplomatic Courier, Here Comes the Groom, The Stars Are Singing, Young at Heart.

O'BRIEN, MARGARET: Actress. b. Los Angeles, Calif., Jan. 15, 1937. Screen debut at 4 in Babes in Arms, Acad. Award best child actress, 1944. Voted one of ten best money-making stars in Motion Picture Herald-Fame Poll 1945–46.
PICTURES INCLUDE: Journey for Margaret, Dr. Gillespie's Criminal Case, Lost Angel, Thousands Cheer, Jane Eyre, The Canterville Ghost, Meet Me in St. Louis, Music for Millions, Our Vines Have Tender Grapes, Three Wise Fools, Unfinished Dance, Tenth Avenue Angel, Secret Garden, Big City, Little Women, Her First Romance, Anabelle Lee, Diabolic Wedding.

O'BRIEN, VIRGINIA: Actress. b. Los Angeles, Apr. 18, 1919. On stage in "Meet the people." Screen debut 1940 in Hullabaloo; now retired.
PICTURES INCLUDE: The Big Store, Lady Be Good, Ringside Maisie, Ship Ahoy, Panama Hattie, DuBarry Was a Lady, Thousands Cheer, Meet the People, Two Girls and a Sailor, The Harvey Girls, Ziegfeld Follies, Till Clouds Roll By, The Showoff, Merton of the Movies.

O'CONNELL, JACK: Producer-Director-Writer-Lyricist. b. Boston. After Germany in WWII got BA Princeton MBA Harvard. After being copy group head at D'Arcy and McCann advertising and doing 500 TV commercials entered feature films working with Fellini on La Dolce Vita, then asst. director to Antonioni on L'Avventura, then writer-producer-director Greenwich Village Story, Revolution, Christa (a.k.a. Swedish Fly Girls), City Women. Features have been invited by critics to represent U.S. at Cannes, Locarno, Berlin and Venice Festivals.

O'CONNOR, CARROLL: Actor. b. New York City, Aug. 2, 1925.

e. University College, Dublin & U. of Montana. Three years with Dublin's Gate Theatre, then N.Y. where stage credits include Ullyses in Nighttown, Playboy of the Western World, The Big Knife; m.p. debut in Fever in the Blood, 1960.
PICTURES INCLUDE: By Love Possessed, Lonely Are The Brave, Cleopatra, In Harm's Way, What Did You Do In The War Daddy?, Hawaii, Not With My Wife You Don't, Waterhole No. 3, The Devil's Brigade, For Love Of Ivy, Kelly's Heroes, Doctors' Wives, Law and Disorder.
TV: US Steel Hour, Armstrong Circle Theatre, Kraft Theatre, All In The Family (Emmy, Golden Globe awards), Of Thee I Sing. Movies: Brass, Convicted.
AUTHOR: Ladies of Hanover Tower (play); Little Anjie Always, The Great Robinson (screenplays). Movies: Brass, Convict.

O'CONNOR, DONALD: Actor. Star of Tomorrow, 1943. b. Chicago, Ill., Aug. 28, 1925. In vaudeville with family and "Sons o' Fun" (Syracuse, N.Y.) before screen debut 1938 in Sing You Sinners; in number other pictures 1938–39 (Sons of the Legion; Tom Sawyer, Detective, Beau Geste, On Your Toes, etc.); in vaudeville 1940–41, then resumed screen career with What's Cookin'?, 1942. Entered armed services, 1943.
PICTURES INCLUDE: Private Buckaroo, Give Out, Sisters, When Johnny Comes Marching Home, It Comes Up Love, Mr. Big, Top Man, Patrick the Great, Follow the Boys, The Merry Monahans, Bowery to Broadway, This Is the Life, Something in the Wind, Are You With It? Feudin', Fussin' and a-Fightin'. Yes Sir, That's My Baby, Francis series, Curtain Call at Cactus Creek, The Milkman, Double Crossbones, Singin' In the Rain, I Love Melvin, Call Me Madam, Walking My Baby Back Home, There's No Business Like Show Business, Anything Goes, Buster Keaton Story, Cry for Happy, That Funny Feeling, That's Entertainment, Ragtime.
TV: Colgate Comedy Hour, 1953–54. Voted best TV performer, M.P. Daily poll, 1953, The Donald O'Connor Show.

OFFENHAUSER, WILLIAM H., JR.: Executive, engineer; b. Brooklyn, N.Y., May 8, 1904; e. Columbia U., RCA, 1929–32; inventor MGM squeezetrack, 1929; contractor, Army Sig. Corps, 1933–34; sales eng., J. A. Maurer, Inc., 1936–39; mgr., Precisions Films Labs., N.Y., & v.p., mem. of bd., J. A. Maurer, 1939–43; project eng., Johns Hopkins U., 1942–43; consultant, Sig. Corps. Photo Center, 1944–45; consultant, film in color TV, CBS, 1946–47, 1949–51; research project, Cornell U. Med. Coll., 1947–49, consultant, Telenews Prod., 1951–52; v.p., Andre Debrie of America, Inc., 1953; ind. consultant, films & TV, 1954. 1960–61, (Photo Staff) M.I.T. Lincoln Laboratory, Lexington, Mass. Author, 16mm Sound Motion Pictures—A Manual; co-author, Microrecording-Industrial and Library Microfilming; ind. consultant, Films, TV, biological Acoustics and Biophysics; 1968, pres. Radio Club of America; 1969–73 Bd. Dir. Radio Club of America.

O'HANLON, GEORGE: Actor. b. B'klyn,. N.Y,. Nov. 23, 1917; e. La Salle Acad., Providence, R.I. p. Sam Rice and Luly Beeson, prof., served in U.S. Air Corps, 1942–45. Appeared in stock, vaudeville and Broadway musicals. On screen first, 1941, New Wine.
PICTURES INCLUDE: The Hucksters, Headin' for Heaven, Triple Cross, Spirit of West Point, Are You With It? star in Joe McDoakes series: Park Row, Cattle Town, Tanks Are Coming, Lion & the Horse, Battle Stations, Million Dollar Duck.
TV: Real George, Life of Riley, Bop Girl, Desilu Playhouse, Pantomime Quiz.

O'HARA, GERRY: Director. b. Boston-Lincs., England 1924. e. St. Mary's Catholic School, Boston. Junior Reporter Boston Guardian. Entered industry in 1942 with documentaries and propaganda subjects. Dir. debut 1963 That Kind of Girl.
PICTURES INCLUDE: Game for Three Lovers; Pleasure Girls (wrote & dir.); Maroc 7; Love in Amsterdam; All the Right Noises (orig. screenplay & dir.); Leopard in the Snow; The Bitch; Fanny Hill.
TV: The Avengers; Man in a Suitcase, Journey into the Unknown, The Professionals (story editor, writer); Special Squad (story consultant).

O'HARA, MAUREEN: Actress. r.n., Maureen FitzSimons. b. Dublin. Aug. 17, 1921. Abbey School of Acting. Won numerous prizes for elocution. Under contract to Erich Pommer-Charles Laughton. Co-starred, Abbey & Repertory Theatre: Jamaica Inn, Mayflower Pictures, 1939; Hunchback of Notre Dame, RKO. In 1940: A Bill of Divorcement, Dance, Girls, Dance, RKO. In 1941: They Met in Argentina, RKO; How Green Was My Valley, 20th-Fox. In 1942: To the Shores of Tripoli, Ten Gentlemen from West Point, The Black Swan.
PICTURES INCLUDE: The Fallen Sparrow, Buffalo Bill, The Spanish Main, Do You Love Me?, Miracle on 34th Street, Foxes of Harrow, The Homestretch, Sitting Pretty, Woman's Secret, Forbidden Street, Sentimental Journey, Sinbad the Sailor, Father Was a Fullback, Comanche Territory, Tripoli, Bagdad, Rio Grande, At Sword's Point, Kangaroo, Flame of Araby, Quiet Man, Against All Flags, Redhead from Wyoming, War Arrow, Fire Over Africa, Magnificent Matador, Lady Godiva, Long Gray Line, Everything But the Truth, Wings of Eagles, The Deadly Companions, Our Man In Havana, Mr. Hobbs Takes a Vacation, McLintock, Spencer's Mountain, The Parent Trap, The Rare Breed, The Battle of Villa Fiorita, How Do I Love Thee:, Big Jake, The Red Pony.

O'HERLIHY, DAN: Actor. b. Wexford Ireland, 1919. e. National U. of Ireland. Actor with Abbey Theatre, Dublin Gate, Langford Prod.; announcer on Radio; Eireann; on Broadway in The Ivy Green.
PICTURES INCLUDE: Odd Man Out, Macbeth, At Swords Point, Actors and Sin, Adventures of Robinson Crusoe, Black Shield of Falworth, Bengal Brigade, Purple Mask, Virgin Queen, That Woman Opposite, City After Midnight, 100 Rifles, The Tamarind Seed, MacArthur.

OHMART, CAROL: Actress. b. Salt Lake City, Utah, June 3. e. Lewis and Clark H.S., Spokane. Newspaper writer, model, radio actress.
TV: Versatile Varieties, Studio One, Philco Playhouse, Colgate Comedy Hour.
THEATRE: On Broadway in Kismet.
PICTURES INCLUDE: Scarlet Hour; Wild Party, House On Haunted Hill, Scavengers.

O'HORGAN, TOM: Director. e. DePaul Univ. At age 12 wrote opera, Doom on the Earth. Is also musician, singer, actor. Responsible for developing many revolutionary off-off Bdwy. artistic innovations in such productions as The Maids, Tom Paine, Futz.
PICTURES INCLUDE: Futz, Rhinoceros.
STAGE: Broadway: Hair, Lenny, Jesus Christ, Superstar, Inner City, Dude.

OHTANI, HIROSHI: Executive. b. Tokyo, Nov. 2, 1910. e. Kobe Commercial C. 1935; entered Shochiku Co., Ltd., 1936; exec. dir. 1937; man. dir. 1944; dir. Taisho-kan Theatre Co., Ltd. 1948; dir. Chuei Co., Ltd. 1953; man. dir. 1953; aud. Schochiku Co., 1954; pres. 1960–62; pres., Chugai motion picture chain. 1962.

O'KEEFE, ALLAN J.: Exhibitor. b. Minneapolis, Minn. e. St. Thomas Coll., St. Paul, Minn.; Univ. of Minnesota, Minneapolis; m. railroading with Soo Line; salesman, Belden-Evans Shirt Co., Minneapolis; Western Theatre Equipment Co., 1919–21; W. W. Hodkinson Corp., 1921; Robertson-Cole, 1922; Goldwyn Cosmopolitan and Metro Goldwyn 1923–24; Producers Distributing Corp. 1925; then br. mgr. Producers Distr. Corp; Pathe Exchange, Inc., Salt Lake City, Utah 1926–30; br. mgr. Pathe and RKO Pathe Dist. Corp., Los Angeles, 1930–31; br. mgr., Universal, Portland, Ore. 1932–33; Los Angeles 1933–May, 1938; west. dist. mgr. 1938; west div. sales mgr. 1943; asst. gen. sales mgr. 1946–50; west coast exhib., 1951–53; v.p. in chge. of sales, Polalite Co., July, 1953. In exhibition since 1953.

O'KEEFE, MICHAEL: Actor. b. Paulland, NJ, 1955. e. New York Univ. On Bdwy. stage in Mass Appeal and Fifth of July.
PICTURES: Gray Lady Down, The Great Santini, Caddyshack, Split Image, Nate and Hayes, Finders Keepers, The Slugger's Wife, The Whoopee Boys.
TELEVISION: A Rumor of War, Harvest Home.

OKON, TED: Producer-director. b. New Kensington, Pa., Oct. 27, 1929. e. U. of Pittsburgh, BA 1949. Started career as radio announcer, disk jockey; John Harris Enterprises, theatres and Ice Capades, 1 year; prod. dir., WDTV-TV, Pittsburgh, formed Togo Productions prod. live and film TV shows: Reach, Yates and Matoon. TV-radio dir. 1956; TV-radio pro. dir. Reach McClinton & Co., 1957. sr. v.p. pro. TV comm. Benton and Bowles Adv. 1958–63; Exec. TV prog. dir. art., Ogilvy, Benson & Mather Adv. 1963–65; v.p. prog. dir. Van Praag Prod.; Exec. prod. Girl Game, TV show, 1966; Pres. Rough & Ready, 1966–69; Pres. prod-dir. Tape 16, Teletronics 1969–70; Pres. 1970's Productions; Exec. prod. Women's Clubhouse, TV show, Pres., exec. prod., Pennysaver Productions, Inc., TV programming syndication. Exec. prod. The Pennysaver Place, Dance Party '76, $50,000 Crossword, Sho-Biz-Quizz, Polka Party, Salsa Time, Northstage Theatre Restaurant.

OLEMBERT, THEODORA: Producer/writer. Doctor of Law Criminology of Paris University. Entered films through documentaries on child delinquency. Worked during the war as assistant to Prof. René Cassin on Franco/British cultural relations including films. Afterwards joined Jean Benoit-Lévy, chief of the United Nations Film Section. Formed Triangle Films Ltd. for international coproductions; associated with l'Editon Française Cinématographique (Paris).
PRODUCED: Leonardo da Vinci, G. B. Shaw, Chopin, Teiva, The Sixth Day of Creation, Salvador Dali, Is Venice Sinking?, Edith Piaf and Corsica. Co-produced: Midnight

Episode, Van Gogh, Moliere, Mont St. Michel and Chinese Theatre. Preparing further films for international releases.

OLIN, MILTON E.: Executive. b. Chicago, Ill., Jan. 25, 1913. e. U. of Chicago, Ph.B., 1934; American Theatre Wing, N.Y., 1946–47. Freelance nightclub MC. radio & TV writer, radio actor; charter member AFRA, Chicago; writer, World Broadcasting System, 1946; radio transcription sales, Ray Block Enterprises & Richard H. Ullman, Inc., 1947–51; div. sales mgr., United Artists TV Corp., 1951–54; TV sales rep., WABC-TV, N.Y., 1954; nat'l sales mgr., Telefilm Enterprises, TV exec., Walt Disney Prod., 1956–60.

OLIVER, ANTHONY: Actor, author. b. July 4, 1923. e. Monmouth, R.A.F., 1940–46; stage debut, 1946; numerous plays; pictures; TV debut, 1946; many TV plays for BBC & ITV. Writes & tells own stories for TV. Authority on antiques. Author of The Victorian Staffordshire Figure; Staffordshire Pottery, The Tribal Art of England, and four novels, The Pew Group, The Property of a Lady, The Elberg Collection, Cover Up.

OLIVIER, LORD. (Sir Laurence Olivier): Actor. b. Dorking, England, May 22, 1907. On stage, London, N.Y. since 1925. Recent plays include, Caesar & Cleopatra, Anthony & Cleopatra, London, 1951, N.Y. 1952; Venus Observed, London 1950; Sleeping Prince, London, 1953; Shakespeare Season, Stratford-upon-Avon, 1955; The Entertainer, London, N.Y., 1957–58; Titus Andronicus European Tour 1957; Coriolanus Stratford-upon-Avon, 1959. Rhinoceros, London, 1960; Becket, N.Y., 1960 & Tour 1961. dir., Chichester festival Theatre; 1962, dir., The Chances, The Broken Heart; Uncle Vanya, dir., acted, 1965; Othello, 1964. dir., National Theatre, 1962; Hamlet, Uncle Vanya. Recruiting Officer 1963–64. Othello Master Builder 1963–65; dir., The Crucible, 1965; Moscow, Berlin, Othello And Love For Love 1965; dir. Juno and the Paycock, 1965–66. Tour of Canada with National Thea. Co. in Love for Love, Dance of Death, Flea in Her Ear, 1967, Home and Beauty, 1969, Shylock in The Merchant of Venice, 1970; Long Day's Journey Into Night, 1972–74; Dir. Amphitryon 38, 1971; Saturday, Sunday, Monday, 1973; The Party, 1973; Eden End, 1974.
PICTURES INCLUDE: As You Like It, Fire Over England, Divorce of Lady X, Wuthering Heights, Rebecca, Pride and Prejudice, That Hamilton Woman, Demi Paradise, Henry V (dir. & cast), Hamlet (prod., dir. & cast), Acad. Award, Best Actor, 1948, Carrie, Beggar's Opera, Richard III (prod., dir. & cast), Prince & the Showgirl, Devil's Disciple, Spartacus, The Entertainer, Term of Trial, Bunny Lake Is Missing, Othello, Khartoum, Shoes of the Fisherman, Oh! What a Lovely War, Battle of Britain, Dance of Death, David Copperfield, Three Sisters, Sleuth, Nicholas & Alexandra, Lady Caroline Lamb, 7% Solution, Marathon Man, A Bridge Too Far, The Betsy, The Boys from Brazil, A Little Romance, Dracula, Clash of the Titans, Inchon, The Jazz Singer, Wagner, The Bounty, Wild Geese II.
TV: John Gabriel Borkman, London. The Moon and Sixpence, N.Y.; The Power & The Glory, N.Y., Uncle Vanya, Long Day's Journey Into Night, 1973, Merchant of Venice, 1973, World at War, 1973, Love Among the Ruins, 1975, Jesus of Nazareth 1976. Prod. and acted in The Collection, Cat on a Hot Tin Roof. Prod. and dir. Hindle Wakes. Prod. and acted in Come Back Little Sheba, Daphne Laureola. Prod. and acted in Saturday Sunday Monday, Brideshead Revisited and King Lear. Actor: The Last Days of Pompeii, Peter the Great.

O'LOUGHLIN, GERALD STUART: Actor. b. N.Y.C., Dec. 23, 1921. e. Blair Academy, Lafayette Coll., U. of Rochester, Neighborhood Playhouse; U.S. Marine, WW II.
THEATRE: Broadway: Streetcar, Shadow of a Gunman, Dark at the Top of the Stairs, A Touch of the Poet, Cook For Mr. General, One Flew Over The Cuckoo's Nest, Calculated Risk. Off Broadway: Who'll Save the Plowboy, Harry, Noon & Night.
PICTURES INCLUDE: Lovers and Lollypops, Cop Hater, Hatful of Rain, Ensign Pulver, A Fine Madness, In Cold Blood, The Valachi Papers, Desperate Characters, The Organization, Twilight's Last Gleaming, Quicksilver.
TV: The Defenders, Ben Casey, Dr. Kildare, 12 O'Clock High, For the People, Going My Way, Naked City, Alcoa Premiere, Child's Cry.

OLSON, DALE C: Executive. b. Fargo, ND, Feb. 20, 1934. e. Portland State Coll. (Oregon). Presently owner, Dale C. Olson & Associates; formerly sn. v.p. & pres., m.p. div., Rogers & Cowan public relations. Journalist on Oregonian Newspaper, West Coast editor, Boxoffice Magazine, 1958–1960; critic and reporter, Daily Variety, 1960–1966; director of publicity, Mirisch Corporation, 1966–1968; Rogers & Cowan, 1968–1985. Past pres., Hollywood Press Club, awarded Bob Yaeger and Les Mason award by Publicists Guild; v.p. Diamond Circle, City Of Hope; delegate for U.S. to Manila International Film Festival.

OLSON, NANCY: Actress. b. Milwaukee, Wis.; e. U. of Wisconsin, Univ. of California, Los Angeles; m. Alan Jay Lerner composer, writer. No prof. experience prior to films.
PICTURES INCLUDE: Union Station, Canadian Pacific, Sunset Boulevard, Mr. Music, Submarine Command, Force of Arms, So Big, Boy From Oklahoma, Battle Cry, Pollyanna, The Absent-Minded Professor, Smith!, Airport 1975, Making Love.

O'NEAL, FREDERICK: Actor-Director-Lecturer. b. Brooksville, Miss., Aug. 27, 1905. e. public schools of Brooksville and St. Louis, Mo., New Theatre School, American Theatre Wing. Acted primarily on stage. Is now pres. of Associated Actors and Artists of America.
PICTURES INCLUDE: Pinky, No Way Out, Something of Value, Anna Lucasta, Take a Giant Step.
TV: Car 54, Where Are You (series, 1961–62).

O'NEAL, PATRICK: Actor. b. Ocala, Fla., 1927. e. Univ. of Fla. Neighborhood Playhouse. In stock cos. before N.Y. TV, 1951.
PICTURES INCLUDE: The Mad Magician, The Black Shield of Falworth, From the Terrace, A Matter of Morals, The Cardinal, In Harm's Way, King Rat, Chamber of Horrors, A Fine Madness, Alvarez Kelly, Matchless, The Assignment, Where Were You When the Lights Went Out?, The Secret Life of an American Wife, Castle Keep, Stiletto, Corky, The Way We Were, The Stepford Wives.
TELEVISION: Dick and the Duchess, Emerald Point NAS.

O'NEAL, RON: Actor. b. Utica, N.Y. e. Ohio State Univ. Spent 8 yrs. at Karamu House in Cleveland (inter-racial theatre) from 1957 to 1966, taking part in 40 plays. 1967–68 spent in N.Y. teaching acting in Harlem. Appeared in all-black revue 1968, The Best of Broadway, then in summer stock. Acted off-Broadway in American Pastorale and The Mummer's Play. 1970 joined Joseph Papp's Public Theatre. Big break came with No Place To Be Somebody, which won him top acting honors: the Obie, the Clarence Derwent, the Drama Desk and the Theatre World Awards.
PICTURES INCLUDE: Move, The Organization, Super Fly, Super Fly TNT, The Master Gunfighter, When a Stranger Calls, The Final Countdown.
TV: The Interns (guest), Playing with Fire (movie).
STAGE: Tiny Alive, The Dream of Monkey Mountain.

O'NEAL, RYAN: Actor, r.n. Patrick Ryan O'Neal. b. Los Angeles, Calif., April 20, 1941. Began as stand-in, then stunt man, then actor in "Tales of the Vikings," series, in Germany, 1959; freelanced in Hollywood; Screen Gems Pilots, Donny Dru, Our Man Higgins, and co-starred in series made from Empire; co-star, Peyton Place, ABC-TV.
PICTURES INCLUDE: The Big Bounce, The Games, Love Story, Wild Rovers, What's Up Doc, Paper Moon, The Thief Who Came To Dinner, Barry Lyndon, Nickelodeon, A Bridge Too Far, The Driver, Oliver's Story, Green Ice, Partners, So Fine, Irreconcilable Differences, Fever Pitch.

O'NEAL, TATUM: Actress. b. Los Angeles, 1964. Daughter of Ryan O'Neal and Joanna Moore. Won A.A. for debut performance in Paper Moon.
PICTURES INCLUDE: Paper Moon, The Bad News Bears, Nickelodeon, International Velvet, Little Darlings, Prisoners, Certain Fury.

O'NEIL, THOMAS F.: Executive. b. Kansas City, Mo., Apr. 18, 1915; e. Holy Cross Coll., 1933–37. Employed by General Tire and Rubber Co., 1937–41; U.S. Coast Guard, 1941–46; v.p., dir., Yankee Network, Boston, 1948–51; pres. chmn. of bd. RKO General, Inc., since 1952. Arranged pubchase RKO Radio by General Teleradio, Inc. from Howard Hughes, July, 1955; chairman of the Board, RKO General, Inc., dir., General Tire & Rubber Co.

O'NEILL, JENNIFER: Actress. b. Rio de Janeiro, Feb. 20, 1949. Model before entering films.
PICTURES: Rio Lobo (debut, 1970), Summer of '42, Such Good Friends, The Carey Treatment, Glass Houses, Lady Ice, the Reincarnation of Peter Proud, Whiffs, Caravans, A Force of One, The Psychic, The Innocent, Steel, Scanners.
TELEVISION: Cover Up (series); Movies: A.D., Chase.

ONTKEAN, MICHAEL: Actor. b. Canada, 1950. e. Univ. of New Hampshire. son of Leonard and Muriel Cooper Ontkean, actors.
PICTURES: The Peace Killers, Pick Up on 101, Necromancy, Hot Summer Weekend, Slap Shot, Voices, Willie and Phil, Making Love, Just the Way You Are.
TELEVISION: The Rookies (series). Movies: The Blood of Others, Kids Don't Tell, The Right of the People.

OPATOSHU, DAVID: Actor. b. N.Y.C., Jan. 30, 1918. e. Morris High School. U.S. Army, 1942–46; played character roles, The Group Theatre at 19; appeared on Broadway.
THEATRE: Me and Molly, Once More With Feeling, Silk Stockings, The Reclining Figure, The Wall, Bravo Giovanni.
PICTURES INCLUDE: Cimmarron, Naked City, The Brothers Karamazov, Exodus, Act of Mercy, Best of Enemies, Enter Laughing, Romance of a Horse Thief.

OPOTOWSKY, STAN: Executive. e. Tulane Univ. Served in U.S. Marine Corps as combat corr. and later joined United Press, working in New Orleans, Denver, and New York. Published own weekly newspaper in Mississippi before returning to N.Y. to join New York Post as mgr. editor and traveling natl. corr. Is also cinematographer and film editor. Joined ABC News as TV assignment editor; named asst. assignment mgr. In 1974 named dir. of operations for ABC News TV Documentaries. In 1975 named dir. of TV News Coverage, ABC News.
AUTHOR: TV: The Big Picture, The Longs of Louisiana, The Kennedy Government, Men Behind Bars.

OPPENHEIMER, GEORGE: Writer. b. New York, N.Y., Feb. 7, 1900; e. Williams Coll., 1916–20; Harvard, 1921. Alfred A. Knopf, publishers, 1921–25; co-founder, Viking Press, 1925–33; WWII, 1942–45; playwright; short stories; radio.
PICTURES INCLUDE: Rendezvous, We Went to College, Libeled Lady, Day at the Races, Married Before Breakfast, Adventures of Don Juan, Anything Can Happen, Tonight We Sing, Decameron Nights.
TV: 30 Topper plays.

OPPENHEIMER, JESS: Producer, director, writer. b. San Francisco, Calif., Nov. 11, 1913. e. Stanford U.; radio, Packard Hour, Fred Astaire, 1937–39; head writer, Screen Guild Program, 1939–40; Writer: Rudy Vallee, John Barrymore Show, 1939–41; head writer, prod., dir., Baby Snooks, 1943–48; writer, prod., dir., Lucille Ball, My Favorite Husband, 1948–51.
TELEVISION: Creator, head writer, prod., I Love Lucy, The Glynis Johns Show. Prod., Get Smart, Gen. Motors 50th Anniversary Program, Danny Kaye Special, Emmy Show. Creator, prod., The Debbie Reynolds Show. Prod., writer: Ford Startime Special, Bob Hope Chrysler Hours (also dir.); creator, prod.-dir., Angel series. Writer, All in the Family.

OPPENHEIMER, PEER J.: Executive e. Georgetown University, UCLA. Founder and pres. of O&O Productions, 1960–64, founder and pres. of HeiRaMatt Productions, 1964. Exec. prod. at CCC Films, Berlin, 1965–66. Pres. of Elite Syncopation, Ltd. London, 1973. Producer of over 22 films including Operation CIA, Lady Hamilton, Kashmir Run, Nashville Girl, Emma Mae, Cassanova and Company. Co-founder and vice-pres. of PRO-International Films, 1975-. West coast editor of Family Weekly since 1954. Member, Writers' Guild of America. Guest lecturer, UCLA.

ORBACH, JERRY: Actor. b. Bronx, NY, Oct. 20, 1935. e. Univ. of Ill., Northwestern Univ. Trained for stage with Herbert Berghof and Lee Strasberg. NY stage debut in Threepenny Opera, 1955.
PICTURES: Please Come Home, The Gang That Couldn't Shoot Straight, A Fan's Notes, Sentinel, Prince of the City, F/X, The Imagemaker.
TELEVISION: Shari Lewis Show, Jack Paar, Bob Hope Presents, Love American Style.

OREAR, RICHARD: Executive. b. Kansas City, MO, June 11, 1911. e. Findlay Engineering Coll. Exhibitor since 1931 in various capacities. 1947, named to board of Commonwelath Theatres; 1955, exec. v.p.; 1959, bd. chmn.

ORKIN, AD: Executive. b. Jackson, Miss., Dec. 7, 1922. e. Univ. of Miss. With Trans World Airlines as flt. eng. 1945–50. Previously co-owner of Orkin Amusements in Jackson. Now owner, Pike Triple Cinema in Troy area. Operates Orkin Badge Co. & Orkin Equipment Co.

ORLEBECK, LESTER: Director, film editor. b. Sheboygan, Wis., June 26, 1907, e. Carroll Coll., Waukesha, Wis. Entered m.p. ind. as lab. tech. with Bennett Laboratories 1925; with Mascot as film ed. 1930. Edited many outdoor & feature pictures including first Gene Autry, Roy Rogers & Don Barry series (Republic). Worked on many Westerns. In 1942 dir. 60 MM Motor, Horsemanship Mounted for U.S. Army. Western films since.

O'ROURKE, JOHN J.: Executive. b. N.Y., N.Y, July 3, 1922. e. City College of New York, 1950. Entered the industry 1939 Music Hall/New York. 20th Century Fox Film Corp. 1941–59, asst. to dir. of exploitation, MGM, 1960–62; asst. exploitation mgr. Astor Pictures 1962–63; exploitation mgr. 1963–67; National dir. of exploitation Avco Embassy Pictures, 1967; national co-ordinator roadshows, United Artists, 1968; asst. roadshow mgr. Universal Pictures. 1969 joined Cinemation Industries as dir. advertising, publicity and exploitation. 1974, v.p., Harry K. McWilliams Assoc. Advertising, 1977, vice pres., Benjamin Philip Associates, Inc., Advertising.

ORR, WILLIAM T.: Executive. b. New York City, Sept. 27, 1917. e. Coburn School, Rumsey Hall, Philips Exeter Academy. Impersonator, Meet the People, revue. Contract, Warner Bros. Joined U.S. Air Force, 1942. Assigned production duties. Air Force's first motion picture unit, 1945. Joined Warner Bros. staff, 1946. Entertained, various night clubs and acting on Broadway stage, New York. Returned to Warner Bros., 1947 as exec. talent dept. and shortly named asst. to Steve Trilling, exec. asst. to Mr. Warner. Chg., studio's TV opers., 1955 as exec. prod. vice-pres., Warner Bros. Pictures, Inc., Nov. 29, 1957–62; vice-pres. in chg. of prod. both features and television, March 1961 to March 1962; vice pres. in chg. of television production, 1962–63; prod., Sex and the Single Girl; asst. to pres., exec. prod., TV div., J. L. Warner, 1963–65; formed Wm. T. Orr Co., 1966, for prods. of M.P.s and TV films.
PICTURES INCLUDE: My Love Came Back, Thieves Fall Out, Navy Blues and Three Sons O'Guns, The Mortal Storm, The Big Street, Unholy Partners, Wicked, Wicked (exec. prod.).

OSBORNE, JOHN: Dramatist. b. London, England, 1929.
AUTHOR: Plays, includ. 1956: Look Back in Anger. 1957: Epitaph for George Dillon. 1958: The Entertainer. 1959: The World of Paul Slickey. 1961: Luther. 1963: Plays for England. 1964: Inadmissible Evidence. Films of his plays include Look Back in Anger, The Entertainer. Film scripts: Tom Jones (Oscar, 1964). Plays: A Patriot for Me, A Bond Honoured, Time Present, The Hotel in Amsterdam, West of Suez, Hedda Gabler (adaptn.).
TV: The Right Prospectus, Very Like A Whale, A Subject of Scandal and Concern.

OSCO, WILLIAM: Producer. b. Akron, OH, Aug. 17, 1948. Pres., General National Enterprises (dist.), since 1967; pres., Bill Osco Productions (films) since 1969; pres., Cybelle Productions (films) since 1979.
PICTURES: Flesh Gordon, Alice in Wonderland, Easter Sunday.

OSGOOD, STANTON M.: Executive. b. Berlin, N.H., e. Dartmouth Coll., B.A. Mgr. Fox Metropolitan Playhouse, Paramount, and worked on short subjects with Fred Waller, 1936–37; market analyst, Young & Rubicam, 1939–41; U.S. Navy, 1942–46; supvr., shorts, RKO Pathe, 1946–48; dir. of TV prod., CBS-TV, 1948–50; NBC, 1950–56, asst. dir., TV oper.; mgr., film prod. & theatre TV: gen. mgr., Paramount Sunset Corp., 1956–58; Ted Bates & Co., adv. agency, 1958–62; bus. mgr., Will Rogers Memorial Hospital, Saranac Lake, N.Y., 1962; special asst. to the president, Pratt Institute, 1969; bond sales prom. rep., U.S. Treasury, Savings Bond Div., 1971.

O'SHEA, MILO: Actor. b. Ireland, 1926. Member of Abbey Players, Dublin, before screen career. On Bdwy. in Staircase, Dear World, The Comedians, A Touch of the Poet, Mass Appeal, etc.
PICTURES: Carry on Cabby, Ulysses, Romeo and Juliet, Barbella, Sacco and Vanzetti, Loot, Arabian Adventure, The Verdict, The Purple Rose of Cairo, etc.
TELEVISION: Two by Forsyth, Ellis Island.

OSMOND, DONNY: Singer/TV Host. b. Ogden, Utah, Dec. 9. 1957. Seventh of 9 children, he was fifth member of family to become professional singer. (Four brothers, Alan, Wayne, Merrill and Jay, are original and present members of Osmond Bros., who originally sang barbershop quartet.) Donny made debut at 4 on Andy Williams Show. Donny has had 12 gold albums. Was co-host of Donny & Marie on TV with sister.

OSMOND, MARIE: Singer/TV Host. b. Ogden, Utah, Oct. 13, 1959. Began career at age of 7 while touring with her brothers. Her first album, Paper Roses, became a gold one. Appeared as co-host with brother Donny on TV's Donny & Marie.

O'SULLIVAN, KEVIN P.: Executive. b. N.Y.C., April 13, 1928. e. Queens College, Flushing, N.Y. Associated with television 33 yrs., initially as a talent; later as businessman. Entered entertainment world after winning first prize in Arthur Godfrey Talent Scouts competition in 1948. 1950—55 professional singer, actor on TV, in theatre, night clubs. 1955–57 on radio-TV promotion staff, Ronson Corp. 1958–61 salesman, Television programs of America. 1961–67 director of program services, Harrington, Righter and Parsons. In 1967 joined ABC Films, domestic sales div. as v.p. & gen. sales mgr. In Jan., 1969 named v.p., gen. mgr., ABC Films, Inc.; in April same yr. named pres. In July 1970 made pres., ABC Int'l. TV, while retaining position as pres., ABC Films. In April, 1973 became pres., chief operating officer, Worldvision Enterprises, Inc., co. formed to succeed ABC Films when FCC stopped networks from TV program dist. Elected chm. & chief exec. officer Worldvision, 1982.

O'SULLIVAN, MAUREEN: Actress. b. Boyle, Eire, May 17, 1911. e. convents in Dublin, London; finishing sch., Paris. On screen numerous pictures, various Hollywood cos. from 191. On many TV shows.
PICTURES INCLUDE: The Big Shot, MGM Tarzan series, Tugboat Annie, The Barretts of Wimpole Street, The Thin Man, David Copperfield, Anna Karenina, Cardinal Richelieu, The Voice of Bugle Ann, A Day at the Races, Big Clock, Bonzo Goes to College, All I Desire, Mission Over Korea,

Duffy of San Quentin, Steel Cage, Never Too Late, Hannah and Her Sisters.
STAGE: The Front Page (1971), No Sex Please, We're British (1973).

OSWALD, GERD: Director. b. Berlin, Germany. Father Richard Oswald, Austrian prod. dir., founder of UFA. Child actor, Vienna 1938; asst. dir., Monogram, Republic, Goldwyn, Paramount; 1949–53, 20th-Fox, prod. mgr., 2nd unit dir., test dir. 1954, 20th-Fox, assoc., prod., Man on a Tightrope, Nightpeople. Prod. Oasis, 1955–58, dir., U.A., A Kiss Before Dying, San Sebastian Film Festival nominee; Brass Legend; Crime of Passion; Fury at Showdown; Valerie; Paris Holiday. 1959–67, dir., Columbia, Screaming Mimi. Prod.-dir., screenplay Germ., prod. The Day the Rains Came; J. Arthur Rank-Allied Artists: Brainwashed, Bombay, & Venice Film Festival nominee; dir., 20th-Fox, The Longest Day (St. Mere-Eglise Seq.). Prod. Dir. Italo-French, Co-prod., The Scarlet Eye; dir., Universal, Agent from H.A.R.M. 1970. Story prod.-dir. Warner Bros. 80 Steps to Jonah, outstanding merit award by motion picture council; 1971 prod.-dir., A.I.P., Bunny O'Hare; 1976, dir. European co-prod.; To The Bitter End.
TV: Ford Theatre, G.E. Hour, Playhouse 90, Perry Mason, Rawhide, Black Saddle, The Virginian, Outer Limits (Soldier episode won HUGO award at world Sci-Fi convention), Fugitive, Blue Light, Felony Squad, Michner's Adventure in Paradise, Star Trek, Shane, Daniel Boone, Gentle Ben, Bonanza, It Takes A Thief, James Garner's Nichols.

O'TOOLE, ANNETTE: Actress. b. Houston, TX, 1953. e. UCLA.
PICTURES: King of the Gypsies, Foolin' Around, Cat People, 48 HRS, Superman III.
TELEVISION: Copacabana.

O'TOOLE, PETER: Actor. b. Ireland, Aug. 2, 1932. Studied at R.A.D.A. Early career with Bristol Old Vic. London Stage in The Long, the Short and the Tall. 1960, with the Stratford-on-Avon Company. Ent. films 1959 in Kidnapped. Partner with Jules Buck, Keep Films, Ltd.
PICTURES INCLUDE: The Savage Innocents, The Day They Robbed the Bank of England, Lawrence of Arabia, Becket, Lord Jim, What's New Pussycat, How to Steal a Million, The Night of the Generals, The Bible, Great Catherine, The Lion in Winter, Goodbye Mr. Chips, Brotherly Love, Murphy's War, Under Milk Wood, The Ruling Class, Man of La Mancha, Rosebud, Man Friday, Foxtrot, Caligula, The Stunt Man, My Favorite Year, Supergirl, Creator, Club Paradise.
TELEVISION: Masada (mini-series), Kim (movie).

O'TOOLE, STANLEY: Producer. Earliest experience with production costs; worked on Cleopatra, Singer, Not the Song, No Love for Johnny, Victim, etc. In 1966 named chief cost acct. for Paramount in U.K.; 1967, promoted to prod. exec. Worked on Downhill Racer, Running Scared, etc. Produced The Last of Sheila in 1972 for W.B.; 1974–75 was in Prague working on Operation Daybreak. Produced The Seven-Per-Cent Solution for Universal. Formed own Martinat Co. and produced for WB The Squeeze. Recent credits: The Boys from Brazil, Nijinsky, Outland, Enemy Mine.

OTWELL, RONNIE RAY: Theatre Executive. b. Carrollton, Ga., Aug. 13, 1929. e. Ga. Inst. Tech. Entered industry as mgr., Bremen Theatre (Ga.), 1950; dir. pub., adv., Martin Theatres, Columbus (Ga.), 1950–63; v.p., dir. Martin Theatres of Ga., Inc., 1963, Martin Theatres of Ala., Inc., 1963; dir. Martin Theatres of Columbus, 1963; sr. v.p., Martin Theatres Companies, 1971. Member: NATO, Ga., NATO, Columbus C of C; Columbus Mus. Arts & Crafts; Assn. U.S. Army.

OWEN, ALUN: Writer. b. Liverpool, Eng., 1925.
STAGE: A Little Winter Love, Maggie May, Progress to the Park, The Rough and Ready Lot, There'll Be Some Changes Made, Norma (Mixed Doubles), Shelter, Fashion of Your Time, The Ladies, Lucia.
TV: The Ruffian, Not Trams to Lime Street, After the Funeral, Lena O My Lena (for ITV's Armchair Theatre); The Rose Affair (two awards, 1961), Ways of Love, You Can't Win 'Em All, A Hard Knock, Dare to be a Daniel, The Stag, The Strain, A Local Boy, Ruth, Funny, Pal, Giants and Ogres, The Piano Player, The Web Flight, Buttons, Lucky, Left. Ronnie Barker and Forget-me-not series, Lady of the Lake, The Look, Passing Through, The Runner, Sea Link, Kisch-Kisch, Colleagues, Francis.
PICTURES INCLUDE: The Criminal, A Hard Day's Night, Minding the Shop, Park People, You'll Be the Death of Me, McNeil, Cornelius, Emlyn.

OWEN, BILL: Actor. b. Acton, Eng., Mar. 14, 1915. Screen debut in Way to the Stars. Numerous TV appearances.
PICTURES INCLUDE: School for Secrets, Daybreak, Dancing With Crime, Easy Money, When the Bough Breaks, My Brother's Keeper, Martha, Parlor Trick, The Roundabout, Trottie True, Once a Jolly Swagman, A Day to Remember, You See What I Mean, Square Ring, Rainbow Jacket, Ship That Died of Shame, Not so Dusty, Davy, Carve her Name with Pride, Carry on Sergeant, Carry on Nurse, Night Apart, Shakedown, Hell Fire Club, Carry on Regardless, Carry on Cabby!, Secret of Blood Island, Georgy Girl, Headline Hunters, O Lucky Man!, Kadoyng, In Celebration, When The Screaming Stopped, Comeback, Laughter House.

OWENS, GARY: Performer, broadcaster. b. Mitchell, S.D., May 10, 1936; e. Wesleyan U. Disc Jockey, KMPC, Hollywood; winner of Gavin Poll, 1966–69; named TV Radio Mirror top D.J. of year, 1970; named top D.J. in U.S. by Billboard, 1971–72; among top three TV announcers in U.S. in 'FAME' poll for three years; regular performer, "Rowan & Martin"s Laugh-In" since inception in 1968.

OWENSBY, EARL: Producer-Actor. b. North Carolina, 1936. Set up his own studio in Shelbyville, NC.
PICTURES: Challenge, Dark Sunday, Buckstone County Prison, Frank Challenge—Manhunter, Death Driver, Wolfman, Seabo, Day of Judgment, Living Legend, Lady Grey.

OXBERRY, JOHN: b. New Rochelle, N.Y., March 17, 1918. Executive. Asst. photog. to Margaret Bourke-White, 1931–32; assoc. A.P. Lane Film Studio, 1932–38; assoc., R. J. Irwin, prod. photog., 1938–41; U.S. Army Signal Corps., 1941–45; cameraman, Tech Film Studio, N.Y., 1945–46; head, camera dept. Mini Toons Inc., 1946–47; pres. Animation Equipment Co., 1947–61; pres., Oxberry Corp., 1962–69; pres. Ox Products, 1971.

P

PAAR, JACK: Actor. b. Canton, O., May 1, 1918; radio announcer in Cleveland & Buffalo; served in U.S. Armed Forces World War II; entertained in Pacific zone with 28th Special Service Div. On radio with own show; m.p. debut in Variety Time, 1948. CBS-TV; Jack Paar Show, NBC-TV.
PICTURES INCLUDE: Walk Softly Stranger, Footlight Varieties, Love Nest, Down Among the Sheltering Palms.

PACINO, AL: Actor. b. New York City, Apr. 25, 1940. Gained attention as stage actor.
STAGE: The Indian Wants the Bronx, (Obie award), Does a Tiger Wear A Necktie? (Tony Award), The Connection, Hello Out There, Tiger at the Gates, The Basic Training of Pablo Hummel (Tony Award).
PICTURES INCLUDE: Panic in Needle Park (debut), The Godfather, Scarecrow, Serpico, The Godfather II, Dog Day Afternoon, Bobby Deerfield, And Justice for All, Cruising, Author! Author!, Scarface, Revolution.

PACKARD, FRED M.: Producer. b. Los Angeles, Calif., March 14, 1919; e. Los Angeles City Coll.; m. Shelagh Mary Rank, d. of J. Arthur Rank, c. Susan & Fred Arthur Rank. Radio commentator, sports and news; personal mgr. Joe Reichman and orch.; adv. pub. rep. Bing Crosby; officer in chge. film ed. dept. & prod. Army films, U.S. Army Pictorial Service in England, France, 1935–41; actor (bit, feat. roles) including East Side of Heaven; film ed. dept. RKO studio; Universal in various dept.; pres. Fred M. Packard Prod., thereafter and since, to Columbia as prod.

PAGE, ANTHONY: Director. b. Bangalore, India, Sept. 21, 1935. e. Oxford. Stage work includes Inadmissible Evidence, Waiting for Godot, A Patriot for Me, Look Back in Anger, Uncle Vanya, Cowardice, etc.
PICTURES: Inadmissible Evidence, Alpha Beta, I Never Promised You a Rose Garden, Absolution, The Lady Vanishes.
TELEVISION: Pueblo, The Missiles of October, The Parachute, FDR—The Last Year, The Patricia Neal Story, Bill, Johnny Belinda, Grace Kelly, Bill—On His Own, Forbidden, etc.

PAGE, GALE: Actress. r.n. Sally Rutter. b. Spokane, Wash., 1918.
PICTURES INCLUDE: Crime School, The Amazing Dr. Clitterhouse, Four Daughters, Heart of the North, You Can't Get Away With Murder, Daughters Courageous, Naughty But Nice, Indianapolis Speedway, Four Wives, A Child is Born, They Drive by Night, Knute Rockne—All American, Four Mothers, Time of Your Life, Anna Lucasta, About Mrs. Leslie.

PAGE, GERALDINE: Actress. b. Missouri, Nov. 22, 1924. m. Rip Torn. After summer stock & off-broadway roles, to Broadway and m.p. Theatre awards include Drama Critics' Circle (2).
STAGE: Summer and Smoke, (revival), Mid-Summer, The Immoralist, The Rainmaker, Separate Tables, Sweet Bird of Youth, Strange Interlude, The Three Sisters, Angela,

Black Comedy, Absurd Person Singular, Clothes for a Summer Hotel, Mixed Couples, Agnes of God. 1984: Mirror Theatre Repertory: Paradise Lost, Inheritors, Rain, Ghosts, Madwoman of Chaillot, Clarence, Vivat Vivat Regina, The Circle.
PICTURES INCLUDE: Hondo, Summer and Smoke, Sweet Bird of Youth, Toys in the Attic, Dear Heart, The Happiest Millionaire, You're a Big Boy Now, Trilogy, Whatever Happened to Aunt Alice, Beguiled, J.W. Coop, Pete 'n' Tillie, The Day of the Locust, Nasty Habits, Interiors, Honky Tonk Freeway, I'm Dancing as Fast as I Can, The Pope of Greenwich Village, The Bride, Flanagan, White Nights, A Trip to Bountiful (Oscar).
TV: The Old Man, Christmas Memory, The Thanksgiving Visitor (Emmy Awards), Barefoot in Athens, The Name of the Game, Look Homeward, Angel, Something for Joey, The Blue and the Gray, The Dollmaker.

PAGE, PATTI: Performer. r.n. Clara Ann Fowler. b. Claremore, Okla. 1927. e. Univ. of Tulsa. Staff performer, radio stat. KTUL, Tulsa; m. Charles O'Curran. Appeared on CBS radio show; star Patti Page Show, TV film series, The Big Record; author, Once Upon a Dream.
PICTURES INCLUDE: Elmer Gantry, Dondi, Boys Night Out.

PAGET, DEBRA: Actress. r.n. Debralee Griffin. b. Denver, Colo., Aug. 19, 1933, e. drama & dancing privately. Stage debut in Marry Wives of Windsor, 1946; in Jeanne D'Arc little theatre prod.; m.p.; debut in Cry of the City, 1948.
PICTURES INCLUDE: House of Strangers, Broken Arrow, Fourteen Hours, Bird of Paradise, Anne of the Indies, Belles on Their Toes, Les Miserables, Stars & Stripes Forever, Prince Valiant, Demetrius & the Gladiators, Princess of the Nile, Gambler from Natchez, White Feather, Seven Angry Men, Last Hunt, Ten Commandments, Tales of Terror, The Haunted Palace.

PAIGE, BOB: Performer. r.n. John Arthur Page. b. Indianapolis, Ind., Dec. 2; e. UCLA. Singer, amateur theatricals, usher Fox West Coast theatres; singer, KGER, Long Beach, Cal., announcer; program dir., KMTR, Hollywood; played films Columbia, Paramount, Universal; 30 films.
TV: Fireside Theatre, Pepsi-Cola Playhouse, Lux Theatre, Studio One, Kraft; 1957, host on Bride and Groom; 1958 co-star Bess Myerson, Big Payoff.

PAIGE, JANIS: Actress (Star of Tomorrow, 1947). r.n. Donna Mae Jaden. b. Tacoma, Wash., Sept. 16, 1923. Sang with Tacoma Opera Co. m.p. debut, 1944, Hollywood Canteen, NY. stage in 1951, and TV in 1956.
STAGE: Two Gals and a Guy, Fugitive Lady, Pajama Game, It's Always Jan.
PICTURES INCLUDE: Of Human Bondage, The Time the Place and the Girl, Two Guys from Milwaukee, Her Kind of Man, Cheyenne, Love and Learn, Wallflower, Winter Meeting, One Sunday Afternoon, Romance on High Seas, House Across the Street, Younger Brothers, Mr. Universe, Remains to be Seen, Please Don't Eat the Daisies, The Caretakers, Welcome to Hard Times.

PAINE, CHARLES F.: Executive. b. Cushing, Texas, Dec. 23, 1920. e. Stephen F. Austin University, pres. Tercar Theatre Company; pres., NATO of Texas, 1972–73. NATO board member, 1973 to present; Motion Picture Pioneers member; Variety Club of Texas member.

PAKULA, ALAN J.: Producer-director. b. New York, N.Y., April 7, 1928. e. Yale Univ. (BA, 1948). Prod. apprentice, MGM, 1950; prod. asst., Para. 1951; prod. Para., 1955. Own prod. co., Pakula-Mulligan Prod. Stage prod. and m.p. dir. prod.
STAGE: Comes a Day, Laurette, There Must Be a Pony.
PICTURES INCLUDE: Fear Strikes Out, To Kill a Mockingbird, Love with the Proper Stranger, Baby the Rain Must Fall, Inside Daisy Clover, Up the Down Staircase, The Stalking Moon, The Sterile Cuckoo, Klute, Love and Pain and the Whole Damned Thing, The Parallax View, All the President's Men, Comes a Horseman, Starting Over (co.-prod., dir.). Roll-over (dir.); Sophie's Choice (s.p., dir., prod.); Dream Lover (co-prod.-dir.).
AWARDS: N.Y. Film Critics for best director, All the President's Men (1976); London Film Critics for best director, Klute (1971).

PALANCE, JACK: Actor. b. Lattimer, Pa., Feb. 18, 1920. e. U. of N. Car. Professional fighter; U.S. Air Corps. Broadway stage and m.p.
STAGE: The Big Two, Temporary Island, The Vigil, Streetcar Named Desire, Darkness at Head.
PICTURES INCLUDE: Flight to Tangier, Man in the Attic, Sign of the Pagan, Silver Chalice, Kiss of Fire, Big Knife, I Died a Thousand Times, Attack!, Lonely Man, House of Numbers, Ten Seconds to Hell, Warriors Five, Barabbas, Contempt, Torture Garden, Kill a Dragon, They Came to Rob Las Vegas, The Desperadoes, Che, The Mercenary, Justine, Legion of the Damned, A Bullet for Rommel, The McMasters, Monte Walsh, Companeros, The Horsemen, The Professionals, Oklahoma Crude, Craze, The Four Deuces, The Diamond Mercenaries, Hawk the Slayer.
TV: Dr. Jekyll and Mr. Hyde, Dracula, Bronk (series), Ripley's Believe It or Not.

PALEY, WILLIAM S.: Executive. b. Chicago, Sept. 28, 1901. e. U. of Penn. Took over operation Columbia Broadcasting System (now CBS, Inc.) as pres. 1928; chairman of the board from January, 1946 to April 1983, when named founder-chm.; built network to leading position and est. innovations in broadcasting. During war on leave to supervise OWI radio in Mediterranean area. Chief of radio of Psychological Warfare Division, SHAEF, 1944–45; Dep. Chief Info. Control Div. of U.S.G.C.C. 1945; Colonel, A.U.S. Deputy Chief Psychological Warfare Division, SHAEF, 1945; pres. & dir., William S. Paley Foundation, Inc.; partner, Whitcom Investment Co.; co-chm., Intl. Herald Tribune; pres. & dir., Greenpark Foundation, Inc. Founder and Chairman of The Board of Trustees of The Museum of Broadcasting; trustee, Emeritus Columbia University; trustee and chairman, emeritus, Museum of Modern Art. Trustee North Shore University Hospital 1949–73, Co-Chairman of the Board, 1954–73. Decorations include the Legion of Merit, Medal for Merit. Legion of Honor, Croix de Guerre with Palm. Chairman of President's Materials Policy Comm., 1951–52, which issued report, "Resources for Freedom."

PALIN, MICHAEL: Actor-Writer. b. Sheffield, Yorkshire, England, May 5, 1943. e. Oxford. Member of Monty Python Flying Circus. On stage with troupe both in London and on Bdwy.
PICTURES: And Now for Something Completely Different, Monty Python and the Holy Grail, Jabberwocky, Life of Brian, Time Bandits, The Missionary (also prod.), Monty Python's The Meaning of Life (also music), A Private Function, Brazil.
TELEVISION: Do Not Adjust Your Set, The Frost Report, Marty Feldman Comedy Machine, How To Irritate People, Pythons in Deutschland, Secrets, Ripping Yarns, etc.

PALLOS, STEVEN: Producer. b. Budapest, Hungary, Journalist before entering m.p. ind. Began prod. & dist. in France & Continental Europe. Entered partnership with Sir Alexander Korda in 1929; later formed with him London Film Prod. From 1943–46 Brit. Army, head Psychological Warfare Br., Film Div., Italy; dir. Pendennis Pictures Corp., Ltd., Gibraltar Prods., Ltd., Britannia Film Distributors, Ltd.
RECENT PICTURES INCLUDE: Where the Spies Are, Captain Nemo & The Underwater City, Catch Me a Spy, The Glorious Musketeers.

PALMER, BETSY: Actress. b. East Chicago, Ind., Nov. 1, 1929. e. Indiana Univ., De Pauw Univ. On stage in The Grand Prize, Affair of Honor, Cactus Flower, etc.
PICTURES: The Long Gray Line, The Tin Star, The Last Angry Man, Mister Roberts, Friday the 13th, Friday the 13th, Part II.
TELEVISION: Studio One, U.S. Steel Hour, Kraft Theatre, etc.

PALMER, GREGG: Actor. r.n. Palmer Lee. b. San Francisco, Calif., Jan. 25, 1927; e. U. of Utah. U.S. Air Force, 1945–46; radio announcer, disc jockey; then to Hollywood; many TV appearances.
PICTURES INCLUDE: Cimarron Kid, Battle at Apache Pass, Son of Ali Baba, Red Ball Express, Francis Goes to West Point, Sally and St. Anne, The Raiders, Back at the Front, Redhead From Wyoming, Column South, Veils of Bagdad, Golden Blade, The All American, Taza Son of Cochise, Magnificent Obsession, Playgirl, To Hell and Back, Creature Walks Among Us, Hilda Crane, Zombies of Mora Tau, Revolt of Fort Laramie, Rebel Set, Thundering Jets, Forty Pounds of Trouble, Night Hunt, The Undefeated, Chisum, Rio Lobo, Big Jake, Providenza (Italy), Ci Risiamo Vero Providenza (Italy & Spain). The Shootist, The Man with Bogart's Face.
TV: Movie of the week: Go West Young Girl, Hostage Heart, True Grit, The Blue and the Gray (mini-series).

PAM, JERRY: Publicist. b. London, England, Oct. 17, 1926. e. Cambridge, London Univ. Reporter, Paris & London; freelance writing, Australia; 1950–53. To U.S. in 1953, on Hollywood Reporter, drama ed. Beverly Hills Citizen, 1953–54; publicist, Moulin Rouge, MGM studios; drama ed., Valley Times 1959–61; partner, Pam and Joseph pub. rel. counsellors; est. Jerry Pam & Associates, pub. rel., April 1965; formed Guttman & Pam, Ltd., 1971. Exec. prod., Highpoint, 1979. Prod., On the Film Scene (weekly series on Z Channel).

PAMPANINI, SILVANA: Actress. b. Rome, Italy, Sept. 25, 1925. e. Academy of St. Cecilia. Studied singing, several concert appearances. Elected Miss Italia of 1946–47; m.p. debut in Secret of Don Giovanni.
PICTURES INCLUDE: Second Ark, Twin Trouble, O.K. Nero, City Stands Trial, A Husband for Anna, Songs of Half a Century, Songs Songs Songs, Matrimony, Enchanting Enemy, A Day in District Court, Loves of Half a Century, Slave of Sin, Orient Express, Merry Squadron, Princess

of the Canary Islands, Mademoiselle Gobette, Don Juan's Night of Love, Roman Tales.

PAN, HERMES: Dance director. b. 1905. In 1935, handled Roberta, RKO stage ensembles. In 1938 won Academy honors for dance direction Damsel in Distress.
PICTURES INCLUDE: Top Hat, Old Man Rhythm, In Person, I Dream Too Much, Follow the Fleet, Swing Time, Shall We Dance, Radio City Revels, Let's Dance, Three Little Words, Excuse My Dust, Texas Carnival, Lovely to Look At, Sombrero, Kiss Me Kate, Student Prince, Hit the Deck, Jupiter's Darling, Meet Me in Las Vegas, Porgy and Bess, Can-Can, Flower Drum Song, Cleopatra, My Fair Lady, Finian's Rainbow, Darling Lilli, The Lost Horizon.
TV: An Evening with Fred Astaire (Emmy Award, choreography), Astaire Time, Sounds of America, Star-times Academy Awards of Songs, Remember How Great, Frances Langford Show.

PANAMA, CHARLES A. (CHUCK): Publicist, b. Chicago, Ill., Feb. 2, 1925. e. Northwestern U., Beloit College, UCLA. Publicist, Los Angeles Jr. Chamber of Commerce; staff So. Calif. sports ed., Los Angeles bureau, INS; pub. 20th Century-Fox Studios; adv. pub. dir., Arcola Pics.; opened L.A. office, John Springer Associates. Assoc. with Jerry Pam & Assoc. Account exec. Rogers, Cowan & Brenner, Inc.; dir. m.p. div., Jim Mahoney & Assoc. v.p. Guttman & Pam, Ltd.; ast. pub. dir., 20th-Fox TV.

PANAMA, NORMAN: Writer, prod., dir. b. Chicago, Ill., April 21. Screen career: wrote, co-prod. & dir., with Melvin Frank, Li'l Abner, Facts of Life, The Road to Hong Kong, Mr. Blandings Builds His Dream House.
PICTURES INCLUDE: My Favorite Blonde, Happy Go Lucky, Star-Spangled Rhythm, Thank Your Lucky Stars, And the Angels Sing, Road to Utopia, Duffy's Tavern, Our Hearts Were Growing Up, Monsieur Beaucaire, It Had to Be You, Return of October, The Reformer and the Redhead, Strictly Dishonorable, Callaway Went Thataway, Above and Beyond, Knock on Wood, White Christmas, Court Jester, Not With My Wife You Don't, How to Commit Marriage, Coffee, Tea, or Me. Wrote and directed: I Will, I Will . . . For Now. Directed, Barnaby and Me; Wrote Fade In—Fade out, The Stewardesses, Li'l Abner, for NBC-TV. Recent works: Co-authored The Glass Bed (novel), and two plays: A Talent for Murder & The Bats of Portobello. 1983: Mrs. Katz and Katz (TV pilot); 1984: Judgment Day (s.p.). 1985: 3 s.p.'s: Cheek to Cheek, The Marathon, Too Much Johnson. 1986: Checkmate!, Donovan.

PANTAGES, CLAYTON G.: Executive. b. Hartford, March 6, 1927. e. Trinity Coll. Served various executive posts for 11 years with 20th Century-Fox; gen. sales mgr. Magna Pictures; Pres., International Coproductions, Inc., S.P. Films, Pantheon Entertainment Ltd., Clayton's Classics.

PAPAS, IRENE: Actress. b. near Corinth, Greece, 1926. Entered dramatic school at 12. At 16 sang and danced in variety shows. Film debut in 1951 Greek film, Lost Angels; 1958 Greek Popular theatre in Athens.
STAGE: The Idiot, Journey's End, The Merchant of Venice, Inherit the Wind, That Summer, That Fall, Iphigenia in Aulis.
PICTURES INCLUDE: Dead City, The Unfaithful, Atilla the Hun, Theodora, Whirlpool, Tribute to a Bad Man, The Guns of Navarone, Antigone (Best Actress Award, Salonika Film Festival), Electra (Best Actress Award, Salonika Film Festival), Zorba the Greek, The Brotherhood, Anne of a Thousand Days, Z, A Dream of Kings, A Ciascuno il Suo, The Odyssey, The Trojan Women, Moses, Mohammed, Messenger of God, Lion of the Desert, Into the Night, The Assisi Underground, Sweet Country.

PARE, MICHAEL: Actor. b. Brooklyn, NY, 1959. Debut as singer-actor in Eddie and the Cruisers (1983). Also in The Philadelphia Experiment and Streets of Fire.

PARIS, JERRY: Producer-Director-Actor. b. San Francisco, CA, July 25, 1925. e. NYC, UCLA. On stage as actor before film acting, production and direction.
PICTURES: Actor: Marty, The Wild One, The Caine Mutiny, The Naked and the Dead, Cyrano De Bergerac, etc. Director: The Grasshopper, Viva Max, How Sweet It Is, Don't Raise the Bridge, Star-Spangled Girl, Police Academy 2—Their First Assignment, Police Academy 3—Back in Training.
TELEVISION: Director: That Girl, The Dick Van Dyke Show, Odd Couple, Happy Days, etc.

PARK, ROBERT H.: Executive. b. Atlanta, Georgia, May 11, 1916. e. University of Texas; Attorney for Jefferson Amusement Co.; now bd. chm., Tercar Theatre Company.

PARKER, ALAN: Director-Writer. b. Islington, London, Feb. 14, 1944. Worked way up in advertising industry from mail room to top writer and director of TV commercials. First feature film was Bugsy Malone (1976), which he both wrote and directed.
PICTURES: Midnight Express, Fame, Shoot the Moon, Pink Floyd—The Wall, Birdy, Angel Heart.
TELEVISION: The Evacuees.

PARKER, BENJAMIN R.: Producer-director. b. New Haven, Conn., Sept. 16, 1909. e. U.C.L.A., Los Angeles and Yale Drama Sch. In m.p. indust. 1939, indep. prod. George Washington Carver. During WW II, dir. 23 training films for Army Air Corps; transferred Signal Corps, Photographic Center, Astoria, L.I., made 39 one-reel musical subjects; many shorts as prod., dir., for General Film prod. Co.

PARKER, ELEANOR: Actress. B. Cedarville, Ohio, June 26, 1922. In Cleveland play group; in summer stock Martha's Vineyard; at Pasadena Community Playhouse.
PICTURES INCLUDE: They Died With Their Boots On, Buses Roar, Mission to Moscow, Between Two Worlds, Very Thought of You, Crime By Night, Last Ride, Never Say Goodbye, Pride of the Marines, Of Human Bondage, Escape Me Never, Woman in White, Voice of the Turtle, Chain Lightning, Caged, Three Secrets, Valentino, Millionaire for Christy, Detective Story, Scaramouche, Above and Beyond, Escape from Fort Bravo, Naked Jungle, Valley of the Kings, Many Rivers to Cross, Interrupted Melody, Man with the Golden Arm, King and Four Queens, Lizzie, Seventh Sin, Home from the Hill, Return to Peyton Place, Madison Avenue, The Oscar, An American Dream, Warning Shot, The Eye of the Cat, The Sound of Music, Sunburn.
TV: Bracken's World, Vanished.

PARKER, FESS: Actor. b. Fort Worth, Tex., Aug. 16, 1925 of Tex., U. of So. Calif. US Navy, 1943–46; national co., Mr. Roberts, 1951; m.p. debut, Untamed Frontier, 1952.
PICTURES INCLUDE: No Room for the Groom, Springfield Rifle, Thunder Over the Plains, Island in the Sky, Kid from Left Field, Take Me to Town, Them, Battle Cry, Davy Crockett, King of the Wild Frontier, Davy Crockett and the River Pirates, Great Locomotive Chase, Westward Ho the Wagons, Old Yeller, The Light in the Forest, The Hangman, The Jayhawkers, Hell Is For Heroes, Smoky.
TV: Mr. Smith Goes to Washington series, Daniel Boone series, Jonathan Winters, Walt Disney presents, Ed Sullivan, Phyllis Diller, Joey Bishop, Dean Martin, Red Skelton, Glen Campbell.

PARKER, JAMESON: Actor. b. Baltimore, Md. e. Beloit College. Professional stage debut in Washington Theatre Club production, Caligula. Acted with Arena Stage in D.C.; worked in dinner theatres and summer stock. Moved to N.Y., working in TV commercials and touring in play, Equus. Feature film debut in The Bell Jar (1979).
PICTURES: A Small Circle of Friends, White Dog.
TELEVISION: Series: Somerset, One Life to Live, Simon and Simon. Movies: Women at West Point, Anatomy of a Seduction, A Caribbean Mystery.

PARKER, SUZY: Actress. r.n. Cecelia Parker. b. San Antonio, Tex. Oct. 28, 1933. e. Schools in N.Y. & Florida. Began career at 17 as fashion model; became known as highest paid fashion model and cover girl in U.S.: to Paris under contract to fashion magazine; m.p. debut as model in Funny Face; signed by 20th-Fox prod. chief Buddy Adler for part opposite Cary Grant in Kiss Them for Me.
PICTURES INCLUDE: Ten North Frederick, The Best of Everything, Circle of Deception, The Interns.

PARKER, WILLARD: Actor. r.n. Worster Van Eps. b. New York City, Feb. 5, 1912. Meter reader; tennis pro; on stage in Johnny Belinda, screen debut in Slight Case of Murder, 1938; in Westerns.
PICTURES INCLUDE: What a Woman, Fighting Guardsman, One Way to Love, Relentless, Wreck of the Hesperus, You Gotta Stay Happy, Calamity Jane and Sam Bass, Bandit Queen, Emergency Wedding, Hunt the Man Down, Caribbean, The Vanquished, Sangaree, Kiss Me Kate, Great Jesse James Raid, The Earth Dies Screaming, Waco, The Great Waltz.

PARKINS, BARBARA: Actress. b. Vancouver, Canada, May 22, 1943.
PICTURES: Valley of the Dolls, Bear Island, The Kremlin Letter, Pupper on a Chain, The Mephisto Waltz, Bear Island.
TELEVISION: Peyton Place (series). Movies: A Taste of Evil, Snatched, Law of the Land, Captains and the Kings, Young Joe, The Forgotten Kennedy, testimony of Two Men, Ziegfield: The Man and His Women, The Critical List, To Catch a King, Calendar Girl Murders, Peyton Place: The Next Generation.

PARKS, BERT: Announcer, m.c. b. Atlanta, Ga, Dec. 30, 1914. Announcer, then chief announcer in Atlanta radio station; announcer, network, N.Y., for Eddie Cantor; m.c. for Xavier Cugat's show; U.S. Army, WWII; radio shows include Break the Bank, Stop the Music, Double or Nothing.
TV: Break the Bank, Stop the Music.

PARKS, GORDON: Director, writer, photographer, composer. Photo-journalist.

AUTHOR: The Learning Tree; A Choice of Weapons; A Poet and His Camera; Whispers of Intimate Things; In Love; Born Black, Moments Without Proper Names, Flavio, To Smile in Autumn, Shannon.
PICTURES INCLUDE: The Learning Tree, Shaft, Shaft's Big Score, Super Cops, Leadbelly.

PARKS, MICHAEL: Actor. b. 1938. Made m.p. debut in Wild Seed, 1964.
PICTURES INCLUDE: Bus Riley's Back in Town, The Bible, The Idol, The Happening, The Last Hard Men, Sidewinder One. ffolkes, Hard Country, Savannah Smiles, King of the City.
TV: Along Came Bronson (series), numerous TV movies: Can Ellen Be Saved?, Savage Bees, Chase.

PARKS, RICHARD: Executive. e. Duke University; University of North Carolina (M.A. in theatre arts). Taught theatre arts at Duke. Associated with Curtis Brown, Ltd., literary agency, for 8 years, specializing in m.p. rights for literary materials and representing authors. Joined United Artists in December, 1978, as exec. asst. to Steven Bach, then snr. v.p. for east coast production. In 1980 promoted to v.p.—production.

PARRISH, ROBERT R.: Director, producer. b. Columbus, Georgia, Jan. 4; actor before joining RKO in 1933, first as assistant director, then film editor. With various companies since, including 20th Century-Fox, Universal, Columbia, United Artists, J. Arthur Rank, etc. Won Academy Award, best film editing, Body and Soul, 1947. U.S. Navy 1941–45; won documentary Academy Award, 1942 and 1943 for Battle of Midway and December 7th. Formed own independent production company, Trimark Productions, Inc., 1955.
PICTURES INCLUDE: City Lights, All Quiet on the Western Front, The Divine Lady, A Double Life, Caught, No Minor Vices, All the King's Men, Cry Danger (dir.), The Mob, San Francisco Story, Assignment–Paris, My Pal Gus, Shoot First, The Purple Plain, Lucy Gallant, Fire Down Below, Saddle the Wind, The Wonderful Country, In the French Style, Up From the Beach, Casino Royale, The Bobo, Duffy, A Town Called Bastard, Flashman.

PARRY, GORDON: Director, producer. b. Aintree, Liverpool, Eng., July 24, 1908; p. Studied electrical eng. before entering m.p. ind. as actor in 1929. Joined Gaumont-British in 1931 as assist. dir. and remained for four years, then prod. mgr. Rock Studios. Returned to GB as assist. to Walter Forde on King of the Damned. Left GB to become prod. mgr. for Soskin Prod. Ltd. and Amalgamated Studios; prod. television in conjunction with E.M.I. Author radio plays and short stories. Unit mgr. Ealing Studios propaganda shorts department. In 1942 under contract to Two Cities Films, 2nd unit.
PICTURES INCLUDE: In Which We Serve, The Demi-Paradise, English Without Tears, The Way to the Stars, Beau Brummell, Bond Street, Third Time Lucky, Now Barabbas, Three Men and a Girl, Midnight Episode, Tom Brown's Schooldays, Night Was Our Friend, Women of Twilight, Innocents of Paris, Front Page Story, Fast and Loose, Yank in Ermine, Sailor Beware, Touch of the Sun, Surgeon's Knife, Tread Softly Stranger, Friends and Neighbors, The Navy Lark.
TV: Robin Hood.

PARSONS, ESTELLE: Actress. b. Marblehead, Mass., Jan. 20, 1927. e. Connecticut College for Women, Bachelor's Degree in Political Science. Attended Boston U. Law School. Helped harvest crops in England with the Women's Land Army. Was active in politics; worked for the Committee for the Nation's Health in Wash. and the Republican Finance Committee in Boston. Was elected to public office in Marblehead, Mass. Joined NBC-TV's Today Show as prod. asst.; then writer, feature producer and commentator. Appeared in two Julius Monk revues, Jerry Herman's Nightcap and the Three-Penny Opera. Dramatic stage debut, Mrs. Dally Has A Lover (won Theatre World Award). Has appeared with the Lincoln Center Repertory Theatre, Mahagonny. Acad. Award, Best Supporting Actress for Bonnie and Clyde.
STAGE: Next Time I'll Sing to You (Obie Award), In the Summer House (Obie Award), Ready When You Are, C.B. Malcolm, The Seven Descents of Myrtle, and Miss Reardon Drinks a Little, The Norman Conquests, Ladies of the Alamo, Miss Margarida's Way, Pirates of Penzance.
PICTURES INCLUDE: Rachel, Rachel, Don't Drink the Water, Strangers, Watermelon Man, I Never Sang For My Father, I Walk the Line, Two People, For Pete's Sake.

PARSONS, LINDSLEY: Executive Vice Pres., Film Finances, Inc. Pres., Completion Service Co., Hollywood. Toronto. b. Tacoma, Wash., Sept. 12. e. U. Calif. (L.A.) On ed. staff City News Service, L.A.: Alhambra Post-Advocate; Calexico Chronicle; Santa Rosa Press Democrat; Humboldt Times; San Marino News (ed. & pub.). Joined Monogram 1931 as pub. dir. in 1933 author s.p. Sagebrush Trails; then wrote orig. s.p. Westerns for Monogram, Republic, Grand Nat'l. In 1939 assoc. prod. Tough Kid; from 1940 prod. numerous westerns; prod. Wayne Morris & James Oliver Curwood series for Allied Artists; prod. Motion Pictures Int'l, 1956–72. Exec. v.p., dir., Film Finances, Inc.
PICTURES INCLUDE: Rocky Rhythm Inn, Casa Manana, Big Timber, Call of the Klondike, Sierra Passage, Yukon, Manhunt, Yellow Fin, Northwest Territory, Desert Pursuit, Torpedo Alley, Jack Slade, Loophole, Cry Vengeance, Finger Man, Return of Jack Slade, Come On, The Intruder, Cruel Tower, Dragon Wells Massacre, Portland Expose, Oregon Passage, Wolf Larsen, Crash Boat, The Purple Gang, Mara of the Wilderness, Good Times, The Big Cube, Bravo Hennessey, Coasts of War.
TV: Gray Ghost TV series.

PARTON, DOLLY: Singer-Composer-Actress. b. Sevierville, TN, Jan. 19, 1946. Gained fame as country music singer, composer and radio and TV personality. Many awards for recordings.
PICTURES: Nine to Five, The Best Little Whorehouse in Texas, Rhinestone.
TELEVISION: Porter Wagoner Show, Cass Walker program, Bill Anderson Show, Wilbur Bros. Show.

PARTRIDGE, DEREK: TV magazine/talk show host, interviewer, newscaster, actor. b. London. Ent. industry 1959 as documentary script writer/assistant director with Film Producers' Guild. 1961–70: Acting in BBC/ITV plays/series. Films: The High Bright Sun, King and Country, Thunderball, Where The Spies Are. Hollywood: TV: Star Trek. Film: The Killing of Sister George. 1976–78: Rhodesian TV: Chief newscaster, host live magazine programme Frankly Partridge, quizmaster The Kwhizz Kids. 1979: Miami: host two daily talk shows and newscaster WKAT/ABC. Films: 1979: The Ivory Ape, 1980: Savage Harvest. 1981–82: TV (Los Angeles): Newscaster/writer/interviewer for Financial News Network. 1982: TV: The Guinness Book of Records Specials (announcer), Ripley's Believe It Or Not! (ABC), The Quest (ABC). Host/producer The Romance of Words. Film: My Tutor. 1983: Film: R.S.V.P. TV: Remington Steele (NBC). Host/interviewer: The Gold Mining Report (KWHY series); Video Aktuell (German TV series); Financial Inquiry (KSCI & SPN series); Hilton Video Magazine; host/presenter Aesop's Fables.

PASSER, IVAN: Director-Writer. b. Czechoslovakia. Began career as writer.
PICTURES INCLUDE: Writer: Loves of Blonde, Fireman's Ball. Director: Intimate Lighting, Born To Win, Law and Disorder, Crime and Passion, The Silver Bears, Cutter and Bone, Creator.

PASTER, GARY M.: Executive. b. St. Louis, Missouri, July 4, 1943. e. University of Missouri—B.A., U.C.L.A., U.S.C.—Graduate School of Business. 1970, joined The Burbank Studios as asst. to the pres. and as treas. 1976 v.p.—administration and chairman of the exec. committee. September, 1977 pres. Board of Directors/Trustees: Permanent Charities Committee of Entertainment Industry, St. Joseph Medical Center Foundation, and The Oakwood School. Member: Academy of Motion Picture Arts and Sciences, Los Angeles Film Development Council, Hollywood Radio and T.V. Society, Advisory Commission—California Motion Picture Council, Academy of Television Arts and Sciences. Advisory bd., Kaufman Astoria Studios, N.Y.

PASTERNAK, JOE: Producer, b. Szilagysomlyo, Hungary, Sept. 19, 1901. 2nd asst. dir. Paramount 1923; asst. dir. Universal (Hollywood), 1926, then prod. mgr. Berlin; made pictures in Vienna and Budapest, returned to Hollywood 1937; assoc. prod. then prod. A "Champion of Champion producers" in Fame Ratings.
PICTURES INCLUDE: Zwei Menschen, Unter Falscher Flagge, Grosse Scehnsucht, Unsichtbare Front, Fraulein Paprika, Gruss Und Gruss, Veronika, Scandal in Budapest, Csibi, Spring Parade, Katherine, Three Smart Girls, 100 Men and a Girl, Mad About Music, That Certain Age, Three Smart Girls Grow up, Destry Rides Again, It's a Date, Nice Girl, It Started With Eve, Presenting Lily Mars, Thousands Cheer, Two Girls and a Sailor, Music for Millions, Thrill of a Romance, Anchors Aweigh, Her Highness and the Bellboy, Two Sisters from Boston, Holiday in Mexico, No Leave No Love, This Time for Keeps, Three Daring Daughters, On an Island With You, Date With Judy, In the Good Old Summertime, Big City, Unfinished Dance, Nancy Goes to Rio, Summer Stock, That Midnight Kiss, Toast of New Orleans, The Great Caruso, Rich, Young and Pretty, The Strip, Merry Widow, Skirts Ahoy!, Because You're Mine, Small Town Girl, Latin Lovers, Easy to Love, Flame and the Flesh, Student Prince, Athena, Hit the Deck, Love Me or Leave Me, Meet Me in Las Vegas, Opposite Sex, 10,000 Bedrooms, This Could Be the Night, Where the Boys Are, Jumbo, A Ticklish Affair, Girl Happy, Penelope.

PATERSON, NEIL: Novelist, screenwriter. b. Scotland, 1916. e. Edinburgh Univ. War Service Lt. R.N.V.R. Early career

as novelist. Awarded Atlantic Award in Literature, 1946. Dir. Grampian TV Chmn. of Production; films of Scotland. Vice-chmn. Scottish Arts Council; Gov. Pitlochry Thea.; Gov. National Film School. Former Gov. British Film Institute. Member Arts Council Gt. Britain.
NOVELS: The China Run, Behold Thy Daughter and Delilah, Man on the Tight Rope.
PICTURES INCLUDE: Man on a Tight Rope, The Little Kidnappers, Woman for Joe, High Tide at Noon, The Shiralee, Innocent Sinners, Room at the Top (s.p. Acad. Award, 1960), The Spiral Road, The Golden Fool, The Forty Days of Musa Dagh, Keeper of My Heart.

PATINKIN, MANDY: Actor. b. Chicago, 1947. e. Univ. of Kansas, Juilliard School (Drama Div.). In regional theatre before coming to New York where played with Shakespeare Festival. Major break came with Evita on Broadway.
PICTURES: French Postcards, Night of the Juggler, The Big Fix, The Last Embrace, Daniel, Yentl, Maxie.
TELEVISION: That Thing on ABC, That 2nd Thing on ABC, Charleston, Taxi, Sparrow, Streets of Gold, Midnight Special, etc.

PATRICK, C. L.: Theatre Executive. b. Honaker, Va., Dec. 6, 1918. Pres. of Fuqua Industries, which owns Martin Theatres and Gulf States Theatres. Prior to this was pres. and chm. of Martin Theatres. Member NATO exec. Comm.; International Ambassador of Variety; Motion Picture Pioneer of the Year in 1976.

PATRICK, GEORGE: Art director, b. Salida, Colo. May 21, 1905. e. U. of So. Calif., 1923–27. Entered m.p. ind. as junior draftsman, First National Pictures, 1928; asst. art dir., art dir. for many prod.; designed, supervised construction of Frontierland section of Disneyland, 1955.
PICTURES INCLUDE: Deadline U.S.A., Beneath the 12-Mile Reef, The Racers.

PATRICK, MICHAEL W.: Executive. b. Columbus, GA May 17, 1950. e. Columbus Col. (BS, 1972). Pres., Carmike Cinemas.
MEMBER: v.p., NATO; pres., Ga. Theatre Owners Assn.; exec. comm., Will Rogers Institute; Variety Intl.; Motion Picture Pioneers.

PATTERSON, RICHARD L.: Executive. b. St. Louis, Mo., November 1924. B.A. U.C.L.A., 1950; graduate work and teaching Theatre Arts Dept., U.C.L.A. until 1952; film dept. and dir. TV until 1955; H.N. Swanson Literary Agency handling TV dept.; head literary dept., Wm. Morris Agency to 1959; chmn., man. dir. Paramount British Pictures, Ltd., 1959; chmn. Seven Arts Prods. (U.K.) Ltd.; dir. Bryanston Seven Arts Ltd., 1961; assoc. Of Human Bondage; prod. The Wild Affair. Joined Christopher Mann Ltd., 1964; int. man. dir., P.L. Representation, 1967; prod. exec. MGM, 1972.

PAUL, M. B.: Cameraman, director. r.n. Morrison Bloomfield Paul. b. Montreal, Canada. Sept. 30. e. De Paul U.; newsreel, publicity picture service; partner, Seymour Studios, 1930–33; film test biz. own studio. Hollywood, 1933–35; prod. adv. films, asst. in N.Y. E.W. Hammons, 1945–47; Acad. Award, one-piece color translucent background system, 1950. Dir. of photography, optical effects, Daystar, United Artists, Outer Limits, 1963; designed, patented, Scenoramic process, 1965. Camera, Paradise Road. Features, Film project supervision A/V consult. Sceno 360 surround system development. Mem. AMPAS, Friars, SMPTE.

PAULEY, JANE: Program Hostess-Reporter. b. Indianapolis, Ind., Oct. 31, 1950. e. Indiana Univ. Involved in Indiana state politics before joining WISH-TV, Indianapolis, as reporter. Co-anchored midday news reports and anchored weekend news reports. Co-anchor of nightly news at WMAQ-TV, NBC station in Chicago. Joined Today show in October, 1976, as featured regular, prior to which had made guest appearances on that program.

PAVAN, MARISA: Actress, r.n. Marisa Pierangeli. b. Cagliari, Sardinia, June 19, 1932; e. Torquado Tasso coll.; s. Pier Angeli, actress. Came to U.S. 1950; m.p. debut in What Price Glory.
PICTURES INCLUDE: Down Three Dark Streets, Drum Beat, Rose Tattoo, Diane, Man in the Gray Flannel Suit, John Paul Jones, Solomon and Sheba, Midnight Story.

PAVLIK, JOHN M.: Executive. b. Melrose, Iowa, Dec. 3, 1939. e. Univ. of Minnesota, B.A. 1963. Reporter, Racine (Wis.) Journal-Times, San Bernardino (Calif.) Sun-Telegram, 1963–66; Writer, News Bureau, Pacific Telephone, Los Angeles, 1966–68; assistant director of public relations, Association of Motion Picture and Television Producers, 1968–72; director of public relations, 1972–78; vice-president, 1978–79; executive administrator, Academy of Motion Picture Arts and Sciences, 1979–82; exec. dir., M.P. & TV Fund, 1982–present; member, board of directors, Permanent Charities Committee of the Entertainment Industries, 1979–84; member, board of directors, Hollywood Chamber of Commerce, 1979–85; vice-president, Los Angeles Film Development Committee, 1977–78, member, executive council, 1974–85; special consultant, California Motion Picture Council, 1974–79.

PAVLOW, MURIEL: Actress. b. June 27, 1924. e. England, France & Switzerland. Stage debut in Dear Octopus, 1938; screen debut in Quiet Wedding.
PICTURES INCLUDE: Night Boat to Dublin, Shop at Sly Corner, It Started in Paradise, The Net (Project M7), Malta Story, Conflict of Wings (Fuss Over Feathers), Doctor in the House, Simon and Laura, Reach for the Sky, Eye Witness, Tiger in the Smoke, Doctor at Large, Rooney, Whirlpool, Meet Miss Marple.

PAY, WILLIAM: Executive. b. London, England; joined London office Quigley Publications. Served in RAF, 1941–46; rejoined Quigley; dir. Burnup Service Ltd., 1951; London news ed., Quigley Pub., 1955. Dir., Quigley Pub. Ltd., 1961; appt. mgr. dir., 1963; mgr. dir., Burnup Company. Appt. Sec. British Kinematograph Sound & TV Society. Conference Co-ordinator biennial Intern. Film & TV Technology Conferences in U.K., 1975–87.

PAYNE, JOHN: Actor. b. Roanoke, Va., 1912. e. Mercersburg Acad., Pa., Roanoke Coll. of Virginia and Columbia. On radio programs. Stage debut, 1973, Good News.
PICTURES INCLUDE: Dodsworth, Wings of the Navy, Indianapolis Speedway, Kid Nightingale, Stardust, Maryland, Great Profile, Tin Pan Alley, King of the Lumberjacks, Tear Gas Squad, Great American Broadcast, Sun Valley Serenade, Week-End in Havana, Remember the Day, To the Shores of Tripoli, Hello Frisco Hello, The Dolly Sisters, Sentimental Journey, Razor's Edge, Wake Up and Dream, Miracle on 34th Street, Larceny, Saxon Charm, El Paso, Crooked Way, Captain China, Eagle and Hawk, Passage West, Crosswinds, Blazing Forest, Caribbean, The Vanquished, Kansas City, Confidential, Raiders of the 7 Seas, 99 River Street, Rails into Laramie, Silver Lode, Hell's Island, Santa Fe Passage, Road to Denver, Tennessee's Partner, Slightly Scarlet, Rebel in Town, Bail Out at 43,000, Hidden Fear.

PAYNE, NORMAN: Artists' and writers' manager. b. London, England. Ent. entertainment ind., 1939. Early career music, then formed talent agency, J.P. Productions, 1945. Later bought by MCA, 1951. Became dir. MCA and head of light ent. for theatres and TV throughout Europe. On MCA terminating reformed agency. TV offices also in Germany & Australia.

PAYNTER, ROBERT: Cinematographer. b. London. e. Mercer School. First job in industry at 15 years as camera trainee with Government Film Dept.
PICTURES: Hannibal Brooks (debut, 1969), The Nightcomers, The Mechanic, Firepower, Superman, Superman II, Trading Places, Superman III.

PEACH, MARY: Actress. b. Durban, South Africa, 1934. Ent. films 1957. TV appearances include Ghosts, The Rat Wife, The Master Builder, Love Story, Hadley, Somerset Maugham, Can You Keep a Secret?, Cat on a Hot Tin Roof, Blind Love, Disraeli, Children at the Gods, Fox.
PICTURES INCLUDE: Room at the Top, Follow That Horse, No Love for Johnnie, A Gathering of Eagles, Ballad in Blue, Scrooge.
RECENT THEATRE: Birthday Run, The Marriage, When the Music Stops, Hilda, Don't Gas the Blacks, Old Times, The Chairman, The Autumn Garden.

PEAKER, E.J.: Actress, singer, dancer. Edra Jeanne Peaker, b. Tulsa, Okla., Feb. 22. e. Univ. of New Mexico, Univ. of Vienna, Austria. Stage debut Bye, By Birdie; m.p. debut Hello, Dolly. Films include All American Boy.
TV: That's Life series, The Flying Nun, That Girl, Movie of the Week, Love American Style, Odd Couple, Police Woman, Rockford Files, Get Christie Love.

PECK, GREGORY: Actor, producer. b. La Jolla, Calif. April 5, 1916; U. Calif.; Neighborhood Playhouse Sch. of Dramatics. On dramatic stage (The Doctor's Dilemma, The Male Animal, Once in a Lifetime, The Play's the Thing, You Can't Take It With You, Sons and Soldiers, etc.); on screen 1944 in Days of Glory. Voted one of ten best Money-Making Stars Motion Picture Herald-Fame Poll, 1947, 1952. Co-prod. and starred in Big Country, for his company, Anthony Productions; prod. the Trial of the Catonsville Nine, The Dove (St. George Productions).
PICTURES INCLUDE: Keys of the Kingdom, Valley of Decision, Spellbound, Yearling, Duel in the Sun, Macomber Affair, Gentleman's Agreement, Paradine Case, Yellow Sky, 12 O'Clock High, Great Sinner, The Gunfighter, Only the Valiant, David and Bathsheba, Captain Horatio Hornblower, World in His Arms, Snows of Kilimanjaro, Roman Holiday, Night People, Man With a Million, Purple Plains, Man in the Gray Flannel Suit, Moby Dick, Designing Woman, The Bravados, Pork Chop Hill, On the Beach, Beloved Infidel,

Guns of Navarone, Cape Fear, To Kill a Mocking Bird, Captain Newman, M.D., Behold a Pale Horse, Mirage, Arabesque, MacKenna's Gold, Stalking Moon, The Chairman, Marooned, I Walk the Line, Shootout, Billy Two Hats, The Omen, MacArthur, The Boys from Brazil, The Sea Wolves.
TELEVISION: The Blue and the Gray, The Scarlet and the Black.

PEERCE, LARRY: Director. b. Bronx, N.Y.
PICTURES INCLUDE: One Potato, Two Potato, The Incident, Goodbye Columbus, The Sporting Club, The Big TNT Show, A Separate Peace, Ash Wednesday, The Other Side of the Mountain, Two Minute Warning, The Other Side of the Mountain—Part II, The Bell Jar, Why Would I Lie?, Love Child, Hard to Hold.
TELEVISION: Love Lives On, I Take These Men, The Fifth Missile.

PELLATT, JOHN: Production Executive. Abandoned school for theatre at age of 14. Became stage manager before serving in H.M. Forces. Then became assistant director for Warner Bros., MGM, London Films, etc. Since 1955 worked as prod. manager/assoc. producer with British Lion, Columbia, Paramount, United Artists, Ivan Tors, American International. Also while assistant gen. prod. mgr. 20th Century Fox, associated with Inn of Sixth Happiness, Roots of Heaven, The Blue Angel, Sons and Lovers, Sink the Bismark.
TV: Series for Incorporated Television Espionage. Worked in Europe, Middle and Far East, India, East and North Africa, Congo, Bahamas, Australia, Hollywood, Southern Africa.
PICTURES INCLUDE: Noose, The Wooden Horse, Silent Dust, Lavender Hill Mob, Man in the White Suit, Ivanhoe, Innocents in Paris, Mogambo, Knights of the Round Table, A Kid for Two Farthings, Oh Rosalinda, The Twelve Days of Christmas, The Captain's Paradise, Zarak Khan, The Green Man, St. Trinians, Only Two Can Play, They're a Weird Mob, Age of Consent, Count Five and Die, Help, The Revolutionary, Wuthering Heights, Elephant Country, Who Slew Auntie Roo, Tower of Evil, The Zoo Gang TV series, Born Free TV series (Kenya), The Diamond Mercernaries (Killer Force in U.S.), One Away. (South & S.W. Africa).

PENN, ARTHUR: Director. b. Philadelphia, Pa., Sept. 27, 1922. e. Black Mountain College, Asheville, N.C., and Universities of Perugia and Florence in Italy. Began as TV dir. in 1953, twice winner of Sylvania Award. Dir. stage plays Two for the Seesaw, Miracle Worker, Toys in the Attic, All the Way Home, Golden Boy. Entered m.p. as dir. of Left-Handed Gun in 1958.
PICTURES INCLUDE: Miracle Worker, Mickey One, The Chase, Bonnie and Clyde, Alice's Restaurant, Little Big Man, Visions of Eight, Night Moves, The Missouri Breaks, Four Friends (also co-prod.), Target.

PENN, CHRISTOPHER: Actor. Brother of actor Sean Penn.
PICTURES: Rumble Fish, All the Right Moves, Footloose, The Wild Life, Pale Rider.

PENN, SEAN: Actor. b. So. Calif., Aug. 17, 1960. Son of actor-director Leo Penn, actress Eileen Ryan. e. Santa Monica H.S. Served as apprentice for two years at Group Repertory Theatre, L.A. Acted in Earthworms, The Girl on the Via Flaminia, etc. First pro appearance as guest star on TV's Barnaby Jones. On Bdwy. in Slab Boys.
PICTURES: Taps (debut), Fast Times at Ridgemont High, Bad Boys, Crackers, Racing with the Moon, The Falcon and the Snowman, At Close Range, Shanghai Surprise.
TELEVISION: Movies: Hellinger's Law, The Killing of Randy Webster. Series: Concrete Cowboys, Barnaby Jones.

PEPPARD, GEORGE: Actor, b. Detroit, Mich., Oct. 1, 1928. e. Dearborn H.S., Carnegie Tech., BFA, Fine Arts. U.S. Marine Corps. Legit. stage debut, Pittsburgh Playhouse, 1949. Worked as mason, construction laborer, fencing instructor, Braddock, Pa. Signed by Sam Spiegel to appear in The Strange One.
STAGE: Girls of Summer, The Pleasure of His Company.
PICTURES INCLUDE: Pork Chop Hill, Home from the Hill, The Subterraneans, Breakfast At Tiffany's, How the West Was Won, The Victors, The Carpetbaggers, The Third Day, Operation Crossbow, The Blue Max, Tobruk, Rough Night in Jericho, P.J., House of Cards, What's So Bad About Feeling Good, Pendulum, Cannon for Cordoba, The Executioner, One More Train to Rob, The Groundstar Conspiracy, Newman's Law, Damnation Alley, Five Days From Home, Your Ticket Is No Longer Valid, Battle Beyond the Stars, Race to the Yankee Zephyr.
TV: Little Moon of Alban, Suspicion, U.S. Steel Hour, Alfred Hitchcock Presents, Matinee Theatre, Alcoa-Goodyear Playhouse, Studio One, Hallmark Hall of Fame, Banacek, The Bravos, Doctors Hospital, Story of Dr. Sam Sheppard, Crisis in Mid-Air, Torn Between Two Lovers, The A Team.

PEPPERCORN, CARL: Executive. b. New York. e. NYU. Ent. film ind. FBO (forerunner of RKO), held var. sls. positions, home office and branches. Lt. Comm. US Navy, WW II; pres. Military Bank of Naples, sales mgr. NY branch RKO; asst. to Eastern sales mgr., RKO; gen'l sales mgr.,. RKO Canada; pres. Dairy-maid Chocolate Co., Toronto; v.p. Fairweather Dept. Stores, Canada; chmn. bd. Andako Mining Co., Canada; v.p. & gen'l sales mgr. Continental Dist. Inc.; v.p. & gen'l sales mgr. Embassy Pictures, Inc.; exec. v.p. and gen'l sales mgr. Cinema V Inc, pres. & sls. mgr., U.M. Film Distributors and Peppercorn-Wormser Film Distributors; Diversified Film Representatives, Inc., Peppercorn Enterprises.

PERAKOS, SPERIE P.: Executive. b. N. Britain, Conn., Nov. 12, 1915. e. Cheshire Acad., Yale, Harvard Law School, Student mgr., Stanley-Warner thtrs., 1939–40; Perakos thtrs., 1940–41; Fellow, Pierson Coll., Yale, 1946–present; Yale Alumni Bd., 1949 to present; Yale Alumni Film Bd. 1952 to present; member Alumni Council for Yale Drama School; past pres. Yale Club of N. Britain, Conn.; dir. of Films & Filmings Seminars, Pierson Coll., Yale; prod. Antigone, 1962; pres. Norma Film Prod., Inc., 1962 to present. Past pres. now chm. Yale's Peabody Museum Associates and member of the University Council of the Peabody Museum. Pres., Perakos Theatres, Conn. Theatre Circuit, Inc.

PERENCHIO, ANDREW J.: Executive. b. Fresno, CA, Dec. 20, 1930. e. Univ. Calif. Vice pres., Music Corp. of America, 1958–62; General Artists Corp., 1962–64; pres., owner, Chartwell Artists, Ltd., theatrical agency, Los Angeles, 1964; pres. & CEO, Tandem Productions, Inc., and TAT Communications Co., 1973–83, when became principal with Norman Lear in Embassy Communications. Holds post of pres. & CEO of Embassy Pictures.

PERKINS, ANTHONY: Actor. b. New York City, Apr. 14, 1932. Columbia U., Rollins College. Broadway stage in Tea and Sympathy. Dr. Steambath, 1970. Wrote s.p. Last of Sheila, 1973.
TV: Kraft Theatre, Studio One, U.S. Steel Hour, Armstrong Theatre.
PICTURES INCLUDE: The Actress, Friendly Persuasion, The Lonely Man, Fear Strikes Out, The Tin Star, This Bitter Earth, Desire Under the Elms, The Matchmaker, Green Mansions, On the Beach, Tall Story, Psycho, Goodbye Again, Phaedra, The Trial, The Fool Killer, The Champagne Murders, Pretty Poison, Catch 22, Someone Behind the Door, Ten Days' Wonder, WUSA, Play It As It Lays, Lovin' Molly, Murder on the Orient Express, Mahogany, Remember My Name, Winter Kills, The Black Hole, ffolkes, Psycho II, Crimes of Passion.
STAGE: Greenwillow, Look Homeward Angel, Steambath, Equus.

PERKINS, JOHN HENRY ROWLAND II: Executive. b. July 10, 1934, Los Angeles. e. Univ. So. Calif., UCLA. Joined William Morris Agency, 1959; exec. in TV dept. In January, 1975, co-founded Creative Artists Agency, of which is senior partner and first pres. Member Hollywood Radio & TV Society since 1964, and Academy of TV Arts & Sciences since 1962.

PERKINS, MILLIE: Actress. b. 1939.
PICTURES: The Diary of Anne Frank, Wild in the Country, Wild in the Streets, Lady Cocoa, Table for Five, At Close Range, Jake Speed.

PERLMUTTER, DAVID M.: Producer. b. Toronto, Canada, 1934. e. University of Toronto. Pres., Quadrant Films Ltd.
PICTURES INCLUDE: The Neptune Factor, 1972; Sunday In The Country, 1973; It Seemed Like A Good Idea At The Time, 1974; Love at First Sight, Find the Lady, 1975; Blood and Guts, The Third Walker, Two Solitudes, 1977; Fast Company, 1978; Double Negative, Nothing Personal, 1979; Misdeal, Love, 1980.

PERMUT, DAVID A.: Producer. b. New York City, Mar. 23, 1954. e. Univ. of Calif. (1972). 1974, pres., Diversified Artists Intl.; 1975, pres., Theatre Television Corp.; 1979, formed Permut Presentations, Inc., of which is pres. Production deals with Columbia Pictures (1979) and Lorimar Productions (1981).
PICTURES: Give 'Em Hell Harry (prod.); Fighting Back (exec. prod.); Love Leads The Way (exec. prod.); Blind Date (prod.); Richard Pryor—Live in Concert (exec. prod.).

PERREAU, GIGI: Actress. r.n. Ghislaine Perreau; b. Los Angeles, Calif. Feb. 6, 1941; sister of Janine Perreau & Richard Miles, prof. m.p. debut in Madam Curie 1943; many stage and TV guest appearances.
PICTURES INCLUDE: Dark Waters, Abigail, Dear Heart, Family Honeymoon, Roseanna McCoy, High Barbaree, Song of Love, Green Dolphin Street, Two Girls and a Sailor, Shadow on the Wall, My Foolish Heart, For Heaven's Sake, Never a Dull Moment, Reunion in Reno, Lady Pays Off, Weekend With Father, Has Anybody Seen My Gal, Bonzo Goes to College, There's Always Tomorrow, Man in the Gray Flannel Suit, Dance With Me Henry, Tammy Tell Me True, Journey to the Center of Time, Hell on Wheels.

PERRIN, NAT: Writer. With Arthur Sheekman wrote series of radio broadcasts for the Marx Brothers. With Sheekman in 1933 wrote additional dialogue on Duck Soup. Par. Collab. s.p. Roman Scandals, many others. CBS-TV West Coast, exec. prod., color programs.
PICTURES INCLUDE: Kid Millions, Rose of the Rancho, Dimples, Pigskin Parade, Stowaway, Don't Tell the Wife, New Faces of 1937, On Again—Off Again, Swing Fever, Whistling in Brooklyn, Abbott and Costello in Hollywood, Song of the Thin Man, Petty Girl, Tell It To The Judge, Miss Grant Takes Richmond, Emergency Wedding.

PERRINE, VALERIE: Actress. b. Phoenix, Sept. 3 1943. e. Univ. of Arizona. Was showgirl in Las Vegas before discovered by agent Robert Walker who got her contract with Universal Pictures. Film debut in Slaughterhouse Five.
PICTURES INCLUDE: The Last American Hero, Lenny (N.Y. Film Critics Award, best supporting actress), W. C. Fields and Me, Mr. Billion, Superman, The Electric Horseman, Can't Stop the Music, Superman II, The Border, Water.
TELEVISION: When Your Lover Leaves.

PERRY, ANTHONY: Producer. b. London, England, 1929. Ent. m.p. ind. 1948 with Two Cities story dept. asst. story ed., Rank Prods. Wrote orig. story and prod. asst. Simba. Prod., The Secret Place in 1957. Created and prod. TV series, Interpol Calling, 1959; founded Eyeline Films, prod. many Brit. prize-winning commercials. Sold Eyeline Films, 1963; wrote, dir. Emma, 1964–65, res. prod. Keep Films/Embassy Prods., London, 1966–67; prod. Dare I Weep, Dare I Mourn, for ABC-TV, and Fernandel TV series. Admin. Yellow Submarine, joined Trickfilm as man. dir. Chmn. Film & TV Copyrights, Ltd.
PICTURES INCLUDE: The Impersonator, Girl on Approval, The Party's Over.

PERRY, EARL: Circuit Executive. b. Aug. 11, 1921. e. Tulane Univ. Spent 4 yrs. as Air Force officer in World War II. Worked for Twentieth Century Fox for four years; then entered exhibition in 1951 as vice pres. and gen. mgr. of Pittman Theatres; in 1966, formed Ogden-Perry Theatres, and as pres., operates theatres in Louisiana, Mississippi, Tennessee, and Florida. Past President of NATO of Louisiana; Past Chief Barker of Variety Club Tent 45.

PERRY, FRANK: Director, producer, writer. served as apprentice, Westport, Conn. Country Playhouse; spent nine years in stock as stage mgr., prod. mgr., and managing director. U.S. Army, 1952–54; director-observer, Actors Studio, 1955; Theatre Guild, 1956–60; s.p. (with Eleanor Perry): Somersault, David and Lisa, and others.
PICTURES INCLUDE: The Swimmer, Ladybug, Ladybug, David and Lisa, Last Summer, Trilogy, Diary of a Mad Housewife, Doc, Play It As It Lays, The Man on the Swing, Rancho Deluxe, Mommie Dearest, Monsignor.

PERSCHY, MARIA: Actress. b. Eisenstadt, Austria, Sept. 23, 1940. e. Max Rheinhardt Seminar (Vienna). Widow of John Melson, writer. Started in 1958 with German film (Nasser Asphalt) and has appeared in over 50 European and U.S. features. Has also appeared on European TV. Recipient of Laurel Award in 1963.
PICTURES INCLUDE: Man's Favorite Sport, Squadron 633, Ride the High Wind, Murders in the Rue Morgue, Last Day of the War, The Desperate Ones, The Tall Woman, Witch Without a Broom, etc.
TV: General Hospital, Hawaii Five-O.

PERSKY, LESTER: Executive. b. New York City, July 6, 1927. e. Brooklyn College. Officer in U.S. Merchant Marine, 1945–48. Founder and pres. of own adv. agency, 1951–1964. Theatrical stage producer, 1966–69. Produced Fortune and Men's Eyes for MGM in 1971. In 1973 creative director and co-owner Persky Bright Org. (owner-financier of numerous motion pictures for private investment group). Films include Last Detail, Golden Voyage of Sinbad, For Pete's Sake, California Split, The Man Who Would be King, The Front, Shampoo. Also Hard Times, Taxi Driver, Missouri Breaks, Bound for Glory, Sinbad and the Eye of the Tiger. Lester Persky Productions, Inc.
PICTURES: Produced Equus, Hair, Yanks, Handcarved Coffins.
TELEVISION: Poor Little Rich Girl (mini-series)

PERSOFF, NEHEMIAH: Actor. b. Jerusalem, Israel, Aug. 14, 1920. e. Hebrew Technical Inst., 1934–37; Actors Studio electrician, 1937–39; signal maint., N.Y.C. Subway, 1939–41.
STAGE: Only in America, Galileo, Richard III, King Lear, Peter Pan, Peer Gynt, Tiger At the Gates, Colombe, Mont Serrat.
PICTURES INCLUDE: Fate is the Hunter, Al Capone, Some Like It Hot, The Harder They Fall, The Badlanders, Men In War, This Angry Age, The Big Show, The Greatest Story Ever Told, The Wild Party, The Power, Mrs. Pollifax—Spy, Red Sky at Morning, Psychic Killer, Voyage of the Damned, Yentl.
TV: Philco-Goodyear Show, Kraft, Producers Showcase, Danger, You Are There, Untouchables, Route 66, Naked City, Wagon Train, Rawhide, Gunsmoke, Thriller, Hitchcock Thriller, Bus Stop, Five Fingers, Mr. Lucky, Sadat.

PERTWEE, JON: TV performer. b. London, July 7, 1919. e. Sherborne, Royal Academy Dramatic Art. Early career, Arts League Traveling Theatre, 5 yrs. repertory; regularly on radio, TV, music hall, cabaret and circus.
PICTURES INCLUDE: Murder At the Windmill, Miss Pilgrim's Progress, Will Any Gentleman?, Gay Dog, It's A Wonderful Life, Mr. Drake's Duck, A Yank in Ermine, Ugly Duckling, Just Joe, Not a Hope in Hell, Nearly a Nasty Accident, Ladies Who Do, Carry on Cleo, I've Gotta Horse, Carry On Cowboy, Carry On Screaming, A Funny Thing Happened On the Way To The Forum, Up in the Air, The Hod, March of the Desert, One of our Dinosaurs is Missing, The House That Dripped Blood, The Island of Young Tigers, The Boys in Blue.
TV: Own series, Sunday Night, London Palladium Compere Variety Show, Doctor Who series, Who Dunnit, Worzel Gummidge.
RADIO: Navy Lark.
STAGE: See You Inside, A Funny Thing Happened On The Way To The Forum, There's A Girl In My Soup, Oh Clarence, My Dear Gilbert, The Bedwinner, Don't Just Lie There, Say Something, Irene, Touch It Light.

PERTWEE, MICHAEL: Writer. b. April 24, 1916. e. Sherborne School and France. Early career, journalist; ent. m.p. ind. 1937. Co-author, co-presentation many BBC plays and serials; many appearances panel games.
PICTURES INCLUDE: Laughter in Paradise, On Monday Next, Top Secret, Happy Ever After, Now and Forever, Against the Wind, Interrupted Journey, The Naked Truth, Too Many Crooks, Bottoms Up, Make Mine Mink, It Started in Naples, In the Doghouse, Mouse on the Moon, Ladies Who Do, Finders Keepers, Strange Bedfellows, A Funny Thing Happened on the Way to the Forum, Salt and Pepper, One More Time, Don't Just Lie There Say Something, Digby the Biggest Dog in the World.
TV: Rainy Day, Strictly Personal, Grove Family, Man in a Moon, The Frightened Man, Yakity Yak (ATV 1956), The Old Campaigner, Terry Thomas series, B and B series, Never a Cross Word, Six of Rix, Men of Affairs.
STAGE: The Four Musketeers, Drury Lane, She's Done It Again, Don't Just Lie There Say Something, Birds of Paradise, A Bit Between the Teeth, Six of One, Ace In A Hole, Find the Lady, Do Not Disturb, Look No Hans!

PESCOW, DONNA: Actress. b. Brooklyn, NY, March 24. e. American Academy of Dramatic Arts. Started career on summer tour in Ah Wilderness in 1975. Did bit in ABC daytime series, One Life to Live. Film debut in Saturday Night Fever (1977). Regular on ABC-TV series, Angie.
TELEVISION: Policewoman Centerfold, Obsessed with a Married Woman.

PETERS, BERNADETTE: Actress. b. New York City, Feb. 28, 1944. Professional debut at age 5 on TV's Horn & Hardart Children's Hours. Stage debut with NY City Center production of The Most Happy Fella. Screen debut, Ace Eli and Rodger of the Skies.
PICTURES INCLUDE: W.C. Fields & Me, Vigilante Force, Silent Movie, The Jerk, Tulips, Pennies from Heaven, Heartbeeps, Annie.

PETERS, BROCK: Actor. b. Harlem, N.Y.C., July 2, 1927. e. Univ. of Chicago. Had numerous featured roles on and off Bdwy. in road and stock cos., nightclubs, TV. Toured with DePaur Infantry Chorus 3 seasons. Made m.p. debut, Carmen Jones, 1955.
PICTURES INCLUDE: Carmen Jones, Porgy and Bess, To Kill a Mockingbird, The L-Shaped Room, The Pawnbroker, Black Girl, Soylent Green, Lost in the Stars.
STAGE: King of the Dark Chamber, Othello, The Great White Hope, Lost in the Stars, Framed.
TELEVISION: The Young and the Restless, It Takes a Thief, Mannix, Mod Squad, etc.

PETERS, JON: Producer. b. Van Nuys, CA, 1947. Started hair-styling business; built it into multi-million-dollar firm before turning film producer. Formed Jon Peters Organization. 1980, joined with Peter Guber and Neil Bogart to form The Boardwalk Co. (now dissolved).
PICTURES INCLUDE: A Star Is Born, The Eyes of Laura Mars, The Main Event, Die Laughing, Caddyshack, Six Weeks, D.C. Cat, Visionquest, Clue (exec. prod.), The Color Purple (exec. prod.).

PETERS, ROBERT C.: Executive. With Paramount Pictures since 1967 holding variety of financial posts: controller, TV div.; v.p., finance-west coast; pres., non-theatrical & educational dist. div. in 1980 appt. snr. v.p. for Paramount, assuming responsibility for all west coast administration, studio operations, post-production, personnel, industrial relations and Paramount Sound Systems, Inc. Continues responsibility for Paramount merchandising and has taken over talent relations.

PETERSEN, WOLFGANG: Director. b. Emden, Germany, Mar. 14, 1941. Career as asst. state director at Ernst Deutsch Theatre in Hamburg before starting to direct for television and later theatrical films.
PICTURES INCLUDE: Black and White Like Day, The Consequence, Das Boot (The Boat), The NeverEnding Story, Enemy Mine.
TELEVISION: Series called Scenes of the Crime, etc.

PETERSON, S. DEAN: Executive. b. Toronto, Canada, December 18, 1923. e. Victoria College, University of Toronto. WWII service RCNVR; 1946 TV newsreel cameraman NBC; founded own production company in 1947; incorporated Dordean Realty Limited to acquire new studios 1959; formed Peterson Production Limited in 1957 to make TV commercials and sponsored theatrical shorts; has international awards as producer, director, director of photography; formed Studio City Limited in 1965 to produce television series and features acquiring an additional studio complex and backlot in Kleinberg, Ontario; 1972 formed SDP Communications Ltd. to package M.P. and TV; 1970 incorporated Intermedia Financial Services Limited to provide specialized financing and consultation to companies in M.P. and TV industries.
Past-President Canadian Film and Television Association, mbr. Variety Club, Tent 28; Canadian Society of Cinematographers; Directors Guild of America, Directors Guild of Canada, SMPTE.

PETERSON, PAUL: Actor. b. Glendale, Calif., Sept. 23, 1945. e. Valley Coll. Mouseketeer (TV).
PICTURES INCLUDE: Houseboat, This Could Be the Night.
TV: The Donna Reed Show, Playhouse 90, Lux Video Theatre, GE Theatre, The Virginian, Ford Theatre, Valentine's Day, Shindig.

PETRIE, DANIEL: Director. b. Glace Bay, Nova Scotia, Nov. 26.
PICTURES INCLUDE: Lifeguard, Buster and Billie; Spy With A Cold Nose; The Idol; Stolen Hours; Raisin in the Sun; The Bramble Bush, The Betsy, Resurrection, Fort Apache, The Bronx, Six Pack, Bay Boy, Half a Lifetime, Square Dance.
THEATRE: Shadow of My Enemy; Who'll Save The Plowboy?; Mornin' Sun; Monoploy, The Cherry Orchard, Volpone, A Lesson from Aloes.
TV FILMS: Sybil, Eleanor and Franklin, Eleanor and Franklin: The White House Years, Silent Night, Lonely Night, Harry Truman, Plain Speaking, The Dollmaker, The Execution of Raymond Graham.

PETROU, DAVID MICHAEL: Writer-Producer. b. Washington, D.C., Nov. 3, 1949. e. Univ. of MD (BA); Georgetown Univ. (MA). Publicity assoc., Psychiatric Institutes of America, Washington, D.C., 1971; assoc. dir. of publicity & film liaison, Random House, 1974; guest lecturer, screen writing & film production, The American University Consortium, Washington, D.C., spring, 1980; Woodrow Wilson Fellowship, 1971. Entered industry in 1975. Joined Salkind Organization in chg. of literary projects. Worked in numerous production capacities on Crossed Swords, Superman, Superman II. 1977, exec. in chg. of literary development, Salkind. Wrote Crossed Swords (1978) and The Making of Superman. Co-authored screenplay, Shoot to Kill. 1978–79, promotional development on Time after Time for Warner Bros.; 1980–83, dir., special projects Joseph Kennedy Foundation. Organized U.S. premiere of Superman II and The Empire Strikes Back; 1983–84, sr. editor for entertainment, Regardie's Magazine; 1984, organized Washington, D.C. premiere of Indiana Jones and the Temple of Doom; 1984–86, sr. exec., p.r. div., Abramson Associates; 1986–present, sr. v.p., Eisner, Held & Petrow, p.r. agency.

PEVERALL, JOHN: Producer. b. Islington, England. Started in entertainment industry in 1945 in mail room of J. Arthur Rank Prods. Promoted to asst. dir. Time out for military service in Royal Air Force Air-Sea Rescue Unit. Resumed career as asst. dir. and unit prod. mgr. on several films produced in Britain and throughout Europe. In 1969 became associated with newly-formed Cinema Center Films as prod. exec. in London. When firm suspended activities became freelance as asst. dir.
PICTURES INCLUDE: Conduct Unbecoming and The Man Who Fell to Earth (both assoc. prod.), The Deer Hunter (prod.).

PEVNEY, JOSEPH: Director, actor. b. New York City; e. N.Y.U., 1933; m. Mitzi Green, former child star; actress, nightclub entertainer. Began career in vaudeville at 13 as jr. mem. song & dance team; later stage in Home of the Brave. US Army ETO WWII.
STAGE: Counsellor at Law, Key Largo, Native Son; (dir.) Swan Song, Let Freedom Sing.
PICTURES INCLUDE: (acting) Nocturne, Outside The Wall, Body & Soul; (dir.) Counsellor at Law, Key Largo, Native Son, Stage Door, Lady from Texas, Meet Danny Wilson, Iron Man, Flesh and Fury, Just Across the Street, Because of You, Desert Legion, It Happens Every Thursday, Back to God's Country, Yankee Pasha, Playgirl, Three Ring Circus, Six Bridges to Cross, Foxfire, Female on the Beach, Away All Boats, Congo Crossing, Tammy and the Bachelor, Man of a Thousand Faces, Cash McCall, Crowded Sky, Night of the Grizzly.

PEYSER, JOHN: Producer, director. b. New York, N.Y., Aug. 10, 1916; e. Colgage U., 1938. In TV ind. since 1939, with Psychological Warfare Div., ETO., WWII; pres. Peypac productions, Madrid.
TV: Director: Hawaii Five-O, Mannix, Movin On, Swiss Family Robinson, Bronk, Combat, Untouchables, Rat Patrol, etc.
FEATURE FILMS: Spain, The Open Door; Kashmiri Run; Honeymoon with a Stranger; Four Rode Out; Massacre Harbor.

PFEIFFER, MICHELLE: Actress. b. Santa Ana, CA, 1957.
PICTURES: Grease II, Scarface, Into the Night, Ladyhawke, Sweet Liberty.
TELEVISION: Delta House, Callie and Son, The Children Nobody Wanted, Splendor in the Grass.

PHILBIN, JACK: Producer. b. Lynn, Mass., e. Boston U., U.C.L.A. Started in Hotel management. Personal mgr., Glenn Miller 1939; Johnny Long 1942; Perry Como, 1944; Jackie Gleason 1948; v.p. General Artists Corp. 3 years; exec. prod., Jackie Gleason Show, Stage Show, The Honeymooners, America's Greatest Bands, CBS prod., The Vic Damone Show, The Big Record, exec. prod. Jackie Gleason American Scene Magazine TV Show, CBS-TV, 1962–63, Jackie Gleason Show 1965–74; Jackie Gleason Specials 1975–1980.

PHILLIPS, BILL: Actor. b. Washington, D.C. e. George Washington U. On N.Y. stage, Alice in Wonderland, Lightnin', etc. On screen 1940 in City for Conquest.
PICTURES INCLUDE: Larceny, Inc, Sergeant York, Action in the North Atlantic, Johnny Come Lately, See Here, Private Hargrove, Thirty Seconds Over Tokyo, Harvey Girls, Holiday in Mexico, Till Clouds Roll By, Sea of Grass, Living in Big Way, Easy Living, Big Jack, Johnny Allegro, Customs Agent, Chain Gang, Bugles in the Afternoon, New York Confidential.

PHILLIPS, D. JOHN: Motion Picture Theatre Consultant. b. New York City. Advertising and publicity mgr. Borden Co. Produce Sales Div., 1933–36; adv. & pub. mgr., Paul R. Dillon Co., Inc., 1936–41. Became field exploitation rep., United Artists Corp., 1941–42; Short Subjects & Paramount News adv. & pub. mgr. Paramount Pictures, 1942–47; exec. dir. Metropolitan Motion Pictures Theatres Assn., 1947–79, New York.

PHILLIPS, JULIA: Producer. b. Brooklyn, N.Y. e. Mt. Holyoke College. Production asst. at McCall's Magazine; later became textbook copywriter for Macmillan. In 1970 she and her husband, Michael, formed a company with actor Tony Bill (Bill/ Phillips Productions) to develop film projects.
PICTURES INCLUDE: Steelyard Blues, The Sting, Taxi Driver, The Big Bus, Close Encounters of the Third Kind.

PHILLIPS, LESLIE: Actor, producer. b. London, April 20, 1924. Early career as child actor. Ent. m.p. ind. 1935.
PICTURES INCLUDE: High Flight, Les Girls, Smallest Show on Earth, Carry on Nurse, King Ferdinand of Naples, This Other Eden, The Navy Lark, Doctor in Love, Please Turn Over, Watch Your Stern, No Kidding, Week-End With Lulu, VIP, Carry on Constable, Raising the Wind, In the Doghouse, Crooks Anonymous, Fast Lady, Father Came Too, Doctor in Clover, You Must Be Joking, Maroc 7, Some Will Some Won't, Doctor in Trouble, The Magnificent 7 & Deadly Sins, Not Now Darling, Don't Just Lie There, Spanish Fly, Not Now Comrade, Out of Africa.
TV: Our Man At St. Marks Impasse, The Gong Game, Time and Motion Man, Reluctant Debutante, A Very Fine Line, The Suit, The Culture Vultures (series), Edward Woodward Show, Casanova 74 (series), Redundant—or the Wife's Revenge. TV film: You'll Never See Me Again, Mr. Palfrey of Westminister.

PHILLIPS, MICHAEL: Producer b. Brooklyn, N.Y., Nov. 10, 1916. Mgr. & prof. pugilist (featherweight), 1930–36. Ent. m.p. ind. as secy to Ray Milland, 1937; apptd asst. dir., U.S. Army Special Service Div., 1942–45; script ed. & prod. activities, Eddie Bracken Radio Prod. until 1949 (orig. & s.p.) Double Cross; formed own prod. co. Demyrtha Prod., Inc. 1950. In 1970 formed prod. co. with wife, Julia, and Tony Bill.
PICTURES INCLUDE: Steelyard Blues, The Sting, Taxi Driver, The Big Bus, Close Encounters of the Third Kind, Heartbeeps, Cannery Row, The Flamingo Kid.

PICERNI, PAUL: Actor. b. New York, N.Y. Dec. 1, 1922. e. Lovola U., Los Angeles. U.S. Air Force 1943–46; head of drama dept. Mt. St. Mary's College, 1949–50; TV credits include Untouchables (co-star).

TV: Philco Playhouse, Climax, Lux, Loretta Young Show, Desilu, Kojak, Mannix, Police Story, Lucy Special, Quincy, Alice, Trapper John, Vegas, Fall Guy, Capitol, Hardcastle & McCormick.
PICTURES INCLUDE: Breakthrough, I Was a Communist for the FBI, Mara Maru, Desert Song, She's Back on Broadway, House of Wax, Shanghai Story, To Hell and Back, Miracle in the Rain, Bobby Ware is Missing, Omar Khayyam, Brothers Rico, Young Philadelphian, The Young Marrieds, The Scalphunters, Airport, Kotch, Beyond the Posiedon Adventure.

PICKER, ARNOLD M.: Executive. b. New York, Sept. 19, 1913; m.; p. Celia and David V. Picker; e. Coll. of City of New York, U. of London; joined Columbia's foreign dept. in June, 1935. Asst. to foreign mgr.; then vice-pres. 1945, Columbia International Corp.; v.p. charge foreign dist., Oct., 1951; exec. v.p. UA, and in charge all distribution, June 1961; chmn. exec. com., 1967. Retired.

PICKER, DAVID V.: Executive. b. New York City, May 14, 1931; e. Dartmouth Coll., B.A., 1953. Father Eugene Picker, exec. Loew's Theatres. Ent. industry in 1956 as adv. pub. & exploitation liaison with sls. dept., United Artists Corp.; exec. v.p. U.A. Records; asst. to Max Youngstein, v.p.; v.p. U.A.; first v.p. UA; pres. 1969 Resigned 1973 to form own production co. In 1976 joined Paramount Pictures as pres. of m.p. div.; v.p., Lorimar Productions; now independent.
PICTURES INCLUDE: Juggernaut, Lenny, Smile, Royal Flash, Won Ton Ton, The One and Only, Oliver's Story, The Jerk, The Man with Two Brains.

PICKER, EUGENE D.: Executive b. New York City, Nov. 17, 1903; married; p. David V. and Celia C. Picker; e. N.Y.U. and School of Business. Started with father in Bronx theatres; joined Loew's Inc., 1920; in charge circuit operations, New York City area, 1945; v.p. Loew's Theatres, Sept. 1954; member bd. of dir., 1956, exec. v.p. Sept. 1958; pres. Loew's Theatres, March 1959. Res. 1961 as pres. Loew's Theatres; joined U.A. as v.p., July 1961. Joined Trans-Lux Corp. as exec. v.p., Jan. 1967; pres. & chief oper. Officer of Entertainment Division of Trans-Lux Corp.; Exec. consultant motion picture industry Jan. 1, 1974 and Pres. E.D.P. Films Inc. as of June 1974; pres. NATO, 1969–71, ch. bd., 1971–72, Bd. dir., Will Rogers Hospital, bd. ch. At present member board of directors, Trans Lux Corp. and Foundation of Motion Picture Pioneers and Broadway Association.

PICKMAN, JEROME: Executive. b. New York, N.Y., Aug. 24, 1916; e. St. John's U.; B'klyn Law Sch. of St. Lawrence U., LL.B. Reporter N.Y. newspapers, 1930–40; adv. dept. 20th-Fox, 1944–46; Eagle-Lion Films, 1947; Paramount, April 1949; v.p., dir., adv. & pub., Paramount Film Dist. Corp., 1951–60; v.p. domestic gen. sls. mgr., Paramount Film Dist. Co., N.Y. till 1962; sls. exec. Columbia Pictures 1963–67; pres. Continental Div. of Walter Reade Org., 1967–70; pres., Levitt-Pickman Film Corp., 1971; snr. v.p., domestic distribution, Lorimar Productions, 1979; pres., Pickman Film Corp., 1982 & COO, Cineworld Enterprises Corp.; pres. Scotti Bros. Pictures, 1985.

PICKMAN, MILTON EUGENE: Executive. b. N.Y.C. e. Columbia U., LL.B; St. Lawrence U. Reporter, Brooklyn Daily Eagle, 1925–29; asst. Florenz Ziegfeld Publicity, 1929–31; mgr. & agent, name bands, 1932–40; exec. M.C.A., 1933–36; U.S. Army, 1942–45; eastern studio rep. & asst. to Harry Cohn, Columbia, 1945; own agency, 1948–51; v.p. & gen. mgr., Wald-Krasna Prod., RKO, 1952; exec. asst. to Jerry Wald, v.p. in charge of prod., Columbia, 1952–54; v.p. of TV prog., Screen Gems Prod.; gen. mgr. Samuel Goldwyn Prod., 1958; prod. exec. and asst. to Buddy Adler, v.p., chg. of prod., 20th Century Fox Studios; exec. v.p., American Entertainment Enterprises.

PICKUS, ALBERT M.: Exhibitor. b. New Haven, Conn., Mar. 20, 1903; e. Washington and Lee U., 1920–24, B.S. Accountant, auditor, New Haven; ent. m.p. ind., 1926; owner, Stratford Theatre, Stratford, Conn.; dir., MPTO of Conn., 1953–59; v.p., TOA, 1953–57; asst. pres. TOA rep. to COMPO, 1957–58; chmn. exec. com. TOA, 1959; exec. com., ACE, 1959; pres. TOA, 1959–61; chmn. of bd., 1962.

PIERCE, FREDERICK S.: Executive. e. Bernard Baruch School of B.A., City College N.Y. Served with U.S. Combat Engineers in Korean War. Associated with Benj. Harrow & Son, CAP, before joining ABC in 1956. Served as analyst in TV research dep.; prom. to supvr. of audience measurements, 1957, named mgr. next year. In 1961 made dir. of research; 1962 dir. of research, sales devel. Named dir. of sales planning, sales devel. April, 1962; elec. v.p., Feb. 1964 and made nat. dir. of sales for TV. In 1968 named v.p., planning; March. 1970 named asst. to pres. In July 1972, named v.p., in chg. ABC TV planning and devel. and asst. to pres. ABC TV, March, 1973. Named sr. v.p., ABC TV, Jan., 1974. Elected pres., ABC Television Division, October, 1974. Now pres. & chief operating off., ABC, Inc.

PIERSON, FRANK: Producer-Director-Writer. b. 1925. Was correspondent for Time Magazine before entering show business as story editor of TV series, Have Gun, Will Travel. Later served as both producer and director for show. Developed a number of properties for Screen Gems before writing theatrical screenplays.
PICTURES INCLUDE: Cat Ballou (co-s.p.), Cool Hand Luke (s.p.), The Anderson Tapes (s.p.), The Looking Glass War, (s.p., dir.), Dog Day Afternoon (s.p.), A Star Is Born (dir., s.p.), King of the Gypsies (dir., s.p.).

PIGOTT-SMITH, TIM: Actor. b. England, 1946. Acted with Bristol Old Vic, Royal Shakespeare Co. On stage in As You Like It, Major Barbara School for Scandal, Sherlock Holmes, The Benefactors, etc.
TELEVISION: The Lost Boys, Henry IV, Day Christ Died, Hunchback of Notre Dame, Fame Is the Spur, Glittering Prizes, The Jewel in the Crown, Dead Man's Folly, etc.

PIKE, JOHN S.: Executive. Joined Paramount Pictures as v.p., video programming; promoted to sr. v.p., video prog. 1984, named sr. v.p., current network programming; 1985, promoted to exec. v.p., Paramount Network TV. 1986, appt. pres., Paramount Network TV Division.

PILCHER, TONY: Executive. b. Boston, England, 1936. e. Shrewsbury School. Ent. m.p. industry 1960 with Anglo-Scottish Pictures. Became prod. exec. 1961, German rep. and exec. 1968. Joined AB-Pathe as German rep., TV and Advertising Films division 1964. TV prod. Heumann Ogilvy & Mather, Frankfurt, 1966; prod. Chambers and Partners; Guild TV; Wace Film, Signal Films, Rayant TV, Filmshop, Europartners 1967 to date.

PILE, SUSAN: Executive. First west coast editor of Interview magazine before entering entertainment industry as media buyer and acct. exec. on m.p. accts for Diener/Hauser/Bates. After 6 years left to become partner in Proper Exposure, specialized mktg. firm in m.p. field. Natl.mag. contact, Universal Pictures; unit publicist for Univesal & Warner Bros. 1980, joined Paramount as dir., west coast adv. & pub. 1981, named v.p., west coast pub. & promo; 1985, sr. v.p., west coast publ, promo. & adv.

PINK, SIDNEY: Producer, director, writer. b. Pitts., Pa., Mar. 6, 1916. e. Univ. of Pitts., B.S., 1934–37; U.S.C., Law, 1940–41 Projectionist, mgr., booker, Warner Bros., Pa., Fox West Coast, United Artists Theatres, Calif. Prod. budget mgr., Something to Sing About and Lost Horizon.
PICTURES INCLUDE: Bwana Devil, Angry Red Planet, Green-Eyed Elephant, Reptilicus, Journey to The Seventh Planet, Operation Camel, Valley of the Swords, Madigan's Millions.

PINSKER, ALLEN: Executive. b. New York City, Jan. 23, 1930. e. N.Y. Univ. Mgr., Hempstead Theatre, 1950. In 1954 joined Island Theatre Circuit as booker-buyer; named head buyer 1958. In 1968 joined United Artists Eastern Theatres as film buyer; head buyer, 1969, v.p., 1970. Named v.p. United Artists Theatre Circuit, 1972. In 1973 named UAET exec. v.p., member bd., 1974.

PINTER, HAROLD: Writer-Director-Actor. b. London, England, Oct. 10, 1930. Began career as actor then turned to writing and direction. Plays include The Birthday Party, The Caretaker, The Homecoming, Landscape, Silence, Old Times, No Man's Land, The Hot House.
PICTURES: The Servant, The Pumpkin Eater, The Quiller Memorandum, Accident, The Go-Between, The Last Tycoon, The French Lieutenant's Woman, Turtle Diary.
TELEVISION: A Night Out, Night School, The Lover, Tea Party, The Basement.

PIROSH, ROBERT: Writer, director, producer. S.p. credits include Battleground (solo orig. s.p. Academy Award winner), Hell Is For Heroes, What's So Bad About Feeling Good, S.P.-dir. credits include Go For Broke, Washington Story, Valley of the Kings.
TV: (Wrote, prod. pilots) Laramie, Combat. (Writer) Hawaii Five-0, Ellery Queen, Mannix, Bonanza, Ironside, The Waltons, Barnaby Jones, The Bold Ones, etc.

PISANO, A. ROBERT: Executive. e. San Jose State Univ.; Univ. of Calif. at Berkeley. Member, State Bar of Calif., Board of Governors of Assn. of Business Trial Lawyers, American Bar Assoc., L.A. County Bar Assoc. Joined O'Melveny & Myers as associate 1969; made partner 1976. 1979–82 headed its Paris office. Returned to L.A. office to handle Paramount Pictures' litigation 1983–84. In 1985 joined Paramount as exec. v.p. & gen. counsel.

PISIER, MARIE-FRANCE: Actress. b. Indochina. First discovered by Francois Truffaut who cast her in L'Amour a Vingt Ans. When film completed returned to school for degree in political science. Continued to work in films.
PICTURES: Trans-Europe Express, Stolen Kisses, Celine

et Julie Vont en Bateau, Cousin Cousine, Souvenirs d'en France, Barocco, The Other Side of Midnight, French Postcards, Chanel Solitaire.

PLACE, MARY KAY: Actress. b. Tulsa, OK, September, 1947. e. Univ. of Tulsa. Worked in clerical jobs before starting to write for TV series (Mary Tyler Moore Show, Phyllis, Maude, MASH, etc.). Turned to acting, appearing in episodes of All in the Family and Mary Tyler Moore Show and as Loretta Haggers on series, Mary Hartman, Mary Hartman (Emmy, best comedy actress).
PICTURES: More American Graffiti (debut), New York, New York, Starting Over, Private Benjamin, Modern Problems, Waltz Across Texas, The Big Chill, Smooth Talk.
TELEVISION: Fernwood 2-Night, Saturday Night Live, The Tonight Show, John Denver Special, etc. Movie: The Girl Who Spelled Freedom.

PLANCK, ROBERT: Cinematographer. b. 1894.
PICTURES INCLUDE: It's Great to be Alive, Life in the Raw, Jane Eyre, Last of the Mohicans, By Secret Command, Canterville Ghost, Secrets in the Dark, Cass Timberlane, It Happened in Brooklyn, Three Musketeers, Luxury Liner, Little Women, Madame Bovary, Summer Stock, Royal Wedding, Texas Carnival, Scandal at Scourie, Torch Song, Rhapsody.
TV: My Three Sons.

PLATT, MILT: Executive. b. New York City. e. CCNY, RCA Institute, Ohio State U.; US Army 1942–46; div. mgr., RKO Radio Pictures until 1957; gen. sls. mgr. Continental Dist., 1957–65; vice-pres. & gen. sls. mgr. Sherpix, 1965; v.p. & gen. sls. mgr., Comet Film Distributors, Inc., 1965; v.p. & sls. mgr., Times Film Corp., 1968. Pres. Eagle Amusement Co., 1970. Appointed member of the Appeals Board of the MPA rating system, 1971; pres. of Pisces Group, Ltd., 1972; v.p. & gen. sls. mgr., International Co-productions, Inc., 1974. pres., Milton Platt Co., 1975. Member governing commettee, IFIDA

PLEASENCE, DONALD: Actor. b. Worksop, England, Oct. 5, 1919. Repertory, first London appearance in Twelfth Night. RAF, WW II. Since London stage, NY stage, ent. m.p, ind. 1953.
STAGE: Vicious Circle, Saint's Day, Hobson's Choice, The Rules of the Game, The Lark, Ebb Tide, The Caretaker, Poor Bitos, The Man in the Glass Booth, Wise Child (N.Y.); voted actor of the year, 1958.
PICTURES INCLUDE: Manuela, The Man in the Sky, Heart of a Child, Tale of Two Cities, Battle of the Sexes, The Shakedown, The Horsemasters, Spare the Rod, No Love for Johnnie, The Caretaker, The Great Escape, The Greatest Story Ever Told, Hallelujah Trail, Fantastic Voyage, Cul-de-Sac, You Only Live Twice, Matchless, 13, Will Penny, Arthur! Arthur, THX 1138, Soldier Blue, Outback, Jerusalem File, Pied Piper, Innocent Bystanders, Death Line, Wedding in White, The Rainbow Boys, The Black Windmill, Journey Into Fear, Escape to Witch Mountain, Hearts of the West, The Devil Within Her, The Last Tycoon, Passover Plot, Trial by Combat, The Eagle Has Landed, Goldenrod, Oh God!, Fear, the Uncanny, Telefon, Escape from New York, Halloween, Halloween II, Terror in the Aisles.
TV: Fate and Mr. Browne, Small Fish are Sweet, The Silk Purse, A House of His Own, The Traitor, The Millionairess, The Cupboard Machinal, The Hatchet Man, The Bandstand, Ambrose, Thou Good and Faithful Servant, Call Me Daddy, Taste, The Fox Trot, Omnibus, Julius Caesar, Occupations, The Joke, The Cafeteria, Hindle Lakes, Master of the Game, Arch of Triumph.

PLESHETTE, EUGENE: Executive. b. Jan. 7, Brooklyn, N.Y. e. CCNY & LaSalle, U., Para. Pict. Acting School; stage actor; assoc. prod. and dir. three off-Broadway plays; treas. and house mgr. N.Y. Paramount; v.p. Reid-Singer Music; exec. mgr. Brooklyn Paramount thea., 1945; mgn. dir. 1953; v.p. in chg. of ABC Merchandising Inc., AB-PT, Inc. and American Broadcasting Co., 1962; exec. v.p., MSG-ABC Prods., Inc. 1965; exec. v.p. Don Reid TV Prod.; 1975, President, Pleshette Associates.

PLESHETTE, SUZANNE: Actress. b. New York, N.Y. Jan. 31, 1937. e. Performing Arts H.S., Finch College, Syracuse U. Broadway debut, Compulsion; m.p. debut Geisha Boy; major TV shows including The Bob Newhart Show, and For Love or Money.
PICTURES INCLUDE: Rome Adventure, The Birds, 40 Pounds of Trouble, Wall of Noise, A Rage to Live, Youngblood Hawke, A Distant Trumpet, The Ugly Dachshund, Bullwhip Griffin, Fate is the Hunter, Mr. Buddwing, Nevada Smith, Blackbeard's Ghost, The Power, If It's Tuesdy This Must Be Belgium, Suppose They Gave a War and Nobody Came, Support Your Local Gunfighter, The Shaggy D.A., Oh, God! Book II.
Stage; The Cold Wind and the Warm, The Golden Fleecing, The Miracle Worker, Compulsion, Two for the Seesaw.

PLESKOW, ERIC: Executive. b., Vienna, Austria. Served as film officer, U.S. War dept., 1946–48; entered industry in 1948 as asst. gen. mgr., Motion Picture Export Association, Germany; 1950–51, continental rep. for Sol Lesser Prods.; joined United Artists in 1951 as Far East Sales Mgr.; named mgr., S. Africa, 1952; mgr., Germany, 1953–58; exec. asst. to continental mgr., 1958–59; asst. continental mgr., 1959–60; continental mgr., 1960–62; v.p. in charge of foreign distribution, 1962; exec. v.p. & chief operating off., Jan. 1, 1973; pres. & chief exec. off., Oct. 1, 1973. Resigned in 1978 to become pres. and chief exec. officer of Orion Pictures Co.; 1982, became pres. & chief exec. off., Orion Pictures Corp.

PLITT, HENRY G.: Executive. b. New York, Nov. 26, 1918. e. Syracuse U. St. Lawrence U. Law School. War service, 6 yrs.; Paramount Pictures International Corp.; United Detroit Theatres; asst. gen. mgr., North Ohio Theatres Corp.; div. mgr., then v.p., Paramount Gulf Theatres, New Orleans; pres. gen. mgr. Paramount Gulf Theatres; pres., ABC Films, 1959–65; Pres. ABC Great States Inc., Great States Theas. 1966; v.p. Prairie Farmer publications, 1971, v.p., ABC Theatre Holdings, Inc.; 1974, purchased Northern Theatre Circuit from American Broadcasting Company, consisting of 127 theatres, naming these theatres Plitt Theatres, Inc., of which he is bd. chmn. 1978, purchased rest of ABC theatres from American Broadcasting Company consisting of 272 screens, and renamed them Plitt Theatres. Sold circuit interest in 1985.

PLUMMER, AMANDA: Actress. b. New York City, March 23, 1957. e. Middlebury Coll. Daughter of Christopher Plummer.
PICTURES: Cattle Annie and Little Britches, Daniel, The Hotel New Hampshire.

PLUMMER, CHRISTOPHER: Actor. b. Toronto, Canada, Dec. 13, 1929. Stage career started with English repertory group visiting Canada; toured U.S. in Nina, 1953; Bway debut in The Constant Wife, 1954; on road and in N.Y. with The Dark is Light Enough; American Shakespeare Festival at Stratford, Conn., in Julius Caesar and The Tempest; Shakespeare Festival at Stratford, Ontario, in Henry V, Twelfth Night, and Hamlet; on Bway in The Lark and Cyrano.
TV: Oedipus Rex, Omnibus, After the Fall, The Shadow Box, The Thorn Birds, Crossings.
PICTURES INCLUDE: Stage Struck, Inside Daisy Clover, The Sound of Music, Triple Cross, The Battle of Britain, The Royal Hunt of the Sun, Lock Up Your Daughters, The Phyx, The Return of the Pink Panther, Conduct Unbecoming, The Man Who Would Be King, International Velvet, The Silent Partner, Murder by Decree, Hanover Street, Somewhere in Time, Eyewitness, The Amateur, Dreamscape, Ordeal by Innocence, Lily in Love, The Boy in Blue.

PODELL, ALBERT N.: Executive. b. New York City, Feb. 25, 1937. e. Cornell U., U. of Chicago. Articles editor, Playboy Magazine, 1959–61; dir. of photog., Argosy Magazine, 1961–64; account exec. on 20th Century-Fox at Diener, Hauser, Greenthal, 1966–68; national advertising dir., Cinema Center Films, 1969; account supervisor on Columbia Pictures at Charles Schlaifer; creator & dir. of Annual Motion Picture Advertising Awards sponsored by Cinema Lodge, B'nai B'rith.

PODESTA, ROSSANA: Actress. b. Tripoli, 1934. Discovered in Italy by French director, Leonide Moguy, who starred her in Tomorrow Is Another Day. For 15 years appeared only in films by her husband, Marco Cicario; now divorced.
PICTURES INCLUDE: Cops and Robbers, La Red, Ulysses, Helen of Troy, Santiago, The Golden Arrow, Il Prete Sposato, Seven Golden Men, Pano, Burro e Marmelate, The Quiet Countrywoman, Sunday Lovers, Stasi.

PODHORZER, MUNIO: Executive. b. Berlin, Germany, Sept. 18. e. Jahn-Realgymnasium. U. of Berlin Medical School. U.S. Army, 1943–47; pres. United Film Enterprises, Inc.; formerly secy.-treas. 86th St. Casino Theatre, N.Y.; former v.p. Atlantic Pictures Corp.; former pres. Casino Films, Inc.; former pres. Film Development Corp.; former rep. Export-Union of the German Film Ind.; former U.S. rep. Franco-London Film, Paris; former pres., Venus Productions Corp.; former U.S. rep. Atlas Int'l Film GmbH, Munich; former U.S. rep. Bavaria Atelier Gesellschaft U.S. past rep. Israfilm Ltd., Tel-Aviv; past rep. Tigon British Film Prod., London; past rep. Elias Querejeta, P.C., Madrid; past rep. Equiluz Films, Madrid, past rep. Airport Cine, Hawaii, Les Films Du Capricorne; Profilmes, Spain; Ligno, Spain; Films D'Alma, France; Intra Films, Italy. Member: Variety Club, Cinema Lodge, B'nai B'rith, Past Board of Governors IFIDA; past pres. CID Agents Assoc. Former gen. foreign sales mgr., theatrical division of National Telefilm Associates. Presently representing Atlas Film+AV, Germany; Barcino Films, S.A., Spain; Eagle Films Ltd., United Kingdom; Les Films Jacques Leitienne, France; Nero Films Classics U.S.A.; Schongerfilm Germany; Profilmes, S.A., Spain; KFM Films, Inc. U.S.A.; Compagnie France Film, Canada; Cia. Iberoamerican de TV, S.A. Spain; V.I.P. Ltd., Israel. Co-chm., entertainment div., United

Jewish Appeal, Federation of Jewish Philanthropies, 1981–83.

PODHORZER, NATHAN: Executive. b. Brody, Poland, Nov. 27, 1919. e. City Coll. of N.Y., Rutgers Univ., U. of So. Calif. U.S. Army, 1942–46; documentary film prod., Israel, 1946–57; vice pres., secy., United Film Enterprises, Inc.

POITIER, SIDNEY: Actor. b. Feb. 24, 1924; e. Nassau. Formed First Artists Prod. Co. Ltd., 1969, with Paul Newman and Barbra Streisand.

STAGE: Lysistrata, Anna Lucasta, Freight.

PICTURES INCLUDE: No Way Out, Cry the Beloved Country, Red Ball Express, Go Man Go, Blackboard Jungle, Good-Bye My Lady, Edge of the City, Something of Value, Porgy and Bess, All the Young Men, Devil at Four O'Clock, A Raisin in the Sun, The Long Ships, Lilies of the Field, Slender Thread, A Patch of Blue, Duel at Diablo, To Sir With Love, In the Heat of the Night, Guess Who's Coming to Dinner, The Lost Man, They Call Me Mister Tibbs, Brother John, For Love of Ivy, Buck and the Preacher, A Sweet December (dir., star), Uptown Saturday Night (dir., star), The Wilby Conspiracy, Let's Do It Again (dir., star), A Piece of the Action (dir., star), Stir Crazy (dir.), Hanky Panky (dir.), Fast Forward (dir.).

POLANSKI, ROMAN: Director/Writer. b. Paris, France, Aug. 18, 1933. Lived in Poland from age of three. Early career, Art School in Cracow; five years State Film College at Lodz. Wrote and dir. Two Men In a Wardrobe, Le Gros et Le Maigre, Mammals. From 1961 wrote and dir. Knife in the Water (Poland), Repulsion, Cul-De-Sac, The Vampire Killers, Rosemary's Baby, Macbeth, What?, Chinatown, The Tenant, Tess, Pirates.

POLIER, DAN A.: Executive. b. Atlanta, Ga. e. Ga. Mil. Acad. and U. of Ill. Sports columnist, Charlotte (N.C.) News; sports editor, army wkly, Yank; entered m.p. industry adv. dept. 20th Century-Fox; head of booking dept. Fox West Coast Theatres; v.p. and director of film buying NT&T Amusement Corp.; v.p. and co-director theatre operations, National General Corp. (formerly NT&T); named v.p. in chg. of production, National General Productions, Inc., 1967. Joined Radnitz/Mattel Productions in 1972 as v.p. in chg. of distribution for Sounder; v.p. Mann Theatres Corp. of Calif., 1973. Rejoined Radnitz/Mattel Productions, 1975, as vice pres. in charge of marketing. Now pres., Knopf/Polier Representation.

POLL, MARTIN H.: Producer. b. New York. e. Wharton School, U. of Pa.; pres. Gold Medal Studios; prod. Love Is a Ball, Sylvia, The Lion in Winter, The Appointment, The Magic Garden of Stanley Sweetheart, The Man Who Loved Cat Dancing, Night Watch, Love and Death (exec. prod.); The Sailor who Fell From Grace with the Sea, Somebody Killed Her Husband, The Dain Curse, Nighthawks, Arthur the King, Gimme an F.

POLLACK, SYDNEY: Director-Producer. b. South Bend, Ind., July 1, 1934. m. Claire Griswold. e. Neighborhood Playhouse, Assistant to Sanford Meisner at Neighborhood Playhouse. Appeared as actor on B'way in A Stone for Danny Fisher, The Dark is Light Enough. As TV actor: Playhouse 90 segments, Shotgun Slade, 15 Ben Caseys, A Cardinal Act of Mercy (won 5 Emmy nominations), The Game on Bob Hope-Chrysler Theatre (won Emmy for direction), Two is the Number. Dir. debut in 1960. Dir. play at UCLA, P.S. 193. Prepared the American version of The Leopard.

PICTURES INCLUDE: The Slender Thread (dir.), This Property is Condemned, The Scalphunters, Castle Keep, They Shoot Horses, Don't They?, Jeremiah Johnson, The Way We Were, The Yakuza, Three Days of the Condor, Bobby Deerfield, The Electric Horseman, Absence of Malice (also prod.); Tootsie (also prod. and actor); Songwriter (prod. only); Out of Africa (also prod.).

POLLEXFEN, JACK: Producer, director, writer. b. San Diego, Calif., June 10, 1918. e. Los Angeles City Coll. Newspaperman, magazine writer, playwright: prod. for RKO, United Artists, Columbia, Allied Artists.

PICTURES INCLUDE: Son of Sinbad, At Swords Point, Secret of Convict Lake, Desert Hawk, Lady in the Iron Mask, Dragon's Gold, Problem Girls, Captive Women, Captain Kidd and the Slave Girl, Neanderthal Man, Captain John Smith and Pocahontas, Return to Treasure Island, Sword of Venus, 1000 Years from Now, Daughter of Dr. Jekyll, Monstrosity, Son of Dr. Jekyll, Mr. Big, Man from Planet X.

POLLOCK, DALE: Executive. e. Brandeis Univ., San Jose State Univ. Began journalistic career in Santa Cruz in early '70s, serving as reporter and film critic for Daily Variety from 1977 to 1980. Then joined Los Angeles Times as film writer, winning paper's Award for Sustained Excellence in 1984. In 1985 left to take post with The Geffen Film Co. as executive in chg. creative development.

POLONSKY, ABRAHAM: Director, writer. b. N.Y.; e CCNY, BA., Columbia Law School. Taught at City College 1932 until war. Wrote s.p. Golden Earrings, I Can Get it For You Wholesale. Wrote novels; The Discoverers, The World Above, The Season of Fear. Wrote orig. story and s.p. Body and Soul; collab. s.p. and directed Force of Evil. Blacklisted from 1951–66. Coll. s.p. Madigan 1968; dir. and s.p. Tell Them Willie Boy is Here, 1970; dir. Romance of a Horse Thief, 1971; Monsignore, 1982.

PONTI, CARLO: Producer. b. Milan, Italy, Dec. 11, 1913. Univ. of Milan 1934. Prod. first picture in Milan, Little Old World; prod. Lux Film Rome; prod. first of a series of famous Toto pictures, Toto Househunting.

PICTURES INCLUDE: A Dog's Life, The Knight Has Arrived. Musolino, The Outlaw, Romanticism, Sensuality, The White Slave, Europe 1951, Toto in Color, The Three Corsairs, Ulysses, The Woman of the River, An American of Rome, Attila, War and Peace, The Last Lover, The Black Orchid, That Kind of Woman, Marriage Italian Style, The Great Spy Mission, Happily Ever After, The Girl and the General, Sunflower, Best House in London, Lady Liberty, White Sister, What?, Andy Warhol's Frankenstein, The Passenger, The Cassandra Crossing, A Special Day.

POOLE, FRANK S.: Executive. b. London, England, 1913. e. Dulwich Coll, 1925–31. Ent. m.p. ind. 1931. Early career with Pathe Pictures, Twickenham Film Distributors, until joining 20th Century Fox as London Branch Office Supervisor 1939. War service 1940–46. Rejoined Fox 1946–53; appt. Leed Branch mgr. 1954–59; supv. 1959–61; asst. sls. mgr., 1961 until joined Rank Film Distrib. as asst. sls. mgr. 1962. Appt. sls. mgr. July 1965, and to board as dir. of sls. Aug. 1965. Appt. gen. mgr. 1968; jnt. man. dir. 1969; appt. man. dir. July 1970; appt. dir. Rank Overseas Film Dist. Ltd., 1972; apptd. co-chmn Fox-Rank Distributors Ltd., Dec. 1972; appt. vice-chairman Rank Film Distributors Ltd. 1977. 1975, elected to Committee of Cinema & TV Veterans. Oct., 1978, retired from Rank Organisation. Appt. chmn., Appeal Tribunal for the Film Industry. Appt. chm., Grebelands Mgt. Committee & to exec. council of CTBF, 1979, assoc. Ceoff Reeve & Associates. 1980, chm. & mng. dir., Omandry Intl. Ltd.

POPE, EDWARD J.: Producer, writer. b. Rye, N.Y., Aug. 3, 1919. e. Western Reserve Academy, 1938; Yale University, 1942. m. H.I.H. Princess Niloufer. World record, all-American swimmer, 1940–42; Commander, USNR, 1942–45; author, History of U.S. Navy, WW II; author, with Marechal Juin, La Defense Nationale, 1946; awarded Exceptional Civil Service Medal; Cross of Malta; Commandante, Grand Order of Merit Italian Republic; Commander, Order of Medjidiye; junior writer, MGM, 1946; prod., writer documentaries, 2 Academy Award nominations, 1947–48; prod. Seaboard Studios, ABC-TV studios, 1949; prod. film seq. Robert Montgomery Presents and 10 Million Bros. (Germany). Producer, Dumont TV, 1950; Auerbach Film Enterprises, 1950–51; ass. prod. 70 US TV films, Europe, 1951–53; v.p., exec. prod. Alpha Omega Films (France), 1954–55; chief int'l and pub. rel. U.S. Defense Dept. Europe, 1956–64; exec. prod., Compagnie Francaise De Coproduction Internationales (France) 1965–69; v.p. General Productions S.A., 1968–69; and Giroux Films, S.A. 1969; associate prod., Sweet Hunter; prod. 12+1; pres., H.I. Management SA (Holiday Inns) Europe.

POPKIN, HARRY M.: Exhibitor, producer. b. N.Y.C., e. Jarvis Collegiate Sch., Toronto, Canada; U. of Cal. Started career as cashier, ticket-seller, asst. to mgr., Gore Bros. Theatre Circuit, Los Angeles; became mgr. & 3 yrs. later theatre owner, L.A.; acq. other theatres, formed Eastland Circuit; purchased Gore Bros. interests; ent. sports world, oper. major auditorium, L.A., San Francisco, Oakland; first m.p. prod. all-Negro films, then, feature picture And Then There Were None; financed other ind. prod. Since 1949 org. ind. prod. unit, Hollywood; world-wide offices.

PICTURES INCLUDE: Impact, Champagne for Caesar, Second Woman, The Well, The Thief, Top Banana.

PORTER, DON: Actor. b. Miami, Okla. e. Oregon Inst. of Tech. Wide theatre work; then m.p, roles. U.S. Army, 3 yrs.

TV: Co-star, Private Secretary, Ann Sothern Show, Gidget, Bionic Woman, Hawaii Five-O, Switch, Love Boat, Three's Company, The President's Mistress, The Murder That Wouldn't Die, The Last Song, Dallas.

STAGE: The Best Man, Any Wednesday, Generation, Plaza Suite, The Price, How To Succeed in Business Without Really Trying, Harvey.

PICTURES INCLUDE: The Racket, The Savage, 711 Ocean Drive, Because You're Mine, Our Miss Brooks, Bachelor in Paradise, Youngblood Hawke, The Candidate, 40 Carats, Mame, White Line Fever, The Last Resort.

PORTER, RAND: Actor/writer/producer. b. Los Angeles, Nov. 9, 1933. e. Tulane Univ. Child actor on stage 1946–50; radio, 1950–51. 1955–64, radio, TV personality. Made films in France and U.S. 1949–56. Producer from 1964–present.

POST, TED: Producer, director. b. Brooklyn, N.Y., dir. many stage plays; dir. CBS-TV Repertoire Thea.; Producer-dir., NBC-TV Coney Island of the Mind.
TV: Studio One, Ford Theatre, Playhouse of Stars, Fred Astaire Show, Gunsmoke, Rawhide, Twilight Zone, Wagon Train, Combat, Peyton Place, Alcoa, Defenders, Route 66, Baretta, and Columbo. Movies: Dr. Cook's Garden, Girls in One Office, Cagney & Lacey, Night Slaves, Five Desperate Women, Stagecoach, etc.
MINI-SERIES: Rich Man, Poor Man.
PICTURES INCLUDE: Go Tell The Spartans, Magnum Force, Hang 'em High, Beneath The Planet of the Apes, The Harrad Experiment, Good Guys Wear Black, Whiffs.

POSTER, STEVEN: Cinematographer. e. L.A. Art Center Coll. Started as commercial cinematographer before moving into feature films.
PICTURES: Blood Beach, Dead and Buried, Spring Break, Strange Brew, Testament, The New Kids, The Heavenly Kid, Blue City, The Boy Who Could Fly, etc.

POTTER, BRIDGET: Executive. Married, author Robert Wool. Served as assoc. prod. of Dick Cavett Show; in chg. TV development for Palomar Pictures Intl. Joined ABC-TV, being named v.p. of prime time program development—east coast. In 1980 appointed v.p., Lorimar Productions, in chg. of m.p. and TV development for east coast.

POTTLE, HARRY: Producton designer. b. London, England, 1925. e. Ealing College of Arts, Fleet Air Arm, 1944–47. Ent. m.p. ind. 1947. Designed Blind Date, 1960. Human Jungle, Avengers (TV series). Art Director, You Only Live Twice, Chitty Chitty Bang Bang, The Adventurers. Production Designer, 39 Steps, Murder by Degree, Bear Island, Matarese Circle, Desert King.

POTTS, ANNIE: Actress. e. Stephens Coll., Missouri. Began acting career in summer stock; on road in Charley's Aunt. Theatrical mp. debut, Corvette Summer (1978).
PICTURES: King of the Gypsies, Heartaches, Stick, Crimes of Passion, Ghostbusters, Pretty in Pink.
TELEVISION: Movies: Flatbed Annie and Sweety Pie, Cowboy, It Came Upon a Midnight Clear, etc.

POUND, LESLIE: Executive. Entered industry in 1943 as reporter on British trade paper, Screen International. Following military service in India and Singapore returned to work for that publication until 1952 when joined Paramount pub. office in London on the The Greatest Show on Earth. Named dir. of adv./pub. in U.K. for Paramount. 1958, retained Para. position when Cinema Intl. Corp. was formed. 1977, joined Lew Grade in ITC Entertainment as worldwide dir. of pub./adv. 1982, intl. pub. chief for Embassy Pictures in Los Angeles. 1983, named Paramount Pictures v.p., intl. mktg. for motion picture div., N.Y.

POWELL, CHARLES, M.: Executive. b. New York, Feb. 17, 1934. B.S. NYU/Journalism. Columbia Pictures National Publicity Manager, National Exploitation Manager, 1959–69. Paramount Pictures, National Publicity Coordinator, 1963–64. WNBC-Radio/TV, Advertising/Promotion Manager 1965. Director adv., pub. for M. J. Frankovich 1969–71. Joined MGM as dir. adv. pub.-expl. in 1972; named div. v.p. & corp. v.p., 1974; Columbia Pictures, v.p. advertising/publicity/exploitation 1975. Universal Pictures, sr. v.p., 1976–80. Powell & Young, m.p. consultants; exec. v.p. & dir., Color Systems Technology, Inc. Board of Governors, Acad. of Motion Picture Arts & Sciences, since 1973. Founder & President, Synagogue for the Performing Arts, L.A and Shofar Synagogue.

POWELL, DILYS C.B.E.: Journalist. b. Bridgenorth, England. e. Bournemouth H.S. & Somerville College, Oxford. Film critic, London Sunday Times 1939–1976; now critic films on TV; Film critic, Punch, frequent broadcaster, author of several books; member of Independent Television Authority, 1954–57. Mem., Cinematograph Films Council, 1965–69. BAFTA Award of Honor.

POWELL, JANE: Actress. r.n. Suzanne Burce. b. Portland, Ore., Apr. 1, 1929. Had own radio program over KOIN, Portland; singer on natl. networks; m.p. debut in Song of the Open Road, 1944, Star of Tomorrow, 1948.
PICTURES INCLUDE: Holiday in Mexico, Three Daring Daughters, Luxury Liner, Date With Judy, Nancy Goes to Rio, Two Weeks With Love, Royal Wedding, Rich Young and Pretty, Small Town Girl, Three Sailors and a Girl, Seven Brides for Seven Brothers, Athena, Deep in My Heart, Hit the Deck, Girl Most Likely, The Enchanted Island.
STAGE: Irene (Broadway, 1974).

POWELL, MICHAEL: Producer-Director-Writer. b. Canterbury, Kent, England, Sept. 30, 1905. Collaborated for many years with Emeric Pressburger in making films.
PICTURES INCLUDE: Writer only: Caste, Park Lane, The Star Reporter, Hotel Splendide, The Fire Raisers, Night of the Party, Lazybones, The Phantom Light, The Man Behind the Mask, etc. Writer-Producer-Director: The Edge of the World, The Spy in Black, The Thief of Baghdad, 49th Parallel, One of Our Aircraft is Missing, The Life and Death of Colonel Blimp, A Canterbury Tale, I Know Where I'm Going, A Matter of Life and Death, Black Narcissus, The Red Shoes, The Small Back Room, Gone to Earth, The Elusive Pimpernel, The Tales of Hoffman, Ill Met by Moonlihgt, Peeping Tom, Honeymoon, The Queen's Guards, They're a Weird Mob, Sebastian (prod. only), Age of Consent, The Boy Turned Yellow.

POWERS, MALA: Actress. r.n. Mary Ellen Powers. b. San Francisco, Calif., Dec. 29, 1921; p. George and Dell Powers, latter, dramatic coach. e. Max Reinhardt Dramatic School, Hollywood, Calif.; U. of Calif., Los Angeles. Pasadena Playhouse in For Keeps, 1946; Distant Isle; Actor's Lab, Hollywood; did considerable radio work.
PICTURES INCLUDE: Outrage, Edge of Doom, Cyrano de Bergerac, Rose of Cimarron, City Beneath the Sea, City That Never Sleeps, Geraldine, Yellow Mountain, Rage at Dawn, Bengazi, Tammy and the Bachelor, Storm Rider, Flight of the Lost Balloon, Daddy's Gone-A-Hunting.

POWERS, C. F. (MIKE) JR: Executive. b. San Francisco, March 6, 1923. e. at Park College, Mo., Columbia University, N.Y, graduated University of Oregon. Entered film business with P.R.C. in Portland, Oregon, 1947. Became Eagle Lion branch mgr. in Portland, 1950, and then United Artists. Moved to Seattle, Wash. as branch mgr. of 20th Century Fox, 1960. Was then western division mgr. for 20th Century Fox until 1967, then western division mgr. for Cinerama till 1973. Became exec. v.p., head film buyer for Robert L. Lippert Theatres, Transcontinental Theatres and Affiliated Theatres until 1978. Became western division mgr. for Filmways Pictures. President of Catholic Entertainment Guild of Northern Calif.; past Chief Barker of Variety Club Tent 32, San Francisco.

POWERS, STEFANIE: Actress. b. Hollywood, CA, Nov. 2, 1942. Theatrical m.p. debut in Among the Thorns. TV debut in The Girl from U.N.C.L.E. series.
PICTURES: Experiment in Terror, McClintock, Warning Shot, Escape to Athena..
TELEVISION: Feather and Father (series), Washington: Behind Closed Doors (mini-series), Hart to Hart (series). Movies: Family Secrets, Mistral's Daughter, Hollywood Wives, Deceptions.

PRAGER, ALICE HEINECKE: Music executive. b. N.Y.C., Aug. 2, 1930; d. Paul and Ruth (Colin) Heinecke; grad. Russell Sage Coll., 1951; grad. study N.Y.U. With SESAC, Inc., N.Y.C., 1946–, now exec. v.p., mng. dir.; pres. The Personal Touch, Inc. Named hon. citizen, Tenn., Fla.; Zonta, International Radio and TV Execs. Soc., Int'l & Am. (mem. adv. bd.) women in radio and TV, A.I.M., Broadcast Pioneers, Advertising Women of N.Y. (Editor, Ad Libber).

PRATLEY, GERALD: Commentator, b. and e. London, Eng. Joined Canadian Broadcasting Corp., 1946; writer, narrator and producer of The Movie Scene and Music from the Films; asst. member British Film Academy, dir. Canadian Film Institute 1953; chairman Toronto and District Film Council 1956; co-dir. & founder A.G.E. Film Society, Toronto; contributor to US and European film journals; film consult., Canadian Centennial Comm. Chmn., Canadian Film Awards; director, Stratford Film Festival; director, Ontario Film Institute, Toronto. Prof. of film, York Univ., Univ. of Toronto. Seneca College, McMaster Univ. Author: Cinema of John Frankenheimer; Otto Preminger; David Lean; John Huston, Torn Sprockets. Mem., classification board, Ontario Theatre branch. 1984, Mem. Advisory boards film depts., Humber College, Ryerson Polytechnical Institute; Mem. order of Canada, 1984.

PRATT, CHARLES A.: Executive. b. Chicago, Oct. 17, 1923. e. Culver Military Academy, 1942; Amherst College, 1949. Worked for General Foods and Alberto-Culver before joining NBC.; pres. Bing Crosby Productions.

PRELOCK, EDWARD P.: Executive. b. Cleveland, Ohio, Sep. 1, 1934. e. University of Kansas, B.A., 1958, J.D., 1963. Defensive end, Cleveland Brown and Saskatchewan Roughriders, 1958; personnel director, Transport Company of Texas, Honolulu, Hawaii, 1959–61; Justice of the Peace, Lawrence Township, Kansas, 1962–63; director of labor relations, Walt Disney Productions, 1964–75; was executive vice-president of Association of Motion Picture and Television Producers (AMPTP), 1975–77; first vice. pres., AMPTP, 1977–; President, Central Casting Corporation, 1976. Chairman of the Board, Contract Services Administration Trust Fund, 1976–; president, Animated Film Producers Association, 1971–; member, board of directors, Permanent Charities Committee of the Entertainment Industries, 1976–; member, board of directors, AMPTP, 1973–.

PRENTISS, PAULA: Actress, r.n. Paula Ragusa. b. San Antonio, Texas, March 4, 1939. e. Northwestern U.; Bachelor degree in drama, 1959; on TV in He & She; on stage in As You Like It, Arf!.

PICTURES INCLUDE: Where the Boys Are, The Honeymoon Machine, Bachelor in Paradise, Man's Favorite Sport, Catch 22, Move, The World of Henry Orient, In Harms Way, What's New Pussycat?, Scraping Bottom, Last of the Red Hot Lovers, The Parallax View, The Stepford Wives, The Black Marble, Buddy, Buddy.

PRESLE, MICHELINE: Actress. r.n. Micheline Chassagne. b. Paris, France, Aug. 22, 1922; e. Raymond Rouleau Dram. Sch. m.p. debut in Je Chante; on stage in Colinette. Am. Stram Gram, Spectacle des Allies; to U.S., 1945.
PICTURES INCLUDE: Jeunes Filles en Detresse, L'Histoire de Rire, La Nuit Fantastique, Felicie Nanteuil, Seul Amour, Faibalas, Boule de Suif, Jeux Sont Faix, Diable au Corps, Under My Skin, American Guerilla in the Phillippines, Adventures of Captain Fabian, Sins of Pompeii, House of Ricordi.

PRESSMAN, EDWARD R.: Producer. b. N.Y.C., ed. Fieldston School. grad., Stanford Univ.; studied at London School of Economics. Began career with film short, Girl, in collaboration with director Paul Williams in London. They formed Pressman-Williams Enterprises.
PICTURES INCLUDE: Out of It, The Revolutionary, Dealing: or the Berkeley to Boston Forty Brick, Lost Bag Blues, Sisters, Badlands (exec. prod.), Phantom of the Paradise; Paradise Alley (exec. prod.); Old Boyfriends (prod.); The Hand (prod.); Conan the Barbarian (exec. prod.); Crimewave (exec. prod.); Plenty (prod.).

PRESSMAN, LAWRENCE: Actor. b. Cynthiana, KY, July 10, 1939. e. Kentucky Northwestern Univ. On Bdwy. in Man in the Glass Booth, Play It Again, Sam, etc.
PICTURES: Man in the Glass Booth, The Crazy World of Julius Vrooder, Hellstrom Chronicle, Shaft, Making It, Nine to Five, Some Kind of Hero.
TELEVISION: Movies; Cannon, The Snoop Sisters, The Marcus-Nelson Murder, Winter Kill, The First 36 Hours of Dr. Durant, Rich Man, Poor Man, Man from Atlantis, Mulligan's Stew, The Trial of Lee Harvey Oswald, The Gathering, Like Mom, Like Me, Blind Ambition.

PRESSMAN, MICHAEL: Producer-Director. b. New York City, July 1, 1950. e. CA Inst. of Arts. Comes from show business family; was actor in college.
PICTURES INCLUDE: The Great Texas Dynamite Chase, The Bad News Bears Breaking Training, Boulevard Nights, Those Lips Those Eyes, Some Kind of Hero, Doctor Detroit.
TELEVISION: Like Mom, Like Me, The Imposter.

PRESTON, ROBERT: Actor. b. Newton Highlands, Mass., June 8, 1918. Pasadena Playhouse, m.p. debut, 1938 in King of Alcatraz.
PICTURES INCLUDE: Illegal Traffic, Disbarred, Union Pacific, Beau Geste, Typhoon, Moon Over Burma, Northwest Mounted Police, New York Town, Macomber Affair, Wild Harvest, Tulsa, Big City, Lady Gambles, Whispering Smith, Blood on the Moon, Sundowners, Best of the Bad Men, My Outlaw Brother, When I Grow Up, Cloudburst, Face to Face (Bride Comes to Yellow Sky), Last Frontier, Dark at the Top of the Stairs, The Music Man, Junior Bonner, Child's Play, Mame, Semi-Tough, "S.O.B.", Victor/Victoria, The Last Starfighter.
STAGE: The Music Man (Tony Award), A Lion in Winter, I Do, I Do (Tony Award), Mack and Mabel, Sly Fox, Theatre Hall of Fame.
TELEVISION: Movies: September Gun, Finnegan Begin Again, Rehearsal for Murder, Outrage.

PREUSTER, CHRISTOPHER W.: Executive. b. Newark, NJ Apr., 16, 1942. e. St. Peters Coll., Jersey City (1960–64). Pub. acct. to many film cos. (UA, Fox, Universal), while with Peat Marwick Mitchell, 1964–67; joined Walter Reade Organization, 1968; named pres. 1984.

PREVIN, ANDRE: Composer, Conductor. b. Berlin, Germany, Apr. 6, 1929; composed and conducted over 50 m.p. scores; currently music director, Pittsburgh Symphony Orchestra, & conductor emeritus of London Symphony Orchestra. Music Director, Royal Philharmonic Orch., from 1985. Guest conductor of most major symphony orchestras in U.S. and Europe.
PICTURES INCLUDE: Three Little Words, Cause for Alarm, It's Always Fair Weather, Bad Day at Black Rock, Invitation to the Dance, Catered Affair, Designing Woman, Silk Stockings, Gigi (Academy Award), Porgy and Bess (Academy Award), Subterraneans, Bells are Ringing, Pepe, Elmer Gantry, Four Horsemen of the Apocalypse, One Two Three, Two for the Seesaw, Long Day's Journey Into Night, Irma LaDouce (Academy Award), My Fair Lady (Academy Award), Goodbye Charlie, Inside Daisy Clover, Fortune Cookie, Thoroughly Modern Millie, Valley of the Dolls, Paint Your Wagon, The Music Lover, Jesus Christ Superstar.

PREVIN, STEVE: Producer, executive. b. New York, 1925. Film editor Universal studios 1941; to Europe 1951 as dir. Foreign Intrigue, TV series. Also dir. TV Sherlock Holmes, Captain Gallant, The Vikings; 1960 joined Disney, dir. Almost Angels, Waltz King, Escapade in Florence; 1965 Eon Productions; London, as TV exec.; joined Paramount in London as European; prod. exec.; 1967, Paramount, London, prod. exec.; 1969, Commonwealth United, London, Eur., prod. exec.; prod. exec. Don't Look Now; '74 from 1975 v.p. in charge of European production Filmways Pictures.

PRICE, FRANK: Executive. b. Decatur, IL, 1930. e. Michigan State Univ., following naval service. Joined CBS in N.Y. in 1951 as story editor and writer. Moved to Hollywood in 1954, serving as story editor first at Screen Gems and then NBC (Matinee Theatre). In 1959 joined Universal as an assoc. prod. and writer. In 1961 named exec. prod. of The Virginian TV series. Appt. exec. prod. of Ironside; later did It Takes a Thief and several World Premiere movies. In 1964 named v.p. of Universal TV; 1971, sr. v.p.; 1974, pres. Also v.p., MCA, Inc. In 1978 left to join Columbia as pres. of new company unit, Columbia Pictures Productions. In 1981 named chm. & CEO of Columbia Pictures. In 1983 joined Universal: named chm., motion picture group, pres. of Universal Pictures, and v.p. of MCA.

PRICE, ROGER: Performer. b. Charleston, W. Va., Mar. 6, 1920; e. U. of Michigan, American Acad. of Art, Max Reinhardt Dramatic Workshop. Appeared at many night clubs, many TV guest appearances; writing credits include the Don Knotts Show, Governor & J.J., Bob Hope, The Partners, The Bluffers. V.P. of Price, Stern, Sloan Publishers.
TV: Toast of the Town, Arthur Godfrey's Friends, Gary Moore Show, This Is Show Business, Jack Parr, Get Smart, Johnny Carson. creator of The Kallikaks (NBC); The Waltons, McMillan and Wife, Mike Douglas.
PICTURES: Mame, Day of the Locust, The Strongest Man in the World, Mixed Company, At Long Last Love, Pete's Dragon, The Devil and Max Devlin, Love on the Run.

PRICE, VINCENT: Actor. b. St. Louis, Mo., May 27, 1911; e. Yale U., U. of London, Nuremberg U.
PICTURES INCLUDE: The Song of Bernadette, Buffalo Bill, The Eve of St. Mark, Wilson, The Keys of the Kingdom, Laura, A Royal Scandal, Leave Her to Heaven, Dragonwyck, Shock, Long Night, Moss Rose, Three Musketeers, Rogues Regiment, The Web, The Bribe, Baron of Arizona, Champagne for Caesar, Bagdad, His Kind of Woman, Adventures of Captain Fabian, Las Vegas Story, House of Wax, Dangerous Mission, Mad Magician, Son of Sinbad, Serenade, While the City Sleeps, Mysterious House of Usher, Return of the Fly, The Bat, The Tingler, House on Haunted Hill, House of Usher, Pit and Pendulum, Tales of Terror, The Mask of the Red Death, War Gods of the Deep, Dr. Gold Foot and the Sex Machine, The House of 1,000 Dolls, More Dead Than Alive, The Oblong Box, Scream and Scream Again, Dr. Phibes, Dr. Phibes Rise Again!, Theatre of Blood, Madman, Scavenger Hunt, House of the Long Shadows.

PRIES, RALPH W.: Executive. b. Atlanta, Ga. August 31, 1919. Graduated Georgia Tech. Pres., MEDIQ/PRN Life Support Services, div. of MEDIQ, Inc. and former President, Ogden Food Service Corporation. Board Member: First Federal Savings & Loan of Philadelphia; National Foundation—March of Dimes; Moss Rehabilitation Hospital; St. Christopher's Hospital for Children; William Likoff Cardiovascular Institute of Hahnemann Medical College and Hospital; Police Athletic League; Motion Picture Pioneers; Board Member and Past International President: Variety Clubs International; Board Member: Will Rogers Hospital, Hahnemann Medical College & Hospital.

PRINCE, HAROLD: Director-Producer. b. New York, N.Y. Jan. 30, 1928. e. Pennsylvania U. Working as stage mgr. for George Abbott on three shows, later co-produced, produced and/or directed the following: The Pajama Game, Damn Yankees, New Girl In Town, West Side Story, Fiorello!, Tenderloin, Take Her, She's Mine, A Call on Kuprin, A Funny Thing Happened on the Way to the Forum, She Loves Me, The Matchmaker (revival), Fiddler On The Roof, Poor Bitos, Baker Street, Flora, The Red Menace, Superman, Cabaret, Zorba, Company, Follies, The Great God Brown, The Visit, Love for Love (the last three all revivals), A Little Night Music, Candide and Pacific Overtures, Side by Side by Sondheim, Some of My Best Friends, On the Twentieth Century and Evita (London, 1978, Broadway 1979, Los Angeles, Australia & Chicago, 1980; Vienna & Mexico City, 1981), Sweeney Todd (Broadway, 1979; London, 1980), Merrily We Roll Along, A Doll's Life, and also directed the operas Ashmadei, Silverlake, Sweeney Todd and Candide for N.Y. City Opera, Girl of Golden West for Chicago Lyric Opera Co. and San Francisco Opera; Willie Stark for Houston Grand Opera; Madame Butterfly for Chicago Lyric Opera and Turandot for Vienna State Opera. In 1984 directed two plays on Bdwy.: Play Memory, End of the World, Directed Grind (Bdwy. 1985); Diamonds (off-Bdwy, 1984).
MOVIES DIRECTED: Something for Everyone and A

Little Night Music. Authored: Contradictions, Notes on Twenty-Six Years in the Theatre (Dodd, Mead & Co., New York, 1974).

PRINCE, WILLIAM: Actor. b. Nichols, N.Y., Jan. 26, 1913; with Maurice Evans, actor, 2 yrs., radio announcer. On N.Y. stage, Ah, Wilderness; m.p. debut in 1943.
STAGE: Guest in the House, Across the Board on Tomorrow Morning, The Eve of St. Mark, John Loves Mary, As You Like It, I Am a Camera, Forward the Heart, Affair of Honor, Third Best Sport, The Highest Tree, Venus at Large, Strange Interlude, The Ballad of the Sad Cafe, Mercy Street.
PICTURES INCLUDE: Destination Tokyo, Cinderella Jones, The Very Thought of You, Roughly Speaking, Objective Burma, Pillow to Post, Lust for Gold, Cyrano de Bergerac, Secret of Treasure Mountain, Macabre, Sacco and Vanzetti, The Heartbreak Kid, The Stepford Wives, Rollercoaster, The Cat from Outer Space, The Promise, Kiss Me Goodbye, Spies Like Us.

PRINCIPAL, VICTORIA: Actress. b. Fukuoka, Japan, Jan 3, 1945. Began dramatic studies with Max Croft in Springfield, MA and with Al Sacks in Miami, FL. Went to New York to become model; left for Hollywood. Film debut in The Life and Times of Judge Roy Bean (1972).
PICTURES INCLUDE: The Naked Ape, Earthquake, I Will, I Will . . . for Now, Vigilante Force.
TELEVISION: Fantasy Island (pilot), Love Story, Love, American Style, Greatest Heroes of the Bible, Dallas. Movies: The Night They Stole Miss Beautiful, Delaney.

PRINE, ANDREW: Actor. b. Jennings, FL, Feb. 14, 1936. e. univ. of Miami. On stage on Look Homeward, Angel, Mind Over Murder, etc.
PICTURES: Advance to the Rear, Company of Cowards, Generation, The Devil's Brigade, Chisum, Grizzly, The Evil, Eliminators.
TELEVISION: Movies: Split Second to an Epitaph, Along Came a Spider, Night Slaves, Wonder Woman, Law of the Land, Tail Gunner Joe, Last of the Mohicans, Christmas Miracle in Caulfield, U.S.A., Donner Pass: The Road to Survival, V: The Final Battle.

PRIZEK, MARIO: TV Producer-director. b. Edmonton, Alberta, Canada, 1922. e. U. of Alberta, U. of British Columbia.
TV: Bamboula, Parade, Socrates, A Month in the Country, The Diary of a Scoundrel, Peer Gynt, Queen After Death, The Unburied Dead, Gianni Schicci (opera), Colombe, Ring Around the Moon, Three Sisters, The Zoo Story, The Dumb Waiter, Gallileo.

PROSKY, ROBERT, Actor. b. Philadelphia. Won TV amateur talent search contest, leading to scholarship with American Theatre Wing. Had leading roles in over 35 stage plays, including Death of a Salesman, Galileo, The Caucasian Chalk Circle, You Can't Take it With You, etc.
PICTURES INCLUDE: Thief, Hanky Panky, Monsignor, The Lords of Discipline, Christine, The Keep, The Natural.
TELEVISION: World War III, The Ordeal of Bill Carny, Lou Grant.

PROVINE, DOROTHY: Actress. b. Deadwood, S.D., Jan. 20, 1937; e. U. of Washington.
TV: The Alaskans, The Roaring 20's.
PICTURES INCLUDE: The Bonnie Parker Story, It's A Mad, Mad, Mad World, Good Neighbor Sam, The Great Race, That Darn Cat, Who's Minding the Mint?

PRYCE, JONATHAN: Actor. b. North Wales, 1947. e. RADA. On stage in Comedians, Taming of the Shrew, Antony and Cleopatra, Comedians, etc.
PICTURES: Voyage of the Damned, Breaking Glass, Loophole, Praying Mantis, The Ploughman's Lunch, Something Wicked This Way Comes, Brazil.
TELEVISION: Comedians, Playthings, Partisans, For Tea on Sunday, Timon of Athens, Murder Is Easy, etc.

PRYOR, RICHARD: Actor. b. Peoria, IL, Dec. 1, 1940. At age 7 played drum with professionals. Appearances on TV (Johnny Carson, Merv Griffin, Ed Sullivan) established him as standup comic. Wrote TV scripts for Lily Tomlin and Flip Wilson; co-author of film, Blazing Saddles. Several albums are best-selling hits.
PICTURES INCLUDE: Actor: Lady Sings the Blues, Bingo Long and the Travelin' All Stars, Silver Streak, Greased Lightning, Which Way Is Up?, Blue Collar, The Wiz, California Suite, Wholly Moses, In God We Trust, Stir Crazy, Bustin' Loose (star, co-prod.), Live on Sunset Strip, Some Kind of Hero, The Toy (also s.p., dir.), Brewster's Millions, Jo Jo Dancer Your Life Is Calling (also prod.-dir.-s.p.), Critical Condition.

PRYOR, THOMAS M.: Journalist. b. New York, NY, May 22, 1912. Joined NY Times, 1929; m.p. dept. 1931 as reporter, editor, asst. film critic; Hollywood bureau chief, corres., NY Times, 1951–59; editor, Daily Variety, 1959.

PTAK, JOHN: Agent. b. San Diego, CA. Graduated UCLA Film Department in 1968. Theatre mgr. and booker for Walter Reade Organization and Laemmle Theatres, 1966–1969. Admin. exec. at American Film Institute's Center for Advanced Studies, 1969–1971. Agent at the International Famous Agency (ICM), 1971–1975. Vice Pres., William Morris Agency, 1976 to present, representing motion picture and television talent. Responsible for the initial representation of such films as Jaws, The Sting, Taxi Driver, Close Encounters of the Third Kind, Coal Miner's Daughter, Airplane, and Gallipoli. Consultant for the National Endowment of the Arts.

PURCELL, PATRICK B.: Executive. b. Dublin, Ireland, Mar. 16, 1943. e. Fordham Univ. (MBA 1973). In pub. & acct., England, 1969–69; acct., Associated Hosp. Service, N.Y.C., 1968–70; joined Paramount Pictures, 1970; v.p., fin., 1980–83; exec. v.p. fin. & admin. 1983–.

PURDOM, EDMUND: Actor. b. Welwyn Garden City, England, Dec. 19, 1924. e. St. Ignatius Coll., London. Played leads, character roles for Northampton Rep. Co., Kettering Rep., two seasons at Stratford-On-Avon; London stage in Way Things Go, Malade Imaginaire, Romeo and Juliet, played in Caesar and Cleopatra, Anthony and Cleopatra, London and N.Y.; TV and radio appearances N.Y. & London.
PICTURES INCLUDE: Titanic, Julius Caesar, Student Prince, The Egyptian, Athena, The Prodigal, King's Thief, Moment of Danger, Rasputin, The Comedy Man, The Beauty Jungle, Don't Open Till Christmas (also dir.).

PURDY, RAI: Producer. b. London, Eng., Nov. 10, 1910; e. Canada. Owned & operated Rai Purdy Prod., Toronto for 12 yrs. Canada's largest ind. radio prod. co.: dir. narr., Out of the Night; C.O. of Canadian Army Shows. Overseas, with rank of Lt. Col., 1950–56 prod. dir. CBS N.Y.; dir. prog. Scottish TV Ltd., Glasgow, 1957–60 TV prod. Toronto, Canada, 1960.

PUTTNAM, DAVID CBE D. Lih.: Producer. b. London, England 1941. e. Michenden School. In advertising before joining VPS/Goodtimes Prod. Co. Dir. of Britain's National Film Finance Corp. Also served on Cinema Films Council and governing council of the British Academy of Film & Television Arts. Governor of National Film School. 1986, appt. Chm. & CEO, Columbia Pictures.
PICTURES INCLUDE: Melody, The Pier Piper, That'll Be The Day, Stardust, Mahler, Bugsy Malone, The Duellists, Midnight Express, Chariots of Fire, Local Hero, Cal, The Killing Fields. The Mission, Defence of the Realm. Co-produced documentaries: Swastika, James Dean—The First American Teenager, Double-Headed Eagle, Brother, Can You Spare a Dime?
TELEVISION INCLUDES: P'Tang Yang Kipperbang, Experience Preferred, Secrets, Those Glory Glory Days, Sharma and Beyond, Winter Flight.

PYKE, REX: Film-Television Producer/Director. Recent productions include Akenfield, Landscape, Eric Clapton's Rolling Hotel, Van Morrison in Ireland and Woodstock in Europe 1979.

Q

QUAID, DENNIS: Actor. b. Houston, TX Apr. 9, 1954. e. Houston Univ. Appeared in Houston stage productions before leaving for Hollywood. Movie debut: September 30, 1955 (1978). On N.Y. stage in True West, 1984.
PICTURES INCLUDE: Crazy Mama, Our Winning Season, Seniors, Breaking Away, Gorp, The Long Riders, All Night Long, Caveman, The Night the Lights Went Out in Georgia, Tough Enough, Jaws 3-D, The Right Stuff, Dreamscape, Enemy Mine.
TELEVISION: Bill: On His Own.

QUAID, RANDY: Actor. b. 1950. Discovered by Peter Bogdanovich while still jr. at Drama Dept. at Univ. of Houston and cast in his The Last Picture Show (1971).
PICTURES INCLUDE: What's Up, Doc?, Paper Moon, Lolly-Madonna XXX, The Last Detail, The Apprenticeship of Duddy Kravitz, Breakout, The Missouri Breaks, Bound for Glory, The Choirboys, Midnight Express, The Long Riders, Heartbeeps, The Wild Life, The Slugger's Wife, Fool for Love.
TELEVISION: A Streetcar Named Desire.

QUALEN, JOHN: Actor. b. Vancouver, B.C., 1899. m. Pearle Larson, 1924. Daughters: Meredith Kilpatrick, Kathleen Roberts, Elizabeth Bacon. e. studied declamation under Eliss Day; bachelor of oratory, also degree in dietetics. Played piano, flute & saxo U.S. phone in concert tours, Canada & On stage in Street Scene, Counsellor at Law, (later in film versions); m.p. debut in Arrowsmith.
TV: Mr. Ed, Andy Griffith Show, Hazel, Danny Thomas Show, Partridge Family.

PICTURES INCLUDE: Casablanca, Adventure, The Fugitive, Grapes of Wrath, My Girl Tisa, Big Steal, Jackpot, Woman on Run, Flying Missile, Belle Le Grand, Hans Christian Andersen, Ambush at Tomahawk Gap, I the Jury, Student Prince, High & the Mighty, Passion, Unchained, Sea Chase, At Gunpoint, The Searchers, Johnny Concho, Country Doctor, Two Rode Together, The Man Who Shot Liberty Valance, The Prize, The Seven Faces of Dr. Lao, Cheyenne Autumn, Sons of Katie Elder, Patch of Blue, Big Hand for the Little Lady, Firecreek, Criss Cross.

QUAYLE, ANTHONY: Actor, stage producer. b. Lancashire, England, 1913. Early career acting Old Vic Co., Elsinore and on tour Continent, North Africa. Army service, 1939–45; joined Stratford Memorial Theatre as director & actor 1948; many plays and acted Shakespearean roles; m.p. debut 1955, Oh Rosalinda; many TV credits in U.S. & England; Moses, David & Saul, Q.B. VII (Emmy). Recent TV: Ice Age, Henry IV, Masada, The Manions of America, The Last Bottle in the World, Testament of John, Lace, Last Days of Pompeii.
PICTURES INCLUDE: Battle of the River Plate, The Wrong Man, No Time for Tears, Woman in a Dressing Gown, The Man Who Would Not Talk, Ice Cold in Alex, Serious Charge, Tarzan's Greatest Adventure, Guns of Navarone, H.M.S. Defiant, Lawrence of Arabia, The Fall of the Roman Empire, East of Sudan, Operation Crossbow, MacKenna's Gold, Before Winter Comes, Anne of a Thousand Days, Everything You Always Wanted to Know About Sex*, Bequest to the Nation, Tamarind Seed, The Eagle Has Landed, Murder by Decree. Dial M for Murder, Key to Rebecca, Quoth the Raven, Oedipus at Colonnus.

QUEEN, ROBERT I.: Writer, author, publicist. b. Aug. 12, 1919; e. CCNY, 1942; reporter, Bronx Home News, 1936–41; information & editorial specialist, U.S. Civil Service (pub. rel.) 1942–55; admin. asst. to pres., Cinema Diorama Adv. Agency in chg., Radio-TV-Press Rel., 1955–56; night copy, headline ed., Journal of Commerce, 1956; dir., Radio-TV 1956–58, Greater New York Fund, writer of GNYF documentaries, GNYF variety shows and panel interview shows. Writer Nick Kenny WABD-TV shows; Operation Maverick, WPIX-TV Army Recruiting Service series; Suspense and The Web shows as free lance writer, CBS Radio Network Press Inf. Dept., copy ed. 1958, 1959 Press Consult. Cong. Alfred E. Santangello, 1960–63; Author: Emigres in Wartime, 1940; Creative PR in Planning Spec. Events Planning Special Events, 1958; co-author with wife, Elephant Comes to Play; own pub. rel. firm, 1955–73; p.r. counsel to NYC Transit Police PBA (1967–69); p.r. counsel-legislative aide, Hon. Thomas J. Manton (D. Queens) 1971; p.r. council, 1971–72, Councilman Morton Povman, 1971; p.r. counsel to State Sen. John R. Dunne (1969–70); teaching consult., Sch. of Contin. Prof. Studies, Pratt Institute; N.Y., N.J. Corres. Press Wire Services, Pub. rel. consultant. 1972, Thomas J. Manton Campaign for Congress; (1973–75) Public Affairs Officer, The Methodist Hospital in Brooklyn and concurrently, Community Relations-Public Relations Aide to State Assemblyman Leonard P. Stavisky, Chairman, Committee on Education; (1973–77) Public Relations Counsel to N.Y. State Senator Jeremiah B. Bloom; 1977 to 1979. Public relations counsel, Jeremiah B. Bloom for Governor Campaign, (1978). P.R. Counsel to N.Y. State Assemblyman Saul Weprin (1979 to date).

QUICK, ROBERT E.: Executive. b. Milwaukee, Wis., Aug. 8, 1917. Joined Loew's Inc., while attending Marquette U.; 1936–42, Loew's Inc., ad sales mgr. booker, apprentice salesman; 1943, adm. asst. Seattle and St. Louis Regional Offices, AAFMPS (formerly Army M.P. Service); 1945, mgr., New Orleans branch. AAFMPS: 1946, gen. man., MIDPAC M.P.S., Hawaii; 1948, ex. asst., HQ AAFMPS, Washington, D.C.; 1949, chief, European M.P.S., Nurenburg, Germany; 1952, dep. chief, AAFMPS Worldwide, Washington, D.C.; 1958, chief, AAFMPS Worldwide.

QUIGLEY, MARTIN, JR.: Educator-writer. b. Chicago, Ill., Nov. 24, 1917. e. A.B. Georgetown Un; M.A., Ed. D, Columbia U., M.P. Herald, Oct. 1939; spcl. ed. rep., M.P. Herald & M.P. Daily, May, 1941; wartime film work in U.S., England, Eire & Italy, Dec. 1941–Oct. 1945; assoc. ed., Quigley Pub., Oct. 1945; ed. M.P. Herald, July, 1949; also edit. dir. of all Quigley Pub., 1956; pres. Quigley Pub. Co., 1964; author, Great Gaels, 1944, Roman Notes, 1946, Magic Shadows—the Story of the Origin of Motion Pictures, 1948. Editor, New Screen Techniques, 1953; m.p. tech. section, Encyclopedia Brit., 1956; co-author, Catholic Action in Practice, 1963. Co-author: Films in America, 1929–69, 1970. Pres., QWS, Inc., educational consultants, 1975–81. Adjunct professor of higher education, Baruch Univ. City of New York. Village of Larchmont, N.Y., trustee, 1977–79; mayor, 1980–84. Board of managers, American Bible Society, 1984–; Religious Education Ass'n., treasurer, 1975–80 & Chairperson, 1981–84; Laymen's Nat'l. Bible Committee, chm. education committee, 1983–; Will Rogers Institute, chm. Health education committee, 1980–.

QUIGLEY, WILLIAM J.: Executive. b. New York City, July 6, 1951. e. Wesleyan Univ. (BA), Columbia Univ., (M.S.) 1983. From 1973 to 1974 was advt. circulation mgr. for Quigley Publishing Co. Taught school in Kenya in 1974; returned to U.S. to join Grey Advt. as media planner. In 1975 joined Walter Reade Organization as asst. film buyer; promoted to head film buyer in 1977. Named v.p., 1982. In 1986 joined Vestron, Inc. as sr. v.p. to establish Vestron Pictures.

QUILLAN, EDDIE: Actor. b. Philadelphia, Pa., March 31, 1907; p. Sarah Owen and Joseph Quillan, professionals; stage training playing in the Quillan act with his family. On the screen in Up and At 'Em.
PICTURES INCLUDE: Night Work, Big Money, A Little Bit of Everything, The Big Shot, Dark Mountain, This Is the Life, Moonlight and Cactus, Song of the Sarong, A Guy Could Change, Sensation Hunters, Sideshow, Brigadoon, Did You Hear the One About the Traveling Saleslady?, Angel in My Pocket, How to Frame a Figg.

QUINE, RICHARD: Actor. b. Detroit, Mich., Nov. 12, 1920. In U.S. Coast Guard during WW II; in vaudeville 6 yrs.; also on radio in 1938. NY stage debut in Very Warm for May, then in My Sister Eileen. First appearance on screen in The World Changes, 1932; variously acted, prod. & dir. many films.
PICTURES INCLUDE: Babes on Broadway, Tish, My Sister Eileen, For Me and My Gal, Dr. Gillespie's New Assistant, Stand By for Action, We've Never Been Licked, Rookie Fireman, Sunny Side of the Street, Purple Heart Diary, Rainbow Round My Shoulder, Sound Off, All Ashore, Cruisin' Down the River, Pushover, So This is Paris, Solid Gold Cadillac, Full of Life, Mad Ball, Drive a Crooked Road, Bell Book and Candle, It Happened to Jane, Strangers When We Meet, The World of Suzie Wong, Notorious Landlady, Paris When It Sizzles, Sex and the Single Girl, How to Murder Your Wife, Synanon. Oh Dad Poor Dad Mama's Hung You In The Closet and I'm Feeling So Sad, Hotel (dir.), A Talent for Loving (dir.), "W" (dir.), Prisoner of Zenda (dir.).
TV: The Jean Arthur Show (exec. prod.).

QUINLAN, KATHLEEN: Actress. b. Pasadena, CA., 1954. Played small role in film, One Is a Lonely Number, while in high school. Also did bit in American Graffiti. Major role debut in Lifeguard (1976).
PICTURES: Airport '77, I Never Promised You a Rose Garden, The Promise, The Runner Stumbles, Sunday Lovers, Hanky Panky, Independence Day, Twilight Zone—The Movie.
TELEVISION: When She Says No (movie).

QUINN, ANTHONY: Actor. b. Mexico, Apr. 21, 1915. Began on screen, 1936 Acad. Award, best supp. actor, Viva Zapata, 1952, Lust for Life, 1956.
PICTURES INCLUDE: Guadalcanal Diary, Buffalo Bill, Irish Eyes Are Smiling, China Sky, Back to Bataan, Where Do We Go From Here?, Black Gold, Tycoon, The Brave Bulls, Mask of the Avenger, The Brigand, World in His Arms, Against All Flags, Ride Vaquero, City Beneath the Sea, Seminole, Blowing Wild, East of Sumatra, Long Wait, Magnificent Matador, Ulysses, Naked Street, Seven Cities of Gold, La Strada, Attila the Hun, Lust for Life, Wild Party, Man from Del Rio, Ride Back, Hunchback of Notre Dame, The River's Edge, Hot Spell, Black Orchid, Last Train From Gun Hill, Warlock, Heller With a Gun, Heller in Pink Tights, Savage Innocents, The Guns of Navarone, Barabbas, Requiem for a Heavy-weight, Behold a Pale Horse, Zorba the Greek, High Wind in Jamaica, The Visit, Guns for San Sebastian, The Secret of Santa Vittoria, A Dream of Kings, Flap, A Walk in the Spring Rain, R.P.M.*, Across 110th Street, Deaf Smith and Johnny Ears, The Don Is Dead, Mohammad, Messenger of God, The Greek Tycoon, Caravans, The Passage, Lion of the Desert.

QUINN, STANLEY J., JR.: Producer, director. b. Brooklyn, N.Y., Mar. 18, 1915; e. Princeton U., 1932–36. Radio writer for Edgar Bergen show; mgr., J. Walter Thompson radio dept. in Australia, 1941–43; war corresp., 1943–45; radio prod. J. Walter Thompson, 1946; prod., dir., Kraft TV Theatre, NBC, 1947–53; ABC, Oct. 1953; vice pres., J. Walter Thompson, June 1954; exec. prod. Lux Video Theatre, 1954; pres. Quinn, McKenney Prod.; v.p. head radio, TV dept., D.C.S.&S.; prod., Grey Adv. for Revlon commercials. Dir. of Admin. MGM-TV Studios 1963–64; dir. Radio-TV Center U. of Conn. 1965–76. Commercial dir. Kraft Foods, 1964–72; Director, Radio/TV Div., CIMT, Univ. Conn., 1976–80. Freelance TV dir., 1980.

R

RABINOVITCH, MARTIN: Executive. b. Winnipeg, Canada, Sept. 25, 1944. e. Bachelor of Science, University of Manitoba, Master of Arts, Psychology, San Diego State University,

Doctor of Philosophy, University of Iowa. Consultant to U. S. Surgeon General's Scientific Advisory Committee on Television and Social Behavior. Entered industry in 1975 as Columbia Pictures-Jack Wodell adv. acc't exec.; as Twentieth Century Fox-Diener/Hauser acc't exec.; later with Disney Productions as dir. of mkt. planning and assoc. producer/mktg.—The Black Hole; v.p. in charge of adv. for Columbia Pictures; v.p./management dir. for Foote, Cone, & Belding Advertising; senior v.p., mktg., Embassy Pictures.

RABINOVITZ, JASON: Executive. b. Boston, MA., e. Harvard College (BA) where elected to Phi Beta Kappa. Following World War II service as military intelligence captain with paratroops, took MBA degree at Harvard Business School in 1948. Started in industry in 1949 as asst. to secty.-treas., United Paramount Theatres. Asst. controller, ABC, 1953; adm. v.p., ABC-TV, 1956; joined MGM as asst. treas., 1957; named MGM-TV gen. mgr., director of business & financial affairs, 1958; treas. & chief financial officer, MGM, Inc., 1963; advanced to financial v.p. & chief fianancial officer, 1967. In 1971 named exec. v.p., Encyclopedia Brittanica Education Corp.; sr. v.p., American Film Theatre, 1974–75. Rejoined MGM as v.p./exec. asst. to the pres., 1976. Elected v.p. finance, 1979; promoted to sr. v.p., finance & corporate admin., MGM Film Co. & UA Prods. Resigned, 1984. Now film & TV consultant and independent producer.

RACKMIL, MILTON R.: Executive. b. New York City. e. NYU Certified Public Accountant prior to assoc. with Brunswick Record Co. 1929; co-founder Decca Records, 1934; pres. Decca Records, 1949; pres. and member of board of dir. Universal Pictures, 1952, after Decca bought controlling stock interest in Universal; pres. emeritus, Universal, 1973.

RADIN, PAUL: Producer. b. N.Y.C. ed. N.Y.U. m. Writer Decla Dunning. After college went in adv. Became v.p. in chg. of m.p. div. of Buchanan & Co. During the war posted in Middle East as film chief for Office of War Information for that area. On return to U.S. assigned by Buchanan to ad campaign for Howard Hughes' The Outlaw. Turned to talent mgr., joining the Sam Jaffe Agency. Then joined Ashley-Famous Agency. Became exec. prod. for Yul Brynner's indep. prod. co. based in Switzerland, with whom made such films as The Journey, Once More with Feeling, Surprise Package.
PICTURES INCLUDE: Born Free, Living Free, Phase IV, The Blue Bird.

RADNER, GILDA: Actress-Writer. b. Detroit, June 28, 1946. Began career as part of Toronto's Second City improvisational group. Moved to New York when John Belushi invited her to work with him on National Lampoon Radio Hour for which she wrote and performed. Soon after joined TV's Saturday Night Live. Appeared in Bdwy. in one-woman show, Gilda Radner—Live from New York, which was filmed for theatrical movie.
PICTURES: First Family, Gilda Live, Hanky Panky, It Came from Hollywood, The Woman in Red, Movers and Shakers, Haunted Honeymoon.

RADNITZ, ROBERT B.: Producer. b. Great Neck, N.Y.; e. U. of Virginia. Taught 2 years at U. of Virginia, then became reader for Harold Clurman; wrote several RKO "This is America" scripts, then to Broadway where co-prod., The Frogs of Spring; prd. The Young and the Beautiful; to Hollywood working at United Artists, then as story consultant for 20th Century-Fox; prod. A Dog of Flanders (1960—first feature), first U.S. film to win Golden Lion Award at Venice Film Festival. Board of Directors, Producer Guild of America: v.p., last 3 years; first producer with retrospective at Museum of Modern Art. First producer honored by joint resolution of both houses of Congress, 1973. Sounder received four Academy Award nominations: best picture, best actor, best actress, best screenplay. Pres. Robert B. Radnitz Productions, Ltd. Vice pres., Producers Guild, 1982, 1984.
PICTURES INCLUDE: Misty, Island of the Blue Dolphins, And Now Miguel, My Side of the Mountain, The Little Ark, Sounder, Where the Lilies Bloom, Birch Interval, Sounder II, A Hero Ain't Nothin' But a Sandwich, Cross Creek (4 AA nominations).
TELEVISION: Mary White (Emmy for teleplay-nominated for best film) Christopher Award for TV special.

RAFELSON, BOB: Producer-Director-Writer. b. N.Y.C., 1935. After Army Service did program promotion for a radio station; then hired by David Susskind to read scripts. Became script supervisor of Play of the Week for Susskind and Ely Landau; wrote 34 adaptations for the series. Joined Screen Gems in California, developing program idea for Jackie Cooper, then head of TV prod. arm of Columbia. Later formed BBS Productions with Burt Schneider and Steve Blauner; their first film, Head.
PICTURES INCLUDE: Head (co-s.p); Five Easy Pieces (co-prod., dir.), The King of Marvin Gardens (prod.-dir.), Stay Hungry (co-prod., co-s.p., dir.), The Postman Always Rings Twice (co. prod.-dir.).

RAFFERTY, FRANCES: Actress. b. Sioux City, Iowa, June 26, 1922; e. U. of California, premedical student UCLA. TV show, December Bridge, CBS.
PICTURES INCLUDE: Seven Sweethearts, Private Miss Jones, Girl Crazy, War Against Mrs. Hadley, Thousands Cheer, Dragon Seed, Honest Thief, Mrs. Parkington, Barbary Coast Gent, Hidden Eye, Abbott and Costello in Hollywood, Adventures of Don Coyote, Money Madness, Lady at Midnight, Old Fashioned Girl, Rodeo, Shanghai Story.

RAFFIN, DEBORAH: Actress. b. Los Angeles, Calif., March 13, 1953. e. Valley College. Was active fashion model before turning to acting when discovered by Ted Witzer. Made m.p. debut in 40 Carats (1973).
PICTURES INCLUDE: The Dove, Once Is Not Enough, The Sentinel, Touched by Love, Death Wish 3.
TELEVISION: Haywire, Threesome, Sparkling Cyanide.

RAGLAND, ROBERT OLIVER: Composer. e. Northwestern Univ., American Conservatory of Music, Vienna Academy of Music. Professional pianist at Chicago nightclubs. In U.S. Navy; on discharge joined Dorsey Bros. Orchestra as arranger. On sls. staff at NBC-TV, Chicago. 1970, moved to Hollywood to become composer for movies; has scored 43 feature films plus many TV movies and series segments. Has also written some 15 original songs.
PICTURES: The Touch of Melissa, The Yin and Yang of Mr. Go, The Thing with Two Heads, Project: Kill, Abby, Seven Alone, The Eyes of Dr. Chaney, Return to Macon County, The Daring Dobermans, Shark's Treasure, Grizzly, Pony Express Rider, Mansion of the Doomed, Mountain Family Robinson, Only Once in a Lifetime, Jaguar Lives, The Glove, Lovely But Deadly, "Q", The Day of the Assassin, A Time To Die, Q, The Winged Serpent, Trial by Terror, The Guardian, Ten to Midnight, Dirty Rebel, Hysterical, Brainwaves, Where's Willie?, The Supernaturals.
TELEVISION: Photoplay's Stars of Tomorrow, Wonder Woman, Barnaby Jones, Streets of San Francisco, High Ice, The Girl on the Edge of Town, The Guardian, etc.

RAGSDALE, CARL V.: Director, producer. b. Illmo, Missouri, May 16, 1925. e. Washington U., St. Louis and Denison U., Ohio. U.S. Navy M.P. Officer, WW II and Korea; CPT, US Naval Reserve. v.p. industrial m.p. prod., Depicto Films, 1954–61; started Carl Ragsdale Associates, 1962; pres. and exec. prod. Sun Dial Films, Inc. 1963–69. Winner of Academy Award for Best Documentary Short of 1966. Nominated for Academy Award for Best Documentary Short of 1967.

RAILSBACK, STEVE: Actor. b. Dallas, TX. Studied with Lee Strasberg. On stage in Orpheus Descending, This Property Is Condemned, Cherry Orchard, Skin of Our Teeth, etc.
PICTURES: The Visitors, Angela, The Stunt Man, Turkey Shoot, The Golden Seal, Deadly Games, Torchlight, Lifeforce.
TELEVISION: Helter Skelter, From Here to Eternity.

RAINES, ELLA: Actress. r.n. Ella Wallace Raines Olds. b. Snoquainde Falls, Wash., Aug. 6, 1921. e. U. Wash. Winner dramatic scholarships; actress little theatre groups; on screen 1943 in Corvette K-225.
PICTURES INCLUDE: Phantom Lady, Enter Arsene Lupin, Hail the Conquering Hero, The Suspect, Strange Affair of Uncle Harry, Time Out of Mind, The Web, Brute Force, Senator was Indiscreet, Impact, Dangerous Profession, Walking Hills, Fighting Coast Guard, Ride the Man Down.

RAKOFF, ALVIN: Producer, director. b. Toronto, Canada. e. Toronto U. Early career as journalist. Dir. in French & U.S. T.V. England, Canada Emmy Award Winner, 1968 for Call Me Daddy. Emmy Award, 1983 for A Voyage Around My Father.
STAGE: Hamlet.
PICTURES INCLUDE: On Friday at 11, The Comedy Man, Crossplot, Hoffman, Say Hello to Yesterday, City of Fire, Death Ship, Dirty Tricks.
TV: The Caine Mutiny Court Martial, Requiem for a Heavyweight, Our Town, The Velvet Alley, A Town Was Turned to Dust, Jokers Justice, Call Me Back, Day Before Atlanta, Heart to Heart, The Seekers, Sweet War Man, The Move after Checkmate, The Stars in My Eyes, Call Me Daddy, Summer & Smoke, Don Quixote, Shadow of a Gunman, The Impeachment of Andrew Johnson, Cheap in August, In Praise of Love, Nicest Man in the World, Dame of Sark, The Kitchen, Romeo and Juliet, Voyage Round my Father, Mr. Halpern and Mr. Johnson, The First Olympics—Athens 1896, Paradise Postponed.

RAKSIN, DAVID: Composer. b. Philadelphia, Pa., Aug. 4, 1912. e. U. of Pennsylvania, studied music with Isadore Freed and Arnold Schoenberg. Composer of music for films, ballet, dramatic and musical comedy, stage, radio and TV, symphony orchestra and chamber ensembles. Arranger of music of Chaplin film, Modern Times; pres. Composers and Lyricists Guild of America, 1962–70; film cartoons include Madeline and The Unicorn in the Garden (UPA), professor of Music and Urban Semester, U.S.C., and Faculty, UCLA School of Music.

PICTURES INCLUDE: Laura, Secret Life of Walter Mitty, Smoky, Force of Evil, Across the Wide Missouri, Carrie, Bad and the Beautiful, Apache, Suddenly, Big Combo, Jubal, Hilda Crane, Separate Tables, Al Capone, Night Tide, Too-Late Blues, Best of the Bolshoi (music for visual interludes), Two Weeks in Another Town, The Redeemer, Invitation to a Gunfighter, Sylvia, A Big Hand for the Little Lady, Will Penny, Glass Houses, What's the Matter with Helen?

TV: Wagon Train, Five Fingers, Journey, Life With Father, Tender is the Night, Father of the Bride, Ben Casey, Breaking Point, Prayer of the Ages, Report from America, Medical Center, The Olympics (CBC).

RALSTON, GIL: Producer, writer. b. Los Angeles, 1912. e. American Acad. N.Y. stage, mgr. Broadway shows, then writer dir., NBC radio; radio dir., exec. prod. Proctor and Gamble, radio shows include Ransom Sherman Show, Junior Miss, Truth or Consequences, Lowell Thomas, Red Skelton Show independent TV prod, packaging firm exec. prod. 1948; exec. prod. CBS-TV dramatic shows, N.Y.; dir. network programs, N.Y. CBS-TV 1956. Exec. prod. High Adventure, 1957; writer, Naked City, Route 66, Ben Casey.

TV: Cavalcade of America, General Electric Theatre, Suspense.

RALSTON, RUDY: Producer. b. Prague, Czechoslovakia, Jan. 30, 1918. e. grad. eng. Realka U. Came to U.S. & joined Consolidated Lab.; exec. Republic Prod.; prod. Republic, 1950.

PICTURES INCLUDE: No Man's Woman, Double Jeopardy, Terror at Midnight, Hell's Crossroads, The Lawless Eighties, Last Stagecoach West, Man Who Died Twice.

RAMPLING, CHARLOTTE: Actress. b. Sturmer, England, Feb. 5, 1946. e. Jeanne D'Arc Academie pour Jeune Filles, Versailles; St. Hilda's, Bushey, England. Ent. m.p. ind. 1966. TV credits include: Six More for BBC, The Superlative Seven—Avenger series, Mystery of Cader Iscom, The Fantasists, What's in it for Henry, Zinotchka, Sherlock Holmes, Infidelities.

PICTURES INCLUDE: The Knack, Rotten to the Core, Georgy Girl, The Long Duel, Sequestro di Persona, The Damned, Three, Ski Bum, Corky, Tis Pity She's a Whore, The Six Wives of Henry VIII, Asylum, The Night Porter, Giordano Bruno, Zardoz, Caravan to Vaccares, Yuppi Dui La Chair De L'orchidee, Farewell My Lovely, Foxtrot, Orca, The Mauve Taxi, Stardust Memories, The Verdicta, Viva La Vie, Angel Heart.

RAMSAY, PATRICK: b. Bristol, Eng., 1926. e. Marlborough College and Jesus College, Cambridge (M.A. History), Eng. Served with Royal Naval Volunteer Reserve (Fleet Air Arm) 1944–46. Joined British Broadcasting Corporation 1949 as a report writer in monitoring service. Became assistant, appointments dept., 1953 and three years later re-joined BBC External Services as senior administrative assistant. In charge of news administration, radio and television 1958 to 1963, helping develop the U.K. regional television news network for BBC. 1963, appointed planning manager (projected arrangements), television. 1966 assistant controller, programme services, television, then assistant controller, program planning, television, from December 1969. Controller, programme services, television, April 1972. Appointed controller, BBC-Scotland, May 1979.

RAND, HAROLD: Executive. b. N.Y., Aug. 25, 1928. e. L.I.U., B.S. 1948–50; City Coll. of N.Y., 1945–46; U.S. Army 1946–48; ent. m.p. ind. 1950, pub. dept. 20th-Fox; variety of posts incl. writer, trade press, newspaper contacts; joined Walt Disney's Buena Vista pub. mgr., 1957; pub. mgr. Paramount Pictures, 1959; formed own pub. rel. firm, 1961; dir. of pub. Embassy Picture Corp. 1962; dir. of world pub. 20th Century Fox 1962; resigned 1963; dir. of adv. & pub., Landau Co., 1963; dir. world pub., Embassy Pictures, 1964; est. Harold Rand & Co., Inc., 1966, pred. of p.r. & mktg. firm. Appt. mktg., dir., Kaufman Astoria Studios, 1984; elected v.p., 1985.

RANDALL, STEPHEN F.: Executive. Held marketing posts with United Vintners and Clorox. Joined Columbia Pictures in 1978 as director of research; named v.p. in 1980 and senior v.p. in 1982. 1983, joined Tri-Star Pictures as snr. v.p. of marketing; promoted to exec. v.p.

RANDALL, TONY: Actor. b. Tulsa, Okla, Feb. 26, 1920. e. Northwestern U. Prof. N.Y. debut as actor in Circle of Chalk; then in Candida and others; U.S. Army 1942–46; radio actor on many shows.

STAGE: Corn is Green, Anthony & Cleopatra, Caesar & Cleopatra, Inherit the Wind, Oh Men Oh Women, Oh Captain, The Sea Gull, The Master Builder.

PICTURES INCLUDE: Oh Men Oh Women, Will Success Spoil Rock Hunter, No Down Payment, The Mating Game, Pillow Talk, Adventures of Huckleberry Finn, Let's Make Love, Lover Come Back, Boys' Night Out, 7 Faces of Dr. Lao, Send Me No Flowers, Fluffy, The Alphabet Murders, Bang! You're Dead, Hello Down There, Everything You Always Wanted to Know About Sex*, Foolin' Around, Scavenger Hunt, The King of Comedy.

TV: One Man's Family, TV Playhouse, Mr. Peepers, Max Liebman Spectaculars, Sid Caesar, Dinah Shore, Playhouse 90, Odd Couple, The Tony Randall Show.

RANDOLPH, ELSIE: Actress, singer. b. London, England, Dec. 9, 1904. London stage debut 1919 in The Girl for the Boy. M.p. debut 1932 in Alfred Hitchcock's Rich and Strange.

STAGE: (London): Battling Butler, Toni, Madame Pompadour, Boodle, Sunny, Peggy-Ann, That's a Good Girl, Follow Through, Wonder Bar, Stand Up and Sing, Mr. Whittington, This'll Make You Whistle, Room for Two, Top Hat and Tails, The Maid of the Mountains, It's Time to Dance, Great Day, Is Your Honeymoon Really Necessary?, No Other Verdict, The Lost Generation, What A Racket!, Lord Arthur Savile's Crime, The Cure for Love (1978).

PICTURES INCLUDE: Brother Alfred, Life Goes On, Rise and Shine, Night of the Garter, Yes, Mr. Brown, That's A Good Girl, This'll Make You Whistle, Smash and Grab, Cheer the Brave, Sky Riders, Frenzy (1972), Charleston (1977).

TV: Harper's West One, Stars and Garters, The Jimmy Logan Show, Fraud Squad, Tales of Piccadilly, Father Brown, Z-Cars, The Coffee Lace, Thriller, Within These Walls (1977), Edward and Mrs. Simpson (1978).

RANSOHOFF, MARTIN: Executive. b. New Orleans, La., 1927. e. grad., Colgate Univ. Adv., Young & Rubicam, 1948–49; slsmn, writer, dir., Gravel Films, 1951; formed own co., Filmways, 1952; industrial films, commercials; formed Filmways TV Prods., Filmways, Inc., Filmways of Calif. chmn., bd. Filmways, Inc., resigned from Filmways in 1972 and formed own independent motion picture and television production company.

TV: Mister Ed, The Beverly Hillbillies, Petticoat Junction, The Addams Family.

PICTURES INCLUDE: The Americanization of Emily, The Sandpiper, Boys Night Out, The Loved One, The Cincinnati Kid, See No Evil, Ten Rillington Place, King Lear, Topkapi, Fuzz, Castle Keep, Ice Station Zebra, Catch 22, Save The Tiger, The White Dawn, Silver Streak (exec. prod.), The Wanderers, Change of Seasons, American Pop, Hanky Panky, Class.

RAPF, MATTHEW: Producer, writer. b. New York City, Oct. 22, 1920; e. Dartmouth Coll., B.A. 1942; p. Harry Rapf, producer. U.S. Navy, World War II as Lt. (j.g.).

PICTURES INCLUDE: Adventures of Gallant Bess s.p., co-prod., assoc. prod., story, The Sellout; prod., Desperate Search, Big Leaguer, Half a Hero.

TV: Loretta Young Show, Frontier, Great Gildersleeve, The Web, Jefferson Drum, Man From Blackhawk, Two Faces West, Ben Casey, Slattery's People, Iron Horse, Young Lawyers, Hardcase, Terror In the Sky, Shadow On the Land, Marcus-Nelson Murders, Kojak, Switch, Doctor's Hospital, Eischied, Oklahoma City Rolls, Gangster Chronicles.

RAPHAEL, FREDERIC: Writer. b. Chicago, 1931. e. Charterhouse, St. John's College, Cambridge. First novel pub., 1956, subsequently, The Earlsdon Way, The Limits of Love, A Wild Surmise, The Graduate Wife, The Trouble With England, Lindmann, Orchestra and Beginners. 1970: Like Men Betrayed. 1971: Who Were You With Last Night. 1972: April, June and November. 1973: Richard's Things. 1975: California Time. 1976: The Glittering Prizes. 1979: Sleeps Six & Other Stories. Ent. m.p. ind., 1956. Several plays for ATV, 1960–62. First feature film credits 1964. Nothing But The Best; 1965, Darling; Ac. Awd. for original screenplay. 1967: Two For The Road, Far From The Madding Crowd. 1971: A Severed Head. 1974: Daisy Miller. 1976: The Glittering Prices, Rogue Male. 1978: Roses, Roses . . . ; School Play, Something's Wrong, The Oresteia of Aeschylus. 1979: From the Greek and An Early Life (plays); Best of Friends (TV); 1981: Richard's Things. Oxbridge Blues, a sequence of plays for BBc-TV, 1984.

RAPHEL, DAVID: Executive. b. Boulogne-s/Seine, France, Jan. 9, 1925; e. University in France. Entered m.p. ind. as asst. to sales mgr. in France, 20th-Fox, 1950–51; asst. mgr. in Italy, 1951–54; mgr. in Holland, 1954–57; asst. to European mgr. in Paris, 1957–59; European mgr. for TV activities in Paris, 1959–61; Continental mgr. in Paris, 1961–64, transferred to N.Y. as vice-pres. in chge. of international sales, 1964; named pres., 20th Century-Fox International, 1973. In Feb., 1975, also appointed senior vice-pres., worldwide marketing, feature film division, for 20th-Fox, headquartered in Los Angeles. In November, 1976, joined ICM, appointed director general of ICM (Europe) headquartered in Paris. In 1979 elected pres. ICM with headquarters in Los Angeles. 1980, formed Cambridge Film Group Ltd.

RAPPER, IRVING: Director. b. London, Eng.; e. New York U., B.A. Assoc. Gilbert Miller in Stage prod. dir. Animal Kingdom, Firebird, Five Star Final, etc.
PICTURES INCLUDE: Shining Victory, One Foot in Heaven, The Gay Sisters, The Adventures of Mark Twain, Rhapsody in Blue, The Corn is Green, Deception; Now, Voyager; Voice of the Turtle, Anna Lucasta, The Glass Menagerie, Another Man's Poison, Forever Female, Bad For Each Other, The Brave One, Marjorie Morningstar, The Miracle, Joseph and His Brethren, Pontius Pilate, The Christine Jorgensen Story, Born Again, Justus.

RAPPOPORT, GERALD J.: Executive-Film Producer. b. New York, N.Y., 1925. e. New York University. U.S. Marine Corps. 1955–1958—pres., Major Artists Representatives Corp.; 1958–1960—director of Coast Sound Services, Hollywood; 1957 to present, pres., Sewan Music Publishers. 1961 to present, repre., major Eastern European film producers. 1970 to present, dir., International Film Exchange Ltd., New York and Paris, and pres. of Family Entertainment Corp.

RATHER, DAN: News Correspondent. Joined CBS News in 1962 as chief of southwest bureau in Dallas. White House Correspondent, 1964 to 1974. Covered top news events, from Democratic and Republican national conventions to President Nixon's trip to Europe (1970) and to Peking and Moscow (1972). Anchored CBS Reports, 1974–75. Presently co-editor of 60 minutes (since 1975) and anchors Dan Rather Reporting on CBS Radio Network (since 1977). Winner of numerous awards, including 5 Emmys. Now anchorman on CBS-TV Evening New.

RAUCHER, HERMAN: Writer. b. Apr. 13, 1928. e. NY Univ. Author of novels—Summer of '42 and Ode to Billy Joe—adapted to films by him.
PICTURES: Sweet November, Hieronymus Merkin, Watermelon Man, Summer of '42, Class of '44, Ode to Billy Joe, The Other Side of Midnight.
TELEVISION: Studio One, Alcoa Hour, Goodyear Playhouse, Matinee Theatre, Master of the Game (Part One).

RAVELO, ROBERT F.: Executive. b. Santiago de Cuba, Oriente, Cuba, Aug. 30, 1947. Emigrated to U.S., 1961. e. Univ. of Connecticut (B.A.). 1966–69, band leader and Latin percussionist. 1969–74, Winchester Intl. Marketing Dept. 1976–77, U.S. Air Force; capt., 1977–81. Entered industry in 1981 as prod. asst. to Robert Towne during filming of Personal Best. Now v.p./sls., v.p. production and operating officer, Arista Films, Inc.

RAVETCH, IRVING: Director, scenarist, producer. m. Harriet Frank.
PICTURES INCLUDE: The Long Hot Summer, The Sound and the Fury, Home from the Hill, The Dark at the Top of the Stairs, Hud, Hombre, The Reivers (also prod.), Conrack (co s.p.), Norma Rae (co.-s.p.), Murphy's Romance (co-s.p.).

RAY, ALDO: Actor. r.n. Aldo DaRe. b. Pen Argyl, Pa., Sept. 25, 1926: e. U. of Calif. U.S. Navy, June, 1944–May, 1946: constable. Crockett, Calif., Nov. 1950–Sept. 1951: m.p. debut in Saturday's Hero.
PICTURES INCLUDE: Star of Tomorrow. 1954: since in Marrying Kind, Pat and Mike, Let's Do It Again, Miss Sadie Thompson, Battle Cry, We're No Angels, Three Stripes in the Sun, Nightfall, Men in War, God's Little Acre, Four Desperate Men, Day They Robbed the Bank of England, Sylvia, What Did You Do in the War Daddy?, To Kill A Dragon, Dead Heat on a Merry-Go-Round, Welcome To Hard Times, The Power, Green Berets, The Violent Ones, Angel Unchained, And Hope To Die, Psychic Killer, Seven Alone, Evils of the Night.

RAY, SATYAJIT: Director-Writer-Composer. b. India, May 2, 1921. Gained international acclaim for his Apu Trilogy in the '50s.
PICTURES: Pather Panchali, The Unvanquished, The Music Room, The World of Apu, The Goddess, Kanchenjunga, The Adventures of Goopy and Bagha, The Adversary, Company Limited, Distant Thunder, The Middle Man, The Chess Player, The Elephant God, The Kingdom of Diamonds, The Home and the World, etc.

RAYBURN, GENE: Performer, b. Christopher, Ill., Dec. 22. e. Knox Coll., Galesburg, Ill. NBC guide; with many radio stations in Baltimore, Philadelphia, N.Y.; U.S. Army Air Force, 1942–45, Rayburn and Finch, show, WNEW, NY., 1945–52; Gene Rayburn Show, NBC radio; TV shows: Many appearances as host-humorist on game shows, variety shows, drama shows. Summer stock: leads in comedies.
BROADWAY: Bye Bye Birdie, Come Blow Your Horn.
TV: Helluva Town, The Match Game, Love Boat, Fantasy Island, Tonite Show.

RAYE, MARTHA: Actress. b. Butte, Mont., Aug. 27, 1916. p. Reed and Hooper, professionals. On stage: sang and did comedy with Paul Ash's orchestra; was in Earl Carroll's Sketch Book; Lew Brown's Calling All Stars. Appeared in night clubs.
PICTURES INCLUDE: Rhythm on the Range, The Big Broadcast of 1937, Hideway Girl, College Holiday, Par, Waikiki Wedding, Mountain Music, Artists and Models, Double or Nothing, Par. Pin Up Girl, Four Jills and a Jeep, Monsieur Verdoux, Pufnstuf, The Concorde—Airport '79.
TV: All Star Revue, Martha Raye Show, NBC, Alice.

RAYMOND, GENE: Actor r. n. Raymond Guion, b. N.Y.C., Aug. 13, 1908. Air Force Reserve, WW II; formed ind. prod. co., Masque Prod., 1949; Broadway starred Shadow of My Enemy, 1957, National Co., The Best Man 1960.
STAGE: Why Not?, The Potters, Cradle Snatchers, Take My Advice, Say When, Mirrors, Jones, Young Sinners.
PICTURES INCLUDE: Personal Maid, Ladies of the Big House, The Night of June 13th, Forgotten Commandments, If I Had A Million, Red Dust, Sadie McKee, Brief Moment, I am Suzanne, Flying Down to Rio, The House on 56th Street, Seven Keys to Baldpate, Hooray for Love, Zoo in Budapest, Behold My Wife, Mr. and Mrs. Smith, Walking On Air, Coming Out Party, Life of the Party, She's Got Everything, The Woman in Red, Ann Carver's Profession, Transient Lady, The Best Man.
TV: Star-host, TV Fireside Theatre and TV Reader's Digest; Lux Video Theatre, Robert Montgomery Presents, Climax, Playhouse 90, Kraft Theatre, Red Skelton, U.S. Steel Hour, Uncle, Girl from Uncle, Laredo, Ironsides, Julia, Judd, etc.

RAYMOND, PAULA: Actress. r.n. Paula Ramona Wright, b. San Francisco, Calif.: e. San Francisco Jr. Coll. 1942. Started career in little theatre groups, San Francisco; leading roles Ah! Wilderness, Peter Pan, other plays; model, Meade-Maddick Agency; TV appearance 1949.
PICTURES INCLUDE: Devil's Doorway, Inside Straight, Duchess of Idaho, Crisis, Grounds For Marriage, Tall Target, Texas Carnival, The Sellout, Bandits of Corsica, City That Never Sleeps, Beast from 20,000 Fathoms, King Richard & the Crusaders, Human Jungle, Gun That Won the West, The Flight That Disappeared, 5 Bloody Graves, Blood of Dracula's Castle.

RAYNOR, LYNN S.: Producer-Production Executive. b. 1940. Produced West Coast premiere of The Balcony by Genet, The Crawling Arnold Review by Feiffer. Joined Television Enterprises, 1965; Commonwealth United, 1968 as business affairs exec. later production supervisor. 1972 opened London branch of the Vidtronics Co. 1974, formed Paragon Entertainment. 1976, producer, PBS. 1977, producer, James Flocker Enterprises. 1979, exec. in charge of production, Lawrance Schiller Productions. 1981, producer, Polygram Pictures; 1984, producer, Newland-Raynor Prods.; 1985, Columbia Pictures TV.
TELEVISION: Waiting for Godot; Camp Wilderness (synd. series); Marilyn, The Untold Story (ABC 3-hour movie); The Execution (NBC); The Pete Gray Story (ABC).
PICTURES: Ghosts That Still Walk, Alien Encounters, Fanny Hill, Dangerously.

REAGAN, RONALD: Actor. b. Tampico, Illinois, Feb. 6, 1911. e. high school and Eureka College; m. Nancy Davis; lifeguard. Wrote weekly sports column for a Des Moines, Iowa newspaper; broadcast sporting events. Signed as actor by Warner Bros. in 1937. In World War II. 1942–45, capt., USAAF. Actor until 1966 on TV as well. Program supvr., General Electric Theatre, Death Valley Days. Gov., California, 1967–74. Businessman and rancher. Elected Pres. of U.S., 1980. Re-elected, 1984.
PICTURES INCLUDE: Love Is On the Air, Submarine D-1, Sergeant Murphy, Swing Your Lady, Accidents Will Happen, Cowboy from Brooklyn, Boy Meets Girl, Girls on Probation, Going Places, Dark Victory, Naughty but Nice, Hell's Kitchen, Kings Row, Juke Girl, Desperate Journey, This is the Army, The Killers, That Hagen Girl, Night Unto Night, Voice of the Turtle, John Loves Mary, Girl from Jones Beach, Hasty Heart, Louisa, Last Outpost, Bedtime for Bonzo, Storm Warning, Hong Kong, She's Working Her Way Through College, Winning Team, Tropic Zone, Law & Order, Prisoner of War, Cattle Queen of Montana, Tennessee's Partner, Hellcats of the Navy, The Killers (1964).

REARDON, BARRY: Executive. Began industry career with Paramount Pictures; named v.p.; left to join General Cinema Theatres Corp. as snr. v.p. Now with Warner Bros. as pres. of domestic distribution co.

REASON, REX: Actor. b. Berlin, Germany, Nov. 30, 1928. e. Hoover H.S., Glendale, Calif. Worked at various jobs; studied dramatics at Pasadena Playhouse.
PICTURES INCLUDE: Storm Over Tibet, Salome, Mission Over Korea, Taza Son of Cochise, This Island Earth, Smoke Signal, Lady Godiva, Kiss of Fire, Creature Walks

Among Us, Raw Edge, Miracle of The Hills, The Rawhide Trail.

REASONER, HARRY: News correspondent. b. Dakota, Iowa. Apr. 17, 1923; e. Stanford Univ., Univ. of Minnesota. Beg. journalism career, reporter, Minneapolis Times 1941–43; U.S. Army, WW II. Ret. to Times, drama critic 1946–48. Author, book, Tell Me About Women, 1946; newswriter, radio station WCCO. CBS affiliate. Minn., 1950–51; writer U.S. Information Agency Manila, 1951–54; news-dir., KEYD-TV (now KMSP-TV). Minn., 1954; Joined CBS News, N.Y., 1956; ABC News 1970–78. Rejoined CBS 1978; co-editor, 60 Minutes.

REDDY, HELEN: Singer. b. Australia, Oct. 25, 1942. Parents were producer-writer-actor Max Reddy and actress Stella Lamond. e. in Britain. Began career at age four as singer and had appeared in hundreds of stage and radio roles with parents by age of 15. Came to New York City in 1966, subsequently played nightclubs, appeared on TV. First single hit record: I Don't Know How To Love Him (Capitol). Grammy Award, 1973, as best female singer of year for I Am Woman. Other Gold singles: Delta Dawn, Leave Me Alone, Angle Baby. Gold Albums: Love Song for Jeffrey, Free & Easy, No Way to Treat a Lady, I Don't Know How To Love Him, Music, Music. Platinum albums: I Am Woman, Long Hard Climb, Helen Reddy's Greatest Hits. Most Played Artist by the music operators of America; American Music Award 1974; Los Angeles Times Woman of the Year (1975); No. 1 Female Vocalist in 1975 and 1976; Record World, Cash Box and Billboard; one of the Most Exciting Women in the World because of her strong convictions, beauty and intelligence—International Bachelor's Society (1976).

PICTURES: Airport 1975 (debut), Pete's Dragon.

TV: David Frost Show, Flip Wilson Show, Mike Douglas Show, etc. The Helen Reddy Show (Summer, 1973, NBC), Permanent host of Midnight Special. Appearances on Tonight Show, Mac Davis Show. Hosted Merv Griffin Show, Sesame St.—Children's Workshop Prod., Tonight Show, Muppet Show.

REDELINGS, LOWELL E.: Columnist & Editor. b. Park Ridge, Ill.; e. U.S.C., B.S. Sports writer Hollywood Citizen-News 1935; sports ed. 1939; film ed. 1943–62; motion picture editor, Evening Outlook, Santa Monica, Feb. 1962–64; Film Columnist, Evening Outlook, to 1965; film drama critic, Los Angeles Herald-Examiner, 1965–66; Holly. Correspondent, Quigley Pub. Co., 1967; 1970–75, amusements ed. Retired.

REDFORD, ROBERT: Actor. b. Santa Monica, Calif., Aug. 18, 1937. University of Colorado, left to travel in Europe, 1957. Attended Pratt Institute and American Academy of Dramatic Arts. m. Lola Van Wangemen.

BROADWAY: Walk-on in Tall Story, also in The Highest Tree, Sunday in New York, Barefoot in the Park.

PICTURES INCLUDE: Warhunt, 1961; Situation Hopeless, But Not Serious, Inside Daisy Clover; The Chase, This Property Is Condemned, Barefoot in the Park, Tell Them Willie Boy is Here, Butch Cassidy and the Sundance Kid, Downhill Racer, The Crow Killer, The Hot Rock, The Candidate, Jeremiah Johnson, The Way We Were, The Sting, The Great Gatsby, The Great Waldo Pepper, Three Days of the Condor, All The President's Men, A Bridge Too Far, The Electric Horseman, Brubaker, The Natural, Out of Africa, Legal Eagles. Director: Ordinary People (AA).

TV: The Iceman Cometh, In the Presence of Mine Enemies, (Playhouse 90).

REDGRAVE, CORIN: Actor. b. London, England, July 16, 1939. e. Cambridge. Son of Sir Michael Redgrave. On stage with England Stage Co., plays including A Midsummer Night's Dream, Chips with Everything, Lady Windermere's Fan, Julius Caesar, Comedy of Errors, etc.

PICTURES: A Man for All Seasons, The Deadly Affair, Charge of the Light Brigade, The Magus, Oh What a Lovely War, When Eight Bells Toll, Serail, Excalibur, Eureka, etc.

REDGRAVE, LYNN: Actress. b. London, England, Mar. 8, 1943. Ent. m.p. and TV, 1962.

PICTURES INCLUDE: Tom Jones, Girl With Green Eyes, Georgy Girl, The Deadly Affair, Smashing Time, The Virgin Soldiers, The Last of the Mobile Hot-Shots, Viva la Muerta Tua, Every Little Crook and Nanny, Everything You Always Wanted to Know About Sex*, The National Health, The Happy Hooker, The Big Bus, Sunday Lovers, Home Front.

TV: Pretty Polly, Ain't Afraid to Dance, The End of the Tunnel, I Am Osango, What's Wrong with Humpty Dumpty, Egg On the Face of the Tiger, Blank Pages, A Midsummer Night's Dream, Pygmalion, Turn of the Screw, William, Vienna 1900, Daft as a Brush, Not For Women Only, Co-host U.S. talkshow (NBC). Movies: Seduction of Miss Leona, Gauguin, Beggerman Thief, Rehearsal for Murder, The Bad Seed, My Two Loves. Series: House Calls, Teachers Only, The Muppet Show.

REDGRAVE, VANESSA: Actress. b. London, England, Jan. 30, 1937. Early career with Royal Shakespeare Company. Ent. m.p. 1958 in Behind the Mask.

TV: A Farewell to Arms, Katherine Mansfield, Playing for Time, My Body, My Child, Three Sovereigns for Sarah, Peter the Great, Second Serve.

STAGE: Daniel Deronda, Cato Street, The Threepenny Opera, Twelfth Night, As You Like It, Taming of the Shrew, Cymbeline, The Sea Gull, The Prime of Miss Jean Brodie, Anthony & Cleopatra, Design for Living, Macbeth, Lady from the Sea.

PICTURES INCLUDE: Morgan, A Suitable Case for Treatment, A Man for All Seasons, Blow-up, Red and Blue, 1967 to Hollywood for Camelot, Charge of the Light Brigade, Isadora, Oh! What a Lovely War, The Seagull, A Quiet Place in the Country, Drop Out, Trojan Women, The Devils, La Vacanza, Mary Queen of Scots, Murder on the Orient-Express, Out of Season, Seven-per-cent Solution, Julia, Agatha, Yanks, Bear Island, Wagner, The Bostonians, Steaming.

REDSTONE, EDWARD S.: Exhib. b. Boston, Mass., May 8, 1928. e. Colgate U., B.A., 1949; Harvard Grad. School of Bus. Admin., M.B.A., 1952; v.p., treas., Northeast Drive-In Theatre Corp.; v.p., Theatre Owners of New England, 1962; chmn., advis. coms., mem. bd. dirs., TOA; gen. conven. chmn., joint convention TOA & NAC, 1962; pres. National Assn. of Concessionaires, 1963; chief barker. Variety Club of New England, 1963; pres., Theatre Owners of New England; gen. chmn., 35th annual reg. convention.

REDSTONE, MICHAEL: Exhibitor. b. Boston, Mass., Apr. 11, 1902. Built first drive-in in N.Y., 1938. Chief Barker of Variety Club of New England, 1957–58; treas. of Jimmy Fund; member of exec. comm. of the Children's Cancer Research Foundation. Chmn. of the board and treas., Northeast Theatre Corp., Boston. Trustee, Combined Jewish Appeal.

REDSTONE, SUMNER MURRAY: Theatre Executive-Lawyer; b. Boston, May 27, 1923; s. Michael and Belle (Ostrovsky) R.; B.A., Harvard, 1944, LL.B., 1947; children Brent Dale, Shari Ellin Korff. Admitted to Mass. Bar 1947; U.S. Ct. Appeals 1st Circuit 1950, 8th Circuit 1957, 9th Circuit 1948; D.C. 1951; U.S. Supreme Ct. 1952; law sec. U.S. Ct. Appeals for 9th Circuit 1947–48; instr. U. San Francisco Law School and labor Management School, 1947; special asst. to U.S. Atty. General, 1948–51; partner firm Ford, Bergson, Adams, Borkland & Redstone, Washington, D.C. 1951–54; exec. v.p. Northeast Drive-In Theatre Corp., 1954–68; pres. Northeast Theatre Corp.—; asst. pres., Theatre Owners America 1960–63, pres. 1964–65; bd. chm., National Association of Theatre Owners 1965–66; dir. ACE Prodns., Inc.; mem. Presidential Advisory Committee John F. Kennedy Center for the Performing Arts; chmn. Jimmy Fund, Boston 1960; met. div. Combined Jewish Philanthropies 1963; sponsor Boston Museum of Science; Trustee Children's Cancer Research Foundation; Art Lending Library; bd. dirs. Boston Arts Festival; v.p., exec. committee Will Rogers Memorial Fund; bd. overseers Dana Farber Cancer Institute; mem. corp. New England Medical Center; Motion Picture Pioneers; bd. mem. John F. Kennedy Library Foundation; 1984–85, 1985–86 State Crusade Chairman American Cancer Society; Board of Overseers Boston Museum of Fine Arts; Professor Boston University Law School 1982–83, 1985–86; Served to 1st Lt. AUS, 1943–45. Decorated Army Commendation medal. Named one of ten outstanding young men Greater Boston Chamber of Commerce 1958; William J. German Human Relations Award Entertainment and Communications Division American Jewish Committee, 1977; 1985 recipient Boston University Law School Silver Shingle Award for Distinguished Public Service; Communicator of the Year B'nai B'rith Communications, Cinema Lodge 1980.

REED, OLIVER: Actor. b. Wimbledon, England, Feb. 13, 1938.

PICTURES INCLUDE: The Rebel, His and Hers, Beat Girl, The Angry Silence, League of Gentlemen, Two Faces of Dr. Jekyll, Sword of Sherwood Forest, Bulldog Breed, Paranoic, No Love for Johnnie, Curse of the Werewolf, Pirates of Blood River, Curse of Captain Clegg, The Damned, The Party's Over, Scarlet Blade, Assassination Bureau, Shuttered Room, The System, Brigand of Kandahar, The Trap, I'll Never Forget What's His Name, Hannibal Brooks, The Jokers, Oliver, The Girl Getters, Women in Love, Take a Girl Like You, The Lady in the Car, Hunting Party, The Devils, Zero Population Growth, Sitting Target, Triple Echo, Fury Rides the Wind, Dirty Weekend, Revolver, Blue Blood, Three Musketeers, Death in Persepolis, Tommy, The Four Musketeers, Ten Little Indians, Royal Flash, Sell Out, Burnt Offerings, The Great Scout and Cathouse Thursday, The Prince and the Pauper, Assault on Paradise, Tomorrow Never Comes, The Big Sleep, The Class of Miss MacMichael, The Broad, Lion in the Desert, Dr. Heckle and Mr. Hype, Condorman, Venom, The Great Question, Deathbite, The Sting II, Masquerade, Second

Chance, Two of a Kind, Christopher Columbus, Black Arrow, Heroine, Spasms.

REED, PETER: Executive. Ent. m.p. ind. 1937. Early career with Union Cinemas, General Film Distributors, Warner Bros. RAF Bomber Command 1939–45. UA Salesman, 1945–50. Paramount, 1950–70. Appt. sales man. Paramount 1963 and to brd. dir. 1966. Formed Carthay Center Distributors Ltd., now NGC Distrs. Ltd., subsidiary of National General Corporation, in May 1970. With NBC withdrawal from UK distribution in 1972, formed Eton Films as ind. venture. 1973; joined Anglo-EMI in exec. capacity. Man. Dir. Cathay Films (UK) Ltd. 1974. UK Rep. Theatrical Dist. N.T.A.

REED, PHILIP: Actor. b. New York City; e. Cornell U. Left coll. in freshman yr. to join Hoboken, N.J. stock co.; later in vaudeville & on N.Y. stage (Grand Street Follies, Grand Hotel, Ziegfeld Follies of 1931, Serena Blandish, Melody, My Dear Children).
PICTURES INCLUDE: Female, The House on 56th Street, Lost Lady, Dr. Monica, Old Acquaintance, People Are Funny, Big Town After Dark, Song of Sheherizade, Pirates of Monterey, Bandit Queen, Tripoli, Davy Crockett, Indian Scout, Target, Take Me to Town, Girl in the Red Velvet Swing, Harem Scarem.

REEVE, CHRISTOPHER: Actor. b. New York City, Sept. 25, 1952. e. Cornell (BA); graduate work at Julliard. National tour with Irregular Verb to Love, co-starring with Celeste Holm. Went to England, visiting repertory theatres; hired for backstage work by Old Vic. Returned to U.S.; played role on daytime TV series, Love of Life. On Bdwy. with Katharine Hepburn in A Matter of Gravity. Theatrical film debut, Gray Lady Down (1978).
PICTURES: Superman, Somewhere in Time, Superman II, Deathtrap, Monsignore, Superman III, The Bostonians, The Aviator, Street Smart.

REEVES, HAZARD, E.: Executive b. Baltimore, Md., July 6, 1906. e. Georgia Inst. of Technology, B.S. 1928; In research eng. dept., Columbia Phonograph Co., 1928; asst. chief eng., Stanley Recording Co., 1929; chief eng., 1930–31; consultant Harvard Film Foundation, 1930–32; chief eng., Standard Sound Co., 1932–33; founder, Reeves Sound Studios, Inc., 1933 (now Cinetel, Inc.); Audio Devices, Inc., 1937; Reeves Industries, Inc., 1946; co-founder, Reeves-Ely Laboratories, Inc., 1942 (now a division of Dynamics Corporation of America); co-founder, 1947, and first pres., Cinerama, Inc.; chmn. bd., Reeves Telecom Corp., Realtron Corp.

REEVES, STEVE: Actor. b. Glasgow, Mont., Jan. 21, 1926. Delivered newspapers. Mr. Pacific, Mr. America, Mr. World, Mr. Universe; ent. theatrical field, Kismet. Appeared The Vamp, With You Were Here.
PICTURES INCLUDE: Athena, Goliath and the Barbarians, Sword of Siracusa, Judos, David and Goliath, Hercules, Giant of Marathon, Last Days of Pompeii, Hercules Unchained, White Warrior, Morgan the Pirate, The Thief of Baghdad, The Trojan Horse, The Private Prince, A Long Ride From Hell.

REGAN, PHIL: Singer and actor. b. Brooklyn, N.Y., May 28, 1906. While a boy was a boatman at Charleston, S.C., navy yard. Was a clerk in an oil company; clerked in different parts of the country, then became a court clerk in New York, finally a detective. After voice was trained, sang for Columbia Broadcasting System. Was signed by WB.
PICTURES INCLUDE: The Key, Housewife, Dames in 1934, Sweet Rosie O'Grady, Swing Parade of 1946, Sunbonnet Sue, Three Little Words.
TV: Many appearances and several radio shows.

REHME, ROBERT G.: Executive. b. Cincinnati, Ohio, May 5, 1935. e. Univ. of Cincinnati. 1953, mgr., RKO Theatres, Inc., Cincinnati; 1961, adv. mgr., Cincinnati Theatre Co.; 1966, dir. of field adv., United Artists Pictures; 1969, named dir. of pub. and ass't gen. sls. mgr., United Artists Pictures; 1972, pres., B&R Theatres and v.p., April Fools Films; 1976, v.p. & gen. sls. mgr., New World Pictures; Feb. 1978, joined Avco Embassy Pictures as snr. v.p. & chief operating officer; Dec. 1978, named exec. v.p.; 1979, named pres., Avco Embassy Pictures, Inc,. 1981, joined Universal Pictures as pres. of distribution & marketing; 1982, named pres. of Universal Pictures; 1983, joined New World Pictures as co-chm. & chief exec. off.

REID, BERYL: Actress. b. Hereford, England, June 17, 1920. Career in radio before London stage debut in revue, After the Show, 1951. Also on stage in The Killing of Sister George, Spring Awakening, Campimello, Born in the Gardens, etc.
PICTURES: The Belles of St. Trinian's, The Extra Day, Inspector Clouseau, The Assassination Bureau, The Killing ofSister George, The Beast in the Cellar, Father Dear Father, No Sex Please We're British, Joseph Andrews, Carry on Emmanuelle, The Doctor and the Devils.

REID, KATE: Actress. b. London, England, Nov. 4, 1930. Performed in stock in Canada and Bermuda. Joined Stratford Shakespeare Festival in Canada to play many roles. On Bdwy. in Dylan, Cat on a Hot Tin Roof, Bosoms and Neglect, Death of a Salesman, etc.
PICTURES: This Property Is Condemned, The Side Glances of a Pigeon Kicker, Andromeda Strain, A Delicate Balance, Equus, Highpoint, Death Ship, Double Negative, Plague, Circle of Two, Atlantic City, The Blood of Others, Heaven Help Us, Fire with Fire.
TELEVISION: Nellie McClung, Crossbar, Robbers Rooftops and Witchers, Death of a Salesman, etc.

REILLY, CHARLES E., JR.: Communications Executive. e. St. Joseph's College, Network Liaison, TV Guide Magazine; asst. to the v.p. & dir., corporate relations, Young & Rubicam, 1964–66; executive dir., National Catholic Office for Radio, 1966–71; Secretary, Catholic Communications Foundation (CCF) 1968–77; exec. v.p., Patrick Carr Associates 1971–73; corp. exec. Communispond Inc. of J. Walter Thompson Co., 1973–76; v.p., Speech Dynamics subsidiary, Ogilvy & Mather International, 1976–77; pres., In-Person Communications Inc. 1977–present.

REILLY, CHARLES NELSON: Actor-Director. b. New York City, Jan. 13. 1931. e. Univ. of Conn. On Broadway mostly in comedy roles before turning to TV and films. Recently directed stage plays.
PICTURES INCLUDE: A Face in the Crowd, Two Tickets to Paris, The Tiger Makes Out, Cannonball Run II.
TELEVISION: Broadway of Lerner and Lowe, Ghost and Mrs. Muir, Dean Martin Show.

REINAUER, RICHARD: Executive. b. Chicago, Ill., April 28, 1926. e. U. of Ill., grad. 1952; prod., dir., free lance, 1952–59; bus. mgr., asst. prod., Showcase Theatre Evanston, 1952; prod., dir., NBC, Chicago, 1953–55; film dir., Kling Studios, 1956; asst. dir., Foote Cone & Belding, 1956–59; dir., radio, TV & m.p., American Medical Assoc., 1959–64; pres., Communications Counselors, 1963–64; exec. dir., TV Arts & Sciences Foundation, 1964; pres., Acad. of TV Arts & Sciences, Chicago Chapter, 1970–72. assoc. prod. & asst. dir. Wild Kingdom & asst. to pres., Don Meier Prods., 1965–present. Member–Illinois Nature Preserve Commission.

REINBERG, DEBORAH: Executive. Attorney in entertainment field for Manatt, Phelps, Rothenberg and Tunney before joining Elektra/Asylum Records as v.p., business affairs. July, 1984, joined Warner Bros. as dir. of music, business & legal affairs. 1985, promoted to newly created position of v.p., business affairs, music.

REINER, CARL: Performer; b. New York, N.Y., March 20, 1923. Comedian on B'way, Call Me Mr., Inside U.S.A., Alive and Kicking; m.p. The Russians are Coming; on TV in Your Show of Shows, first Bob Hope Show, Caesar's Hour; Sid Caesar Invites You, 1958; prod.-writer, The Dick Van Dyke Show, CBS (Emmy Award-writing Comedy) 1961–62. Prod., The New Dick Van Dyke Show 1973; Heaven Help Us, 1975–76.
PICTURES INCLUDE: The Gazebo, writ. orig. s.p. The Thrill of It All, dir. co-author & co-prod. The Comic; Generation. A Performer: It's a Mad, Mad, Mad, Mad World; Happy Anniversary, Gidget Goes Hawaiian, The End. Co-author & dir: Enter Laughing; Dir: Where's Poppa, Oh, God!, The One and Only, The Jerk, Dead Men Don't Wear Plaid (s.p. & actor), The Man with Two Brains (co-s.p.-dir.), All of Me (dir.), Summer Rental (dir.).
RECORDINGS: Carl Reiner and Mel Brooks, The 2000 Year Old Man, The 2001 Year Old Man, 2013 Year Old Man.
AUTHOR: Enter Laughing, Something Different, B'way.

REINER, ROB: Actor-Writer-Director. b. 1945. Son of actor/writer/director Carl Reiner. Worked as actor with regional theatres and improvisational comedy troupes. Breakthrough as actor came in 1971 when signed by Norman Lear for All in the Family on TV, playing Mike Stivic (Meathead). Directorial debut with This Is Spinal Tap, 1984.
PICTURES: This is Spinal Tap (co-s.p., dir., act.); The Sure Thing (dir.), Stand By Me (dir.).

REINHARDT, GOTTFRIED: Producer, writer. b. Berlin, Germany, p. Max Reinhardt, noted theatrical prod.; Else Reinhardt, actress; brother, Wolfgang Reinhardt, prod.; e. Berlin. Began career at 19 as asst. to prod. Ernst Lubitsch, father's friend, with m.p. Design For Living; asst. to Walter Wanger; later to Bernard H. Hyman (Saratoga; San Francisco). Wrote orig. story, I Live My Life, The Great Waltz; collab. Bridal Suite; book for NY musicals, Rosalinda, Helen of Troy. U.S. Army service, Signal Corps. 1942–46.
PICTURES INCLUDE: Comrade X, Rage in Heaven, Two-Faced Woman, (co-prod.) Homecoming, Command Decision, The Great Sinner, The Red Badge of Courage, Invitation, Young Man With Ideas, (dir. 2 seq.) Story of Three Loves, Betrayed, Town Without Pity, Hitler: The Last Ten Days (prod., co. s.p.).

REINHART, ALICE: Actress. b. San Francisco, Calif., May 6 Legit. theatre work, 1928–49; appeared in stock, numerous Broadway plays; radio work since 1930; shows include Woman in My House, The Whistler, Life Can Be Beautiful, many other shows on all networks; on stage, American Dream in Hollywood.
TV: Stage 13, Man Behind the Badge, Big Town, O. Henry Series, Dragnet, Crusader, The Donna Reed Show.
PICTURES INCLUDE: Lieutenant Wore Skirts, The Iron Sheriff, Bachelor Flat.

REINHOLD, JUDGE: Actor. b. Wilmington, DL. e. Mary Washington Coll., North Carolina School of Arts. Acted in regional theatres before signed to TV contract at Paramount. Theatrical film debut in Running Scared, 1979.
PICTURES: Stripes, Thursday the Twelfth, Fast Times at Ridgemont High, Gremlins, Beverly Hills Cop, Roadhouse, Head Office, Off Beat, Ruthless People.
TELEVISION: Wonder Woman, Magnum P.I., The Survival of Dana, Brothers and Sisters, A Step Too Slow, The Willmar Eight, Booker.

REISENBACH, SANFORD E.: Executive. e. N.Y. University. Associated with Grey Advertising for 20 years; exec. v.p. and pres. of Grey's leisure/entertainment division in N.Y. In August, 1979, joined Warner Bros. as exec. v.p. in chg. of worldwide adv. & pub.; named pres., worldwide adv. & pub., 1985.

REISNER, ALLEN: Director. b. N.Y.C.
FEATURES: The Day They Gave Babies Away; St. Louis Blues.
FEATURES FOR TV: The Captain and the Kings; Mary Jane Harper Cried Last Night, Your Money or Your Wife; To Die in Paris; The Cliff; Skag; They're Playing Our Song; The Gentleman From Seventh Avenue; Escape of Pierre Mendes-France; Deliverance of Sister Cecelia; The Sound of Silence.
TV FILM SERIES: Murder She Wrote, Twilight Zone, Hardcastle & McCormick, Airwolf, The Mississippi, Hawaii Five-O, Blacke's Majic, Last Electric Knight, etc.
LIVE TV SERIES: Playhouse 90, Studio One, Climax, United States Steel Hour, Suspense, Danger, etc.

REISNER, DEAN: Writer. Began career as director: Bill and Coo, 1947. Has collaborated on following screenplays, among others: Coogan's Bluff, Dirty Harry, Play Misty for Me.

REISS, JEFFREY C.: Executive. b. Brooklyn, N.Y., April 14, 1942. e. Washington Univ., St. Louis (B.A., 1963). Consultant at N.Y. Univ. and Manhattanville College and instructor at Brooklyn College before entering industry. Agt. in literary dept. for General Artists Corp., 1966. Supervised development in N.Y. of Tandem Prods. for Norman Lear, 1968. Produced off-Bdwy. plays 1968–70. Dir. of progm. devel. for Cartridge TV, Inc. (mfg. of video-players-recorders) 1970–73. Joined ABC Entertainment as director of network feature films, 1973–75. Founder and pres., Showtime Entertainment (pay TV), 1976–80. Co-founder, pres., & CEO, Cable Health Network, 1981–83. in March, 1983, named vice chm. & CEO, Cable Health Network. Chm & CEO, Reiss Media Enterprises, 1984; founder & pres., Request Television (pay-per-view svc.), 1985.

REISS, STUART A.: Set decorator. b. Chicago, Ill., July 15, 1921. e. L.A. High Sch., 1939. Property man, 20th-Fox, 1939–42; U.S. Army Air Corps, 1942–45; set decorator, 20th-Fox since 1945; 6 Acad. nom.; 2 Acad. Awards, Diary of Anne Frank & Fantastic Voyage.
PICTURES INCLUDE: Titanic, How to Marry a Millionaire, Hell and High Water, There's No Business Like Show Business, Soldier of Fortune, Seven Year Itch, Man in the Grey Flannel Suit, Teen Age Rebel, What a Way to Go, Doctor Doolittle, Fantastic Voyage, Oh God!, Swarm, Beyond the Poseidon Adventure, Carbon Copy, All the Marbles, The Man Who Loved Women, Mickey and Maude, A Fine Mess.

REISZ, KAREL: Director. b. Czechoslovakia, 1926. e. Britain. Wrt. Technique of Film Editing for British Film Academy. Worked with British Film Institute and National Film Library, 1954; co. dir. (with Tony Richardson) Momma Don't Allow, 1957; prod. Every Day Except Christmas, 1958; dir. We Are the Lambeth Boys, 1959–60; dir. Saturday Night & Sunday Morning, 1962; prod. This Sporting Life, 1963; dir. Night Must Fall, 1966; dir. Morgan, 1968; dir. Isadora; The Gambler. Dir. On the Road. (BBC-TV). Dir. Rag Soldiers (U.S. Title: Who'll Stop the Rain) (1978), The French Lieutenant's Woman, 1981 (also co-prod.), Sweet Dreams, 1985.

REITMAN, IVAN: Producer-Director. b. Czechoslovakia, Oct. 26, 1946. e. McMaster Univ.
PICTURES: Foxy Lady, Cannibal Girls, Shivers, Death Weekend, Blackout, Animal House (prod.); Meatballs (prod.-dir.); Stripes (prod.-dir.); Heavy Metal (prod.); Spacehunter (prod.); Ghostbusters (prod.-dir.); Legal Eagles (prod.-dir.).
TELEVISION: The Delta House.

RELPH, MICHAEL: Producer, director, writer, designer. 1942 art dir. Ealing Studios then assoc. prod. to Michael Balcon on The Captive Heart, Frieda, Kind Hearts and Coronets, Saraband (also designed: nominated Oscar). 1948 appt. producer and formed prod/dir. partnership Basil Dearden (until 1972). 1971–76 Governor Brit. Film Institute. Chairman B.F.I. Prod. Board. Chairman Film Prod. Assoc. of G.B., member Films Council.
PICTURES INCLUDE: (For Ealing) The Blue Lamp (Brit. Film Academy: Best Brit. Film 1950), I Believe in You, The Gentle Gunman, The Square Ring, The Rainbow Jacket, Out of the Clouds, The Ship That Died of Shame, Davy (for Brit. Lion), The Smallest Show on Earth. (For Rank) Violent Playground, Rockets Galore (Island Fling U.S.), Sapphire (Brit. Film Academy: Best Brit. Film 1959), 1960 Founder Dir. Allied Film Makers: Prod. The League of Gentlemen, Man in the Moon (Co-author S.P.), Victim, Life For Ruth (Walk in the Shadow U.S.). Also produced: Secret Partner (For M.G.M.), All Night Long (For Rank), The Mind Benders (For Anglo). A Place To Go (Author S.P.) For United Artist Produced: Woman of Straw (Co-author S.P.) Masquerade (Co-author S.P.) For Paramount produced, wrote and designed The Assassination Bureau. For E.M.I. produced The man Who Haunted Himself (Co-author S.P.). 1978, exec. in chg. prod., Kendon Films, Ltd. exec. prod., Scum, 1982, co-prod., An Unsuitable Job for a Woman. 1984, exec. prod.: Treasurer Houses of Britain; TV series, proc., Heavenly Pursuits, 1985–86.

RELYEA, ROBERT E.: Producer. b. Santa Monica, Calif., May 3, 1930. e. UCLA (B.S., 1952). In Army 1953–55. Entered industry in 1955. Started production of films in 1968 with Bullitt.
PICTURES INCLUDE: Bullitt, The Reivers, Day of the Dolphin.

REMBUSCH, TRUEMAN T.: Exhibitor. b. Shelbyville, Ind., July 27, 1909; f. Frank J. Rembusch, pioneer exhibitor; e. Notre Dame U. Sch. of Commerce, 1928; m. Mary Agnes Finneran. Ent. m.p. ind., 1928, servicing sound equip., father's circuit; became mgr., 1932; elect. bd. of dir., Allied Theatre Owners of Ind., 1936–45, pres. 1945–51, 1952–53; dir. chmn. Allied TV Committee, 1945–50; pres. Allied States Assn., 1950–51; 1952, named by Allied as one of triumvirate heading COMPO; elected chmn. Joint Com. on Toll TV, 1954; Nov. 1953 named by Gov. of Indiana as dir. State Fair Board. Currently pres. Syndicate Thea., Inc., Franklin, Ind. member, In Notre Dame Club of Indianapolis (Man of Yr., 1950); BPOE, Antelope Club, 4th Degree K of C, Meridian Hills Country Club, Marco Island Country Club. American Radio Relay League (amateur & commerce, licenses); OX5 Aviation Pioneers; awarded patent, recording & counting device, 1951; dir. Theatre Owners of Indiana; dir. to NATO; dir. NATO member ad hoc comm; 1972 chair., NATO Statistical Committee; presently ch., trade practice comm.; 1976–NITE Award service to Independent Exhibition.

REMICK, LEE: Actress. b. Boston, Dec. 14, 1937. e. Miss Hewitt's Sch., Barnard Coll. Started in summer stock; on tour in Jenny Kisses Me, The Seven Year Itch, Paint Your Wagon; first N.Y. stage appearance, Be Your Age; major TV shows incl. Studio 1, Playhouse 90, Armstrong Circle Theatre; m.p. debut in A Face in the Crowd.
PICTURES INCLUDE: The Long Hot Summer, Anatomy of a Murder, Wild River, Sanctuary, Experiment in Terror, The Days of Wine and Roses, The Wheeler Dealers, Travelin' Lady, Baby the Rain Must Fall, Hallelujah Trail, Hard Contract, A Severed Head, Sometimes A Great Notion, A Delicate Balance, Hennessy, The Omen, Telefon, The Medusa Touch, The Europeans, The Competition, Tribute.
TELEVISION: Movies: A Good Sport, The Gift of Love, Mistral's Daughter, Rearview Mirror, Toughlove.

REMSEN, BERT: Actor. b. Glen Cover, NY, Feb. 25, 1925. e. Ithaca Coll.
PICTURES: Pork Chop Hill, Kid Galahad, Moon Pilot, Brewster McCloud, Thieves Like us, Baby Blue Marine, McCabe and Mrs. Miller, Sweet Hostage, Nashville, The Awakening Land, California Split, Tarantulas, A Wedding, Buffalo Bill and the Indians, The Rose, Uncle Joe Shannon, Carny, Borderline, Second Hand Hearts, Joni, Inside Moves, Looking to Get Out, Sting II, Code of Silence, Stand Alone.

RESNAIS, ALAIN: Director. b. Cannes, France, 1922. Began career as asst. dir. to Nicole Vedres on compilation of film for Paris 1900. During '50s worked as asst. editor and editor; experimented with making his own 16mm films. Did series of shorts on various painters, culminating with documentary on Van Gogh (1948), which he co-directed with Robert Hessens, with whom he later filmed Guernica. Co-directed The Statues Also Die with Chris Marker.
PICTURES INCLUDE: Night and Fog, Hiroshima, Mon Armour, Last Year at Marienbad, Muriel, La Guerre Est Finie, Je t'Aime, Je t'Aime, Stavisky, Providence, Mon Oncle d'Amerique.

RESNICK, JOEL H.: Executive. b. New York City. e. Univ. of Pennsylvania (B.A., 1958); New York Law School; 1961, admitted to N.Y. State Bar. In 1962 received Masters of Law degree in taxation. 1961–66 served as associate with New York law firm, Phillips, Nizer, Benjamin, Krim & Ballon. Was in-house counsel to United Artists Corp. 1967, joined UA as spec. asst. to the snr. v.p. & gen. mgr. 1970, moved to American Multi-Cinema, Inc., Kansas City, as asst. to pres. 1972, named v.p. in chg. development; 1976, promoted to v.p. in chg. film development. 1977, named exec. v.p. 1983, elected exec. v.p. & dir., AMC Entertainment. 1984, appt. to office of pres. as chm. & CEO, film mktg. 1986, resigned to join Orion Pictures as chm. Has served as co-chairman NATO trade practices comm. since 1979. In 1982 elected pres., NATO; 1984, became chm. NATO bd.

RETCHIN, NORMAN: Writer, producer. b. Chicago. May 6, 1919. e. U. of Pa., 1940. U.S. Air Force, 1943–45; J. Walter Thompson adv. agency, 1946–51; story ed. & assoc. prod. Screen Televideo Co., 1951–55; story ed. Clover Prod. 1955; stage, orig. bk. and lyrics, The Genius Farm; TV, orig. prod., The Untouchables.
PICTURES INCLUDE: Uranium Boom, (collab.) Leather Saint, Ride Out for Revenge, Mission Mars, Into Thin Air, (orig. story).

RETTIG, TOMMY: Actor. b. Jackson Heights, N.Y., Dec. 10, 1941; on stage in Annie Get Your Gun; TV series, Lassie.
PICTURES INCLUDE: Gobs and Gals, Paula, Lady Wants Mink, 5000 Fingers of Dr. T., So Big, River of No Return, The Raid, The Egyptian, The Cobweb, At Gunpoint.

REVERE, ANNE: Actress. b. New York City, June 25, 1907; e. Wellesley Coll., B.A., m. Samuel Rosen, director. On stage, Stuart Walker Stock Co., 1928–29, Double Door, 1933–34. Children's Hour, 1934–37, org. & dir. Surry Theat., Maine, N.Y., 1936–39; Acad. Award best supporting role (National Velvet), 1945.
PICTURES INCLUDE: Double Door, Howards of Virginia, Men of Boys Town, Remember the Day, Star Spangled Rhythm, Song of Bernadette, National Velvet, Keys of the Kingdom, Sunday Dinner for a Soldier, Dragonwyck, Forever Amber, Body and Soul, Gentleman's Agreement, Place in the Sun, Great Missouri Raid, Tell Me That You Love Me Junie Moon, Birch Interval.

REVILL, CLIVE: Actor. b. Wellington, New Zealand, Ent. m.p. ind. 1965.
STAGE: Irma La Douce, The Mikado, Oliver, Marat/Sade, Jew of Malta, Sherry, Chichester Season, The Incomparable Max (N.Y.), Sherlock Holmes (NY), Lolita (NY), Pirates of Penzance (LA).
PICTURES INCLUDE: Bunny Lake is Missing, Once Upon a Tractor, Modesty Blaise, A Fine Madness, Kaleidoscope, The Double Man, Fathom, Italian Secret Service, Nobody Runs Forever, Shoes of the Fisherman, Assassination Bureau, The Private Life of Sherlock Holmes, The Buttercup Chain, A Severed Head, Boulevard de Rhum, Avanti!, Flight to the Sun, The Legend of Hell House, The Little Prince, The Black Windmill, Ghost in the Noonday Sun, One of Our Dinosaurs Is Missing, Galileo, Matilda, Zorro, The Gay Blade.
TV: Chicken Soup with Barley, Volpone, Bam, Pow, Zapp. Candida, Platonov, A Bit of Vision, Mill Hill, The Piano Player, Hopcroft in Europe, A Sprig of Broome, Ben Franklin in Paris, Pinocchio, The Great Houdini, Show Business Hall of Fame, Feather and Father, Winner Take All, The New Avenger, Licking Hitler, Columbo, Centennial, A Man Called Sloane, Nobody's Perfect, Marya, Moviola, Diary of Anne Frank, Mikado, The Sorcerer (London), Wizards & Warriors (Los Angeles), George Washington.

REY, FERNANDO: Actor. b. Spain, Sept. 20, 1917. r.n. Fernando Casado Arambillet. e. Madrid School of Architecture. Dubbed dialogue of foreign films into Spanish before beginning acting career.
PICTURES INCLUDE: Welcome Mr. Marshall, The Adventurers, The French Connection, The Discreet Charm of the Bourgeoisie, French Connection II, That Obscure Object of Desire, Quintet, Rustler's Rhapsody, etc.
TELEVISION: A.D.

REYNOLDS, BURT: Actor/Director. b. Waycross, Ga., Feb. 11, 1936. Former Fla State U football star, won fame as actor on TV in series: Riverboat, Gunsmoke, Hawk and Dan August.
PICTURES INCLUDE: Armored Command, Angel Baby, Operation CIA, Navajo Joe, Impasse, Shark, Sam Whiskey, 100 Rifles, Fade-In, Skullduggery, Everything You Wanted To Know About Sex, Fuzz, Deliverance, Shamus, White Lightning, The Man Who Loved Cat Dancing, The Longest Yard, W.W. & The Dixie Dancekings, At Long Last Love, Hustle, Lucky Lady, Gator (dir.-star), Silent Movie, Nickelodeon, Smokey & The Bandit, Semi-Tough, The End (dir-star), Hooper, Starting Over, Rough Cut, Smokey & The Bandit II, Cannonball Run, Paternity, Sharky's Machine (dir.-star), The Best Little Whorehouse in Texas, Best Friends, Stroker Ace, The Man Who Loved Women, Cannonball Run II, Stick (also dir.), City Heat.

REYNOLDS, CLARKE: Writer, producer. b. Bklyn, N.Y. e. U. of Missouri; pub. rel. NYC, pub. rel on WAAM-TV, Baltimore.
PICTURES INCLUDE: Disc-Jockey, Shotgun, Chisera, Gunmen of Laredo, Imperial Venus, Gunfighters of Casa Grande, Gringo, Genghis Khan, Son of a Gunfighter, The Viking Queen, The Viscount, Warhead, Shalako, The Marauders, The Red Sun, Private Navy, Operation Thunderbolt (Oscar nominee), Cruise Missile, Night Games.
TV: Celebrity Playhouse, Playhouse 90, Damon Runyon Theatre, Cheyenne, 20th Century-Fox Hour, Lux Video Hour, West Point, Whiplash, Playhouse 90, Walter Winchell File, Wells Fargo, Tombstone Territory, The Texan, Peter Gun, Wagon Train, U.S. Marshall, Zane Grey Theatre, Broken Arrow (pilot), The Beachcomber, The Deputy, The Investigators, Cain's Hundred, Created Man Without a Gun.

REYNOLDS, DEBBIE: Actress. r.n. Mary Frances Reynolds. b. El Paso, Tex., April 1, 1932. e. Burbank & John Burroughs H.S., Burbank, Calif. With Burbank Youth Symphony during h.s.; beauty contest winner (Miss Burbank) 1948, signed by Warner Bros.; on stage in Personal Appearances, Blis-Hayden Theater, Star of Tomorrow, 1952.
PICTURES INCLUDE: The Daughter of Rosie O'Grady, Three Little Words, Two Weeks With Love, Mr. Imperium, Singing in the Rain, Skirts Ahoy, I Love Melvin, Give a Girl a Break, Affair of Dobie Gilllis, Susan Slept Here, Athena, Hit the Deck, Tender Trap, Catered Affair, Bundle of Joy, Tammy and the Bachelor, The Mating Game, Say One for Me, It Started With a Kiss, The Gazebo, The Rat Race, Pleasure of His Company, Second Time Around, How the West Was Won, Goodbye Charlie, The Unsinkable Mollie Brown, The Singing Nun, Divorce, American Style, What's The Matter With Helen?, That's Entertainment!
TV: The Debbie Reynolds Show.
STAGE: Irene.

REYNOLDS, JOYCE: Actress. b. San Antonio, Texas, Oct. 7, 1924; e. UCLA. School plays including role of Alice in Alice in Wonderland at UCLA, contracted by Warner Bros. in 1942, appearing in Yankee Doodle Dandy, George Washington Slept Here, Mark Twain, Constant Nymph, Janie, Always Together, Wallflower, Girl School, Dangerous Inheritance.

REYNOLDS, MARJORIE: Actress. b. Buhl, Idaho, Aug. 12, 1921. On screen as child 1923 & later (Scaramouche, Svengali, Revelation, etc.).
PICTURES INCLUDE: Murder in Greenwich Village (1937), College Humor, Holiday Inn, Star-Spangled Rhythm, Dixie, Ministry of Fear, Up in Mabel's Room, Three Is a Family, Duffy's Tavern, Bring on the Girls, Meet Me on Broadway, Heaven Only Knows, Bad Men of Tombstone, Great Jewel Robber, Rookie Fireman, Home Town Story, No Holds Barred, Models, Inc., Silent Witness.
TV: The Life of Riley (series).

REYNOLDS, SHELDON: Writer, producer, director. b. Philadelphia, Pa., 1923. e. NYU. Radio-TV writer; programs include My Silent Partner, Robert Q. Lewis Show, We the People, Danger; writer, prod., dir. Foreign Intrigue film; prod. dir. s.p. collab. story, Foreign Intrigue.

REYNOLDS, STUART: Producer. b. Chicago, Ill., March 22, 1907. e. Chicago law schools. Adv. exec., Lord and Thomas, BBD & O. General Mills; sales exec. Don Lee-Mutual; formed Stuart Reynolds Prod., TV films. Now motion picture & TV program consultant.
TV: General Electric Theatre, Cavalcade of America, Your Jeweler's Showcase, Wild Bill Hickok. Producer and worldwide distributor of educational/training films; Eye of the Beholder.

RICH, DAVID LOWELL: Director. b. New York City, Aug. 31, 1920. Started career on live television inNew York: Studio One, Playhouse, etc. 1950, left for Hollywood to work on TV series: Naked City, Route 66, etc.
PICTURES: Senior Prom, Hey Boy, Hey Girl, Have Rocket Will Travel, Madame X, The Plainsman, Rosie, A Lovely Way To Die, Eye of the Cat, Concorde—Airport '79, Chu Chu and the Philly Flash.
TELEVSION: Movies include See How They Run, Marcus Welby, M.D., The Mask of Sheba, The Sheriff, All My Darling Daughters, The Judge and Jake Wyler, Brock's Last Case, Crime Club, Satan's School for Girls, Sex Symbol, The Daughters of Joshua Cabe Return, You Lie So Deep My Love, Ransom for Alice, Telethon, Little Women, The Hearst and Davies Affair, His Mistress, Scandal Sheet, etc.

RICH, IRENE: Actress. b. Buffalo, N.Y. Oct. 13, 1897. e. St. Margaret's Episcopal School; painting. Real estate saleswoman; stock farmer; on radio, in night clubs, vaudeville.
PICTURES INCLUDE: Exalted Flapper, Lady Windemere's Fan, Lost Lady, Craig's Wife, They Had to See Paris, So

This is London, Down to Earth, That Certain Age, Mortal Storm, Lady in Question, Queen of the Yukon, Keeping Company, This Time for Keeps, Angel and the Badman, Calendar Girl, New Orleans, Fort Apache, Joan of Arc.

RICH, JOHN: Producer-Director. b. Rockaway Beach, N.Y., July 6, 1925. e. U. of Michigan, B.A., Phi Beta Kappa, 1948; M.A. 1949 Sesquicentennial Award, 1967; bd. of dir., Screen Dir. Guild of America, 1954–1960; v.p. 1958–1960 Founder-Trustee, Producers-Directors Pension Plan, chmn. of bd. 1965, 1968, 1970; treasurer, Directors Guild of America, 1966–67; v.p. 1967–72.
TV: Academy Awards, The Dick Van Dyke Show, 1963; All in the Family, 1972 (director); All in the Family, 1973 (producer); Directors Guild Award, Most Outstanding Directorial Achievement, 1971. Christopher award: Henry Fonda as Clarence Darrow, 1975. NAACP Imog. Award, 1974; Golden Globe Awards, All in the Family, 1972–73.
PICTURES INCLUDE: Boeing-Boeing; The New Interns; Wives and Lovers; Roustabout; Easy Come, Easy Go.

RICH, LEE: Producer. b. Cleveland, OH. e. Ohio Univ. Adv. exec.; resigned as sr. v.p., Benton & Bowles, to become producer for Mirisch-Rich TV, 1965. Resigned 1967 to join Leo Burnett Agency. Left to form Lorimar Productions in 1969 and served as pres. until 1986 when left to join United Artists as chm. & CEO.
PICTURES: Executive Producer: The Man, Who Is Killing the Great Chefs of Europe?, Marriage Is Alive and Well, The Big Red One.
TELEVISION INCLUDES: Executive Producer: Helter Skelter, The Waltons, Sybil, Eric, Green Eyes, The Blue Knight, The Long Journey Back, Kaz, Eight is Enough, Dallas, Some Kind of Miracle, Mr. Horn, Studs Lonigan, A Man Called Intrepid, Big Shamus, Little Shamus, Young Love, First Love, Mary and Joseph—A Story of Faith, Knots Landing, Skag, Flamingo Road, Reward, Willow B—Women in Prison, Joshua's World, A Perfect Match, Secret of Midland Heights.
AWARDS: Honorary doctorate in communications, Ohio Univ., 1982; Distinguished Citizenship Award, Southwestern Univ. School of Law, 1983; named Man of Year by Beverly Hills Lodge of B'nai B'rith, 1983.

RICHARD, CLIFF: Singer and actor. b. 1940. Ent. show business 1958 in TV series Oh Boy. Other TV includes Sunday Night at the London Palladium, several Cliff Richard Shows; film debut in Serious Charge, 1959; star, play Aladdin, London Palladium Theatre, 1964–65. Top British Singer, 1960–71. Stageplays: Five Finger Exercise (1970), The Potting Shed (1971). Twice rep. U.K. in Eurovision Song Contest. 3 BBC TV series plus doc. series. 29 silver discs, 10 gold discs for single record releases.
PICTURES INCLUDE: Expresso Bongo, The Young Ones, Summer Holiday, Wonderful Life, Voted top box-office Star of Grt. Britain, 1962–63, 1963–64. Finder's Keepers, Two a Penny, Take Me High.

RICHARDS, BEAH: Actress. b. Vicksburg, MS. e. Dillard Univ. On Bdwy. in The Miracle Worker, A Raisin in the Sun, etc.
PICTURES: Take a Giant Step, The Miracle Workers, Guess Who's Coming to Dinner, Heat of the Night, Hurry Sundown, Great White Hope, Mahogany.
TELEVISION: Movies: Footsteps, Outrage, A Dream for Christmas, Just and Olds Sweet Song, Ring of Passion, Roots II—The Second Generation, A Christmas without Snow.

RICHARDS, DICK: Producer-Director-Writer. b. New York City, 1936. in U.S. Army as photo-journalist; worked for Life, Look, Time, Esquire, etc. as photographer. Won over 100 int'l. awards, for commercials and photographic art work.
PICTURES: The Culpepper Cattle Co. (p., d., s.p.), Rafferty and the Gold Dust Twins (d.), Farewell, My Lovely (d.), March or Die (p., d., s.p.), Man, Woman and Child (d.).

RICHARDS, JEFF: Actor. r.n. Richard Mansfield Taylor. b. Portland, Ore. Nov. 1. e. Tacoma, Wash. H.S., U.S.C. served in U.S. Navy, 1943–46; professional baseball.
PICTURES INCLUDE: Kill the Umpire, Tall Target, The Strip, Angels in the Outfield, The Sellout, Above and Beyond, Desperate Search, Code Two, Big Leaguer, Crest of the Wave, Seven Brides for Seven Brothers, Many Rivers to Cross, The Marauders, It's A Dog's Life, Waco, Johnny Belinda.

RICHARDS, THOMAS LLOYD: Producer-Writer. b. Cardiff, Wales. Entered industry in London at Stoll Studios in 1926, working in production and as 3rd asst. director. Named 1st asst. dir. for producer Herbert W. Wilcox, going to Hollywood to work on Wilcox films starring Anna Neagle: No, No, Nanette, Nurse Edith Cavell, Sunny, and Irene. Worked for RKO Studios as 1st asst. dir., acting in that capacity; for Without Reservations, etc. Joined Four Star Productions (TV producers) as v.p. in chg. prod. Produced 24 in Untouchables series at Desilu. Prod. assoc. of many TV special and features for TV; also special consultant to producers of TV series and mini-series.

RICHARDSON, TONY: Director. b. Shipley, Yorks; England, 1928. e. Wadham Coll., Oxford, where he dir. number prod. for O.U.D.S. Began career with BBC TV and directed such plays as Othello and The Gambler. In 1955 joined English Stage Co. as Assoc. Artisitic Dir. Started with Look Back in Anger, Member of the Wedding, 1958 at Shakespeare Memorial Theatre. 1960, N.Y. co-dir., A Taste of Honey. Recent stage work, dir., Seagull and St. Joan of the Stockyards, Threepenny Opera, I Claudius. Ent. m.p. ind. 1958 to dir. prod. Look Back in Anger, The Entertainer, 1959–60; prod. Saturday Night and Sunday Morning.
PICTURES INCLUDE: A Taste of Honey, Loneliness of the Long Distance Runner, Tom Jones, The Loved One, Mademoiselle, The Sailor from Gibralter, Red and Blue, Charge of the Light Brigade, Laughter in the Dark, Hamlet, Ned Kelly, A Delicate Balance, Dead Cert, Joseph Andrews, The Border, The Hotel New Hampshire (also s.p.).

RICHMAN, MARK: Actor. b. Philadelphia, Pa. Stage credits incl. End as a Man, Masquerade, The Zoo Story, Detective Story, Rose Tattoo.
PICTURES INCLUDE: Friendly Persuasion, Dark Intruder, Agent for H.A.R.M., For Singles Only.
TV: Cain's Hundred.

RICHMOND, TED: Producer. b. Norfolk. Va., June 10, 1912; e. Mass. Inst. Tech. Ent. m.p. ind. as publicity dir., RKO Theats.; later mgr. Albany dist. Pub. dir. Fabian circuit, N.Y.: Paramount upper N.Y. state theats.; Grand Nat'l Pictures. Author Grand Nat'l series Trigger Pal, Six Gun Rhythm. Formed T. H. Richmond Prods., Inc., 1941.
PICTURES INCLUDE: Hit the Hay, The Milkman, Kansas Raiders, Shakedown, Smuggler's Island, Strange Door, Cimarron Kid, Bronco Buster, Has Anybody Seen My Gal, No Room for the Groom, Weekend with Father, The Mississippi Gambler, Desert Legion, Column South, Bonzo Goes to College, Forbidden, Walking My Baby Back Home, Francis Joins the Wacs, Bengal Brigade, (Formed Copa Prod. with Tyrone Power, 1954) Count Three and Pray, Nightfall, Abandon Ship, Solomon and Sheba, Charlemagne. Formed Ted Richmond Prod. Inc. for MGM release, 1959. Reactivated Copa Prod. Ltd., England, 1960. Produced for MGM: Bachelor in Paradise, Advance to the Rear; for Paramount, Pancho Villa; for Mirisch-U.S., Return of the 7; Independent, Red Sun; Producer, Pappillon-Allied Artists, various distributors.

RICHTER, W. D.: Writer. b. Connecticut. e. USC Film School.
PICTURES: Slither, Peeper, Nickelodeon, Invasion of the Body Snatchers, Dracula, Brubaker, All Night Long, Adventures of Buckeroo Banzai (prod.-dir.).

RICKERT, JOHN F.: Executive. b. Kansas City, Mo. e. Univ. So. Calif. Joined Universal Pictures in 1951; left in 1957 to start independent productions From 1960 to 1968 handled indep. roadshow distribution (4-walling). In 1959 formed CineWorld Corporation, natl. dist. co., of which he is pres. In 1975–76 did tax shelter financing for 13 films. Currently involved in distribution, production packaging and intl. co-production as pres. of Coproducers Corp.

RICKETSON, FRANK H., JR.: Executive. b. Leavenworth, Kan. e. U. Ky., LL.B. U. Denver. On ed. staff Kansas City Star, The Denver Post. Member exploitation Dept., Famous Players-Lasky Corp., 1921–24. Pres. Consolidated Theatres 1924 to 1929, Pres. Fox Inter-Mountain Theatres, 1934 to 1957, v.p. & gen. mgr. of Theatre Operations, National Theatres, Inc., 1956–58. Author of The Management of Motion Picture Theatres, Europe after the Marshall Plan, Opportunity Needs a Selling, Gems from a Thousand Sources. Retired director, Public Service Co. of Colorado, Continental Airlines, United Banks of Colorado, Cheyenne Newspapers Inc., Frontier Broadcasting Co., honorary bd. Central City Opera House Assn., Denver Museum of Natural History, first individual elected to Rocky Mountain Motion Picture Association Hall of Fame.

RIEGERT, PETER: Actor. b. New York City, 1948. e. Univ. of Buffalo. Brief stints as teacher, social worker before turned actor, off-off Bdwy. Debuted on Bdwy. in Dance with Me. First film in short, A Director Talks About His Film.
PICTURES: National Lampoon's Animal House, Head Over Heels, Local Hero. Anne and Joey.
TELEVISION: Ellis Island, News at Eleven.

RIFKIN, HARMON "BUD": Theatre Executive. b. Springfield, MA, Apr. 1, 1942. e. Clark Univ. (AB, 1964); Boston Coll. Graduate School of Business Admin. (MBA, 1967). Worked for Rifkin Theatres while student; upon graduation continued in film and equipment purchasing and financial management for circuit. 1972, co-founded Cinema Centers Copr. & Theatre Management Services; currently pres. of Cinema Centers with responsibility for new theatre development and general operations.
MEMBER: Exec. Comm., Natl. Assoc. of Theatre Owners. Past program chm., v.p., pres. & chm. of Theatre Owners of New England.

RIFKIN, JULIAN: Exhibitor. b. Boston, May 26, 1915. e. MIT. Member bd. of dir. Allied States Assoc.of M.P. Exhibitors, and Theatre Owners of America. Pres. Theatre Owners of New England 1961–63. Chairman bd. Theatre Owners of New England. 1964–65. Past pres. Allied Artists Corp. of New England. Pres., 1968–69, chmn. of bd. Nat'l Assoc. of Theatre Owners, 1970. Pres. Rifkin Theatres. Pres. Cinema Centers Corp. Chm. NATO Code and Rating Comm., 1968–79. Received Sherrill C. Corwin Memorial Award, 1985.

RIGG, DIANA: Actress. b. Doncaster, England. July 20, 1938. Formerly with the Royal Shakespeare Co. at Aldwych Theatre, 1962–64. Ent. TV in The Avengers series, 1965. Ent. films 1967.
PICTURES INCLUDE: The Assassination Bureau, On Her Majesty's Secret Service, The Great Muppet Caper, Evil Under the Sun.

RINGWALD: MOLLY: Actress. b. Sacramento, CA, 1968. Daughter of jazz musician Bob Ringwald; began performing at age 4 with his Great Pacific Jazz Band. Professional debut at 5 in stage play, The Glass Harp. Appeared in TV's New Mickey Mouse Club, a West Coast stage production of Annie and in TV series, The Facts of Life, before theatrical film debut in Tempest (1982).
PICTURES: Sixteen Candles, The Breakfast Club, Pretty in Pink.
TELEVISION: Surviving (movie).

RISI, DINO: Director. b. Italy, 1916. Studied medicine but left for film job as assistant on Mario Soldati's Giacomo L'Idealista. Interned in Switzerland in World War II. Returned home to make documentaries and short films before directing Vacanze col Gangster in 1952.
PICTURES INCLUDE: Sign of Venus, Poveri ma Bellis, Il Sorpasso, Scent of a Woman, Sunday Lovers.

RISSIEN, EDWARD L.: Executive. b. Des Moines, IA. e. Grinnell Coll., Stanford Univ. (B.A., 1949). Army Air Force, World War II. Bdwy. stage, mgr., 1950–53; v.p., Mark Stevens. Prods., 1954–56; prod., v.p., Four Star, 1958–60; prog. exec., ABC-TV, 1960–62; v.p., Bing Crosby Prods., 1963–66; v.p., Filmways TV Prods.; assoc. producer, Columbia, 1968–69; indep. producer, 1970; prod., WB, 1971; exec. v.p., Playboy Prods., 1972–80; consultant & indep. prod., 1981–82; sr. consultant, cable, Playboy Prods., 1982–85; pres., Playboy Programs, 1985–present.
PICTURES INCLUDE: Snow Job (prod., WB); Castle Keep (exec. prod.); Julius Vrooder (prod., Fox); Saint Jack (exec. prod.).
TELEVISION: Minstrel Man (exec. prod., CBS); A Whale for the Killing (exec. prod., ABC); Ocean View Park (exec. prod., ABC); Big Bob Johnson (exec. prod., NBC).

RISSNER, DANTON: Executive. b. New York City, March 27, 1940. Began as agent with Ashley Famous (later Intl. Famous), 1967-69. In 1969 joined Warner Bros. as v.p., chg. European prod.; 1970, moved to United Artists as v.p., chg. European prod. 1973, named v.p. in chg. East Coast & European prod. for UA; 1975, v.p. in chg. of world-wide prod. Resigned 1978 to enter ind. prod.; Exec. v.p., 20th Century-Fox. Produced Up the Academy in 1977. 1984, joined UA as sr. v.p., motion pictures.

RITCHIE, MICHAEL: Director. b. Waukesha, Wisc., 1938. e. Harvard Univ. where he directed first production of Arthur Kopit's play, Oh Dad, Poor Dad, Mama's Hung You in the Closet and I'm Feeling So Sad. Professional career began as ass't. to Robert Saudek on Ford Foundation's Omnibus TV series. Later became assoc. prod. and then dir. on Saudek's Profiles in Courage series. Then had dir. assignments on top series (Man from U.N.C.L.E., Dr. Kildare, The Big Valley, Felony Squad).
PICTURES INCLUDE: Downhill Racer, Prime Cut, The Candidate, Smile (also prod.), The Bad News Bears, Semi-Tough, An Almost Perfect Affair, The Island, Bette Midler's Divine Madness, The Survivors, Fletch, Wildcats, The Golden Child.
TELEVISION: Man from U.N.C.L.E., Dr. Kildare, The Big Valley, Felony Squad, Run for Your Life, The Outsider (pilot).

RITT, MARTIN: Dir. b. N.Y., N.Y. Mar. 2 e. Elon Coll., Burlington, Ky, Started as actor in Golden Boy. N.Y. stage; studied acting under Elia Kazan; dir. stage; Mr. Peebles and Mr. Hooker, The Man, Set My People Free, A View From the Bridge, N.Y.; acted in 150 and dir. 100 TV dramas.
TV: Danger.
PICTURES INCLUDE: Edge of the City (first screen dir.), No Down Payment, The Long Hot Summer, The Black Orchid, The Sound and the Fury, Adventures of a Young Man, Hud (also co-producer), The Outrage, Spy Who Came In From the Cold, Hombre, The Brotherhood, The Molly Maguires, The Great White Hope, Sounder, Pete 'n' Tillie, Conrack, The Front, Casey's Shadow, Norma Rae, Back Roads, Cross Creek, Murphy's Romance. Acted: End of the Game, The Slugger's Wife.

RITTER, JOHN: Actor. b. Hollywood, Sept. 17, 1948. Father was late Tex Ritter, country-western star. Married, actress Nancy Morgan. Attended Hollywood High School. Interest in acting began at Univ. of So. Calif. in 1968. Appeared with college cast at Edinburgh Festival; later with Eva Marie Saint in Desire under the Elms. Gained fame as star of TV series, Three's Company.
PICTURES: Americathon, Hero at Large, Wholly Moses, They All Laughed.
TELEVISION: Movies: Leave Yesterday Behind, In Love with an Older Woman, Love Thy Neighbor, Letting Go.

RIVE, KENNETH: Executive. b. London, England, July 26, 1919. Early career as actor, radio compere, theatrical agent. Served in Intell. Corps. during WWII. After demob. theatre sup. and gen. man. cinema co. promoted dir. 1947. Started in continental exhibition forming Gala Film Distrib. Ltd., 1950. Now man. dir. Gala Film Dist., Carlton & Majestic Cinemas & Dance Hall Ltd., Cosmopolitan Film Dist. Ltd., Gala-Jacey Enterprises Ltd., Berkeley & Continentale (Holdings) Ltd., Gala TV Prod. Ltd., Galaworldfilm Prod. Ltd., Gala Maintenance Ltd.; 1966, Gala Co-Productions, Ltd., Gala Int'l Film & TV Enterprises, Ltd. Film Industry Defence Org., Malta United Film Corp. Ltd., Children's Film Foundation Ltd., International Films Theatre Ltd. Director, Video Copyright Protection Society, Ltd.
PICTURES INCLUDE: During One Night, The Boys, Devil Doll, Curse of Simba.

RIVERA, GERALDO: TV Reporter. b. N.Y.C., July 4, 1943. e. Univ. of Arizona, Columbia School of Journalism. Started legal career than switched to journalism, making several TV documentaries on such subjects as institutions for retarded, drug addiction, migrant workers, etc. Joined WABC-TV, New York, in 1970.
TV: Geraldo Rivera: Good Night America; Good Morning America (contributor). 20/20.

RIVERS, JOAN: Actress-Writer-Director. b. New York City, June 8, 1933. Most of career on TV and in nightclubs; as of 1983 sole substitute guest host for Johnny Carson. 1986, started own TV talk show on Fox Network.
PICTURES: The Swimmer (act.); Rabbit Test (act., dir., s.p.); Uncle Sam (act.); The Muppets Take Manhattan (act.).

RIVKIN, ALLEN: Writer, producer. b. Hayward, Wis., Nov. 20, 1903. Newspaperman, novelist, playwright. Authored 85 s.p. including Farmer's Daughter, Battle Circus, Prisoner of War, Joe Smith American, Eternal Sea, Big Operator.
TV: Prod. Troubleshooters series, 1960 Democratic Nat'l Convention; author (with Laura Kerr) Hello, Hollywood; past pres. scr. br. and currently dir. pub. rel., WGAW, liaison rep., Legal Advisory Committee on m.p. & TV of the American Bar Assn. Recipient of Morgan Cox and Valentine Davies Awards.

RIVKIN, JOE: Production executive. b. Hartford, Conn. Exploit. dir., Pathe, also artist mgr. then to Hal Roach. In armed services Pres. Carthay Prod., v.p. gen. mgr. Wald & Krasna Prod., 1951; talent exec. Allied Artists Pictures. Now with Wm. Morris Agency.

RIX, BRIAN: C.B.E. Actor, manager. b. Yorkshire, England, 1924. e. Bootham Sch., York. Ent. m.p. ind. 1951.
TV: Farces, 1956–72, over 80. Men of Affairs (series); A Roof over My Head (series).
PICTURES INCLUDE: Reluctant Heroes, What Every Woman Wants, Up to His Neck, Dry Rot, Wanted on Voyage, And the Same to You, The Night We Dropped a Clanger, The Night We Got the Bird, Nothing Barred, Don't Just Lie There Say Something!

ROACH, HAL, JR.: President, owner Hal Roach Studios. Unit mgr. 20th Century-Fox, 1944–45; gen. mgr., Rainbow Prod., 1945–46. Member of Acad. of M.P. Arts & Sciences, M.P. Producers Assoc., Pres. Alliance of TV Film Producers; treas. & bd. member and former pres. of Acad. of TV Arts & Sciences; pres. Rabco Corp., Hal Roach Prod., chmn. exec. officer, dir., F. I. Jacobs, Detroit; past chmn. bd., Mutual Broadcasting System, bd. member, Vitapix Corp.; gen. exec., TV Prod., Seven Arts Associated.
PICTURES INCLUDE: Block Heads, A Chump at Oxford, One Million B.C., Road Show, All American Co-ed, Calaboose, Prairie Chickens, Army Training films, Physical Education & Military Training, Military Justice of Court Martials, Fighting Man series.
TV: Stu Erwin Show, Racket Squad, Public Defender, My Little Margie, Passport to Danger, Screen Directors Playhouse, Stories of John Nesbitt, Code 3, Charlie Farrell Show, Gale Storm Show, Blondie, Forest Ranger.

ROBARDS, JASON, JR.: Actor. b. Chicago, July 26, 1922. Served in Navy during WW II. Studied acting at Acad. of Dramatic Arts. Began with Children's World Theatre, radio parts, asst. stage mgr. on Stalag 17. First major break 1953 in play American Gothic, followed by The Iceman Cometh, Long Day's Journey into Night, Toys in the Attic. After the Fall, others; to Hollywood, 1958.

PICTURES INCLUDE: The Journey, By Love Possessed, Long Day's Journey Into Night, Tender is the Night, Act One, A Thousand Clowns, Any Wednesday, The St. Valentine's Day Massacre, The Night They Raided Minsky's, Hour of the Gun, The Loves of Isadora, Once Upon a Time in the West, Ballad of Cable Hogue, Fools, Johnny Got His Gun, Murders in the Rue Morgue, Pat Garrett and Billy the Kid, All the President's Men, Julia, Comes a Horseman, Hurricane, Raise the Titanic! Caboblanco, Something Wicked This Way Comes, Square Dance.
TV: Washington: Behind Closed Doors, The Day After, The Atlanta Child Murders, Sakhorov, Johnny Bull, The Long Hot Summer.

ROBBIE, SEYMOUR MITCHELL: Producer, director.
TV: Studio One, Omnibus, Play of the Week, Jackie Gleason Show, The Man From U.N.C.L.E., Eleventh Hour, Dupont Show of the Week, F Troop, Mr. Roberts, Amos Burke, Honey West, Disney Wonderful World of Color, Felony Squad, Lost in Space, Name of the Game, Hawaii Five-O, It Takes a Thief, High Chapparal, Mannix, Mission: Impossible, Cannon (TV film), F.B.I., Mod Squad, Streets of San Francisco, Kojak, Moving On, Murder She Wrote.
PICTURES INCLUDE: C.C. & Company, Marco Polo.

ROBBINS, BURTON: Exec. Chm. & chief exec. officer, National Screen Service Corp. b. New York City.

ROBBINS, MATTHEW: Writer-Director. e. Univ. of S. Calif. School of Cinema. Writes scripts in collaboration with Hal Barwood, Robbins branching out into directing also with Corvette Summer in 1978.
PICTURES INCLUDE: Scripts, all with Barwood: The Sugarland Express, The Bingo Long Traveling All-Stars and Motor Kings, Corvette Summer (also dir.); Dragonslayer (also dir.).

ROBERT, PATRICIA HARRISON: Executive. b. Atlanta, Ga., March 31, 1939. e. Manhattanville College of the Sacred Heart, Ecole Francaise (Paris), U. of Virginia Graduate School. Dir. of pub. & pub. relations, Gerald Rafshoon Advertising, 1965–69; drama critic, Atlanta Magazine, 1965–68; drama critic, feature writer, The Atlanta Constitution, 1968–69; asst. to publicity director, The Walter Reade Organization, 1969–70; director of publicity—public relations, Radio City Music Hall, 1970. Became Director of Advertising—Public Relations, July, 1973; appt. v.p., 1976. Named east coast pub. dir., Universal Pictures, 1983. In 1984 appt. v.p., pub., Orion Pictures Dist. Corp.

ROBERTS, CURTIS: Producer. b. Dover, England. e. Cambridge U. Child actor. England, Germany; numerous pictures for Rank Org.; prod. England, on Broadway in Gertie, Island Visit; co-prod. on Broadway, Horses in Midstream, Golden Apple, Tonight or Never; tour and N.Y. 1965, The Journey, B'way, 1965. Now pres., CGC Films, Munich.
TV: Rendezvous, Deadly Species, Top Secret, The Ilona Massey Show, When In Rome, Ethan Frome, Black Chiffon.
PICTURES INCLUDE: An Actress in Love, La Die, Hypocrite, Jet Over the Atlantic, The Vixen, Farewell Party, Polly's Return, Rain Before Seven, Halloween, Malaga, My Dear Children, Bus Stop, Eve Arden Show.
BOOKS: History of Summer Theatre, The History of Vaudeville, Other Side of the Coin, 1969, History of Music (Popular) 1900–70. 1970, History of English Music Halls (1972), Latta (1972). Then There Were Some (1979), I Live to Love (1985), Gabor the Merrier (1986).
TOURS: Blithe Spirit, Showboat, Kiss Me Kate, Generation, The Camel Bell, Farewell Party, Twentieth Century, Great Sebastians, Goodbye Charlie, Time of the Cuckoo, Under Papa's Picture, Everybody's Gal, Divorce Me Darling, Gingerbread Lady, September Song, 1975, Same Time Next Year, Funny Girl, Pal Joey, South Pacific, It girl, Fanny (& Bdwy.), 1984–85. Breaking Up the Act (pre-Bdwy.).

ROBERTS, ERIC: Actor. b. Biloxi, MS, April 18, 1956. Father founded Actors and Writers Workshop in Atlanta (1963). Eric began appearing in stage prods. at age 5. Studied in London at Royal Academy of Dramatic Arts, 1973–74. Returned to US to study at American Academy of Dramatic Arts. On stage in Rebel Women, Streetcar Named Desire, etc.
PICTURES: King of the Gypsies (debut, 1978), Raggedy Man, Star 80, The Pope of Greenwich Village, The Coca Cola Kid, Runaway Train, Nobody's Fool.
TELEVISION: Paul's Case, Miss Lonelyhearts, etc.

ROBERTS, LYNNE: Actress (also know as Mary Hart); b. El Paso, Tex., Nov. 22, 1922. e. Lawler Prof. Sch. On stage prior to screen debut in Dangerous Holiday, 1937.
PICTURES INCLUDE: My Buddy, Big Bonanza, Girls of the Big House, The Chicago Kid, Winter Wonderland, Eyes of Texas, Sons of Adventure, Timber Trial, Trouble Preferred, Madonna of the Desert, Secret Service Investigator, Call of Klondike, Blazing Sun, Great Plane Robbery, The Blazing Forest, Because of You, Port Sinister.

ROBERTS, MARGUERITE: Writer. b. Clarks, Neb. m. John Sanford, novelist.
PICTURES INCLUDE: Honky Tonk, Dragon Seed, Ziegfeld Girl, Sea of Grass, If Winter Comes, Ambush, Escape, Soldiers Three, Diamond Head, Love Has Many Faces, Five Card Stud, Norwood, Shootout, Red Sky At Morning, True Grit.

ROBERTS, PERNELL: Actor. b. Waycross, GA, May 18, 1930. e. Univ. of Maryland. Left college to begin working with summer stock companies, joining Arena Stage in Washington, D.C. In 1952 began appearing off-Bdwy. in New York; made Bdwy. debut in 1958 in Tonight in Samarkand. Film debut in Desire Under the Elms (1958).
PICTURES: The Sheepman, Ride Lonesome, etc.
TELEVISION: Series: Bonanza, Vegas, Trapper John M.D. Movie: High Noon Part II: The Return of Will Kane.

ROBERTS, STEPHEN: Executive. b. 1939. Started career at Columbia Pictures Industries in 1958; 1967, moved to intl. sls. div. of 20th Century-Fox. Named pres. of two Fox units: intl. theatres div. and licensing corp. In 1977 appt. pres. of Fox telecommunications div. and in 1979 chm. of Fox Video (formerly Magnetic Video). In 1982 named pres. of new CBS-Fox Co., video cassette and disc firm.

ROBERTS, TONY: Actor. b. New York City, Oct. 22, 1939. e. Northwestern Univ. On Bdwy. in Play It Again Sam, Promises Promises, Barefoot in the Park, Absurd Person Singular, Sugar, Doubles, etc.
PICTURES: Million Dollar Duck, The Star Spangled Girl, Play It Again Sam, Serpico, The Taking of Pelham One Two Three, Lovers Like Us, Annie Hall, Just Tell Me What You Want, Stardust Memories, A Midsummer Night's Sex Comedy, Amityville 3-D, Key Exchange, Hannah and Her Sisters.
TELEVISION: The Lindbergh Kidnapping Case, Girls in the Office, If Things Were Different, The Way They Were, A Question of Honor, etc.

ROBERTS, WILLIAM: Writer-Producer. b. Los Angeles. e. USC.
PICTURES INCLUDE: The Mating Game, The Magnificent Seven, Wonderful World of the Brothers Grimm, Come Fly With Me, The Devil's Brigade, The Bridge At Remagen, One More Train to Rob, Red Sun, The Last American Hero, Posse, Ten to Midnight.
TV: created Donna Reed Show.

ROBERTSON, CLIFF: Actor. b. La Jolla, Calif., 1925.
STAGE: Mr. Roberts, Late Love, The Lady and the Tiger, The Wisteria Tree, Orpheus Descending.
TV: Philco-Goodyear, Studio One, Robert Montgomery presents; Man Without a Country (movie); Washington: Behind Closed Doors; Falcon Crest.
PICTURES INCLUDE: Picnic, Autumn Leaves, Battle of the Coral Sea, As the Sea Ranges, Underworld, USA, The Big Show, Gidget, All in a Night's Work, The Interns, PT 109, The Best Man, 633 Squadron, Masquerade, The Honey Pot, The Devil's Brigade, Charly, (Academy Award, Best Actor, 1969), Too Late the Hero, The Great Northfield, Minnesota Raid, J. W. Coop (director, actor); Man On a Swing, Three Days of the Condor, Midway, Shoot, Class, Brainstorm, Star '80.

ROBERTSON, DALE: Executive, actor, producer (Star of Tomorrow, 1951), r.n. Dayle; b. Oklahoma City, Okla., July 14, 1923; e. Oklahoma Military Coll. Prof. prizefighter; U.S. Army Sept. 1942–June 1945; m.p. debut in Fighting Man of the Plains.
PICTURES INCLUDE: Caribou Trail, Two Flags West, Call Me Mister, Take Care of My Little Girl, Golden Girl, Lydia Bailey, Return of the Texan, Outcasts of Poker Flat, O. Henry's Full House, Farmer Takes a Wife, Gambler from Natchez, Sitting Bull, Son of Sinbad, Day of Fury, Law of the Lawless, Blood on the Arrow, The Walking Major, The Coast of Skeleton, The One-Eyed Soldier, The Last Ride of the Daltons, Dakota Incident, View from the Terrace, Fast and Sexy, Hell's Canyon.
TELEVISION: (series) Wells Fargo, The Iron Horse, Death Valley Days, Hollywood Palace. (films) Melvin Purvis, Kansas City Massacre.

ROBIN, DANY: Actress. b. Paris, France. Dancer since child. Played at the opera; acted on stage in Paris, then m.p.
PICTURES INCLUDE: Thirst of Men, Naughty Martine (L'Eventail); American Language debut in Act of Love, 1954. Holiday for Henrietta, Topaz.

RODDAM, FRANC: Director. b. 1946, England. Studied at London Film School; spent two years as adv. copywriter/prod. with Ogilvy, Benson, Mather before joning BBC as documentary filmmaker. Feature film debut, Quadrophenia.
PICTURES: The Lords of Discipline, Rain Forest, The Bride.
TELEVISION: The Family, Mini, Dummy, Aufwiedersehen Pet.

RODDENBERRY, GENE: Producer—Writer. b. El Paso, EX,

Aug, 19, 1921. Was airline pilot and LAPD sergeant.
PICTURES: Pretty Maids All in a row (p., s.p.). Star Trek—The Motion Picture.
TELEVISION: Star Trek (creator-prod.), Questor, The Lieutenant, Genesis 2.

RODGERS, GABY: Actress. b. Frankfort, Germany, Mar. 29, 1928; e. Mt. Holyoke Coll., 1944–48. Barter Theatre Award, 1950; summer stock, many TV shows.
TV: Suspense, Philco Playhouse, Danger, Robert Montgomery, Pulitzer Prize Playhouse, Kraft TV Theatre, Omnibus.
PICTURES INCLUDE: Kiss Me Deadly.

ROEG, NICHOLAS: Director-Cameraman. b. London Aug. 15, 1928. Entered film industry through cutting rooms of MGM's British Studios, dubbing French films into English. Moved into prod. as clapper boy and part of photographer Freddie Young's crew. Next became camera operator (Trials of Oscar Wilde, The Sundowners). Had first experience as cameraman on TV series (Police Dog and Ghost Squad). Feature film debut as cameraman on Doctor Crippen. Debut as director on Performance; co-directed with Donald Cammell. First solo dir. film, Walkabout.
PICTURES INCLUDE: Cameraman: The System, Every Day's a Holiday, The Caretaker, Nothing But the Best, A Funny Thing Happened on the Way to the Forum, Fahrenheit 451, Far from the Madding Crowd, Petulia. Director-Cameraman: Performance (co.-dir.), Walkabout, Don't Look Now, The Man Who Fell To Earth, Bad Timing, Eureka. Director: Insignificance.

ROGELL, ALBERT S.: Producer and director. b. Oklahoma City, Okla., Aug. 21, 1901; e. public school and h.s., Spokane, Wash., Washington State Coll.; m. Irma Warner; camera man; cutter, titler, author, dir. Has been assoc. with First Nat'l, Universal, FBO and Tiffany. Ent. m.p. ind. 1916 with Washington M.P. Co., Spokane. Went to Hollywood, 1917, as assist. to George Loane Tucker, prod. of The Miracle Man; joined Andrew J. Callahan Prod. In 1921 made Hollywood's first coop. film, costing $1,200 which C.B.C. bought; prod. Hallroom Boys series for Columbia. Then joined Western Pictures Exploitation Co. In 1925 joined Universal for two years, dir. 8 pic. a year; to First Nat'l & dir. Shepherd of the Hills, Aloha, Mamba, Tiffany Tip Off.
PICTURES INCLUDE: Magnificent Rogue, Earl Carroll, Sketchbook, Heaven Only Knows, Song of India, Northwest Stampede, Admiral Was a Lady, Shadow of Fear.
TV: Ford Theatre, 20th Century Hour, Broken Arrow, etc.

ROGERS, CHARLES (BUDDY): Actor. b. Olathe, Kan., Aug. 13, 1904; m. Mary Pickford; p. Maude & Bert Henry Rogers; e. U. of Kansas, and was trained for screen in Paramount Picture School. Appeared in Fascinating Youth and others. In armed services WW II. In 1945 named v.p. & treas. Comet Prods., Inc. Assoc. prod. Sleep My Love, 1950, pres. PRB, Inc., prod. radio, video shows.
PICTURES INCLUDE: Wings, My Best Girl, Get Your Man, Abie's Irish Rose, The Lawyer's Secret, Road to Reno, Working Girls, This Reckless Age, Best of Enemies. Fox: Take a Chance, Dance Band, Old Man Rhythm, One In a Million, Let's Make a Night of It, This Way Please, Golden Hoofs, Mexican Spitfire's Baby, Sing for Your Supper, Mexican Spitfire at Sea, Mexican Spitfire Sees a Ghost, Don't Trust Your Husband.

ROGERS, FRED: Television Host & producer. b. Latrobe, PA, 1928. e. Rollins College (BA, music composition). In 1951 served as asst. prod. of NBC-TV's The Voice of Firestone and NBC-TV Opera Theatre. Later promoted to network floor dir., supervising Your Lucky Strike Hit Parade, Kate Smith Hour, etc. In Nov., 1953, joined WQED-TV in Pittsburgh, educational TV station, to handle programming. In 1954 started Children's Corner series, writing, producing and performing; it ran 7 years. In 1963 was ordained minister of Presbyterian Church, dedicated to working with children and families through TV. Same year introduced character of Mister Rogers on Canadian Bdctg. Corp. of 15-min. daily program. Ran for one year—was similar in content to present half-hour program, Mister Rogers' Neighborhood. In 1964 programs were incorporated into larger, half-hour format on ABC affiliate in Pittsburgh. In 1966, 100 programs acquired by Eastern Educational Network, broadcast in Pittsburgh, and seen for first time in other cities. Program now carried over 270 PBS stations.
AWARDS: George Foster Peabody, NET Special, Saturday Review TV, General Federation of Women's Club, Ralph Lowell, Gabriel, many honorary doctoral degrees from universities. Emmy—(1980) Outstanding Individual Achievement in Children's Programming; Abe Lincoln Distinguished Communications Recognition Award. Odyssey Award, 1981; Ohio State Award, 1983; Christopher Award, ACT Awards, 1984; Emmy, 1985.

ROGERS, GINGER: Actress. r.n. Virginia Katherine McMath; b. Independence, Mo., July 16, 1911. On stage in vaudeville, m.p. theat. presentations & musical comedy (Girl Crazy;). On screen from 1930. Academy Award, best performance by an actress. 1940 (Kitty Foyle, RKO Radio); voted among ten best Money-Making Stars in M.P. Herald-Fame Poll 1935, '37. In numerous pictures including Young Man of Manhattan, Gold Diggers of 1933, and others.
PICTURES INCLUDE: 42nd Street, Flying Down to Rio, The Gay Divorcee, Top Hat, Swing Time, The Story of Irene & Vernon Castle, Having Wonderful Time, Bachelor Mother, Tom Dick & Harry, Vivacious Lady, Stage Door, Primrose Path, Kitty Foyle, Roxie Hart, The Major & the Minor, Once Upon a Honeymoon, Lady in the Dark, Tender Comrade, I'll be Seeing You, Week-End at the Waldorf, Heartbeat, Magnificent Doll, It Had to Be You, Barkeleys of Broadway, Perfect Strangers, Groom Wore Spurs, Storm Warning, We're Not Married, Dream Boat, Monkey Business, Forever Female, Black Widow, Twist of Fate, Tight Spot, First Traveling Saleslady, Oh! Men, Oh! Women, Teenage Rebel, Harlow, The Confession.
TV: Como Show, Pontiac, Pat Boone, Dinah Shore, Bob Hope, Ed Sullivan, Hollywood Palace, Chrysler, Steve Allen, Jack Benny, Cinderella.

ROGERS, HENRY C.: Publicist. b. Irvington, N.J., April 19, 1914; e. U. of Pa., 1934, bd. chm., Rogers & Cowan, Inc.

ROGERS, JOHN W.: Producer. b. Buffalo, N.Y. 1916; p. Charles R. Rogers, prod.; e. U.S.C., 2nd asst. dir., 20th-Fox, then asst. dir., 5 yrs.; assoc. prod., Pine-Thomas prod.; U.S. Army, 4 yrs.; indep. Prod.; assoc. prod., U-I, 1951; prod., 1952.
PICTURES INCLUDE: Powers Girl, Fabulous Dorseys, Buccaneer's Girl, Iron Man, Raging Tide, Here Come the Nelson's, Red Ball Express; prod., Spirit of West Point, Law and Order, War Arrow, Ride Clear of Diablo, Black Horse Canyon.

ROGERS, KENNY: Singer-Actor-Songwriter. b. Crockett, TX, Aug. 21, 1938. Country and Western singer. On screen in Six Pack.
TELEVISION: Many specials and Movies: Kenny Rogers as The Gambler, Coward of the County, The Gambler—The Adventure Continues, Wild Horses, etc.

ROGERS, LAWRENCE H., II: Executive, b. Trenton, N.J. Sept. 6, 1921; e. Princeton U. 1942, U.S. Army, 1942–1946; WSAZ, Huntington, W. Va. Radio & TV, V.P. & Gen. Mgr., 1949–55; WSAZ, Inc., President, 1955–59; Taft Broadcasting Co., v.p., 1959–63; Taft Broadcasting Co., President, 1963–76. Vice Chairman, Hanna-Barbera Productions, L.A., Calif. and Cinemobile Systems, Hollywood. Director: Cine Artists International, Hollywood; Cincinnati Financial Corp.; Inter-Ocean Insurance Co., Cinti.; Cardinal Fund, Ohio; Federal Reserve Bank of Cleveland, Cincinnati Branch; Theater Development Fund, New York; Greater Cincinnati Foundation; Rockford College, Rockford, Ill.

ROGERS, PETER: Executive. b. Rochester, Eng., Feb. 20, 1916; e. Kings School, Rochester, Journalist and in theatre and BBC; joined G. W. H. Productions 1941 as script writer; with Gainsborough Studios; asst. scenario ed. to Muriel Box; assoc. prod.; personal asst. to Sydney Box 1949.
PICTURES INCLUDE: Dear Murderer, Holiday Camp, When the Bough Breaks, Here Come the Huggetts, Huggetts Abroad, Vote for Huggett, It's Not Cricket, Marry Me, Don't Ever Leave Me, Appointment with Venus (Island Rescue), The Clouded Yellow, The Dog and the Diamonds (Children's Film Found.), Up to His Neck, You Know What Sailors Are, Cash on Delivery, To Dorothy A Son, Gay Dog, Circus Friends, Passionate Stranger, After the Ball, Time Lock, My Friend Charles, Chain of Events, Carry on Sergeant, Flying Scott, Cat Girl, Solitary Child, Carry On Teacher, Carry On Nurse, Carry On Constable, Please Turn Over, Watch Your Stern, The Tommy Steele Story, The Duke Wore Jeans, No Kidding, Carry On Regardless, Raising the Wind, Twice Around the Daffodils, Carry on Cruising, The Iron Maiden, Nurse on Wheels, Carry on Cabby, This is My Street, Carry On Jack, Carry On Spying, Carry On Cleo, The Big Job, Carry on Cowboy, Carry on Screaming, Don't Lose Your Head, Follow that Camel, Carry on Doctor, Carry on Up the Khyber, Carry on Camping, Carry on Assault, Carry on Henry, Quest, Revenge, Carry on At Your Convenience, All Coppers Are . . . Carry on Matron, Carry on Abroad, Bless This House, Carry on Girls, Carry on Dick, Carry on Behind, Carry on England, The Best of Carry On, Carry on Emmannuelle.
TV: Ivanhoe series, Carry on Laughing, Carry on Laughing (2), What a Carry on (2).

ROGERS, RICHARD H.: Executive. b. New York, Jan. 26, 1926. e. Colby Coll., Waterville, Me. Served in U.S. Army during WW II with Engineers. Joined Ziv TV in research and asst. to film ed. on Yesterday's Newsreel, 1948; sales dept., 1949; Flamingo Films, handling midwest sales, 1950; R. Monroe Prod., sales mgr. of TV properties, 1952; southeastern sales mgr. Sterling TV, 1954; PR dept., Shell Oil, 1955; acct. exec. Modern Talking Picture Service,

1957; elected v.p. and eastern sales mgr., 1962; v.p. for theatre division, 1965. Pres. of RHR Filmedia, Inc.

ROGERS, RODDY: Producer. b. Philadelphia; e. St. George's School. R.I.; U. of Pa. asst. acct. exec., Gray & Rogers Adv. Agency, Phila., 1946–48; stage mgr. and lighting coordinator at WFIL-TV, 1948; operations correlator, 1949; prod., dir., 1950; exec. prod. for WFIL-TV, 1951, prod. dir. Paul Whiteman TV Teen Club for ABC and Youth on the March, both on ABC-TV; dir. TV prod., WFIL-TV, 1953, mgr. radio, TV prod., Ward Wheelock Co., New York, 1954; prog. prod., radio-TV account supervisor N. W. Ayer & Son, 1955, N.Y.; chge. network sup. Ayer, N.Y. 1958; v.p., mgr. home office Ayer, 1959, pres. Agency Services Co.; pres. E. H. Rogers & Co., 1969.

ROGERS, ROY: Actor. Family name originally Leonard Slye. b. Cincinnati, O. Nov. 5, 1911. Radio singer; many m.p. from 1937. Voted No. 1 Money-Making Western Star in M.P. Herald-Fame, 1943–54 inclusive; also voted one of ten best money-making stars in 1945, '46. Acting & prod. TV films, 1952 with wife, Dale Evans; one-hour spectaculars, Chevy Show, 1959–60; contracted for several TV specials and for nationwide appearances with Roy Rogers touring show in Canada & U.S., 1962; State Fairs, Rodeo's since 1962; TV series.

PICTURES INCLUDE: Under Western Stars, The Old Barn Dance, Rep. in 1938; Billy the Kid Returns, Come On Rangers, Rough Riders, Round-Up, Frontier, Pony Express, Southward Ho!, In Old Caliente, Wall Street Cowboy, Heart of the Golden West, Sunset Serenade, Son of Paleface.

ROGERS, TED: Producer. b. Cleveland, O., Oct. 21, 1920. e. Cornell U.; dir. prog.; prod. I.T.C.

ROGERS, WILL, JR.: Actor. b. New York, N.Y. Oct. 20, 1912; p. late Will Rogers, actor; e. Stanford U., 1935. Publisher, ed., Beverly Hills Citizen; for. corresp.; elected congressman from Calif.; U.S. Army, WW II; m.p. debut in Story of Will Rogers, since in Eddie Cantor Story, Boy From Oklahoma.

ROHM, MARIA: Actress. b. Vienna, Austria, 1949. Early career with Burgtheater in Vienna. Ent. TV 1963, Films 1966. Films incl: Million Eyes of Sumuru, Five Golden Dragons, House of a Thousand Dolls, 99 Women, Blood of Fu Manchu, Justine, Venus in Furs, Eugenie, Black Beauty, Treasure Island, Call of the Wild, The Assassin Is Not Alone, Ten Little Indians, End of Innocence. Flight to Hell, TV Series, Quatermain, White Stallion (assoc. producer) and Black Arrow.

ROIZMAN, OWEN: Cinematographer.

PICTURES INCLUDE: The French Connection, Play it Again, Sam, The Heartbreak Kid, The Exorcist, Network, Straight Time, Three Days of the Condor, The Electric Horseman, Absence of Malice, Tootsie, Vision Quest.

ROLAND, GILBERT: Actor. r.n. Luis Alonso. b. Juarez, Mexico, Dec. 11, 1905; p. Mr. & Mrs. Francisco Alonso, father a bull-fighter in Spain. e. private schools in Mexico.

PICTURES INCLUDE: Captain Kidd, Pirates of Monterey, Dude Goes West, Malaya, We Were Strangers, Crisis, The Furies, The Torch, Bullfighter and Lady, Mark of Renegade, Ten Tall Men, My Six Convicts, Glory Alley, Miracle of Fatima, Apache War Smoke, Bad & the Beautiful, Thunder Bay, Diamond Queen, Beneath the 12-Mile Reef, French Line, Underwater, The Racers, That Lady, Treasure of Pancho Villa, Guns of the Timberland, The Wild Innocents, Eyes of Father Thomasino, The Big Circus, Samar, Cheyenne Autumn, The Reward, High Chaparral, Christian Licorice Store, Islands in the Stream, Caboblanco, Barbarosa.

TV: Bonanza, Alfred Hitchcock Presents, The FBI, Gunsmoke, The Fugitive, etc.

ROLEY, SUTTON: Director. b. Belle Vernon, Pa. Made dir. debut in live TV on Lights Out. Directed many live NBC-TV shows in "golden days" including Macbeth, with Judith Anderson and Maurice Evans. Moved to L.A.: joined Ziv-UA and wrote, produced and directed Target. Was asst. prod. on Men of Annapolis.

PICTURES INCLUDE: Chosen Survivors.

TELEVISION: The Fugitive, Name of the Game, Gunsmoke, Rawhide, Mannix, Mission Impossible, Lost in Space, Bonanza, The Invaders, and many TV feature films.

ROLLE, ESTHER: Actress. b. Pompano Beach, Fla., Nov. 8. e. New School for Social Research. One of original members of Negro Ensemble Co. in N.Y. Has appeared both off and on Bdwy and in several TV series.

TELEVISION: Guest roles in N.Y.P.D., Like It Is, The Winners. Regular on series: Maude, Good Times. Film: I Know Why the Caged Bird Sings.

ROLLINS, HOWARD E., JR.: Actor. b. Baltimore, MD, 1951. e. Towson State Coll. On stage in Traps, Streamers, Medal of Honor Rag, etc.

PICTURES: Ragtime, The House of God, A Soldier's Story.

TELEVISION: The Edge of Night, King, Roots—The Next Generation, Member of the Wedding, My Old Man, A Doctor's Story, He's Fired She's Hired, etc.

ROLLINS, JACK: Executive. Joined in partnership with Charles H. Joffe (see bio) to set up management-production org. Involved in production of many Woody Allen films with Joffe.

TV: Dick Cavett Show (exec. prod.).

ROMAN, LAWRENCE: Writer. b. Jersey City, N.J., May 30, 1921. e. UCLA, 1943.

PICTURES INCLUDE: (collab.) Drums Across the River, Vice Squad, (collab.) Naked Alibi, (collab.) One Desire, Man From Bitter Ridge, (s.p.) Kiss Before Dying, The Sharkfighters, (s.p.) Slaughter on Tenth Avenue, The Swinger, Author B'way play & collab. s.p. Under the Yum Yum Tree, Author B'way play P.S. I Love You. s.p. Paper Lion, collab. Red Sun, orig. s.p. A Warm December; wrote play, Buying Out, prod. in Buffalo, N.Y.; wrote play Crystal, Crystal Chandelier, prod. in Stockbridge, Mass. McQ, (orig. s.p.) The Mayflower Number; (orig. s.p.) Abracadabra (org. s.p.), Skeletons (orig. s.p.); Lovers Three (orig. s.p.). Broadway play: If! If! If!, Omar Bradley (TV special movie), Anatomy of an Illness (TV movie) based on Norman Cousin's book; Badge of the Assassin (TV movie based on Robert Tanenbaum's book); Alone Together (Bdwy. play).

ROMAN, RUTH: Actress. b. Boston, Mass., Dec. 23, 1924. p. professionals; e. Girls H.S., Boston; Bishop Lee Dramatic Sch. Started career with little theatre groups: New Eng. Repertory Co., Elizabeth Peabody Players. Screen debut in Universal serial, Queen of the Jungle, then minor roles; author stories, The Whip Son, The House of Seven Gables.

PICTURES INCLUDE: Good Sam, Belle Starr's Daughter, Whip Son, House of Seven Gables, The Window, Champion, Barricade, Beyond the Forest, Always Leave Them Laughing, Colt .45, Three Secrets, Dallas, Strangers on a Train, Tomorrow is Another Day, Invitation, Starlift, Mara Maru, Young Man With Ideas, Blowing Wild, Far Country, Shanghai Story, Tanganyika, Down Three Dark Streets, Joe Macbeth, Bottom of the Bottle, Great Day in the Morning, Rebel in Town, Bitter Victory, Look in Any Window, Miracle of the Cowards (Spanish prod.), Love Has Many Faces.

TV: Naked City, Route 66, The Defenders, Breaking Point, Eleventh Hour, Producers Showcase, Dr. Kildare, The Long Hot Summer, Go Ask Alice (movie).

ROMERO, CESAR: Actor. b. New York City, Feb. 15, 1907; e. Collegiate Sch., Riverdale Country Sch. In U.S. Coast Guard, WW II. In 1927 on N.Y. stage.

PICTURES INCLUDE: Wintertime, Coney Island, Captain from Castile, Show Them No Mercy, Beautiful Blonde from Bashful Bend, Deep Waters, That Lady in Ermine, Diamond Jim Brady, Clive of India Metropolitan, Weekend in Havana, Springtime in the Rockies, Tales of Manhattan, Tall, Dark and Handsome, Once a Thief, The Jungle, Lost Continent, FBI Girl, Happy Go Lovely, Scotland Yard Inspector, Prisoners of the Casbah, Shadow Man, The Americano, Vera Cruz, The Racers, Leather Saint, Ocean's 11, The Computer Wore Tennis Shoes, Madigan's Millions, Now You See Him, Now You Don't, The Spectre of Edgar Allan Poe, The Strongest Man in the World, Carioca Tiger, The Story of Father Kino, Lust in the Dust.

ROONEY, ANDY: Writer-Director-Actor. b. Albany, NY, Jan. 14, 1920. e. Colgate Univ. Started career as writer for Arthur Godfrey then for Garry Moore, Sam Levenson, Victor Borge, etc. Produced, directed and performed in documentaries, including Black History—Lost, Strayed or Stolen, An Essay on War, In Praise of New York City, Mr. Rooney Goes to Work, etc. Regularly appears on 60 Minutes (CBS).

ROONEY, MICKEY: Actor. r.n. Joe Yule, Jr.; b. Brooklyn, N.Y., Sept. 23, 1922; son of Joe Yule & Nell Carter, vaudeville performers. U.S. Army, WW II; in vaudeville during early infancy with parents and others before m.p. debut and after; from age of 5 to 12 created screen version of Fontaine Fox newspaper comic character Mickey McGuire in series of short subjects of that title, also appeared in number of features (Not to be Trusted, Orchids and Ermine, The King, etc.). Adopting name of Mickey Rooney, ret. to vaudeville; resumed screen career 1934. Special Academy Award 1940; for Andy Hardy characterization; voted among first ten Money-Making Stars in M.P. Herald-Fame Poll. 1938–43.

PICTURES INCLUDE: The Strip, Sound Off, Off Limits, All Ashore, Slight Case of Larcency, Drive a Crooked Road, Bridges at Toki-Ri, Atomic Kid, Twinkle in God's Eye, Bold and the Brave, Magnificent Roughnecks, The Last Mile, Big Operation, Private Lives of Adam and Eve, Platinum High School, King of the Roaring 20's, Breakfast at Tiffany's, It's a Mad, Mad, Mad, Mad World, Everything's Ducky. The Secret Invasion, The Extraordinary Seaman, The Comic, The Cockeyed Cowboys of Calico County, Skidoo, Pulp, Richard, B.J. Presents, That's Entertainment!, The Domino Principle, Pete's Dragon, The Black Stallion, Arabian Adventure.

TV: Playhouse 90, Pinocchio, Eddie, Somebody's Waiting, The Dick Powell Theater, Mickey, Bill, Bill: On His Own.

ROONEY, PAT: Performer stage, nightclubs, pictures. Producer. e. Denver Univ.; Santa Monica College; Univ. Cal. Los Angeles; Marquette Univ. Entertainer vaudeville, theatres, stage, TV and pictures. Captain U.S. Army Air Corps. during Korean War. Entertained troops Far East Commands. Producer, 1960, C.B.S. Films Inc., producing TV pilots and series. 1962, formed Pat Rooney Prods. with Del E. Webb, hotel and construction exec. 1963–68, producer for Jerry Buss Prods. c/o Paramount Pictures, Hollywood, making feature films.
MAJOR PICTURES INCLUDE: Dime With A Halo, Danger Pass, Caged, Law of the Lawless, Requiem for a Gunfighter, Bounty Killer, Young Once, Hells Angels, Fools, Christmas Couple, Black Eye, Jan and Dean.

ROOT, WELLS: Writer. b. Buffalo, N.Y. e. Yale, Drama ed., NY World; dramatic and film critic, Time mag.; fiction, articles, various magazines; many TV dramas, various programs.
PICTURES INCLUDE: I Cover the Waterfront, Tiger Shark, Bird of Paradise, Prisoner of Zenda, Magnificent Obsession, Texas Across the River.

ROSE, ALEX: Producer. r.n. Alexandra Rose. Started in m.p. distribution with Medford Films, marketing low-budget pictures. Later became asst. sls. mgr. for New World Pictures, working in all phases of distribution. In 1972 met Tamara Asseyev and joined her in co-producing, starting with Drive-In, released by Columbia.
PICTURES INCLUDE: With Tamara Asseyev: Drive-In, I Wanna Hold Your Hand, Big Wednesday, Norma Rae.

ROSE, DAVID: Composer, conductor. b. London, England, June 15, 1910. To U.S. 1914; studied music, Chicago Coll. of Music; pianist with Chicago orchestras; staff arranger for several radio stations; mus. dir., West Coast network; while in U.S. Army, comp. dir. of Winged Victory; songs include Holiday for Strings, Our Waltz.
PICTURES INCLUDE: Texas Carnival, Rich Young & Pretty, The Clown, Bright Road, Jupiter's Darling, Port Afrique.
TV: Musical dir., Red Skelton Show; composer-conductor, Bonanza. Emmy, Fred Astaire special.

ROSE, DAVID E.: Producer. b. Kansas City, Mo., 1895. Ent. industry in 1930 in assoc. Douglas Fairbanks; v.p. gen. mgr. United Artists Studios; same posts with Goldwyn. Prod. and dir. UA Corp. unitl 1938 when he went to England to become chmn., man. dir. of all Paramount companies in Great Britain; currently prod. as David E. Rose Productions, Inc.
PICTURES INCLUDE: Island of Desire, Sea Devils, End of the Affair, Port Afrique, The Safecracker, The House of the Seven Hawks.

ROSE, JACK: Writer. b. Warsaw, Poland, Nov. 4, 1911; e. Ohio U. 1934, B.A. m. Audrey Mary Rose, writer, prod. Paramount Pictures, L.A.
PICTURES INCLUDE: Ladies Man, Sorrowful Jones, The Great Lover, It's A Great Feeling, Pale Face, My Favorite Brunette, Road to Rio, Daughter of Rosie O'Grady, Always Leave Them Laughing, On Moonlight Bay, Riding High, I'll See You in My Dreams, Room for One More, April in Paris, Trouble Along the Way, Living it Up, Seven Little Foys, Houseboat, Five Pennies, Beau James, It Started in Naples, Double Trouble, Papa's Delicate Condition, Who's Got the Action?, Who's Been Sleeping in My Bed?, A Touch of Class, the Duchess and the Dirtwater Fox, Lost and Found, The Great Muppet Caper.

ROSE, REGINALD: Writer, b. New York, 1921. e. C.C.N.Y. Worked as clerk, publicist, Warner Bros.; adv. acct. exec., copy chief; US Air Force, WW II; first TV play, Bus to Nowhere, 1951; since then numerous TV plays, Studio One, other programs.
PICTURES INCLUDE: Crime in the Streets, 12 Angry Men, The Man in the Net, Somebody Killed Her Husband, The Wild Geese, The Sea Wolves, Whose Life Is It Anyway?, Wild Geese II.
TELEVISION: Studs Lonigan.

ROSE, STEPHEN: Executive. Entered m.p. industry in 1964 with Columbia Pictures; named adv. dir. In 1970 joined Cinema V Distributing, Inc. as dir. of adv.; left in 1971 to take post at Cinemation Industries, where was named v.p. and bd. member. In 1975 joined Paramount Pictures as dir. of adv.; promoted to v.p./adv. In 1979 formed Barrich Prods. with Gordon Weaver. In Feb., 1982, rejoined Paramount as v.p., mktg; 1983, named v.p. of mktg. for Paramount; sr. v.p., mktg., 1983. Resigned in 1984 to form Barrich Marketing with Gordon Weaver.

ROSE, SYDNEY: Producer. b. 1939. Ent. ind. 1956 as free-lance writer/photographer, 1959–61: publicity director Films de France Ltd. 1961–3: independent film publicist. 1963–8: Artistes' management company in association with Frankie Vaughan. 1968: Formed independent artistes' agency. 1970–4: Executive agent M.A.M. Agency Ltd. 1975: Independent film producer. 1977: Exec. prod., The Kids are Alright. 1979: Co-prod., Five Star Five.

ROSE, WILLIAM: Screen writer. b. Jefferson City, U.S.A. Ent. m.p. ind. in Britain, 1947.
PICTURES INCLUDE: Gift Horse (Glory at Sea), Genevieve, The Maggie (High and Dry), Touch and Go, The Ladykillers, Man in the Sky, Davy, The Smallest Show on Earth, It's a Mad, Mad, Mad, Mad, World, The Russians are Coming, The Russians are Coming, The Flim Flam Man, Guess Who's Coming to Dinner, The Secret of Santa Vittoria.

ROSENBERG, FRANK P.: Producer–Writer. b. New York City, Nov. 22, 1913. e. Columbia U., N.Y.U. Joined Columbia 1929; writer m.p. & radio; exploit, mgr., 1941; apptd. national dir. adv., publicity, exploitation, Columbia Pictures Feb. 1944. Pub. dir. M.P. Victory Loan, 1945; dir. pub. Columbia Pictures Studios, Hollywood, Jan. 1946. Resigned 1947 to enter production. Co-prod. Man Eater of Kumaon. Collab. adapt., assoc. prod. Where the Sidwalk Ends.
PICTURES INCLUDE: Secret of Convict Lake, Return of the Texan, The Farmer Takes a Wife, King of the Khyber Rifles, Illegal, Miracle in the Rain, Girl He Left Behind, One-Eyed Jacks, Critic's Choice, Madigan, exec. prod., The Steagle, prod. The Reincarnation of Peter Proud; sole adaptation, Gray Lady Down.
TV: Exec. prod. and prod. for Schlitz Playhouse programs during 1957–58; prod., The Troubleshooters; exec. prod., Arrest and Trial, 1963–64; exec. prod. Kraft Suspense Theatre, 1964–65; v.p. MCA Universal 1964; pres., Cutlass Prods., Inc.

ROSENBERG, GRANT E.: Executive. Started career in research dept., NBC; 1977, joined Paramount in research and later in development; 1984, v.p., dramatic develp.; then sr. v.p., develp., for TV group, Paramount. 1985, named sr. v.p., network TV for Walt Disney Pictures.

ROSENBERG, MARK: Executive. Started career in magazine publishing field in New York. Adv. exec. with Seiniger & Associates; agent in m.p. dept. of IFA (later became ICM). With literary agency of Adams, Ray, Rosenberg. In 1978 joined Warner Bros., as v.p., prod.; in 1980 promoted to snr. v.p. of prod.; 1983, pres., W B theatrical production division. 1986, partner with Sydney Pollack in Mirage Prods.

ROSENBERG, RICHARD K.: Executive. b. Paterson, NJ, Apr. 4, 1942. e. Indiana Univ. 1966–77 corp. & entertainment atty. for many major corps. & celebrities. 1974, produced Alice, Sweet Alice, debut film of Brooke Shields. Formed RKR Entertainment Group in 1977, with its subsidiaries, RKR Releasing, Inc., RKR Artists & RKR Prods.
PICTURES: Alice Sweet Alice, Hell's Angels Forever, Search for the Mother Lode, The Wild Duck.
PUBLICATIONS: Entertainment Industry Contracts, 1986.

ROSENBERG, RICK: Producer. b. Los Angeles. e. L.A. City College, UCLA. Started career in mail room of Columbia Pictures, then asst. to prod. Jerry Bresler on Major Dundee and Love Has Many Faces. Asst. to Col. v.p., Arthur Kramer. Was assoc. prod. on The Reivers and in 1970 produced first feature, Adam at Six A.M., with Bob Christiansen, with whom co-produced all credits listed below.
PICTURES INCLUDE: Adam at Six A.M., Hide in Plain Sight.
TV: Features: Suddenly Single, The Glass House, A Brand New Life, The Man Who Could Talk to Kids, The Autobiography of Miss Jane Pittman, I Love You . . . Goodbye, Queen of the Stardust Ballroom, Born Innocent, A Death in Canaan, Strangers, Robert Kennedy and His Times, Kids Don't Tell, As Summers Die.

ROSENBERG, STUART: Director-Producer. b. New York City, 1927. e. New York University.
PICTURES INCLUDE: Murder, Inc., Cool Hand Luke, The April Fools, WUSA, Pocket Money, The Laughing Policeman, The Drowning Pool, Voyage Of The Damned, The Amityville Horror, Brubaker, The Pope of Greenwich Village. Has made over 300 TV shows for such series as The Untouchables, Naked City, The Defenders, Espionage. Chrysler Theatre, Emmy Award, 1962.

ROSENFELT, FRANK E.: Executive. b. Peabody, Mass., Nov. 15, 1921. e. Cornell Univ. (B.S.) & Cornell Law School (L.L.B.). Served as atty. for RKO Radio Pictures, before joining MGM in 1955 as member of legal dept. Appt. secty. in 1966. Named v.p., gen. counsel in 1969 and pres. in 1973. In 1974 also named chief exec. officer. Bd. chm. & chief exec. officer, MGM; now vice chm., MGM/UA Entertainment Co. Member: Bd. of Governers, Academy of M.P. Arts & Sciences.

ROSENFIELD, JONAS, JR.: Marketing Consultant. b. Dallas, Texas. e. U. of Miami, A.B. In U.S. Navy, World War II.

Warner Bros. advertising copy department, adv. mgr. Walt Disney, Adv. copywriter Donahue & Coe. Advertising copy chief 20th Century-Fox. Pres. N.Y. Screen Publicists Guild. In July 1942, ex-officio member industry's War Activities Committee. In 1945 apptd. asst. adv. mgr., 20th Cent.-Fox; adv. mgr., 1949–51; dir. of pub. rel. for Italian Films Export 1952; v.p. chg. adv. prom., pub. IFE Releasing Corp., 1953–55; exec. asst. to Paul Lazarus; v.p., of Columbia Pictures, 1955; exec. in chg., avd., pub. expl., Columbia, 1958; v.p. in chg. adv. pub. expl. Columbia, 1960; elected v.p., Columbia Int'l Pictures Corp., 1962; elected gen. exec. officer, Columbia Pictures, 1962; vice president, worldwide advertising, publicity and promotion, Twentieth Century-Fox, 1963–77; film mktg. consultant, 1977–78; lecturer in mktg., University of So. Calif., 1978–79; v.p. in chg. of worldwide mktg., Melvin Simon Productions, 1979. In 1980 named snr. v.p.; 1981, joined Filmways Pictures as exec. v.p., worldwide adv./pub., promo. 1982, film mkt. consultant, lecturer adjunct, U.S.C. School of Cinema & TV; 1983, exec. dir., American Film Mktg. Assn.; 1985, pres. AFMA.

ROSENSTEIN, GERTRUDE: Director. b. New York, N.Y. e. Barnard Coll., B.A. Neighborhood Playhouse. exec. asst. to George Balanchine & Lincoln Kirstein, NYC Ballet. Assoc. with Gian Carlo Menotti, Festival of Two Worlds, Spoleto, Italy.
TV: Assoc. dir., NBC Opera, Emmy Awards, news programs, election coverages, Kennedy Memorial Mass; dir., Concentration; TV staff dir., NBC. Now free-lance director.

ROSENTHAL, BUD: Executive. b. Brooklyn, N.Y., Mar. 21, 1934. e. Brooklyn College, B.A. 1954, New York U.; U.S. Army, 1954–56; college correspondent, N.Y. Times; ent. m.p. ind. as associate editor, Independent Film Journal, 1957. Joined Columbia Pictures publicity dept. as trade paper contact and news writer, 1959, newspaper and syndicate contact 1960; appointed national publicity mgr., Columbia Pictures Corp., 1962–67; asst. prod. Something For Everyone; pub. dir., Anderson Tapes, Such Good Friends; story ed. and casting dir., Sigma Prods., 1972–75; associate producer, Broadway play, Full Circle, 1973, assoc. prod., Rosebud, 1974; dir. intl. press relations, The Bluebird, 1975; Warner Bros. project coordinator, Superman, 1977–79; Superman II, 1980–81; Superman III, 1982–83; Columbia Pictures intl. mktg. coordinator, Ghostbusters, 1984–85; Tri-Star intl. mktg. coordinator, Labyrinth, 1986.

ROSENTHAL, JANE: Executive. e. Brown Univ., New York Univ. (BA). Original producer of Actor Studio prod., The Best Little Whorehouse in Texas; also served as asst. to dir. of off-Bdwy. & Bdwy. versions of same play. Joined CBS Entertainment 1977 as editor in program practices; 1978 moved to prog. dept.; promoted to prog. exec., mini-series (LA). 1979, named assoc. dir., motion pictures for TV; promoted to dir.; 1984, joined Universal Pictures as v.p., prod. 1985, appt. v.p., prod., for M.P. & TV div., Walt Disney Prods.

ROSENTHAL, RICK: Director. b. New York City, June 15, 1949. Launched career as filmmaker-in-residence with New Hampshire TV Network. Moved to Los Angeles to study at American Film Institute where filmed Moonface, 1973. Theatrical feature debut: Halloween II, 1981.
PICTURES: Bad Boys, American Dreamer.
TELEVISION: Fire on the Mountain, Code of Vengeance, Secrets of Midland Heights.

ROSENTHAL, ROBERT M.: Producer. b. N.Y.C., Dec. 28, 1936. e. Lawrence Academy, Mass., 1952–56. U. of Penn., The Wharton School, 1956–60. Pictorial Officer, Prod.-dir. for U.S. Army Signal Corp., 1960–62; Chief, U.S. Army Production Facilities, France, 1961–62. Production mgr., Gurney Productions Inc., 1963; comptroller, Jalor Productions Inc., 1964; pres. Rosenthal Productions Inc., 1964; prod. Lieut. Wolf, I Wonder Why, Been Down So Long It Looks Like Up To Me. Producer/atty.-at-law, Southwestern Univ. School of Law, 1973–76. Pres., Bel Air Broadcasting Corp., 1984.

ROSI, FRANCESCO: Director. b. Naples, Italy, 1922. Apprenticed as asst. to Visconti and Antonioni; directed first feature La Sfida (The Challenge) in 1958.
PICTURES INCLUDE: Salvatore Giuiliano, Hands Over the City, More Than a Miracle, Just Another War, Lucky Luciano, The Mattei Affair, Eboli, Three Brothers.

ROSS, DIANA: Singer-Actress. b. Detroit, Mich., Mar. 26, 1944. Formed musical group at age 14 with two friends, Mary Wilson and Florence Ballard. In 1960 they auditioned for Berry Gordy, head of Motown Record Corp. and were hired to sing backgrounds on records for Motown acts. After completing high school, the trio was named the Supremes and went on tour with Motor Town Revue. Over period of 10 yrs. Supremes had 15 consecutive hit records and once had five consecutive records in no. one spot on charts. In 1969 Diana Ross went on her own, appearing on TV and in nightclubs. Made film debut in Lady Sings the Blues, 1973.
PICTURES INCLUDE: Lady Sings the Blues, Mahogany, The Wiz.
TV: Diana! (spec.).

ROSS, FRANK: Producer-writer. b. Boston, Mass., Aug. 12, 1904; e. Exeter and Princeton. President, Frank Ross Inc. In 1939, asst. prod. Of Mice and Men, UA, Roach. In 1941, producer, The Devil and Miss Jones, RKO. Co-author of story and s.p. The More the Merrier. Spec. Acad. Award (1945) for prod. The House I Live In, short subject on tolerance.
PICTURES INCLUDE: The Lady Takes a Chance, Flame and the Arrow, The Lady Says No, The Robe, Demetrius and the Gladiators, Rain of Ranchipur, Kings Go Forth, Mr. Moses, Maurie (prod.).

ROSS, HERBERT: Director, b. New York City, May 13. Resident Choreographer A.B.T., Choreographer on Broadway for I Can Get It For You Wholesale, Tovarich, Anyone Can Whistle, Do I Hear a Waltz, On a Clear Day You Can See Forever, The Apple Tree. Broadway Director: Chapter Two. I Ought To Be in Pictures. Ent. m.p. ind. as choreographer/musical sequences dir.
PICTURES INCLUDE: As Director/Choreographer: Funny Girl. As director: Goodbye Mr. Chips, The Owl and the Pussycat, Play It Again, Sam, The Last Of Sheila (produced and directed), Funny Lady, The Sunshine Boys, The Seven-Per-Cent Solution (produced and directed), The Turning Point (produced and directed), The Goodbye Girl, California Suite, Nijinsky, Pennies from Heaven (prod.-dir.), I Ought To Be in Pictures (prod.-dir.), Max Dugan Returns (prod.-dir.), Footloose, Protocol.
TV: Bell Telephone Hour, Fred Astaire Special.

ROSS, KATHARINE: Actress. b. Los Angeles, Calif., Jan. 29, 1943. e. Santa Rosa College. Joined the San Francisco Workshop, appeared in The Devil's Disciple, The Balcony, 1962, poetry festival. TV debut, 1962 in Sam Benedict segment.
TV: Doctors at Work, World Premiere, The Longest Hundred Miles, Ben Casey, The Bob Hope-Chrysler Theatre, The Virginian, Wagon Train, Kraft Mystery Theatre, the Lieutenant, The Road West, Secrets of a Mother and Daughter. Acted in the UCLA theatre Arts prod. of King Lear.
PICTURES INCLUDE: Shenandoah, Mister Buddwing, The Singing Nun, Games, The Graduate (nom. for Acad. Award, Best Actress; voted Most Promising Female Newcomer, Golden Globe Award), Hellfighters, Butch Cassidy and the Sundance Kid, Tell Them Willie Boy is Here, They Only Kill Their Masters, The Stepford Wives, Voyage of the Damned, The Betsy, The Swarm, The Legacy, The Final Countdown, Wrong Is Right.

ROSS, KENNETH: Writer. b. London, Sept. 16, 1941.
TV: The Roundelay, ATV Network, 1963. The Messenger, CBC Network, 1966.
THEATRE: The Raft, Hampstead Theatre, London, 1964. Under The Skin, Citizens' Theatre, Glasgow, 1968. Mr. Kilt & The Great I Am, Hampstead Theatre, London, 1970.
PICTURES INCLUDE: Entered industry 1970. Brother Sun, Sister Moon, 1970. Slag, 1970. Original story and screenplay, The Reckless Years, 1971. Abelard & Heloise, 1971. The Day of the Jackal (nominated for Writers' Guild, SFTA, and Golden Globe Awards), 1971–72. The Devil's Lieutenant, 1972. The Odessa File (nominated for Writers' Guild Award), 1973–74. Original story and screenplay, Quest, 1974–75. Original story and screenplay, Lorenzo The Magnificent, 1975.

ROSS, LANNY: Singer. M.C., Actor. b. Seattle, Washington, Jan. 19, 1906; e. Yale 1928. Columbia Law, Juilliard, 1933. AAU title 1927–28; qualified 1928 Olympics, Star of Showboat NBC 1932–37; retired from track to sing. Town Hall debut, 1936; Showboat, 1932–36. Radio; Packard Mardi Gras, Hit Parade Franco American, Camel Caravan; U.S. Army, Major 1943–46; Ivory Show. First musical show on TV Swift Show 1947–49. Concert Tour of U.S. 1949–54. WCBS Radio, The Lanny Ross Show 1954–61, Telephone Hour, 1963; Today Show, 1964; Les Crane Show, 1965; Joe Franklin, 1973, Salvation Army Banquet, Palm Beach, 1973–75. Records include Jolly Doctor Dolliwell, Silver Dollar Country Album.
PICTURES INCLUDE: Melody in Spring, College Rhythm, The Lady Objects, Stage Door Canteen.

ROSSO, LEWIS, T.: Executive. b. Hoboken, N.J., Feb. 3, 1911. Ent. m.p. ind. 1930; prod. & mgt. for Consolidated Film Ind., 1930–44; Republic Prod., 1944–50; prod. mgr. Republic, 1950–55; asst. sec'y and asst. treas. Republic Pictures Corp., 1959; exec. asst. to exec. prod. mgr., 20th Century-Fox Films, 1960; plant mgr., Samuel Goldwyn Studios, 1961–71; exec. admin. asst. plant mgr., The Burbank Studios, 1972–86.

ROTH, CY: Writer, producer, director. b. Chicago, Ill., Mar. 16, 1912; e. U. of Calif. at L.A. Formed and headed Cy Roth Productions, later formed and was pres. Saturn Films, Inc.
PICTURES INCLUDE: Flight to Outer Space, Caballero

Jones, Spanish Territory, Top Secret, Solar Rescue, Crawling Hand, Stone Dragon, Battle at Silver Pass, Passport to Freedom, Danger at Ghost Town; dir. Combat Squad; prod. dir. s.p. Air Strike, Fire Maidens of Outer Space.
TV: Prod., dir., writer. Adventures of Rainbow Riley; writer, Central Allied Intelligence, Tokyo Police, Attack Squadron, The Twisted Black Cross; dir., Rheingold Theatre, Outlaw Queen; prod., dir., s.p., Attack Squadron, Nuremberg, Growing Wild; prod., dir. Horrors of the Black Forest. Heads C.R. Ent.

ROTH, PAUL A.: Executive, born Asheville, N.C., March 28, 1930. U. of N.C., A.B. Political Science 1948–51. George Washington Univ. Law School 1951–52. U.S. Army 1952–55. Dist. Mgr. Valley Enterprises, Inc. 1955–56. Vice Pres. Roth Enterprises, Inc. 1956–65. Pres. Roth Enterprises, Inc. 1965–present. President NATO of Virginia 1971–73. Chairman of Board NATO of Virginia, 1973–75. Member National NATO Board, 1971–present. Executive Committee NATO of Metro-D.C. 1970–present. Variety Club Tent 11 Board Member 1959–65. President National NATO, 1973–75; chairman National NATO board of directors 1975–77. Co-Chairman Motion Picture Energy Conservation Council, 1973–present. Member Foundation Motion Picture Pioneers, 1973–present. Director & advisory committee, Will Rogers Hospital, 1973–present. Trustee American Film Institute, 1973–75. President, Valley Lanes, Inc., 1975–present. Director, First Fidelity Bank, 1984–present. Director, Metro Mortgage Acceptance Corp., 1984–present. Vice-pres., CAPA, Ltd., 1976–present.

ROTH, RICHARD A.: Producer. b. Bev. Hills, 1943. e. Stanford U. Law School. Worked for L.A. law firm before beginning film career as lawyer and literary agent for Ziegler-Ross Agency. In 1970 left to develop s.p. Summer of '42 with Herman Raucher.
PICTURES INCLUDE: Summer of '42, Our Time, The Adventures of Sherlock Holmes Smarter Brother, Julia, Outland.

ROTHKIRCH, Dr. EDWARD v.: Producer. b. July 30, 1919; e. Friedrich Wilheim U., Berlin; Rockhurst Coll., Midwestern College. Prod. asst., research, Pan American Prod., 1941; research Pacific Films, 1942; U.S. Air Force, 1942–44; asst. prod., Pan American Productions, 1945; analyst, Cambridge Prod., 1947; assoc. prod., Pentagon Films, 1949; assoc. prod., Reelestic Pictures, 1950; assoc. prod. Cambridge-Meran Prod. Co., 1951; assoc. exec. prod., Cambridge Prod., 1954; also v.-p. Continental Prod. Services; assoc. exec. prod. Trinity Hill Productions, produced Pan-American Highway 1954, The Keepers TV series, 1953–58, Famous Women of the Bible, 1955–58; To the Stars TV series, 1954–58; also sec.-treas. Crusader Records and v.p. Orbit Records. Member of many professional societies, director International Association of Independent Producers, presently Executive Producer—Galaxie Productions, and Encore Records also Executive Editor, Intercontinental Media Services, Ltd.

ROTHMAN, FRANK: Executive. b. Los Angeles, Dec. 24, 1926. e. Univ. So. Cal. (LLB, 1951). Mmb. Calif. Bar. Dept. city atty., City of Los Angeles, 1951–55; law firm, Wyman, Bautzer, Rothman, Kuchel & Silbert, Los Angeles, 1956–82; chmn. bd., MGM/UA Entertainment Co., 1982–86. Now partner in law firm.

ROTHMAN, MO: Executive. b. Montreal, Canada, Jan. 14, 1919. Royal Canadian A.F. Student trainee, Universal, India; mgr., Malaysia; mgr. prod. Worldwide Rep. for Edward Small, 1950; sales mgr. UA for Continent, Near East, 1955; Cont'l mgr., 1957; v.p. int'l oper., 1960; exec. v.p., Columbia Pict. Int'l, 1960; v.p. world distrib. 1966; exclusive rights all media, Chaplin Pictures, 1971.

ROTUNNO, GIUSEPPE: Cinematographer. Gained fame as leading cinematographer of Italian films working with Federico Fellini. Also worked for Lina Wertmuller and Luchino Visconti. Later worked in Hollywood.
PICTURES: Scandal in Sorrento, White Nights, Anna of Brooklyn, The Naked Maja, The Angel Wore Red, Rocco and His Brothers, The Best of Enemies, The Leopard, Yesterday, Today and Tomorrow, Anzio, The Secret of Santa Vittoria, Satyricon, Sunflower, Carnal Knowledge, Man of La Mancha, The Stranger, The Organizer, Juliet of the Spirits, Fellini's Roma, Amarcord, Casanova, Orchestra Rehearsal, City of Women, Love and Anarchy, All Screwed Up, A Night Full of Rain, The Bible, All That Jazz, Rollover.

ROUNDTREE, RICHARD: Actor. b. New Rochelle, N.Y. July 9, 1942. e. Southern Illinois University. Former model, Ebony Magazine Fashion Fair; joined workshop of Negro Ensemble Company, appeared in Kongi's Harvest, Man, Better Man, Mau Mau Room; played lead role in Philadephia road company of The Great White Hope before film debut.
PICTURES INCLUDE: Shaft, Shaft's Big Score, Shaft in Africa, Charley One-Eye, Earthquake, Man Friday, Diamonds, Escape to Athena, An Eye for an Eye, The Winged Serpent, Inchon, The Graduates of Malibu High, City Heat.
TV: Shaft (series, 1973), Firehouse (movie), Roots, A.D., The Fifth Missile.

ROURKE, MICKEY: Actor.
PICTURES: Fade to Black, Body Heat, Diner, Eureka, Rumblefish, The Pope of Greenwich Village, 9½ Weeks, Year of the Dragon, Angel Heart.

ROUSE, RUSSELL: Prod., dir., writer. b. New York City. ed. U.C.L.A. Formed Greene-Rouse Prods. with Clarence Greene. Acad. Oscar co-orig. story Pillow Talk. Acad. award nom. co-orig. s.p. The Well. 2 Writers Guild nominations. Writers Guild award outstanding teleplay: One Day In The Life of Ivan Denisovitch.
PICTURES INCLUDE: Prod., collab. s.p. The Town Went Wild. Orig. story Yokel Boy. Collab. orig. s.p. The Home Front, D.O.A. Co-author Pillow Talk. Dir. and collab. s.p. The Well, The Thief, Wicked Woman, New York Confidential, Fastest Gun Alive, House of Numbers, Thunder in the Sun, A House Is Not A Home, The Oscar, Dir. Caper of the Golden Bulls. Dir. and collab. Prod.-writer T.V. series: Tightrope.

ROWAN, DANIELLE: Executive. Began career with Paramount Pictures 1980; asst. to pres. & gen. s.s. mgr. Canadian operations. 1984, transferred to N.Y. as asst. to sr. v.p., dist. 1985, appt. exec. administrator dist./mktg.

ROWE, ROY: Owner-operator, Rowe Amusement Co., Burgaw, N.C. b. Burgaw, May 29, 1905; e. U. of No. Car. Eng. instructor, private bus. coll., 1926–29; Publix Sch. for Mgrs., N.Y., 1930–31; mgr. theatres, Spartanburg, S.C.; Greensboro & Raleigh, N.C.; mgr., Warner Theatre, Pittsburgh, Pa., 1931–34; city mgr. for Warner Theatres, Washington, Pa., 1934–35; opened own theatres in N.C. 1935; member N.C. Senate, 1937, 1941, 1945, 1949, 1957, 1965; House of Rep., 1943; Major, Civil Air Patrol, WWII; pres. Carolina Aero Club, 1943–44; chmn. N.C. Aeornautics Comm., 1941–49; dir. Theatre Owners No. & So. Car. 1943–45; pres., Theatre Owners of S.C. & N.C. 1944–45; pres., Assn. of Governing Boards of State Universities, 1964. Owned and operated motel, Carolina Beach, N.C., 1965–67., Rowe Insurance Agency, 1967–69. Mem. Exec. Bd., U. of N.C. Trustees, 1969. Principal Clerk N.C. Senate 1969–75. Retired. Now water color artist and world traveller.

ROWLAND, ROY: Director. b. New York City, Dec. 31; e. U. of So. California (law). Script clerk; asst. dir.; asst. to late W. S. Van Dyke on Tarzan pictures; dir. of shorts, "How to" Benchley series; Crime Does Not Pay series. Pete Smith Specialties.
PICTURES INCLUDE: Think First, Stranger in Town, Lost Angel, Our Vines Have Tender Grapes, Tenth Avenue Angel, Night patrol, Ski Soldier, Boys' Ranch, Romance of Rosy Ridge, Killer McCoy, Scene of the Crime, Outriders, Excuse My Dust, Two Weeks With Love, Bugles in Afternoon, 5000 Fingers of Dr. T. Affair with a Stranger, The Moonlighter, Witness to Murder, Rogue Cop, Many Rivers to Cross, Hit the Deck, Meet Me in Las Vegas, Slander, Somewhere I'll Find Him, Gun Glory, The Seven Hills of Rome, The Girl Hunters, Gunfighters of Casa Grande, They Called Him Gringo, Tiger of the Seven Seas, Thunder Over the Indian Ocean.

ROWLAND, WILLIAM: Producer, director. b. Philadelphia, Pa., Sept. 12, 1900; e. U. of Pa. Actor: vaude., prod.; play prod.; author; prod. shorts, Universal, 1931–32; prod. features Moonlight and Pretzels, Take a Chance, Sweet Surrender, I Loved an Actress; prod., dir. in chge. Spanish prod., RKO, 1937; Spanish Acad. Award for best prod., dir., Perfidis, 1939; won highest Spanish awards for prod. dir., author, Harvest of Hate, 1940; prod. dir., Int'l Forum series, Follies Girl.
PICTURES INCLUDE: Song for Miss Julie, Flight to Nowhere, Women in the Night.

ROWLANDS, GENA: Actress. b. Cambria, Wisc. June 19, 1936. e. Univ. of Wisc. Came to New York to attend American Academy of Dramatic Arts, where met and married John Cassavetes. Made Bdwy. debut as understudy and then succeeded to role of the Girl in The Seven Year Itch. Launched as star with part in The Middle of the Night, which she played 18 mos. Then brought to Hollywood to make film debut in The High Cost of Living (1958).
PICTURES INCLUDE: Lonely Are the Brave, The Spiral Road, A Child Is Waiting, Tony Rome, Faces, Minnie and Moskowitz, A Woman Under the Influence, Two Minute Warning, The Brink's Job, Gloria, Tempest, Love Streams, Light of Day.
TV: The Philco TV Playhouse, Studio One, Alfred Hitchcock Presents, Dr. Kildare, Bonanza, The Kraft Mystery Theatre, Columbo. Movies: Question of Love, Strangers: The Story of a Mother & Daughter, An Early Frost.

ROWLEY, JOHN H.: Executive. b. San Angelo, Tex., Oct. 6, 1917. e. U. of Tex., 1935–39. v.p. United Artists Communications, Inc., Rowley United Div.: past president, NATO of Texas; past Int'l Chief barker, Variety Clubs Int'l; past pres., TOA; pres., Variety Foundation of Texas.

ROYLE, SELENA: Actress. b. New York City, Nov. 6, 1904; d. Edwin Milton Royle & Selena Fetter, pro. Made debut on N.Y. stage, 1921 in Launcelot & Elaine. Has appeared in numerous N.Y. prod.; on radio starred in Woman of Courage, Kate Hopkins, and many others. On screen 1941 in Stage Door Canteen.
PICTURES INCLUDE: The Sullivans, Mrs. Parkington, This Man's Navy, Main Street After Dark, Courage of Lassie, Green Years, Gallant Journey, No Leave, No Love, Night and Day, Summer Holiday, Wild Harvest, Cass Timberlane, Smart Woman, You Were Meant for Me, Joan of Arc, You're My Everything, My Dream Is Yours, Bad Boy, Big Hangover, Branded, Dammed Don't Cry, The Heiress, He Ran All the Way, Come Fill the Cup, Robot Monster, Murder Is My Beat.

ROZSA, MIKLOS: Composer. b. April 18, 1907, Budapest, Hungary. e. Leipzig Conservatory. Wrote great number of symphonic and chamber music works. Composed music for many m.p. In 1936, Knight Without Armor, Acad. Award best music scoring for drama or comedy (Spellbound) 1945; best music scoring for drama or comedy (Double Life) 1947; Ben-Hur, 1959. Pres., Screen Composers Assn. 1956. Cesar of French Academy for Providence, 1978.
PICTURES INCLUDE: Jungle Book, Thief of Bagdad, Double Idemnity, The Killers, Madame Bovary, The Lost Weekend, Spellbound, Asphalt Jungle, Quo Vadis, Ivanhoe, Julius Caesar, Story of Three Loves, Plymouth Adventure, Young Bess, Knights of the Round Table, A Time to Love and a Time to Die, The World the Flesh and the Devil, Ben Hur, Lust for Life, Something of Value, King of Kings, El Cid, Sodom and Gomorra, The VIP's, The Power, The Green Berets, The Private Life of Sherlock Holmes, Sinbad's Golden Voyage, Providence, Secret Files of J. Edgar Hoover, Fedora, Last Embrace, Time After Time, Eye of the Needle, Dead Men Don't Wear Plaid.

RUBIN, STANLEY: Producer, writer. b. New York, N.Y. Oct. 8, 1917; ed. UCLA, 1933–37. Phi Beta Kappa. Writer—radio, magazines, pictures, 1937–41; U.S. Army Air Force, 1942–45; writer, prod., owner, Your Show Time, Story Theatre TV series; producer, RKO, 20th-Fox, U.I.
PICTURES INCLUDE: The Narrow Margin, My Pal Gus, Destination Gobi, River of No Return, Destry, Francis in the Navy, Behind the High Wall, Rawhide Years, Promise Her Anything, The President's Analyst, The Take.
TV: Ghost and Mrs. Muir, Bracken's World, The Man and the City.

RUDDY, ALBERT S.: Producer. b. Montreal, Canada, March 28, 1934. e. U. of So. Calif., B.S. in Design, School of Architecture, 1956.
PICTURES INCLUDE: The Wild Seed (Pennebaker); prod.; Little Fauss & Big Halsey (Alfran Prods.), Paramount Studios Prod.; Making It (Alfran Prods.—for 20th Century Fox); prod. The Godfather (Albert S. Ruddy Production, Inc. for Paramount). 1974; The Longest Yard, Coonskin, both for Para. 1978: Matilda. 1981: The Cannonball Run. 1982; Megaforce. 1984: Lassiter, Cannonball Run II.

RUDIE, EVELYN: Actress, Singer, Songwriter. r.n. Evelyn Rudie Bernauer, b. Hollywood, Calif. March 28. e. Hollywood H.S., U.C.L.A. At 19, after childstar career in TV and films, stage debut at Gallery Theatre in Hollywood as songwriter, musical director, choreographer and star performer: Ostrogoths and King of the Schnorrers. Currently Producer, Artistic Director at Santa Monica Playhouse; founder of own repertoire Company; among major productions: Backstreet, Dreamplay, and musicals Anatol-Anatol, Attorney at Love, Author-Author, The Alchemist, etc. Screen debut as child performer Daddy Longlegs. Received Emmy Nomination for first TV leading role, Eloise, Playhouse 90, 1956.
PICTURES INCLUDE: The Wings of Eagles, Gift of Love. Filmdom's Famous Fives critics award, 1958.
TV: Hostess with the Mostess, Playhouse 90, Dinah Shore, Red Skelton Show, George Gobel Show, Omnibus, Matinee Theatre, Hitchcock presents, Gale Storm Show, Jack Paar, Wagon Train, G.E. Theatre, 77 Sunset Strip, etc.

RUDIN, SCOTT: Executive. b. New York City, Feb. 14, 1958. Began career as prod. asst. on Bdwy. for producers Kermit Bloomgarden, Robert Whitehead, Emmaneul Azenberg; then casting director. 1984, became producer for 20th Century Fox; named exec. v.p. prodn.; 1986, appt. pres. prodn., 20th-Fox.

RUDOLPH, ALAN: Director-Writer. b. Los Angeles, 1948. Son of Oscar Rudolph, TV director of '50s and '60s. Began in industry doing odd jobs in Hollywood studios. In 1969 accepted for Assistant Director's Training Program sponsored by the Director's Guild. Worked with Robert Altman on California Split and The Long Goodbye (asst. dir.) and co-writer on Buffalo Bill and the Indians.
PICTURES: Welcome to L.A. (debut as dir.), Remember My Name, Roadie, Endangered Species, Songwriter, Choose Me, Trouble in Mind, Made in Heaven.

RUGOLO, PETE: Composer, arranger. b. Sicily, Italy, Dec. 25, 1915. To U.S., 1919; e. San Francisco State Coll., Mills Coll., Oakland. Armed Forces, 1942–46; pianist, arr. for many orch. including Stan Kenton; m.p. and TV.
PICTURES INCLUDE: The Strip, Skirts Ahoy, Glory Alley, Latin Lovers, Easy to Love, Jack the Ripper.
TV: Richard Diamond, The Thin Man, Thriller.

RULE, ELTON H.: Executive. b. Stockton, CA, 1917. e. Sacramento Coll. With Amer. Bdg. Cos., Inc., since 1952; gen. sls. mgr., KABC-TV, 1953–60; gen. mgr., 1961–68; pres., ABC TV Network 1968–70; group v.p. Am. Bdg. Cos. Inc., 1969–72; pres., ABC div. 1970–72; pres., chief operating officer, mem. exec. comm., Amer. Bdg. Cos., 1972–83; vice chm., Amer. Bdg. Cos., Inc. & member exec. comm., 1983–84. Formed Rule/Starger Productions with Martin Starger.

RULE, JANICE: Actress. b. Cincinnati, O., Aug. 15, 1931; e. Wheaton & Glenhart H.S., Glen Ellyn, Ill. Dancer 4 yrs. in Chicago & New York nightclubs; stage experience in It's Great To Be Alive, as understudy of Bambi Lynn; in chorus of Miss Liberty; Picnic, 1953. Screen debut, Goodbye My Fancy.
PICTURES INCLUDE: Starlift, Holiday for Sinners, Rogue's March, Woman's Devotion, Gun for a Coward, Subterraneans, Invitation to a Gunfighter, The Chase, Welcome to Hard Times, The Ambushers, Kid Blue, 3 Women, Missing.

RUNCIMAN, ALEX: Director-producer. b. Santa Cruz, Calif., May 30, 1924. e. U. of So. Calif., B.A., 1949; M.A., 1951; Ph.D., 1959. Served in U.S. Army, 1943–46; radio work, 1946–49; in prod. department, CBS, 1953; staff dir., 1954; has dir. panel, news, educational, variety programs, Television Journal, 1959–60; prod. Eye on St. Louis, 1960–61; prod. award-winning public service programs; Host of Metroplex Series, 1963.

RUSH, BARBARA: Actress. b. Denver, Colo. Jan. 4, 1930. e. U. of Calif. First stage appearance at age of ten, Loberto Theatre, Santa Barbara, Calif., in fantasy, Golden Ball; won acting award in coll. for characterization of Birdie, (The Little Foxes); scholarship, Pasadena Playhouse Theatre Arts Coll.
PICTURES INCLUDE: The First Legion, Quebec, Molly, When Worlds Collide, Flaming Feather, Prince of Pirates, It Came From Outer Space, Taza Son of Cochise, Magnificent Obsession, Black Shield of Falworth, Captain Lightfoot, Kiss of Fire, World in My Corner, Bigger Than Life, Oh Men! Oh Women!, Harry Black and the Tiger, The Young Philadelphians, Bramble Bush, Strangers When We Meet, Come Blow Your Horn, Robin and the Seven Hoods, Hombre, Airport, The Man, Superdad, Can't Stop the Music, Summer Lovers.

RUSH, HERMAN: Executive. b. Philadelphia, PA, June 20, 1929. e. Temple Univ., Headed Flamingo Telefilms, Inc. 1957–60; 1960–71, pres., television div. of Creative Mgt. Assoc. Pres., Herman Rush Assoc. Inc., 1971–77. In 1977–78 chmn bd., Rush-Flaherty Agency, Inc. In 1970 headed Marble Arch TV. In 1980 named pres., Columbia TV; 1984, named pres. of newly formed Columbia Pictures TV Group.

RUSH, RICHARD: Director, producer, writer; wrote, dir. prod., Too Soon To Love (U.I.), 1960; Of Love and Desire (Fox), 1963; dir. A Man Called Dagger (MGM) 1965; dir. Fickle Finger of Fate, 1966; dir. Thunder Alley, 1966; dir. Hell's Angels on Wheels, 1967; dir. wrote Psych-Out, 1967; dir. Savage Seven, 1968; dir., prod. Getting Straight (Columbia), 1970, dir. prod. Freebie and the Bean (Warner Bros.) 1974; dir., prod. wrote, The Stunt Man (Fox), 1980 (AA nominations for best dir., s.p.).

RUSSELL, CHARLES W.: Producer, b. N.Y.C., Mar. 31, 1918. Actor, m.p. & radio.
PICTURES INCLUDE: The Purple Heart, The Late George Apley.
TV: CBS-TV prod., You Are There, Danger.

RUSSELL, EDWARD: Executive. b. Chicago, June 12, 1945. e. Columbia Coll. Started with industry in Chicago as asst. adv. mgr. for Plitt Theatres, 1968–70; asst. adv. mgr., midwest div., MGM, 1970–72; midwest adv. mgr., United Artists, 1972–74; midwest adv. mgr., Filmways (AIP), 1974–77; in 1977 made natl. dir. of cooperative adv. & field promo. for Filmways; promoted in 1980 to exec. asst. to the v.p. of worldwide adv., promo., pub. Member: Academy of M.P. Arts & Sciences.

RUSSELL, JACK: Performer. b. Saratoga Spr., N.Y., Sept. 22, 1919. e. Rollins College, 1945–47. U.S. Air Force, 1940–45; appeared in B'way shows including: Sleepy Hollow, Heaven on Earth, As the Girls Go, Alive & Kicking; many nightclubs as singer; on NBC-TV opera, Pagliacci, 1951; guest star

N.Y.C. Opera, 1953; featured aqua show, A Night in Venice, 1952–53; singer, Your Show of Shows, NBC-TV, 1950–53.

RUSSELL, JANE: Actress. b. Bemidji, Minn., June 21, 1921; e. Max Reinhardt's Theatrical Workshop & Mme. Ouspenskaya. Photographer's model; m.p. debut in Outlaw, 1943.
PICTURES INCLUDE: Young Widow, Paleface, Montana Belle, His Kind of Woman, Double Dynamite, Macao, Son of Paleface, Las Vegas Story, Gentlemen Prefer Blondes, French Line, Underwater, Gentlemen Marry Brunettes, Foxfire, Tall Men, Hot Blood, Revolt of Mamie Stover, Fuzzy Pink Nightgown, Darker Than Amber, Born Losers, Fate Is The Hunter, Waco.

RUSSELL, JOHN: Actor. b. Los Angeles, Calif., Jan. 3, 1921; e. U. of Calif. Served in U.S. Marine Corps. 1942–44, as 2nd Lt. m.p. debut in Frame-Up.
PICTURES INCLUDE: Story of Molly X, Gal Who Took the West, Slattery's Hurricane, Yellow Sky, Sitting Pretty, Forever Amber, Somewhere in the Night, Within These Walls, Don Juan Quilligan, Bell for Adano, Barefoot Mailman, Man in the Saddle, Hoodlum Empire, Oklahoma Annie, Fair Wind to Java, Sun Shines Bright, Jubilee Trail, Hell's Outpost, Last Command, Rio Bravo, Yellowstone Kelly, Fort Utah.

RUSSELL, KEN: Director. b. Southampton, England, 1927. e. Walthamstow Art School. Early career as dancer, actor, stills photographer, TV documentary film-maker. Ent. TV ind. 1959. Made 33 documentaries for BBC-TV.
PICTURES INCLUDE: Prokofiev, Elgar, Bartok, The Debussy films, Isadora Duncan, Song of Summer—Delius, Dance of the Seven Veils, French Dressing, Billion Dollar Brain, Women in Love, The Music Lovers, The Devils, The Boy Friend, Savage Messiah, Mahler, Tommy, Lisztomania, Valentino, Altered States, Crimes of Passion.

RUSSELL, KURT: Actor. b. Springfield, MA, March 17, 1951.
PICTURES: The Absent-Minded Professor, Follow Me Boys, The Horse in the Grey Flannel Suit, Charley and the Angel, Superdad, Used Cars, Escape from New York, The Fox and The Hound (voice only), The Thing, Silkwood, Swing Shift, The Mean Season, The Best of Times, Big Trouble in Little China.
TELEVISION: Series: Travels of Jamie McPheeter, The Quest. Movie: Elvis.

RUSSELL, ROBERT: Performer. b. Passaic, N.J., Baritone, Philadelphia Grand Opera Co.; then radio work as quiz master, m.c., singer, gagwriter, composer, writer spec. material; m.c., writer, composer, dir. eleven Miss America pageants; staged, wrote, dir. five Miss Universe pageants.
TV: Birthday Party, Bonny Maid Show, It's in the Bag, Toast of the Town, Live Like a Millionaire; now m.c. Stand Up and Be Counted, CBS-TV; pres. Pageant Productions, Inc.

RUSSELL, THERESA: Actress. b. San Diego, CA, 1957. e. Burbank High School. Studied at Actors' Studio in Hollywood. Professional film debut in The Last Tycoon (1977).
PICTURES: Straight Time, Bad Timing/A Sensual Obsession, Eureka, The Razor's Edge, Insignificance.
TELEVISION: Blind Ambition (mini-series).

RUTHERFORD, ANN: Actress. b. Toronto, Canada, 1924. Trained by mother (cousin of Richard Mansfield); with parents in stock as child; later on Los Angeles radio programs. Screen debut, 1935.
PICTURES INCLUDE: Laramie Trail, Happy Land, Bermuda Mystery, Two O'Clock Courage, Bedside Manner, The Madonna's Secret, Murder in the Music Hall, Secret Life of Walter Mitty, Operation Haylift, Adventures of Don Juan, They Only Kill Their Masters.

RYAN, ARTHUR N.: Executive. Joined Paramount in N.Y. in 1967 as asst. treas; later made dir. of admin. and business affairs, exec. asst. to Robert Evans and asst. scty. In 1970 appt. v.p.-prod. adm. In 1975 named senior v.p. handling all prod. operations for Paramount's m.p. and t.v. divisions, including supvr. of physical prod., business affairs, studio operations and coordination with co.'s creative personnel and filmmakers. Named asst. to the Chairman and Chief Executive Officer 1976; Chairman and President Magicam, Inc.; Chairman Fortune General Corp.; Chairman Paramount Communications; co-chm. of scholarship comm. of Academy of Motion Picture Arts and Sciences; trustee of Univ. Film Study Center in Boston. Joined Technicolor in August 1976 as pres., chief operating officer and director; vice chm., 1983–85; chm. & CEO, 1985 to date. Chairman Technicolor Audio-Visual Systems International, Inc.; director Technicolor S.P.A.; director Technicolor, Film International; and chairman of executive committee, Technicolor Graphis Services, Inc.; director, Technicolor, Inc.; chairman, Technicolor Fotografica, S.A.; Chairman Technicolor Film International Service Company, Inc.; director and Deputy Chairman Technicolor Limited; chm. & dir., The Vidtronics Company, Inc.; chm. & CEO, Compact Video, Inc., 1984 to date; dir, Four Star Int'l., 1983 to date; dir., MacAndreus & Forbes Grays, Inc. 1985 to date; Permanent charities committee of the Entertainment Industry; Hollywood Canteen Foundations. Vice-Chm. & Dir., Calif. Institute of Arts. Trustee: Motion Picture & Television Fund. In 1985 named chm., Technicolor.

RYAN, MITCHELL: Actor. b. Louisville, Ky. was New York stage actor working off-Bdwy. for Ted Mann and Joseph Papp; on Bdwy. in Wait Until Dark. Member of Arena Stage group in Washington.
PICTURES INCLUDE: Monte Walsh, The Hunting Party, My Old Man's Place, High Plains Drifter, The Friends of Eddie Coyle, Magnum Force.

RYAN, PEGGY: Actress, r.n. Margart Irene Ryan. b. Long Beach, Calif., August 28, 1924. Before entering pictures appeared in vaudeville; on TV in Hawaii Five-O.
PICTURES INCLUDE: Top of the Town, The Women Men Marry, The Flying Irishman, She Married a Cop, Girls Town, Miss Annie Rooney, Private Buckaroo, Give Out, Sisters, Top Man, Mr. Big, Patrick the Great, The Merry Monahans, Follow the Boys, Babes on Swing Street, Bowery to Broadway, Merrily We Sing, That's the Spirit, This Is the Life, Here Come the Co-eds.
STAGE: Everybody, Men in Her Diary, Shamrock Hill, There's a Girl in My Heart, All Ashore.

RYAN, SHEILA: Actress. r.n. Katherine Elizabeth McLaughlin; b. Topeka, Kansas, June 8, 1921; e. Le Conte Jr. H.S., Hollywood H.S.
PICTURES INCLUDE: Something for the Boys, The Caribbean Mystery, Lone Wolf in London, Cobra Strikes, Caged Fury, Western Pacific Agent, Mask of the Dragon, Jungle Manhunt, On Top of Old Smokey, Pack Train.

RYDELL, MARK: Producer-Director-Actor. b. 1934. Studied acting with Sanford Meisner of N.Y. Neighborhood Playhouse. Became member of Actors Studio. Was leading actor for six years on daytime CBS serial, As The World Turns. Made Broadway debut in Seagulls over Sorrento and film bow in Crime in the Streets. Went to Hollywood as TV director (Ben Casy, I Spy, Gunsmoke, etc.). Theatrical feature debut: The Fox. Partner with Sidney Pollack in Sanford Prods., film, TV prod. co.
PICTURES INCLUDE: Director: The Fox, The Receivers, The Cowboys, Cinderella Liberty (also prod.), Harry and Walter Go To New York, The Rose, On Golden Pond, The River. Actor: The Long Goodbye.

RUTHERFORD, ANN: Actress. b. Toronto, Canada, 1924. Trained by mother (cousin of Richard Mansfield); with parents in stock as child; later on Los Angeles radio programs. Screen debut, 1935.
PICTURES INCLUDE: Laramie Trail, Happy Land, Bermuda Mystery, Two O'Clock Courage, Bedside Manner, The Madonna's Secret, Murder in the Music Hall, Secret Life of Walter Mitty, Operation Haylift, Adventures of Don Juan, They Only Kill Their Masters.

RYAN, ARTHUR N.: Executive. Joined Paramount in N.Y. in 1967 as asst. treas; later made dir. of admin. and business affairs, exec. asst. to Robert Evans and asst. scty. In 1970 appt. v.p.-prod. adm. In 1975 named senior v.p. handling all prod. operations for Paramount's m.p. and t.v. divisions, including supvr. of physical prod., business affairs, studio operations and coordination with co.'s creative personnel and filmmakers. Named asst. to the Chairman and Chief Executive Officer 1976; Chairman and President Magicam, Inc.; Chairman Fortune General Corp.; Chairman Paramount Communications; co-chm. of scholarship comm. of Academy of Motion Picture Arts and Sciences; trustee of Univ. Film Study Center in Boston. Joined Technicolor in August 1976 as pres., chief operating officer and director; vice chm., 1983–85; chm. & CEO, 1985 to date. Chairman Technicolor Audio-Visual Systems International, Inc.; director Technicolor S.P.A.; director Technicolor, Film International; and chairman of executive committee, Technicolor Graphis Services, Inc.; director, Technicolor, Inc.; chairman, Technicolor Fotografica, S.A.; Chairman Technicolor Film International Service Company, Inc.; director and Deputy Chairman Technicolor Limited; chm. & dir., The Vidtronics Company, Inc.; chm. & CEO, Compact Video, Inc., 1984 to date; dir, Four Star Int'l., 1983 to date; dir., MacAndreus & Forbes Grays, Inc. 1985 to date; Permanent charities committee of the Entertainment Industry; Hollywood Canteen Foundations. Vice-Chm. & Dir., Calif. Institute of Arts. Trustee: Motion Picture & Television Fund. In 1985 named chm., Technicolor.

RYAN, MITCHELL: Actor. b. Louisville, Ky. was New York stage actor working off-Bdwy. for Ted Mann and Joseph Papp; on Bdwy. in Wait Until Dark. Member of Arena Stage group in Washington.
PICTURES INCLUDE: Monte Walsh, The Hunting Party, My Old Man's Place, High Plains Drifter, The Friends of Eddie Coyle, Magnum Force.

RYAN, PEGGY: Actress, r.n. Margart Irene Ryan. b. Long Beach, Calif., August 28, 1924. Before entering pictures appeared in vaudeville; on TV in Hawaii Five-O.
PICTURES INCLUDE: Top of the Town, The Women Men Marry, The Flying Irishman, She Married a Cop, Girls Town, Miss Annie Rooney, Private Buckaroo, Give Out, Sisters, Top Man, Mr. Big, Patrick the Great, The Merry Monahans, Follow the Boys, Babes on Swing Street, Bowery to Broadway, Merrily We Sing, That's the Spirit, This Is the Life, Here Come the Co-eds.
STAGE: Everybody, Men in Her Diary, Shamrock Hill, There's a Girl in My Heart, All Ashore.

RYAN, SHEILA: Actress. r.n. Katherine Elizabeth McLaughlin; b. Topeka, Kansas, June 8, 1921; e. Le Conte Jr. H.S., Hollywood H.S.
PICTURES INCLUDE: Something for the Boys, The Caribbean Mystery, Lone Wolf in London, Cobra Strikes, Caged Fury, Western Pacific Agent, Mask of the Dragon, Jungle Manhunt, On Top of Old Smokey, Pack Train.

RYDELL, MARK: Producer-Director-Actor. b. 1934. Studied acting with Sanford Meisner of N.Y. Neighborhood Playhouse. Became member of Actors Studio. Was leading actor for six years on daytime CBS serial, As The World Turns. Made Broadway debut in Seagulls over Sorrento and film bow in Crime in the Streets. Went to Hollywood as TV director (Ben Casy, I Spy, Gunsmoke, etc.). Theatrical feature debut: The Fox. Partner with Sidney Pollack in Sanford Prods., film, TV prod. co.
PICTURES INCLUDE: Director: The Fox, The Receivers, The Cowboys, Cinderella Liberty (also prod.), Harry and Walter Go To New York, The Rose, On Golden Pond, The River. Actor: The Long Goodbye.

S

SACKHEIM, WILLIAM B.: Producer-Writer. b. Gloversville, NY, Oct. 31, 1919. e. UCLA. Sr. v.p., Rastar Films. Joined Universal TV 1981 as creative consultant.
PICTURES: Smart Girls Don't Talk, One Last Fling, A Yank in Korea, Paula, Reunion in Reno, The Human Jungle, Border River, Chicago Syndicate, Art of Love, The In-Laws, The Competition, First Blood, The Survivors (prod.), No Small Affair (prod.).

SACKS, SAMUEL: Attorney, agent. b. New York, N.Y., March 29, 1908. C.C.N.Y., St. John's Law School, LL.B., 1930. Admitted Calif. Bar, 1943; priv. prac., law, N.Y. 1931–42; attorney, William Morris Agency, Inc., Sept. 1942; head of west coast TV business affairs, 1948–75. bd. of dir., Alliance of Television Film Producers, 1956–60. L.A. Copyright Society Treasurer, Beverly Hills Bar Assn., Los Angeles Bar Assn., American Bar Assn.; Academy of TV Arts & Sciences; Hollywood Radio & TV Society. Pres. Adat Shalom Synagogue, 1967–69, chmn. of bd., 1969–71; pres., American Field Service West L.A. Chapter 1970–72, United Synagogue of America (Pacific Southwest region), v.p., 1974–86. Counsel, entertainment field, Simon & Sheridan, 1975–86, Los Angeles Ctizens' Olympic Committee. Arbitrator for Screen Actors Guild, Assn. of Talent Agents and American Arbitration Assn. Chm. Task Force Project Caring; board of dir., Jewish Family Service of L.A.; exec. comm., Congregational Cabinet University of Judaism, 1975 to date.

SAFER, MORLEY: News Correspondent. b. Toronto, 1931. e. Univ. of Western Ontario. Started as corresp. and prod. with Canadian Broadcasting Corp. Joined CBS News as head of Saigon Bureau, 1965. Chief of CBS London bureau 1967–70. Joined 60 minutes as co-editor in Dec., 1970.

SAFFLE, M. W. "BUD": Executive. b. Spokane, Wash., June 29, 1923. e. Univ. of Wash. In service 1943–46. Started in m.p. business as booker, 1948. Entire career with Saffle Theatre Service as buyer-booker; named pres. in 1970. Also pres. of Grays Harbor Theatres, Inc., operating theatres in Aberdeen, Wash. Also operates d.i. in Centralia, Wash. On bd. of NATO of Wash. for 15 yrs; pres. of same for 2 terms and secty.-treas. 6 yrs. Elected to National NATO bd. in 1972. Founder of Variety Tent 46, serving as chief barker three times.

SAFIR, SIDNEY: Executive. b. Vienna, Aust., Feb. 2, 1923. e. London U. Ent. m.p. ind. 1940, Shipman & King Cinemas; RKO Radio Picture, 1941; salesman, British Lion, 1943; European sls. mgr., Lion Int'l, 1958; gen. sls. mgr. Lion Int'l, 1960; president, Lion Int'l Inc., 1965; man. dir. Lion Int'l Ltd. 1969; dir., British Lione Film Ltd., 1972.

SAGAL, BORIS: Director. b. Russia, Oct. 18, 1923. e. UCLA, Harvard Law School, Yale School of Drama. Married Marge Champion.
PICTURES: Dime with a Halo, Twilight of Honor, Girl Happy, Made in Paris, The Thousand Plane Raid, Mosquito Squadron, The Omega Man, etc.
TELEVISION: Movies: U.M.C., Destiny of a Spy, Night Gallery, The D.A.: Murder One, The Movie Murderer, Hauser's Memory, The Harness, The Failing of Raymond, Hitched, Deliver Us from Evil, Indict and Convict, A Case of Rape, The Greatest Gift, The Dream Makers, The Runaway Barge, Man on the Outside, The Oregon Trail, Rich Man, Poor Man, Mallory: Circumstantial Evidence, Sherlock Holmes in New York, The Moneychangers, The Awakening Land, Ike: The War Years, The Diary of Anne Frank.

SAGANSKY, JEFF: Executive. b. 1953. Joined CBS 1976 in bdcst. finance; 1977, NBC, assoc. in pgm. devlpt.; 1977, mgr. film pgms.; 1978, dir. dramatic dvlpt.; 1978, v.p., dvlpt. David Gerber Co.; 1981, returned to NBC as series devlp. v.p.; 1983, snr. v.p. series pgming.; 1985, joined Tri-Star Pictures as pres. of production.

SAINT, EVA MARIE: Actress. b. Newark, N.J., July 4, 1924. e. Bowling Green State U., Ohio. Radio, TV actress; on Broadway in Trip to Bountiful; m.p. debut in On the Waterfront (Acad. Award, best supporting actress, 1954).
PICTURES INCLUDE: That Certain Feeling, Raintree County, Hatful of Rain, North by Northwest, Exodus, All Fall Down, Grand Prix, The Stalking Moon, Loving, Cancel My Reservation, Nothing in Common.
TV: How the West Was Won, Fatal Vision.

ST. JACQUES, RAYMOND: Actor-Director. Began career as actor, asst. dir. and fencing dir. for American Shakepeare Festival, Stratford, Conn. Made prof. acting debut in off-Bdwy. play, High Name Today. Made m.p. debut, Black Like Me, 1964.
PICTURES INCLUDE: The Pawnbroker, The Comedians, Mr. Moses, Madigan, Mister Buddwing, The Green Berets, Uptight, If He Hollers Let Him Go, Change of Mind, Cotton Comes to Harlem, Cool Breeze, Come Back Charleston Blue, Book of Numbers (also dir. debut), Lost in the Stars, The Evil That Men Do.
STAGE: The Blacks, Night Life, The Cool World, Seventh Heaven.

ST. JAMES, SUSAN: Actress. b. Los Angeles, Aug. 14, 1946. e. Conn. College for Women. Was model for six years; then signed to contract by Universal Pictures.
TELEVISION: The Name of the Game (series), McMillan & Wife (series), numerous shows.
PICTURES INCLUDE: What's So Bad About Feeling Good?, Jigsaw, P.J., Where Angels Go . . . Trouble Follows, Magic Carpet, Outlaw Blues, Love at First Bite, How to Beat the High Cost of Living, Carbon Copy.

ST. JOHN, BETTA: Actress. b. Hawthorne, Calif., Nov. 26. B'way debut in Carousel; then in South Pacific in N.Y. & London; m.p. debut in Dream Wife; since many more m.p., TV films.
PICTURES INCLUDE: All the Brothers were Valiant, The Robe, Dangerous Mission, Saracen Blade, Student Prince, Law vs. Billy the Kid, Alias John Preston, Naked Dawn, Tarzan and the Lost Safari, High Tide at Noon, City of the Dead.

ST. JOHN, JILL: Actress. b. Los Angeles, Aug. 19, 1940. On radio series One Man's family. Television debut, A Christmas Carol, 1948. Theatrical film debut, Summer Love, 1957.
PICTURES: The Remarkable Mr. Pennypacker, Holiday for Lovers, the Roman Spring of Mrs. Stone, Tender Is the Night, Come Blow Your Horn, Who's Been Sleeping in My Bed?, Honeymoon Hotel, The Oscar, Banning, Tony Rome, Diamonds Are Forever.
TELEVISION: Fame Is the Name of the Game, Dupont Theatre, Fireside Theatre, Emerald Point NAS, etc.

ST. JOHNS, RICHARD R.: Executive Producer. b. Los Angeles, CA. e. Stanford University, B.A. 1953; Doctorate of Jurisprudence, Stanford Law School 1954. Joined law firm O'Melveny & Meyers 1954, specializing in entertainment law. 1963 became partner in law firm. 1968 became senior v.p., Filmways, Inc., becoming president and chief operating office in 1969. 1972, formed Richard R. St. Johns and Associates, independent management and packaging firm. Formed Guinness Film Group in 1975, branching out into full-scale motion picture production.
PICTURES: (exec. prod.): The Uncanny, Death Hunt, Matilda, The Silent Flute (Circle of Iron), Nightwing, The Wanderers, The Mountain Men, The Final Countdown, A Change of Seasons, Dead & Buried, American Pop and Venom, Fire and Ice.

SAKS, GENE: Director—Actor. b. N.Y.C., Nov. 8, 1921. e. Cornell Univ. m. actress Bea Arthur. Attended Dramatic Workshop of the New School for Social Research. Active in off-Broadway in 1948–49, forming cooperative theatre group at Cherry Lane Theatre. Joined Actor's Studio, followed by touring and stock. Also appeared in live TV dramas (Philco Playhouse, Producer's Showcase). Directed many Broadway plays before turning to film direction with Barefoot in the Park (1967).

PICTURES INCLUDE: Director: Barefoot in the Park, The Odd Couple, Last of the Red Hot Lovers, Mame, Cactus Flower. Actor: A Thousand Clowns, Prisoner of Second Avenue, The One and Only, Lovesick, The Goodbye People, Brighton Beach Memoirs.

BROADWAY: Director; Enter Laughing, Nobody Loves an Albatross, Generation, Half a Sixpence, Mame. Actor: Middle of the Night, Howie, The Tenth Man, A Shot in the Dark, A Thousand Clowns, Same Time, Next Year.

SALANT, RICHARD S.: Executive. b. New York, N.Y., Apr. 14, 1914; e. Harvard Coll. A.B., 1931–35; Harvard Law Sch., 1935–38; Atty. Gen.'s Com. on Admin. Procedure, 1939–41; Office of Solicitor Gen., U.S. Dept. of Justice, 1941–43; U.S. Naval Res., 1943–46; assoc., Roseman, Goldmark, Colin & Kave, 1946–48; then partner, 1948–51; pres. CBS news div., 1961–64; v.p. special asst. to pres. CBS, Inc., 1951–61, 1964–66; pres., CBS news div., 1966; mem. bd. of dir., CBS, Inc. 1964–69; vice chm., NBC bd., 1979–81; sr. adviser, 1981–83; pres. CEO, National News Council, 1983–84. Retired.

SALE, RICHARD: Writer, director. b. New York, N.Y., Dec. 17, 1911; e. Washington & Lee, 1934; m. Irma Foster, designer. Author novels, over 400 published stories; honor roll Best Short Stories, 1935; ent. m.p. ind. with Paramount, 1944; member: WGAW, DGA: Acad. of M.P. Arts & Sciences, Authors League of Amer., BMI: pres. Voyager Films, Inc.; v.p. Libra Productions, Inc.

PICTURES INCLUDE: Strange Cargo, Rendezvous with Annie, Spoilers of the North, Campus Honeymoon, Lady at Midnight, Calendar Girl, Inside Story, Dude Goes West, Mother Is a Freshman, Father Was a Fullback, When Willie Comes Marching Home, Mr. Belvedere goes to College, Ticket to Tomahawk, I'll Get By, Driftwood, Meet Me After the Show, Half Angel, Let's Make It Legal, Girl Next Door, My Wife's best Friends, Let's Do It Again, Torpedo Run, French Line, Suddenly, Women's World, Gentlemen Marry Brunettes, Abandon Ship, The Oscar, The White Buffalo, The President's Wife a.k.a. Assassin.

SALETRI, FRANK R.: Producer-Director-Writer. b. Chicago, Jan. 20, 1928. Is criminal trial lawyer, member of State of Calif. bar. Heads FRSCO Prods., Ltd., m.p. prod.

PICTURES INCLUDE: Black Frankenstein—Blackenstein (s.p., prod.); Black the Ripper (s.p., dir.); The Return of the Ghost of the Son of the Bride of the House of Frankenstein, 1984 (s.p., dir.), The Skid Row Slasher, s.p., dir; The Secret of the Maltese Falcon, s.p., dir; Annually prod., s.p. & dir. for The Academy of Science Fiction, Horror and Fantasy Films. Annually prod., s.p. & dir. for The Annual Count Dracula Society 'Ann Radcliffe' Awards. (Both are documentaries).

SALKIND, ALEXANDER: Producer. b. Danzig/Gdansk, of Russian extraction. Grew up in Berlin where father, Miguel, produced films. Went to Cuba with father to assist him in film production. First solo venture a Buster Keaton comedy, 1945. Returned to Europe where made many pictures in Spain, Italy, France and Hungary.

PICTURES INCLUDE: The Three Musketeers, The Four Musketeers, Superman, Supergirl, Santa Claus.

SALKIND, ILYA: Producer. Mexico City. e. Univ. of London. Grew up in many countries as father, Alexander, produced films. First film job as production runner on The Life of Cervantes for father. Was assoc. prod. on Light at the Edge of the World.

PICTURES: The Three Musketeers, The Four Musketeers, Superman, Superman II (exec. prod.).

SALKOW, SIDNEY: Director, writer. b. New York City, June 16, 1911; e. City Coll. N.Y., B.A. Harvard Law Sch. Stage dir. & prod. asst. number N.Y. dram. prods. (Dir. Bloodstream, Black Tower, etc.) and mgr. summer theat. From 1933 variously dialogue dir., assoc. dir., writer & dir. numerous pictures Paramount, Universal, Republic, Columbia, etc.; dir. number of pictures in Lone Wolf series (for Columbia), Tillie the Toiler, Flight Lieutenant, etc. In armed service, WW II.

PICTURES INCLUDE: Millie's Daughter, Bulldog Drummond at Bay, Admiral Was a Lady, Fugitive Lady, Golden Hawk, Scarlet Angel, Pathfinder, Prince of Pirates, Jack McCall Desperado, Raiders of the 7 Seas, Sitting Bull, Robbers' Roost, Shadow of the Eagle, Las Vegas Shakedown, Toughest Man Alive, Chicago Confidential, Iron Sheriff, Great Sioux Massacre, Martin Eden.

TV: Created, prod. dir., This is Alice series for Desilu, Lassie, Fury, Wells Fargo series. Headed prod. for F&F Prod. in Rome, 1967–71.

SALMI, ALBERT: Actor. b. Coney Island, N.Y., 1928. After serving in World War II, studied—1948–54—with Dramatic Workshop, American Theatre Wing, Actors Studio. Appeared in many off-Bdwy. plays and live TV prods. Big hit on Bdwy. in Bus Stop. Other plays include The Rainmaker and The Brothers Karamazov. Has appeared in over 20 feature films and over 200 TV shows.

PICTURES INCLUDE: The Lawman, Something Big, The Deserter, The Crazy World of Jules Vrooder, Empire of the Ants, Dragonslayer, Love Child, Hard to Hold.

TV: Gunsmoke, Barnaby Jones, etc. Movie: Dress Gray.

SALT, WALDO: Writer. b. Chicago, Ill., Oct. 18, 1914. e. Stamford U., 1934, A.B. Taught dramatics & music, Menlo Jr. Coll., 1935; served as civilian consultant writer, Army films, OWI Overseas Film Burea, 1945.

PICTURES INCLUDE: Shopworn Angel, Tonight We Raid Calais, Rachel & the Stranger, M, Wild Man of Borneo, Mr. Winkle Goes to War, The Flame & the Arrow, Midnight Cowboy, Gang That Couldn't Shoot Straight, Serpico, The Day of the Locust, Coming Home.

SALTER, HANS J.: Composer, conductor. e. U. Acad. of Music, Vienna-Austria, Mus. dir.: Volksopera, Vienna; State Oper. Berlin; Metropole Theatre, Berlin; comp., cond., UFA, Berlin, 1929–33; European br., Universal, 1934–36; to U.S., Univ. 1938–47, 1950–52, wrote over 150 scores.

PICTURES INCLUDE: It Started With Eve, His Butler's Sister, Scarlet Street, Magnificent Doll, The Spoilers, Frenchie, Flesh and Fury, Golden Horde, The Sign of the Ram, Frightened City, Ghost of Frankenstein, Black Friday, House of Frankenstein, The Wolfman, Hold That Ghost, The Invisible Man Returns, the Mummy's Hand, Man-Eater of Kumaon, This Island Earth, Tomahawk, The Battle of Apache Pass, Please Believe Me, Apache Drums, Untamed Frontier, Lover Come Back, Thunder on the Hill, Bend of the River, Against All Flags, Black Shield of Falworth, Sign of the Pagan, Far Horizons, Man Without a Star, Wichita, Autumn Leaves, Red Sundown, Hold Back the Night, Rawhide Years, The Oklahoman, Three Brave Men, Pay the Devil, Law of the Trigger, Female Animal, Raw Wind in Eden, The Wild and the Innocent, Bat Masterson Story, Man in the Net, Come September, Follow That Dream, If a Man Answers, Bedtime Story, The Warlord, Beau Geste, Return of the Gunfighter.

TV: Wichita Town, Laramie, The Law and Mr. Jones, The Virginian, Wagon Train, Lost in Space, Maya.

SALTZMAN, HARRY: Producer. Lowndes Productions, Ltd. b. October, 1915. St. John, N.B., Canada. Ent. film ind. 1945. Chm. bd., H.M. Tenment, Ltd., London.

PICTURES INCLUDE: The Iron Petticoat, Look Back in Anger, The Entertainer, Saturday Night, Sunday Morning, Billion Dollar Brain, Battle of Britain, Nijinsky. Also co-producer of 10 James Bond films.

SALVATORI, RENATO: Actor. b. Italy, Mar. 20, 1934.

PICTURES: The Girls on the Spanish Steps, Big Deal on Madonna Street, Rocco and His Brothers, Two Women, The Organizer, One Out of Three, The Harem, Z, State of Siege, The Burglars, Lighthouse at the End of the World, Todo Modo, The Gypsy, Luna, Lost and Found, Illustrious Corpses, etc.

SALZBURG, JOSEPH S.: Producer, editor. b. New York, N.Y., July 27, 1917. Film librarian, then rose to v.p. in chge. of prod., Pictorial Films, 1935–42; civilian chief film ed. U.S. Army Signal Corps Photo Center, 1942–44; U.S. Army Air Forces, 1944–46; prod. mgr., Pictorial Films, 1946–50; prod. mgr. Associated Artists Prod., then M.P. for TV, 1950–51; org. m.p. prod. & edit. service for theatrical, non-theatrical & TV films; prod. mgr., dir. of films oper., official Films. Oct. 1956; prod. sup. tech. dir. Lynn Romero Prod. features and TV; assoc. prod. Lynn Romero Prod. TV series, Counterthrust; v.p., sec'y, B.L. Coleman Assoc., Inc. & Newspix, Inc. 1961; pres. National Production Assoc., Inc. 1962, chief of production, UPI Newsfilm, 1963. Prod. a/c Fred A. Niles Comm. Center, 1966. Appt. v.p., F.A. Niles Communications Centers Inc., N.Y., 1969. In 1979 appointed in addition exec. producer & gen. mgr., F. A. Niles Communication centers Inc., N.Y. studio.

SALZBURG, MILTON J.: Producer. b. New York N.Y., Dec. 17, 1912. Book publishing field, N.Y.; film librarian; ed. instructional film, Dealers in Death; founder & pres. Pictorial Films, Inc., prod. instructional & topical shorts; pres. Academic Film Co. & Academic Prod. of Hollywood; sold Pictorial to Pathe Industries, remaining as pres., 1945; pres. 1946; sales mgr., Post Pictures, 1946; re-purchased Pictorial Films & pres. Nov. 1961; pres. Cornell Films; prod., Pattern for Survival, documentary film & Target: U.S.A., industrial film; pres. Novel Films, Dec. 1952; pres. Award TV Corp. (prod. Jimmy Demaret Golf series, Golden Era of Boxing), pres. Birad Corp., prod. dist. educat. films, 1960 pres. Productions Unlimited, Inc., producers of 16 mm educational films. Prod. 1963 Life Cycle of WASP, Cine Golden Eagle, Pre-Historic Animals, 1965 Story of Rice. Prod. Instincts of an Insect which has won Blue Ribbon, American Film Festival; Chris Award, Columbus Film Festival; Golden Eagle at Cine; Silver Hugo at Chicago Film Festival. 1967, v.p. & gen. sales mgr., Fleetwood Films, 1970, pres. Non-Theatrical Div., United Productions of America, DEI Industres, Inc. Left UPA in 1971 to reactivate Productions Unlimited, Inc., producing shorts and supplying films to govt. agencies.

SAMPSON, LEONARD E.: Exhibitor. b. New York, N.Y. Oct., 1918. e. CCNY (B.B.A. '39). Entered m.p. industry as stagehand helper and usher, Skouras Park Plaza, Bronx 1932–36; asst. mgr. Gramercy Park, 1937–38; mgr., 5th Avenue Playhouse, 1939–41; mgr., Ascot Bronx, 1941–42. In Army 1942–46. On return entered into partnership with cousin Robert C. Spodick in Lincoln, a New Haven art house. Organized Nutmeg Theatres, operating 6 art and conventional theatres in Conn., associated with Norman Bialek in Westport and Norwalk. Sold Nutmeg in 1968 to Robert Smerling. Retains partnership with Spodick in New Haven's York Sq., Lincoln, and Crown. Built Groton, Conn., Cinemas I and II in 1970 and Norwich, Conn., Cinema I & II, 1976 and acquired Village Cinemas I and II, Mystic, in association with Spodick and William Rosen. Acquired Westerly Cinema I & II, 1982.

SAMUELS, ABRAM: Executive. b. Allentown, Pa., Sept. 15, 1920. e. Lehigh U. U.S. Army 1942–46; pres. Automatic Devices Co. 1946–76; named bd. chmn. in 1976.

SAMUELSON, DAVID W.: F.R.P.S., F.B.K.S., B.S.C.: Executive. b. London, England, 1924. Son of early producer G. B. Samuelson. Joined ind. 1941 with British Movietone News. Later film cameraman, 1947. Left Movietone 1960 to join family company, Samuelson Film Service Ltd. Dir., Samuelson Group Plc, 1958–84. Past president British Kinematograph Sound & TV Soc., Chmn, Inc. Ass. Kine. Mans.; chm., London Intl. Film School. Author of Motion Picture Camera and Lighting Equipment, Motion Picture Camera Techniques, Motion Picture Camera Data, Samuelson Manual of Cinematography, and Cinematographers Computer Program. Currently consultant on technology film making, author, lecturer.

SAMUELSON, PETER GEORGE WYLIE: Producer. b. London, England, October 16, 1951. Masters Degree: English Literature, Cambridge University. Early career as interpreter and production assistant. Production Manager: 1973, Speed Merchants. 1974, High Velocity. 1975, One by One. 1976, Return of the Pink Panther. 1977, Sante Fe 1836. 1978, A Man, a Woman and a Bank. 1979–84, exec. v.p., Interscope Communications, Inc. Pres., Starlight Foundation. Director, Friends of British Academy, Filmex. 1985–86, pres., Film Associates, Inc.
RECENT PICTURES: Revenge of the Nerds (exec. prod., 1984); Turk 182 (exec. prod., 1985).

SAMUELSON, SYDNEY: C.B.E., B.S.C., Hon. F.B.K.S., Executive. b. London, England, 1925. Early career as cinema projectionist, 1939–42; Gaumont British News, 1942–43; Royal Air Force, 1943–47; asst. cameraman, cameraman, director/cameraman until 1960; founded Samuelson Film Service, 1955; now chmn. and chief executive, Samuelson Group plc; (man. dir., Panavision Corp. of Calif. Ltd. 1965). Trustee and chmn. board of management, British Academy of Film and Television Arts (chmn. of Council 1973–76). Pres. & sr. Trustee Cinema & Television Benevolent Fund (1983–86). Member of Executive, Cinema & Television Veterans (pres. 1980–81); assoc. member, American Society of Cinematographers. Hon. Tech. Adviser, Royal Naval Film Corp. Hon. member, Guild of British Camera Technicians (1986); Member, British Society of Cinematographers. (governor, 1969–79; 1st vice pres., 1976–77).

SANDERS, DENIS: Writer-producer-director, executive SRS Productions. b. New York City, Jan. 21, 1929. e. UCLA (M.A. 1954). Awards include 2 Academy Awards, A Time Out of War 1954; Czechoslovakia, 1968 in 1970. Made over 70 documentaries including Trial: City and County of Denver v.s. Lauren R. Watson; Arbitration: The Truth of the Matter.
FEATURES INCLUDE: Elvis, That's The Way It Is, MGM: Soul To Soul, Cinerama; One Man's Way, UA: War Hunt, UA: Crime and Punishment, USA.

SANDERS, NAT: Executive. b. New York City, Mar 4, 1892; e. C.C.N.Y., 1912. Publicity dir. & pub. rel. counsel; independent business mgr. for m.p. stars and directors; with sales dept. Commonwealth Pictures, Inc.; gen. mgr. Sanders Films; gen. mgr. Film Alliance of U.S. Inc.; pres. The Baker's Wife, Inc.; pres. Leo Films, Inc.; vp. English Films, Inc.; pres. Film Renters, Inc.; gen. mgr., United Motion Pictures Org., gen. mgr., Times Film Corp.; southern dist. rep: Lopert Films, Inc., Janus Films, Inc., Audubon Films, Continental Distribution Corp., Mishkin Motion Pictures, Inc,; member: M.P. Pioneers, Variety Clubs International Sect'y, National Assoc. M.P. Ind., Motion Picture Pioneers of Florida.

SANDERS, TERRY BARRETT: Producer, director, writer. b. New York, Dec. 20, 1931. e. UCLA, 1951; Co-prod., photographed, A Time Out of War, 1954. Academy award best two-reel subject, and won first prize Venice Film Festival, etc.; co-wrote The Day Lincoln Was Shot, CBS-TV; s.p. The Naked and the Dead; prod. Crime and Punishment—USA., prod. War Hunt; prod. and dir. Portrait of Zubin Mehta for U.S.I.A. Assoc. dean, Film School, Calif. Instit. of the Arts.
TV: Prod. dir., Hollywood and the Stars, The Legend of Marilyn Monroe, National Geographic Society specials, The Kids from Fame, Film Bios Kennedy Center Honors; exec. v.p., American Film Foundation.

SANDRICH, JAY: Director. b. Los Angeles, Feb. 24, 1932. e. UCLA.
PICTURES: Seems Like Old Times.
TELEVISION: Movies: The Crooked Hearts, What Are Best Friends For? Series: Mary Tyler Moore Show (Emmy), Soap, Phyllis (pilot), Tony Randall Show (pilot), Bob Newhart Show (pilot), Benson (pilot), Packy, Insight/Checkmate, etc.

SANDS, ERNEST: Executive. b. Newark, N.J., May 5, 1924. e. NYU, B.S., 1947. Sales exec., Warner Bros., 1947–59; film buyer, Fabian Theatres, 1960–61; gen. sales mgr., Astor Pic., 1962; gen. sales mgr., Allied Artists, 1963–64; asst. gen. sales mgr., Paramount, 1965; v.p. asst. gen. sales mgr., Paramount, Resigned 1969. Ivan Tors Films, Inc., sales exec., 1970; v.p. gen. sales mgr., Cannon Releasing Corp., 1970–73; Sands Film Co. Inc. president, March, 1973. Distributor and Producer's Representative.

SANDS, JOHNNY: Actor. r.n. John Harp; b. Lorenzo, Tex., Apr. 29, 1927. Started in school plays; screen debut in Stranger 1946.
PICTURES INCLUDE: Till the End of Time, Affairs of Geraldine, Born to Speed, Blaze of Noon, Bachelor and the Bobby-Soxer, Fabulous Texan, Admiral Was a Lady, Lawless, Two Flags West, Aladdin and His Lamp, Basketball Fix.

SANDS, TOMMY: Singer. b. Chicago, Aug. 27, 1937; e. Schools there and Greenwood, La. Father, Benny Sands, pianist with stage bands. Started career as guitar player, singer when 10, at KWKH station, Shreveport, followed by other radio app.; TV with Ernie Ford, then Kraft TV show The Singin' Idol; recording contract won him million record sales of "Teen Age Crush."
PICTURES INCLUDE: Sing Boy Sing, Mardi Gras, Love in a Goldfish bowl, Babes in Toyland, The Longest Day.

SANFORD, CHARLES: Musical Director. b. June 17, 1905, N.Y.C. Has been conducting since age of 15; asst. Cond. NY Hippodrome; district musical supervisor, RKO; conducted various shows, assoc. cond. to Alexander Smallens, Porgy and Bess.
TV: Musical dir., Admiral Broadway Review, 1948; Your Show of Shows, 1950–54; Bob Hope, 1950–51; Elgin American Show, 1950; Beatrice Lillie Show, 1950–51; Max Liebman Presents, 1954–56; Producer's Showcase, 1957–58; Jerry Lewis, Patrice Munsel Shows; 1959–60 Max Liebman Specials, Phil Silvers, Sid Caesar Specials.

SANFORD, ISABEL: Actress. b. New York City, Aug. 29. e. Textile High School, Evander Childs High School. Began acting in elementary school and continued through high school. Joined American Negro Theatre (then The Star Players) which disbanded in World War II. Latter associated with YWCA project and off-Bdwy. plays. Bdwy. debut in The Amen Corner.
PICTURES: Guess Who's Coming to Dinner, Pendulum, Stand Up and Be Counted, The New Centurions, Love at First Bite.
TELEVISION: Series: The Carol Burnett Show, All in the Family, The Jeffersons, etc. Movie: The Great Man's Whiskers.

SANGER, GERALD: (C.B.E., J.P.): Director, British Movietone News, Ltd. b. Su-biton, Eng., May 23, 1898; married. e. Shrewsbury School and Kebie Coll., Oxford. Lieut., Royal Marines, 1917–19. Secretary of Hon. Esmond Harmsworth, M.P. (Lord Rothermere), 1921–29. Ed. Brit. Movietone News, 1929–53; dir., Assoc. Newspapers Ltd., 1944–63; F. Hewitt & Son (1927) Ltd. 1954; News Holdings Ltd., 1954; Associated-Rediffusion Ltd., 1954–56; Daily Mail & Gen. Trust Ltd., 1963.

SANGSTER, JIMMY: Producer, director, screenwriter. Ent. m.p. ind. 1943. Prod. man. for Break in the Circle, Men of Sherwood Forest, X the Unknown.
PICTURES INCLUDE: Man on the Beach, The Curse of Frankenstein, The Trollenberg Terror, The Georkel, The Blood of the Vampire, Dracula, Intent to Kill, The Revenge of Frankenstein, Jack the Ripper, The Mummy, The Brides of Dracula, The Man Who Could Cheat Death, The Siege of Sydney Street, The Criminal, The Hell Fire Club, See No Exit, 1960 prod. and scripted Taste of Fear for Hammer Films 1961. Prod. The Savage Guns; 1962; prod. s.p. Maniac, Nightmare, Devil Ship Pirates; prod. Hysteria, s.p., The Giants, Paranoiac, 1963; s.p. Brainstorm, 1964; prod., s.p. The Nanny, s.p. Deadlier Than the Male, The Bridge of Newgate Jail, 1965; 1966 s.p. Java Weed, s.p. The Anniversary. 1967 prod. 1968 s.p. Doubled in Diamonds, Hide and Seek, Foreign Exchange, Private I (prod.) 1969; s.p. The Killing Game, The Claw, Touchfeather. 1970

wrote, prod. dir. The Horror of Frankenstein; dir. Lust for a Vampire, 1971; co-wrote s.p. Gingerbread House, Murder by Month Club, A Taste of Evil, The Goldfish Bowl, s.p. prod., dir. Fear in the Night, 1971. 1973: Screenplay: The Fairytale Man. 1974: s.p. The Monstrous Defect. 1977: s.p. The Legacy. 1980: s.p., Phobia.
TV: Writing credits include: Motive for Murder, The Assassins, I Can Destroy the Sun, 1972, exec. story consultant Screen Gems-NBC short story series, McCloud, Banacek, Cannon, Ironside, etc. 1977–78; prod. CBS series, Young Dan'l Boone; worte & produced pilot for CBS: Ebony Ivory and Jade; wrote pilot for ABC: Adventure (Columbia TV); wrote pilot for NBC: Murder in Music City; The Concrete Cowboys (CBS-movie); Holiday (CBS pilot); Once Upon a Spy (ABC-movie), No Place To Hide (CBS-movie; writer/prod./dir., Ripley's Believe It or Not (ABC).

SANSOM, LESTER A.: Producer. b. Salt Lake City, Utah. e. University of Utah. Radio singer under name of Jack Allen, 1930; ent. m.p. ind. in editorial dept., Fox Film Corp., Dec. 1931; served in U.S. Navy as head of film library, Washington, D.C., 1942–45; head of edit. dept. & post-prod., Allied Artists, since 1953; assoc. prod. Skabenga; prod., co-writer, Battle Flame; assoc. prod. Hell to Eternity, exec. prod. The Thin Red Line, prod. Crack in the World; prod. Bikini Paradise, Battle of the Bulge, Custer of the West, Co-prod., Krakatoa—East of Java; exec. prod. 12+1.

SAPERSTEIN, HENRY G.: Executive. b. Chicago, Ill., June 2, 1918. e. U. of Chicago. Theatre owner, Chicago, 1943–45; pres. Television Personalities, Inc., 1955–67 Mister Magoo, Dick Tracy, TV shows, 1960–62; 1960–67 Glen Films, Inc.; prod., All-Star Golf, 1958–62; prod. Championship Bowling, 1958–60; prod. Ding Dong School, 1959–60; pres. owner, UPA Pictures, Inc., prod. Gay Purr-ee, animated features. Mr. Magoo, Dick Tracy cartoon series, Mr. Magoo's Christmas Carol. Prod. War of the Gargantuas, Invasion of the Astros, What's Up, Tiger Lily?, T-A-M-I, T.N.T. Show, Turnon, Tune In Drop Out, 1968; Hell in the Pacific. Pres. Screen Entertainment Co., Benedict Pictures Corp., United Prod. of America; pres. H. G. Saperstein & Associates. Producer: The Vaudeville Thing; Tchaikovsky Competition, Gerald McBoing Boing Show.

SARAFIAN, RICHARD C.: Director. b. New York City. Studied medicine and law before entering film industry with director Robert Altman doing industrial documentaries. Made documentaries before starting TV career.
TV: Gunsmoke, Bonanza, Guns of Will Sonnet, I Spy etc.
PICTURES: Andy (debut, 1965), Run Wild, Run Free, Ballad of a Badman, Fragment of Fear, Man in the Wilderness, Vanishing Point, Lolly Madonna (XXX), The Man Who Loved Cat Dancing, The Next Man (also prod.), Sunburn, The Bear.

SARANDON, CHRIS: Actor. b. Beckley, WV, July 2, 1942. e. Univ. of West Va.
PICTURES: Dog Day Afternoon, Lipstick, The Sentinel, Cuba, Atlantic City, USA, The Osterman Weekend, Protocol, Fright Night.
TELEVISION: You Can't Go Home Again, The Day Christ Died, A Tale of Two Cities, This Child Is Mine, etc.

SARANDON, SUSAN: Actress. b. New York, 1946. e. Catholic University. Came to New York to pursue acting, first signing with Ford Model Agency. Made film debut in Joe. Also appeared on TV in A World Apart series. Co-produced film, The Last of the Cowboys.
PICTURES INCLUDE: The Great Waldo Pepper, The Rocky Horror Show, Lovin' Molly, The Front, Porgy Page, Dragonfly, Walk Away Madden, The Other Side of Midnight, Pretty Baby, King of the Gypsies, Loving Couples, Atlantic City, Tempest, The Hunger, The Buddy System.
TELEVISION: Who Am I This Time, A.R., Mussolini and I.

SARGENT ALVIN: Writer. Began career as writer for TV, then turned to theatrical films.
PICTURES INCLUDE: The Stalking Moon, Gambit, The Sterile Cuckoo, The Effect of Gamma Rays on Man in the Moon Marigolds, Love and Pain (and the whole damn thing), Julia, Bobby Deerfield, Straight Time, Ordinary People.

SARGENT, DICK: Actor. b. Carmel, CA, 1933. Veteran of over 140 TV shows, 17 feature films and four TV series.
PICTURES: Captain Newman, M.D., Operation Petticoat, Mardi Gras, Bernadine, Hardcore, etc.
TELEVISION: Bewitched.

SARGENT, JOSEPH: Director. b. Jersey City, NJ, 1925.
PICTURES INCLUDE: The Taking of Pelham One, Two, Three, MacArthur, Goldengirl, Coast to Coast.
TV: The Marcus-Nelson Murders (Emmy award for tv movie that was pilot for Kojak series), The Night That Panicked America, Sunshine, Tribes, Hustling, Terrible Joe Moran, Choices of the Heart (also prod.), Space, Love Is Never Silent, Passion Flower.

SARLUI, ED: Executive. b. Amsterdam, Holland, Nov. 10, 1925. Owner, Peruvian Films, S.A.; pres., Radio Films of Peru, S.A.; pres. Bryant Films Educatoriana, S.A.; partner, United Producers de Colombia Ltd.; pres. Royal Film N.V.; pres., United Producers de Centroamerica, S.A.; pres. United Producers de Mexico, S.A.; pres., United Producers Int'l, Inc., Continental Motion Pictures, Inc.

SARNOFF, ROBERT W.: Executive. b. New York, N.Y., July 2, 1918; Harvard U., B.A., 1939; Columbia Law Sch. 1940. In office of Coordinator of Info., Wash., D.C., Aug. 1941; the U.S. Navy, Mar. 1942; asst. to publisher, Gardner Cowles, Jr., 1945; mem. of staff Look Mag., 1946, with NBC, 1948–65; pres., Dec. 1955–58; chmn. bd., 1958; bd. of dir. RCA, 1957; chmn bd. chief exec. officer, NBC, 1958–65; pres. RCA, 1966; Chief Exec. Officer, 1968; bd. chmn., 1970–75. Mem., TV Pioneers, 1957; pres., 1952–53; International Radio & TV Society, Broadcasters Committee for Radio Free Europe. Am Home Products, Inc., dir., of Business Committee for the Arts.

SARNOFF, THOMAS W.: Executive. b. New York, N.Y., Feb. 23, 1927. e. Phillips Academy, Andover, Mass., 1939–43, Princeton U., 1943–45, Stanford U. grad. 1948, B.S. in E.E., Grad School of Bus. Admin. 1948–49. Sgt., U.S. Army Signal Corps, 1945–46; prod. & sales, ABC-TV, Hollywood, 1949–50; prod. dept. MGM, 1951–52; asst. to dir. of finance and oper., NBC, 1952–54; dir. of prod. and bus. affairs, 1954–57; vice pres., prod. and bus. affairs, 1957–60; v.p. adm. west coast, 1960–62; v.p. west coast, 1962; exec. v.p. 1965–77; bd. of dir., NBC prods 1961–77; bd of dir. Hope Enterprises 1960–75; dir. NABCAT, Inc. 1967–75; dir. Valley County Cable TV, Inc. 1969–75; Pres. NBC Entertainment Corp. 1972–77; Pres. Sarnoff International Enterprises, Inc. 1977–81; pres., Sarnoff Entertainment Corp., 1981–; exec. v.p., Venturetainment Corp., 1980–. Past pres. Research Foundation at St. Joseph Hospital of Burbank; past pres. Permanent Charities of the Entertainment Ind.; past ch. bd. of trustees, National Acad. of TV Arts and Sciences.

SARRAZIN, MICHAEL: Actor. r.n. Jacques Michel Andre Sarrazin. b. Quebec, Canada, May 22, 1940. Began acting at 17 on CBC TV; signed by Universal, 1965, appearing on several TV shows.
PICTURES INCLUDE: Gunfight in Abilene (debut), The Flim-Flam Man, The Sweet Ride, Journey to Shiloh, A Man Called Gannon, Eye of the Cat, In Search of Gregory, They Shoot Horses, Don't They?, The Pursuit of Happiness, Sometimes a Great Notion, Believe in Me, Harry in Your Pocket, For Pete's Sake, The Reincarnation of Peter Proud, Scaramouche, The Gumball Rally, Caravans, The Seduction, Fighting Back, Joshua Then and Now.
TV: Chrysler Theatre, The Virginian, World Premiere.

SASSOWER, HARVEY L.: Advertising director. b. N.Y., July 28, 1945. e. CCNY (B.A. in adv.); 1968 asst. to adv. mg., United Artists. 1969, asst. to adv. dir., 20th Century-Fox, 1969, appointed adv. mgr. of ABC Pictures Corp., dir. of adv., ABC Pictures, 1970; pres., Universal Spectrum, Inc. (design & adv. studio). Art director; author.

SAUL, OSCAR: Writer. b. Brooklyn, N.Y., e. B'klyn Coll. Co-author play, Medicine Show; m.p. ed., U.S. Public Health Svce; numerous radio and tv plays.
PICTURES INCLUDE: collab. s.p., Once Upon a Time, Strange Affair; collab. story, Road House, Lady Gambles; s.p., Woman in Hiding, Secret of Convict Lake; adapt., Streetcar Named Desire; collab. sp. p., Thunder on the Hill, Affair in Trinidad; prod., Let's Do It Again; collab. s.p. Helen Morgan Story; s.p. Joker Is Wild; collab. story Naked Maja; collab. s.p. Second Time Around, Major Dundee; s.p. The Silencers; collab. s.p. Man and Boy. Novel: The Dark Side of Love (NBC movie). 1984, adapted A Streetcar Named Desire (ABC-TV).

SAUNDERS, DAVID: Executive. b. 1943. e. George Washington Univ. (BA); Univ. of Michigan Law School. Member of NY and Calif. bar groups. 1974, joined LA law firm of Mitchell, Silberberg & Knupp as specialist in entertainment law. 1979–81, exec. v.p., business affairs, PolyGram Pictures. 1981, v.p., business affairs, CBS Theatrical Films. 1983, named snr. v.p., 20th Century-Fox Productions, responsible for supervising production and development of feature films.

SAVAGE, DAVID: Executive Producer & Advertising Executive b. New York, N.Y., March 17, 1929. e. Rochester Institute of Technol. In research development & testing div., Eastman Kodak Co., 2 yrs.; adv. mgr. asst. nat'l sales mgr., Official Films; org., film dept. mgr. WCBS-TV; dir. of film procurement, CBS; mgr. of film procurement, NBC; mgr. planning, merchandising, Recorded Tape Dept., RCA Records; promo. mgr., special products mktg. RCA Records Div.; v.p., operations, Wunderman, Rilotto, & Kline, 1970; pres., Response Industries, Inc., (adv. agency), 1973 which became affiliate of McCann Erickson, and was sr. v.p. of McCann Erickson in addition to continuing as pres. of R.I. Pres., Mattel Direct Marketing, 1982.

SAVAGE, JOHN: Actor. Studied at American Academy of Dramatic Arts. In Manhattan organized Children's Theatre Group which performed in Public Housing. Has appeared in many plays both on and off Bdwy. Won Drama Circle Award for performance in One Flew Over the Cuckoo's Nest in Chicago and Los Angeles.
PICTURES: Bad Company, Steelyard Blues, All the Kind Strangers, The Deer Hunter, Hair, The Onion Field, Cattle Annie and Little Britches, Inside Moves, The Amateur, Brady's Escape, Maria's Lovers.
STAGE: Fiddler on the Roof, Ari, Siamese Connections, The Hostage, American Buffalo.
TELEVISION: Eric, Gibbsville (series), The Nairobi Affair (movie).

SAVALAS, TELLY: Actor. b. Garden City, N.Y., Jan. 21, 1924. r.n. Aristotle Savalas, e. Col. Univ. (B.S.). Joined Information Services of State Dep't.; made exec. dir. Then named sr. dir. of news, special events for ABC, where created Your Voice of America series. Acting career began with debut in Bring Home a Baby on Armstrong Circle Theatre TV.
PICTURES INCLUDE: Birdman of Alcatraz, Young Savages, Cape Fear, Man from the Diner's Club, Battle of the Bulge, Greatest Story Ever Told, Beau Geste, Dirty Dozen, Buona Sera, Mrs. Campbell, Crooks and Coronets, Kelly's Heroes, On Her Majesty's Secret Service, Killer Force, Lisa and the Devil, Capricorn One, Escape to Athena, Beyond the Posidon Adventure, Cannonball Run II.
TELEVISION: Mongo's Back in Town (movie), Visions (movie), The Marcus-Nelson Murders (movie), Kojak (series).

SAWELSON, MEL: Executive b. Los Angeles, Calif., Sept. 5, 1929. e. USC 1947–48, UCLA 1948–49. Entered M.P. industry in 1947; mgr., Acme Film Laboratories, Inc., 1952; pres. Sports-TV; 1957–59; produced, Olympic Films, International Olympic Organization, 1956; produced, Big 10 Hilites, PCC Hilites, All American Game of the Week, 1957–59; 1st m.p. lab. exec. to install videotape, 1959; created Acme-chroma process of transferring color videotape to film; pres., Acme Film & Videotape Labs., 1967–71; v.p. Consolidated Film Industries, 1971, exec. v.p. 1972; pres., Glen Glenn Sound Co., 1972.

SAWYER, DIANE: News Correspondent and Anchor. b. Glasagow, KY, Dec. 22, 1945. e. Wellesley College. Studied law before deciding on career in TV. Worked for Nixon Administration in press office from 1970–74; assisted Nixon in writing memoirs, 1975–78. Joined CBS News as reporter in Washington bureau in 1978; named correspondent in 1980. Served as CBS State Dept. correspondent 1980–81. Joined Charles Kuralt as co-anchor of the weekday editions of CBS Morning News in 1981. In 1984 switched to 60 Minutes.

SAXON, JOHN: Actor. b. Brooklyn, N.Y., Aug. 5, 1935. Model; m.p. debut: Running Wild. On TV in Scarecrow and Mrs. King.
PICTURES INCLUDE: The Unguarded Moment, Rock Pretty Baby, Summer Love, The Restless Years, The Reluctant Debutante, Cry Tough, Portrait in Black, The Unforgiven, The Plunderers, Posse from Hell, War Hunt, Nightmare, Evil Eye, For Singles Only, Joe Kidd, Enter The Dragon, Black Christmas, Strange Shadows in an Empty Room, The Electric Horseman, Wrong Is Right, The Big Score, Nightmare on Elm Street, Fever Pitch.

SAYLES, JOHN: Writer-Director. b. Schnectady, NY, Sept. 28, 1950. e. Williams Univ. Wrote two novels: Pride of the Bimbos (1975) and Union Dues (1978); also The Anarchist's Convention, collection of short stories. First screenplay: Piranha (1978). Directed plays off-Bdwy.
PICTURES: Battle Beyond the Stars (s.p.), Lady in Red (s.p.), Return of the Secaucus Seven (s.p., dir.), Alligator (s.p.), The Howling (s.p.), The Challenge (co-s.p.), Lianna (s.p., dir.), Baby, It's You (s.p., dir.), The Brother from Another Planet (s.p., dir., editor), The Clan of the Cave Bear (s.p.).

SCARDINO, DON: Actor. b. Canada. On Bdwy. in Godspell, King of Hearts, Johnny No Trump, As You Like It, etc.
PICTURES: The People Next Door, Homer, Squirm, Cruising, He Knows You're Alone.

SCARWID, DIANA: Actress. b. Savannah, GA. Went to N.Y. after high school to attend American Academy of Dramatic Arts and Pace Univ. Member of National Shakespeare Conservatory (Woodstock, N.Y.) and worked in regional theatres before moving to Hollywood 1976. Motion picture debut in Pretty Baby, 1978.
PICTURES: Inside Moves, Honeysuckle Rose, Mommie Dearest, Rumble Fish, Strange Invaders, Silkwood, The Ladies Club.
TELEVISION: Gibbsville (series), Studs Lonigan (mini-series), and films: The Guyana Tragedy, The Glitter Palace, Battered.

SCHAEFER, CARL: Publicist, b. Cleveland, Ohio, Sept. 2. e. U.C.L.A., contr. to mag., including Vanity Fair, Hollywood Citizen-News, 1931–35; Warner Bros., 1935.; Huesped de Honor, Mexico, 1943; OSS WWII, 1944–45; Int'l Comt. AMPS, chmn. 1966–67; Italian Order of Merit, 1957; Chevalier de l'ordre de la Couronne, Belgium, 1963. Pres., Foreign Trade Assn. of Southern Calif., 1954; chmn. of bd., 1955; British-American C. of C., Dir., 1962; Chevalier French Legion d'Honneur, 1955; Comm. Hollywood Museum; dir., International Relations, Warner Bros. Seven Arts Int'l Corp., 1960; formed own firm, Carl Schaefer Enterprises, 1971. Dir. pub. rel., British-American Chamber of Commerce, 1971; dir. pub. rel. Iota International Pictures, 1971; dir. pub. rel. Lyric Films International, 1971; bureau chief (Hollywood) Movie/TV Marketing, 1971; managing dir., International Festival Advisory Council, 1971; dir. pub. rel. & adv. Francis Lederer Enterprises (Inc. American National Academy of Performing Arts, and Canoga Mission Gallery) 1974; West Coast rep. Angelika Films of N.Y. 1974, Hwd. rep Korwitz/Geiger Products. 1975–; Hwd. corresp. Movie News, S'pore, & Femina, Hong Kong, 1974–; member Westn. Publications Assn. 1975–; field rep. Birch Records 1975; Hollywood rep Antena Magazine, Buenos Aires; dir pub rel Style Magazine. Coordinator Hollywood Reporter Annual Key Art Awards; coordinator Hollywood Reporter Annual Marketing Concept Awards; executive committee & historian ShoWest; Mbr., National Panel of Consumer Arbitrators, 1985; Hollywood Corr., Gold Coast Times of Australia, 1986.

SCHAEFER, JACK: Writer. b. Cleveland, O., Nov. 19, 1907. e. Oberlin Coll., Columbia U. edit. & pub., Theatre News, 1935–40, The Movies, 1939–41.
AUTHOR: Short stories for TV anthologies; Shane, First Blood, Jeremy Rodock, Company of Cowards, Monte Walsh, The Great Endurance Horse Race.

SCHAFER, NATALIE: Actress. b. New York City, Nov. 5. e. Merrill School and Hamilton Institute.
B'WAY: Lady in the Dark, Susan and God, The Doughgirls.
PICTURES INCLUDE: Marriage is a Private Affair, The Snake Pit, Molly and Me, Dishonored Lady, Susan Slade, 40 Carats, The Day of the Locust.
TV: I Love Lucy, Route 66, 77 Sunset Strip, Thriller, The Beverly Hillbillies, Gilligan's Island.

SCHAFFNER, FRANKLIN: Director. b. Tokyo, Japan, May 30, 1920; e. Franklin & Marshall Coll. U.S. Navy, W.W. II; Dir. Person to Person, Studio One. Kaiser-Aluminum Hour, Playhouse 90; Emmy Best dir. 1945–55.
PICTURES INCLUDE: The Stripper, 1962, The Double Man, The Best Man, Planet of the Apes, Patton, Nicholas and Alexandra, Papillon, Islands in the Stream, The Boys from Brazil, The Sphinx, Yes, Giorgio.

SCHATZBERG, JERRY: Director. b. N.Y.C. Early career in photography as asst. to Bill Helburn.
PICTURES INCLUDE: Puzzle of a Downfall Child, Panic in Needle Park, Scarecrow, Sweet Revenge (prod.-dir.), The Seduction of Joe Tynan, Huckleberry Rose, Misunderstood, No Small Affair, Street Smart.

SCHEFFER, STEVE: Executive. e. Harvard Business School (1966). Home Box Office exec. v.p. of film programming and prod.; exec. v.p. for HBO theatrical film subsidiary, Silver Screen Partners.

SCHEIDER, ROY: Actor. b. Orange, N.J., 1932. e. Franklin and Marshall College where he won the Theresa Helburn Acting Award twice. First professional acting in N.Y. Shakespeare Festival 1961 prod. of Romeo and Juliet. Became member of Lincoln Center Repertory Co. and acted with Boston Arts Festival, American Shakespeare Festival, Arena Stage (Wash. D.C.) and American Repertory Co.
PICTURES INCLUDE: Loving, Paper Lion, Stiletto, Star!, Puzzle of a Downfall Child, Klute, The French Connection, The Outside Man, The Seven Ups, The Inheritor, Sheila Levine, Jaws, Marathon Man, Sorcerer, Jaws II, Last Embrace, All That Jazz, Stall of the Night, Blue Thunder, 2010, 52 Pick-up, The Men's Club.
TV: Hallmark Hall of Fame, Studio One, N.Y.P.D.
STAGE: Richard III, Stephen D, Sergeant Musgrave's Dance, The Alchemist, Betrayal.

SCHELL, MARIA: Actress. b. Vienna, 1926. Sister of Maximillian Schell. Made debut at 12 in Swiss film, The Gravel Pit. Subsequently appeared in many British and American films.
PICTURES: Angel with a Trumpet, The Heart of the Matter, So Little Time, The Magic Box, The Brothers Karamazov, The Hanging Tree, Cimarron, The Odessa File, Voyage of the Damned, The Twist, Superman, 1919.

SCHELL, MAXIMILIAN: Actor. b. Vienna, Dec. 8, 1930.
TV: Shows include: Playhouse 90, Judgment at Nuremburg, The Fifth Column, Turn The Key Deftly. Mini-Series: Peter the Great.
PICTURES INCLUDE: Children, Mother and the General, The Young Lions, Judgment at Nuremburg, Five Finger Exercise, The Condemned of Altona, Return from the Ashes, The Deadly Affair, Counterpoint, The Desperate

Ones, The Castle, Krakatoa East of Java, The Odessa File. Dir., starred First Love; The Man in the Glass Booth (actor), End of the Game (dir., co-prod.), St. Ives, A Bridge Too Far, Cross of Iron, Julia, Players, The Black Hole, The Chosen, The Assisi Underground.
TELEVISION: The Fifth Column, The Diary of Anne Frank, Peter the Great, etc.

SCHENCK, AUBREY: Producer. b. Brooklyn, N.Y., Aug. 26, 1908; e. Cornell U.; N.Y.U. With law firm of O'Brien, Driscoll & Raftery; buyer & attorney for Natl. Theatres, 1936; prod. for 20th Century-Fox 1945; exec. prod. Eagle Lion 1946; contract prod. Universal Internatl. 1948; Aubrey Schenck Productions, Inc.
PICTURES INCLUDE: Shock, Johnny Comes Flying Home, Strange Triangle, Repeat Performance, T-Men, Mickey, It's a Joke Son, Trapped, Port of New York, Wyoming Man, Undercover Girl, Fat Man, Target Unknown; formed own co. to prod. War Paint, Beachhead. Also: Yellow Tomahawk, Shield for Murder, Big House, U.S.A., Crime Against Joe, Emergency Hospital, Ghost Town, Broken Star, Rebels in Town, Pharaoh's Curse, Three Bad Sisters, Fort Yuma, Desert Sands, Quincannon, Frontier Scout, Black Sheep, Hot Cars, War Drums, Voodoo Island, Revolt at Fort Laramie, Tomahawk Trail, Untamed Youth, Girl in Black Stockings, Bop Girl Goes Calypso, Up Periscope, Violent Road, Reckless, Frankenstein 1970, Wild Harvest, Robinson Crusoe On Mars, Don't Worry, Ambush Bay, Kill a Dragon, Impasse, More Dead Than Alive, Barquero, Daughters of Satan.
TV: Miami Undercover, series.

SCHEPISI, FRED: Producer-Director-Writer. b. Melbourne, Australia, Dec. 26, 1939.
PICTURES: The Priest (d.), The Devil's Playground (d., p., s.p.), The Chant of Jimmie Blacksmith (d., p., s.p.), Barbarosa (d.), Iceman (d.), Plenty (d.).

SCHERICK, EDGAR J: Executive Producer. e. Harvard Univ.; elected to Phi Beta Kappa. Introduced Wide World of Sports on TV thru his co., Sports Programs, Inc. Was v.p. in chg. of network programming at ABC-TV. Pres. of Palomar Pictures Int'l. Now independent producer.
PICTURES INCLUDE: For Love of Ivy, The Birthday Party, Take the Money and Run, They Shoot Horses, Don't They?, The Killing of Sister George, Sleuth, The Heartbreak Kid, Law and Disorder, The Stepford Wives, I Never Promised You a Rose Garden, I'm Dancing As Fast As I Can, Shoot the Moon, White Dog, Reckless, Mrs. Soffel.

SCHERMER, JULES: Associate producer. In 1942: True to the Army, Henry Aldrich, Editor, Par. In 1943: Henry Aldrich Gets Glamour, Par.; collab. s.p. The Sullivans.
PICTURES INCLUDE: Framed, Man From Colorado, Criss-Cross, Illegal Entry, Union Station, Pride of St. Louis, Lydia Bailey, Pickup on South Street, Pushover, Carthay Center Prods. Inc., 1965. Prod., A Dream of Kings.

SCHIAVONE, JAMES: Executive. b. Niagara Falls, N.Y., Nov. 14, 1917. e. U. of Michigan. Started career as newspaperman; general manager WWJ-AM-FM-TV, Detroit, 1952–68; v.p.-gen. mgr., KSAT-TV, San Antonio, Tex., 1969–present.

SCHICK, ELLIOT: Executive. b. Brooklyn, N.Y., Dec. 24, 1924. e. Brooklyn Coll. (B.A.), New School for Social Research (drama workshop, directing 1945–46). Author of book for Ballet Theatre, Manfred; book, The Administration of the Economic and Social Council. 1942–48, prod. & dir. radio shows for WNYC, N.Y.C., composed and arranged music for radio and stage production; 1946–48; dialogue director, Republic Studios; 1948–50, prod. & dir. TV shows and commercials, Nova Productions; 1950–51, editor, United Nations Film Div.; 1951–53, editor, Candid Camera; 1953–55, asst. studio mgr., American Natl. Studios; 1955–56, prod. & dir. live and video tape shows for KCET; 1969, asst. dir., Tora, Tora, Tora; 1969–72, prod. mgr. for features: 3 in the Attic, Up in the Cellar, Bunny O'Hare, Honkers, Hickey and Boggs, Kansas City Bomber, White Lightning; 1973–77 spvr. prod. for AIP on Sugar Hill, Return to Macon County, Cooley High, Futureworld, Island of Dr. Moreau in 1977 joined EMI Films, Inc. as v.p. prod.; 1978, exec.-in-chg.-prod., Deer Hunter; 1980, produced The Earthling; 1981, prod., Private Benjamin (TV series), supvr. prod., Pippin (TV); Blue Skies Again (exec.-in-chg.-prod.); 1982, Fools Die (prod.); 1983, Fast Eddie (prod.); 1984, Marie (exec. prod.); 1985, Cherry-2000 (co-prod.), 1986, Masters of the Universe (co-prod.).

SCHIFRIN, LALO: Composer, b. Buenos Aires. Father was conductor of Teatro Colon in B.A. for 30 years. Schifrin studied with Juan Carlos Paz in Arg. and later Paris Cons. Returned to homeland and wrote for stage, modern dance, TV. Became interested in jazz and joined Dizzie Gillespie's band in 1962 as pianist and composer. Settled in L.A.
PICTURES INCLUDE: The Cincinnati Kid, The Liquidator, Cool Hand Luke, The President's Analyst, The Fox, Kelly's Heroes, Magnum Force, Man on a Swing, The Four Musketeers, Voyage of the Damned, The Eagle Has Landed, Rollercoaster, The Manitou, Boulevard Nights, Escape to Athena, The Amityville Horror, The Nude Bomb, The Competition, Caveman, Buddy, Buddy, Amityville II: The Possession, The Sting II, The Osterman Weekend, Sudden Impact, The Mean Season, The New Kids.
TELEVISION: Hollywood Wives, A.D., Private Sessions.

SCHILLER, FRED: Playwright, screen & TV writer. Awarded: New York Literary Prize, for McCall magazine story Ten Men and a Prayer. National Member of Smithsonian Institution, Member of Societé Des Auteurs et Compositeurs Dramatiques. Member of Los Angeles World Affairs Council. Formerly chief corres. European Newspaper Feature Services. Honored by the Univ. of Wyoming for literary achievements with a special Fred Schiller Collection for their library.
PICTURES FOR: MGM, Columbia, RKO, Republic and Henri Sokal Films, Paris.
TELEVISION: Wrote some 53 TV plays for all major networks. Adapted G.B. Shaw play, The Inca of Jerusalem, presented by NBC as special. Wrote TV special: Demandez Vicky! for Paris and Finder BitteMelden! for Austrian TV.
STAGE: Come On Up (U.S.), Anything Can Happen (London), Demandez Vicky (Paris), Finder Please Return (Athens, Madrid), Finder Bitte Melden (Berlin, Baden-Baden, and Vienna). Peter Sellar production at Kennedy Center, Come on Up; a Mae West revival.

SCHILLER, LAWRENCE J.: Producer-Director. b. New York City, Dec. 28, 1936. Photo-journalist with Life Magazine & Saturday Evening Post, 1958–70; collaborated on numerous books including three by Norman Mailer: The Executioner's Song, Marilyn, and The Faith of Graffiti; Muhammad Ali with Wilfrid Sheed; Minamata with Eugene Smith.
PICTURES: The Man Who Skied Down Everest (editorial concept & direction); Lady Sings the Blues, Butch Cassidy & the Sundance Kid (conceived and executed special still montages & titles); The American Dreamer (prod./dir.).
TELEVISION: Hey, I'm Alive (prod./dir.); Producer: The Trial of Lee Harvey Oswald, The Winds of Kitty Hawk, Marilyn, The Untold Story, An Act of Love, Child Bride of Short Creek. 1983: The Executioner's Song (prod. & dir.).

SCHIMMEL, HERBERT D.: Executive. b. New York, N.Y., October 15, 1927. e. University of Pennsylvania, Wharton School. C.P.A., partner with M. Schimmel and Co. prior to entering m.p. industry in 1966 as treasurer, Europix Consolidated Corp.; pres., 1968; pres., Europix International Ltd., 1971.

SCHINE, G. DAVID: Executive. Film exhibitor until 1966 in New York, Ohio, Kentucky, Maryland, Delaware, and West Virginia. Exec. prod. of French Connection, 1971. Writer, prod., dir. of That's Action!, 1977. Chief Exec. officer of Schine Productions (production) and Epic Productions (distribution), Visual Sciences, Inc., High Resolution TV, Inc., and Studio Television Services, Inc.

SCHLAIFER, CHARLES: Executive. President, Charles Schlaifer and Company, Inc., advertising agency with offices in New York and Los Angeles. b. Omaha, Nebr. Reporter Daily News, World-Herald, (Omaha). In 1930 apptd. adv. mgr. Paramount theatres, Omaha; then of Publix theats., Omaha; then of Tri-State circuit, Neb., Iowa; 1936–42 managing dir. United Artists Theats., San Francisco; advisor, nat'l adv., United Artists prod. In 1942 apptd. adv. mgr. 20th Cent.-Fox; named asst. dir. adv., publicity, & exploitation, 1944; appt'd. dir. of advertising, publicity, exploitation and radio, 1945. Resigned 20th-Fox post, Feb. 1, 1949, to establish own adv. agency. Pres., Charles Schlaifer & Co., Inc. Chmn. advertising advisory council, MPAA; instructor at New School of Social Research, N.Y., on m.p.; revised m.p. adv. code; permanent chmn. first MPAA pub rel. com. Member; Nat'l Advisory Mental Health Council to U.S. Surgeon General; vice-chmn. bd. of gov., Nat'l Assn. of Mental Health. Lecturer, writer on adv. & mental health bd. of gov., Menninger Foundation; founder, co-chmn., Nat'l Mental Health Comm., secy., treas., Joint Comm. on Mental Illness & Health; expert witness Congress, govt. hearings. Elected Hon. Fellow of the Amer. Psychiatric Assn., 1959; V. chmn., trustee in chg., Mental Health and Mental Retardation Facilities, N.Y. State, 1964; secy., treas., Joint Commission Mental Health for Children; vice chmn. bd. Foundation for Child Mental Welfare, 1963. Member bd. trustees Research Foundation 1966. Member White House Conference on the Handicapped, 1952–65; elected honorary fellow, Post Graduate Psychiatric Institute, 1968. Hon. Doctor of Letters, John F. Kennedy College, Wahoo, Neb., 1969; Chmn. N.Y. State Health and Mental Hygiene Facilities Improvement Corp., 1970; Hon. Fellow—American Ortho Psychiatric Assoc., 1970; Hon. Fellow British Royal Society of Health. Wisdom Award Hon. Wisdom Mag., 1969; social conscience award Karen Horney Clinic, 1972. Chairman, New York State Facilities Development Corp., 1973–; Advisory Council to the National Institute of Mental Health & to the Surgeon General of the U.S. 1976–.

SCHLANG, JOSEPH: Executive. b. N.Y.C. Feb. 24, 1911, e. N.Y.U. Owner and leader in N.Y.C. real estate, and exec.

dir. of many enterprises. Pres. of International Opera Co. & Opera Presentations, Inc. Has produced two weekly radio programs: Opera Stars of Tomorrow and 100 & More Ways to Improve N.Y.C. since April, 1973. Opera Presentations, Inc., a non-profit corp. distributes and exhibits opera, ballet and art films throughout America and the school system. Over 100 cultural films owned by Schlang are supplied to Opera Presentations free to use.

SCHLESINGER, JOHN: Director. b. London, England. 1960: Wrote and dir. Terminus for British Transport Films (Golden Lion, best doc., Venice); The Class. Some episodes The Valiant Years series.
PICTURES INCLUDE: 1961: A Kind of Loving (Golden Bear, Berlin); 1962–63; Billy Liar; 1964–65; Darling (New York Film Critics Award); 1966–67: Far From the Madding Crowd. 1968: Midnight Cowboy (Best dir. and film, S.F.T.A. and 'Oscars'), 1970: Sunday, Bloody Sunday (Best dir. and film, S.F.T.A.), Visions of Eight (sequence), The Day of the Locust, Marathon Man, Yanks, Honky Tonk Freeway, The Falcon and the Snowman (also co-prod.).
TELEVISION: Separate Tables, An Englishman Abroad (BAFtA award).
OPERA: Les Contes d Hoffmann (Royal Opera House 1981); SWET award; Der Rosenkavalier (Royal Opera House 1984).
THEATRE: No Why (RSC), 1964; Timon of Athens (RSC), 1965; Days in the Trees (RSC), 1966; I And Albert (Piccadilly Theatre), 1972; Heartbreak House (NT), 1975; Julius Caesar (NT), 1977; True West (NT), 1981.

SCHLONDORFF, VOLKER: Director. b. Wiesbaden, Germany, Mar. 31, 1939. Studied in France, acquiring degree in political science in Paris. Studied at French Intl. Film School before becoming asst. to Jean-Pierre Melville, Alain Resnais, and Louis Malle Debut film, Der Junge Torless (Young Torless), 1965.
PICTURES: A Degree of Murder, 1966; Michael Kohlhass, 1968; The Sudden Fortune of the Poor People of Kombach, 1970; Die Moral der Rugh Halbfass, 1971; A Free Woman, 1972; The Lost Honor of Katharine Blum, 1975; Le Coup de Grace, 1976; Valeska Gert, 1977; The Tin Drum, 1979; Swann in Love, 1985.

SCHLOSSBERG, JULIAN: Producer-Distributor-Director-Radio Host. b. N.Y.C. Jan. 26, 1942. e. N.Y.C. Joined ABC-TV network 1964 as asst. acct. rep.; named act. rep. 1965; 1966, joined Walter Reade Organization as asst. v.p. chg. of TV; 1969, moved to WRO Theatre Div.; 1970, joined faculty of School of Visual Arts; 1971 named v.p. of WRO Theatres; 1972, Jan., 1976, joined Paramount Pictures as v.p. in charge of feature film acquisition. Since 1978 pres. & owner of Castle Hill Productions; 1974, prod. & moderated An Evening with Joseph E. Levine at Town Hall, N.Y.C.; 1974 to 1980, host of radio show Movie Talk on WMCA (N.Y.C.), WMEX (Boston), WICE (Providence) and WHT (N.Y.)..
PICTURES INCLUDE: Ten from Your Show of Shows, No Nukes, Going Hollywood—The 30's, Hollywood Ghost Stories.
THEATRE: It Had To Be You, An Evening with Nichols and May (Rainbow Room, N.Y.C., 1983).
TELEVISION: The Best of Steve Allen.

SCHLOSSER, HERBERT S.: Executive. b. Atlantic City, N.J. e. Princeton U., Yale Law. Joined law firm of Phillips, Nizer, Benjamin, Krim & Ballon, 1954; attorney, California National Productions (subsidiary of National Broadcasting Company) 1957; v.p. & gen. mgr., 1960; director, talent & program administration, NBC television network, 1961; v.p., talent & program admin., 1962; v.p. programs, west coast, 1966–72; exec. v.p., NBC-TV, 1972; president, NBC Television Network, 1973, pres. & chief operating officer, NBC, April 1, 1974–76; Pres. & chief executive officer, 1977–78; exec. V.P. RCA 1978–85; sr. advisor, entertainment & broadcasting, Wertheim & Co., 1986.

SCHLUSSELBERG, MARTIN: Film Executive. b. Sept. 1936. e. Yeshiva Univ. Booking clerk. UA. 1956; head booker, Citation Films, 1958; head booker, Desilu Dist., Co., 1961; head booker, and asst. to gen. sls. mgr., Medallion Pictures Corp., 1963; World Ent. Corp., 1966, Sales Mgr.; Crystal Pictures, 1978, sls. mgr., v.p.

SCHMIDT, WOLF: Producer-Distributor. b. Freiburg/Br., Germany, June 30, 1937. Came to U.S. 1962 as free-lance journalist. Started producing in 1969, distributing independently since 1972. Now heads Kodiak Films.
PICTURES INCLUDE: Ski Fever (prod.), Stamping Ground (co-prod.), Young Hannah (exec. prod.), Things Fall Apart (prod.),The Passover Plot (prod.), Run For the Roses (co-prod.).

SCHMOELLER, DAVID: Writer-Director. b. Louisville, KY, Dec. 8, 1947. e. Universidad de Las Americas (1967–69; Univ. of Texas (BA; MA 1969–74). Wroter and directed 7 short films while studying at Univ. Texas; won 27 intl. awards. In Hollywood spent 6 months working as intern to Peter Hyams on film, Capricorn One. Now heads own co., The Schmoeller Corp.
PICTURES: Tourist Trap (debut as dir.); The Seduction (Dir., s.p.); Crawlspace (dir., s.p.). As writer only: The Day Time Ended, Seven Doors, The Presence, The Peeper, Soliders of Paradise, Last Chance Romance, Thrill Palace, Warriors of the Wind (Eng. adaptation), Prison Planet, Cafe Americano, Ghost Town, etc.
TELEVISION: James at 15 (s.p.); Kid Flicks (cable; s.p., prod.).
NOVEL: The Seduction.

SCHNEER, CHARLES H.: Producer, b. Norfolk, Va., May 5, e. Columbia College; pres., Morningside Prods. Inc. & Pictures Corp.; 1956. Founded Andor Films 1974.
PICTURES INCLUDE: Prod. The 3 Worlds of Gulliver, The 7th Voyage of Sinbad, I Aim at the Stars, Face of a Fugitive, Good Day for a Hanging, Battle of the Coral Sea, Tarawa Beachhead, Mysterious Island, Jason and the Argonauts, First Men In The Moon, Half A Sixpence, Land Raiders, Valley of Gwangi, The Executioner, The Golden Voyage of Sinbad, Sinbad & The Eye of the Tiger, Clash of the Titans.

SCHNEIDER, DICK: Prod.-dir. b. Cazadero, Calif., Mar. 7; e. Coll. of the Pacific; U.S. Navy, WWII. Winner of 3 Emmys.
TV: Dough Re Mi, NBC-TV, Wide Wide World, NBC-TV, Colgate Comedy Hours, Beatrice Lilly & Jackie Gleason Comedy Hours, Henry Morgan Show, Kate Smith Show, Big Story, Treasury Men in Action, Doorway to Danger, Today Show, Home, Tonight Show, General Mills Circus; dir. coverage of political conventions; dir. NBC-TV coverage, Princess Margaret's Wedding and Paris Summit conference; dir. Eleanor Roosevelt Specials, 1959–60; Something Special 61, At This Very Moment, Inauguration, Gemini, Emmys, 1962, 1963, 1964; Papal Mass for all networks at Yankee Stadium, 1965–66; 1966–67 Tonight Show, Orange Bowl, Macy's Parade; Jr. Miss Pageant; 1967–70 College Queen, Emmy Award. Prod.; Macy's Parade, 1968–69 Orange Bowl Parade, 1968–69; Prod.-dir., NBC Expt. in TV, New Communication; prod., Big Sur; prod.-dir., Jr. Miss Pageant, 1968–69; dir. Dream House, ABC; dir. Who, What or Where, NBC; produced in 1970: Macy's Parade, Junior Miss, Orange Bowl Parade. 1971–79 Macy's Parade, Stars and Stripes; in 1972: Post Parade, Stars and Stripes 1973–75; Rose Parade 1974–81; Salute to Sir Lew; Jeopardy; NBC Star Salute, 1980; Emmy winner, 1980; Rose Parade, 1981-84; Star Salute, 1981; UCP Telethons, 1981-86. Macy's Parade, 1980–85; Diabetes Telethon, 1983; NBC Affiliate Convention, 1980–85; 1986, People's Choice, Jeopardy.

SCHNEIDER, JOHN: Actor. b. Mount Kisco, NY, Apr. 8. Active in drama club in high school in Atlanta. Got job as fashion model and played guitar and sang own compositions in various Atlanta clubs. Active in local community theatre. Summer stock in New Hampshire.
PICTURES INCLUDE: Smokey and the Bandit, Million Dollar Dixie Deliverance, Eddie Macon's Run, Cocaine Wars.
TELEVISION: Dukes of Hazzard; John Schneider—Back Home. Movies: Dream House, Happy Endings, Stagecoach.

SCHNEIDER, JOHN, A.: Exec. b. Chicago, Ill., Dec. 4, 1926. e. Notre Dame, B.S. U.S.N.R., 1943–47, Exec. assignments with CBS-TV, in Chicago and New York City 1950–58; VP, gen. mgr. WCAU-TV, Philadelphia 1958–64; WCBS-TV, New York City 1964–65; pres. CBS-TV Network 1965–66; pres. CBS/Broadcast Group 1966–69, 1971–77; exec. VP CBS Inc. 1969–71, TV and MP consultant 1977–79; consultant WCI, 1979; pres., CEO Warner Amex Satellite Entertainment Corp., 1980.

SCHNEIER, FREDERICK: Executive. b. New York, N.Y., May 31, 1927; e. N.Y. Univ., 1951, bus. admin., N.Y.U. Grad. Sch., MBA, 1953. Dir. Sls. planning, Mutual Broadcasting System, 1947–53; media research dir., RKO Teleradio, 1953–55; RKO Teleradio Advisory Comm., 1955–56; exec. staff RKO Teleradio & dir., marketing services, 1956–58; exec. vice-pres., Showcorporation, 1958–71; v.p. TV programming, RKO General, 1972–1973; v.p.; Hemdale Leisure Corporation, 1973–79; Viacom Enterprises v.p., feature films, 1979; sr. v.p., program acquisitions & motion pictures, 1980–83; snr. v.p., acquisitions, Showtime/The Movie Channel, 1983–85; currently sr. v.p. program acquisitions, program enterprises.

SCHNUR, JEROME: Producer-director. b. N.Y.C., July 30, 1923; e. Carnegie Tech. Film prod. & dir. many indep. cos., 1939–43; prod., dir., training films, U.S. Air Force 1943–46; indep. film prod., Hollywood, 1946–50: on bd. of dir., Alson Prod., Inc. & Burwood Pictures Corp.; prod., dir., CBS-TV, N.Y., 1950–51; prod., dir., Goodson-Todson Prod., 1951–56; pres., Holiday Prod., indep. TV prod., 1956; Metropole Prod., indep. film prod., 1956; exec. prod. chg. creative prog. Frank Cooper Assoc., 1958; pres., Jerome Schnur Prods., Inc. Packager and Producer TV and Film.
TV: It's News to Me, Two for the Money, The Name's the Same, What's My Line, Beat the Clock, Robert Q.

Lewis Show, Judge for Yourself, Holiday film series, Fred Allen Show, Dotto, Make the Connection, Scene of the Crime, Who Pays, Shari Lewis Show, Bell Telephone Hour, U.S. Steel Spec., Private Eye—Private Eye, exec. prod., United Fund Simulcast This Is My Town; writer, dir., Mark of Cain, CBS-TV, Chronicle, Science Special, Tomorrow Was Yesterday; dir., L'Enfance du Christ, CBS-TV; exec. prod., Supermarket Sweep, ABC-TV; dir., Michelangelo's Pauline Chapel. CBS News spec.; dir., Jeptha's Daughter. St. Joan. TV ballet specials. Exec. Prod. Everybody's Talking; dir. Missions of San Antonio; Light in the Wilderness, and David Wept (all CBS). Exec. Prod. Politithon 1970—PBS. Exec. Prod. & Dir. "Threatened Paradise" (PBS) "A Time To Live" (PBS) 1972; Director "Questions of Abraham" Special Contata (CBS) "American Ballet Theatre Special" (PBS) "Luther" (CBS) 1973. Exec. prod., Musical Chairs, Strategy, others, 1974; Director, Joffrey ballet, PBS special; dir. Jerusalem Symphony, CBS spec.; 1977; dir. Song of Songs, CBS spec., 1978, Director, All Star-Jazz Show, CBS Special 1976. Recipient 1970–71 Peabody Award, 1970–71 Saturday Review Award, 1972 Emmy Citation; 1975 Ohio State Award.

SCHOENFELD, JOE: Executive. b. June 2, 1907. New York City. e. New York City Schools. Reporter, Hearst newspapers, 1924–32; reporter & editor, Variety, 1932–43 William Morris Agency, 1944–50; editor, Daily Variety, 1950–59; M.P. agency exec., William Morris, 1959–74. Retired.

SCHOENFELD, LESTER: Executive. b. Brooklyn, N.Y., Dec. 6, 1916; e. C.C.N.Y., 1934–38, Asst. mgr., Randforce Amusement, 1936–38; mgr., Rugoff & Becker circuit, 1938–47; mgr., Golden & Ambassador Theatres, 1948; print & sales dept., Film Classics, 1948–50; chg. of Theatrical, non-theatrical & TV dist., Brit. Info. Serv.; est. Lester A. Schoenfeld Films, 1958; Schoenfeld Films Distributing Corp., 1960.

SCHONFELD, NORMAN J.: Theater Executive, b. Newark, N.J., June 25, 1934, e. University of PA, BA 1955, Captain, U.S.A.F., 1957, sls. rep. Bache & Co. 1963, v.p. Tiger Films, Inc., 1966 founder and president, Wood Theater Group.

SCHORR, DANIEL: Television News Correspondent. b. New York City, Aug. 31, 1916. e. CCNY. Started with various news services and newspapers. Joined CBS in 1953 on special assignment; 1955, reopened CBS bureau in Moscow; 1958–60, roving assignment; 1960–1966, chief German Bureau; 1966–76, chief of Washington Bureau; 1979, Public Radio and TV; 1980, correspondent for Cable News Network.

SCHRADER, PAUL: Writer. b. Grand Rapids, Mich., 1946. e. Columbia Univ., U.C.L.A. (Master's in Cinema). Served as film critic for L.A. Free Press and Cinema 1970, 1971, 1972. First screenplay was The Pipeliner (unproduced).
PICTURES INCLUDE: The Yakuza, Taxi Driver, Close Encounters of the Third Kind, Rolling Thunder, Blue Collar (co-s.p., dir). Hardcore (s.p., dir.), Old Boyfriends (co-s.p.), American Gigolo (s.p., dir.), Raging Bull (co-s.p.), Cat People (dir.), Mishima (co-s.p., dir.), Light of Day (dir.).

SCHRODER, RICKY: Actor. b. Staten Island, NY, April 3, 1970. Started modelling while only four months; did many TV commercials before theatrical film debut in The Champ (1979) at age nine.
PICTURES: The Last Flight of Noah's Ark, The Earthling.
TELEVISION: Silver Spoon (series). Movies: Little Lord Fauntleroy, Two Kinds of Love, A Reason to Live.

SCHULBERG, BUDD WILSON: Writer. b. New York City, Mar. 27, 1914; son of B. P. Schulberg, prod.; e. Dartmouth Coll. Publicist, Paramount Pictures, 1931; writer for screen from 1932; addit. dial., A Star is Born; collab. s.p., Little Orphan Annie; orig. & collab. s.p., Winter Carnival. Weekend for Three; collab. orig., City Without Men; adap. Government Girl. Armed services World War II. Author, 3 best-selling novels including The Disenchanted. Harder They Fall; story, s.p. On the Waterfront (Acad. Award & Writers Guild Award, 1954), Face in the Crowd, Wind Across the Everglades. Recent books: Everything That Moves (novel), Moving Pictures: Memories of a Hollywood Prince; play and TV production of What Makes Sammy Run? Teleplay: A Question of Honor and documentary, Joe Louis: For All Time (1985—Cine Golden Eagle). Non-fiction books; Writers in America, Swanwatch; Loser and Still Champion: Muhammad Ali.

SCHULMAN, JOHN A.: Executive. e. Yale University; law degree from Boalt Hall, Univ. of Calif. at Berkeley, 1972. Founding partner in Beverly Hills law firm, Weissmann, Wolff, Bergman, Coleman & Schulman in 1981 after nine years with firm of Kaplan, Livingston, Goodwin, Berkowitz and Selvin. Joined Warner Bros. 1984 as v.p. & gen. counsel, reporting to Barry Meyer, exec. v.p.

SCHULMAN, WILLIAM B.: Advertising executive. b. Dayton, O., July, 2, 1916; e. Ohio State U., B.A., 1940; Columbia U. Lieut. Comm. U.S. Navy. WWII. In 1945 with Universal home office exploitation dept.; New England pub. and exploitation mgr., Universal. 1946. Became dir. adv. publ. & exploit., member bd. dir. Realart Pictures; gen. mgr. Screen Ad Adv. Agency, Inc.; adv. mgr. Sharmark Ent. Inc.

SCHUMAN, EDWARD L.: Executive vice president & partner, Quartet Films. b. Lisbon, Conn., Sept. 3, 1916. e. Wayne Univ., 1932–34, Univ. of Michigan, 1934–37. Mathematician, 1937–51, assistant actuary, Detroit City Employees Pension Fund. Pres., Studio Theatre Corp, Detroit, 1951 to 1975; pres., Studio 8 Theatre Corp., Detroit, 1953 to 1975; secy.-treas., Studio New Center Theatre Corp. of Detroit, 1975; v.p. and gen. mgr. Art Theatre Guild, 1954–60; v.p. Rugoff Theatres, N.Y., 1960–1963. V.p. and bd. member, Walter Reade Organization 1975: Associate producer Broadway play, Same Time Next Year, The Comedians, and Anna Christie, Assoc. prod. of First Monday in October. Co-prod., Torch Song Trilogy in London.

SCHUTE, MARTIN: Producer. Began as asst. dir. to Lewis Milestone; then graduated to prod. supervisor on Gentlemen Marry Brunettes for United Artists in 1955. Spent 3 years with Columbia Pictures in London. Became gen. mgr. of Otto Preminger's production co. during making of Exodus.
PICTURES INCLUDE: The Cardinal (assoc. prod.), Bunny Lake is Missing (assoc. prod.), Maroc 7 (exec. prod.), The Lion in Winter (prod. exec.), Macho Callahan (co-prod.), Miss Julie (co-prod.), Not Now Darling (co-prod.), The Tempter (co-prod.), Not Now Comrade (prod.), Silver Bears (exec. prod.).

SCHWARTZ, BERMUDA: Publicist. b. Deal, N.J., July 30, e. Seton Hall University; grad. Transylvania University, Newspaper editor, radio personality, Ice Capades; Mutual Radio Network; Broadway publicity; head, Schwartz, O'Heney, Thompson Inc., N.Y. pub./rel. firm. Motion picture publicity, Studio City, North Miami, Fla., Ivan Tors, Miami, Fla.

SCHWARTZ, BERNARD: Producer. Brought to Hollywood by the late Howard Hughes to watch his film interests; Schwartz teamed with atty. Greg Bautzer to package movie deals for clients. Re-cut number of Buster Keaton's silent movies into documentary anthologies (The Golden Age of Comedy, When Comedy Was King, etc.). Subsequently made TV series, One Step Beyond, followed by The Wackiest Ship in the Army, Miss Teen International specials, etc. Named pres. Joseph M. Schenck Enterprises, for which made Journey to the Center of the Earth, Eye of the Cat, A Cold Wind in August, I Passed for White, The Shattered Room, Trackdown. Presently partnered with Alan Silverman of Essaness Theatres. 1979, produced Coal Miner's Daughter. 1985, co-exec. prod., St. Elmo's Fire.

SCHWARTZ, LESLIE R.: Exhibitor. b. New York City, June 7, 1915; e. Lehigh U., 1937. Entered m.p. ind. with Century Theatres Construction Co., 1937–39; film buyer, Century Theatres, 1940–42; personnel exec. 1942–43; U.S. Army service, 1943–45; with Andrews, Inc., Century Theat. concessions, 1945–48; apptd. gen. theatre mgr. 1948; pres., 1955. Member: Pi Lambda Phi; North Shore Country Club; pres., Metropolitan Motion Picture Assn., 1960–62; pres., 1955–present.

SCHWARZENEGGER, ARNOLD: Actor. b. Graz, Austria, July 30, 1947. Was Mr. Universe.
PICTURES: Stay Hungry, Pumping Iron, The Villain, Conan the Barbarian, Conan the Destroyer, Terminator, Red Sonja, Commando, Raw Deal, Predator.
TELEVISION: The Jayne Mansfield Story.

SCOFIELD, PAUL: Actor. b. Hurstpierpoint, England, Jan. 21, 1922. Gained greatest fame on London stage doing much Shakespeare and modern plays, including Staircase and Desire Under the Elms.
PICTURES INCLUDE: That Lady, Carve Her Name with Pride, The Train, A Man for All Seasons (Oscar, 1966), King Lear, Scorpio, A Delicate Balance.

SCOGNAMILLO, GABRIEL A.: Art director. b. New York, N.Y., Oct. 27, 1906; e. Royal Acad. of Fine Arts, Italy, 1922–25; N.Y. Sch. of Fine & Applied Arts, France, 1925. Architectural designer; stage scenery; Paramount, Long Island, 1928; Braunberger-Richebe Studios, Paris, 1930–33; MGM, 1934; in armed forces, 1942–46; returned to MGM, 1946.
PICTURES INCLUDE: Man Proof, Babes on Broadway, Thousands Cheer, Great Caruso, Lovely to Look At, Story of Three Loves, Latin Lovers, Strange Lady in Town, World of Tomorrow (Disneyland).
TV: Ozzie & Harriet, Westinghouse Playhouse, MGM-TV.

SCOLA, ETTORE: Director. b. Trevico, Italy, May 10, 1931. e. Univ. of Rome. Began career 1947 as journalist; 1950, wrote for radio shows. Began career as script writer 1954; debut as director, 1964. Has directed or co-directed 20 films, all of which he also scripted or co-wrote. Also has written 50 other scripts, mostly comedies, for other directors.

PICTURES: Let's Talk about Women, Economical Crisis, One Sketch, The Archdevil, Will Your Heroes Find Their Friends Who Disappeared So Mysteriously in Africa?, Inspector Pepe, Pizza Triangle, Excuse Me My Name Is Rocco Papaleo, The Greatest Evening of My Life, We All Loved Each Other So Much, Down and Dirty, Signore e Signori Buonanotte, A Special Day, Viva Italia, Chi Si Dice a Roma, The Terrace, Passion of Love, The Night of Varennes, Le Bal, Macaroni.

SCORSESE, MARTIN: Writer-Director-Editor. b. N.Y.C., Nov. 17, 1942. Began career while film arts student at N.Y. Univ., doing short, It's Not Just You, Murray.
PICTURES INCLUDE: Editor: Woodstock, Medicine Ball Caravan, Elvis. Director: Who's That Knocking at My Door?, Boxcar Bertha, Mean Streets (also co-s.p.), Alice Doesn't Live Here Anymore, Taxi Driver, New York, New York, The Last Waltz (also actor), Raging Bull, King of Comedy, After Hours, The Color of Money.

SCOTT, GEORGE C.: Actor, Director. b. Wise, Va., Oct. 18, 1927. Served 4 years Marine Corps. e. University of Missouri, appeared in varsity productions, summer stock, Shakespeare.
THEATRE: Off-Broadway in Richard III, As You Like It, Children of Darkness, Merchant of Venice, Desire Under the Elms, Antony and Cleopatra; Broadway in Comes a Day, The Andersonville Trial, The Wall, The Little Foxes, Plaza Suite, Uncle Vanya, director All God's Chillun Got Wings, director-actor Death of a Salesman, Sly Fox.
PICTURES INCLUDE: Film debut in Hanging Tree, 1959. Anatomy of a Murder, The Hustler, List of Adrian Messenger, Dr. Strangelove, The Bible, Film-Flam Man, Patton, They Might Be Giants, The Last Run, Hospital, The New Centurions, Oklahoma Crude, The Day of the Dolphin, The Hindenburg, Islands in the Stream, Crossed Swords, Movie Movie, Hardcore, The Changeling, The Formula, Taps, Firestarter.
Director-Actor, Rage; Director-Producer-Actor, The Savage is Loose.
TV: Major TV playhouses including Dupont Show of the Month, Playhouse 90, Hallmark Hall of Fame, Kraft Theatre, Omnibus, Armstrong Theatre, Play of the Week, NBC Sunday Showcase, Dow Hour of Great Mysteries, Esso Theatre; East Side, West Side series; The Crucible, Jane Eyre, The Price, Fear on Trial, Beauty and the Beast; directed The Andersonville Trial, A Christmas Carol, China Rose, Choices. Mini-Series: Mussolini—The Untold Story.

SCOTT, GORDON: Actor. r.n. Gordon M. Werschkul. b. Portland, Ore., Aug. 3, 1927. e. Oregon U. U.S. Army, 1944–47; then worked as fireman, cowboy, life guard; signed by Sol Lesser Prod. for role of Tarzan; debut in Tarzan's Hidden Jungle; since in: Tarzan and the Lost Safari, Tarzan's Greatest Adventure, The Tramplers.

SCOTT, GORDON L. T.: Producer. b. Edinburgh, Scotland, January 3, 1920. e. George Watson's Boys College. Served H.M. Forces 1939–46. Ent. m.p. ind. 1946 as 3rd asst. dir. with Ealing Studios. 1948: 1st asst. dir. on Passport to Pimlico, Train of Events; joined Associated British 1949 and worked on The Dancing Years, The Franchise Affair, Laughter in Paradise, Angels One Five, Isn't Life Wonderful, Will Any Gentleman, Rob Roy; 1953 prod. man. The Weak and the Wicked, It's Great To Be Young, The Dam Busters; 1956 appt. production exec. asst.; prod. Look Back in Anger, Sands of the Desert, Petticoat Pirates, The Pot Carriers, The Punch & Judy Man, Crooks in Cloisters, Forbush and the Penguins, Voices, The Maids, Snow Children, Out of Season, Hedda, The Abbess. Left Associated British 1969. Currently freelance. Recent Prods: Spectre Hanover Street, Friend or Foe, Tightrope to Terror, Lace, Haunters of the Deep, Out of the Darkness.
TV: (Prod): International Detective Series, The Avengers, Pathfinders, The Maids, Snow Children, A Man Called Intrepid, Undying Love, The Eye of the Yemanja.

SCOTT, J.C.: Executive. e. UCLA. Worked as prod. asst. on The Waltons and prod. coordinator for America at the Movies; two years at Intl. Creative Mgt. She joined Edward S. Feldman Co. at 20th-Fox as dir. of creative affairs; then v.p. of creative affairs for Marvin Worth Prods. Left to join Walt Disney Pictures 1983 as exec. asst. to Richard Berger, pres. 1984, promoted to v.p., m.p. prod.

SCOTT, MARGARETTA: Actress. b. London, England, Feb. 13, 1912; e. Conv. of Holy Child, London; Royal Acad. Dram. Art. In provincial rep. prior to London debut 1929 in, Her Shop; thereafter in numerous London productions. Screen debut 1934.
TV & PICTURES INCLUDE: Fanny by Gaslight, Man from Morocco, The First Gentleman, Mrs. Fitzherbert, Calling Paul Temple, Case of Shirley Yorke, Where's Charley, Landfall, Last Man to Hang, Town on Trial, Devil's General, Mayerling Story, You Never Can Tell, Long Sunset, The Heiress, Henry IV of Pimandello, Adventure Story, Second Mrs. Tanquery, Queen in Hamlet, Maigret, The Weather in the Streets, Member of the Family, Nicked at the Bottle, End of Term, File on Harry Jordan, The Importance of Being Earnest, Mr. Aitch, Upstairs and Downstairs, Elizabeth R., The Poisoning of Charles Bravo, The Duchess of Duke Street, What Every Woman Knows, All Creatures Great and Small, Tales of the Unexpected, Murder Trap, Racing Game, Together.

SCOTT, MARTHA: Actress. b. Jamesport, September 22, 1916; e. U. Michigan. In little theatres over U.S.; summer stock N.Y.; on radio with Orson Welles; film debut in "Our Town" 1940.
PICTURES INCLUDE: Cheers for Miss Bishop, They Dare Not Love, One Foot in Heaven, In Old Oklahoma; Hi Diddle Diddle; So Well Remembered, When I Grow Up, Desperate Hours, Ten Commandments, Airport 1975, Turning Point.
PLAYS INCLUDE: Soldier's Wife, Voice of the Turtle, The Number, Male Animal, Remarkable Mr. Pennypacker.

SCOTT, MORTON W.: Executive. b. San Francisco, Calif., Jan. 17; e. Stanford U. Pres., Studio City Television Productions, Inc.

SCOTT, RANDOLPH: Actor. b. Orange Co., Va., Jan. 23, 1903; e. U. of No. Car. On stage west coast; m.p. debut in Sky Bridge, 1931.
PICTURES INCLUDE: Roberto, Follow the Fleet, My Favorite Wife, Trail Street, The Gunfighters, Christmas Eve, Albuquerque, Return of the Bad Men, Coroner Creek, Canadian Pacific, Fighting Man of the Plains, Doolins of Oklahoma, Walking Hills, Cariboo Trail, The Nevadan, Colt .45, Sugarfoot, Sante Fe, Fort Worth, Man in the Saddle, Starlift, Carson City, Man Behind the Gun, Hangman's Knot, Thunder Over the Plains, Stranger Wore a Gun, Riding Shotgun, Bounty Hunter, Ten Wanted Men, Rage at Dawn, Tall Man Riding; act., assoc. prod., Lawless Street, Westbound, The Name's Buchanan. Ride Lonesome, Comanche Station, Ride the High Country.
One of Top Ten Money-Making Stars, M.P. Herald-Fame Poll, 1950–53. Retired.

SCOTT, RIDLEY: Director. b. England.
PICTURES: The Duellists, Alien, Blade Runner, Legend.

SCOTT, TONY: Director. Began career in tv commercials, being partnered with his brother Ridley in prod. co. Winner of numerous Clios, Gold & Silver Lions, and other awards. Entered m.p. industry 1972, directing half-hr. film, One of the Missing, for British Film Institute and Loving Memory, 1-hr. feature for Albert Finney.
PICTURES: The Hunger, Top Gun.

SCOTT, WALTER M.: Set decorator. b. Cleveland, Ohio, Nov. 7, 1906. e. U.S.C., 1929; Chouinard School of Art. Interior decorator, Fred B. Martin Co., 1929–30, asst. mgr., United Studios, 1930–31; joined Fox Film Corp., 1931; asst. set decorator, 1932; set decorator, 1933; set decorator, 20th Century-Fox, 1935; supervising set decorator, 1952–72. Now consultant decorator for Fox.
PICTURES INCLUDE: Twenty-one Academy Nominations —6 oscars for Robe, King and I, Diary of Ann Frank, Cleopatra, Fantastic Voyage, Hello, Dolly, On Board of Governors of the Academy of Motion Picture Arts and Sciences 1968–76, 1980–81, 1981–85.

SCULLY, JOE: Talent Executive-Casting Director-Producer. b. Kearney, N.J., March 1, 1926. e. Goodman Memorial Theatre of the Art Institute of Chicago, 1946. m. Penelope Gillette. Daughter, Samantha. Acted until 1951. CBS-TV, N.Y. Casting Dir., Danger You Are There, Omnibus, The Web, 1951–56. 1956–60, CBS-TV, Associate Prod., Studio One, Dupont Show of the Month, Playhouse 90. 1962–64, CBS Stations Div. KNXT, Producer, Repertoire Workshop. 1965–70 Casting Dir. 20th Century-Fox Films. 1970–74 Independent Casting Director. 1974–75 Universal TV, Casting Dir. 1975, NBC-TV Manager, Casting & Talent. 1978, Re-established Joe Scully-Casting independent Service to the industry. 1983, casting director, Walt Disney Pictures.
PICTURES INCLUDE: Hello Dolly, In Like Flint, Valley of the Dolls, Planet of the Apes, The Flim-Flam Man, Sounder, Lady Sings the Blues, Play It As It Lays, The Stone Killer, Parallax View, Lifeguard, Man in the Glass Booth, Middle Age Crazy, Death Wish II.
TV: Peyton Place, Room 222, Pilots: Julia, The Ghost & Mrs. Muir. 1970, Joe Scully Casting, Indep., The Bill Cosby Show, 1971: TV Feature, Thief, Missiles of October, Earth II; Series, Search, Bonanza, Nichols, Snoop Sisters, Columbo, Switch, McMillian & Wife, Tales of the Unexpected, Gone are the Dayes (Disney Channel, 1983).

SCULLY, PETER R.: Producer. b. Arlington, Mass., June 14, 1920; e. Mass. Inst. of Tech., 1939. With Ross Federal Research Corp. N.Y. (consumer studies) 1939–40; studied, Feagin School Dramatic Art. N.Y., to Universal as contract actor, then film ed., 1940–41; U.S. Marine Corps until 1945; film ed. Univ-Internat'l 1945–48; became m.p. prod. indep. cos., releasing through Monogram Prod., Inc. (Mayfair

Pictures, Inc. & Motion Pictures, Inc.).
PICTURES INCLUDE: Father's Wild Game, Father Takes The Air, Son of Belle Star.

SCUSE, DENNIS GEORGE (M.B.E.): Executive. g. Ilford, England, May 19, 1921. e. Park School; Mercers' School, London. British Army, Royal Artillery, 1939; command entertainment officer, Ceylon Army, 1941–42; joined British Army Broadcasting Service, Italy, 1944–46; overseas div., BBC, 1947; loaned to Forces Broadcasting Service, Middle East, 1948–50; dir., British Forces network, Germany, 1950–57; ret., BBC-TV, senior planning asst., Jan. 1958; chief asst., light entertainment dept., BBC-TV, 1960; apptd., chief asst. (TV) BBC N.Y. office, Sept. 1960; apptd., BBC rep. in U.S., July, 1962; gen. mgr., Television Enterprises, 1963; gen. mgr., Radio Enterprises 1968.

SEALEY, PETER S.: Executive, b. 1941. e. Univ. of Fla. (BS, economics), Yale Univ. Graduate School (Master of industrial admin.). Now exec. v.p., Columbia Pictures Industries. Came to post from Coca-Cola Co., CPI parent, where was v.p. & mgr. of its marketing operations dept. Responsible for long-range planning at CPI and corporate mktg. dir., handling personnel, administrative services and corporate communications. Joined Coca-Cola Co.. 1969; named v.p., mgr. of mktg. planning dept., 1976–79. 1979–82, v.p. & mktg. dir. of The Wine Spectrum, Coca-Cola subsidiary. 1982, elected v.p. of Coca-Cola and named mgr. of corporate mktg. operations. Prior to joining Coca-Cola was mktg. planning acct. exec. for Coca-Cola with McCann-Erickson Advertising, 1967–69. Prior to that associated with Quakers Oats Co., 1966–67; 1963–66, with foods division of Procter & Gamble Co.

SECOMBE, SIR HARRY, C.B.E.: Singer, comedian, actor. b. Swansea, Wales, Sept. 8, 1921; e. m.p. debut, Penny Points to Paradise, 1951; awarded, C.B.E., 1963. 1963–64: London stage starring in Pickwick. 1965: same role New York stage. 1967–68 The Four Musketeers, 1975 The Plumber's Progress.
PICTURES INCLUDE: Forces Sweetheart, Down Among the Z Men, Trilby, Davy, Jet Storm, Oliver, The Bed Sitting Room, Song of Norway, Rhubarb, Doctor in Trouble, The Magnificent Seven Deadly Sins, Sunstruck.
TV: Numerous appearances, incl. own series: Secombe and Friends, The Harry Secombe Show, Secombe with Music. Also special version, Pickwick. Author of Twice Brightly, Goon for Lunch, Katy and the Nurgla, Welsh Fargo, Goon Abroad, The Harry Secombe Diet Book, Introduced Highways (series).

SEGAL, GEORGE: Actor. b. N.Y., N.Y., Feb. 13, 1934. m. Marion Sobol. e. Columbia U. 1955. B.A. Worked as janitor, ticket-taker, soft-drink salesman, usher and under-study at N.Y.'s Circle in the Square theatre. Acting debut: Downtown Theatre's revival of Don Juan.
THEATRICAL CREDITS INCLUDE: 1956 revival: The Iceman Cometh, N.Y. Shakespeare Festival's Antony and Cleopatra, Leave It To Jane, The Premise (satiric improvisational revue), Rattle of a Simple Man, The Knack.
Formed a nightclub singing act with Patricia Scott. Record album of ragtime songs and banjo music: The Yama, Yama Man. Dir. debut: Bucks County Playhouse prod. Scuba Duba.
TV: Death of a Salesman, Of Mice and Men, The Desperate Hours, The Cold Room, The Zany Adventures of Robin Hood, Not My Kid.
PICTURES INCLUDE: The Young Doctors (1961), The Longest Day, Act One, The New Interns, Invitation to A Gunfighter, Ship of Fools, King Rat, The Lost Command, Who's Afraid of Virginia Woolf? (Acad. Award nom.), The Quiller Memorandum, The St. Valentine's Day Massacre, Bye Bye Braverman, No Way to Treat a Lady, The Southern Star, The Bridge at Remagen, The Girl Who Couldn't Say No, Loving, The Owl and the Pussycat, Where's Poppa?, Born to Win, Hot Rock, A Touch of Class, Blume in Love, The Terminal Man, California Split, The Black Bird, Russian Roulette, The Duchess and the Dirtwater Fox, Fun with Dick and Jane, Rollercoaster, Who Is Killing the Great Chefs of Europe?, Lost and Found, The Last Married Couple in America, Carbon Copy, Stick.

SEGAL, MAURICE: Publicist. b. New York, N.Y., July 22, 1921; e. C.C.N.Y., 1937–41. Entered m.p. ind., adv. dept., 20th Fox, 1941–42; U.S. Army 1942–46; feature writer, pub. dept., 20th Fox, April, 1946; asst. to dir., adv., pub., Century Circuit, 1947; press book dept., Paramount, 1949; trade press rep. 1950; trade press rep. RKO Radio, Nov. 1952; res. to join Richard Condon-Kay Norton, publicists, May, 1953; adv., pub. dept., U-I. Sept. 1954; asst. pub. mgr., United Artists Apr. 1957. Hollywood pub.-exploit., coordinator, 1958; exec. in chg. of M.P. press dept., Universal City Studios, 1966; West Coast adv.-pub. dir., National Gen. Pictures, 1971; Pres., Maurice E. Segal Co., 1974; div., West Coast operations, Charles Schlaifer & Co., 1976; v.p., Max Youngstein Enterprises, 1979; exec. v.p., Taft Intl. Pictures, 1980; pres. Maurice E. Segal Co., 1982.

SEIDMAN, LLOYD: Adv. exec. b. Brooklyn, N.Y., 1913. e. Columbia U., B.A., 1932; NYU School Business Administration. adv. dept., Montgomery Ward; M.P. dept., Lord & Thomas Adv. Agency, 1935; Donohue & Coe, 1936; v.p., 1942–61; pres., Educ. Science Div., U.S. Industries Inc., 1961; v.p., West, Weir & Bartel, 1963–65; exec. staff, v.p., Charles Schlaifer & Co., 1965; acct. superv. adv., Loew's Theatres; Jack Tinker & Partners, 1968; acct. superv. CBS Films (Cinema Center Films); vice-president, 1969, Blaine-Thompson Company.

SELBY, DAVID: Actor. b. Morganstown, W. Va. e. W. Va. Univ. Acted in outdoor dramas in home state and did regional theatre elsewhere. Was ass't. instructor in lit. at So. Ill. Univ.
PICTURES INCLUDE: Up the Sandbox, Super Cops, Lady in Blue, Night of Dark Shadows, Rich Kids, Rich and Famous.
TV: Dark Shadows (series), Washington: Behind Closed Doors, Telethon, Family, Falcon Crest, etc.

SELF, WILLIAM: Producer. b. Dayton, Ohio, June 21, 1921. e. Univ. of Chicago, 1943; prod.-dir., Schlitz Playhouse of Stars, 1952–56; prod., The Frank Sinatra Show, 1957; exec. prod., CBS-TV, The Twilight Zone, Hotel De Paree. 1960–61 exec. prod., 20th Century-Fox TV. Hong Kong, Adventures in Paradise, Bus Stop, Follow The Sun, Margie; v.p. in chg. of prod., 20th Century-Fox TV, 1962; exec. v.p., 1964. Pres., FOX TV 1969; v.p. 20th Century Fox Film Corp., 1969; pres. of William Self Productions, Inc., partner, Frankovich/Self Productions; 1975; vice-pres., programs, Hollywood CBS Television Network, 1976; 1977, v.p. motion pictures for television and miniseries, CBS Television Network; 1982, pres., CBS Theatrical Films. In 1985, pres., William Self Prods. in association with CBS Prods.

SELIG, ROBERT WILLIAM: Exhibitor. b. Cripple Creek, Colo., e. U. of Denver, 1932, B.A.; Doctorate, 1959. Consultant, Pacific Theatres. Lifetime Trustee, U. of Denver. Member Kappa Sigma, Omicron Delta Kappa, Beta Gamma Sigma; Nat'l Methodist Church Foundation; Pres., Theatre Association of California; board of directors Los Angeles Chamber of Commerce; chm., ShoWest Conventions.

SELLARS, ELIZABETH: Actress. b. Glasgow, Scotland, May 6, 1923; e. Queenswood, Hatfield. Memb. Lincolns Inn. Stage debut with Wilson Barrett Co. in Laburnum Grove, Glasgow.
PLAYS INCLUDE: Remarkable Mr. Pennypacker, South Sea Bubble, Tea & Sympathy, The Sound of Murder; 1960–61: Stratford upon Avon.
PICTURES INCLUDE: m.p. debut in Floodtide. Also: Madeleine, Prime of Miss Jean Brodie, Guilt Is My Shadow, Cloudburst, Hunted (Stranger in Between), Night Was Our Friend, Gentle Gunman, Long Memory, Barefoot Contessa, Desiree, Prince of Players, Three Cases of Murder, Last Man to Hang, Man in the Sky, The Shiralee, Jetstorm, The Day They Robbed the Bank of England, The Moment of Truth, Middle of Nowhere, 55 Days at Peking, The Chalk Garden, The Hireling.
TV: Many appearances include: Still Life, Too Late for the Mashed Potato, Harbour Island, The Happy Ones, The Sound of Murder, R 3 (series), Family Christmas, Person to Person, Person Unknown, Shades of Greene, Beasts, Last Love, Disraeli, Voyage Round My Father, Winter Sunlight.

SELLECK, TOM: Actor. b. Detroit, Jan. 29, 1945. e. USC.
PICTURES: Daughters of Satan, Myra Breckenridge, Midway, Seven Minutes, Coma, High Road to China, Lassiter, Runaway.
TELEVISION: Bracken's World, Countdown at the Superbowl, The Sacketts, Gypsy Warriors, Boston and Kilbride, The Concrete Cowboys, Magnum, P.I.

SELLER, THOMAS: Writer. b. San Francisco, Calif. e. Stanford U., Yale Drama School. Armed Forces, World War II; contract writer. MGM, 8 years.
PICTURES INCLUDE: Andy Hardy Meets Debutante, Tish, The Man From Down Under, The Black Arrow.
TV WRITER FOR: Rawhide, Laramie, Combat, Private Secretary, The Ann Sothern Show, Playhouse of Stars, Riverboat, The Tall Man, Death Valley Days, Cimarron City, Cavalcade of America, The Lone Ranger, The Stu Erwin Show, Walt Disney's Wonderful World of Color, The FBI, Bonanza, The Virginian, Kentucky Jones.

SELLERS, ARLENE: Producer. In partnership as attorneys in L.A. for 20 years with Alex Winitsky before they turned to financing and later production of films.
PICTURES INCLUDE: (co-prod. with Winitsky) End of the Game, The Seven-Per-Cent Solution, Cross of Iron, Night Calls, Silver Bears, Cuba, Blue Skies Again, Scandalous, Swing Shift, Bad Medicine.

SELTZER, JULES: Executive. b. New York City, Sept. 4, 1908; e. U. of Penn. Adv. and pub. depart., Fox Theatres Corp., Roxy Theatre, N.Y. District pub. Publix Theatres, Florida. Publ. depart., Warner Brothers Theatres, Philadelphia, for seven years. In 1937; Quigley Silver Showmanship Awards winner. Adv. and pub. dir., Warner Brothers theatres, Philadelphia, for two years, then pub. representative for Hal Roach. In 1940; joined Western Advertising. Resigned March, 1943, to join U.S. Navy. Returned to Hal Roach Studios dir. pub., 1945: 20th-Fox Studios, 1949. Retired 1973.

SELTZER, WALTER: Executive. b. Philadelphia, Pa., Nov. 7, 1914; e. U. of Penn.; married. Publicity man for Warner Bros. Theatres, Philadelphia; Fox West Coast Theatres; to Hollywood with MGM 1936–39; Columbia, 1940–41. Enlisted U.S. Marine Corp., 1941–44. Pub. dir., Hal Wallis, 1945–54; v.p. in chg. adv & pub., Hecht-Lancaster Orgn., Feb., 1954–55; assoc. prod., The Boss; partner, Glass-Seltzer, pub. rel. firm; v.p. & exec. prod, Pennebaker Production. 1982, v.p., M.P. & TV Fund.
PICTURES INCLUDE: One-Eyed Jacks, Shake Hands With the Devil, Paris Blues, The Naked Edge, Man in the Middle, Wild Seed, War Lord, Beau Geste, Will Penny, Number One, Darker Than Amber, The Omega Man, Skyjacked, Soylent Green, The Cay, The Last Hard Men.

SEMEL, TERRY: Executive. b. New York City, Feb. 24, 1943. e. C.C.N.Y. (MBA, 1967). Was with C.P.A. accounting firm 1965–66. Entered ind. with Warner Bros. in 1966 as br. mgr., New York, Cleveland, Los Angeles. From 1971 to 1973 was domestic sls. mgr. for CBS—Cinema Center Films. In 1973 joined Buena Vista as v.p., gen. sls. mgr. In 1975 went to Warner Bros. as v.p., gen. sls. mgr. In 1978 named exec. v.p. and chief operating officer. Now pres., WB.

SEMPLE, LORENZO, JR.: Writer.
PICTURES: Pretty Poison, Marriage of a Young Stockbroker, The Drowning Pool, Three Days of the Condor, King Kong, Hurricane, Flash Gordon, Never Say Never Again, Sheena.
TELEVISION: Rearview Mirror.

SEN, BACHOO: Producer/director/distributor. Born 1934, Calcutta, India. Entered industry 1950 in India and 1958 in U.K. Director of English Film Co. Ltd., English Film Co. (Exports) Ltd. and English Film Co. (Productions) Ltd. 1968: Produced: Her Private Hell, Loving Feeling. 1969: Produced: Love Is A Splendid Illusion. 1972: Sex Is Beautiful, Love-Hungry Girls. 1973: Tenderness. 1975: Adam and Nicole, The Intruders. 1970: Formed The English Film Co. 1974: Chief exec. & man. dir, Superground, Ltd.

SENDREY, ALBERT: Music composer, arranger, conductor. b. Chicago, Ill., 1921; e. Trinity Coll. Music, London, U.S.C., Paris & Leipzig Conservatories. Winner, Chi. Symphony Orch. prize for First Symphony, 1941; 1948, Reichhold Award Detroit Symph. Orch. for 2nd Symphony. Ohio Sesquicentenn. Award for Overture, Johnny Appleseed, 1953; One Act Opera: The Telltale Stones, 1964; arr., Mary Martin at Radio City Music Hall, 1965. Compose, arr., orch. for many plays, films and TV.
MEMBER: M.P. Academy, ASCAP, CLGA, ASMA, TV Academy.
BROADWAY: orch., arr.: Peter Pan, Ziegfeld Follies, New Faces, At the Grand, Pink Jungle, The Great Waltz, Turn to the Right.
PICTURES INCLUDE: The Yearling, Three Musketeers, Father's Little Dividend, Duchess of Idaho, Royal Wedding, Easy to Love, Great Caruso, American in Paris, Brigadoon, Athena, Finian's Rainbow, Guys and Dolls, Meet Me in Las Vegas, Opposite Sex, High Society, Raintree County, Let's Be Happy, Ride the High Country, Hallelujah Trail, The Hook, The Comancheros, Nevada Smith, The Oscar, Thoroughly Modern Millie, Hello Down There, Private Navy of Sgt. O'Farrell, Hard Times, Soul of Nigger Charley.
TV: comp. music: Laramie, Wagon Train, Ben Casey, Wolper Documentaries, Americans Abroad, J. F. Kennedy Anthology; Youn Man from Boston, collab. with Harry Sukman, High Chaparral, Bonanza (with D. Rose), The Monroes, Ken Murray's Hollywood, SWAT collab. B. de Vorzon, Hard Times, collab.

SERNAS, JACQUES: Actor-Producer. b. Lithuania, July 30, 1925. Became naturalized French citizen, studying medicine in Paris. Was amateur boxer when heard Jean Gabin needed an acting boxer for The Mirror, in which he made professional debut as actor. Has appeared in over 80 films, made in recent years primarily in Italy, now his home.
PICTURES INCLUDE: Lost Youth, The Golden Salamander, Helen of Troy, Jump into Hell, The First Night, La Dolce Vita, 55 Days in Peking, F.B.I.: Operation Baalbeck (also prod.), Operation Gold in the Balearic Islands (also prod.), Super Fly TNT.
TV: The School of the Painters of Paris (prod. only), The 18th Century Seen Through Its Famous Painters (prod. only), The Red Triangle (Ital. series).

SERPE, RALPH B.: Producer. b. Portland, Me., Dec. 23, 1914; e. Columbia U. Ind. thea. agent, 1936. U.S. Army, Spec. Services, 1942. v.p., Scalera Films, 1946; v.p., Italian Films Export, 1948; U.S. rep., assoc. prod., exec. asst., Dino De Laurentiis, 1952.
PICTURES INCLUDE: War and Peace, Ulysses, The Tempest, Under Ten Flags, Yovanka, Barabbas, The Bible, Drum, The Brinks' Job.

SEVAREID, ERIC: News commentator. b. Velva, N.D., Nov. 26, 1912; e. U. of Minn., Paris. Started career as reporter: Minneapolis Journal, Paris Herald Tribune, United Press; joined CBS radio news staff in Paris at outbreak of World War II; with CBS radio, TV since; nat. corres; retired (1977).
BOOKS: author: Not So Wild a Dream, In One Ear, Small Sounds in the Night, This is Eric Sevareid.

SEVERINO, JOHN C.: Executive. b. New Haven, CT. e. Univ. of Connecticut. Joined ABC in 1965 as acct. exec. for WABC-TV; later served in various positions for ABC-TV Spot Sales in N.Y. and Chicago. In 1968 named sls. mgr., WLS-TV, Chicago; promoted to gen. sls. mgr., WXYZ-TV, Detroit, 1969. Returned to Chicago station in 1974 as v.p., gen. mgr. In 1974 named v.p., gen. mgr. of KABC-TV, Los Angeles. In 1981 named pres. of ABC Television.

SEWALL, BARBARA JEAN: Public Relations. b. Holly, Colo., Jan. 6; e. LACC, UCLA. pub. dir. & adv. mgr., Saks Fifth Ave., Beverly Hills; owner-publicity agency representing actors, independent production cos. & , Hollywood Athletic Club; RKO, Samuel Goldwyn Prods., Inc., MGM, Edward Small Prod., Warner Bros., 20th Century-Fox, Lowell Thomas, Cinerama, VideoTravel.

SEYMOUR, ANNE: Actress. b. New York City, Sept. 11, 1909. On many radio programs, including Story of Mary Marlin, Grand Hotel, etc.
PICTURES: All the King's Men, The Whistle at Eaton Falls, Man on Fire, Pollyanna, Desire Under the Elms, Gift of Love, Home from the Hill, Misty, Good Neighbor Sam, Mirage, How To Succeed in Business without Really Trying, Fitzwilly, Stay Away, Joe, Hearts of the West, etc.
TELEVISION: Empire, General Hospital. Movies: I Never Said Goodbye, The Last Survivors, James at 15, Studs Lonigan, The Miracle Worker, Angel on My Shoulder, etc.

SEYMOUR, DAN: Actor. b. Chicago, Ill., Feb. 22, 1915. Performer burlesque, nightclubs. Stage, screen and TV actor.
PLAYS: Rain, Amphitryon 38, Room Service, and others.
PICTURES INCLUDE: Casablanca, To Have and Have Not, Confidential Agent, Intrigue, Key Largo, Johnny Belinda, Rancho Notorious, Maru Maru, Glory Alley, Face to Face, The System, Second Chance, Big Heat, Human Desire, Moonfleet, Buster Keaton Story, Sad Sack, Watusi, Return of the Fly, Leader of the Pack, The Mummy, The Way Things Were, Soft Touch, Escape from Witch Mountain, Rainbow Island.
TV: Casablanca, Restless Gun, Perry Mason, Untouchables, Holiday Inn, This Gun for Hire, 77 Sunset Strip, Hawaiian Eye, Get Smart, My Mother The Car, Batman, U.N.C.L.E., Beverly Hillbillies, Voyage to the Bottom of the Sea, My Favorite Martian, Don't Eat the Daisies, The Bob Hope Show, Kojak, The Chase, Barbary Coast, Fantasy Island.

SEYMOUR, JANE: Actress. b. England, Feb. 15, 1951. r.n. Joyce Frankenberg. Dancer with London Festival Ballet at 13. Theatrical film debut, Live and Let Die (1973). On Bdwy. in Amadeus.
PICTURES: Sinbad and the Eye of the Tiger, Battlestar Galactica, Oh, Heavenly Dog, Somewhere in Time, Lassiter.
TELEVISION: Movies: Frankenstein: The True Story, Captains and the Kings, Benny and Barney: Las Vegas Undercover, Seventh Avenue, Killer on Board, The Four Feathers, The Awakening Land, Love's Dark Ride, Dallas Cowboys Cheerleaders, East of Eden, The Haunting Passion, Dark Mirror, The Sun Also Rises, Obsessed with a Married Woman, Crossings.

SEYRIG, DELPHINE: Actress. b. Beirut, Lebanon, 1932. Formal dramatic training in Paris; later at Actors Studio, N.Y.
PICTURES: Pull My Daisy, Last Year in Marienbad, Muriel, La Musica, Accident, Mr. Freedom, Stolen Kisses, Daughters of Darkness, Peau d'Ane, The Discreet Charm of the Bourgeoisie, The Day of the Jackal, The Black Windmill, Aloise, Doll's House, Dear Michael, Le Dernier Cri, India Song, Faces of Love, Le Chemin Perdu, I Sent a Letter to My Love.

SHABER, DAVID: Screenwriter. b. Cleveland. e. Western Reserve Univ., Yale, Taught at Allegheny College on speech and drama dept. Contributor to Cosmpolitan, Life, Esquire; had several short stories in O'Henry prize collections. Also wrote dramas (Shake Hands with the Clown, The Youngest Shall Ask, etc.). First screenplay was Such Good Friends

for Otto Preminger.
PICTURES INCLUDE: The Last Embrace, The Warriors, Those Lips, Those Eyes, Night Hawks, Rollover.

SCHAFER, MARTIN: Executive. e. UCLA. Attorney-at-law. Served as producer on Modern Romance & The Awakening before joining Embassy Pictures as prod. exec. 1983; promoted to pres., prod. 1985, named exec. v.p., prod., for 20th Century Fox.

SHAFTEL, JOSEF: Producer, director, writer. b. Cleveland, Ohio, 1919. Early career violinst, musician, newspaper correspondent, photographer, screen writer, director. Ent. m.p. ind. 1949.
PICTURES INCLUDE: prod: Man Who Watched the Trains Go By, Naked Dawn, No Place to Hide, Naked Hills, The Biggest Bundle of Them All, The Bliss of Mrs. Blossom, The Last Grenade, Goodbye Gemini, Say Hello to Yesterday, The Statue, The Trojan Women, Soul to Soul, Assassination of Trotsky, Where Does it Hurt?, Redneck, Alice's Adventures in Wonderland.
TV: 1962–63 prod: The Untouchables.

SHAGAN, STEVE: Writer. b. New York City. Apprenticed in little theatres, film lab chores, stagehand jobs. Wrote, produced and directed film short, One Every Second; moved to Hollywood in 1959. Was IATSE man, working as grip, stagehand, electrician to support film writing. Was freelance advertising man and publicist; produced "Tarzan" TV show. In 1968 began writing and producing two-hour films for TV.
PICTURES INCLUDE: Save the Tiger (prod., s.p.-AA nomination—WGA award, best original s.p.), Hustle (s.p.), Voyage of the Damned (co.-s.p.-AA nomination), The Formula (s.p., prod.).
TV: Writer-producer: River of Mystery, Spanish Portrait, Sole Survivor, A Step Out of Line, etc.
BOOKS: Save the Tiger, City of Angels, The Formula, The Circle, The Discovery, Vendetta.

SHALIT, GENE: b. N.Y.C., 1932. e. Univ. of Illinois. Started as free-lance writer; joined NBC Radio Network, working on Monitor. Has been book and film critic, sports and general columnist. In January, 1973 replaced Joe Garagiola as featured regular Today Show.

SHAPIRO, BYRON M.: Executive b. Hill City, Minn., Aug. 15, 1918. e. Univ. of Minn. (graduated 1940). Served in U.S. Army Air Corp., 1941–44. Entered m.p. industry as booker with Columbia in Minneapolis, 1944, later becoming branch mgr. in Des Moines (1951), St. Louis (1957), Minneapolis, (1958). Named western div. mgr. for Columbia in 1966. In 1974 appt. MGM v.p. domestic dist; 1982, v.p. dir. exhibitor relations, MGM; 1984, v.p., dist. exec., Tri-star Pictures.

SHAPIRO, IRVIN: Executive. Formerly newspaperman; m.p. reviewer; director of national publicity campaigns. Publicity, RKO; active in ind. dist. & in export & import. Now pres., Films Around the World, Inc.; Filmworld Export Corp. which represents leading film producers and distributors throughout the world.

SHAPIRO, JACOB: Executive. b. Harbin, China, Aug. 26, 1928; e. Gakushuin Univ. (Peers' School), Tokyo, Japan, B.A. Pol. Sci. Joined Columbia Pictures Intl., N.Y., 1961; Japan sales manager, 1961–65; Puerto Rico gen. mgr., 1965–68; appointed Japan and South Korea gen. mgr., Columbia, 1968; from 1970 became Columbia supv. for Philippines as well as gen. mgr. Japan and South Korea until Feb. 1981; from 1981 v.p. Far East and Australasia, Twentieth Century Fox, Los Angeles.

SHAPIRO, KEN: Producer-Director-Writer-Actor. b. New Jersey, 1943. e. Bard College. Was child actor on tv and teacher in Brooklyn before opening "world's first video theatre" in East Village of Manhattan: Channel One, 90 mins. of TV lampoons and original material shown on TV monitors to live audience. Took 16 mm material on college dates with success, culminating in feature film: The Groove Tube (1974).
PICTURE: Modern Problems (s.p., dir.).

SHAPIRO, ROBERT K.: Executive. b. New York, N.Y., Feb. 12; e. CCNY. St. John's Coll. Usher, Rialto Theatre, N.Y., 1928; chief of service, 1929; Paramount Theatre, N.Y., 1930; treas. asst. mgr., Rivoli, Criterion, B'klyn Paramount Theatres, 1930–33; treas., Paramount Theatre, 1933; asst. mgr., 1936; house mgr., 1941; mgr., 1945; exec. mgr., 1953; managing dir., 1954; coord., TV network progs., Western Div., American Broadcasting, 1964. Member: Variety Club of N.Y.; past pres., Cinema Lodge, B'nai B'rith, Trustee Agva Youth Fund; pres., Metropolitan Motion Picture Theatres Assn., 1962–64, Head of Int. Motion Pic. Div. 1974.

SHAPIRO, ROBERT W.: Producer. b. Brooklyn, N.Y., 1938. Joined William Morris Agency, Inc., 1958. dir. and head of motion picture dept., William Morris Agency (UK) Ltd., 1969; man. dir., 1970. 1974 vice president William Morris, Inc. In March, 1977 joined Warner Bros. as exec. v.p. in chg. of worldwide production. 1981, named WB pres., theatrical production div. Resigned 1983 to produce films for WB. In 1985 produced Pee-Wee's Big Adventure.

SHARAFF, IRENE: Costume Designer. b. 1910. Long career on stage and in films. Winner of Tony, two Donaldson Awards, five Academy Awards and 16 Oscar nominations. Has worked on more than 30 motion pictures.
PICTURES INCLUDE: Meet Me in St. Louis, Hello, Dolly, Guys and Dolls, Call Me Madam, Yolanda and the Thief, Brigadoon, Porgy and Bess, Flower Drum Song, The Best Years of Our Lives, The Taming of the Shrew, A Star is Born (1954). Oscar winners include An American in Paris, The King and I, West Side Story, Cleopatra, Who's Afraid of Virginia Woolf?, Mommie Dearest.

SHARE, MICHAEL: Executive. Began career with Paramount Pictures 1974 as booker in Indianapolis. 1975–76 appt. salesman; 1976–77 sls. mgr. in Philadelphia; 1977, Cincinnati branch mgr.; 1980, Chicago branch mgr. 1985, promoted to v.p., eastern div.

SHARIF, OMAR: Actor. b. Alexandria, Egypt, April 10, 1932. r.n. Michel Shahoub; e. Victoria College, Cairo. pres. of College Dramatic Society; m. Faten Hamama. Starred in 21 Egyptian and two French films prior to Lawrence of Arabia.
PICTURES INCLUDE: The Blazing Sun, 1955 (debut), Goha, 1959, Lawrence of Arabia, Ghengis Khan, The Fall of the Roman Empire, The Yellow Rolls-Royce, Behold a Pale Horse, Doctor Zhivago, Night of the Generals, More Than a Miracle, McKenna's Gold, Che!, Funny Girl, The Appointment, Mayerling, The Horsemen, The Burglars, The Tamarind Seed, The Mysterious Island of Captain Nemo, Juggernaut, Funny Lady, Crime and Passion, The Baltimore Bullet, Green Ice.
TELEVISION: The Far Pavillions, Pleasure Palace, Peter the Great, Harem.

SHARKEY, RAY: Actor. b. Red Hook, Brooklyn, New York, 1952. Began on TV, guesting in Kojak, Police Story, Barney Miller, etc. Also performed on stage in Los Angeles. Theatrical movie debut in Hot Tomorrows in 1976.
PICTURES: Who'll Stop the Rain?, Heartbeat, Willie and Phil, The Idolmaker, Love and Money, Some Kind of Hero, Body Rock, Wise Guys.
TELEVISION: Behind Enemy Lines.

SHARP, ALAN: Writer. b. Glasgow, Scotland. Writes western screenplays.
PICTURES INCLUDE: The Hired Hand, Ulzana's Raid, Billy Two Hats, Night Moves, The Osterman Weekend, Little Treasure (also dir.).

SHARP, DON: Writer, director. b. Hobart, Tasmania, Australia, 1922. Early career as actor in Australia. Ent. m.p. ind. in England with Group Three as screenwriter, 1951. Began directing 1955 with doc. children's films, 2nd unit work and filmed TV series.
PICTURES INCLUDE: Kiss of the Vampire, It's All Happening, Devil Ship Pirates, Witchcraft, Those Magnificent Men in Their Flying Machines (2nd unit), Curse of the Fly, The Face of Fu Manchu, Rasputin—The Mad Monk, Our Man in Marrakesh, The Brides of Fu Manchu, Rocket to the Moon, Taste of Excitement, The Violent Enemy, Puppet on a Chain, Psychomania, Dark Places, Callan, Hennessy, The Four Feathers, The 39 Steps, Bear Island.
TELEVISION: Ghost Squad, The Champions, The Avengers, House of Horror, Q.E.D., A Woman of Substance, Tusitala, Hold the Dream.

SHATNER, WILLIAM: Actor. b. Montreal, Mar. 22, 1931. e. McGill Univ. Toured Canada in various stock, repertory companies. Bdwy. debut, Tamburlaine the Great (1956).
PICTURES INCLUDE: The Brothers Karamazov, Judgment at Nurembergm The Explosive generation, The Intruder, The Outrage, Big Hot Mama, Dead of Night, The Devil's Rain, Kingdom of the Spiders, Star Trek—The Motion Picture, The Kidnapping of the President, Star Trek II: The Wrath of Khan, Airplane II: The Sequel, Star Trek III: The Search for Spock, Star Trek IV: The Voyage Home.
TELEVISION: Star Trek, The Statesman, The Bastard, Disaster on the Coastline, The Baby Sitter, Andersonville, T.J. Hooker, Secrets of a Married Man, North Beach of Rawhide.

SHAVELSON, MELVILLE: Writer, director. b. B'klyn. N.Y., April 1, 1917; e. Cornell U. 1937, A.B. Radio writer: We The People, Bicycle Party, 1937, Bob Hope Show, 1938–43. Screen writer; apptd. prod., Warner Bros, 1951. Conceived for TV: Make Room for Daddy, My World and Welcome To It. Author: book, How To Make a Jewish Movie. Lualda, The Great Houdinis, The Eleventh Commandment, Ike. Pres., Writers Guild of America, West, 1969–71, 1979–81, 1985–; Pres., Writers Guild Foundation 1978–86.
PICTURES INCLUDE: Princess & The Pirate, Wonder Man, Kid From Brooklyn, Sorrowful Jones, It's a Great

Feeling, Daughter of Rosie O'Grady, Always Leave Them Laughing, Where There's Life, On Moonlight Bay, I'll See You in My Dreams, Room For One More, April in Paris, Trouble Along the Way, Living It Up, Seven Little Foys, Beau James, Houseboat, It Started in Naples, The Five Pennies, On the Double, The Pigeon That Took Rome, A New Kind of Love, Cast a Giant Shadow, Yours Mine and Ours, The War Between Men and Women, Mixed Company.
TV FEATURES: The Legend of Valentino, The Great Houdinis, Ike, The Other Woman, Deceptions.

SHAW, EDWARD S.: Producer-Actor-Executive. b. Buffalo, N.Y., July 13, 1939. e. El Camino College. Began as child actor on radio, joined CBS-TV in 1957, then owner/president of p.r./adv. firm under his own banner.
PICTURES INCLUDE: Actor; Sergeant Rutledge, Claudell English, Palm Springs Weekend, Rise & Fall of Legs Diamond, PT-109, Critics Choice. Production: Assoc. prod. Harlow, Give'em Hell Harry; Exec. prod. Half A House, Aftermath; Co-prod., Hollywood Knight, Lady Taxi Driver; Prod., The Josephine Baker Story.

SHAWLEE, JOAN: Actress. b. Forest Hills, N.Y., March 5, 1929; e. Calif. & N.Y. high schools. Powers model, night club entertainer.
PLAYS: By Jupiter, Connecticut Yankee in King Arthur's Court.
TV: Abbott and Costello TV show, series: Aggie.
PICTURES INCLUDE: Marrying Kind, Something for the Birds, Conquest of Space, A Star is Born, Francis Joins the Wacs, Some Like it Hot, The Apartment, Critic's Choice, Irma LaDouce, All the Fallen Angels, Tony Rome, Live a Little, Love a Little, Willard, One More Train To Rob.

SHAWN, DICK: Actor. r.n. Richard Schulefand. b. Buffalo, N.Y., December 1, 1929. e. U. of Miami. Actor, play: For Heaven's Sake, Mother, A Funny Thing Happened on the Way to the Forum. Worked night club circuit, 5 yrs.
PICTURES INCLUDE: Wake Me When It's Over, It's a Mad Mad Mad Mad World, The Producers, The Happy Ending, Love at First Bite, Angel.
TV: Max Liebman TV Spectaculars, Mary (series).

SHAYE, ROBERT: Executive. b. Detroit, MI, Mar. 4, 1939. e. Michigan Univ. (BBA); Columbia Univ. Law. Pres. & CEO, New Line Cinema.

SHAYNE, ROBERT: Actor. b. Yonkers, N.Y. On N.Y. stage, on screen 1943 in Shine on Harvest Moon.
PLAYS: Claudia, Night of January 16th, Both Your Houses, Yellow Jack, Whiteoaks, Without Love, etc.—70 in all
PICTURES INCLUDE: Mr. Skeffington, Christmas in Connecticut, Welcome Stranger, Neanderthal Man, North by Northwest, The Arrangement, Tora Tora Tora, Barefoot Executive, Million Dollar Duck—96 in all.
TV: Marcus Welby, M.D., Doris Day Show, S.W.A.T., Emergency, Superman series—350 segments in all.

SHEAFF, DONALD J.: Executive. b. Oct. 23, 1925; e. U.C.L.A., 1948, Pierce College, 1957. Served 4 yrs. during WW II in Navy Air Corps in South Pacific. 1946, joined Technicolor Motion Picture Div. in supervisory capacity; 1957, lab. supervisor, Lookout Mountain Air Force Station, handling Top Secret film for Air Force and Atomic Energy Commission. Est. and org. the installation of Vandenberg Air Force Base Lab. facilities, which Technicolor designed. 1961 joined Panacolor Corp., 1963; joined Pacific Title and Art Studio in charge of color control for special effects and titles. Returned to Technicolor Corp. 1966, app't. Plant Mgr. of Television Div., Oct. 1966, V.P. & Gen. Mgr. of the Television Div., July, 1973 appt v.p. & gen. mgr., Motion Picture Division; 1976; mgr., special visual effects, Universal City Studios. Member: SMPTE, Nat'l Academy of Television Arts & Sciences. Has conducted scientific seminars for SMPTE.

SHEDLO, RONALD: Producer. b. Los Angeles, 1940. Secretary to Errol Flynn, 1956. Asst. prod. Strangers in the City, 1961. Prod. The Whisperers, 1966. Prod. The Reckoning, Day of Locust, Letters from Frank, Back Roads. Now with Rastar Prods. as exec. prod.

SHEEDY, ALLY: Actress. b. New York City, June 13, 1962. e. USC. Daughter of literary agent Charlotte Sheedy. At age 12 wrote children's book, She Was Nice to (ulp) Mice; later pieces in The New York Times, The Village Voice, Ms. Film debut in Bad Boys, 1983.
PICTURES: WarGames, Oxford Blues, The Breakfast Club, St. Elmo's Fire, Twice in a Lifetime, Blue City, Short Circuit.
TELEVISION: Episodes of Hill Street Blues.

SHEELER, MARK: Actor. r.n. Morris Sheeler. b. New York, N.Y., April 24, 1923; e. UCLA. Disc jockey 1942–48. Air Corp. Photog. during war. Voices, animated cartoons, commercials. M.p. debut in Born Yesterday.
PLAYS: Hillbarn Thea., Calif.: Harvey, The Happy Time, Time of Your Life, Amphitryon 38, Send Me No Flowers, The Gazebo, etc.
PICTURES INCLUDE: The High and the Mighty, Blood Alley, It Came From Beneath the Sea, Apache Warrior, Tank Battalion, P.O.W., Book of Israel, Why Must I Die?, Irma La Douce, The Raven, Elmer Gentry, How the West Was Won, Mary Poppins, Unsinkable Molly Brown, Sound of Music, After the Fox, Elmer Gantry, See the Man Run, Capricorn I, Damien, Omen II, The Hand, Blue Thunder.
TV: Hitchcock Presents, Kraft Thea., Day in Court, Defenders, East Side, West Side, Dr. Kildare, The Fugitive, Mr. Ed, Jack Benny Show, Life of Riley, Man from Uncle, Doctors & the Nurses, The Invaders, Batman, Here's Lucy, Dennis the Menace, Andy Griffith, Marcus Welby, Banachek, Moses the Lawgiver, All My Children, Kojak, Charlie's Angels, Police Woman, The Tonight Show, Mash, Fantasy Island, Photo Clinic (PBS), The C.C. Connection, Nero Wolfe, House Calls, China Smith, Highway Patrol, Three's Company, Ike: The War Years, Cagney and Lacey, Barnaby Jones, Mike Hammer, Trapper John.

SHEEN, CHARLIE: Actor. Son, Martin Sheen. Made debut as extra in TV movie, The Execution of Private Slovik (starring father) and as extra in Apocalypse Now (also starring father).
PICTURES: Grizzly II—The Predator, The Red Dawn, Lucas, Platoon, Ferris Buehler's Day Off, The Wraith.
TELEVISION: Movies: Silence of the Heart, The Boys Next Door.

SHEEN, MARTIN: Actor. r.n. Ramon Estevez. b. Dayton, O., Aug. 3, 1940.
PICTURES INCLUDE: The Subject Was Roses, The Incident, Catch 22, No Drums, No Bugles, Rage, Pickup on 101, Badlands, The Cassandra Crossing, The Little Girl Who Lives Down the Lane, Apocalypse Now, The Final Countdown, Gandhi, That Championship Season, Enigma, Man, Woman and Child, The Dead Zone, Firestarter.
TELEVISION: Movies: That Certain Summer, Letters for Three Lovers, The Execution of Private Slovik, The California Kid, The Missiles of October, Sweet Hostage, The Guardian, The Atlanta Child Murders, Consenting Adult, Shattered Spirits, News at Eleven, Out of the Darkness, Samaritan.

SHEFFER, CRAIG: Actor. b. York, PA. e. East Strousberg Coll., PA. Started career in tv commercials; in soap opera, One Life to Live. On off-Bdwy. stage in Fresh Horses and on and off-Bdwy. in Torch Song Trilogy.
PICTURES: That Was Then . . . This Is Now, Fire with Fire.

SHEFFIELD, JOHN: Actor. b. Pasadena, Calif., April 11, 1931; e. UCLA. Stage debut at 7 in On Borrowed Time. Created screen role of Tarzan's son; in Tarzan pictures since.
PICTURES INCLUDE: Babes in Arms, Little Orvie, Bomba series, creating name part in Million Dollar Baby, Knute Rockne, Roughly Speaking, Cisco Kid.
TV: series: Bantu the Zebra Boy.

SHEFTER, BERT: Composer, conductor. b. Russia, May 15, 1904; e. Carnegie Inst. of Tech., Curtis Inst., Damrosch Inst. Member of piano team, Gould & Shefter, on radio & in theatres; org. own band; concert pianist; comp., cond. for many films and TV.
PICTURES INCLUDE: compose, conduct: Tall Texan, No Escape, Great Jesse James Raid, Sins of Jezebel, The Big Circus, The Fly, Lost World, Jack the Giant Killer, Monkey on My Back, Cattle King, Curse of the Fly, Last Man on Earth, Voyage to the Bottom of the Sea, The Bubble, Dog of Flanders.
TV: Written shows for Sunset Strip, Surfside, Hawaiian Eye, Maverick, Sugarfoot, Lawman, Bourbon St., Roaring 20's.

SHEINBERG, SIDNEY JAY: Executive. b. Corpus Christi, TX, Jan. 14, 1935. e. Columbia Coll. (Ab, 1955; LLB, 1958). Admitted to Calif. bar, 1958; assoc. in law U. Cal. Sch. Law, Los Angeles, 1958–59; Joined MCA, Inc, 1959. Pres., TV div., 1971–74; exec. v.p., parent co., 1969–73. Named MCA pres. & chief oper. off., 1973.

SHELDON, DAVID: Director-Writer-Producer. b. New York City. e. Yale Univ., School of Drama (M.F.A.), Principia College (B.A.), Actors Studio (directors unit). Directed N.Y. & L.A. companies of The Star Spangled Girl, Alley Oop, Jimmy Shine, etc. Mgn. dir., The Gateway Playhouse in N.Y. where produced & directed over 50 plays and musicals. From 1972–74 was exec. in chg. of development at American Intl. Pictures supervising various production & post-production aspects of such films as Dillinger, The Frogs, Macon County Line, Slaughter, Dr. Phibes, Boxcar Bertha, Heavy Traffic, etc.
PICTURES INCLUDE: Producer-Writer, Sheba, Baby, Grizzly, The Evil, Project: Kill. Producer: Just Before Dawn. Director: Timelapse, Lovely But Deadly. Writer: The Predator.

SHELDON, JAMES: Director. b. New York, N.Y.; e. U. of N.C. Page boy, NBC; announcer-writer-dir., NBC Internat'l Div.;

staff dir., ABC radio; staff prod. dir., Young & Rubicam; free lance prod. dir. of many programs live tape and film, N.Y. and Hollywood.

TV: prod., dir.: Mr. Peepers, Armstrong Circle Theatre, Robert Montgomery Presents, Schlitz Playhouse, West Point, Zane Grey Theatre, The Millionaire, Desilu Playhouse, Perry Mason, Twilight Zone, Route 66, Naked City, The Virginian, Alfred Hitchcock Presents, Fugitive, Espionage, Defenders, Nurses, Bing Crosby Show, Family Affair, Wonderful World of Disney, Man From UNCLE, Felony Squad, That Girl, Ironside, My World and Welcome To It, To Rome With Love, Owen Marshall, Room 222, Gidget Grows Up (ABC Movie), Apple's Way, Love American Style, McMillan and Wife, Sanford and Son, Ellery Queen, Rich Man, Poor Man II, Family, MASH, Switch, Loveboat, With This Ring (ABC Movie), Sheriff Lobo, Gossip Columnist (movie), Knott's Landing, The Waltons, 240-Robert, Nurse, Dukes of Hazard, Todays F.B.I., McLain's Law, 7 Brides for 7 Brothers, Lottery, Partners in Crime, Jessie, Half Nelson, Stir Crazy, The Equalizer, Sledge Hammer.

SHELDON, SIDNEY: Writer-Producer-Novelist. b. Chicago, Feb. 11, 1917. e. Northwestern Univ. Novels made into films include Other Side of Midnight, Bloodline, Naked Face. Awards: Oscar, Writers Guild, Tony, Edgar.

PICTURES INCLUDE: Bachelor and the Bobbysoxer, Easter Parade, Annie Get Your Gun, Dream Wife, Jumbo, Pardners, You're Never Too Young, Birds and the Bees, Three Guys Named Mike, Remains To Be Seen, Gambling Daughters, Dangerous Lady.

TELEVISION: Created Patty Duke Show; Created and produced I Dream of Jeannie, Nancy and created Hart to Hart. Novels made into mini-series: Rage of Angels, Master of the Game.

NOVELS: The Naked Face, The Other Side of Midnight, A Stranger in the Mirror, Bloodline, Rage of Angels, Master of the Game, If Tomorrow Comes.

SHENSON, WALTER: Producer. b. San Francisco, Calif., e. Stanford U., Calif.; Ent. m.p. ind. 1941; studio exec., writing, prod., prom. shorts, trailers, Columbia; sup. publ., expl., London, Columbia European production, 1955.

PICTURES INCLUDE: prod.: The Mouse That Roared, A Matter of Who, The Mouse on the Moon, A Hard Day's Night, Help!, 30 is a Dangerous Age, Cynthia, Don't Raise the Bridge Lower the River, A Talent for Loving, Welcome to the Club (prod.-dir.), The Chicken Chronicles (co-prod.).

SHEPARD, SAM: Writer-Actor. b. Fort Sheridan, Ill, Nov. 5, 1943. Grew up in California, Montana and South Dakota. Lives near San Francisco, where, in addition to writing, runs a drama workship at the Univ. of California at Davis. Recipient of Brandeis Univ. Creative Arts Citation (1976) and American Academy of Arts and Letters Award (1975).

PLAYS INCLUDE: Cowboys and Rock Garden (double bill), Chicago, Icarus' Mother, and Red Cross (triple bill—1966 Obie Award), La Turista (1967 Obie), Forensic and the Navigators, Melodrama Play, Tooth of Crime (1973 Obie), Back Dog Beast Bait, Operation Sidewinder, 4-H Club, The Unseen Hand, Mad Dog Blues, Shaved Splits, Rock Garden, Curse of the Starving Class (1978 Obie), Buried Child, etc.

ACTOR: Days of Heaven, Resurrection, Raggedy Man, Frances, The Right Stuff, Country, Fool for Love.

SCREENPLAY: Paris, Texas, Fool for Love.

SHEPHERD, CYBILL: Actress-singer. b. Memphis, Tenn., Feb. 18, 1950. e. Hunter Col., NYU, USC. Was fashion model before acting debut in 1971. Debut record album, Cybill Does It . . . To Cole Porter (Paramount), 1974.

PICTURES INCLUDE: The Last Picture Show (debut), The Heartbreak Kid, Daisy Miller, At Long Last Love, Taxi Driver, Special Delivery, Silver Bears.

TELEVISION: Yellow Rose, Secrets of a Married Man, Moonlighting, Seduced, The Long Hot Summer.

SHEPHERD, RICHARD: Producer. b. Kansas City, Mo., June 4, 1927. e. Stanford Univ. In U.S. Naval Reserve, 1944–45. Entered ent. field as exec. with MCA, 1948, functioning in radio, TV, and m.p. fields until 1956, with time out for U.S. Army, 1950–52. In 1956 became head of talent for Columbia Pictures. In 1962 joined CMA talent agency on its founding, becoming exec. v.p. in chg. of m.p. div. Left to join Warner Bros. in Aug., 1972, as exec. v.p. for prod. Resigned Oct. 1, 1974 to become indep. prod. In 1976 named MGM sr. vp. & worldwide head of theatrical prod.

PICTURES INCLUDE: Twelve Angry Men, The Hanging Tree, The Fugitive Kind, Breakfast at Tiffany's (prod.), Alex and the Gypsy, Robin and Marian, Volunteers, The Hunger.

SHER, JACK: Writer, producer, director. b. Minneapolis, Minn. e. U. of Minnesota. Syndicated newspaper columnist; contrib. mag. articles (fiction & non-fiction). U.S. Army, WW II.

BROADWAY: The Perfect Setup, 1963.

BOOKS: author: The Cold Companion, 12 Sports Immortals, 12 More Sports Immortals.

PICTURES INCLUDE: collab. s.p.: My Favorite Spy, Off Limits; s.p.: Kid from Left Field; addit. dial.: Shane; s.p., collab. story: World in My Corner; collab. s.p.: Walk the Proud Land, Joe Butterfly; s.p., dir.: Four Girls in Town; s.p., dir.: Kathy O, The Wild and the Innocent; collab. s.p., dir.: 3 Worlds of Gulliver; collab. s.p.: Paris Blues; s.p., dir.: Love in a Goldfish Bowl; s.p.: Critic's Choice; collab. s.p.: Move Over Darling, produced and wrote "Goodby Raggedy Ann" produced "Slither."

SHER, LOUIS K.: Executive. b. Columbus, Ohio, Feb. 25, 1914; e. Ohio State Univ., 1933. Exec., Stone's Grills Co., 1934–37; owned & operated, Sher Vending Co., 1937–43. U.S. Army, 1943–46. V.p., Sons Bars & Grills, 1947–54; org. & pres. Art Theatre Guild, 1954; opened art theatres for first time in many cities, org. opera film series, film classic series and similar motion picture activities in many cities. Org., Film Festival at Antioch Coll., 1960; pioneer in fighting obscenity laws in Ohio; operates 25 theatres in midwest and western states. Co-producer of the musical broadway production Shenandoah and American Dance Machine. Produced film, Deathmask.

SHERAK, THOMAS: Executive. b. Brooklyn, NY June 22, 1945. e. NY Community Coll. (mktg. degree). 1967–69, US Army, Specialist E5 Sgt.; 1970, began career in m.p. industry, Paramount Pictures sls. dept.; 1974, R/C Theatres, booking dept.; 1977, joined General Cinema Theatres as district film buyer; 1978, promoted to v.p., films; 1982, promoted to v.p. head film buyer; 1983, joined 20th Century Fox as pres., domestic dist. & mktg.; 1985, pres., domestic dist.

SHERDEMAN, TED: Writer, producer, director. b. Lincoln, Neb.; e. U. of Nebraska, Creighton U.

PICTURES INCLUDE: Lust For Gold, Scandal Sheet, Breakthrough, Retreat Hell, Winning Team, Eddie Cantor Story, Riding Shotgun, Them, McConnell Story, Toy Tiger, Away All Boats, Maracaibo, St. Louis Blues, Hell to Eternity, A Dog of Flanders, The Big Show, Misty, Island of the Blue Dolphins, And Now Miguel, My Side of the Mountain, Latitude Zero.

TV: Wagon Train, Zane Grey, Californians, Astronaut, Hazel, Men Into Space, My Favorite Martian, Bewitched, Family Affair, The Monroes, Flying Nun.

SHERMAN, AL: Producers Representative, Film and public relations consultant. b. New York. N.Y., April 27; e. Columbia U., CCNY. Film & pub. consultant, Royal Norwegian Information Service, Wash., D.C.; Wash.; pres. Sherman Films, Inc.; American rep., Films of Scotland, Edinburgh, Scotland; Patria Film Prods. Ltd., London; British Films Ltd., London. Member: Silurians; Educational Film Library Association; American Federation of Film Societies; M.P. Pioneers, American Film Institute.

SHERMAN, GEORGE: Director. b. New York City, 1908.

PICTURES INCLUDE: The Bandit of Sherwood Forest, Red Canyon, Yes Sir That's My Baby, Sword in the Desert, Comanche Territory, Sleeping City, Spy Hunt, Tomahawk, Target Unknown, Golden Horde, Steel Town, Raging Tide, Against All Flags, Battle at Apache Pass, The Lone Hand, Veils of Bagdad, War Arrow, Border River, Johnny Dark, Dawn at Socorro, Chief Crazy Horse, Count Three and Pray, Treasure of Pancho Villa, Comanche, Reprisal, Flying Fontaines, Enemy General. Formed Shergari Corp. with F. H. Ricketson, Jr., and Ted R. Gamble made For the Love of Mike; dir.: Panic Button, Wounds of Hunger, Jacquin Murieta, Smokey, Big Jake. In 1976 wrote, produced, and directed Artie-Charley and Friend, indep. feature.

TV: Prod. and/or dir. for 20th Century-Fox, and NBC, CBS. 1978, prod., Little Mo (TV movie NBC), Man O'War and Trudy (TV movie ABC).

SHERMAN, RICHARD M.: Composer, lyricist. b. New York, N.Y., June 12, 1928; e. Bard Coll. B.A. 1949. Info. & Educ. Br., U.S. Army, 1953–55. Songwriter, composer, Walt Disney Prods.

SONGS: Things I Might Have Been, Tall Paul, Christmas in New Orleans, Mad Passionate Love, Midnight Oil, You're Sixteen, Pineapple Princess, Let's Get Together, Maggie's Theme, Chim Chim Cheree, Comedy Album: Smash Flops.

PICTURES INCLUDE: Nightmare, The Cruel Tower, Absent Minded Professor, The Parent Trap, Big Red, The Castaways, Moon Pilot, Bon Voyage, Legend of Lobo, Summer Magic, Miracle of the White Stallions, The Sword in the Stone, Merlin Jones, Mary Poppins, Those Calloways, The Monkey's Uncle, That Darn Cat, Symposium of Popular Songs, Winnie the Pooh, Bedknobs & Broomsticks, Tom Sawyer (s.p. and score.), Huckleberry Finn.

TV: Wonderful World of Color, Bell Telephone Hour.

SHERMAN, ROBERT B.: Composer, lyricist, b. New York, N.Y., Dec. 19, 1925; e. Bard Coll., B.A., 1949. U.S. Army, WWII, 1943–45. Songwriter, 1952–60; pres., Music World Corp., 1958; songwriter, composer, Walt Disney, 1960–65.

SONGS: Things I Might Have Been, Tall Paul, Young & In Love, Midnight Oil, Pineapple Princess, You're 16, Let's Get Together, Maggie's Theme, Chim Chim Cheree.

PICTURES INCLUDE: Absent Minded Professor, The Parent Trap, Big Red, The Castaways, Moon Pilot, Bon Voyage, Legend of Lobo, Miracle of the White Stallions, Summer Magic, The Sword in the Stone, Merlin Jones, Mary Poppins, Those Calloways, The Monkey's Uncle, That Darn Cat, Winnie the Pooh, Symposium of Popular Songs, Bedknobs & Broomsticks, Tom Sawyer (s.p. and score.), Huckleberry Finn.
TV: Wonderful World of Color, Bell Telephone.

SHERMAN, ROBERT M.: Executive. Entered ind. as agent for MCA; later joined Arthur P. Jacobs pub. rel. firm. Became acc't. exec. when Jacobs merged with Rogers & Cowan. In 1964 joined CMA; 1967 made v.p. in m.p. div., serving both in London and Hollywood. In 1972 formed own prod. co., Layton Prods., with first film, Scarecrow for WB. In 1973 prod. Night Moves, also for WB. In 1974 named v.p., prod., for 20th-Fox. Returned to independent prod.: The Missouri Breaks, Convoy, Oh God! You Devil, etc.

SHERMAN, SAMUEL M.: Producer, director, writer. b. New York, N.Y., e. CCNY, BA. Entered m.p. ind. as writer, cameraman, film ed., neg. & sound cutter; nat'l mag. ed., Westerns Magazine 1959; pres., Signature Films; prod., dir., TV pilot, The Three Mesquiteers, 1960; prod., Pulse Pounding Perils, 1961; helped create, ed., dir., Screen Thrills Illustrated; exec. prod., Screen Thrills; v.p., Golden Age Films, 1962; prod., Joe Franklin's Silent Screen, 1963; N.Y. rep., Victor Adamson Productions; owns world rights; The Scarlet Letter; 1965; N.Y. rep., Tal prods., Hlywd.; adv. & pub. Hemisphere Pictures; ed., autobiog., Joe Bonomo; prod., writer, Chapln's Art of Comedy, The Strongman; prod., Hollywood's Greatest Stuntman; story adapt., Fiend With the Electronic Brain. 1967, prod. Spanish version Chaplin Su Arte Y Su Comedia; tech. consul., Hal Roach Studios, NBC, Music from the Land; 1968, N.Y. rep. East West Pict. of Hollywood. 1968, N.Y. rep., Al Adamson Prods. of Hollywood; post-prod'n consultant: The Fakers, Creatures of the Prehistoric Planet; sales U.K. of U.S. product; promo. consultant, Love is a Woman, Blood Fiend, Brides of Blood, The Gastly Ones. 1969, post prod'n and promo. consultant, Blood Demon, Mad Doctor of Blood Island. Ed.-in-chief, bk., The Strongman. Prod'n consultant, Satan's Sadists, The Blood Seekers. Pres., Independent-International Pictures Corp., assoc. prod. Horror of the Blood Monsters, Blood of Ghastly Horror; Producer-Writer Brain of Blood; prod. supervisor Dracula vs. Frankenstein; Exec. prod. Angels, Wild Women; pres., Producers Commercial Productions Inc.; producer-writer, The Naughty Stewardesses; producer, Girls For Rent; producer TV special, Wild Wild World of Comedy; executive producer, The Dynamite Brothers; producer-writer, Blazing Stewardesses; production consultant, In Search of Dracula; executive producer, Cinderella 2000; producer & orig. story, Team-Mates; Chairman of Creditors' Committee, Allied Artists Television Corp.; president, Independent-International Entertainment, TV div. Independent-International Pictures Corp. Pres., Technovision Inc.; pres., Super Video, Inc.; dir-s.p., Raiders of the Living Dead.

SHERMAN, VINCENT: Director. b. Vienna, Ga., July 16, 1906; e. Oglethorpe U. B.A. Writer, actor, dialogue dir., then prod. dir.
PICTURES INCLUDE: Dir.: Underground, Saturday's Children, Flight from Destiny, Old Acquaintances, In Our Time, Mr. Skeffington, Pillow to Post, Nora Prentiss, The Unfaithful, Adventures of Don Juan, Somewhere in the City, Hasty Heart, Damned Don't Cry, Harriet Craig, Goodbye, My Fancy, Lone Star, Assignment—Paris; prod. dir.: Affair in Trinidad, The Young Philadelphians, The Naked Earth, Second Time Around.
TV: 25 episodes of Medical Center; 3 Westside Medical; 6 Baretta; 4 Waltons; 2 Doctors Hospital; The Last Hurrah (movie); Women at West Point (movie); The Yeagers (pilot), Bogey, The Dream Merchants.

SHERRIN, NED: Producer, director, writer. Early career writing plays and musical plays. Prod., dir., ATV Birmingham, 1955–57; prod., Midlands Affairs, Paper Talk, etc. Joined BBC-TV 1957 and produced many TV talk programmes. Novels: (with Caryl Brahms) Cindy-Ella or I Gotta Shoe (also prod. as stage play), Rappell 1910, Benbow Was His Name.
TV: England: prod.: Ask Me Another, Henry Hall Show, Laugh Line, Parasol. Assoc. prod.: Tonight series. Little Beggars, 1962; prod., creator: That Was The Week That Was, 1962–63; prod., dir.: Benbow Was His Name (co-author), 1964; Take a Sapphire (co-author), The Long Garden Party, The Long Cocktail Party. ABC of Britain revue. Prod., dir.: thrice-weekly series Not So Much a Programme, More a Way of Life, 1964–65. Appearances inc. Your Witness, Quiz of The Week, Terra Firma, Who Said That, The Rather Reassuring Programme, Song by Song.
PICTURES INCLUDE: prod.: The Virgin Soldiers (with Leslie Gilliat), Every Home Should Have One, Up Pompeii, Girl Stroke Boy (co-author with Caryl Brahms), Up the Chastity Belt, Rentadick, The Garnet Saga, Up the Front, The National Health, The Cobblers of Umbridge (dir. with Ian Wilson).

SHERWOOD, MADELINE: Actress. b. Montreal, Canada, Nov. 13, 1922. On Bdwy. in Sweet Bird of Youth, Invitation to a March, The Crucible, Inadmissible Evidence, All Over, etc.
PICTURES: Baby Doll, Cat on a Hot Tin Roof, Sweet Bird of Youth, The 91st Day, Hurry Sundown, Pendulum, Wicked, Wicked.
TELEVISION: The Flying Nun, Rich Man, Poor Man, Nobody's Child.

SHIELDS, BROOKE: Actress. b. New York City, May 31, 1965. Discovered at age 11 months by photographer Francesco Scavullo to pose in Ivory Snow ads. Later became Breck girl in commercials; appeared in Richard Avenon's Colgate ads for 3 yrs.
PICTURES INCLUDE: Alice Sweet Alice (Communion), Pretty Baby, Tilt, King of the Gypsies, Wanda Nevada, Just You and Me, Kid, The Blue Lagoon, Endless Love, Sahara.
TV: The Prince of Central Park, After the Fall, Wet Gold.

SHIELDS, WILLIAM A.: Executive. b. New York City, 1946. e. El Camino College and California State College. Entered the motion picture industry in 1966 when he went to work for Pacific Theatres. Other industry affiliations included: MGM sales department, Los Angeles and Denver, 1970; New World Pictures, Western Division manager, 1972; branch manager, 20th Century-Fox, Washington, 1973; New York district manager, 20th Century-Fox, 1973–75. Joined Mann Theatres Corporation of California as head booker in 1975. Gen. sls. mgr., Far West Films, 1977–79; joined Avco Embassy as Western div. mgr., promoted to asst. gen. sls. mgr., 1980; promoted to v.p.-gen. sls. mgr., January, 1981. In 1983 joined New World Pictures as exec. v.p., world-wide mktg. & acquisitions. Promoted to pres., w-w sls. & mktg., 1985.

SHIKATA, MASAO: Executive. b. Kyoto, Japan, Apr. 22, 1918. e. Naniwa Commercial College. Chm., Sansha Electric Manufacturing Co. Ltd., Tokyo and Osaka, makers of power semiconductors & applied electronic equipment; pres. Japan Motion Picture Equipment Manufacturers & Suppliers Assoc.; v.p., Japan Machinery Design Center; v.p., Japan Optical Industry Assoc.; director, Federation of Japanese Film Industries Inc.

SHIMA, KOJI: Director. b. Japan. Entered m.p. ind. as actor, 1930; then asst. dir., director. Dir., Daiei M. P. Co. (now defunct). Presently indep. director.
PICTURES INCLUDE: Golden Demon, Phantom Horse.

SHINBACH, BRUCE D.: Executive. b. South Bend, Ind., June, 1939. e. Univ. of Colorado, (B.A. 1963), N.Y. Institute of Finance, Northwestern Univ. (M.A., 1965). Stockbroker for Harris, Upham & Co., 1964, shopping center developer, Dixie Associates, 1966 to present. Pres., Monarch Theatres.

SHIPMAN, BARRY: Writer. b. S. Pasadena, Cal., Feb. 24, 1912. Parents professional. M.p. writer since 1936. U.S.M.C.R. photog. officer 1942–46. 43 sole s.p. credits including Montana Territory for Col., 1946–52.

SHIPMAN, KENNETH: Producer. b. London, England, 1930. Electro-mechanical engineer, entered m.p. ind. as assistant dir., Riverside Studios, 1949; mgr., Southhall Studios; dept. chmn., Bryanston Films; formed Kenneth Shipman Productions, 1964; prod., The System, exec. prod., Burke and Hare, Au Pair Girls.

SHIRE, DAVID: Composer. b. Buffalo, NY, July 3, 1937
PICTURES INCLUDE: Farewell My Lovely, The Conversation, All the President's Men, Saturday Night Fever, Old Boyfriends, Norma Rae, The Night the Lights Went Out in Georgia, Only When I Laugh, Paternity, The World According to Garp, Max Dugan Returns, 2010, Return to Oz, Short Circuit, 'night, Mother.
TELEVISION: Raid on Entebbe, Do You Remember Love.

SHIRE, TALIA: Actress. b. New York City, April 25, 1946. Raised on road by her father, arranger-conductor Carmine Coppola, who toured with Broadway musicals. After 2 yrs. at Yale School of Drama she moved to L.A. where appeared in many theatrical productions. Is sister of Francis Ford Coppola.
PICTURES INCLUDE: The Dunwich Horror, Gas-s-s, The Christian Licorice Store, The Outside Man, The Godfather, The Godfather, Part II, Rocky, Old Boyfriends, Rocky II, Windows, Rocky III, Rocky IV, RAD.
TV: Rich Man, Poor Man, Kill Me If You Can.

SHIVAS, MARK: Producer/Director. TV credits incl: Presenter of Cinema. The Six Wives of Henry VIII, Casanova, The Edwardians, The Evacuees, The Glittering Prizes, Abide With Me, Rogue Male, 84 Charing Cross Road, The Three

Hostages, She Fell Among Thieves, Professional Foul, Telford's Change, On Giant's Shoulders, Winston Churchill: The Wilderness Years, The Price, What If it's Raining? Film: Producer; Richards' Things, Moonlighting, A Private Function. Exec. Prod.: Bad Blood.

SHONFELD, PHIL: Executive. Began career in sls. dist. at Universal Pictures. Later asst. to western sls. mgr. for National General and western dist. mgr. for Buena Vista. Joined Warners in November, 1976 as asst. to v.p. & gen. sls. mgr. In 1979 promoted to v.p.—sls. admin., continuing to head playdate and contract depts. while becoming involved in all aspects of sls. dept.

SHORE, DINAH: Singer. r.n. Frances Rose Shore. b. Winchester, Tenn., Mar. 1, 1917; e. Vanderbilt U., B.A. 1939; m. George Montgomery. Became singer WNEW, N.Y., 1938; joined NBC as sustaining singer, 1938; started contract RCA-Victor, 1940; star Chamber Music Soc. of Lower Basin St. program, 1940; joined Eddie Cantor radio pgm., 1941; star own radio program, General Foods, 1943; entertained troops European Theatre of operations, 1944; radio program, Procter & Gamble. Star TV show, Chevrolet, 1951–61; Dinah Shore Specials, 1964–65. 1969: Dinah Shore Special, Like Hep. 1970–71: Dinah's Place, Dinah!

AWARDS: Awarded New Star of Radio Motion Picture Daily Poll and World Telegram-Scripps-Howard Poll, 1940; Best Popular Female Vocalist M.P. Daily Fame's Annual Poll Radio and TV 1941–61; Michael Award Best Female Vocalist, Radio and TV, 1950, 51, 52; Billboard Award; Favorite Female Vocalist in radio, 1949; Billboard Award Favorite Female Vocalist in records, 1947; Gallup Poll One of Most Admired Women in the World, 1958–61; 6 Emmy Awards 1954 to 59. Recording of songs by Decca; Los Angeles Times Woman of the Year Award, 1957; TV-Radio Mirror mag. award, best female singer, radio, 1952, 53, 56, 57, 58; TV-Radio Mirror mag. award, TV's Best Musical Variety Show, 1956, 58, 59; Peabody TV Award, 1957; Fame's Critics' Poll, Best Female Vocalist, 1958, 63; Hollywood Foreign Press Assn's Golden Globe Award, 1959; Radio-TV Daily, Female Vocalist of the Year, 1949, 56.

SHORE, SIG: Producer. b. New York City. Served as navigator in Air Force, World War II. First job in films in pub. dept. at Warner Bros. Formed own ad agency on West Coast; then turned to TV production with The Errol Flynn Theatre. Engaged by David O. Selznick Films to dist. its films to TV outlets. Entered theatrical distribution, importing Hiroshima, Mon Amour, The 400 Blows, etc. In mid-50s became involved in cultural exchange program of US State Dept., importing and distributing Soviet films. Returned to TV production, turning out over 250 shows, including The Outdoor World for Shell Oil. Headed co. for Ivan Tors which made Flipper, Daktari, Gentle Ben series. In 1970 formed Plaza Pictures for theatrical dist.

PICTURES INCLUDE: Super Fly, Super Fly TNT, That's The Way of the World, Sudden Death. (s.p.-dir.).

SHOWALTER, MAX: Actor, composer. s.n. Casey Adams. b. Caldwell, Kans., June 2, 1917; e. Caldwell H.S.; Pasadena Playhouse. Composed background music for films: Vicki, Return of Jack Slade. Arrangements for records.

BROADWAY: Knights of Song, Very Warm for May, My Sister Eileen, Showboat, John Loves Mary, Make Mine Manhattan, Lend an Ear.

PICTURES INCLUDE: Always Leave Them Laughing, With a Song in My Heart, What Price Glory, My Wife's Best Friend, Niagara, Destination Gobi, Dangerous Crossing, Vicki, Night People, Naked Alibi, Never Say Goodbye, Bus Stop, Down Three Dark Streets, Designing Woman, Female Animal, Voice In the Mirror, The Naked and the Dead, It Happened in June, Elmer Gantry, Return to Peyton Place, Summer and Smoke, Music Man, Smog, Bon Voyage, My Six Loves, Lord Love a Duck, The Anderson Tapes, Sixteen Candles.

SHULER, LAUREN: Producer. b. Cleveland, OH, June 23, 1949. Began filmmaking career as camera-woman in TV production, 1972; producing film, Amateur Night at the Dixie Barr and Grill for NBC.

PICTURES: Mr. Mom, Ladyhawke, St. Elmo's Fire, Pretty in Pink.

SHULL, RICHARD: Actor. b. Evanston, IL, Feb. 24, 1929. e. State Univ. of Iowa. US Army, 1953. NY stage debut in Minnie's Boys, 1970. Film debut in The Anderson Tapes, 1971.

PICTURES: B.S. I Love You, Such Good Friends, Slither, Hail to the Chief, The Black Bird, Cockfighter, Hearts of the West, The Fortune, Dreamer, Wholly Moses, Heartbeeps, Spring Break, Lovesick, Unfaithfully Yours, Splash, etc.

TELEVISION: Holmes & Yoyo, Rockford Files, Good Times, Love American Style, Hart to Hart, Lou Grant, etc.

SHULMAN, MAX: Writer. b. St. Paul, Minn., March 14, 1919; e. U. of Minn., B.A., 1942.

NOVELS: Barefoot Boy with Cheek, Feather Merchants, Zebra Derby, Sleep Till Noon, Rally Round the Flag Boys.

BROADWAY: Barefoot Boy with Cheek, Tender Trap.

PICTURES INCLUDE: collab. story: Always Leave Them Laughing; Collab. story, s.p.: Confidentially Connie; story, s.p.: Affairs of Dobie Gillis, Half a Hero.

TV: Creator: The Many Loves of Dobie Gillis.

SHURPIN, SOL: Executive. b. New York, N.Y., Feb. 22, 1914; e. Pace Institute, 1936. Law stenog., 1932–33; Joe Hornstein, Inc., 1933–41; National Theatre Supply, 1941–48; purchased interest in Raytone Screen Corp., became v.p., 1948; pres., Raytone, 1952; pres., Technikote Corp., which succeeded Raytone Screen, 1956–present; sole owner, Technikote Corp., 1962.

SHUTT, BUFFY: Executive. Joined Paramount 1973 as member of NY pub. staff; 1975, natl. mag. contact. 1978, named dir. of pub.; later exec. dir. of pub. Promoted 1980 to v.p., pub. & promo. Resigned to join Time-Life Films; returned to Paramount in 1981 as v.p. & asst. to pres. of Motion Picture Group. 1984, appt. exec. v.p.-mktg. for M.P. Group, Paramount. 1986, resigned.

SIDARIS, ANDY: Producer, director. b. Chicago, Ill., Feb. 20, 1932. e. Southern Methodist University, B.A. in Radio-TV. Began television career in 1950 in Dallas, Texas as a director at station WFAA-TV; now pres., The Sidaris Company.

PICTURES INCLUDE: Dir., Stacey, The Racing Scene, M*A*S*H football sequences, Seven (prod.-dir.).

TV: Dir., The Racers/Mario Andretti/Joe Leonard/Al Unser, ABC's Championship Auto Racing, ABC's NCAA Game of the Week, 1972 Summer Olympics, 1968 Summer Olympics (won Emmy Award), Wide World of Sports, The Racers/Craig and Lee Breedlove, dir.: The Burt Reynolds Late Show, dir., Kojak episode, Nancy Drew, Dukes of Hazzard.

SIDNEY, GEORGE: Director, producer. b. New York, N.Y. 1916; son of L. K. Sidney, veteran showman and v.p. MGM and Hazel Mooney, actress. From 1932 at MGM as test, second unit and short subjects dir. Several Academy Awards for shorts, Our Gang Comedies, Pete Smith etc. In 1941 made feature dir., MGM. Pres., Director's Guild of America, 16 yrs; spec. presidential assignment to Atomic Energy Commission and U.S. Air Force; 1961–66, Pres., Hanna-Barbera Productions; Doctorate of Science Hanneman Medical University and Hospital. Mem. ASCAP. Pres., Directors, Inc., since 1969; v.p., Directors Foundation; v.p., R.W. Griffith Foundation; life mem., ACTT (England) and DGA.

PICTURES INCLUDE: dir., prod.: Free and Easy, Pacific Rendezvous, Pilot No. 5, Thousands Cheer, Bathing Beauty, Anchors Aweigh, Harvey Girls, Cass Timberlane, Three Musketeers, Red Danube, Key to the City, Annie Get Your Gun, Holiday in Mexico, Show Boat, Scaramouche, Young Bess, Kiss Me Kate, Jupiter's Darling, Eddie Duchin Story, Jeanne Eagels, Pal Joey, Who Was That Lady, Pepe, Bye Bye Birdie, A Ticklish Affair, Viva Las Vegas, Who Has Seen the Wind?, U.N. special; The Swinger, Half a Sixpence.

SIDNEY, SYLVIA: Actress. b. New York, N.Y., Aug. 8, 1910; e. Theatre Guild School. On stage, then screen debut in Through Different Eyes.

PLAYS: Nice Women, Crossroads, Bad Girl, The Gentle People, etc.

PICTURES INCLUDE: City Streets, Five Minutes from the Station, Ladies of the Big House, Confessions of a Co-Ed, An American Tragedy, The Miracle Man, Merrily We Go to Hell, Madame Butterfly, Blood on the Sun, Mr. Ace, Searching Wind, Love from a Stranger, Les Miserables, Violent Saturday, Behind the High Wall, Summer Wishes, Winter Dreams, I Never Promised You a Rose Garden, Damien-Omen II, Hammett.

TV: Movies: Raid on Entebbe, Finnegan Begin Again, An Early Frost.

SIEGEL, DON: Director. b. Chicago, Ill., Oct. 26, 1912; e. Jesus Coll., Cambridge U. (England). Has appeared with the Royal Academy of Dramatic Arts, London, and Contemporary Theatre Group, Hollywood. Joined Warner Bros. as asst. film librarian, 1934; became asst. cutter and head of insert dept. Organized montage dept.; wrote and dir. all montages.

PICTURES INCLUDE: dir.: Star in the Night and Hitler Lives (two Academy Awards for distinctive achievement for shorts, 1945). dir.: The Verdict, Night Unto Night, Big Steal, Duel at Silver Creek, No Time For Flowers, Count the Hours, China Venture, Riot in Cell Block 11, Private Hell 36, Annapolis Story, Invasion of the Body Snatchers, Madigan, Coogan's Bluff, Two Mules for Sister Sara, The Beguiled, Dirty Harry; appeared in Play Misty for Me, Charley Varrick, Black Windmill, The Shootist, Telefon, Escape from Alcatraz, Rough Cut, Jinxed.

SIEGEL, SIMON B.: Financial vice-president, treas., American Broadcasting Paramount Theatres & mem. bd. of dir. Started career in ind. 1929, comptroller's staff Paramount

Pictures, Inc.; asst. to comptroller of the company's theatre div., 1941; comptroller, 1949; joined United Paramount Theatres, 1950; in 1953 named treasurer when ABC & UPT were merged; named financial v.p. and treas., 1957; exec. vice-pres., ABC-Paramount Theatres.

SILBERKLEIT, WILLIAM B.: Executive. e. New York University, Full Colonel, USAF. Pres., Tommy J Productions, independent producer: Bonnie's Kids, Roommates, Centerfold Girls, Linda Lovelace for President, Alice Cooper's Welcome to My Nightmare, A Woman for All Men. In 1975 became chm. and co-founder of Pro-International Films. Executive producer for PRO-International Films. Executive producer for PRO-International: Young Lady Chatterly, Once Upon a Girl, Detroit 9000, Emma Mae.

SILLIPHANT, STIRLING: Executive-Writer. b. Detroit, Mich., Jan. 16, 1918. e. U. Southern California, B.A., 1938; married. On pub. staff, Walt Disney Productions, Burbank 1938–41; 1941–42, exploit. & pub., Hal Horne Org. for 20th Century-Fox in New York & other key cities, 1942–43, asst. to Spyros P. Skouras. U.S. Navy, World War II. Since 1946, 20th-Fox; in chge. special events and promotions, June 1949; apptd. Eastern pub. mgr. Aug, 13, 1951; prod., Joe Louis Story; co-prod., collab. s.p., 5 Against the House; screenwriter, producer, Naked City, Route 66, The Slender Thread, In the Heat of the Night; s.p., Marlowe; collab., s.p., The Liberation of L. B. Jones; s.p., A Walk in the Spring Rain; p., Shaft, Shaft in Africa, (s.p.). The New Centurions (s.p.), The Poseidon Adventure, (s.p.), The Towering Inferno (s.p.),The Killer Elite (co.-s.p.), The Enforcer (co.-s.p.), Telefon (co-s.p.), The Swarm, When Time Ran Out.

SILVA, HENRY: Actor. b. Puerto Rico, 1928.
PICTURES: Viva Zapata, Crowded Paradise, A Hatful of Rain, The Bravados, Green Mansions, Cinderfella, The Manchurian Candidate, Johnny Cool, The Return of Mr. Moto, The Reward, The Plainsman, The Hills Ran Red, Buck Rogers in the 25th Century, Thirst, Virus, Alligator, Sharkey's Machine, Cannonball Run II, Lust in the Dust, Code of Silence.

SILVER, JOAN MICKLIN: Writer-Director. b. Omaha, Nebr., 1935. e. Sarah Lawrence College. Began career as writer for educational films. Original s.p., Limbo, purchased by Universal Pictures. In 1972 Learning Corp. Of Am. commissioned her to write and direct a 30-min. documentary, The Immigrant Experience. Also wrote and directed two children's films for same co. First feature was Hester Street, which she wrote and directed.
PICTURES INCLUDE: Hester Street (s.p., dir.); Bernice Bobs Her Hair (short, s.p.-dir., later shown on TV), Between the Lines (dir.); Head Over Heels (s.p., dir.).
TELEVISION: Finnegan Begin Again (dir.).

SILVER, LEON J.: Executive. b. Boston, Mass., March 25, 1918. e. U. of So. Calif., 1935–38. Independent prod. of short subjects, 1939; story analyst, Paramount, 1940, film writer, U.S. Army Pictorial Service, 1941–45; free lance writer, 1946; film writer. prod., U.S. Public Health Service, 1946–51, asst. chief, foreign film prod., U.S. Dept. of State, 1951–54; acting chief, domestic film prod., U.S. Information Agency, 1955. Division Chief, Worldwide Documentary Film & Television Product, U.S. Information Agency, Apr. 6, 1968, 1978 to present, sr. advisor IV, film production. Resigned, 1980. Now TV network writer-producer-novelist.

SILVER, MILTON: Advertising executive. b. New York City. U.S. Army World War I. Co-ed. Who's Who on Screen and Little Movie Mirror books; co-author Broadway stage production, The Mystery Ship; dir. adv., exploit., Universal Pictures, trailer ed, adv. manager, National Screen Service; exec. asst. to dir. adv. pub. Republic Pictures; to Souvaine Selective Pictures as adv., pub. dir., 1951; adv. pub. dept. United Artists 1953. Free lance writer since 1960.

SILVER, PAT: Writer. co-s.p., Wizard of Baghdad, Pirates of Tortuga, orig. story, s.p., 7 Woman From Hell, The Golden Touch, Dare To Be Free; prod., Ghost Town.
TV: Mables Fables Series, Rescue 8, New Breed, Shannon, Paladin.

SILVER, RAPHAEL D.: Producer. b. Cleveland, Ohio, 1930. e. Harvard College and Harvard Graduate School of Business Adm. Is pres. of Midwestern Land Devel. Corp. and Hodgson Houses, Inc. In 1973 formed Midwest Film Productions to produce Hester Street, written and directed by his wife, Joan Micklin Silver. Also distributed film independently. Also produced Between the Lines, directed by wife. Directed On the Yard.

SILVER, RON: Actor. b. New York City, July 2, 1946. e. Univ. of Buffalo. Trained for stage at Herbert Berghof Studios and Actors Studio. NY stage debut in Kasper and Public Insult, 1971. Film debut in Semi-Tough, 1977. TV debut in Rhoad, 1976.
PICTURES: Silent Rage, Best Friends, The Entity, Lovesick, Silkwood, Garbo Talks, Goodbye People.
TELEVISION: Hill Street Blues, Stockard Channing Show, Mac Davis Show, Bakers Dozen. Movies: Betrayal, Word of Honor, etc.

SILVERMAN, FRED: b. N.Y.C. Sept., 1937. e. Syracuse Univ., Ohio State (Master's in TV and theatre arts). Joined WGN-TV, indep. sta. in Chicago. Came to N.Y. for exec. post at WPIX-TV, where stayed only six weeks CBS-TV hired him as dir. of daytime programs. Named v.p.—programs June, 1970. In May, 1975 left CBS to become pres., ABC Entertainment. In June, 1978, named pres. and chief exec. officer of NBC. Now independent producer.

SILVERMAN, JIM: Executive. b. Des Moines, IA, June 26, 1950. e. Univ. of Hawaii (BA, 1972); Taiwan Natl. Univ., (foreign langauge study, 1973). Exec. v.p. & co-founder, Commtron Corp., division of Bergen Brunswig Corp., 1975–83; pres. & founder, Continental Video, Inc., division of Cinema Group, Inc.

SILVERMAN, RON: Producer-writer. b. Los Angeles, Calif., June 13, 1933. e. UCLA, 1951–53, U. of Arizona, 1953–55; reporter reviewer, Daily Variety, 1957–61; asst. to prod.-dir. Mark Robson, Red Lion Films, 20th Century-Fox, 1961–62; assoc. prod., Daystar Productions, 1961; v.p., 1964; assoc. prod. Crackerby TV series, 1965. Prod. exec., Warner Bros. TV, 1966; prod. & exec. Ted Mann Prods., 1967.
PICTURES INCLUDE: Buster and Billie (prod.), 1974, Lifeguard, Brubaker.
TV: Wild Wild West (writer), 1967.

SILVERMAN, SYD: Executive. b. N.Y., Jan. 23, 1932. e. The Manlius School, 1946–50; Princeton Univ., 1950–54. Lt., U.S. Army, 1954–56. Publisher, Variety and Daily Variety, executive editor, Weekly Variety.

SILVERS, SID: Actor, writer, song writer. b. Brooklyn, N.Y., Jan. 1, 1908. On stage with Phil Baker for 7 yrs., as stooge & collab., many songs; began screen writing, 1930; Oh, Sailor, Behave; Follow The Leader, Par.
PICTURES INCLUDE: (collab. story, s.p. & appeared) Bottoms Up, Born To Dance; (collab. s.p. & appeared) Broadway Melody of 1936, (collab. story) Broadway Melody of 1938; (collab. music) Walking On Air; (add. dial. & appeared) 52nd Street; (collab. s.p.) Kentuky Kernels, The Gorilla, The Fleet's In, For Me and My Gal. Collab. s.p., Two Tickets to Broadway; collab. story, The Stooge.

SILVERSTEIN, ELLIOT: Director. b. Boston, Aug. 3, 1927. e. Boston Coll., Yale. Started career on television.
PICTURES: Cat Ballou, The Happening, A Man Called Horse, Deadly Honeymoon, The Car.
TELEVISION: Belle Sommers, Betrayed by Innocence.

SILVERSTEIN, MAURICE: Executive. b. Syracuse, N.Y., March 1, 1912; booker, salesman, MGM domestic dep't; International Dep't, MGM; supervisor Southeast Asia Hdqts. Singapore, MGM, 1938–42; OWI chief, film distribution for Europe, hdqts. London, during World War II; asst. sales supervisor, Far East, MGM; regional director, Latin America, 1947; liaison exec. to handle independent productions MGM, 1956; vice-pres., MGM International, 1957; first vice-pres., 1958; pres., MGM International, 1963; vice-pres., parent company, Metro-Goldwyn-Mayer Inc. 1970; Silverstein Int'l Corp., pres.

SILVESTER, VICTOR: (O.B.E.) Musical director. b. Wembley, England. e. St. John's Leatherhead, John Lyons, Harrow. Exclusive BBC contract; with his orchestra, Records exclusively for Pye Records.

SIMMONS, JEAN: Actress. b. London, Jan. 31, 1929. e. Aida Foster Sch., London. m. Richard Brooks, director, writer. Screen debut 1944, in Give Us the Moon. Voted one of top ten British money-making stars in M.P. Herald-Fame Poll, 1950–51.
PICTURES INCLUDE: Mr. Emmanuel, Kiss the Boys Goodbye, Sports Day, Caesar and Cleopatra, Way to the Stars, Great Expectations, Hungry Hill, Black Narcissus, The Women in the Hall, Blue Lagoon, Hamlet, Adam and Evalyn, Trio, So Long as the Fair, Cage of Gold, The Clouded Yellow, Androcles and the Lion (U.S. film debut), Angel Face, Young Bess, Affair with a Stranger, The Actress, The Robe, She Couldn't Say No, A Bullet Is Waiting, The Egyptian, Desiree, Footsteps in the Fog, Guys and Dolls, Hilda Crane, This Could Be the Night, Until They Sail, Home Before Dark, Spartacus, The Grass Is Greener, All the Way Home, Elmer Gantry, Divorce American Style, Rough Night in Jericho, The Happy Ending (Acad. Award nom.).
TELEVISION: Beggarman Thief, Valley of the Dolls, The Thorn Birds (Emmy award), North & South Book II.

SIMMONS, JOHN: Producer, director, writer, creative consultant. e. St. Clement Danes, the Univ. of London, the Temple. Assoc. with many adv. doc. feature & TV films. Numerous International Festival awards, incl. Oscar nomin.; creative dir., Cinevista Ltd.; wrote, The Blue Bird, Loganberry Fair (lyrics, etc.), devised adv. campaigns, The Guns of Navarone, Summer Holiday; creative dir., John Simmons Creative Consultants Ltd. Join The Tea Set, Shell, Ovaltine, Waddington, Tide, Terylene, Marks & Spencer, Schweppes, Crown, Cleveland, Gold Camera Award (1st Place) for The Bosch Equation, U.S. Int. Ind. Film Festival, 1974. 1st Prize San Francisco Fest. 1975. Dev. & Dir. Cinema Ad. Awards, 1976. Corr. to Fin. Times, Variety, Campaign etc. Gold Camera Award 1977 for Stop Her, Silver Award, New York Fest. Consultant, Rank Advertising Awards (cinema) and commercial radio. Best radio commercial Award 1977. Award, Cannes 1978, 'A Clear Edge.'

SIMMONS, STANLEY: Producer, director. b. New York City, May 8, 1915. e. McBurney Preparatory School. Entered m.p. ind. 1930; pres. own distributing co.; advance man on roadshow m.p. 5 yrs.; ed. Hollywood shorts & features; apptd. managing dir. Amer. Museum of Natural History's exhibit at N.Y. World's Fair; film ed.; prod.-dir. Carnival in Brazil, 1941; served in U.S. Army 1942–45, as prod.-dir. ed. over 100 documentaries & head of special trailer dept. ETO; supvr. color Western feature series; prod. head of Realart Productions, Inc.; lab & exchange rep. for Soundies Distributing Corp.; prod. mgr. North Amer. Video Productions, Inc.

PICTURES INCLUDE: (prod.-dir. for video) It's a Woman's World series, Album of Songs (musical series), spots for Life Cigarettes and others. 9 Acapello musicals.

SIMMS, FRANK: Announcer. b. Tulsa, Okla., June 8, 1921. e. U. of Tulsa, 1946. Radio announcer, U.S. Air Force, WWII; announcer, KVOO, Tulsa, to N.Y., 1953.

TV: I Love Lucy, My Little Margie, Public Defender, Garry Moore Show.

SIMON, MELVIN: Executive. b. N.Y.C., Oct. 21, 1926. e. City College, New York (BBA, 1949); graduate work at Indiana Univ. Law School. Owns and operates, in partnership with two brothers, over 90 shopping centers in U.S. In 1978 formed Melvin Simon Productions, privately owned corp., to finance films. Dissolved Co. in 1983.

MEMBER: Friars Club; N.Y. div.; 1978, v.p., In-tl. Council of Shopping Centers; 1978, commerce and industry chm. of muscular dystrophy; mem. bd., Indiana Repertory Theatre 1978, corporate sponsor: Indianapolis 500 Festival, Indianapolis Museum of Arts, Indianapolis Children's Museum; Indianapolis Zoological Society.

SIMON, NEIL: Playwright. b. Bronx, N.Y., July 4, 1927. Wrote comedy for radio with brother, Danny, also TV scripts for Sid Caesar, Red Buttons, Jackie Gleason.

PLAYS INCLUDE: Barefoot in the Park, The Odd Couple, Sweet Charity, The Star Spangled Girl, Plaza Suite, Promises, Promises, The Last of the Red Hot Lovers, The Gingerbread Lady. Adapted several of own plays to screen and wrote original s.p.s, The Out-of-Towners, and The Slugger's Wife.

PICTURES: Sunshine Boys, Murder by Death, The Goodbye Girl, The Cheap Detective, California Suite, Seems Like Old Times, Only When I Laugh (also co-prod.).

SIMON, PAUL: Singer-Composer-Actor. b. Newark, NJ, Nov. 8, 1942. Teamed with Art Garfunkel, writing and performing own songs; they parted in 1970 to go separate ways. Reunited for concert in New York, 1982, which was televised on HBO.

PICTURES: The Graduate (songs), Annie Hall (actor), One Trick Pony (s.p., act., comp.)

TELEVISION: The Paul Simon Special (Emmy), Home Box Office Presents Paul Simon.

SIMONE, SIMONE: Actress. b. April 23, 1914, Marseilles, France. Played in many films in Europe, among them Les Beaux Jours, and Lac aux Dames. On stage in Toi C'est Moi, and others.

PICTURES INCLUDE: Girl's Domitory, Ladies in Love, Seventh Heaven, Love and Kisses, Josette, Johnny Doesn't Live Here Any More, Silent Bell, Temptation, Harbor, Lost Women, La Ronde, Pit of Loneliness, Le Plaisir.

SIMPSON, DON: Producer. b. Anchorage, Alaska, Oct. 29, 1945. e. Univ. of Oregon (Phi Beta Kappa, 1967). Began career in industry as acct. exec. with Jack Woodel Agency, San Francisco, where supervised mktg. of Warner Bros. films. Recruited by WB in 1971 as mktg. exec. specializing in youth market; oversaw Woodstock, Clockwork Orange, Billy Jack, etc. Co-writer on low-budget films, Aloha, Bobby and Rose (Columbia) and Cannonball (New World). Joined Paramount as prod. exec. 1975; promoted 1977 to v.p., prod. Named sr. v.p. of prod., 1980; pres. of world-wide prod., 1981. Formed Simpson/Bruckheimer Prods. 1983, entering into exclusive deal with Paramount to develop and produce for m.p. and TV divisions.

PICTURES: Flashdance, Thief of Hearts, Beverly Hills Cop, Top Gun.

SIMPSON, GARRY: Producer, director, writer. e. Stanford U. Major shows with NBC-TV: Jimmy Durante Show, Armstrong Circle Theatre, Ed Wynn Show, Philco TV Playhouse, Ballet Theatre. Awards: Academy of TV Arts & Sc., Sylvania. Documentary film writer-producer awards: International Film & TV Festival, Chicago Film Festival, Broadcast Media Awards. Currently, pgm mgr., Vermont Ed. TV Network.

SIMPSON, O.J.: Actor. b. San Francisco, July 9, 1947. r.n. Orenthal James Simpson. e. Univ. of Sou. Calif. Was star collegiate and professional football player.

PICTURES: The Towering Inferno, The Klansman, Killer Force, Cassandra Crossing, Capricorn One, Firepower, Hambone & Hillie.

TELEVISION: Movies: Roots, A Killing Affair, Goldie and the Boxer (also exec. p.), Detour to Terror (exec. p.), The Golden Moment—An Olympic Love Story.

SIMS, JOAN: Actress. b. London, England, 1930.

PICTURES INCLUDE: Dry Rot, Off the Record, No Time for Tears, Just My Luck, The Naked Truth, The Captain's Table, Passport to Shame, Emergency Ward 10, Most of the 'Carry On' films, Doctor in Love, Watch Your Stern, Twice Round the Daffodils, The Iron Maiden, Nurse on Wheels, Doctor in Clover, Doctor in Trouble, The Garnett Saga, Not Now Darling, Don't Just Lie There Say Something, Love Among the Ruins, One of Our Dinosaurs Is Missing, Till Death Us Do Part, The Way of the World, Deceptions.

TELEVISION: Born and Bred, Worzel Gummidge, Ladykillers, Crown Court, Cockles, Fairly Secret Army, Tickle on the Tum, Miss Marple: A Murder Is Announced, Hay Fever, In Loving Memory, Drummonds, Farrington of the F.O., Dr. Who.

SINATRA, FRANK: Actor, singer. b. Hoboken, N.J., 1915. Sportswriter; then singer on radio various N.Y. stations; joined Harry James orchestra, later Tommy Dorsey. On screen 1943 in Reveille with Beverly. Spec. Academy Award 1945 for acting in The House I Live In, short subject on tolerance; Academy Award 1953.

PICTURES INCLUDE: Higher and Higher, Step Lively, Anchors Aweigh, It Happened in Brooklyn, Till the Clouds Roll By, Miracle of the Bells, Kissing Bandit, Take Me Out to the Ball Game, On the Town, Double Dynamite, Meet Danny Wilson, From Here to Eternity (Acad. Award. best supporting actor, 1953), Suddenly, Young at Heart, Not as a Stranger, Guys and Dolls, Tender Trap, Man With the Golden Arm, Johnny Concho, High Society, Around The World in 80 Days, Pride and the Passion, The Joker is Wild, Pal Joey, Kings Go Forth, Some Came Running, A Hole in the Head, Never So Few, Ocean's 11, Devil at Four O'Clock, Sergeants 3, The Manchurian Candidate, Come Blow Your Horn, The List of Adrian Messenger, 4 for Texas, Robin and the Seven Hoods, None But the Brave (dir.), Von Ryan's Express, Marriage on the Rocks, Cast a Giant Shadow, Assault on a Queen, The Naked Runner, Tony Rome, The Detective, Lady in Cement, Dirty Dingus Magee, That's Entertainment!, The First Deadly Sin.

TV: The Frank Sinatra Show, numerous specials, etc. Won both an Emmy and a Peabody Award. Hersholt Humanitarian Award, 1971. 1977: Contract on Cherry Street (movie).

SINCLAIR, ANDREW: Director, writer. Early career as novelist and historian, playwright. Published 18 books in U.K., U.S.A. Entered m.p. ind. 1968.

PICTURES INCLUDE: s.p.: Before Winter Comes, Adventures in the Skin Trade, The Voyage of the Beagle, You?; dir., writer: The Breaking of Bumbo, 1970; dir., writer: Under Milk Wood, 1971; prod. Malachi's Cove, 1973; Tuxedo Warrior, 1982; Writ. The Representative, The Scarlet Letter; Martin Eden.

SINCLAIR, MARY: Actress. r.n. Mary Cook. b. San Diego, Nov. 15. Model; summer stock; TV debut, CBS, 1949. Screen debut in Arrowhead, 1953.

TV: Fireside Theatre, Studio One, Suspense, Pulitzer Prize Playhouse. Under contract CBS TV, 1951.

SINDEN, DONALD: Actor. b. Plymouth, England, Oct. 9, 1923. Stage debut 1941 in fit-up shows; TV debut 1948; screen debut in 1953, Cruel Sea.

PICTURES INCLUDE: The Cruel Sea, Mogambo, A Day to Remember, You Know What Sailors Are, Doctor in the House, The Beachcomber, Mad About Men, An Alligator Named Daisy, Black Tent, Eyewitness, Tiger in the Smoke, Doctor at Large, Rockets Galore, The Captain's Table, Operation Bullshine, Your Money or Your Wife, The Siege of Sydney Street, Twice Around the Daffodils, Mix Me a Person, Decline and Fall, The Island at the Top of the World.

TV: Bullet in the Ballet, Road to Rome, Dinner With the Family, Odd Man In, Love from Italy, The Frog, The Glove, The Mystery of Edwin Drood, The Happy Ones, The Comedy of Errors, The Wars of the Roses, The Red House, Blackmail, A Bachelor Gray, Our Man at St. Marks (3 series), The Wind in the Tall Paper Chimney, A Woman Above Reproach, Call My Bluff, Relatively Speaking, Father Dear Father, The 19th Hole, Seven Days in the Life of

Andrew Pelham (serial), The Assyrian Rejuvenator, The Organization (serial), The Confederacy of Wives, Tell It to the Chancellor, Two's Company (4 series), All's Well That Ends Well, Never the Twain (4 series).

SINGER, A: Chairman-Managing Director, White City Films Ltd. b. Bradford, York, CBE England, Jan. 21, 1927; e. Giggleswick High School, Bradford Grammer Sch. Entered m.p. ind. 1943; dir. 8 films; worked as unit mgr. in Austria; TV as BBC prod., 1949; prod. 80 programs of events and features. Joined Scottish Region 2-year attachment. N.Y. office, BBC as TV officer working with American TV networks and local stations, Oct., 1953; ret. to London, 1956; prod. BBC-TV, Eye on Research and Science Intl. series; Asst. Head Outside Broadcasts 1959; exec. producer for E.B.U.; on first programme exchange between Europe and America 1962; Head of Outside Broadcasts Feature and Scientific Programmes, 1963. Head of features group, BBC Television, 1967. Controller BBC 2, 1974. Managing Director, BBC Radio, 1978. Managing Director, BBC Television, 1982.

SINGER, LORI: Actress. b. Corpus Christi, TX. Sister of actor Marc Singer. Concert cellist while in teens. Won starring role in TV series Fame (1981). Motion picture debut in Footloose (1984).
PICTURES: The Falcon and The Snowman, The Man with One Red Shoe, Trouble in Mind.

SINGER, MARC: Actor. b. Vancouver, B.C., Canada. Trained in summer stock and regional theatre.
PICTURES: Go Tell the Spartans, If You Could See What I Hear, The Beastmaster.
TELEVISION: Roots II, 79 Park Avenue, Journey from Darkness, The Contenders, For Ladies Only, Her Life as a Man, "V" (movie and series).

SINGER, MAURICE: Executive. Producer for Home Box Office with these titles: HBO v.p. of motion picture production and pre-production; HBO Film Licensing, v.p. in charge of production. Is also ranking west coast exec. for Silver Screen Partners, HBO subsidiary originating theatrical features.

SINGLETON, PENNY: Actress. r.n. Dorothy McNulty. b. Philadelphia, PA, September 15, 1908; e. Columbia U. First Broadway success came as top comedienne in Good News., exec. pres. AGVA.
PICTURES INCLUDE: Innumerable films in Blondie series; Young Widow.

SINN, ROBERT S.: Executive. b. Philadelphia, Pa., March 9, 1930; e. U. of Pa., A.B., M.S. Pres., Ultronic Systems Corp., 1960–70; chmn., The Wall Street Venture Capital Corp.; chmn., Microwave Semiconductor Corp.; chmn., Medical Electroscience & Pharmaceuticals Inc.; backer, Joe. Founder GSF Productions, Inc.

SIODMAK, CURT: Director. e. U. of Zurich. Engineer, newspaper reporter, writer in Berlin; novelist, including "F.P.1 Does Not Answer," adapt. 1932 for Ufa. Originals and screenplays in France and England including France (Le Bal), Transatlantic Tunnel, GB.
PICTURES INCLUDE: In U.S. originals and screenplays, many pictures including Her Jungle Love, Aloma of the South Sea, Par.; Invisible Woman; basis: Son of Dracula; s.p.: The Mantrap; (orig.) House of Frankenstein; collab. orig. s.p.: Shady Lady; s.p.: Beast with Five Fingers; collab. s.p., story: Berlin Express; collab. s.p.: Tarzan's Magic Fountain, Four Days Leave; dir.: Bridge of the Gorilla; collab. s.p., dir.: The Magnetic Monster; s.p.: Riders to the Stars; story, s.p.: Creature with the Atom Brain; story: Earth vs. the Flying Saucers.

SIPES, DONALD: b. 1928. Executive. Attorney. Worked for talent agencies early in career; also for NBC and CBS networks as business affairs official. Joined MCA Inc. in 1975, becoming pres. of its Universal TV unit in 1978 and corporate v.p. in June, 1981. In November, 1981, named MGM Film Co. pres. and chief operating officer. 1983, named UA Corp. Chm & CEO. In 1984, pres., Lorimar Dist. Group.

SIRK, DOUGLAS: Director, writer. b. Denmark, April 26, 1900; e. U. Hamberg, Munich. Prod. for UFA, stage actor & producer, newspaperman. From 1944, dir., Hollywood.
PICTURES INCLUDE: Sleep My Love, Lured, Slightly French, Shockproof, Mystery Submarine; prod. dir.: The First Legion; dir.: Thunder on the Hill, Lady Pays Off, Weekend With Father, Has Anybody Seen My Gal?, No Room for the Groom, Meet Me at the Fair, Take Me to Town, All I Desire, Taza Son of Cochise, Magnificient Obession, Sign of the Pagan, Captain Lightfoot, There's Always Tomorrow, All That Heaven Allows, Battle Hymn, Written on the Wind, A Time to Love and a Time to Die, Imitation of Life.

SKELTON, RED: Actor, comedian. r.n. Richard Skelton. b. Vincennes, Ind. July 18, 1913. Joined medicine show at 10; later in show boat stock, minstrel shows, vaudeville, burlesque, circus. Screen debut 1939 in Having Wonderful Time. On radio from 1936. Red Skelton Show, TV, since 1950. Composer of music, writer of short stories and painter.
PICTURES INCLUDE: Flight Command, Lady Be Good, The People vs. Dr. Kildare, Whistling in the Dark, Whistling in Dixie, Ship Ahoy, Maisie Gets Her Man, Panama Hattie, Du Barry Was a Lady, Thousands Cheer, I Dood It, Whistling in Brooklyn, Bathing Beauty, Ziegfeld Follies, Fuller Brush Man, Southern Yankee, Neptune's Daughter, Yellow Cab Man, Three Little Words, Watch the Birdie, Excuse My Dust, Texas Carnival, Lovely to Look At, The Clown, Half a Hero, Great Diamond Robbery, Public Pigeon No. 1, Those Magnificent Men in Their Flying Machines.

SKILES, MARLIN: Composer. b. Harrisburg, Pa., Dec. 17, 1906; e. Froehlich Sch. of Music, Harrisburg. Pianist for several dance orch.; mus. dir., pianist, arr. for Paul Whiteman, Irving Aaronson, others; to Hollywood, 1932; comp., arr. for radio & many m.p.
PICTURES INCLUDE: com., arr.: Over 21, Jolson Story, Gilda, Tonight and Every Night, Dead Reckoning, Callaway Went Thataway, Rose Bowl Story, Battle Zone, The Maze, Fighter Attack, Pride of the Blue Grass, Arrow in the Dust, Dial Red O, Annapolis Story, many Bowery Boys features, Sudden Danger.

SKIRBALL, WILLIAM N.: Exhibitor. b. Homestead, Pa. Began career with Metro in Des Moines & Chicago; states rights distrib., Cleveland; assoc. with brother, Jack H. Skirball (of Skirball-Manning prod. team), educational films br. mgr.; also brother of Joseph Skirball, first nat'l franchise owner, Pittsburgh. Currently partner Skirball Bros. circuit (10 theatres, Ohio), hdqts., Cleveland, Ohio.

SKLAR, MICHAEL: Producer. b. Philadelphia, e. Temple U. Beg. career in broadcasting field, free lancing, scrip writer, radio: Grand Central, First Nighter, Superman, 1939; producer, ed., writer, WMCA, N.Y., Five Star Final; joined CBS-TV, 1948 You Are There; New World A'Coming, 1947 radio prod.; wrote-prod., The Greatest Drama, series of film biog. of famous people, Fox Movietone; Eye on the World, Talkaround, The Good Morning Show, CBS-TV; prod., New Frontiers, 1956; prod., Conquest, 1957 presented in co-operation with the American Assoc. for the Advancement of Science, 1960; prod., writer, Intertel, U.S.A. 1961–62; Britain Postscript to Empire, Mexico—The Unfinished Revolution; prod., writer, Exploring The Universe, 1962; prod., Mayer-Sklar Prods., 1962–63; prod., writer, Intertel, U.S.A., 1964; This Question of Color; prod. exec., Confidential—For Women, 1966, prod., How it Happened.

SKOLIMOWSKI, JERZY: Director. b. Poland, 1938.
PICTURES: Identification Marks—None, Walkover, The Barrier, The Departure, Hands Up, Dialogue, The Adventures of Gerard, Deep End, King Queen Knave, The Shout, Circle of Deceit (act.), Moonlighting (also s.p., prod.); Success Is the Best Revenge, The Lightship. Actor: White Nights.

SLATER, DAPHNE: Actress. b. Bayswater, London, England, March 3, 1928; e. Haberdashers' Askes Sch.; Royal Acad. Dramatic Arts. Stage debut: The Rising Generation, 1945; several plays including King Lear; m.p. debut in Courtneys of Curzon Street, 1947; TV debut for BBC in I Want To Be An Actor, 1946.
TV: Emma, Shout Aloud Salvation, All the Year Round, They Fly by Twilight, Pride and Prejudice, The Affair at Assino, Beau Brummell, Jane Eyre, Precious Bane, The Dark Is Light Enough, Mary Rose, Julius Caesar, Berkeley Square, Less Than Kind, The Burning Glass, Persuasion, The Winslow Boy, She Stoops to Conquer, Nothing to Pay, The Father, The Bald Prima Donna, The Big Breaker, The Cocktail Party, Photo Finish, The Seagull, Love Story, Emergency Ward 10, Jackanory, The First Freedom, Man of Our Times, The Jazz Age, Callan, The Piano Tuner, Happy Ever After, The Pretenders, Virtue, Elizabeth R, The Staff Room, Footprints in the Sand.

SLATZER, ROBERT FRANKLIN: Writer, Director, Producer, Author; b. Marion, Ohio; April 4, 1927; e. Ohio State Univ., UCLA, 1947; Radio news commentator sportscaster, wrote radio serials; adv. dir., Brush-Moore Newspapers; feature writer, Scripps-Howard Newspapers; adv. exec., The Columbus Dispatch; syndicated columnist, New York Journal-American; wrote several guest columns for Walter Winchell and Dorothy Kilgallen; author of several western short stories and novels; wrote, directed, produced many industrial films, documentaries, sports specials and commercials; 1949–51, writer for Harry "Pop" Sherman Productions, Monogram Pictures, Republic Studios, Eagle-Lion Films; 1951, publicist, Hope Enterprises; Pub. Dir., Paramount Pictures; 1952, personal manager to Marilyn Monroe, Ken Maynard, James Craig, Gail Russell and other stars; 1953, story editor and assoc. prod., Joe Palooka Productions; 1953–54, staff writer Universal Studios, RKO Radio Pictures, MGM, Columbia and Paramount Studios; 1958, formed Robert F.

Slatzer Productions; 1960, exec. in chg. of prod., Jaguar Pictures Corp.; 1963–65, president Slatzer Oil & Gas Company; 1966–67, board director, United Mining & Milling Corp.; 1967–70, wrote and directed several feature films; 1970–74, exec., Columbia Pictures Corp.; 1974, resumed producing and financing features and television films; 1976, honored as "Fellow", Mark Twain Institute.
PICTURES INCLUDE: White Gold, The Obsessed, Mike and the Heiress, Under Texas Skies, They Came To Kill, Trail of the Mounties, Jungle Goddess, Montana Desperado, Pride of the Blue, Green Grass of Wyoming, The Naked Jungle, Warpaint, Broken Lance, Elephant Walk, South of Death Valley, The Big Gusher, Arctic Flight, The Hellcats, Bigfoot, John Wayne's 'No Substitute for Victory', Joniko—Eskimo Boy, Operation North Slope, Don't Go West, Mulefeathers, The Unfinished, Single Room Furnished, Viva Zapata, Inchon.
TELEVISION: The Great Outdoors, Adventures of White Arrow, Let's Go Boating, The Joe Palooka Story, Amos & Andy, I am the Law, Files of Jeffrey Jones, Fireside Theatre, The Unser Story, Year of Opportunity (Award winning spec.), The Big Ones, Ken Maynard's West, Where are They Now?, The Groovy Seven, The Untouchables, The Detectives, Wild Wild West, Wagon Train, Playhouse 90, Highway Patrol, David Frost Special, Today Show.
AUTHOR: (novels) Desert Empire, Rose of the Range, Rio, Rawhide Range, The Cowboy and the Heiress, Daphne, Campaign Girl, Scarlet, The Dance Studio Hucksters, Born to be Wild, Single Room Furnished, The West is Still Wild, Gusher, The Young Wildcats; (Biographies) The Life and Curious Death of Marilyn Monroe, The Life and Legend of Ken Maynard, Who Killed Thelma Todd?, The Duke of Thieves, Bing Crosby—The Hollow Man, Duke, The Life and Times of John Wayne.

SLAVIN, GEORGE: Writer. b. Newark, N.J., 1916; e. Bucknell U., Drama Dept., Yale U.
PICTURES INCLUDE: story, collab. s.p., Intrigue; collab. story, Woman on Pier 18; collab. s.p., The Nevadan, Mystery Submarine; collab. story & s.p. Peggy, Red Mountain, City of Bad Men; collab. story, Weekend with Father, Thunder Bay, Rocket Man; collab. story, collab. s.p., Smoke Signal, Uranium Boom; collab. s.p., Desert Sands.

SLOAN, JOHN R.: Producer. e. Merchiston Castle, Edinburg, 1932–39; asst. dir. and prod. man. Warners, London, Hollywood; 1939–46, Army Service.
PICTURES INCLUDE: Sea Devils, The End of the Affair, Port Afrique, Abandon Ship, The Safecracker, Beyond this Place, The Killers of Kilimanjaro, Johnny Nobody, The Reluctant Saint, The Running Man, The Last Command, To Sir With Love, Fragment of Fear, Dad's Army, Lord Jim, No Sex Please, We're British, The Odessa File, Force 10 From Navarone, The Children's Story.

SLOCOMBE, DOUGLAS: Cinematograper. b. England, 1913. Former journalist.
PICTURES: Dead of Night, The Captive Heart, Hue and Cry, The Loves of Joanna Godden, It Always Rains on Sunday, Saraband for Dead Lovers, Kind Hearts and Coronets, Cage of Gold, The Lavender Hill Mob, The Man in the White Suit, The Titfield Thunderbolt, Man in the Sky, The Smallest Show on Earth, Tread Softly, Stranger, Circus of Horrors, The Young Ones, The L-Shaped Room, Freud, The Servant, Guns at Batashi, A High Wind in Jamaica, The Blue Max, Promise Her Anything, The Vampire Killers, Fathom, Robbery, Boom, The Lion in Winter, The Italian Job, The Music Lovers, Murphy's War, Jesus Christ Superstar, The Great Gatsby, Rollerball, Hedda, Nasty Habits, Julia, Lost and Found, Nijinsky, Raiders of the Lost Ark, Never Say Never Again, Indiana Jones and the Temple of Doom.
TELEVISION: Love Among the Ruins, The Corn Is Green, etc.

SMAKWITZ, CHARLES A.: e. Syracuse University, named by Warner Bros. as dist. mgr. Albany, Troy and Utica, and named as zone mgr. Warner Bros., New York State Theatres. Made zone mgr. of Stanley Warner Theatres for the State of New Jersey and New York State Theatres added to N.J. Zone and made headquarters in Newark, N.J. in 1955, transferred to New York City home office as national director of public relations, publicity, advertising for Stanley Warner Corp. nation-wide. In the various areas was Mayor's Rehabilitation and Urban Development Com. of Albany, State Albany Chairman War Activities Committee, National Public Dir. Red Cross Fund Organized Albany V.C. Tent #9 and served as Chief Barker 3 years, 1949–1952, elected National Representative V.C. of America. Member N.Y. State Program and Planning Committee, Pres. Heart Assn. of Albany County, N.J. State Chairman Nat. Conf. of Christian and Jews 1955–62. Organized and Pres. of Syr. Un. of Greater, N.Y. Served as v.p. of V.C. of N.Y. Assistant to Spyros R. Skoveas 1969–71, served as International-Ambassador at large of V.C. International Consultant exhibition, production, promotion, real estate and public relations.

SMIGHT, JACK: Director. b. Minneapolis, Minn., 1926.
PICTURES INCLUDE: I'd Rather Be Rich, The Third Day, Harper, Kaleidoscope, The Secret War of Harry Frigg, No Way to Treat a Lady, Strategy of Terror, The Illustrated Man, The Travelling Executioner, Rabbit Run, Dr. Frankenstein, Frankenstein: The True Story, Airport 1975, Midway, Damnation Alley, Fast Break, Loving Couples, Number One with a Bullet.
TV: Banacek, Columbo, etc.

SMITH, ALEXIS: Actress. b. Penticton, Can., June 8, 1921; e. Los Angeles City Coll. In summer stock British Columbia; star in coll. prod., Night of January 16th; in m.p. for Warner Bros.
PICTURES INCLUDE: Smiling Ghost, Dive Bomber, Steel Against the Sky, Gentlemen Jim, Thank Your Luck Stars, Constant Nymph, Conflict, Adventures of Mark Twain, Rhapsody in Blue, Horn Blows at Midnight (Star of Tomorrow, 1943), One More Tomorrow, Night and Day, Of Human Bondage, Stallion Road, Two Mrs. Carrolls, Woman in White, Decision of Christopher Blake, Whiplash, South of St. Louis, Any Number Can Play, One Last Fling, Undercover Girl, Wyomying Hall, Montana, Here Comes the Groom, Cave of the Outlaws, Turning Point, Split Second, Sleeping Tiger, Eternal Sea, The Young Philadelphians, Once Is Not Enough, The Little Girl Who Lives Down the Lane, Casey's Shadow, Tough Guys.
BROADWAY: Follies, 1971, Platinum, 1978.
TELEVISION: Movies: A Death in California, Dress Gray.

SMITH, A. BERKELEY: TV commentator, producer. b. Bournemouth, Eng., Dec. 8, 1918. e. Blundell's Sch., St. Andrews U. Royal Artillery, 1939–46; lecture tour, U.S., 1945; prod.-comment., BBC North American service, 1946; to U.N. Assembly, New York, for BBC home service, 1949; TV as BBC outside broadcasts prod., 1949; devised, prod. sports & farming series with other documentaries; Comm. State Occasions. Theatre Shows, etc., 1951; prod. Show Places series; prod. exchange program from R.T.F. Paris; commentator Coronation & all State visits, 1953; prod. Arenascope, programs radio show, 1954; asst. head TV outside broadcasts. Feb. 1955; head outside broadcasts Southern Television Ltd., 1958; asst. Con. Programs, 1961; Con. Programs (Southern TV Ltd), 1964; dir. Southern TV, 1965, Left Dec. 75, Dir. ITV Prog. Planning, 1976.

SMITH, CHARLES MARTIN: Actor. b. 1955. e. Calif. State Univ. f. is animation artist Frank Smith.
PICTURES INCLUDE: The Culpepper Cattle Company, Fuzz, The Spikes Gang, American Graffiti, More American Graffiti, Never Cry Wolf, Starman.
TELEVISION: The Brady Bunch, Monte Nash.

SMITH, CONSTANCE: Actress. r.n. Constance Smyth. b. Limerick, Ire.; e. St. Louis Covent. Began career as model for Noel Mayne; winner of beauty contest Screen Magazine. Free-lance actress, studios in Eng., prior to Hollywood m.p. debut in The Mudlark.
PICTURES INCLUDE: Brighton Rock, Now Barrabas, Trottie True, Murder at the Window, Blackmail, The Perfect Woman, Room to Let, The 13th Letter, I'll Never Forget You, Red Skies of Montana, Treasure of the Golden Condor, Lure of the Wilderness, Taxi, Man in the Attic, Big Tipoff.

SMITH, HOWARD K.: News commentator. b. Ferriday, La., May 12, 1914. e. Tulane Univ., 1936. Heidelberg U., Germany; Oxford U., Rhodes Scholarship. United Press, London, 1939; United Press Bureau, Copenhagen; United Press, Berlin, 1940; joined CBS News, Berlin corr., 1941. Reported on occupied Europe from Switzerland to 1944; covered Nuremberg trials, 1946; ret. to U.S., moderator, commentator or reporter, CBS Reports, Face the Nation, Eyewitness to History, The Great Challenge, numerous news specials. Sunday night news analysis. CBS News Washington corr., 1957; chief corr. & mgr., Washington Bureau, 1961; joined, ABC News, Jan. 1962. News and Comment, ABC news. Anchorman and Commentator, ABC Evening News. Author: Last Train from Berlin, 1942, The State of Europe, 1949. Washington, D.C.—The Story of Our Nation's Capital, 1967.

SMITH, HY: Executive. b. New York City, June 3, 1934. e. Baruch School, CCNY, BBA. Joined Paramount Pictures 1967, foreign ad.-pub coordinator; 1969-joined United Artists as foreign ad.-pub mgr., named int'l. ad.-pub dir., 1970; named v.p.; intl. adv.-pub. 1976; Appointed vice pres. worldwide Advertising, publicity and promotion, July 1978; 1981, named first v.p., adv./pub./promo; 1982, joined Rastar Films as v.p., intl. project director for Annie. 1983, joined United Intl. Pictures as sr. v.p., adv/pub, based in London. 1984, named sr. v.p., mktg.

SMITH, JACLYN: Actress. b. Houston, Texas, Oct. 26, 1947. Started acting while in high school and studied drama and psychology at Trinity Univ. in San Antonio. Appeared in many commercials as model.
PICTURES INCLUDE: Bootleggers, The Adventures, Deja

Vu.
TV: McCloud, Get Christy Love, The Rookies, World of Disney, Switch, Charlie's Angels (regular). Movies: The Night They Saved Christmas, Sentimental Journey, Florence Nightingale, George Washington.

SMITH, JACQUELINE: Executive. b. Phila., Pa., May 24, 1933. e. Antioch College, 1954. m. William Dale Smith, novelist (pseudonym David Anthony). Actress, Bermudiana Theatre in Bermuda, The Antioch Theatre in Ohio and several little theatres in Washington, D.C.; with the Stanford U. Players. Did research and writing for RCA, worked as a nursery school teacher and directed Little Theatre groups in the West Coast area. 1957: wrote and produced over 100 weekly children's programs at KPIX, San Francisco. Promotion director at WPIX-TV, N.Y. Worked with CBS TV Network for over 5 yrs. as general prog. exec. and exec. prod. of CBS West Coast Daytime Programs. Currently director of special projects at Warner Bros. Television Dept. and executive producer of Warner Bros. Animation Division.

SMITH, JOSEPH P.: Executive. b. Bklyn, N.Y. e. Columbia Univ. Started career Wall Street; joined RKO Radio Pictures, served in sales and managerial posts; exec. vice-pres., Lippert Productions, Hollywood; vice pres., Telepictures, Inc., formed and pres., Cinema-Vue Corp.; pres., Pathe Pictures, Inc., Pathe News, Inc.

SMITH, MAGGIE: Actress. b. Ilford, England, Dec. 28, 1934. Early career Oxford Playhouse. Numerous TV appearances Britain, America.
PICTURES INCLUDE: Nowhere to Go, The V.I.P.s, Young Cassidy, Othello, The Honey Pot, Hot Millions, The Prime of Miss Jean Brodie (Acad. Award, Best Actress), Oh What a Lovely War, Love and Pain, Travels with my Aunt, Murder by Death, Death on the Nile, California Suite (AA), Clash of the Titans, Quartet, Evil Under the Sun, Better Late Than Never, The Missionary, A Private Function, Lily in Love, A Room with a View.

SMITH, MAURICE: Producer, director, writer. b. London, England, May 12, 1939. e. St. Ignatius College. Prior to entering m.p. industry, worked in bank in England, on newspaper in Canada, pool hustler, general contractor in Los Angeles, Calif.
PICTURES INCLUDE: The Glory Stompers, Scream Free, Cycle Savages, Hard Trail, Diamond Stud, Love Swedish Style, November Children, How Come Nobody's On Our Side, Joys of Jezebel.

SMITH, ROGER: Actor. b. South Gate, Calif., Dec. 18, 1932. e. U. of Arizona, started career at age 7, one of the Meglin Kiddies, appearing at the Mayan Theater, Wilshire, Ebell.
PICTURES INCLUDE: No Time to Be Young, Crash Landing, Operation Madball, Man of a Thousand Faces, Never Steal Anything Small, Aunti Mame, Rogues Gallery.
TV: The Horace Heidt Show, Ted Mack Original Amateur Hour, 77 Sunset Strip, writer, ABC-TV, sings, composes, American folk songs.

SMITH, WILLIAM: Actor. b. Columbia, MO, May 24, 1932.
PICTURES INCLUDE: Twilight's Last Gleaming, The Frisco Kid, Any Which Way You Can.
TELEVISION: Rich Man, Poor Man, Hawaii 5-0, The Jerk Too.

SMOLEN, DONALD E.: Executive. b. New York City, Aug. 10, 1923; e. NYU 1943, Pratt Institute 1947, Ecole Des Beaux Arts 1949, Art dept. Fox, 1940–41; art dept. Kayton Spiero Advtg., 1942; illustrator designer, Gilbert Miller Studios 1946–49; free lance illustrator, designer, 1951–65 servicing such accounts as UA, Fox, Warner Bros., TWA, Ford Motors; dir. of adv., UA. Resigned 1974 to form own co., Donald E. Smolen and Associates, consultant for m.p. adv.; 1975 merged to form Smolen, Smith and Connolly, advertising and marketing consultants to m.p. industry. Created ad campaigns for All the Presidents' Men, Fiddler on the Roof, Rocky, Superman, Star Wars.

SNAPER, WILBUR: Exhibitor. b. Perth Amboy, N.J., Oct. 30, 1911. e. Yale U. 1933, N.J. Law, 1935. Pres. Snaper Theatres, New York, nat'l pres. Allied States Assn.; partner 1957. Member: Yale Club, Variety Club, N.Y. Bridge Club; pres. Triangle Theatres; pres., AIT Theatres, N.J.; pres. Triangle Theatres.

SNELL, PETER R. E.: Producer. b. 1941. Prod.: 1967: Winters Tale, Some May Live, A Month in the Country, Carnaby 68. 1968: Subterfuge. 1969–70: Juliet Ceasar, Goodbye Gemini. 1971: Anthony and Cleopatra. 1972: The Wicker Man. Appt. head of prod. and man. dir. British Lion 1973. Joined Robert Stigwood group 1975. Hennessy. 1976: Returned to indep. prod. 1978: Bear Island. 1981: Motherlod. 1982: Appt. chief exec., Britannic Film & Television Ltd. 1985, purchased British Lion Film Prods., Ltd. from Thorn/EMI. Produced Lady Jane, Turtle Diary.

SNODGRESS, CARRIE: Actress. b. Chicago, Ill., Oct 27, 1945; e. Northern Illinois U. Acted with Goodman Theatre where plays include All Way Home, Oh What a Lovely War, Caesar and Cleopatra and Tartuffe (Sarah Siddons Award, 1966).
PICTURES INCLUDE: Rabbit, Run, Diary of a Mad Housewife, The Fury, A Night in Heaven, Murphy's Law.
TV: World Premier (Silent Night, Lonely Night, The Whole World Is Watching), The Outsider, The Virginian, Judd for the Defense, Medical Center, Marcus Welby, M.D.

SNOWDON, LEIGH: Actress. b. Memphis, Tenn., June 28, 1932. e. Lambeth College, Jackson, Tenn. Model, TV appearances.
PICTURES INCLUDE: Kiss Me Deadly, All That Heaven Allows, Francis in the Navy, Rawhide Years, Square Jungle, Creature Walks Among Us, Outside the Law.

SNYDER, TOM: Newscaster, show host. b. Milwaukee, May 12, 1936. e. Marquette Univ. First job in news dept. of WRIT, Milwaukee. Subsequently with WSAV-TV, Savannah; WAII-TV, Atlanta; KTLA-TV, Los Angeles; and KYW-TV, Philadelphia, before moving to KNBC in Los Angeles in 1970 as anchorman for weeknight newscast. Named host of NBC-TV's Tomorrow program in Oct., 1973, and moved to N.Y.C. in Dec., 1974, at which time began as anchorman of one-hour segment of NewsCenter 4. In Aug., 1975, inaugurated the Monday-thru-Friday editions of NBC News Update, one-minute prime time news spot. Host for Tomorrow talk show.

SNYDER, WILLIAM L.: Producer, executive. b. Baltimore, Md., Feb. 14, 1920; e. B.A. The John Hopkins U., 1940. Lt. Comnder., U.S. Navy WWII, 1941–45. Established Rembrandt Films, N.Y.C., 1948 as importer and dist. of foreign films. Co-prod. White Mane (UA, dom.), winner Cannes Fest. Grand Prize, seven other int'l awards, 1945. Prod. 13 Tom & Jerry Cartoons (MGM) and more than 100 Miss Nightingale, She, Little Lord Fauntleroy, The Secret Army (2 series). Popeye and Krazy Kat cartoons for U.S. TV plus number cartoons (Para.)., 1956. Won Academy Award for cartoon Munro (Para.), 1961. Rec'd Academy nominations for Self Defense for Cowards (1962), The Game (1963), How to Avoid Friendship (1964) and Nudnik (1965). Prod. cartoon feature Alice in Paris (Childhood Prodns.), 1966. Prod. I a Woman II, 1968 (Chevron Picts.), and The Daughter (Chevron Picts.), 1970.

SOADY, WILLIAM C.: Executive. Career with Universal Pictures started in 1970 when named Toronto branch mgr.; promoted to v.p. & gen. sls. mgr. of Universal Film (Canada) in 1971. Promoted to v.p. & gen. sls. mgr., Universal Pictures, 1981, in New York, relocating to L.A. in 1981. In 1983 named pres. of Universal Pictures Distribution, new dist. div. of Universal.

SOAMES, RICHARD: Executive. b. London, England, 1936. Joined Film Finances Ltd. 1972; Appt. director Film Finances Ltd., 1977: Appt. man. dir. 1979. Appt. pres. Film Fimances Canada Ltd. 1982: Appt. pres., Film Finances Inc.

SOBLE, RON: Actor. b. Chicago, March 28, 1932. e. Univ. of Michigan. Served U.S. Army, 11th Airborne, in Japan. Studied acting in New York and was member of Jose Quintero's Circle in the Square Players. Acted in such plays as Romeo and Juliet, Murder in the Cathedral, The Petrified Forest; prod. assoc. on TV series Suspense and Danger, and appeared in 56 series. Co-star in The Monroes TV show.
PICTURES INCLUDE: Navajo Run, Al Capone, The Cincinnati Kid, Joe Kidd.

SOFAER, ABRAHAM: Actor. b. Rangoon, Burma, Oct. 1, 1896. Stage debut 1921 in Chas. Doran Shakespeare Co.'s first London appearance, Glorianna, 1925; starred in several London productions & subsequently Old Vic & Stratford-on-Avon; broadcaster & TV star; played in many British films; Broadway stage and films in Hollywood.
PICTURES INCLUDE: His Majesty O'Keefe, Elephant Walk, The Naked Jungle, Out of the Clouds, Bhowani Junction, Sinbad, King of Kings, Head.

SOHMER, STEVE: Executive. b. 1942. 1977–82, v.p., adv./promo. CBS-TV. 1982, joined NBC as v.p. of adv./creative svcs. Promoted to exec. v.p., 1984. In 1985 joined Columbia Pictures as pres. & chief oper. officer.

SOKOLOW, DIANE: Executive. b. New York City. e. Temple Univ. M. Mel Sokolow. 1975, v.p., East Coast operations, for Lorimar; with Warner Bros. 1977–81; served as v.p. of East Coast production. Left to form The Sokolow Co. with husband, Mel, to produce films. 1982, returned to WB as v.p., East Coast prod. 1984, joined Motown Prods. as exec. v.p.

SOLDATI, MARIO: Director. b. Turin, Italy, 1906. e. Superior Institute of the History of Art, Rome. Lecturer, Columbia U.; author of America First Love, other books; m.p. dir. since 1939.

PICTURES INCLUDE: O.K. Nero, Wayward Wife, Stranger's Hand, Don Juan's Night of Love.

SOLO, ROBERT H.: Producer. Early career as agent with Ashley-Famous; later production as exec. asst. to Jack Warner and Walter MacEwen at Warner Bros. In London prod. Scrooge for Cinema Center Films, 1970; co-prod. The Devils, 1971; 1971, named WB v.p., foreign production 1974, named exec. v.p., prod. at Burbank Studio. Now indep. prod. Invasion of the Body Snatchers, 1978, for United Artists; The Awakening (EMI-Orion), 1980; I, The Jury (American Cinema), 1981; Bad Boys, 1983.

SOLOMON, FLORENCE: Executive. b. New York City. e. Hunter College. Research mgr., Ligon Johnson's copyright title search firm, 1937–65; dir. for research, Entertainment Copyright Research Co., Inc., 1965–1968; ASCAP (Music Index-Library) 1968–present. Pres. Cinema History Correspondent Society assoc. ed. TV Movies, research associate, The Great Movie Series, The Slapstick Queens, The Paramount Pretties, The MGM Stock Co.; The RKO Gals, The Glamour Girls, The Great Spy Pictures, Actors' Television Credits, 1950–1972; Good Dames, Hollywood's Great Love Teams, Liza! Elvis!, The Debonairs, The Swashbucklers, Hollywood Players: The Forties, The Great Gangster Pictures, Hollywood Players: The Thirties, The Great Western Pictures, the All-Americans, Leading Ladies, The Great Science Fiction Pictures, Hollywood Character Actors, Film Actors Guide: Western Europe, Hollywood on Hollywood, Hollywood Beauties, The Funsters, The Forties Gals, Actors TV Credits: Supplement I, The Hollywood Regulars, Best of MGM: The Golden Years.

SOLOMON, MICHAEL JAY: Executive. b. Jan. 20, 1938. e. Emerson in Boston; N.Y.U. Evening School of Commerce while working at first job with United Artists in 1956. Became student booker. Hired by Seymour Florin as booker for one year; returned to UA in intl. dept. January, 1960 went to Panama as asst. to mgr. of Central America. Transferred to Bogota after one yr.; made mgr. of UA in Peru and Bolivia. In 1964 joined MCA Latin American div., reorganizing office in Mexico and later opening office in Brazil. Made v.p., 1968, of MCA-TV. Supervised Latin American and Caribbean div., 1973 made head of feature film sales to tv stations internationally while still supervising MCA business in Latin America. Resigned 1977 to form Michael Jay Solomon Films International, Inc. & Solomon International TV Newsletter. In 1978 formed Telepictures Corporation to distribute films worldwide and enter production. Was chm. & CEO. In 1986 merged with Lorimar to form Lorimar—Telepictures. Is member of 4-man office of the pres. Co. is a leading supplier of tv programs world-wide, produces films, has video co. & ad agency; bought MGM studios.
MEMBER: Vice-pres., N.Y. World TV Festival; bd. of dir., Intl. Council of NATAS; chm., Intl. Comm. of NATPE; bd., AFMA; bd., U.S. Magazine.

SOLOMON, T. G.: Executive. b. Jan. 5, 1920, e. LSU, 1941. Chairman of Board to Gulf States Theatres, New Orleans, LA, operating theatres in Louisiana, Mississippi, and Texarkana; Past chm. and past pres. of the National Association of Theatre Owners. Past chief barker, Variety Tent 45; past pres., Mississippi Theatre Owners; past pres., Texas Theatre Owners; chm., Lousiana Film Commission; past pres., Louisiana Theatres Assn.

SOLT, ANDREW: Writer. b. Budapest, Hungary, June 7, 1916; e. St. Stephen's Coll.
PICTURES INCLUDE: They All Kissed the Bride, Without Reservations, Joan of Arc, Little Women, Jolson Story, In a Lonely Place, Thunder on the Hill, Lovely to Look At; orig. s.p. For the First Time.
TV: Hitchcock Presents, Ford Theatre, Douglas Fairbanks Presents, Wire Service, General Electric Theatre, BBC and Stuttgart TV.
STAGE: 1973, Geld In Der Tasche, produced by Theatre am Kurfurstendamm, West Berlin.

SOLTZ, CHARLENE E.: Executive. b. New London, Conn. Director of press relations for Motion Picture Association of America, Inc.

SOMERS, SUZANNE: Actress. b. San Bruno, CA, Oct. 16, 1946. e. Lone Mountain, San Francisco College for Women. Pursued modeling career; worked as regular on Mantrap, syndicated talk show. Did summer stock and theatrical films. Wrote books: Touch Me Again, Some People Live More Than Others. Biggest TV success in Three's Company series.
PICTURES: Bullitt, Daddy's Gone A-Hunting, Fools, Magnum Force, American Graffiti, Yesterday's Hero, Nothing Personal.
TELEVISION: One Day at a Time, Lotsa Luck, The Rockford Files, Starsky & Hutch, The Rich Little Show, Battle of the Network Stars, Us Against the World, Love Boat, etc. TV movies: Happily Ever After, The Princess and the Lumberjack, Zuma Beach, Ants, Hollywood Wives.

SOMMER, ELKE: Actress. b. Germany, 1941. To Britain 1956 English. Ent. films in Germany, 1958, and since made films in Germany and Italy incl. Friend of the Jaguar, Traveling Luxury, Heaven and Cupid, Ship of the Dead. 1960: made debut in Birtish films.
PICTURES INCLUDE: Don't Bother to Knock, The Victors, The Money Trap, Love the Italian Way, A Shot in the Dark, The Venetian Affair, Deadlier Than the Male, Frontier Hellcat. Under contract to ABPC; The Corrupt Ones, The Wicked Dreams of Paula Schultz, They Came to Rob Las Vegas, The Wrecking Crew, Baron Blood, Percy, Zeppelin, Ten Little Indians, Lisa and the Devil, The Prisoner of Zenda, The Astral Factor, Lily in Love.
TELEVISION: Jenny's War, Peter the Great.

SOMMER, JOSEF: Actor. b. Greifswald, Germany, June 26, 1934. e. Carnegie-Mellon Univ. Studied at American Shakespeare Festival in Stratford, CT, 1962–64. US Army, 1958–60. NY stage debut in Othello, 1970. Film debut in Dirty Harry, 1971.
PICTURES: The Front, Close Encounters of the Third Kind, Oliver's Story, Hide in Plain Sight, Reds, Independence Day, Absence of Malice, Hanky Panky, Still of the Night, Rollover, Sophie's Choice (narrator), Silkwood, Iceman, D.A.R.Y.L., Target, etc.
TELEVISION: Morning Becomes Electra, The Scarlet Letter, Saigon, Sparkling Cyanide, etc.

SONDHEIM, STEPHEN: Composer-Writer. b. New York City, March 22, 1930. e. Williams Coll. Bdwy work: West Side Story, Gypsy, A Funny Thing Happened on the Way to the Forum, Anyone Can Whistle, Do I Hear a Waltz?, Company, Follies, A Little Night Music, Pacific Overtures, Sweeney Todd, Merrily We Roll Along, Sunday in the Park with George.
PICTURES: The Last of Sheila (s.p.), Stavisky (score), A Little Night Music, Reds (score).

SONENFELD, OTTO: Producer, distributor. Former br. mgr., RKO, Czechoslovakia, ind. prod. German & Czech films, latter including Erotikon (silent), Ecstasy, first with Hedy Lamarr, Revolution of Blood and Mud, first Czech feature-length doc.; first Israeli prod. Adama (Tomorrow is a Wonderful Day); oper. as Forum Films, hdqts., Tel-Aviv;. Also rep. Korda-London Film, London & Lux Films, Rome and Israel; member Int'l Fed. of Film Prod., Paris.

SORIANO, DALE: Publicist, b. Brooklyn, N.Y. Ent. m.p. Ind. as a reelboy in projection room, later usher, sign painter, manager, film booker stagehand (NBC-CBS-ABC). Orchestra leader, director of info. for various N.Y.C. depts., licenses, real estate, law, public events and firearms control board. Publicist for Americana festivals, various veteran organizations. V.F.W., A.L., D.A.V., C.W.V. and Army & Navy Union and many philanthropic organizations. World War II served with 1st Marine Div. U.S.M.C. in S.W. Pacific thea. of opera. 1960–68 v.p. Publicists Association, I.A.T.S.E. conducted many TV and vet columns for the Brooklyn Eagle and independent newspapers. Show*Biz column 1st for the Brooklyn Daily Bulletin. Also stage, records, movies, radio and TV Editor. Pres. of Lighthouse Productions and pres. of Flatlands Chamner of Commerce; pres. National Council of Civic Assn. Member of Motion Picture Pioneers, National Publicists Association, and American Newspaper Guild.

SORVINO, PAUL: Actor. b. New York City, 1939. Acted on Bdwy.; broke into films with Where's Poppa in 1970.
PICTURES: Day of the Dolphin, Made for Each Other, The Gambler, A Touch of Class, Oh, God, Bloodbrothers, Slow Dancing in the Big City, The Brink's Job, Lost and Found, Cruising, I, The Jury, That Championship Season, Off the Wall, Turk 182, The Stuff.
TELEVISION: Seventh Avenue, Tell Me Where It Hurts, Chiefs, Surviving, With Intent to Kill.

SOTHERN, ANN: Actress. b. Valley City, N.D., Jan. 23, 1923; e. Washington U.; p. Annette Yde-Lake, opera singer. On stage, in m.p. since 1934.
PICTURES INCLUDE: Let's Fall in Love, Melody in Spring, Three Hearts for Julia, Swing Shift Maisie, Cry Havoc, Thousands Cheer, Maisie series, April Showers, Letter to Three Wives, Judge Steps Out, Words and Music, Nancy Goes to Rio, Blue Gardenia, Lady in a Cage, Sylvia, Chubasco, The Killing Kind, Golden Needles, Crazy Mama, The Manitou.
TV: Private Secretary, Ann Sothern Show, Captain and the Kings.

SOUL, DAVID: Actor. b. Chicago, Aug. 28, 1943. Attended several colleges but gave up studies to pursue a career in music. Made 25 singing appearances on The Merv Griffin Show where was spotted and given screen test. Signed contract with Screen Gems and given starring role in ABC-TV series, Here Come the Brides.
PICTURES INCLUDE: Johnny Got His Gun, Magnum Force, Dog Pound Shuffle.
TV: Guest Star: The Streets of San Francisco, Cannon,

Medical Center, The Rookies, Ironside, Star Trek, McMillan and Wife, Dan August, Circle of Fear, Owen Marshall, Counselor at Law. Movies: The Disappearance of Flight 412, Intertect, Movin' On, Little Ladies of the Night, The Fifth Missile. Series: Starsky and Hutch, Yellow Rose.

SPACEK, SISSY: Actress. b. Quitman, TX, Dec. 25, 1950. Christened Mary Elizabeth. Cousin of actor Rip Torn. Was photographic model; attended acting classes in New York under Lee Strasberg.
PICTURES INCLUDE: Prime Cut (debut), Ginger in the Morning, Badlands, Carrie, Welcome to L.A., 3 Women, Heart Beat, Coal Miner's Daughter, Raggedy Man, Missing, The River, Marie, Violets Are Blue, 'night, Mother, Crimes of the Heart.
TV: The Girls of Huntington House, The Migrants, Katherine (all TV movies), two episodes of The Waltons.

SPALLA, JOSEPH SALVATORE "RICK": Executive, producer. b. Sandusky, Ohio, May 22, 1923. e. Ohio State U. 1943 and 1946; U. of So. Calif., B.A., 1953. m. Shirley Egland. Studied voice while teenager, soloist with Sandusky High a cappella choir, Ohio State U. Chorus and Men's Glee Club & OSU Symphonic Choir. To Hollywood, 1946, as City Messenger. Member, Screen Extras Guild, Screen Actors Guild. Co-owner of cab co. 1953–54, cameraman with Hollywood Prod. Co., travel series: The Open Road and document series, Before Your Eyes. 1954–56, one of the founders, prod. head and v.p., Bill Burrud Prod., Inc. Started half-hour weekly series, Wanderlust (later syndicated as Vagabond). Prod. supervisor and co-creator of Assignment America, 1956–57, v.p. and gen. mgr. of Jet TV and Film Prods., Inc. Exec. prod. of TV: The Open Road. Creator and exec. prod. of High Road to Danger, 1957–62, formed RSVP, Rick Spalla Video Productions. Prod. Those Faraway Places, Enchanted Lands. Created series, Guest Shot, 1962–67, formed Hollywood Newsreel Syndicate, Inc., sub. of RSVP; created, prod. Hollywood Backstage TV series, prod., dir. Hollywood's Fantastic Artists and Models Ball (TV special); producer-director of TV series, Portrait of a Star, (12 hour-long specials) also TV series Holiday on Wheels. Owns millions of feet of film on stars, newsreel, travelogue footage etc. Producer of TV commercials and industrial films.

SPANO, VINCENT: Actor. b. New York City, Oct. 18, 1963. Film debut in Over the Edge (1978).
PICTURES: Rumblefish, The Black Stallion Returns, Baby It's You, Alphabet City, Maria's Lovers, Creator.
TELEVISION: Search for Tomorrow, The Gentleman Bandit, Senior Trip.

SPARKS, ROBERT: Producer. b. West Union, Ohio; e. U. of Cincinnati Law School; assoc. prod. Para., 1932; story ed., RKO, 1935; prod. Columbia, 1938; U.S.M.C., 1942; Univ., 1946; exec. prod. RKO, 1947; exec. prod. CBS TV network, 1955–59; dir. syndication, Screen Gems, Hollywood, 1959–62; exec. prod., CBS, 1962; exec. prod., MGM TV, 1963.

SPEARS, JR., HAROLD T.: Executive. b. Atlanta, GA, June 21, 1929. e. Univ. of Ga. (1951). With Floyd Theatres, Lakeland, FL., since 1953; now pres.

SPECKTOR, FREDERICK: Executive. b. April 24, 1933, Los Angeles. e. Univ. of So. Calif., UCLA. M.P. agent, Ashley Famous Agency, 1962–64; Artists Agency Corp., 1964–68; exec. M.P. dept., William Morris Agency, 1968–78; exec. Creative Artists Agency, 1978–present.

SPELLING, AARON: Executive. b. Dallas, TX, Apr. 22, 1928. Was actor/writer before becoming producer at Four Star in 1957. In 1967, formed Thomas/Spelling Productions to produce several series and movies, including Mod Squad. In 1969, formed his own company, Aaron Spelling Productions, and then in 1972, partnered with Leonard Goldberg to produce The Rookies, Charlie's Angels, Fantasy Island, Starsky and Hutch, Hart to Hart, T.J. Hooker, and under own company banner, Love Boat, Vega$, Dynasty, Matt Houston, Hotel, The Colbys, Life with Lucy, and over 103 movies for television.

SPENGLER, PIERRE: Producer. b. Paris, 1947. Went on stage at 15; returned to language studies at Alliance Française. Entered film industry as production runner and office boy. Teamed for first time with friend Ilya Salkind on The Light at the Edge of the World, produced by Alexander Salkind.
PICTURES INCLUDE: Bluebeard, The Three Musketeers, The Four Musketeers, Crossed Swords, Superman, Superman II, Superman III, Santa Claus.

SPENSER, JEREMY: Actor. b. Ceylon, 1937; e. Downshill School, Farnham, England. Ent. films 1947 in Anna Karenina.
PICTURES INCLUDE: It's Great To Be Young, The Prince and the Showgirl, Wonderful Things, Ferry to Hong Kong, Roman Spring of Mrs. Stone, Vengeance, King and Country, He Who Rides a Tiger.

SPERLING, MILTON: Producer. b. New York City. e. C.C.N.Y., Shipping clerk Paramount Newsreel; messenger boy, Paramount, Astoria studio; script clerk, United Artists studio, Hollywood, secy. to Darryl Zanuck, Warner Bros.; secy. to Hal B. Wallis, assoc. prod., Edward Small Prod.; asst. to Winfield Sheehan, Fox Films; screen writer 20th-Fox, Four Sons, Sing, Baby, Sing, Thin Ice, Cisco Kid; apptd. prod.; served in U.S. Marines as Capt. 3½ yrs; prod. Sun Valley Serenade, Hello, Frisco, Hello, Crash Dive, Rings on Her Fingers; To the Shores of Tripoli; Iwo Jima; documentary m.p.; org. & pres. of U.S. Pictures, 1945.
PICTURES INCLUDE: Cloak and Dagger, Pursued, Three Secrets, The Enforcer, Distant Drums, Retreat Hell, Blowing Wild, prod. collab. story & s.p. Court Martial of Billy Mitchell; supv. prod. Top Secret Affair, prod., Marjorie Morningstar; prod. collab. s.p. The Bramble Bush; prod. collab. s.p., Merrill's Marauders; collab. prod. s.p. Battle of the Bulge; prod., collab. Captain Apache.
TV: Black Market Baby (MOW, ABC), Brave New World (exec. prod., NBC. mini-series); The Dream Merchants (exec. prod., OPT series). Supervising Producer: Deadly Intentions (ABC mini), Promises to Keep (MOW, ABC).

SPEWACK, BELLA: Writer. b. Hungary, 1899. e. Washington Irving H.S., 1917. m. Samuel Spewack, 1922; writer. Reporter N.Y. Call, N.Y. Mail, N.Y. World, N.Y. Evening World; feature writer, N.Y. Herald Tribune, N.Y. Times; nat'l pub. dir. Camp Fire Girls, then Girl Scouts; asst. to husband for corr. for N.Y. World, Russia 1922–26; author plays with husband include: Solitaire Man, Poppa, War Song, Clear All Wires, Spring Song, Boy Meets Girl, Leave It to Me, Kiss Me Kate, My Three Angels, Festival. Member: Dramatists Guild; SWG; pres., N.Y. Girls Scholarship Fund.
PICTURES INCLUDE: Clear All Wires, Boy Meets Girl, Cat and the Fiddle, Rendezvous, The Nuisance, Three Loves of Nancy, My Favorite Wife, When Ladies Meet, Weekend at the Waldorf, Move Over Darling, We're No Angels (based on play My Three Angels).
TV: Mr Broadway, Kiss Me Kate, My Three Angels, The Enchanted Nutcracker, Kiss Me Kate, BBC.

SPIEGEL, LARRY: Producer-Writer-Director. b. Brooklyn, New York. e. Ohio Univ. With CBS-TV 1960–66; Benton & Bowles, 1966–67; Wells, Rich, Green, 1967–71; BBD&O, 1972–73.. Now co-heads Spiegel-Bergman Productions.
PICTURES INCLUDE: Hail (s.p.); Book of Numbers (s.p.); Death Game (prod.); Stunts (prod.); Spree (direc./s.p.); Phobia (prod.); Reno: The First Adventure (prod.); Dove Against Death (prod.).
TV: Alexander (s.p., prod.); Incredible Indelible Magical Physical Mystery Trip (s.p.); Bear That Slept Through Christmas (s.p.); Never Fool With A Gypsy Ikon (s.p.); Mystery Trip Through Little Red's Head (s.p.); Planet of The Apes (animated) (s.p.); Jan Stephenson Golf Video (prod.).

SPIEGEL, TED: Publicist. b. New York City. e. N.Y.U., B.S. 1948. Joined Columbia Pictures 1948 in adv. copy, exploitation, pub. depts.; foreign public rel., Columbia International 1956. Spec. adv., pub. rep., Kingsley Int'l Pictures, 1960; spec. asst. to pres. Kingsley Int'l Pictures, 1962; mgr. dir., theatre operations, The Landau Co., 1963; pub. exec., Embassy Pics. Corp., 1964; dir. pub., Avco Embassy Pictures, 1968. In 1976 joined A. Stirling Gold as dir. adv./pub. relations. In 1978 named acct. exec. for Solters & Roskin.

SPIELBERG, STEVEN: b. Cincinnati, Dec. 18, 1947. e. Calif. State Coll. Made home movies as child; completed first film with story and actors at 12 yrs. old in Phoenix. At 13 won film contest for 40-min. war movie, Escape to Nowhere. At 16 made 140-min. film, Firelight. At CSC made five films. First professional work, Amblin', 20 min. short which led to signing contract with Universal Pictures.
TV: Duel, Something Evil.
PICTURES INCLUDE: The Sugarland Express; Jaws; Close Encounters of The Third Kind; I Wanna Hold Your Hand (exec. prod.); 1941; Used Cars (exec. prod.); Raiders of the Lost Ark; Poltergeist (prod.-s.p.); E.T.: The Extra-Terrestrial (dir.); Twilight Zone—The Movie (prod.-dir.); Indiana Jones and the Temple of Doom (dir.); Gremlins (exec. prod.).; Goonies (exec. prod.); Back to the Future (exec. prod.); The Color Purple (co-prod.-dir.); Young Sherlock Holmes (co-prod.).

SPIER, WILLIAM: Producer, director, novelist, radio-TV writer; m. June Havoc. Network exec., producer; prod. radio shows including March of Time, Columbia Work Shop, Adventures of Sam Spade, Philip Morris Playhouse, Suspense; co-dir. film, Lady Possessed.
TV: The Clock, 1951; Fred Waring, Omnibus, 1952–53; Medallion Theatre, Willy, 1954–55; Perry Mason, 1956; scripts for Omnibus, The Clock, 20th Century-Fox Hour, The Lineup, Reader's Digest, Passing Parade, Alfred Hitchcock, Steve Canyon, Peter Gunn, Desilu, Playhouse 90, The Untouchables, 77 Sunset Strip, Bourbon Street, Dragnet, Richard Diamond, CIC, The Islanders, Thin Man, etc.

Winner of Peabody Award, Look Magazine, Mystery Writers of America, Writers' Guild Award, best hour script of 1961.

SPIKINGS, BARRY: Executive. b. 1939. Ent. m.p. ind. 1963. Jnt. Mang. Dir. British Lion Films Ltd., 1975. Co-prod. Conduct Unbecoming, Man Who Fell to Earth, 1976. Appt. jnt. man. dir. EMI Films Ltd., 1977. Prod. The Deer Hunter, Convoy. 1979, appt. chm. & chief exec., EMI Film & Theatre Corp.; chm. & chief exec, EMI Films, Ltd., chm. EMI Cinemas, Ltd.; chm., Elstree Studios, Ltd. Chm. EMI-TV Programs, Inc., 1980, appt. chm. chief exec., EMI Films Group.

SPIRA, STEVEN S.: Executive. e. City College, New York; Benjamin Cardozo School of Law. Associated 10 years with N.Y. law firm, Monasch, Chazen & Stream. 1984, joined 20th Century Fox as sr. counsel; 1985, to Warner Bros. Now WB v.p., studio business affairs.

SPIRES, JOHN B.: Executive. b. New York, N.Y. e. N.Y.U. Assistant manager Tribune Theatre, N.Y., 1934–36; Paramount Pictures lab., 1936–42; Capt. U.S. Army, 1942–46; Major U.S. Reserves, 1946–48; foreign rep., RKO, Europe, 1946; asst. foreign mgr., United World Films, 1947–48; in charge 16mm foreign oper., Universal 1949; asst. to European gen. mgr., Universal International, 1950; European gen. mgr., Continental Europe, Near East, Universal International, 1955; gen. mgr., foreign film sales, MCA-TV, 1958; dir., TV sis., 1964; named v.p. of MGM-TV, 1973; snr. v.p., MGM-TV, UK, Europe, MGM-TV, 1961; dir., Int'l TV sis., MGM-TV, 1978. Founded Phoenix Intl. TV Associates, 1980; pres., Phoenix Intl.

SPITZ, HENRY: Producer. b. Paterson, N.J., Mar. 4, 1905. e. N.Y.M.A. Gen. mgr., Quackenbush Dept. Stores; on bd. Preakness Hill Country Club & Barnet Memorial Hosp.; v.p. Marshall-Matherson dept. store, 1930–34; ent. m.p. ind. as prod. & bus. mgr., Cameo, 1935; assoc. prod., Cameo-Imperial Pictures, 1936; asst. prod. mgr. & asst. dir. Conn Prod.; asst., prod. mgr. Universal.
PICTURES INCLUDE: I Demand Payment, High Hat, Here's Flash Casey, Headleys at Home, Hawaiian Nights, Private Affairs; assoc. prod. Two Dollar Bettor, Sabre Jet, Commanche.

SPITZ, JAMES R.: Executive. Began career in industry 1962 with Warner Bros., working way thru sls. dept. and holding various positions such as booker and office mgr. in New York, San Francisco, Salt Lake City, Seattle and Kansas City. Appt. branch mgr. of WB Seattle-Portland branch; then L.A. branch mgr. Worked at United Artists 1972–77, first as L.A. branch mgr. and then western div. mgr. Joined Avco Embassy as asst. gen. sls. mgr., 1979. In 1980 left to go to Columbia Pictures as v.p. & gen. sls. mgr. In 1981 promoted to pres. of Columbia Pictures' domestic distribution.

SPITZER, MARIAN: Writer. b. New York City. e. NYU. m. Harlan Thompson, writer. Was reporter on Brooklyn Times, then N.Y. Globe, in dramatic dept. Did publicity for B.F. Keith Circuit, Shubert & Edgar Selwyn. First short story pub. in 1924 by Smart Set. Novels include Who Would Be Freed? and A Hungry Young Lady. Was in editorial dept. Fox, then contract writer. Became asst. to chmn. of ed. board. Paramount.
PICTURES INCLUDE: Dolly Sisters, Look for the Silver Lining.

SPIVAK, LAWRENCE E.: TV-radio producer. b. New York City, 1900. e. Harvard U. LL.D. (hon.) Wilberforce U.; Litt. D. (hon.) Suffolk U. L.H.D. (hon.) Tampa U. Began as bus. mgr., Antiques Mag., 1921–30; asst. to the pub., Hunting and Fishing, Nat. Sportsman mags., 1930–33; bus. mgr., American Mercury, 1934–39; pub., 1939–44; editor, pub., 1944–50; founder, pub. until 1954, Ellery Queen's Mystery Mag., The Mag. of Fantasy and Science Fiction, Mercury Mystery Books, Bookseller Mysteries, Jonathan Press Books; producer, panel member, TV program, Meet the Press. Recipient two Peabody Awards. Winner of Emmy Award for outstanding achievement in Coverage of Special Events and Honor Award from University of Missouri for Distinguished Service in Journalism.

SPODICK, ROBERT C.: Exhibitor. b. New York City, Dec. 3, 1919; e. CCNY, 1940; ent. m.p. ind. as errand boy Skouras Park Plaza, Bronx 1932–33; reel boy, asst. mgr., Loew's Theatres; mgr., Little Carnegie and other art theatres; exploitation man, United Artists. Acquired Lincoln, New Haven art house in 1945 in partnership with cousin Leonard E. Sampson; developed Nutmeg Theatre circuit, which was sold in 1968 to Robert Smerling. Now operates in Groton, CT., Cinemas I and II; Norwich Cinemas I and II, Village Cinemas I, II and III in Mystic in Partnership with Sampson and William Rosen, and Westerley Triple Cinemas in Rhode Island; also York Square Triple Cinemas in New Haven. Pres., Allied of Conn., 1962–64; Pres. NATO of Conn. 1968–73. Past chm. exec. comm., Conn. Ass'n of Theatre Owners.

SPRADLIN, G.D.: Actor. b. Oklahoma. Started career as lawyer and active in local politics before turning to acting. Joined Oklahoma Repertory Theatre in 1964. Film debut in Will Penny.
PICTURES INCLUDE: Monte Walsh, Tora! Tora! Tora!, The Hunting Party, The Godfather, Part II, North Dallas Forty, MacArthur, Wrong Is Right, The Formula, Apocalypse Now, The Lords of Discipline.
TELEVISION: Space.

SPRINGER, PAUL D.: Executive. e. Brooklyn Law School. Served as assoc. for N.Y. law firm, Johnson and Tannebaum. Later with legal dept. of Columbia Pictures. 1970, joined Paramount Pictures N.Y. legal dept. 1985, promoted to sr. v.p., chief resident counsel, responsible for all legal functions for corp. on east coast. Mbr., N.Y. Bar.

SPRINGFIELD, RICK: Actor-Singer-Songwriter. b. Australia, Aug. 23, 1949.
PICTURES: Battlestar Galactica, Hard to Hold (act., addl. music).
TELEVISION: General Hospital, An Evening at the Improv, Countdown '81.

SPRINGSTEEN, R. G.: Director. b. Tacoma, Wash., Sept. 8, 1904; e. U. Washington. With Universal Studios 1930; asst. dir. Fox; asst. dir. & dir. Republic.
PICTURES INCLUDE: Out of the Storm, Hellfire, Red Menace, Singing Guns, Honeychile, Toughest Man in Arizona, Gobs & Gals, Perilous Journey, Geraldine, I Cover the Underworld, Cross Channel, When Gangland Strikes, Come Next Spring, Track the Man Down, Secret Venture, Double Jeopardy, Johnny Reno, Red Tomahawk.

STACK, ROBERT: Actor. b. Los Angeles, Calif., Jan. 13, 1919; e. U. So. Calif.; dramatic school. In U.S. Armed Forces, WW II.
PICTURES INCLUDE: First Love, When the Daltons Rode, Mortal Storm, Little Bit of Heaven, Nice Girls, Badlands of Dakota, To Be or Not To Be, Eagle Squadron, Men of Texas, Fighter Squadron, Date With Judy, Miss Tatlock's Millions, Mr. Music, Bullfighter and the Lady, My Outlaw Brother, Bwana Devil, War Paint, Conquest of Cochise, Sabre Jet, Iron Glove, High & the Mighty, House of Bamboo, Good Morning Miss Dove, Great Day in the Morning, Written on the Wind, John Paul Jones, Last Voyage, Killers of Killimanjaro, The Caretakers, The Corrupt Ones, Story of a Woman, 1941, Airplane!, Uncommon Valor, Big Trouble.
TV: The Untouchables, Name of the Game, George Washington, Hollywood Wives.

STAHL, AL: Executive. Syndicated newspaper cartoonist; asst. animator, Max Fleischer, gag ed. Terrytoons; U.S. Signal Corps; opened own studios, 1946; prod. first animated TV cartoon show; pres., Animated Prod., prod. live and animated commercials; member of bd. NTFC.

STALLONE, SYLVESTER: Actor-Writer. b. New York City, July 6, 1946. After high school taught at American College of Switzerland instructing children of career diplomats, young royalty, etc. Returned to U.S. in 1967 and graduated form Univ. of Miami in 1969. Came to New York to seek acting career, taking part-time jobs, including usher for Walter Reade Theatres. Then turned to writing, selling several TV scripts. Back to acting with lead role in The Lords of Flatbush.
PICTURES INCLUDE: Capone, Death Race 2000, Rocky (also s.p.), F.I.S.T. (actor, co. s.p.), Paradise Alley (actor, s.p., dir). Rocky II (actor, s.p., dir.), Nighthawks, Victory, Rocky III (s.p.-dir.-actor); First Blood (co-s.p.-actor), Staying Alive (p., dir., s.p.); Rhinestone (actor, co-s.p.); Rambo: First Blood Part II (actor, co-s.p.); Rocky IV (s.p.-dir.-actor); Cobra (s.p.-actor).

STAMP, TERENCE: Actor. b. London, England, 1938. After stage experience. Alfie On Broadway. Recent stage: Dracula, The Lady from the Sea.
PICTURES INCLUDE: Billy Budd, Term of Trial, The Collector, Modesty Blaise, Far from the Madding Crowd, Poor Cow, Blue, Tales of Mystery, Theorem, The Mind of Mr. Soames, A Season in Hell, Hu-Man, The Divine Creature, Strip-Tease, Superman, Meetings With Remarkable Men, The Thief of Baghdad, Together, Superman II, Death in the Vatican, The Hit, Link, Legal Eagles.

STANDER, LIONEL: Actor. b. New York City. e. coll.; N.Y. stage, 1952. On TV in Hart to Hart.
PICTURES INCLUDE: Scoundrel, Page Miss Glory, Gay Deception, Music Goes 'Round, Mr. Deeds Goes to Town, Meet Nero Wolfe, Guadalcanal Diary, Big Show-Off, Specter of the Rose, In Old Sacramento, Kid From Brooklyn, Gentleman Joe Palooka, Pal Joey, Mad Wednesday, Call Northside 777, Unfaithfully Yours, Trouble Makers, Two Gals and a Guy, St. Benny the Dip, Cul de Sac, A Dandy in Aspic, The Gang That Couldn't Shoot Straight, Pulp, The Black Bird, The Cassandra Crossing, New York, New York, Matilda, 1941.

STANFILL, DENNIS C: Executive. b. Centerville, Tenn., April 1, 1927; e. Lawrenceburg H.S.; B.S., U.S. Naval Academy, 1949; M.A., Oxford U. (Rhodes scholar) 1953; L.H.D. (hon.) U. South Carolina. Corporate finance specialist, Lehman Brothers 1959–65; v.p. finance, Times Mirror Company, Los Angeles, 1965–69; exec. v.p. finance, 20th Century-Fox Film Corp., 1969–71, pres., 1971, chmn. bd./chief exec. officer, 1971–81; pres., Stanfill, Doig & Co., venture capital firm, 1981–.

STANG, ARNOLD: Performer, b. Chelsea, Mass., Sept. 28, 1927. Radio, 1935–50; on B'way, in five plays and in m.p. and short subjects; guest appearances on TV shows.
TV: Milton Berle, Danny Thomas, Perry Como, Ed Sullivan, Red Skelton, Frank Sinatra, Wagon Train, Top Cat, Batman, Bonanza, Bob Hope, Danny Kaye, Broadside, Jackie Gleason, Emergency, Feeling Good, Chico & The Man, Super Jaws & Catfish, Busting Loose, Flying High, Robert Klein Specials.
PICTURES INCLUDE: Man with the Golden Arm, The Wonderful World of the Brothers Grimm, It's a Mad, Mad, Mad, Mad World, Pinocchio in Outer Space, Dondi, Alakazam the Great, Hello Down There, Skidoo, Walt Disney's Aristocats, Raggedy Ann & Andy, Gang That Couldn't Shoot Straight, We Go Pogo, That's Life.

STANLEY, KIM: Actress. b. Tularss, NM, Feb. 11, 1925. r.n. Patricia Reid.
PICTURES: The Goddess, Seance on a Wet Afternoon, Frances, The Right Stuff.
TELEVISION: Clash by Night, The Travelling Lady, A Cardinal Mercy, Cat on a Hot Tin Roof.

STANLEY, PHYLLIS: Actress. b. London, England, Oct. 30. e. Beauclair Sch., London. On London stage in 1932–35.
STAGE: The Miracle, Words & Music, The Town Talks, Oh! You Letty, Happy Returns, Lights Up.
PICTURES INCLUDE: Side Street Angel (m.p. debut), St. Martin's Lane, Jeannie, One Exciting Night, Next of Kin, The Case of Lady Brooke, Lovely to Look At, Take Me To Town, Her 12 Men, Strange Lady in Town, Black Sleep, Seventh Veil.
TV: Fireside Theatre, Ford Theatre, Four Star Playhouse (Schlitz Playhouse, Lux Video Theatre, Matinee Theatre).

STANTON, HARRY DEAN: Actor. b. Kentucky, July 14, 1926. Acting debut at Pasadena Playhouse. Theatrical film debut in Tomahawk Trail (1957).
PICTURES INCLUDE: The Proud Rebel, Pork Chop Hill, A Dog's Best Friend, Cool Hand Luke, Kelly's Heroes, Two-Lane Blacktop, Pat Garrett and Billy the Kid, Dillinger, Zandy's Bride, The Godfather Part II, Rancho Deluxe, Farewell, My Lovely, The Missouri Breaks, Private Benjamin, Escape from New York, Young Doctors in Love, Tough Enough, Christine, Paris Texas, One Magic Christmas, Pretty in Pink, Fool for Love.

STANWYCK, BARBARA: Actress. r.n. Ruby Stevens; b. Brooklyn, N.Y., July 16, 1907. Film debut, Locked Door, 1929.
PICTURES INCLUDE: Ladies of Leisure, Night Nurse, So Big, Bitter Tea of General Yen, Brief Moment, Woman in Red, Annie Oakley, Plough and the Stars, Stella Dallas, Mad Miss Manton, Union Pacific, Golden Boy, Meet John Doe, Two Mrs. Carrolls, B.F.'s Daughter, Sorry, Wrong Number, Lady Gambles, East Side, West Side, Thelma Jordan, The Furies, No Man of Her Own, to Please a Lady, Man With a Cloak, Clash by Night, Jeopardy, All I Desire, Titanic, Blowing Wild, The Moonlighter, Executive Suite, Witness to Murder, Violent Men, Double Indemnity, Ball of Fire, Cattle Queen of Montana, Escape to Burma, There's Always Tomorrow, Maverick Queen, These Wilder Years, Crime of Passion, Trooper Hook, Forty Guns, Walk on the Wild Side, Roustabout, The Night Walker.
TV: Guest, Jack Benny, Ford, Zane Grey, Alcoa-Goodyear; 4 yrs., 1965–69, The Big Valley, The Thorn Birds (Emmy award), The Colbys.

STAPLETON, JEAN: Actress. b. New York City, Jan. 19, 1923. e. Wadleigh High School. Summer stock in New Hampshire, Maine, Mass., and Penna. First Broadway appearance in In the Summer House.
PICTURES: Damn Yankees, Bells Are Ringing, Something Wild, Up the Down Staircase, Cold Turkey, Klute, The Buddy System.
TV: All in the Family. Movies: Eleanor: First Lady of the World, A Matter of Sex, Dead Man's Folly.

STAPLETON, MAUREEN: Actress. b. Troy, N.Y., June 21, 1925. Studied acting with Herbert Berghof in N.Y. in 1944 and became member of Actors Studio. Broadway debut, 1946, in The Playboy of the Western World. Other early roles in: Antony and Cleopatra, Detective Story, The Bird Cage. Became a star in 1951 in The Rose Tattoo and later acted in 27 Wagons Full of Cotton, Orpheus Descending, The Glass Menagerie. m.p. debut 1949 in Lonelyhearts. Recent play: Gingerbread Play (Tony Award), 1970–71.
PICTURES INCLUDE: Fugitive Kind, View form the Bridge, Bye Bye Birdie, Airport, Plaza Suite, Interiors, The Runner Stumbles, On the Right Track, Reds, Johnny Dangerously, Cocoon, The Money Pit, Made in Heaven.
TV: Movies: Tell Me Where It Hurts, Queen of the Stardust Ballroom, Cat on a Hot Tin Roof, Family Secrets, Sentimental Journey.

STARGER, MARTIN: Executive. e. N.Y. City Coll. Serviced in U.S. Army Signal Corp., where prod. training films. Joined BBDO, starting in TV prod. dept.; later made v.p. & assoc. dir. of TV. Joined ABC in April 1966, as v.p. of programs, ABC-TV, East Coast. In March, 1968, prom. to v.p. and natl prog. dir; in 1969 named v.p. in chg. progr. Named pres., ABC Entertainment, July 17, 1972. In June, 1975 formed Marstar Productions Inc., M.P. & TV production company of which he is pres. In March 1978 formed Marble Arch Productions, of which he is pres. In 1984 produced Mask.

STARK, RAY: Producer. e. Rutgers U. Began career after WWII as agent handling radio scripts, and later literary works for such writers as Costain, Marquand and Hecht. Joined Famous Artists Agency, where he represented such personalities as Marilyn Monroe, Kirk Douglas and Richard Burton; in 1957, resigned exec. position to form Seven Arts Prods. with Eliot Hyman, serving as exec. v.p. and head of production until July, 1966, when he left to take on personal production projects, including Reflections in a Golden Eye and Funny Girl.
PICTURES: The Sunshine Boys, Robin and Marian, Murder by Death, Casey's Shadow, The Cheap Detective, California Suite, The Electric Horseman, Chapter Two, Seems Like Old Times, Annie, The Slugger's Wife.

STARK, WILBUR: Producer-Director. b. New York City, Aug. 10, 1922. e. Columbia Univ. Started career as actor, Brooklyn Academy Players; slsm. & producer radio station WMCA-NY, 1942–46; for 18 yrs. producer-director of theatrical feature films and over 1500 live dramas and over 300 TV movies, including 81 for CBS as producer (directing over 30).
PICTURES: The Thing (exec. prod.); The Cat People, (exec. consultant); My Lover, My Son (prod., story); Vampire Circus (prod., story); The Love Box (prod., dir. s.p.); A Policeman's Lot (prod., dir); All I Want Is You, and You . . . (prod.).
TELEVISION: Newsstant Theatre, ABC: Rocky King, Detective, Dumong; Modern Romances with Martha Scott, NBC; Truse Story, NBC, Col. Humphrey Flack, My Father Is a Detective, etc.

STARR, EVE: Columnist. b. Chicago, Ill., May 1. e. Columbia Univ., Miami Univ., Julliard Sch. of Music. Radio-TV playwright, feature writer, actress. Hollywood foreign correspondent; m.p. writer, newspapers, mags.; m.p. columnist, Hollywood Citizen-News; Daily syndicated TV column, Inside TV—General Features Synd.; feature column, Tell It To Eve, International Newspapers; Traveling With Eve, Nat'l Syndicated Travel Column.

STARR, RINGO: Singer-Musician-Songwriter. b. Liverpool, England, July 7, 1949. Member of The Beatles.
PICTURES ALONE: Actor: The Last Waltz, Sextette, The Kids Are Alright, Caveman, Give My Regards to Broad Street.
TELEVISION: Actor: Princess Daisy.

STEEL, ANTHONY: Actor. b. London, Eng., May 21, 1920; e. private schools, South Ireland & Cambridge. Film debut in Saraband for Dead Lovers.
PICTURES INCLUDE: Portrait from Life, Christopher Columbus, Helter Skelter, Poet's Pub, The Blue Lamp, The Wooden Horse, Laughter in Paradise, The Mudlark, Where No Vultures Fly (Ivory Hunter), Another Man's Poison, Emergency Call, Something Money Can't Buy, The Planter's Wife (Outpost in Malaya), Malta Story, Master of Ballantrae, Albert, R.N. (Break to Freedom), West of Zanzibar, Sea Shall Not Have Them, Passage Home, Storm Over the Nile, Black Tent, Checkpoint, Valerie, A Question of Adultery, Harry Black, Honeymoon, The Switch, The Mirror Crack'd.

STEEL, DAWN: Executive. Joined Paramount Pictures 1978 as dir. of merchandising and licensing; promoted 1979 to v.p. 1980, named v.p., production; 1983, promoted to sr. v.p. 1985, named pres., prod.

STEELE, TOMMY: Performer. b. London, 1936. Early career Merchant Navy. First TV and film appearances, 1956. Composed and sang title song for The Shiralee. Recent Stage Musical: Singin' in the Rain, London Palladium, 1983.
PICTURES INCLUDE: Kill Me Tomorrow, The Tommy Steele Story, The Duke Wore Jeans, Tommy the Toreador, Light Up the Sky, It's All Happening, The Happiest Millionaire, Half A Sixpence, Finian's Rainbow, Where's Jack?
TV: Tommy Steele Spectaculars, Richard Whittington Esquire (Rediffusion), Ed Sullivan Show, Gene Kelly Show, Perry Como Show, Twelfth Night, The Tommy Steele Hour,

Tommy Steele in Search of Charlie Chaplin, Tommy Steele And A Show, Quincy's Quest.

STEENBURGEN, MARY: Actress. b. Newport, AZ, 1953. Studied at Neighborhood Playhouse.
PICTURES: Goin' South, Time after Time, Melvin and Howard (AA), Ragtime, A Midsummer Night's Sex Comedy, Cross Creek, One Magic Christmas.
TELEVISION: Tender Is the Night.

STEIGER, ROD: Actor. b. Westhampton, N.Y., Apr. 14, 1925; e. Westside H.S., Newark, N.J. Served in U.S. Navy, then employed in Civil Service; studied acting at N.Y. Theatre Wing Dramatic Workshop Actors' Studio; numerous TV plays; on Broadway in ANTA prod. of Night Music; m.p. debut in On the Waterfront.
PICTURES INCLUDE: Big Knife, Oklahoma! Court Martial of Billy Mitchell, Jubal, Harder They Fall, Back from Eternity, Run of the Arrow, Unholy Wife, Al Capone, Seven Thieves, The Mark, Reprieve, 13 West Street, Hands Upon the City, The Time of Indifference, The Pawnbroker, In the Heat of the Night, The Girl and the General, No Way to Treat a Lady, And There Came a Man, The Illustrated Man, Three Into Two Won't Go, Duck, You Sucker, Happy Birthday, Wanda June, Waterloo, The Lolly-Madonna War, Lucky Luciano, Hennessy, W. C. Fields and Me, F.I.S.T., The Amityville Horror, Lion of the Desert, Cattle Annie and Little Britches, The Chosen, The Naked Face.
TELEVISION: Race to the Pole, Hollywood Wives, etc.

STEIN, JOSEPH L.: Attorney. b. Portland, Me.; e. NYU, NYU Law Sch., LL.B. Admitted to N.Y. Bar. Specialist in copyright and m.p. law . Member of Sargoy & Stein, New York until Dec. 1970 when he retired, becoming counsel to firm. Compilers and annual revisers of U.S. Copyright Law Digest for Martindale-Hubbell Law Directory. Special counsel nationally for ten major m.p. dist. cos. in copyright & dist. matters. Former member: American Bar Assn. and of its Copyright Subsection's Committees on Anti-Trust Matters, 1951–54, on Copyright Office Affairs. 1953–55, 1959–63, 1966–67, on Copyright Law Revision, 1955–56, 1963–65, on Int. Copyrights, 1956–57, 1966–67, on Cooperation with Other Sections, 1956–57, on authors, 1959–61, and on Related Rights, 1957–59; American Patent Law Assn.: American Judicature Society; National Panel of Arbitrators of American Arbitration Assn.; American Society of International Law; American Foreign Law Soc.; Assn. of the Bar of City of New York; N.Y. County Lawyers' Assn.; N.Y. State Bar Assn.; Fed. Bar Assn. of N.Y., N.J. & Conn.; dir., N.Y. Tuberculosis & Health Assn., Inc.

STEIN, RONALD: Composer, conductor, pianist, teacher, filmmaker. b. St. Louis, Mo., April 12, 1930. e. Washington Univ., St. Louis, 1947–51, Yale Univ., New Haven, 1951–52, U.S.C., Los Angeles, 1960–63 U.S. Army, 1952–54. Music director's asst. Municipal Opera, St. Louis, 1950–51, 1954; asst. music dir., Greek Theatre, 1955; assoc. mus. dir., Phoenix Star Theatre, 1964; asst. prof. of music, Calif. State Univ. at Northridge, 1960–61; 83 m.p. scores since 1955; Documentary film director, writer, editor, photographer. U.S. Educational Films (Administrator). Professor of Music, Univ. Colorado, 1980–85; v.p. creative affairs, Techrev Communications.
PICTURES INCLUDE: The Littlest Hobo, Raymie, Legend of Tom Dooley, A Man Called Dagger, Premature Burial, Of Love and Desire, Dime With A Halo, Psych-Out, Dementia 13, The Rain People, Getting Straight, The Prisoners, Stalemate, Frankenstein's Great Aunt Tillie. Dateline Yesterday TV series, (Editorial Supervisor). National Parks—A Road For The Future (Photographer, Editor), The Eye of The Mind (Writer, Director).

STEINBERG, HERB: b. New York, N.Y. July 3, 1921; e. CCNY, 1937–41. Capt. U.S. Army, 1942–46; pub. PRC, 1946, Eagle Lion, 1946–49, Paramount 1949; pub. mgr. 1951; expl. mgr., 1954; studio adv. & pub. dir., 1958; exec. chg. of spec. proj., press dept., Universal City Studio, 1963; v.p., Universal Studio Tours, 1971; 1974 v.p., MCA Recreation Services. Appt. to California Tourism Commission, 1984.

STEINMAN, MONTE: Executive. Joined Paramount Pictures 1980 as sr. financial analyst. Series of promotions followed, culminating in appt. as dir. of financial planning of Gulf & Western's Entertainment and Communications Group, in February, 1984. In 1985, named exec. dir., financial planning.

STELLOFF, SKIP: Producer. b. N.Y.C., Aug. 10, 1925, e. U.S. Naval Academy; U.S. Navy, 1943–51; WWDC Radio, Wash., D.C., 1951–52; Ziv Television, 1952–56; sls. mgr., C&C Television, 1956–58; pres., Heritage Productions, 1958–60.

STEMBLER, JOHN H.: Executive. b. Miami, Fla., Feb. 18, 1913; e. U. of Florida Law School, 1937. Asst. U.S. att., South. dist. of Fla., 1941; U.S. Air Force, 1941–45; pres. Georgia Theatre Co., 1957; named chm., 1983; NATO member exec. comm. and past pres.; Major Gen. USAF (Ret); past bd. chm., National Bank of Georgia.

STEMBLER, WILLIAM J.: Executive. b. Atlanta, GA Nov. 29, 1946. e. Westminister Schools (1964); Univ. of Florida (1968); Univ. of Ga. Law School (1971). 1st. lt. USA Army, 1971; capt., U.S. Army Reserve; resigned 1976. Enforcement atty., SEC, Atlanta office, 1972–73; joined Georgia Theatre Co., 1973; pres. since 1983.
MEMBER: bd. of dir., Natl. Bank of Ga.; bd. of dir., & v.p., NATO, 1983–present; mbr., NATO OF Ga. & past-pres., 1983–85.

STEPHEN, SUSAN: Actress. b. London, Eng., July 16, 1931; e. Eastbourne and Royal Acad. of Dramatic Art. Screen debut in His Excellency, 1951.
PICTURES INCLUDE: Stolen Face, Treasurer Hunt, Father's Doing Fine, Luxury Girls, The Red Beret (Paratrooper), House Across the Lake, Private Man, Golden Ivory, For Better For Worse, As Long As They're Happy, Value for Money, His Excellency, Pacific Destiny, Barretts of Wimpole Street, Carry on Nurse.
TV: Little Women, Birdcage Room, No Hero, Pillars of Midnight.

STERLING, JAN: Actress. r.n. Jane Sterling Adriance. b. April 3, 1923. e. Private tutors; Fay Compton Sch. of Dramatic Art, London. N.Y. stage debut: Bachelor Born.
STAGE: Panama Hattie, Present Laughter, John Loves Mary, Two Blind Mice, Front Page, Over 21, Born Yesterday.
PICTURES INCLUDE: Johnny Belinda (debut), Appointment with Danger, Mating Season, Union Station, Skipper Surprised His Wife, Big Carnival, Caged, Rhubarb, Flesh and Fury, Sky Full of Moon, Pony Express, The Vanquished, Split Second, Alaska Seas, High & the Mighty, Return From the Sea, Human Jungle, Women's Prison, Female on the Beach, Man with the Gun, 1984, The Harder They Fall, Love in a Goldfish Bowl, The Incident, The Minx.

STERLING, ROBERT: Actor. r.n. William Sterling Hart; b. Newcastle, Pa., Nov. 13, 1917; e. U. of Pittsburgh; m. Anne Jeffreys, actress. Fountain pen salesman, day laborer, clerk, industrial branch credit mgr., clothing salesman on West Coast; served as pilot-instructor U.S. Army Corps. 3 yrs.
PICTURES INCLUDE: Blondie Meets the Boss, Only Angels Have Wings, Manhattan Heartbeat, Yesterday's Heroes, Gay Caballero, Penalty, I'll Wait for You, Get-Away, Ringside Maisie, Two-Faced Woman, Dr. Kildare's Victory, Johnny Eager, This Time for Keeps, Somewhere I'll Find You, Secret Heart, Roughshod, Bunco Squad, Sundowners, Show Boat, Column South.
TV: Topper.

STERN, ALFRED E. F.: Public relations executive. b. Boston, Mass., Aug. 4. e. Boston U. Reporter, editor, Lowell Sun, Quincy Patriot-Ledger, Dartmouth News; publicist, RKO Radio Pictures, 1946–54; publicity dir., 1955; West Coast publicity dir., NTA, 1958; own public relations org., Alfred E. F. Stern Co., Inc., 1960.

STERN, DANIEL: Actor. b. Bethesda, MD, 1957.
PICTURES: Breaking Away, It's My Turn, One-Trick Pony, Stardust Memories, I'm Dancing As Fast As I Can, Blue Thunder, Get Crazy, Hannah and Her Sisters.

STERN, EDDIE: Film buyer. b. New York City, Jan. 13, 1917. e. Columbia Sch. of Journalism; head film buyer and booker, specializing in art theatres, for Rugoff and Becker, N.Y.; Captain, USAF; joined Wometco Ent. in 1952 as asst. to film buyer; v.p. motion picture theatre film buying and booking, Wometco Enterprises, Inc. Retired from Wometco 1985. Now handling film buying and booking for Theatres of Nassau, Ltd.

STERN, EZRA E.: Attorney. b. New York, N.Y., Mar. 22, 1908. e. Southwestern U. 1930, LL.B.; pres., Wilshire Bar Assn. Former legal counsel for So. Calif. Theatre Owners Association. Member: Calif. State Bar; member, Int'l Variety Clubs; former chief barker, Variety Club So. Calif. Tent 25; pres., Variety Int'l Boys' Club; board of dir., Los Angeles Metropolitan Recreation & Youth Services Council; bd. of trustees, Welfare Planning Council, Los Angeles Region; former mem. Los Angeles Area Council, Boys' Club of America; pres., Variety International Boys' Club 1976–77 and 1979–80. Member bd., Will Rogers Institute, M.P. Pioneers. 1984, honored by Variety Boys and Girls Club as founder of youth recreational facility.

STERN, STANLEY L.: Executive. b. Philadelphia, Dec. 31, 1917. Major, USAF, World War II & Korea. Entire working career with Wometco Enterprises, starting as usher in 1933. Served as theatre mgr., m.p. booker, in chg. of real estate and insurance, before taking over Wometco Theatre Division in 1973. Elected v.p., 1959, sr. v.p., in 1967, dir. in 1972. Placed in chg. Wometco Entertainment Division, 1976. Named pres., Wometco Theatres, 1982. Retired in 1985.

MEMBER: VCI, Tent 33, Motion Picture Pioneers; v.p. and dir., NATO. Bd. member, Dade County Chapter, Red Cross.

STERN, STEWART: Writer. b. New York, N.Y., Mar. 22, 1922. e. Ethical Culture Schools, 1927–40; U. of Iowa, 1940–43; Rifle Squad Leader, S/Sgt. 106th Inf. Div., 1943–45; actor, asst. stage mgr., The French Touch, B'way, 1945–46; dialogue dir. Eagle-Lion Studios, 1946–48. 1948 to date: screenwriter.
TV: (Plays) Crip, And Crown Thy Good, Thunder of Silence, Heart of Darkness, Sybil.
PICTURES INCLUDE: Teresa, Benjy (orig. s.p.) Rebel Without a Cause, The Rack, The James Dean Story, The Outsider, The Ugly American, Rachel, Rachel, The Last Movie, Summer Wishes—Winter Dreams (orig. s.p.).

STERNAD, RUDOLPH: Producer, designer, art director. b. N.Y., Oct. 6, 1905. e. Cooper Union Inst., 1922–23; Beaux Arts, 1924; Chouinand, 1925; arch. designer, Society M.P. Art Directors; designer, MGM, Fox, United Artists, Univ. Studios, 1926–34; art dir., 20th-Fox, Old Chicago, Suez, etc. 1934–40; art dir. Columbia Studios, More the Merrier, Talk of the Town, Craig's Wife, 1001 Nights, You Were Never Lovelier, etc.; prod. designer, Stanley Kramer Prod., 1948–62.
PICTURES INCLUDE: Champion, Home of the Brave, The Men, Cyrano de Bergerac, High Noon, Death of a Salesman, Four Poster, Caine Murder, Not as a Stranger, The Defiant Ones, On the Beach, Judgment at Nuremberg, Pressure Point, A Child Is Waiting, It's a Mad, Mad, Mad, Mad World.

STEVENS, ANDREW: Actor. b. Memphis, Tenn., 1956. Son of actress Stella Stevens. e. Memphis Messick H.S. Studied acting with Strasberg, David Craig, Vincent Chase, and Robert Easton. Began on TV, later playing in feature films.
PICTURES INCLUDE: Shampoo, Day of the Animals, Vigilante Force, The Boys in Company C, The Fury, Death Hunt, The Seduction.
TV: Adam-12, Apple's Way, The Quest, Police Story, Shazan, Once an Eagle (mini-series), Oregon Trail, Pumper One. Movies: S Secrets, The Last Survivors, The Werewolf of Woodstock, The Bastard (mini-series), The Rebels (mini-series), Beggarman Thief, Topper, Emerald Point NAS, Hollywood Wives.

STEVENS, CONNIE: Actress. r.n. Concerta Ann Ingolie. b. Brooklyn, N.Y., August 8, 1938. e. Sacred Heart Academy, Hollywood Professional School; began career as winner of several talent contests in Hollywood; prof. debut, Hollywood Repertory Theatre's prod. Finian's Rainbow; recordings include: Kookie, Kookie, Lend Me Your Comb, 16 Reasons, What Did You Make Me Cry For, From Me to You, They're Jealous of Me, A Girl Never Knows.
PICTURES INCLUDE: Eighteen and Anxious, Young and Dangerous, Drag Strip Riot, Rock-a-Bye Baby, Parish, Susan Slade, Palm Springs Weekend, Cruise A-Go-Go, The Grissom Gang, Last Generation, Grease 2.

STEVENS, CRAIG: Actor. b. Liberty, Mo.; e. U. Kansas. Played in coll. dramatics. On screen 1941 in Affectionately Yours.
PICTURES INCLUDE: Since You Went Away, The Doughgirls, Roughly Speaking, Too Young to Know, Humoresque, The Man I Love, That Way With Women, Night Unto Night, Love and Learn, Lady Takes a Sailor, Phone Call from a Stranger, French Line, Where the Sidewalk Ends, Duel on the Mississippi, The Name's Buchanan, Gunn, Limbo Line, The Snoop Sisters, "S.O.B.".
TV: Lux Video Theatre, Four Star Playhouse, Loretta Young Show, Schlitz Playhouse, Peter Gunn, Dinah Shore, Ernie Ford Shows, Chevvy Show, Summer on Ice, Person to Person, Man of the World series (ATV England); Mr. Broadway, The Millionaire, Name of the Game, The Bold Ones.
STAGE: Here's Love, King of Hearts, Plain and Fancy, Critics Choice, Mary Mary; Nat. Co. Cactus Flower.

STEVENS, GEORGE, JR.: Director—Writer—Producer. b. Los Angeles, Calif., Apr. 3, 1932, e. Occidental College, 1949–53, B.A., 1st Lieut. U.S. Air Force; TV dir., Alfred Hitchcock Presents, Peter Gunn, 1957–61; prod. asst. Giant Productions, 1953–54; prod. asst. Mark VII, Ltd., 1956–57; assoc. prod., dir., The Diary of Anne Frank, 1957–59; assoc. prod., dir., The Greatest Story Ever Told, 1959–62; dir. M.P. Service, U.S. Information Agency 1962–67; chmn., U.S. deleg. to Film Festivals at Cannes (1962, 1964), Venice (1962, 1963), Moscow (1963); prod. John F. Kennedy; Years of Lightning, Day of Drums. Founding director, American FilmInstitute, 1967–79; co-chm., American Film Institute, 1979 to present. Producer, America at the Movies (1976). Executive producer of The American Film Institute's Salute to James Cagney for which he was awarded an Emmy by National Academy of Television Arts and Sciences on May 19, 1975; producer/writer, American Film Institute's Salutes, 1973–84; executive producer, The Stars Salute America's Greatest Movies, 1977; producer/writer, The Kennedy Center Honors, 1978–85; producer/writer, America Entertains Vice Premier Deng, 1978. Exec. prod./s.p., Christmas in Washington, 1982–83; dir./writer/prod., George Stevens: A Filmmaker's Journey, 1984.

STEVENS, K. T.: Actress, r.n. Gloria Wood. b. Hollywood, Calif.; e. U. So. Calif.; d. late Sam Wood, director.
STAGE: You Can't Take It With You, The Man Who Came to Dinner, My Sister Eileen, Nine Girls, St. Joan.
PICTURES INCLUDE: (debut) Peck's Bad Boy, The Great Man's Lady, 1942; Nine Girls, Address Unknown, Kitty Foyle, Harriet Craig, Vice Squad, Tumbleweed, Missile to the Moon.

STEVENS, LEE: President, Chief Executive Officer, William Morris Agency, Inc. b. March 10, 1930, New York City. e. NYU School of Commerce, grad. 1951 BS; NYU Law School, grad. 1957, Jurist Doctor, member of NY bar. With William Morris Agency 33 years.

STEVENS, LESLIE: Executive, writer, producer, director. b. Wash., D.C., Feb. 3, 1924. e. Westminister School, London, Yale Drama School, American Theatre Wing, N.Y.C. Sold first play, The Mechanical Rat at 15; wrote six plays for summer stock groups, 1941–42; U.S. Air Force, 1943; pres., exec. prod. Daystar Prods.; writer, producer, director, film TV and features.
STAGE: Bullfight (off B'way) 1953–54; wrote, Broadway: Champagne Complex, 1954; The Lovers, 1956; The Marriage-Go-Round, 1958; The Pink Jungle, 1959.
TV: For Playhouse 90: Invitation to a Gunfighter, Charley's Aunt, Rumors of Evening, The Violent Heart, Portrait of a Murderer, The Second Man; Kraft TV Theatre, Duel; Four Star Playhouse, Award, Producers Showcase, Bloomer Girl; created, prod., dir. Stoney Burke, ABC series, 1962, created, prod., dir. Outer Limits, pilot It Takes a Thief; exec. prod. series, ABC; prod.-writer pilot McCloud, NBC; exec. prod. series; exec. prod. Men From Shiloh series; exec. prod., writer-dir., Name of the Game, Warner Bros. (Leslie Stevens Productions), 1971, prod.-writer, pilot of Search, exec. prod. of NBC: series creator, CATV series Movie of Today, Paperback Playhouse, Earthside Missile Base. Exec. prod., Universal Studios, Invisible Man, 1975. Supervising prod. Gemini Man, 1976 pilot and series.
PICTURES INCLUDE: author, The Left-Handed Gun 1958; co-prod.-wrote-dir. Private Property 1959; wrote, The Marriage-Go-Round 1960; wrote-prod.-dir. Hero's Island 1961.

STEVENS, MARK: Actor. r.n. Richard Stevens. b. Cleveland, Ohio, Dec. 13, 1922. e. privately; Beaux Arts and Sir George Williams Sch. of Fine Arts, Montreal. Had varied career before appearing on stage and radio in Canada; later joined station WAKB in Akron; then prod. mgr., WJW, Akron. Screen debut in Objective Burma.
PICTURES INCLUDE: God Is My Co-Pilot, Pride of the Marines, From This Day Forward, The Dark Corner, I Wonder Who's Kissing Her Now, Between Midnight and Dawn, Katie Did It, Little Egypt, Reunion in Reno, Mutiny, Big Frame, Torpedo Alley, Jack Slade, Cry Vengeance, Timetable, September Storm, Fate Is the Hunter, Frozen Alive, Sunscorched.
TV: Martin Kane, NBC; Big Town, NBC; prod., starred, script. Formed Mark Stevens Prod., Mark Stevens Television Prod., 1955.

STEVENS, STELLA: Actress. b. Hot Coffee, Mississippi, Oct. 1, 1938. e. Attended Memphis State University. Modeled in Memphis when she was discovered by talent scouts. Was briefly a term contract actress at 20th Century-Fox, later under exclusive contract to Paramount, then Columbia.
PICTURES INCLUDE: Say One For Me, The Blue Angel, Li'l Abner, Too Late Blues, Man Trap, The Courtship of Eddie's Father, The Nutty Professor, Advance to the Rear, Synanon, The Secret of My Success, The Silencers, The Ballad of Cable Hogue, Stand Up & Be Counted, Slaughter, The Poseidon Adventure, Arnold, Las Vegas Lady, Cleo Jones and the Casino of Gold, Nickelodeon, The Manitou, Wacko, Chained Heat, The Longshot.
TV: Five episodes of Ben Casey.

STEVENSON, PARKER: Actor. b. Philadelphia, June 4, 1953. e. Princeton Univ. Began professional acting career by starring in film, A Separate Peace, while high school senior, having attracted attention through work on TV commercials.
PICTURES INCLUDE: A Separate Peace (debut), Our Time, Lifeguard, Stroker Ace, Stitches.
TV: The Streets of San Francisco, Gunsmoke, Hardy Boys Mysteries. Guest and host on several talk shows and specials. Mini-Series: North & South Book II.

STEWART, ELAINE: Actress. b. Montclair, N.J., May 31, 1929. Usherette & cashier, m.p. theatre, Montclair; model, Conover Agcy., 1948; many TV shows; screen debut in Sailor Beward; Star of Tomorrow, 1954.
PICTURES INCLUDE: Sky Full of Moon, The Bad and the Beautiful, Desperate Search, Code Two, Slight Case of Larceny, Young Bess, Take the High Ground, Brigadoon,

Adventures of Hajji Baba, Tattered Dress, Rise and Fall of Legs Diamond, Most Dangerous Man Alive.

STEWART, HUGH: Producer. b. Falmouth, Cornwall, Dec. 14, 1910. e. Clayesmore School, St. John's College, Cambridge; ent. m.p. ind. 1932; editor, Gaumont British, 1932.
PICTURES INCLUDE: Man Who Knew Too Much, London Films: Dark Journey, Storm in a Teacup, Action for Slander, South Riding, Q Planes, Spy in Black. Army Service, 1939–45. Co-producer with Frank Capra of Anglo-US War Film, Tunisian Victory; True Glory. An Ideal Husband, Trottie True, Night Without Stars, Long Memory, Up to His Neck, Man of the Moment, Up in the World, Just My Luck, Innocent Sinners, The Square Peg, Follow a Star, Make Mine Mink, The Bulldog Breed, In the Doghouse, On the Beat, A Stitch in Time, The Intelligence Men, The Early Bird, That Riviera Touch, The Magnificent Two, All at Sea, Mr. Horatio Knibbles, Anoop and The Elephant, The Flying Sorcerer, The Chiffy Kids (two series), High Rise Donkey.

STEWART, JAMES: Actor. b. Indiana, Pa., May 20, 1908. e. Mercersburg Acad.; Princeton U. With Falmouth Stock Co., Cape Cod; on N.Y. stage in Goodbye Again; stage mgr. for Camille with Jane Cowl (Boston). Won Acad. Award for best performance 1940; joined U.S. Air Force 1942, commissioned Col. 1944. Voted one of top ten money-making stars; M.P. Herald-Fame poll, 1950, 52, 54, 57; No. 1 Money-Making Star, 1955. 1968, Screen Actors Guild Award. Mem.: Bd. of Trustees, Princeton U. Trustee, Claremont College; exec. bd. of Los Angeles Council of Boy Scouts of America, bd. of dirs., Project Hope.
STAGE: Spring in Autumn, All Good Americans, Yellow Jack, Journey at Night, Harvey.
PICTURES INCLUDE: Murder Man, Rose Marie, Wife vs. Secretary, Next Time We Love, Speed, Gorgeous Hussy, Born to Dance, Seventh Heaven, You Can't Take It With You, Vivacious Lady, Mr. Smith Goes to Washington, Philadelphia Story, It's A Wonderful World, Destry Rides Again, Shop Around the Corner, Mortal Storm, It's a Wonderful Life, Magic Town, Call Northside 777, Rope, You Gotta Stay Happy, Stratton Story, Malaya, Winchester '73, Broken Arrow, Harvey, Jackpot, No Highway in the Sky, Greatest Show on Earth, Carbine Williams, Bend of the River, Naked Spur, Thunder Bay, Glenn Miller Story, Far Country, Rear Window, Strategic Air Command, Man From Laramie, Man Who Knew Too Much, Spirit of St. Louis, Night Passage, Vertigo, Bell, Book and Candle, FBI Story, The Mountain Road, Two Rode Together, Man Who Shot Liberty Valance, Mr. Hobbs Takes a Vacation, How the West Was Won, Take Her, She's Mine, Cheyenne Autumn, Dear Brigitte, Shenandoah, The Rare Breed, Flight of the Phoenix, Firecreek, Bandolero, Cheyenne Social Club, Fool's Parade, That's Entertainment, The Shootist, Airport '77, The Big Sleep.
TV: Hawkins, 1973; Right of Way, 1984.

STEWART, JAMES L.: Executive. e. Univ. of So. Calif. (BA in cinema-TV and MBA in finance). Worked for two years in sales for CBS Radio Network—West Coast. Spent four years with MGM in promotion and marketing. With Walt Disney Prods. for 12 years, functioning in marketing, management and administrative activities; named v.p.-corp. relations & admin. asst. to pres. In 1978 joined in formation of Aurora Pictures, of which is exec. v.p., secty., & COO.
PICTURES: Exec. Prod.: Why Would I Lie?, The Secret of NIMH, Eddie and the Cruisers, Heart Like a Wheel, East of the Sun, West of the Moon, Maxie.

STEWART, KEN: Executive. First affiliated with Universal as asst. to head of trailers dept. Joined Paramount in 1981 as member of West Coast pub. dep.; later administrator, audio visual Services. 1984, appt. exec. dir. of creative services (New York).

STEWART, MARILYN: Public Relations Executive. b. New York City. e. Hunter College. Entered Ind. as scty. in 1960 to Si Seadler, MGM dir. of adv. Promoted in 1963 to asst. to Seadler. Left in 1964 to become prom.-pub. dir. for Verve/Folkways Records; duties also included a&r and talent scouting. In 1966 joined 20th-Fox as radio/tv pub. coordinator. In 1969 went to Para. Pictures as mag. pub. coordinator. Following year named worldwide director of pub. for Para., including creation of overall mkt. concepts, becoming 1st woman to be appointed to that position at major co. Campaigns included Love Story and The Godfather. In 1972 opened own consulting office specializing in m.p. marketing and p.r. Headquarters in N.Y.; repr. in L.A. Has represented American Film Theatre, The Lords of Flatbush, Bang the Drum Slowly, The Kids Are Alright, Autumn Sonata, The Tin Drum, L.A. Film Exposition, Michael Moriarty, Fred Schepisi, Lucasfilm, etc.

STEWART, MARTHA: Actress. r.n. Martha Haworth, b. Bardwell, Ky., Oct. 7, 1922; m. Joe E. Lewis, prof. vocalist, Glenn Miller and Claude Thornhill bands; appeared in Copacabana, N.Y.; star Lucky Strike Hit Parade, 1943. On screen first, 1945 Doll Face.
PICTURES INCLUDE: Johnny Comes Flying Home, I Wonder Who's Kissing Her Now, Daisy Kenyon, Are You With It?, Convicted, In a Lonely Place, Aaron Slick from Punkin Crick.

STEWART, PEGGY: Actress. b. West Palm Beach, Fla., June 5, 1923; in 1933 was champion swimmer, Georgia; acq. honors in horseback riding. Taught riding in Calif. at age of 14. On San Francisco stage: Great American Family, Goodnight Ladies.
PICTURES INCLUDE: Wells Fargo, That Certain Age, Back Street, All This and Heaven Too, Pride of Maryland, The Longhorn, Vengeance Trail, Kansas Territory, Montana Incident, The Way West, The Animals, Pickup on 101.

STIGWOOD, ROBERT: Executive. b. Adelaide, Australia, 1934. e. Sacred Heart College. Began career as copywriter for Aust. ad agency; at 21 left home for England. Series of first jobs led to his opening a London theatrical agency. Began casting commercials for TV; produced records for clients. Became first independent record producer in Great Britain. In mid '60s joined forces with Brian Epstein, manager of Beatles, to become co-mgr. of NEMS Enterprises. At Epstein's death formed own company, launching careers of such artists as Bee Gees, Cream, etc. Moved into theatre production in London: Hair, Jesus Christ Superstar, Pippin, Oh! Calcutta!, Evita. Entered film production with Jesus Christ Superstar. Formed RSO Records in 1973.
PICTURES INCLUDE: Jesus Christ Superstar, Tommy, Saturday Night Fever, Grease, Sgt. Pepper's Lonely Hearts Club Band, Moment by Moment, Times Square (co.-prod.), The Fan, Grease 2, Staying Alive.

STING: Musician-Actor. b. Newcastle-Upon-Tyne, England, 1951. r.n. Gordon Matthew Summer. e. Warwick Univ. A schoolteacher before helping form rock group, The Police.
PICTURES: Quadrophenia, Brimstone and Treacle, Dune, Plenty, Bring on the Night.

STOCKWELL, DEAN: Actor. b. Hollywood, Calif., Mar. 5, 1936. p. Harry and Betty Veronica Stockwell; e. L.I. public schools and Martin Milmore, Boston. On stage in Theatre Guild prod. Innocent Voyage. Has appeared on radio in Death Valley Days and Dr. Christian.
PICTURES INCLUDE: (debut) Anchors Aweigh, The Valley of Decision, Abbott and Costello in Hollywood, The Green Years; named in 1949 M.P. Herald-Fame Stars of Tomorrow poll; Home Sweet Homicide, The Mighty McGurk, The Arnelo Affair, The Romance of Rosy Ridge, Song of the Thin Man, Gentleman's Agreement, Deep Waters, Down to Sea in Ships, Boy with Green Hair, Secret Garden, Happy Years, Kim, Stars in My Crown, Cattle Drive, Compulsion, Sons and Lovers, Long Day's Journey Into Night, Psych-out, The Dunwich Horror, The Last Movie, The Loners, Paris, Texas, Dune, To Live and Die in L.A.

STODDARD, BRANDON: Executive. e. Yale Univ., Columbia Law School. Was program ass't. at Batton, Barton, Durstine and Osborn before joining Grey Advertising, where was successively, program operations supvr., dir. daytime programming, v.p. in chg. of TV, radio programming. Joined ABC in 1970; named v.p. daytime programs for ABC Entertainment, 1972; v.p. children's programs, 1973. Named v.p., motion pictures for TV, 1974. In 1976 named v.p., dramatic programs and motion pictures for television. In June, 1979, named pres., ABC Motion Pictures. In 1985 appt. pres., ABC Entertainment.

STOLBER, DEAN: Executive. b. Philadelphia, Penna., Sept. 2, 1944. e. Harvard (A.B., 1966); NYU School of Law (J.D., 1969). Acted on Broadway and in TV before starting career in law and business affairs in films. 1979, sr. v.p., business affairs, for United Artists Corp.; 1981 named exec. v.p.; 1982, sr. v.p., MGM/UA Entertainment Co.

STOLNITZ, ART: Executive. b. Rochester, N.Y. March 13, 1928. e. University of Tennessee. LLB, 1952; U.S. Navy Air Force. Legal dept., William Morris Agency, 1953, dir. business affairs, ZIV, 1959; dir. new program development, ZIV-United Artists, 1960; literary agent, MCA, 1961; dir. business affairs, Selmur Productions, Selmur Pictures, 1963; v.p. ABC Pictures, 1969; v.p. Metromedia Producers Corporation, 1970, executive v.p. Metromedia Producers Corporation; 1975 exec. v.p. and prod. Charles Fries Prods. 1976, prod. Edgar J. Scherick Productions; 1976–77 prod., Grizzly Adams (TV); 1977; v.p. business affairs, Warner Bros.-TV; 1980, snr. v.p., business affairs.

STOLOFF, VICTOR: Producer, writer, director, editor; e. French Law U. Ac. Fines Arts. Prod. dir. writer of award winning documentaries (Warner Bros. release); Prod. dir. writer first U.S. film made in Italy, When in Rome; First U.S. film made in Egypt; Collaborator William Dieterle films; Contract; writer, dir. to Sidney Buchman, Columbia, S.p. Volcano, The Sinner, Shark Reef.
TV: Ford Theatre, Lloyd Bridges series, NBC, National Velvet, CBS High Adventure, with Lowell Thomas, Journey

Around the World, Prod. Writ. Of Love and Desire; producer-director, Intimacy, Prod. on location 22, Hawaii Five-O, The 300 Year Weekend, Why? Director (orig. s.p.) Created Woman of Iran, first of TV series. 1977: producer-director: The Washington Affair.

STOLTZ, ARNOLD T.: Publicity executive. b. New York; e. Washington, U., St. Louis. Worked as reporter, publicity adv. man, 1933–37. Was pub. dir. and mgr., Warner and Loew theatres. Was radio commentator under name of Solly Wood. Pen name, Franc Arnold. Winner Quigley Silver Grand Award for exploitation, 1941. In 1942 named exploitation mgr., United Artists. In July, 1945 named natl. dir. and pub. PRC Pictures; then sales rep. Resigned 1947 to enter prod.; exec. prod. Movie Star, American Style. Joined Famous Players Corp.; adv., pub. dir., 1965; v.p. & gen sales mgr., 1966. pres. Movie-Rama Color Corp., 1967; exec. prod. Tell Me in the Sunlight, The Golden Poodle.

STONE, ANDREW L.: Producer, director. b. Calif., July 16, 1902; e. U. Calif. Ent. ind. 1918 at Universal San Francisco exch.; later author, prod., dir. series of pictures for Paramount; prod., dir. for Sono-Art; 1932–36. org. and oper. Race Night company; prod., dir., The Girl Said No, 1936; Stolen Heaven, Say It in French, The Great Victory Herbert, Magician Music, 1940. Dir. Stormy Weather; formed Andrew Stone Prods., 1943.

PICTURES INCLUDE: Hi Diddle Diddle, Sensations of 1945, Bedside Manner, Bachelor's Daughter, Fun on a Weekend, Highway 301, Confidence Girl, Steel Trap, Blueprint for Murder, Night Holds Terror, Julie, Cry Terror, The Decks Ran Red, The Last Voyage, Ring of Fire, Password is Courage, Never Put It in Writing, Secret of My Success, Song of Norway, The Great Waltz.

STONE, BURTON J.: Executive. b. Feb. 16, 1928; e. Florida So. Coll; Pres., Deluxe Laboratories, Inc. and Deluxe Laboratories. Was film ed., Hollywood Film Co. 1951–53; serv. mgr., sales mgr. and gen. mgr., Consolidated Film Inds., 1953–61; nat'l sales mgr., Movielab, 1961–63; pres., All Service Film Laboratories, 1963–68; v.p. Technicolor, Inc., 1968–70. Pres., Precision Film Labs., 1970–78.

MEMBER: Board of directors, Will Rogers Hospital; member, Academy of M.P. Arts & Sciences; assoc. member, American Society of Cinematographers; member, SMPTE; trustee, Motion Picture Laboratory Technicians Local 702 IATSE, Pension and Welfare Fund; member, Cinema Lodge, B'nai B'rith, Variety Club 1035, N.Y., Motion Picture Pioneers. University Film Producers, Association of Cinema Laboratories.

STONE, EZRA C.: Actor, director, writer, producer, teacher, farmer. b. New Bedford, Mass., Dec. 2, 1917; e. American Acad. of Dramatic Arts, N.Y., 1934–35; actor: National Junior Theatre, 1931; WCAU, Phila., 1930–34; vaudeville, Steel Pier, Atlantic City, N.J., 1931–32; YW & YMHA & Plays & Players Productions, Phila., 1928–30; Broadway: Parade, Ah Wilderness, Oh Evening Star, Three Men on a Horse, Room Service, Brother Rat; created Henry Aldrich, What a Life, The Alchemist, She Stoops to Conquer; prod. asst. to George Abbott, 1935–40; created Henry Aldrich on radio's Aldrich Family, 1938; starred, Those Were the Days, Paramount, 1939, This is the Army, Warners 1943, USAAF, 1941–45; directed on Broadway: See My Lawyer, 1939, Reunion in New York, 1940.

STAGE: This is the Army, 1942, January Thaw, 1946, At War With the Army, 1949, To Tell You the Truth, 1947, Me and Molly, 1948, Wake Up Darling, 1956, Make a Million, 1958, The Man That Corrupted Hadleyburg, 1951, The Pink Elephant, 1953, Dear Ruth, 1961; Come Blow Your Horn, 1962, God Bless Our Bank, Fallen Angels, 1963; Finishing Touches (1978); Dracula—The Vampire King (1978); Sweet Land (exec. prod., dir.); Centennial Celebration of Founding Newtown, PA (actor).

PICTURES INCLUDE: (docum.) I.B.M., American Heart Assn. Chapman Coll., University of Judaism, Jewish Theological Seminary; dir. live action sequences for The Daydreamer; The Forty Million (producer, director, co-narrator).

TV: Aldrich Family, Danny Thomas, Ed Wynn, Ezio Pinza, Martha Raye, Fred Allen, Herb Shriner, Life With Father, Sid Caesar, Joan Davis, dir. Joe and Mabel, prod., dir. Bachelor Father, Angel, The Hathaways, spec. Affairs of Antol, Shari Lewis, Bob Hope, My Living Doll, Munsters, Karen, Tammy, O.K. Crackerby, Please Don't Eat the Daisies; dir., writer Woody Allen pilot, Loredo, Pistols & Petticoats, Petticoat Junction, Phyllis Diller Show, Lost in Space, Tammy Grimes show, Julia, Flying Nun, Debbie Reynolds, The Jimmy Stewart Show, Lassie, Sandy Duncan Show, Tribute to the Lunts, Love American Style, Bob Newhart, Space Academy, Munster's Revenge, Quincy, ABC Circle Playhouse Project UFO, Actor, (PBS Paul Muni, biography film). Did 300 docmentary films for IBM. Has over 25 intl. film awards; Grand Prize, Barcelona Int'l Film Festival.

AUTHOR: Coming Major, 1945, co-author; Deems Taylor; Puccini Opera, 1951; contributor to: Variety, Magazine Digest, N.Y. Post; Equity Magazine, etc. Teacher: American Acad. Dramatic Arts, assoc. dir., American Theatre Wing; American College Theatre Festival, Princeton, Yale, U.C.L.A.: pres./dir., David Library of Amer. Revolution.

STONE, MARIANNE: Actress. b. London, England. Studied Royal Acad. of Dramatic Art, making her first appearance West End stage in The Kingmaker, 1946. Since then has appeared in numerous films.

TV: Maigret, Bootsie and Snudge, Jimmy Edwards Show, Wayne and Schuster Show, Roy Hudd Show, Harry Worth Show, Steptoe and Son, Informer, Love Story, Father Dear Father, Bless This House, The Man Outside, Crown Court, Public Eye, Miss Nightingale, She, Little Lord Fauntleroy, The Secret Army (2 series), Shillingbury Tale, The Bright Side (series).

PICTURES INCLUDE: Brighton Rock, Seven Days to Noon, The Clouded Yellow, Wrong Arm of the Law, Heavens Above, Stolen Hours, Nothing But the Best, Curse of the Mummy's Tomb, Hysteria, The Beauty Jungle, A Hard Day's Night, Battle of a Simple Man, Echo of Diana, Act of Murder, Catch Us If You Can, You Must Be Joking, The Countess from Hong Kong, The Wrong Box, To Sir With Love, 1967–68; The Bliss of Mrs. Blossom, Here We Go Round the Mulberry Bush, Carry on Doctor, The Twisted Nerve, The Best House in London, Oh! What a Lovely War, 1970; The Raging Moon, There's a Girl in My Soup, All the Right Noises, Assault, Carry On at Your Convenience, All Coppers Are . . ., Carry on Girls, Penny Gold, The Vault of Horror, Percy's Progress, Confessions of a Window Cleaner, Carry on Dick, That Lucky Touch, Sarah, Carry on Behind, Confessions From a Holiday Camp, The Chiffy Kids, What's Up Superdoc?; The Class of Miss McMichael, The Human Factor, Dangerous Davies, Funny Money. Recent TV: The Balance of Nature, Always, Hammer House of Mystery & Suspense, Teny on the Fence.

STONE, OLIVER: Director-Writer. b. New York City, Sept. 15, 1946. e. Yale Univ., NYU.

PICTURES: Seizure (dir., s.p.), Midnight Express (s.p.—AA), The Hand (dir., s.p.), Conan the Barbarian (s.p.), Scarface (s.p.).

STONE, PETER: Writer. b. Los Angeles, Feb. 20, 1930. Won Oscar in 1964 for Father Goose; Emmy for segment of The Defenders.

PICTURES INCLUDE: Charade, Arabesque, Mirage, Sweet Charity, The Taking of Pelham One Two Three, 1776 (adapted own stage musical book to screen), Silver Bears, Who Is Killing the Great Chefs of Europe?, Why Would I Lie?

STONE, ROBERT L.: Executive. e. Williams College; joined U.S. Air Force, 1942. Awarded Distinguished Flying Cross & Air Medal with eight Oak Leaf clusters, earned while flying 40 combat missions in the Pacific. Began business career 1946 as staff assoc. with Cresal, McCormick and Paget. 1952, joined ABC as acct. exec. of TV network sales; 1953 named dir. of TV production services. 1955, gen. mgr. WABC-TV, New York; 1947, v.p. in chg. of station. 1959, joined NBC as v.p., opns. & engineering; promoted to v.p. and gen. mgr., TV network, in 1960. Pres. of radio div. & exec. v.p., 1971; elected member of NBC board. 1972, elected chm & CEO, Hertz Corp; named pres., 1973. In 1978 appt. exec. v.p., Columbia Pictures Industries.

STONEMAN, JAMES M.: Executive. b. Jan. 16, 1927. Pres., Interstate Theatres Corp., Boston. 1985, pres., Theatre Owners of New England.

STOREY FREDERICK: Executive. b. Columbus, Georgia, Nov. 12, 1909. e. Georgia Tech. Adv. staff Atlanta Journal, 1933–38; adv. staff C. P. Clark Adv. Agcy., 1938; partner 1940; U.S. Navy, 1941–46; staff Georgia Theatre Co., 1946; v.p. 1947–52. Founded Storey Theatres Inc., Atlanta, Ga.; 1952, now bd. chm. (formerly pres.) of Georgia State Theatres; dir. numerous theatre cos.; v.p. dir., Motion Picture Theatre Owners of Georgia, member, NATO, member, pres., advisory council. Dist. Alumnus award, Ga. Tech, 1979.

STORKE, WILLIAM F.: Producer. b. Rochester, N.Y. e. Univ. of Calif. In Navy in World War II. First position with NBC Hollywood guest relations staff, 1948. Moved to continuity acceptance dept. as comm. editor. Prom. to asst. mgr, comm. supvr. before joining NBC West Coast sales dept., 1953. Transferred to N.Y. as progr. acct. exec., 1955; named administrator, participating prog. sales, Nov., 1957. Named dir., participating program sales, 1959. Named dir., program adm., NBC-TV, Jan., 1964; in Feb. elected v.p., program adm. In 1967 named v.p., programs, East Coast; Nov. 1, 1968, appt. v.p., special programs, NBC TV Network; 1979, pres., Claridge Group, Ltd.; exec. v.p. Entertainment Partners, Inc., NYC, 1982–. Producer: film Oliver Twist, 1982, To Catch A King, 1983, A Christmas

Carol, 1984; The Last Days of Patton, 1985; A Special Friendship, The Ted Kennedy Jr. Story, 1986.

STORM, GALE: Actress. r.n. Josephine Cottle. b. Bloomington, Texas, April 5, 1922. In high school became interested in dramatics. To films, 1940.
PICTURES INCLUDE: Between Midnight and Dawn, Underworld Story, Curtain Call at Cactus Creek, Al Jennings of Oklahoma, Texas Rangers, Woman of the North Country.
TV: My Little Margie, Oh Susanna, radio show.

STOSSEL, JOHN: News Correspondent. e. Princeton Univ. Started as producer-reporter with KGW-TV in Portland, OR. Joined WCBS-TV in New York as investigative reporter and consumer editor, winning 15 local Emmy Awards. In June, 1981 joined ABC-TV, appearing on Good Morning America and 20/20 as consumer editor. Also provides twice-weekly consumer reports on ABC Radio Information Network. Author: Shopping Smart (1982).

STRADLING, HARRY, JR.: Cinematographer. b. New York City, Jan. 7, 1925. Son of Harry Stradling, British-born cinematographer who worked extensively in U.S.
PICTURES: Welcome to Hard Times, Support Your Local Sheriff, The Mad Room, Something Big, Fools Parade, The Way We Were, Bite the Bullet, Airport 77, Midway, The Big Bus, Born Again, Convoy, Go Tell the Spartans, Prophecy, S.O.B., Buddy, Buddy, The Pursuit of D.B. Cooper, Micki and Maude.

STRAIGHT, BEATRICE: Actress. b. Old Westbury, N.Y. 1918. Trained in classics; won Tony award early in career for best actress in Arthur Miller's The Crucible. Many films and TV programs.
PICTURES: Patterns, The Nun's Story, Phone Call from a Stranger, Network (AA), The Promise, The Formula, Endless Love, Poltergeist, Power.
STAGE: A Streetcar Named Desire, Phedre, The Heiress, Ghosts, The Lion in Winter, etc.
TELEVISION: Beacon Hill, Robert Kennedy and His Times, Under Seige, etc.

STRASBERG, SUSAN: Actress. b. New York City, May 22, 1938.; e. there. Parents: Lee Strasberg, stage dir. & dir. of Actors Studio, and Paula Miller, actress. Made stage debut in off-Bdwy. production of Maya; on TV in series, The Marriage, The Duchess and the Smugs, Catch a Falling Star; starred on Bway. in The Diary of Anne Frank.
PICTURES INCLUDE: Picnic, Stage Struck, Scream of Fear, Adventures of a Young Man, The Trip, Psych-Out, The Name of the Game Is Kill, Rollercoaster, The Manitou, In Praise of Older Women, The Delta Force.

STRASSBERG, STEPHEN: Publicist. b. New York, N.Y.; e. C.C.N.Y., B.S.S., joined Loew's Inc., 1940; served in U.S. Army, WW II; publicist with Republic Pictures, 1946–49; asst. nat'l adv. dir., Film Classics, 1949–50; pub. dir., Eagle Lion Classics, 1950; publicist Lopert Films, Inc., 1951; dir. of adv., pub., Imperial Films, 1953; pub. dir., WABC, WABC-TV, N.Y., 1955; asst. dir., Press Information; ABC, 1957; dir. press info. ABC-TV Network, 1958; dir., News Information, ABC-TV Network, 1975.

STRATTON, JOHN: Actor. b. Clitheroe, England, 1925; e. Royal Grammar School, Clitheroe. Early career in repertory; m.p. and TV debut 1948.
TV: The First Mrs. Fraser, The Confidential Clerk, Adams Apple, You Know What People Are (series). Death of a Salesman, Quatermass in The Pit, The Wind and the Rain, The Secret Kingdom, Kipps, The Dobson Fund, The Problem of Mary Winshaw, A Perfect Woman, Climate of Fear, Thank You and Goodnight, What's In It for Walter, A Free Weekend, Workshop Limits, 24 Hour Call, 2 Cars, The Odd Man, It's Dark Outside, For the West, Man in Room 17, Julie's Gone, The Trouble Shooters, Turn out the Lights, Mr. Rose, The Black Doctor, Sir Arthur Conan Doyle, The Newcomers, Tickle Time, Letters from the Dead, Z Car, Wanted Single Gentleman, Softly Softly, Fall of the Goat, City '68, Artist in Crime, The First Lady, Print and Be Damned, The Expert, Resurrection (serial), Sherlock Holmes, Measure of Malice, The Elusive Pimpernel (serial), The Pallisers, Fall of the Eagles, Clayhanger, Trinity Tales, Witch of Pendle, When We Are Married, Just William, Backs to the Land, Forget Me Not, A Superstition, The Professionals, Mill on the Floss, , The Good Companions, Great Expectations, The Forgotten Story, The Tales of Beatrix Potter, My Cousin Rachel, Dr. Who: Juliet Brajo.
PICTURES INCLUDE: Small Back Room, Seven Days to Noon, Appointment With Venus (Island Rescue), Happy Family, Cruel Sea, Long Arm, Man In the Sky, Seven Waves Away (Abandon Ship), The Challenge, Strangler's Web.

STRAUSS, JOHN: Publicist. b. N.Y. Apr. 2, 1913; e. Yale U., B.A., 1935. Securities trader & analyst, Mabon & Co., N.Y. 1935–41; New Eng. factory rep., Star Rubber Co., 1941; city sales rep., W. B., Buffalo, 1941–45; unit pub., W.B., Burbank, 1945; asst. pub. dir., PRC., 1946; unit pub., Enterprise Prod., 1946–47; pub., Columbia Studios, 1947–48; Pres., McFadden, Strauss & Irwin, Inc., pub. rel. counsellors for personalities, m.p. TV & indust. accts., Los Angeles, New York, Palm Springs, London, Paris.

STRAUSS, PETER: Actor. b. Croton-on-Hudson, N.Y., 1947. e. Northwestern Univ. Spotted at N.U. by talent agent and sent to Hollywood. Debut in Hail Hero (1969). Has acted at Mark Taper Theatre in Dance Next Door, The Dirty Man.
PICTURES: Hail, Hero!, Soldier Blue, The Trail of the Catonsville Nine, The Last Tycoon, Spacehunter.
TELEVISION: Man Without a Country, Attack on Terror, The Forgotten Kennedy, Heart of Steel, Under Siege. Mini-Series: Rich Man, Poor Man, Masada, Kane & Abel, Tender Is The Night.

STRAUSS, PETER E.: Executive. b. Oct. 7, 1940. e. Oberlin College, London School of Economics, Columbia University School of Law (L.L.B., 1965). Vice pres., University Dormitory Development Co., 1965–68; v.p., Allart Cinema 16, 1968–69; v.p. Production, Allied Artists Pictures Corp., 1970; June 14, 1974 elected exec. v.p. Joined Rastor Films; left to become independent.

STRAUSS, RICHARD: b. Chicago, Ill.; e. Northwestern U., Fordham U., Univ. of Illinois (also graduate work U. of Ill., U.S.C.), Northwestern. President of Bevelite-Adler Co. Past pres. TESMA; bd. secty. TEA, Calif. Sign Ass'n.; Exhibit rules of Nat'l Electric Sign Ass'n.; Variety Club, life member; bd. of dir., National Electric Sign Assn.

STREEP, MERYL: Actress. b. Bernardsville, N.J. April 22, 1949. Gained fame on N.Y. stage in such plays as Trelawny of the Wells, The Taming of the Shrew, The Cherry Orchard, Happy End, etc.
PICTURES: Julia, Manhattan, The Deer Hunter, The Seduction of Joe Tynan, Kramer vs. Kramer (AA, best supporting actress, 1979), The French Lieutenant's Woman, Still of the Night, Sophie's Choice, Silkwood, Falling in Love, Plenty, Out of Africa, Heartburn.
TELEVISION: Holocaust, The Deadliest Season.

STREISAND, BARBRA: Singer, actress. b. New York, April 24, 1942. e. Erasmus H.S., Brooklyn. Appeared in New York night clubs. On Broadway in I Can Get It For You Wholesale, debut 1962; Funny Girl.
PICTURES INCLUDE: (debut) Funny Girl, Hello Dolly, On A Clear Day You Can See Forever, The Owl and the Pussycat, What's Up Doc?, Up the Sandbox, The Way We Were, For Pete's Sake, Funny Lady, A Star Is Born, (star, prod.), The Main Event (star, co-prod.), All Night Long, Yentl (prod., dir., co.s.p., star).
TV: My Name is Barbra, Color Me Barbra, Bell of 14th Street, A Happening in Central Park.

STRICKLYN, RAY: Actor. b. Houston, Texas, October 8; e. University of Houston.
PLAYS INCLUDE: Broadway debut in Moss Hart's The Climate of Eden. Tour: Stalag 17. Off-B'way: The Grass Harp. Alley Theatre, Houston: Mourning Becomes Electra, Long Day's Journey Into Night, etc. Los Angeles: Starred in Compulsion and The Caretaker.
FILMS INCLUDE: The Proud and the Profane, Crime In the Streets, Somebody Up There Likes Me, Catered Affair, The Last Wagon, Return of Dracula, 10 North Frederick, The Remarkable Mr. Pennypacker, The Big Fisherman, The Plunderers, The Lost World, Young Jesse James, Track of Thunder, Arizona Raiders, Shuffle.
AWARDS: Broadway Theatre World Award; two Hollywood Foreign Press Golden Globe nominations (10 North Frederick and The Plunderers).

STRITCH, ELAINE: Actress. b. Detroit, MI, Feb. 2, 1926. Major career on stage.
PICTURES: The Scarlet Hour (debut, 1955), Three Violent People, A Farewell to Arms, The Perfect Furlough, Who Killed Teddy Bear?, Sidelong Glances of a Pigeon Kicker, The Spiral Staircase, Providence.
TELEVISION: My Sister Eileen (series), Two's Company, Kennedy Center Tonight, Follies in Concert, etc.

STROCK, HERBERT L.: Prod.-writer, dir., film editor. b. Boston, Mass., Jan. 13, 1918. e. Univ. of So. Calif., A.B., M.A. in Cinema; prof., of Cinema, Univ. of So. Calif., 1941. Started career, publicity leg man, Jimmy Fidler, Hollywood columnist; editorial dept., MGM, 1941–47; pres., IMPPRO, Inc., 1955–59; assoc. prod.-supv. film ed., U.A.; dir., AIP; dir., Phoenix Films. Pres., Herbert L. Strock Prods.
PICTURES INCLUDE: Storm Over Tibet, Magnetic Monster, Riders to the Stars, The Glass Wall, Gog, Battle Taxi, Donovan's Brain, Rider on a Dead Horse, Devil's Messenger, Brother on the Run, One Hour of Hell, Witches Brew, Blood of Dracula, I Was a Teenage Frankenstein, The Crawling Hand. Director; Soul Brothers Die Hard, Monstroids. Writer-film editor, Hurray for Betty Boop (cartoon). Sound Effects editor on Katy Caterpillar (cartoon feature). Director: Witches' Brew. Editor: Night Screams.
TV: Highway Patrol, Harbor Command, Men of Annapolis,

I Led Three Lives, The Veil, Dragnet, 77 Sunset Strip, Maverick, Cheyenne, Bronco, Sugarfoot, Colt 45, Science Fiction Thea., Seahunt, Corliss Archer, Bonanza, Hallmark Hall of Fame, The Small Miracle, Hans Brinker, The Inventing of America (specials) for World Vision Intl.; What Will We Say to a Hungry World (5 hr. Telethon), They Search for Survival (special). NBC specials, Flipper (series). Documentaries: Atlantis, Legends, UFO Journals, UFO Syndrome, Legend of the Lochness Monster, China-Mao to Now, El-Papa—Journey to Tibet.

STRONG, JOHN: Producer-Director-Writer-Actor. b. New York City, Dec. 3. e. U. of Miami, Cornell U., (BS architectural engineering). Began acting in small role in film Duel in the Sun; on B'way in Annie Get Your Gun and understudy for James Dean in Immoralist. Appeared in many radio and TV serials, regular on Captain Video and the Video Ranger, later under contract as actor to Universal and Warner Bros.
PICTURES INCLUDE: Perilous Journey (exec. prod., writer), Eddie & the Cruisers (superv. prod.), Heart Like a Wheel (superv. prod.), For Your Eyes Only (writer), The Earthling (prod.), The Mountain Men (actor, prod.), Savage Streets (prod.).
TELEVISION: The John Strong Show (host, exec. prod.), The Nurse (special, writer), McCloud (prod., writer), The Thrill of the Fall (prod.), Search (prod., writer, 2nd unit dir.), Outer Limits (exec. chge. prod.), Name of the Game (exec. chge. prod.), I Spy (writer), Love American Style (writer), All in the Family (writer), Changes (prod., dir., writer), Charlie's Angels (writer), Hawaii Five 'O' (writer). Member, Writers Guild America West, Directors Guild of America, Producers Guild of America, Dramatists Guild.

STROSS, RAYMOND: Producer, exhibitor. b. Leeds, England, May 22, 1916. e. Abington, Oxford. Ent. m.p. ind. 1933, worked at Sound City, other studios as exec. until 1938; then prod., exhibitor; formed Raymond Stross Theatres; re-entered production, 1950.
PICTURES INCLUDE: Hell is Sold Out, Tall Headlines, Man Who Watched the Trains Go By, Rough Shoot (Shoot First), Star of India, Jumping for Joy, As Long as They're Happy, An Alligator Named Daisy, A Touch of the Sun, The Flesh is Weak, A Question of Adultery, The Angry Hills, A Terrible Beauty, The Mark, Very Edge, The Leather Boys, Ninety Degrees in the Shade, The Fox, I Want What I Want, The Woman Who Rode Away.

STROUD, DON: Actor. b. 1937.
PICTURES: Madigan, Games, What's So Bad About Feeling Good?, Coogan's Bluff, Bloody Mama, Explosion, Von Richtofen and Brown, Tick Tick, Tick, Joe Kidd, Scalaway, The Killer Inside Me, The Choirboys, The House by the Lake, The Buddy Holly Story, The Amityville Horror, The Night the Lights Went Out in Georgia, Search and Destroy, Striking Back, Sweet Sixteen.

STRUTHERS, SALLY: Actress. b. Portland, OR, July 28, 1948.
PICTURES INCLUDE: The Phynx, Charlotte, Five Easy Pieces, The Getaway.
TELEVISION: Summer Bros. Smothers Show, Tim Conway Comedy Hour, All in the Family (series). Films: The Great Houdinis, Aloha Means Goodbye, Hey, I'm Alive.

STULBERG, GORDON: Executive. b. Toronto, Canada, Dec. 17, 1923; e. U. of Toronto, B.A., Cornell Law, LLB. Was assoc. & member, Pacht, Ross, Warne & Bernhard; ent. m.p. ind. as exec. asst. to v.p., Columbia Pictures Corp., 1956–60; v.p. & chief studio admin. off., 1960–67; pres. of Cinema Center Films (div. of CBS) 1967–71; pres. 20th Century-Fox, Sept. 1971–75; 1980, named pres. & chief operating officer, PolyGram Pictures. Member of N.Y. & Calif. bars.

STURGES, JOHN ELIOT: Director. b. Jan. 3, Oak Park, Ill. e. Marin Jr. Coll. asst. in blueprint dept., RKO-Radio Pictures, 1932; art dept; asst. film ed.; prod. asst., David O. Selznick; film ed.; Captain, Air Corps, WW II; directed, edited, 45 documentaries, training films.
PICTURES INCLUDE: The Man Who Dared, Shadowed, Alias Mr. Twilight, For the Love of Rusty, Keeper of the Bees, Best Man Wins, Sign of the Ram, The Walking Hills, The Capture, Mystery Street, Right Cross, The Magnificent Yankee, Kind Lady, The People vs. O'Hara, The Girl in White, Jeopardy, Fast Company, Escape from Fort Bravo, Bad Day at Black Rock, Gunfight at the O.K. Corral, The Old Man and the Sea, Last Train from Gun Hill, Never So Few, The Magnificent Seven, By Love Possessed, Sergeants Three, A Girl Named Tamiko, The Great Escape, The Satan Bug, Hallelujah Trail, Hour of the Gun, Ice Station Zebra, Marooned, Joe Kidd, McQ, The Eagle Has Landed.

STURGIS, NORMAN: Director, actor, writer. b. Dallas, Tex. 1922; prod., Your Navy Sings, Evanston; TV dir. Space X, Theaterama, Plays Anthology, The Viewers, TV commercials, educational films and newsfilms.
TV: The Web, Gunsmoke, Twilight Zone, Alcoa Goodyear Theatre, Bat Masterson, The Untouchables.
PICTURES INCLUDE: Solid Gold Cadillac, Bernardine, Mardi Gras, Compulsion.

STYNE, JULE: Composer, producer, r.n. Jules Stein. b. London, Eng. To U.S. as a child; guest piano soloist with Chicago Symph. Orch. at 8; played with many dance bands; gen. mus. dir. Granada & Marbro Theat., Chicago; vocal coach, arranger, conductor & comp. for several m.p. studios; entertainment consult.
SONGS: I've Heard That Song Before, It's Magic, I'll Walk Alone, It's Been a Long, Long Time; Let It Snow, 3 Coins in the Fountain (Acad. Award in collab. Sammy Cahn, 1954), People.
STAGE: High Button Shoes, Gentlemen Prefer Blondes, Two on the Aisle, Hazel Flagg, Gypsy, Sugar, Peter Pan, Bells Are Ringing, Funny Girl, Hallelujah Baby (Tony Award).
PICTURES INCLUDE: Kid from Brooklyn, It Happened in Brooklyn, Romance on the High Seas, It's a Great Feeling, West Point Story, Meet Me After the Show, Living It Up, My Sister Eileen.

SUBOTSKY, MILTON: Writer, producer. b. New York, 1921. Early career studying engineering. Wrote, dir. and edited doc. & educational films. Ent. m.p. ind. 1938. Wrote and prod. live TV programmes 1941. Wrote & prod. TV film series Junior Science 1954. Wrote & co-prod. Rock, Rock, Rock; Jamboree, The Last Mile, in USA. In England: City of the Dead, It's Trad Dad, Just for Fun, Dr. Terror's House of Horrors, Dr. Who and The Daleks, Daleks' Invasion Earth 2150 A.D., The Skull, The Psychopath, The Deadly Bees, The Terrornauts, They Came From Beyond Space, Torture Garden, Danger Route, The Birthday Party, Thank You All Very Much (Brit. title: A Touch of Love), Scream and Scream Again, The Mind of Mr. Soames, The House That Dripped Blood, I Monster, What Became of Jack and Jill, Tales From the Crypt, Asylum, Vault of Horror, And Now the Screaming Starts, Madhouse, From Beyond the Grave, The Beast Must Die, The Land That Time Forgot, At The Earth's Core, The Uncanny, Dominique, The Martian Chronicles, The Monster Club, Cat's Eye, Maximum Overdrive. TV series: Classic Fairy Tales.

SUCHER, HENRY: Writer. b. New York City, Sept. 3, 1900; e. N.Y.U. With A.E.F., WW I. M. Pearl Krex, Reporter, N.Y. Globe, then mag. ed. (Nugents, Garment Weekly, The Brooklynite); publicity adv. copywriter; contrib. light satirical verses and humorous bits to the Sat. Eve. Post, Colliers, The New Yorker and other nat'l mags. Began screen career 1941 with collab. orig. s.p. The Miracle Kid. In 1942 wrote Soundies for Roosevelt-Coslow-Mills Corp. Wrote serials, Jack Holt, G. Man, and others for Larry Darmoor at Columbia Studios. Contract writer, Eagle-Lion Studios.
PICTURES INCLUDE: Captive Wild Woman, The Mummy's Tomb, Mug Town, The Mummy's Ghost (adapt. & collab. orig.), The Frozen Ghost, Jungle Woman, Your Fate Is In Your Hands, Lines of Destiny; short subjects released by RKO; now v.p. Edward Finney Prod., v.p. Boots and Saddles Pictures, Inc.

SUCHITZKY, PETER: Cinematographer. Spent long time in Latin America as documentatory cinematographer. Later made commercials in France, England, and U.S. First feature It Happened Here (1962).
PICTURES: Lisztomania, Valentino, Leo the Last, Privilege, Charlie Bubbles, That'll Be the Day, The Rocky Horror Picture Show, The Empire Strikes Back, Krull, Falling in Love.

SUGAR, JOSEPH M.: Executive. b. New York City. e. N.Y.U. Ent. m.p. ind. 1938 in contract dept., Republic Pictures; ent. U.S. Army Air Forces, 1942; asst. contract mgr. PRC, then mgr.; when PRC merged with Eagle Lion continued as mgr. contract dept.; then exec. asst. to dist. v.p.; to U.A.N.Y. exchange, Jan. 1, 1953; v.p. sales, Magna Theatre Corp., 1959; member: Cinema Lodge, B'nai B'rith; road show mgr., 20th Century-Fox, 1962; v.p. chg. dom. distrib., 1963; exec. v.p. Warner-Seven Arts, 1967; pres Cinerama Rel. Corp., 1968; pres., Gamma III Dist. Co., 1975; May, 1976: Joe Sugar, Inc., pres.; 1978, joined AIP as exec. v.p., worldwide sls. and pres. of AIP Distributing Co. which became Filmways Pictures. 1982, pres., Joe Sugar, Inc; 1983, named exec. v.p., domestic distribution, Embassy Pictures.

SUGARMAN, HAROLD: Executive. b. New York City, Oct. 17, 1905; m.; e. New York Univ. Joined Paramount foreign sales dept., 1927. In charge foreign versions and adapt. at Paramount Astoria studio, Long Island City, 1928–31. Dist. mgr., UA Latin American distribution 1932–36. Prod. ind. pictures in Hollywood, 1936–40. Org. and head Universal Studio foreign dept., 1941–46. Transf. to Universal New York office, 1946 to org. and head 16 mm. overseas oper. Apptd. v.p. in chge. of export, United World Fillms, Inc., 1947; apptd. superv. So. Europe, Universal-International, hdqts., Rome, Italy, 1950; prod. & sales exec. Archer Television Prod., 1952. dist. & prod. exec. dir., of Chancellor Films.

SUHOSKY, BOB: Publicist. b. Philadelphia, Pa., Nov. 23, 1928. Marine Corps 1946–57; 20th Century Fox Television, publicist, 1959, publicity director, 1964–70; pres. Bob Suhosky Assoc., public relations, 1971–77. Chairman, Suhosky & Hardiman Public Relations, 1977 to date. Wrote s.p. for Lone Star Girls (theatrical film) and Code R (TV).

SULLIVAN, BARRY: Actor. r.n. Patrick Barry. b. New York, N.Y., Aug. 29, 1912; e. N.Y.U., Temple U. Usher in theat.; buyer for dept. stores; N.Y. stage: The Man Who Came to Dinner, Brother Rat, Idiot's Delight, The Land Is Bright, Caine Mutiny Court Martial, etc.
PICTURES INCLUDE: Woman of the Town, Lady in the Dark, Rainbow Island, Two Years Before the Mast, And Now Tomorrow, Duffy's Tavern, Three Guys Named Mike, Cause for Alarm, Grounds for Marriage, Life of Her Own, Nancy Goes to Rio, Inside Straight, Payment on Demand, Mr. Imperium, No Questions Asked, Unknown Man, Skirts Ahoy, The Bad and the Beautiful, Jeopardy, Cry of the Hunted, China Venture, Loophole, Her 12 Men, Miami Story, Playgirl, Queen Bee, Texas Lady, Maverick Queen, Strategic Air Command, Purple Gang, Seven Ways from Sundown, Light in the Piazza, War Lords of Outer Space, Stage to Thunder Rock, Buckskin, Tell Them Willie Boy Is Here, Earthquake, The Human Factor, Oh, God!, Caravans.

SULLIVAN, J. CHRISTOPHER: Actor. b. Greenville, TX, Sept. 15, 1932. e. Prairie View A & M Univ.; Sorbonne (Paris); Univ. of Texas. Ph.D. Stage debut in The Sign in Sidney Brustein's Window. Also appeared in Hatful of Rain, Anna Lucasta, Ceremonies in Dark Old Men, Dark of the Moon, Take a Giant Step, Therese. First black to teach at any predominantly white university in the south; as an instructor of speech and communications at Univ of Texas (Austin) 1964.
PICTURES INCLUDE: Night Call Nurses, The Venetian Affair, The Lost Man, Body Heat, Black Starlet, The Black Gestapo, The Happy Ending, D.C. Cab.
TELEVISION: The White Shadow, Jeffersons, Good Times, One Day at a Time, General Hospital, Serpico, Starsky & Hutch, Death Flight, McClain's Law, Growing Pains, etc.

SULLIVAN, REV. PATRICK J., S.J., S.T.D.: Provost, Graduate Center at Tarrytown, Fordham Univ. b. New York, N.Y., March 25, 1920; e. Regis H.S.: Georgetown U., A.B., 1943; Woodstock Coll. M.A., 1944; Fordham U., 1945–47; S.T.L. Weston Coll., 1947–51; S.T.D. Gregorian U. (Rome), 1952–54; Prof. of Theology, Woodstock Coll., 1954–57; Consultor, Pontifical Commission for Social Communications.

SUMMERFIELD, ELEANOR: Actress. b. London, Eng., Mar. 7, 1921. Stage debut in Cornelius, 1939; screen debut in London Belongs to Me (in U.S.A., Dulcimer Street), 1947.
PICTURES INCLUDE: Take My Life, All Over the Town, No Way Back, The Third Visitor, Scrooge, Laughter in Paradise, Mandy, Top Secret, Isn't Life Wonderful, Street Corner (Both Sides of the Law), Face the Music, Murder by Proxy, Lost, It's Great to Be Young, Odongo, No Road Back, A Cry from the Streets, The Millionairess, Spare the Rod, Don't Bother to Knock, Petticoat Pirates, On the Fiddle, Act of Mercy, On the Beat, The Running Man, The Yellow Hat, Private Eye, Foreign Exchange, Some Will, Some Won't, Watcher in the Woods.
TV: (BBC, indep.) My Wife's Sister, The Two Charles (series), The Invasion, Dickie Henderson Shows, Night Train to Surbiton, Many A Slip, World of Wooster, David Copperfield, The Suede Jacket, Haunted, You're Lovely in Black, Misleading Cases, East of Eden, Tennis, Elbow, Foot Game, Murder at the Panto, Now Take My Wife, Madly in Love, Kate, Simon Fenton's Story, Kept on a String, Password, Husband of the Year, The Overnight Bag, The Rather Reassuring Show, Murder at the Wedding, Pig in the Middle.

SUNDBERG, CLINTON: Actor. b. Appleton, Minn., Dec. 7; e. Hamline U. Teacher of English literature; in New England stock cos.; on London and N.Y. stage.
STAGE: Silent Witness, She Loves Me Not, Boy Meets Girl, Room Service, Arsenic and Old Lace, Over 21, Diary of Anne Frank, Mary, Mary.
PICTURES INCLUDE: Undercurrent, Undercover Maisie, Living in a Big Way, Song of Love, Hucksters, Kissing Bandit, Easter Parade, Good Sam, Date With Judy, Words and Music, Command Decision, In the Good Old Summertime, Key to City, Annie Get Your Gun, Toast of New Orleans, Fat Man, As Young as You Feel, Belle of New York, Girl Next Door, Main Street to Broadway, The Caddy, Birds and the Bees, Wonderful World of Brothers Grimm, How the West Was Won.

SUNSHINE, MORTON: Honorary Executive Vice President, Variety Clubs Intl.–1984 special consultant; SInternational Executive Director, Variety Clubs International, 1975 to present. b. Brooklyn, N.Y., Sept. 20, 1915. B.S. in S.S. (1935), LL.B. (1938), J.S.D. (1939); admitted to N.Y. Bar 1939. Federal Bar 1941. Practicing attorney, 1941–44; Federal investigator with U.S.C.S.C. 1944–45; business mgr., Independent Theatre Owners Assn. 1945–46; exec. dir. since 1946; member COMPO tax & legis. com., 1950; sp. rep. Org. of M.P. Ind. of City of N.Y., 1952–55; exec. coord. Tony Awards dinner Amer. Theatre Wing, 1958–60, Sophie Tucker Golden Jubilee; ind. trib. to Jimmy Durante; Will Rogers; A. Montague; Herman Robbins; S. H. Fabian; Rodgers-Hammerstein; Eric Johnston; Diamond Jubilee, Stagehands, 1962. Danny Thomas; indus. pub. rel. consultant; exec. coord. IFIDA Int'l Film Awards Dinners; pres. cabinet, Nat'l Assn. of Theatre Owners, Exec. dir., Variety Club of N.Y., 1970; Consultant to American Film Institute, 1973–75; executive director, Motion Picture Pioneers, 1970–75; Editor-Publisher, Independent Film Journal, 1947–75.

SURTEES, BRUCE: Cinematographer. Son of Robert L. Surtees.
PICTURES INCLUDE: Play Misty for Me, Dirty Harry, The Great Northfield Minnesota Raid, The Beguiled, High Plains Drifter, Blume in Love, Joe Kidd, Lenny (A.A. nomination), Leadbelly, Sparkle, Big Wednesday, Escape from Alcatraz, Firefox, Inchon, Honkytonk Man, Bad Boys, Risky Business, Sudden Impact, Tightrope, Beverly Hills Cop, Pale Rider, Psycho III, Out of Bounds.

SUSSKIND, DAVID: Producer—TV Talk Show Host. b. New York City, Dec. 19, 1920. Producer of TV shows, founder of production co., Talent Associates; host of own syndicated interview program (The David Susskind Show; formerly called Open End.) Notable for producing TV adaptations of famous plays; Glass Menagerie, The Crucible, Death of a Salesman, etc. In 1970 Norton Simon, Inc. acquired his co., renaming it Talent Associates—Norton Simon for theatrical as well as TV film production. Sold in 1977 to Time-Life Films.

SUTHERLAND, DONALD: Actor b. St. John, New Brunswick, Canada, July 17, 1934. m. Shirley Douglas, actress. e. U. of Toronto. At 14 became a radio announcer and disc jockey. Worked in a mine in Finland. Theatre includes: The Male Animal (debut), The Tempest (Hart House Theatre, U. of Toronto), Two years at London Acad. of Music and Dramatic Art. Spent a year and a half with the Perth Repertory Theatre in Scotland, the repertory at Nottingham, Chesterfield, Bromley and Sheffield. London stage debut: August for the People.
STAGE: On a Clear Day You Can See Canterbury, The Shewing Up of Blanco Posnet, The Spoon River Anthology.
PICTURES INCLUDE: The Castle of the Living Dead, Dr. Terror's House of Horrors, The Dirty Dozen, Oedipus the King, Interlude, Joanna. The Split, Start the Revolution Without Me, The Act of the Heart, M*A*S*H*, Kelly's Heroes, Little Murders, Alex in Wonderland, Klute, F.T.A., Steelyard Blues, Lady Ice, Don't Look Now, S*P*Y*S*, The Day of the Locust, Casanova, The Eagle Has Landed, 1900, National Lampoon's Animal House, Invasion of the Body Snatchers, Murder by Decree, The Great Train Robbery, Nothing Personal, Ordinary People, Gas, Eye of the Needle, Threshold, Crackers, Ordeal by Innocence, Heaven Help Us, Revolution.
TV: (British) Gore Vidal's Marching to the Sea, Albee's The Death of Bessie Smith, Hamlet at Eisinore, The Saint, The Avengers, Gideon's Way, The Champions, The Winter of Our Discontent.

SUTTON, JAMES T.: Executive. b. Calif., Sept. 13 e. Columbia U.; film inspector, U.S. Government; overseas m.p. service, WW II; co-owner, gen. mgr., Hal Davis Studios; hd. TV commercial div., Allan Sandler Films; Academy Art Pictures; pres., chmn. of bd., exec. prod., Royal Russian Studios, Inc., western hemisphere div.; pres. exec. prod. Gold Lion Prods., Inc.; pres. exec. prod. James T. Sutton-John L. Carpenter Prods.; pres., exec. dir., Airax Corp.; pres. of Skyax (div. of Airax).

SUZMAN, JANET: Actress. b. Johannesburg, South Africa, Feb. 9, 1939. e. Kingsmead Coll., Univ. of Witwaterstrand. Joined the Royal Shakespeare Co. in 1962. London stage debut in The Comedy of Errors.
PICTURES: A Day in the Death of Joe Egg, Nicholas and Alexandra, The Black Windmill, Nijinsky, Priest of Love.
TELEVISION: The Three Sisters, Hedda Gabler, The House on Garibaldi Street, The Zany Adventures of Robin Hood.

SWALLOW, NORMAN: Producer. b. Manchester, Eng., Feb. 17, 1921. e. Manchester Grammar Sch., Keble Coll. (Oxford U.). British Army 1941–46; BBC as writer-prod. of docum., 1946; wrote 3 docum. films, 1948; TV as docum. prod., 1950; prods. include American Looks at Britain, with Howard K. Smith for CBS, Wilfred Pickles at Home series; orig. Speaking Personally series with appearance of people like Bertrand Russell; co-prod. TV coverage of Britain's general election, 1951; ed. prod. BBC monthly prog. Special Inquiry,

1952–56; World is Ours, 1954–56; study tour Middle East, India, Pakistan, Ceylon, 1956–57; writer, prod. Line of Defense, I Was a Stranger; asst. head films for BBC, 1957; writer-prod., On Target, 1959; apptd. chief asst. (doc. & gen.), BBC-TV, 1960; asst. editor, Panorama, BBC-TV, 1961. Joined Denis Mitchell films, May 1963; writer, prod., Pomp and Pageantry, The Right to Health, A Wedding on Saturday, 1964; The End of a Street, 1964; exec. prod., Report from Britain, 1964; writer, prod., Youth, British, Football; co-prod. This England. prod. A Railwayman for Me, 1966; co-prod. Ten Days That Shook the World, 1967. Co-prod. The Long Bridge, 1968. prod., dir., The Three Happiest Years; exec. prod. Omnibus series, 1968–70. Writer, prod., dir. To Leningrad With Love; exec. prod. Omnibus Series, 1968–72. Writer, co-prod. Eisenstein, 1970. BBC-TV Head of Arts Features 1972–74. Prod.-dir. series A Lasting Joy 1972. Exec. prod. Granada TV since 1974 of The Christians, This England, Clouds of Glory. Winner Desmond Davis Award (UK) 1977. Exec. prod. A Conductor At Work, A Pianist At Work, 1981. Prod., A Lot of Happiness (1982 Emmy Award). Freelance producer/director since 1985. The Last Day for BBC-TV, 1986.

SWAYZE, JOHN CAMERON: Reporter, commercial spokesman. b. Wichita, Kansas, Apr. 4, 1906; e. Univ. of Kansas; Anderson-Milton Dramatic Sch. Reporter and ed., Kansas City, Mo. Journal-Post; news dept. KMBC, Kansas City; head of news, NBC western network, Hollywood; NBC radio news reports, N.Y.C.; covered political conv. TV 1948–52; began News Caravan on NBC in 1949–56; panel mem. Who Said That, 1949–51; Watch the World on NBC-TV, 1948–50; Sightseeing With The Swayzes (with family) NBC-TV, 1953; news program, ABC, 1957. Host: Circle Theatre, NBC, and panel member, To Tell the Truth, CBS. Voted best news commentator, M.P. Daily TV Poll, 1951–55.
MEMBER: Lambs Club; National Press Club, Washington, Greenwich, Conn., CC.

SWAYZE, PATRICK: Actor. b. Houston, TX. 18. Began as dancer appearing in Disney on Parade on tour. On Bdwy. in Goodtime Charley, Grease, etc.
PICTURES: Skatetown USA, The Outsiders, Uncommon Valor, Red Dawn, Grandview USA, Youngblood.
TELEVISION: The New Season, Pigs vs. Freaks, The Comeback Kid, The Return of the Rebels, The Renegades.

SWEDROE, JEROME D.: Executive. b. N.Y.C., September 7, 1925. e. NYU, B.S. Entered industry 1949 bookkeeping dept. Skouras Theatres Corp. Advanced through dept. to Comptroller in March 1962 and v.p. June 1964. Appointed exec. v.p. in charge operations of the chain, name had been changed to United Artists Eastern Theatre Circuit, Inc., in April, 1967; promoted v.p. parent company, UATC, January 1968. Resigned to join Cinecom March 3, 1969. Elected director Aug. 1969; joined Redstone Management Co., June, 1971; named v.p., operations, U.S. Cinema Corp., December, 1971, consultant October, 1973.

SWERLING, JO: Writer. b. Russia, Apr. 8, 1897. Newspaper & mag. writer; author vaude. sketches; co-author plays, The Kibitzer, Guys and Dolls.
PICTURES INCLUDE: s.p., The Kibitzer, Guys and Dolls; s.p.; Platinum Blonde, Washington Merry-Go-Round, Dirigible, Man's Castle; collab. s.p., Whole Town's Talking; s.p., No Greater Glory, Pennies from Heaven, Double Wedding, Made for Each Other; collab. s.p., The Westerner; s.p., Confirm or Deny, Blood and Sand; collab. s.p., Pride of the Yankees; story, Lady Takes a Chance; s.p., Crash Dive, Lifeboat, Leave Her to Heaven, Thunder in the East.
TV: collab. The Lord Don't Play Favorites, NBC.

SWIFT, ALLEN: Performer. b. New York City, Jan. 16, 1924; Actor vaudeville, legitimate stage, radio and TV shows, including Bob Hope, Eddie Cantor, Jackie Gleason shows; voices for Mighty Mouse and UPA features and commercials; now announcer-master of ceremonies.

SWIFT, DAVID: Producer, director, writer. b. Minneapolis, 1919. Served with 8th Air Force in England, WW II. Entered m.p. ind. in Walt Disney animation dept. After service, comedy writer for radio. Later, starting in 1949, TV drama writer for Philco Playhouse, Studio One, Kraft Theatre, Omnibus. Created Mr. Peepers, Jamie. Writer-dir. Playhouse 90, Rifleman, Wagon Train, Climax, others. First feature film Pollyana (writer-dir.).
PICTURES INCLUDE: The Parent Trap, The Interns, Love Is a Ball, Under the Yum Yum Tree; pr.-dir.-writer, Good Neighbor Sam, How to Succeed in Business Without Really Trying, Candleshoe.

SWIFT, LELA: Director.
TV: Studio One, Suspense, The Web, Justice, Dupont Show of the Week, Purex Specials For Women, (Emmy Award) Dark Shadows, Norman Corwin Presents, ABC Late Night 90 min. Specials, ABC Daytime 90 min. Play Break. Won three Emmy awards for best director of day-time serial: Ryan's Hope (1977, 1979, 1980). Monitor award for best director of a daytime serial: Ryan's Hope, 1985.

SWIMMER, SAUL: Producer-director. b. Uniontown, Pa. e. Carnegie Tech Drama Dept. Producer-director of Melephant. Winner, Gold Leaf Venice Award, 1959. Director: Force of Impulse. Exec. prod. The Wounds of Hunger; prod. dir. Around the World of Mike Todd (Embassy Pictures TV Special, 1967), 1965–67; TV series development for Screen Gems. Advisor: CBS-TV Children's Film Festival (1967). In Charge of Production: Mrs. Brown, You've Got a Lovely Daughter, Only Lovers Left Alive; Stranger in the Night.
PICTURES INCLUDE: Cometogether (co-prod., dir.), The Concert for Bangladesh (dir.), Blindman (prod.).

SWINK, ROBERT E.: Film editor, Director. b. Rocky Ford, Colo., June 3, 1918; married. Joined editorial dept., RKO Radio, 1936; apptd. film ed., 1941. In U.S. Army Signal Corps, 1944–45; supv. editor, Fox studio. Edited numerous productions.
PICTURES INCLUDE: Detective Story, Carrie, Roman Holiday, Desperate House, Friendly Persuasion, The Big Country, The Diary of Anne Frank, The Young Doctors, The Children's Hour, The Best Man, The Collector, How To Steal A Million, Flim Flam Man, Funny Girl, The Liberation of L. B. Jones, The Cowboys, Skyjacked, Lady Ice, Papillion, Three the Hard Way, Rooster Cogburn, Midway, Islands in the Stream, Gray Lady Down, The Boys From Brazil, The In-Laws, Going in Style, The Sphinx.

SWISS, FERN: Executive. Executive director-financial planning for Motion Picture Group of Paramount Pictures. Joined co. in 1979 as financial analyst and advance to controller-TV in 1983. Named to present post, 1984.

SWIT, LORETTA: Actress. b. Passaic, NJ, Nov. 4, 1937. Stage debut in Any Wednesday. Toured in Mame for year. Arrived in Hollywood in 1969 and began TV career. Theatrical film debut in Stand Up and Be Counted, 1972.
PICTURES: Freebie and the Bean, Race with the Devil, "S.O.B.", Beer.
TELEVISION: MASH, Gunsmoke, Mannix, Hawaii Five-O, Mission: Impossible, The Doctors, Cade's County. Films: Shirts/Skin, Coffeeville, Valentine, Mirrors, Mirror, The Walls Came Tumbling Down, First Affair, The Execution.

SWOPE, HERBERT BAYARD, JR.: Director, producer, commentator. b. N.Y. e. Horace Mann Sch., Princeton Univ. U.S. Navy, 1941–46; rejoined CBS-TV as remote unit dir., 1946 directing many "firsts" in sportscasting; winner, Variety Show Management Award for sports coverage & citation by Amer. TV Society, 1948; joined NBC as dir., 1949; prod. dir., 1951; Lights Out, The Clock, The Black Robe, dir., Robert Montgomery Presents; winner, Sylvania, 1952. TV Award Outstanding Achievement in Directorial Technique; became executive producer, NBC-TV in charge of Wide, Wide, World; directed Arsenic & Old Lace on Best of Broadway, CBS-TV, 1955; dir. Climax, CBS-TV, Film prod., 20th Century-Fox, Hilda Crane, Three Brave Men, True Story of Jesse James, The Bravados, The Fiend who Walked the West; 1960–62; exec. prod. 20th-Fox TV; Many Loves of Dobie Gillis, Five Fingers; dir. co-prod. on Broadway, Step On A Crack, Fragile Fox, Fair Game for Lovers. 1970–72 exec. at NYC Off-Track Betting Corp. 1973–74; vice-president, Walter Reade Organization, Inc.; 1975–76 producer-host, This Was TV, Growth of a Giant; 1976 to present commmentator, Swope's Scope, (radio—WPBR-AM)); Critic (TV); Herbert Swope Interviews (WPTV, Palm Beach).

SYKES, ERIC: Scriptwriter, comedian. b. Oldham, England, 1924. Early career actor; ent. TV industry, 1948; wrote first three series, BBC's Educating Archie and radio, TV comedy series for Frankie Howard, Max Bygraves, Harry Secombe. BBC panel show member. Longterm contract ATV, 1956; own BBC series, 1958–65, Sykes Versus TV, The Frankie Howard Show; Sykes and a Big, Big Show, 1971, 1978 19th Year BBC-TV series. Toured extensively in Big Bad House. 1977 Summer Show Sykes. 1978 Tour of Sykes to Rhodesia, Australia, Canada, The Plank, Rhubarb. Toured one man show, 1982. Time and Time Again, 1983; Run for Your Wife (London & Canada).
PICTURES INCLUDE: Watch Your Stern, Invasion Quartet, Village of Daughters, Kill or Cure, Heavens Above, The Bargee, One Way Pendulum, Those Magnificent Men in Their Flying Machines, Rotten to the Core, The Liquidator, Spy With The Cold Nose. 1967, Dir. s.p. The Plank, Shalako, The Monte Carlo Rally, Theatre of Blood.
TELEVISION: Varying specials, remade The Plank, If You Go Down to the Woods Today, Cannon and Ball Show, It's Your Move.

SYLBERT, ANTHEA: Executive. b. New York. e. Barnard (B.A.); Parsons School of Design (M.A.). Early career in costume design with range of Bdwy., off-Bdwy. and m.p. credits (Rosemary's Baby, F.I.S.T., Shampoo, The Fortune, A New Leaf, The Heartbreak Kid. Two A.A. nominations for creative costume designs for Julia and Chinatown. Joined Warner

Bros. in October, 1977, as v.p., special projects, acting as liaison between creative executives, production dept., and creative talent producing films for company. In October, 1978, named v.p., production (projects included One Trick Pony, Personal Best, etc.). In March, 1980 appointed v.p.—production, for United Artists, working on Stab, Jinx, etc. For Warner Bros.: Swing Shift, Protocol, Wildcats.

SYMS, SYLVIA: Actress. b. London, 1934. e. Convent and Grammar Schools. Film debut, 1955, My Teenage Daughter.
PICTURES INCLUDE: No Time for Tears, Birthday Present, Woman in a Dressing Gown, Ice Cold in Alex, The Devil's Disciple, Moonraker, Bachelor of Hearts, No Trees in the Street, Ferry to Hong Kong, Expresso Bongo, Conspiracy of Hearts, The World of Suzie Wong, Flame in the Streets, Victim, Quare Fellow, Punch & Judy Man, The World Ten Times Over, East of Sudan, The Eliminator, Operation Crossbow, The Big Job, Hostile Witness, The Marauders, The White Cold, Danger Route, Run Wild, Run Free, The Desperados, The Tamarind Seed, Give Us This Day, There Goes the Bride.
TV: The Human Jungle (series), Something to Declare, The Saint (series), The Baron (series), Bat Out of Hell, Department in Terror, Friends and Romans, Strange Report, Half-hour Story, The Root of All Evil, The Bridesmaid, Clutterbuck, Movie Quiz, My Good Woman, Looks Familiar, Love and Marriage, The Truth About Verity, I'm Bob, He's Dickie, Blankety Blank, The Story of Nancy Astor, Give Us a Clue, Sykes, Crown Court, A Murder Is Announced, Murder at Lynch Cross.

T

TAFFNER DONALD L.: Executive. b. New York City. e. St. Johns University. William Morris Agency, 1950–59; Paramount Pictures. 1959–63; D. L. Taffner Ltd., 1963-present.

TAKEI, GEORGE: Actor. b. Los Angeles, April 20. e. University of Calif., UCLA. Professional debut in Playhouse 90 production while training at Desilu Workshop in Hollywood. Gained fame as Sulu in Star Trek TV series. Co-author of novel, Mirror Friend, Mirror Foe.
PICTURES: Ice Palace, A Majority of One, Hell to Eternity, An American Dream, Walk, Don't Run, The Green Berets, Star Trek—The Motion Picture, Star Trek II: The Wrath of Khan, Star Trek III: The Search for Spock.
TELEVISION: Perry Mason, Alcoa Premiere, Mr. Novak, The Wackiest Ship in the Army, I Spy, Magnum PI, Trapper John, MD, etc.

TALBOT, JOSEPH T. (Brud): Producer-Director-Actor. b. NYC, Sept. 16, 1938. e. Deerfield Academy, University of Virginia, Welsh Drama Workshop. Co-producer, actor: Force of Impulse, 1961; Without Each Other, 1962; Wounds of Hunger, 1963; co-star, Finger on the Trigger, 1964; Production supervisor TV special "Around the World of Mike Todd." 1965. Producer, Soundblast '66, musical spectacular Yankee Stadium, 1966. Producer-director TV commercials & documentaries, Filmex, Inc., 1966–69. Producer-director TV Documentary, The Singlehanders. President Dana Films Ltd., 1969–72; prod. Run Before the Wind, (Official m.p. rep. to Bicentennial Council of the Thirteen Original States), 1972–73 Executive in charge of Production Cinemation Industries; 1976–78 pres., Truesdale Pictures Ltd.
OTHER PICTURES:: The Case of the Smiling Stiff (prod., dir.); The Black Pearl (co.-prod.); Willie Sutton, Bank Robber (Prod.).

TALBOT, LYLE: Actor. r.n. Lysle Hollywood. b. Pittsburgh, Pa., Feb. 8, 1904. In Army Air Corps, World War II. First screen appearance in Vitaphone short; then in Love Is A Racket, 1932.
PICTURES INCLUDE: Up in Arms, Sensations of 1945, One Body Too Many, Dixie Jamboree, Gambler's Choice, Strange Impersonation, Vicious Circle, Mutineers, Sky Dragon, The Jackpot, Sea Tiger, Down Among the Sheltering Palms, Star of Texas, Capt. Kidd & the Slave Girl, Tobor the Great, Steel Cage, There's No Business Like Show Business, Jail Busters, Sudden Danger.
MEMBER: Masonic Lodge (Shriner), Lambs, Masquers, American Legion.

TAMBLYN, RUSS: Actor b. Los Angeles, Calif., Dec. 30, 1935. e. No. Hollywood H.S. West Coast radio shows; on stage with little theatre group; song-and-dance act in Los Angeles clubs, veterans hospitals.
PICTURES INCLUDE: Boy with Green Hair, Reign of Terror, Samson and Delilah, Deadly Is the Female, Kid from Cleveland, Captain Carey, U.S.A., Father of the Bride, As Young as You Feel, Father's Little Dividend, Winning Team, Retreat Hell, Take the High Ground, Seven Brides for Seven Brothers, Many Rivers to Cross, Hit the Deck, Last Hunt, Fastest Gun Alive, Young Guns, Don't Go Near the Water, Peyton Place, High School Confidential, Tom Thumb, Cimarron, West Side Story, Wonderful World of the Brothers Grimm, The Haunting, Long Ships, Son of Gunfighter, The Last Movie.

TANDY, JESSICA: Actress. b. London, Eng., June 7, 1909; wife of Hume Cronyn. On London, N.Y. stage, 1928–42.
THEATRE: N.Y. stage. Streetcar named Desire, Hilda Crane, The Four Poster, Coward In Two Keys; The Way of the World, Eve and A Midsummer Night's Dream at Stratford Festival 1976, Canada; limited tours of Many Faces of Love 1974, 75, 76 and for CBC, Canada 1977; performed in The Gin Game, Long Wharf Thea., New Haven, Conn. June 1977; Long Day's Journey Into Night, Theatre London, London, Canada 1977. Appeared in The Gin Game, Pulitzer Prize Winning Play, at The Golden Thea. N.Y.C. 1977–78, and toured with it in U.S., Toronto, London and U.S.S.R., 1979 and Long Day's Journey Into Night Foxfire, Stratford Festival 1980, Rose Cort, NYC 1981; Foxfire, Guthrie Theatre, Minneapolis 1981 and NYC in 1982–83; The Glass Menagerie, NYC, 1983.
PICTURES INCLUDE: The Green Years, Forever Amber, A Woman's Vengeance, September Affair, The Desert Fox, Adventures of a Young Man, Butley, A Light in the Forest, The Birds, Honky Tonk Freeway, Still of the Night, The World According to Garp, Best Friends, The Bostonians.

TANEN, NED: Executive. b. Los Angeles. e. UCLA (law degree). Joined MCA, Inc. 1954; Appd. v.p. in 1968. Brought Uni Records, since absorbed by MCA Records, to best-seller status with such artists as Neil Diamond, Elton John, Olivia Newton-John. First became active in theatrical film prod. in 1972. In 1975 began overseeing feature prod. for Universal. In 1976 named pres. of Universal Theatrical Motion Pictures, established as div. of Universal City Studios to encompass all theatrical film prod. activities. Left in 1982 to become independent producer. 1985, joined Paramount Pictures as pres. of Motion Picture Group.

TANKERSLEY, ROBERT K.: Executive. b. Decatur, Ill., July 31, 1927. In U.S. Navy, 1945–46; Marine Corps, 1949–55. With Natl. Theatre Supply as salesman in Denver 13 yrs. 1959 to present, pres. Western Service & Supply, Denver, theatre equip. form. Also is pres. theatre chain, Theatre Operators, Inc., Bozeman, Mont. Member: Theatre Equipment Assn. (past pres.), National NATO (presently dir.), Rocky Mt. Motion Picture Assn. (past pres.), SMPTE, Motion Picture Pioneers.

TANNER, WINSTON R.: Exhibitor. b. Appomattox, Va., Feb. 10, 1905. e. U. of Richmond. Entered m.p. ind., 1939 as asst. to owner, mgr. Free State Victoria Theatres, Kenbridge, Va.; dir. partner Kendig-Tanner Theatres, 1942; bought partner's interest in 1957; operator Tanner Theatres 7 houses, in Va.; operates Winston R. Tanner booking-buying service.

TAPLIN, JONATHAN: Producer. b. Cleveland, OH, July 18, 1947. e. Princeton Univ.
PICTURES: Mean Streets, The Last Waltz, Carny, Under Fire, Baby, My Science Project.
TELEVISION: Six episodes of Shelly Duvall's Faerie Tale Theatre.

TAPS, JONIE: Producer. Executive. Columbia Studio.
PICTURES INCLUDE: Jolson Story, Down to Earth, Thrill of Brazil. Produced: When You're Smiling, Sunny Side of Street, Sound Off, Rainbow Round My Shoulder, All Ashore, Cruisin' Down the River, Drive a Crooked Road, Three for the Show, Bring Your Smile Along, He Laughed Last, Shadow on the Window.
MEMBER: Friars Club, Hillcrest Country Club.

TARADASH, DANIEL: Writer. Director. b. Louisville, Ky., Jan. 29, 1913. e. Harvard Coll., BA, 1933; Harvard Law Sch., LL.B., 1936. Passed N.Y. Bar, 1937; won nationwide playwriting contest, 1938; U.S. Army W.W. II.
PICTURES INCLUDE: collab. s.p. Golden Boy, A Little Bit of Heaven, Knock on Any Door; s.p., Rancho Notorious, Don't Bother to Knock, From Here to Eternity (Acad. Award 1953); Desiree; collab. story, s.p. and dir., Storm Center; s.p., Picnic, Bell Book and Candle. The Saboteur Code Name—Morituri; col. s.p. Hawaii; collab. s.p. Castle Keep, s.p. Doctors' Wives; Collab. s.p. The Other Side of Midnight. Pres. Screen Writers Branch, WGA, 1955–56; v.p., Writers Guild of America, West 1956–59; mem. Writers Guild Council, 1954–65; mem., bd. of govnrs. M.P. Acad. of Arts & Sciences, 1964–74, and v.p. 1968–70; chmn., trustee, Producers-Writers Guild Pension plan 1960–73. Mem. Bd. of Trustees of American Film Institute 1967–69. WGA's Valentine Davies Award, 1971. Pres., Academy M.P. Arts & Sciences, 1970–73, member of Board of Trustees, Entertainment Hall of Fame Foundation. Member, Public Media General Programs panel for the National Foundation for the Arts, Pres. Writers Guild of America, West, 1977–79. Nat'l. chm., Writers Guild of America, 1979–81.

TARNOFF, JOHN B.: Producer. b. New York City, Mar. 3, 1952. e. UCLA (motion pictures & TV, 1973–74); Amherst College (BA, 1969–73). Named field exec. with Taylor-Laughlin Distribution (company arm of Billy Jack Enterprises) 1974; left in 1975 to be literary agent with Bart/Levy, Inc.; later with Michael Levy & Associates, Paul Kohner/Michael Levy Agency; Headed TV dept., Kohner/Levy, 1979. Joined MGM as production exec., 1979; v.p., development, 1979–80; sr. v.p. production & devel., 1981–82; exec. v.p., Kings Road Prods., 1983–84; v.p., prod., Orion Pictures Corp., 1985; exec. prod., Out of Bounds, Columbia Pictures, 1986.

TARTIKOFF, BRANDON: Executive. b. New York City, 1949. e. Yale Univ. Started TV career in 1971 in promo. dept. of ABC affiliates in New Haven, Ct. Joined promo. staff at ABC affiliate in Chicago. In 1976 went to New York, with ABC-TV as mgr., dramatic development; moved to NBC Entertainment in Sept., 1977, as dir., comedy programs. In 1978 appt. v.p., programs, West Coast, NBC Entertainment; 1980, named pres. of that division.

TASCO, RAI: Actor, announcer. r.n. Ridgeway Tasco. b. Boston, Mass., Aug. 12, 1917. e. Boston English High. 1935. U.S. Army, 1935–45. Grad., Cambridge School of Radio & TV, New York, 1950. Appeared in most TV and radio dramatic shows, and stage plays, New York and Hollywood; Broadway stage & films; dramatic instructor.

TATUM, DONN B.: Executive. b. Los Angeles, January 9, 1913. e. Stanford, Oxford. Director, retired chm. & chief exec., Walt Disney Co. 1943, lawyer, RCA and ABC. 1949, v.p., counsel, Dir. of Don Lee Companies. Gen. Mgr., KABC, dir. of Television, Western Division ABC. 1956, prod. business mgr. for Walt Disney Productions; exec. v.p. Disneyland, v.p. TV sales; v.p. and adm. asst. to pres. and exec. comm.; exec. v.p.; president; now Member of Bd. of Dir.; a director of Greyhound Corp; director and chm. John Tracy Clinic; dir. & v.p. Community Building Funds of So. Calif.; trustee of Calif. Institute of the Arts, the Salk Institute & the St. John's Hospital Foundation; overseer, Huntington Library.

TAVERNIER, BERTRAND: Director-Writer. b. Lyon, April 25, 1941. After 2 yrs. of law study, quit to become film critic. Partner for 6 yrs. with Pierre Rissient in film promotion company, during which time he studied all aspects of film-making. Debut picture: The Watchmaker of St. Paul (aka The Clockmaker) in 1974.
PICTURES INCLUDE: Let Joy Reign Supreme (dir., co-writer), The Judge and the Assassin, Spoiled Children, Deathwatch, A Week's Vacation, Clean Slate, Mississippi Blues, A Sunday in the Country, 'Round Midnight.

TAYLOR, ANTHONY: Producer. b. Los Angeles, Calif., Feb. 5, 1931. e. U. of So. Cal.; USAF 1954–56; mem. Chicago Board of Trade, 1962–65; columnist, L.A. Herald Examiner, 1964–65; also mem. N.Y. Mercantile Exchange, Chicgo Mercantile Exchange; partner commodity Futures Co., Westwood, Calif.; 1966, produced feature Incubus; 1966, award for motion picture excellence, San Francisco Int'l Film Festival; 1967, award Incubus, Cork Int'l Film Festival, Ireland; 1968: prod. feature, Possession.

TAYLOR, DELORES: Actress-Writer. b. Winner, So. Dak. e. Univ. of So. Dak., studying commercial art. m. Tom Laughlin. First TV experience was heading art dept. at RCA wholesale center in Milwaukee. Made feature film debut as actress in Billy Jack in 1971. Wrote s.p. with husband for that and the sequel, The Trial of Billy Jack, under pseudonym Teresa Christina.
PICTURES INCLUDE: Billy Jack, The Trial of Billy Jack.

TAYLOR, DON: Actor-Director. b. Freeport, Pa., Dec. 13. e. Pennsylvania State Univ. Appeared in Army Air Corps' Winged Victory; on stage & screen; author short stories, radio dramas, one-act plays, TV shows, both ½ hour and hour.
PICTURES INCLUDE: Actor: Girl Crazy, Naked City, For the Love of Mary, Battleground, Father of the Bride, Father's Little Dividend, Submarine Command, Flying Leathernecks, Blue Veil, Japanese War Bride, Stalag 17, The Girls of Pleasure Island, Destination Gobi, Johnny Dark, I'll Cry Tomorrow, Bold and the Brave. Director: Jack of Diamonds, Five Man Army, Escape from The Planet of the Apes, Tom Sawyer, Echoes Of A Summer, The Great Scout and Cathouse Thursday, The Island of Dr. Moreau, Damien-Omen II, The Final Countdown.
TELEVISION: Director: He's Not Your Son, My Wicked Wicked Ways, Secret Weapons, Going for the Gold.

TAYLOR, ELIZABETH: Actress. b. London, Eng.., Feb. 27, 1932; e. Bryon House, London, When 3 years old danced before Princess Elizabeth, Margaret Rose. Came to U.S. on outbreak World War II. In 1943–44 screen debut Lassie Comes Home.
PICTURES INCLUDE: National Velvet, Life with Father, Cynthia, Courage of Lassie, Little Women, White Cliffs of Dover, Jane Eyre, Date With Judy, Conspirator, Big Hangover, Father of the Bride, Father's Little Dividend, Love Is Better Than Ever, Place in the Sun, Ivanhoe, The Girl Who Had Everything, Rhapsody, Elephant Walk, Beau Brummell, Last Time I Saw Paris, Giant, Raintree Country, Suddenly, Last Summer, Butterfield 8, Cleopatra, The V.I.P.'s, The Night of the Iguana, Who's Afraid of Virginia Woolf, The Taming of the Shrew, The Sandpiper, Doctor Faustus, The Comedians, Reflections In A Golden Eye, Boom!, Secret Ceremony, The Only Game in Town, X, Y, and Zee, Hammersmith Is Out, Night Watch, Ash Wednesday, That's Entertainment!, The Driver's Seat, The Blue Bird, A Little Night Music, The Mirror Crack'd.
TELEVISION: Movies: Divorce His, Divorce Hers, Victory at Entebbe, Repeat Performance, Between Friends, Malice in Wonderland.

TAYLOR, KENT: Actor. r.n. Louis Weiss. b. Nashua, Iowa, May 11, 1907. In many feature productions from 1931.
PICTURES INCLUDE: Merrily We Go to Hell, Blonde Venus, Death Takes a Holiday, Mrs. Wiggs of the Cabbage Patch, Alaska, Bomber's Moon, Roger Touhy—Gangster, Notorious Gentleman, Dangerous Millions, Deadline for Murder, Second Chance, Crimson Key, Half Past Midnight, Western Pacific Agent, Payment on Demand, Playgirl, Slightly Scarlet, Track the Man Down, Secret Venture, Ghost Town, Iron Sheriff.
TV: Boston Blackie.

TAYLOR, LAWRENCE: Writer. b. Atlanta, Ga.; e. Northwestern U., '33. Reporter, dramatic critic, foreign correspondent 1934–40; writer radio, m.p., 1940–42; U.S.A.F., 1942–45; writer, m.p. story consultant. TV since 1945, U.S. and England.
PICTURES INCLUDE: Dixie Jamboree, Philco Vance's Secret Mission, Devil Ship, Bulldog Drummond Strikes Back; (story basis) Lady Without a Passport; (collab. s.p.) Jackie Robinson Story, Candelario (coll. with son, Heath).

TAYLOR, MICHAEL: Executive. b. New York City, March 28. Joined United Artists in 1973 as trainee. Named asst. to v.p. in chg. of production, 1975. Appointed exec. in chg. of production in London, where worked in acquisition and production of properties, working on such pictures as The Spy Who Loved Me, Valentino, The Pink Panther Strikes Again, etc. Left U.A. to form Taylor/Wigutow Productions in 1977. Produced Last Embrace, The Pursuit of D. B. Cooper. In 1982 joined Orion Pictures as exec. asst. to pres; made corporate v.p., 1984.

TAYLOR, RENEE: Actress-Writer. b. March 19, 1945. Wife of actor Joseph Bologna, with whom she collaborates in writing. Their Bdwy. plays include Lovers and Other Strangers.
PICTURES: Actress: The Last of the Red Hot Lovers, The Errand Boys, The Detective, The Producers, A New Leaf, Lovers and Other Strangers (also s.p.), Made for Each Other (also s.p.), Lovesick.
TELEVISION: Writer: Acts of Love and Other Comedies (Emmy), Paradise, Calucci's Department, The American Dream Machine, etc.

TAYLOR, ROD: Actor. b. Sydney, Australia, Jan. 11, 1929. e. Fine Arts College. Started out as artist then turned to acting on stage. After co-starring in film Long John Silver, to Hollywood in 1954. First film The Virgin Queen, followed by Giant, Separate Tables and Step Down to Terror. Also made a number of TV appearances. Formed own company, Rodler, Inc., for TV-film production.
PICTURES INCLUDE: Ask Any Girl, The V.I.P.'s, The Birds, Sunday in New York, Young Cassidy, The Time Machine, Seven Seas to Calais, A Gathering of Eagles, 36 Hours, Do Not Disturb, The Glass Bottom Boat, Hotel, Chuka, Dark of the Sun, The Hell with Heroes, Zabriskie Point, The Train Robbers, Trader Horn, The Deadly Trackers, A Time To Die, On the Run.
TELEVISION: Cry of the Innocent, Charles and Diana, Masquerade.

TAYLOR-YOUNG, LEIGH: Actress. b. Washington, D.C., Jan. 25, 1945. e. Northwestern Univ.
PICTURES: I Love You, Alive B. Toklas, The Big Bounce, The Adventurers, The Buttercup Chain, The Horseman, The Gang That Couldn't Shoot Straight, Soylent Green, Can't Stop the Music, Looker, Secret Admirer, Jagged Edge.
TELEVISION: Peyton Place (series), Marathon.

TEITELBAUM, PEDRO: Executive. b. Porto Alegre, Rio Grande Do Sul, Brasil, Nov. 21, 1922. e. Colegio Uniao, Brasil, 1942 (CPA); Univ. of Porto Alegre, Brasil, 1945 (economics & business admin.) 1939; Columbia Pictures; 1943, Warner Brothers; 1958, Latin-American supervisor for Republic Pictures; 1957, producer, distributor, exhibitor in Brasil; 1968, area supervisor for United Artists; 1973, v.p. intl. sales; 1975, v.p. international sales & distribution; 1976, senior v.p. and foreign manager. In Jan., 1977, joined CIC as senior exec. v.p. Named pres., July, 1977.

TELLER, IRA Executive, b. New York, N.Y., July 3, 1940. e. CCNY 1957–61; NYU Graduate Sch. of Arts, 1961–62; publicist, Pressbook Dept., 20th Century Fox., 1961–62; asst. to adv. mgr., Embassy Pictures Corp., 1962–63; asst. adv. mgr., Columbia Pictures Corp., 1963; adv. mgr., Columbia Pictures Corp., 1964, 1964–65; asst. to chmn. of bd., Diener, Hauser, Greenthal Agy., 1966; adv. mgr., 20th Century-Fox, 1966–67; 1967, adv. dir. 20th Cent.-Fox.; Dir. of Adv., Nat'l General Pictures Corp., 1969; eastern dir., adv.-pub., 1972; National Director, Adv-Pub., 1973; Bryanston Distributors, Inc. v.p. adv.-pub., 1974; Cine Artists Pictures Corp. v.p. adv-pub., 1975; Lorimar Productions, v.p., adv.-marketing, 1976–77. 1977-present, pres. Ira Teller and Company, Inc.

TEMPLE, SHIRLEY JANE: Actress. b. Santa Monica, Calif., April 23, 1929. In 1932 screen debut, Red Haired Alibi. In 1933 To the Last Man; then leading figure in Baby Burlesque series Educational shorts until Stand Up and Cheer (1934), which resulted in career as child star.

PICTURES INCLUDE: Baby Takes a Bow, Bright Eyes, Now I'll Tell, Change of Heart, Little Miss Marker, Now and Forever, The Little Colonel, Our Little Girl, Curly Top, The Littlest Rebel, Captain January, Poor Little Rich Girl, Dimples, Stowaway, Wee Willie Winkle, Heidi, Rebecca of Sunnybrook Farm, Little Miss Broadway, Just Around the Corner, Little Princess, Susannah of the Mounties, The Blue Bird, Young People. In 1941 Kathleen. In 1942 Miss Annie Rooney. Voted one of ten best Money-Making Stars in Motion Picture Herald-Fame Poll, 1934–39. Since You Went Away, I'll Be Seeing You, Kiss and Tell, That Hagen Girl, Honeymoon, Fort Apache, Bachelor and the Bobby-Soxer, Mr. Belvedere Goes to College, Adventure in Baltimore, Story of Seabiscuit, Kiss for Corliss.

TV: Hostess, fairy tale series.

TENNANT, VICTORIA: Actress. b. London, England, Sept. 30, 1953. e. Central School of Speech & Drama. Daughter of ballerina Irene Baronova and talent agent Cecil Tennant.

PICTURES: The Ragman's Daughter, The Speckeld Band, The Killing, Strangers Kiss, Horror Planet, All of Me.

TELEVISION: Winds of War, Dempsey, Chiefs.

TENNANT, WILLIAM: Executive. Partner in literary agency of Ziegler, Ross, and Tennant. Turned to m.p. production with Cleopatra Jones for Warner Bros., following with writing and producing of sequel, Cleopatra and the Casino of Gold. In 1975 joined Columbia Pictures as v.p.-prod., headquartering at Burbank Studios. Named pres., Casablanca Filmworks; now pres., PolyGram Pictures m.p. division..

TERRY, SIR JOHN: Film Consultant. b. London, England, 1913; e. Mill Hill School. Early career as solicitor. Entered m.p. ind. Film Producers Guild 1946–47; then legal dept. Rank Organization until 1949; joined National Film Finance Corporation; its chief solicitor 1949–57; sec., 1956–57; man. dir., 1958–78.

TESICH, STEVE: Writer. b. Yugoslavia. e. Indiana Univ., Columbia. Came to U.S. at age 14. While doing graduate work in Russian literature at Columbia left to begin writing. Taken up by American Place Theatre which did his play, The Carpenters, in 1970 and then six others. Wrote screnplays; first produced was Breaking Away, 1979; then Four Friends, 1981; The World According to Garp, 1982; Eleni, 1985.

TETZLAFF, TED: Director. b. Los Angeles, Calif., June 3, 1903. Joined camera dept. Fox Studios, became first cameraman; dir., 1940; served in U.S. Air Corps as a Major, World War II.

PICTURES INCLUDE: cameraman: Enchanted Cottage, Notorious; dir.: World Premiere, Riffraff, Fighting Father Dunne, Window, Johnny Allegro, Dangerous Profession, Gambling House, White Tower, Under the Gun, Treasure of Lost Canyon, Terror on a Train, Son of Sinbad.

TEWKESBURY, JOAN: Writer. e. Univ. of So. Calif. Directed and choreographed Little Theatre prods. in L.A. area; taught in theatre arts depts. of three universities: Univ., of So. Calif., Immaculate Heart and Mount St. Mary's. Became script supvr. for Robert Altman on McCabe & Mrs. Miller.

PICTURES INCLUDE: Thieves Like Us (co. s.p.), Nashville, (s.p.), Old Boyfriends (dir.), A Night in Heaven (s.p.).

THACHER, RUSSELL: Producer-Writer. b. Hackensack, N.J. e. Bucknell Univ., N.Y.U. Author of novels: The Captain, The Tender Age, A Break in the Clouds. Editor Omnibook Magazine, 1946–58; Book of the Month Club, 1958–63. Exec, story editor, MGM, 1963–69. Exec. prod., MGM, 1969–72. Dri., creative affairs, Samuel Goldwyn Co., 1983–84.

PICTURES INCLUDE: Travels with My Aunt (assoc. prod.), Soylent Green, The Cay, Last Hard Men, The Golden Seal (assoc. prod.), Once Bitten (assoc. prod.).

THALHIMER, JR., MORTON G.: Theatre Executive. b. Richmond, Va., June 27, 1924. e. Dartmouth Coll. (1948, B.A.); Univ. of Va. (1959). Naval aviator in World War II. Joined Century Theatres as trainee 1948; Jamestown Amusement, 1949–50. Now pres. Neighborhood Theatre, Inc. Charter member of Theatre Owners of America; continuing member and v.p. of NATO, served on finance comm. and Trade Practice comm. bd. member and past president of NATO of Va. (1973–75.) Mem. Variety Club Int'l., Tent 11; patron life member, Variety Club of Israel, Tent 51.

THATCHER, HEATHER: Actress. b. London, England. London stage debut in Girl From Ciro's 1916. Entered m.p. ind. as extra in 1916.

PLAYS: Naughty Princess, Sally, Constant Wife, School for Husbands, Lucky Break, Full House.

PICTURES INCLUDE: (Hollywood pictures since 1936): Hour of Thirteen, Duel in the Jungle.

THAXTER, PHYLLIS: Actress. b. Portland, Me., Nov. 20, 1921; e. St. Genevieve School, Montreal. Screen debut in Thirty Seconds Over Tokyo.

PICTURES INCLUDE: Week-End at the Waldorf, Bewitched, Tenth Avenue Angel, Sign of the Ram, Blood on the Moon, The Breaking Point, Fort Worth, Jim Thorpe—All American, Come Fill the Cup, She's Working Her Way Through College, Operation Secret, Springfield Rifle, Women's Prison, World of Henry Orient, Superman.

TV: Wagon Train, Alfred Hitchcock, Twilight Zone, Purex Specials For Women, Playhouse 90, The Fugitive, Defenders, Three Sovereigns for Sarah, etc.

THEODORAKIS, MIKIS: Composer. b. Greece, 1925.

PICTURES: Eva, Night Ambush, Shadow of the Cat, Phaedra, Five Miles to Midnight, Zorba the Greek, The Day the Fish Came Out, The Trojan Women, State of Siege, Serpico, Iphigenia.

THINNES, ROY: Actor. b. Chicago, April 6, 1938.

PICTURES: Journey to the Far Side of the Sun, Charlie One-Eye, Airport 75, The Hindenburg.

TELEVISION: Series: The Long Hot Summer. Movies: The Other Man, The Psychiatrist: God Bless the Children, Black Noon, The Horror at 37,000 Feet, The Norliss Tales, Satan's School for Girls, Death Race, The Manhunter, Secrets, Code Name: Diamond Head, From Here to Eternity, The Return of the Mod Squad, etc.

THOMAS, BILL: Fashion designer. b. Chicago, Ill., Oct. 13, 1921; e. U.S.C., A.B. 1941. Art Center, Los Angeles, 1941. Started career as designer on assignment to USO shows; Theatre Royale, Brisbane, Australia; from duty with U.S. A.F., 1941–46. Asst. to Irene, Irene Inc., 1948; asst. costume designer MGM Studios 1947–48; U-I Studios 1949–59; currently free lance.

PICTURES INCLUDE: High Time, Beloved Infidel, By Love Possessed, Babes in Toyland.

THOMAS, DANNY: Actor. r.n. Amos Jacobs. b. Deerfield, Mich., Jan. 6, 1914. Night club entertainer; on radio and TV, films.

TV: Own TV show, The Danny Thomas Show, CBS-TV, 1953–64; NBC-TV specials 1964–66, Danny Thomas Show, 1967–68; CBS-TV Specials 1967 & 1970. Make Room for Grandaddy series 1970–71, ABC-TV; The Practice, 1976–77; NBC-TV.

PICTURES INCLUDE: Unfinished Dance, Big City, Call Me Mister, I'll See You in My Dreams, Jazz Singer.

THOMAS, GERALD: Producer, director. b. Hull, England, 1920. Entered m.p. industry 1946.

PICTURES INCLUDE: Tony Draws a Horse, Appointment With Venus, Venetian Bird, Sword and the Rose, A Day to Remember, Mad About Men, Doctor in the House, Above Us the Waves, A Novel Affair, After the Ball, Timelock, Vicious Circle, Chain of Events, Solitary Child, The Duke Wore Jeans, Carry On Sergeant, Carry on Nurse, Carry on Teacher, Please Turn Over, Carry on Constable, Watch Your Stern, No Kidding, Carry on Regardless, Raising The Wind, Twice Around the Daffodils, Carry on Cruising, The Iron Maiden, Nurse on Wheels, Call Me a Cab, Carry on Jack, Carry on Spying, Carry On Cleo, The Big Job, Carry On Cowboy, Carry on Screaming, Don't Lose Your Head, Follow That Camel, Carry on Doctor, Carry On Up The Khyber, Carry on Up the Jungle, Carry on Loving, Carry on Camping, Carry On Again, Doctor, Carry On, Henry, Carry On At Your Convenience, Carry On Matron, Carry on Abroad, Bless This House, Carry On Girls, Carry on Dick, Carry On Behind, Carry On England, That's Carry On, Carry On Emmannuelle.

TV: Prod. and dir. Rob Roy, serial; The Second Victory. Prod. Carry on Christmas for Thames TV. Prod., Carry On Laughing for ATV. Dir. Best of Carry On. Prod. Odd Man Out, series for Thames TV. Dir., Carry on Laughing, Just for Laughs, Comedy Tonight (Canada), What a Carry On.

THOMAS, HARRY E.: Exhibitor. b. Monroe, La., May 22, 1920; e. L.S.U. 1938–41. Psychological Branch of Army Air Force, 1942–46. Past pres., secy., and treas. of NATO of Mississippi. Dir. of Design & Const. & Sec. Gulf State Theatres Inc. Retired 1978.

THOMAS, HOWARD: Executive. b. CWM. Monmouthshire. Entered m.p. ind. in 1944. Newspaper columnist & feature writer; adv. copywriter; writer of revue sketches, books, radio plays; mgr., sponsored radio dept., London Press Exchange, Ltd.; BBC prod. & orig. The Brains Trust. Prod.-in-chief, Associated British-Pathe, Ltd.; managing dir., ABC Television Ltd., 1956. Appt. dir., Associated British Picture Corp., 1964; div. dir., EMI, Ltd., 1970; man. dir., Thames TV, 1968–74; Thames TV Int. Ltd., pres., Cinema TV Veterans, 1979–80. Dir., Argus Press Ltd., T.I.E. Television Ltd.

THOMAS, MARLO: Actress. b. Detroit, Nov. 21, 1938. f. is Danny Thomas. e. U. of Southern Calif. Started career with small TV roles, summer stock. Appeared in London stage prod. of Barefoot in the Park. Debut in own TV series, That Girl, 1966. Most Promising Newcomer Awards from both "Fame" and "Photoplay."

PICTURES INCLUDE: Jenny, Thieves.

TELEVISION: Movies: The Lost Honor of Kathryn Beck (also exec. prod.), Consenting Adult, Nobody's Child.

THOMAS, PHILIP MICHAEL: Actor. b. Columbus, OH, May 26, 1949. e. Oakwood Coll.

PICTURE: Black Fist.

TELEVISION: Miami Vice.

THOMAS, RALPH: Director. b. Hull, Yorkshire, England, Aug. 10, 1915; e. Tellisford College, Clifton and Universtiy College, London. Journalist in early career, entered m.p. ind. 1932 as film ed.; service with 9th Lancers, 1939–45; then film director.

PICTURES INCLUDE: prod.: The Clouded Yellow, Appointment with Venus (Island Rescue), Day to Remember, Travellers' Joy, Venetian Bird, Once Upon a Dream, Doctor in the House, Mad about Men, Above Us the Waves, Doctor At Sea, Iron Petticoat, Checkpoint, Doctor at Large, Campbell's Kingdom, A Tale of Two Cities, The Wind Cannot Read, The 39 Steps, Upstairs and Downstairs, Conspiracy of Hearts, Doctors in Love, No Love for Johnnie, No, My Darling Daughter, A Pair of Briefs, The Wild & The Willing, Doctor in Distress, Hot Enough for June, The High Bright Sun, Agent 008½, Doctor in Clover, Deadlier Than the Male, Nobody Runs Forever, Some Girls Do, Doctor in Trouble, Percy, Quest, The Love Ban, Percy's Progress, A Nightingale Sang in Berkeley Square, Pop Pirates.

THOMAS, RICHARD: Actor. b. N.Y.C., June 13, 1951. e. Col. Univ. Made TV Debut at age 7 and featured in several series.

PICTURES INCLUDE: Last Summer, Red Sky at Morning, The Todd Killings, Cactus in the Snow, You'll Like My Mother, September 30th, 1955.

TELEVISION: Medical Center, Marcus Welby, M.D., The F.B.I., The Waltons (regular). Movies: The Fifth of July, The Master of Ballantrae, Hobson's Choice, Final Jeopardy.

THOMAS, ROBERT G. ("BOB"): Producer-Director. b. Glen Ridge, N.J., July 21, 1943. e. Univ. of Bridgeport, Fairleigh Dickinson Univ. Produced educational radio programs, 1962, WPKN-FM. Asst. stage manager at Meadowbrook Dinner Theatre, 1963. In March, 1964 began career as TV cameraman for New York stations. Worked both full-time and free-lance for major TV and video tape studios. In January, 1968, started Bob Thomas Productions and began producing business/sales films and TV commercials. Has 8 awards from natl. film festivals; nominated for 5 Emmys for TV series called The Jersey Side he produced for WOR-TV.

PICTURES: Shorts: Valley Forge with Bob Hope, New Jersey—200 Years. Road-Eo '77.

TV: The Jersey Side (talk/entertainment), Jersey People (weekly talk/entertainment program); $10,000 Touchdown (game show). Sir Reginald and the 3rd Dimension (Children's Show) 3-D Television—for local TV station promotion "The First Annual Comedy Awards" (TV Special).

THOMAS, ROBERT J. ("BOB"): Columnist, Associated Press, Hollywood. b. San Diego, Cal., Jan. 26, 1922; p. George H. Thomas, publicist; e. U. of Calif., L.A. Joined Associated Press staff, Los Angeles, 1943; corr. Fresno, 1944; Hollywood since 1944. Writer mag. articles; appearances, radio; orig. story Big Mike.

BOOKS: author: The Art of Animation, King Cohn, Thalberg, Selznick, Winchell, Secret Boss of California, The Heart of Hollywood, Howard, The Amazing Mr. Hughes, Weekend '33, Marlon, Portrait of the Rebel as an Artist, Walt Disney, An American Original; Bud and Lou, The Abbott and Costello Story; The Road to Hollywood (with Bob Hope); The One and Only Bing, Joan Crawford; Golden Boy: The Secret Life of William Holden; Astaire: The Man, The Dancer; I Got Rhythm; The Ethel Merman Story.

THOMOPOULOS, ANOTHONY D.: Executive. b. 1938. e. Georgetown Univ. Began career in broadcasting at NBC, 1959, starting as mailroom clerk and moving to radio division in prod. & admin. Shortly named to post in International Division Sales, involved with programming for stations and in developing TV systems for other nations. Joined Four Star Entertainment Corp. as dir. of foreign sales, 1964; named v.p., 1965; exec. v.p., 1969. In 1970 joined RCA SelectaVision Div. as dir. of programming. In 1971 joined Tomorrow Entertainment as v.p. In 1973 joined ABC as v.p., prime-time programs in N.Y.; 1974, named v.p., prime-time TV creative operations, ABC Entertainment. In 1975 named v.p. of special programs, ABC Entertainment; 1976 made v.p., ABC-TV, assisting pres. Frederick S. Pierce in supervising all activities of the division. In Feb., 1978 named pres. of ABC Entertainment. In June 1983 promoted to be pres., ABC Broadcast Group in chg. all TV & radio operations. 1986, pres. & COO, United Artists Corp.

THOMPSON, CARLOS: Actor. b. Buenos Aires, Argentina, June 7; e. National U., Buenos Aires. Stage & screen actor in Argentina; Hollywood m.p. debut in Fort Algiers, 1953.

PICTURES INCLUDE: Flame and the Flesh, Valley of the Kings, Magic Fire.

THOMPSON, J. LEE: Writer, Director, Producer. On Brit. stage; writer of stage plays including: Murder Without Crime, Cousin Simon, Curious Dr. Robson (collab.) Thousands of Summers, Human Touch. Writer and m.p. director.

PICTURES INCLUDE: The Yellow Balloon, Weak and the Wicked, Yield To The Night, Woman In The Dressing Gown, Ice Cold in Alex, No Trees in the Street, Tiger Bay, I Aim at the Stars, The Guns of Navarone, Taras Bulba, Cape Fear, Kings of the Sun, What A Way to Go, John Goldfarb, Please Come Home, Return From the Ashes, MacKenna's Gold, Battle for the Planet of the Apes, Before Winter Comes, Country Dance, Conquest of the Planet of the Apes, Huckleberry Finn, The Reincarnation of Peter Proud, St. Ives, The White Buffalo, The Greek Tycoon, The Passage, Caboblanco, Happy Birthday To Me, The Ambassador, The Evil That Men Do, King Solomon's Mines, Murphy's Law.

THOMPSON, JACK: Actor. b. Sydney, Australia, Aug. 31, 1940. e. Queensland Univ. Joined drama workshop at school; first part was in TV soap opera as continuing character.

PICTURES INCLUDE: A Sunday Too Far, The Chant of Jimmie Blacksmith, Breaker Morant (Australian award), The Earthling, The Club.

THOMPSON, MARSHALL: Actor. r.n. James Marshall Thompson; b. Peoria, Ill., Nov. 27, 1926. e. Occidental Coll., L.A. In school dramatics; studied for clergy; wrote play Faith, prod. by Westwood Players; in Westwood Players as actor; m.p. debut in Reckless Age, 1944.

PICTURES INCLUDE: They Were Expendable, Gallant Bess, Valley of Decision, Homecoming, B.F.'s Daughter, Words and Music, Command Decision, Roseanna McCoy, Battleground, Dial 1119, Devil's Doorway, Mystery Street, Tall Target, Basketball Fix, My Six Convicts, Rose Bowl Story, The Caddy, Battle Taxi, Port of Hell, Cult of the Cobra, Crashout, To Hell and Back, Clarence, The Cross-eyed Lion, Around the World Under the Sea, White Dog.

THOMPSON, SADA: Actress. b. Des Moines, Sept. 27, 1929. e. Carnegie Inst. of Technology, Pittsburgh. First N.Y. stage appearance in Under Milkwood with Dylan Thomas. Bdwy. career has produced many awards topped by The Effects of Gamma Rays, for which she won Obie, Drama Desk, Variety Poll.

TV: Sandburg's Lincoln, The Entertainer, Our Town, Princess Daisy. Series: Family (regular).

THOMSON, ALAN: Studio Publicity manager, EMI Elstree Studios Ltd. e. in Scotland. Early career in Glasgow with his father, well-known cinema manager. Ent. journalism on staff film magazine, other Scottish publications. Ent. m.p. with Associated British Productions 1953. Appt. studio pub. mgr. 1956.

THORPE, RICHARD: Director. b. Hutchinson, Kan., Feb. 24, 1896; m. Belva Kay, prof. In vaudeville, stock & musical comedy, 1915–18. Now retired.

PICTURES INCLUDE: cast, Torchy Comedies, Three O'Clock in the Morning, Burn 'Em Up Barnes, Flame of Desire; dir. since 1933. dir., Night Must Fall, Ivanhoe, Double Wedding, Crowd Roars, Earl of Chicago, Huckleberry Finn, White Cargo, Two Girls and a Sailor, Sun Comes Up, Big Jack, Challenge to Lassie, Malaya, Black Hand, Three Little Words, Vengeance Valley, The Great Caruso, Unknown Man, It's a Big Country, Carbine Williams, Prisoner of Zenda, The Girl Who Had Everything, All the Brothers Were Valiant, Knights of the Round Table, Student Prince, Athena, Quentin Durward, The Prodigal, The Tartars, Honeymoon Machine, Horizontal Lieutenant, Follow The Boys, The Truth About Spring, That Funny Feeling, Scorpio Letters, Last Challenge, Retired.

THULIN, INGRID: Actress, director. b. Solleftea, Sweden, Jan. 27, 1929. m. Harry Schein, founder and head of Sweden's Film Institute. Made acting debut at 15 at the Municipal Theatre in Norrkoping. Studied at Stockholm's Royal Dramatic Theatre. Worked with Malmo repertory. Appeared on Swedish stage in Gigi, Peer Gynt, Two for the Seesaw, Twelfth Night, Miss Julie. Has directed plays in Stockholm. N.Y. stage debut, 1967: Of Love Remembered.
PICTURES INCLUDE: For Ingmar Bergman: Wild Strawberries, Brink of Life (Best Actress Award, Cannes Film Festival), The Magician, Winter Light, The Silence, The Hour of the Wolf, The Ritual, Night Games, The Bathers, Adelaide, La Guerre Est Finie, The Four Horsemen of the Apocalypse, Return From Ashes, The Damned, Cries and Whispers, Moses, The Cassandra Crossing, Madame Kitty, After the Rehearsal. Dir. short film: Devotion.

THUNA, LEONORA: Writer-Producer. b. May 3, 1929. e. Hunter Coll. (AB, 1951). Is produced playwright, author of The Natural Look (Broadway, 1967); Show Me Where the Good Times Are (1970); Let me Hear You Smile (1973) and other plays and musicals off-Bdwy. and on tour.
TELEVISION: Family Secrets (movie; s.p., co-prod.); The Natural Look (s.p., prod., pilot); I Know Why the Caged Bird Sings (s.p.); Madam (movie). Wrote episodes of Family, Lou Grant, and In the Beginning and worked on Starting Fresh (prod.); Grandpa Goes to Washington (co-exec. prod.); Angie (exec. prod.); The Goodtime Girls (co-creator & supvr. prod.). Also writer for Broadway variety special for Entertainment Channel.
PICTURE:How to Beat the High Cost of Living (story).

THURSTON, CAROL: Actress. b. Forsyth, Mont.; e. Montana U.; Bliss-Hayden School of Acting. With father in amateur theatricals prior to screen debut.
PICTURES INCLUDE: Swamp Fire, Jewels of Brandenburg, Last Round-Up, Rogue's Regiment, Arctic Manhunt, Apache Chief, Flaming Feather, Arctic Flight, Conquest of Cochise, Killer Ape, Yukon Vengeance.

TIERNEY, GENE: Actress. b. Brooklyn, N.Y., Nov. 20, 1920; e. St. Margaret's School, Brilmont, Switzerland; Miss Farmer's School, Farmington, Conn.
PICTURES INCLUDE: Return of Frank James, Hudson's Bay, Tobacco Road, Belle Starr, Sundown, Shanghai Gesture, Son of Fury, Heaven Can Wait, Laura, Bell for Adano, Leave Her to Heaven, Dragonwyck, Razor's Edge, Ghost and Mrs. Muir, Iron Curtain, That Wonderful Urge, Whirlpool, Where the Sidewalk Ends, Night and the City, Mating Season, On the Riviera, Secret of Convict Lake, Way of a Gaucho, Close To My Heart, Plymouth Adventure, Never Let Me Go, Personal Affair, The Egyptian, Black Widow, Left Hand of God, Advise & Consent.

TIERNEY, LAWRENCE: Actor. b. Brooklyn, N.Y., Mar. 15, 1919; e. Manhattan Coll. Track athlete (natl. championship Cross Country Team, N.Y. Athletic Club). On stage as actor. Screen debut 1943 in The Ghost Ship.
PICTURES INCLUDE: Youth Runs Wild, Dillinger, Mama Loves Papa, Badman's Territory, Step By Step, San Quentin, Devil Thumbs a Ride, Born to Kill, Bodyguard, Kill or Be Killed, Best of the Bad Men, Shakedown, Greatest Show on Earth, Hoodlum, Bushwackers, Steel Cage, Custer of the West, Such Good Friends, Midnight, Prizzi's Honor.

TIFFIN, PAMELA: Actress. b. Oklahoma City, Okla., Oct. 13, 1942. Hunter College. Started modeling as a teeenager. Film debut in Summer and Smoke.
PICTURES INCLUDE: One Two Three, State Fair, Come Fly With Me, For Those Who Think Young, The Pleasure Seekers, The Hallelujah Trail, Harper, Paranoia, Kiss The Other Sheik, Viva Max.
PLAY: Dinner at Eight.

TILLY, MEG: Actress. b. California. Raised in Victoria, B.C., where began acting and dancing in community theatrical prods. while in high school. To New York at 16; appeared on TV in Hill Street Blues.
PICTURES: Tex (debut), Psycho II, One Dark Night, The Big Chill, Rest in Peace, Impulse, Agnes of God, Off Beat.

TINKER, GRANT A.: Executive. b. Stamford, Conn., Jan. 11, 1926. e. Dartmouth College, 1947. m. Mary Tyler Moore. Joined NBC radio prog. dept. 1949. In 1954 with McCann-Erickson ad agency, TV dept. In 1958, Benton & Bowles Ad Agency, TV dept. From 1961–66 with NBC, v.p., programs, West Coast; v.p. in chg. of programming, N.Y., 1966–67. Joined Universal Television as v.p., 1968–69; 20th-Fox, v.p., 1969–70. Became pres. MTM Enterprises, Inc. 1970. Named NBC bd. chm. & CEO, 1981.

TINLING, JAMES: Director. b. Seattle, Wash., May 8, 1889; e. U. Washington. Started in m.p. as prop boy for Century Studios; wrote comedies 2 yrs.; stunt man; dir.
PICTURES INCLUDE: Silk Legs, Don't Marry, Very Confidential, Exalted Flapper, True Heaven, Words and Music, Fox, Flood, Mr. Moto's Gamble, Boy Friend, Riders of the Purple Sage, Crime Buster, Rendezvous, Deadline for Murder, Strange Journey, Dangerous Millions, Roses Are Red, Second Chance, Night Wind, Trouble Preferred, Tales of Robin Hood.
TV films.

TISCH, LAURENCE A.: Executive. b. Bklyn, N.Y., March 5, 1923. e. N.Y. Univ., 1941; Univ. of Pa. Wharton School, 1942; Harvard Law School, 1946. pres. Tisch Hotels, Inc., 1950–59; pres. Americana Hotel, Inc., Miami Beach, 1956–59; Chmn. of bd. and chief executive officer of Loews Corp since 1960. Also chmn. of bd. of CNA Financial Corp since 1947.

TISCH, PRESTON ROBERT: Executive. b. Bklyn., N.Y., April 29, 1926. e. Bucknell U. Lewisberg, Pa., 1943–44; B.A., U. Mich., 1948. Pres. Loew's Corporation.

TISCH, STEVE: Producer. e. Tufts Univ. Worked during school breaks for John Avildsen and Fred Weintraub. Signed upon graduation as exec. asst. to Peter Guber, then prod. head at Columbia Pictures. Entered producer ranks with Outlaw Blues (1977), collaborating with Jon Avnet with whom formed Tisch/Avnet Prods.
PICTURES: Risky Business, Deal of the Century, Soul Man.
TELEVISION: Homeward Bound, No Other Love, Prime Suspect, Something So Right, The Burning Bed (exec. prod.)

TOBACK, JAMES: Writer-Producer-Director. b. New York City, 1944. e. Harvard. Taught literature at City College of New York; contributed articles and criticism to Harper's, Esquire, Commentary, etc. Wrote book Jim, on actor-athlete Jim Brown (1971). First screenplay, The Gambler, filmed in 1974.
PICTURES: Fingers (s.p., dir.); Love and Money (s.p., dir., prod.).

TODD, ANN: Actress. b. 1909. e. Central School of Speech Training & Dramatic Art. Autobiography: The Eighth Veil, 1980.
BRITISH STAGE PLAYS INCLUDE: Service, When Ladies Meet, Man in Half-Moon Street, Peter Pan, Brit., Lottie Dundass.
PICTURES INCLUDE: Squeaker, Seventh Veil, Perfect Strangers, Gaiety George, Hollywood debut in Paradine Case. Ret. to theatre Feb., 1951 in stage version, Seventh Veil, So Evil My Love; Old Vic. Theatre, 1954–55: Doctor's Dilemma, Four Winds, Duel of Angels, One Woman's Story, Daybreak, Madeleine, The Sound Barrier, Green Scarf, Time Without Pity, Taste of Fear, Son of Captain Blood, Ninety Degrees in The Shade, The Human Factor.
TV: Many appearances and TV films, New York, Hollywood, The Paradine Case, So Evil My Love. London incl.: Camille, The Vortex, The Door, Snows of Kilimanjaro, TV film, Hollywood. 1964: Prod., travelogue in Nepal, Love Story, Makes own Diary Documentaries and appears in them. Films for cinema and TV incl. Thunder in Heaven, Thunder of Gods, Thunder of Kings. Persian Fairy Tale. Free in the Sun, Thunder of Silence. Recent TV appearances, The Last Target, Maelstrom series, The McGuffon.

TODD, RICHARD: Actor. b. Dublin, Eire, June 11, 1919. e. Shrewsbury. In repertory, 1937; founder-member, Dundee Repertory Theatre, 1939; distinguished war service, 1939–46; Dundee Repertory, 1946–48; screen debut, 1948; For Them That Trespass, 1948. 1970 Founder-Director Triumph Theatre Productions.
PICTURES INCLUDE: The Hasty Heart, Lightning Strikes Twice (USA), Robin Hood, The Venetian Bird, Sword and the Rose, Rob Roy, A Man Called Peter (USA), Virgin Queen (USA), The Bed, Dam Busters, D-Day the Sixth of June (USA), Marie Antoinette, Yangtse Incident, Chase a Crooked Shadow, The Naked Earth, Danger Within, The Long the Short and the Tall, The Hellions, Never Let Go, The Longest Day, The Boys, The Very Edge, exec. prod., star own prod. Don't Bother to Knock, Operation Crossbow, Coast of Skeletons, Asylum, The Big Sleep, House of the Long Shadows.
STAGE: 1966–67, An Ideal Husband; 1967–68, Dear Octopus. Co-founder, Triumph Theatre Prods., Ltd. plays since 1970: Roar Like a Dove, Grass Is Greener, The Marquise, 1972. (USA). Sleuth, 1972–73 (England and Australia). Murder by Numbers 1973, The Hollow Crown (with RSC), 1974–75, Equus. 1975, On Approval, Quadrille, 1977; This Happy Breed, 1980; The Business of Murder, 1981–86 in London.

TODMAN, HOWARD: Executive. b. N.Y.C., Nov. 24, 1920; e. Hamilton College 1941; dir. business affairs, Goodson-Todman Productions; treas., Goodson-Todman Associates, inc.; v.p. & treas., Goodson-Todman Enterprises, Ltd.; Treasurer, Peak Prods., Inc.; Treas. Goodson-Todman Bcstg. Inc.; v.p. Price Productions, Inc.; v.p. Celebrity Productions, Inc.; chm., N.Y. Cancer Crusade, radio & TV.

TOGNAZZI, UGO: Actor. b. Cremona, Italy, March 23, 1922. Graduate of law. Started entertainment career in 1945 as

comic in music hall revues. Film career began in 1950 with Les Cadets de Gascogne. Has produced four films and a detective series for TV. Also acted on stage.
PICTURES INCLUDE: His Women, The Fascist, Queen Bee, The Magnificent Cuckold, Question of Honor, Barbarella, Property Is No Longer a Theft, La Cage aux Folles, La Cage aux Folles II, Sunday Lovers, Tragedy of a Ridiculous Man, La Cage aux Folles 3: The Wedding.

TOKOFSKY, JERRY H.: Executive. b. New York City, Apr. 14, 1936. e. NY Univ. (BS, journalism, 1956); N.Y. Law (1959). Entered William Morris Agency while at NYU 1953, working in night club dept. to live TV. Moved to Beverly Hills office, 1959. Joined Columbia Pictures, as prod. v.p., 1963–70. Now producer & exec. v.p., Zupnik Enterprises, Inc.
PICTURES: Producer: Where's Poppa, Born to Win, Paternity, Dreamscape, Fear City, Wildfire.

TOM, C. Y.: Cinematographer and distributor. b. Toy Shan, Kwangtung, China, Nov. 6, 1907; graduated N.Y. Institute of Photography 1926; photographed newsreels for The Great Wall Film Co. of Shanghai; in New York, 1926–29; in charge of production, Shanghai, 1929–32. Studied production techniques in Hollywood. Toured Europe, managing Chinese vaudeville, 1934–35. Studio mgr. and dir. photography for Chi Ming Motion Picture Co., 1935–41. President, Chinamerica Film Exchange and Chinamerica Film Studio, Hong Kong and Shanghai. Distributor, Monogram, Film Classics and Telenews, Hong Kong, Macao and China; asst. man. dir., Capitol Theatre, Hong Kong, 1948–59.

TOMBRAGEL, MAURICE: Writer.
PICTURES INCLUDE: Legion of Lost Flyers, Horror Island, Mutiny in the Arctic, Two Senoritas from Chicago, Lone Wolf in Mexico, Return of the Whistler, Prince of Thieves, The Creeper, Highway 13, Thunder in the Pines, Sky Liner, Arson Inc., Motor Patrol, Fort Bowie, Moon Pilot, s.p. Monkeys Go Home; v.p. Running Wild, Golden Circle Prods., 1973.
TV: Wild Bill Hickock, Stories of the Century, Annie Oakley, Soldiers of Fortune, Western Marshal, Wyatt Earp, Frontier Doctor, Texas Rangers, Sergeant Preston, Adventures of Jim Bowie, Bat Masterson, Walt Disney's Elfego Baca, John Slaughter TV series, Life of Johann Strauss, Escapade in Florence, Bristle Face. Gallegher series, The Tenderfoot series. For Disney, The Treasure of San Marco (2 parts), The Gentle Ben Series.

TOMLIN, LILY: Actress. b. Detroit, Sept. 1, 1939. Wayne State Coll. Started inventing characters for comedy sketches in college, used them in cafe and night club dates. In December, 1969, first appeared on Laugh-In, TV series, gaining national attention.
TV: Laugh-In, The Lily Tomlin Show, Lily.
PICTURES INCLUDE: Nashville, The Late Show, Moment by Moment, Nine to Five, The Incredible Shrinking Woman, All of Me.
RECORDS: This Is a Recording, And That's The Truth.

TOMLINSON, DAVID: Actor. b. May 17, 1917; e. Tonbridge Sch. On stage first, 1934 in "Outward Bound." Screen debut, 1938, "Name, Rank and Number."
PICTURES INCLUDE: Way to the Stars, School for Secrets, Quiet Wedding, Miranda, Easy Money, Sleeping Car to Trieste, Chiltern Hundreds, So Long at the Fair, Wooden Horse, Broken Journey, Hotel Sahara, Castle in the Air, Made in Heaven, Landfall, Three Men in a Boat, Carry on Admiral, Up the Creek, Further Up the Creek, Follow That Horse, Tom Jones, Mary Poppins, The Truth About Spring, City in the Sea, The Liquidator, The Love Bug, Bed Knobs & Broomsticks, From Hong Kong with Love, Wambling Free, Dominique, Fiendish Plot of Dr. Fu Manchu.

TOOMEY, REGIS: Actor. b. Pittsburgh, Pa., Aug. 13, 1902; e. U. Pittsburgh; Carnegie Inst. of Technology (drama); on N.Y. & London stage 5 yrs; film debut in Alibi, 1929.
PICTURES INCLUDE: Spellbound, Big Sleep, Her Sister's Secret, Guilty, High Tide, Magic Town, Bishop's Wife, Boy With Green Hair, Mighty Joe Young, Come to the Stable, Cry Danger, Tall Target, People Against O'Hara, Show Boat, My Six Convicts, Battle at Apache Pass, Just For You, My Pal Gus, Never Wave at a Wac, It Happens Every Thursday, High and the Mighty, Top Gun, Guys and Dolls, Great Day in the Morning, 3 for Jamie Down, Dakota Incident, Warlock, Guns of the Timberland, The Day of the Gun, The Last Sundown, Journey to the Bottom of the Sea, Man's Favorite Sport, Peter Gunn, Change of Habit, Run Shadow Run, The Carey Treatment.
TV: Four Star Theatre, December Bride, Hey Mulligan, Dodsworth, Richard Diamond (series), Shannon (series), Burke's Law (series), Petticoat Junction (series).

TOPOL: Actor. b. Israel, 1935. r.n. Chaim Topol. On Bdwy. in Fiddler on the Roof.
PICTURES: Cast a Giant Shadow, Sallah, Before Winter Comes, Fiddler on the Roof, Follow Me, Galileo, Flash Gordon, For Your Eyes Only.
TELEVISION: House on Garibaldi Street, The Winds of War.

TORME, MEL: Singer, actor. b. Chicago, Ill., Sept. 13, 1925. Singing debut at age of 4; won radio audition 1933; on radio; composed song "Lament to Love"; with Chico Marx's orchestra as drummer, arranger & vocalist 1942; served in U.S. Army, World War II; m.p. debut in "Higher and Higher" 1943; org. vocal group "Meltones"; many recordings; in night clubs.
PICTURES INCLUDE: Pardon My Rhythm, Good News, Let's Go Steady, Janie Gets Married, Night and Day, Good News, Words and Music, Duchess of Idaho, Girls Town, Walk Like a Dragon.

TORN, RIP: Actor. b. Temple, Tex., Feb. 6, 1931. e. Texas A&M, Univ. of Texas. Served in army. Signed as understudy for lead in Cat on a Hot Tin Roof on Broadway.
PICTURES INCLUDE: Baby Doll, A Face in the Crowd, King of Kings, The Cincinnati Kid, You're a Big Boy Now, Beach Red, Sol Madrid, Beyond the Law, Coming Apart, Maidstone, Tropic of Cancer, Payday, Crazy Joe, Birch Interval, The Man Who Fell to Earth, Nasty Habits, Coma, The Seduction of Joe Tynan, One Trick Pony, First Family, The Beastmaster, Jinxed, Airplane II: The Sequel, Cross Creek, Misunderstood, Songwriter, Flashpoint, City Heat, Summer Rental, Beer, Extreme Prejudice.
TELEVISION: The Execution, When She Says No, The Atlanta Child Murders.

TOTTER, AUDREY: Actress. b. Joliet, Ill., Dec. 20, 1923. In many stage plays. On radio 1939–44; film debut in "Main Street" 1944.
PLAYS INCLUDE: Copperhead, Stage Door, Late Christopher Bean, My Sister Eileen.
PICTURES INCLUDE: Her Highness and the Bellboy, Dangerous Partners, Sailor Takes A Wife, Cockeyed Miracle, Lady in the Lake, High Wall, Beginning or the End, Unsuspected, Alias Nick Beal, Saxon Charm, Any Number Can Play, Tension, Set-Up, Under the Gun, Blue Veil, Sellout, F.B.I. Girl, Assignment-Paris, My Pal Gus, Woman They Almost Lynched, Cruisin' Down the River, Man in the Dark, Mission Over Korea, Champ for a Day, Massacre Canyon, Women's Prison, A Bullet for Joey, Vanishing American, Chubasco.
TV: Medical Center, City Killer.

TOWERS, CONSTANCE: Actress. b. Whitefish, MT, May 20, 1933. e. Julliard School of Music. Stage work on Broadway and tour.
PICTURES: Horse Soldiers, Sergeant Rutledge, Fate Is the Hunter, Shock Corridor, Naked Kiss, The Spy, Sylvester.
TELEVISION: Series: Love Is a Many Splendored Thing, Capitol. Mini-Series: On Wings of Eagles.

TOWERS, HARRY ALAN: Executive and producer. b. London, England, 1920. Prod. and wrote: 1963: Sanders of the River; 1964: Code Seven Victim Five.
PICTURES INCLUDE: City of Fear, Mozambique, Coast of Skeletons, Sandy the Seal, 24 Hours to Kill, The Face of Fu Manchu, Ten Little Indians, Marrakesh, Circus of Fear, The Brides of Fu Manchu, Sumuru, Five Golden Dragons, The Vengeance of Fu Manchu, Jules Verne's Rocket to the Moon, House of a Thousand Dolls, The Face of Eve, Blood of Fu Manchu, 99 Women, Girl From Rio, Marquis de Sade's Justine, Castle of Fu Manchu, Venus in Furs, Philosophy in the Boudoir, Eugenie, Dorian Gray, Count Dracula, The Bloody Judge. Black Beauty, Night Hair Child, The Call of the Wild, Treasure Island, White Fang, Death in Persepolis, Ten Little Indians, End of Innocence, Black Cobra, Black Velvet-White Silk, Night of The High Tide, King Solomon's Treasure, Shape of Things to Come, Klondike Fever, Fanny Hill, Frank and I, Black Venus, Christmas, Black Arrow, Pompeii, Love Circles, Lightning—The White Stallion, Land of the Amazon Queens.

TOWNE, ROBERT: Writer-Director-Producer. Was member of Warren Beatty's production staff on Bonnie and Clyde and made contributions to that screenplay.
PICTURES INCLUDE: Villa Rides, The Tomb of Ligeia, The Last Detail, Chinatown, Shampoo (co-s.p.), The Yazuka (co.-s.p.), Personal Best (s.p., prod., dir.).

TOWNSEND, CLAIRE: b. New York City, Feb. 20, 1952. e. Princeton. Joined 20th Century-Fox in 1976; named west coast story editor & v.p, creative affairs. Left in 1978 to go to United Artists, where named v.p. of production, responsible for managing the acquisition, development and production of feature films. Now independent producer.

TOWNSEND, LEO: Writer. b. Faribault, Minn., May 11, 1908; e. Minnesota U. Formerly radio and feature story magazine writer. In 1942 collab. s.p., It Started With Eve, collab. orig. s.p. Seven Sweethearts.
PICTURES INCLUDE: The Amazing Mrs. Halliday, Can't Help Singing, Chip Off the Old Block, Night and Day, Southside E-1000, One Big Affair, Dangerous Crossing, Siege at Red River, A Life in the Balance, White Feather,

Running Wild, Fraulein, The Black Hand, Shadow On the Window, Flight to Hong Kong, That Way With Women, Seven Sweethearts, I'd Rather Be Rich, Bikini Beach, Beach Blanket Bingo, How to Stuff a Wild Bikini, Fireball 500.
TV: Jane Wyman Theatre, Wagon Train, Maverick, 77 Sunset Strip, Hawaiian Eye, Dinah Shore Chevy Show, Shirley Temple Show, Perry Mason, Bourbon Street Beat, Beulah, Bachelor Father, Surfside Six, Destry, Patty Duke Show, Gidget, Man From U.N.C.L.E., My Three Sons, The Munsters, Batman, Andy Griffith Show, Bewitched.

TOWNSEND, PAULINE SWANSON: Writer. b. Athen, Ohio, e. Ohio University. Former Hollywood head of Tom Fizdale and Robert S. Taplinger p.r. agencies. Fiction and non-fiction writer for most national magazines.
TV: Death Valley Days, Patty Duke Show, Gidget, The Munsters, Batman, Andy Griffith Show, Bewitched.

TOYE, WENDY: Director. e. privately. Early career, ballet actress, dir., plays and musicals; entered m.p. industry 1952; dir., Stranger Left No Card (Award winning Short Cannes Festival 1953).
PICTURES INCLUDE: Three Cases Of Murder, Teckman Mystery, Raising A Riot, On The 12th Day (Nom. Best Short America 1955), All For Mary, True as a Turtle, We Joined The Navy, The Kings Breakfast.
STAGE: As You Like It, Majority Of One, Fledermaus, Orpheus in the Underworld, La Vie Parisienne, Virtue in Danger, Midsummer Night's Dream, Robert & Elizabeth, On the Level. Dir., Tribute to Noel Coward, Phoenix Th., Great Waltz, Soldiers Tale, Show Boat, Cowardly Custard, Stand and Deliver, She Stoops to Conquer, R Loves J, The Confederacy, Italian Girl in Algiers, Made in Heaven, Follow the Star, Make Me a World, Oh Mr. Porter, Once More With Music, Colette, Gingerbread Man, The Mikado, This Thing Called Love. Assoc. prod., Singing in the Rain, London Palladium; Noel & Gertie (Monte Carlo & Canada), Barnum (assoc. prod., Manchester), Madwoman of Chaillot (Canada), Kiss Me Kate (dir., choreographer, Copenhagen).
TV: Esme Divided, Chelsea at Nine, Orpheus in the Underworld, The Soldiers Tale, Cliff in Scotland, Girls Wanted, Istanbul, A Goodley Manor for a Song, Girls, Girls, Girls, All Star Golden Gala ATV, Follow the Star, Tales from the Unexpected, Stranger in Town, Trial by Jury.
OPERAS: Seraglio, Don Pasquale, The Impresario, Italian Girl in Algiers, The Merry Widow, Orpheus in the Underworld.

TRAMBUKIS, WILLIAM J.: Executive. b. July 26, 1926. Began career as usher with Loews in Providence, R.I. 1941. Served 1943–46 with Navy Seabees. Recipient of Quigley Awards. Managed/supervised Loews Theatres in several New England cities, Harrisburg, Pa., Syracuse, Rochester, Buffalo, N.Y., Washington, D.C., Richmond, Norfolk, Va., Toronto, Canada, Atlanta, Ga. Appt. Loews NorthEastern Division mgr. 1964, Loews gen. mgr. 1975: v.p. in 1976; sr. v.p., 1985.

TRAVANTI, DANIEL J.: Actor. b. Kenosha, WI, March 7, 1940. e. Univ. Wisconsin.; Yale School of Drama. On stage in Twigs, Othello, etc.
PICTURE: St. Ives.
TELEVISION: Hill Street Blues, A Case of Libel, Adam, Aurora, Murrow.

TRAVERS, BILL: Actor, Producer, Director. b. Newcastle-on-Tyne, England. Actor in repertory co.; London stage in Cage Me a Peacock, Damask Cheek, Square Ring, I Captured the Castle, 1961; A Cook for Mr. General (Broadway); Royal Shakespeare Theatre Co., 1962. Abraham Cochrane, 1964. Peter Pan, 1970.
PICTURES INCLUDE: Square Ring, Romeo and Juliet, Geordie, Footsteps in the Fog, Bhowani Junction, Barretts of Wimpole Street, Smallest Show on Earth, Seventh Sin, Passionate Summer, Bridal Path, Gorgo, The Green Helmet, Two Living—One Dead, Born Free, Duel at Diablo, A Midsummer Night's Dream, Ring of Bright Water, Boulevard du Rhum, The Belstone Fox.
TV: A Cook for the General (Kraft), Episode, A Giant Is Born (U.S.A.), Espionage, Rawhide, CBS Voice of America (Rome), Lorna Doone, The Admirable Crichton. Producer/Director/Writer: The Lions Are Free, An Elephant Called Slowly, The Lion at Worlds End, Christian the Lion, Wild Dogs of Africa, Baboons of Gombe, The Hyena Story, Deathtrap, Lions of the Serengeti, River of Sand, Bloody Ivory, Sexual Encounters of the Floral Kind.

TRAVIS, J. MARK: Executive. b. Los Angeles, March 7, 1953. e. Yale. 1971, v.p., Sackheim Agency; 1973, pres., Entertainment 4; 1975, chm., CEO, Theatre Television Corp.; 1977, pres., Special Event Entertainment; 1979, Columbia Pictures—Travis Productions; 1980, Lorimar Productions—Travis; 1983, pres. & CEO, Movie Music Co., Inc.
PICTURES: Give 'em Hell Harry (prod.); Stop the World I Want to Get Off (prod.), Richard Pryor Live in Concert (prod.); Fighting Back (exec. prod.).

TRAVIS, RICHARD: Actor. r.n. William Justice. b. Carlsbad, N.M., Apr. 17, 1913. Started career in radio as announcer, sportscaster; writer and publisher of Cinemag. (theatrical tabloid); 3 yrs. U.S. Army.
PICTURES INCLUDE: The Man Who Came To Dinner, Postman Didn't Ring, Big Shot, Escape from Crime, Busses Roar, Truck Busters, Mission to Moscow, Last Ride, Jewels of Brandenburg, Alaska Patrol, Sky Liner, Operation Haylift, Passage West, Roaring City, Mask of Dragon, Lost Women, Girl in the Red Velvet Swing, Speed to Spare, Pier 21, Fingerprints Don't Lie, Annapolis Story, City of Shadows.
TV: Lucky Strike Theatre, Racket Squad, Lone Ranger, Schlitz Playhouse, Loretta Young Show, Treasury Men in Action, Pepsi Cola Playhouse, Ray Milland Show, Pride of the Family, The Falcon, Fury, Crossroads; host-narrator, Code 3, Missile to the Moon.

TRAVOLTA, JOHN: Actor. b. Englewood, N.J., Feb. 18, 1954. Quit school at 16 to pursue theatre career; first stage role in Who Will Save the Plowboy? Did off-Bdwy prod. of Rain; next to Broadway in Grease. Toured with latter for 10 months. Also in Over Here on Bdwy. with Andrew Sisters for 10 months.
PICTURES INCLUDE: Carrie, Saturday Night Fever, Grease, Moment by Moment, Urban Cowboy, Blow Out, Staying Alive, Two of a Kind, Perfect.
TV: Emergency, Owen Marshall, The Rookies, Medical Center, Welcome Back, Kotter (regular). Movie: The Boy in the Plastic Bubble.

TREEN, MARY LOU: Actress. b. St. Louis, Mo.; p. Helen Sullivan Treen, prof.; e. Ramona Convent; Denishawn School; Marion Morgan Dancers. With Fachon & marco revuew; on circuits; in early Bryan Foy short subjects; on stage in Little Boy Bluew In; screen debut in Hot Tires.
PICTURES INCLUDE: Happiness Ahead, Strange Impersonation, From This Day Forward, She Wouldn't Say Yes, One Exciting Week, Let's Live a Little, The Stooge, Sailor Beware, Let's Do It Again, The Caddy, When Gangland Strikes, Birds and the Bees, Rockabye Baby, Paradise Hawaiian Style.

TREMAYNE, LES: Actor. b. London, England, Apr. 16, 1913; Northwestern U., Chicago Art Institute; Columbia, UCLA. First professional appearance in British mp., 1916, with mother; stock, litte theatres, vaudeville, 1925–40; entered radio field, 1931; numerous shows on all networks.
SHOWS INCLUDE: Woman in My House (with wife, Alice Reinheart), Errand of Mercy, Your Are There, One Man's Family, Heartbeat Theatre, The First Nighter (lead 7 yrs.); on Broadway in Heads or Tails, Detective Story.
TV: Lux Video Theatre, 20th Century-Fox Hour, Navy Log, One Man's Family, Meet Mille, The Millionaire, The Whistler, Truth or Consequences, NBC Matinee, The Girl, O'Henry series, Rin Tin Tin, Bachelor Father, The Texan, Adventures of Ellery Queen, Court of Last Resort, Rifleman, State Trooper, Rescue 8, June Allyson-Dupont Show, Wagon Train, M Squad, Hitchcock Presents, Mr. Ed., Perry Mason.
PICTURES INCLUDE: The Racket, Blue Veil, Francis Goes to West Point, It Grows on Trees, I Love Melvin, Under the Red Sea, Dream Wife, War of the Worlds, Susan Slept Here, Lieutenant Wore Skirts, Unguarded Moment, Everything But the Truth, Monolith Monsters, Perfect Furlough, North by Northwest, Say One for Me, The Gallant Hours, The Angry Red Planet, The Story of Ruth.
Blue ribbon award for best perf. of the month for A Man Called Peter; dir. Hollywood Repertory Theatre, 1957; pres. Hollywood Actors' Council, 1951–58; chmn. Actors Div. workshop com. Acad. TV Arts & Sciences; Member of The Workshop Comm. of the Hollywood M.P. & TV Museum Commission.

TREVOR, CLAIRE: Actress. b. New York City, 1909. e. Amer. Acad. of Dram. Arts; Columbia U.; m. Milton H. Bren. On Broadway in Party's Over, Whistling in the Dark, Big Two.
PICTURES INCLUDE: Life in the Raw, Last Trail, Mad Game, Jimmy and Sally, Stagecoach, Allegheny Uprising, Dark Command, Murder, My Sweet, Johnny Angel, Crack-Up, Bachelor's Daughters, Born to Kill, Raw Deal, Valley of the Giants, Babe Ruth, Velvet Touch, Key Largo (Acad. Award), Lucky Stiff, Best of the Bad Men, Border Line, Hoodlum, Empire, Hard, Fast and Beautiful, My Man and I, Stop, You're Killing Me, Stranger Wore a Gun, High and the Mighty, Man Without a Star, Luch Gallant, The Mountain, Marjorie Morningstar, Two Weeks in Another Town, The Stripper, How to Murder Your Wife, Capetown Affair, Kiss Me Goodbye.
TV: Dodsworth (Academy Emmy).

TREXLER, CHARLES B.: Exhibitor. b. Wadesboro, N.C., Feb. 8, 1916. From 1937 to Nov. 1948 was practicing CPA except for 2 yrs. in U.S. Army in World War II. Joined Stewart & Everett Theatres in 1948 as controller. In March, 1953 named gen. mgr.; Jan. 1, 1954, exec. v.p., treas.; May, 1962 named pres.; Feb. 1, 1983, named bd. chm. Retains title as bd. chm., NATO of North and South Carolina; v.p. & bd. mbr., National NATO.

TRIKONIS, GUY: Director. b. New York City. Started career in chorus of West Side Story on Bdwy. Turned to direction, making low-budget "weekenders" (films shot in 12 days only on weekends).
PICTURES: Moonshine County Express, The Evil Touched by Love, Take This Job and Shove It.
TELEVISION: Dark Side of Terror, Dressed To Kill, The Last Convertible (final three hours).

TRINDER, TOMMY: TV performer. b. London, March 24, 1909. Early career, music halls. Starred London Palladium 1939, Top Of The World 1940, Best Bib and Tucker 1942, Happy And Glorious 1944, Here, There And Everywhere 1947, Fancy Free 1951, Variety and several Command Performance shows. Entered m.p. industry 1936.
PICTURES: Almost A Honeymoon, Laugh It Off, Sailors Three, The Foreman Went To France, Champagne Charlie, Fiddlers Three, Bitter Springs, You Lucky People.
TV: Master of Ceremonies, Sunday Night At The London Palladium (ATV), My Wildest Dream, BBC, The Trinder Box.

TRINTIGNANT, JEAN-LOUIS: Actor. b. Aix-en-Provence, France, Dec. 11, 1930. m. Nadine Marquand. Theatre debut: 1951, To Each According to His Hunger. Then Mary Stuart, Macbeth (at the Comedie de Saint-Etienne). 1955 screen debut.
PICTURES INCLUDE: Si Tous Les Gars Du Monde, La Loi Des Rues, And God Created Woman, Club De Femmes, Les Liaisons Dangereuses, L'Ete Violent, Austerlitz, La Millieme Fenetre, Plein Feux Sur L'Assasin, Cceur Battant, L'Atlantide, The Game of Truth, Horace 62, Les Sept Peches Capitaux (7 Capital Sins), Le Combat Dans L'Ile, The Easy Life, Il Successo, Nutty, Naughty Chateau, Les Pas Perdus, La Bonne Occase, Mata-Hari, Meurtre A L'Italienne, La Longue Marche, Le 17eme Ciel, Un Jour A Paris, Is Paris Burning?, The Sleeping Car Murder, A Man and a Woman, Enigma, Safari Diamants, Trans-Europ Express, Mon Amour, Mon Amour, Un Homme A Abattre, La Morte Ha Fatto L'Uovo, Les Biches, Grand Silence, Z, Ma Nuit Chez Maud (My Night at Maud's), The Conformist, The Crook, Without Apparent Motive, The Outside Man, The French Conspiracy, Les Violons du Bal, The Sunday Woman, Under Fire, Femme de Personne.

TROELL, JAN: Writer-Director-Cinematographer. b. Sweden, 1931. Was teacher before entering industry. In early 60s photographed Bo Widerberg's first film, The Pram. Became apprentice in TV; made m.p. debut as director in 1965 with Stay in the Marshland.
PICTURES INCLUDE: Here Is Your Life, Eeny, Meeny, Miny, Mo., The Emigrants, The New Land, Zandy's Bride, Hurricane.

TROSPER, GUY: Writer. b. Lander, Wyo. Started as reader, Samuel Goldwyn; then story ed.; screen writer since 1941.
PICTURES INCLUDE: collab. s.p., Stratton Story; s.p., Devil's Doorway, Inside Straight; story; Pride of St. Louis; collab. s.p., Many Rivers to Cross; s.p., The Americano, Girl He Left Behind.

TRYON, TOM: Actor. b. Hartford, Conn., Jan. 14 1926. e. Yale U. Served in U.S. Navy, World War II, studied at Art Students League; with Cape Playhouse, Dennis, Mass., as set painter, asst. stage mgr., actor; prod. asst., CBS; then TV actor.
PLAYS INCLUDE: Wish You Were Here, Cyrano de Bergerac, Richard III.
PICTURES INCLUDE: m.p. debut in Scarlet Hour; since in Screaming Eagles, Three Violent People, Moon Pilot, Marines Let's Go, The Cardinal, The Glory Guys, The Horsemen.
AUTHOR: The Other, Crowned Heads.

TSUKASA, YOKO: Actress. b. Tottori, Japan, Aug. 20, 1934. e. Kyoritsu College; joined Toho Studio 1954 after period as magazine cover girl.
PICTURES INCLUDE: Don't Die My Darling, Blue Beast, Eternity of Love, End of Summer, Three Treasures, Yojimbo (The Bodyguard), Women of Design.

TUCKER, FORREST: Actor. b. Plainfield, Ind., Feb. 12, 1919; e. George Wash. U., Wash., D.C. Screen debut, 1940, in The Western, foll. by 42 feature roles, 1940–51, first starring role, Rock Island Trail, Rep., 1950. Star of Tomorrow, 1952. Member: Masquers Club of Hollywood, Lakeside Golf.
PICTURES INCLUDE: The Yearling, The Howards of Virginia, Never Say Goodbye, Warpath, Sands of Iwo Jima, Oh! Susanna, Crosswinds, Fighting Coast Guard, Wild Blue Yonder, Flaming Feather, Bugles in the Afternoon, Hoodlum Empire, Montana Belle, Hurricane Smith, Ride the Man Down, San Antone, Flight Nurse, Pony Express, Jubilee Trail, Laughing Anne, Trouble in the Glen, Rage at Dawn, Vanishing American, Finger Man, Night Freight, Paris Follies of 1956, Break in the Circle, Counterplot, The Night They Raided Minsky's, Auntie Mame, Barquero, Chisum, The Wild McCullocks.
TV: Crunch and Des, F Troop; Rad. Show: WCFL, Chicago.
Chicago Co., Plaza Suite, Oct. 1968 to June, 1969. Now assoc. prod. Drury Lane Theatre, Ill. Mem., Lambs Club, Friars Club, N.Y. Opened Nat'l Co., Music Man, L.A., on tour.

TUCKER, MELVILLE: Executive. b. New York City, Mar. 4, 1916; e. Princeton U. Asst. purchasing agent Consolidated Laboratories, N.Y., 1934–36; sound effects & picture ed., Republic Productions, Inc. 1936–8; then asst. production mgr. & first asst. dir., 1938–42; served in U.S. Army 1942–46; asst. prod. Republic 1946; assoc. producer, 1947–52; prod., Universal 1952–54; prod. exec. v.p., Universal, 1955–70; prod.-Verdon Prods., 1971–present.
PICTURES INCLUDE: The Missourians, Thunder in God's Country, Rodeo King and the Senorita, Utah Wagon Train. U-I prod., 1953: Drums Across the River, Black Shield of Falworth; production exec. U-I, 1954–71. prod., Verdon Prod., prod. A Warm December, 1972; prod., Uptown Saturday Night, Producer, Let's Do It Again, 1975; prod., A Piece of the Action, 1977; exec. prod., Stir Crazy, 1980; Hanky Panky, 1982; Fast Forward, 1985.

TUCKERMAN, DAVID R.: Executive. b. Perth Amboy, NJ Nov. 9, 1946. e. Monmouth College (FLU, 1967–70; BSBA). Entered industry with A.I.T. Theatres, 1967; gen. mgr., Music Makers Theatres, 1973; v.p., Leigh Group, MMT, head film buyer, 1976; sr. v.p., MMT, 1980.
MEMBER: SMPTE, Variety Int., MPBC, AFI.

TUGGLE, RICHARD: Director-Writer. Wrote screenplays before directorial debut with Tightrope (1984) which he also wrote. Previous work includes s.p. for Escape from Alcatraz.

TULIPAN, IRA H.: Publicist. b. New York City. e. N.Y.U. 1934, B.S. Entered m.p. ind. as theatre mgr., Boston, 1934; pub. dept. Warner Bros. home office, 1935–40; joined 20th Century-Fox 1942; U.S. Army service 1943–46; returned to Fox upon disch., feature writer, press book ed.; trade paper contact; newspaper contact; pub. mgr. 1955; ass't. dir. adv. pub. expl. Columbia Pictures. 1960; exec. adm. asst. to adv., publ., v.p., Columbia, 1963; dir. overseas prod. pub., 1966. Returned to U.S. in 1978 as eastern pub.-coordinator.

TUNBERG, KARL: Writer. b. Spokane, Wash. From 1937 collab. many Hollywood s.p.
PICTURES INCLUDE: You Can't Have Everything, My Lucky Star, Hold That Co-Ed, Down Argentine Way, Yank in the RAF. In 1942 (collab. s.p.) My Gal Sal, Orchestra Wives, Lucky Jordan, (collab. s.p.) Dixie, Standing Room Only, Bring on the Girls; (prod. & collab. s.p.) Kitty; (prod.) You Gotta Stay Happy; (collab. s.p.) Love That Brute, Night Into Morning, Law and the Lady, Because You're Mine, Scandal at Scourie, Valley of the Kings; s.p. Beau Brummell, Scarlet Coat, Seventh Sin, Ben Hur, s.p. Count Your Blessings; s.p. Libel, Taras Bulba; s.p., I Thank A Fool; s.p. The Seventh Dawn, Harlow (story); col. s.p., Where Were You When the Lights Went Out?

TUNE, TOMMY: Actor-Dancer. b. Wichita Falls, TX, Feb. 28, 1939. Began professional career dancing in choruses of Bdwy. shows (Baker Street, A Joyful Noise, How Now Dow Jones, etc.). Signed by 20th-Fox and cast in Hello, Dolly!
PICTURE: The Boy Friend.
STAGE: Performer: Seesaw, My One and Only. Director: The Club, Cloud 9, The Best Little Whorehouse in Texas, Nine. Choreographer: A Day in Hollywood/A Night in the Ukraine.
TELEVISION: Dean Martin Presents the Golddiggers.

TUNICK, IRVE: Writer. b. New York, N.Y.; e. N.Y.U. and Georgetown U. Commenced writing career with radio scripts; later senior writer (TV) for Cavalcade of America and You Are There, stories produced by Studio One and Armstrong Circle Theatre; five radio and TV scripts won Peabody Awards; script editor for Princess Pictures 1953–55; orig. s.p. for Lady of Vengeance; s.p. for High Hell.

TURMAN, LAWRENCE: Producer. b. Los Angeles, Nov. 28, 1926. e. UCLA. In textile business 5 years, then joined Kurt Frings Agency; left in 1960 to form Millar-Turman Prods.
PICTURES INCLUDE: (prod.) The Young Doctors, I Could Go on Singing, The Best Man. Formed own prod. co., Lawrence Turman, Inc., to make The Flim-Flam Man, The Graduate, Pretty Poison, The Drowning Pool, First Love, Heroes, Walk Proud, Caveman (co-prod.), The Thing, Second Thoughts (co-prod., dir.), Mass Appeal (co-prod.), The Mean Season (co-prod.), Short Circuit (co-prod.), Running Scared (co-prod.).

TURNER, CLIFFORD: Producer. b. Leeds, England, 1913. ent. m.p. industry as cutting room asst. Gaumont British. Edited number early British pictures, before going to Hollywood in 1935. Subsequently edited for Warners, Columbia, Universal, Fox. Returned to England 1948 to edit The Small Back Room. Dir. and exec. producer since 1950 in Hollywood and New York. Formed Boulevard Film Productions Ltd., Screen Biographies International Inc., Television Enterprises Inc. Four Against the Bank of England. 1972: Utrillo. 1975, Rose of Cimarron, 1976 Mystery of the General Grant; La Cicatrice, The Valadon Story, Streets of Montmartre. Recent production: The Murderess.

TURNER, KATHLEEN: Actress. b. Springfield, MO, June 19, 1954. e. Univ. Maryland. Starred in NBC soap opera, The Doctors; on Bdwy. stage in Gemini. Theatrical film debut in Body Heat, 1981.
PICTURES: The Man With Two Brains, Romancing the Stone, Crimes of Passion, A Breed Apart, Prizzi's Honor, Jewel of the Nile, Peggy Sue Got Married.

TURNER, LANA: Actress. b. Wallace, Idaho, Feb. 8, 1920; p. Virgil Turner, prof.
PICTURES INCLUDE: They Won't Forget, Great Garrick, Adventures of Marco Polo, Love Finds Andy Hardy; Rich Man, Poor Girl; Dramatic School, Calling Dr. Kildare, These Glamour Girls, Dancing Coed. Two Girls on Broadway, We Who Are Young, Ziegfeld Girl, Dr. Jekyll and Mr. Hyde, Johnny Eager, Slightly Dangerous, Youngest Profession, Marriage Is a Private Affair, Keep Your Powder Dry, Week-End at the Waldorf, Postman Always Rings Twice, Green Dolphin Street, Cass Timberlane, Homecoming, Three Musketeers, Life of Her Own, Mr. Imperium, The Merry Widow, Bad & the Beautiful, Latin Lovers, Flame & the Flesh, Betrayed, The Prodigal, Sea Chase, Rains of Ranchipur, Diane, Lady and the Flyer, Imitation of Life, Portrait in Black, By Love Possessed, Bachelor in Paradise, Who's Got the Action?, Love Has Many Faces, Madame X, The Big Cube, Persecution, Bittersweet Love.
TV: The Survivors.

TURNER, TED: Executive. b. Cincinnati, OH., Nov. 19, 1938. Began career in Savannah in family's outdoor adv. business, selling space on billboards. Bought co. in 1963 and in 1970 entered broadcasting with purchase of a failing TV station in Atlanta which he turned into WTBS, a "superstation" which in 1985 reached 80% of U.S. homes equipped with cable. 1980, established CNN a 24-hr. cable news service. Co-owner two professional sports teams in Atlanta: Braves (baseball) and Hawks (basketball).

TURNER, TINA: Singer-Actress. b. Brownsville, TX, Nov. 26, 1939. r.n. Annie Mae Bullock. Previously married to Ike Turner and appeared with him on road in Ike and Tina Turner Revue. Many hit records.
PICTURES: Gimme Shelter, Soul to Soul, Tommy, Sound of the City, Mad Max Beyond Thunderdome.

TUSHINGHAM, RITA: Actress. b. Liverpool, England, 1942. Student at Liverpool Playhouse, Motion pic. debut 1961 in A Taste of Honey.
PICTURES INCLUDE: The Leather Boys, A Place to Go, Girl With Green Eyes, The Knack, Dr. Zhivago, The Trap, Smashing Time, Diamonds for Breakfast, The Guru, The Bedsitting Room, Straight on 'til Morning, Situation, Instant Coffee, The Human Factor, Rachel's Man, The Slum Boy, Green Eyes, The Black Journal, Bread, Butter and Jam, Mysteries, Felix Krull, Lady Killers, The Spaghetti Thing, Seeing Red.

TUTIN, DOROTHY: Actress. b. London, Eng., Apr. 8, 1930; e. St. Catherine's School Bramley, Guildford (Surrey). Stage debut in The Thistle & the Rose, 1949.
PLAYS INCLUDE: Much Ado About Nothing, The Living Room, I Am a Camera, The Lark, Wild Duck, Juliet, Ophelia, Viola, Portia, Cressida, Rosalind, The Devils, Once More With Feeling, The Cherry Orchard, Victoria Regina—Portrait of a Queen, Old Times, Peter Pan, What Every Woman Knows, Month in the Country, Macbeth, Antony and Cleopatra, Undiscovered Country, Reflections, After the Lions, Ballerina, A Kind of Alaska, Are You Sitting Comfortably?
PICTURES INCLUDE: Screen debut in The Importance of Being Earnest. Also: The Beggar's Opera, A Tale of Two Cities, Cromwell, Savage Messiah, The Shooting Party, Murder with Mirrrso.
TV: Living Room, Victoria Regina, Invitation to a Voyage, Antigone, Colombe, Carrington V.C., The Hollow Crown, Scent of Fear, From Chekhov With Love, Anne Boleyn in The Six Wives of Henry VIII, Flotsam and Jetsam, Mother & Son, South Riding, Willow Cabins, Ghosts, Sister Dora, The Double Dealer, The Combination, La Ronde, Tales of the Unexpected, 10 Downing Street, Life After Death, King Lear, Landscape, The Father, The Demon Lover, Robin Hood.

TWAIN, MICHAEL: Actor-director. b. Nov. 1, 1939, New York City. e. Ohio State University. Served U.S. Army. While studying with Lee Strasberg, worked as private detective, school teacher. Made stage debut City Center, 1956, in Mr. Roberts. Became village coffee house and club comedian 1968 to 1972.
PICTURES INCLUDE: Marriage Italian Style (voice only); American Soap, Blood Bath, Up! the Girls, F.I.S.T.
TELEVISION: The Silent Drum, Starsky & Hutch, Wonder Woman, Streets of San Francisco, Soap, Lou Grant, Diff'rent Strokes, Nurse, Stalk the Wild Child, The Courage and the Passion, Eischied.

TWIGGY: Recording Artiste. b. London, Sept. 19, 1949. r.n. Leslie Hornby. m. actor Michael Witney. At 17 regarded as world's leading high fashion model. Made m.p. debut in The Boy Friend (1971). Starred in many London West End Shows, including Cinderella and Captain Beaky Presents. Star of Broadway and touring stage productions of Funny Face. 1983: Broadway Musical, My One and Only
TV: Hosted and starred in major American & British music shows including Twiggy (UK), Twiggy and Friends (UK), and Juke Box (US), Pygmalion (England).
PICTURES INCLUDE: W, There Goes the Bride, The Blues Brothers, The Doctor and the Devils, Club Paradise.

TWYMAN, ALAN P.: Executive. b. Dayton, Ohio, May 30, 1934. e. Univ. of Cincinnati. Twyman Films, Inc. sales 1958, vice pres.-pres., 1975. NAVA board of directors, 1964–69; pres. 1970, chm. of bd., 1972. In 1983 left to form own co., Alan Twyman Presents.

TYLER, BEVERLY: Actress. r.n. Beverly Jean Saul. b. Scranton, Pa., July 5, 1928; e. Scranton H.S. Church choir singer; on radio, TV.
PICTURES INCLUDE: Green Years, My Brother Talks to Horses, Beginning or End, The Palomino, The Fireball, Cimarron Kid, Battle at Apache Pass.

TYRRELL, SUSAN: Actress. b. San Francisco, 1946. Made first prof. appearance with Art Carney in summer theatre tour prod. of Time Out for Ginger. Worked in off-Bdwy. prods. and as waitress in coffee house before attracting attention in Lincoln Center Repertory Co. prods. of A Cry of Players, The Time of Your Life, Camino Real.
PICTURES INCLUDE: The Steagle, Shoot Out, Fat City, Catch My Soul, Islands in the Stream, Andy Warhol's Bad, I Never Promised You A Rose Garden, Another Man, Another Chance, September 30, 1955, Angel, Avenging Angel, Flesh and Blood.
TELEVISION: If Tomorrow Comes.

TYSON, CICELY: Actress. b. New York City, Dec. 19, 1933. e. NYU. Studied at Actor's Studio.
PICTURES INCLUDE: A Man Called Adam, The Comedians, The Heart Is a Lonely Hunter, Sounder, A Hero Ain't Nothin, But a Sandwich, The Concorde—Airport '79.
TELEVISION: The Autobiography of Miss Jane Pittman, Roots, East Side, West Side, A Woman Called Moses, King, Playing with Fire, Acceptable Risks, Samaritan.

U

UGGAMS, LESLIE: Singer. b. New York, May 25, 1943. e. Professional Children's Sch., grad., 1960. Juilliard. Beg. singing career age 5. TV debut: age 7, Johnny Olsen's TV kids. Records for Columbia Records.
STAGE: Hallelujah Baby.
RADIO: Peter Lind Hayes-Mary Healy Show, Milton Berle, Arthur Godfrey, Star Time.
TV: Milton Berle Show, Name That Tune, Jack Paar Show, Garry Moore, Sing Along With Mitch.

ULLMANN, LIV: Actress. b. Japan of Norwegian parents, Dec. 16, 1939. Accompanied parents to Canada when World War II began and later returned to Norway. Was catapulted to fame in a succession of Swedish films directed by Ingmar Bergman.
PICTURES INCLUDE: Swedish: Persona (debut), Hour of the Wolf, Shame, The Passion of Anna, The Emigrants, Cries and Whispers; American: The Devil's Imposter (formerly Pope Joan), Lost Horizon, 40 Carats, Zandy's Bride, The Abdication, Face to Face, A Bridge Too Far, The Serpent's Egg, Autumn Sonata, The Wild Duck, Bay Boy.

UNGER, ANTHONY B.: Executive-Producer. b. New York, Oct. 19, 1940. e. Duke Univ. and Univ. of Southern Calif. Prod. ass't Third Man, TV series, 1961. v.p. Unger Productions, Inc., 1964; v.p. Landau-Unger Co., Inc., 1965; v.p. Commonwealth United Entertainment in London, 1968; pres., Unger Prods. Inc., 1978–present.
PICTURES INCLUDE: 1966: assoc. prod., The Desperate Ones. 1968: assoc. prod., The Madwoman of Chaillot. 1969: exec. prod., The Battle of Neretva, The Magic Christian, Julius Caesar. 1970: exec. prod., The Devil's Widow. 1973: exec. prod., Don't Look Now; 1980: prod., The Unseen; 1982: prod., Silent Rage.

UNGER, KURT: Producer. b. Berlin, Jan. 10, 1922. Entered ind. in 1939 in chg. m.p. entertainment British troops in Middle East. Subsequently distributor for United Artists Corp. in Israel and Italy.

PICTURES INCLUDE: Judith, Best House in London, Puppet on a Chain, Pope Joan (The Devil's Imposter).

UNGER, STEPHEN A.: Executive. Started as independent prod. and dist. of theatrical and TV films. In June, 1978, joined Universal Pictures Intl. Sales as foreign sls. mgr. Named v.p. Universal Theatrical Motion Pictures in 1979, responsible for licensing theatrical or TV features not handled by C.I.C. in territories outside U.S. & Canada. In 1981 joined CBS Theatrical Films as int'l. v.p., sls.; 1982–present, pres., Unger Int'l. Distributors, Inc.

URICH, ROBERT: Actor. b. Toronto, Ohio, Dec. 19, 1947. e. Florida State Univ. (BA in radio and TV communications). Appeared in university plays. Was sales account executive at WGN Radio, Chicago, before turning to stage acting.
TELEVISION: The FBI, Gunsmoke, Kung Fu, Marcus Welby, MD, S.W.A.T., Bob & Carol & Ted & Alice, Soap, Tabitha, The Love Boat, Vega$, Princess Daisy, Invitation to Hell, Mistral's Daughter, His Mistress, Scandal Sheet, Young Again.
PICTURES: Magnum Force, Endangered Species, The Ice Pirates, Turk 182.

URQUHART, ROBERT: Actor, writer. b. Scotland, October 16, 1922; e. George Heriots, Edinburg. Served in Merchant Navy 1938–45; stage debut, Park Theatre, Glasgow; screen debut: You're Only Young Twice, 1951.
PICTURES INCLUDE: Isn't Life Wonderful, The House Of The Arrow, Knights Of The Round Table, Happy Ever After (Tonight's The Night), Golden Ivory, The Dark Avenger, You Can't Escape, Yangtse Incident, Curse of Frankenstein, Dunkirk, The Trouble with Eve, Danger Tomorrow, Foxhole in Cairo, Murder in Mind, The Bulldog Greed, 55 Days At Peking, The Break, Murder at the Gallup, The Syndicate, The Limbo Line, The Looking Glass War, Brotherly Love (Country Dance).
TV: Tamer Tamed, Infinite Shoeblack, Morning Departure, The Human Touch, The Iron Harp, Sleeping Clergyman, The Naked Lady, For Services Rendered, The Bright One, Jango, Murder Swamp, She Died Young, Plane Makers series, Reporter, Inheritors series; 1976 series: Mr. Goodall, The Nearly Man, The Button Man, Happy Returns, Endless-Aimless.
AUTHOR: (Wrote TV) House of Lies, End of the Tether, Landfall, The Touch of a Dead Hand.

USLAN, MICHAEL E.: Producer-writer. b. Bayonne, N.J., 1951. e. Indiana U. AB, MS, JD. Wrote 12 books, including Dick Clark's 1st 25 Years of Rock 'n Roll; 1976–80 atty. with United Artists; Produced with Benjamin Melniker: Three Sovereigns for Sarah (American Playhouse/Goldcrest Films); Swamp Thing (UA/Embassy); Television's Greatest Bits (RCA/Syndicast); Dinosaucers (Columbia Pictures TV/RCA); in progress: Batman (WB).

USTINOV, PETER: Actor, writer, dir. b. London, Eng., Apr. 16, 1921; e. Westminster Sch. In Brit. Army, World War II. On Brit. stage from 1937. Screen debut 1941 in Brit. picture Mein Kampf, My Crimes.
PICTURES INCLUDE: The Goose Steps Out, One of Our Aircraft Is Missing, Let the People Sing, The Way Ahead, The True Glory, (collab. s.p.) The Way Ahead; (wrote, dir. & co-prod.) School for Secrets, Vice Versa; (adapt., dir., co-prod.) Private Angelo, Odette, Quo Vadis, Hotel Sahara, The Egyptian, Beau Brummell, We're No Angels, Lola Montez, The Spies, An Angel Flew Over Brooklyn, The Sundowners, Spartacus; prod.., scripted, acted, Romanoff and Juliet; dir., prod./scpt., acted, Billy Budd, Topkapi, John Goldfarb Please Come Home; prod. dir., Lady L., Blackbeard's Ghost, The Comedians, Hot Millions, Viva Max. Dir. and acted, Hammersmith Is Out, acted Big Truck, Poor Clare, Logan's Run, Treasure of Matecumbe, One of Our Dinosaurs Is Missing, Le Taxi Mauve, The Last Remake of Beau Geste, Doppio Delitto, Death on the Nile, Charlie Chan and the Curse of the Dragon Queen, The Great Muppet Caper, Evil Under the Sun. Dir., prod., starred in Memed My Hawk.
STAGE: Romanoff and Juliet, N.Y., London; and 17 other plays. Dir., acted, Photo Finish; wrote, Life In My Hands, The Unknown Soldier and His Wife, Half Way Up The Tree, King Lear, Beethoven's Tenth, etc.
RECENT TV: The Well Tempered Bach, 13 at Dinner, Deadman's Folly, Peter Ustinov's Russia, World Challenge.

V

VACCARO, BRENDA: Actress. b. Brooklyn, N.Y., Nov. 18, 1939. e. Thomas Jefferson High School, Dallas; studied two yrs. at Neighborhood Playhouse in N.Y. Was waitress and model before landing first Bdwy. role in Everybody Loves Opal. Toured in Tunnel of Love and returned to N.Y. for role in The Affair. Won Tony for best supporting actress in Cactus Flower.
PICTURES INCLUDE: Midnight Cowboy (debut), I Love My Wife, Summertree, Going Home, Once Is Not Enough, Airport '77, House by the Lake, Capricorn One, The First Deadly Sin, Zorro, the Gay Blade, Supergirl, Water.
TV: The F.B.I., The Name of the Game, The Helen Reddy Show, The Shape of Things (special), Sunshine (tv movie), etc.

VADIM, ROGER: Director-Writer. b. Paris, 1928. r.n. Roger Vadim Plemiannikow.
PICTURES: Futures Vedettes (s.p.). Writer-Director: And God Created Woman, Heaven Fell That Night, Les Liaisons Dangereuses, Warriors Rest,Vice and Virtue, La Ronde, The Game is Over. Director: Barbarella, Pretty Maids All in a Row, Don Juan, Night Games, A Faithful Woman, Hot Touch.

VAJNA, ANDREW: Executive. b. Budapest, Hungary, Aug. 1, 1944. e. UCLA. Exhibitor and dist. of feature films since 1970. Formed Carolco Service, Inc. (foreign sls. org.), 1977. Pres., American Film Mkt. Assn., 1983.
PICTURES: Exec. Prod.: The Silent Partner, The Changeling, Suzanne, The Amateur, Your Ticket Is No Longer Valid, Carbon Copy, First Blood, First Blood Part II.

VALE, EUGENE: Writer. b. April 11, 1916. e. Zurich, Switzerland. m. Evelyn Wahl. Story and s.p., The Second Face, The Shattered Dream, 1954 SWG award nom., best written telefilm; The Dark Wave. 1957, m.p. academy award nominations.
PICTURES: A Global Affair, Francis of Assissi, The Bridge of San Luis Rey.
TV: Four Star Playhouse, Fireside Theatre, 20th Century Fox Hour, Schlitz Playhouse, Hollywood Opening Night, NBC, Crusader, Lux Video Theatre, Danger, CBS, Chevron Theatre, Douglas Fairbanks, Pepsicola Playhouse, Waterfront, Christophers, Cavalcade of America, Hallmark Hall of Fame.
AUTHOR: Technique of Screenplay Writing.

VALENTI, JACK J.: Executive. b. Sept. 5, 1921. e. Univ. of Houston, B.A., 1946; Harvard, MBA, bus. admin., 1948. Air force pilot in European theatre, WWII; adv. and pub. rel. exec. in Houston; special asst. and advisor to Pres. Lyndon B. Johnson, 1963–66; pres., MPAA; elected pres., MPAA, MPEA and AMPTP, June, 1966.

VALENTINE, KAREN: Actress. b. Sebastopol, CA, May 25, 1947.
PICTURES: Forever Young, Forever Free, Hot Lead and Cold Feet, The North Avenue Irregulars.
TELEVISION:Series: Room 222 (Emmy), Karen, My Friend Tony, Hollywood Squares, Laugh-In, The Bold Ones, Sonny and Cher. Movies: Gidget Grows Up, The Daughters of Joshua Cabe, Coffee, Tea or Me?, The Girl Who Came Gift-Wrapped, The Love Boat, Having Babies, Murder at the World Series, Return to Fantasy Island, Go West, Young Girl, American 2100, Only the Pretty Girls Die, Muggable Mary, He's Fired; She's Hired, A Fighting Choice.

VALLI, ALIDA: Actress. b. Pola, Italy, May 31, 1921. e. M.P. Academy, Rome (dramatics); m. Oscar de Mejo, pianist-composer. In Italian m.p.; won Venice Film Festival Award in "Piccolo Monde Antico" (Little Old World).
PICTURES INCLUDE: Vita Ricomincia, Giovanna; to U.S. 1947; U.S. m.p. debut in Paradine Case, 1947; later pictures: Miracle of the Bells, The Third Man, Walk Softly Stranger, White Tower, Lovers of Toledo, Stranger's Hand, The Castilian, Ophelia, Spider's Stratagem, The Cassandra Crossing, Susperia, 1900, Luna.

VALLIN, RICK: Actor. b. Russia; son of Nedja Yatsenko, ballerina. In stage stock, radio; joined Pasadena Playhouse, 1942. Screen debut 1942.
PICTURES INCLUDE: King of the Stallions, Nearly Eighteen, Corregidor, Lady from Chungking, A Night for Crime, Panther's Claw, Northwest Outpost, Two Blondes and a Redhead, Jungle Jim, Shamrock Hill, Comanche Territory, Aladdin and His Lamp, Magic Carpet, Woman in the Dark, Jungle Manhunt, Strange Fascination, Voodoo Tiger, Star of Texas, many Westerns, Bowery to Bagdad, Treasure of Ruby Hills, Dial Red O.

VALLONE, RAF: Actor. b. Turin, Italy, Feb. 17, 1916. e. U. of Turin. Newspaper writer; m.p. debut in Bitter Rice.
PICTURES INCLUDE: Under the Olive Tree, Anna, Path of Hope, White Line, Rome 11 O'Clock, Strange Deception, Anita Garibaldi, Daughters of Destiny, Teresa Raquin, Riviera, The Secret Invasion. 1961: Two Women, El Cid, A View From the Bridge, Phaedra, Kiss The Girls and Make Them Die, The Desperate Ones, The Cardinal, The Italian Job, The Kremlin Letter, Summertime Killer, Rosebud, The Human Factor, The Other Side of Midnight, The Greek Tycoon, Lion of the Desert.

VAN CLEEF, LEE: Actor. b. Somerville, N.J., Jan. 9, 1925. e. Somerville H.S., 1942. Joined U.S. Navy, 1942; asst. mgr. in summer camp, public accountant; then joined little theatre group.

PICTURES INCLUDE: High Noon, Beast from 20,000 Fathoms, Vice Squad, The Nebraskan, Gypsy Colt, Arrow in the Dust, Yellow Tomahawk, Dawn at Socorro, Princess of the Nile, Ten Wanted Men, The Conqueror, Big Combo, Treasure of Ruby Hills, I Cover the Underworld, Road To Denver, Posse from Hell, The Man Who Shot Liberty Valance, A Man Alone, Vanishing American, Tribute to a Bad Man, For a Few Dollars More, The Good, The Bad and The Ugly, The Big Gundown, Death Rides a Horse, Day of Anger, Barquero, El Condor, The Magnificent Seven Ride, Return of Sabata, Escape from New York.

VAN DEVERE, TRISH: Actress. b. Englewood Cliffs, NJ, March 9, 1945. e. Ohio Wesleyan. Wife of actor George Scott. On Bdwy. in Sly Fox, Tricks of the Trade, etc.
PICTURES: Where's Poppa?, The Last Run, One Is a Lonely Number, The Day of the Dolphin, The Savage is Loose, Fifty-Two Pickup, Movie, Movie, The Changeling, The Hearse.
TELEVISION: Mayflower—The Pilgrim's Adventure, All God's Children, Haunted.

VAN DOREN, MAMIE: Actress. r.n. Joan Lucille Olander. b. Rowena, S.D., Feb. 6, 1933. e. Los Angeles High Sch. Secy. law firm, L.A.; prof. debut as singer with Ted Fio Rita orch.
THEATRE: Appeared in many stock plays incl.: Once in a Lifetime, Boy Meets Girl, Come Back Little Sheba.
PICTURES INCLUDE: (m.p. debut) Forbidden; All American, Yankee Pasha, Francis Joins the Wacs, Ain't Misbehavin, Second Greatest Sex, Running Wild, Star in the Dust, Untamed Youth, Girl in Black Stockings, Teachers Pet, The Navy Vs. The Night Monsters.

VAN DYKE, DICK: Actor. b. West Plains, Mo., Dec., 18, 1925. U.S.A.F., WWII. partner, ad. agency, nightclub acts: Merry Mutes, Eric and Van.
THEATRE: The Girls Against the Boys, Bye Bye Birdie.
PICTURES INCLUDE: Bye Bye Birdie, Mary Poppins, What a Way to Go. The Art of Love, Lieutenant Robinson Crusoe, Divorce American Style, What's New Fitzwilly?, Chitty Chitty Bang Bang, Some Kind of Nut, The Comic, Cold Turkey, The Runner Stumbles.
TV: The Merry Mute Show, The Music Shop, The Dick Van Dyke Show (variety prog.), Cartoon Theater, The New Dick Van Dyke Show, The Carol Burnett Show, Found Money (movie).

VAN FLEET, JO: Actress. b. Oakland, Calif., 1922. e. College of the Pacific. Neighborhood Playhouse.
THEATRE: On Broadway in Winter's Tale, Whole World Over, Closing Door, King Lear, Flight into Egypt, Camino Real, Trip to Bountiful (Tony Award); Look Homeward Angel (Critics Award); The Glass Menagerie; Off Broadway: The Alligators, Oh Dad, Poor Dad, Mama's Hung You In The Closet and I'm Feeling So Sad.
PICTURES INCLUDE: East of Eden (Academy Award, best supporting actress, 1955); I'll Cry Tomorrow (Look Award), Rose Tattoo, This Angry Age, King and Four Queens, Gunfight at the OK Corral; Wild River, Cool Hand Luke, I Love You, Alice B. Toklas, Gang Who Couldn't Shoot Straight, The Tenant.
TELEVISION: Cinderella, Bonanza, Mod Squad, Power, etc.

VANGELIS: Composer-Conductor. Full name: Vangelis Papathanassiou. b. Greece. Formed band Formynx in Greece; then Aphrodite's Child in Paris.
PICTURES: Chariots of Fire (Oscar), Missing, Blade Runner, The Bounty, Wonders of Life, Wild and Beautiful.

VAN HEUSEN, JIMMY: Composer. b. Syracuse, N.Y., Jan. 26, 1919. e. Syracuse U. Pianist with publishing houses; songs for many m.p. including Sunday, Monday or Always, Swinging on a Star (Acad. Award 1944), Sunshine Cake, etc.
PICTURES INCLUDE: Road to Rio, Emperor Waltz, Connecticut Yankee, Mr. Music, Riding High, Road to Bali, Little Boy Lost, All the Way (Academy Award), Call Me Irresponsible (Academy Award), won Emmy for Love and Marriage; Songwriters Hall of Fame.

VANOCUR, SANDER: News Commentator. b. Cleveland. e. Northwestern Univ. Began career as journalist in London; joined NBC in 1957, hosting First Tuesday series. Resigned in 1971 to be correspondent of the National Public Affairs Center for PBC. In 1977 joined ABC News as v.p., special reporting units.

VAN PALLANDT, NINA: Actress. b. Copenhagen, Denmark, July 15, 1932. e. Univ. of So. Calif. Returned to Denmark where married Baron Frederik Van Pallandt with whom she had appeared as folk singer throughout Europe. Made 3 films with him; went on world tour together. Now divorced. Has appeared in New York as singer.
PICTURES: The Long Goodbye, A Wedding, Quintet, American Gigolo, Cloud Dancer, Cutter and Bone.
TELEVISION: The Sam Shepherd Murder Case.

VAN PATTEN, DICK: b. N.Y.C., Dec. 9, 1928. Began career as child actor with Bdwy. debut at 7 yrs., playing son of Melvyn Douglas in Tapestry in Gray. Has worked since in stage, radio, TV, films.
PICTURES INCLUDE: Making It, Joe Kidd, Soylent Green, Dirty Little Billy, Westworld, Gus, Treasure of Matecumbe, High Anxiety.
TV: Series: Mama, The Partners, The New Dick Van Dyke Show, Eight Is Enough. Guest Roles: Arnie, The Rookies, Cannon, Banyon, The Little People, The Streets of San Francisco, When Things Were Rotten.
STAGE: The Lady Who Came to Stay, O Mistress Mine, On Borrowed Time, Ah, Wilderness, Watch on the Rhine, The Skin of Our Teeth, Kiss and Tell, Mister Roberts, I Was Dancing.

VAN PATTEN, JOYCE: Actress. b. New York City, March 9, 1934.
PICTURES: The Goddess, I Love You Alice B. Toklas, Something Big, Thumb Tripping, Mikey and Nicky, The Falcon and the Snowman, St. Elmo's Fire.
TELEVISION: Many specials and Movies: Shadow of Fear, The Martian Chronicles, Eleanor First Lady of the World, Bus Stop, In Defense of Kids, Malice in Wonderland, etc.

VAN PEEBLES, MELVIN: Director, writer, composer. Was navigator-bombardier in Air Force, drove cable car in San Francisco.
AUTHOR: A Bear for the F.B.I., Don't Play Me Cheap (play) won 1st prize, Belgian Festival; and photo-essay book on cable cars. Albums of his own music: Brer Soul, Ain't Supposed to Die a Natural Death. Composed music for Watermelon Man.
PICTURES INCLUDE: The Story of a Three-Day Pass, Watermelon Man, Sweet Sweetback.
MEMBER: French Director's Guild; one of first Black directors to be member of Directors Guild of America.
STAGE: Ain't Supposed to Die a Natural Death, Don't Play Us Cheap.

VAN PRAAG, WILLIAM: Executive, Producer, Director, Writer, Editor. Advertising Consultant. b. N.Y.C., Sept. 13, 1924. e. CREI, Columbia Univ.; U.S. Army, 1942. Paramount, 1945; Brandt Bros. Prods., 1946; NBC, 1947; v.p. Television Features, 1948. Devlpd. vidicon system in m.p. prod., 1949. Started, pres., Van Praag Prod. Inc. 1951. Formed Ernst-Van Praag, Inc. 1971, a communications and marketing counseling firm (N.Y., Brussels, Tokyo). Pres., International Film, TV and A-V Producers Ass'n, 1969, Creator of Van-O-Vision. Winner of commercial, short subject and feature theatrical awards. Author of Color Your Picture, Primer of Creative Editing, and Van Praag's Magic Eye. Past pres., Film Producer's Ass'n, mem. DGA, SAG, 71 IATSE, National Academy of TV Arts and Sciences, International Radio and TV Executive Society and Soc. of MP and TV Engineers.

VAN RIKFOORD, HAROLD C.: Producer. b. New York, Jan. 1, 1935. e. Bryant H.S., grad., 1952; N.Y. Univ. Errand boy, stage mgr., N.Y., 1954–57. Co-prod. two Broadway plays. Prod., The Long Ride Home, Rome, 1957; prod., short subject films; prod., Moment of Crisis, 1959; prod., television pilot films; exec. prod., Jonathan Shields Prod.

VAN THAL, DENNIS: Executive. b. London, June 4, 1909. e. University College. Early career musical dir.; war service, Royal Navy; entered m.p. industry 1946; casting dir. Pinewood Studios; dir., Myron Selznick Ltd.; joined dir. Alexander Korda as prod. exec., 1953; apptd. dir., Big Ben Films, 1955; joined Ealing Films, 1956; prod. assoc. Anastasia; assoc. prod. The Admirable Crichton, Barnacle Bill, The Scapegoat; mgr. dir. London Management, Ltd.

VANCE, LEIGH: Scriptwriter and producer. b. Harrogate, England. Early career; reporter, critic. Ent. TV 1951, then films, many TV scripts; 1961, won Edgar Allan Poe Award, 1969 brought to Hollywood by Paramount. In 1973 exec. story consultant and producer, Cannon; 1974, exec . story consultant, Caribe; 1975, prod., Bronk. 1976: Exec. prod., Baretta & Switch, 1977–78: Prod., Switch; 1981, Prod., Phoenix; 1983, Prod., Hart to Hart.
PICTURES INCLUDE: The Flesh Is Weak, Heart of a Child, Picadilly Third Stop, Women Shall Weep, The Shakedown, Eyes of Youth, The Frightened City, It's All Happening Dr. Crippen, Outcast, Walk Like A Man, Cross Plot, Tall Cool Girl, The Black Windmill.
TV: Mannix, Mission Impossible, many pilots and movies-of-the-week. The Avengers, The Saint, Cannon, Caribe, Bronk, Baretta, Switch, The Phoenix, Hart to Hart.

VARDA, AGNES: Photographer-Director-Writer. b. France, 1928. Started as still photographer for The Theatre National Populaire de Jean Vilar. Became a photo-journalist. In 1954 wrote and directed first film, La Pointe Courte. Afterwards made both documentaries and features.
PICTURES INCLUDE: Cleo from 5 to 7, Le Bonheur, Les Creatures, Lion's Love, One Sings, The Other Doesn't.

VARSI, DIANE: Actress. b. San Francisco,1938.
PICTURES: Peyton Place, Ten North Frederick, From Hell to Texas, Compulsion, Sweet Love, Bitter, Wild in the Streets, Killers Three, Bloody Mama, Johnny Got His Gun, I Never Promised You a Rose Garden.
TELEVISION: The People (movie).

VAUGHN, ROBERT: Actor. b. New York City, Nov. 22, 1932. Played Napoleon Solo in The Man From U.N.C.L.E. TV series.
CREDITS: Hell's Crossroads, No Time to Be Young, Unwed Mother, Good Day for a Hanging, The Young Philadelphians, The City Jungle (Acad. Award nom.), The Magnificent Seven, The Big Show, The Caretakers, To Trap a Spy, The Spy With My Face , One Spy too Many, The Venetian Affair, How to Steal the World, Bullitt, The Bridge at Remagen, The Mind of Mr. Soames, If It's Tuesday, This Must Be Belgium, Julius Caesar, The Statue, The Clay Pigeon, One of Our Spies Is Missing (TV, Great Britain), The Spy in the Green Hat (TV, Great Britain), The Towering Inferno, Starship Invasions, S.O.B., Superman III, The Delta Force, Black Moon Rising.
AUTHOR: Only Victims, 1972.
TV: Washington: Behind Closed Doors, The Blue and the Gray, Evergreen, International Airport, Murrow, Prince of Bel Air.

VEITCH, JOHN: Executive. b. New York City, June 22, 1925. Started production career as asst. director and moved through ranks as prod. mgr., assoc., prod., prod., second unit dir., and exec. prod. mgr. Appointed Columbia Pictures exec. asst. prod. mgr., 1961; became exec. prod. mgr., 1963. Named v.p. & exec. prod. mgr., 1966; promoted in 1977 to exec. v.p. & exec. prod. mgr. of world-wide productions. In 1979 named pres. of Columbia Pictures Productions. Resigned 1983 to be consultant and independent producer exclusively for Columbia.

VELAISE, ROBERT: Executive. e. Zurich U.; ent. production 1957; formed Vauban Productions of Paris, Robert Velaise Productions, Ltd., of London, 1961; prod., Les Oeufs de l'Autruche, Nina, Geliebte Hochstaplerin, Give Me Ten Desperate Men, The Wrong Arm of the Law, The Go-Between.

VELAZCO, ROBERT E.: r.n. Emil Velazco, Jr. b. Dallas, Texas, Jan 1, 1924. e. Columbia Univ., Business Administration 1942–43. Started in film business with father, Emil Velazco, 1942. Following yrs. worked for Emil Velazco, Inc., NTA, Ross Gaffney, Inc. During this time worked on over 8,500 productions from 5 sec. to feature films. In charge of Velazco, Inc., Kansas City, Mo., 1947–49. Owner and pres., Musifex Co., Inc., 1958. Opened Musifex Inc. Arlington, Va., 1972. Two films scored by Velazco nominated for Academy Award, 1978 and 1980. In 1983 expanded into video tape music editing and video mixing.

VELDE, DONALD L.: Executive. b. Tremont, Ill., Sept. 10, 1902. e. Bradley Prep, Swarthmore Coll. Paramount Pictures, 1922–40; National Screen Service, 1940–48; chairman, Donald L. Velde, Inc. Retired.

VELDE, JAMES R.: Executive. b. Bloomington, Ill., Illinois Wesleyan Univ. Entered m.p. ind. as night shipper Paramount ex. Detroit, 1934; then city salesman, office mgr. until joining Army, 1943, rejoining same ex. upon dischge., 1946; to Paramount, Washington as Baltimore city salesman, same yr.; br. mgr. Selznick Rel. Org. Pittsburgh, 1948; salesman Eagle-Lion Classics, Pittsburgh, 1949; br. mgr. ELC, Des Moines, 1949; br. mgr., ELC, Detroit, 1950; west coast dist. mgr., United Artists, April, 1951; Western div. mgr. UA, 1952; gen. sales mgr., 1956; v.p., 1958; dir., UA, 1968; sr. v.p., 1972. Retired, 1977.

VENTURA, LINO: Actor. b. Italy, 1918. French resident since age of 8. Was professional wrestler until injury ended career in ring. First acting appearance in Touchez pas au Grisbi (1953) opposite Jean Gabin. Veteran of over 50 films.
PICTURES: Marie Octobre, Crooks in Clover, Les Aventuriers, The Valachi Papers, Wild Horses, Sunday Lovers, etc.

VEREEN, BEN: Singer-Dancer-Actor. b. Miami, FL, Oct. 10, 1946. On stage in Sweet Charity, Jesus Christ Superstar, Pippin (Tony), etc.
PICTURES: Gasss, Funny Lady, All That Jazz, The Zoo Gang.
TELEVISION: Movies: Louis Armstrong—Chicago Style, Roots, Ten Speed and Brown Shoe. Specials: Ben Vereen—His Roots, Uptown—A Tribute to the Apollo Theatre, Ellis Island, A.D.

VERNON, ANNE: Actress. r.n. Edith Antoinette Alexandrine Vignaud. b. Paris, Jan. 24. e. Ecole des Beaux Arts, Paris. Worked for French designer; screen debut in French films; toured with French theatre group; first starring role, Le Manneuin Assassine 1948.
PICTURES INCLUDE: Ainsi Finit La Nuit, A Warning to Wantons, Patto Col Diavolo, A Tale of Five Cities, Shakedown, Song of Paris, Edward and Caroline, Terror on a Train.

VERNON, JOHN: Actor. b. Canada, 1936. e. Banff School of Fine Arts, RADA.
PICTURES: Point Blank, Justine, Topaz, One More Train to Rob, Dirty Harry, Charlie Varrick, The Black Windmill, Fear Is the Key, Cat and Mouse, Brannigan, The Outlaw Josey Wales, Angela, A Special Day, National Lampoon's Animal House, Fantastica, Crunch, Herbie Goes Bananas, Chained Heat, Curtains, Savage Streets, Doin' Time.
TELEVISION: Movies: Trial Run, Escape, Cool Million, Hunter, The Questor Tapes, Mousey, The Virginia Hill Story, The Imposter, Swiss Family Robinson, The Barbary Coast, Matt Helm, Mary Jane Harper Cried Last Night, The Sacketts, The Blue and the Gray etc.

VERONA, STEPHEN: Director. e. School of Visual Arts. Directed some 300 commercials before turning to feature films in 1972, which he wrote as well.
PICTURES: Pipe Dreams, Boardwalk.

VETTER, RICHARD: Exec. b. San Diego, Calif., Feb. 24, 1928. e. Pepperdine Coll., B.A., 1950; San Diego State Coll., M.A., 1953, U.C.L.A., Ph.D., 1959. U.S. Navy: aerial phot., 1946–48, reserve instr., San Diego County Schools, 1951–54; asst. prof., audio-vis. commun., U.C.L.A., 1960–63. Inventor, co-dev., Dimension 150 Widescreen Process. 1957–63: formed D-150 Inc., 1963; exec. v.p. mem.: SMPTE, Technical & Scientific Awards Committee, AMPAS.

VICTOR, JAMES: Actor. r.n. Lincoln Rafael Peralta Diaz. b. Santiago, Dominican Republic, July 27, 1939. e. Haaren H.S., NYC. Studied at Actors Studio West. On stage in Bullfight, Ceremony for an Assassinated Blackman, Latina, The Man in the Glass Booth, The M.C., I Gave You a Calender, etc.
PICTURES: Fuzz, Rolling Thunder, Boulevard Nights, Defiance, Losin' It, Borderline.
TELEVISION: Series: Viva Valdez, Condo. Many appearances on specials. Movies made-for-TV: Robert Kennedy and His Times, Twin Detectives, The Hound of Hell, etc.
AWARDS: Cleo (1975) for Mug Shot; L.A. Drama-Logue Critics Award (1980) for Latina; Golden Eagle Award (1981) for consistent outstanding performances in motion pictures.

VIETHEER, GEORGE C.: Executive. b. New York, N.Y., Feb. 27, 1910. e. Norwich U., B.S., 1932; Syracuse U, M.S., 1933. U.S. Army officer, 1933–37; chief service bureau, later Wash. rep. Panama Canal & R.R. Co., 1937–41; deputy dir., personnel, Office of Emergency Mgt., 1941–43; U.S. Army, 1943–46; mem., Nat'l Comm. on Manpower Shortages, 1946; deputy dir., personnel, U.S. Dept. of Commerce, 1946–50; U.S. rep. to U.N. Public Admin. Conf., 1950; deputy asst. admin. Econ. Stab. Agency, 1951; mgr., Washington office, MPAA, 1952; subsequently v.p., MPEAA and also v.p. American Motion Picture Export Co. (Africa) and v.p., Afram Films, Inc. Author: various pubs., articles on bus. mgt. Retired since 1977.

VILAS, WILLIAM H.: Executive. e. Harvard U.: U. Minnesota, B.A. Dunwoody Institute. In adv. & sales management; wrote, prod. or supervised over 100 productions for TV, industrial or theatre release; organized & supervised film training projects for U.S. Armed Forces, World War II: v.p., Wilding Pictures Prod.; special consultant for OSS; prod. of theatrical, TV & non-theatrical m.p. For pub. rel.; recent TV: Terry and the Pirates, series on film, dir., motion picture & television dept. & account exec., J. M. Mathes, Inc., N.Y.; chmn. bd. gov. Yankee Highway Assn.; dir. Citizens Assn. of Conn.; pub. Brotherhood Press. Clubs; Pequet Yacht, Southport, Conn., Harvard, New Canaan, Conn.

VILLECHAIZE, HERVE: Actor. b. Paris, France, April 23, 1943. Sought career as artist, studying in Paris and then coming to New York to the Art Students League. Studied acting with Julie Bovasso. First film, The Guitar, shot in Spain. On Broadway in Elizabeth the First and Gloria and Esperenze. Also performed mime in N.Y. City Opera productions.
PICTURES: Hollywood Blvd. No. 2, Hot Tomorrow, The Man with the Golden Gun, Crazy Joe, The Gang That Couldn't Shoot Straight, Seizure, The One and Only, Forbidden Zone.
TELEVISION: Fantasy Island (regular).

VINCENT, JAN-MICHAEL: Actor. b. Denver, Colo., July 15, 1944. e. Ventura City (Calif.) College as art major. Joined National Guard. Discovered by agent Dick Clayton. Hired by Robert Conrad to appear in his film, Los Bandidos, made in Mexico. Signed to 6-mo. contract by Universal, for which made Journey to Shiloh. Then did pilot TV movie for 20th-Fox based on Hardy Boys series of book. Originally called self Michael Vincent; changed after The Undefeated.
PICTURES INCLUDE: Los Bandidos, Journey to Shiloh, The Undefeated, Going Home, The Mechanic, The World's

Greatest Athlete, Buster and Billie, Bite the Bullet, White Line Fever, Baby Blue Marine, Vigilante Force, Shadow of the Hawk, Damnation Alley, Big Wednesday, Hooper, Defiance, Hard Country, The Last Plane Out.

TV: Lassie, Bonanza, The Banana Splits Adventure Hour, The Survivors (series), Tribes (movie released theatrically abroad), The Catcher (movie), Sandcastle (movie). Airwolf (series).

VINCENT, JR., FRANCIS T: Executive. Exec. v.p. of The Coca-Cola Company and pres. & CEO of its entertainment business sector. e. Also is chm. & CEO of Columbia Pictures Industries, Inc. appt. pres. CEO, 1978. Williams College, Yale Law School. 1969–78, partner in law firm of Caplin & Drysdale, specializing in corporate banking and securities matters. 1978, assoc. dir. of, Division of Corporation Finance of Securities & Exchange Commission. Trustee of Williams College & The Hotchkiss School. Memb er of board of dir. of The Coca-Cola Bottling Co. of New York.

VINCENT, JUNE: Actress. r.n. Dorothy June Smith. b. Harrods, Ohio, 1919. Concert pianist; photographer's model. On dramatic stage, The Family. Screen debut Second Honeymoon, 1937.

PICTURES INCLUDE: The Climax, Ladies Courageous, Can't Help Singing, Shed No Tears, Creeper, Counterspy Meets Scotland Yard, Secrets of Monte Carlo, Colorado Sundown, Night Without Sleep, Wac from Walla Walla, Clipped Wings, City of Shadows.

VINCENT, KATHARINE: Actress. r.n. Ella Vincenti. b. St. Louis, Missouri, May 28, 1919. e. Two years of high school, left in 1937 to go on the stage. m. Pandeno Descanto, producer.

THEATRE: Broadway shows include: Love or Bust, 1938; Could She Tell?, 1939; Banners of 1939; Czarina Smith, 1940. Numerous road show tours.

PICTURES INCLUDE: Peptipa's Waltz, 1942 (debut), Error in Her Ways, 1943, Skin Deep, 1944, The Hungry, Voodoo Village, Welcome to Genoa, 1950, Unknown Betrayal, 1956, The Hooker, 1962 (Descanto films).

TV: The Untouchables, Moses, The Lawgiver.

VINER, MICHAEL: Producer-Writer. b. 1945. e. Harvard, Georgetown. Served as aide to Robert Kennedy; was legman for political columnist Jack Anderson. Settled in Hollywood, where worked for prod. Aaron Rosenberg, first as prod. asst. on three Frank Sinatra films; then asst. prod. on Joaquin Murietta. In music industry was record producer, manager, executive, eventualy heading own division, at MGM. Debut as writer-producer in 1976 with TV special, Special of the Stars. Theatrical film debut as prod.-co-writer of Touched by Love, 1980.

VITALE, JOSEPH A.: Actor. b. New York City, Sept. 6, 1901. In 1924, on dramatic stage (Hold on to Your Hats, Page Miss Glory, All Editions, I'd Rather Be Right, Common Ground). Screen debut, 1943.

PICTURES INCLUDE: None But the Lonely Heart, Lady Luck, Road to Rio, Where There's Life, Connecticut Yankee, Illegal Entry, Red Hot and Blue, Paleface, Fancy Pants, My Friend Irma Goes West, Stop You're Killing Me, Stranger Wore a Gun, Square Jungle, Rumble On the Docks, Apache Rifles.

TV: Climax, Lineup, Bengal Lancers, Wagon Train, Schlitz Playhouse, Cimmaron City, Telephone Time, Wyatt Earp, Rawhide, Red Skelton, The Thin Man, M Squad, Dawson, Ben Casey, Empire, Hazel, Mr. Ed, To Rome With Love, Fisherman's Wharf (pilot).

VITALE, MILLY: Actress. b. Rome, Italy. July 16, 1938. e. Lycee Chateaubriand, Rome. Has appeared in numerous Italian films.

PICTURES INCLUDE: The Juggler, Seven Little Foys, Breath of Scandal.

VITTI, MONICA: Actress. b. Italy, 1933. r.n. Monica Luisa Ceciarelli.

PICTURES: L'Avventura, La Notte, L'Eclipse, Dragees du Poivre, The Nutty, Naughty Chateau, The Red Desert, Modesty Blaise, The Chastity Belt, Girl with a Pistol, The Pacifist, Duck in Orange Sauce, An Almost Perfect Affair, The Mystery of Oberwald, The Flirt.

VOGEL, JESSE: Writer, Composer. b. New York, N.Y., Oct. 24, 1925. e. CCNY, B.S.Sc., 1947; Paris Conservatory of Music, 1949; dir., Vogel Films, Paris, post-production services, English and Foreign versions. Screenplays: Carmen, Baby; Therese and Isabelle. Produced: Who's Harriet? My Pleasure Is My Business.

VOHS, JOAN: Actress. r.n. Elinor Joan Vohs. b. St. Albans, L.I., N.Y., July 30, 1931; e. Andrew Jackson H.S., Professional Children's School. Radio City Music Hall Rockette at 16; Bdwy play; Parlor Story; many TV shows.

TV: Readers Digest, Stage Seven, Dear Phoebe, Ray Bolger Show, Robert Cummings Show, Stage 7, Frontier, Schlitz Playhouse, Lux Video Theatre.

PICTURES INCLUDE: My Dream Is Yours, Girl from Jones Beach, Inspector General, Yes Sir That's My Baby, Vice Squad, Fort Ti, Crazylegs, Sabrina, Cry Vengeance, Fort Yuma, Terror at Midnight.

VOIGHT, JON: Actor. b. Yonkers, N.Y. Dec. 29, 1938. e. Archbishop Stepinac High School, White Plains, N.Y.: Catholic University, Bachelor of Fine Arts Degree, 1960; studied acting at the Neighborhood Playhouse and in private classes with Stanford Meisner, four yrs. Off-Broadway in: A View From the Bridge (revival), 1964. Won the Theatre World Award for Broadway prod. That Summer, That Fall. Played Romeo, San Diego Shakespeare Festival.

TV: Public Broadcast Lab.'s The Dwarf, also Gunsmoke, Cimarron Strip.

PICTURES INCLUDE: Fearless Frank, Hour of the Gun, Midnight Cowboy (Acad. Award nom., Best Actor), Out of It, Catch 22, The Revolutionary, All American Boy, Deliverance, Conrack, The Odessa File, End of the Game, Coming Home, The Champ, Lookin' To Get Out (also co-s.p.), Table for Five, Runaway Train, Desert Bloom.

VOLONTE, GIAN MARIA: Actor. b. Milan, April 9, 1933. e. Rome's National Academy of Dramatic Art (1957 graduate). Entered on professional theatrical career, playing Shakespeare and Racine, along with modern works, Sacco and Vanzetti and The Deputy. On TV in Chekov's Uncle Vanya and Dostoyevsky's The Idiot. First major film roles in Un Uomo da Bruciare (1961) and Il Terrorista (1963). Called self John Welles in credits for "spaghetti westerns."

PICTURES INCLUDE: For a Fistful of Dollars, For a Few Dollars More, Investigation of a Citizen Above Suspicion, The Working Class Goes to Heaven, Wind from the East, Sacco and Vanzetti, L'Attenat, Slap the Monster on Page One, Just Another War, The Mattei Affair, Lucky Luciano, Eboli, The Death of Mario Ricci.

VON SYDOW, MAX: Actor. b. Lund, Sweden, April 10, 1929. m. Keratin Olin, actress, 1951. Theatrical debut in a Cathedral School of Lund prod. of The Nobel Prize. Served in the Swedish Quartermaster Corps two yrs. Studied at Royal Dramatic Theatre School in Stockholm. Tour in municipal theatres. Has appeared on stage in Stockholm, London, Paris and Helsinki in Faust, The Legend and The Misanthrope. 1954 won Sweden's Royal Foundation Cultural Award.

PICTURES INCLUDE: Wild Strawberries, Brink of Life, The Magician, The Seventh Seal, The Virgin Spring, Through a Glass Darkly, Winter Light, Hawaii, The Greatest Story Ever Told, The Reward, Hour of the Wolf, Shame, The Kremlin Letter, The Passion of Anna, The Immigrants, Night Visitor, The Emigrants, The New Land, Three Days of The Condor, Voyage of the Damned, Exorcist II: The Heretic, March or Die, Flash Gordon, Victory, Conan The Barbarian, Never Say Never Again, Dreamscape, Dune, Code Name: Emerald, Hannah and Her Sisters.

TELEVISION: Samson and Delilah.

VONDERHAAR, RAYMOND T.: Executive. b. Rugby, No. Dak., Nov. 1, 1919. e. St. Cloud State. Spent entire career in exhibition. Pres., Allied Theatre Assn., 1963–64; pre., NATO North Central States, 1965–76; National NATO bd., 1965–84; also memb. exec. comm. 1965–84; NATO No. Central, chm., 1976–84.

VON ZERNECK, FRANK: Executive. b. New York City, Nov. 3, 1940. e. Hofstra Coll. (1962). Has produced plays in New York, Los Angeles, and on national tour and over 30 films for American TV. Mid-'70s founded (with Robert Greenwald) Moonlight Prods. Devised "Portrait" film genre for TV movies: Portrait of a Stripper, Portrait of a Mistress, Portrait of a Centerfold, etc. Also produced 21 Hours at Munich, Dress Gray, Miracle on Ice.

Past chm. of California Theatre Council; former officer of League of Resident theatres; active member of Producers Guild of America and League of New York Theatres & Producers; bd. of gov., Producers Guild of America.

VORHAUS, BERNARD: Director. In 1933, wrote and directed Money for Speed (UA-British).

PICTURES INCLUDE: 1934, directed The Ghost Camera (Radio-British), Crime on the Hill (BIP) and Night Club Queen (Universal-British); 1935; Broken Melody (APD), Blind Justice (Universal-British), Ten Minutes Alibi (BL), Street Song (Radio-British). In 1936; directed Last Journey, Twickenham; Dark World, Fox British. Associate producer Broken Blossoms; director, Dusty Ermine, Twickenham; Cotton Queen, Rock Studios, Bury Me Dead, Winter Wonderland, The Spiritualist, So Young, So Bad, Pardon My French.

W

WADLEIGH, MICHAEL: Director. b. Akron, Ohio, Sept. 24, 1941. e. Ohio State U., B.S., B.A., M.A., Columbia Medical School. Directed Woodstock.

WAGGONER, LYLE: Actor, b. Kansas City, Kan., April 13, 1935. e. Washington Univ., St. Louis, Was salesman before becoming actor with road co. prod. of Li'l Abner. Formed own sales-promo co. to finance trip to Calif. for acting career in 1965. Did commercials, then signed by 20th-Fox for new-talent school.
TELEVISION: The Carol Burnett Show, It's Your Bet (Host), The New Adventures of Wonder Woman.
PICTURES: Love Me Deadly, Journey to the Center of Time, Catalina Caper, Surf II.

WAGNER, JANE: Writer-Director. b. Morristown, TN, Feb. 2, 1935. Bdwy. work includes Appearing Nitely and The Search for Signs of Intelligent Life in the Universe—both starring Lily Tomlin.
PICTURES: Moment by Moment (s.p., dir.); The Incredible Shrinking Woman (exec. prod., s.p.).
TELEVISION: Lily, Lily Tomlin, People, Lily—Sold Out, Lily for President?, etc.

WAGNER, LINDSAY: Actress. b. Los Angeles, June 22, 1949. Appeared in school plays in Portland, Oregon; studied singing and worked professionally with rock group. In 1968 went to L.A. and decided to make acting her career. Signed to Universal contract in 1971.
PICTURES INCLUDE: Two People, Paper Chase, Second Wind, Nighthawks, Martin's Day.
TV: The F.B.I., Owen Marshall, Counselor at Law, Night Gallery, The Bold Ones, Marcus Welby, M.D., The Rockford Files, The Six Million Dollar Man, The Bionic Woman, Two Kinds of Love, Passions, Child's Cry, Convicted, This Child Is Mine, Young Again.

WAGNER, RAYMOND JAMES: Producer. b. College Point, L.I., N.Y., Nov. 3, 1925. e. Middlebury College & Williams College. Joined Young & Rubicam, Inc., as radio-TV commercial head in Hollywood, 1950–59. Head of pilot development, Universal Studios, 1960–65. Produced Petulia for Warner Bros. (1967) and was exec. prod. of Loving for Columbia (1969). V.p. of production (features) for MGM, 1972–79. Presently independent producer for 20th Century-Fox. 1985, produced Code of Silence (Orion).

WAGNER, ROBERT: Actor. b. Detroit, Feb. 10, 1930; e. Saint Monica's H.S. Film debut, Halls of Montezuma.
PICTURES INCLUDE: The Frogmen, Let's Make It Legal, With A Song in My Heart, What Price Glory, Stars and Stripes Forever, The Silver Whip, Titanic, (Star of Tomorrow, 1953). Beneath the 12-Mile Reef, Prince Valiant, Broken Lance, White Feather, Kiss Before Dying, The Mountain, True Story of Jesse James, Stopover Tokyo, The Hunters, In Love and War, Say One for Me, Between Heaven and Hell, All the Fine Young Cannibals, Sail a Crooked Ship, The Longest Day, The War Lover, The Condemned of Altona, Harper, Banning, The Biggest Bundle of Them All, Don't Just Sit There, Winning, The Towering Inferno, Midway, The Concord—Airport '79, Curse of the Pink Panther, I Am the Cheese.
TV: Series: It Takes A Thief, Switch, Hart to Hart. Movies: Pearl, Cat on a Hot Tin Roof, To Catch a King.

WAHL, KEN: Actor. b. Chicago, 1957. no acting experience when cast for Orion's The Wanderers in 1978.
PICTURES: Fort Apache, The Bronx, Race for the Yankee Zephyr, Running Scared, Jinxed, The Soldier, Purple Hearts.
TELEVISION: The Dirty Dozen: The Next Mission, Double Dare, The Gladiator.

WAITE, RALPH: Actor. b. White Plains, NY, June 22, 1929. e. Bucknell Univ., Yale Univ. Social Worker, publicity director, assistant editor and minister before turning to acting. Appeared in many Bdwy. plays, including Hogan's Goat, The Watering Place, Trial of Lee Harvey Oswald, etc., and off-Bdwy. and regional theatres. Biggest success on TV in The Waltons. Is founder of the Los Angeles Actors Theatre. Wrote, produced, directed and acted in theatrical film, On the Nickel.
PICTURES: Five Easy Pieces, Lawman, The Grissom Gang, Dime Box, The Sporting Club, etc.
TELEVISION: Series: The Waltons, The Mississippi. Movies: Red Alert, The Secret Life of John Chapman, Ohms, Angel City, A Good Start, Crime of Innocence, etc. Mini-series: Roots.

WAITE, RIC: Cinematographer. Photographed more than 40 movies-of-the-week for TV, 1979–83. Theatrical film debut, The Other Side of the Mountain (1975).
PICTURES: On the Nickle, The Long Riders, The Border, Tex, 48 Hrs., Footloose, Brewster's Millions, Cobra.

WAKELY, JIMMY: Actor, singer, songwriter. b. Mineola, Ark., Feb. 16, 1914. Began as farmer, then singer, radio, Oklahoma City, Decca recordings. Author lyrics & music numerous hillbilly songs (Too Late, I'll Never Let You Go). Screen debut 1939 in Saga of Death Valley; collab. on music Six Lessons from Madame La Zonga, 1941, From 1939 in many Westerns various cos. (Paramount, Universal, Republic, etc.); producing Westerns independently; act., Marshal's Daughter, Arrow in the Dust.

WALD, MALVIN: Writer, producer. b. New York City, N.Y., Aug. 8. e. Brooklyn College, B.A., J.D. Woodland University College of Law, graduate work Columbia U., New York University U.S.C. Newspaper reporter and editor, publicist, social worker, radio actor. Screenplays and original stories for Columbia, 20th-Fox, UA, MGM, WB; U.S. Air Force; tech. sgt., wrote 30 documentary films for film unit.
PICTURES INCLUDE: The Naked City (Acad. Award nomination, best story); Behind Locked Doors, The Dark Past, Ten Gentlemen from West Point, The Powers Girl, Two in a Taxi, Undercover Man, Outrage, On the Loose; (assoc. producer and sec.-treas., Filmakers Pictures, Inc.); Battle Taxi, Man on Fire, Al Capone, Venus in Furs. In Search of Historic Jesus. Legend of Sleepy Hollow. Shorts: An Answer, Employees Only (Academy Award nomin., best sht. doc.), Boy Who Owned a Melephant (Venice Children's Film Festival gold medal), Unarmed in Africa, The Policeman, James Weldon Johnson, Me An Alcoholic?. Problem Solving, Managerial Control.
TV: Many credits including Playhouse 90, Hollywood: The Golden Years, The Rafer Johnson Story, D-Day, Project: Man in Space, Tales of Hans Christian Andersen, Biography of A Rookie, Alcoa-Goodyear Hour, Climax, Shirley Temple Storybook, Life of Riley, Peter Gunn, Perry Mason, Dobie Gillis, Combat, Moonport (U.S.I.A.; prod., writer), Daktari, (Associate Prod.) Primus, California Tomorrow, prod. Mod Squad, Untamed World, Around the World of Mike Todd, The Billie Jean King Show, Life and Times of Grizzly Adams, Mark Twain's America, Greatest Heroes of the Bible, Littlest Hobo. Rich Little's You Asked For It. Exec. prod., 20th Century Fox TV Documentary Unit, 1963–64 writer-prod. U.S.I.A., 1964–65; writer-prod., Ivan Tors Films, 1965–69; prof., U.S.C., School of Cinema, UCLA, 1983–85 bd. or dir.; Writer's Guild of America, Acad. of Motion Picture Arts and Sciences, co-author of book, Three Major Screenplays. Contributor to books, American Screenwriters, Close-Ups. Published s.p., Naked City. Consultant, Natl. Endowment for Humanities and Corp. for Public Broadcasting. Visiting professor, Southern Illinois Univ. Pre-selection judge, Focus writing awards. Media & prod. consultant, Apache Mountain Spirit (PBS); actor-playwright, Group Repertory Theatre.

WALD, RICHARD C.: Executive. b. New York City. e. Columbia College, Clare College (Cambridge). Joined the New York Herald Tribune in 1951 as Columbia College correspondent; religion editor, political reporter; foreign correspondent (London, Bonn), 1959–63; associate editor, 1963–65; managing editor from 1965 until paper ceased publication in 1966; Sunday editor, World Journal Tribune, 1966; managing editor, Washington Post, 1967; vice president, Whitney Communications Corp., 1967–68; joined National Broadcasting Company as vice president, NBC News, 1968; exec. v.p., 1972; president, NBC News, 1973; sr. v.p., ABC News, 1978.

WALDMAN, WALTER: Publicist. b. New York City. e. CCNY, Columbia U. Newspaper reporter; magazine writer; radio-television-film critic; radio news writer, Current Events, Triangle Publications; The Bronx Home News; Grolier Society; Netherlands Information Bureau, station WLIB; free-lance New York Times and New York Herald Tribune; writer, press book dept., 20th Century-Fox; copy writer, advertising dept., Republic Pictures; writer, Variety, Box office Magazine; publicity writer, copy chief, publicity dept., Paramount Pictures; publicity copy chief, contact, MGM/United Artists Entertainment Co.

WALKEN, CHRISTOPHER: Actor. b. Astoria, N.Y., Mar. 31, 1943. Began career in off-Bdwy. musical revue, Best Foot Forward, starring Liza Minnelli. Continued in musicals until cast in original Bdwy. production of The Lion in Winter, winning Clarence Derwent Award for performance as King Philip. Switched to dramatic roles, winning Obie Award for title role in Kid Champion and Theater World Award for performance in N.Y. City Center revivial of Rose Tattoo. 1984 stage appearance, Hurlyburly (NYC).
PICTURES INCLUDE: The Anderson Tapes (debut), Next Stop, Greenwich Village, Roseland, Santa Fe–1936, The Sentinel, Annie Hall, The Deer Hunter, Heaven's Gate, The Dogs of War, Pennies from Heaven, Brainstorm, The Dead Zone, A View to a Kill, At Close Range.

WALKER, CLINT: Actor. b. Hartford, Ill., May 30, 1927. e. schools there. Joined Merchant Marine 1944, worked as sheet metal worker, carpenter, other jobs in Alton, Ill.; set out with wife and infant daughter for oil fields in Texas; decided to try acting. Got screen test at Paramount Studios for Cecil B. De Mille; later landed contract to star in Cheyenne TV films at Warner.
PICTURES INCLUDE: Fort Dobbs, Yellowstone Kelly, None But the Brave, Pancho Viva, Maya, Night of the Grizzly, Gold of the Seven Saints, Send Me No Flowers, The Dirty Dozen, The Great Bank Robbery, Sam Whisky, More Dead Than Alive, etc.

WALKER, E. CARDON: Executive. b. Rexburg, Idaho, Jan. 9, 1916. e. UCLA, Los Angeles; B.A. 1938. Four years Officer,

U.S. Navy, Started with Walt Disney Productions 1938; camera, story, unit director short subjects, budget control. Headed, 1950, adv. & pub. 1956, v.p. in chg. of adv. & sales. 1960 member bd. of dir. & exec. comm. 1965 v.p., mkt. 1967 exec. v.p. operations 1968, exec. v.p. and chief operating officer; pres., 1971; Nov. 1976 pres. and chief executive officer; June, 1980, named bd. chm. & chief executive officer; May, 1983, became chm. of exec. committee, which position he retained until Sept. 1984. Remains a board member.

WALKER, KATHRYN: Actress. b. Philadelphia. e. Wells College, Harvard. Studied acting at London Academy of Music and Dramatic Art on Fulbright Fellowship. Stage roles include part in Private Lives with Elizabeth Taylor and Richard Burton.
PICTURES: Rich Kids, Slap Shot, Neighbors, D.A.R.Y.L.
TELEVISION: Family Reunion, FDR: The Final Years, Special Bulletin, O Youth and Beauty, The Adams Chronicles, etc.

WALKER, NANCY: Actress-Director. b. Philadelphia, May 10, 1922. As child toured Europe with her parents, The Barto and Mann vaudeville team. Pursued career as serious vocalist until George Abbott steered her toward comedy when she auditioned for Broadway prod., Best Foot Forward. Directed film, Can't Stop the Music (1980).
STAGE: On the Town, Barefoot in the Park, Phoenix '55, Fallen Angels, Copper and Brass, Pal Joey, Wonderful Town, Girls Against the Boys, Look Ma, I'm Dancing, Along Fifth Avenue, Lucky Me.
PICTURES INCLUDE: Best Foot Forward, Girl Crazy, Broadway Rhythm, Meet the People, Stand Up and Be Counted, Forty Carats, Won Ton Ton, Murder by Death.
TV: Nearly every major TV show, plus series: McMillan & Wife, Rhoda, The Nancy Walker Show, Blansky's Beauties.

WALLACE, CHARLES: Producer, writer, director. b. Temple, Texas, May 5, 1930. e. New Mexico Military Institute; Arizona State Univ. Ent. industry, announcer engineer, KTYL, Phoenix, 1948; prod. dir., KVAR, Phoenix, 1950; prod. dir., Wide Wide World, NBC-TV, 1955–58; prod. dir., writer, NBC News overseas, U.S. Air Force Power for Peace, 1956; assoc. prod. writer, Twenty-Six Men, ABC-TV, 1958; prod. dir., writer, American Pauses spectaculars, CBS-TV Zane Grey Theatre, Johnny Ringo, Wyatt Earp, Robert Taylor Show, 1959; prod. writer, Four Star pilots, Hardcase-Yuma, 1959; writer, Wells Fargo, NBC-TV, Ichabod and Me, 1960; writer, Death Valley Days, U.S. Air Force Classified Documentaries; writer, Screen Gems, Whirlpool pilot, 1961; prod., Lum 'n Abner, Four Star TV, 1962.

WALLACE, IRVING: Writer. b. Chicago, Ill., March 19, 1916. e. Williams Inst., Berkeley, Calif., 1935–36. For. correspondent in Japan & China, Liberty Mag., 1940; U.S. Army doing m.p. & photog.; covered France, Germany, Spain for Sat. Evening Post, Collier's, Reader's Digest, 1946, 1947, 1949, 1953.
AUTHOR: The Fabulous Originals, 1955; The Square Pegs, 1957; The Sins of Philip Fleming, 1959; The Fabulous Showman, 1959; The Chapman Report, 1960; The Twenty-Seventh Wife, 1961; The Prize, 1962; The Three Sirens, 1963; The Man, 1964; The Sunday Gentleman, 1965; The Plot, 1967. The Writing of One Novel, 1968; The Seven Minutes, 1969; The Nympho and Other Maniacs, 1971; The Word, 1972, The Fan Club, 1974; The People's Almanac, 1975; The R Document, 1976.
PICTURES INCLUDE: story, collab. s.p., West Point Story; s.p., Meet Me at the Fair; collab. s.p. Desert Legion, Gun Fury; collab. story and s.p., Split Second; s.p., The Burning Hills, Bombers B-52; novel (basis for film), The Chapman Report, The Prize, The 7 Minutes, The Man.

WALLACE, JEAN: Actress. b. Chicago, Oct. 12, 1930. As teenager signed by Paramount as contract player and studied at Actors Laboratory (Method School) in Hollywood. Later, switched to 20th Century-Fox. In 1951 went to Argentina to star in first film, Native Son. Board of Directors Permanent Charities Committee and (Womens Auxiliary), Antans (The Womens Auxiliary of the American National Theater and Academy); hospitality chm., Beverly Hills P.T.A. Member, So. Calif. Motion Picture Council and recipient of its Bronze Halo Award of Special Merit. Mbr., L.A.D.I.E.S.
PICTURES INCLUDE: Storm Fear, The Big Combo, The Man on the Eiffel Tower, The Devil's Hairpin, Maracaibo, The Sword of Lancelot, Beach Red, No Blade of Grass. bd. of dir. of Screen Smart Set.

WALLACE, MIKE: TV commentator, interviewer. b. Brookline, Mass., May 9, 1918. e. Univ. of Michigan; 1939. Night Beat, WABD, N.Y., 1956; The Mike Wallace Interview, ABC, 1956–58; Newspaper col., Mike Wallace Asks, N.Y. Post, 1957–58; News Beat, WNTA-TV, 1959–61; The Mike Wallace Interview, WNTA-TV, 1959–61; Biography, 1962; correspondent, CBS News, 1963, CBS Radio; Personal Closeup, Mike Wallace at Large; Co-editor, 60 Minutes, CBS News.

WALLACH, ELI: Actor. b. Brooklyn, N.Y., Dec. 7, 1915. e. U. of Texas. Capt. in Medical Admin. Corps during WW II. After college acting, appeared in Summer stock. Made Broadway debut in Skydrift, 1945, followed by Antony & Cleopatra, The Rose Tattoo, Major Barbara, Rhinoceros, Luv. Charter member, Actors Studio in 1947.
PICTURES INCLUDE: first film Baby Doll. Also: The Magnificent Seven, Seven Thieves, The Misfits, The Victors, Hemingway's Adventures of A Young Man, How the West Was Won, Act One, Genghis Khan, The Moonspinners, Lord Jim, How to Steal a Million, The Good, the Bad and the Ugly, The Tiger Makes Out, Band of Gold, How to Save a Marriage and Ruin Your Life, A Lovely Way to Die, Ace High, The Brain, Zigzag, The People Next Door, Romance of a Horse Thief, Cinderella Liberty, Crazy Joe, Movie Movie, The Hunter, Sam's Son, Tough Guys.
TV: Studio 1, Philco Playhouse, Playhouse 90; Won Emmy for A Poppy Is Also a Flower, Anatomy of an Illness, Murder: By Reason of Insanity.

WALLACH, GEORGE: Producer, writer, dir. b. New York, N.Y., Sept. 25, 1918; e. N.Y.U. Actor in theatre & radio 1938–45; U.S. Navy 1942–45; supvr. radio-TV Div. of Amer. Thea. Wing 1946–48; dir., WNEW, 1947–48; prod./div., Wendy Barrie Show, 1948–49; prod.-dir. for WNBC-WNBT, 1950; Dir., news, spec. events WNBT-WNBC, 1951–52; prod. mgr., NBC Film Div. since 1953; CBS-TV; formed George Wallach Prod., 1956; prod. dir. It Happened in Havana, appt. TV officer, U.S.I.A., 1957. Film-TV officer American Embassy, Bonn, Germany, 1961. Film-TV officer American Embassy; Tehran, Iran, 1965–66; m.p. Prod. Officer, JUSPAO, American Embassy, Saigon, 1966; prod.-dir.-wr., Greece Today, 1967–68. Exec. prod.-dir., George Wallach Productions, spec. doc., travel, and industrial films, chairman, Film-TV Dept., N.Y. Institute of Photography, 1968–75; Prof. film-TV-radio, Brooklyn Coll., 1975–80; presently special projects officer, DGA, N.Y.
PICTURES INCLUDE: NBC-producer. Inner Sanctum, The Falcon, His Honor Homer Bell, Watch the World; assoc. prod., prod. mgr., Bwana Devil; dir., Wanted, CBS-TV series.

WALLIS, HAL B.: Producer. b. Chicago, Ill., Sept. 14, 1899. m. Martha Hyer, actress. Entered m.p. ind. 1922, learning exhib. & distrib. as mgr. Los Angeles theat. Later in pub. dept., Warner Bros. Then variously with Principal Pictures Corp.; First Nat'l (studio mgr., prod. mgr.); Warner Bros. in chge. prod. From 1933 prod. many features; established Hal Wallis Prods., 1944. Academy-Irving Thalberg Award, 1938, 1943. Partner with Joseph Hazen in Wallis-Hazen Prod. rel. via Paramount. Wallis-Hazen dissolved June 1953.
PICTURES INCLUDE: Little Caesar, Five Star Final, Dawn Patrol, Midsummer Night's Dream, The Story of Louis Pasteur, Anthony Adverse, Zola, Jezebel, King's Row, Sergeant York, The Male Animal, In This Our Life, Yankee Doodle Dandy, Desperate Journey, Now Voyager, Casablanca, Saratoga Trunk, Love Letters, The Affairs of Susan, You Came Along, Strange Love of Martha Ivers, Searching Wind, Sorry Wrong Number, The Accused, Bitter Victory, The Furies, Desert Fury, I Walk Alone, Rope of Sand, My Friend Irma, My Friend Irma Goes West, Dark City, September Affair, Red Mountain, That's My Boy, The Stooge, Peking Express, Sailor Beware, Jumping Jacks, Come Back Little Sheba, Scared Stiff, Cease Fire, Money from Home, About Mrs. Leslie, Three Ring Circus, Rose Tattoo, Artists and Models, Hollywood or Bust, The Rainmaker, Gunfight at the OK Corral, Loving You, Wild Is the Wind, Sad Sack, Last Train from Gun Hill, Don't Give Up the Ship, Hot Spell, King Creole, Career, Visit to A Small Planet, All In A Night's Work, G.I. Blues, Summer and Smoke, Blue Hawaii, A Girl Named Tamiko, Girls! Girls! Girls!, Wives & Lovers, Fun in Acapulco, Becket, Roustabout, The Sons of Katie Elder, Boeing-Boeing, Easy Come, Easy Go, Barefoot in the Park, 5 Card Stud, True Grit, Norwood, Anne of the Thousand Days, Red Sky at Morning, Shoot Out, Mary, Queen of Scots, The Partner with Joseph Hazen in Wallis-Hazen Prod. rel. via Public Eye, The Nelson Affair, The Don Is Dead, Rooster Cogburn.

WALSH, DERMOT: Actor, playwright. b. Dublin, Eire, Sept. 10, 1924; e. St. Mary's Coll., University Coll., Four Courts (Dublin), Abbey School of Acting. With Longford Productions. Dublin Gate Theatre, screen debut in Hungry Hill 1947.
PICTURES INCLUDE: Jassy, Mark of Cain, To the Public Danger, My Sister and I, Third Time Lucky, Torment, Frightened Many, Ghost Ship, Counterspy, Floating Dutchman, Straw Man, Blue Parrot, On the Night of the Full Moon, Bond of Fear, The Hide-Out, On the Stroke of Nine, Sea Fury, Sea of Sand, The Bandit, The Flesh and the Fiends, Shoot to Kill, The Challenge, The Clock Struck Three, Tarnished Heroes, Tell Tale Heart, The Breaking Point, The Trunk, Bedelia, Woman of Mystery, Chain of Events, The Crowning Touch, Make Mine a Million, Crash Dive, The Witness, Emergency, The Cool Mikado, The

Switch, Echo of Diana, Infamous Conduct.
TV: Richard The Lionheart (series), Too Late for the Mashed Potato, Court Martial, Love Me Like A Brother, Softly Softly.

WALSH, M. EMMET: Actor.
PICTURES: Midnight Cowboy, Stiletto, Alice's Restaurant, End of the Road, The Traveling Executioner, Little Big Man, Cold Turkey, Loving, The Jerk, Straight Time, Back Roads, Reds, The Escape Artist, Blade Runner, Silkwood, Blood Simple, The Pope of Greenwich Village, Missing in Action, The Best of Times, Wildcats, Critters.
TELEVISION: High Noon Part II, Hellinger's Law, Night Partners, You Are the Jury, The Deliberate Stranger, Resting Place, etc.

WALSH, RICHARD F.: President Emeritus International Alliance Theatrical Stage Employees and M.P. Machine Operators. b. Brooklyn, N.Y., 1900. In 1917 became apprentice stage electrician; 1920 full member Local 4, Brooklyn stagehand union IATSE & MPMO. Stage electrician various theatres. In 1924 elected pres. Local 4. 1926 business agent: 1934 int'l vice-pres. IATSE & MPMO; Nov., 1941 named pres. by exec. board; elected pres. by convention June, 1942; re-elected International pres. by convention thereafter; v.p., AFL-CIO, 1956. ch. of bd., Will Rogers Hospital, pres., Union Label Dept, retired as IATSE president in 1974.

WALSTON, RAY: Actor-Director. b. New Orleans, Louisiana, Nov. 22, 1918. Dir. of Bdwy-musical, Damn Yankees, 1974.
TV: You Are There, Producers Showcase, There Shall Be No Night, Studio One, Playhouse 90, My Favorite Martian, The Fall of the House of Usher.
PICTURES INCLUDE: South Pacific, Damn Yankees, Kiss Them For Me, Say One for Me, The Tall Story, The Apartment, Portrait In Black, Convicts Four, Wives and Lovers, Who's Minding the Store, Kiss Me Stupid, Caprice, Paint Your Wagon, The Sting, Popeye, Fast Times at Ridgemont High, Johnny Dangerously, RAD.

WALTER, JESSICA: Actress. b. Brooklyn, N.Y., Jan. 31, 1944. e. High School of Performing Arts. Studied at Bucks County Playhouse and Neighborhood Playhouse. Many TV performances plus lead in series, For the People. Broadway debut in Advise and Consent, 1961. Also, Photo Finish (Clarence Derwent Award), Night Life, A Severed Head.
PICTURES INCLUDE: Lilith, The Group, Grand Prix, Bye Bye Braverman, Number One, Play Misty For Me, Going Ape, The Flamingo Kid.
TV: Love of Life, Ironside, Amy Prentiss, The Execution.

WALTERS, BARBARA: TV Personality. b. Boston, 1931. e. Sarah Lawrence Coll. Began working in TV right after graduation. Joined Today in 1961 as writer, making occasional on-camera appearances. In 1963 became full-time on camera. In April, 1974, named permanent co-host. Also hosts own synd. prog., Not for Women Only. In 1976 joined ABC-TV.

WANAMAKER, SAM: Actor, stage producer, film director. b. Chicago, 1919. e. Drake University. On Braodway stage as actor, producer, presenter. Hollywood films incl.: My Girl Tisa. British films incl: Give Us This Day, Mr. Denning Drives North. London West End stage: Winter Journey, The Big Knife, The Threepenny Opera, The Rainmaker, 1955: starred in film The Secret. 1956–58; Acting, producing London and Liverpool stage. 1959–60: Acting at Stratford-on-Avon. Numerous TV plays incl.: The Big Wheel, The White Death and dir. A Young Lady of Property, 1960: Film, The Criminal. 1961–62: Acting on New York stage in The Far Country. TV productions: The Defenders, Oedipus Rex, etc. Film: Taras Bulba. 1963: prod. dir. Children From Their Games, N.Y. stage.
TV: CBS special, Russian Self Impressions. Man of World, TV series. 1962: Stage, Washington D.C., Rhinoceros, Arms and The Man. Opera productions, King Priam, Forza Del Destino, etc. 1963: Dir., A Case of Libel (N.Y.). TV: Espionage, Outer Limits. Film: Man in the Middle (London). 1964–65: Acted in Macbeth (Chicago) and films, Those Magnificent Men in Their Flying Machines, The Spy Who Came In From The Cold, The Warning Shot, The Day The Fish Came Out, Voyage of the Damned. Dir. The Executioner. Dir. several The Defenders TV series (N.Y.), 1968; The Eliminator, The Chinese Visitor. 1971; Catlow. 1972; Sinbad and the Eye of the Tiger, 1977; Founder and exec. dir. Globe Playhouse Trust; starred BBC film Arturo Ul. 1973. Dir. Sydney Opera House Opening. War & Peace. 1974. Acted in The Law. Prod. Bankside Festival. U.S. Tour Shakespeare's globe. 1980: Private Benjamin, The Competition, San Francisco Opera, Aida, 1981, Oedipus Rex, Boston Symphony, 1982. 1983–84: Films, The Aviator, Irreconcilable Differences. TV films: The Ferret, Heartsounds, The Berrengers, The Ghost Writer.

WARBURTON, JOHN: Actor. b. Liverpool, Eng., e. Oxford U. With British Army, World War I; then on stage Liverpool Repertory Theatre. To U.S. 1920.
STAGE: Journey's End, Bird In the Hand, Dishonorable Lady.
PICTURES INCLUDE: on screen 1933 in Cavalcade. Also: Chi Ci, Becky Sharp, Sisters, Saratoga Trunk, The White Cliffs, Marriage Is a Private Affair, Confidential Agent, Living in a Big Way, City Beneath the Sea, East of Sumatra, Royal African Rifles.

WARD, BURT: Actor/Executive. b. Los Angeles, CA, July 6, 1946. Is pres. of Entertainment Management Corp. and Entertainment Licensing Corp., fan club and merchandising companies, respectively.
TV: Batman.

WARD, DAVID S.: Writer-Director. b. Oct. 24, 1945. e. Univ. of So. Calif. where attended film school. First script was Steelyard Blues produced at Warner Bros. in 1972 by producers Michael and Julia Phillps.
PICTURES: The Sting (s.p.); Cannery Row (s.p., dir.); The Sting II (s.p.).

WARD, FRED: Actor. b. 1943. Studied at Berghoff Studio. On stage in The Glass Menagerie, One Flew over the Cuckoo's Nest, etc.
PICTURES: No Available Witness, Tilt, Escape from Alcatraz, Southern Comfort, Timerider, The Right Stuff, Silkwood, Uncommon Valor, Swing Shift, Uforia, Secret Admirer, Remo Williams: The Adventure Begins.

WARD, RACHEL: Actress. b. London, 1957. m. actor Bryan Brown. Top model before becoming actress. Studied acting with Stella Adler and Robert Modica; numerous commercials on TV.
PICTURES: Night School, Three Blind Mice, Sharkey's Machine, Dead Men Don't Wear Plaid, Against All Odds, The Final Terror.
TELEVISION: The Thorn Birds, Fortress.

WARD, SARAH E.: Executive. b. Warrenton, VA., April 5, 1920. 1949–1962, office clerical positions with RKO, 20th Century-Fox, Todd AO Corp; v.p. sales mgr. for Europix Consolidated Corp., 1968; v.p.—sec'y for Europix International Ltd., 1971.

WARD, SIMON: Actor. b. London, England, 1941. Ent. ind. 1964.
PICTURES: If, Frankenstein Must Be Destroyed, I Start Counting, Young Winston, Hitler—The Last Ten Days, The Three Musketeers, The Four Musketeers, Children of Rage, Deadly Strangers. All Creatures Great & Small, Aces High, The Battle Flag, Holocaust 2000, Zulu Dawn, Supergirl.
TELEVISION: Spoiled, Chips with Everything, The Corsican Brothers, etc.

WARDEN, JACK: Actor. b. Newark, N.J., Sept. 18, 1920. With Margo Jones theatre in Dallas.
TV: Philco Goodyear Producer's Showcase, Kraft, Raid on Entebbe, Robert Kennedy and His Times, Hobson's Choice, A. D.
THEATRE: View from the Bridge, Very Special Baby.
PICTURES INCLUDE: From Here to Eternity, 12 Angry Men, Edge of the City, Bachelor Party, Escape from Zahrain, The Thin Red Line, Summertree, Who Is Harry Kellerman?, The Sporting Club, Welcome to the Club, Billy Two Hats, The Apprenticeship of Duddy Kravitz, Shampoo, All the President's Men, Heaven Can Wait, Death on the Nile, And Justice for All, Being There, The Great Muppet Caper, Carbon Copy, So Fine, The Verdict, Crackers, The Aviator.

WARNER, DAVID: Actor. b. Manchester, England, 1941. Made London stage debut in Tony Richardson's version of A Midsummer Night's Dream. Four seasons with Royal Shakespeare Co.
PICTURES INCLUDE: Tom Jones, Morgan, Work Is a Four Letter Word, The Bofors Gun, The Fixer, The Seagull, Michael Kohlhaas, The Ballard of Cable Hogue, Perfect Friday, Straw Dogs, A Doll's House, Tales from the Crypt, Providence, Cross of Iron, Silver Bears. The Concorde—Airport '79, Time After Time, The Island, Time Bandits, Tron, The Company of Wolves.

WARNER, JACK JR.: Producer. b. San Francisco, Calif., Mar. 27, 1916; p. Jack L. Warner, and Mrs. Albert S. Rogell; e. Beverly Hills High Sch., B.A., U of Southern Calif. Entered Warner New York office studying distrib. and exhib. for 1½ years. Transferred to prod. dept. at West Coast studios, then to short subject dept. as assoc. prod. As Reserve Officer called to active duty in 1942 and served as combat photo unit officer in 164th Signal Photo Co. for one year. Transf. to Signal Corps Photographic Center, Astoria, N.Y., where participated in prod. Army Signal Corps Training Films. Was asst. to chief of training films prod. In 1944 assigned to Hq. First U.S. Army Group to assist in planning combat photography for invasion of Europe. Until cessation of hostilities was asst. chief Photo Branch Office of Chief Signal Officer in 12th Army Group and on fall of Germany was on staff of General Eisenhower in Frankfurt as asst. and acting photo officer, Office of the Chief Signal Officer, Theatre Service Forces European Threatre (TSFET). Released from active duty April 20, 1945. Commissioned Lt. Col. Signal Corps Reserve. In

1947 with Warner Bros. Pictures Distrib. Corp., making survey of exhib. and distrib. as related to prod.; liaison between Warner and Assoc. Brit. Pictures on The Hasty Heart, 1948–49; org. Jack M. Warner Prod., Inc., 1949; first film, The Man Who Cheated Himself, distrib. by 20th Cent.-Fox; prod. dept., Warner Bros., 1951; prod. exec. Warners 1953. In charge of TV film prod. for Warners 1955; exec. in charge of television comm. and ind. film dept., Warner Bros. 1956; v.p., Warner Bros. Pictures, Inc., Jan. 1958; Warner association terminated Jan. 1959. Reactivated independent motion picture company Jack M. Warner Prod. Future activities production of feature television and industrial films; pres., Jack Warner Prods., Inc., prod. theatrical films, 1961; prod., dir., Brushfire; Commissioned Colonel, Signal Corps. U.S. Army Reserve, 1962; 1977–78: Producer, TV series & films for theatrical and TV, Jack Warner Pdns; writer, 1979–81. Author: Bijou Dream (novel, 1982).

WARREN, CHARLES MARQUIS: Director, producer, writer b. Baltimore, Md.; e. McDonogh School (Maryland), Baltimore City College. Commander U.S. Navy, World War II; then to Hollywood. Writer for screen, magazines; author of books.
BOOKS INCLUDE: Only the Valiant, Valley of the Shadow, Wilderness, Deadhead, History of American Dental Surgery.
PICTURES INCLUDE: Only the Valiant, Beyond Glory, Redhead and the Cowboy, Streets of Laredo, Springfield Rifle, Day of the Evil Gun, Little Big Horn, Hellgate, Pony Express, Arrowhead, Flight to Tangier, 7 Angry Men, Trooper Hook, Tension at Table Rock, Cattle Empire, Charro!, Down to the Sea, Time of the Furies, Copper Sky, Ride a Violent Mile, Blood Arrow, The Unknown Terror.
TV: Creator of Gunsmoke, Rawhide, Gunslinger, and the Virginian, series as well as prod.-dir.-writer. Exec. prod. on Iron Horse series.

WARREN, GENE: Executive. b. Denver, Co., Aug. 12, 1916. Pres. of Excelsior Prods., production co. specializing in special effects and animation. Has headed 2 other cos. of similar nature over past 20 years, functioning at various times as prod., dir., studio prod. head and writer. Producer-Director of following shorts: The Tool Box, Suzy Snowflake, Santa and the Three Dwarfs, Land of the Midnight Sun and these documentaries/training films: Mariner I, Mariner III, Apollo, U.S. Navy titles.
Special effects on theatrical features including. Black Sunday, McNamara's Band, Satan's School for Girls, My Name Is John, The Power, 7 Faces of Dr. Lao, Wonderful World of the Brothers Grimm, The Time Machine, Tom Thumb, etc. TV series include The Man from Atlantis, Land of the Lost, Star Trek, Outer Limits, Twilight Zone, Mission Impossible, etc.

WARREN, LESLEY ANN: Actress. b. New York City, Aug. 16, 1946. Studied ballet under Stella Adler. Big break came in Cinderella on stage, where seen by Disney scout. Film debut in The Happiest Millionaire.
PICTURES: Victor/Victoria, Race to the Yankee Zephyr, A Night in Heaven, Songwriter, Choose Me, Clue.
TELEVISION: Mini-series: Beulah Land, Pearl, 79 Park Avenue, Evergreen. Movies: Portrait of a Stripper, Betrayal.

WARRICK, RUTH: Actress. b. St. Louis, June 29. In 1941: "Citizen Kane," "Obliging Young Lady," RKO; "The Corsican Brothers," UA-Small. In 1942: "Journey Into Fear," RKO. In 1943: "Forever and a Day," RKO. On TV in Peyton Place, All My Children.
PICTURES INCLUDE: The Iron Major, Secret Command, Mr. Winkle Goes to War, Guest in the House, China Sky, Driftwood, Daisy Kenyon, Arch of Triumph, The Great Dan Patch, Make Believe, Ballroom, Three Husbands, Let's Dance, One Too Many, Roogie's Bump.

WASHBURN, DERIC: Writer. b. Buffalo, N.Y. e. Harvard Univ. (English lit.). Has written number of plays, including The Love Nest and Ginger Anne.
PICTURES: Silent Running (co-s.p.), The Deer Hunter, The Border.

WASILEWSKI, VINCENT, T.: Executive. b. Athens, Ill. e. Univ. of Ill., Coll. of Engineering, 1940; U.S. Air Force, Sept. 1942–Oct. 1945; ret. to Univ. of Ill., bachelor degree in political science, 1948, degree of Doctor of Jurisprudence, 1949; admitted to the Illinois Bar, 1950; joined staff of the National Association of Broadcasters, Oct. 12, 1949; chief attorney, Feb. 1953; mgr., government relations, Aug. 1955; v.p., governmental affairs, NAB, June 1960; exec. v.p., NAB, Aug. 1961; pres., Jan. 1965–Sept. 1982; partner, Dow, Lohnes & Albertson, Oct. 1982.

WASSERMAN, DALE: Writer, producer. b. Rhinelander, Wis., Nov. 2, 1917. Stage: lighting designer, dir., prod.; dir. for. attractions, S. Hurok; began writing, 1954. Founding member & Trustee of O'Neill Theatre Centre; Artistic Director Midwest Playwrights Laboratory; member Motion Picture Academy; awards include Emmy, Tony, Critics Circle (Broadway), Outer Circle; Writers Guild, etc.
TV: The Fog, The Citadel, The Power and the Glory, Engineer of Death, The Lincoln Murder Case, I Don Quixote, Elisha and the Long Knives, and others.
PLAYS: Livin' the Life, 998, One Flew Over the Cuckoo's Nest, The Pencil of God, Man of La Mancha, Play With Fire.
PICTURES INCLUDE: Cleopatra, The Vikings, The Sea and the Shadow, Quick, Before It Melts, Mister Buddwing, A Walk With Love and Death, Man of La Mancha.

WASSERMAN, LEW: Chairman of the bd., Chief Executive Officer, MCA, Inc., Universal City, Calif.

WASSON, CRAIG: Actor-Musician. b. Eugene, OR, March 15, 1954. On stage in Godspell, All God's Chillun Got Wings, Death of a Salesman, The Glass Menagerie, etc.
PICTURES: Actor: The Boys in Company C (also music), Go Tell the Spartans, The Outsider, Carny, Schizoid, Night at O'Rears, Ghost Story, Second Thoughts, Four Friends, Body Double, The Men's Club.
TELEVISION: Actor: Phyllis, Baa Baa Black Sheep, Serpico, Skag, Why Me?, etc.

WATERHOUSE, KEITH: Writer. b. Leeds, England, 1929. Early career as journalist, novelist. Author of There is a Happy Land, Billy Liar, Jubb, The Bucket Shop. Ent. m.p. ind. 1960, s.p. (with Willis Hall).
PICTURES INCLUDE: Whistle Down The Wind, A Kind of Loving, Billy Liar, Man in the Middle, Pretty Polly, Lock Up Your Daughters, The Valiant, West Eleven.
TV: (series): Inside George Webley, Queenie's Castle, Budgie, Billy Liar, There is a Happy Land.

WATERS, GEORGE, W.: Writer, producer, executive. b. Washington, D.C., Dec. 24, 1908; e. Catholic Univ. of America, 1923. Reporter, Times-Herald, Wash., D.C., 1923–25; Reporter, state ed., Washington Evening Star, 1925–30; City ed., Wash. Times-Herald, 1936–43; city ed., Miami Daily News, 1943–47; dir. of publicity Int'l Polo, Miami Seahawks pro football team, night clubs, etc., 1950; senatorial accts., press relations, Wash., D.C., 1950–55; co-author, assoc. prod., Tank Battalion, 1958; co-author, pictures: Speed Crazy, Why Must I Die?
TV: Scene of the Crime; Segments; Violence Comes Easy, Collector's Item. Georgetown Films.

WATERSTON, SAM: Actor. b. Cambridge, Mass., Nov. 15, 1940. e. Yale Univ. Began acting on stage in New York (Indians, Halfway Up a Tree, The Trial of the Catonsville Nine) and in Los Angeles (Meeting by the River, Volpone, etc.). Won Drama Desk Award as best actor for role in Joseph Papp production of Much Ado About Nothing (1972–73 Broadway season).
PICTURES INCLUDE: Three, Savages, The Great Gatsby, Rancho Deluxe, Journey into Fear, Capricorn One, Interiors, Heaven's Gate, The Killing Fields, Just Between Friends.
TV: Much Ado About Nothing, The Glass Menagerie, Emerald Point NAS, Dempsey, Love Lives On, Finnegan Begin Again, The Fifth Missile.

WATKINS, GRATH: Actor. b. London, Aug. 8, 1922. e. University College School. Served in Royal Air Force 1944–45. Entered films in 1945 with role in The Captive Heart.
PICTURES INCLUDE: Bedelia, Gaiety George, A Matter of Life and Death, The Hanging Judge, Goodbye Mr. Chips, Cromwell, The Rise and Fall of Michael Rimmer, Virgin Witch, Fright, Naughty, Twins of Evil, Mary, Queen of Scots, Steptoe and Son, Henry VIII, Cinderella, The Omen.
TV: People in Conflict (Canada).

WATLING, JACK: Actor. b. Chingford, London, Eng., Jan. 13, 1923. e. Italia Conti Stage Sch. Stage debut in Where the Rainbow Ends, 1936; m.p. debut in 60 Glorious Years, 1937.
PICTURES INCLUDE: Goodbye, Mr. Chips, We Dive at Dawn, Day Will Dawn, Demi Paradise, Way Ahead, Journey Together, Easy Money, Winslow Bay, Quartet, Courtneys of Curzon Street, Once a Sinner, Naked Heart, White Corridors, Under Capricorn, Private Information, Father's Doing Fine, Meet Mr. Lucifer, Trouble in The Glen, Sea Shall Not Have Them, Confidential Report, Admirable Crichton, A Night to Remember, Sink the Bismarck, The Night We Sprang A Leek, Nearly A Nasty Accident, Mary Had A Little, Three On A Spree, Edgar Wallace, The Nanny, 11 Harrow House.
TV: Crime on My Hands, No Medals, Disturbance, Manor at Northstead, Devil Makes Three, Aren't We All, World of Tim Fraser, No Hiding Place, Zero I, Hancock Half Hour, Anna Karenina, Both Ends Meet, Loyalties, Ghost Squad, Tales of Mystery, Boyd Q.C., The Planemakers, Love Story, Six of the Best, The Power Game, Dixon of Dock Green, Mickey Dunne, Emergency Ward 10, Dr. Who, Softly Softly, No That's Me Over Here, The Power Game, The Pathfinders, Spike Milligan, The Mackinnons, Many Wives of Patrick, The Cedar Tree, The Doctors' Daughters.

WATTLES, JOSHUA S.: Executive. Now sr. atty. for Paramount Pictures, working with Richard Zimbert, sr. v.p. & gen.

counsel. Prior to joining para. legal dept. in 1981 was atty. in office of gen. counsel at ASCAP. Member N.Y. and Calif. bars.

WAX, MO.: Publisher and editor of Film Bulletin. b. Philadelphia. e. Villanova U. Also pres., Audienscope, Inc., Entertainment research organization.

WAYLAND, LEN: Actor. b. California, Dec. 28. e. Junior College, Modesto, California. Wrote, prod. weekly radio series 1939–41, KPAS, KTRB, Calif. Service, radar navigator, 1941–45; en. theatre, Tobacco Road, 1946; 1973, formed Len Wayland Prods. for production of theatrical pictures and TV series. In 1976–77: produced/directed. Don't Let It Bother You. 1978, pro./dir., You're not there yet, for own company.
THEATRE: Played summer and winter stock 1947–49. B'way, Streetcar Named Desire, 1949, and tour; toured as lead, Heaven Can Wait, 1951; My Name Is Legion, 1952–53; toured, Love of Four Colonels, 1953, Stalag 17, 1954. Lead, NBC-TV serial, A Time to Live, 1954. NBC-TV First Love, 1955; Armstrong Circle Theatre, Justice, Sgt. Bilko, Kraft Theatre, etc., 1956–58; NBC-TV, Dr. Weaver, From These Roots, 1958–61. Off Broadway prod., USA, 1960; on Broadway; A Man For All Seasons, 1962.
TV: Profiles In Courage, Dr. Kildare, Gunsmoke, Slattery's People, Ben Casey, A Noise in The World, 1967, Love Is A Many Splendored Thing, 1969; Dragnet, Outsider, 1970; Ironside, Name of the Game, The Bold Ones, Daniel Boone, The Virginian, Project U.F.O., Sam, The Blue and the Gray.

WAYNE, DAVID: Actor, r.n. Wayne McKeekan; b. Traverse City, Mich., Jan. 30, 1916; e. Western Michigan, 1936; in marionette shows, 1937.
THEATRE: Finian's Rainbow, Mister Roberts, Teahouse of the August Moon.
PICTURES INCLUDE: Portrait of Jennie, Adam's Rib, Reformer and the Redhead, My Blue Heaven, Stella, M, Up Front, As Young As You Feel, With a Song in My Heart, Wait 'Til the Sun Shines, Nellie; Down Among the Sheltering Palms, The I Don't Care Girl, We're Not Married, O. Henry's Full House, Tonight We Sing, How to Marry a Millionaire, Hell and High Water, Tender Trap, Last Angry Man, The Big Gamble, The Andromeda Strain, The African Elephant (narrator), Huckleberry Finn, The Front Page, The Apple Dumpling Gang, Finders Keepers.

WAYNE, JOEL: Executive. Began career with Grey Advertising; in 17 years won many awards (60 Clios, 25 NY Art Director Club Awards, etc.). Was exec. v.p. & creative dir. of agency when left in 1979 to join Warner Bros. as v.p., creative adv. 1986, named v.p., worldwide creative adv.

WAYNE, MICHAEL A.: Executive. r.n. Michael A. Morrison. b. Los Angeles, Calif., Nov. 23, 1934. f. John Wayne. e. Loyola H.S., Loyola Univ., B.B.A. Asst. dir., various companies, 1955–56; asst. dir., Revue Prods., 1956–57; pres. Batjac Prods, and Romina Prods., 1961; asst. to producer: China Doll, 1957; Escort West, 1958; The Alamo, 1959; prod., McClintock, 1962; co-prod., Cast Giant Shadow, 1965; prod. The Green Berets, 1967; exec. prod. Chisum, 1968; prod. Big Jake, 1970; prod. The Train Robbers, 1972; prod. Cahill, U.S. Marshall, 1972, exec. prod. McQ, 1973, Brannigan, 1974.

WAYNE, PATRICK: Actor. b. July 15, 1939. Son of John Wayne. Made film debut at age 11 in Rio Grande.
PICTURES INCLUDE: The Searchers, The Alamo, The Comancheros, McClintock, The Bears and I, Mustang Country, Sinbad and the Eye of the Tiger, The People Time Forgot, Rustler's Rhapsody.

WEAKLAND, KEVIN L.: Actor-Consultant-Producer. b. Philadelphia, Aug. 14, 1963. e. Holy Family College. 1977, free lance actor; 1982 film consultant; 1984, formed co. to serve all facets of entertainment industry. Continues as actor. 1985, producer & promoter of concerts also.

WEAVER, DENNIS: Actor, director. b. Joplin, Mo., June 4, 1925. e. Univ. of Oklahoma, B.A. fine arts, 1948.
TV: Chester, in Gunsmoke, 1955–64; title role, Kentucky Jones, NBC series, 1964–65; Gentle Ben, 1967–69; McCloud, 1970–76, The Forgotten Man, Duel, The Rolling Man, The Great Man's Whiskers, McCloud, (1970–77), Terror on the Beach, Intimate Strangers (ABC) 1977, Pearl (1978), Centennial (1978); Stone (series, 1979–80). Movies: Amber Waves, Dr. Mudd, Cocaine: One Man's Seduction, Go for the Gold. Emerald Point NAS (series, 1983–84).
PICTURES INCLUDE: Duel at Diablo, Way Way Out, Gentle Giant, A Man Called Sledge, What's the Matter with Helen?, The Gallant Hours, Mission, Batangas.

WEAVER, FRITZ: Actor. b. Pittsburgh, Jan. 19, 1926. e. Univ. of Chicago. On stage in Chalk Garden, Miss Lonelyhearts, All American, Shot in the Dark, Baker Street, Child's Play (Tony), The Price, etc.
PICTURES: Demon Seed, Marathon Man, Black Sunday, The Day of the Dolphin, The Guns of August, The Big Fix, Creepshow, Power.
TELEVISION: Movies: The Borgia Stick, Berlin Affair, heat of Anger, The Snoop Sisters, Hunter, The Legend of Lizzie Borden, Captains Courageous, Holocaust, The Hearst and Davies Affair, A Death in California. Mini-Series: Dream West.

WEAVER, MARJORIE: Actress. b. Grossville, Tenn., Mar. 2, 1913; e. U. of Kentucky, Indiana U. Played with McCauley Stock Co.; Billy Rose's Shrine Minstrels. In 1936 appeared in China Clipper, WB; from 1937 in many 20th Century-Fox pictures.
PICTURES INCLUDE: Let's Face It, Pardon My Rhythm, You Can't Ration Love, The Great Alaskan Mystery, Shadows of Suspicion, Fashion Model, Leave It to Blondie, We're Not Married.

WEAVER, SIGOURNEY: Actress. b. New York City, 1949. e. Stanford and Yale. Daughter of Sylvester "Pat" Weaver, former NBC pres. Mother, actress Elizabeth Inglish (one-time contract player for Warner Bros.). After college formed working partnership with fellow student Christopher Durang for off-Bdwy. improvisational productions. First professional appearance on stage in 1974 in The Constant Wife with Ingrid Bergman. Theatrical film debut in Alien (1979).
PICTURES: Eyewitness, The Year of Living Dangerously, Deal of the Century, Ghostbusters, A Woman or Two, Aliens, Half Moon Street.
TELEVISION: Somerset, The Sorrows of Gin.

WEAVER, SYLVESTER L., JR.: Executive. b. Los Angeles, Calif., Dec. 21, 1908; e. Dartmouth Coll. CBS, Don Lee Network, 1932–35; Young & Rubicam adv. agency, 1935–38; adv. mgr., American Tobacco Co., 1938–47; v.p. Young & Rubicam, 1947–49; joined NBC as v.p., chg. TV, 1949; appt'd v.p. chg. NBC Radio & TV networks, 1952; vice-chmn. bd., NBC, Jan., 1953; pres., NBC, Dec., 1953; bd. chmn., Dec. 1955; own firm, 430 Park Avenue., N.Y.C., 1956; chmn. of bd. McCann-Erickson Corp. (Intl.), 1959; pres., Subscription TV, Inc. Comm. Consultant in Los Angeles, Cal. and President, Weaver Productions, Inc.

WEBB, JERRY: Editor. b. Indianapolis, Ind. Feature editor, supervision, Fox Studio, 1929–33; 20th Century-Fox, 1934–57. supv. film editor, Bonjour Tristese, London, 1957; film editor, Yovanka, Under Ten Flags, Roma, 1959–60; Esther and The King, Roma, 1960; Lion of Sparta, Athens, London, 1961; supv. editor, Damon & Pythias, Roma, 1962. 1964 entered commercial field. 1968: invented new anamorphic method of photography and printing of film: Vertiscope.

WEBB, ROBERT A.: Film editor, writer. b. Springfield, Ill., May 27, 1911. Film editor, Goldwyn, 20th-Fox; served 3½ years with John Ford's Naval Photog. Unit & headed film editorial unit at Nurnberg Internat'l Military Trials; ed. many short film sketches, Omnibus (TV), 1953; ed., Patti Page Shows. Member: M.P. Film Editors, Soc. of M.P. Film Editors, Acad. of TV Arts & Sciences.

WEBB, ROBERT D.: Director.
PICTURES INCLUDE: assoc. prod., Lure of the Wilderness; dir., Glory Brigade, Proud Ones. Prod., dir.: Threshold of Space, Seven Cities of Gold, Beneath the 12 Mile Reef, White Feather, The Jackals, Capetown Affair, Love Me Tender, The Way to the Gold.

WEBBER, ROBERT.: Actor. b. Santa Ana, Calif., Oct. 14. e. Belmont High, Van Nuys High, Compton Jr. Coll. USMC, 1943–45. Summer stock. Co-starred, Wonderful Town, American Pavilion, Brussels World Fair, 1958.
THEATRE: Two Blind Mice, Goodbye My Fancy, Royal Family, No Time for Sergeants, Orpheus Descending, Fair Game, A Loss of Roses, Period of Adjustment.
PICTURES INCLUDE: Highway 301, Twelve Angry Men, The Stripper, The Sandpiper, The Third Day, Harper, The Silencers, The Hired Killer, Dead Heat on a Merry-Go-Round, Don't Make Waves, The Dirty Dozen, The Big Bounce, The Great White Hope, The French Mistress, $(Dollars), Every Man Is My Enemy, Bring Me the Head of Alfredo Garcia, Midway, Casey's Shadow, The Choirboys; The Revenge of the Pink Panther, Ten, Private Benjamin, S.O.B., Sunday Lovers, Wrong Is Right, Who Dares Wins, Wild Geese II.
TV: Over 400 shows from 1947 through 1985.

WEBSTER, DAVID: Resident Associate, Carnegie Endowment, Washington, D.C. b. Taunton, England, 1931. Joined BBC Extend Services News in 1953. Moved to BBC Television Current Affairs 1959 and worked on Face to Face and Lifeline before going to Panorama in 1959. Panorama producer until start of BBC-2 in 1964, when he left to run Enquiry, Encounter on BBC-2. Returned to Panorama as Deputy Editor, becoming Editor in 1967. Appt. Assistant Head of Current Affairs Group, Television 1970. For five years (1971–76) BBC rep. in the USA. Chairman of the International Council of the National Academy of Television Arts and Sciences 1974–75. In 1976 returned to England to become the BBC's Controller of Information Services.

Appt. Director, Public Affairs 1977 and a member of board of management. Appointed BBC dir. for U.S., 1981. Retired, 1985.

WEBSTER, M. COATES: Writer. b. East Orange, N.J. December 15, 1906. e. U. Pa., Wesleyan U. On stage 8 yrs. Wrote 3 novels (published) Showboy, Derelict Alley, Strange Fraternity.
PICTURES INCLUDE: Klondike Kate; collab., story, s.p., Adventures of a Rookie; (s.p.) Blonde Ransom; (collab. s.p.) Jungle Captive; (s.p.) Strange Confession, I'll Remember April, Song of Arizona, Frisco Tornado, Rough Riders of Durango, Desert of Lost Men, Captive of Billy the Kid, Leadville Gunslinger, Montana Belle.

WEDGEWORTH, ANN: Actress. b. Abilene, TX, Jan. 21, 1935. e. Univ. of Texas. On stage in Thieves, Blues for Mr. Charlie, Chapter Two, etc.
PICTURES: Handle with Care, Thieves, Bang the Drum Slowly, Scarecrow, Law and Disorder, Dragon Fly, The Birch Interval, No Small Affair, Sweet Dreams, The Men's Club.
TELEVISION: The Edge of Night, Another World, Somerset, All That Glitters, Three's Company, Filthy Rich, Right to Kill?, etc.

WEILER, GERALD E.: Producer. b. Mannheim, Germany, May 8, 1928. e. Harvard, 1946–48; Columbia, B.S., 1949–51; NYU Grad. Sch., 1951–53; writer, WHN, N.Y. writer, sports ed., news ed., Telenews Prod., Inc., 1948–52; asst. to prod., Richard de Rochemont, Vavin, Inc., 1952; U.S. Army, 1953–55; v.p., 1955–73; President, Weiler Communications Inc. 1973.

WEINBLATT, MIKE: Television Executive. e. Syracuse Univ. Served in Army as counter-intelligence agent, mostly in Japan (1952–53). Joined NBC in 1957; has headed two major TV network functions—talent/program admin. & sls. Joined network business affairs dept. in 1958 as mgr., business affairs, facilities operations; rose to post of director, pricing & financial services before moving to sales in November, 1962, as mgr., participating program sales. Named v.p., eastern sales, NBC-TV, 1968. Named v.p., talent & program admin., October, 1968; promoted to v.p. sales, February, 1973. January, 1975 named snr. v.p., sales; later became exec. v.p. Appointed exec. v.p. & gen. mgr. of NBC TV network in August, 1977. 1983, joined Showtime/Movie Channel as pres. & chief oper. off. 1984, pres., Multi Media Entertainment.

WEINSTEIN, HENRY T.: Executive Producer. b. New York, N.Y. e. C.C.N.Y., Carnegie Institute of Technology. Dir. of: the Brattle Theatre, Theatre in the Round, Houston, Texas. Prod. for The Theatre Guild, N.Y. Producer, 20th Century-Fox, M.G.M. Executive in charge of production, American Film Theatre, Skyield Productions. Currently, executive vice president in charge of production, Cannon Films.
PICTURES INCLUDE: Tender is the Night, Joy in the Morning, Cervantes, Madwoman of Chaillot, The Battle of Neretva, Magic Christian, A Delicate Balance, The Homecoming, The Iceman Commeth, Lost in the Stars, Butley, Luther, Rhinoceros, Galileo, The Man in the Glass Booth, In Celebration, Runaway Train.
TV: Play of the Week series, prod.

WEINSTEIN, PAULA: Independent Producer. Partnered with Gareth Wigan in WW Productions at Warner Brothers. Started as theatrical agent with William Morris and International Creative Management. With Warner Brothers, 1976–78 as production v.p.: left to go to 20th Century-Fox in same capacity. Named Fox snr. v.p., worldwide production. In 1980 appointed v.p., production, the Ladd Company. 1981, joined United Artists as pres., motion picture div. In 1983, began own production company at Columbia Pictures, also serving as a consultant for Columbia.

WEINTRAUB, FRED: Executive, producer. b. April 27, 1928, Bronx, N.Y. e. U. of Pennsylvania Wharton School of Business, Owner of The Bitter End Coffeehouse to 1971. Personal management, Campus Coffee House Entertainment Circuit; TV Production Hootenanny, Popendipity; syndicated TV show host: From The Bitter End; motion picture production; v.p., creative services, Warner Bros. 1969, executive in charge of Woodstock; producer motion pictures, Weintraub-Heller Productions, 1974, Enter The Dragon, Rage, Black Belt Jones, Truck Turner, Golden Needles, Animal Stars, Hot Potato, The Ultimate Warrior, Dirty Knights Work, Those Cuckoo Crazy Animals, Crash, Outlaw Blues, The Pack, The Promise, Tom Horn, Battle Creek Brawl, Force: Five, High Road to China, Out of Control.

WEINTRAUB, JERRY: Producer. b. New York City, Sept. 26, 1937. Sole owner and chm. of Management Three, representing entertainment personalities, including John Denver, John Davidson, Frank Sinatra, Neil Diamond, etc. Also involved with Intercontinental Broadcasting Systems, Inc. (cable programming) and Jerry Veintraub/Armand Hammer Prods. (production co.). 1985, named United Artists Corp. chm. Resigned, 1986.
PICTURES: Nashville, Oh, God!, Cruising, All Night Long, Diner, The Karate Kid.

WEINTRAUB, SY: Executive. b. New York City, 1923. e. Univ. of Missouri (B.A., Bach. of Journalism, 1947); graduate of American Theater Wing. Started career in 1949 forming with associates a TV syndication co., Flamingo Films, Inc., which merged with Associated Artists to form Motion Pictures for Television, Inc., largest syndicator at that time. He originated Superman and Grand Ol'Opry series for TV. In 1958 bought Sol Lesser Prods., owners of film rights for Tarzan, and began producing and distributing Tarzan films through Banner Productions, Inc. Also formerly chmn. of bd. of Panavision, Inc.; bd. mem. and pres. of National General Television Corp., and pres. of KMGM-TV in Minneapolis. In 1978 named chm. of Columbia Pictures Industries' new Film Entertainment Group, also joining Office of the Chief Executive of CPI.

WEIR, PETER: Director-Writer. b. Sydney, Australia, Aug. 8, 1944.
PICTURES: First prof. credit: director-writer of Michael, an episode of the feature, Three To Go (1970). Writer-Director: The Cars That Ate Paris, The Last Wave, The Plumber. Director only: Picnic at Hanging Rock, Gallipoli, The Year of Living Dangerously, Witness, Mosquito Coast.

WEIS, DON: Writer, director, producer. b. Milwaukee, Wis., May 13, 1922; e. U. of Southern Calif. No prior bus. experience.
PICTURES INCLUDE: (dial. dir.) Body & Soul, Red Pony, Champion, Home of the Brave, The Men; (dir.) Letter From a Soldier, sequence in It's a Big Country, Bannerline, Just This Once, You for Me, I Love Melvin, Remains To Be Seen, A Slight Case of Larceny, Half a Hero, Affairs of Dobie Gillis, Adventures of Haiji Baba, Ride the High Iron, Catch Me If You Can, Gene Krupa Story, Critic's Choice, Looking for Love, The King's Pirate, Repo.
TV: Dear Phoebe. Best TV director, 1956, 1958. Screen Dir. Guild, The Longest Hundred Miles, It Takes a Thief, Ironside, M.A.S.H., Happy Days, Planet of the Apes, Bronk, Petrocelli, The Magician, Mannix, Night Stalker, Barbary Coast, Courtship of Eddie's Father, Starsky & Hutch, Hawaii Five-O, Chips, Charlie's Angels, Love Boat, Fantasy Island.

WEIS, JACK: Producer-Director-Writer-Cinematographer-Film Editor. b. Tampa, Fla., October 1, 1932. e. Notre Dame (BS); Master Univ. of Chicago. Was in U.S. Air Force six yrs. Founded Associated Productions/Associated Advertising Productions, Inc. in New Orleans in Aug., 1967, and has been involved in over 120 films and approx. 1,500 commercials. Produced, directed and wrote original s.p.s. for several HEW youth rehabilitation pictures. Member: Cinematography Local 666, Chicago IATSE; Film Editor Local 780, IATSE, Chicago; Directors Guild of America; Writers Guild of America.
PICTURES INCLUDE: Quadroon (dir.), Storyville (prod., dir., s.p.), Damballa (prod., dir., s.p.); creature from Hony Island Swamp (prod.-dir., s.p.); Lehia (prod., dir., camera), You Never Gave Me Roses, (s.p., prod., dir.); The Perfect Circle (TV-s.p., prod., dir.); Crypt of Dark Secrets (prod., dir., s.p.); Mardi Gras Massacre, prod., dir., s.p., editor).

WEISBERG, BRENDA: Writer. b. Rowne, Poland. Magazine writer, social service, public health, drama instructor. Married to the late Morris Meckler.
PICTURES INCLUDE: s.p., China Sky; s.p., When a Girl's Beautiful, Burning Cross, Port Said, Rusty series, Girl's School; collab. s.p., Isle of Samoa; collab. orig., Reunion in Reno, Alias Mr. Twilight, King of the Wild Horses, Little Tough Guy, s.p. Shadowed. Collaborator, Scarlet Claw, Ding Dong Williams, Babes On Swing Street, Weird Woman, The Mummy's Ghost, The Mad Ghoul, Keep 'Em Slugging, Mug Town, Tough As They Come, Mob Town, There's One Born Every Minute, Hit the Road, Sing Another Chorus, You're Not So Tough.
TV: Fireside Theatre, Philco Theatre, Matinee Theatre.
AUTHOR: U (short stories), Woman's Home Companion, Collier's. American Mercury (Mencken's) Plain Talk, Forum.

WEISER, MARTIN: Publicist. b. New York City, Oct. 18, 1916. e. U. of Rochester, 1936. Pub. dept. Warner Bros., N.Y.C., 1936–40; exploitation dir., western states, 1940–45; studio exploitation head, 1945–50; adv. pub. head, Lippert Pictures, 1950. Partner, Weiser and Thomas, Inc., 1954; pres., Marty Weiser Co., prom. Columbia Studio, 1959; Pub. dept., Warner Bros. Studios, 1961; Paramount Studios, 1962; asst. ad. pub. dir., Allied Artists Pictures, 1963; studio exploitation director Warner Bros. 1964; west coast advertising and exploitation co-ordinator for Warner Bros. Inc., 1973.

WEISS, STEVEN ALAN: Executive. b. Glendale, CA, Oct. 19, 1944. e. Los Angeles City Coll. (AA, 1964); Univ. of So. Calif. (BS, 1966); Northwestern Univ. (BS, 1967); LaSalle Extension Univ., (JD 1970). U.S. Navy-San Diego, Great Lakes, Vallejo & Treasure Island, 1966–67; shipyard liaison

officer, Pearl Harbor Naval Shipyard, US Navy, 1970; gen. mgr., Adrian Weiss Prods., 1970–74; organized Weiss Global Enterprises with Adrian Weiss 1974 for production, acquisition & distribution of films. Purchased with Tom J. Corradine and Adrian Weiss from the Benedict E. Bogeaus Estate nine features, 1974. Secty./treas. of Film Investment Corp. & Weiss Global Enterprises. (Cos. own, control or have dist. rights to over 300 features, many TV series, documentaries, etc.)
MEMBER: Natl. Assn. of TV Program Executive Intl.; National Cable TV Assn.; American Film Institute.

WEISSMAN, MURRAY: Executive. b. New York City, Dec. 23. e. U. of Southern California. Promotion mgr., TV Guide, 1952; asst. publicity director, KABC-TV, 1953–60; asst. dir. of press info., CBS, 1960–66; mgr., TV press dept., Universsal Studio, 1966–68; executive in charge of m.p. press dept., Universal Studios & asst. secy., Universal Pictures, 1968–76; marketing exec., Columbia Pictures, 1976–77; vice pres. of advertising & publicity, Lorimar Productions, 1977; vice pres., ICPR Public Relations Company, 1978–81; now principal, Murray Weissman & Associates.

WEISSMAN, SEYMOUR J.: Executive, producer, director. Weissman Franz Productions. b. Brooklyn, N.Y., May 28, 1931. e. Kenyon Coll., Eng. Lit., A.B., 1953; Univ. of Southern Calif., Cinema, 1955. Unity Films, 1954; Henry Strauss & Co., 1954; Dir. of motion pictures, White Sands Proving Grounds, N.M., 1954–55; M.P.O., 1955; Coleman Prod., 1956; prod. dir., Dynamic Films, Inc., 1958–59; prod., dir., Viston Assoc., 1959–64; dir., VPI Prods., 1966.

WEITMAN, ROBERT M.: Executive. b. New York City, August 18, 1905. e. Cornell University. Attended Paramount Managers' Training School. Assigned to Rialto Theatre, assistant manager, in 1926. Promoted to manager, Brooklyn Paramount. City manager of New York Paramount Public Theatres. Appointed managing director of New York Paramount Theatre in 1935. Managing dir. of N.Y. and Brooklyn Paramount Theatres. Vice-pres. United Paramount Theatres, supervising southern and Philadelphia houses; v.p. American Broadcasting-Paramount Theatres, Inc. in chge. of programming and talent; v.p. in charge of program development, CBS TV, 1956; v.p. chge. prod. MGM-TV, 1960; v.p. in chg. prod., MGM, Inc., 1962; member MGM bd. directors; resigned MGM, July, 1967; v.p. in charge of studio production, Columbia, July, 1967. Dec., 1969 formed own prod. company.

WEITZNER, DAVID: Executive. b. New York, Nov. 13, 1938. e. Michigan State U. Entered industry in 1960 as member Columbia Pictures adv. dep't; later with Donahue and Coe as ass't exec. and Loew's Theatres adv. dep't; later with Embassy Pictures, adv. mgr.; dir. of adv. and exploitation for Palomar Pictures Corp.; v.p. in charge of adv., pub., and exploitation for ABC Pictures Corp.; v.p., entertainment/leisure div., Grey Advertising; v.p., worldwide adv., 20th Century Fox; exec. v.p. adv./pub./promo., Universal Pictures; exec. v.p., mktg. & dist., Embassy Pictures; 1985, joined 20th Century-Fox Films as pres. of mktg. Resigned, 1986.

WELCH, RAQUEL: Actress. r. n. Raquel Tejada. b. Chicago, Ill., Sept. 5, 1942. e. La Jolla H.S. Fashion and photographic modeling. Co-hostess. Hollywood Palace.
PICTURES INCLUDE: Roustabout, A House is Not a Home, Swinging Summer, Fantastic Voyage, Shoot Louder . . . I Don't Understand, One Million Years B.C., Fathom, Bedazzled, The Biggest Bundle of Them All, The Queens, Bandolero, Lady in Cement, 100 Rifles, Flare Up, The Magic Christian, Myra Breckinridge, Hannie Caulder, Kansas City Bomber, Fuzz, The Last of Sheila, The Three Musketeers, The Four Musketeers, The Wild Party, Mother, Jugs and Speed, Crossed Swords.

WELCH, ROBERT L.: Producer, writer. b. Chicago, Ill., Nov. 23, 1910. e. Northwestern U., U. of Illinois. In stock as actor-prod. Hedgerow Theatre, Phila.; with Pasadena Community Playhouse & Padua Hills Theatre; on radio wrote & prod. Kate Smith, Fred Allen & Jack Benny shows, originated Henry Aldrich shows with Young & Rubicam, N.Y.; prod. all U.S. Armed Forces radio shows, World War II; writer-prod. Paramount Pictures Corp.
PICTURES INCLUDE: (collab. s.p.) Variety Girl; (prod.) Paleface, Sorrowful Jones, Top O' the Morning, Fancy Pants, Mr. Music, The Lemon Drop Kid, Son of Paleface. Writer, dir., prod., NBC-TV, 1953.
MEMBER: Lambs, AMPAS, Screen Writers Guild, Producers Guild, American Legion.

WELD, TUESDAY: Actress. b. New York, Aug. 27, 1943. e. Hollywood Professional School. Began modeling at 4 yrs. Film debut, Rock, Rock, Rock.
PICTURES INCLUDE: Rally Round The Flag, Boys! The Five Pennies, The Private Lives of Adam and Eve, Return to Peyton Place, Wild in the Country, Bachelor Flat, Lord Love a Duck, Pretty Poison, I Walk the Line, A Safe Place, Play It As It Lays, Looking for Mr. Goodbar, Who'll Stop the Rain, Thief, Author! Author!, Once Upon a Time in America
TV: The Many Loves of Dobie Gillis, Winter of Our Discontent, Seduced and Swindled.

WELDEN, BEN: Actor. b. Toledo, Ohio, 1901. First appeared on the stage in 1926 at the Central Park Theatre, New York; then on London stage. Has appeared in many British and Hollywood film productions.
PICTURES INCLUDE: It's in the Bag, Appointment With Murder, Search for Danger, Fighting Fools, Sorrowful Jones, Tales of Robin Hood, All Ashore, Killers from Space, Steel Cage, Ma and Pa Kettle at Waikkii, Hidden Guns.

WELDON, JOAN: Actress. b. San Francisco, Calif., Aug. 5, 1933. e. San Francisco Conservatory of Music, U. of Calif. at Berkeley, City Coll. in San Francisco. Sang in chorus of San Francisco Grand Opera Co.; then L.A. Civic Light Opera Co.; m.p. debut in The System, 1953.
PICTURES INCLUDE: So This Is Love, Stranger Wore a Gun, The Command, Riding Shotgun, Them, Deep in My Heart.

WELK, LAWRENCE: Orchestra leader. b. Strasburg, N.D., March 11, 1903. Played accordion community dances, church socials, etc. Started own group. Biggest Little Band in America. Played hotels, ballrooms, music became known as Champagne Music. Signed Aragon Ballroom, Pacific Ocean Park, Calif., 1951, with weekly television show. Champagne Music Makers, ABC-TV, July 2, 1955; The Lawrence Welk Show, ABC; signed lifetime contract, Hollywood Palladium, July 1961. Recording: Calcutta, 1961; syndicated network show started 1971.

WELLER, PETER: Actor. b. Wisconsin. Acting since 10 years old. e. North Texas State Univ. Studied at AADA with Uta Hagen. Member, Actor's Studio.
PICTURES: Butch and Sundance: The Early Years, Just Tell Me What You Want, Shoot the Moon, Of Unknown Origin, Vera, Buckeroo Banzai, Firstborn.
TELEVISION: Two Kinds of Love (movie), Lou Grant, The Silence, Exit 10, Earring.
STAGE: Sticks and Bones, Streamers, Summer Brave, Macbeth, The Wool-Gatherers, etc.

WELLS, FRANK G.: Executive. b. March 4, 1932, Calif. e. Pomona College, 1949–53; Oxford U., 1953–55; Rhodes Scholarship Jurisprudence; U.S. Army, Infantry first lieutenant, 1955–57; Stanford Law School, 1957–59; joined Gang, Tyre & Brown (entertainment industry law firm) 1959; partner, 1962–69; mem., State Bar of Calif., American Bar Assoc., Los Angeles County Bar Assoc., vice chm., Warner Bros. Inc.; 1985, pres. & COO, Walt Disney Prods., Inc.

WELSH, CHARLES L.: b. New York, N.Y., June 7, 1906. e. Morris H.S., 1923. Press dept., N.Y. Hippodrome, 1919; B.F. Keith's Theats., 1921–29; United Trailer Svce., 1930; Meyer-Rigger Lab., 1931; partner Welgot Trailer Svce., 1932; mgr. special film div. Nat'l Screen Service, 1959. Pres., Summit Screen Service, 1967.

WENDERS, WIM: Director. b. Dusseldorf, Germany, 1945. Studied film from 1967 to 1970 at Filmhochschule in Munich. Worked as film critic. In 1967 made first short films (Schauplatze) and three others before first feature, Summer in the City, in 1970.
PICTURES INCLUDE: Die Angst Des Tormanns Beim Elfmeter, The Scarlet Letter, Aus Der Familie Der Panzerechsen, Falsche Bewegung, Alice in the Cities, The Goalie's Anxiety at the Penalty Kick, Kings of the Road, The American Friend, Paris, Texas, Tokyo-Ga.

WERNER, PETER: Producer-Director. b. New York City, Jan. 17, 1947. e. Dartmouth Coll.
PICTURES: In the Region of Ice, Don't Cry It's Only Thunder.
TELEVISION: Producer: Battered, Barnburning, Learning in Focus. Director: Aunt Mary, Hard Knox, I Married a Centerfold, Women in Song, Sins of the Father.

WERTHEIMER, THOMAS: Executive. Exec. v.p., MCA, Inc.; director and officer of subsidiaries. Member exec. committee.

WERTMULLER, LINA: Writer-Director. b. Rome. After graduating high school enrolled in drama school. Began working in theatre in 1951; spent decade doing everything from puppetry to stage managing to writing and directing for radio and TV. Began film career as asst. to Fellini on 8½ in 1962. Following year wrote and directed first film, The Lizards. Had big TV success with series called Gian Burasca and then returned to theatre for a time.
PICTURES: This Time, Let's Talk About Men, The Seduction of Mimi, Love and Anarchy, All Screwed Up, Swept Away, Seven Beauties, A Night Full of Rain, A Joke of Destiny, Sotto Sotto.

WESTCOTT, HELEN: Actress. r.n. Myrthas Helen Hickman. b. Hollywood, Calif; e. L. A. Jr. Coll., 1946. In play The

Drunkard, at 7, for 9 yrs.; many radio shows.
PICTURES INCLUDE: Midsummer Night's Dream (as child), Adventures of Don Juan, Girl from Jones Beach, Mr. Belvedere Goes to College, Whirlpool, Dancing in the Dark, The Gunfighter, Three Came Home, Secret of Convict Lake, Phone Call from a Stranger, Return of Texan, With a Song in My Heart, Loan Shark, A&C Meet Dr. J. & Mr. H., Charge at Feather River, Hot Blood, The Last Hurrah.

WESTON, JACK: Actor. b. 1915. Began career in 1934 in children's division of Cleveland Playhouse. In Army in World War II. Success came in Broadway hit, Season in the Sun. Was frequent performer in top TV shows during 1950s. Film debut in Stage Struck in 1958.
PICTURES INCLUDE: Stage Struck, Please Don't East the Daisies, All in a Night's Work, The Honeymoon Machine, It's Only Money, Palm Springs Weekend, The Incredible Mr. Limpet, Mirage, The Cincinnati Kid, Wait Until Dark, The Thomas Crown Affair, The April Fools, Cactus Flower, A New Leaf, Fuzz, Marco, Gator, The Ritz, Cuba, The Four Seasons, The Longshot, RAD.
TELEVISION: Studio One, Philco Theatre, Kraft Playhouse, Rod Browning of the Rocket Rangers.

WESTON, JAY: Producer. b. New York City, March 9, 1929. e. NYU. Operated own pub. agency before moving into film prod. In 1965 launched Weston Production; sold orig. s.p., The War Horses, to Embassy Pictures; acquired and marketed other properties. Became prod. story exec. for Palomar-ABC Pictures in 1967.
PICTURES INCLUDE: For Love of Ivy (co-prod.), Lady Sings the Blues (co-prod.), W.C. Fields and Me, Chu Chu and the Philly Flash, Buddy, Buddy.
STAGE: Does a Tiger Wear a Necktie (co-prod.).

WESTON, ROBERT R.: Executive. b. N.Y., e. Peekskill Military Acad., Fordham Univ., Publicity dir., WFUV-FM, 3 yrs.; copy writer, Columbia Pictures, asst. accnt. exec., Donahue & Coe, asst. adv. mgr., United Artists adv. dir., Embassy Pictures, v.p., asst. to exec. v.p.; v.p. asst. to pres., resigned to become independent film producer, 1971. Presently pres., Harold Robbins Int'l., film prod. co. Prod.: The Betsy.

WEXLER, HASKELL: Cinematographer, director. b. Chicago, 1926. Photographed educational and industrial films before features.
PICTURES INCLUDE: The Savage Eye, The Bus, The Hoodlum Priest, Angel Baby, A Face In the Rain, America, America, The Best Man, The Loved One, Who's Afraid of Virginia Woolf, In the Heat of the Night, The Thomas Crown Affair. Co-produced, directed, wrote, Medium Cool. 1972: Trial of Catonsville Nine, Interview Allende. American Graffiti, One Flew Over the Cuckoo's Nest, Introduction to the Enemy, Bound for Glory, Days of Heaven, Lookin' to Get Out, Coming Home, The Man Who Loved Women. Director-Writer: Latino.

WHEELER, LYLE: Art director. b. Woburn, Mass., Feb. 12, 1905; e. U. So. Calif. Mag. illustrator, industrial designer before entering m.p. ind. as art dir. of Garden of Allah. In 1944 apptd. supervising art dir. 20th Century-Fox. Academy Award, in collab. art-direction black & white for Anna and the King of Siam; Gone With the Wind, color art dir., collab., The Robe, 1953. Love Is a Many-Splendored Thing, Daddy Longlegs, The Diary of Anne Frank (AA, 1959), Journey to the Center of the Earth, The Cardinal.

WHITE, BETTY: Actress. b. Oak Park, IL, Jan. 17, 1924. Wife of late Allen Ludden. Began on radio in Blondie, The Great Gildersleeve, This Is Your F.B.I. Moved into TV with live local show, L.A.
TELEVISION: Life with Elisabeth (Emmy), Tonight Show, Mary Tyler Moore Show (Emmy), The Pet Set, Macy's Thanksgiving Parade, The Betty White Show, The Best Place To Be, The Gossip Columnist, The Carol Burnett Show, Mama's Family.

WHITE, JESSE: Actor. b. Buffalo, N.Y., Jan. 13, 1919; e. Akron, O., H.S. Did odd jobs, then salesman; radio, vaudeville, burlesque, nightclubs and little theatre work; Broadway stage debut in Moon is Down, 1942; other shows include Harvey, Born Yesterday, etc. Has appeared on numerous radio and TV shows, regular on Danny Thomas, Ann Southern Shows.
PICTURES INCLUDE: Harvey, Death of a Salesman, Callaway Went Thataway, Million Dollar Mermaid, Witness to Murder, Forever Female, Not As a Stranger, Bad Seed, Back from Eternity, Designing Woman, Marjorie Morningstar, Legs Diamond, Fever in the Blood, Sail a Crooked Ship, It's Only Money, The Yellow Canary, It's a Mad, Mad, Mad, Mad World, Looking For Love, A House Is Not a Home, Bless the Beasts and Children, The Cat from Outer Space.

WHITE, LAWRENCE R.: Executive. b. 1926. e. Syracuse U. Began career as producer-director for the Dumont Television Network in 1948. Dir. of programming, Benton & Bowles, Inc., 1951; joined CBS TV network as v.p., daytime programming, 1959; dir. of program development, CBS, 1963; joined NBC television network in 1965 as v.p., daytime programs; v.p. programs, east coast, 1969; v.p. programs, NBC-TV, 1972; ind. prod. affiliated with CPT, 1975. Resigned 1980 to become independent producer.
TELEVISION: The Blue and the Gray, The Master of Ballantrae.

WHITE, LEONARD: Producer, director, actor. b. Sussex, Eng. TV dir., prod., CBS-TV (Canada), T.W.W. Ltd. T.T. TV & ABC-TV; Jupiter Thea., Inc.; Crest Theatre; Royal Alexandra Thea.; Toronto Thea., 1953–57. England, Playhouse, Oxford, Perth Repertory Thea., Hornchurch, Guilford Repertory Thea. Belgrade Thea., Coventry. Actor: U.S.A. debut in A Sleep of Prisoners, 1951–52; London West End. In the White Devil, He Who Gets Slapped, Macbeth, Still She Wished for Company, Point of Departure.
PICTURES INCLUDE: The Dark Man, The Large Rope, River Beat, Hunted, Martin Luther, Passage Home, Breakout, Circumstantial Evidence, At the Stroke of Nine, etc.
TV: All networks, G. Britain and CBC (Canada). Prod., ABC-TV, 1960–68. Inside Story series, Armchair Mystery Thea., series. Police Surgeon series, The Avengers, series, Out of This World, series, Armchair Theatre series. Prod., 1968–69; prod., Thames Television, 1969–70. Drama consultant CBC-TV Toronto.

WHITE, PAUL: Executive, producer, director. b. New York, N.Y.; e. Columbia U. Worked for N.Y. Times, Wide World Pictures; managing ed., Nation-Wide News Service; ed.-publisher of "Key Magazine"; home office exec. Paramount Pictures. Author, alone & in collab., books including I Find Treason. Served in U.S. Marine Corps as officer-in-chg. combat photography in the Pacific WWII, prod. & dir. wire recording of first sound ever made of actual war conditions under battle fire in the Marshalls. Joined David O. Selznick as gen. mgr. of European operations 1946; formed own co., Paul White Productions, Inc. 1948; v.p. & dir., Procter Prod., Inc.; pres., PSI-TV 1953. Joined Subscription TV 1958 as v.p. in chg. pgmg; pioneer cablevision and Pay-TV; pres. MCI; created 11 audio-visual inventions; 1973 Paul White Enterprises (consultants). Clients: RCA; Impresario S. Hurok; Radix Intl. Corp.; Motivational Systems, Inc.; Holographics R&D; Liberty Mint. Chm. exec. comm. The Education Guild; 1979–80, bd. chm. Holoptic 3-D Film Systems; mem. bds. Hi-Tech Industries, Inc.; Creative Holographics, U.K.; 1984, co-founder & chm., Holoptics Network Intl. N.Y./London, viz. Dimensional Imaging: Holography; Linear Optics; 3-D Systems for TV, Motion Pictures, Stills, (co-inventor) pat pend anti-counterfeit ID labeling system with visible 3-D or animated tickets, labels, etc., invisibly encoded inside label, which portable mini computer can decode & display essential readout info re product, i.e. TV sets, hi-tech equipment, records, toys, wearing apparel, etc.
PICTURES INCLUDE: Battle of the Marshalls, Saipan, Tinian, To the Shores of Iwo Jima, Song of Siam, Pearl of the Orient, Land of Fair Dinkum, Unusual Sports, Flying Doctor.
TV: Series Created and/or supervised incl.: Playhouse of Stars, China Smith, Play of The Week, Orient Express, prod. & dir. "The Keys to Peace" (Pope Paul's U.S. Visit); exec. prod. two 90-min TV Specials, "The Bolshoi Ballet" Bicentennial project; OP Sail 1976, The Tall Ships; Creative & technical svcs. for 3-D TV & multi-graphic applications.

WHITE, ROY B.: Executive, exhibitor. b. Cincinnati, Ohio. e. University of Cincinnati. Flight engineer, U.S. Air Force during World War II; worked in sales department of 20th Century-Fox, 1949–52; began in exhibition, 1952; past pres., Mid-States Theatres; pres., R. M. White Management, Inc.; past president, National Association of Theatre Owners, past Chairman of the Board, National Association of Theatre Owners: Board of Trustees—American Film Institute; Board of Directors NATO of Ohio, v.p., Motion Picture Pioneers Foundation; Will Rogers Hospital, Nat'l. Endowment for Arts.

WHITELAW, BILLIE: Actress. b. Coventry, England. Acted on radio and television since childhood. Winner of the TV Actress of the Year; Variety Club Actress of the Year 1960. British Academy Award 1969. U.S. National Society of Film Critics Award for Best Supporting Actress, Variety Club, 1977. Evening News, Best Film Actress, 1977.
STAGE: 3 years with National Theatre of Great Britain. Revue: England, My England. Stage plays include: Progress to the Park, A Touch of the Poet, Othello, Trelawney of the Wells, After Haggerty, Not I, Alphabetical Order, Footfalls, Molly, The Greeks, Happy Days, Passion Play, Rockaby (also in N.Y. and Adelaide Festival), Tales from Hollywood.
PICTURES INCLUDE: No Love for Johnnie, Mr. Topaze, Hell Is a City, Payroll, Charlies Bubbles, The Adding Machine, Twisted Nerve, Start the Revolution Without Me, Leo the Last, Eagle in a Cage, Gumshoe, Frenzy, Nightwatch, The Omen, The Water Babies, A Tale of Two

Cities, An Unsuitable Job for a Woman, Slayground, Shadey, The Chain.

TV: Over 100 leading roles incl. No Trains to Lime Street, Lady of the Camelias, Resurrection, The Pity of it All, You and Me, A World of Time, Dr. Jekyll and Mr. Hyde, Poet Game, Sextet (8 plays for BBC), Wessex Tales, The Fifty Pound Note, Supernatural (2 plays), Three plays by Samuel Beckett, Eustace and Hilda, The Oresteia of Aeschylus, The Haunted Man, Private Schultz, Jamaica Inn, Rockaby, Camille.

WHITFIELD, RICHARD ALLEN: Producer-Executive. b. Goldsboro, N.C., 1946. e. Univ. of North Carolina. Adv. writer-producer for American Brands, Pepsicola, 1970–73; TV-film producer, industrial-educational, 1973–77; v.p., adv., Independents International Films, Inc., distributor, 1978; v.p.-producer, Rick Friedberg & Associates, 1979; pres. Golden Image Motion Picture Corp., feature production, 1980.

PICTURES INCLUDE: K-GOD (exec. prod.), Used Cars (video segments prod.), Bones of Peking (prod.).

WHITMAN, STUART: Actor. b. San Francisco, Calif., Feb. 1, 1926. e. Los Angeles City Coll. Army Engineers June 1945 to Sept. 1948, Engineers at Fort Lewis, Wash.; while in army, became light heavyweight boxer. Studied drama, L.A. City Coll., 2 yrs.; attended Ben Bard's training sch. for actors, became member of Chekhov group, and Arthur Kennedy famed local Stage Society. Joined tent show, Here Comes Mr. Jordan, then TV and pictures.

PICTURES INCLUDE: When Worlds Collide, The Day The Earth Stood Still, China Doll, Darby's Rangers, Johnny Trouble, Hell Bound, Seven Men from Now, No Sleep Till Dawn, Ten North Frederick, These Thousand Hills, The Deck Ran Red, The Sound and The Fury, Hound Dog Man, The Story of Ruth, Murder, Inc., Francis of Assisi, The Fiercest Heart, The Mark, The Comancheros, Reprieve, The Day and the Hour, Signpost to Murder, Rio Conchos, Sands of Kalahari, An American Dream, Last Escape, Last Generation, Night of the Lepus, Crazy Mama, Call Him Shatter, Las Vegas Lady, Strange Shadows in an Empty Room, Butterfly, Gayana-Cult of the Damned, Deadly Intruder.

TV: The Crowd Pleaser (Alcoa-Goodyear), Highway Patrol, Dr. Christian, Hangman's Noose (Zane Grey), The Last Convertible, Condominium.

WHITMORE, JAMES: Actor. r.n. James Allen Whitmore, Jr. b. White Plains, N.Y., Oct. 1, 1921. e. Yale U. In Yale Drama School players; co-founder Yale radio station, 1942; U.S. Marine Corps, World War II; in USO, in American Wing Theatre school, in stock. Broadway debut in Command Decision, 1947; m.p. debut in Undercover Man. Star of Tomorrow.

PICTURES INCLUDE: Battleground, Asphalt Jungle, Next Voice You Hear, Mrs. O'Malley and Mr. Malone, Outriders, Please Believe Me, Across the Wide Missouri, It's a Big Country, Because You're Mine, Above and Beyond, Girl Who Had Everything, All the Brothers Were Valiant, Kiss Me Kate, The Command, Them, Battle Cry, McConell Story, Last Frontier, Oklahoma, Face of Fire, Eddie Duchin Story, Who Was That Lady?, Black Like Me, Chuka, Water Hole No. 3, Nobody's Perfect, Planet of the Apes, Madigan, The Split, Guns of the Magnificent Seven, Chato's Land, Where the Red Fern Grows, Give 'em Hell, Harry, The Serpent's Egg, The First Deadly Sin.

TV: The Law and Mr. Jones, Celebrity.

WHITTAKER, WILLIAM: Producer. Entered m.p. ind. as asst. dir. prod. man. with Gaumont British 1932. War service 1939–45. Joined Associated British Picture Corporation as prod. man 1946 Producer 1954. From 1960 Con. of AB Productions. 1970: independent producer.

PICTURES INCLUDE: (From 1946) prod.: Dam Buster, No Time for Tears, Ice Cold in Alex, The Rebel, The Cracksman, The Bargee, Mister Ten Per Cent, Judith, Universal Soldier.

WICKES, MARY: Actress. e. Washington U., Doctor of Arts (hon.), 1969.

THEATRE: (B'way) The Man Who Came to Dinner, Town House, Stage Door, Danton's Death. Dramatic & musical comedy stock includes: St. Louis Municipal Opera, Starlight Theatre, Houston Music Theatre.

PICTURES INCLUDE: The Man Who Came to Dinner, Now, Voyager, White Christmas, The Music Man, The Trouble With Angels, Where Angels Go Trouble Follows, Napoleon and Samantha, Snowball Express, Touched by Love.

TV: The Halls of Ivy, The Danny Thomas Show, Dennis the Menance, Bonino, Hitchcock Presents, Studio One, Playhouse 90.

WIDMARK, RICHARD: Actor. b. Sunrise, Minn., Dec. 26, 1914. e. Lake Forest U. Instructor, 1938. On radio, then stage, films.

PICTURES INCLUDE: Kiss of Death, Cry of the City, Road House, Street With No Name, Yellow Sky, Down to the Sea in Ships, Slattery's Hurricane, Night and the City, Panic in the Streets, No Way Out, Halls of Montezuma, The Frogmen, Red Skies of Montana, Don't Bother to Knock, O. Henry's Full House, My Pal Gus, Destination Gobi, Pickup on South Street, Take the High Ground, Hell & High Water, Broken Lance, Prize of Gold, The Cobweb, Backlash, Last Wagon, Saint Joan, Warlock, Kingdom of Man, The Long Ships, Run for the Sun, The Alamo, Judgment at Nuremberg, How the West Was Won, The Way West, Madigan, Death of a Gunfighter, When The Legends Die, Murder on the Orient Express, Twilight's Last Gleaming, The Domino Principle, Rollercoaster, Coma, The Swarm, Hanky Panky, The Final Option, Against All Odds.

WIDOM, DIANE: Executive. Held marketing positions with Warner Bros., in New York, London & Burbank, for 10 years prior to joining 20th Century Fox in 1980 as West Coast pub. dir. 1982, named dir. of natl. mag. pub. & special photography. Promoted to natl. pub. dir. 1985, named v.p., pub., Fox m.p. div.

WIENER, JACK: Executive. b. Paris, France, June 8, 1926. Pub. rep., MGM, New Orleans, Jacksonville, Fla., 1952–56; joined Columbia Pictures Int. Corp., 1956, continental publicity mgr., Columbia, Paris; v.p., Columbia Pics. Int'l. 1966; continental prod. exec., 1968; v.p. Columbia Pictures Corp., 1970. In 1972 became indep. prod., making Vampira, The Eagle Has Landed, Escape to Athena, Green Ice, F/X.

WIESEN, BERNARD: Producer, Director, Executive. b. New York City, Oct. 6. e. College of the City of New York (B.B.A.) Pasadena Playhouse College of Theatre (Master of Theatre Arts), Dramatic Workshop of New School.

PICTURES INCLUDE: Producer-Director: Fear No More. Asst. Director on films, including The King and I, The Left Hand of God, The Rains of Ranchipur, To Catch a Thief, The Trouble with Harry, Fear No More.

TV: Director: How to Marry A Millionaire, Valentine's Day. Assoc. Producer: Valentine's Day, Three on an Island, Cap'n Ahab, Sally and Sam. Assoc. Prod.: Daniel Boone. Producer/Director: Julia, Co-Producer-Director: The Jimmy Stewart Show. Prod. Exec.: Executive Suite (pilot). Exec. Paramount TV, director of current programming.

STAGE: First Monday in October (Bdwy.)—co. prod.

WIESENTHAL, SAM: Executive. b. New York, N.Y., Jan. 26, 1909; e. N.Y.U., 1929. In story dept., Universal Pictures 1929–31; asst. to pres., 1931–39; v.p., gen mgr. & dir. of General Service Studios & producing companies since 1942, exec. v.p., assoc. producer many films. pres., Olympic Prod., 1964.

PICTURES INCLUDE: Bridge at San Luis Rey, Dark Waters, The Macomber Affair, Cry Danger, with W. R. Frank; Second Chance (RKO) The Americano, Bengazi, Tension at Table Rock, The Day They Gave Babies Away, The Jack Dempsey Story.

WIEST, DIANNE: Actress. b. Kansas City, MO. e. Univ. of Maryland. Studied ballet but abandoned if for theatre. Did regional theatre work (Yale Repertory, Arena Stage) and performed with N.Y. Shakespeare Festival. Plays include Heartbreak House, The Hostage, Julius Caesar, Our Town, Ashes, Three Sisters, Old Times, After the Fall, etc. Film debut in I'm Dancing As Fast As I Can (1982).

PICTURES: Independence Day, Footloose, Falling in Love, The Purple Rose of Cairo, Hannah and Her Sisters.

TELEVISION: The Wall, The Face of Rage.

WILCOX, CLAIRE: Actress. b. Toronto, Canada, 1955. Photographer's model, 3 yrs. of age; appeared on numerous national magazine covers; TV commercials; signed contract, Curtis Enterprises.

PICTURES INCLUDE: 40 Pounds of Trouble, Wives and Lovers.

TV: Harris Versus the World.

WILD, JACK: Actor. b. Lancashire, England, 1952. m.p. debut in Oliver, 1968. To Hollylwood 1969 to star in H. R. Pufnstuf TV series for Krofft Television Productions. Under contract to Hemdale Group.

PICTURES INCLUDE: Pufnstuf, Oliver!, Swalk, Fight of the Doves, Pied Piper, The 14.

TV: Our Mutal Friend, The Government Inspector.

WILDE, ARTHUR L.: Executive. b. San Francisco, Calif., May 27, 1918. S.F. Daily News; Matson Lines; pub. dept., Warner Bros., 1936; dir. exploitation, CBS; pub. dir., Hal Wallis Prod.; pub. dept., Paramount; pub., Hecht-Hill-Lancaster; v.p., Arthur Jacobs, public rel.; Blowitz-Maskell Publicity Agency; pub. dir., C. V. Whitney Pictures; gen. v.p., 1958; owner, pub.-ad. agency, The Arthur L. Wilde Co., 1961–65; freelance publicist, 1965–66; pub. rel. consultant, Marineland of Florida, 1965; unit publicity dir., United Artists, National General, Paramount, 1966–69; free lance publicity, 1971; unit publicist, MGM, Paramount, United Artists, 1972–74; staff position; Features Publicity at Paramount Pictures, 1973. Free lance unit publicist again in 1976 at Universal, Paramount and Lorimar Productions. 1978–79, Columbia Pictures & Universal Studios; 1980, Marble Arch. Prods. & Northstar Intl. Pictures; 1981, studio pub. mgr., 20th Century-Fox; recently staff unit publicist for 20th-Fox; 1984, free lance unit publicist for feature films.

WILDE, CORNEL: Actor, producer, director, author. b. New York, Oct. 13, 1918; e. Columbia & City Coll., N.Y. Art Sch., Budapest; Columbia Med. School; studied drama with Strasberg, Bulgakov, Chekov. First screen role, 1941, High Sierra.
STAGE: Moon Over Mulberry Street, Love is Not So Simple, Daughters of Altreus, Having a Wonderful Time, Romeo & Juliet.
PICTURES INCLUDE: Wintertime, A Song to Remember, The Perfect Snob, A Thousand and One Nights, Leave Her to Heaven, Bandit of Sherwood Forest, Centennial Summer, Forever Amber, The Homestretch, It Had to be You, Walls of Jericho, Roadhouse, Four Days Leave, Two Flags West, Greatest Show on Earth, At Sword's Point, Saadia, Passion, Woman's World, Big Combo, Scarlet Coat, Hot Blood, Star of India, Beyond Mombasa, Omar Khayyam, Edge of Eternity, Constantine the Great; act., prod., dir.: Storm Fear, Maracaibo; act., prod., dir., cowriter: The Devil's Hairpin, The Sword of Lancelot; act., prod., dir.: The Naked Prey; act., prod., dir., co-author s.p.: Beach Red; prod., dir., co-author s.p.: No Blade of Grass; prod., dir., act., screenplay: Sharks' Treasure; actor: The Fifth Musketeer.

WILDER, BILLY: Producer, director, writer. b. Austria, June 22, 1906. Newspaperman active Vienna, Berlin; then author screen story People on Sunday, s.p.: Emil and the Detectives (in Museum of Modern Art), UFA. Wrote, dir., Mauvaise Graine, Paris. To Hollywood 1934, (collab. s.p.) Bluebeard's Eighth Wife, Ninotchka, What a Life, Midnight, Arise My Love, Ball of Fire, Hold Back the Dawn. Head Film Section, Psych. Warfare Div., U.S. Army, 1945, Am. Zone, Germany.
PICTURES INCLUDE: (collab. s.p., dir.) The Major and the Minor, Five Graves to Cairo, Double Indemnity, The Emperor Waltz, A Foreign Affair. Academy Award for dir., best s.p. (collab.) for Lost Weekend, 1945. Academy Award for best story & s.p. (collab.) for Sunset Boulevard, 1950; (collab. s.p., dir., prod) The Big Carnival, Stalag 17, Sabrina, Love in the Afternoon, Some Like it Hot, The Apartment (Academy Award for best direction, best story, and s.p., best picture, 1960); One, Two, Three, Irma La Douce; (collab. s.p., dir. co-prod.) Seven Year Itch; (collab., dir.) Spirit of St. Louis; (collab. s.p. & dir.) Witness for the Prosecution; (prod. dir., collab.) Kiss Me, Stupid, The Fortune Cookie, The Private Life of Sherlock Holmes, Avanti, The Front Page, Fedora, Buddy, Buddy (co-s.p., dir.).

WILDER, GENE: Actor. b. Milwaukee, Wis., 1935. e. University of Iowa. Joined Bristol Old Vic company in England, became champion fencer; in New York, worked as chauffer, fencing instructor, etc. Before N.Y. off-Broadway debut in Roots.
BROADWAY: The Complaisant Lover, Mother Courage, Luv.
PICTURES INCLUDE: Bonnie and Clyde, The Producers, Start the Revolution Without Me, Quacsker Fortune Has an Uncle in the Bronx, Willie Wonka and the Chocolate Factory, Everything You Always Wanted to Know About Sex*, Blazing Saddles, Rhinoceros, Young Frankenstein, The Little Prince, Adventures of Sherlock Holmes Smarter Brother (s.p., dir., star), Silver Streak, The World's Greatest Lover (s.p., dir., star), The Frisco Kid, Stir Crazy, Sunday Lovers, (dir., s.p., act.), Hanky Panky, The Woman in Red (dir., s.p., act.), Haunted Honeymoon (dir., s.p., act.).

WILDER, W. LEE: Producer, director. b. Austria; e. U. Vienna. Awards: First prize 1950 Venice Film Festival musical documentary category.
PICTURES INCLUDE: The Vicious Circle, Shadows of Fire, The Pretender, Once A Thief, Three Steps North, Phantom from Space, Killers from Space, Snow Creature, Big Bluff, Manfish, Man Without a Body, Fright, Spy in the Sky, Bluebeard's Ten Honeymoons.

WILK, TED: Theatrical agent. b. Minneapolis, Minn., Jan. 5, 1908. e. U. of Mich., 1926–30. Publix Theatres, Duluth, Minn., 1930; Warner Bros., Minneapolis, 1932–33; Film Daily, Hollywood, 1934–40; U.S. Army, 1941–46; Lou Irwin agency 1946–61; Ted Wilk Agency, since 1961.

WILKINSON, ROBERT: Executive. Came to Universal in 1941 as student booker in Memphis branch. Spent 4 years in Marines; then returned to Memphis as salesman, branch mgr.; later mgr. of Dallas branch, then district and regional mgr. Named Universal asst. gen. sls mgr. in 1964. Appt. exec. v.p. in chg of domestic dist. in 1978.

WILLIAMS, BERT: Executive, actor. b. Newark, N.J., April 12, 1922. e. USC Navy, 1942–45. Summer Stock, 1940–41; world's prof. diving champion, 1945–48; star diver, Larry Crosby, Buster Crabb, Johnny Weismuller, Dutch Smith Shows, 1945–48; writer, asst. prod., Martin Mooney Prods., PRC, Goldwyn Studios; pres., Bert Prods., Bert Williams Motion Picture Producers and Distributors, Inc. Member, M.P. Academy of Fine Arts & TV Academy of Arts & Science.
THEATRE: roadshow plays include: Cat on a Hot Tin Roof, Hamlet, Run From The Hunter, Sugar and Spice, Hope Is a Thing Called Feathers, 69 Below, Tribute.
PICTURES INCLUDE: Actor, Angel Baby; prod., dir., actor, The Nest of the Cuckoo Birds; actor, Around the World Under the Sea; s.p. auth. Deathwatch 28; dir., Twenty Eight Watched, prod. dir. Adventure To Treasure Reef. s.p. Knife Fighters. orig. story & s.p.; Black Freedom; A Crime of Sex; The Masters (actor). Crazy Joe, Serpico, Lady Ice, The Klansman, Report to the Commissioner, Tracks, All the President's Men, From Noon Till Three. (all actor), While Buffalo (actor), Helter Skelter (actor), Shark Bait (writer), The Big Bus (actor). Actor: Wanda Nevada, Horn, Sunnyside, Cuba, The Last Resort, The All Night Treasure Hunt. Recent acting: Tom Horn, Kill Castro, Midnight Madness, The All-American Hustler, 10 to Midnight, Police Academy 2, One More Werewolf Picture, Murphy's Law, Cobra (actor).
TV: Flipper, Sea Hunt, prod., Speargun, Gentle Ben, The Law (pilot) and Police Story (actor). Recent actor: Get Christy Love, General Hospital, Columbo, Brenner for the People (actor), Mayday 40,000 Feet (actor) Jigsaw John (Blue Knight episode). Actor: Police Woman, Chips, Mobil One, Street Killing, East of Eden, Rose for Emily, Brett Maverick, Today's F.B.I. etc. Produced, directed & wrote pilot, Fifth St. Gym. Appeared on Mike Douglas Show & Johnny Carson Show, Tales on Dark Side, The Last Car, This Is the Life, Deadly Intentions, Tales on the Dark Side, The Last Car, Divorce Court, etc.

WILLIAMS, BILL: Actor. r.n. William Katt. b. Brooklyn, N.Y. e. Pratt Inst., Brooklyn. In U.S. Army, World War II. Began as professional swimmer; later with Municipal Opera House, St. Louis; then on vaudeville tour, U.S. & England. Screen debut 1944 in "Murder in the Blue Room."
PICTURES INCLUDE: Thirty Seconds Over Tokyo, Those Endearing Young Charms, Blue Blood, Great Missouri Raid, Operation Haylift, Cariboo Trail, Havana Rose, Rose of Cimarron, Son of Paleface, Bronco Buster, Pace That Thrills, Torpedo Alley, Racing Blood, Outlaw's Daughter, Apache Ambush, Hell's Horizon, Wiretapper, Broken Star, Dogs Best Friend, Buckskin, Tickle Me, Scandalous John.

WILLIAMS, BILLY DEE: Actor. b. New York City, April 6, 1937. Studied acting with Paul Mann and Sidney Poitier at actor's workshop in Harlem. Was child actor; Broadway adult debut in The Cool World in 1961.
STAGE: A Taste of Honey, Hallelujah, Baby.
PICTURES INCLUDE: The Last Angry Man (debut), The Out-of-Towners, The Final Comedown, Lady Sings the Blues, Hit! Mahogany, The Bingo Long Travelling All-Stars, The Empire Strikes Back, Nighthawks, Return of the Jedi, Marvin and Tige, Fear City, Number One with a Bullet.
TV: Brian's Song, The Glass House, Chiefs and appearances on series: The F.B.I., The Interns, Mission Impossible, Mod Squad. Movie: The Right of the People.

WILLIAMS, BOB: Writer. b. Sioux Falls, S.D., Oct. 19, 1913.
PICTURES INCLUDE: collab. s.p., Treat 'Em Rough, Overland Mail Robbery, Pride of the Plains, Youth on Trial, Sergeant Mike; s.p., Lone Texas Ranger, Trail to Vengeance, many Westerns; collab. s.p., Stage to Tucson.

WILLIAMS, CARA: Comedienne. r.n. Bernice Kamiat. b. Brooklyn, N.Y. e. Hollywood Professional Sch.; ent. ind., 20th Century Fox, child actress.
PICTURES INCLUDE: Boomerang, Something For the Boys, Meet Me In Las Vegas, Never Steal Anything Small, The Defiant Ones, The Man From the Diners' Club, Doctors' Wives.
TV: Pete and Gladys, Alfred Hitchcock Presents, Desilu Playhouse, The Jackie Gleason Show, Henry Fonda Special, The Cara Williams Show.

WILLIAMS, CARL W.: Executive. b. Decatur, Ill., March 9, 1927. e. Illinois State Normal U., B.S., 1949; UCLA, M.A., 1950. dir. adv. photo., Clark Equipment Co., 1951–54; film dir., WKAR-TV, E. Lansing, Mich., 1954–56; Prod., dir., Capital Films, E. Lansing, Mich., 1957; dir., A-V Laboratory, UCLA, 1957–63; co-dev. Dimension 150 Widescreen process, 1957; formed D-150 Inc., 1963; Filbert Co., 1970, v.p., 1977; v.p., Cinema Equipment Sales of Calif., Inc., 1986.
MAMPAS, SMPTE, AFI.

WILLIAMS, CHARLES: Actor, writer. b. Albany, N.Y., Sept. 27, 1898. Appeared on stage in "Rio Rita," dialogue for vaudeville and stage. To Fox Studios, Hollywood, 1931. In 1933 appeared in Gambling Ship. In 1935 collab. music and lyrics, Gigolette; collab. orig. s.p. Arm of the Law, Midnight Limited.
PICTURES INCLUDE: The Girl from Monterey, Where Are Your Children? (collab. orig. & s.p.) Hollywood and Vine; (cast) End of the Road, Identity Unknown, Doll Face, Heldorado, Due Goes West, Grand Canyon.

WILLIAMS, CINDY: Actress. b. Van Nuys, Calif., Aug. 22, 1947. e. L.A. City Coll. Appeared in high school and college plays; first prof. role in Roger Corman's film Gas. Made TV debut in Room 222 and had continuing role.
PICTURES INCLUDE: Beware the Blob, Drive, He Said, The Christian Licorice Store, Travels with My Aunt, American Graffiti, The Conversation, Mr. Ricco, The First Nudie Musical, More American Graffiti, Uforia.
TV: Episodes of The Funny Side, The Neighbors, Barefoot in the Park, My World and Welcome to It, Love, American Style, Nanny and the Professor, The Bobby Sherman Show—Getting Together; Laverne and Shirley. Movies: The Migrants, Helped Wanted: Kids.

WILLIAMS, DERICK: Cinematographer. b. Nottingham, Eng., 1906. e. Brighton Coll.; Nottingham U. Cinematog., 1929; first cameraman & experimental work on Evans color process, 1930; head camera dept., Gainsborough Pictures, 1932; org. camera dept. Nat'l Studios, Sydney, Austrailia, 1935.
PICTURES INCLUDE: In Which We Serve, Way Ahead, Way to the Stars, Beware of Pity, For Them That Trespass, Lady Possessed; mgr. dir., Derick Williams Prod., Ltd.; Voice of London, Ltd.

WILLIAMS, DIAHN: Actress. b. Gainesville, Fla., June 30. e. Univ. of Miami (BA, psychology, speech), also attended Univ. of Florida, UCLA. m. Thomas J. McGrath, prod. & atty. Started as fashion model in New York, France, Germany. Top woman exec. as assoc. dir. of pub. rel. at Chesebrough-Ponds, 1971–72.
PICTURES INCLUDE: Chair de Poule, Another Nice Mess, Deadly Hero.
TV: Harry's Girls (series, 1963–64), Somerset (series, 1973–74) and guest-starred in many TV shows, including I Spy, Get Smart, Tarzan, Here Comes the Brides, Andy Griffith Show, G.E. Theatre, etc.

WILLIAMS, ELMO: Film editor. b. Oklahoma City, Okla., Apr. 30, 1913. Film editor 1933–39, with British & Dominion Studio, England. Since then with RKO-Radio as film editor for numerous major productions; Academy Award, best film ed. (collab.) High Noon, 1952; dir. film ed., Tall Texan; prod. dir., ed., The Cowboy; ed., 20,000 Leagues Under the Sea; dir. Apache Kid; second unit dir., film ed. The Vikings; dir. 2nd Unit DFZ prod., The Big Gamble; assoc. prod., The Longest Day; mgr., dir., 20th Century Fox Prod. Ltd. Producer: Tora! Tora! Tora! v.p., worldwide production, 20th Century-Fox Film 1971. President Ibex Films. Exec. v.p., Gaylord Prods., 1979; promoted to pres., worldwide prods.
TV: co-prod. dir., Tales of the Vikings.

WILLIAMS, ESTHER: Actress. b. Los Angeles, Calif., Aug. 8, 1923. e. U. of So. Calif. Swimmer San Francisco World's Fair Aquacade; professional model. On screen 1942 in Andy Hardy Steps Out.
PICTURES INCLUDE: A Guy Named Joe, Bathing Beauty, Thrill of a Romance, This Time for Keeps, Ziegfeld Follies, Hoodlum Saint, Easy to Wed, Fiesta, On an Island With You, Take Me Out to the Ball Game, Neptune's Daughter, Pagan Love Song, Duchess of Idaho, Texas Carnival, Skirts Ahoy!, Million Dollars Mermaid, Dangerous When Wet, Easy to Love, Jupiter's Darling, Unguarded Moment, the Big Show. Voted one of Top Ten Money-Making Stars in M.P. Herald-Fame poll, 1950.

WILLIAMS, GEORGE EMLYN: (C.B.E.) Writer, actor, producer. b. Mostyn, Flintshire, Wales, Nov. 26, 1905. e. Christ Church, Oxford, M.A., LL.D. (Hon.). On London stage from 1927 (And So to Bed, The Case of the Frightened Lady, Wild Decembers, Night Must Fall, The Corn is Green, etc.); also author many plays (Glamour, The Late Christopher Bean, Night Must Fall, He Was Born Gay, The Corn is Green, The Light of Heart, etc.). Began Brit. screen career 1932 as actor in The Case of the Frightened Lady; Friday the Thirteenth, Evergreen, This England, In 1945 on Brit. stage; author & cast the Wind of Heaven, Trespass, Accolade, Charles Dickens Mixed Bill & Bleak House, Someone Waiting.
PICTURES INCLUDE: Broken Blossoms, The Citadel, Jamaica Inn, The Stars Look Down, The Girl in the News, Major Barbara, You Will Remember, Hatter's Castle, Last Days of Dolwyn, Three Husbands, Scarf, Another Man's Poison, Ivanhoe, Deep Blue Sea, I Accuse, Beyond This Place, The Wreck of the Mary Deare, The L-Shaped Room, The Eye of the Devil.
TV: The Winslow Boy, The Defenders, Yob and Nabob, The Burning Bush, The Deadly Game, Rumpole of the Bailey.
BOOKS: George, Beyond Belief, Emlyn, Doctor Crippen's Dairy, Headlong.

WILLIAMS, JOBETH: Actress. b. Texas. e. Brown Univ. With repertory companies in Rhode Island, Philadelphia, Boston, Washington, D.C., etc. Spent over two years in New York-based daytime serials, Somerset and The Guiding Light. Theatrical film debut in Kramer Vs. Kramer, 1979.
PICTURES INCLUDE: Stir Crazy, The Dogs of War, Poltergeist, Endangered Species, The Big Chill, American Dreamer, Teachers, Desert Bloom, Poltergeist II.
TV: Fun and Games, Feasting with Panthers, Jabberwocky, The Day After, Adam, Kids Don't Tell.

WILLIAMS, JOHN: Composer. b. New York City, Feb. 8, 1932. e. UCLA, Juilliard School. Worked as session musician in '50s; began career as film composer in late '50s. Considerable experience as musical director and conductor as well as composer.
PICTURES INCLUDE: I Passed for White, Because They're Young, The Secret Ways, Bachelor Flat, Diamond Head, Gidget Goes to Rome, The Killers, None But the Brave, John Goldfarb Please Come Home, The Rare Breed, How To Steal A Million, The Plainsman, Not with My Wife You Don't, Penelope, A Guide for the Married Man, Fitzwilly, Valley of the Dolls, Daddy's Gone A-Hunting, Good-bye Mr. Chips (mus. supvr. & dir.), The Reivers, Jane Eyre, Fiddler on the Roof (musc. dir.). The Cowboys, Images, Pete 'n' Tillie, The Poseidon Adventure, Tom Sawyer (musc. supvr.), The Long Goodbye, The Man Who Loved Cat Dancing, The Paper Chase, Cinderella Liberty, Conrack, The Sugarland Express, Earthquake, The Towering Inferno, The Eiger Sanction, Jaws, Family Plot, The Missouri Breaks, Midway, Black Sunday, Star Wars, Encounters of the Third Kind, The Fury, Jaws II, Meteor, Quintet, Dracula, Radiers of the Lost Ark; E.T.: The Extra-Terrestrial, Return of the Jedi, Indiana Jones and the Temple of Doom, The River, Space Camp.
TV: Once Upon a Savage Night, Sergeant Ryker, Heidi.

WILLIAMS, MURIEL: Actress. e. Leland Powers Dramatic School, Boston. Played in stock. Cape Playhouse, Dennis, Mass.; with nat'l co. Autumn Garden, Heaven Can Wait; with late husband formed model, prod. agency, Hart Model Agency; commentator for fashion shows.
TV: frequent appearances; series: Brighter Day, CBS-TV.

WILLIAMS, OSCAR: Writer-Producer-Director. e. San Francisco State Univ., getting degree in film, TV. Was director's intern on The Great White Hope (directed by Martin Ritt) through the American Film Institute.
PICTURES INCLUDE: The Final Comedown (s.p., prod. dir.); Black Belt Jones (s.p., assoc. prod.) Five on the Black Hand Side (dir.), Truck Turner (s.p.), Hot Potato (s.p., dir.).

WILLIAMS, PAUL: Composer. b. Omaha. Sept. 19, 1940. Began career at studios as set painter and stunt parachutist. Bit and character parts in commercials followed. Seen briefly in The Chase and The Loved One. Became song writer, collaborating briefly with Biff Rose and later with Roger Nichols, with whom wrote several best-sellers, including We've Only Just Begun, Rainy Days and Mondays, Just an Old-Fashioned Love Song, etc.
PICTURES INCLUDE: Cinderella Liberty (score), Phantom of the Paradise (actor, score), Bugsy Malone (score), A Star Is Born (songs), Smokey and the Bandit, Part III (actor).

WILLIAMS, PAUL: Director. First gained attention as director of film short, Girl, which won Golden Eagle award. Made in collaboration with producer Edward R. Pressman, with whom he formed Pressman-Williams Enterprises.
PICTURES INCLUDE: Out of It, The Revolutionary, Dealing: or the Berkeley to Boston Forty Brick, Lost Bag Blues, Nunzio.

WILLIAMS, RICHARD: Producer-painter-film animator. b. March, 1933, Toronto, Canada. Entered industry in 1955. Founded Richard Williams Animation Ltd. in 1962, having entered films by producing The Little Island (1st Prize, Venice Film Festival) in 1955. His company produces TV commercials, entertainment shorts and animated films. Also designed animated feature titles for such films as What's New Pussycat?, A Funny Thing Happened On The Way To The Forum, Casino Royale, etc. (20 feature titles in 6 years). 1969: Animated sequences: Charge of the Light Brigade (Woodfall). 1971: A Christmas Carol, animated TV special for ABC-TV. His company makes TV commercials for England, America, France and Germany. His films have won awards at Festivals at Venice, Edinburgh, Mannheim, Montreal, Trieste, Melbourne, West Germany, New York, Locarno, Vancouver, Philadelphia, Zagreb, Hollywood, Cork, Los Angeles. 1973: Won Hollywood Oscar, Best Cartoon.

WILLIAMS, ROBERT: Actor. b. Glencoe, Ill.; Dartmouth U., B.A. Member: Psi Upsilon, Dartmouth Club, University Club (Chicago).
THEATRE: Burlesque, Strictly Dishonorable, Let Freedom Ring, Sailor Beware, Room Service, Eve of St. Mark.
PICTURES INCLUDE: The Girl in the Case, Secret Command, That Wonderful Urge, Apartment for Peggy, Dark Past, It Happens Every Spring, Oh, You Beautiful Doll, The Lawless, Mister 880, Groom Wore Spurs.

WILLIAMS, ROBERT X., JR.: Exhibitor, attorney. b. Taylor, Miss., Nov. 16, 1900. e. U. of Miss. Law Sch.; m. owner

& mgr. Lyric Theatre, Oxford, Miss. since 1917; active in oper. to prevent adverse legislation (theatres); del., Nat'l Democratic Conventions, Phila. & Chicago; chmn. campaign funds for Democratic Party, 2nd Congressional Dist., Miss.; chmn. Roosevelt Electors of Oxford; treas. Pat Harrison campaign, Lafayette Co.; pres. De Soto Memorial Highway Assn. of Miss.; secy.-treas. Jackson to Jackson Highway Ass'n.

MEMBER: MPTO of Ark., Miss. & Tenn. (pres.); MPTO of Miss. (pres.); mayor, City of Oxford; Rotary (dir. Oxford); Shriner; Soldiers of Soil Div. of Lafayette Co. (sgt.); U. of Miss. Alumni Assn., 2nd Congressional Dist. (chmn.).

WILLIAMS, ROBIN: Actor—Comedian. b. Chicago, July 21, 1952. e. Claremont Men's College (Calif.), College of Marin (Calif.), studying acting at latter. Continued studies at Julliard in New York. As San Francisco club performer appeared at Holy City Zoo, Intersection, the Great American Music Hall and The Boardinghouse. In Los Angeles performed as stand-up comedian at Comedy Store, Improvisation, and The Ice House. First TV appearance on Laugh In, followed by The Great American Laugh Off.

TELEVISION: Mork and Mindy, America Tonight, Ninety Minutes Live, The Alan Hamel Show, E.T. & Friends.

PICTURES: The Last Laugh, Popeye, The World According to Garp, The Survivors, Moscow on the Hudson, The Best of Times, Club Paradise.

WILLIAMS, ROGER: Pianist, concert-film-TV personality. b. Omaha, Oct. 1, 1926. e. Drake U., Idaho State Coll. Hon. Ph.D. Midland and Wagner Colls. Served U.S. Navy WWII. Appeared as guest artist in number of films. Public debut on TV's Arthur Godfrey Talent Scouts and Chance of a Lifetime. Other TV appearances include Ed Sullivan, Hollywood Palace, Kraft Summer Series, Celanese Special. Tours in addition to U.S. and Australia. Concert Halls—Japan, Mexico, Union of South Africa. Recorded 75 Albums, Kapp (now MCA) Records, with sales over 15 million albums.

WILLIAMS, TREAT: Actor. b. Rowayton, Conn. e. Franklin and Marshall College. Landed role on Bdwy. in musical, Over There! also played leading role in Grease on Bdwy. Film debut in The Ritz.

PICTURES: Deadly Hero, The Eagle Has Landed, Hair, 1941, Why Would I Lie?, The Pursuit of D. B. Cooper, Prince of the City, Once Upon a Time in America, Flashpoint, Smooth Talk, The Men's Club.

TELEVISION: Movies: Dempsey, A Streetcar Named Desire.

WILLIAMS-JONES, MICHAEL: Executive. b. England, June 3, 1947. Joined United Artists as trainee, 1967; territorial manager, South Africa, 1969; territorial manager, Brazil, 1971; territorial manager, England, 1976; appt. v.p., continental European manager, 1978; sr. v.p. foreign manager, 1979; In 1982 joined United Intl. Pictures as sr. v.p. intl. sls., based in London. 1984, named pres. UIP motion picture group.

WILLIAMSON, FRED: Actor-Director-Writer. b. Gary, Ind., March 5, 1937. e. Northwestern Univ. Spent 10 yrs. playing pro football before turning to acting.

PICTURES INCLUDE: M*A*S*H*, Tell Me That You Love Me, Junie Moon, The Legend of Nigger Charley, Hammer, Black Caesar, The Soul of Nigger Charley, Hell Up in Harlem, That Man Bolt, Crazy Joe, Three Tough Guys, BLACK Eye, Three the Hard Way, Bucktown, Vigilantes, 1990: The Bronx Warriors; The Big Score (dir., actor); The Last Fight (dir., actor); Foxtrap (prod., dir., actor).

TV: Julia (series), Police Story, Monday Night Football.

WILLIAMSON, NICOL: Actor. b. England, Sept. 14, 1938. Has played many classical roles with Royal Shakespeare Co., including Macbeth, Malvolio, and Coriolanus. Starred on Broadway in Inadmissible Evidence; musical debut in Rex.

PICTURES INCLUDE: Six Sided Triangle, Inadmissible Evidence, The Bofors Gun, Laughter in the Dark, The Reckoning, Hamlet, The Jerusalem File, The Seven-Per-Cent Solution. The Goodbye Girl (cameo), The Cheap Detective, The Human Factor, Excalibur, Venom, I'm Dancing As Fast As I Can, Return to Oz.

TELEVISION: Passion Flower, Lord Mountbatten.

WILLIAMSON, PATRICK: President-Columbia Pictures International Corp., New York Apptd. June 1978. b. England, Oct. 1929. Joined Columbia Pictures London office 1944—career spanned advertising & publicity responsibilities until 1967 when apptd. managing director Columbia Great Britain in 1971. Also man. dir. on formation of Columbia-Warner. Promoted to executive position in Columbia's home office, New York, April, 1973 and headed international operations since Feb. 1974. Vice pres., Coca-Cola Export Corp., April, 1983; exec. v.p. Columbia Pictures Industries, 1985; director, CPI, 1985.

WILLIS, GORDON: Cinematographer. Acted two summers in stock at Gloucester, MA, where also did stage settings and scenery. Photographer in Air Force; then cameraman, making documentaries. In TV did commercials and documentaries.

PICTURES INCLUDE: End of the Road, Loving, The Landlord, Little Murders, Bad Company, Klute, Up the Sandbox, The Paper Chase, The Godfather, The Parallax View, The Godfather, Part II, All the President's Men, September 30, 1955, Annie Hall, Comes a Horseman, Interiors, Pennies from Heaven, A Midsummer Night's Sex Comedy, Perfect, Zelig, The Purple Rose of Cairo, The Money Pit. Director: Windows (1980; debut).

WILLIS, TED: Screenwriter and dramatist. b. England, Jan. 13, 1918.

PICTURES INCLUDE: The Blue Lamp (orig. treatment), Good-Time, Trouble in Store, One Good Turn, Top of the Form, Up to His Neck, Woman in a Dressing Gown, The Young and the Guilty, Great to Be Young, No Trees in the Street, The Horsemasters, Flame in the Streets, Bitter Harvest, The Naked Sun, Mrs. Harris M.P., Spy on Ice, Mrs. Hams Goes to New York.

TV: Dixon of Dock Green, Big City, Look in Any Window, Strictly for the Sparrows, Scent of Fear, Inside Story, Hot Summer Night, Sergeant Cork, The Four Seasons of Rosie Carr, The Sullivan Brothers, Knock On Any Door, Virgin of the Secret Service, Crime of Passion, Black Beauty, Hunter's Walk, Valley of the Kings, A Place for Animals, The Campbells in Canada.

WILSON, ELIZABETH: Actress. b. Grand Rapids, MI, April 4, 1925. On Bdwy. in Picnic (debut, 1953), The Desk Set, The Tunnel of Love, Little Murders, Dark of the Moon, Sticks and Bones (Tony), Uncle Vanya, Morning's at Seven, etc.

PICTURES: Little Murders, Day of the Dolphin, Man on the Swing, Nine to Five, The Increditble Shrinking Woman, Grace Quigley, Where Are the Children?.

TELEVISION: Doc, Million Dollar Infield.

WILSON, FLIP: Performer. b. Newark, N.J. Dec. 8, 1933. r.n. Clerow Wilson. Left school at 16 to join Air Force; played clubs in Fla. & Bahamas until 1965 when guest appearance on NBC began; The Flip Wilson Show debuted 1970–71 season, NBC.

PICTURE: The Fish That Saved Pittsburgh.

WILSON, HUGH: Producer-Director-Writer. b. Miami Beach, FL, Aug. 21, 1943. Gained fame for creating, writing, producing and directing TV series, WKRP in Cincinnati. Feature film dir. debut with Police Academy (1984).

PICTURES: Stroker Ace (s.p.), Police Academy (dir.), Rustler's Rhapsody (s.p./dir.).

WILSON, NORMAN: (OBE). Editor. b. Edinburgh, Scotland. ed. The Living Cinema, formerly ed. Cinema Quarterly; assoc. ed. World Film News; author scripts for British documentaries and book Presenting Scotland: A Film Survey; attached to British Ministry of Information, World War II; ed. Film Forum, Documentary. Chmn. Edinburgh Film Guild, Edinburgh International Film Festival, 1947–60; Films of Scotland Com.; Governor, Brit. Film Inst.

WILSON, RICHARD: Producer, director. b. McKeesport, Pa., Dec. 25, 1915. e. Denver U. actor, announcer, Denver radio stations; radio actor, N.Y.; actor, asst. stage mgr., stage mgr., prod. asst. with Mercury Theatre, 1937–38; mgr., prod., summer theatres, 1939–40; assoc. with all Orson Welles films & radio shows to 1951; U.S. Air Force, 1942–45; assoc., prod., then prod., U-I.

PICTURES INCLUDE: assoc. prod., Lady from Shanghai, Macbeth, Ma and Pa Kettle on Vacation, Ma and Pa Kettle Go to Waikiki, Redhead from Wyoming; prod., Ma and Pa Kettle at Home, Golden Blade, Man with a Gun, Kettles in the Ozarks; dir. The Big Boodle; co-writer, dir. Man with a Gun; co-writer, dir., Raw Wind in Eden; dir., Al Capone; collab. s.p., dir. Invitation to a Gunfighter, Three in the Attic (prod.-dir.).

WILSON, SCOTT: Actor. b. Atlanta, Ga., 1942. Was college athlete on basketball scholarship when injured and had to leave school. Moved to L.A. and enrolled in local acting class. Made film debut, In Cold Blood, 1968.

PICTURES INCLUDE: The Grissom Gang, The Gypsy Moths, Castle Keep, In the Heat of the Night, The New Centurions, Lolly-Madonna XXX, The Great Gatsby, The Aviator, A Year of the Quiet Sun, Blue City.

WILSON, WARREN: Writer, producer. b. Boston, Mass., May 11, 1909. On stage under name Warren Burke. Began writing for screen 1941; screenplay Blondie Goes to College, Col. in 1942; Tanks a Million, UA; Sing Your Worries Away, RKO; Helzapoppin, Strictly in the Groove.

PICTURES INCLUDE: (collab., s.p.) She Gets Her Man; (story, prod.) Her Lucky Night; (collab. s.p.) If You Knew Susie; (org. s.p.) Square Dance Katy; (s.p.) Big Timber.

WINCER, SIMON: Director. b. Australia. Directed over 200 hours of dramatic programs for Australian TV, including Cash and Company, Tandarra, Ryan, Against the Wind,

The Sullivans, etc. Exec. prod. of The Man from Snowy River, top-grossing theatrical film in Australia.
PICTURES: Snapshot, Harlequin, Phar Lap, D.A.R.Y.L.

WINCHELL, PAUL: Perfomer. b. New York, N.Y., 1924. e. School of Industrial Arts. At 13 won first prize Major Bowes Radio Amateur Hour; signed by Ted Weems; created Jerry Mahoney when 17; ventriloquist & star own Paul Winchell-Jerry Mahoney show, NBC-TV.

WINDSOR, MARIE: Actress. b. Maryvale, Utah, Dec. 11, 1924. r.n. Emily Marie Bertelson. Winner of beauty contests, including Miss Utah. Worked as telephone girl, dancing teacher. Trained for acting by Maria Ouspenskaya.
PICTURES INCLUDE: Song of the Thin Man, Force of Evil, Dakota Lil, Little Big Horn, The Narrow Margin, The Eddie Cantor Story, The Bounty Hunter, Swamp Woman, The Killing, The Story of Mankind, Critics Choice, Mail Order Bride, Chamber of Horrors, Support Your Local Gunfighter, One More Train To Rob, Cahill, U.S. Marshall, The Outfit, Freaky Friday.

WINELAND, FRED L.: Theatre Executive. b. Washington, D.C., 1926. e. Southeastern Univ. (1957). Pres., Wineland Theatres, circuit which owns and operates two Maryland drive-ins, three Maryland indoor multi-cinemas and two Virginia multi-cinemas.

WINFIELD, PAUL: Actor. b. Los Angeles, 1940. e. UCLA.
PICTURES: The Lost Man, RPM, Brother John, Sounder, Gordon's War, Conrack, Justle, Damnation Alley, The Greatest, A Hero Ain't Nothin' But a Sandwich, Twilight's Last Gleaming, Carbon Copy, Star Trek II—The Wrath of Khan, White Dog, On the Run, Mike's Murder, Go Tell It on the Mountain, The Terminator, Blue City.
TELEVISION: King, Backstairs at the White House, Angel City, Key Tortuga, The Sophisticated Gents, Dreams Don't Die, Sister Sister, The Blue and the Gray, For Us the Living, Under Siege.

WINGER, DEBRA: Actress. Began career in TV series Wonder Woman; also featured in TV film, Special Olympics. Feature film debut: Slumber Party (1976).
PICTURES: Thank God, It's Friday, French Postcards, Urban Cowboy, Cannery Row, An Officer and a Gentleman, Mike's Murder, Terms of Endearment, Legal Eagles, Made in Heaven.

WINITSKY, ALEX: Producer. In partnership as attorneys in L.A. for 20 years with Arlene Sellers before they turned to financing and later production of films.
PICTURES INCLUDE: (co-prod. with Winitsky) End of the Game, The Seven-Per-Cent Solution, Cross of Iron, Night Calls, Silver Bears, Cuba, Blue Skies Again, Scandalous, Swing Shift, Bad Medicine.

WINKLER, HENRY: Actor. b. New York City, Oct. 30, 1945. e. Emerson College, Yale School of Drama. Appeared with Yale Reportory Co.; returned to N.Y. to work in radio. Did 30 TV commercials before starring in The Great American Dream Machine and Masquerade on TV.
PICTURES INCLUDE: The Lords of Flatbush (debut), Crazy Joe, Heroes, The One and Only, Night Shift.
TV: The Mary Tyler Moore Show, The Bob Newhart Show, The Paul Sand Show, Rhoda, Happy Days (regular), Laverne & Shirley. Movie: Katherine.

WINKLER, IRWIN: Producer. b. N.Y.C. e. N.Y. Univ. With I. Robert Chartoff formed production co., Chartoff-Winkler Prods. All films co-produced with Chartoff.
PICTURES INCLUDE: Double Trouble, Point Blank, The Split, They Shoot Horses, Don't They?, The Strawberry Statement, Leo The Last, Believe in Me, The Gang That Couldn't Shoot Straight, The New Centurions, Up the Sandbox, The Mechanic, Busting, SPY's, The Gambler, Breakout, Rocky, Nickelodeon, New York, New York, Valentino, Comes a Horseman, Uncle Joe Shannon, Raging Bull, True Confessions, Rocky III, Author! Author!; Right Stuff, Rocky IV.

WINNER, MICHAEL: Producer, director, writer. b. London, Eng. 1935. e. Cambridge U.; ent. m.p. ind. as columnist, dir., Drummer Films.
TV: White Hunter series, Dick and the Duchess series.
PICTURES INCLUDE: orig. s.p., Man With A Gun; prod. dir., writ., Shoot to Kill, Swiss Holiday, Climb Up the Wall, Out of the Shadow, Some Like it Cool, Girls, Girls, Girls, It's Magic, Behave Yourself; formed, Scimitar Films; prod. dir., Haunted England, Play It Cool, The Cool Mikado; dir., West 11; co-prod., dir., The System; co-author, dir. You Must Be Joking; co-prod. author. dir. The Jokers; prod. dir. I'll Never Forget What's 'Is Name; prod. dir., Hannibal Brooks, The Nightcomers, Chato's Land; dir. The Mechanic, Scorpio, The Stone Killer 1973, Death Wish, (prod. dir.), 1974 Won Ton Ton, The Dog That Saved Hollywood (prod., dir.), 1975. Prod. dir. The Sentinel, 1976, The Big Sleep, 1977; Firepower, 1978; Death Wish II, 1982; The Wicked lady (also co-s.p.), 1983; Scream for Help (prod., dir.); Death Wish 3 (prod., dir.), 1984.

WINTERS, DEBORAH: Actress. b. Los Angeles. e. Professional Children's School, New York City, began studying acting with Stella Adler at age 13. Acting debut at age six in TV Commercials.
CREDITS: Me, Natalie, Hail Hero!, The People Next Door, Kotch, The People Next Door (TV production) Class of '44.

WINTERS, DAVID: Choreographer, actor, director. b. London, April 5. Acted in both Broadway and m.p. version of West Side Story. Directed and acted in number of TV shows. Choreography credits include films Viva Las Vegas, Billie, Send Me No Flowers, Tickle Me, Pajama Party, Girl Happy, The Swinger, Made in Paris, Easy Come, Easy Go, Was choreographer for TV series Hullabaloo and Steve Allen Show, and several TV specials.

WINTERS, JERRY: Producer, director. b. Waterbury, Conn., Aug. 18, 1917. e. Antioch College, B.A., 1940. Photog., 1940–42; U.S. Air Force, 1942–46; photog., Hollywood, 1946–47; prod. assoc. Tonight on Broadway, CBS-TV, 1949; assc. prod., College Bowl, ABC-TV, 1950–51; in charge N.Y. film prod., Television Varieties, Inc., 1951–54; Production head Eldorado Int'l Pictures Corp., 1964–67; vice president, Edutornics Corp., 1968; pres. Giralda Pros., 1971.
PICTURES INCLUDE: prod., Renoir; prod.-dir., Herman Melville's Moby Dick, Speak to Me Child; prod; English version, The Loves of Liszt.

WINTERS, JONATHAN: Perfomer. b. Dayton, Ohio, Nov. 11, 1925. e. Kenyon College. Disc jockey, Dayton and Columbus stations; night club comedian.
TV: And Here's the Show, Columbus—TV, NBC Comedy Hour, Jonathan Winters Show, NBC-TV.
PICTURES INCLUDE: It's A Mad, Mad, Mad, Mad World, The Loved One, Viva Max, The Fish That Saved Pittsburgh, The Longshot.

WINTERS, RICHARD J.: Executive. b. New York City, Oct. 3, 1928. e. Columbia Univ. Started in film industry in 1952 in pub. dep't., RKO Pictures; joined 20th-Fox in 1954 in pub. dept., first as nat'l. mag. contact then dir. of special events; went to MGM 1957 as nat'l. mag. contact, named N.Y. pub. mgr., 1959; nat'l. pub. dir., 1961; in 1969 named nat'l. pub. dir. for Columbia Pictures. Worked on production pub. assignments for MGM and Paramount in 1972. Named nat'l. dir. adv.-pub.-prom., Paramount TV, 1973; promoted to exec. dir. adv./pub./promo., 1977.

WINTERS, ROLAND: Actor. b. Boston, Mass., Nov. 22, 1905. Appeared on stage and in stock, 1923–33; numerous radio programs, 1933–47. On screen in 13 Rue Madaleine, Return of October. Starred as Charlie Chan in pictures for Monogram.
PICTURES INCLUDE: West Point Story, Follow the Sun, Inside Straight, She's Working Her Way Through College, Jet Pilot, So Big.

WINTERS, SHELLEY: Actress. r.n. Shirley Schrift. b. St. Louis, Mo., Aug. 18, 1922. e. Wayne U. Clerked in 5 & 10 cent store; in vaudeville; on dramatic stage (Conquest, Night Before Christmas, Meet the People, Rosalinda, etc.). On screen 1944 in Nine Girls, Sailor's Holiday. N.Y. stage; A Hatful of Rain, Girls of Summer, Minnie's Boys.
PICTURES INCLUDE: Double Life, Cry of the City, Larceny, Take one False Step, Johnny Stool Pigeon, Great Gatsby, South Sea Sinner, Winchester '73, Place in the Sun, Untamed Frontier, My Man and I, Tennessee Champ, Executive Suite, Saskatchewan, Playgirl, Mambo, Night of the Hunter, I Am a Camera, Big Knife, Treasure of Pancho Villa, I Died a Thousand Times, Cash on Delivery, Diary of Anne Frank, Young Savages, Lolita, Chapman Report, A House is Not a Home, A Patch of Blue, Alfie, Enter Laughing, The Scalphunters, Wild in the Streets, Buena Sera Mrs. Campbell, The Mad Room, Bloody Mama, What's the Matter with Helen?, The Poseidon Adventure, Cleopatra Jones, Something To Hide, Blume in Love, Diamonds, Next Stop Greenwich Village, The Tenant, Pete's Dragon, City on Fire, "S.O.B.", Over the Brooklyn Bridge, Ellie, Deja Vu, The Delta Force.

WINTMAN, MELVIN R.: Theatre Executive, b. Chelsea, MA. e. Univ. of Mass., Northeastern Univ. (degree of juris doctor). Major, infantry, AUS, World War II. Attorney. Now consultant & dir., General Cinema Corp.; formerly exec. v.p., GCC and pres., GCC Theatres, Inc., Boston. Dir. Will Rogers Memorial Fund. Former pres. Theatre Owners of New England (1969–70); past dir. NATO (1969–70); treas., Nat'l Assoc. of Concessionaires (1960).

WISBERG, AUBREY: Writer, producer, director. b. London, Eng., Oct. 20; e. Columbia U. Newspaper writer, radio, TV dramatist U.S. Eng., Australia, radio diffusionist, Paris, France. Author novels Bushman at Large, Patrol Boat 999, This Is the Life; plays Virtue, Inc., Whiphand.
PICTURES INCLUDE: s.p., prod. The Man From Planet X, Captive Women, Sword of Venus, The Neanderthal

Man, Capt. John Smith & Pocahontas, Problem Girls, Dragon's Gold, Capt. Kidd & the Slave Girl, Return to Treasure Island, Murder is My Beat, The Women of Pitcairn Island, Port Sinister, Submarine Raider, Counter Espionage, Escape in the Fog, U-Boat Prisoner, Power of the Whistler, Adventures of Rusty, After Midnight, The Wreck of the Hesperus, The Big Fix, Betrayal from the East. The Falcon's Adventure, Son of Sinbad, At Swords Point, Hit Parade, They Came to Blow Up America, Bombers Moon, Rendezvous 24, The Lady in the Iron Mask, The Steel Lady, Treasure of Monte Cristo, Road to the Big House, The Burning Cross, St. Montana Mike, Casanova's Big Night, So Dark the Night, The Desert Hawk, s.p. Just Before Dawn, Out of the Depths, Target Minus Forty, Mission Mars, Ride the Wild Wind, Hercules in N.Y., Evil in the Blood.

WISDOM, NORMAN: Actor, singer, comedian. Musical and legit. b. London, Eng. Many London West End Stage shows including Royal Command Performances. New York Broadway shows include Walking Happy and Not Now Darling. Two Broadway awards. Films include Trouble in Store (Academy Award) and 19 others mostly for the Rank Organization and United Artists. Latest American film, The Night They Raided Minsky's.

WISE, ROBERT: Producer, director. b. Winchester, Ind., Sept. 10, 1914; e. Franklin Coll., Franklin, Ind. No prior bus. experience. Ent. m.p. ind. in cutting dept. RKO, 1933; sound cutter, asst. ed.; film ed., 1939; dir., 1943; to 20th Century-Fox, 1949; ass'n. Mirisch Co. independent prod. 1959; assn. MGM independent prod., 1962; assn. 20th Century Fox Independent Prod. 1963. Partner, Filmakers Group, The Tripar Group.
PICTURES INCLUDE: The Body Snatchers, Blood on the Moon, The Set Up, Day the Earth Stood Still, Captive City, So Big, Executive Suite, Helen of Troy, Tribute to a Bad Man, Somebody Up There Likes Me, Until They Sail, Run Silent Run Deep, I Want to Live, Odds Against Tomorrow, West Side Story, Two For the Seesaw, The Haunting, The Sound of Music, The Sand Pebbles, Star!, The Andromeda Strain, Two People, The Hindenburg, Audrey Rose, Star Trek.

WISEMAN, JOSEPH: Actor. b. Montreal, Canada, 1918. Began acting in the thirties, including Bdwy. stage, radio, m.p. and later TV.
PICTURES INCLUDE: Viva Zapata, Les Miserables, The Silver Chalice, The Garment Jungle, Dr. No, Bye Bye Braverman, The Night They Raided Minsky's, The Valachi Papers, The Apprenticeship of Duddy Kravitz, The Betsy.
STAGE: King Lear, Golden Boy, The Diary of Anne Frank, Uncle Vanya, The Last Analysis, Enemies, etc.

WITHERS, GOOGIE: Actress. b. Karachi, India, Mar. 12, 1917. Trained as a dancer under Italia Conti, Helena Lehmiski & Buddy Bradley; stage debut Victoria Palace in Windmill Man, 1929. Best Actress Award, Deep Blue Sea, 1954. Began screen career at 18. TV also. Theatrical tours Australia, Sun Award, Best Actress, 1974.
PICTURES INCLUDE: Traveler's Joy, Night and the City, White Corridors, Derby Day, Devil on Horseback, Safe Harbor, Nickel Queen.
STAGE: (Britain) Winter Journey, Deep Blue Sea, Hamlet, Much Ado About Nothing. (Australian) Plaza Suite, Relatively Speaking, Beckman Place, Woman in a Dressing Gown, The Constant Wife, First Four Hundred Years, Roar Like a Dove, The Cherry Orchard, An Ideal Husband. (London) Getting Married, Exit the King. (New York) The Complaisant Lover, Chichester Festival Theatre and Haymarket, London, in The Circle, The Kingfisher, Importance of Being Earnest, The Cherry Orchard, Dandy Dick, The Kingfisher (Australia), Time and the Conways (Chichester), School for Scandal (London), Stardust (UK tour).
TV: Series, Within These Walls.

WITHERS, JANE: Actress. b. Atlanta, Ga., 1927. By 1934 attracted attention as child player on screen, after radio appearance in Los Angeles and experimental pictures parts, in 1934 in Fox production Bright Eyes, Ginger; thereafter to 1942 featured or starred in numerous 20th-Fox prod. Voted Money-Making Star M.P. Herald-Fame Poll 1937, 1938.
PICTURES INCLUDE: North Star, Johnny Doughboy, My Best Gal, Faces in the Fog, Dangerous Partners, Affairs of Geraldine, Danger Street, Giant, The Right Approach, Captain Newman.

WIZAN, JOE: Executive. Started in industry as agent for William Morris Agency. Left to form London Intl. Artists, Ltd. in association with Richard Gregson, Alan Ladd, Jr. and Mike Gruskoff. When firm dissolved joined Creative Management Associates as v.p. in chg. of creative services. In 1969 formed own indep. prod. co. 1981, named pres., CBS Theatrical Film Div. 1982, returned to 20th Century-Fox as independent producer. 1983, named pres., 20th-Fox Prods.; Resigned in 1984.
PICTURES: Jeremiah Johnson, Junior Bonner, Prime Cut, The Last American Hero, Audrey Rose, Voices, And Justice for All, Best Friends, Unfaithfully Yours, Two of a Kind.

WIZEMAN, JR. DONALD G.: Executive. b. Fort Smith, Ark., Nov. 17, 1944. e. Old Dominion Univ. Formed Wizeman & Associates, Ltd. Advertising Agency and Artus Specialty Company in 1967; is pres. of both. In 1971 formed Filmakers, Ltd. which also heads.
PICTURES INCLUDE: Moonchild (exec. prod.), Come Out of the Bathroom Hannibal Fry (exec. prod.).

WOLCOTT, JAMES L.: Executive. b. Wilmington, Del. e. Williams Coll., Harvard Bus. Sch.; Wilmington Trust Co., banking dept.; Fox Film Corp. New York legal dept.; Fox Movietonews cutter, asst. ed. short subjects dept.; Fox Film Corp. publicity dept.; DeLuxe Lab.; 20th Century-Fox Studios asst. dir., head of test dept.; March of Time prod. mgr., ed. board; Audience Research, Inc. v.p. and gen. mgr.; Pathe Laboratories, Inc. sales v.p., exec. v.p. and director; Pathecolor, Inc. pres. and director; Transamerica Releasing Corp. pres. and director; Dorado Int'l Corp. pres. and director; James Wolcott Productions, Inc. pres. and director.

WOLF, EMANUEL, L.: Executive b. Brooklyn, N.Y., Mar. 27, 1927. e. Syracuse U.B.A., 1950; Maxwell School, Syracuse U. M.A. 1952; Maxwell Scholar in Public Admin.-Economics; Chi Eta Sigma (Econ. Hon.). 1952–55. Management consultant, exec. office of Secretary of Navy & Dept. of Interior, Wash., D.C. 1956. National dir. of Program & Admin. of a Veterans Org. 1957–61. Pres. E. L. Wolf Associates, Washington, D.C. 1961–Jan. 1965. Treasurer, Kalvex, Inc. Dec. 1962. Director Kalvex, Inc. March 1963. Dir. Allied Artists Pictures Corp., Jan. 1965. Pres. Kalvex, Inc. April 1966–present, pres. & chmn. of the Bd. Kalves, Inc.; Chmn. of the Bd. Vitabath, Inc.; Chmn. of the Bd. Lexington Instruments; pres. & chairman of the Bd. Pharmaceutical Savings Plan, Inc. Syracuse U. Corporate Advisory Board, American Committee for the Weizmann Institute of Science (Bd. of Directors). Pres. and Chmn. of Bd., Allied Artists Pictures Corp: January, 1976: pres., bd. chm. & chief executive officer of Allied Artists Industries Inc., created by Merger of Allied Artists Pictures Corp., Kalvex Inc. and PSP, Inc. 1985, formed independent prod. co., Mended Dreams, Inc.

WOLF, HERBERT: Producer. b. New York, N.Y., July 11, 1917. e. N.Y.U., 1937. Radio & TV prod. Wolf Presentations, Inc.
TV: (N.Y.) Masquerade Party, Break the Bank, Hold That Note, Keep Talking, Window Shopping.

WOLF, THOMAS HOWARD: TV news exec. b. New York, N.Y., April 22, 1916; e. Princeton, B.A., magna cum laude, 1937. Time & Life Mag. 1937–39; 1937–39 NEA (Scripps-Howard) 1940–46; European mgr., NEA, 1942–46. War correspondent, ETO, MTO) NBC radio correspondent, Paris, 1944–45; co-owner, pres., Information Prod., Inc. founded 1951; co-owner, chairman. Butterfield & Wolf, Inc. founded 1955; prod. CBS series. Tomorrow, 1960; exec. prod., CBS daily live Calendar Show, 1961–62; senior prod., ABC News Report, 1963; exec. prod., ABC Scope, 1964–66. v.p. dir. of TV Documentaries, 1966; v.p., dir. of TV Public Affairs, 1974; dir. TV Cultural Affairs, 1976.

WOLFF, LOTHAR: Producer, director, president: Lothar Wolff Productions Inc. b. Bromberg, Ger. Asst. prod., March of Time WWII; Officer in Charge, U.S. Coast Guard M.P. section; head, Marshall Plan film section, Paris, 1949–50; M.P. advisor to Indonesian Govt. 1953–55; v.p. & prod., Louis de Rochemont Assoc.; prod. & co-author, Martin Luther, produced: Question Seven, 13 half hour Planet Earth and five Year of the Quiet Sun Films (Natl Academy of Sciences), Fortress of Peace (Swiss Govt. Cinerama); assoc. prod. Lost Boundaries, Walk East on Beacon, Windjammer, Roman Spring of Mrs. Stone. Series executive producer for Time-Life Films (The World We Live In; Other People, Other Places; Wild, Wild World of Animals). Editorial Director, I Sought my Brother, Harvard U./WQED; Producer, The Joy of Bach, Lutheran Film Associates, a 60-minute special. Three astronomy films for Educational Dept. of National Geographic; 1 hr. special, The Sky's the Limit, for Cable-TV div. of National Geographic.

WOLFSON, RICHARD: Executive. b. New York City, Jan. 7, 1923. e. Harvard Coll. Yale Law School, 1945–47, law sect'y to Justice Wiley Rutledge, U.S. Supreme Court; law instructor at NYU Law School; later received Guggenheim Fellowship; 1952, joined Wometco Ent. as counsel and asst. to pres.; named v.p. and dir. in 1959 and senior v.p. in 1962; named exec. v.p. and general counsel in 1973; named chm., exec. comm., 1976; co-author of Jurisdiction of the Supreme Court of the United States and author of articles in various legal publications. Retired from Wometco 1982; counsel, Kreeger & Kreeger, Miami.

WOLPER, DAVID L.: Producer. b. New York, N.Y., Jan. 11, 1928. e. Drake U., U. of So. Calif., Treas., Flamingo Films,

1948; merged with Associated Artist to form M.P. for TV, Inc., acting as v.p. in chge of West Coast oper., 1950; v.p. reactivated Flamingo Films, 1954; also pres. Harris-Wolper Pictures, Inc.; pres. Wolper Prod. 1958; pres. Dawn Prod.; v.p. Bd. Dir. Metromedia, 1965; pres. Wolper Pictures Ltd. 1967; ch. of bd. Wolper Prod., Inc., 1967; pres. Wolper Pictures, 1968; pres. Wolper Productions, 1970; pres. & ch. of bd. of dir. The Wolper Organization, Inc., 1971; consultant to Warner Bros. & Warner Communications. Pres., David L. Wolper Prods., Inc. 1977; married Gloria Diane Hill, July 11, 1974.

TV & M.P.: The Race For Space, 1958; Story of . . . series, 1962–63; Biography series, 1962–63; Hollywood and the Stars series, 1963–64; The Making of the President, 1960, 1964, 1968; Men in Crisis series, 1964; Four Days in November feature, 1965; National Geographic Society Specials, 1965–68, 1971–75; The March of Time series, 1965–66; The Rise and Fall of the Third Reich, 1967–68; The Undersea World of Jacques Cousteau, 1967–68; If It's Tuesday, This Must Be Belgium feature, 1968; Plimpton specials, 1970–72; Say Goodbye, 1971; Willy Wonka and the Chocolate Factory feature, 1971; Appointment With Destiny series, 1971–73; Visions of Eight feature, 1973; American Heritage specials, 1973–74; Primal Man specials, 1973–75; Get Christie Love series, 1974; Judgment specials, 1974; Birds Do It, Bees Do It feature, 1974; Chico and the Man series, 1974–; Smithsonian Specials, 1974–; Sandburg's Lincoln, 1974–76; Welcome Back, Kotter series, 1975–; I Will Fight No More, Forever, 1975; Collison Course, Victory at Entebbe, 1976; Roots, 1977; Roots: The Next Generation, 1978; Moviola, 1980; Agatha Christie: Murder Is Easy, 1981; Casablanca, 1982; The Thorn Birds, 1983.

WOODHAM-SMITH GEORGE IVON: Solicitor. b. London, England, Dec. 20, 1895. 1st Lt., Machine Gun Corps., Brit. Army, World War I, studied law; also journalist. Since 1928 partner in Richards Butler & Co., London law firm. In charge of legal work for the Rank Orig.

WOODLAND, NORMAN: Actor. b. Dusseldorf, Germany March 16, 1910; e. Edward VI School. Stratford-on-Avon. Spent several years in repertory cos.; joined BBC 1939 and spent 6 yrs. as commentator; stage career largely assoc. with Shakespearean and classical plays; TV appearances; screen debut in Hamlet.

PICTURES INCLUDE: Escape, I Know You, All Over the Town, Background, Romeo and Juliet, Master Plan, Richard III, Teenage Daughter, Guilty, No Road Back, The Bandit, Rough and the Smooth.

WOODS, DONALD: Actor. b. 1906.

PICTURES INCLUDE: Watch on the Rhine, Roughly Speaking, 13 Ghosts, Kissin' Cousins, Moment to Moment, A Time to Sing.

STAGE: Two for the Seesaw, L.A., 1961; Rosmersholm, NYC, 1962; One by One, NYC, 1964; Soldier, You Can't Take It With You, Chicago, 1969; Twelfth Night, Assassination 1865; Chicago, 1969–71.

TV: G.E. Theatre, Wagon Train, Thrillers, Sunset Strip, Ben Casey, Laramie, The Rebel, The Law and Mr. Jones, The Roaring 20's, Wild Wild West, Bonanza.

PICTURES: The Way We Were, Alex and the Gypsy, The Choirboys, The Onion Field, The Black Marble, Eyewitness, Captured, Fast Walking, Videodrome, Against All Odds, Once Upon a Time in America, Cat's Eye, Joshua Then and Now, Salvador.

TELEVISION: Movies: All the Way Home, The Great American Tragedy, The Disappearance of Aimee, Raid on Entebbe, Billion Dollar Bubble, Badge of the Assassin. Mini-series: Holocaust.

WOODS, JAMES: Actor. b. Vernal UT, Apr. 18, 1947. e. MIT. Left college to pursue acting career in New York; appeared off-Bdwy. in Borstal Boy, Conduct Unbecoming, Saved, etc. Also in Trial of the Catonsville Nine, Moonchildren, Green Julia, Finishing Touches, etc. Feature film debut in Visitors (1971).

PICTURES: The Way We Were, Alex and the Gypsy, The Choirboys, The Onion Field, The Black Marble, Eyewitness, Captured, Fast Walking, Videodrome, Against All Odds, Once Upon a Time in America, Cat's Eye, Joshua Then and Now, Salvador.

TELEVISION: Movies: All the Way Home, The Great American Tragedy, The Disappearance of Aimee, Raid on Entebbe, Billion Dollar Bubble, Badge of the Assassin. Mini-series: Holocaust.

WOODWARD, EDWARD: O.B.E. Actor, Singer. b. Croydon, England, 11 LPs. 1 Gold Disc.

TV: Sword of Honour, Callan series. Over 300 TV plays latest: Bassplayer and Blonde, Saturday, Sunday, Monday, 1990 series, Nice Work, Rod of Iron, The Trial of Lady Chatterly's Lover, Wet Job—Callan Special, Churchill: The Wildnerness Years, Blunt Instrument, Killer Contact. Television Actor of the Year, 1969–70; also Sun Award Best Actor 1970, 71, 72.

PICTURES INCLUDE: Becket, File on the Golden Goose, Murders in the Rue Morgue, Julius Caesar, The Listener, Young Winston, Sitting Target, Hunted, Wicker Man, Callan, Stand Up Virgin Soldiers, Breaker Morant, The Appointment, Who Dares Wins, Forever Love, Merlin and the Sword, Champions, A Christmas Carol, King David.

THEATRE: 16 West End Plays and Musicals. Latest: On Approval, Richard III, The Assassin.

WOODWARD, JOANNE: Actress. b. Thomasville, Ga., Feb. 27, 1930. e. La. State U. Studied at Neighborhood Playhouse Dramatic Sch. m. Paul Newman, N.Y.; appeared in many TV dramatic shows; on B'way in Picnic; m.p. debut in Count Three and Pray.

PICTURES INCLUDE: Kiss Before Dying, Three Faces of Eve (Academy Award 1957, best actress); Long Hot Summer, No Down Payment, Rally Round the Flag Boys, The Sound and the Fury, From the Terrace, Fugitive Kind, Paris Blues, The Stripper, A New Kind of Love, Signpost to Murder, A Big Hand for the Little Lady, Rachel, Rachel (Acad. Award nom.); Winning, WUSA, The Effect of Gamma Rays on Man-in-the-Moon Marigolds, Summer Wishes, Winter Dreams, The Drowning Pool, The End, Harry and Son.

TV: Movies: Sybil, See How She Runs, Passions, Do You Remember Love.

WOODY, CHESTER F.: Actor. b. Zoar Valley, Colo., Aug. 13, 1934; e. U. of Colo. Writer, stories, songs, lyrics used on radio, TV.

PICTURES INCLUDE: The Glenn Miller Story, The Mob, Monsters of the Deep, Hit the Deck, The Rangers, The Big Circus, Gangland, Adventure Is our Destiny, Freed, Distant Field Are Greener, And Now My Love, Murder at Midnight, The Queen's Guard, Look Back and Cry.

WOOLF, SIR JOHN: Chairman Romulus Films, Ltd. Chm., British and American Film Holdings, Plc.

PICTURES INCLUDE: Pandora and the Flying Dutchman, African Queen, Moulin Rouge, Beat the Devil, Carrington V.C., I am a Camera, Sailor Beware, Three Men in a Boat, The Story of Esther Costello, Room at the Top, The L-Shaped Room, Life At The Top, Oliver! (Oscar for best film 1969), The Day of the Jackal, The Odessa File.

WOPAT, TOM: Actor. b. Lodi, WI, Sept. 9, 1951. e. University of Wisconsin. Left school to travel for two years with rock group as lead singer and guitarist. Spent two summers at Barn Theater in Michigan. Came to New York; off-Bdwy. in A Bistro Car on the CNR. On Bdwy. in hit play, I Love My Wife. Now star of TV's The Dukes of Hazzard.

WORMSER, RICHARD: Writer. b. New York, N.Y., Jan. 30, 1908. e. Princeton U. Publicist. 1927–32; fiction writer, Street & Smith, 1932–34; freelance fiction writer, 1934–41; forest officer. U.S. Forest Service. 1941–45; then free lance m.p., magazine writer; novels include Pass through Manhattan, Lonesome Quarter, Road to Carmichael's.

PICTURES INCLUDE: s.p., In Self Defense; collab. orig., The Showdown; orig. s.p. Fort Dodge Stampede.

WORTH, IRENE: Actress. b. Nebraska, June 23, 1916. Bdwy. debut in The Two Mrs. Carrolls, after which went to London where made her home. Appeared with Old Vic and Royal Shakespeare Co.; returned to U.S. to appear on Bdwy. in the Cocktail Party, Toys in the Attic, Sweet Bird of Youth, Cherry Orchard; etc.

PICTURES: Orders to Kill (British AA as best actress), King Lear, Nicholas and Alexander, Rich Kids, Eyewitness, Deathtrap, Fast Forward.

TELEVISION:: The Lady from the Sea, The Duchess of Malfi, The Way of the World, Prince Orestes, etc.

WORTH, MARVIN: Producer-Writer. b. Brooklyn, NY. Jazz promoter and manager before starting to write special material for Alan King, Buddy Hackett, Joey Bishop.

PICTURES: Writer: Boys Night Out, Three on a Couch, Promise Her Anything. Producer: Where's Poppa?, Lenny, Fire Sale, The Rose, Up the Academy, Unfaithfully Yours, Rhinestone, Falling in Love.

TELEVISION: Steve Allen Show, Jackie Gleason, Milton Berle Show, Colgate Comedy Hour, Judy Garland Show, etc.

WOWCHUK, HARRY N.: Actor, Writer, Photographer, Producer, Executive. b. Phila. Pa. Oct. 16, 1948. e. Santa Monica City College, U.C.L.A. Theater Arts, 1970. Started film career as actor, stunt-driver-photographer. T.V. and commercial credits include: Warner Bros.; Columbia Records; R.C.A.; Playboy Magazine: T.V. Guide; Seal Test; Camel Cigarettes; Miller High Life; American Motors; Camera V; A&W Rootbeer; Harold Robbins Productions. Former exec. v.p. International Cinema, in charge of prod. and distribution; V.P. J. Newport Film Productions; pres., United West Productions.

PICTURES INCLUDE: The Lost Dutchman, Las Vegas Lady, This Is A Hijack, Tidal Wave, Tunnel Vision, Incredible 2-Headed Transplant, Jud, Bad Charleston Charlie, Some Call It Loving, Summer School Teachers, Five Minutes of

Freedom, Pushing Up Daisies, Money-Marbles-Chalk, The Models, Love Swedish Style, Up-Down-Up, Sunday's Child, Soul Brothers, Freedom Riders, Perilous Journey, Claws of Death, Georgia Peaches.

WOWCHUK, NICHOLAS: Executive, Producer, Writer, Editor, Financier. b. Philadelphia, Pa. e. St. Basil's College, U.C.L.A. Founder-publisher: All-American Athlete Magazine; Sports and Health Digest; The Spectator. Former sports writer: Phila. Evening Public Ledger; Phila. Daily Record; Phila. Inquirer. Founder & board chairman: Mutual Realty Investment Co.; Mutual Mortgage Co., Beverly Hills, Calif. President: Mutual General Films, Bev. Hills, Calif.; Abbey Theatrical Films, N.Y.C.; Mutual Film Distribution Co.; Mutual Recording & Broadcasting Enterprises.
PICTURES INCLUDE: Exec. Prod.: Perilous Journey; Incredible 2-Headed Transplant; Pushing Up Daisies; Money-Marbles-Chalk; Five Minutes Of Freedom; The Campaign; Claws of Death. Prod.: Scorpion's Web; Pursuit; Brave Men; Sea of Despair; The Hetman; Cossack's In Battle; The Straight White Line; Tilt, Rooster, To Live . . . You Gotta Win.

WRAY, FAY: Actress. b. Alberta, Canada, Sept. 10, 1907. m. Robert Riskin, writer. On stage in Pilgrimage Play, Hollywood, 1923; m.p. debut in Gasoline Love; thereafter in many m.p. for Paramount to 1930; then in films for various Hollywood and Brit. prod.
PICTURES INCLUDE: King Kong, Small Town Girl, Treasure of the Golden Condor, Rock Pretty Baby, Tammy, Out of Time, The Cobweb, Summer Love.
TV: Pride of the Family, ABC-TV.

WRIGHT, BASIL: Producer and director. b. London, June 12, 1907. Educated at Sherborne school, Corpus Christi College, Cambridge. Assistant, 1929, to John Grierson and was associated with him in creation of "documentary" film in England.
PICTURES INCLUDE: The Country Comes to Town, O'er Hill and Dale, Windmill in Barbadoes, Cargo from Jamaica, and Liner Cruising South for Empire Marketing Bd. in 1931–33. In 1934 made The Song of Ceylon and awarded First Prize and Prix de Gouvernement at Brussels Film Festival in 1935. With Henry Watt directed Night Mall for GPO Film Unit, under prod. of John Grierson. In 1937 founded Realist Film Unit. Exec. prod., Film Centre, Ltd., 1939–44. In 1945, prod. in chge, Crown Film Unit. In 1946 adv. to Dir. Gen. of M.O.I.; prod. dir. Waters & Time for Festival of Britain, 1950–51; made World Without End for Unesco 1953: with Gladys Wright prod. The Immortal Land and Greek Sculpture; prod. dir. A Place for Gold, 1960, 1962–68 Lecturer at U. of C., Los Angeles, 1974, published The Long View (a history of world cinema). 1975 Guest of Honour Melbourne Film Festival; 1975–76 Lecture Tour USA, Canada. 1977–78 Visiting Lecturer Temple Univ., Philadelphia.

WRIGHT, ROBERT C.: Executive. President and Chief Exec. Off., NBC Bdcst. Co., as of September 1986. 1969, joined General Electric; lawyer in plastics div. Later moved into product & sls. management in that div. 1980, moved to Cox Cable as pres. Returned to GE 1983 heading small appliances div.; moved to GE Financial Services & GE Credit Corp. as pres., which posts he held when named head of NBC following purchase of NBC's parent RCA by GE.

WRIGHT, TERESA: Actress. b. New York City, Oct. 27, 1918. m. Divorced from Niven Busch and Robert Anderson. Ent. m.p. 1941, The Little Foxes, Goldwyn-RKO. In 1942: Pride of the Yankees, Goldwyn-RKO, Mrs. Miniver, MGM Acad. Award 1942 supporting role (Mrs. Miniver).
PICTURES INCLUDE: Shadow of a Doubt, Casanova Brown, Best Years of Our Lives, Trouble with Women, Pursued, Imperfect Lady, Enchantment, The Capture, The Men, Something to Live For, California Conquest, Steel Trap, Count the Hours, The Actress, Track of the Cat, Hail Hero, The Happy Ending, Roseland, Somewhere in Time.
STAGE: Tours: Mary, Mary, Tchin-Tchin, The Effect of Gamma Rays on Man-in-the-Moon Marigolds, Noel Coward in Two Keys, The Master Builder. Regional Theatre: Long Day's, Journey into Night, You Can't Take It With You, All The Way Home, Wings. New York: Life with Father, Dark at the Top of the Stairs, I Never Sang for My Father, Death of a Salesman, Ah, Wilderness!, Morning's at Seven (Broadway and London).

WRIGHT, TONY: Actor. b. London, Dec. 10, 1925. Stage debut in repertory, South Africa; screen debut; Flanagan Boy, 1951.
PICTURES INCLUDE: A Toi De Jouer Callaghan, Plus De Whiskey, Pour Callaghan (France), Jumping for Joy, Jacqueline, Tiger in the Smoke, Seven Thunders, Broth of a Boy, Faces in the Dark, In the Wake of a Stranger, Journey to Nowhere, The Liquidator.
TV: Compact, Marriage Lines, No Hiding Place, The Saint, Mystery Theatre, Curtains for Sheila, Crossroads, Make Me A Widow, Wednesday's Train, Onedin Line, 6 Saints, Persuaders, The Jensen Code, Follow Me, Kidnapped.

WUNSCH, ROBERT J.: Executive. e. Yale. Literary agent—first with Adams, Ray & Rosenberg; later with Intl. Famous Agency. Entered indep. motion picture production; co-producer of Slap Shot, and exec. producer of Defiance. Named dir. of motion pictures for TV at CBS. Left to join United Artists as v.p., production, West Coast, in June, 1979.

WYATT, JANE: Actress. b. Aug. 10, 1913, New York: e. Miss Chapin's School, Barnard College; m. Edgar B. Ward. Joined Apprentice School, Berkshire Playhouse, Stockbridge, Mass. Understudied in Tradewinds and The Vinegar Tree. Appeared in Give Me Yesterday and the Tadpole. In 1933 succeeded Margaret Sullivan in Dinner at Eight. m.p.: New York stage, The Autumn Garden, 1951; other plays, The Bishop Misbehaves, Conquest, Eveninsong, The Mad Hopes.
PICTURES INCLUDE: Great Expectations, The Navy Comes Through, The Kansan, None But the Lonely Heart, Boomerang, Gentlemen's Agreement, No Minor Vices, Bad Boy, Canadian Pacific, Pitfall, Task Force, Our Very Own, My Blue Heaven, Man Who Cheated Himself, Criminal Lawyer, Lost Horizon, Never Too Late, Treasure of Matecumbe.
TV: Father Knows Best, winner 3 Emmy Awards (6 yrs.), Bob Hope Chrysler Theater, The Virginian, Wagon Train, U.S. Steel Hour, Bell Telephone Hour, Hostess moderator, Confidential For Women, My Father My Mother. Guest star—Star Trek, Barefoot in the Park Pilot CBS-TV, The Ghost and Mrs. Muir, Here Come the Brides, Love American Style, ABC Movie of Week, Guest star, the Men of Shiloh, Alias Smith and Jones, Kraft Music Hall; co-star, Hollywood TV Theater, Katherine (guest star), Tom Sawyer; Father Knows Best Reunion, A Love Affair, Amelia Earhart, Superdome, Fantasy Island, Love Boat, The Nativity, The Millionaire.

WYMAN, JANE: Actress. r.n. Sarah Jane Fulks. b. St. Joseph, Mo., Jan. 4, 1914. In 1936: My Man Godfrey, U; Cain and Mabel, Smart Blonde, Warner. From 1937 in many Hollywood pictures. In 1942: Larceny, Inc., My Favorite Spy, Footlight Serenade. Voted one of top ten money-making stars in M.P. Herald-Fame poll 1954. TV shows: Fireside Theatre, Falcon Crest.
PICTURES INCLUDE: Princess O'Rourke, Doughgirls, Make Your Own Bed, Crime by Night, Lost Weekend, One More Tomorrow, Night and Day, The Yearling, Cheyenne, Magic Town; academy award, best actress, Johnny Belinda, 1948, Three Guys Named Mike, Here Comes the Groom, Blue Veil, Just for You, Story of Will Rogers, Let's Do It Again, So Big, Magnificent Obsession, Lucy Gallant, All That Heaven Allows, Miracle in the Rain, Pollyanna, Holiday for Lovers, Bon Voyage, How to Commit Marriage.

WYMAN, THOMAS H.: Executive. b. 1931. Joined CBS, Inc. in 1980 as pres. & chief exec. Now chm. Prior career as chief exec. of Green Giant Co.; became v. chm. of Pillsbury Co. when it acquired Green Giant in 1979.

WYMORE, PATRICE: Actress. b. Miltonvale, Kans., Dec. 17, 1926. p. James A. Wymore, oper. exhib. film delivery service throughout Kans.; ret. Began career as child performer, tent shows, county fairs, vaudeville; later, toured night clubs in middle west, own song & dance act; modelled, Chicago understudy Betty Bruce, U Up in Central Park, played role Hollywood Bowl; then, NY stage, Hold It! All For Love; radio & TV roles.
PICTURES INCLUDE: Screen debut: Tea for Two, 1950, then Rocky Mountain, I'll See You In My Dreams, Star-Lift, Big Trees, Man Behind the Gun, She's Working Her Way Through College, She's Back on Broadway, Chamber of Horrors.

WYNN, KEENAN: Actor. b. New York City, July 27, 1916. s. of Ed Wynn (died June 19, 1966). e. St. John's Military Acad. New York stage, radio stock in Skowhegan, Me.
PICTURES INCLUDE: See Here, Private Hargrove, Since You Went Away, Marriage Is a Private Affair, Between Two Women, The Clock, Without Love, Week-End at the Waldorf, What Next Corporal Hargrove?, The Hucksters, B.F.'s Daughter, Three Musketeers, Neptune's Daughter, Annie Get Your Gun, Three Little Words, Royal Wedding, Kind Lady, Angela in the Outfield, Texas Carnival, Phone Call from a Stranger, Fearless Fagan, Sky Full of Moon, Desperate Search, Battle Circus, Code Two, All the Brothers Were Valiant, Kiss Me Kate, Long Long Trailer, Tennessee Champ, Men of the Fighting Lady, Glass Slipper, The Marauders, Running Wild, Man in the Gray Flannel Suit, Shack Out on 101, Johnny Concho, Great Man, Some Came Running, A Hole in the Head, King of the Roaring Twenties, Absent-Minded Professor, Warning Shot, Welcome to Hard Times, The War Wagon, Point Blank, Finian's Rainbow, McKenna's Gold, Smith, Once Upon a Time in

the West, 80 Steps to Jonah, Cancel My Reservation, Pretty Maids All in a Row, The Animals, B.J. Presents, The Mechanic, Snowball Express, Wild in the Sky, Herbie Rides Again, Nashville, The Devil's Rain, The Shaggy D.A., Orca, Just Tell Me What You Want, Best Friends.

WYNN, MAY: Actress. r.n. Donna Lee Hickey. b. New York, Jan. 8, 1930; e. Newtown H.S., Elmhurst, L.I. Model; Chorus girl, then singer, dancer; played bits in Hollywood; then The Caine Mutiny, They Rode West, Violent Men.

WYNN, TRACY KEENAN: Writer. b. Hollywood, CA, Feb. 28, 1945. Fourth generation of show business; son of actor Keenan Wynn; grandson of Ed Wynn; great-grandson of Frank Keenan Wynn, Irish Shakespearean actor who made Bdwy. debut in 1880.
PICTURES INCLUDE: The Longest Yard, The Deep (co. s.p.).
TV: The Glass House, Tribes, The Autobiography of Miss Jane Pittman, The Drowning Pool, Quest.

WYNNE, DONALD. Production executive and writer. b. Surrey, England 1918. Early career: actor, camera prod. assistant. Ent. m.p. industry 1935; served in Army 1938–46; since prod. man., assoc, prod. Concanen, Nettlefold, Pan Productions.
PICTURES INCLUDE: Fabian of the Yard series, On Such a Night, prod. sup. Rank Screen Services. Wrote, dir. prod. for African Film Prod. in S. and E. Africa; Donald Wynne Prods. Ltd.

WYNTER, DANA: Actress. b. London, England. June 8, 1930. e. Rhodes U. On stage in London; TV appearances include Robert Montgomery Show, Suspense, Studio One, U.S. Steel Hour.
PICTURES INCLUDE: Invasion of the Body Snatchers, View from Pompey's Head, D-Day, The Sixth of June, Something of Value, Fraulein, Shake Hands with the Devil, In Love and War, Sink the Bismarck, The List of Adrian Messenger, Airport.
TV: Playhouse 90, Dick Powell Show, Wagon Train, Virginian, Burkes Law, Bob Hope Presents, Alfred Hitchcock, Twelve O'Clock High, The Rogues, Ben Casey, FBI Story, My Three Sons, Wild Wild West, The Man Who Never Was, The Royal Romance of Charles and Diana.

Y

YABLANS, FRANK: Executive. B. Brooklyn, N.Y. Aug. 27, 1935. Ent. m.p. ind. as Warner Bros. booker, 1957. Warner Bros. salesman in N.Y., Boston, Milwaukee, Chicago, 1957–59. Milwaukee br. mgr. Buena Vista, 1959–66. Midwest sales mgr., Sigma III, 1966. Eastern sales mgr., 1967, sales v.p. 1968. V.P. general sales mgr., Paramount Pic. Corp., 1969; v.p.-dist., April 1970; sr. v.p.-mkt., Oct., 1970; exec. v.p., April 1971; named pres. May, 1971. In Jan., 1975, became an independent producer, his company called, Frank Yablans Presentations Inc. 1983, MGM/UA Entertainment Co. as bd. chm. & chief oper. off. Held titles of bd. chm. & chief exec. off. with both MGM and UA Corp when resigned, 1985. Same year teamed with PSO Delphi to form Northstar Entertainment Co.
PICTURES: Silver Streak (exec. prod.), The Other Side of Midnight (prod.), The Fury (prod.), North Dallas Forty (prod.-co-s.p.), Mommie Dearest (prod.-co-s.p.); Monsignor (co.-prod).

YABLANS, IRWIN: Executive. b. Brooklyn, N.Y. Began career in industry at WB in 1956 after two-yr. stint in Germany with U.S. Army. Held m.p. sales posts in Washington, D.C., Albany, Detroit, Milwaukee and Portland. In 1962 joined Paramount as L.A. mgr.; in 1964 made western sales mgr. In 1972 entered production as assoc. prod. on Howard W. Koch's Badge 373. First prod. on own: The Education of Sonny Carson (1974). Pres. of Compass Int'l. Pictures. Exec. v.p., low budget films, Lorimar Productions. Resigned June, 1984. In 1985 named chm., Orion Pictures Distributing Corp.
PICTURES: Halloween, Roller Boogie (both exec. prod.), Roller Boogie (exec. prod., story), Fade To Black (story). Produced Seduction and Tank (producer).

YATES, PETER: Producer, director. b. July 24, 1929. Ent. m.p. ind. as studio manager and dubbing asst. with De Lane Lea. Asst. dir. The Entertainer, The Guns of Navarone, A Taste of Honey. Stage: dir. The American Dream, The Death of Bessie Smith, Passing Game, Interpreters.
TV: Danger Man (Secret Agent), The Saint (series).
PICTURES INCLUDE: Summer Holiday, One Way Pendulum, Robbery, Bullitt, John and Mary, Murphy's War, The Hot Rock, The Friends of Eddie Coyle, For Pete's Sake, Mother, Jugs and Speed, The Deep, Breaking Away, Eyewitness, Krull, The Dresser, Eleni.

YORDAN, PHILIP: Writer. b. Chicago, Ill. e. University of Ill., B.A., Kent Coll. Law, LL.D. Author, producer, playwright (Anna Lucasta). Began screen writing 1942 with collab. s.p. Syncopation.
PICTURES INCLUDE: Unknown Guest, Johnny Doesn't Live Here, When Strangers Marry, Dillinger (Acad. Award nomination), Whistle Stop, The Chase, Suspense; play & s.p. Anna Lucasta, House of Strangers; s.p. Edge of Doom; collab. s.p. Detective Story, (Acad. Award nomination) Mary Maru, s.p., Houdini, Blowing Wild; collab. s.p., Man Crazy, Naked Jungle; s.p., Johnny Guitar; story, Broken Lance (Acad Award 1954); adapt. Conquest of Space; collab. s.p. Man from Laramie, Last Frontier; prod. s.p. Harder They Fall, Men In War, No Down Payment, God's Little Acre; s.p. Bravados, Time Machine, The Day of the Outlaw, Studs Lonigan, King of Kings; collab., El Cid, 55 Days at Peking, Fall of the Roman Empire; prod., Crack in the World, Battle of the Bulge, Royal Hunt of the Sun, Brigham, Cataclysm, Night Train to Terror, Satan's Warriors, Cry Wilderness.

YORK, DICK: Actor. r.n. Richard Allen York. b. Fort Wayne, Ind., Sept. 4, 1928. e. De Paul U. Drama School. Appeared on radio shows; commercial m.p. actor; on Broadway in Tea and Sympathy, Bus Stop; TV appearances.
TV: Omnibus, Robert Montgomery Show, Mr. D.A., The Web, Wagon Train, Alfred Hitchcock, Twilight Zone, Route 66, Going My Way, Bewitched.
PICTURES INCLUDE: Inherit the Wind, Cowboy, They Came to Cordura, My Sister Eileen, Three Stripes in the Sun.

YORK, MICHAEL: Actor. b. Fulmer, England, March 27, 1942. Early career with Oxford University Dramatic Society and National Youth Theatre; later Dundee Repertory, National Theatre.
TV: The Forsyte Saga, Rebel in the Grave, Great Expectations, Jesus of Nazareth, True Patriot, Much Ado About Nothing, A Man Called Intrepid, The Phantom of the Opera, The Master of Ballantrae, Space, For Those I Loved, The Far Country.
STAGE: Any Just Cause, Hamlet, Outcry (Broadway), Ring Round The Moon (Los Angeles), Bent, Cyrano De Bergerac, The Little Prince.
PICTURES INCLUDE: The Taming of the Shrew, Accident, Red and Blue, Smashing Time, Romeo and Juliet, The Strange Affair, The Guru, Alfred The Great, Justine, Something for Everyone, Zeppelin, La Poudre D'Escampette, Cabaret, England Made Me, Lost Horizon, The Three Musketeers, Murder on the Orient Express, The Four Musketeers, Conduct Unbecoming, Logan's Run, Seven Nights in Japan, The Last Remake of Beau Geste, The Island of Dr. Moreau, Fedora, The Riddle of the Sands, The White Lions, Final Assignment, Success Is the Best Revenge, Dawn.

YORK, SUSANNAH: Actress. b. London, Jan. 9, 1942. Ent. TV 1959. Appearances include: The Crucible The Rebel and the Soldier, The First Gentleman, The Richest Man in the World. Ent. films in 1960. Wrote two books: In Search of Unicorns and Lark's Castle.
PICTURES INCLUDE: Tunes of Glory, There Was a Crooked Man, Greengage Summer, Freud, Tom Jones, While the Tiger Sleeps, The Seventh Dawn, Scene Nun—Take One, Sands of Kalahari, Scruggs, Kaleidoscope, A Man for All Seasons, Sebastian, The Killing of Sister George, Oh What a Lovely War, The Battle of Britain, Lock Up Your Daughters, They Shoot Horses Don't They? (Acad. Award nom.), Brotherly Love, Zee & Co., Happy Birthday Wanda June, Images, The Maids, Gold, Conduct Unbecoming, Heaven Save Us From Our Friends, Sky Riders, The Silent Partner, Superman, The Shout, Superman II, Falling in Love Again, Alice Loophole, The Awakening.
TV: Slaughter of St. Teresa's Day, Kiss On A Grass Green Pillow, Fallen Angles, Prince Regent, Second Chance, Betjeman's Briton, We'll Meet Again, A Christmas Carol, Star Quality.
STAGE: A Cheap Bunch of Flowers, Wings of the Dove, Singular Life of Albert Nobbs, Man and Superman, Mrs. Warren's Profession, Peter Pan, The Maids, Private Lives, The Importance of Being Earnest, Hedda Gabler (New York), Agnes of God, The Human Voice. Produced The Big One, a Variety Show for Peace, 1984. Penthesilea, Fatal Attraction, The Apple Cart, Private Treason.

YORKIN, BUD: Producer-director. r.n. Alan "Bud" Yorkin. b. Washington, Pa., Feb. 22, 1926. e. Carnegie Tech., Columbia U. U.S. Navy, 1942–45; prod., dir., NBC-TV.
TELEVISION: Song at Twilight, Martin & Lewis Show, Abbott and Costello Show, Ritz Bros. Show, Spike Jones Show; writer, prod. dir., Tony Martin Show, 1954–55; dir., George Gobel Show, 1954–55; prod. dir., The Ernie Ford Show 1956–57; owner. co-prod. All In The Family; Sanford and Son; Maude; Good Times; What's Happening!!; Carter Country.
PICTURES: Dir. Never Too Late; Divorce American Style; Inspector Clouseau; prod.-dir. Start the Revolution Without

Me; Thief Who Came to Dinner, Twice in a Lifetime; co-prod.-dir. Come Blow Your Horn; exec.-prod. The Night They Raided Minsky's; Cold Turkey, Deal of the Century.

YOSHISAKA, KIYOJI: Executive. b. Shanghai, China 1908. e. Thomas Hambury College, Shanghai. Ent. ind. 1930 RCA Victor of China, 1932 Victor Talking Machine, 1938 Manchuria Talking Machine, 1940 Victor of Japan. Left Photophone Div. of Victor in 1950 for Tokyo Theatre Supply 1950–58; 1959–63 Rhythm Friend Corp.; exec. dir.s Nichior 1964–66; became consultant Nihon Eiga Shizai 1966 and after name changed to Toshiba Photo Phone became mgr. trade. div. 1969 then dir. and gen. mgr. of trade div. in 1970. Retired.

YOUNG, ALAN: Actor. r.n. Angus Young; b. North Shield, Northumberland, England, Nov. 19, 1919. Sign painter; cartoonist, acted first as monologuist at 13 years in Canada; radio comedian 10 yrs. in Canada and U.S.; served in Canadian Navy as sub-lt. 1939–42; wrote, dir. and acted in comedy broadcasts; TV: Alan Young Show, Mister Ed; m.p. debut in Margie 1946.
PICTURES INCLUDE: Chicken Every Sunday, Mr. Belvedere Goes to College, Aaron Slick from Punkin Crick, Androcles and the Lion, Gentlemen Marry Brunettes, Tom Thumb, Time Machine, The Cat from Outer Space.

YOUNG, BUDDY: Executive. b. New York City, June 15, 1935; e. CCNY, UA publicity dept. 1952; asst. pub. mgr., UA 1963; pub. dir. Fox, Oct. 1965; west coast coordinator of adv. and publicity UA. In 1975 joined Columbia Pictures as worldwide dir. of adv.-pub.-exp. In 1976 named MGM adv.-pub. co-ordinator. Joined Universal Pictures in 1976 as dir. of pub. & promo. promoted to v.p., of advertising, publicity and promotion; 1980, partner in m.p. consulting firm, Powell & Young; 1983, pres. & dir., Color Systems Technology, Inc..

YOUNG, BURT: Actor-Writer. b. N.Y.C., April 30, 1940. Worked at variety of jobs (boxer, trucker, etc.) before turning to acting and joining Actor's Studio. Appeared in off-Bdwy. plays which led to Hollywood career.
PICTURES INCLUDE: Cinderella Liberty, The Gambler, The Killer Elite, Chinatown, Rocky, The Choirboys, Convoy, Uncle Joe Shannon (actor, s.p.), All the Marbles, Rocky III, Lookin' To Get Out, Amityville II: The Possession, Over the Brooklyn Bridge, Once Upon a Time in America, The Pope of Greenwich Village, Rocky IV, Back to School.
TV: M*A*S*H, Baretta, etc.

YOUNG, CARROLL: Writer. b. Cincinnati, Ohio. e. St. Xavier Coll. Publicist for Pathe Studios, Fox West Coast Theatres, RKO Studios, MGM, 1930–35; story ed. Sol Lesser Prod., Ernst Lubitsch Prod., 1936–40; asst. to exec. prod., RKO, 1941; U.S. Army Air Force, 1942–44.
PICTURES INCLUDE: story, collab. s.p. Tarzan Triumphs; story, Tarzan's Desert Mystery; story, s.p. Tarzan and Leopard Woman, Tarzan and Mermaids; s.p. many in Jungle Jim series, Hidden City, The Jungle; story, Lost Continent; collab. s.p. Tarzan and the She-Devil; story s.p. Cannibal Attack; collab. story & s.p. Apache Warrior; collab. s.p. She-Devil, The Deerslayer; collab. s.p. Machete.

YOUNG, FREDDIE: Cinematographer. b. 1902. Ent. m.p. ind. 1917. Early career as cameraman and directing for Gaumont Film Co., British and Dominion Film Corp., MGM British, Army Training Films, now freelance.
PICTURES INCLUDE: Victoria The Great, Sixty Glorious Years, Nell Gwyn, Goodbye Mr. Chips, Edward My Son, Ivanhoe (Oscar Nom.), Bhowani Junction, Greengage Summer, Lawrence of Arabia (Oscar award), Macbeth, Doctor Zhivago (Oscar award), The Deadly Affair, You Only Live Twice, Battle of Britain, Ryan's Daughter (Oscar), Nicholas and Alexandra (Oscar Nom.), Luther, The Tamarind Seed, Great Expectations, The Blue Bird, Permission to Kill, The Man In the Iron Mask, Rough Cut, Stevie, Bloodline, Richard's Things, Arthur's Hallowed Ground (dir.).

YOUNG, IRWIN: Executive. b. N.Y.C. e. Perkiomen School, Lehigh Univ., B.S., 1950. Pres., Du Art Film Laboratories, Inc.

YOUNG, LORETTA: Actress. r.n. Gretchen Young; b. Salt Lake City, Utah, Jan. 6, 1913. e. Ramona Convent, Alhambra, Calif. Immaculate Heart College, Hollywood. After small part in Naughty But Nice, lead in Laugh Clown, Laugh. Played in almost 100 films. Won Academy Award best perf. (Farmer's Daughter) 1947; NBC-TV Loretta Young Show, 1953–61; CBS-TV New Loretta Young Show 1962; won TV Acad. Awards, 1954–56–59. Has won innumerable other awards.

YOUNG, ROBERT: Actor. b. Chicago, Ill., Feb. 22, 1907. Star numerous pictures before and after sound; from 1932 in many productions, various Hollywood producers; star. weekly TV show, Father Knows Best.
PICTURES INCLUDE: Claudia, Sweet Rosie O'Grady, The Canterville Ghost, Secrets in the Dark, The Enchanted Cottage, Those Endearing Young Charms, Claudia and David, Lady Luck, They Won't Believe Me, Crossfire, Sitting Pretty, Adventures in Baltimore, And Baby Makes Three, Bride for Sale, Second Woman, That Forsyte Woman, Goodbye My Fancy, Half-Breed, Secret of the Incas.
TV: Marcus Welby, M.D.

YOUNG TERENCE: Director, writer, b. Shanghai, China, June 20, 1915; e. Cambridge U. Served with Guards Armoured Div. WWII; ent. m.p. ind. 1936 at BIP Studios.
PICTURES INCLUDE: On the Night of the Fire, On Approval, Dangerous Moonlight, Theirs is the Glory, dir., Corridor of Mirrors, One Night With You, Woman Hater, They Were Not Divided, The Valley of the Eagles, Red Beret (Paratrooper), That Lady, Safari, Storm Over the Nile, Action of the Tiger, Serious Charge, Black Tights, Dr. No. From Russia With Love, Moll Flanders, Thunderball, Triple Cross, The Rover, Wait Until Dark, Mayerling, The Christmas Tree, The Red Sun, Grand Slam, The Valachi Papers, War Goddess, The Klansman, Jackpot, Bloodline, Inchon, The Jigsaw Man.

YOUNGSTEIN, MAX E.: Executive. b. 1913. e. Fordham U. Member New York Bar. Former motion picture executive with United Artists and Paramount. Motion picture consultant and independent producer. Member, Producers Guild. Pres., Max E. Youngstein Enterprises.
PICTURES: Young Billy Young, Best of Cinerama, Man in the Middle, Fail Safe, The Money Trap, The Dangerous Days of Kiowa Jones, Welcome to Hard Times.

YULIN, HARRIS: Actor. On Bdwy. in Watch on the Rhine, A Lesson from Aloes, etc.
PICTURES: Doc, The Midnight Man, Night Moves, Steel, Scarface.
TELEVISION: The Thirteenth Day—The Story of Esther, When Every Day Was the Fourth of July, Last Ride of the Dalton Gang, Robert Kennedy and His Times.

Z

ZADORA, PIA: Singer-Actress. b. New York City, 1954. e. High School of Professional Arts. On stage in Henry Sweet Henry. Singer in nightclubs and has appeared on numerous talk and variety TV shows.
PICTURES: Butterfly, Fakeout, The Lonely Lady.

ZAENTZ, SAUL: Producer. b. Passaic, NJ.
PICTURES: One Flew Over the Cuckoo's Nest (Oscar), Three Warriors, The Lord of the Rings, Amadeus.

ZAMPA, LUIGI: Director. b. Rome, Italy, 1905. Playwright studied at Experimental Film Center, Rome, 1935–1938; script writer, director.
PICTURES INCLUDE: American on Vacation, To Live in Peace, Difficult Years, Angelina, The White Line, City on Trial, Two Gentlemen in a Carriage, His Last 12 Hours, We Women, Woman of Rome, Art of Getting Along.

ZAMPI, GIULIO: Associate producer. b. London, Eng., Sept. 29, 1923; p. Mario Zampi; e. Rome U. Ed. to Marcel Varnel, then to Mario Zampi; dir. of Anglofilm Ltd.& Transocean Films Ltd.
PICTURES INCLUDE: Phantom Shot, Fatal Night, Shadow of the Past, Come Dance with Me, Third Time Lucky, Laughter in Paradise, Top Secret, I Have Chosen Love, Happy Ever After (Tonight's the Night), Now and Forever, The Naked Truth, Too Many Crooks, Bottoms Up, Five Golden Hours.

ZANNELLA, MICHAEL: Executive. Began career in entertainment industry with The Tonight Show; head talent coordinator for 13 years. Special assignments included assoc. prod., The Dick Cavett Show; creative consultant for Good, Morning America, David Frost Show, Hot Hero Sandwich. Creative consultant for talent dept.; head of NBC Saturday Night Live. 1985, joined Paramount Pictures as dir., talent; for M.P. Group.

ZANUCK, RICHARD DARRYL: Executive, b. L.A., Calif., Dec 13, 1934; e. Stanford U. 1952–56; f. Darryl Zanuck. Story dept., 20th Century Fox, 1954; N.Y. pub. dept., 1955; asst. to prod., Island in the Sun, 1957; The Sun Also Rises, 1956; v.p. Darryl F. Zanuck Prod. 1958; prod. Compulsion, 1959, DFZ Prod., 20th Century Fox; prod., Sanctuary, 1961; prod., The Chapman Report, 1962; asst. to prod., The Longest Day, 1962; president's prod. rep., 20th Century Fox Studio, 1963; v.p. charge prod., 20th Fox; pres., 20th Fox TV exec. v.p. chge. prod., 20th Fox, 1967. 1968: Chmn. of Bd., Television div., 20th Century Fox, 1969: Pres., 20th Century Fox Film Corp. Joined Warner Bros., March 1971, as sr. exec. v.p.; Resigned July, 1972 to form Zanuck-Brown Production Company, Universal Pictures. Films under Z/B Company released: Sssssss, 1973; The Sugarland Express, 1974; Willie Dynamite, 1973; The Sting, 1973; The Black Windmill, 1974, The Girl from

Petrovka, 1974; The Eiger Sanction, 1975; Jaws, 1975; MacArthur, 1977; Jaws 2, 1978; The Island, 1980; Neighbors, 1981; The Verdict, 1982. Joined 20th Century-Fox, 1980–83. To Warner Bros., 1983. 1985 films: Cocoon, Target. To MGM Entertainment, 1986.

ZEFFIRELLI, FRANCO: Director. b. Italy, Feb. 12, 1923. Was stage director before entering film industry.
PICTURES INCLUDE: The Taming of the Shrew, Romeo and Juliet, Brother Sun, Sister Moon, The Champ, Endless Love, La Traviata, Otello.

ZEMECKIS, ROBERT: Director-Writer. b. Chicago 1952. e. USC's School of Cinema. At USC wrote, produced and directed a 14-minute film, A Field of Honor, which won special jury award at Second Annual Student Film Awards sponsored by M.P. Academy of Arts & Sciences, plus 15 international honors. Has film editing background, having worked as cutter on TV commercials in Illinois. Also cut films at NBC News, Chicago, as summer job. After schooling went to Universal to observe on set of TV series, McCloud. Wrote script for that series in collaboration with Bob Gale. Turned to feature films, directing I Wanna Hold Your Hand and co-writing s.p. with Gale and co-writing 1941 with him.
PICTURES: Used Cars, Romancing the Stone, Back to the Future.

ZENS, WILL: Producer-director. b. Milwaukee, Wis., June 26, 1920. e. Marquette Univ. and Univ. of Southern Calif., BA, MA. Wrote, produced and directed many TV shows. Formed Riviera Productions in 1960 to produce theatrical motion pictures.
TV: Punch & Trudy, Your Police, Aqua Lung Adventures.
PICTURES INCLUDE: Capture That Capsule, The Starfighters, To the Shores of Hell, Road to Nashville, Hell on Wheels, From Nashville with Music, Yankee Station, Help Me . . . I'm Possessed!

ZETTERLING, MAI: Actress, director. b. Sweden, May 24, 1925. e. Ordtuery Sch. & Theater Sch. First m.p.: Sweden, Frenzy. Has made numerous stage and screen appearances since in Sweden. British screen debut, Frieda. Since 1969 directing plays & films in Sweden. Won Golden Lion at Venice in 1964 for The War Game.
PICTURES INCLUDE: Bad Lord Byron, Quartet, Portrait from Life, Romantic Age, Blackmailed, Hell is Sold Out, Desperate Moment, Knock on Wood, Dance Little Lady, Prize of Gold, Seven Waves Away (Abandon Ship), The Truth About Women, Jetstorm, Faces in the Dark, Piccadilly Third Stop, Offbeat, Only Two Can Play, The Main Attraction. 1965–66 wrote, dir. Loving Couples, Night Games. 1968: Dr. Glas, The Girls, The Rain Hat, We Have Many Names.
TV: Idiot's Delight, Mayerling, Doll's House, Dance of Death, etc. dir, doc. for BBC and in Sweden. Wrote and dir. Scrubbers, Amorosa.

ZIEFF, HOWARD: Director. b. Los Angeles, 1943. Started as artist and photographer, working as newsreel photographer for L.A. TV station. Went to N.Y. to do still photography; became top photo artist in advertising. Turned to film direction with Slither in 1972.
PICTURES INCLUDE: Slither, Hearts of the West, House Calls, The Main Event, Private Benjamin, Unfaithfully Yours.

ZIFFER, FELIX C.: Lawyer. b. Staniscawow, Poland. Aug. 8, 1930. e. Yale U., 1947–51; Columbia U. Law School, 1952–55; law practice, since 1955; rep. many firms in music & records fields inc. United Artists (spec. counsel), J. Arthur Rank Organization (gen. counsel); pres., International Entertainment Corp.

ZIFKIN, WALTER: Executive. b. July 16, 1936. New York City. e. UCLA A.B. 1958; USC LL.B. 1961. CBS legal dept., 1961–63; William Morris Agency 1963–present; exec. vice-pres.

ZIMBALIST, EFREM, JR.: Actor. b. New York, Nov. 30, 1923. Fay School, Southboro, Mass., St. Paul's, Concord, N.H., Yale. Studied drama, Neighborhood Playhouse, N.Y. Stage debut, The Rugged Path. Shows with American Repertory Theatre; Henry VIII, Androcles and the Lion, What Every Woman Knows, Yellow Jack, Appeared, Hedda Gabler. Co-prod., The Medium, The Telephone, The Consul, (Critics Award, Pulitzer Prize) Barrymore Theatre. m.p. debut, House of Strangers. Gave up acting after death of his wife and served as asst. to father, Curtis Institute of Music for 4 years. Returned to acting, stock co., Hammonton, N.J., 1954. Appeared in TV series.
TV: Philco, Goodyear Playhouse, U.S. Steel Hour, Maverick, 77 Sunset Strip, The FBI.
PICTURES INCLUDE: Bomber B-52, Band of Angels, The Deep Six, Violent Road, Girl on the Run, Too Much Too Soon, Home Before Dark, The Crowded Sky, A Fever in the Blood, By Love Possessed, Chapman Report, The Reward, Harlow (electronovision), Airport 1975.

ZIMBERT, RICHARD: Executive. Member, California bar. Has been with Paramount Pictures in executive capacities since 1975. In 1985 named exec. v.p. of co.

ZINNEMANN, FRED: Director. b. Vienna, Austria, Apr. 29, 1907; e. Vienna U. (law). Studied violin as a boy; after law, studied photographic technique, lighting & mechanics (Paris); asst. cameraman 1 yr. Paris; came to U.S. 1929; extra in m.p. All Quiet on the Western Front, 1930; asst. to Berthold Viertel, script clerk & asst. to Robert Flaherty, 1931; dir. Mexican documentary The Wave; short subjects dir., MGM, winning Academy Award for That Mothers Might Live, 1938; feature dir. 1941; winner of first Screen Directors' Award 1948 with The Search. 4 N.Y. Film Critics Awards; 2 Director's Guild Annual Awards; 4 Acad. Awards. Other awards: Gold Medal City of Vienna, Donatello Award (Italy), Order of Arts & Letters (France), Golden Thistle Award (Edinburgh, Scotland), etc.
PICTURES INCLUDE: The Seventh Cross, The Search, The Men, Teresa, High Noon (N.Y. Film Critics Award), Benjy, short for L.A. Orthopedic Hosp. for which Academy Award, best doc. short, 1951; Member of the Wedding; From Here to Eternity (Acad. Award, best dir., 1953, N.Y. Film Critics Award, Director's Guild Award), Oklahoma, Hatful of Rain, Nun's Story (N.Y. Film Critics Award), Sundowners, Behold a Pale Horse, A Man for All Seasons, (Oscars for best picture & direction) Day of the Jackal, Julia, Five Days One Summer.

ZINNEMANN, TIM: Producer. Began career industry as film editor; then asst. dir. on several films. Production mgr. for several projects; assoc. prod. on The Cowboys and Smile. Produced Straight Time for Warners with Stanley Beck.
PICTURES: A Small Circle of Friends, The Long Riders, Tex, Impulse, Fandango.
TELEVISION: The Jericho Mile (ABC).

ZITO, JOSEPH: Director. b. New York City, May 14, 1946. e. City Coll. New York.
PICTURES: Abduction, The Prowler, Friday the 13th: The Final Chapter, Missing in Action, Invasion U.S.A., Spider-Man.

ZOUARY, MAURICE H.: Executive. b. Brooklyn, N.Y., July 17, 1921; e. Sch. of Industrial Design & Art, 1937; Trans-Lux Theatres, 1941; U.S. Armed Forces, 1943; production, acct. exec. ad agencies; Bud Gamble Prod., 1948; TV dept., Edward S. Kellogg Agency, L.A.; formed Zouary TV-Film Prod., 1950; prod. supvr. Films for Industry, 1950–52; TV prod., Grey Adv. Agency, 1952–54; prod, new commercials div., Guild Films, 1955–56; prod. Dore Prod., 1956–57; reactivated Zouary TV Film Prod., 1957; formed Filmvideo Releasing Corp. film stock shot library, 1957. Prod.: Freedom (feature film); Prod. Kiddie Camera (TV series); Prod.: The Vaudevillains (TV special); Prod.: Dr. DeForest. In 1975 formed TV National Releasing Corp., supplier of TV programming. Wrote and produced two cassettes for Movietronics: Buster Keaton & The First Sound of Movies—The Case for Dr. Lee DeForest.

ZSIGMOND, VILMOS: Cinematograher. b. Hungary. e. National Film School. Began career photographing Hungarian Revolution of 1956. Later escaped from Hungary with friend Laszlo Kovacs, also a cinematographer.
PICTURES: McCabe and Mrs. Miller, Images, Deliverance, Scarecrow, The Long Goodbye, Cinderella Liberty, Sugarland Express, Obsession, Close Encounters of the Third Kind, The Deer Hunter, Heaven's Gate, Jinxed, Table for Five, No Small Affair, The River, Real Genius.

ZUCKER, DAVID: Producer-Director-Writer. b. Milwaukee, WI, Oct. 16, 1947. e. University of Wisconsin, majoring in film. With brother, Jerry, and friend Jim Abrahams founded the Kentucky Fried Theatre in Madison in 1979 and wrote script for film of that name released in 1977. Trio followed this with Airplane (1980) which they wrote and jointly directed while serving as executive producers.
PICTURES: Top Secret (co-dir., co-s.p.); Ruthless People (co-dir.).

ZUCKER, JERRY: Producer-Director-Writer. b. Milwaukee, WI, Mar. 11, 1950. e. University of Wisconsin, majoring in film. With brother, David, and friend Jim Abrahams founded the Kentucky Fried Theatre in Madison in 1979 and wrote script for film of that name released in 1977. Trio followed this with Airplane! in 1980 which they wrote and jointly directed and served as executive producers.
PICTURES: Top Secret (co-dir., co-s.p.); Ruthless People (co-dir.).

ZUGSMITH, ALBERT: Producer, director, writer. b. Altantic City, N.J., April 24, 1910. e. U. of Va. Pres. Intercontinental Broadcasting Corp.; ed. publ. Altantic City Daily World; v.p. Smith Davis Corp.; Chmn of bd., Continental Telecasting Corp., Television Corp. of America; assoc. ed. American Press; pres. World Printing Co.; exec. CBS; pres. American Pictures Corp.; pres. Famous Players Int'l Corp.
PICTURES INCLUDE: Written on the Wind, Man in the Shadow, Red Sundown, Star in the Dust, Tarnished Angels, The Incredible Shrinking Man, The Girl in the Kremlin, The Square Jungle, Female on the Beach, Touch of Evil, Captive Women, Sword of Venus, Port Sinister, Invasion

U.S.A., Top Banana, Paris Model, Slaughter on Tenth Avenue, The Female Animal, High School Confidential, Night of the Quarter Moon, Beat Generation, The Big Operator, Girls Town, Violated!, Platinum High School, Private Lives of Adam and Eve, Dondi, College Confidential, Confessions of an Opium Eater, The Great Space Adventure, On Her Bed of Roses, Fanny Hill, The Rapist! author, Private Lives of Adam and Eve, The Beat Generation, How to Break Into the Movies, The Chinese Room, Street Girl, The President's Girl Friend, The Phantom Gunslinger, Sappho, Darling, Menage A Trois, Two Roses and a Goldenrod, The Friendly Neighbors, Why Me, God?, Tom Jones Rides Again, etc.

Services

Advertising, In-Theatre 311
Advertising & Publicity Representatives 320
Animals and Trainers 311
Animation 311
British-Based Companies .. 334
Camera Sales, Rentals, Repairs 311
Checking Theatre Attendance 312
Colorization by Computer . 312
Commercial Jingles 312
Completion Guarantees and Bonding 312
Consultants 312
Costumes and Uniforms .. 312
Cutting Rooms 312
Distributors of 16mm Films 339
Editing Equipment 313
Editing Services 313
Film Carriers 313
Film Distributors 302
Film Preservation 308
Film Processing, Labs, Raw Stock, Preservation . 307
Film Storage 310
Financing Companies and Banking Services 315
Government Film Bureaus . 337
Lighting Equipment 315
Manufacturers and Services 322
Manufacturers and Services By Product Classification 330
Market Research 315
Merchandisers 315
Music, Music Libraries, Music Cutting 315
Photo Reproduction Labs . 308
Properties and Scenery ... 316
Raw Stock Manufacturers . 310
Refreshment Products and Equipment 328
Rental Studios and Production Facilities 316
Screening Rooms 316
Slides-Telops 317
Sound and Recording Services 317
Special Effects 318
Stock-Shot Film Libraries . 310
Stop Watches 318
Studio Equipment 326
Subtitles 318
Talent and Literary Agencies 319
Theatre Supply Dealers ... 332
Trailers 318

Film Distributors in Key Cities

ATLANTA

Alliance International, 161 Spring St., NY 30303; (404) 524-7579.
Atlantic Releasing Corp., 220 Northlake Pkwy., Suite 288, Tucker, GA 30084; (404) 491-7766
Bradley Films, 1876 De Foor Ave., N.W., 30318; (404) 352-3316. Gordon Bradley.
Buena Vista Distribution Co., 1190 W. Druid Hill Dr., P.O.B. 10517, 30329; (404) 634-6525.
Chappell Releasing Co., 2814 New Spring Rd. 30339; (404) 432-3361. Wayne Chappell, pres.
Clark Film, Inc., 2200 Northlake Pkwy., Tucker, GA 30084; (404) 491-7766. Lewis Owens.
Clark Film Releasing Co., 161 Spring St., NW, 30303; (404) 524-6588.
Columbia Pictures, 2600 Century Parkway, N.E., 30345; (404) 325-9525. Henry Harrell, mgr.
Craddock Films, Inc., Atlanta Film Bldg., 161 Spring St., N.W.; Suite 417; (404) 523-5653.
General Film Distributing, 3950 Peachtree Rd., N.E. 30319; (404) 261-5363. C. L. Autry.
Harnell Independent Productions, 6065 Roswell Rd., 30328; (404) 256-3464. Walter Powell, gen. sls. mgr.
MGM/UA Motion Picture Distribution, 401 W. Peachtree, N.E., Suite 1760, 30308; (404) 552-6386. R. Tarwater, Mgr.
New World Pictures, 3301 Buckeye Rd., 30341; (404) 458-0975. Walter Powell.
Orion Pictures Distribution Corp., 1675 Paces Ferry Rd., Suite 220, 30303; (404) 434-0500, Glenn Simonds, mgr.
Paramount Pictures Corp., 2200 Century Parkway, #810, 30345; (404) 325-7674. M. V. McAfee.
R.S. Films, Inc., 1455 Tullie Circle, N.W., 30329; (404) 325-0690.
Toddy Pictures Co., Box 150, 30301; (404) 355-9654. Ted Toddy, pres.
Transvue Pictures Corp., 161 Spring St., N.W.; Tel: (404) 523-6566.
Twentieth Century-Fox, 2200 Century Parkway, 30345; (404) 321-1178. Jerry Smith.
Universal Film Exchange, 6060 McDonough Dr., Norcross GA 30091; (404) 448-8032. Mark Gaines, Mgr.
Warner Bros., 2600 Century Pkwy., 30345; (404) 325-0301. Barry Nelson.

BOSTON

Association Films, 410 Great Road, Littleton, MA 01460; (617) 486-3518.
Atlantic Releasing Corp., 585 Boylston St., 02116; (617) 266-5400.
Buena Vista Distribution Co., 990 Washington St., Dedham, MA, 02026; (617) 426-9360. Joe Foley, Mgr.
Columbia Pictures Corp., 20 Park Plaza, 02116. (617) 426-8980; Gasper Urban, mgr.
Ellis Gordon Films, 46 Church St., 02116; (617) 542-5550. Ellis Gordon, mgr.
Lockwood & Friedman Film Corp., 430 Park Sq. Bldg., 02116; (617) 482-9717.
MGM/UA Motion Picture Distribution, Park Square Bldg., 31 St. James Ave., 02116; (617) 426-6540. Joseph Griffin, br. mgr.
New England Film Distributing, 31 St. James Ave., 02116; (617) 482-9025.
Orion Pictures Distribution Corp., 31 St. James Ave., 02116; (617) 542-0677. Beth Weiner, mgr.
Paramount Film Distributing Corp., 31 St. James Avenue, 02116; (617) 426-1070. Joe Rathgeb.
Jud Parker Films, 46 Church St., 02116; (617) 542-0744.
Topar Films, Inc., 771 Truman Parkway, Hyde Park, MA 02136; (617) 361-1640.
20th Century-Fox, 545 Boylston St., Suite 1101, 02116; (617) 267-4800. Morris Birnbaum.
Universal Film Exchanges, Inc., 44 Winchester St., 02116; (617) 426-8760. Joan Corrado, mgr.
Warner Bros. Pictures Dist. Corp., 330 Stuart St., 02116; (617) 482-3290. Jeff Goldstein, mgr.

BUFFALO

Frontier Amusement Corp., 505 Pearl St., 14202; (716) 854-6752. Mannie Brown, pres.
MGM/UA Motion Picture Distribution, 300 Delaware Ave., 14202; (716) 854-1500. William Abrams, br. mgr.
Paramount Pictures, Inc., 300 Delaware Ave., 14202; (716) 856-3758. Anthony J. Mercurio, mgr.
20th Century-Fox, 300 Delaward Ave., 14202; (716) 852-0784. John Serfustino, mgr.
Universal Film Exchange, 1314 Peppertree Dr., Derby, NY 14047; (716) 947-4218

CHARLOTTE

Atlantic Releasing Corp., 230 S. Tyron St., 28202; (704) 376-5549
Buena Vista Dist. Co. Inc., 230 S. Tryon St., 28202; (704) 373-0724. Jack Kirby.
Carolina Booking Service, 291 S. Church St., 28202; (704) 375-7787. Frank Lowry.
Carolina Film Service Inc., 5012 Hovis Rd.; (704) 394-3129. E. J. Poole (ship); Marg. Miller (off.)
Charlotte Booking Service, N.W. Bank Bldg., 28230; (704) 376-5569. J R McClure.
Cinema Film Distributing, 222 S. Church, 28201; (704) 332-8539. Ron Witherspoon.
Clark Film Inc., 230 S. Tryon St., 28202; (704) 376-5569. Bob McClure, branch mgr.
Columbia Pictures Corp., 201 S. College St., 28244; (704) 375-0705. Ed. McLaughlin.
Dominant Pictures Co., 1400 Charlotte Plaza, 28244; (704) 375-0705. Harry Kerr, mgr.
Galaxy Films, 222 S. Church St., 28202; (704) 372-6747. W. R. James, mgr.
Howco Exchange, 301 So. McDowell, 28204; (704) 834-8510. J. Francis White.
International Amusement Corp., 222 So. Church St., 28202; (704) 332-4163.
JACO Productions, 222 So. Church St., 28202; (704) 375-2519. K. Rogers, Charlie Mincey, branch mgrs.
MGM/UA Motion Picture Distribution, 230 So. Tyron St., 28202; (704) 332-5070. D. Gurin, mgr.
Paramount Film Dist. Corp., 230 S. Tryon St., 28202; (704) 374-0193. Joe L. Cutrell, mgr.
Premier Pictures, 221 S. Church St., 28202; (704) 332-5101. Jerry Helms.
Pyramid Films, 221 S. Church St., 28202; (704) 333-2894.
Queens City Advertising & Amusement, Inc., 221 So. Church St., 28202; (704) 375-4419. Hugh M. Sykes, Jr.
20th Century-Fox Film Corp., 230 So. Tryon St., 28202; (704) 332-7101. Larry Jameson.
Universal Film Exchanges, Inc., See Atlanta.
Variety Films, Inc.,221 S. Church St., 28202; (704) 374-1611. Bob McClure, mgr.

CHICAGO

Apache Films, 32 W. Randolph, 60601; (312) 782-5620. Harry Goodman.
Atlantic Releasing Corp., 9575 W. Higgins Rd., Suite 602, Rosemont, IL 60018; (312) 692-2300
Azteca Films, Inc., 1233 S. Wabash Ave., 60605; (312) 922-6186. Edward G. Edwards, br. mgr.
Buena Vista Distribution Co. Inc. 8550 W. Bryn Mawr Ave., 60631; (312) 693-8580.
Don Buhrmester & Assoc., Inc., 203 N. Wabash Ave., 60601; (312) 782-0988. Don Buhrmester.
Clark Service, Inc., 2265 W. St. Paul Ave.; (312) 342-3140. Jack Bailey.
Columbia Pictures Corp., O'Hare Atrium Office Center, 2800 R River Road, Des Plaines, IL 60018; (312) 699-6800. Gene Gibbons.
Dudelson Film Distributing, 1325 S. Wabash Ave., 60605; (312) 922-3546. Moe Dudelson.
Empire Pictures, 999 East Touhy Ave., Des Plaines, IL 60018; (312) 699-1055. Neil W. Wise.
Gilbreth Film Co., 32 West Randolph St., 60601; (312) 726-6220. Jack Gilbreth.
J.M.G. Film Co., 32 West Randolph St., 60601; (312) 346-6916. Virgil Jones.
Kaplan-Continental Pictures, 203 No. Wabash Ave., 60601; (312) 782-8413. Sam Kaplan.

William Lange & Associates, 32 West Randolph St., 60601; (312) 332-1734. Bill Lange.
Modern Talking Picture Service, 2020 Prudential Plaza; (312) 337-3252. Edwin Swanson, vice pres.
Modern TV, 1587 Elmhurst Rd., Elk Grove Village, IL 60007; (312) 593-3256.
Paramount Pictures Corp., 111 E. Wacker Dr., 60601; (312) 565-1990. Vicchi Burns, br. mgr.
Select Film Co., 32 West Randolph St., 60601; (312) 236-1233. Sam Seplowin.
Teitel Film Corp., 333 S. Michigan, 60601; (312) 346-2566. Chas Teitel, bd. chmn.
Topar Films, Inc. 345 Fullerton Parkway, 60614; (312) 348-0210. John McLaurin.
Twentieth Century-Fox Film Corp., 1100 Woodfield Rd., Schaumbury, IL, 60195. Ray Russo.
United Film Distribution Co., Suite 420, 625 Plainfield Rd., Willowbrook, IL 60521; (312) 789-1444. Sharon McAndrews, mgr.
Universal Film Exchanges, 425 N. Michigan Ave., 60611; (312) 822-0513. W. Gehring, mgr.
Warner Bros. Dist. Corp., 1111 East Touhy Ave., Des Plaines, IL 60018; (312) 296-5070. Seymour Hite, div. mgr.

CINCINNATI

Buena Vista Distribution Co., Inc., 636 Northland Rd., 45240; (513) 742-0900. Norma Wethington, mgr.
J.M.G. Film Co., 636 Northland Blvd., 45240; (513) 851-9933. Jay Goldberg, mgr.
MGM/UA Motion Picture Distribution, 35 E. 7th St., 45202; (513) 241-1546. Frank Morris, br. mgr.
MYCO Films, 617 Vine St., 45202; (513) 579-8090. Jo Harrison.
Paramount Pictures Corp., 414 Walnut St., 45202. Clark Woods.
Regency Film Distributing, 617 Vine St., 45202; (513) 621-2955. William Blum.
C. J. Ruff Film Distributing Co., 1620 Harrison Ave., 45214; (513) 921-8200.
Edward Salzberg, Inc., 35 East Seventh St., 45202; (513) 241-3671.
20th Century-Fox Film Corp., 617 Vine Street, 45202; (513) 241-6460. Anthony Knollman.
Universal Film Exchanges, Inc., 4440 Lake Forest Dr., Blue Ash, OH 42542; (513) 733-3821. D. Coons, br. mgr.
Warner Bros. Dist. Corp., 120 E. 4th St., 45202; (513) 241-6824. Andrew Silverman.

CLEVELAND

Academy Film Service, Inc. 2108 Payne Ave., 44114; (216) 696-0661. Blair Mooney, pres. M. M. Blaettner, mgr.
Cine-Pix, 2108 Payne Ave., 44114; (216) 781-0622. Jack Kaufman.
Columbia Pictures Corp., 3 Commerce Park Square, 23200 Chagrin Blvd., 44122; (216) 292-3610. David Spero.
Imperial Pictures, 2108 Payne Ave., 44114; (216) 621-9376.
MGM/UA Motion Picture Distribution, 29001 Cedar Rd., Lyndhurst, OH 44124; (216) 461-1266. D. Buckley, mgr.
Selected Pictures Corp., 29001 Cedar Rd., Lyndhurst, OH 44124; (216) 461-9770. Jay Schultz, pres.
States Film Service, Inc., Warner Bldg., 2336 Payne Ave.; (216) 771-3723. Harry Lyman, mgr.
20th Century-Fox Film Corp., 29001 Cedar Rd., Lyndhurst, OH 44124; (216) 461-4977. William Anderhalt.
Universal Film Exchanges Inc., 1435 E. 17 St., 44114; (216) 771-0413. J. Ryan, br. mgr.

DALLAS

American National Enterprises, 11422 Harry Hines Blvd., 75231; (214) 243-5171. A. H. Watts.
Atlantic Releasing Corp., 700 S. Story Rd., Suite 1021, Irving, TX 75060; (214) 259-3636
Buena Vista Distribution, 10300 N. Central Expressway, 75206; (214) 363-9494.
Columbia Pictures, 12770 Merit Dr., 75251; (214) 770-4220. John A. Lundin, mgr.
Crump Distributors, Inc. 1712 Commerce St., 75201; (214) 741-3370. Jim Crump.
Dal Art Film Exchange, 8235 Douglas St. 75225; (214) 987-2161. Fred Beiersdorf, pres.
Dimension General Eric Distributing, 10830 N. Central Expressway, 72531; (214) 692-7744. Eric Deneve, Don Scruggs.
Empire Pictures, 10300 North Central Expressway Bldg., 75231; (214) 739-6966. Dale Smith.
Film Booking Service, 500 So. Ervay, Suite 603, 75201; (214) 744-3165. Bennie Lunch.
G&M Film Distributors, 500 So. Ervay St., 75201; (214) 748-7093. Frank Meyers, Jake Guiles.
Jaco Productions, 500 So. Ervay St., 75201; (214) 748-6145. Bill Hill.
MGM/UA Motion Picture Distribution, Suite 438, 6060 N. Central Expressway, 75206; (214) 692-0777. Enoch Stevens, mgr.
Major Film Distributors, 1907 Elm St., 75201; (214) 744-4069. Jack Durrell.
Orbit Films, 4411 N. Central Exp. 75205; (214) 522-7780. Al Weiner.
Orion Pictures Distribution Corp., 7557 Rambler Rd., 75231; (214) 363-7800. Kenneth Durbin, mgr.
Paramount Pictures, 8350 N. Central Expressway, 75206; (214) 369-4600. Don Wallace.
R.S. Films, Inc., 6060 N. Central Expressway, 75206; (214) 368-8083.
Sack Amusement Enterprises, 1710 Jackson St., 75201; (214) 742-9445.
Southern Enterprises, 2344 Farrington St., 75207; (214) 634-2690. Carl Sims, gen. mgr.
Starline Pictures, 3220 Lemmon West, 75204; (214) 522-8300. James Prichard.
Topar Films, Inc., 1 No. Park East; (214) 691-7660. M. Parker, J. Kauffman.
Twentieth Century-Fox, 1400 S. Griffin, 75215; (214) 565-0221.
United Film Distribution Co., 314 South Harwood St., 75201; (214) 747-1822. Sara Murray, mgr.
Universal Film Exchanges, Inc., 7502 Greenville Ave., 75231; (214) 360-0022. E. Harris, br. mgr.
Variety Film Distributors, 4308 N. Central Expressway, 75206; (214) 827-7800. Vern Fletcher.
Warner Bros. Distributing Corp., 7424 Greenville Ave., 75231; (214) 691-6101. Jackie Stanley.

DENVER

Buena Vista Dist. Co., Inc., 6000 E. Evans Ave., P.O.B. 24006, 80222; (303) 757-7841. Pat Halloran.
Columbia Pictures Industries, 600 S. Cherry St., 80222; (303) 394-2602. Sherman Wood, br. mgr.
Crest Films, 1860 Lincoln St., 80203; (303) 623-1221. Jack Felix, branch mgr.
J&B Independent Films, 1860 Lincoln, 80203; (303) 255-0495.
McGee Film Distributing, 655 S. Alton Way; (303) 343-3413.
Mountain States Film Dist., 2145 Broadway; (303) 623-1377. David Inget.
Paramount Pictures Corp., 158 Fillmore St., 80206; Robert Fox.
20th Century-Fox Film Corp., 55 Steele St.
Universal Film Exchanges, Inc., 600 S. Cherry St., 80222; (303) 329-3476. Ron Miller, mgr.
Warner Bros. Dist. Corp., 88 Steele St., 80203; (303) 355-4431. Ralph Albi.

DES MOINES

Columbia Pictures Corp., 1501 Ingersoll Ave., 50309; (515) 243-0105. Judith Marsh.
D&D Enterprises, Inc., 311 Eleventh St., 50309; (515) 288-6006.
D&H Distributors, P. O. Box 4907, 50306; (515) 276-4263. Dick Haes.
MGM/UA Motion Picture Distribution, 1213 Grand Ave., 50309; (515) 283-0481. George Bloxham.
McCulloch Film Distributing, 500-A Produce Bank Bldg. 55403; (612) 333-2281. Stan McCulloch, owner.
Paramount Film Distributing Corp., 1535 Linden St., 50309; (515) 288-3638. Charles A. Caliguiri, br. mgr.
Producers Distributing Co., 1219 Paramount Bldg., 50309; (515) 282-5157. Ken Weldon, Mike Weldon.
20th Century-Fox Film Corp., 3737 Woodland Ave., 50265; (515) 223-9606. Mary Ann Shaughnessy.

DETROIT

Columbia Pictures Corp., 27700 Northwestern Hwy., 48034; (313) 352-9110, Jonathan Sands.
D&R Distributors, 13131 Fenkell Ave., 48277; (313) 491-2180. Al Dezel, George Rossman.
Gail Film Distributors, 16300 W. 9 Mile Road, Southfield, MI 48075; (313) 557-5024. Arthur Weisberg, pres.
J.M.G. Films, 2330 Greenfield Road, Oak Park, 48237; (313) 968-0500.
Levin Film Distributors, 29501 Greenfield Rd., Southfield, MI, 48072; (313) 559-1101. Nate Levin.
Orion Pictures Distribution Corp., 24700 Northwestern Hwy., Southfield, MI 48075; (313) 358-0733. Linda Victel, mgr.
Paramount Pictures, 23300 Greenfield Rd., Oak Park, 48237; (313) 968-8137. Robert Weiss.
R. Distributors, 13131 Fenkell, 48227; (313) 491-2180.

Regency Film Distributing, 24655 Southfield Road, Southfield, 48075; (313) 354-3245. Herb Gillis.
C. J. Ruff Films, 23300 Greenfield Road, Oak Park, 48237; (313) 968-7770. Dennis Glenn.
Twentieth Century-Fox, Southfield Office Plaza, 17117 W. 9 Mile Road, Southfield, MI 48075; (313) 569-3110.
Universal Film Exchanges, Inc., 225 E. Brown St., Birmingham, MI 48011; (313) 540-9744. D. Gonda.
Warner Bros. Dist. Corp. 24700 Northwestern Hwy., Southfield, MI 48075; (313) 353-9690. Don E. Martin, br. mgr.

HONOLULU, HI

Hawaii Nichibel Film Co. Inc., 728 9th Ave., 96816; (808) 737-3455.
Pacific Motion Picture Co. Ltd., 1190 Nuuanu Ave., 96817; (808) 538-1035.

HOUSTON, TX

Conner, Charles M. Productions, 4713 Braeburn Drive, Bellaire, TX; (713) 668-9900.

INDIANAPOLIS

Howco Films, 6385 N. Park Ave., 46220; (317) 251-5070. R. V. Jones.
Paramount Pictures, Inc., 428 Illinois Bldg.; 634-7563. John Kane, mgr.
Universal Film Exchange (See Cincinnati)
W.D. Releasing, 505 Investors Trust Bldg., 26204; (317) 635-4372.
Zipp Film Distributors, 718 N. Senate Ave.; (317) 632-6873.

JACKSONVILLE, FL

Atlantic Releasing Corp., 905 North St., 32211; (904) 721-2112
Buena Vista Distribution Co., Inc., 9550 Regency Blvd., 32211; (904) 724-7002. Bob Pollard, mgr.
Clark Film Releasing, 905 North St., 32211; (904) 721-2122. Harry Clark, pres. Belton Clark, gen. mgr.
Columbia Pictures Corp., 9550 Regency Sq. Blvd., 32211; (904) 725-8891. Terry H. Tharpe.
Paramount Film Dist. Corp., 9550 Regency Square Blvd., 32211; (904) 725-6470. Al Stout, mgr.
South Eastern Entertainment, 10348 Atlantic Circle, 32216; (904) 356-7216. Robert Capps.
20th Century-Fox Film Corp., One Regency Place, 32211; (904) 725-0993. Charles Jones, mgr.
United Film Distribution Co., 9333 Atlantic Blvd., 32211; (904) 725-4077. Richard Settoon, mgr.
Universal Film Exchanges, Inc., (See Atlanta)
Warner Bros. Pictures Dist. Corp., (See Atlanta)

KANSAS CITY, MO

Atlantic Releasing Corp., 3859 W. 95 St., Overland, KS 66206; (913) 381-2058
Buena Vista Distribution Co., 4220 Johnson Dr., Shawnee Mission, KS 66205; (913) 362-9500. Doug Finlay, mgr.
Columbia Pictures Corp., 3130 Broadway; 64111; (816) 561-3021. James Donlon, mgr.
Marcus Film Distributing, 3773 W. 95th St., Overland Park, KS, 66206; (913) 381-6222. Ben Marcus, pres.
Mercury Film Co., 3865 W. 95th St., KS, Overland Park, 66206; (913) 383-3880. Bev. Miller.
Midwest Films, 3879 W. 95th St., Shawnee Mission, KS 66206; (913) 381-2058. Gene Irwin.
Orion Pictures Distribution Corp., 3101 Broadway, 64111; (816) 932-6500. Jack Klug, mgr.
Paramount Pictures Corp., 4200 Johnson Dr., Shawnee Mission, KS, 66205; (913) 831-9212. Mike Klein, br. mgr.
Thomas/Shipp Film Distributing, 207 Westport Rd., 64111; (816) 561-0202. Howard Thomas, John Shipp.
20th Century-Fox Film Corp., 406 W. 34th St., 64111; (816) 531-6211. Neill Blatt, br. mgr.
United National Distributors, 1703 Wyandotte, 64108; (816) 474-5330. Gene Irwin.
Universal Film Exchanges, Inc., 1700 Wyandotte St., 64108;;(816) 421-5624. S. Miller, br. mgr.

LOS ANGELES

Amerikana Film Co., 6255 West Sunset Blvd., L.A. 90046; (213) 464-3131.
Atlantic Releasing Corp., 8265 Sunset Blvd., Suite 104, L.A. 90046; (213) 650-2550.
Azteca Films, Inc., 555 N. La Brea Ave., 90036; (213) 938-2413.
BFA Educational Media, 2211 Michigan Ave., Santa Monica, 90212; (213) 829-2901.
Seymour Borde Associates, 1800 N. Highland Ave., Hollywood, CA 90028; (213) 461-3936.
Buena Vista Dist. Co. Inc., 350 S. Buena Vista St., Burbank, 91521; (213) 841-1000.
Carlyle Films Ltd., 6430 Sunset Blvd., 90028; (213) 466-0864.
Cavalcade Pictures, Inc., 8950 Venice Blvd., 90034; (213) 836-2048.
Columbia Pictures, Corp., 8671 Wilshire Blvd., 90211; (213) 657-6410. Richard Sands.
Cori Films International, 2049 Central Park East #1200, 90067; (213) 557-0173.
Counselor Films, 8816 Sunset Blvd, L.A.; 90069; (213) 659-5720.
Crest Film Distributors, 116 No. Robertson Blvd., 90052; (213) 652-8844. J. Persell.
Crown International Pictures, 292 S. La Cienega Blvd., B.H. 90211; (213) 657-6700.
Empire Pictures, 1551 N. La Brea Ave., 90028; (213) 850-6110. Jim Rogers.
Favorite Films of California, Inc., 292 La Cienega Blvd., B.H.; (213) 657-6700.
Film Investment Corp. 333 S. Beverly Drive, B.H., 90211; (213) 553-5806.
Hollywood International Film Corp. of America, 1044 S. Hill St., L.A. 90015; (213) 749-2067.
International Film Enterprises, Inc., 721 North La Brea Ave., 90038; (213) 655-2534.
MGM/UA Motion Picture Distribution, 116 No. Robertson Blvd., 90048; (213) 657-7000. Robert Wood, mgr.
Manson International, 9145 Sunset Blvd., 90069; (213) 273-8640. Michael F. Goldman, pres.
National Telefilm Associates, Inc., 12636 Beatrice St., 90066; (213) 306-4040.
Orion Pictures Distribution Corp., 11500 W. Olympic Blvd., 90064; (213) 473-5073. Bob Humak, mgr.
Paramount Film Dist. Corp. 9440 Santa Monica Blvd., Beverly Hills, 90210; (213) 550-8600. Walter Lange.
Services Marketing & Distribution Co., P.O. Box 85, Ross, CA 94957.
Summit Film Distributors, 116 No. Robertson Blvd., 90048; (213) 652-7702.
Toho Co., Ltd., 2049 Century Park E, 90067; (213) 277-1081.
Topar Films, Inc., 18321 Ventura Blvd., Tarzana, CA 91356; (213) 881-9115.
Tower Film Co., 8400 W. Sunset Blvd., L.A. 90069; (213) 654-4414.
Twentieth Century-Fox Film Corp., 9440 Santa Monica Blvd., 90210 (213) 550-1044. Donna Littman.
United Film Distributing Co., 6380 Wilshire Blvd., Suite 1111, 90048; (213) 655-5044. Steven Naify, mgr.
Universal Film Exchanges, Inc., 8901 Beverly Blvd., 90048; (213) 550-7461. J. Finn, mgr.
Warner Bros. Pictures Distribution Corp., 8484 Wilshire Blvd., 90211; (213) 653-9600. Shirley Becker.

MEMPHIS

Blue Ribbon Pictures, 942 Normandy Ave., 38137; (901) 683-3949.
Clark/Pabst Films, Inc., 1188 Perkins Rd. S. 38117; (901) 683-8182.
Dimension General, 138 Huling St., 38102; (901) 278-4442. Jeff Williams.
Don Kay Enterprises, 138 Huling St., 38102; (901) 527-4023. Fordyce Kaiser, branch mgr.
Paramount Pictures, 100 N. Main St., 38103; (901) 527-9575. Tom Donahue.
Starline Pictures, 100 N. Main Bldg., 38103; (901) 527-9424. Bailey Prichard, owner.
Tab Films, 1364 No. Watkins, 38108; (901) 274-6491. Charles Arendall.

MILWAUKEE

Independent Film Distributor, 6421 Milwaukee Ave.; 771-9470. Fern Anderson, mgr.
Mescop Distributing, 9235 W. Capitol Dr., 53222; (414) 466-1700. Fred Florence, pres.

MINNEAPOLIS

Buena Vista Distribution Co., Inc., 6950 Wayzata Blvd., Golden Valley, MN 55426; (612) 546-8533.

Columbia Pictures Corp., 711 Hennepin Ave., 55403; (612) 333-6227. Gary Wiebusch.
Independent Film Distributors, 2249 Pennsylvania Ave., So.; 545-7015. Abbott Swartz, owner.
William H. Lange & Associates, 54 W. Randolph St., 60601; (312) 322-1734. Bill Lange.
MGM/UA Motion Picture Distribution, 711 Hennepin Ave., 55403; (612) 333-7276. Walter Badger, mgr.
McCulloch Film Distributing, 500-A Produce Bank Bldg., 55403; (612) 333-2281. Stan McCulloch, owner.
Mid West Entertainment, 704 Hennepin Ave., 55043; (612) 332-3303. James Payne.
Paramount Pictures Corp., 6950 Wayzata Blvd., 55426; (612) 544-0112. Forrie Myers, br. mgr.
Twentieth Century-Fox, 600 S. County Rd., #18 Suite, St. Louis Park, 55426; (612) 546-1240. Aaron Rosen, mgr.
Universal Film Exchanges, Inc., 6800 Shingle Creek Parkway, 55430; (612) 566-9620. Frank Zanotti, br. mgr.
Viking Films, 1228 Wagon Wheel Rd., Hopkins, Minn., 55343; (612) 933-4508. Jack Kelvie.
Warner Bros. Dist. Corp., See Chicago

NEW ORLEANS

Atlantic Releasing Corp., 5515 Pepsi St., Jefferson, LA 701213; (504) 733-3555
Blue Ribbon Pictures, Inc., International Trade Mart, Suite 1400, 2 Canal St., 70130; 522-8788-89. George Pabst, owner.
Clark/Pabst Film, Inc., P.O. Box 7865, Metairie, LA, 70010; (504) 733-3555.
Columbia Pictures Corp., Heritage Plaza, 111 Veterans Blvd., Metairie, LA 70005; (504) 529-2461. Kenneth Newbert.
I.F.I. Films, 4117 Heaslip Ave., Metairie, LA 70011; (501) 837-6106.
Jaco Productions, 822 Peroido, 70112; (504) 524-4218. Ken Rodgers.
MGM/UA Motion Picture Distribution, 4900 Veterans Memorial Blvd., Metaire, LA 70002; (504) 885-7333. Greg Potash.
Paramount Pictures Corp., 3525 N. Causeway Blvd., Metairie, 70002; (504) 837-7751. Norman Shindler.
Southern Film Distributing, 143 N. Rampart St., 70112; (504) 837-5200.
Twentieth Century-Fox Distrib. Corp., 3829 Veterans Memorial Blvd., Metairie, LA 70002; (504) 455-2632. Jeff Lee, br. mgr.
Universal Film Exchanges, Inc., 734A Martin Behrman Ave., Metairie, LA 70005; (504) 837-2631. N. Gazaway, mgr.

NEW YORK

Atlantic Releasing Corp., 475 Park Ave. South, 32nd Floor, 10016; (212) 213-3232
Bedford Entertainment, 51 East 42 St., 10017; (212) 697-6188.
Buena Vista Distribution Co., 477 Madison Ave., 10022; (212) 593-8900.
Challenge Film Corp., 444 Madison Ave., 10022.
Cinevista Releasing, 347 West 39 St., 10018; (212) 947-4373.
Columbia Pictures, 1700 Broadway, 10019; (212) 765-5860. Joseph Curtin.
Films, Inc., 440 Park Ave. South, 10016; (212) 889-7910.
First Run Features, 153 Waverly Place, 10011; (212) 243-0600.
Grange Communications, Inc., 45 West 60 St., 10023; (212) 582-4261.
Gray City, Inc., 853 Broadway, 10001; (212) 473-3600.
Independent International Pictures Corp., 223 State Hwy. #18, East Brunswick, NJ 08816; (201) 249-8982.
Italtoons Corp., 32 West 40 St., 10018; (212) 730-0280.
ITM Releasing Corp., 321 W. 44 St., 10036; (212) 582-6946.
Marvin Films, 221 W. 47 St., 10036; (212) 397-3555. Marvin Friedlander, pres.
Marvin Films, Inc., 1560 Broadway, 10019; (212) 575-7753.
Miramax Films, 211 West 56 St., 10019; (212) 247-4264.
Orion Pictures Distribution Corp., 9 West 57 St., 10019; (212) 980-1117. Robert Schein, mgr.
Paramount Film Distributing Corp., 1 Gulf & Western Plaza, 10023; (212) 333-7000. Pam Pritzler.
Platinum Pictures, Inc., 264 West 35 St., 10001; (212) 244-1518.
Promovision International Films, Ltd., 347 West 39 St., 10018; (212) 947-4373.
Sandcastle #5 Productions, 128 Central Park South, 10020; (212) 582-2970.
Third World Newsreel, 160 Fifth Ave., 10010; (212) 243-2310.
Times Film Corp., 144 West 57 St., 10019; (212) 757-6980.
20th Century-Fox Film Corp., 40 W. 57 St. 10019; (212) 977-5500. Leo Fisch, mgr.
United Film Dist. Co., 11 Middleneck Rd., Great Neck, NY 11021; (212) 895-7100. R. Hassanein.
Universal Film Exchanges, Inc., 445 Park Ave., 10022; (212) 759-7500. A. Quaedvlieg, mgr.
Warner Bros. Distributing Corporation, 75 Rockefeller Plaza, 10019; (212) 484-6230. Charles Barcellona.

OKLAHOMA CITY

Conner, Charles M., Productions, 4713 Braeburn Dr., Bellaire, TX; (713) 668-9945.
MGM/UA Motion Picture Distribution, 2000 Classen Blvd., 73106. (405) 528-2888. T. Dyksterhuis.

PHILADELPHIA

Alan Pictures, 900 Kings Highway North, Cherry Hill, NJ 08034; (215) 561-0800. Alan Strulson, pres.
Buena Vista Distribution, One Cherry Hill, Cherry Hill, NJ 08002; (609) 779-8804.
Capital Film Exchange, 309 N. 13th St. 19107; (215) 567-2698.
Columbia Pictures Corp., 1700 Market St., 19103; (215) 568-3889. Lewis O'Neil.
MGM/UA Motion Picture Distribution, 1612 Market St., 19103; (215) 563-9500. H. Brillman, sls. mgr.
Magill Films, 1612 Market St., 19103; (215) 563-7428. Mort Magill.
M.Y. Film Co., 1518 Walnut St., 19102; (215) 732- 6543. Emanuel Youngerman, pres.
Paramount, Fox Bldg., 1612 Market St., 19103; (215) 567-3672. Ralph Garman, br. mgr.
Twentieth Century-Fox Film Corp., 1429 Walnut St., 19102; (215) 568-7030. Louis Korte, br. mgr.
United Film Distribution Co., 2201 Route 38, Suite 230, Cherry Hill, NJ 08002; (215) 563-5827. Ed Potash, mgr.
Universal Film Exchanges, 1165 Marlkress Rd., Cherry Hill, NJ 08003; (609) 424-5045. P. Ciccotta, mgr.
Warner Bros. Pictures Dist. Corp., 1800 J.F. Kennedy Blvd., 19103. (215) 557-7030. William Waynberg.

PITTSBURGH

Paramount Pictures, Inc., Fulton Bldg., 107 6th St.; 281-9270. Don Hicks, mgr.
MGM/UA Motion Picture Distribution, Fulton Bldg., 107 Sixth St. 15222; (215) 471-8960. David Litto, mgr.
Screenguild Pictures, 415 Van Braam, 15219; (412) 281-1630. William Jenkins.
Wheeler Films, 107–6 St., 15222; (412) 471-8225.

ST. LOUIS

Kemp Film Distributors Corp., 539 No. Grand Blvd., 63103; (314) 535-1159. Stan Smith.
Paramount Pictures Corp., 539 N. Grand, 63103; (314) 533-4231. Barry Florin.

SALT LAKE CITY

Embassy Pictures, 2095 Douglas St. 84015; (801) 487-4700. Lyle Livsey, br. mgr.
MGM/UA Motion Picture Distribution, P.O. Box 11525, 84147; (801) 532-1224. Robert Loftis.
Twentieth Century-Fox Film Corp., 88 Steel St., 80206; (801) 363-3908. Gordon Larsen.

SAN FRANCISCO

Buena Vista Dist. Co., Inc., 1323 Columbus Ave., 94133; (415) 441-7114. James Nocella, mgr.
Cardinal Films, 1255 Post St., 94102; (415) 776-2626. R. Stafford.
Columbia Pictures, 595 Market St., 94105; (415) 546-7211. James Goldschlager.
MGM/UA Motion Picture Distribution, 681 Market St., 94105; (415) 441-5500. Mike Musarra.
Orion Pictures Distribution Corp., 15 Dorman Ave., 941 24; (415) 550-2200. Robert Coley, mgr.
Pacific Film Enterprises, 1 Hallidie Plaza, 94102; (415) 479-8223. Paul Williams.
Paramount Pictures, Inc., 1700 Montgomery St., 94111; (415) 433-8660. Larry St. John
Ted Reisch Enterprises, 1325 Laurel St., San Carlos, 94070; (415) 593-7060.
Twentieth Century-Fox Film Corp., 605 Market St., 94105; (415) 495-0211. J. Edward Shugrue, mgr.
United Film Distributors Co., 172 Golden Gate Ave., 94102; (415) 928-3200. Steven Naify, mgr.

Universal Film Exchange, 693 Sutter St., 94102; (415) 776-3660. R. Taylor, mgr.

Warner Bros. Pictures Distributing Corp., 150–4th St., 91403; (415) 543-8015. Mike Timko.

SEATTLE

Buena Vista Dist. Co. Inc., 975 John St., 98109; (206) 624-0186. Homer Schmitt, br. mgr.

MGM/UA Motion Picture Distribution, 225-108th Ave., N.E. Bellevue, WA 98004. S. Amato, mgr.

Paramount Pictures Corp., 975 John St., 98109; (206) 747-1176. Joe Vigil.

Parnell Film Distributors Inc., 10245 Main St., Bellevue, WA 98004; (206) 455-2632.

Twentieth Century-Fox Film Corp., 100 W. Harrison St., 98119; (206) 282-3335. William Robinson.

Universal Film Exchange Inc., 2401 Second Ave., 98121; (206) 623-6823. J. Kitts.

WASHINGTON, DC

Association-Sterling Films, 1701 N. Fort Meyer Drive, Arlington, VA; 525-4475. C. Edgar Bryant, sales mgr.

Buena Vista Dist. Co., 5205 Leesbury Pike, Falls' Church, VA 22041; (703) 931-6876.

Columbia Pictures Corp., 2011 I St., N.W., 20006; (202) 466-6570. Glenn Abrams, br. mgr.

Empire Pictures, 450 Maple Ave., East, Vienna, VA 22180; (703) 255-0655. John Nau.

Key Theatre Ent., 1325½ Wisconsin Ave., N.W., 20007; (202) 965-4401. David Levy.

MGM/UA Motion Picture Distribution, 7315 Wisconsin Ave., N.W., 20014; (301) 652-6658. Herbert Schwartz, mgr.

Orion Pictures Distribution Corp., 5205 Leesburg Pike, Falls Church, VA 22041; Jerry Sandy, mgr.

Paramount Film Dist. Co., 5249 Duke St., Suite 306, Alexandria, VA 22304; (703) 751-1733. Claudia Unger.

Twentieth Century-Fox Film Corp., 1156 15th Street, Suite 701, N.W.; (202) 223-6320. Francis X Gornley, br. mgr.

Universal Film Exchanges, Inc., P.O.B. 706, Riverdale, MD, 20737; (301) 699-3200. Steve Turner, br. mgr.

Warner Bros. Dist. Corp., 1700 Rockville Pike, Rockville, MD 20852; (301) 230-1324. Daniel Chinich.

Wheeler Films, 4701 42nd St. N.W., 20016; (202) 244-1500. Ross Wheeler, Sr.

Film Processing, Raw Stock, Preservation, Storage

Film Labs, Processing

ATLANTA

CINEMA PROCESSORS, INC., 2156 Faulkner Rd., 30324; (404) 633-1448.
COLOR-GRAPHIC, 3184 Roswl Rd., N.W., 30305; (404) 233-2174.
SOUTHERN FILM LAB INC., 2381 John Glenn Dr., Chambler, GA 30341; (404) 458-0026.
WOMETCO & CO. FILM LABS, INC., 3630 Peachtree Rd., N.W., 30305; (404) 233-5387.

BOSTON

CINE SERVICE LABORATORIES, INC., 51 Kondazian St.; Watertown 02172; (617) 926-0210.
D-4 FILM STUDIOS, INC., 109 Highland Ave., Needham Hts., MA 02194; (617) 444-0226.
FILM SERVICE LAB, 62 Berkeley St., 02116; (617) 542-1238.
MASTER MOTION PICTURE CO., 50 Piedmont St., 02116; (617) 426-3592.
SPORTS FILM LAB, 361 W. Broadway, 02127; (617) 268-8388.

CHICAGO

ASTRO COLOR LAB, 61 W. Erie, 60610; (312) 280-5500.
CINEMA VIDEO PROCESSORS, 211 East Grand Ave., 60611; (312) 527-4050.
COLBURN LABORATORY, GEORGE W., INC., 164 North Wacker Drive, 60606; (312) 332-6286.
DOUGLAS FILM INDUSTRIES, INC., 10 W. Kinzie, 60630; (312) 664-7455.
EAGLE FILM LABORATORY, INC., 4971 N. Elston, 60630; (312) 282-7161.
EDITEL, INC., 301 E. Erie (312) 440-2360.
ESKAY FILM SERVICE, INC., 540 N. Lakeshore, 60611; (312) 467-6250.
SUPERIOR BULK FILM CO., 442 N. Wells; SUperior 7-4448.
TITLE-CRAFT, 2722 W. Lawrence, 60625; (312) 271-5731.

CINCINNATI

CINCINNATI FM LABS, 3705 Lonsdale St., 45227; (513) 271-5540.
FILM ART, INC., 2436 Vine St., 45220; (513) 621-4930.
MARATHON MOVIE LABORATORY, 2436 Vine St., 45219; (513) 621-5313.

CLEVELAND

FILM LAB SERVICE, 4117 Prospect Ave., 44103; (216) 881-4511.

COLUMBIA, SC

SOUTHEASTERN FILM COMPANY, 3604 Main St., 29203; (803) 252-3753.

COLUMBUS, OH

JOHN R. BENNETT, 2553 Cleveland Ave., 43211; (614) 263-7007.

DALLAS

PSI FILM LAB., 3011 Diamond Park Dr., 75247; (214) 631-5670.
SOUTHWEST FILM LABORATORY, INC., 3024 Fort Worth Ave., 75211; (214) 331-8347.

DAYTON

FILM ASSOCIATES, INC., 4600 S. Dixie Ave., 45439; (513) 293-2164.

DETROIT

DYNAMIC FILM SERVICE, 3028 E. Grand Blvd.; (313) 873-4720.
FILM CRAFT LAB., INC., 66 Sibley, 48201; (313) 962-2611.
THE JAM HANDY ORGANIZATION, 2792 E. Grand Boulevard, 48211; (313) 845-2450.
PRODUCERS COLOR SERVICE, 2921 E. Grand Blvd.; (313) 874-1112.

HOLLYWOOD-LOS ANGELES

AMERICAN FILM IND., 1138 N. La Brea Ave., Hollywood 90038; (213) 467-1118.
AUDIO VISUAL HEADQUARTERS CORP., 515 S. Olive St., L.A. 90013; (213) 629-3661.
CINEMA RESEARCH CORP., 6860 Lexington Ave., L.A. 90038; (213) 460-4111.
CINE-CRAFT INC., 13062 Saticoy, North Hollywood 91605; (818) 765-1414.
CINESERVICE, INC., 6518 Santa Monica Blvd., 90038; (213) 463-3178.
COLOR REPRODUCTION COMPANY, 7936 Santa Monica Blvd., Los Angeles 90046; 654-8010.
CONSOLIDATED FILM INDUSTRIES, 959 No. Seward St., Los Angeles 90038; (213) 462-3161.
CREST NATIONAL FILM & VIDEO LABS, 1141 N. Seward St., L.A. 90038; (213) 462-3073.
DELUXE GENERAL INC., 1546 N. Argyle Ave., Hollywood CA 90028; (213) 462-6171; 1377 N. Serrano Ave., Hollywood, CA 90027; 462-6171.
EASTMAN KODAK LABORATORY 1017 N. Las Palmas Ave., Los Angeles 90038; (213) 465-7151.
FILMSERVICE & VIDEO LABS, INC., 6327 Santa Monica Blvd., Hollywood 90038; (213) 464-5141.
FLORA COLOR, 1715 N. Mariposa St., Hollywood 90027; (213) 663-2291.
FOTO-KEM INDUSTRIES, INC., 2800 W. Olive Ave., Burbank, 91505; (213) 846-3101.
HOLLYWOOD FILM ENTERPRISES, INC., 6060 Sunset Blvd., Los Angeles 90028; (213) 464-2181.
MANN, HAL, 7070 Santa Monica Blvd., Hollywood, CA 90038; (213) 466-3231.
MGM/UA ENTERTAINMENT CO. LABS., INC 10202 W. Washington Bl. C.C. 90230; (213) 558-5050.
METRO-KALVAR, INC., 8927 W. Exposition Bl. L.A. 90034; (213) 870-1602.
MOVIELAB-HOLLYWOOD, INC., 6823 Santa Monica Blvd., Los Angeles 90038; (213) 469-2211.
NEWSFILM LABORATORY, INC., 516 N. Larchmont Bl., LA 90004; (213) 462-6814.
PACIFIC TITLE AND ART STUDIO, 6350 Santa Monica Blvd., Los Angeles 90038; (213) 464-0121.
PEERLESS FILM PROCESSING CORP., 730 Salem, Glendale; (213) 242-2181.
RANK FILM—TECHNICAL SERVICES, 1015 N. Cahuenga Blvd., Hollywood 90038; (213) 469-9094.
REVERSALS UNLIMITED ENTERPRISES, 7052 Santa Monica Blvd., L.A. 90038. (213) 469-2731.
TECHNICOLOR INC., (Professional Film Division), 4050 Lankershim Bl., North Hollywood, 91608; (818) 769-8500.
UNITED COLOR LAB. INC., 835 N. Seward 90038; (213) 461-9921.
UNIVERSAL FACILITIES RENTAL DIVISION, 100 Universal City Plaza, Universal City, CA 91608; (818) 508-3000.
YALE LABS, 1509 N. Gordon St., L.A., 90028; (213) 464-6181.

HOUSTON

A-V CORP., 2518 No. Blvd., 77006; (713) 523-6701.
THE PHOTOGRAPHIC LABORATORIES, 1926 W. Gray, 77019; (713) 529-5846.

INDIANAPOLIS, IND.

FILMCRAFT LABORATORIES, 5323 W. 86th St., 46268; (317) 299-7070.

MEMPHIS, TENN.

MOTION PICTURE LABORATORIES, INC., 781 S. Main St.; 38106. (901) 774-4944.

MIAMI, FLA.

CAPITAL FILM LABORATORIES, INC., 1998 N.E. 150 St., 33161; (305) 949-4252.

MILWAUKEE, WISC.

CENTRAL FILM LABORATORY & PHOTO SUPPLY, 1003 North Third St., 53203; (414) 272-0606.

NEW ORLEANS

PAN AMERICAN FILMS, 822 N. Rampart St., 70116; (504) 522-5364.

NEW YORK CITY

ACCURATE FILM LABS, 45 W. 45th St., 10036; (212) 730-0555.
BEBELL INC., 416 W. 45th St., New York 10036; (212) 245-8900.
BERKEY FILM PROCESSING, 77 E. 13 St., 10003. (212) 475-8700.
CINEFFECTS LAB, 115 West 45th St., 10036; (212) 575-5151.
CINELAB CORP., 475 Tenth Ave., 10019; (212) 244-7400.
CONTROL FILM SERVICE, 321 W. 44th St., 10036; (212) 245-1574.
DELUXE GENERAL INC., 630 Ninth Ave., 10036; (212) 489-8800.
DU-ART FILM LABORATORIES, 245 W. 55th St., 10019; (212) 757-4580.
FILMTRONICS LABS, 231 West 54th Street, 10019; (212) 586-3150.
GUFFANTI FILM LABORATORIES INC., 630 Ninth Ave., 10036; (212) 265-5530.
HBO STUDIO PRODS., 120 East 23 St., 10010; (212) 477-8600.
HUEMARK FILMS INC., 277 East 44th Street, 10017; (212) 986-5066.
J & D LABS INC., 12 West 21st St., 10010; (212) 691-5613.
KIN-O-LUX, INC., 17 West 45th Street, 10036; (212) 869-5595.
MAGNO SOUND & VIDEO, 212 West 48th St., 10036; (212) 757-8855.
MEDIA FILM SERVICES, INC., 351 West 52nd Street, 10019; (212) 581-4995.
MOVIELAB INC., 619 W. 54th St., 10019; (212) 586-0360.
PRECISION FILM & VIDEO LABS, 630 Ninth Ave., 10036; (212) 489-8800.
QUALITY FILM LABORATORIES CO., 619 W. 54th St., 10019; (212) 586-4912.
RAPID FILM TECHNIQUE, INC., 37-02 27th Street, L.I. City, 11101; (212) 786-4600.
TVC IMAGE TECHNOLOGY, 311 W. 43rd St., New York, 10036; (212) 397-8600.
TECHNICOLOR INC., 321 W. 44th St., 10036; **U.S. PHOTO EQUIPMENT,** 40-13 104th St., Corona, 11368; (212) 672-3140.

NIAGARA FALLS, N.Y.

NIAGARA PHOTO CENTER, 726 Division Ave. 14305; (716) 285-2914.

OMAHA

CORNHUSKER FILM PROCESSING LAB., 1817 Vinton St.; 341-4290.

PHILADELPHIA

NEWS REEL LABORATORY, 1733 Sansom St., Philadelphia 3; RIttenhouse 6-3892. Louis W. Kellman, pres.

PITTSBURGH

MOTION PICTURE FILM SERVICES, 401 Fort Pitt Blvd., Pittsburgh 15219; (412) 566-2222.
WRS MOTION PICTURE LAB., 210 Semple St., Pittsburgh 15213; (412) 683-6300.

PORTLAND ORE.

FORDE MOTION PICTURE LABS., 2153 NE Sandy Blvd., 97232; (503) 234-0553.
KING FILM LAB., 1501 SW Jefferson St., 97201; (503) 224-8620.

SALT LAKE CITY, UTAH

STOCKDALE & CO., INC.—PHOTO-TECH. LAB., 200 E. 1st South St.; 521-3505.

SAN FRANCISCO

ALPHA CINE LABORATORY, N.C., 1500 16th St., No. 200, 94103; (415) 864-1888.
DINER/ALLIED FILM & VIDEO, 620 Third St., 94107; (415) 777-1700.
HIGHLAND LABS., 90 Tehama St., 94105; (415) 986-5010.
MONACO LABORATORIES, INC., 234 Ninth St., 94103; (415) 864-5350.
MULTICHROME LABORATORIES, 760 Gough St., 94102; (415) 431-6567.
PALMER, W. A., FILMS, INC., 611 Howard St., 94105; (415) 986-5961.

SEATTLE, WASH.

ALPHA CINE LABORATORY, 1001 Lenora St., 98121; (206) 682-8230.
FORDE MOTION PICTURE LABORATORY, 306 Fairview Ave. N., 98109; (206) 682-2510.

SHREVEPORT, LA.

DELTA FILMS, 327 Market Street, 71101; (318) 423-2679.

SPRINGFIELD, MASS.

BAY STATE FILM PRODUCTIONS, INC., 35 Springfield St., Agawarm 01101; (413) 734-3164.

TAMPA, FLA.

BEACON FILM LABORATORY, 3705 N. Nebraska Ave.; Tel.: (813) 248-4935.

Film Preservation

THE CINECURE COMPANY, 1112 Lancaster Ave., Rosemont Pennsylvania, PA 19010; (215) 527-1855 Walter E. Shank, pres.
THE DURAFILM CO., 137 No. La Brea Ave., Hollywood, CA 90036; (213) 936-1156. Madelon Cohen, pres.
FILMLIFE INCORPORATED, Filmlife Bldg., 141 Moonachie Road, Moonachie, NJ 07074; (201) 440-8500. Marvin A. Bernard, bd. chm. & pres.
FILMTREAT INTERNATIONAL CORP., 42-24 Orchard St., Long Island City, NY 11101; (212) 784-4040. Y. W. Mociuk, pres. (See display ad on page 309.)
PEERLESS FILM PROCESSING CORPORATION, 42-24 Orchard St., Long Island City, NY 11101; (212) 784-4040. Y. M. Mociuk, pres.
RESEARCH TECHNOLOGY, INC., 4700 Chase Ave., Lincolnwood, IL 60646; 677-3000.

Photo Reproduction Labs

APCO-APEDA PHOTO CO., INC., 250 West 54th St., NY 10019, NY; (212) 586-5755.
BEBELL INC., 416 West 45th St., New York 10036; (212) 245-8900. 16mm. 35mm. reversal processing, black & white and color release prints. Slides and slide films, camera masters, dupes. Giant size color prints, plus transparencies.
FRANKLIN PHOTOS, INC., 353 West 48th St., N.Y., NY 10036; (212) CI 6-4255.

Film Storage Vaults

ATLANTA

ATLANTA FILM SERVICE, 161 Spring St., N.W.; Tel.: 524-5380. Geoffrey Tyers, pres., R. D. (Curly) Burns, mgr.
BENTON FILM FORWARDING CO., 168 Baker St., N.W.; 577-2821. William B. Langston, mgr.

HOLLYWOOD-LOS ANGELES

(Hollywood studios have own storage vaults)

BEKINS VAN AND STORAGE COMPANY, 1025 North Highland Avenue; (213) 466-9271.
BONDED SERVICES, INC., 8290 Santa Monica Blvd., 90046; (213) 654-7575.
CONSOLIDATED FILM INDUSTRIES, 959 No. Seward Street, Hollywood CA 90038; (213) 462-3161. (Stores only film which Consolidated Laboratory is handling.)
EVCO REFRIGERATED FILM VAULTS, 838 N. Seward, Hollywood, 90038; (213) 464-9252.
HOLLYWOOD FILM CO., 956 N. Seward St. 90038; (213) 462-3284.
HOLLYWOOD VAULTS, INC., 742 N. Seward St., Hollywood 90038; (213) 461-4646.
PRODUCERS FILM CENTER, 948 N. Sycamore Ave., 90038; (213) 851-1122.

NEW YORK CITY

BEKINS ARCHIVAL SERVICES, INC., 609 W. 51 St., 10019; (212) 489-7890.
BONDED SERVICES, 2050 Center Ave., Ft. Lee, NJ 07024; (201) 592-7808.
BONDED FILM STORAGE, 550 Main Street, NJ 07024; (212) 557-6732.
RAPID FILM TECHNIQUE, INC., 37-02 27 St., L.I. City 11101; (212) 786-4600.
TAPE-FILM INDUSTRIES, 619 W. 54th St., 10019; (212) 708-0500.

Raw Stock Manufacturers

AGFA-GEVAERT, INC., MOTION PICTURE PRODUCTS DIVISION. (Manufacturer, distributor 35mm 16mm color, black, white raw stock. Executive offices: 275 North St., Teterboro, NJ 07608; (201) 288-4100; (212) 563-5500.
BRANCHES:
San Francisco, 94010: 1633 Old Bayshore Highway, Burlingame, CA; (415) 692-2432.
Los Angeles, 90067: 1801 Century Park East; (213) 552-9622.
EASTMAN KODAK CO., 343 State St., Rochester, NY; Tel.: (716) 325-2000. 1901 W. 22nd St., Oakbrook, IL 60521; Tel.: (312) 654-5300. 6706 Santa Monica Blvd., Hollywood, CA; Tel.: (213) 464-6131. 1133 Ave. of Americas, New York City 10036; Tel.: (212) 262-6000.
FUJI PHOTO FILM U.S.A., INC., (distributor of Fuji Professional Motion Picture Film) 350 Fifth Ave., N.Y., NY; 736-3335.
GAF CORP., Binghamton, NY 13902; (607) 729-6555.
GEVAERT COMPANY OF AMERICA, INC., (see Agfa-Gevaert).
ILFORD, INC., 70 W. Century Rd., Paramus, NJ 07562; (201) 265-6000.
3M COMPANY (MINNESOTA MINING & MANUFACTURING CO.), Photographic Products Division, manufacturer and distributor of Ferrania 3M motion picture films; 2501 Hudson Rd., St. Paul, Minn. 55101, (612) 733-0020; 845 Third Ave., New York, NY, (212) LT-1-1416; 6023 So. Garfield Ave., Los Angeles, CA 90022, (213) 685-9600.
RESEARCH TECHNOLOGY, INC., 4700 Chase Ave., Lincolnwood, IL 60646; (312) 677-3000.

Stock-Shot Film Libraries

HOLLYWOOD-LOS ANGELES

EVCO LIBRARY, 838 N. Seward, Hollywood 90038; (213) 464-9252.
SHERMAN GRINBERG FILM LIBRARIES, INC., 1040 N. McCadden Pl., Hollywood, CA 90038; (213) 464-7491.
METRO-GOLDWYN-MAYER, 10202 W. Washington Blvd., Culver City, CA 90230; (213) 836-3000.
PRODUCERS LIBRARY SERVICE, 7325 Santa Monica Blvd., Hollywood 90046; (213) 851-2201.
ALLAN SANDLER FILM LIBRARIES, INC., 1001 No. Poinsetta Place, Hollywood; (213) 876-2021.
TRANS AMERICA FILM CORP., 1680 Vine St., L.A. 90028; 466-7575.
UNITED AIRLINES, (stock footage), 626 Wilshire Blvd., L.A. 90017; (213) 482-2000.
UNIVERSAL CITY STUDIOS, 100 Universal City, 91608; (213) 985-4321.

NEW YORK CITY

ARCHIVE FILM PRODUCTIONS, INC., 530 W. 25 St., NYC 10001; (212) 620-3955.
FOTOSONIC INC., 15 West 46 St., 10036; (212) JU 6-0355.
HEARST METROTONE NEWS, 235 E. 45 St. 10017; (212) 682-7690.
MOVIETONEWS, INC. FILM LIBRARY, (Subsidiary of 20th Century Fox), 1345 Avenue of the Americas, 10019; (212) 397-8548.
MUSEUM OF MODERN ART FILM LIBRARY, 11 West 53 Street, 10019; (212) CIrcle 5-8900.
SHERMAN-GRINBERG FILM LIBRARIES, INC., 630 Ninth Avenue, NY 10036; (212) 765-5170.
STOCK SHOTS TO ORDER, 521 Fifth Ave., New York, NY 10017; (212) 682-5844.
STRATFORD INTERNATIONAL FILM SEARCHERS, INC., 250 West 57 St.; (212) 586-3828.
TELENEWS FILM CORP., 235 E. 45 St., 10019; (212) 682-5600.

Services for Producers

Advertising, In-Theatre

MOONDIAL MANUFACTURING CORP. (dba) Barnett Film Service, 8969 Sunset Blv., Hollywood, CA 90069; (213) 271-4448. Gabriel Barnett, pres.; Matilda Barnett, v.p.; Morton Bregman, sec.-treas. (Sponsored theatre clocks especially designed and perfected for advertising use in motion picture theatres.)
MOVIE MEDIA NETWORK, INC., 2600 Douglas Road, Coral Gables, FL 33134; (305) 448-0008. David I. Weiss, pres. (National program of in-theatre poster advertising; company installs posters of products and services for the general consumer public on the walls of theatre lobbies)

Animals and Trainers

EAST COAST

ANIMAL ACTORS INTERNATIONAL, INC., R.D. 3 Box 221, Washington, NJ 07882; (201) 689-7539. Professionally trained animals for all media, natural filming lociations.
ANIMAL TALENT SCOUTS, INC., 331 W. 18 St., New York, NY 10011; (212) 243-2700.
DAWN ANIMAL AGENCY, 160 W. 46 St., New York, NY 10036; (212) 757-9396.

WEST COAST

ANIMAL ACTORS OF HOLLYWOOD, 864 W. Carlisle Rd., Thousand Oaks, CA 91361; (805) 495-2122.
ANIMAL TRAINERS UNLIMITED, 12617 Foothill Blvd., Sylmar, CA 91342; (213) 896-0068.
LION ANIMAL RENTAL, Box 259, Ventura, CA 93001; (805) 648-6550.
PUMA PAW RANCH, P.O. Box 606, Rifle, CO 81650; (303) 625-2786.
WORKING WILDLIFE, Box 65, Acton, CA 93510; (805) 947-4041.

Animation

CALIFORNIA

BOSUSTOW, STEPHEN, PRODUCTIONS, 1649 Eleventh St., Santa Monica, CA 90404; (213) 394-0218.
HANNA BARBERA, 3400 West Cahuenga Blvd., Hollywood, CA 90028; (213) 466-1371.
IMAGINATION INC., 443 Jackson St., San Francisco, CA; (415) 433-5480.
MONTROY SUPPLY CO., 4165 Beverly Blvd., Hollywood, CA; (213) 662-2111.
QUARTET FILMS, INC., 5631 Hollywood Blvd., Los Angeles Ca 90046; (213) 464-9225.
RUBY-SPEARS PRODUCTIONS, 3400 Cahuenga Blvd., W. Los Angeles, 90068; (213) 764-7700.
THOMAS BROTHERS, 30 Berry St., San Francisco, CA 94107; (415) 664-1901.

NEW YORK

ANIMATED CAMERA WORKSHOP, 51 East 42 St., N.Y., NY 10017; (212) 687-5009.
ANIMATED PRODUCTIONS, INC., 1600 Broadway, N.Y. NY 10019; (212) 265-2942.
BEBELL & BEBELL COLOR LABORATORIES, INC., 416 West 45 St., N.Y., NY 10036; (212) 245-8900.
ELINOR BUNIN PRODUCTIONS, INC., 30 East 60 St., N.Y., NY 10022; (212) 688-0759.
CLARK, IAN 229 E. 96 St., New York, NY 10028; (212) 289-0998.
CREATIVISION, INC., 295 West 4 St., N.Y., NY 10012; (212) 924-3935.
GRANATO ANIMATION PHOTOGRAPHY INC., 15 West 46 St., N.Y., NY 10036; (212) 869-3231.
HARVEY FAMOUS CARTOONS, 15 Columbus Circle, N.Y., NY 10024; (212) 582-2244.
HUBLEY STUDIO, 815 Park Ave., N.Y., NY 10021; (212) 744-8050.
LEO ANIMATION CAMERA SERVICE, 15 West 46 St., N.Y., NY 10036; (212) 582-2525.
NATIONAL SCREEN SERVICE BORP., TV & INDUSTRIAL FILMS DIVISION, 1600 Broadway, N.Y., NY 10019; (212) CI 6-5700.
THE OPTICAL HOUSE, 25 West 45 St., N.Y., NY 10036; (212) 757-7840.
OVIATION FILMS, 33 W. 46 St., N.Y., NY 10036; (212) 581-4406.
RAINBOW FILM EFFECTS, INC., 45 West 45 St., N.Y., NY 10036; (212) CO 5-2942.
TELEMATED M.P., 51 East 42, N.Y., NY 10017; (212) 682-3434.
ZEPLIN PRODUCTIONS, 850 Seventh Ave., N.Y., NY 10019; (212) 582-6633.

Camera Sales, Rental, Repairs

NEW YORK

ARRIFLEX CO. OF AMERICA, P.O. Box 1050, Woodside, NY 11377; (212) 932-3403.
CAMERA MART, INC., 465 West 55th St., 10019; (212) 757-6977.
CAMERA SERVICE CENTER 625 W. 54th St., 10019; (212) 757-0906.
F&B/CECO/SOS, 315 W. 43rd St., New York 10036; (212) 586-1420.
FILM EQUIPMENT RENTAL CO., 707 11th Ave., 10019; (212) 245-4800.
GENERAL CAMERA, 471 11th Ave., 10018; (212) 594-8700.
NATIONAL CINE EQUIPMENT, INC., 4140 Austin Blvd., Island Park; (212) 799-4602.
OLDEN CAMERA & LENS CO., INC., 1265 Broadway; (212) 725-1234.
RANK PRECISION INDUSTRIES, 260 N. N. Route 303, West Nyack, NY 10994; (914) 353-1914.
ROSS-GAFFNEY, 21 W. 46 St., 10036; (212) 719-2744.
WILLOUGHBY CAMERA STORES, 110 W. 32 St., 10001; (212) 564-1600.

HOLLYWOOD

AKKAD INTERNATIONAL PRODS. INC., 8730 Sunset Blvd., CA 90069; (213) 657-7670.
AREMAC CAMERA CO., 5609 Sunset Blvd., L.A. 90028; (213) 469-2988.
ARMISTEAD, MARK INC., 1041 N. Formosa, L.A. 90046; (213) 467-6181.
BACH AURICON, INC., 6950 Romaine St., Hollywood 90038; (213) 462-0931.
BELL & HOWELL, 623 Rodier Drive, Glendale, CA; (213) 245-6631.
BIRNS & SAWYER, 1026 N. Highland Ave., Hollywood 90038; (213) 466-8211.
F&B/CECO/SOS, 7051 Santa Monica Blvd., L.A. 90038; (213) 466-9361.
GALLI, HERMAN, CAMERA SERVICE, 6804 Melrose Ave., L.A. 90038; (213) 931-4111.
GORDON ENTERPRISES, 5362 N. Cahuenga Blvd., N. Hollywood 91601; (213) 985-5500.
HOLLYWOOD CAMERA, 1255 No. La Brea Ave., 91603; (213) 783-1134.
HOLLYWOOD FILM CO., 956 Seward St., Hollywood, 90038; (213) 462-3824.

KENWORTHY SNORKEL CAMERA SYSTEMS INC., P.O. Box 49851, L.A. 90049; (213) 476-4100.
MOLE-RICHARDSON CO., 937 N. Sycamore Ave., Hollywood, 90038; (213) 851-0111.
OPTICAL CAMERA SERVICE, 507 W. Colorado Blvd., Glendale, CA 91204; (213) 246-0995.
PILL, JACK & ASSOCIATES INC., 6370 Santa Monica Blvd., Hollywood, CA 90038; (213) 466-5391.
TECH-CAMERA RENTALS, INC., 6370 S. Monica Blvd., 90038; (213) 466-3238.
UPS STUDIO RENTALS, 6561 Santa Monica Blvd., Hollywood, CA 90038; (213) 461-1442.

Checking Theatre Attendance

CERTIFIED MARKETING SERVICES, INC., 120 N. Main St., New City, NY 10956; (914) 638-1021. National field interviews; in-theatre and telephone. William P. Smith, pres.
DI-AN RESEARCH, INC. Kinderhook, NY 12106; (518) 758-1492. Theatre checking; industry research. Joe Sugar, pres.
DALE SYSTEM INC., 1101 Stewart Ave., Garden City, NY 11530; (516) 794-2800. Harvey Yaffe, pres.
THEATRE CONSULTANTS OF AMERICA, P.O. Box 1293, Hurst, TX 76053; (817) 656-1998.

Colorization by Computer

COLOR SYSTEMS TECHNOLOGY, INC., 7080 Hollywood Blvd., Los Angeles, CA 90028; (213) 469-1801.

Commercial Jingles

AEOLUS PRODUCTIONS, INC., 119 West 57th St., N.Y., NY 10019; (212) 541-9388.
FAILLACE PRODUCTIONS, 207 East 45th Street, New York, NY; 687-9080. Tony Faillace.
MAMORSKY, ZIMMERMANN & HAMM, INC., 56 West 45th St., N.Y., NY 10036; (212) 986-1084.
MUSIC MAKERS, INC., 200 Central Park So., N.Y., NY 10019; (212) 245-3737.

Completion Guarantees and Bonding

THE COMPLETION BOND CO., INC., 9601 Wilshire Blvd., 90210; (213) 859-8300.
MOTION PICTURE GUARANTORS, INC., Head Office: 43 Britain St., Toronto, Canada, M5A 1R7; (416) 361-1664. Telex: CA 065-24697. Provides completion guarantees for motion pictures, TV series and TV movies throughout the world, for producers and major banks, studios, and investors. Branch offices: Sydney: Level 3, MLC Centre, Sydney, NSW 2000, (02) 235-2736, Telex: AA 23917; Montreal, (514) 286-4022; Calgary: (403) 236-3025; Vancouver: Suite 3E, 111–18th St., West Vancouver, B.C. (604) 926-0392 and (604) 224-0520. See listing in Corporations.
WORLDWIDE COMPLETION SERVICES, INC., 900 Sunset Blvd., 90069, (213) 276-4084; New York office: 888 Seventh Ave., 10106, (212) 489-7439. Services include payroll, cash flow projections, budget analysis, accounting, etc.

Consultants

AMERICAN FILM PRODUCTIONS INC., 1540 Broadway, N.Y., NY 10019; (212) 582-1900.
BROADCAST INFORMATION BUREAU, 30 East 42 St., N.Y., NY 10017; (212) 687-1668.
DALE SYSTEM INC., 200 Garden City Plaza, Garden City, NY 11530; (516) 741-2070. Harvey Yaffe, pres.
FILM COUNSELORS, INC., 500 Fifth Ave., N.Y., NY 10022; (212) 736-7220.
FILM PLANNING ASSOCIATES, INC., 305 East 46 St., N.Y., NY 10017; (212) 725-9316.
NATIONAL SCREEN SERVICE CORP., TV & INDUSTRIAL FILMS DIVISION, 1600 Broadway, N.Y., NY 10019; (212) CI 6-5700.
RADIO FEATURES, INC., 527 Madison Ave., N.Y., NY 10022; (212) EL 5-4616.
ROSS-GAFFNEY, 21 West 46 St., N.Y., NY 10036; (212) JU 2-3744.
THEATRE CONSULTANTS OF AMERICA, P.O. Box 1293, Hurst, TX 76053; (817) 656-1998.

Costumes & Uniforms

NEW YORK

ANIMAL COSTUME CO., 236 West 55 Street, 10019; (212) 245-5199.
BROOKS-VAN HORN COSTUME CO. INC., 117 West 17 St., 10011; (212) 989-8000.
CHENKO STUDIO, 108 W. 45 St., 10036; (212) 582-1646.
EAVES COSTUME COMPANY, INC., 151 W. 46 St., 10019; (212) 757-3730.
KARINSKA, MME., 6 West 61 St., 10023; (212) 247-3341.

WEST COAST

A-CINEMA HOLLYWOOD COSTUMERS, 5514 Hollywood Blvd., 90028; (213) 464-9894.
ACUNA, FRANK, 8212 Sunset Blvd., L.A. 90046; (213) 656-1413.
ADELE'S OF HOLLYWOOD, 5059 Hollywood Blvd., L.A., 90038; (213) 662-2231.
IC COSTUME RENTALS, 6121 Santa Monica Blvd., L.A. 90038; (213) 496-2056.
TUXEDO CENTER, 7360 Sunset Blvd., L.A., 90046; (213) 874-4200.
WESTERN COSTUME CO., 5335 Melrose Ave., Hollywood, CA 90038; (213) 469-1451.

Cutting Rooms

LOS ANGELES

F&B/CECO EDITING CENTER, 7051 Santa Monica, L.A., CA 90038; (213) 466-9361.
HORIZONTAL EDITING STUDIOS, 6253 Hollywood Blvd., Hollywood, CA 90028; (213) 461-4643.

NEW YORK

ANIMATED PRODS., INC., 1600 Broadway, New York, NY 10019; (212) 265-2942.
CAMERA MART, THE, 456 W. 55 St., New York, NY 10019; (212) 757-6977.
CINERGY COMMUNICATIONS CORP., 321 W. 44 St., 10036; (212) 582-2900.
CRITERION FILM LABORATORIES, INC., 415 West 55 St., 10019; (212) 265-2180.
DE LUXE GENERAL INC., 630 Ninth Ave., New York, NY 10036; (212) 489-8800; 1546 N. Argyle Ave., L.A. 90038; (213) 462-6171.
MOVIELAB THEATRE SERVICE, 619 West 54 Street, New York, NY 10019; (212) 586-0360; 6823 Santa Monica Blvd., L.A.; (213) 469-5981.

PREVIEW HOUSE, 7655 W. Sunset Blvd., L.A., 90046; (213) 876-6600.
PREVIEW THEATRE, 1600 Broadway, New York, NY 10019; (212) 246-0865.
ROSS-GAFFNEY, INC., 21 West 46 St., New York, NY 10036; (212) 582-3744.

Editing Equipment

CIRO EQUIPMENT CORPORATION, 6820 Romaine St., Hollywood, CA; (213) 467-1296. (8, 16, 35 & 70mm self-perforating film splicers and splicing tape) Barry Green, pres.
CAMERA MART, INC., 456 W. 55th St., 10019; (212) 757-6977.
EASY EDIT, 630 Ninth Ave., 10036; (212) 541-9664.
LAUMIC CO., INC., 306 E. 39th St., 10016; (212) 889-3300.
KLM ASSOCIATES INC., 11810 Charen Lane, Potomac, MD; (301) 299-7259. (sells and rents film editing equipment; horizontal editing tables and related hardware) Mar McElroy, pres.
MAYSLES FILM, INC., 250 W. 54th St., 10010; (212) 582-6050.
TWENTY-FOURTH FRAME, 303 Depot, N.W., P.O. Box 2167, Christiansburg, VA 24073; (703) 382-4135. (manufactures 35mm, 16mm, two-picture 3-sound, 8-plate flatbed editing machines) Ike Jeanes, owner.

Editing Services

LOS ANGELES

ARRIFLEX CORP., 600 N. Victory Blvd., Burbank, CA 91502; (818) 841-7070.
BRAVERMAN PRODUCTIONS, INC., 1237 Seventh St., Santa Monica, CA 90401; (213) 451-9762.
COMPACT VIDEO SERVICES, INC., 2813 West Alameda Ave., Burbank, CA 91005; (213) 843-3232.
CREATIVE FILM ARTS, 7026 Santa Monica Blvd., Los Angeles, 90038; (213) 466-5111.
FILM CORE, 849 Seward St., Hollywood, 90038; (213) 464-7303.
FILM PLACE, THE, 1311 N. Highland Ave., L.A. 90028; (213) 464-0116.
HOLLYWOOD ASSOCIATES, INC., 2800 W. Olive Ave., Burbank, CA 91505; (818) 841-4136.
IMAGE TRANSFORM LAB., 3611 N. San Fernando Blvd., Burbank, CA 90038; (818) 841-3812.
KEM EDITING SYSTEMS, 7237 Santa Monica Blvd., L.A. 90066; (213) 850-0200.
MGM/UA ENTERTAINMENT CO. STUDIOS, 10202 W. Washington Blvd., Culver City, CA 90230; (213) 558-5000.
MOTION PICTURE RECORDING, INC., 7060 Hollywood Blvd., Hollywood 90028; (213) 462-6987.
NEW WORLD PICTURES POST PRODUCTION, 650 N. Bronson Ave., L.A. 90004; (213) 461-3217.
PARAMOUNT STUDIOS, 5555 Melrose Ave., Hollywood 90038; (213) 468-5000.
RIVIERA PRODUCTIONS, 6610 Selma St., L.A. 90028; (213) 462-8585.
SCREEN IMAGES, INC., 1041 N. Orange Dr., Hollywood 90038; (213) 462-4383.
UNIVERSAL FACILITIES RENTAL DIVISION, 100 Universal City Plaza, Universal City 91608; (818) 508-3000.

NEW YORK

ANI-LIVE FILM SERVICE, INC., 45 W. 45 St. 10036; (212) 819-0700.
ANIMATED PRODS., INC., 1600 Broadway, 10019; (212) 265-2942.
ANOTHER DIRECTION, 252 E. 51 St., 10022; (212) 753-8250.
JERRY BENDER EDITORIAL, 26 E. 36 St., 10016; (212) 686-7407.
BERGMAN FILM ASSOCIATES, INC., 235 E. 49 St., 10017; (212) 751-4143.
BERT'S PLACE, 141 E. 44 St., 10017; (212) 682-5891.
CHANNEL FILMS, INC., 45 W. 45 St., 10036; (212) 586-4311.
CHUNG GROUP, INC., 48 East 50 St., 10022; (212) 832-0530.
CINE METRIC, INC., 290 Madison Ave., 10017; (212) 532-4140.
DJM FILMS, INC., 4 E. 46 St., 10017; (212) 687-0111.
DOUBLE IMAGE, INC., 124 E. 40 St., 10016; (212) 687-3605.
EDIFILM/EDITAPE, The Penthouse, 205 E. 42 St., 10017; (212) 697-7185.
EDITORS HIDEAWAY, INC., 595 Madison Ave., 10022; (212) 759-1105.
HARVEY'S PLACE, 919 Third Ave., 10022; (212) 688-5510.
NEW YORK FILM EXPERIENCE, 329 E. 50 St., 10022; (212) 753-9420.
ROSS-GAFFNEY, INC., 21 West 48 St., 10036; (212) 719-2744.
PHOTOSONIC EDITING, IND., 429 Lexington Ave., 10017; (212) 586-0355.
THE SPOT SHOP, 243 E. 49 St., 10017; (212) 758-4149.

Film Carriers

ALBANY

CLARK SERVICE, INC., 24 North Third St., 12204; (518) 434-1289. John Pemberton, mgr.
FIRLIK EXPRESS SERVICE, INC., 141 South Hawk St., 12204; (518) 463-3712. John Firlik, pres.
WESCO FILM SERVICE, INC., 24 N. Third St., 12204; (518) 434-1289. John Pemberton.

ATLANTA

BENTON FILM FORWARDING CO., INC., 168 Baker St., N.W., 30313; (404) 577-2821.
THEATRES SERVICE CO., 830 Willoughby Way, N.E., 30313; (404) 577-2821. W. B. Langston.

BOSTON

NFS OPERATING CORP., 20 Freeport Way, Dorchester, MA 02122; (617) 288-1600.

BUFFALO

WESCO FILM SERVICE, INC., 108 Gruner Rd., 14225; (716) 897-0467. Robert Neffke.

CHARLOTTE

CAROLINA FILM SERVICE, INC., 522 Penman St., P.O. Box 30845, 28230; (704) 333-2115. Ernest J. Poole.
CAROLINA DELIVERY SERVICE CO., INC., 1336 S. Graham St., 28230; (704) 333-5196.

CHICAGO

ALLIN EXPRESS SERVICE, 2101 S. Peoria, 60608; (312) 666-5407. J. B. Allin, owner.
CLARK FILM SERVICE, 222 No. Laflin St., 60607; (312) 829-3700. William Saley.
EMERY AIRFREIGHT, Chicago O'Hare Airport, 60666; (312) 686-7300. George Brown, mgr.
LAVIN BROS. FILM DELIVERY SERVICE, 6328 N. Richmond Ave.; (312) 274-6450. William Lavin and Lewis Lavin, owners.
NOVO AIR FREIGHT, 2707 Coyle Ave., 60607; (312) 593-7300. Donald C. Galloy, v.p. central region; Sid Weintraub, city mgr.

CINCINNATI

CLARK FILM SERVICE, 421 Bauer St., 45214; (513) 621-4240. Harry Jansen.
STATES FILM SERVICE, INC., 421 Bauer St., 45214; (513) 621-4240. Harry Jansen, mgr.

CLEVELAND

CLEVELAND FILM SERVICE, INC., 2336 Payne Ave., 44114; (216) 771-3723. John Remec.
STATES FILM SERVICE, INC., 2336 Payne Ave., 44114; (216) 771-3723. Harry Lyman, mgr.; K. Wessel, owner.

DALLAS

CENTRAL SHIPPING & INSPECTION, 2500 S. Harwood, 75215; (214) 421-5411. Wallace Jack, mgr.

DENVER

DENVER SHIPPING AND INSPECTION, 2118 Stout St., 80205; (303) 222-5616. Alan Castle, mgr.

DES MOINES

IOWA FILM DEPOT, 3123 Delaware Ave., 50316; (515) 265-1469. Robert Boots, mgr.
KING, H. W. DELIVERY SERVICE, 1320 Grand Ave., 50316; (515) 243-5269. Floyd L. King, mgr.

DETROIT

NFS OPERATING CORPORATION, 6111 Concord Ave., 48211; (313) 923-2150. Ed McCauley.

INDIANAPOLIS

BRADFORD FILM TRANSIT CO., 718 N. Senate Ave., 46202; (317) 636-2800. Don A. Pierce.
CLARK FILM SERVICE, 429 N. Senate Ave., 46204; (317) 638-3531. George Davenport.
INDIANA TRANSIT SERVICE, 4300 W. Morris St., 46241; (317) 241-9321. Wm. R. Smith, mgr.

JACKSONVILLE, FL

JACKSONVILLE FILM SERVICE, INC., 2208 W. 21 St., 32209; (904) 355-5447. Bert D. Benton.

KANSAS CITY, MO

CENTRAL SHIPPING & INSPECTION, 120 West 17th Ave. 64108; (816) 471-0884. Abbot Sher.
INDEPENDENT FILM SHIPPERS, 1800 Central, 64108; (816) 471-3348.

LOS ANGELES

AIR SEA FORWARDERS, 9009 La Cienega Blvd., L.A. 90045; (213) 776-1611.
BARNETT INTERNATIONAL FORWARDERS, INC. OF CALIF., 8635 Aviation Blvd., Inglewood, 90301; (213) 776-1178.
BARNETT/NOVO INTERNATIONAL CORP., P.O. Box 91100, Worldway Postal Center, Los Angeles, CA 90009.
BLISS FILM DELIVERY, 1120 S. Second St., Alhambra, CA; (213) 282-9532.
GARDNER'S DELIVERY SERVICE, INC., 11229 S. Prairie, Inglewood, CA; (213) 978-9018.
GILBOY, INC., 8401 Clauson Ave., Pico Rivera, CA 90606; (213) 949-9397. James Hunter, Mgr.
NOVO INTERNATIONAL CORP., 8635 Aviation Blvd., Inglewood, 90301; (213) 776-1178.

MEMPHIS

FILM TRANSIT, INC., 291 Hernando St., 38118; (901) 525-6894. Guilbert Brandon, president.
MEMPHIS FILM SERVICE, INC., 3931 Homewood Rd., 38118; (901) 365-7550. A. S. Crews.

MILWAUKEE

FILM CENTER, INC., 333 No. 25th St., 53233; (414) 342-3717. Oliver Trampe, mgr.
MILWAUKEE FILM CENTER, INC., 333 No. 25th St., 53233; (414) 344-0300. John Prostinak.

MINNEAPOLIS

CENTURY MOTOR FREIGHT, INC., 3245-4th St. S.E. 55414; (612) 645-9484. Steve Bonello, pres.
HYMAN FREIGHTWAYS, INC., 2690 Prior Ave. N., St. Paul; 633-7310. Eugene Pikovsky, pres.
INDEPENDENT FILM SERVICE, INC., 245 Second Ave. No., 55401; (612) 335-2203. Jim Perrin.
TWIN CITY FREIGHT, 2280 Ellis, St. Paul, 55414; (612) 645-3661. W. E. Elshotz, Sr., pres.

NEW HAVEN

NEW HAVEN FILM SERVICE, 90 Woodmont Rd., 06460, Milford; (203) 878-1465. William Rosen.

NEW ORLEANS

FILM INSPECTION SERVICE, INC., 2411 Edenborn Ave., Metairie, LA 70001; (504) 833-5552. Dan Brandon.
NOVO AIR FREIGHT, 2411 Edenboro Ave., Metairie, LA, 70001; (504) 837-0922.

NEW YORK CITY

BONDED FILM DISTRIBUTORS, 550 Main St., Ft. Lee, NJ 07024; (212) 557-6738. Mike Berg.
HUDSON FILM DELIVERY CORP., 560 Main, Fort Lee, NJ 07024; 201-947-5200.
STATE FILM DELIVERY, 560 Main, Fort Lee, NJ 07024; (201) 947-5200.
RAPID FILM DISTRIBUTORS, INC., 37-02 27th St., Long Island City, 11101; (212) 786-4600.
TRANS-WORLD INTERNATIONAL INC., 767 Fifth Ave.; 755-9415.

OKLAHOMA CITY

MISTLETOE EXPRESS SERVICE, INC., 111 N. Harrison 73125; (405) 236-1482. Jack LaMonte, mgr.
OKLAHOMA CITY SHIPPING & INSPECTION, 8009 S. West 7th St., 73125; (405) 235-2553. Charles Baird.

OMAHA

OMAHA FILM DEPOT, 1441 N. 11th St., 68102; (404) 342-6576. Charles Janousek.

PHILADELPHIA

INTERNATIONAL FILM SERVICE, INC., 130 Ferry Ave., Camden, NJ 08104; (215) 232-3500. Stanley Adleman.
STATES FILM SERVICE, INC., 130 Ferry Ave., Camden, NJ 08104; (215) LO 30303. Meyer Adelman.

PITTSBURGH

KALLY EXPRESS EXHIBITORS SERVICE, 239 Calmar Dr., Verona, PA 15147; (412) 731-9018. Ed M. Duva, owner.
PITTSBURGH FILM SERVICE, Building 16, Nichol Ave., McKees Rocks, 15136; (412) 771-2665. John Callahan, mgr.

PORTLAND, OR

LOVETT INTERSTATE THEATRE SERVICE, 935 N.W. 19th Ave., 97210; (503) 224-6108. J. G. (Jack) Lovett, mgr.
PORTLAND NATIONAL FILM SERVICE, 2369 N.W. Quimby St., 97210; (503) 224-6205. Cathy Slade.

ST. LOUIS, MO

KAHAN FILM DISTRIBUTORS, 3974 Page Blvd., 63113; (314) 371-6572. Meyer Kahan, mgr.
LEWTON FILM SERVICE INC., 12721 San Clemente, 63113; (314) 739-0717.

SALT LAKE CITY, UT

NFS OPERATING CORP., 190 N. 640 West, North Salt Lake, 84054; (801) 292-7626. Rulon Hammer.

SAN FRANCISCO

FILM MESSENGER SERVICE, 215 Golden Gate Ave.; 431-4074. Stan Draper, owner.
NFS OPERATING CORP., 35 Guy Place, 94105; (415) 362-2182. Donna Primeau.

SEATTLE

LOCAL FILM DELIVERY, INC., 900 Maynard South, 98134; (206) 682-6663. Chas. D. Lawson, pres.
SEATTLE NATIONAL FILM SERVICE, 900 Maynard Ave., So., 98134; (206) 682-6685. Norman Jones.

WASHINGTON, DC

HIGHWAY DISTRIBUTION SERVICE, 15113 Old Marlboro Pike, Upper; Marlboro, MD 20772; (301) 952-1320. John Hinner.
MOLITCH FILM SERVICE, 3194 Bladensburg Rd., N.E. 20018; (202) 526-0733. Dan McClafferty.

Financing Companies & Banking Services

BANK OF AMERICA, 555 S. Flower St., Los Angeles, CA 90071; (213) 228-4096.
CINEMA GROUP, 8758 Venice Blvd., Los Angeles, CA 90212; (213) 204-0102.
CITICORP, 444 S. Flower St., Los Angeles, CA 90071; (213) 745-3500.
CITY NATIONAL BANK, 400 N. Roxbury Dr., Beverly Hills, CA 90210; (213) 550-5696.
FIRST LOS ANGELES BANK, 9595 Wilshire Blvd., Beverly Hills, CA 90212; (213) 557-1211.
MERCANTILE NATIONAL BANK, 1840 Century Park East, Los Angeles, CA 90067; (213) 277-2265.
SKOURAS PICTURES, INC., 415 N. Crescent Dr., Beverly Hills, CA 90210; (213) 859-7727.
THIRD EYE PRODUCTION CO., 100 S. Doheny Dr., Los Angeles, CA 90048; (213) 858-4939.
WELLS FARGO BANK, 9600 Santa Monica Blvd., Beverly Hills, CA 90210; (213) 550-2262.

Lighting Equipment

BARDWELL & McALLISTER, 7269 Santa Monica Blvd., Hollywood, CA 90038; (213) 876-4133.
BATES LIGHTING CO., 1215 Bates Ave., L.A. 90029; (213) 661-1262.
BIRNS & SAWYER, 1026 N. Highland Ave., L.A. 90038; (213) 466-8211.
BERKEY-COLORTRAN, INC., (A division of Berkey Photo, Inc.), 1015 Chestnut St., Burbank, CA 91502; (213) 843-1200; 842 Broadway, N.Y.; 475-8700. (Berkey Photo).
BLAKE FILMS, 104 West Concord, St., Boston, MA 02118; (617) 267-7713.
BOKEN, INC., 349 West 48th St., N.Y., NY 10036; (212) LT 1-5626.
THE CAMERA MART, 456 West 55th St., N.Y., NY 10019; (212) 757-6977.
F&B/CECO/SOS, 315 W. 43rd St., N.Y. 10036; (212) 586-1420; 7051 Santa Monica Blvd., 90038; (213) 466-9361.
ALAN GORDON ENTS., CO., 5342 Cahuenga, No. Hollywood, CA; (213) 985-5500.
LEONETTI CINE RENTALS, 5609 Sunset Blvd., L.A., CA 90028; (213) 469-2987.
LIGHTING & PRODUCTION EQUIPMENT, INC., 1081 Memorial Drive, S.E. (rear) Atlanta, GA 30316; (404) 681-0130. W. Bruce Harlan, pres.
LOS ANGELES STAGE LIGHTING CO. LTD., 1451 Venice Blvd., L.A., CA 90006; (213) 384-1241.
MOLE-RICHARDSON CO., 937 N. Sycamore Ave., L.A. 90038; (213) 851-0111.
CHARLES ROSS, INC., 333 W. 52nd St., N.Y., NY 10019; (212) CI 6-5470.
TIMES SQUARE THEATRICAL & STUDIO SUPPLY CORP., 318 West 47th St., New York, NY 10019; (212) 245-4155.

Market Research

MARKET RESEARCH CORP. OF AMERICA, 122 E. 42nd St., New York, NY 10017, (212) 953-7240; 624 South Michigan Ave., 60605, (312) 939-1500.
NIELSEN, A. C., CO., Nielsen Plaza, Northbrook, IL 60062, (312) 498-6300; 1290 Ave. of Americas, N.Y., NY 10019, (212) 956-2500.
OPINION RESEARCH CORP., Research Park, Princeton, NJ 08540; (212) 489-1955.
POLITZ, ALFRED, RESEARCH INC., 300 Park Ave., So., N.Y., NY 10010; (212) 982-7600.
THE PULSE, INC., 730 5th Ave., N.Y., NY 10019; (212) 586-3316.
ROPER ORGANIZATION, THE, 1 Park Ave., N.Y., NY 10017; (212) 679-3523.
SAN FRANCISCO RESEARCH GROUP, 2200 Sacramento St., Suite 1206, San Francisco, CA 94115.
SINDLINGER & CO., INC., Harvard & Yale Aves., Swarthmore, PA 19081; (215) 544-9000.
STARCH INRA HOOPER, INC., East Boston Post Rd., Mamaroneck, NY 10543; (914) 698-0800.
TRENDEX, INC., 477 Madison Ave., New York, NY 10017; (212) 752-7160.
VIDEODEX, INC., 342 Madison Ave., New York, NY 10017; (212) 687-8837.

Merchandisers

DISNEY, WALT, PRODUCTIONS, (Character Merchandising Division), 477 Madison Ave., N.Y., NY 10022; (212) 593-8900.
HARVEY FAMOUS CARTOONS, 15 Columbus Circle, N.Y., NY 10024; (212) 582-2244.
HODGE CO., MARGARET, 488 Madison Ave., N.Y., NY 10022; (212) 758-9230.

Music, Music Libraries and Music Cutting

ARIES SOUND INTERNATIONAL, 245 E. 63 St., N.Y., NY 10021; (212) 838-4940.
EMIL ASCHER, INC., 666 Fifth Ave., N.Y., NY 10019; (212) 581-4504.
AUDIO DIRECTORS, INC., 325 West 19 St., N.Y., NY 10011; (212) 924-5850.
CHAPELL MUSIC LIBRARY, 810 Seventh Ave., New York, NY 10019; (212) 977-7213.
CORELLI-JACOBS FILM MUSIC INC., 25 West 45 St., N.Y., NY 10036; (212) 586-6673.
DE WOLFE MUSIC LIBRARY, 25 W. 45 St., N.Y., NY 10036; (212) 586-6673.
EDWARDS, CLEVE (composer-producer), 311 Pall Mall St., Columbia, SC 29201; (803) 252-3504.
FILM SCORES BY JERRY MARKOE, 11 Fort George Hill 13c, New York, NY 10040; (212) 567-6223. Jerry Markoe, composer-conductor.
FILMSOUNDS, INC., 128 East 41 Street, N.Y., NY 10017; (212) 867-0330.
MacGREGOR, C. P., CO., 729 South Western Ave., Los Angeles 90005; (213) 384-4191.
MEDIA IN MUSIC, 34 Starlight Lane, Levittown, N.Y. 11756; (516) 731-8735. Howard Lerner, President.
MUSIC FOR FILMS INC., 49 West 45 St, N.Y., NY 10036; (212) 247-3577.
MUSIC HOUSE INC., 16 East 48 St., N.Y., NY 10017; (212) 758-7773.
M.S.T.S. MUSIC, 1600 Broadway, N.Y., NY 10019; (212) 246-4687.
PIC COLOR CORP., 25 W. 45 St., New York, NY 10036; (212) 575-5600.
PICTURE SCORES, INC., 115 West 45 St., N.Y., NY 10036; (212) JU 6-1845.
ROSS-GAFFNEY, INC., 21 W. 46 St., N.Y., 10036; (212) 582-3744.
SCORE PRODUCTIONS, INC., 249 East 49 St., N.Y., NY 10021; (212) 751-2510.
THOMAS BROTHERS, 30 Berry St., Los Angeles, CA 94107; (415) 664-1901.
VALENTINO, THOMAS J., INC, 150 W. 46 St., N.Y., NY 10036; (212) 246-46675.

Properties and Scenery

BASCH, JOS, GALLERIES CO., 5755 Santa Monica Blvd., Hollywood, 90038; (213) 463-5116.
CINEMA MERCANTILE CO., 5857 Santa Monica Blvd., L.A. 90038; (213) 467-1151.
CINEMA PROPS CO., 6161 Santa Monica Blvd., Hollywood, 90038; (213) 464-3191.
FANTASY FAIR, 4310 San Fernando Rd., Glendale, CA; (213) 245-7367.
FLORA SET, INC., 127 Camino De Las Colinas, Redondo Beach, CA 90277. Specializes in artificial foliage.
GROSH, R. L. (Scenic Studios), 4114 Sunset Blvd.; L.A. CA, 90028; (213) 662-1134.
HOUSE OF PROPS, 1117 Gower St., Hollywood, CA; 463-3166.
MGM/UA ENTERTAINMENT CO., 10202 West Washington Blvd., Culver City, CA 90230; (213) 836-3000.
OMEGA STUDIO RENTALS, 5757 Santa Monica, Blvd., L.A., 90038; (213) 466-8201.
ROSCHU, 6514 Santa Monica Blvd., L.A. 90038; (213) 469-2749.
SILVESTRI STUDIOS, 1733 Cordova, Hollywood; (213) 735-1481.
WOOLF BILLY HOUSE OF MOTION PICTURE ACCESSORIES, INC., 1112 N. Beachwood Dr., Hollywood; (213) 469-5335.

Rental Studios and Production Facilities

ATLANTA

LIGHTING & PRODUCTION EQUIPMENT, INC., 1081 Memorial Drive, S.E. (rear), 30316; (404) 681-0130.

LOS ANGELES

R. L. BEVINGTON, INC., 146 N. LaBrea Ave., 90036; (213) 937-0546.
BURBANK STUDIOS, 4000 Warner Blvd., Burbank, CA 91522; (213) 843-6000.
CARTHAY STUDIOS, INC., 5903-07 W. Pico Blvd., L.A. 90035; (213) 938-2101.
CBS/FOX STUDIOS, 4024 N. Radford Ave., N. Hollywood, CA 91604; (818) 760-5000.
CINEMOBILE SYSTEMS, INC., 11166 Gault St., No. Hollywood; (213) 764-9900.
COLUMBIA PICTURES CORP., Colgems Sq. Burbank, 91505; (213) 843-6000.
CULVER CITY STUDIOS, INC., 9336 W. Washington 90230; (213) 871-0360.
FALCON STUDIOS, 5526 Hollywood Blvd., L.A. 90028; (213) 462-9356.
F&B/CECO OF CALIFORNIA, INC., 7051 Santa Monica Blvd., Hollywood 90038; (213) 466-9361.
GOLDWYN, SAMUEL STUDIOS, 10203 Santa Monica Blvd., L.A. 90067; (213) 851-1234.
HOLLYWOOD GENERAL STUDIOS, 1040 N. Las Palmas Ave., L.A., 90038; (213) 552-2255.
MGM/UA ENTERTAINMENT CO., 10202 W. Washington Blvd., Culver City, CA 90230; (213) 836-3000.
MOLE-RICHARDSON CO., 937 N. Sycamore Ave., L.A. 90038; (213) 654-3060.
PARAMOUNT PICTURES CORP., 5555 Melrose Ave., 90038; (213) 468-5000.
PRODUCERS STUDIO, INC., 650 North Bronson Ave., Los Angeles 90004; (213) 466-8111.
U.P.A. PICTURES, INC., 4440 Lakeside Drive, Burbank, CA, 91505; (213) 849-6666.
UNIVERSAL CITY STUDIOS, 100 Universal City Plaza, Universal City Plaza, Universal City, 91608; (213) 985-4321.

MIAMI

LUKE MOBERLY STUDIOS AND PRODUCTIONS, 4810 S.W. 54, Ft. Lauderdale, FL; Tel.: 581-7508.

NEW YORK

BOKEN SOUND STUDIO, 513 West 54th St., NY 10019; (212) 581-5507.
CINEMOBILE SYSTEMS, INC., 601 West 29th St.; (212) 695-7585.
DIRECTORS STUDIO, 527 West 4th St., 10036; (212) 581-2050.
EAST COAST TELEPRODUCTION, 3200 Expressway Dr., So., Central Islip, NY 11722; (516) 582-6700.
HBO STUDIO PRODS., 120 East 23rd St., 10010; (212) 477-8600.
KAUFMAN ASTORIA MOTION PICTURE AND TELEVISION PRODUCTION CENTER, 34-31 35th Ave., Astoria 11106; (212) 392-5600.
METROPOLIS STUDIOS, 31 Union Square West, #1300, New York, NY 10003; (212) 620-0222.
NATIONAL SCREEN SERVICE CORPORATION, TV AND INDUSTRIAL FILMS DIVISION, 1600 Broadway, New York, NY 10017; (212) 246-5700.
NATIONAL VIDEO CENTER/RECORDING STUDIOS, INC., 460 West 42 St., New York, NY 10036; (212) 279-2000.
PRODUCTION CENTER, 221 West 26th St., 10001; (212) 675-2211.
REEVES TELETAPE, 708 Third Ave., 10017; (212) 573-8600.
SILVERCUP STUDIOS, INC., 42–25 21st St., Long Island City, NY 11101; (212) 784-3390.
TITRA SOUND CORPORATION, 1600 Broadway, NY 10019; (212) PL 7-6681.
TVC VIDEO, 225 East 43rd St., 10017; (212) 599-1616.
UNITED FILM ENTERPRISES, INC., 1546 Broadway, New York, NY 10036; (212) 586-1442.

TAMPA, FLORIDA

POST PRODUCTION SERVICES, 3808 San Nicholas St.; (813) 253-0402.

Screening Rooms

ATLANTA

ATLANTA PREVIEW THEATRE, 161 Spring St., N.W.; (404) 523-0663.
20th-CENTURY FOX EXCHANGE, 2200 Century Parkway, 30345; (404) 321-1178.

BOSTON

E.M. LOEW THEATRES, 164 Tremont St., Boston, 02111; (617) 482-9200.
UNIVERSAL, 44 Winchester St., 02116; (617) 426-8760.

CHICAGO

H. & E. BALABAN THEATRES, 190 North State St., Chicago 60601; (312) 372-2262.
CHICAGO INTERNATIONAL FILM FESTIVAL, 235 Eugenie, Chicago 60614; (312) 644-3400.
DOUGLAS FILM INDUSTRIES, 10 W. Kinzie, 60610; (312) 664-7455.
ESSANESS THEATRES CORPORATION, 54 West Randolph, Chicago 60601; (312) 332-7465.
UNIVERSAL FILM EXCHANGES, INC., 425 North Michigan Avenue, Chicago 60601; (312) 822-0513.

CINCINNATI

20TH CENTURY-FOX FILM CORP., 617 Vine St., 45202; (513) 241-6460.

DENVER

THE FLICK THEATRE, Larimer Sq., 80202; (303) 244-9155.
THE SCREENING ROOM, 1245 Champa St., 80204; (303) 892-0987.
THEATRE AT THE COURT, 1776 Grand St., 80203; (303) 861-2000.

KANSAS CITY

COMMONWEALTH THEATRES, 215 W. 18th St., 64108; (816) 471-2390.
DICKINSON OPERATING CO., 5913 Woodson Rd., Mission, KS 66202; (316) 432-2234.

LOS ANGELES

ACADEMY AWARD THEATRE, 8949 Wilshire Blvd., Beverly Hills, 90211; (213) 278-8900.
AIDIKOFF, CHAS., SCREENING ROOM, 9255 W. Sunset Blvd., 90069; (213) 274-0866.
BEVERLY HILLS SCREENING ROOM, 8949 Sunset Blvd., Beverly Hills, CA 90069; (213) 550-9839.
BURBANK STUDIOS, 4000 Warner Blvd., Burbank, CA 91522; (213) 954-6000.
CENTRE FILMS INC., 1103 N. El Centro Ave., Hollywood 90038; (213) 466-5123.
CONSOLIDATED FILM INDUSTRIES, 959 Seward St., L.A. 90038; (213) 462-3161.
DE LUXE GENERAL, 1546 N. Argyle Ave., L.A. 90028; (213) 462-6171.
DIRECTORS GUILD OF AMERICA, 7950 W. Sunset Blvd., Los Angeles 90046; (213) 656-1220.
HOLLYWOOD SCREENING ROOM, 1800 N. Highland Ave., Suite 511, Hollywood 90028; (213) 466-1888.
MARTIN NOSSECK PROJECTION THEATRE, 9118½ Sunset Blvd., Hollywood, 90069; (213) 275-3037.
PREVIEW HOUSE, 7655 S. Sunset Blvd., L.A. 90046; (213) 876-6600.
JOE SHORE'S SCREENING ROOM, 9229 W. Sunset Blvd., L.A. 90046; (213) 274-4888.

MILWAUKEE

CENTRE THEATRE BLDG., 212 W. Wisconsin Ave., 53203; (608) 272-6020.
RKO-STANLEY WARNER THEATRES, INC., 5341 W. Fond du Lac Avenue (Capitol Court Theater); (608) 871-2213.

NEW YORK

(All major producers-distributors have screening rooms at their home offices in New York for their own use. Most also have screening room facilities at their New York exchanges).

CINE-METRIC THEATRE INC., 290 Madison Ave., 10017; (212) 532-4140.
FIFTH AVENUE SCREENING ROOM, 4 West 56th St., 10019; (212) 541-5454.
MAGNO PARK AVE., 445 Park Ave., 10019; (212) 757-8855.
MOVIELAB THEATRE SERVICE, INC., 619 W. 54th St., 10019; (212) 586-0360.
PRECISION FILM LABS' SCREENING THEATRE, 630 Ninth Avenue; 489-8800.
PREVIEW THEATRE, 1600 Broadway, 10019; (212) 246-0865.
RIZZOLI SCREENING ROOM, 712 5th Ave., 10019; (212) 397-3738.
ROSS-GAFFNEY INC., 21 W. 46 St., 10036; (212) 582-3744.
WESTSIDE SCREENINGS, INC., 311 West 43rd St., 10036; (212) 246-3838.

SAN FRANCISCO

MOTION PICTURE SERVICE CO., 125 Hyde St., 94107; (415) 673-9162.
THOMAS BROTHERS, 30 Berry St., 94107; (415) 664-1901.

TAMPA

POST PRODUCTION SERVICES, INC., 3808 San Nicholas St.; (813) 253-0400.

WASHINGTON

CAPITAL FILM LABORATORIES, INC., 470 "E" St., S.W., 20002; (202) 347-1717.
KOSTER FILM FACILITIES, INC., 1017 "E" St., S.W., 20002; (202) 544-4410.

Slides-Telops

BEBELL, INC., 416 W. 45th St., N.Y., NY 10036; (212) 245-8900.
TWO BY TWO SLIDES, INC., 2 West 45 St., 10036; (212) 972-0744.

Sound and Recording Services

HOLLYWOOD

ALTEC SERVICE CORP., 1515 S. Manchester Ave., Anaheim; (714) 774-2900.
ARTISAN SOUND RECORDERS, 1600 N. Wilcox Ave., Hollywood 90028; (213) 461-2751.
AUDIO EFFECTS COMPANY, 1600 N. Western Ave., Hollywood 90027; (213) 469-3692. (Complete recording services).
BURBANK STUDIOS, THE, 4000 Warner Blvd., Burbank, CA 91522; (213) 843-6000.
CINESOUND, 915 North Highland Ave., Hollywood, CA 90038; (213) 464-1155.
COLUMBIA PICTURES TELEVISION, 300 S. Colgens Square, Burbank, 91522; (213) 954-6000.
CONSOLIDATED FILM INDUSTRIES, 959 N. Seward St., L.A. 90038; (213) 462-3161.
DOLBY LABORATORIES, Hollywood Film Support, 6671 Sunset Blvd., Suite 1591, Hollywood, CA 90028; (213) 464-4596.
GLEN GLENN SOUND CO., 6624 Romaine St., Hollywood 90038; (213) 469-7221.
INDEPENDENT PRODUCERS SERVICE, 7370 Melrose Ave., Hollywood 90046; (213) 655-3599.
MGM/UA ENTERTAINMENT CO., 10202 W. Washington Blvd., Culver City 90230; (213) 836-3000.
NEWJACK SOUND RECORDERS, 1717 N. Highland Ave., L.A. 90038; (213) 466-6141.
PARAMOUNT RECORDING STUDIOS, 5451 Marathon St., Hollywood, 90038; (213) 46137170.
PRODUCERS SOUND SERVICE, INC., 3610 West Magnolia Blvd., Burbank 91505; (818) 841-4887.
QUALITY SOUND, 5625 Melrose Ave., 90038; (213) 467-7154.
RYDER SOUND SERVICES, INC., 1611 Vine St., Hollywood; (213) 469-3511.
SCOTTSOUND, INC., 6110 Santa Monica Blvd., 90038; (213) 462-6981.
TODD-AO SOUND RECORDING SCORING, 1021 N. Seward St., Hollywood, 90038; (213) 463-1136.
TV RECORDERS, 6054 Sunset Blvd., Hollywood; (213) 469-8201.
UNIVERSAL CITY STUDIOS, 100 Universal City, Plaza, UC 91608; (213) 985-4321.
WARNER HOLLYWOOD STUDIOS, 1041 N. Formosa, Los Angeles, 90046; (213) 650-2500.

NEW YORK

ADD SOUND, INC., 16 W. 46 St., 10036; (212) 575-0719.
AQUARIUS TRANSFER, 12 E. 46 St., 10017; (212) 581-0123.
AURA RECORDING, INC., 136 W. 52nd St., 10019; (212) 582-8105.
DOLBY LABORATORIES, New York Film Support, 342 East 55 St., #6D, 10022; (212) 759-4511.
HIT FACTORY, THE, INC., 353 W. 48 St., 10036; (212) 581-9590.
IMAGE SOUND STUDIO, INC., 1619 Broadway, 10036; (212) 581-6717.
MAGNO SOUND, INC., 212 W. 48th, 10036; (212) 757-8855.
MUSIC SOUND TRACK SERVICE, 1600 Broadway, 10019; (212) CIrcle 6-4687-8.
NATIONAL RECORDING STUDIOS, 730 Fifth Ave., 10019; (212) 757-6440.
RKO SOUND STUDIOS, 1440 Broadway, 10018; (212) 564-8000.
ROSS-GAFFNEY, INC., 21 W. 46th St., 10018; (212) 582-3745.
SOUND SHOP, THE, 304 E. 44 St., 10017; (212) 757-9800.
TITRA SOUND CORP., 1600 Broadway, 10019; (212) 757-6681.
THOMAS J. VALENTINO, 151 West 46th St., 10036; (212) 246-4675.

SAN FRANCISCO

DOLBY LABORATORIES, Head Office & U.S. Sales, 100 Potrero Ave., 94103; (415) 558-0200. Telex: 34409.
THOMAS BROTHERS, 30 Berry St., 94107; (415) 664-1901.

WASHINGTON, DC

BYRON MOTION PICTURES INC., 65 K St., N.E., 20002; (202) 783-2700.
CAPITAL FILM LABORATORIES, INC., 470 E. St., S.W., 20024; (202) 347-1717.

Special Effects

NEW YORK

ACTION PRODUCTIONS, INC., 16 West 46 St., New York, NY 10036; (212) 391-2747.
ANIMATED CAMERA WORKSHOP, 51 East 42 St., N.Y., NY 10017; (212) 687-5009.
ANIMATED PRODUCTIONS, INC., 1600 Broadway, New York NY 10019; (212) 265-2942.
EUE/SCREEN GEM PRINTS, 222 East 44 St., New York, NY 10017; (212) 867-43030.
EXCEPTIONAL OPEICALS, INC., 17 East 45 St., New York, NY 10017; (212) 972-1760.
FILM OPTICALS, INC., 144 East 44 St., New York, NY 10017; (212) 697-4744.
I.F. STUDIOS, INC., 328 East 44 St., New York, NY 10017; (212) 683-4747.
MINI-EFFECTS, INC., 15 West 44 St., New York, Ny 10036; (212) 869-0370.
NATIONAL SCREEN SERVICE CORP., TV & INDUSTRIAL FILMS DIVISION, 1600 Broadway, New York, NY 10019; (212) 246-5700.
OPTICAL HOUSE, INC., 25 West 45 St., New York, NY 10036; (212) 757-7840.
PROFESSIONAL OPTICALS, INC., 20 East St., New York, NY 10017; (212) JU 2-0650.
RAINBOW FILMS EFFECTS, INC., 45 West 45 St., New York, NY 10036; (212) 247-1676.
TRI-PIX FILM SERVICE, INC., 49 West 45 St., New York, NY 10036; (212) JU 2-0650.
WORLD EFFECTS, INC., 20 East 46 St., New York, NY 10017; (212) 687-7070.

HOLLYWOOD

ANDERSON, HOWARD A., CO., Main Office: Paramount Studios, 5451 Marathon St., Hollywood, CA 90038; (213) 463-2336.
BRAVERMAN PRODS., INC., 8961 Sunset Blvd., L.A. 90069; (213) 278-5444.
CINEMA SERVICE, INC., 5725 Santa Monica Blvd.; (213) 462-1376.
COAST SPECIAL EFFECTS, 4907 N. Lankershim Blvd., N. Hollywood, 91602; (213) 876-2021.
CONSOLIDATED FILM INDUSTRIES, 959 N. Seward St., 90038; (213) 462-3161.
FILM EFFECTS OF HOLLYWOOD, 1140 N. Citrus, Hollywood; (213) 469-5808.
MERCER RAY & CO., 4241 Normal Ave.; (213) 663-9331.
MODERN FILM EFFECTS, 6824 Melrose Ave., 90030; (213) 938-2155.
OPTICAL PRINT SERVICES, INC., 1132 N. Vine St., Los Angeles, 90028; (213) 462-7446.
PACIFIC TITLE & ART STUDIO, 6350 Santa Monica Blvd., Los Angeles 90038; (213) 464-0121.
VIDEOTAPE ENTERPRISES, 8610 Sunset Blvd., Los Angeles, 90069; (213) 659-4801.

Stop Watches

DUCOMMUN, M., CO., 48 Main St., Warwick, NY 10990; (914) 986-5757.
MARCEL WATCH CORP., 1180 Sixth Ave., N.Y., NY 10036; (212) 245-3355.
RACINE, JULES & CO., 85 Executive Rd., Elmsford, NY 10523; (914) 592-4760.

Sub-titles

WHITE ROSE CAPTION, INC., Sundvall Bldg., 83-90 Broadway, Elmhurst, Queens, NY 11373; (212) 271-3388. Negative subtitle cards—super-imposed negative and traslations in most languages for motion pcitures and TV. Ms. Rose Robles, pres.

Trailers

ATLANTA

CINEMA CONCEPTS THEATRE SERVICE, INC., P.O. Box 720576, Atlanta 30328; (404) 396-1055.

NATIONAL SCREEN SERVICE, 1325 Logan Circle, N.W.; 351-1416. Robert Sedlak, br. mgr.

CHICAGO

FILMACK CORP., 1327 S. Wabash Ave., 60605; (312) 427-3395. Joseph R. Mack, pres.

KANSAS CITY, MO

NATIONAL SCREEN SERVICE CORP., 1800 Baltimore Ave., 64108; 842-5893. William Lustig, sls. mgr.
UNIVERSAL IMAGES, LTD., 9504 E. 63rd Street, Kansas City, MO 64133; (816) 358-6166. Garrett Tuck, president.

LOS ANGELES

COMING ATTRACTIONS, 6671 Sunset Blvd., 90028; (213) 469-1207.
LAJON PRODUCTIONS, INC., 2907 W. Olive Ave., Burbank, CA 91505; (213) 841-1440.
NATIONAL SCREEN SERVICE, 2001 S. La Cienega Blvd., 90034; 836-1505. Robert Young, br. mgr.
UTA, INC., 1658 Cordova St., 9007; (213) 734-0510. Joan Atamian Bodin, pres.

NEW YORK CITY

NATIONAL SCREEN SERVICE, 1600 Broadway, 10019; (212) 246-5700.
TFI, 619 West 54th St., 10019; (212) 708-0500.

PHILADELPHIA

NATIONAL SCREEN SERVICE, 130 Ferry Ave., Camden, NJ 08104. Wm. Gwiazdowski, br. mgr.

Talent and Literary Agencies

HOLLYWOOD

(Where two letters are given for zip code the first three are 900. Telephone area code is 213, unless otherwise indicated.)

ABRAMS-RUBALOFF & ASSOC., INC.,
8075 West 3rd (48), 935-1700
AGENCY FOR PERFORMING ARTS,
9000 Sunset Blvd., #.315 (69), 273-0744
AIMEE ENTERTAINMENT ASSOCIATES,
13749 Victory Blvd., Van Nuys, CA (91401), 994-9354
ALVARADO, CARLOS,
8820 Sunset Blvd. (69), 652-0272
AMARAL/MURPHY AGENCY,
1000 Riverside Dr., Toluca Lake (91602), (818) 980-1013
AUER, MILES BOHM,
8344 Melrose Ave., Suite 29 (69), 653-8105
BARSKIN AGENCY,
11240 Magnolia Blvd., No. Hollywood (91601), (818) 985-2992
BLAKE AGENCY, LTD.,
409 N. Camden Dr., BH (91602), 278-6885
BLANCHARD, NINA,
1717 N. Highland (28), 462-7341
BREWIS AGENCY, ALEX,
4721 Laurel Canon Blvd., No. Hollywood (91607), (818) 509-0831
CALDER AGENCY,
4150 Riverside Dr., Burbank (91505), (818) 845-7434
CAREY-PHELPS-COLVIN,
121 N. Robertson, (90211), 659-6671
CENTURY ARTISTS, LTD.,
9744 Wilshire Blvd., BH (90212), 273-4366
CHARTER MGMT.,
9000 Sunset Blvd. (69), 278-1690
COMMERCIALS UNLTD.,
7461 Beverly Blvd. (36), 937-2220
CONTEMPORARY-KORMAN,
132 Lasky Dr., BH (90212), 278-8250
COUGLIN AGENCY, KERWIN,
2221 W. Olive, Burbank (91506), (818) 848-7929
CUMBER, LIL,
6515 Sunset Blvd. (28), 469-1919
CUNNINGHAM & ASSOC.
261 S. Robertson, BH (90211), 855-1700
DIAMOND ARTISTS, LTD.,
9200 Sunset Blvd. (69), 278-8146
EISENBACH-GREENE-DUCHOW, INC.,
760 N. La Cienega Blvd. L.A. (69), 659-3420
ENTERTAINMENT ENTERPRISES,
1680 Vine St. (28), 462-6001
FELBER, WM.,
2126 Cahuenga Blvd. (68), 466-7627
FIELDS ASSOC., JACK,
9255 Sunset Blvd. (69), 278-1333
FRINGS, KURT,
415 N. Crescent Dr., BH (90210), 274-8881
GARRICK, DALE,
8831 Sunset Blvd. (69), 657-2661
GERSH AGENCY, PHIL,
222 N. Canon Dr., BH (90210), 274-6611
GIBSON, J. CARTER,
9000 Sunset Blvd (69), 274-8813
GORDEAN AGENCY, INC.,
809 N. Foothill Rd., BH (90210), 273-4195
GREENVINE AGENCY,
9021 Melrose Ave. (69), 278-5800
GREEN AGENCY, IVAN,
1888 Century Park East (67), 277-1541
GROSSMAN & ASSOCIATES,
211 S. Beverly Dr. (90212), 550-8127
HAMILBURG, MITCHELL,
292 S. La Cienga, BH (90211), 657-1501
HECHT, BEVERLY,
8949 Sunset Blvd. (69), 278-3544
HUNT, GEORGE B.,
8350 Santa Monica Blvd. (46), 654-6600
INGERSOLL, GEORGE,
6513 Hollywood Blvd. (28), 874-6434
INT'L CREATIVE MANAGEMENT,
8899 Beverly Blvd. (48), 550-4000
KELMAN, TONI AGENCY,
7813 Sunset Blvd. (46), 851-8822
KING AGENCY, HOWARD,
118 S. Beverly Dr., BH, (69) 858-8048
KOHNER, PAUL,
9169 Sunset Blvd. (69), 550-1060
LAZAR, IRVING PAUL,
211 S. Beverly Dr., BH, 275-6153
LEONETTI, CAROLINE,
6526 Sunset Blvd. (28), 463-5610
LONGNECKER, ROBERT,
11704 Wilshire (25), 477-0039
LYONS, GRACE,
204 S. Beverly Dr. (90212), 652-5290
McHUGH AGENCY, JAMES,
8150 Beverly Blvd. (48), 651-2770
McMILLIAN, HAZEL,
126 N. Doheny Dr. (90211), BH, 276-9823
MESSENGER, FRED,
8235 Sunset Blvd. (46), 654-3800
MISHKIN AGENCY,
9255 Sunset Blvd. (69), 274-5261
MORRIS, WILLIAM,
151 El Camino Dr., BH (90212), 274-7451
PEARSON, BEN,
606 Wilshire Blvd. Santa Monica (90401), 451-8414
PREMIERE ARTISTS & PROD.
6399 Wilshire Blvd. (48), 651-3545
PRESCOTT, GUY,
8920 Wonderland Ave. (46), 656-1963
RAPER ENTERPRISES AGENCY,
9441 Wilshire Blvd. (12), 273-7704
ROBINSON-WEINTRAUB & ASSOCIATES,
8428 Melrose Place (69), 653-5802
RUSH, ART,
10221 Riverside Dr., No. Hwd. (91602), 985-3033
SACKHEIM AGENCY,
9301 Wilshire Blvd., BH (90210), 858-0606
SANDERS AGENCY, NORAH,
1100 Glendon Ave. (24), 824-2264
SCHWARTZ & ASSOC., DON,
8721 Sunset Blvd. (69), 657-8910
SHAW, GLENN,
3330 Barkam Blvd. (68), 851-6262
SHERRELL AGENCY LEW,
7060 Hollywood Blvd. (28), 461-9955
TANNEN & ASSOC. HERB,
6640 Sunset Blvd. (28), 466-6191
TOBIAS & ASSOCIATES,
1901 Ave. of Stars (67), 277-6211
WEINER, JACK,
8721 Sunset Blvd. (69), 652-1140
WEVER, WARREN,
1104 S. Robertson Blvd. (35), 276-7065
WOSK AGENCY, SYLVIA,
435 S. La Cienega (48), 274-8063
WRIGHT ASSOC., ANN,
8422 Melrose Pl. (69), 655-5040

NEW YORK

(Where two letters are given for zip code the first three are 100. Area telephone code is 212.)

AGENCY FOR PERFORMING ARTS,
888 Seventh Ave. (10106), 582-1500.
ALEXANDER INC., WILLARD,
660 Madison Ave. (21), 751-7070
AMERICAN-INT'L TALENT
166 W. 125 St. (27), 663-4626
ANDERSON, BEVERLY,
1472 Broadway, Ste. 806 (36), 944-7773
ASSOCIATED BOOKING CORP.,
1995 Broadway (23), 874-2400
ASTOR, RICHARD,
1697 Broadway (19), 581-1970
CASE, BERTHA,
345 W. 58 St. (19), 541-9451
COLEMAN-ROSENBERG AGCY.,
667 Madison Ave. (21), 838-0734

COOPER ASSOC., BILL,
224 West 49 St. (19), 307-1100
DEACY, JANE,
300 E. 75 St. (21), 752-4865
DIAMOND ARTISTS, LTD.,
119 W. 57 St. (19), 247-3025
DRAPER, STEPHEN AGENCY,
37 W. 57 St. (19), 421-5780
GAGE GROUP, THE,
1650 Broadway (19), 541-5250
HARTIG, MICHAEL,
114 East 28 St. (22), 684-0010
HENDERSON/HOGAN AGENCY,
200 W. 57 St. (19), 765-5190
HUNT, DIANA,
44 W. 44 St. (36), 391-4971
INT'L CREATIVE MANAGEMENT,
40 W. 57 St. (19), 556-5600
JACOBSON/WILDER, INC.,
419 Park Ave. S. (16), 686-6100.
JAN J. AGENCY,
224 E. 46 St. (17), 490-1875
JORDAN, JOE TALENT AGCY.,
200 West 57 St., (19), 582-9003
KENNEDY ARTISTS REP.,
237 West 11 St. (19), 675-3944
KROLL LUCY,
390 West End Ave. (24), 877-0627
LARNER, LIONEL LTD.,
850 7th Ave. (19), 246-3105
LEIGH ENTERPRISES, LTD., SANFORD,
440 East 62 St. (22), 752-4450
LEWIS ASSOC., LESTER,
110 West 40 St. (18), 921-8370
McDERMOTT, MARGE,
216 E. 39th (16), 889-1583
MARTINELLI MANAGEMENT,
888 8th Ave. (36), 977-7166
MORRIS AGENCY, WM.,
1350 Ave. of Americas (19), 586-5100
OPPENHEIM-CHRISTIE ASSOC.,
565 5th Ave. (17), 661-4330
OSCARD/FIFI AGENCY,
19 W. 44th St. (36), 764-1100
OSTERTAG, BARNA,
501 Fifth Ave. (17), 697-6339
PITT AGENCY, JOEL,
144 W. 57th St. (19), 765-6373
PREMIER TALENT ASSOC.,
3 E. 54th (22), 758-4900
RUBENSTEIN, BERNARD,
215 Park Ave., S. (16), 460-9800
RYAN, CHARLES VERNON,
200 W. 57th (19), 245-2225
SCHULLER AGENCY, WM.,
667 Madison Ave. (22), 758-1919
SILVER, MONTY,
200 W. 57th (19), 765-4040
STROUD MGMT.,
18 E. 48th St. (17), 688-0226
TALENT REPS., INC.,
20 E. 53rd St. (22), 752-1835
THOMAS, MICHAEL,
18 East 53 St. (22), 421-1461
TROY, GLORIA TALENT AGENCY,
1790 Broadway (19), 582-0260
WATERS AGENCY, BOB,
510 Madison Ave. (22), 593-0543
WOLTERS, HANNS,
10 West 37 St. (18), 714-0100
WRIGHT REPS., ANN,
13 E. 57th St. (22), 832-0110

Advertising & Publicity Representatives

HOLLYWOOD-LOS ANGELES-BEVERLY HILLS

(Area code is 213 unless otherwise indicated.)

ABRAMS, BOB, AND ASSOCIATES, 2030 Prosser Ave., Los Angeles 90025; 475-7739.
BARLOR ASSOCIATES, 428 North Palm Dr., Beverly Hills; 278-1998.
BRAVERMAN-MIRISCH, INC., 9255 Sunset Blvd., Los Angeles 90069; 274-5204.
BROCATO & KELMAN, INC., 8425 W. 3rd St., Los Angeles 90048; (213) 653-9570.
DICK BROOKS UNLIMITED, 9465 Wilshire Blvd., Beverly Hills, CA 90212; (213) 273-8477.
BYOIR, CARL, AND ASSOCIATES, INC., 900 Wilshire Blvd., Los Angeles 90019; 627-6421.
DRUXMAN, MICHAEL B. & ASSOCIATES, 8831 Sunset Blvd., Los Angeles 90069; 652-5592.
EDELMAN, DANIEL, INC., 1925 Century Park East, Los Angeles 90067; 553-1560.
FRANKEN PUBLIC RELATIONS, 8530 Wilshire Blvd., B.H. 90021; 655-9326.
GELFOND, FORDON AND ASSOCIATES, 9808 Wilshire Blvd., Beverly Hills 90212; 273-1440.
GUTTMAN & PAM LTD., 120 El Camino Drive, Beverly Hills, 90212; 278-6775.
HANSON & SCHWAM, 9229 Sunset Blvd., Los Angeles 90069; 278-1255.
HARSHE-ROTMAN & DRUCK, INC., 3345 Wilshire Blvd., Los Angeles 90010; 385-5271.
LEE & ASSOCIATES, 8727 West 3rd, Los Angeles 90048; 278-5300.
LEWIS & ASSOCIATES, 3600 Wilshire Blvd., Los Angeles 90010; 739-1000.
LIBERMAN, FRANK, AND ASSOCIATES, 9021 Melrose Ave., Los Angeles 90069; 278-1993.
MAHONEY/WASSERMAN & ASSOCIATES, 117 N. Robertson Blvd., Los Angeles 90048; (818) 788-0164.
McKENZIE, KING & GORDON, 1800 N. Argyle, Hollywood 90028; (213) 466-3421.
MILLER, RENEE PUBLIC RELATIONS, 1313 Foothill Blvd., Suite 8, La Canada, CA 91011; 952-2022.
ROGERS & COWAN, 1000 Santa Monica Blvd., Los Angeles, 90067; 201-8800.
TAMKIN ASSOCIATES, INC., 1122 Robertson Blvd., 90035; (213) 275-6122.
THOMPSON, J. WALTER CO., 10100 Santa Monica Blvd., Los Angeles, 90067; 553-8383.

NEW YORK

(First three letters of zip code are 100 and area code is 212, unless otherwise indicated)

AYER, INC., N.W., 1345 Ave. of Americas, 10105; 708-5000.
BATES & CO., INC., TED, 1515 Broadway, (36), 869-3131.
BATTEN, BARTON, DURSTINE & OSBORNE, INC., 383 Madison Ave., (17); 355-5800.
BECK, MEYER P., 1700 Broadway, (19); 957-9750.
BENTON & BOWLES, INC., 909 Third Ave., (22); 758-6200.
BYOIR, CARL & ASSOCIATES, INC., 380 Madison Ave., (36); 986-6100.
DAVIS, AL, PUBLICITY, 6 East 39, (16); 725-0850.
EISEN, MAX, 234 West 44th St., (36); 391-1072.
GIFFORD/WALLACE, INC., 1211 Park Ave.; 427-7600.
GOODMAN, FRANK, 1776 Broadway, (19); 246-4180.
GREY ADVERTISING AGENCY, 777 Third Ave., (17); 546-2000.
MARCH FIVE, INC. 30 East 42nd St., (16); 687-3484.
MASLANSKY-KOENIGSBERG, INC., 545 Madison Ave., (22); 759-5202.
POST, MYRNA ASSOCIATES, 145 East 49 St., (22); 935-7122.
ROFFMAN, RICHARD H., ASSOCIATES, 697 West End Ave., (23); 749-3647.
ROGERS & COWAN, INC., 122 East 42 St., (16); 490-8200.
RUDER, FINN & ROTMAN, INC., 110 East 59th St.; 593-6400.
SCHLAIFER & CO., INC., CHARLES, 150 East 58th St., 10155; 688-1510.
SACCI PUBLIC RELATIONS, 40 East 49th St., 10017; (212) 486-5336
SOLTERS, ROSKIN, AND FREIDMAN, INC., 45 West 34th St., (36); 947-0515.
WAX, MORTON D. PUBLIC RELATIONS, 1650 Broadway, (19); 247-2159.
WOLHANDER, JOE, ASSOCIATES, INC., 11 West 30 St., (01); 947-6015.
YOUNG & RUBICAN INTERNATIONAL, 285 Madison Ave., (17); 210-3000.

Equipment and Supplies

* MANUFACTURERS & SERVICES

* STUDIO EQUIPMENT

* REFRESHMENT PRODUCTS, EQUIPMENT

* MANUFACTURERS & SERVICES (By Product Classification)

* THEATRE SUPPLY DEALERS

Manufacturers & Services

A-Wagner Zip Change, Inc.

(formerly WAGNER Sign Service)
3100 Hirsch Street, Melrose Park, IL 60160; Tel.: (312) 681-4100.

WAGNER brand slotted dimensional marquee letters in 4", 6", 8", 10" and 17" letters in red, green, blue or black plastic. Wagner brand marquee background with stainless steel frames and unbreakable Enduronamel Panel Assembly, low cost metal marquee for 8" or larger letters, ready to install. Zip-Change plastic or metal flat marquee letters in 6", 8", 10", 12", 15", 17", and 24". Letter changing Mechanical Hands. Letter storage cabinets. Rating Units (PG, R, G). Alumabar letter track. Sell thru theatre suppliers only.

Altec Lansing Corp.

10500 W. Reno, Oklahoma City, OK 73128.

Manufacturers of amplifiers, loudspeakers, electronic devices, microphones and transformers "Voice of the theatre" speaker systems.

American Desk Manufacturing Co.

P.O. Box 429, Temple, TX; Tel.: (817) 773-1776.

Manufacturers of theatre seating.

American Playground Device Co.

Main Offices: 1801-1831 So. Jackson, P.O. Drawer 2599, Anderson, IN 46011; Tel.: (317) 642-0288.

Branch Offices: Nahma Blvd., Nahma, MI 49864; Tel.: (317) 642-0288.

Manufacturers of playground equipment, park benches, picnic tables, charcoal grills, flood lights and swimming pool equipment for drive-in theatres, and bicycle racks for theatres. Complete line of American approved extra-heavy-duty Park, Picnic, Playground, Swimming Pool, Beach and Dressing Room Equipment.

American Seating Company

901 Broadway, N.W., Grand Rapids, MI 49504; Tel.: (616) 456-0600.

(District offices in principal cities)

Manufacturers of auditorium and theatre chairs and portable stacking chairs.

ASC Technical Services Corp. (formerly Altec Service Corporation)

Executive offices: P.O. Box 706, Piano, TX 75074; (214) 422-2160. J. B. Waddell, pres.; R. V. Gandolfi, v.p.

Nationwide sound service and full booth maintenance.

National Director of Field Operations: Lamar Michael, 5857 N. Winthrop, Indianapolis, IN; (317) 257-1807.

Atlantic Audio Visual Corp.

630 Ninth Avenue, New York, NY 10036.

Projection system for mini or maxi theatres. Exclusive U.S. Distributors of Zeiss Ikon Projection Equipment.

Automatic Devices Co.

2121 South 12th St., Allentown, Pa. 18103; Tel.: (215) 797-6000.

Manufacturers of stage, television, drapery and cubicle hardware.

Ballantyne of Omaha, Inc.

(See Strong International)

Bauer Division, AIC Photo, Inc.

168 Glen Cove Road, Carle Place, NY 11514.

Super 8 movie cameras and projectors, 16 mm projectors.

Bevelite-Adler

14824 South Main Street, Gardena, CA 90248; Tel.: (800) 421-1256, (213) 321-5641.

Changeable Marquee letters: "Snap Lok" - "Pronto Glo" - "Regency" - 3"* - 4" - 6" - 8" - 10" - 12" - 15"* - 17" - 24". Red, Black, Blue, Green, White for Snap Lok. Pronto, Regency. Brite Glo is Black/Clear or Black/Yellow. Background support available in complete Stainless steel frames or stainless steel, plastic or aluminum track for self mounting. Pronto change arms and storage cabinets for Pronto and Brite Glo.

* Only in Pronto Style

Brandt, Inc.

705 12th St., Watertown, WI 53094; Tel.: (414) 261-1780.

Manufacturers of coin sorting and counting machines, automatic coin wrappers, currency and document counters.

Bulletin & Directory Board Mfg. Co.

2317 West Pico Blvd., Los Angeles, CA 90006; (213) 382-1147.

Manufacturer of changeable letter boards, magnetic & write-on boards, cork & chalk boards, glass cases/indoor & outdoor free-standing & wall mounted.

Canrad-Hanovia, Inc.

(See Strong International)

CEMCORP (Consolidated Engineering & Manufacturing Corp.)

1515 Melrose Lane, P.O. Box 105, Forest Hill, MD 21050; (301) 838-0036 and (301) 879-3022.

Manufacturers and designers of ticket issuing equipment: "Automaticket" line, including Ticketaker control boxes, drive-in equipment, ticket control systems and TIM/100, complete box office control system.

Century Projector Corporation

1690 Oak, Lakewood, NJ; (201) 367-4434.

Manufacturers and distributors of motion picture equipment.

Christie Electric Corp.

20665 Manhattan Place, Torrance, CA 90501; (213) 320-0808.

Tom Christie, pres.; Fred Benjamin, sr. v.p.; Lynn Shubert, v.p.; Jack Kline, natl. sls. mgr.

Manufacturers of Xenolite consoles (lamphouse, rectifier power supply and projector based housed in one unit), dual sound system, and automatic system.

Cinema Film Systems, Inc.

950 E. Renwick Road, Glendora, CA 91740; (213) 963-6049 and (213) 335-1402. Telex: 67-4668.

Ron E. Offerman, pres.; Richard E. Niccum, sr. v.p.

Manufacture a complete line of projection booth equipment, including platters (3-stack, 5-stack and 35/70), lamphouses, consoles, sound, automation, dimmers, reel arms and projectors. Act as National Sales Representatives for D.O. Industries (KOWA), North American Philips Lighting and Ultra Sound low voltage aisle lighting.

Cinematograph International, Inc.

341 W. 44th St., New York, NY 10036; Tel.: (212) 246-6285.

Distributors of automated theatre equipment and supplies; Cinemeccanica Victoria 70/35mm projectors in U.S.; complete Drive-In theatre equipment; projection-sound equipment and supplies; speaker systems; projection arclamps-rectifiers-generators; Xenon light systems; stage lighting, spotlighting, stage draperies; auditorium seats, carpets; display frames, marquee letters, box office equipment; equipment for Studios, Schools, Auditoriums.

Cinemeccanica U.S., Inc.

5475-115th Ave., North, Clearwater, FL 33520; (813) 577-3211. Victor Nicelli, pres.; Thomas H. Brenner, gen. mgr.

Distributor of Cinemeccanica projection and sound equipment.

Dolby Laboratories Inc.

731 Sansome St., San Francisco, CA 94111; Tel.: (415) 392-0300.

Manufacturer of a full line of equipment for motion picture sound.

Econo-Pleat—Phil Sperling

(A division of Eastwest Carpet Mills)

2664 So. La Cienga Blvd., Los Angeles, CA 90034; Tel.: (213) 871-1690.

Manufacturers of acoustical fabric wall coverings.

EPRAD, Inc.

P.O. Box 73, Rossford, OH 43460; (1) (800) 782-0170; (1) (419) 666-3266.

Manufacturers/suppliers of a complete range of motion picture theatre booth equipment & accessories, including Starscope/Starlet/Galaxy series SVA sound processors and power amps, Universal Xenon lamp houses and consoles, Sword and DBL-MUT large reel film handling devices, and Co-Operator automation sysems.

Forest Bay Construction Corp.

2 Lawson Ave., East Rockaway, NY 11518; Tel: (516) 599-0070.

Experts in theatre design.

Glatz-Jacobsen Theatre Design Consultants, Inc.

1420 Vance St., Suite 100, Lakewood, CO 80215; (303) 238-6415.

Architects for motion picture theatres design, remodeling, interior redecorating.

Goldberg Brothers, Inc.

P.O. Box 38819, Denver, CO 80217; (303) 321-1099.

Manufacturers of motion picture film accessories, including reels, cans, cases, splicing equipment, auomatic rewinds, film rack & cabinets, video tape reels, box office & lobby accessories.

Griggs International Inc.

805 E. 4th St., Belton, TX 76513; (817) 939-3761.

Manufacturers of conventional and Push-Back theatre chairs, lobby and office furniture.

Gulistan Carpet, Division of J. P. Stevens & Co., Inc.

1185 Avenue of the Americas, New York, NY 10036; Tel.: (212) 575-2282.

Manufacturers of Gulistan carpets.

Heywood-Wakefield Company

National Sales Office, Public Seating Division: 3010 Tenth St., Menominee, MI 49858.

Manufacturers of theatre seating and lounge furniture.

Hurley Screen Corp.

A subsidiary of CEMCORP. 1610 Robin Circle, P.O. Box 217, Forest Hill, MD 21050; (301) 836-9333 and 879-6757.

Manufacturers of custom-made motion picture screens and frames, including Superglo, pearlescent; Silverglo, aluminized; MW-16, matte white; glassmatte, beaded and rear projection surfaces. Frames in wood, steel, aluminum, and rope and pulley style.

Hussey Manufacturing Co., Inc.

One Dyer St., North Berwick, ME 03906; Tel.: (207) 676-2271.

Manufacturers of theatre seating.

The Imperial Electric Company

64 Ira Avenue, Akron, OH 44309; Tel.: (216) 253-9126.

Indiana Cash Drawer Company

P.O. Box 236, Shelbyville, IN 46176; Tel.: (317) 398-6643.

Manufacturers of cash drawers.

International Cinema Equipment Company

6750 N.E. 4th Court, Miami, FL 33138; (305) 756-0699. Telex: 522071 INT CINEMA MIA

Sells, services and distributes all type of 16/35 mm and 70mm projection and sound equipment, representing all major manufacturers of this type of equipment. (Is parent company of Westar Sales and Services Mfg. in the United Kingdom. See listing in British-based Equipment/Services)

Irwin Seating Company

3251 Fruitridge Road, P.O. Box 2429, Grand Rapids, MI 49501; Tel.: (616) 784-2621.

Manufacturers of theatre seating.

Kalart Victor Corporation

Hultenius Street, Plainville, CT 06062; Tel.: (203) 747-1663.

Manufacturers of audio-visual equipment and educational television systems including: 16mm sound and silent motion picture projectors: Tele-Beam large screen TV projectors; 16mm TV projectors; Kalart Victor overhead and opaque projectors; 16mm TV uniplex film chain; Craig film editing and viewing equipment for super 8mm and 16mm film.

K-Hill® Signal Company, Inc.

326 West Third St., Uhrichsville, OH 44683; Tel.: (614) 922-0421.

Manufacturers of drive-in traffic counters. "One way" for box office and flashing light for "exit" sneak-in protection.

Kinotone, Inc.

257 Tenth Avenue, Paterson, NJ 07524; Tel.: (201) 279-9700.

Distributors of projection and sound equipment.

Kneisley Electric Company

2501-9 Lagrange Street, P.O. Box 4692, Toledo, OH

43620; Tel.: (419) 241-1219.

Manufacturers of silicon rectifiers for carbon arcs; also power supplies and lamphouses for Xenon lamps. Silicon replacement stacks for selenium rectifiers, "sil-tubes" (silicon tubes) to replace gas-filled tubes in rectifiers and in exciter lamp supplies. Silicon exciter lamp suppliers, Xenon conversions for 16mm projectors, slide projectors, and for strong trouper. Xenon conversions for carbon arc lamphouses. Xenon "super-spot" lamp and Xenon conversion for strong follow spots.

Kollmorgen Corporation

347 King St., Northampton, MA 01060; Tel.: (413) 586-2330.

Manufacturers of special optics, and optical instruments.

Koneta Matting Division

700 Lunar Drive, Wapakoneta, OH 45895; Tel.: (419) 738-2155.

Manufacturers of rubber and vinyl entrance mats and matting, nylon top-vinyl back wipe off mats.

LaVezzi Precision, Inc.

900 North Larch Avenue, Elmhurst, IL 60126; Tel.: (312) 832-8990.

Manufacturers of parts for projector mechanisms and soundheads, including complete intermittent movement assemblies. Also special high precision machine parts for all types of motion picture equipment.

Manko Fabrics Company, Inc.

50 West 36th Street, New York, NY 10018; Tel.: (212) OX 5-7470.

Specialists in manufacturing seat covers, backs, etc. Large inventory nylons, vinyls, mohair fabrics.

The Marble Company, Inc.

P.O. Box 160080, 421 Hart Lane, Nashville, TN 37216; (615) 227-7772.

National manufacturer of Marble "Double Eagle" carbons, X-Cel Xenon bulbs and products, projections lens, projection reflectors, and Exciter lamps.

Massey Seating Company, Inc.

100 Taylor Street, Nashville, TN 37208; (615) 242-2561.

Manufacturers of theatre seating, polyurethene foam cushions, tailored upholstery units and general seating supplies. Products distributed by leading theatre equipment dealers.

Miracle Equipment Co.

Box 275, Grinnell, IA 50112; Tel.: (515) 236-7536.

Manufacturers of drive-in playground equipment, outdoor fiberglass picnic tables and benches. Also coin-operated carousels, stadium seating, water slides, and liter-liminaters (trash receptacles).

National Ticket Company

1650 Broadway, New York, NY 10019; (212) 757-1426.

Ticket printers to theatres; roll-machine-reserved.

Neumade Products Corporation

720 White Plains Rd. or P.O. Box 568, Scarsdale, NY 10583; Tel.: (914) 725-4900. PLANT: 2485 Walden Ave., Buffalo, NY 14225; Tel.: (716) 684-0051.

Manufacturers of motion picture, audio visual, and television equipment and accessories, 8mm, 70mm, 35mm, and 16mm fields.

Nick Mulone & Son

Pittsburgh St., Cheswick, PA 15024; Tel.: (412) 274-6646 or 274-5994.

Manufacturers of wide screen frames, all types.

Novelty Scenic Studios

40 Sea Cliff Ave., Glen Cove, NY 11542; Tel.: (718) 895-8668, (516) 671-5940.

Stage curtains and drapes, wall coverings, tracks and stage equipment.

Optical Radiation Corporation

1300 Optical Drive, Azusa, CA 91702; Tel.: (213) 969-3344.

Manufacturer of ORCON lamphouses, OPTIMAX consoles, Xenon bulbs, automation sound systems, and platters. Also exclusive North American distributor of ISCO projection lenses.

Osram Corporation

P.O. Box 7062, Jeanne Drive, Newburgh NY 12550; (914) 564-6300.

U.S. distributor of OSRAM theatre Xenon bulbs.

Panavision, Inc.

18618 Oxnard St., Tarzana, CA 91356.

Manufacturers and lessors of motion picture processes—Ultra Panavision 70, Super Panavision 70, Panavision 70 and Panavision 35.

Perey Turnstiles

535 Fifth Avenue, New York, NY 10017; (212) 599-0077.

Manufacturers of theatre turnstiles. Application engineering available.

Poblocki and Sons

620 South First St., Milwaukee, Wis. 53204; Tel.: (414) 273-3333.

Manufacturers of marquees and canopies, signs, poster cases, etc.

Prestoseal Manufacturing Corp.

545 Meacham Ave., Elmont, NY 11003; Tel.: (516) 488-1155.

Manufacturers of motion picture and microfilm splicers.

Projected Sound, Inc.

469 Avon Ave., P.O. Box 112, Plainfield, Ind. 46168; Tel.: (317) 839-4111.

Manufacturers and suppliers of In-Car Speakers, Junction Boxes, cone units and component parts.

RCA

30 Rockefeller Plaza, New York, NY 10020; Tel.: (212) 689-7200.

RCA Service Company, Cherry Hill Offices, Camden, NJ 08101; Tel.: (609) 963-8000.

Theatre Service Field Offices

JERSEY CITY, 43 Edward J. Hart Road, Liberty Industrial Park; W. P. Browski, mgr.
CLEVELAND, OH, 20338 Progress Drive, Strongsville, OH; M. J. Duffield, mgr.
ATLANTA, 4508 Bibb Blvd., Tucker, GA; L. N. Howard, mgr.
SKOKIE, IL, 7620 Gross Pointe Rd.; R. H. Bunting, mgr.
HOLLYWOOD, 1501 Beach St., Montebello, CA; M. B. Solomon Jr., mgr.

Schneider

400 Crossways Drive, Woodbury, NY 11797; (516) 496-8500.

Manufacturers of the CINELUX-ULTRA motion picture projection lenses and CINELUX-ULTRA wide angle lenses with focal lengths from 26mm to 150 mm Cinelux Anamorphic 2× for Cinema-Scope.

Selby Industries, Inc.

P.O. Box 277, Richfield, OH 44286; Tel.: (216) 659-6631.

Manufacturers and erectors of drive-in screen towers and prefabricated box offices; drive-in design consultants; speaker posts; canopies, and fencing.

Simplex Projector Co.

(Division of National Screen Service Corp.)

1600 Broadway, New York, NY 10019; (212) 245-6900.

Richard J. Green, vice pres. & gen. mgr.

Product: Simplex projection equipment.

Soundfold, Inc.

Box 2125, Dayton, OH 45429; (513) 228-3773 and (513) 293-2671.

Manufacturers of Soundfold, the original patented pleated acoustical wallcovering system. Soundfold also carries a wide variety of fabrics and colors; pleated trim; decorative wall carpet; fiberglass insulation; and Soundfold II high tech acoustical wall panels with an N.R.C. rating of .87.

Stewart Filmscreen Corp.

1161 W. Sepulveda Blvd., Torrance, CA 90502; Tel.: (213) 326-1422.

Manufacturers of complete line of Stewart seamless, professional projection screens for front and rear projected backgrounds of all sizes. Also makers of blue screens for travelling matte process.

Strand Century, Inc.

20 Bushes Lane, Elmwood Park, NJ 07407; Tel.: (201) 791-7000.

18111 S. Santa Fe Ave., Rancho Dominguez, CA; (213) 637-7500.

Manufacturers of studio, stage and auditorium lighting fixtures and all types of dimmer control equipment.

Strand Lighting (Rank Strand Limited)

P.O. Box 51, Great West Road, Brentford, Middlesex, England TW8 9HR. Tel: 01-568 9222. Telex: 27976. Cables: Rankaudio Brentford.

Strong International

1712 Jackson St., Omaha, NE 68102; (402) 342-4444.

Marketing Division for:

Canrad, Inc., 100 Chestnut St., Newark, NJ 07105; (201) 589-4300.

Ballantyne of Omaha, Inc., 1712 Jackson St., Omaha, NE 68102; (402) 342-4444.

Strong Electric, 1712 Jackson St., Omaha, NE 68102; (402) 342-4444.

Manufacturers of Canrad projection bulbs, Simplex & Ballantyne projectors, soundheads, automation, sound systems, pedestals, Strong lamphouses and consoles with associate power supplies, Tufcold and silver reflectors and Strong follow spotlights.

Systems & Products Engineering Company

709 North 6th St., Kansas City, KS 66101; (913) 321-3978.

Manufacturers of 35 & 70MM Platter Systems, Analog Light Dimmers, Automation, 35 & 35-70MM Split Film Cue Detectors, Reel Arms, Emergency Paging Systems and Drive-In Theatre Products.

Technikote Corporation

63 Seabring Street, Brooklyn, NY 11231; Tel.: (718) MAin 4-6429/6430. (See ad on page 433).

Manufacturers of seamless projection Screens—Anti-static XR-171 Pearlescent Dust-resistant screen, Jetwhite screen, Lenticolar screens, Hilux metallic screen, Matte white screen; drive-in screen paints, wood & metal screen frames; rope and pulley screens.

Theatrical Electronics

Box 706, Matthews, NC 28105.

Reel brackets, rewinds plastic reels, sankor lens, rebuilt used equipment and platters. Everything for the booth.

Union Carbide Corp.—Carbon Products Division.

J-4 Old Ridgebury Rd., Danbury, CT 06817; (203) 794-3617.

Sales Office: P.O. Box 94617, Cleveland, OH 44101; (800) 342-3698.

In Europe: Union Carbide Europe S.A., Rue Pedro-Meylan 5, CH-1211, Geneva 17, Switzerland; Tel.: (022) 47.44.11.

Manufacturers of carbons for brushes, carbon, graphite and metal-graphite for electric motors, generators and converters.

Williams Screen Company

1674 Summit Lake Blvd., Akron, OH 44314; Tel.: 745-0521.

Manufacturers of projection screens.

Edw. H. Wolk, Inc.

1241 S. Wabash Ave., Chicago, IL 60605; Tel.: (312) WE 9-2720-21-22(-)45.

Manufacturers of replacement parts for all American made projectors, arc lamps and sound reproducers, 26½" Reel Arms for regular and automated projection. Deluxe & "Moto-Matic" Hand Rewinders. "Solfonic" Solar Cells & Power Pacs. Distributor of Naren Spot Lights, Ex-Cell Sand/Water Urns, G.E. & Westinghouse Projection and Exciter Lamps, Cetron Photo-Electric Cells, Bausch & Lomb Glass Silvered Reflectors & "Wolk" Rectifier Bulbs; Sav-A-Reel kits.

Studio Equipment

Ampex Corporation

U.S. SALES OFFICES:

California: 401 Broadway, Redwood City, CA 94063; Tel.: (415) 367-2296 and 500 Rodier Drive, Glendale, CA 91201; (818) 240-5000.

Georgia: 1872 Montreal Road, Tucker, GA 30084; (404) 491-7112.

Illinois: 719 West Algonquin Road, Arlington Heights, IL 60005; (312) 593-6000.

Maryland: 10215 Fernwood Road, Bethesda, MD 20034; (301) 530-8800.

New Jersey: 5 Pearl Court, Allendale Industrial Park, Allendale, NJ 07401; (201) 825-9600.

Texas: 3353 Earhart Drive, Carrollton, TX 75006; (214) 960-1162.

Utah: 2880 South Main St., Suite 111, Salt Lake City, UT 84115; (801) 487-8181.

Washington: 628 Industry Drive, Tukwila, WA 98188; (206) 575-0156.

Audio/Video recording equipment for industry/studios/radio & TV stations.

Amusement Supply Co.

208 West Montcalm, Detroit 48201; (313) 961-3440.

R. Ruben, owner.

Automatic Devices Co.

2121 South 12th St., Allentown, PA 18103; Tel.: (215) 797-6000.

Manufacturers of stage and drapery hardware.

BHP, Inc.

1800 Winnemac Ave., Chicago, IL 60640; (312) 989-2140.

Professional motion picture film printers, film/video tape editing systems, and related accessories for motion picture film and video laboratories.

Bach Auricon, Inc.

6950 Romaine St., Hollywood, CA 90038; (213) 462-0931.

Manufacturers of "Filmagnetic" sound-on-film recording equipment and "Auricon" motion picture cameras.

The Camera Mart, Inc.

456 W. 55th St., New York, NY 10019; Tel.: (212) PLaza 7-6977.

Sale & Rental of motion picture and TV equipment, both film & videotape.

CECO, Inc.

440 West 15th St., New York, NY 10001; (212) 206-8280.

Rental, sale and service of photographic equipment for motion picture and TV studios. Manufacturer of professional tripods, tripod heads, editing viewers, camera motors, editing tables and other professional motion picture production equipment. Distributor for Hajnal Snorkel lens systems. Camera towers to 75 ft. (mobile); lighting towers to 125 ft. (mobile).

Digital Entertainment Corporation

Quad Eight/Westrex

(Member of Mitsubishi Pro Audio Group)

International Headquarters: 225 Parkside Dr., San Fernando, CA 91340; (818) 898-2341.

Offices of Digital Entertainment: 555 West 57 St., New York, NY 10019; (212) 713-1600; 2200 Hillsboro Road, Nashville, TN 37212; (615) 298-6613.

Products include digital tape recorders; audio mixing consoles; magnetic film recorders; reproducers; photographic film sound recorders.

Fiberbilt Cases, Inc.

601 West 26th St., New York, NY 10001; (800) 847-4176 and (212) 675-5820.

Manufacturers of cases and trunks for all types of motion picture equipment; also film cases.

Jack A. Frost

234 Piquette Avenue, Detroit, MI 48202; Tel.: 873-8030.

Studio and motion picture lighting equipment. HMI lights—temporary power—transformers.

Grosh Scenic Studios

4114-4122 Sunset Blvd., Hollywood, CA 90029; Tel.: (213) 662-1134.

Design, manufacture and installation of theatrical stage draperies; custom and standard theatrical hardware.

Kliegl Bros. Universal Electric Stage Lighting Company, Inc.

32-32 48th Ave., Long Island City, NY 11101; Tel.: (212) 786-7474.

Manufacturers of Klieglights and lighting control equipment for TV studios, stage, auditorium and architectural lighting specialties.

Magnasync-Moviola Corp.

5539 Riverton Avenue, North Hollywood, CA 91601; (213) 763-8441. Telex: 67-3199 MAGNA/MOVIS LAS.

Manufacturers and marketers of Videola film-to-video transfer and broadcast equipment. Microprocessor controlled Multi-channel voice logging recorders.

OXBERRY Div. of Richmark Camera Service Inc.

180 Broad St., Carlstadt, NJ 07072.

Manufacturers of Animation Stands, Optical Printers, Media Pro Equipment, Registration devices, etc.

RCA

30 Rockefeller Plaza, New York, NY 10020; Tel.: (212) 598-5900.

Commercial Communications Systems Division, Broadcast Systems, Front and Cooper St., Camden, NJ 08102; Tel.: (609) 963-8000.

Commerical Communications Systems Division, Photophone Systems, 2700 West Olive Ave., Burbank, CA 91505; Tel.: (213) 849-6741.
Complete theatre service.

Ringold Theatre Equipment Co.

6504 28th St., S.E. Grand Rapids, MI 49506; (616) 975-2684; Nights: (616) 949-0124. Paul Voudouris, president.
Branch Offices: 30948 Ford Rd., Garden City, MI 48135; (313) 522-4650. Harry Russell, mgr.

Ritter Co. Studio Equipment

3325 Cahuenga Blvd., Hollywood, CA 90068; Tel.: (213) 851-3325.

Gas and Electric Wind Machines.

Roctronics Entertainment Lighting and Special Effects, Inc.

100-MPA Roctronics Park, Pembroke, MA 02359; (617) 826-8888.

Designers, manufacturers and sellers of entertainment lighting electronics (dimmers and color synthesizers) and special effects (foggers, bubblers, stroboscopes, laser beam scanners, large screen video, animated displays).

Charles Ross, Inc.

333 West 52nd St., New York, NY 10019; Tel.: (212) 246-5470.

Rental, sale and service of motion picture and TV lighting, grip equipment and generators. Distributors of Mole-Richardson Co. products in the State of New York.

Tru-Roll Corporation

622 Sonora Ave., Glendale, CA 91201; Tel.: (213) 243-9567 and 245-5741.

Designers and manufacturers of custom and standard theatrical hardware. Curved and straight drapery tracks, contour drapery rigging, motion picture screen frames, top and side screen masking rigging motors and controls, motorized revolving stages, motorized bandwagons, orchestra enclosures, sliding panels, disappearing motion picture screens.

XETRON Corporation

10 Saddle Road, Cedar Knolls, NJ 07927; (201) 267-8200.

Lorraine Carbons—Carbon electrodes for all motion picture applications—Xetron Products—Professional 16, 35, 70MM projection equipment and accessories manufactured by Prevost S.P.A. Xetron Xenon lamphouses, consoles, bulbs, film transports, electronic dimming systems, 16MM and 35MM projection lenses. HMI, HID, HQI,—Ballast and starters manufactured by IREM. 16MM and 35MM Prevost flat bed editing tables.

Refreshment Products and Equipment

Bagcraft Corporation of America

10 Minue St., Carteret, NJ 07008; (201) 969-1234.

Manufacturers of popcorn packaging; foil and wax sandwich wraps and bags; french fry, hero, pizza slice packaging; over 150 stock food service packages.

Paul F. Beich Co.

Bloomington, IL 61701; Tel.: (309) 828-1311.

Manufacturers of 10¢ Bike Whiz. Complete line of other 10¢ bars and 15¢ Milk Chocolate caramel filled shells.

Blevins Popcorn Co.

Popcorn Village, Memphis, TN 38117; 813 Ridge Lake Blvd., P.O. Box 171233; Tel.: (901) 761-2062.

Processing Plants in Ridgway, IL and North Bend, NE

Concession supply branches in Atlanta, GA 30325: P.O. Box 20176 Sta. N., 2023 Hills Ave., N.W.; Cincinnati, OH 45246: 11699 Chesterdale Rd.; Dallas, TX 75042: P.O. Box 25264, 2729 Market St.; Houston, TX 77018: P.O. Box 10243, 202 W. 38th St.; Jacksonville, FL 32205: P.O. Box 2752, 5599 Commonwealth Ave.; Louisville, KY 40214: 6224 Strawberry Lane; Memphis, TN 38116: P.O. Box 16834, 3070 Fleetbrook Dr.; Miami, FL 33166: 7760 N.W. 62nd St.; Nashville, TN 37228: P.O. Box 90766, 744 Freeland Station Rd.; New Orleans, LA 70181: P.O. Box 10585, 1017 Jefferson Hwy.; Omaha, NE 68102: P.O. Box 1282, 1009 Capitol Ave.; Tampa, FL 33605: P.O. Box 5461, 1212 N. 39th St.; West Terre Haute, IN 47885: Highway 40 West.

Warehouses in Little Rock, AR, Knoxville, TN & North Loup, NE

Processors of raw popcorn and distributors of all high profit concession supplies and equipment.

Canada Dry Corp. (Syrup Division)

100 Park Ave., New York, NY 10017; Tel.: (212) LE 2-4300.

Manufacturers of beverage syrups: Ginger Ale, Cola, Tahitian Treat, Hi-Spot Orange, Cactus Cooler, Root Beer and others.

Castleberry's Food Co.

Box 1010, August, GA 30903.

Fast foods, sauces, packed foods.

Coca-Cola USA

P.O. Drawer 1734, Atlanta, GA 30301; Tel.: (404) 676-2121.

Manufacturers of soft drink syrups, Coca-Cola, Tab, Sprite, Fanta flavors, Fresca.

Delmonte Franchise Beverages, USA

2600 Century Parkway, Atlanta, GA 30345; (404) 321-1776. A division of General Cinema Corp.

Suppliers of Sunkist Orange Soda Fountain syrup, bottles, cans.

Dr Pepper Company

5523 East Mockingbird Lane, P.O. Box 225086, Dallas, TX 75265; Tel.: (214) 824-0331.

Manufacturers of Dr Pepper and Sugar-Free Dr Pepper concentrates and fountain syrups.

Goetze's Candy Co., Inc.

3900 E. Monument St., Baltimore, MD 21205.

Candy designed exclusively for theatres; 3½oz. 12 pack.

Greer Enterprises, Inc.

281 N. Grant Ave., Columbus, OH 43215; Tel.: CA 1-3245. Factory and Sales: 31 Chicago St., Quincy, MI 49082; Tel.: (517) 639-9825.

Manufacturers of combination frankfurter barbecue unit and bun warmer, Glenray manufacturers of Moist Heat Portable Steam Table (steamette).

Henry Heide, Inc.

P.O. Box 271, New Brunswick, NJ 08903; Tel.: (201) 846-2400.

Manufacturers of candy—Jujyfruits, Jujubes, Chocolate Flavor Babies, Candy Corn, Red Hot Dollars, Gummi Bears, and drops.

Hershey Foods Corp. Hershey Chocolate and Confectionery Division

19 East Chocolate Avenue, Hershey, PA 17033; Tel.: (717) 534-4200.

Manufacturers of chocolate and cocoa.

M. J. Holloway & Company

308 West Ontario, Chicago, IL 60610; Tel.: (312) 642-2700.

Manufacturers of candy—Milk Duds, Slo-Poke and Black Crow Suckers, Hi-noon bars, Zooper Dooper bars.

Hollywood Brands, Inc.

A subsidiary of Consolidated Foods Corp.

836 South Chestnut Street, Centralia, IL 62801; Tel.: (618) 532-4767.

Manufacturers of Pay Day, Butternut, Milk Shake, and Zero.

James River Corp.

605 Kuebler Road, Easton, PA 18042; (215) 250-1400.

Manufacturers of paper products: plates, cups, bowls, towels, tissues, etc.

Jet Spray Corp.

P.O. Box 8250, 825 University Ave., Norwood, MA 02062; (617) 769-7500.

Manufacturers of visual display, electrically refrigerated carbonated and non-carbonated beverage dispensers, hot chocolate dispensers, freeze-dried coffee dispensers, coin operated coffee and chocolate dispensers, instant mashed potato dispensers, hot and cold tea dispenser.

Manley, Inc.

1920 Wyandotte, Kansas City 8, MO (Mail: P.O. Box 1006, Kansas City, MO 64141; Tel.: (816) 421-6155.

Manufacturers of popcorn machines and theatre concession stands. Sale of popcorn.

M & M/Mars

High Street, Hackettstown, NJ 07840.

Manufacturers of M & M's Plain Chocolate Candies, Milky Way Milk Chocolate Bar, M & M's Peanut Chocolate Candies, 3 Musketeers bar, Snickers, Mars Almond, Mars Double Crunch, Sprint Chocolate Wafer, Snickers Peanut Munch, Milky Way Dark Chocolate Bar.

The Nestlé Company, Inc.

100 Bloomingdale Rd., White Plains, NY 10605; (914) 682-6000.

Manufacturers of movie snacks: Raisinets, Goobers, Sno Caps, CRUNCH, Superior Milk Chocolate, Superior Milk Chocolate with Almonds, $100,000 Bar and Bit-O-Honey.

Ogden Food Service

One Bills Drive, Orchard Park, NY 14127; (716) 649-6780.

Ogden Foods, Inc.

3660 S. Lawrence St. Philadelphia, PA 19148.

Operators of Theatre Food Concessions—both Indoor Houses and Drive-Ins.

Pepsi-Cola Company

Purchase, NY.

Manufacturers of Pepsi-Cola syrup and bottlers of Pepsi-Cola, Diet-Pepsi, Teem.

Peter Paul Codbury, Inc.

New Haven Road, Naugatuck, CT 06770.

Manufacturers of candy; Mounds, Almond Joy, York Peppermint Patties, Codbury chocolate.

H. B. Reese Candy Company, Inc., Subsidiary of Hershey Chocolate Co.

Hershey, PA 17033; Tel.: (717) 534-4100.

Manufacturers of Peanut Butter Cups.

Rowe International, Inc.

75 Troy Hills Road, Whippany, NJ 07981; Tel.: (201) 887-0400.

Manufacturers of Automatic Venders, music systems and bill and coin changers.

Royal Crown Cola Co.

Gould Center East Tower, Suite 500, 2550 Golf Road, Rolling Meadows, IL 60008; (312) 981-4000.

Branch: 1000 Tenth Ave., P.O. Box 1440, Columbus, GA 31994; Tel.: (404) 571-6451.

Manufacturers of soft drinks.

Scotsman Ice Systems

505 Front St., Albert Lea, MN 56007; (507) 373-3961.

Manufacturers of Scotsman ice cube and flake machines, combination ice machines and drink dispensers.

The Seven-Up Company

121 South Meramec, St. Louis, MO 63105; (314) 889-7777.

7UP and Diet 7UP are available in bottles, cans, pre-mix, and post-mix from the local 7UP Bottling company. The 7UP Bottler is a source for pre-mix and post-mix dispensing equipment and bottle and can venders.

Simonin's C. F. Sons, Inc.

Tioga & Belgrade Streets, Philadelphia, PA 19134; Tel.: (215) GA 6-2300.

Manufacturers of popcorn oils and colored and flavored seasonings.

Smithfield Ham & Products Company

Smithfield, VA 23430; Tel.: (804) 357-2121.

James River brand beef barbeque, pork barbeque and hot dog chili.

Stein Industries, Inc.

22 Sprague Avenue, Amityville, NY 11701; (516) 789-2222.

Manufacturers and designers of concession stands, popcorn warmers, display frames, doormen's boxes, and box offices.

Virga's Pizza Crust Company

2236 Conner Street, New York, NY 10466; Tel.: XX 4-9100.

Frozen pizza and ingredients.

Manufacturers and Services By Product Classification

Animation Equipment
Oxberry Berkey Technical

Attraction Advertising Equipment
A-Wagner Zip Change
Bevilite-Adler

Beverages and Beverage Dispensers
Canada Dry Corp.
Coca-Cola USA
Dr Pepper Co.
Jet Spray Corp.
Manley, Inc.
Pepsi-Cola Co.
Royal Crown Cola Corp.
Seven-Up Company
Sunkist Soft Drinks
Vendo Co.

Camera Equipment
Bell & Howell Company
Camera Mart, Inc.
CECO, Inc.
Mauer, J. A., Inc.
Mitchell Camera Corp.
Oxberry Berkey Technical

Candy and Candy Machines
Beich, Paul F., Co.
Heide, Henry, Inc.
Hershey Chocolate Corp.
Holloway, M. J. Co.
Hollywood Brands, Inc.
M&M/Mars
Quaker City Chocolate & Confectionery Co., Inc.
H. B. Reese Candy
Vendo Co.

Carbons, Carbon Savers & Carbon Coolers
The Marble Co., Inc.
Union Carbide Corp.
Xetron

Coin Changing Machines
National Rejectors, Inc.

Concession Stands
Stein Industries, Inc.

Cups & Trays
American Can Company
Continental Can Co.
Lily-Tulip Cup Corp.

Curtains and Curtain Controls and Acoustical Drapes
Automatic Devices Co.
Econo-Pleat
Novelty Scenic Studios
Soundfold, Inc.

Drive-In Admissions Control
Eprad
K-Hill Signal Corp.

Drive-In Screens and Towers
Ballantyne of Omaha
Selby Industries, Inc.
Technikote

Equipment Cases
Fiberbilt, Division of Ikelheimer-Ernst, Inc.

Film Editing
A.V.E. Corporation

Film Splicers
Prestoseal Mfg. Corp.

Floor Coverings
Gulistan Carpet
Koneta Matting
Smith, Alexander, Inc.

Food and Food Concessions Suppliers
Castleberry's Food Co.
Rowe Mfg. Co.
Smithfield Ham & Products Co.
Stein Industries, Inc.
Tri-State Refreshments, Inc.
Vendo Co.
Virga's Pizza Crust Company

Food Equipment
Greer Enterprises, Inc.

In-Car Speakers and Heaters
Ballantyne of Omaha
Eprad, Inc.
The Marble Co., Inc.
Projected Sound, Inc.

Interior Decoration
Novelty Scenic Studios

Lenses, Projection
Atlantic Audio Visual Corp.
Cinema Film Systems, Inc.
Kollmorgen Corp.
The Marble Co., Inc.

Panavision, Inc.
Schneider Corp. of America

Lighting Equipment, Studio
Kliegl Bros. Universal Electric Stage Lighting Co., Inc.
Charles Ross, Inc.

Playground Equipment
American Playground Device Co.
Herschell, Allan, Co., Inc.
Miracle Space Equipment Co.

Popcorn Machines and Supplies
Blevins Popcorn Co.
Manley, Inc.
Rex Packaging
Simonin's, C. F. Sons, Inc.
Stein Industries, Inc.

Projection Light Equipment
Ballantyne of Omaha
Canrad Hanovia, Inc.
Cinema Film Systems, Inc.
Imperial Electric Co.
The Marble Co., Inc.
Kneisley Electric Co.
Optical Radiation Corp.
Osram Sales Corporation
RCA
Rank Organisation
Strong Electric Co.
Xetron

Projection Room Accessories
Neumade Products Corp.
Theatre Equipment Co.

Projectors and Parts
A.V.E. Corporation
Ballantyne of Omaha
Century Projector Corp.
Cinema Film Systems, Inc.
Kinotone, Inc.
La Vezzi Machine Works
National Theatre Supply
RCA
Simplex Equipment Corp.
Edward H. Wolk

Recording Equipment
Ampex Corporation
Bach Auricon, Inc.
Magnasync Corp.
Maurer, J. A., Inc.
RCA
Reeves Equipment Corp.
S.O.S. Photo-Cine-Optics, Inc.
Westrex-Litton Industries, Inc.

Screen Frames
Stewart Filmscreen Corp.

Screens and Screen Paint
Hurley Screen Co.
Stewart Filmscreen Corp.
Technikote Corp.
Williams Screen Co.

Seating for Auditoriums
American Desk Co.
American Seating Co.
Griggs Int'l. Inc.
Heywood-Wakefield Co.
Irwin Seating Co.
Mannk Fabrics Co., Inc.
Massey Seating Co.

Sound Equipment
Altec-Lansing
Ballantyne of Omaha
Century Projector Corp.
Cinema Film Systems, Inc.
Cinematograph International, Inc.
Kinotone, Inc.
RCA
Simplex Equipment Corp.
Westrex-Litton Industries, Inc.

Spotlights
Kneisley Electric Co.
Strong Electric Co.

Stage Lighting
Century Strand, Inc.
Kliegl Bros.

Studio Lighting
Century Strand, Inc.
Frost Inc., Jack A.
Charles Ross, Inc.

Theatre Design
Forest Bay Construction

Ticket Machines and Boxes
Eprad

Theatre Supply Dealers

ALABAMA

Birmingham

QUEEN CONCESSION SUPPLY CO., 2409 First Ave., North 35203; (205) 251-8665.

ARIZONA

Phoenix

ARIZONA THEATRE EQUIPMENT, 1410 E. Washington, 85026; (602) 437-0215.

CALIFORNIA

Culver City

BUDD THEATRE SUPPLY, INC., 8537 West Washington Blvd., 90230; (213) 870-9301.

Inglewood

CARTER EQUIPMENT CO., LTD., 15430 Condon Ave., Lawndale, CA 90260; (213) 772-1177.

Los Angeles

AUTOMATIC DEVICES CO., 553 Oak Knoll Ave., Pasadena 91109; (213) 681-4338.
BARRETT-ROBINSON CO., 9165 Las Tunas Dr., Temple City 91780; (213) 285-1229.
FILBERT, JOHN P., 1100 Flower, Glendale; 247-6550.
GROSH, SCENIC STUDIOS, 4114 Sunset Blvd.; (213) 662-1134.
HARRAH'S THEATRE SERVICE & SUPPLY, INC., 624 So. San Fernandino Blvd., Burbank, CA 91502; (818) 842-5111.
NATIONAL THEATRE SUPPLY, 2001 S. La Cienega Blvd. 90034; (213) 838-1821.
OLESEN CO., 1535 Ivar Ave., L.A.; (213) 461-4631.
PEMBREX THEATRE SUPPLY, 1100 Flower, Glendale 91209; (213) 247-6550.
THEATRE UPHOLSTERING CO., 1338 W. 24th, L.A.; 734-0740.

San Francisco

PACIFIC THEATRE EQUIPMENT CO., 142 Leavenworth St., 94101; (415) 771-2950.

COLORADO

Denver

MID-CONTINENT THEATRE SUPPLY, 6743 East 50th Ave., Commerce City, CO 80022; (303) 289-5727. Dick Lutz, mgr.
WESTERN SERVICE & SUPPLY, 4081 South Eliot St., Englewood, CO 80110; (303) 762-8100. R. K. Tankersley, mgr.

DISTRICT OF COLUMBIA

Washington

BEN LUST, 623 Sligo Ave., Silver Spring, MD 20910; (301) 589-6606. Irwin Lust, pres.
R&S THEATRE SUPPLY CO., 4701 42nd St., N.W.; (202) 244-1500.
WILMO CORP., 3322 M St., N.W., 20013; (202) 337-6680.

FLORIDA

Jacksonville

JACKSONVILLE FILM SERVICE, INC., 2208 West 21st, 32209; (904) 355-5447.

Miami

JOE HORNSTEIN, INC., 759 W. Flagler St., 33152; (305) 545-5842.

GEORGIA

Albany

DIXIE THEATRE SERVICE & SUPPLY, 1010 N. Slappey Dr., 31701.

Atlanta

AMERICAN THEATRE SUPPLY, P.O. Box 54553, 30303; (404) 875-3167.
CAPITAL CITY SUPPLY, 2124 Jackson Parkway, N.W., 30304; (404) 792-9424.
NATIONAL THEATRE SUPPLY, 1325 Logan Circle, N.W., 30318; (404) 351-1419.

Savannah

RHODES SOUND & PROJECTION SERVICE, 218 E. 56th St., 31401.

ILLINOIS

Chicago

NATIONAL THEATRE SUPPLY (National Screen Service), 1322 S. Wabash Ave., 60605; (312) 427-8211.

IOWA

Des Moines

MTS NORTHWEST SOUND, INC., 1005 High St., 50309; (515) 243-6520.

KENTUCKY

Louisville

FALLS CITY THEATRE EQUIPMENT, 427 S. Third St., 40201.
HADDEN THEATRE SUPPLY, 909 Emerson Ave., P.O. Box 4151, 40201.

LOUISIANA

New Orleans

NATIONAL CINEMA SUPPLY CORP., 5624 Jefferson Hwy., Harahan, LA 70123.
SOUTHERN THEATRE SUPPLY, INC., 3822 Airline Highway, Metairie; (504) 831-1001.

MASSACHUSETTS

Boston

MAJOR THEATRE EQUIPMENT CORP., 28 Piedmont St., 02116; (617) 542-0445 or 542-6797.

MICHIGAN

Detroit

ALTEC SERVICE CO., 401 Commerce Bldg., 48403; (313) 963-3180.
AMUSEMENT SUPPLY CO., 208 W. Montcalm, 48043; (313) WO 1-3440.
NORTHWEST STUDIOS, INC., 36419 Groesbeck Highway, Mt. Clemens, MI 48043; (313) 792-1380.

Garden City

RINGOLD THEATRE EQUIPMENT CO., 30948 Ford Road; (313) 522-4650.

Grand Rapids

RINGOLD THEATRE EQUIPMENT CO., 6504–28 St., S.E., 49506; (616) 957-2684.

MINNESOTA

Minneapolis

MTS NORTHWEST SOUND, INC., 51 Glenwood Ave., 55403; (612) 332-1166.

MISSOURI

Kansas City

MID CONTINENT THEATRE SUPPLY, 1800 Wyandotte, 64108; (816) 221-0480.
NATIONAL THEATRE SUPPLY, 1800 Baltimore, 64108; (816) 221-9858.

St. Louis

RINGOLD CINEMA EQUIPMENT CORP., 4547 Green Park Rd., 63123; (314) 487-3283.

NEBRASKA
Omaha
SLIPPER THEATRE SUPPLY, INC., 1502 Davenport St., 68102; (402) 341-5715.

NEVADA
Las Vegas
PEMBREX THEATRE SUPPLY CO., 3519 Algonquin Dr., 89109; (702) 735-5542.

NEW JERSEY
Camden
NATIONAL THEATRE SUPPLY CO., 130 Ferry Ave., 08104; (609) 962-9200.

NEW YORK
Albany
ALBANY THEATRE SUPPLY, 443 N. Pearl St.; (518) 465-8894. Jack McGrath.
Buffalo
THEATRE EQUIPMENT & SERVICE CO., 688 Main St., 14202; (716) 854-1736.
Kingston
SUMMIT ENTERPRISES, Gov. Clinton Hotel; (914) 338-5095.
Tarrytown
MOTION PICTURE ENTERPRISES, P.O. Box 276, 10591; (212) 245-0969. Herbert R. Pilzer, pres.
New York City
CAPITOL MOTION PICTURE SUPPLY, CORP., 630 Ninth Ave.; (212) 757-4510.

JOE HORNSTEIN, INC., 341 W. 44th St., 10036; (212) 246-6285.

STAR CINEMA SUPPLY, 217 W. 21st Street, 10011; (212) 675-3515.

NORTH CAROLINA
Charlotte
AMERICAN THEATRE SUPPLY CO., 529 S. Tryon St., 28202; (704) 333-5076.

CHARLOTTE THEATRE SUPPLY CO., 704 Morris St., 28233; (704) 333-9651.

WIL-KIN, INC., 800 S. Graham St., 28202; (704) 333-6101.
Greensboro
STANDARD THEATRE SUPPLY CO., 125 Higgins St., 20660; (919) 272-6165.

OHIO
Cleveland
OHIO THEATRE SUPPLY CO., 7976 Broadview Rd., 44101; (216) 526-2783.

OKLAHOMA
Oklahoma City
OKLAHOMA THEATRE SUPPLY, 628 W. Sheridan Ave., 73125; (405) 236-8691.

PENNSYLVANIA
Philadelphia
BLUMBERG BROS., 1305 Vine St., 19104; (215) 925-7240.
Pittsburgh
NATIONAL THEATRE SUPPLY, 107 6th St. (Fulton Bldg.), 15233; (412) 471-4630.

THEATRE EQUIPMENT & SERVICE CO., 100 Lighthill St., 15233; (412) 322-4600 or (412) 322-0320.

TENNESSEE
Memphis
TRI-STATE THEATRE SUPPLY, 151 Vance Ave., 38101; (901) 525-8249.
Nashville
CAPITAL CITY SUPPLY CO., INC., 6028 Neighborly Ave., 37209; (615) 256-0347.

MID-SOUTH THEATRE SERVICE, 439 Brewer Drive, 37209; (615) 832-5660.

TEXAS
Dallas
MODERN SALES & SERVICE, 2200 Young St., 75247; (214) 747-3191.

TEXAS INTERNATIONAL THEATRE SUPPLY, 7138 Envoy Court, 75247; (214) 634-7150.
Houston
SOUTHWESTERN THEATRE EQUIPMENT, 500-C North Shepherd Dr., 77007; (713) 861-3344.
San Antonio
INDEPENDENT THEATRE SUPPLY, 2750 E. Houston, 78205.

TEXAS THEATRE SUPPLY, 915 S. Alamo St., 78205; (214) 222-1002.

UTAH
Salt Lake City
CLACO EQUIPMENT & SERVICE, 1212 South State St., 84111; (801) 355-1250.

UNIVERSAL THEATRE SUPPLY, 264 East First South St.; (801) 328-1641.

VIRGINIA
Alexandria
STANDARD THEATRE SUPPLY CO., 82 South Early St., 22304; (703) 370-4500.
Roanoke
PERDUE MOTION PICTURES EQUIPMENT, INC., 2315 Williamson Rd., N.E., 24012; (703) 366-0295.
Norfolk
1540 Norview Ave., 23513; (804) 855-8029.

WASHINGTON
Seattle
BROCKLIND'S INC., 901 Olive Way, 98109; (206) MU 2-5898.

BURNS, S. F. & CO., INC., 2319 2nd; (206) 624-2515.

FACTORY DIRECT DRAPERIES INC., 8300 Aurora N; LA 5-7932.

FAIRBANKS HARLAN CO., 1405 Elliott W; 284-7420.

NATIONAL THEATRE SUPPLY CO., 2413 2nd Ave., 98121; (206) 624-7710.

WEST VIRGINIA
Charleston
MOORE THEATRE EQUIPMENT, 213 Delaware Ave. P.O. Box 782, 25301; (304) 344-4413.

WISCONSIN
Milwaukee
HARRY MELCHER ENTERPRISES, 3607 W. Fond Du Lac Ave., 53220; (414) 442-5020.

British-Based Equipment/Services

ACMADE INTERNATIONAL
Oakside Oxford Road, Uxbridge, Mddx. UB9 4DX (0895-36313) Telex: 8954606.

AEG-TELEFUNKEN (UK) LTD.
217 Bath Road, Slough, Berks. SL1 4AW (2-872101).

AGFA-GEVAERT LTD.
Great West Road, Brentford, Middx: (OL 560 2131).

AKG ACOUSTICS LTD.
191 The Vale, London, W3 7QS (01 749 2042).

AMPEX INTERNATIONAL
Acre Road, Reading, Berks, (0734 85200).

ARRI (G.B.) LTD.
The Movie House, 2/3 Airlinks, Spitfire Way, Heston, Middx (01-848 8881).

ASTON ELECTRONIC DEVELOPMENTS LIMITED
125 Deepcut Bridge Road, Deepcut, Camberley, Surrey (02516 6221).

AUDIX LTD.
Station Road, Wenden, Saffron Walden, Essex.

AUDIO KINETICS
Kinetic House, Theobald St., Boreham Wood, Herts. (01-953 8118).

AV DISTRIBUTORS (LONDON) LTD.
21-22 St. Albans Place, Upper Street, Islington Green London N1 ONX (01-226-1508).

BALLANCROFT FILM & TV EQUIPMENT CO, LTD.
292 Worton Road, Isleworth, Middlesex, (01-560 494).

F.W.O. BAUCH LTD.
49 Theobald Street, Boreham Wood, Herts. (01-953 0091).

BELL & HOWELL LTD.
Alperton House, Bridgewater Road, Wembley, Middlesex HA0 1EG (01-902 8812).

ROBERT BOSCH LTD.
PO Box 166, Rhodes Way, Watford. (0923 44233).

BRABURY ELECTRONICS LTD.
Smirham Bridge, Hungerford, Berks. RG17 1$OQU (04886 5511).

BOSTON INSULATED WIRE (UK) LTD.
1 Canbury Park Road, Kingston-upon-Thames, Surrey. (01-5463384).

CINEFOCUS LTD
1 Pavilion Parade, Wood Lane, London, W12 0HQ. (01-743 2552).

DOEL ENGINEERING LTD.
Station Road, Hatfield Peverel, Chelmsford, Essex CM3 2DX (0245 380151) Telex: 987562 CHOCHAC.

DOLBY LABORATORIES INC.
346 Clapham Road, London SW9 9AP (01-720 1111).

EDRIC AUDIO VISUAL LTD.
34-36 Oak End Way, Gerrards Cross, Bucks. SL9 8BR (02813 84646 and 86521).

ELECTROSONIC LTD.
815 Woolwich Road, London, SE7 8LT (01 855 1101).

ELF AUDIO VISUAL LTD.
836 Yeovil Road, Trading Estate, Slough, Berks. (75-36123).

ENGLISH ELECTRIC VALVE COMPANY LIMITED
Chelmsford, Essex CM1 2QU, (0245 61777).

EVERSHED POWER-OPTICS LTD.
Bridge Wharf, Bridge Road, Chertsey, Surrey T16 8LJ (09328-61181).

FUJI PHOTO FILM (UK) LTD.
125 Finchley Road, Swiss Cottage, London, NW3 6JH (01-586 5900).

FUTURE FILM DEVELOPMENTS
114 Wardour Street, London W1A 3DG. (01-434 3344) Telex: 21624 ALOF FED G.

GEC (LAMPS AND LIGHTING) LTD.
PO Box 17, East Lane, Wembley, Middlesex HA9 7PG (01-904 4321).

GORDON AUDIO VISUAL LTD.
28 Market Place, Oxford Circus, London W1N 8PH (01-580 9191).

HARKNESS SCREENS LTD.
The Gate Studios, Station Road, Boreham Wood, Herts. (01-953 3611).

HAYDEN LABORATORIES LTD.
Chiltern Hill, Chalfont St. Peter, Bucks. 9UG (0753 888447).

HITACHI DENSHI (UK) LTD.
13-14 Garnick Industrial Centre, Garnick Road, Hendon, NW9 (01-202 4311. Ext. 216.)

INDEPENDENT CAMERA AND EQUIPMENT CO. LTD.
60 Farringdon Road, London EC1R 3BP (01-251 3885).

INTERNATIONAL VIDEO CORPORATION (UK) LTD.
10 Portman Road, Reading, Berks, RG3 1JR, (0734 585421).

JOE DUNTON CAMERAS LTD.
Wycombe Road, off Benesford Avenue, Wembley, Middlesex HA0 1QN. (01-903 7933)

KADEK VISION
P.O. No. 21, Shepperton Studio Centre, Studios Road, Shepperton, Middlesex TW17 0QD. (093 2866941).

KEM ELECTRONIC LTD.
24 Vivian Avenue, London NW4 3XP (01-202 0244).

KODAK LTD.
P.O.Box 66, Kodak House, Station Road, Hemel Hempstead, Herts. (0442-62331).

LEE COLORTRAN
85 Barlby Road, London W10 5HH. (01-968 9616.)

LEE ENTERPRISES LTD.
128 Wembley Park Drive, Wembley, Middlesex (01-969 9521).

LEE FILTERS LTD.
Walworth Industrial Estae, Andover, Hants SP10 5AN (0264-66245).

LIPSNER-SMITH CO. LTD.
Unit 7, Cowley Mill Trading Estate, Longbridge Way, Uxbridge, Middlesex (89 52191).

3M UK LTD.
3M HOUSE, P.O. Box 2, Bracknell, Berks. RG12 1JU (0344 26726).

MARCONI COMMUNICATION SYSTEMS LTD.
Marconi House, New Street, Chelmsford, Essex CM1 1PL. (0245 53221).

NEILSON-HORDELL LTD.
Central Trading Estate, Staines, Middlesex (81-56456).

NEVE ELECTRONICS INTERNATIONAL
Cambridge House Melbourn, Nr. Royston, Herts: SG8 6AU (0763 60776).

OPTICAL & TEXTILE LTD.
22-26 Victoria Road, New Barnet, Herts. EN4 9PF. (01-441 2199).

OSRAM (GEC) LTD.
P.O. Box 17, East Lane, Wembley, Middlesex HA9 7PG. (01-904 4321).

JOHN PAGE LTD.
Wesley House, 75 Wesley Avenue, London, N.W. 10. (01 961 4181).

P.A.G. FILM LTD., & P.A.G. POWER LTD.
565 Kingston Road, London SW20 85A (01-543 3131).

PHOTOGRAPHIC ELECTRICAL CO. LTD.
71 Dean Street, London W1V 6DE. (01-437 4633).

PHOTOMEC (LONDON) LTD.
(Humphries Group) Valley Road Industrial Estate, St. Albans, AL3 6NU, Herts. (56 50711).

PYE TVT LTD.
(The Broadcasting Company of Phillips)
PO Box 41, Coldhams Lane, Cambridge, CB1 3JU, (0223 45115).

RANK AUDIO VISUAL
P.O. Box 70, Great West Road, Brentford, Middlesex TW8 9HR (01-568 9222).

RANK CINTEL
Watton Road, Ware, Hertfordshire, (0920 3939).

RANK FILM LABORATORIES LTD.
North Orbital Road, Denham, Uxbridge, Middlesex UB9 5HQ (01-332 2323).

RANK TAYLOR HOBSON

P.O. Box 36, 2 New Star Rd., Leicester LE4 7SQ (Leicester 763771).

RANK VIDEO SERVICES LTD.

Phoenix Park, Great West Road, Brentford, Middlesex TW8 9PL. Tel: 01-568 4311. Telex 22345

RCA INTERNATIONAL LTD.

Lincoln Way, Windmill Road, Sunbury-on-Thames, Middlesex (76 85511).

SAMCINE SALES LTD.

303 Cricklewood Broadway, London NW2 6PQ (01-450-4557).

SAMUELSON GROUP PLC

303-315 Cricklewood Broadway, London NW2 6PQ. (01-452 8090).

SAMUELSON SIGHT & SOUND LTD.

303-315 Cricklewood Broadway, London NW2 6PQ (01-452 8090).

SCREEN ELECTRONICS LTD.

19 Anson Road, Martlesham Heath, Nr. Ipswich, Suffolk. (0473 623748) Telex 988732.

SHURE ELECTRONICS LTD.

Eccleston Road, Maidstone, Kent, ME15 6AU (0622 59881).

SONY BROADCAST LTD.

Belgrave House, Basing View, Basingstoke, Hants. RG21 2LA (0256 55011).

SOUND ASSOCIATES LTD.

56 Ayres Street, London, SW1 1EU. (01-403 5348.)

STRAND LIGHTING

P.O. Box 51, Great West Road, Brentford, Middlesex TW8 9HR. (01-568 9222)

SYLVANIA LIGHTING

Otley Road, Charlestown Shipley, West Yorkshire, BD17 7SN (0274 595921).

TECHNOVISION

Unit 4 St. Margarets Business Centre, Middlesex TW1 1JN. (01-891 5961).

THOMSON-CSF ELECTRONIC TUBES LTD.

Ringway House, Bell Road, Daneshill, Basingstoke.

THORN EMI LAMPS AND COMPONENTS LTD.

Miles Road, Mitcham, Surrey CR4 37X (01-640 1221)

THORN EMI PLC

THORN EMI House, Upper St. Martin's Lane, London, WC2H 9ED Tel: 01-836 2444 Telex Thorn London 24184/5.

VALIANT ELECTRICAL WHOLESALE CO

20 Lettice Street, Fulham, London SW6 (01-736 8115).

W. VINTEN LTD.

Western Way, Bury St. Edmunds, Suffolk IP33 3TB. (0284-2121).

WESTAR SALES & SERVICES LTD.

Unit 7, Cowley Mill Trading Estate, Longbridge Way, Ubridge, Middlesex UB8 2YG. (0895 34429) Telex: 8954 169.

WOTAN LAMPS LTD

1 Gresham Way, Durnsford Road, London, SW19 8HU (01-947 1261)

ZONAL LTD

Holmethorpe Avenue, Redhill, Surrey, RH1 2NX (0737 67171)

Government Film Bureaus

DEPARTMENT OF AGRICULTURE:

U.S. Department of Agriculture Video & Film Division, Washington, D.C. 20250. Larry A. Quinn, acting chief, Video & Film Division.

USDA films are available through the cooperating extension libraries of the Land Grant Universities and are included in their respective catalogs. (USDA no longer issues a film catalogue.) Prints of the USDA films or replacement footage can be purchased from the National Audiovisual Center (NAC), General Services Administration, Washington, D.C. 20409. Contact NAC Sales Branch for prices and ordering procedures at (301) 763-1891. NAC rents 16mm films for a nominal fee and offers preview prints of selected titles. The Reference Section will direct inquirers to the closest free loan source, either commercial service or regional Federal agency loan library. NAC will also provide specialized research, using master data files of all available AV materials produced by the U.S. Government. Printed information lists, brochures, and catalogs listing titles by subject, media, or Federal agencies, are available. Call (301) 763-1896.

DEPARTMENT OF COMMERCE:

International Trade Administration, Office of Service Industries, 14th and E Streets, N.W., Washington, DC 20230; (202) 377-4581. Theodore A. Nelson.

This division studies and reports statistics of the industry at home and abroad. The material gathered is published in department reports and is used with information from other industries to help fulfill the function of "representing business to the government and the Government to business."

DEPARTMENT OF DEFENSE

The Pentagon Building, Washington, DC 20301-1400. Assistant Secretary of Defense (Public Affairs) Michael I. Burch.

Special Assistant (Audiovisual): M. Donald E. Baruch, Room 2E789, 685-2936: Acts on all requests for Department of Denfence assistance from any segment of the motion picture and television industry concerned with dramatic productions and documentaries not dealing with news.

Radio-Television Branch: LCol. Daniel Braun, Rm 2E765, 695-0168. Responds to request for DOD assistance from major television/radio networks and other news documentary film/video productions. Arranges technical aspects of news conferences and media coverage at the Pentagon.

Media Support: M. Ed Michaelski, Rm 2E773, 697-1252. Obtains and releases Department of Defense still and motion picture/video to news and other media outlets.

DEPARTMENT OF THE ARMY

Office Chief of Public Affairs, Los Angeles Branch, Chief, COL Rolf G. Schmitz, 11000 Wilshire Blvd., Suite 10104, Los Angeles, CA 90024-3688; (213) 209-7621).

Marine Corps Public Affairs Office, Los Angeles, California: MAJ Fred C. Peck, 11000 Wilshire Blvd., Suite 10113, Los Angeles, CA 90024-3688; (213) 209-7272.

Department of the Navy, Navy Office of Information, West: LCDR Connie Haney, Director, 11000 Wilshire Blvd., Suite 11100, Los Angeles, CA 90024-3688; (213) 209-7481.

Department of the Air Force, Western Region Office of Public Affairs: COL Leo M. Terrill, Chief, 11000 Wilshire Blvd., Suite 10114, Los Angeles, CA 90024-3688; (213) 209-7511.

DEPARTMENT OF TRANSPORTATION

Coast Guard Public Affairs Liaison Office, Los Angeles: CAPT Donald J. Aites, 11000 Wilshire Blvd., Suite 10125, Los Angeles, CA 90024-3688; (213) 209-7817.

DEPARTMENT OF HEALTH AND HUMAN SERVICES:

330 Independence Avenue, S.W., Washington, DC 20201. (202) 245-6296.

Information Office: 963-4568. Sanford H. Winston, director; York Onnen, asst. director; Harry Bell, dir., (Audio Visual Services), 963-5319.

Health Services & Mental Health Administration: Dr. Vernon E. Wilson, administrator: Edward J. McVeigh, Director of Information; 443-2086.

HS and MHA produces and distributes film, audio and video tape, and multi-media materials on problems of mental and physical health by a combination of contract and in-house facilities.

National Institutes of Health: Dr. Robert S. Stone, Director; Storm Whaley, Associate Director for Communications, 496-4461.

NIH's Audio Visual facilities are responsible for the production and distribution of motion pictures, slides and other materials depicting biomedical research and its implications.

Environmental Protection Agency: William D. Ruckelshaus, administrator, 755-2700; Thomas Hart, dir. of public affairs, 755-2700; Luke C. Hestor, films, 443-4804.

EPA produces films on the environment and information lists for the public.

SOCIAL SECURITY ADMINISTRATION:

John A. Svahm, Commissioner; Russell R. Jalbert, asst. commr., Public Affairs (301) 594-1990; Robert Fenwick, Audio Visual Staff Chief, 944-5587.

SSA produces and distributes films for use throughout the country describing social security and its benefits.

SOCIAL AND REHABILITATION SERVICE:

James S. Dwight, Administrator; Robert A. Wilson, Director of Public Affairs, 962-4655.

SRS produces and distributes films on a wide variety of subjects, such as social welfare services. Medicaid, rehabilitation, juvenile delinquency and related topics.

OFFICE OF EDUCATION:

Terrel H. Bell, commissioner; Anne Graham, chief, office of public affairs, 254-5800.

Audio-Visual division: The Office of Public affairs is responsible for clearance and monitoring of all motion picture and other audio-visual materials generated by OE contracts with, or grants to companies or non-profit organizations and Institutions. Distribution of these materials is made through the National Audio-Visual Center (located at the National Archives and Records Services) or by special arrangements with producers. Public use of OE audiovisual materials is approved by the HEW Office of Public Affairs.

Caption films division: Malcom Norwood, asst. chief, 963-5230. This division purchase already produced films and captions them for use by the deaf.

DEPARTMENT OF THE INTERIOR

Bureau of Mines, Motion Picture Booking Section. 4800 Forbes Ave. Pittsburgh, Pa. 15213: Tel.: 412-621-4500. This is the main distributing center; however copies of some films are deposited at cooperating educational film distribution centers throughout the country.

The Bureau maintains a library of motion pictures depicting mining and metallurgical operations and related manufacturing processes. They are loaned free of charge, except for return postage (book rate) to educational institutions, industries, training workers, engineering, and scientific societies, civic and business associations, and other responsible organizations. The cost of production is paid by co-operating industrial concerns but the pictures do not carry trademarks, trade names or other direct advertising materials. William Gage, (202) 634-1335, officer in charge Bureau of Mines Audio-Visual Programs, Washington, is in charge of production.

DEPARTMENT OF JUSTICE:

Constitution Avenue and 10th Street, N.W., Washington D.C. 20530.

William French Smith, Attorney General; Terence B. Adamson, Director of Public Information; 739-2014.

SMITHSONIAN INSTITUTION:

Washington, DC 20560, 628-4422.

S. Dillon Ripley, secretary; Nazaret Cherkezian, Telecommunications coordinator, 381-2414.

Coordinates production on all motion picture and TV filming.

DEPARTMENT OF STATE:

21st Street and Virginia Avenue, Washington, D.C. 20503. George Schultz, Secretary of State.

OFFICE OF MEDIA SERVICES

Paul E. Auerswald, director, 632-2083. Provides State Department assistance on film and TV production. Produces an average of one film a year on foreign policy subjects and distributes them for public service TV and classroom use.

OFFICE OF INTERNATIONAL TRADE:

Dept. of State; 632-2543.

(Concerned with commercial aspects of film industry, trade treaties, quotas, restrictions, etc.)

EXECUTIVE AGENCIES

FEDERAL COMMUNICATIONS COMMISSION:

1919 M St., N.W., Washington, D.C. 20054—Mark Fowler, Chairman; William A. Russell, Jr., Public Information Officer. (202) 632-7260.

Charged with regulating interstate and foreign communications including radio, television, satellite, cable and wire services. Licenses all standard, FM, and television broadcasting stations and services.

FEDERAL TRADE COMMISSION:

Sixth Street and Pennsylvania Avenue, N.W., Washington, D.C. 20580—David A. Clanton, chairman; Theodore O. Cron, director of information. 523-3625.

Administraters statues designed to promote fair competition; institutes proceeding to prevent unfair or deceptive practices, combinations in restraint of trade, false advertising, and illegal price discrimination. Supervises associations of exporters under the Export Trade Act.

SECURITIES AND EXCHANGE COMMISSION:

500 N. Capital St., Washington, D.C. 20549; Harold M. Williams, chairman; George A. Fitzsimmons. Secretary (information), 755-1160.

Registers security offerings and supervises exchange trading in securities.

U.S. INFORMATION AGENCY:

1750 Pennsylvania Avenue, N.W., Washington, D.C. 20547—John E. Reinhardt, director. (202) 724-9042.

Motion Picture and Television Service: 376-7806. McKinney Russell, assistant director; Stanley Moss, deputy assistant director. Certifies exemption of import duties if film is educational in nature.

USIA produces and acquires about 200 film and television documentaries annually for information and cultural programs in 117 countries. In addition, close to 350 targeted, and 150 worldwide new clips are made for use on foreign television. These are seen abroad in commercial theatres, in television, in schools and community centers, and by clubs, universities, and other audiences.

LIBRARY OF CONGRESS

10 First Street, S.E., Washington, D.C. 20540. 202-426-5000. Daniel J. Boorstin, Librarian of Congress; Mrs. Mary C. Lethbridge, Information Officer, 202-426-5108.

This agency serves as the national library and includes the U.S. Copyright Office as one of its departments. In addition to registering films for copyright and publishing a record of copyright registrations, the Library catalogs motion pictures and filmstrips, publishes printed catalog cards, book catalogs and machine-readable tapes for such materials, collects current film selectively, maintains an extensive archive of motion pictures from 1894 to date, and provides related bibliographic services.

Copyright Office—Barbara Ringer, Register of Copyrights.

Robert D. Stevens, Chief of the Copyright Cataloging Division, 703-557-8715, supervises the preparation of the semi-annual *Catalog of copyright Entries: Motion Pictures and Filmstrips,* which is distributed by the Superintendent of Documents, Government Printing Office, Washington, D.C. 20402. This publication contains descriptive data for all theatrical and nontheatrical pictures registered for copyright during each 6-month period and includes renewal registrations.

Processing Department—Joseph H. Howard, Director.

Vivian L. Schrader, Head of the Audiovisual Section of the Descriptive Cataloging Division, 202-426-5238, supervises the cataloging of approximately 5,000 motion pictures, filmstrips, and sets of slides and transparencies a year, largely on the basis of information supplied by producers and media libraries.

Research Department—Alan Fern, Director.

Motion Picture Section in the Prints and Photographs Division, 202-426-5840, which has custody of the Library's collection of over 60,000 motion pictures. The collection is primarily an archive. It contains educational, scientific, religious, industrial, and documentary films, as well as newsreels and features. Chiefly American, it includes German, Italian, and Japanese films, and in it are historically important films preserved by the Library from the early days of the motion-picture industry. Since 1942, about 1,500 representative titles a year have been retained.

Distributors of 16mm Feature Films

Following is a listing of distributors having substantial selections of 16mm films for lease or rental. Additionally, some of the companies may have prints available for outright purchase. Inquiries for catalogs listing complete product should be made to the addresses given below.

BENCHMARK FILMS
145 Scarborough Road, Briarcliff Manor, NY 10510.

BLACKHAWK FILMS
Box 3990, Davenport, IA 52808.

BUDGET FILMS
4590 Santa Monica Boulevard, Los Angeles, CA 90029.

CAROUSEL FILMS
241 East 34 St., New York, NY 10016.

COLUMBIA PICTURES
711 Fifth Avenue, New York, NY 10022.

CORINTH FILMS
410 East 62nd St., New York, NY 10021.

DISNEY PRODUCTIONS
500 South Buena Vista St., Burbank, CA 91521.

FILM CLASSIC EXCHANGE
1914 S. Vermont Avenue, Los Angeles, CA 90007.

FILM-MAKERS COOPERATIVE
175 Lexington Avenue, New York, NY 10016.

FILMS INCORPORATED
1144 Wilmette Ave., Wilmette, IL 60091.

GROVE PRESS, INC. FILM DIVISION
196 West Houston, New York, NY 10014.

HISTORICAL FILMS
Box 46505, Hollywood, CA 90046.

HURLOCK CINE-WORLD, INC.
13 Arcadia Rd., Old Greenwich, CT 06870.

IFEX FILMS/INTERNATIONAL FILM EXCHANGE LTD.
201 West 52 St., New York, NY 10019.

INSTITUTIONAL CINEMA, INC.
10 First, Saugerties, NY

IVY FILM
165 West 46 St., New York, NY 10036.

JANUS FILMS
888 Seventh, Avenue, New York, NY 10106.

MOVIE WONDERLAND
6166 Glen Tower, Hollywood, CA 90028.

MUSEUM OF MODERN ART FILM LIBRARY
11 West 53rd Street, New York, NY 10019.

NEW LINE CINEMA
575 Eighth Ave., New York, NY 10003.

NEW YORKER FILMS
16 West 61st St., New York, NY 10023.

PARAMOUNT NON-THEATRICAL
5451 Marathon St., Hollywood, CA 90038.

PAULIST PRODUCTIONS
P.O. Box 1057, Pacific Palisades, CA 90272.

PYRAMID FILMS
2801 Colorado Ave., Santa Monica, CA 90404.

RADIM FILMS, INC.
1034 Lake St., Oak Park, IL 60301.

REPUBLIC PICTURES CORPORATION
12636 Beatrice St., Los Angeles, CA 90066.

ROA'S FILMS
1696 No. Astor Street, Milwaukee, Wisc. 53202.

STANDARD FILM SERVICE
14710 W. Warren Avenue, Dearborn, MI 48120.

SWANK MOTION PICTURES
201 S. Jefferson Ave., St. Louis, MO 63166.

"THE" FILM CENTER
915 12th Street N.W., Washington, D.C. 20005.

TRANS-WORLD FILMS
332 S. Michigan Ave., Chicago, IL 60604.

TWYMAN FILMS, INC.
Box 605, Dayton, OH 45401.

UNITED FILMS, INC.
1122 South Cheyenne, Tulsa, OK 74119.

WARNER BROS., INC.
Non-Theatrical Division, 75 Rockefeller Plaza, New York, NY 10019.

ON MICROFILM

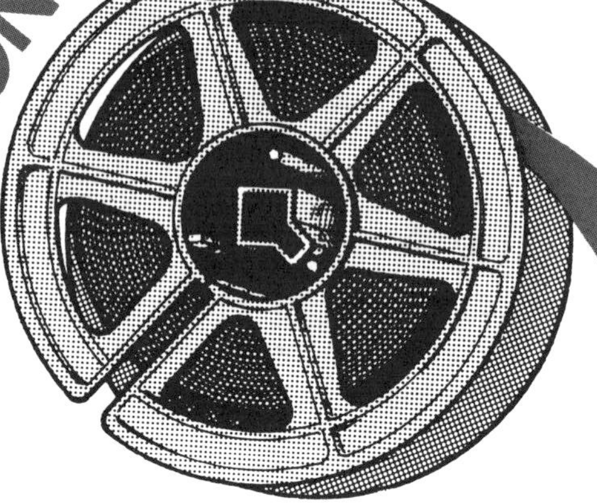

MOTION PICTURE HERALD

MOTION PICTURE DAILY

These historically invaluable trade journals of the Motion Picture industry published by Quigley Publishing Company from 1915 to 1972 have been recorded on microfilm by Brookhaven Press and are now available for immediate delivery.

MOTION PICTURE HERALD
1915-1972 (77 reels)

MOTION PICTURE DAILY
1930-1972 (39 reels)

For price and further information
call (608) 781-0850
or order from:

BROOKHAVEN PRESS
Box 1653
La Crosse, WI 54601

SPECIFICATIONS: 35mm positive microfilm, silver halide at a reduction of approximately 17X (meeting ANSI/NMA standards).

Home Video

Statistics

Freedom of choice—the control of one's own viewing habits—has been the major impact of home video on the leisure-time industry in America. Owners of videocassette recorders can view what they want when they want and are no longer subject to the programming schedules of the television networks and cable stations. The VCR owner is able to watch yesterday's motion pictures today (by renting or owning vintage Hollywood films, foreign features and television product, as well as films released theatrically as recently as six months ago) and today's television programming tomorrow—along with how-to tapes, music videos and home movies.

Time shifting, the ability of the viewer to tape a show for later viewing (as well as eliminating commericals—by editing them out or fast forwarding past them) is the most common usage of VCRs. One can watch one program while taping another, or tape with the tv set off and nobody home. One can select entertainment or instruction from the more than 50,000 prerecorded tapes now available from the more than 30,000 video specialty stores, supermarkets, hardware stores and libraries. There are more than 40 brands of VCRs with 150 models now available. Home video has had a revolutionary effect on the entertainment habits of the nation.

Video History

1923: Though the patent for a video-camera-like device was filed in Germany one hundred years ago, the first practical product was devised by Vladimir Zworykin, a Russian/American immigrant in 1923.

1938: A primitive video disk was on sale in Selfridges of London.

Post World War II: With the development in the early 1930s of an electronic television signal and the audio tape recorder, and their coming into broadcast use in the mid-1940s, it was not long before experiments (by Ampex and RCA in the US, and BBC and Decca in Great Britain) in recording television shows and playing them back were made in earnest. Freeing directors to edit or re-shoot and attempting to loosen the stranglehold live television broadcasting imposed on the medium, the first recorders were longitudinal machines that looked like audio recorders and used large reels of tape at high speeds.

Early 1955: BBC went on the air with its VERA (Vision Electronic Recording Apparatus) with a head gap of 20 microns and a tape speed of 200 inches per second. A reel about 5 feet in diameter was needed for taping a half-hour program.

April 1956: An American company, Ampex, produced the first working video recorders for broadcast use, using four (quad) recording heads on a rotating drum, and two-inch wide magnetic tape which was reusable. They were first used over the air at CBS's Hollywood studios in November, 1956. (A more portable system using narrower tape and a helical scan system had been patented in Germany in 1953, but the prototypes were far too expensive and difficult to use; a tape could be used only once, and each time it was used the machine had to be cleaned of tape particles.)

1967: A Japanese company, Sony, introduced the first transportable video system which used reel-to-reel tape and recorded in black and white only.

1970: Home video arrived when the first

video cassette systems were produced, in the Philips Video Cassette Recorder or VCR. (Philips had also developed and licensed the compact audio cassette.) Sony introduced its ¾-inch U-Matic format intended for professional use in the film and television industries.

1972: Philips launched its N1500, the first video recorder with a tuner-timer, making domestic video recording a reality.

Late 1975: Sony introduced the Betamax system, utilizing narrower ½-inch tape (the narrower tape size resulted in lowered costs of recording and recorders). An optional timer was included to enable a viewer to tape even when he was not at home and offered the capability of recording one program while watching another. The cost was approximately $2,200 for a recorder with TV set. Blank tape cost $20.

1976: Cartrivision, V-Cord, and VHS (Video Home System) introduced systems incompatible with Betamax machines. The first two fell by the wayside while VHS (backed by Matsushita Electronics Corporation) emerged as the challenger to Sony's Betamax by making it possible to record up to 2 hours of broadcast material for the first time. Magnavox came out with a video disk machine, strictly a playback system which used a disc similar in size and substance to a record album that is "read" by a laser beam. RCA manufactured a rival, incompatible videodisc system.

1977: The video software market was born when a small midwestern company called Magnetic Video Corporation licensed 50 feature-length films from 20th Century-Fox and released them for sale on Beta and VHS formats at retail prices of $49.95 to 79.95.

1983: Paramount Pictures paved the way for burgeoning cassette sales when it lowered the price of some of its strongest titles to $39.95 from $79.95. Other prerecorded cassette distributors soon followed suit.

Jan. 1984: United States Supreme Court, after lengthy consideration of a suit brought by MCA Inc and Walt Disney Productions against Sony, ruled that home taping of broadcast programming is not a violation of copyright laws, in effect legitimizing what viewers were already doing.

Facts and Statistics

- While the Japanese and Koreans dominate the hardware market of the video industry, American producers, distributors, and marketers and retailers fill the programming needs of the ever expanding industry.
- Estimates regarding the number of United States households that currently own a VCR vary between 33% and 40%. Media analyst Paul Kagan anticipates that by the early 1990s, 70% of US homes will have a VCR.
- Electronic Industries Association (EIA) figures show that 11.5 million VCRs were sold in 1985, while 7.62 million were sold in 1984. The EIA calculates that 50 million prerecorded video cassettes were sold in 1985, up 127% over 1984's 22 million units.
- Prerecorded videocassettes doubled both in dollar sales ($8 billion) and unit sales (53 million) in 1985 and were expected to rise again in 1986 to 75 million units worth $2.3 billion; blank videocassette sales, after climbing 20% in 1985 to $925 million, were expected to pass the $1 billionmark in 1986 with 220 million units sent to dealers.
- Camcorder sales were expected to rise nearly 90% to 750,000 units in 1986 while sales of color video cameras fell 18% to 405,000 units in 1985 and are expected to fall again to 350,000 units in 1986. (EIA)
- A 1984 A.C. Nielsen survey revealed

that the average user spends 6 to 9 hours a week recording and playing back programming off the air. Soap operas are the most frequently taped shows (accounting for 27.2% of the total recording time) followed by movies (17.1%), dramatic shows (14.5%), and comedy (8.9%).

- The May 1986 A.C. Nielsen report indicated that recording with the set turned off is responsible for the greatest portion of total VCR recording. Viewing and recording the same channel simultaneously accounts for less than one-third of total recording time. Approximately 15% of all recording is done while viewing one channel and recording a different channel.
- While film companies are enjoying healthy growth from selling videocassettes, they are prohibited by law from garnering any of the rental revenues. The First Sale Doctrine states that once the cassette is sold to the retailer, the merchant can rent the cassette as many times as he can without giving back any royalties to the producers.

FIGURE 3

TOTAL FACTORY SALES OF VIDEOCASSETTE RECORDERS

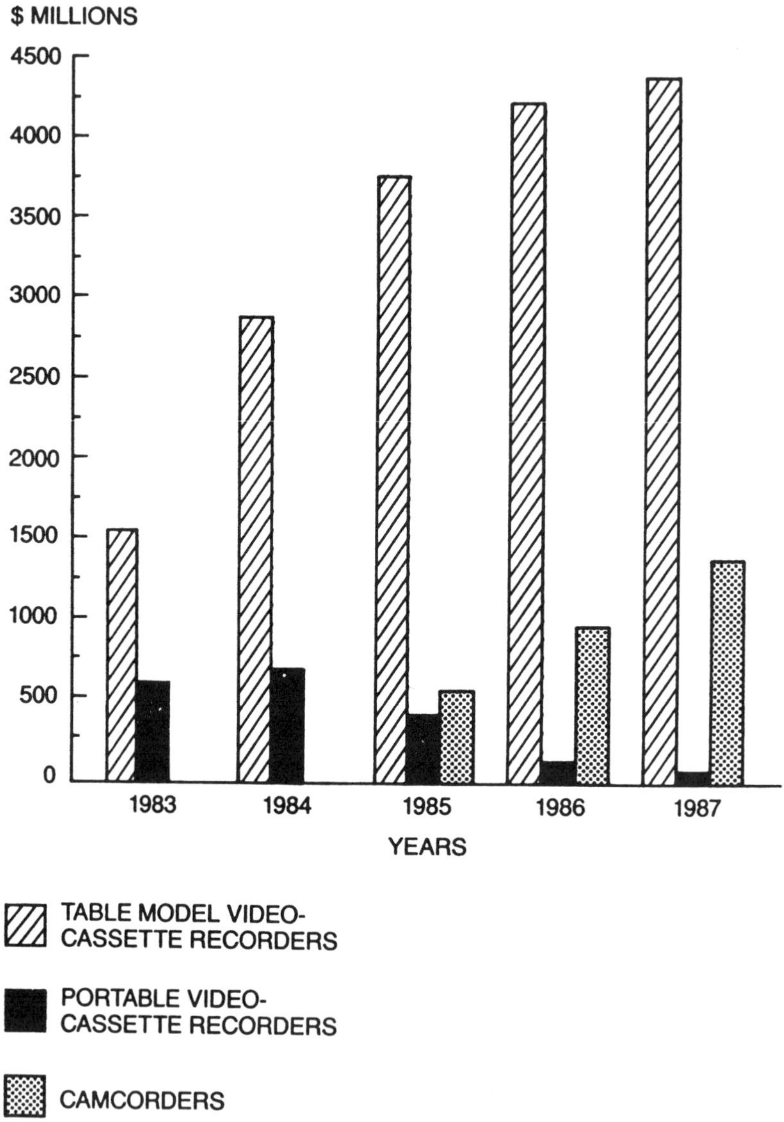

From Tables 7, 8, and 9

Source: Electronic Industries Association

VIDEOCASSETTE RECORDERS

TABLE 7
TABLE MODEL VIDEO-CASSETTE RECORDERS

	Total Sales to Dealers in Units (Thousands)	Total Factory Sales in Dollars (Millions)	Average Value (Dollars per Unit)
1982	1,599	na	na
1983	3,354	1,575	470
1984	6,731	2,898	431
1985	10,750	3,771	351
1986 (proj.)	12,000	4,235	353
1987 (est.)	12,400	4,400	355

TABLE 8
PORTABLE VIDEOCASSETTE RECORDERS
(Excluding Camcorders)

	Total Sales to Dealers in Units (Thousands)	Total Factory Sales in Dollars (Millions)	Average Value (Dollars) per Unit)
1982	436	na	na
1983	737	587	796
1984	885	687	776
1985	586	402	686
1986 (proj.)	200	120	600
1987 (est.)	100	55	550

TABLE 9
CAMCORDERS

	Total Sales to Dealers in Units (Thousands)	Total Factory Sales in Dollars (Millions)	Average Value (Dollars) per Unit)
1985	517	565	1,093
1986 (proj.)	1,000	975	975
1987 (est.)	1,500	1,380	920

TABLE 10
TOTAL VIDEOCASSETTE RECORDERS
(Sum of Tables 7, 8 and 9)

	Total Sales to Dealers in Units (Thousands)	Total Factory Sales in Dollars (Millions)	Average Value (Dollars per Unit)
1980	805	621	771
1981	1,361	1,127	828
1982	2,035	1,303	640
1983	4,091	2,162	528
1984	7,616	3,585	471
1985	11,853	4,738	400
1986 (proj.)	13,200	5,330	404
1987 (est.)	14,000	5,840	417

Source: Electronic Industries Association

OTHER VIDEO PRODUCTS

TABLE 11

COLOR VIDEO CAMERAS
(Excl. Camcorders)

	Total Sales to Dealers in Units (Thousands)	Total Factory Sales in Dollars (Millions)	Average Value (Dollars) per Unit)
1980	114	na	na
1981	190	147	774
1982	296	232	784
1983	414	303	732
1984	489	355	726
1985	395	228	577
1986 (proj.)	150	85	570
1987 (est.)	75	40	500

TABLE 12

VIDEODISC PLAYERS*

	Total Sales to Dealers in Units (Thousands)	Total Factory Sales in Dollars (Millions)	Average Value (Dollars per Unit)
1980 (est.)	40	na	na
1981	157	55	350
1982	223	54	242
1983	307	81	264
1984 (est.)	200	45	230
1985 (est.)	200	45	230
1986 (est.)	200	45	230
1987 (est.)	200	45	230

*Non-commercial.

TABLE 13

VIDEOCASSETTE PLAYERS

	Total Sales to Dealers in Units (Thousands)	Total Factory Sales in Dollars (Millions)	Average Value (Dollars per Unit)
1985 (est.)	125	22	175
1986 (est.)	125	22	175
1987 (est.)	100	15	150

Source: Electronic Industries Association

BLANK VIDEOCASSETTES

	Sales to Dealers in Units (Thousands)	Factory Sales in Dollars (Millions)
1982	33,529	357
1983	75,003	580
1984	166,371	931
1985	293,659	1,285

Home Video Outlook

By William Gallagher
President, Home Video Division
MGM/UA Home Entertainment Group

I'm firmly convinced we are all fortunate to be associated with a dynamic growth industry built on a solid foundation and guaranteeing those who are willing to work for it a solid profitable future!

How can I say this so positively? Because I speak from experience and plain common sense.

There are close to one hundred million American and Canadian homes equipped with well over 200 million television monitors—so far, more than 35% of these homes own a VCR—but we all know that without resorting to fancy growth graphs that these numbers are changing dramatically as of now. It is my estimation that by 1987 mid-year, we will have equipped 50% of all North American homes with VCRs—homes and people that automatically become videocassette customers—potential customers for every videocassette that has been released since the early 1980s—that is a solid future for good catalog product! We are guaranteeing relief for the weary North American TV viewers who have been literally saturated with lackluster programs to watch for the past 20 years—the VCR is changing all that—the entertainment starved consumer now knows he can program his own living room with the kind of entertainment he wants when he wants it!

Here's an interesting analogy to the growth of the video industry—the phonograph industry! It provides a perfect comparison.

Edison invented the phonograph record in 1879—then Marconi invented the long wave radio in 1920 which gave the American public automatic access to free music. This meant the end to any future growth in the record industry! Right? Wrong—not so—America heard the music they liked on radio but could only have it whenever they wanted to. Then in the mid-1940s TV arrived and this exciting medium developed artists who were originally recording artists and the record industry continued to have unparalleled growth!

Now there's more new and exciting technology all around us so let them increase the cable audience—refine the Pay-TV program schedules on HBO, Showtime and Cinemax—develop the pay-per-view technology that dealers have been told is a threat to their future—and yet, only if one owns a VCR and a videocassette of "The Wizard of Oz" can he or she enjoy this great program in your living room whenever *you* wish! The record industry withstood all the challenges of technology and the prognostications of gloom (the financial wizards), and is still a $5 billion industry today—simply offering the music the consumer wants when they want it!

The video industry is built on just as solid a foundation—it has the entertainment you want—when you want it. It must evolve from the currently rental only world to a solid sell through industry and/or rental if you wish for the titles you don't wish to own.

We haven't the space here to examine just how this evolution will come about, but mass production technology will spawn lower prices and mass marketing techniques will inspire the video enthusiast to want to own a collection of his or her favorite programs and exercise their right to rent or buy those titles they want when they want to see them. The future for those with vision is sound.

Home Video Producers

Budget Video Inc.

(D/B/A Hollywood Home Theatre)
1540 N. Highland Ave., Suite 110, Hollywood CA 90028; (213) 466-0121, (213) 466-0127. Organized 1979. (Dealer, distributor, retailer of video cassettes and laser discs.)

PRESIDENT
Larry S. Fine
VICE PRESIDENT
Stephen Stumbris

CBS/Fox Video

1211 Avenue of the Americas, New York, NY 10036; (212) 819-3200. (Subsidiary of CBS, Inc./20th Century Fox)

PRESIDENT
Lawrence B. Hilford
PRESIDENT, CONSUMER PRODUCT DIVISION
Leonard White
VICE PRESIDENT, SALES
Bob De Lellis

Embassy Home Entertainment

1901 Avenue of the Stars, Los Angeles, CA 90069; (213) 553-3600. Organized 1982. (Videocassette marketing and distribution company.)

CHIEF EXECUTIVE OFFICER
Andre Blay
PRESIDENT, PRODUCTION & PROGRAMMING
Richard B. Childs
PRESIDENT, EHE INTERNATIONAL
Alan Kaupe
SENIOR VICE PRESIDENT, DISTRIBUTION
Rand Bleimeister
SENIOR VICE PRESIDENT, ACQUISITIONS & PRODUCTION
Al Eicher
SENIOR VICE PRESIDENT, CFO
Jeff Della Betta
BRANCHES
7 United States, 1 Canada, 1 Germany, 1 Japan, 1 London

HBO/Cannon Video

1370 Avenue of the Americas, New York, NY 10019; (212) 977-8990, (800) 648-7650. Subsidiary of The Cannon Group.

CHIEF EXECUTIVE OFFICER
Frank O'Connell
PRESIDENT
Nicholas Santrizos
VICE PRESIDENT, MARKETING
Jay Press

Karl/Lorimar Home Video Inc.

899 W. 16th St., Newport Beach, CA 92663; (714) 642-1148. 17942 Cowan Ave., Irvine, CA 92714; (714) 474-0355.

PRESIDENT
Stuart Karl

Key Video

1211 Avenue of the Americas, New York, NY 10036; (212) 819-3200; (619) 459-0500. Subsidiary of CBS/Fox Video.

PRESIDENT
Herb Fischer

Lightning Video

1011 High Ridge Rd., Stamford, CT 06905; (203) 322-8720. (Subsidiary of Vestron.)

VICE PRESIDENT
Gordon Bossin

MCA Distributing Corp.

70 Universal City Plaza, 3rd Floor, Universal City, CA 91608; (818) 777-4000. (Distributor of pre-recorded video cassettes and records.) A division of MCA/Universal.

SENIOR VICE PRESIDENT, DISTRIBUTION
John Burns
VICE PRESIDENT, VIDEO DISTRIBUTION
Louis Feola
VICE PRESIDENT, VIDEO PRODUCTS
Neil Hartley
Branches
REGIONAL VIDEO DIRECTOR (EAST)
Bill Hickman
REGIONAL VIDEO DIRECTOR (MIDWEST)
Janis Durr
REGIONAL VIDEO DIRECTOR (SOUTHEAST)
Roger Mill
REGIONAL VIDEO DIRECTOR (WEST)
Steve Garwood

MGM/UA Home Entertainment Group, Inc.

1350 Avenue of the Americas, New York, NY 10019; (212) 408-0600; (800) 468-7600.

BOARD OF DIRECTORS: Fred Benninger, Syemour Leslie, Lee Rich, Frank Rothman, Sidney Sapsowtz, Walter M. Sharp, Stephen D. Silbert

EXECUTIVE COMMITTEE: Seymour Leslie, Lee Rich, Sidney H. Sapsowitz

OFFICERS

CHAIRMAN OF THE BOARD OF DIRECTORS, PRESIDENT AND CHIEF EXECUTIVE OFFICER
Seymour Leslie
PRESIDENT, HOME VIDEO DIVISION
William P. Gallagher
SENIOR VICE PRESIDENT—FINANCE
Thomas P. Carson
SENIOR VICE PRESIDENT AND GENERAL COUNSEL—ENTERTAINMENT
William Allen Jones
VICE PRESIDENT
Kathleen A. Coughlan
VICE PRESIDENT, LICENSING DIVISION
William F. Dennis
VICE PRESIDENT
Walter C. Hoffer
VICE PRESIDENT—FINANCE AND TREASURER
Lawrence K. Stern
VICE PRESIDENT—TAXES
Daniel Taylor
CORPORATE CONTROLLER
Barbara Benely

MGM/UA Home Video Division

PRESIDENT
William P. Gallagher
SENIOR VICE PRESIDENT, BUSINESS AND LEGAL AFFAIRS
Alan A. Benjamin
VICE PRESIDENT, TECHNICAL OPERATIONS
Peter G. Anderson
VICE PRESIDENT, MGM/UA HOME VIDEO U.K.
Chris Collins
VICE PRESIDENT, CREATIVE SERVICES
Jack Heller
VICE PRESIDENT—FINANCIAL PLANNING AND OPERATIONS
Jeffrey D. Ivers
VICE PRESIDENT, SALES AND MARKETING
Saul H. Melnick
VICE PRESIDENT, INTERNATIONAL MARKETING
Michael O. Murphy

Media Home Entertainment, Inc.

5730 Buckingham Parkway, Culver City, CA 90230; (213) 216-7900, (800) 421-4509. (Subsidiary of A. Heron International Co.)

PRESIDENT
Ron A. Safinick
VICE PRESIDENT, SALES
Alan Ostroff

New World Video

1440 S. Sepulveda Blvd., 2nd floor, Los Angeles, CA 90025; (213) 444-8100. Organized 1974.

PRESIDENT
Paul Culberg
VICE PRESIDENT, ACQUISITIONS & DEVELOPMENT
Roy Cox
VICE PRESIDENT, SALES & MARKETING
David Pierce

Nostalgia Merchant

5730 Buckingham Parkway, Culver City, CA 90230; (213) 216-7900, (800) 421-4509. (Subsidiary of Media Home Entertainment.)

VICE PRESIDENT, SALES
Alan K. Ostroff

Paramount Home Video

5555 Melrose Ave., Los Angeles, CA 90038; (213) 468-5000.

VICE PRESIDENT, MARKETING
Eric Doctorow
VICE PRESIDENT, ADVERTISING
Hollace Brown
VICE PRESIDENT, GENERAL MANAGER
Tim Clott

Playhouse Video

1211 Avenue of the Americas, New York, NY 10036; (212) 819-3238.

Prism Entertainment Corporation

1875 Century Park, Suite 1010, Los Angeles, CA 90067; (213) 277-3270. Organized 1983. (Home video distribution.)

CHAIRMAN—DIRECTOR
Paul Levinson
PRESIDENT—DIRECTOR
Barry Collier
SENIOR VICE PRESIDENT
Robin Montgomery
VICE PRESIDENT—DIRECTOR
Earl Rosenstein
BOARD OF DIRECTORS
Robert Borcharnt

RCA/Columbia Pictures Home Video

2901 W. Alameda Ave., Burbank, CA 91505; (818) 954-4950.

PRESIDENT
Robert Blaitner
CUSTOMER CONTACT
Vallery Kountze
Gary Khamars

RKO Home Video

(Subsidiary of RKO Pictures)
1900 Avenue of the Stars, Suite #1562, Los Angeles, CA 90067; (213) 277-3133. Organized 1983. (Ancillary distribution—home video and cable.)

VICE PRESIDENT
Ellen S. Wander
NATIONAL MARKETING MANAGER, ANCILLARY DISTRIBUTION
Robert D. Lazarus
MARKETING COORDINATOR
Maggie Leatherman
BOARD OF DIRECTORS
C. Robert Manby (Chairman); Mark Seiler (President)

Republic Pictures Corporation

12636 Beatrice St., Los Angeles, CA 90066; (213) 306-4040. Organized 1952. (Film and video distribution.)

PRESIDENT
A.W. Groskopf
VICE PRESIDENT
Nick Draklich
CONTROLLER
Alex Tovar
BOARD OF DIRECTORS
George Hatch (Chairman of the Board); Robert Magness (Board Member); Paul J. O'Brien (Treasurer)

Sony Video Communications

(Division of Sony Corp. of America)
Sony Dr., Park Ridge, NJ 07656; (201) 930-1000.

CORPORATE PRESIDENT
Kenji Tamiya
PRESIDENT
Philip J. Stack
VICE PRESIDENT, SALES
Robert Mueller
NATIONAL SERVICE MANAGER
Philip Hart

Trans World Entertainment

6430 Sunset Boulevard, Suite 505, Hollywood, CA 90028; (213) 461-0467. Organized 1983. (Production of feature films, sales of all media worldwide, domestic video distribution.)

CHAIRMAN
Moshe Diamant
PRESIDENT
Sunil R. Shah

U.S.A. Homevideo

7920 Alabama Ave., Canoga Park, CA 91304-4991; (818) 888-3040, (800) 423-7455. (Subsidiary of International Video Entertainment.)

SENIOR VICE PRESIDENT & GENERAL MANAGER
Len Levy
NATIONAL SALES MANAGER
David Solomon

Vestron Video

60 Long Ridge Rd., P.O. Box 40000, Stamford, CT 06907; (203) 968-0000.

CHAIRMAN, VESTRON, INC.
Austin O. Furst
PRESIDENT, VESTRON, INC.
Jon Peisinger
EXECUTIVE VICE PRESIDENT, CHIEF FINANCIAL OFFICER
Stephen Einhorn
SENIOR VICE PRESIDENT, FEATURE FILM PROGRAMMING
Ruth Vitale
VICE PRESIDENT, FEATURE FILM PROGRAMMING
Lawrence Kesanoff
VICE PRESIDENT, FEATURE FILM ACQUISITIONS
C.J. Kettler
DIRECTOR, FILM ACQUISITIONS AND ACQUISITION PLANNING
Anne Heekin-Canedy
VICE PRESIDENT, FILM EVALUATION
Nana Greenwald
VICE PRESIDENT, PROGRAMMING DEVELOPMENT
Michael Wiese
DIRECTOR OF SPECIALITY PROGRAMS
Melissa Hoffman
MANAGER OF ORIGINAL PROGRAMMING
Jeffrey Peisch
DIRECTOR FILM ACQUISITIONS
Anne Templeton
MANAGER, FILM ACQUISITIONS
Susan Grosoff
VICE PRESIDENT/FILM EVALUATION
Nana Greenwald

Vidamerica Inc.

235 E. 55 St., New York, NY 10022; (212) 355-1600. (Subsidiary of Video Corp., of America.)

Walt Disney Home Video

500 S. Buena Vista St., Burbank, CA 91521; (818) 840-1859.

PRESIDENT
Jim Jimirro
VICE PRESIDENT, RETAIL PROD.
Ben Tenn
MARKETING
Richard Fried

Walt Disney Educational Media Co.

500 S. Buena Vista St., Burbank, CA 91521; (818) 840-1000. (Division of Walt Disney Productions.)

MARKETING COORDINATOR
Linda Capuano

Warner Home Video Inc.

4000 Warner Blvd., Burbank, CA 91522; (818) 954-6000. Organized 1979. (Brings the motion picture and entertainment-media productions of Warner Bros. Inc. to the prerecorded home video marketplace.) A subsidiary of Warner Bros. Inc., a Warner Communications company.

PRESIDENT
Warren N. Lieberfarb
VICE PRESIDENT/GENERAL MANAGER
Edward J. Byrnes
VICE PRESIDENT/WORLDWIDE PLANNING AND OPERATIONS
James F. Cardwell
VICE PRESIDENT/MARKETING
Barbara O'Sullivan
DIRECTOR OF PROGRAMMING
Elyse Eisenberg
PUBLICITY AND PROMOTIONS MANAGER
Michael Finnegan

Production Companies

ABC Video Enterprises
2040 Avenue of the Stars, Los Angeles, CA 90067; (213) 557-6600. Subsidiary of American Broadcasting Co., Inc.

PRESIDENT
Herb Granath
MARKETING & SALES
Marvinia Hunter

AEF Entertainment
3807 Dickerson Rd., Nashville, TN 37207; (615) 868-2040. Organized 1965. (Provides programming for commercial, cable television, along with educational markets. Also provides home video programming.)

CHIEF EXECUTIVE OFFICER
Robert Springer
PRESIDENT
James Springer
SECRETARY—TREASURER
Nancy Springer
BOARD OF DIRECTORS
Robert Springer, James Springer, Nancy Springer
Branches
Nashville, TN; Beverly Hills, CA

A & M Video
1416 N. La Brea Ave., Hollywood, CA 90028; (213) 469-2411.

DIRECTOR OF VIDEO
Sherry Marsh

A M Productions Home Video
46 South De Lacey Ave., Suite 15, Pasadena, CA 91105; (818) 449-0683.

ANE Home Video
106 West, 2950 South, Salt Lake City, UT 84115; (801) 486-3155.

ARC Video, Inc.
88 Lexington Ave., Suite 3-K, New York, NY 10016; (212) 725-5530. Organized 1976. (Produces performing arts TV programming—education/informational/performance-oriented.)

CO-DIRECTOR/TECHNICAL DIRECTOR
Jeff Bush
CO-DIRECTOR/ARTISTIC DIRECTOR
Celia Ipiotis

AVG Inc./SQN Corp.
27 Dryden Lane, Providence, RI 02904; (401) 521-3143. Organized 1971. (Audio/video producing, manufacturing, marketing of quality children's, instructional, music, self-help audio, videocassettes, compact discs.)

CHAIRMAN & CHIEF EXECUTIVE OFFICER
Samuel S. Attenberg
PRESIDENT & C.O.O.
Joan Grow
BOARD OF DIRECTORS
Samuel S. Attenberg, Joan Grow, Richard Carbeau
AFFILIATIONS
VSDA, ABA, NACS

AVS, Inc.
4600 Maryland, Room #13, St. Louis, MO 63108; (314) 361-7072. (Consultants and producers of video and audio.)

PRESIDENT
Susan Meryl Greenberg

Academy Home Entertainment, Inc.
341 N. Maple Dr., Suite 406B, Beverly Hills, CA 90210; (213) 858-6007, (800) 972-0001.

PRESIDENT
Roger M. Reese

Acorn Sports, Inc.
5816 Shakespeare Rd., Columbia, SC 29204; (803) 735-0733. Organized 1981. (Golf videos.)

PRESIDENT
D. Swing Meyer

Active Home Video
9300 W. Pico Blvd., Los Angeles, CA 90035; (213) 274-8233. Organized 1984. (Video production and distribution.)

PRESIDENT
Ron Levanson
VICE PRESIDENT, MARKETING
John Levin
VICE PRESIDENT, ACQUISITIONS
Rana Arons
EXECUTIVE VICE PRESIDENT
Kip Morrison

Admit One Video Presentations
311 Adelaide St. East, Toronto, Canada M5A 1N2; (416) 863-9316. Organized 1981. ("B" movies, schlock horror, classics.)

PRESIDENT
Andrew S. Hermant
VICE PRESIDENT
Len Curtis
OPERATIONS
Joe Mancuso
AFFILIATIONS
Manta Film Productions Ltd., Manta Sound Company

Adventures in Cassettes
1401-B West River Rd., North, Minneapolis, MN 55411; (800) 328-4818. (Division of Metacom, Inc.)

PRESIDENT
Jim McCann

Aero/Space Visuals Society
13547 S.E. 27th Place, Suite 3A2, Bellevue, WA 98005; (206) 881-2661, (800) 225-AERO. Organized 1978. (Produces educational and documentary videos.)

Alamance Co.
8306 Wilshire Blvd., Suite 361, Beverly Hills, CA 90211; (213) 931-6335.

PRESIDENT
Peter Bieler

Alameda County Office of Education
313 West Winton Ave., Hayward, CA 94544-1198; (415) 887-0152 (ext 211).

All Seasons Entertainment
18121 Napa St., Northridge, CA 91325; (818) 886-8680, (800) 423-5599. Organized 1984. (Acquisition of home video rights for various general release programming, manufacture and distribution, "in house" duplication and production.)

PRESIDENT
Fred Hirsch
VICE PRESIDENT
Dwight Krizman
AFFILIATIONS
V.S.D.A.

Lewis Allen/Peter Newman Productions
1500 Broadway, Suite 2805, New York, NY 10036; (212) 221-2400. Organized 1983. (Film and television production.)

PARTNERS
Lewis Allen
Peter Newman
HEAD OF PRODUCTION
Walker Stuart
ADMINISTRATIVE ASSOCIATE
Deborah Stillwell
AFFILIATIONS
Guadalupe Productions, 2700 Bee Cave Rd., Austin, TX 78746

Alpine Film & Video Exchange
1024 N. 250 East, P.O. Box 1254, Orem, UT 84057; (801) 226-

8209. (Science and educational videos.)
PRESIDENT
Lorie Fowlker

Alti Corporation

3333 N. Torrey Pines Court, Suite 320, La Jolla, CA 92037; (619) 452-7703.

American Educational Films

3807 Dickerson Rd., P.O. Box 8188, Nashville, TN 37207; (800) 822-5678.
PRESIDENT
James Springer

American Home Video Library

1500 Broadway, Suite 1807, New York, NY 10036; (212) 869-2616.

American Humanist Association

Television Dept., P.O. Box 146, Amherst, NY 14226-0146; (716) 839-5085.

American National Enterprises, Inc.

106 W. 2950 South, Salt Lake City, UT 84115; (801) 486-3155. Organized 1965. (Film production and distribution to the world market.)
PRESIDENT
Hal Brown
CHIEF EXECUTIVE OFFICER
Neil Rosenstein
VICE PRESIDENT, ADMINISTRATION
Beth Zimmerman
VICE PRESIDENT, BUSINESS AFFAIRS
Bonnie L.W. Mitchell
CONTROLLER
Larry Whitlock
VICE PRESIDENT, PRODUCTION
George Gale
BOARD OF DIRECTORS
Neil Rosenstein, Hal Brown, McNeil Fiske, Aaron Grunfeld, Floyd Sassa
BRANCHES
Suites 217-219, 5858 Hollywood Blvd., Hollywood, CA 90026; (213) 467-2490

American Red Cross

Production Center, 5816 Seminary Rd., Falls Church, VA 22041; (703) 379-8160. (Health, science and safety videos.)

American Sports Network, Inc.

8926 Valley Blvd., P.O. Box 6100, Rosemead, CA 91770; (818) 572-4727. Organized 1976. (Sports production/video, television and cable.)
PRESIDENT
Louis Zwick

American Video

4660 Maryland Ave., St. Louis, MO 63108; (314) 361-7072.
PRESIDENT
Geoffrey S. Simril

American Video Works

Box 333, Evanston, IL 60204; (312) 328-0400. Organized 1979. (Home video.)
CHIEF EXECUTIVE OFFICER
Graham Carlton
VICE PRESIDENT
Mike Rodgers

Amrit Productions Inc.

206 West 99 St., Room 5D, New York, NY 10025; (212) 663-6933. Organized 1982. (Produces and distributes film, video and how to tapes.)
PRODUCER/DIRECTOR/PRESIDENT
Tirlok Malik
DIRECTOR/VICE PRESIDENT
Chander Malik
BRANCHES
Amrit Productions Inc., H-58 Shiva Jee Park, New Delhi 11006, India

Amstar Productions

2020 Avenue of the Stars, Suite 240, Century City, CA 90067; (213) 556-1325.
PRESIDENT
R.J. Barich

Anti-Defamation League of B'Nai B'rith

823 United Nations Plaza, Audio-Visual Dept., New York, NY 10017; (212) 490-2525.
MARKETING DIRECTOR
Carolyn Gold

Morris Anton Associates

301 W. 22 St., New York, NY 10011; (212) 989-2098.
PRESIDENT
Morris Anton

Appalshop, Inc.

306 Madison St., Whitesburg, KY 41858; (606) 633-0108. Organized 1969. (Documents and presents history, culture and social issues of rural America.)

Armour Productions

1030-B North Grove St., Anaheim, CA 92806; (714) 630-3042.
PRESIDENT
Ron Armour

Artmusic, Inc.

248 Sackett St., Brooklyn, NY 11231; (718) 624-3506. Organized 1980. (Presents and produces TV series/PBS video exhibitions and large scale music events.)
PRESIDENT
Wendy Chambers
SECRETARY
Tim Jensen
VICE PRESIDENT
Barbara Mayfield
BOARD OF DIRECTORS
Kelly Knauer, Andy Feigenbaum

Asia Society

725 Park Ave., New York, NY 10021; (212) 288-6400.

Atlantic Film

102 Harbor Rd., Kittery Point, ME 03905; (207) 439-3739. (Outdoor and educational videos.)

Atlantis Productions, Inc.

1252 La Granada Dr., Thousand Oaks, CA 91362; (805) 495-2790. Organized 1952. (Production and distribution of motion pictures in film and video.)
PRESIDENT
Dr. J. Michael Hagopian
VICE PRESIDENT
Becci Meadors

Aura Productions

7911 Willoughby Ave., Los Angeles, CA 90046; (213) 656-9373.
PRESIDENT
Richard Bock

Avant Communications, Inc.
36 W. 44 St., Room 707, New York, NY 10036; (212) 759-3051.
PRESIDENT
Allan Stanley

Avetka Productions Inc.
164 Madison Ave., 4th floor, New York, NY 10016; (212) 686-4550. Organized 1982. (Video production and computer animation.)
PRESIDENT
Maria Avgerakis
VICE PRESIDENT & CREATIVE DIRECTOR
George Avgerakis

BFA Educational Media
468 Park Avenue South, New York, NY 10016; (212) 684-5910, (800) 221-1274. (Subsidiary of Phoenix Films Inc.)
PRESIDENT
H. Gelles

Baffico/Breger Video
915 Broadway, Room 1602, New York, NY 10010; (212) 254-3900. Organized 1983. (Produces cooking videos and PBS series "Madeleine Cooks.")
PRESIDENT
Sue Breger
PRODUCER/DIRECTOR
Charles Pinsky
ASSOCIATE
Barbara Prisco

Bandera Enterprises Inc.
Box 1107, Studio City, CA 91604; (818) 985-5050.
PRESIDENT
Don Flagg

Barnholtz Organization
10966 Le Conte Ave., Suite D., Westwood, CA 90024;, (213) 208-6444.
PRESIDENT
Barry Barnholtz

Barr Films
P.O. Box 5667, Pasadena, CA 91107;, (818) 793-6153.
PRESIDENT
Donald Barr
VICE PRESIDENT
John S. Dyas

Norman Beerger Productions
3217-A29, Arville St., Las Vegas, NV 89102-7612;, (702) 876-2328. Organized 1984. (Produces and distributes wilderness home video programs.)
OWNER
Norman Beerger

Best Film & Video Corporation
98 Cutter Mill Rd., Great Neck, NY 11021;, (516) 487-4515.
PRESIDENT
Roy B. Winnick

Blackhawk Films, Inc.
1 Old Eagle Brewery, Davenport, IA 52802;, (319) 323-9736. Organized 1927.
PRESIDENT
Ted Ewing

Michael Blackwood Productions
251 W. 57 St., Room 427, New York, NY 10019;, (212) 247-4710. (Produces and distributes documentaries on 20th-Century fine artists and performing artists.)
PRESIDENT
Michael Blackwood

Les Blank's Flower Films and Video
10341 San Pablo Ave., El Cerrito, CA 94530;, (415) 525-0942. Organized 1967. (Seeks out and documents America's vanishing minority cultures, their music and traditions.)
PRODUCER/DIRECTOR/CAMERA
Les Blank
DISTRIBUTION MANAGER
Susan Kell
FOLKLORIST/2nd CAMERA
Christine Simon
EDITOR
Maureen Gosling

Bodacious Films
2022 Day St., Ann Arbor, MI 48104;, (313) 663-6928.
PRESIDENT
Peg Dice

Book-of-the-Month Club, Inc.
485 Lexington Ave., New York, NY 10017; (212) 867-4300.
DIRECTOR OF VIDEO DIVISION
George Spitzer

Bookshelf Video
301-B West Dyer Rd., Santa Ana, CA 92707; (714) 556-7918.
PRESIDENT
Mike Kahled
VICE PRESIDENT, MARKETING
Katherine Rice

Bosustow Productions
2207 Colby Ave., West Los Angeles, CA 90064; (213) 478-0821.

Britannica Video
425 North Michigan Ave., Chicago, IL 60611; (800) 558-6968, (312) 321-6841.

Broadcast Quality Inc.
7800 S.W. 57th Ave., Suite 219, South Miami, FL 33142; (305) 665-5416.
PRESIDENT
David Clarke

Broadman
127 Ninth Ave. N., Nashville, TN 37234; (615) 251-2561. (800) 251-3225, (800) 342-0021. (Tennessee).

Brooklyn College
Dept. of Television and Radio, 018 Whitehead Hall, Bedford Ave. H., Brooklyn, NY 11210; (718) 780-5555.
PRESIDENT
Robert C. Williams

Bullfrog Films, Inc.
Oley, PA 19547; (215) 779-8226. Organized 1973. (Distributes programs for personal self-reliance—how-to's on gardening, home improvements, energy-saving, etc.—and environmental responsibility.)
PRESIDENT
John Hoskyns-Abrahall
SECRETARY & TREASURER
Winifred Scherrer
PROMOTIONS MANAGER
Chris Everly
CUSTOMER SERVICE MANAGER
Steve Jarrett
BOARD OF DIRECTORS
John Hoskyns-Abrahall, Winifred Scherrer

CBS Video Club/CBS Video Library
1400 N. Fruitridge Ave., Terre Haute, IN 47811, and 1211 Avenue of the Americas, New York, NY 10036; (212) 975-4875. (Subsidiary of Columbia House, a division of CBS Inc.)
VICE PRESIDENT, MARKETING
Brian Wood

CBS Worldwide Enterprises
51 W. 52 St., New York, NY 10019; (212) 975-4515. (Subsidiary of CBS Broadcast Group, CBS Inc.)

CC Studios/Children's Circle
389 Newtown Turnpike, Weston, CT 06883; (203) 222-0002. Organized 1963. (Produces and markets home audio/video cassettes to consumers; adaptations of children's books.)
PRESIDENT & TREASURER
Morton Schindel
VICE PRESIDENT
Katharine Gordon
SECRETARY
Elisabeth Rommel
ASSISTANT TREASURER
Betsy Rhines
BOARD OF DIRECTORS
Morton Schindel, Paul Schindel, Elisabeth Rommel
AFFILIATIONS
Weston Woods; Georgetown Studios

CVI/Cirace Video International
2300 S. 9th St., Room 136, Arlington, VA 22204; (703) 486-1555, (800) 222-3992. Organized 1980. (Television production company.)
PRESIDENT
Robert H. Cirace
VICE PRESIDENT
Verdine O. Palmer
SECRETARY & TREASURER
Debra D. Palmer
BOARD OF DIRECTORS
Robert H. Cirace, Verdine O. Palmer, Wendie L. Wachtel, Barry B. Wright, Cherry Wyman
AFFILIATIONS
Majority stockholder in Uplink Corp., Satellite Service Company

Cable Video
Country Club Station, Box 7171 Kansas City, MO 64113; (913) 362-2804. (Subsidiary of Cable Films.)
PRESIDENT
Herbert Miller

Calypso Video, Inc.
2040 Reynolds Rd., Southwyck Center, Toledo, OH 43614; (419) 865-4169.
PRESIDENT
C. Opfermann

Candlelight Studios
P.O. Box 627, Little River, CA 95456; (707) 937-5424. Organized 1981. (Provides fine art instruction for all ages on videotape.)
PRESIDENT
E. John Robinson
MANAGER
Jon Harwood

Cape Cod Writers' Conference
309 Green Dunes Drive, Box 111, West Hyannisport, MA 02672; (617) 775-4811, summer: (617) 384-0425. Organized 1963. (Promotes writing through video, audio, conferences and writer-in-the-schools.)
EXECUTIVE DIRECTOR
Marion Vuilleumier
PRESIDENT
Katherine Fitzgerald
VICE PRESIDENT
Dr. Gerald Leinwand
SECRETARY & CLERK
Marian Logan
TREASURER
Olive St. Germaine
REGISTRAR
Mattie MacFadden
BOARD OF DIRECTORS
Marion Vuilleumier, Katherine Fitzgerald, Dr. Gerald Leinwand, Marian Logan, Olive St. Germaine, Mattie MacFadden
AFFILIATIONS
Cape Arts Workshops, Box 12, Cummaquid, MA 02637

Caravatt Communications, Inc.
49 Riverside Ave., Westport, CT 06880;, (203) 227-0775.
PRESIDENT & CHIEF EXECUTIVE OFFICER
Paul J. Caravatt, Jr.
DIRECTOR OF OPERATIONS
Paul F. Schucker
DIRECTOR OF MARKETING
David Wood
PROJECT DIRECTORS
Jane Scarpellino
Thomas Duggan
BOARD OF DIRECTORS
Wm E. Chambers (Pres., Norman Craig & Kummel, Ret.); Robert Morse, (Pres., Morse Williams, NYC); Peter Winslow (Ex. VP, Monz Cabot, Boston); Munanar Hidaya Halah (Pres. Consultancy & Mgt., NYC)

Catholic Television Network/Bay Area Dioceses
324 Middlefield Rd., Menlo Park, CA 94025; (415) 326-7850.
GENERAL MANAGER
Tom Bellick

Centron Films
65 East South Water St., Chicago, IL 60601; (312) 977-4000, (800) 621-2131. (Programs distributed by MTI Teleprograms, Inc.)

Doris Chase Productions
222 W. 23 St., Room #722, New York, NY 10011; (212) 243-3700. Organized 1972. (Produces for television, film and video art.)
AFFILIATIONS
Museum of Modern Art, Coe Films Women Make Movies, Video Data Bank, Coronet Films

Children's Video Library
P.O.. Box 4995, 1011 High Ridge Rd., Stamford, CT 06907; (203) 968-0100.

Christ for the Nations Inc.
P.O. Box 24910, Dallas TX 75224; (214) 376-1711.
DIRECTOR
Gene Steiner

Christian Media
P.O. Box 748, 924 24th St., Suite 7, Ogden, UT 84402; (801) 399-4006.
PRESIDENT
Joe Burdett

Christophers
12 E. 48 St., New York, NY 10017; (212) 759-4050.
DIRECTOR
Rev. John Catoir

Chronicle Video Cassettes
9000 Sunset Blvd., Suite 415, Los Angeles, CA 90069; (213) 858-0141.
PRESIDENT
Bill Hickey

Churchill Films, Inc.
662 N. Robertson Blvd., Los Angeles, CA 90069; (213) 657-

5110. Organized 1964. (Educational producers and distributors—documentary, theatrical, television.)
PRESIDENT
George McQuilkin
VICE PRESIDENTS
Robert B. Churchill
Robert L. Glore
BOARD OF DIRECTORS
George McQuilkin, Robert B. Churchill, Robert L. Glore

Cinema Guild
1697 Broadway, Suite 802, New York, NY 10019; (212) 246-5522. (Subsidiary of Document Associates, Inc.)
PRESIDENT
Philip Hobel
GENERAL MANAGER, MARKETING & SALES
Gary Crowdus

Cinema Products
P.O. Box 594, Tujunga, CA 91042; (818) 352-2243.
PRESIDENT
Bob Krasnow

Cinemagreats
15825 Rob Roy Drive, Oak Forest, IL 60452; (312) 687-7881.

Circle Video Productions
2901 W. 16th St., Indianapolis, IN 46222; (317) 638-1066.

Classic Family Entertainment
6649 Odessa Ave., Van Nuys, CA 91406; (818) 780-7100.
PRESIDENT
Sidney Niekerk

Coast Telecourses
11460 Warner Ave., Fountain Valley, CA 92708-2597; (714) 241-6109. (Educational videos.)

Color Leasing, Inc.
330 Route 46, Fairfield, NJ 07006; (201) 575-1118, (212) 662-2655. Organized 1966.
PRESIDENT
Taul Berberian

Columbia School of Biblical Education (Video Department)
7435 Monticello Road, Columbia, SC 29203; (803) 754-4100, ext. 131. (Provides quality Biblical teaching on video.)
DEAN OF COLUMBIA SCHOOL OF BIBLICAL EDUCATION
Dr. Jim Wenger
DIRECTOR, CSBE Video Ministries
Rick H. Byers

Comet Video
2320 Cotner Ave., Los Angeles, CA 90064; (213) 477-8055.
PRESIDENT
Jim Silverman

Comex Systems
The Mill Cottage, Mendham, NJ 07945; (201) 234-1616.
VICE PRESIDENT
Loe Brovalowski

Communicorp, Inc.
805 S. Main St., Suite 6, Lombard, IL 60148; (312) 629-7070. Organized 1983. (Video production of corporate, sports, health-care and consumer videos.)
PRESIDENT
John F. Moran, Ph.D.
VICE PRESIDENT
Timothy Bukowski
PRODUCTION MANAGER
Andy Lock
AFFILIATIONS
Independently produces video. Consumer marketing done by AmbreCorp.

Compuvid
815 N. Royal St., Alexandria, VA 22314; (703) 683-3234. (Computer and educational videos.)

Concepts Unlimited
600 S. Main St., Oshkosh, WI 54901; (414) 426-0863.
PRESIDENT
M.J. Beckman

Concordia Publishing House
3558 S. Jefferson, St. Louis, MO 63118-3968; (314) 664-7000.
PRESIDENT
Ralph Beinke

Continental Video, Inc.
2320 Cotner Ave., Los Angeles, CA 90064; (213) 477-8055.
PRESIDENT
Jim Silverman

Cornell University Audio Visual Center
8 Research Park, Ithaca, NY 14850; (607) 256-2090. Organized 1929. (Provides educational programs to Cooperative Ext. agents so they can provide information to consumers.)
AFFILIATIONS
Consortium of University Film Centers, Educational Film Library Association

Coronet Films
108 Wilmont Rd., Deerfield, IL 60015; (312) 940-1260.
CO-CHAIRMEN
R. Robert Whitworth
Lloyd Singer

Courier Productions
P.O. Box 291285, Los Angeles, CA 90010; (213) 937-2848.
PRESIDENT
Linda D. Roberts

Covenant Video
3200 W. Foster Ave., Chicago, IL 60625; (312) 478-4676; (800) 621-1290. (Religious videos.)
PRESIDENT
Stan Torgerson

Creative Tax Planning Association
225 Broadway, Suite 1100, New York, NY 10007; (212) 227-4000.
OWNER
Howard Einbinder

Creative Visions Video
721 S. San Pedro St., Los Angeles, CA 90014; (213) 623-9254, (800) 421-8528. (Subsidiary of Image Laboratories, Inc.)
PRESIDENT
Robert Hoffman

Crown Video
One Park Ave., New York, NY 10016; (212) 532-9200.

Crystallus Films, Inc.
11 Fayette St., Cambridge, MA 02139; (617) 492-6739. Or-

ganized 1979. (Produces and distributes films and television works of artistic and educational interest.)

PRESIDENT
Elliot Hoffman

A.S. Csaky Motion Picture and Video Productions

420 Legato Terrace, Silver Spring, MD 20901; (301) 681-3333 and 681-3390. Organized 1968. (Develops, produces and distributes motion picture and video productions and screenplays nationally and internationally.)

CHAIRMAN OF THE BOARD & PRESIDENT
A.S. Csaky
VICE PRESIDENT, PRODUCTION
Ramzi D. Seikaly
VICE PRESIDENT, SCREENPLAY DEVELOPMENT
Bud Fleischer
VICE PRESIDENT, TRAVEL MANAGEMENT
Albert Cambata
VICE PRESIDENT, PUBLIC RELATIONS
Cecilia Korda-Bros
VICE PRESIDENT, SALES & MARKETING
Catherine White
GRAPHICS DIRECTOR
Juan Chavarria
BRANCHES
Washington, DC, New York, NY

Cunningham Dance Foundation, Inc.

463 West St., New York, NY 10014; (212) 255-3130. (Cultural and arts videos.)

Custom Films/Video, Inc.

11 Cob Drive, Westport, CT 06880; (203) 226-0300. Organized 1962. (Produces film and video.)

PRESIDENT
Lester S. Becker

Cycle Vision Tours, Inc.

1020 Green Valley Rd. NW, Albuquerque, NM 87107; (505) 345-5217. Organized 1983. (Production and marketing of the videocycle series. Video exercise programs for exercise bicycles.)

PRESIDENT
George L. Dixon, Jr., M.D.
VICE PRESIDENT
Margery M. Dixon
MARKETING DIRECTOR
Mark S. Lange
OPERATIONS
Martha D. Lange
BOARD OF DIRECTORS
George L. Dixon, Jr., M.D., Margery M. Dixon, Mark S. Lange, Martha D. Lange
AFFILIATIONS
Video Software Dealers Assoc., National Bicycle Dealers Assoc., National Sporting Goods Assoc.

Czar Productions, Inc.

39 Princeton St., West Hartford, CT 06110; (203) 233-2034.

PRESIDENT
Gene Czarnecki

Damon & Grace Corporation

P.O. Box 1767, East Lansing, MI 48823; (517) 337-7471. Organized 1972. (Videos to better the quality of life for individuals through behavior modification.)

PRESIDENT
Grace A. Reinbold
VICE PRESIDENT
Jay M. Reinbold
BRANCHES
38 Music Square East, Suite 219, Nashville, TN 37203

Dawn's Video

519 W. Foothill, Suite C, Rialto, CA 92376; (714) 874-1414. Organized 1980. (Video specialty store.)

OWNER
Gregory C. George
BRANCHES
2085 E. Highland Ave., San Bernadino, CA 92404; (714) 864-3113
9725 Sierra, Fontana, CA 92335; (714) 350-8833
267 E. 40th, San Bernadino, CA 92404; (714) 883-5737
1330 Massachusetts Ave., Riverside, CA 92507; (714) 784-1414

Daya, Inc.

36 Weston Rd., Westport, CT 06880; (203) 226-1964. (Needlecraft and educational videos.)

De Luz Video

P.O. Box 1431, Fallbrook, CA 92028; (619) 433-7220. Organized 1978. (Produces railroad home video tapes, VHS only.)

OWNER & PRESIDENT
Frank C. Boulter
PRODUCER & CAMERAMAN
Edward F. Boulter

Development Communications Incorporated

815 N. Royal St., Alexandria, VA 22314; (703) 638-3100. Organized 1978. (Training tapes.)

PRESIDENT
Welby A. Smith, Jr.
VICE PRESIDENT
Lawrence M. Franks
SECRETARY-TREASURER
Elizabeth P. Smith
BOARD OF DIRECTORS
Welby A. Smith, Jr., Lawrence M. Franks, Betsy P. Smith
AFFILIATIONS
ITVA, Dept. of Defense QVPL, ADPA, ASTD, Washington Film Council

Dial Productions

3220 Colony View, Malibu, CA 90265; (213) 456-6980.

PRESIDENT
Charlotte Dial

Digital Touch Ltd.

303 W. 42 St., Suite 4034, New York, NY 10036; (212) 246-3811, ext. 683. Organized 1985. (Multi-media development and production.)

PRESIDENT
Jeffrey Selig
VICE PRESIDENT
Bruce E. Colfin
COUNSEL
Jeffrey E. Jacobson
BOARD OF DIRECTORS
Jeffrey Selig, Bruce E. Colfin, J.E. Jacobson
BRANCHES
Boston
AFFILIATIONS
AES

Direct Broadcast Programs, Inc.

22761 Pacific Coast Highway, Malibu, CA 90265; (213) 456-7071. (Subsidiary of Video Connection of America.)

VICE PRESIDENT, MARKETING
Raphael Knier

Direct Video

1800 N. Higland Ave., #709, Los Angeles, CA 90028; (818) 506-7470.

Discount Video Tapes, Inc.

3717 W. Clark Ave., Suite B, Burbank, CA 91505; (818) 843-3366. Organized 1979. (Specializing in rare and unusual pre-recorded videos. Retail and wholesale.)

PRESIDENT
Woody Wise

Dobovan Productions

1370 Kapiocani Blvd., Suite 101A, Honolulu, HI 96814.

PRESIDENT
John B. Dobovan

Double Vision Video Productions

410 South St., Sacramento, CA 95814; (916) 448-8220. (Instructional videos.)

Dudkowski-Lynch Associates, Inc.

150 Shoreline Highway, Bldg. E, Mill Valley, CA 94941; (415) 332-5825. Organized 1974. (Video production and post-production.)

PRESIDENT
Ed Dudkowski
VICE PRESIDENT
Marijane Lynch

EDC Publishing

8141 E. 44th St., Tulsa OK 74105; (918) 622-4522. (Subsidiary of Educational Development Corp.)

PRESIDENT
John O. Whitney

Eagle Productions Ltd.

7860 Mission Center Court, Suite 106, San Diego, CA 92108; (619) 297-8870.

Echo Film Productions

Box 4692, Aspen, CO 81612; (303) 925-5605. Organized 1968. (Sports films, environmental documentaries, adventure films, new age health and arts.)

OFFICERS
Wilk Wilkinson
Tulasi Wilkinson
Jama Wilkinson
AFFILIATIONS
AFI, 659

Educational Cable Consortium Inc.

24 Beechwood Rd., Summit, NJ 08701; (201) 277-2870. (Family-oriented educational videos.)

EXECUTIVE DIRECTOR
Kate Wood

Educational Dimensions Group

792 Pacific St., Stamford, CT 06904; (203) 327-4612.

PRESIDENT
Richard A. Byrnes

Educational Video, Inc.

31800 Plymouth Rd., Livonia, MI 48150; (313) 661-0163. Organized 1983. (Production and marketing of original pre-recorded videocassettes.)

PRESIDENT
Robert Tollini
VICE PRESIDENTS
Pamela Bonk
Petra Pepellashi

Electronic University

P.O. Box 938, Pt. Reyes Station, CA 94956; (415) 663-9102. (Subsidiary of Electronic Educational Programs.)

PRESIDENT
Mark Watts

Emory Medical Television Network

1440 Clifton Rd., N.E., Atlanta, GA 30322; (404) 329-5697. (A subsidiary of Emory University School of Medicine.)

MARKETING & SALES
Alan S. Kaminsky

Enter-Tel, Inc.

24400 Chagrin Blvd., Beachwood, OH 44122; (216) 831-6940.

Environmental Video, Inc.

1116 8th St., Room B, P.O. Box 577, Manhattan Beach, CA 90266; (213) 546-4581. Organized 1981. (Manufactures and produces pre-recorded videocassettes for the home video market.)

PRESIDENT
James R. Spencer

Epic Pictures

1940 South Cotner Ave., Los Angeles, CA 90025; (213) 273-8477.

Episcopal Radio-TV Foundation, Inc.

3379 Peachtree Rd., N.E., Suite 610, Atlanta, GA 30326; (404) 233-5419

Equinox Entertainment Corp.

2423 Wilcox Dr., Norman, OK 73069; (405) 360-6595.

PRESIDENT
Jerry Colclazier

Esquire Publishing Corp.

2 Park Ave., New York, NY 10016; (212) 561-8226.

Event Video

P.O. Box 3733, Ventura, CA 93003; (805) 642-1838. (Holistic health and how-to videos.)

PRESIDENT
Bill Peay

Everything Video

P.O. Box 313, New Brunswick, NJ 08903; (201) 753-5826. Organized 1982. (Production of railroad videos and distribution of rare historical railroad video tapes.)

PRESIDENT
Norman Skolnick
VICE PRESIDENT
Murray Skolnick

Eye Contact, Inc.

1431 Center St., Oakland, CA 94610; (415) 836-1180. Organized 1982. (Provides multilingual production services in film and video.)

PRESIDENT
Carla Itzkowich
VICE PRESIDENT
Norma Armon
AFFILIATIONS
Division of Catalyst Production Services

Eye Contact, Inc.

1755 Seaview Terrace, Los Angeles, CA 90046; (213) 850-0294.

FFH Video

743 Alexander Rd., Princeton, NJ 08540; (609) 452-1128.

PRESIDENT
Harold Mantell

FJC-Intellimedia, Inc.

P.O. Box 6632, Syracuse, NY 13217-6632; (315) 472-3442.

PRESIDENT
Joseph Crisafulli

Family Home Entertainment

7920 Alabama Ave., Canoga Park, CA 91304; (818) 888-3040; (800) 423-7455. (Children's video.)

SENIOR VICE PRESIDENT & GENERAL MANAGER
Len Levy

Ferde Grofe Films

3100 Airport Ave., Santa Monica, CA 90405; (213) 397-7524. (800) 854-0561, ext. 925. (Science and educational films.)

Festival Films

2841 Irving Ave. South, Minneapolis, MN 55408; (612) 870-4744.

Four Point Entertainment, Inc.

3575 Cahuenga Blvd. West, Room 600, Los Angeles, CA 90068; (213) 850-1600. Organized 1984. (Television production, videocassette production, home video distribution.)

PRESIDENT
Ron Ziskin
CHAIRMAN
John LaCapra
EXECUTIVE VICE PRESIDENTS
Joseph Benti
Shukri Ghalayini

Fox/Lorber Associates, Inc.

432 Park Avenue South, New York, NY 10016; (212) 686-6777.

PRESIDENT
Richard Lorber

Freewheelin' Films Ltd.

P.O. Box 599, Aspen, CO 81611; (303) 925-2640. (Sports and educational videos.)

DIRECTOR
Rodney Jacobs

GN Communications, Ltd.

1723 Howard St., Evanston, IL 60202; (312) 864-0075. Organized 1984. (Sells video tapes of special interest programming to the television and home market.)

PRESIDENT
Steven Polydoris
AFFILIATIONS
Chicago Film and Video, American Film & Video Network

Gateway Films Inc.

Box A, Lansdale, PA 19446; (215) 584-1893. Organized 1972. (Motion picture production and distribution.)

PRESIDENT
A. Kenneth Curtis

Genesis Project, Inc.

630 Fifth Ave., Suite 1510, New York, NY 10020; (212) 399-1020, (800) 336-4545. (Religious videos.)

PRESIDENT
Michael Manuel

Glenn Video Vistas

6924 Canby Ave., Suite 103, Reseda, CA 91335; (818) 981-5506. Organized 1980. (Sale of videotapes.)

OWNER/MANAGER
Murray Glass
AFFILIATIONS
Glenn Photo Supply

Global Village

454 Broome St., New York, NY 10013; (212) 966-7526.

Golden Bay Video

61 Camino Alto, Suite #108, Mill Valley, CA 94941; (415) 381-2566. Organized 1982. (Video production.)

PRESIDENT
Vinton W. Medbury, Jr.

Golden Classics Media

419 W. Walnut, Gardena, CA 90248; (213) 516-0315. (Subsidiary of See Hear Industries.)

PRESIDENT
Raymond Jacobs

Golden Productions

9022 Leatrice Dr., Little Rock, AR 72207; (501) 224-4479. Organized 1983. (Education and training programs for mental health professionals.)

PRESIDENT
Dr. Kenneth M. Golden

Gorgon Video

15825 Rob Roy Dr., Oak Forest, IL 60452; (312) 687-7881. (Horror videos.)

PRESIDENT
Jaffa Ali

Gospel Films, Inc.

P.O. Box 455, Muskegon, MI 49443; (616) 773-3361.

PRESIDENT
Rev. Billy Zeoli

Gospel Video

9929 Venice Blvd., Los Angeles, CA 90034;, (213) 204-3397.

Granada TV International

1221 Avenue of Americas, Suite 3468, New York, NY 10020;(212) 869-8480.

UNITED STATES MANAGER
Leica Maw
SALES EXECUTIVE
Alison Brantley
BOARD OF DIRECTORS
Barrie Heads (Managing Director); Vivien Wallace (Director of Sales); Patrick Rickenberg (Director of Development).
BRANCHES
36 Golden Square, London W1, England; 01-734-8080.
18 Rue Volney, Paris 75002, France; 4261 7910 (Sales manager: Sara De St. Hubert)

Grand Award Video Inc.

2170 W. Broadway, Room 526, Anaheim, CA 92801; (714) 995-0707. Organized 1983. (Manufacturer of video pre-recorded software and TV's wide screen.)

PRESIDENT
Jeffrey M. Scheirer
VICE PRESIDENT
Harry F. Scheirer
BOARD OF DIRECTORS
Jeffrey Scheirer, Harry F. Scheirer

Grass Roots Network, Inc.

70 Pacific Ave., Aspen, CA 81612; (303) 925-8000.

DIRECTOR
Greg Poschman

Gravity Sports Films, Inc.

1591 So. 1100 E., Salt Lake City, Utah 84105; (801) 485-3702. Organized 1980. (Video production and distribution on sports subjects.)

PRESIDENT
Ronald S. Rossi
SECRETARY & TREASURER
Wanda Padgett
BOARD OF DIRECTORS
Ronald Rossi, Bruce Stafford, Wanda Padgett
AFFILIATIONS
Gravity Sports Video, Birkland, Ontario

Great Mountain Productions

233 Broadway, Suite 3715, New York, NY 10279; (212) 227-5820. (Educational and children's videos.)

Green Mountain Post Films

37 Ferry Rd., P.O. Box 229, Turners Falls, MA 01376; (413) 863-4754.

PRESIDENT
Daniel Keller

Ham Mastertapes

136 E. 31 St., New York, NY 10016; (212) 685-7844. (How-to videos concerning ham radios.)

PRESIDENT
Larry Horne

Harmony Vision

116 N. Robertson Blvd., Suite 701, Los Angeles, CA 90048; (213) 652-8844. (Music and concert videos.)

PRESIDENT
Jerry Percell

Hartly Film Foundation, Inc.

Cat Rock Road, Cos Cob, CT 06807; (203) 869-1818. Organized 1970. (Produces educational films.)

PRESIDENT
Elda Hartley
VICE PRESIDENT
James Porter
OFFICE MANAGER
Barbara LaRosa

Health Media of America, Inc.

11300 Sorrento Valley Rd., #250, San Diego, CA 92121; (619) 453-3887.

PRESIDENT
Robert H. Garrison, Jr.

Henwood Cinema Video

106 North Keswick Ave., Glenside, PA 19038; (215) 884-7533. Organized 1976. (Television programming of motion pictures and videocassette programming of feature films.)

PRESIDENT
Alan Henwood, Jr.
SALES MANAGER
Mary Henwood
OFFICE MANAGER
Margaret Jones
ASSISTANT SALES MANAGER
Ann Miller

Hewlett-Packard

1819 Page Mill Rd., Palo Alto, CA 94304; (415) 857-2381. (How-to and educational videos.)

Alfred Higgins Productions Inc.

9100 Sunset Blvd., Los Angeles, CA 90069; (213) 272-6500.

PRESIDENT
Jim Novak

High Gate Pictures

16 W. 61 St., New York, NY 10023; (212) 397-9330.

PRESIDENT
William F. Deneen

Don L. Higley & Associates

4930 Sawyer Ave., Santa Barbara, CA 93103; (805) 684-9515. (Sports, How-to, educational videos.)

PRESIDENT
Don L. Higley

Hollywood Home Theatre

1540 N. Highland Ave., #110, Hollywood, CA 90028; (213) 466-0121, (213) 466-0127.

PRESIDENT
Larry S. Fine

Hollywood International Film Corporation of America

1044 South Hill St., Los Angeles, CA 90015; (213) 749-2067. Organized 1969. (Film production and distribution.)

PRESIDENT
Efrain Tobalina
VICE PRESIDENT
Maria-Pia Tobalina

Hot Licks Productions, Inc.

P.O. Box 337, Pound Ridge, NY 10576; (914) 763-8013. Organized 1979. (Produces video and audio music instruction.)

PRESIDENT
Arlen Roth
VICE PRESIDENT
Deborah Roth
BOARD OF DIRECTORS
Arlen Roth, Deborah Roth
AFFILIATIONS
Labtek in U.K., Music Sales in Australia and New Zealand

Houghton Mifflin Company

One Beacon St. (executive offices); 2 Park St. (trade and dictionary divisions), Boston, MA 02108; (617) 725-5000. (Birdwatching and general entertainment videos.)

PRESIDENT
Richard W. Young

How To Video Corp.

606 N. Main St., Ashland City, TN 37015; (615) 792-4472, 792-4417.

PRESIDENT
Jerry Hooker

Hyde Park Media

7158 Lee St., Chicago, IL 60648; (312) 967-7666.

PRESIDENT
A.E. De Bartolo

IRS Video

633 N. La Brea, Los Angeles, CA 90036; (818) 508-1657. (Music videos.)

Icarus Films

200 Park Avenue South, Suite 1319, New York, NY 10003; (212) 674-3375.

Image Magnetic Associates, Inc.

5514 Satsuma Ave., North Hollywood, CA 91601; (818) 762-3993.

PRESIDENT
David Allen

Images Video & Film Archive, Inc.

300 Phillips Park Road, Mamaroneck, NY 10543; (914) 381-2994.

PRESIDENT
Robert A. Harris
VICE PRESIDENT—ACQUISITIONS, ARCHIVAL FILM MATERIALS
Audrey E. Kupferberg
MANAGER—VIDEO DISTRIBUTION
Joanne Lawson

Imperial Video Corp.

106A Benkert St., Bethpage, NY 11714; (516) 935-5050, (800) 645-5060.

PRESIDENT
B. Rubinowitz

Impulse Entertainment
1665 12th St., Santa Monica, CA 90404; (213) 450-2527.
PRESIDENT
Randi Freeman

Increase Video
8265 Sunset Blvd., Suite 105, Los Angeles, CA 90046; (213) 654-8808.
PRESIDENT
Howard Silvers
VICE PRESIDENT
Arny Schorr

Innovations In Video
8448 Reseda Blvd., Suite 101, Northridge, CA 91324; (818) 701-1423, (800) 624-9327 (CA), (800) 227-1586.

Instant Replay Video Magazine
2951 S. Bayshore Dr., Miami, FL 33133; (305) 448-7088.
PRESIDENT
Charles Azar

Instructional Video Cassette Corp.
2035 S. 7th St., Philadelphia, PA 19148; (215) 271-1500.

Intercollegiate Video Clearing House
P.O. Drawer 33000R, Miami, FL 33132; (305) 221-8383. (Educational and how-to videos.)
DIRECTOR
Dr. Thomas Stroh

International Historic Films, Inc.
3015 W. 59th St., Chicago, IL 60629; (312) 436-8051. Organized 1976. (Distribution and production of military and political features and documentaries. Also distribution of Eastern European films. Provides stock footage to producers. Sales and rental of films on videocassette through store and direct mail internationally. Videocassettes available on NTSC, PAL and SECAM videostandards.)
PRESIDENT
Peter Bernotas
AFFILIATIONS
Lithuanian Historical Society

International Marketing Services Inc.
2170 W. Broadway, Bldg. 522, Anaheim, CA 92804; (714) 891-6015.
VICE PRESIDENT
Jeff Scheirer

International Sunday School Lesson, Inc.
P.O. Box 2711, Lubbock, TX 79408; (806) 741-1015. Organized 1976. (Exegetical verse-by-verse Bible teaching using historical-grammatical hermeneutics.)
FOUNDER & HOST
Rev. Bob Utley
OFFICE MANAGER
Vernon Odom
AFFILIATIONS
Member of National Religious Broadcasters

Ivy Video
165 W. 46 St., New York, NY 10036; (212) 382-0111. (Subsidiary of Multi-Media Entertainment, Inc.)
PRESIDENT
Sidney Tager

JEF Films Inc.
Film House, 143 Hickory Hill Circle, Osterville, MA 02655; (617) 428-7198. Organized 1973. (Production and distribution of films, TV shows and video programs throughout the world.)
PRESIDENT
Jeffrey H. Aikman
VICE PRESIDENT
Elsie Aikman
SECRETARY & TREASURER
Donald Aikman
MARKETING MANAGER
Jo-Anne Polak
SALES
Janie Barber
BOARD OF DIRECTORS
Jeffrey H. Aikman, Elsie Aikman, Donald Aikman
BRANCHES
Film Classic Exchange, Los Angeles, CA
JEF Films Inc.—England, Canada, Australia, Japan, China, Netherlands, New Zealand, Scandinavia, Norway, Denmark, Germany, Sweden, Hong Kong, Iceland, Fiji, Ireland, Scotland, Wales
AFFILIATIONS
Owner of Film Classic Exchange (founded 1916), VIP Video, XTC Video, JEF Video Line

JMJ Productions
P.O. Box 4449, Hollywood, FL 33083; (305) 652-3952. (Railroad related documentaries.)
PRESIDENT
Morry Farcus

Stefaan Janssen Studio
4615 N. Lincoln Ave., Chicago, IL 60625; (312) 728-9277. Organized 1983. (Sells and produces special interest programs for the home video market.)
OWNER
Stefaan Janssen
AFFILIATIONS
Member: VSDA; Center for New Television; AIFV

Johansen Video Productions
1121 First Ave., Suite 400, Denver, CO 80206; (303) 333-8777. Organized 1978. (Creates and sells video productions.)
PRESIDENT
David A. Johansen
VICE PRESIDENT
William D. Peterson
AFFILIATIONS
Production facilities with Multi Vision of Denver

K-Video Productions
157 Wiltshire Rd., Claymont, DE 19703; (302) 798-2229. Organized 1980. (Educational tapes, corporate and private videos.)
PRESIDENT
John Kay
VICE PRESIDENT
Stan Kay
SECRETARY & TREASURER
Charmaine Imburgia
AFFILIATIONS
DBE, GWVCB, Delaware State Chamber of Commerce

Kalmbach Publishing Co.
1027 N. 7th St., Milwaukee, WI 53233; (414) 272-2060.
PRESIDENT
James J. King.

Kartes Productions Inc.
10 East 106th St., Indianapolis, IN 46280; (317) 844-7403, (800) 582-2000

Keep the Faith Inc.
810 Belmont Ave., North Haledon, NJ 07508; (201) 423-5395, (800) 221-1564. (Religious videos.)

Allan Keith Productions, Inc.
630 Ninth Ave., Suite 714, New York, NY 10036; (212) 246-0239. Organized 1961. (Produces educational subjects—film and video—speech, make up, sex equity, auto body repair, etc.)
PRESIDENT

Allan Keith
VICE PRESIDENT
Michael Keith
SECRETARY
Laurie Schilling

Kennen Publishing

150 Shoreline Highway, Bldg. E., Mill Valley, CA 94941; (415) 332-5828. (How-to computer videos.) (Subsidiary of Dudkowski-Lynch Assoc. Inc.)

PRESIDENT
Ed Dudkowski

King of Video

3529 S. Valley View Blvd., Las Vegas, NV 89103; (800) 634-6143m (702) 362-2520.

GENERAL MANAGER
Robert Hillman

Walter J. Klein Company, Ltd.

6311 Carmel Road, Box 2087, Charlotte, NC 28211-2087; (704) 542-1403. Organized 1946. (Production and distribution of sponsored films and tapes.)

PRESIDENT
Walter J. Klein
VICE PRESIDENT
Richard A. Klein
SECRETARY
Elizabeth G. Klein
TREASURER
Betsy J. Klein
BOARD OF DIRECTORS
Walter J. Klein, Richard A Klein, Elizabeth G. Klein, Betsy J. Klein
BRANCHES
Seven Devils, NC

Kultur International Films Ltd.

121 Highway #36, Suite 326, West Long Branch, NJ 07764; (201) 229-2343. Organized 1980. (Performing arts programs on homevideo and Russian cultural programs for broadcast and cable.)

PRESIDENT
Dennis M. Hedlund
VICE PRESIDENT
Pearl Lee
PUBLICITY DIRECTOR
Jean Dalrymple
SALES MANAGER
Dudley Smith
SALES ADMINISTRATOR
Lynn Hager
DIRECTOR OF OPERATIONS
Austin Culter

Learn Incorporated

113 Gaither Drive, Mt. Laurel, NJ 08054; (609) 234-6100. Organized 1968. (Publishes and markets "How to" video programs and audio programs with print materials.)

PRESIDENT
Bruce E. Corley
EXECUTIVE VICE PRESIDENT
Nate Rosenblatt
VICE PRESIDENT, FINANCE
Lynn Weaver

Learning Corporation of America

1350 Avenue of the Americas, New York, NY 10019; (212) 397-9360. (A division of Simon & Schuster Inc.)

Legalvision, Inc.

%Jacobson & Colfin, 150 Fifth Ave., Room 1103, New York, NY 10011, (212) 691-5630. Organized 1982. (Produces educational and instructional videotapes for attorneys and businesses.) Distributed by Totaltape Publishers.

Leisure Time Products/3M

(See 3M)

Life Video Gospel Association

1435 Central Ave., College Place, WA 99324; (509) 522-0784. Organized 1979. (Produces and distributes religious videotapes.)

PRESIDENT
Donald M Vories
TREASURER
Walter Anderson
SECRETARY
Jeanne Vories
BOARD OF DIRECTORS
Donald M. Vories, Walter Anderson, Jeanne Vories, Fred E.J. Harder, Vernon Shafer, Paul Turpel, Frank Salt, D.K. Smith, James Hannum

Ligonier Valley Study Center

Stahlstown, PA 15687; (412) 593-6102, (800) 435-4343. (Religious videos.)

EXECUTIVE VICE PRESIDENT
Ralf Verrman

The Little Red Filmhouse

P.O. Box 691083, Los Angeles, CA 90069; (213) 653-0407. Organized 1975. (Producers and distributes film and video programming.)

PRESIDENT
Larry Klingman
VICE PRESIDENT
Anette Klingman

Llamavision

P.O. Box 50859, Tucson, AZ 85703; (602) 293-8088. Organized 1984. (Video production from script to finished product, travel videos, Third World, How-To)

PRESIDENT
Gerald D. Harwood, Ph.D.
VICE PRESIDENT
Sarajean A. Harwood
AFFILIATIONS
Bastet Productions and Video Safari's International

MMI Video Incorporated

425 N. Michigan Ave., Room 915, Chicago, IL 60611; (312) 644-2775. Organized 1983. (Produces and markets behavioral modification, self-help, and heatlh related videocassettes.)

PRESIDENT
Mitchell Morris

MPI Home Video

15825 Rob Roy Drive, Oak Forest, IL 60452; (312) 687-7881. (Production and distribution of programming for home video.)

PRESIDENT
Waleed B. Ali
VICE PRESIDENT
Malik B. Ali
MARKETING DIRECTOR
Jaffer Ali
BOARD OF DIRECTORS
Waleed B. Ali, Malik B. Ali, Jaffer Ali

Macmillian Video

866 Third Ave., New York, NY 10022; (212) 702-3241, 702-2000. (Children's and educational videos.)

EXECUTIVE PRODUCER
James P. Macquire

Magic Window

2901 West Alameda Ave., Burbank, CA 91505; (818) 954-4950. (A division of RCA/Columbia.) (Children's videos.)

Magna Systems, Inc.

West Countyline 95, Barrington, IL 60010; (312) 382-6477. Organized 1978. (Produces and markets video learning programs.)

PRESIDENT
Wilbur S. Edwards
TREASURER
James F. Griffin

SECRETARY
John Kearney
BOARD OF DIRECTORS
Wilbur S. Edwards, James F. Griffin, John Kearney

Magnum Entertainment

9301 Wilshire Blvd., Room 602, Beverly Hills, CA 90210; (213) 278-9981. Organized 1984. (Manufactures pre-recorded videocassettes for home use.)

PRESIDENT
Ed Walsh
DIRECTOR OF MARKETING & SALES
Thomas K. Rooney
ADVERTISING MANAGER & DIRECTOR OF PROMOTIONS
Eve Kemp
OFFICE MANAGER
Susan Sennett
COORDINATOR OF SALES
Jamie Massalas
COORDINATOR OF ADVERTISING
Sue Singer
AFFILIATIONS
VSDA, NAVD, NAD

Mercedes Maharis Productions

712 Wilshire Blvd., Santa Monica, CA 90401; (213) 393-5800. (Horse-related educational and how-to videos.)

PRESIDENT
Mercedes Maharis

Major League Baseball Productions

1212 Avenue of the Americas, New York, NY 10036; (212) 921-8100. Subsidiary of Major League Baseball Promotion Corp.

PRESIDENT
Joe Podesta

Maljack Productions, Inc.

15825 Rob Roy Dr., Oak Forest, IL 60452; (800) 323-0442. (Educational and documentary videos.)

Manta Film Productions Ltd.

311 Adelaide St. E., Toronto, Ontario, Canada M5A IN2; (416) 863-9316. (Nostalgia, cult, and classic videos.)

The Market Place

4112 Marsh Ave., Rockford, IL 61111, (815) 877-1514. Organized 1985. (Videocassette distribution of inspirational programs to the home and church markets. Children's programs, music concert videos, financial planning seminar.)

PRESIDENT
Max Anderson

Market W Productions, Inc.

3309 Caminito Gandara, San Diego, CA 92037; (619) 587-0514. Organized 1984. (Video production and marketing.)

PRESIDENT
Lois Winsen

Mass Media Video Ministries

2116 North Charles St., Baltimore, MD 21218; (301) 727-3270. Organized 1964. (A nationwide agency providing the educational and religious communities and other service organizations quality video programs.)

PRESIDENT
Clifford J. York
VICE PRESIDENT & TREASURER
Janice P. York
BOARD OF DIRECTORS
Clifford J. York, Janice P. York

Master Arts Video

11549 Amigo Ave., Northridge, CA 91326;, (818) 368-9220. Subsidiary of Multiple Development Corp. (Martial arts feature films.)

PRESIDENT
Joseph A. Pershes

MasterVision

969 Park Ave., Suite 8R, New York, NY 10028; (212) 879-0448. Organized 1980. (Special interest videocassettes and cultural and educational disc programming.)

PRESIDENT
Richard Stadin

Mattingly Productions, Ltd.

10100 Main St., Fairfax, VA 22031; (703) 385-6625. Organized 1971. (Video production and training services.)

PRESIDENT
E. Grayson Mattingly
VICE PRESIDENT
Suzanne Fisher Mattingly
SECRETARY & TREASURER
William E. Mattingly
BOARD OF DIRECTORS
E. Grayson Mattingly, Suzanne Fisher Mattingly, William E. Mattingly

Cameron McKay Productions, Inc.

1011 N. Cole Ave., Hollywood, CA 90038; (213) 463-6073.

PRESIDENT
Cameron McKay

Medallion Productions

4909 Wyandotte, Kansas City, MO 64112; (816) 753-3358.

PRESIDENT
Rebecca B. Newman

Media Bus, Inc.

P.O. Box 718, Woodstock, NY 12498; (914) 679-7739.

PRESIDENT
Bart Friedman

Media Concepts, Inc.

559 49th Street South, St. Petersburg, FL 33707; (813) 321-2122. Organized 1974. (Video production and speciality house.)

PRESIDENT
Charles W.R. (Bob) Skidmore
VICE PRESIDENT
John P. Gallagher
GENERAL MANAGER
Richard E. Smith
BRANCHES
Fort Myers, FL; Naples, FL

Mediacast TV

300 W. Washington, Chicago, IL 60606; (312) 332-3288.

PRESIDENT
Tom Edinger

Meeting House Productions

Mennonite Church and Schuylkill Roads, Spring City, PA 19475; (215) 948-4800. (Family entertainment.)

Metacom Audio Publishing Group

1401-B West River Road North, Minneapolis, MN 55427; (612) 588-2781. Organized 1970. (Manufactures and distributes—primarily through direct mail—audio and video cassettes of subliminal self help and public domain movies.)

PRESIDENT
James I. McCann
EXECUTIVE VICE PRESIDENT/GENERAL MANAGER
Phillip T. Levin
VICE PRESIDENT OF FINANCE/CONTROLLER
David Benson

Metro Video Productions

36 Virginia Ave., Edgewater, MD 21037; (307) 261-7660. Organized 1981. (Video production and post production facility.)

PRESIDENT
Thomas Kreazburg
VICE PRESIDENT

Troy J. Jones
TREASURER
Dan Wolf

Metropolitan Museum of Art

Fifth Ave. and 82 St., New York, NY 10028; (212) 879-5500. (Art-related videos.)

Midnight Video

8750 Holloway Dr., Los Angeles, CA 90069; (213) 659-4347. (Horror films.)

Mike Milkovich Enterprises

4505 W. 78th St., Prairie Village, KS 66208; (913) 341-1421.

Mindware Video Programming

P.O. Box 641, Kalaheo, HA 96741; (808) 332-9242. Organized 1976. (Produces stress reduction videos.)

PRESIDENT
Terry Kamen
AFFILIATIONS
Nebulae Productions

Arthur Mokin Productions, Inc.

2900 McBride La., Santa Rosa, CA 95401; (707) 542-4868.

PRESIDENT
William Mokin

Monterey Home Video

7920 Alabama Ave., Canoga Park, CA 91304-4991; (818) 888-3040, (800) 423-7455. Subsidiary of International Video Entertainment.

PRINCIPAL
Scott Mansfield
SENIOR VICE PRESIDENT & GENERAL MANAGER
Len Levy

Morcraft Films Inc.

837 N. Cahuenga Blvd., Hollywood, CA 90038; (213) 464-2009. Organized 1976. (Restoring, re-releasing and printing old public domain films, cartoons and newsreels.)

PRESIDENT
D.W. Morgan
VICE PRESIDENT
W.H. Morgan
SECREATRY & TREASURER
Charles Kirkwood

Morris Video

936 Hermosa Ave., First Floor, Hermosa Beach, CA 90254; (213) 374-4984. Organized 1984. (Produces and distributes quality information and entertainment video.)

PRESIDENT & C.E.O.
Dawn Morris
VICE PRESIDENT & C.F.O.
George Morris, Ph.D.
BOARD OF DIRECTORS
Dawn Morris, George Morris, Ph.D., George Bott, David Van Horn.
BRANCHES
663 The Village, Redondo Beach, CA 90277; (213) 374-4984.

Mossman Williams Productions

Box 7135, Kansas City, MO 64113; (816) 363-4352; (816) 921-3845.

PRESIDENT
Wade Williams

Motor Cycle Video

P.O. Box 0550, 316 Hennessee St., Lakeland, FL 33802-0550; (813) 686-9380.

PRESIDENT
James W. Elbon, Jr.

Movie Buff Video

250 W. 95 St., New York, NY 10025; (212) 666-0331. (Subsidiary of Manhattan Movietime.)

Movie Merchants, Inc.

3254 Youngfield St., Wheat Ridge, CO 80033; (303) 234-9282.

PRESIDENT
Shelley Gooch

Multi-Video Inc.

1424 E. Independence Blvd., Charlotte, NC 28205; (704) 334-3862. (Educational and music videos.)

Muppet Home Video

117 E. 69 St., New York NY 10021; (212) 794-2400.

DIRECTOR
Bob Lilianfeld

Music Media

5730 Buckingham Parkway, Culver City, CA 90230; (213) 216-7900, (800) 421-4509. Subsidiary of Media Home Entertainment.

VICE PRESIDENT, SALES
Alan Ostroff
VICE PRESIDENT, MARKETING
Jack Bernstein

NFL Films

330 Fellowship Rd., Mt. Laurel, NJ 08054; (609) 778-1600. Organized 1961. (Produces programming for the National Football League.) A subsidiary of the NFL.

PRESIDENT
Ed Sabol
EXECUTIVE VICE PRESIDENT
Steve Sabol
DIRECTOR OF VIDEO SALES
David Grassman

NSI Video

736 Longfellow Ave., Hermosa Beach, CA 90254; (213) 374-7476. Subsidiary of Native Son International.

PRESIDENT
Gerard Ravel

N.T.S.C. Video Co., Inc.

1780 Broadway, Suite 1100, New York, NY 10019; (212) 315-3550, (800) 228-1717. Subsidiary of Telefilm Co., Inc.

PRESIDENT
Tom Ward
VICE PRESIDENT
Daniel Brookshire

National Film Board of Canada

1251 Avenue of the Americas, 16th floor, New York, NY 10020; (212) 586-5131. (Film agency of Canada. Produces and distributes motion pictures.)

National Geographic Television

1145 17th St., N.W., Washington, D.C. 20036; (212) 857-7680. Organized 1965.

VICE PRESIDENT, DIRECTOR OF EDUCATIONAL FILMS
Dennis B. Kane
BOARD OF DIRECTORS
Gilbert M. Grosvenor (President); Melvin M. Payne (Chairman of the Board)
BRANCHES
New York Explorer Office: 1600 Broadway, Suite 310, New York, NY 10019.

National Golf Foundation

200 Castlewood Dr., North Palm Beach, FL 33408; (305) 844-2500. (Sports videos.)

Natural Reflections Video

P.O. Box 476, Coloma, CA 95667; (916) 621-1771. Organized 1980. (Broadcast productions—industrial, prime-time specials, home video productions—specializes in white water productions.)

PRESIDENT
Michael Dennis

Nebulae Productions

400 E. 85 St., New York, NY 10021; (212) 697-9800. Organized 1978. (Produces and distributes nature, relaxation and self-help video programs.)

PRESIDENT
Terry Kamen
VICE PRESIDENT
Roy Kamen

Sara Needham Gallery

Mink Hollow Road, Lake Hill, NY 12448; (914) 679-2807. Organized 1970. (Presents to the general public, knowledge of artist, writer, philosopher, Sara Needham, founder of Disabled Friends of Ulster County.)

CHIEF EXECUTIVE OFFICER
Sara Needham
BOARD OF DIRECTORS
Sara Needham, Henry Needham
BRANCHES
Woodstock, NY; Charleston, SC

New Age Video Inc.

1500 Broadway, New York, NY 10036; (212) 869-2616. (Educational, sports, music and dance videos.)

New Breed Music

P.O. Box 661, Pomona, CA 91768; (714) 623-1999.

PRESIDENT
Jesse Mac Lynum, Jr.

New Liberty Films

1805 W. Magnolia Blvd., Burbank, CA 91506; (818) 842-6167. (Educational and sports videos.)

New Mode Media

One Park Ave., Old Greenwich, CT 06870; (203) 637-3616. (Division of Listening Library, Inc.)

PRESIDENT
Anthony Ditlow

New Orleans Video Access Center

2010 Magazine St., New Orleans, LA 70130; (504) 524-8626. (Cultural/arts and educational videos.)

PRESIDENT
Adelle Badeaux

New Video Center, Inc.

276 Third Ave., New York, NY 10003; (212) 473-6000.

VICE PRESIDENT, ACQUISITIONS
Mike Tollack

New York Times Productions

130 Fifth Ave., New York, NY 10011; (212) 645-3000. Organized 1978. (Produces programming for home video, network and syndication domestically and internationally.) A division of The New York Times Syndication Sales Corporation, an affiliate of *The New York Times* Company.

CHAIRMAN
Arthur Ochs Sulzberger
VICE CHAIRMAN
Sydney Gruson
PRESIDENT
Sam Summerlin
EXECUTIVE PRODUCER
Ted Harbert

Nightingale-Conant Corp.

7300 N. Lehigh Ave., Niles, IL 60648; (312) 467-0300. (Self-help and psychology videos.)

Northeast Productions, Inc.

1450 Penobscot Bldg., Detroit, MI 48226; (313) 963-2257.

PRESIDENT
W. Beauford

Nova Video Art

10583 Felton Way, Cupertino, CA 95014; (408) 725-0708. Organized 1983. (Produces instructional dance videotapes—e.g., "Learn Classical Ballet and Enjoy It".)

OWNER/PRODUCER
Lilia Peloquin
MARKETING DIRECTOR
Mike Peloquin
GRAPHIC DESIGNER/NARRATOR
Katalin Maritza Balogh
AFFILIATIONS
Video Productions: Vertex Video Associates
Music: Silver Label Recording Co.

Ocean Video Inc.

#601, 4605 Lankershim Blvd., North Hollywood, CA 91602; (818) 506-3216. (Martial arts videos.)

VICE PRESIDENT
Aaron Yeung

O'Neil and Jeffries Film Productions

3855 Lankershim Blvd., North Hollywood, CA 91604; (818) 760-6666. (Subsidiary of Jeffries Film Int'l.)

PRESIDENT
Hugh Jeffries

Optical Programming Associates

11812 San Vicente Blvd., Suite 200, Los Angeles, CA 90049; (213) 207-4355. Subsidiary of MCA Home Video. Organized 1980. (Produces interactive Laser discs.)

BUSINESS MANAGER
Ira Roth

Original Face Video

P.O. Box 447, Grass Valley CA 95945; (916) 272-3568.

PRESIDENTS
Johanna Luther
Joseph Tiefer

Pacific Arts Video Records

26382 Carmel Rancho Lane, Carmel, CA 93923; (408) 624-4704.

PRESIDENT
David Bean

Paragon Video Productions

3529 S. Valley View Blvd., Las Vegas, NV 89103; (702) 362-2520, (800) 634-6143. Subsidiary of King of Video.

PRESIDENT
Steve Vincent
DIRECTOR, MARKETING
Michael Henry
DIRECTOR OF SALES
Barry Martin

Parent's Magazine Enterprises

685 Third Ave., New York, NY 10017; (212) 878-8700. (How-to videos.) Subsidiary of Gruner & Jahr, U.S.A., Inc.

Pat Film & Video Services Inc.

630 Ninth Ave., 5th floor, New York, NY 10036; (212) 247-0900. Organized 1964. (Production and distribution of television shows and commercials.)

PRESIDENT
Peter M. Piech
EXECUTIVE VICE PRESIDENT
Ervin Rosenfeld
VICE PRESIDENT/GENERAL MANAGER
Andrew Cuomo
ASSISTANT GENERAL MANAGER
Peter Elonomos
CONTROLLER
Tahlr Rasheed
SECRETARY/TREASURER
Charles Haydon

Peak Performance Inc.

P.O. Box 2829, Duxbury, MA 02332; (617) 837-3398. (Sports and how-to videos.)

PRESIDENT
John Gillis

Pelican Films

3010 Santa Monica Blvd., Suite 400, Santa Monica, CA 90404; (213) 399-3753.

Penguin Video Productions

P.O. Box 65157, Los Angeles, CA 90065; (213) 222-2707.

PRESIDENT
Kim Dunnahoo

Phipps and Company Productions

5807-E. S. Garnett Rd., Tulsa, OK 74146; (918) 250-7371. (Educational and sports videos.)

PRESIDENT
Terry L. Phipps

Phoenix Films Inc.

468 Park Avenue South, New York, NY 10016; (212) 684-5910.

PRESIDENT
H. Gelles

Pola Productions, Inc.

18662 MacArthur Blvd., Room 200, Irvine, CA 92715; (714) 752-5700. Organized 1984. (Video production/distribution.)

PRESIDENT
James Polakof
EXECUTIVE DIRECTOR
Pepper Stone
PUBLIC RELATIONS DIRECTOR
Priscilla McMurtry
BRANCH
San Francisco

Polygram Video Music U.S.

810 Seventh Ave., New York, NY 10019; (212) 399-7069. Subsidiary of Polygram Records, Inc.

VICE PRESIDENT
Len R. Epand

Prince Leopard Film Productions, Inc.

307 E. 93rd St., Suite 3E, New York, NY 10128; (212) 505-5508. Organized 1984. (Special interest home video tapes, programming and production.)

PRESIDENT
Sylvia Grodin
VICE PRESIDENT
Lenny Grodin
PRODUCTION COORDINATOR
Arietta Venizelos

Producers Consortium

337 E. 1165 N., Orem, Utah 84057; (801) 224-5407; (801) 226-8209. Organized 1985. (Produces and distributes film and video productions.)

PARTNERS
R. Conrad Teichert
P. Michael J. Karr
BOARD OF DIRECTORS
R. Conrad Teichart, P. Michael J. Karr
AFFILIATIONS
Kappa Tau Alpha, AFI, IFPA, SMPTE

Producers International Corporation

3921 N. Meridian St., Indianapolis, IN 46208; (317) 924-5163. Organized 1968. (Business communications producer. Carries "Jerry Yeagley's Fundamentals of Soccer" for the home video market.)

DIRECTOR OF MARKETING
Lori A. Feeney

Progress Research, Inc

355 Grand Ave., Oakland, CA 94610; (415) 832-0305. (How-to, sports.)

PRESIDENT
Richard E. Johnson

Public Access Producers Association

2652 N. Winchell, Portland, OR 97217; (503) 289-2309.

DIRECTOR
R.S. Kolemaine

Public Production Group

1346 Connecticut Ave. N.W., Suite 918, Washington, DC 20036; (202) 775-8733. (Educational and public interest videos.)

PRESIDENT
Sam Love

PyraVid International

61 Camino Alto, #108, Mill Valley, CA 94941; (415) 381-2567.

PRESIDENT
L. Lee Buschel

Quadrus Media Ministry Inc.

128 Kishwaukee St., Rockford, IL 61104; (815) 987-3970, (800) 435-4489. (Children's and educational.)

PRESIDENT
Joe Musser

RCA Videodiscs

P.O. Box 91079, 7900 Rockville Rd., Indianapolis, IN 46224; (317) 273-3640.

RICON Enterprises

5863 Village Forest Court, Houston, TX 77092; (713) 683-0105. Organized 1983. (Production and distribution of videos about the space shuttle program and other NASA projects.)

OWNER
Richard C. Colton

RKM Video Publishing Co.

8899 Beverly Blvd., 102, Los Angeles, CA 90048; (213) 274-8072. (How-to and diet videos.)

PRESIDENT
Alan Riseman

RMI Media Productions, Inc.

2807 W. 47 St., Shawnee Mission, KS 62205;, (913) 262-3974. (Instructional videos.)

PRESIDENT
David L. Little

Random House, Inc.

201 E. 50 St., New York, NY 10022; (212) 751-2600. Organized 1955. (Publishing company.)

EXECUTIVE VICE PRESIDENT, HOME VIDEO
Gerald Harrison
CREATIVE DIRECTOR, HOME VIDEO
Sharon Lerner
MAREKTING DIRECTOR
Robert Singer
VICE PRESIDENT, SALES
Edward Martin

Ravenswood Productions
4822 Mindora Dr., Torrance, CA 90503; (213) 375-5801.
PRESIDENT
James Sudalnik

Reader's Digest
Pleasantville, NY 10570; (914) 769-7000. (How-to, sports, educational and children's videos.)

Reeves Corporate Services
708 Third Ave., 11th Floor, New York, NY 10017; (212) 573-8570. Subsidiary of Communications Corp. (Educational, science and business-related videos.)
PRESIDENT
Webster F. Golinkin

Rego Irish Records and Tapes, Inc.— Rego Video
64 New Hyde Park Rd., Garden City, NY 11530; (516) 328-7800. Organized 1974. (Manufactures and distributes Irish recordings. Also manufactures and imports Irish videos.)
PRESIDENT
Patrick J. Noonan
VICE PRESIDENT
Margaret E. Noonan
MANAGER
Vincent Mitchell
AFFILIATIONS
Paddy Noonan Entertainments, Inc.

Research Press
2612 North Mattis, Box 3177, Champaign, IL 61821; (217) 352-3273. (Pyschology and educational videos.)
PRESIDENT
Ann Wendel

Rhapsody Films Inc.
P.O. Box 179, New York, NY 10014; (212) 243-0152. Organized 1982. (Distributes jazz and blues films for all markets— television, home video and non-theatrical.)
PRESIDENT
Bruce Ricker

Rhino Video
1201 Olympic Blvd., Santa Monica, CA 90404, (213) 450-6323; (Horror feature films.)
PRESIDENT
Randi Freeman

Ed Rich Productions Inc.
1950 S. Ocean Dr., Hallandale, FL 33009; (305) 454-8068.
PRESIDENT
Ed Rich

Rizzoli/A.C. Video
597 Fifth Ave., New York, NY 10017; (212) 223-0100. Organized 1985.
DIRECTOR
John Brancati

Rocky Mountain Motion Pictures
P.O. Box 2850, Park City, UT 84060; (801) 649-1030. (Sports videos.)
PRESIDENT
Dean Lyras

Rodale Press Inc.
33 East Minor St., Emmaus, PA 18049; (215) 967-5171.

Sagebrush Productions
1940 South Cotner Ave., Los Angeles, CA 90025; (213) 479-0946.

Saturn Productions, Inc.
1780 Broadway, Suite 1100, New York, NY 10019; (212) 489-2460. Organized 1984. (Pre-recorded videocassettes.) Parent company is Telefilm Inc.
PRESIDENT
Tom Ward
VICE PRESIDENT
Daniel Brookshire
NATIONAL SALES DIRECTOR
Jeff Montaigne

Sea-TV
1639 Chapel St., New Haven, CT 06511; (203) 624-2318. Organized 1983. (Marketing and production of nautical video cassettes.)
PRESIDENT
Charles P. Croft
BOARD OF DIRECTORS
Herb Hild

See Hear Industries
419 W. Walnut, Gardena, CA 90248; (213) 516-0315. Division of RJA Inc.
PRESIDENT
Raymond L. Jacobs

Select-A-Tape
8756 Holloway Drive, Los Angeles, CA 90069; (213) 657-2706, (800) 421-4465. (Distributes midnight videos [horror films] and adult films.)
PRESIDENT
Alan Roberts

Self Improvement Video, Inc.
Suite 283, 77 Ives Street, Providence, RI 02906; (401) 351-7676. Organized 1983. (Produces and markets home video programming.)
PRESIDENT
John R. Koenig
VICE PRESIDENT
Maria P. Koenig
BOARD OF DIRECTORS
John R. Koenig, Maria P. Koenig, A. Bill Comeau
AFFILIATIONS
Engaged in joint ventures with Creative Services Source, Inc.

Serendipity Communications
101 Southwestern Blvd., #210, Sugar Land, TX 77478; (713) 242-6999.
PRESIDENT
Fred R. Brison

Sherwood Video Production Co.
Box 14212, 676 North St. Clair St., Suite 1716, Chicago, IL 60611, (312) 275-9191. (Educational videos.)
PRESIDENT
Barry Torman

Shokus Video
P.O. Box 8434, Van Nuys, CA 91409, (818) 704-0400. Organized 1979. (Preservation of vintage TV films and kinescopes in the public domain.)
PRESIDENT

Stuart Shostak
COORDINATOR
Juli Sebera
AFFILIATIONS
AFTRA (since 1982), VSDA 1981-85

Single Concept Films

2 Terrain Dr., Rochester, NY 14618, (716) 442-9740. (Educational and medical videos.)

PRODUCER
Jack Ruda

Snoopy's Home Video Library

5730 Buckingham Parkway, Culver City, CA 90230, (213) 216-7900; (800) 421-4509. (Children's videos.) Subsidiary of Media Home Entertainment.

Society of Manufacturing Engineers

1 SME Dr., P.O. Box 930, Dearborn, MI 48121, (313) 271-1500.

PRESIDENT
William Hilty
MARKETING & SALES
Vince Cini

Sonoma Video Productions

1717 Darby Rd., Sebastopol, CA 95472, (707) 829-0127. (Producer of instructional and travel video programs.)

PRESIDENT
Michael Heumann
PRODUCTION MANAGER
Gene Lambert

Sony Video Software

9 W. 57th St., New York, NY 10019, (212) 418-9473. (Subsidiary of Sony Corp. of America.)

DIRECTOR VIDEO SOFTWARE
John O'Donnell
MARKETING & SALES
Andrew Schofer

Spectrum Video

18121 Napa St., Northridge, CA 91325, (818) 886-8680, (800) 423-5599. (Acquisition and production of alternative non-theatrical, how-to programming for distribution to home video market place.)

PRESIDENT
Fred Hirsch
VICE PRESIDENT
Dwight Krizman
AFFILIATIONS
V.S.D.A.

Sperry Corporation Information Group

P.O. Box 2191, Princeton, NJ 08540, (201) 329-3899; (800) 222-0966. (Science and how-to videos.)

Sports Films & Talents, Inc.

12755 State Highway 55, Minneapolis, MN 55441, (612) 540-5972. (Sports videos.)

Sports World Cinema

P.O. Box 17022, Salt Lake City, UT 84117, (801) 486-3925.

PRESIDENT
Gary B. Ewing

Spotlight Video

12636 Beatrice St., Los Angeles, CA 90066, (213) 306-4040. (Subsidiary of Public Pictures Home Video Co.)

SENIOR VICE PRESIDENT
Nick Draklich

Star Video Productions

10701 Wilshire Blvd., Room 2001, Los Angeles, CA 90024, (213) 470-6522. Organized 1980. (Production and distribution of How-to home videos.)

PRESIDENT
Alfredo Ringel
EXECUTIVE VICE PRESIDENT
Deborah Taper Ringel

Martha Stuart Communications, Inc.

Box 246, 2 Anthony St., Hillsdale, NY 12529, (518) 325-3900. (Educational and general interest videos.)

PRESIDENT
Martha Stuart
MARKETING & SALES
Victoria Simons

Sun Video

15 Donnybrook Dr., Demarest, NJ 07627, (201) 784-0662. Organized 1979. (Home videocassette production and distribution.)

CO-PRESIDENTS
Henry J. Stern
Serafim Karalexis
BOARD OF DIRECTORS
Henry J. Stern, Serafim Karalexis

Sun West Video Services

950 Hampshire Rd., #108, Westlake Village, CA 91361, (805) 495-3082.

PRESIDENT
King Hempel

Supervideo

417 Colorado Ave., Santa Monica, CA 90401, (213) 394-9696. (Subsidiary of Exploration in Video.)

PRESIDENT
Nissim Raphael

SyberVision Systems, Inc.

6066 Civic Terrace Ave., Newark, CA 94560, (415) 790-3637. Organized 1977. (Produces self-achievement and sports video and audio tapes.)

PRESIDENT
Michael Doepke
CO-FOUNDERS
Steven DeVore
Nasser Hamedani
VICE PRESIDENT, FINANCE
John Heinke
VICE PRESIDENT, OPERATIONS
Regan Jones
VICE PRESIDENT, PRODUCT DEVELOPMENT
Howard Jamison
AFFILIATIONS
Professional Ski Instructors of America, Direct Marketing Association, National Sporting Goods Association, International Tape/Disc Association, Video Software Dealers Association

Syndistar, Inc.

648 Hickory Ave., New Orleans, LA 70123, (504) 737-4486. Organized 1979. (Produces and distributes information films and video.) Affiliations: ICIA, USDA.

PRESIDENT
Greg Fox
VICE PRESIDENT, SALES & MARKETING
Ralph Behrman
VICE PRESIDENT, OPERATIONS
Norman Landry
VICE PRESIDENT, PRODUCTION
David Lussier

TV Collector

P.O. Box 188, Needham, MA 02192, (617) 583-0459. (Old television programs and nostalgia.)

PRESIDENTS
Stephen W. Albert
Diane L. Albert

TV Sports Scene, Inc.

(TVSS, Inc.)
5804 Ayrshire Blvd., Minneapolis, MN 55436, (612) 925-9661. Organized 1970. (TV program distribution, national and international.)

PRESIDENT & CHAIRMAN OF THE BOARD
Donald L. Herrick
VICE PRESIDENT
Robert C. Bruce
SECRETARY & TREASURER
Barbara Conley
BOARD OF DIRECTORS
Donald L. Herrick, Robert C. Bruce, Barbara Conley
AFFILIATIONS
Owner of U.S. Television Communications, Inc. (USTC)
Owner—Division Northwest Advertising & Marketing
Owner—Division MED TV
Owner—Division Consumer Products Division TV Sports Scene, Inc.

Telecine Spanish Video

2151 Belmont Ave., New York, NY 10457, (212) 798-7028.

PRESIDENT
Peter Velez
MARKETING AND SALES
Ed Freeberg

Telefilm Co. Inc./Saturn Productions Inc.

1780 Broadway, Room 1100, New York, NY 10019, (212) 489-2460. Organized 1981. (Theatrical, television, cable Saturn Productions pre-recorded videocassettes.)

PRESIDENT
Tom Ward
VICE PRESIDENT
Daniel Brookshire

Telequest Inc.

14 Washington Road, Princeton JCT, NJ 08550, (609) 799-2105. Organized 1977. (Film and video production for broadcast and industry.)

PRESIDENT
Richard Blofson
VICE PRESIDENT
Sam Russell
SECRETARY/TREASURER
Scott Nielsen

Telstar Inc.

366 N. Prior Ave., St. Paul MN 55104 (612) 644-4726. Organized 1968. (Produces and markets video training and instructional materials to industry, home and education.)

PRESIDENT
J.K. Wasley
VICE PRESIDENT
Bob Miller
BOARD OF DIRECTORS
J.K. Wasley, Bob Miller

3M Company/Leisure Time Products

3M Center, Building 223-3S-03, St. Paul, MN 55144; (612) 733-4751. (Sportsman's video collection.)

PROJECT MANAGER
Howard West
SALES MANAGER
Jeff Hagman
MARKETING COORDINATOR
Carol Bystrzycki

Thriller Video

7920 Alabama Ave., Canoga Park, CA 91304-4991; (818) 888-3040, (800) 423-7455. (Subsidiary of International Video Entertainment.)

SENIOR VICE PRESIDENT & GENERAL MANAGER
Len Levy
NATIONAL SALES MANAGER
David Solomon

Touchstone Home Video

500 S. Buena Vista St., Burbank, CA 91521; (818) 840-6056. Subsidiary of Walt Disney.

DIRECTOR, NATIONAL SALES
Dick Longwell

Tournament Video Tapes

1615 W. Burbank Blvd., Burbank, CA 91506; (213) 843-0373. Division of Richard J. Soltys Productions. (Sports business videos.)

PRESIDENT
Richard J. Soltys

Two Star Films Inc.

Box 495, St. James, NY 11780; (516) 584-7283.

UC Video

425 Ontario St. S.E., Minneapolis, MN 55414; (612) 376-3333. (Cultural/arts educational videos.)

EXECUTIVE DIRECTOR
Tom Borreys

Understanding Personal Computers

P.O. Box 5849, Stanford, CA 94305; (415) 494-3737. (How-to videos.)

PRESIDENT
Colin Mick

Unicorn Video Inc.

20822 Dearborn St., Reseda, CA 91311; (818) 407-1333. Organized 1981. (Manufactures pre-recorded cassettes.)

PRESIDENT
Joanne Goldstein
VICE PRESIDENT
Edward Goldstein
SECRETARY & TREASURER
Anita Goldstein

United Artists

(see MGM/UA Entertainment Group)

United Entertainment, Inc.

4111 So. Darlington St., Suite 600, Tulsa, OK 74135; (918) 622-6460. Organized 1983. (Manufactures and distributes pre-recorded video.)

PRESIDENT
Bill Blair
EXECUTIVE VICE PRESIDENT
Robert Blair
NATIONAL DIRECTOR, SALES & MARKETING
Rick Buehler
BRANCHES
18178 Mollie Lane, Yorba Linda, CA 92686
245 Unquowa Rd. #133, Fairfield, CT 06430

Universal

(see MCA Home Video)

Upswing Artists Management, Ltd.

%Jacobson and Colfin, 150 Fifth Ave., Room 1103, New York, NY 10011; (213) 691-5630. Organized 1979. (Produces music video.)

PRESIDENT
Martin Steckler
VICE PRESIDENT
Bruce Colfin
BOARD OF DIRECTORS
Martin Steckler, Bruce E. Colfin
AFFILIATIONS
Performance Video

V.C.I. Home Video

6535 E., Skelly Dr., Tulsa, OK 74145; (918) 622-6470; (800) 331-4077. Subsidiary of United Entertainment, Inc. (How-to, adult, religious and science fiction videos.)

PRESIDENT
Bill Blair

VC II Home Video

13402 Wyandotte Ave., North Hollywood, CA 91605; (800) 221-4274. Organized 1978. (Acquires program licensing for video distribution. Produces, manufactures and distributes [worldwide] theatrical, cable and video.)

CHIEF OPERATING OFFICER
Rudy Sutton
MARKETING DIRECTOR
Dave Stevens
ACQUISTIONS
Mike Fredrychs

VCL Communications, Inc.

2980 Beverly Glen Circle, Westwood, CA; (213) 474-4225.

PRESIDENT
Annie Frank

VIP Video

143 Hickory Hill Circle, Osterville, MA 02655; (617) 428-7198. Subsidiary of JEF Films.

PRESIDENT
Jeffrey H. Aikman
MARKETING & SALES
Elsie Aikman

Van Dam Productions

15 Van Dam St., New York, NY 10013; (212) 807-1877. Subsidiary of Teleculture, Inc.

PRESIDENT
Jordan Bock

Vanguard Video

6535 E. Skelly Dr., Tulsa, OK 74145; (918) 622-6460; (800) 331-4077. Subsidiary of United Entertainment.

PRESIDENT
Bill Blair

Vencompass, Inc.

155 West Eighth St., Erie, PA 16501; (814) 453-7704. Organized 1983. (Produces educational corporate videos.)

PRESIDENT/CHAIRMAN OF THE BOARD
Pamela J. Venable
SECRETARY
Atty. John Leemhuis
TREASURER
John Petersen
BOARD OF DIRECTORS
Thomas L. Venable

Vidcrest

12023 Lorne St., North Hollywood, CA 91605;, (213) 654-8808.

PRESIDENT
Robert Weinbach

Video Action

237 Ogden Ave., Jersey City, NJ 07307; (201) 792-3833. (Health videos.)

OWNER
Bob Brennan

Video Action

708 W. First St., Los Angeles, CA 90012; (213) 687-8262. Organized 1981. (Video production and distribution.)

OWNER (PARTNER)
Leslie T. Hamasaki
OWNER (PARTNER)
Ruth Watanabe
OPERATIONS MANAGER
Gregg S. Yokoyama

Video Aided Instruction, Inc.

182 Village Rd., East Hills, NY 11577; (516) 621-6176. Organized 1983. (Produces instructional, educational videocassettes.)

PRESIDENT
Peter Lanzer
VICE PRESIDENT
Mona Lanzer
BOARD OF DIRECTORS
Peter Lanzer, Mona Lanzer

Video Arts International, Inc.

2112 Broadway, Room 401, New York, NY 10023; (212) 799-7798. Organized 1983. (Manufactures home videocassettes.) Distributed exclusively in the U.S. and Canada by RCA/Ariola International

PRESIDENT
Ernest J. Gilbert
VICE PRESIDENT, MARKETING
Glenn A. Smith
DIRECTOR CONSUMER MARKETING
Marc E. Jacoby

Video Associates

5419 Sunset Blvd., Los Angeles, CA 90027; (213) 463-3255. Organized 1978. (Post production company.)

PRESIDENT
Donald Penfield
VICE PRESIDENT, SALES
Declan M. Kavanagh
VICE PRESIDENT, OPERATIONS
Marga Tamplin
VICE PRESIDENT, MARKETING
Sharon Popp
CHIEF FINANCIAL OFFICER
Andrew Shaddock
BOARD OF DIRECTORS
Donald Penfield

Video City Productions

4266 Broadway, Oakland, CA 94611; (415) 428-0202. Organized 1983. (Manufactures and distributes pre-recorded VHS and Beta film product.)

MARKETING DIRECTOR
Bob Brown
OTHER COMPANY OWNED LABELS:
Combat Video, Art House Video, Chop 'Em Ups Video

Video Craft

141 E. 55 St., New York, NY 10022; (212) 688-1276. (How-to, educational videos.)

PRESIDENT
Lee Craft

Video Dynamics

Box 20330, Jackson, MS 39209; (601) 373-7717, (800) 647-2284. (Children's, educational and religious.)

PRESIDENT
Pat Robinson
MARKETING & SALES
Steve Robinson

Video Educational Systems

619 E. Nine Mile Rd., Hazel Park, MI 48030; (313) 541-1000. (Subsidiary of Gemini School of Fine Art and Airbrushing.)

PRESIDENT
Donald J. Davenport

Video Gems

731 North La Brea Ave., Los Angeles, CA 90038; (213) 932-2385. Organized 1979. (Manufacturer and distributor of pre-recorded videocassettes.)

PRESIDENT

Joseph Infante
VICE PRESIDENT
Vivienne Infante

Video Image, Inc.

4400 Will Rogers Parkway, Suite 103, Oklahoma City, OK 73108, (405) 942-6564. (Children's, how-to and educational videos.)

PRESIDENT
Jerome Welch

Video International Publishers, Inc.

118 6th St. So., Great Falls, MT 59405; (406) 727-7133. Organized 1980. (Production and distribution of corporate communication, educational and how-to video programming.)

PRESIDENT
James M. Colla
VICE PRESIDENT
Penny L. Adkins
SECRETARY/TREASURER
Penny L. Adkins

Video Knowledge Inc.

29 Bramble Lane, Melville, NY 11747; (516) 367-4250.

PRESIDENT
Sally Dubrowsky
VICE PRESIDENT
Ed Dubrowsky
BOARD OF DIRECTOR
Geoffrey S. Dubrowsky, Robin Sims

Video Latino

409 N. Figueroa, Wilmington, CA 90744; (213) 549-4490. (Spanish language general interest videos.)

PRESIDENT
Russell C. Greene

Video Library

4152 Woodruff Ave., Lakewood, CA 90713; (213) 420-8383.

OWNER
Debbie Cantril

Video Library of Arts

716 S. Main, Broken Arrow, OK 74012; (918) 251-0466. Division of Ken Meyer Productions.

PRESIDENT
Ken Meyer

The Video Naturals Company

2590 Glen Green, Suite #6, Los Angeles, CA 90068; (213) 469-0019. Organized 1982. (Produces and distributes "mood videos" for the home video market.)

PRESIDENT/OWNER
Steve Siporin
AFFILIATIONS
Distributors: Videotakes; Norstar; Metro Video

Video Presentations, Inc.

2326 Sixth Ave., Room 230, Seattle, WA 98121; (206) 728-9241. Organized 1979. (Video off-line editing, production and duplication services in prof. BETA, ¾" U-matic and VHS.)

PRESIDENT
H.V. Wright
VICE PRESIDENT
Nancy L. Wright

Video Properties, Inc.

33 E. 68 St., New York, NY 10021; (212) 570-1200.

PRESIDENT
John A. Friede

Video Reel, Inc.

7009 Owensmouth Ave., Suite 201, Canoga Park, CA 91303; (818) 710-1823. Organized 1983. (Produces and duplicates how-to sports videos.)

PRESIDENT
Robert Mann
VICE PRESIDENT
Bonnie Krolop
TREASURER
Robert Mann
SECRETARY
Bonnie Krolop
BOARD OF DIRECTORS
Robert S. Mann, Bonnie L. Krolop
AFFILIATIONS
Recording Association of America

Video Research

18 Ellery St., Cambridge, MA 02138; (617) 576-0864. Organized 1983. (Home video product development.)

PRESIDENT
David Burke
EXECUTIVE VICE PRESIDENT
Fred Surr
VICE PRESIDENT, FINANCE
Jane Lytle-Manns
VICE PRESIDENT, MARKETING
Bitsy McKay
BOARD OF DIRECTORS
David Burke, Fred Surr, Lila Hexner, Barry Unger, Judy Obermayer

Video Sports Productions

1704 Sweeney, Las Vegas, NV 89104; (702) 384-7514. (Golf and other sports videos.)

PRESIDENT
C.A. Montana

Video Tech

19346 Third N.W., Seattle, WA 98177; (206) 546-5401.

PRESIDENT
Eugene Ekblad

Video Travel, Inc.

153 W. Fourth St., Williamsport, PA 17701; (917) 326-6525. (Sports, how-to and travel videos.)

PRESIDENT
Larry Seaman

Video Unlimited, Inc.

10931 N. 56 St., Temple Terrace, FL 33617; (813) 985-3866.

PRESIDENT
Deborah A. Mellor
VICE PRESIDENT
Walter I. Van Horn

Video Visa Inc.

9200 Sunset Blvd., Suite 824, Los Angeles, CA 90069; (213) 859-8987. Subsidiary of Televisa SA.

Video Vision Associates, Inc.

7 Waverly Place, Madison NJ 07940; (201) 377-0302. (Educational, science and entertainment videos.)

PRESIDENT
William Clark

Video Yesteryear

Box C, Sandy Hook, CT 06482. Organized 1978.

PRESIDENT
Jon Sonneborn

Videodisc Publishing Inc.

381 Park Avenue South, #1601, New York, NY 10016; (212) 685-5522.

MARKETING MANAGER
Steve Sagman

Videofashion

One West 37 St., 5th floor, New York, NY 10018; (212) 869-4666. Organized 1976. (World's first "Videomagazine." Produces and distributes 40 programs each year of fashion and lifestyle videos.)

CHAIRMAN & PRESIDENT
Nicholas Charney
INTERNATIONAL DISTRIBUTION
Marlene B. McGinnis

Videograph

2833 25th St., San Francisco, CA 94110; (415) 282-6001. (English and Spanish health and educational videos.)

PRESIDENT
Jim Locker

Videologue Marketing Corp.

3409 Avenue H, Brooklyn, NY 11210; (718) 377-3194; (800) 431-9300.

Videotakes, Inc.

220 Shrewsbury Ave., Red Bank, NJ 07701; (201) 747-2444. Organized 1982. (Marketing of non-feature film videocassettes.)

PRESIDENT
Joe Kennedy, 509 Fisk Ave., Brielle, NJ 08730
SECRETARY
Jenny Peters, 26 W. 83 St., New York, NY 10024

Vidmark

2450 Wilshire Blvd., Suite 1, Santa Monica, CA 90403; (213) 829-4359, (800) 424-7070, (800) 351-7070.

PRESIDENT
Mark Amin

Vision Productions

7475 Callaghan Rd., Room 202, San Antonio, TX 78229; (512) 349-6229. (Complete video production, location up to three cameras, A/B" Roll, 3/4" editing.)

OWNER
William T. Skinner II

Vision Productions, Ltd.

311 E. 6th St., #2, Moscow, ID 83843; (208) 883-0105. Organized 1979. (Video production and marketing.)

PRESIDENT
John A.L. Francis
VICE PRESIDENT
E.A. Francis

Weiss Global Enterprises

2055 Saviers Rd., Suite 12, Oxnard, CA 93033; (805) 486-4495.

PRESIDENT
Adrian Weiss
SECRETARY & TREASURER
Stephen A. Weiss

Western Film & Video, Inc.

30941 W. Agoura Rd., Building 302/304, Westlake Village, CA 91361; (818) 889-7350. Organized 1974. (Motion picture laboratory and complete video-tape facility. Productions, duplication, editing, film to tape X-fers and standards conversions.)

PRESIDENT & CHIEF EXECUTIVE OFFICER
Gary R. Guenot
VICE PRESIDENT
Christopher Beck
SECRETARY & TREASURER
Jim Guenot
BRANCHES
Video Magic (mail-order software)
AFFILIATIONS
Part of the Westlake Media Center

Western Publishing Company, Inc.

1220 Mound Ave., Racine, WI 53404; (414) 633-2431. Subsidiary of Mattel Inc. (How-to, children's, educational.)

PRESIDENT
Joseph Marino
VICE PRESIDENT, SALES
William Nahikian

Westlamb Associates

2781 Las Ramblas, Suite 200, Mission Viejo, CA 92691; (714) 643-9031.

PRESIDENT
James Polakof

Weston Woods Studios, Inc.

389 Newton Turnpike, Weston, CT 06883; (800) 243-5020; (203) 226-3355. Organized 1956. (Producer of audiovisual adaptations of children's picture books.)

PRESIDENT
Morton Shindel
SECRETARY
Elisabeth Rommel
TREASURER
Morton Schindel

Wild Wing Productions

7240 Valjean Ave., Van Nuys, CA 91406; (818) 994-4955. Organized 1984. (Creates and produces original home video programming in how-to, children's, educational and entertainment categories.)

PRESIDENT & CHIEF EXECUTIVE OFFICER
Drew Michaels
VICE PRESIDENT & DIRECTOR OF MARKETING
Shar Kanan
BOARD OF DIRECTORS
Drew Michaels, Chairman of the Board, Chief Executive Officer, President; John Smart, Director; Shar Kanan, Vice President, Director of Marketing, Director; Warren R. Kaufman, Director; Kathryn G. Grossman, Director.
AFFILIATIONS
Association of Visual Communicators

Wilderness Video

P.O. Box 2175, Redondo Beach, CA 90278; (213) 542-5813. Organized 1982. (Produces wilderness videos of national parks.)

OWNER
R.W. Glusic

Wade Williams Productions

5500 Ward Parkway, Kansas City, MO 64113; (816) 523-2699. Organized 1980. (Production and distribution of science fiction motion pictures and home videos.)

PRESIDENT
Wade Williams
VICE PRESIDENT
Brian Mossman
SECRETARY
Ben Mossman

Windward Video

P.O. Box 613, Paia, Maui, HI 96779; (808) 579-9313. (Educational videos.)

PRESIDENT
Jerry Rochford

Wizard Video Inc.

1551 N. La Brea Ave., Los Angeles, CA 90028; (213) 850-6563.

Wombat Productions

(Division of CorTech, Inc.)
250 West 57 St., Suite 916, New York, NY 10019; (212) 315-2502. Organized 1970. (Produces and distributes educational films and documentaries.)

PRESIDENT
Gene Feldman
EXECUTIVE VICE PRESIDENT
Suzette Winter

VICE PRESIDENT, MARKETING
Stephen Janson

Wonderland Video

3529 S. Valley View Blvd., Las Vegas, NV 89103; (702) 362-2520; (800) 634-6143. (Children's videos.) Subsidiary of King of Video.

PRESIDENT
Steve Vincent

Wooden Boat Publications, Inc.

Naskeag Rd., Brooklin, ME 04616; (207) 359-4651. (Wooden boat construction and repair.)

PRESIDENT
Jonathan Wilson

World Premiere Home Video

3125 W. Burbank Blvd., Burbank, CA 91505; (818) 843-0949, (800) 437-9063.

VICE PRESIDENT & GENERAL MANAGER
Wendy Marino

World Research Inc.

Campus Studies Institute Division, 11722 Sorrento Valley Rd., San Diego, CA 92121; (619) 276-9620.

PRESIDENT
Dan T. Loerff

World Video Enterprise, Inc.

6736 Laurel Grove Ave., North Hollywood, CA 91606; (818) 764-1194. Subsidiary of World Video Enterprises.

PRESIDENT
Roy Horam

World Video Pictures

12401 Wilshire Blvd., Suite 102, Los Angeles, CA 90025; (213) 820-6100. (Formerly Program Hunters.)

PRESIDENT
George Atkinson

Worldvision Home Video, Inc.

660 Madison Ave., New York, NY 10021; (212) 832-3838. (Subsidiary of Taft Broadcasting.)

PRESIDENT
Tom Devlin

Xerox Information Resources Group

One Pickwick Plaza, P.O. Box 6710, Greenwich, CT 06836; (203) 625-5634. (Subsidiary of Xerox Corp.)

PRESIDENT
William J. Senter

Wholesale Distributors

A.C. Video Distribution, Inc.
P.O. Box 8522, New York, NY 10150, (212) 223-0100, ext. 46. Subsidiary of Rizzoli/A.C. Video.

AW Industries
8415 Ardmore Rd., Landover, MD 20785, (301) 322-1000.

Acorn Sports, Inc.
5816 Shakespeare Rd., Columbia, SC 29204, (803) 735-0733. Organized 1981. (Golf videos.)

PRESIDENT
D. Swing Meyer

Admit One Video Presentations
311 Adelaide St. East, Toronto, Canada M5A 1N2, (416) 863-9316. Organized 1981. ("B" movies, schlock horror, classics.)

PRESIDENT
Len Curtis
OPERATIONS
Joe Mancuso
AFFILIATIONS
Manta Film Productions, Ltd., Manta Sound Company

Adult Video Corp.
18121 Napa St., Northridge, CA 91325, (800) 886-8680; (800) 423-5599.

PRESIDENT
Fred M. Hirsch
MARKETING & SALES
Tony Marino

Adventures in Cassettes
1401-B W. River Rd., N., Minneapolis, MN 55411, (800) 328-4818. Division of Metacom, Inc.

PRESIDENT
Jim McCann

Aero-Space Visuals Society
1720 130 Avenue, N.E., Bellevue, WA 98005, (206) 881-9444. Subsidiary of Energy Sciences Corp.

Allied Video Distributors
106A Benkert St., Bethpage, NY 11714, (516) 935-5050; (800) 645-5060.

PRESIDENT
B. Rubinowitz
MARKETING & SALES
Beatrice Berg

AmbreCorp, Incorporated
805 S. Main St., Suite 5, Lombard, IL 60148, (312) 629-7070. Organized 1985. (Distributes or obtains video distribution rights to works produced by independent video producers.)

PRESIDENT
John F. Moran, Ph.D.
VICE PRESIDENT
Edward Guy
BRANCHES
California Office: 3134 Big Springs Ave., Simi Valley, CA 93063
AFFILIATIONS
Distributors for Communicorp Video and More Music Inc.

American Medical Association
535 N. Dearborn, Chicago, IL 60610, (312) 645-4986.

American National Enterprises, Inc.
106 W. 2950 South, Salt Lake City, UT 84115, (801) 486-3155. Organized 1965. (Film production and distribution to the world market.)

PRESIDENT
Hal Brown
CHIEF EXECUTIVE OFFICER
Neil Rosenstein
VICE PRESIDENT, ADMINISTRATION
Beth Zimmerman
VICE PRESIDENT, BUSINESS AFFAIRS
Bonnie L.W. Mitchell
CONTROLLER
Larry Whitlock
VICE PRESIDENT, PRODUCTION
George Gale
BOARD OF DIRECTORS
Neil Rosenstein, Hal Brown, McNeil Fiske, Aaron Grunfeld, Floyd Sassa
BRANCHES
Suites 217-219, 5858 Hollywood Blvd., Hollywood, CA 90026, (213) 467-2490

American Video Tape
1116 Edgewater Ave., Ridgefield, NJ 07657, (201) 941-4404.

Anti Defamation League of B'Nai B'rith
823 United Nations Plaza, New York, NY 10017, (212) 490-2525.

Arizona Peddler
790 S. Main, Cottonwood, AZ 86326.

PRESIDENT
Jack Poland

Artec Distributing, Inc.
One Pine Haven Shore Rd., Shelburne, VT 05482, (802) 985-9411. (Provides software and support services to video retailers.)

CHIEF OPERATING OFFICER
Martin Gold
CHIEF FINANCE OFFICER
Howard Goldberg
VICE PRESIDENT, OPERATIONS
Matt Brown
VICE PRESIDENT, SALES
Ken Miller
VICE PRESIDENT, FINANCE
Gerry Lawrence
VICE PRESIDENT, DATA PROCESSING
Greg Kasto
BRANCHES
Canton, MA; Middletown, CT
AFFILIATIONS
V.S.D.A., NAVD

Atlantis Productions, Inc.
1252 La Granada Dr., Thousand Oaks, CA 91362; (805) 495-2790. Organized 1952. (Production and distribution of motion pictures in film and video.)

PRESIDENT
Dr. J. Michael Hagopian
VICE PRESIDENT
Becci Meadors

BFA Educational Media
468 Park Avenue South, New York, NY 10016; (212) 684-5910. Subsidiary of Phoenix Films Inc.

PRESIDENT
H. Gelles
MARKETING & SALES
Robert Dunlap

Bandera Enterprises, Inc.
Box 1107, Studio City, CA 91604; (818) 985-5050.

PRESIDENT
Don Flagg

Barr Films
P.O. Box 5667, Pasadena, CA 91107;, (818) 793-6153.

PRESIDENT
Donald Barr
VICE PRESIDENT
John S. Dyas

Beacon Films
1250 Washington St., P.O. Box 575, Norwood, MA 02062;, (617) 762-9316.
PRESIDENT
Robert Vale

Bee Gee Records & Tapes, Inc.
10 Northway Lane, N. Latham, NY 12110; (518) 785-1122. Subsidiary of Bee Gee Distributing Corp.

Norman Beerger Productions
3217-A29, Arville St., Las Vegas, NV 89102-7612; (702) 876-2328. Organized 1984. (Produces and distributes wilderness home video programs.)
OWNER
Norman Beerger

Bellevue Home Entertainment Inc.
9 Brockhouse Rd., Toronto, Ontario, Canada M8W 2W8; (416) 259-8411, (416) 259-6692. Subsidiary of Astral Bellevue Pathe Inc.
PRESIDENT
Harold Greenberg
MARKETING & SALES
Steve Ferguson
Isar Klaiman

Blackhawk Films, Inc.
One Old Eagle Brewery, Davenport, IA 52802; (319) 323-9736. Organized 1927.
PRESIDENT
Ted Ewing

Michael Blackwood Productions
251 W. 57 St., Room 427, New York, NY 10019; (212) 247-4710. (Produces and distributes documentaries on 20th-Century fine artists and performing artists.)
PRESIDENT
Michael Blackwood

Les Blank's Flower Films and Video
10341 San Pablo Ave., El Cerrito, CA 94530; (415) 525-0942. Organized 1967. (Seeks out and documents America's vanishing minority cultures, their music and traditions.)
PRODUCER/DIRECTOR/CAMERA
Les Blank
DISTRIBUTION MANAGER
Susan Kell
FOLKLORIST/2nd CAMERA
Christine Simon
EDITOR
Maureen Gosling

Blank Tape Supply
2800-M Door Ave., Fairfax, VA 22031; (703) 698-7077, (800) 722-3300. Organized 1979. (Wholesale audio, video and computer products.)
PRESIDENT
Bob Vanjani
VICE PRESIDENT
Gayle Vanjani

Bullfrog Films, Inc.
Oley, PA 19547; (215) 779-8226. Organized 1973. (Distributes programs for personal self-reliance—how-to's on gardening, home improvements, energy-saving, etc.—and environmental responsibility.)
PRESIDENT
John Hoskyns-Abrahall
SECRETARY & TREASURER
Winifred Scherrer
PROMOTIONS MANAGER
Chris Everly
CUSTOMER SERVICE MANAGER
Steve Jarrett
BOARD OF DIRECTORS
John Hoskyns-Abrahall, Winifred Scherrer

CC Studios/Children's Circle
389 Newtown Turnpike, Weston CT 06883; (203) 222-0002. Organized 1963. (Produces and markets home audio/video cassettes to consumers; adaptations of children's books.)
PRESIDENT & TREASURER
Morton Schindel
VICE PRESIDENT
Katharine Gordon
SECRETARY
Elisabeth Rommel
ASSISTANT TREASURER
Betsy Rhines
BOARD OF DIRECTORS
Morton Schindel, Paul Schindel, Elisabeth Rommel
AFFILIATIONS
Weston Woods; Georgetown Studios

Cable Films & Video
#7171 County Club Station, Kansas City, MO 64113; (913) 362-2804. Organized 1976. (Film classics distribution to cable TV and video.)
PRESIDENT
Herb Miller
GENERAL MANAGER
Todd Randall
AFFILIATIONS
NCTA, NATPE, National Academy of TV Arts & Sciences, Mid-America Cable TV Association

Calypso Video, Inc.
2040 Reynolds Rd., Southwyck Center, Toledo, OH 43614; (419) 865-4169.
PRESIDENT
C. Opfermann

Capezio Ballet Makers
33 W. 60 St., 8th Floor, New York, NY 10023; (212) 247-7660.

Caravatt Communications, Inc.
49 Riverside Ave., Westport, CT 06880; (203) 227-0775.
PRESIDENT & CHIEF EXECUTIVE OFFICER
Paul J. Caravatt, Jr.
DIRECTOR OF OPERATIONS
Paul F. Schucker
DIRECTOR OF MARKETING
David Wood
PROJECT DIRECTORS
Jane Scarpellino
Thomas Duggan
BOARD OF DIRECTORS
Wm. E. Chambers (Pres., Norman Craig & Kummel, Ret.); Robert Morse, (Pres., Morse Williams, NYC); Peter Winslow (Ex. VP, Monz Cabot, Boston); Munanar Hidaya Halah (Pres., Consultancy & Mgt., NYC)

Cassette Express
3123 Sylvania Ave., Toledo, OH 43613; (419) 472-7727. Subsidiary of Video Connection.
PRESIDENT
John Day

Catalina Video Distributing
6611 Santa Monica Blvd., Los Angeles, CA 90038; (213) 485-9105, (800) 421-3269.

Century Distributing West, Inc.
16153 Cohasset St., Van Nuys, CA 91406; (818) 786-2846, (800) 423-2304.

Century East Distributors
85 E. Hoffman Ave., Lindenhurst, NY 11757; (516) 957-5520, (800) 221-6922. Subsidiary of JCP Associates.

Champions on Film and Video
745 State Circle, Box 1941, Ann Arbor, MI 48106; (313) 761-5176.

PRESIDENT
Donald N. Canham

Cinema Concepts, Inc.

2461 Berlin Turnpike, Newington, CT 06111; (203) 667-1251. Organized 1971. (Non-theatrical distribution of entertainment motion pictures in 16 mm, Beta, VHS, U-Matic, 8 mm to school, libraries and home market. Mail-order plus three retail stores.)

PRESIDENT
Joel G. Jacobson
VICE PRESIDENT
Susan G. Jacobson
BRANCHES
Porter Plaza, Main St., Old Saybrook, CT 06475; (203) 388-1481
Rt. 72 Plaza, 859 Mill St., East Berlin, CT 06023; (203) 828-1815
AFFILIATIONS
Video Software Dealers Association (Joel Jacobson is a Board Director of CT Chapter)

The Cinema Guild

1697 Broadway, Room 802, New York, NY 10019; (212) 246-5522. Organized 1975. (Film and video distribution.)

PRESIDENT
Philip S. Hobel
VICE PRESIDENTS
Gary Crowdus
Mary-Ann Hobel
DISTRIBUTION MANAGER
Eva Jakubowski

City One Stop

2551 S. Alameda St., Los Angeles, CA 90058; (213) 234-3336. Subsidiary of Show Industries.

PRESIDENT
Lou Fogelman

Coast Video Distributor, Inc.

620 Paula Ave., Glendale, CA 91201; (818) 500-0114, (800) 32-COAST.

PRESIDENT
Gil Padilla

Coast to Coast Family Video Inc.

85 E. Hoffman Ave., Lindenhurst, NY 11757; (516) 957-5520, (800) 221-6922.

MARKETING MANAGER
Michelle Gordon

Commtron Corp.

1501 50 St., Suite 300, West Des Moines, IA 50265; (515) 224-1784. Subsidiary of Bergen Brunswig Corp.

NATIONAL SALES MANAGER
Tim Shannahan

Concord Video

900 Sunset Blvd., Suite 603, Los Angeles, CA 90069; (213) 271-5705.

Corinth Films & Video

410 E. 62 St., Room 701, New York, NY 10021; (212) 412-4770. Organized 1977. (Film and video distribution.)

PRESIDENT
John M. Poole V
SENIOR VICE PRESIDENT
Peter J. Meyer
VICE PRESIDENT, SALES
Matthew Curtis
VICE PRESIDENT, MARKETING & PUBLICITY
Henry Baker
TECHNICAL DIRECTOR
Richard Evangelista
COMPTROLLER
Tom Sabo

Courier Productions

P.O. Box 291285, Los Angeles, CA 90010; (213) 937-2848. Subsidiary of LDR, International.

PRESIDENT
Linda D. Roberts

Covenant Video

3200 W. Foster Ave., Chicago, IL 60625; (312) 478-4676, (800) 621-1290.

PRESIDENT
Stan Torgerson

Creative Visions Video

72 S. San Pedro St., Los Angeles, CA 90014; (213) 623-9254, (800) 421-8528. Subsidiary of Image Laboratories, Inc.

PRESIDENT
Robert Hoffman

A.S. Csaky Motion Picture and Video Productions

420 Legato Terrace, Silver Spring, MD 20901; (301) 681-3333 and 681-3390. Organized 1968. (Develops, produces and distributes motion picture and video productions and screenplays nationally and internationally.)

CHAIRMAN OF THE BOARD AND PRESIDENT
A.S. Csaky
VICE PRESIDENT, PRODUCTION
Ramzi D. Seikaly
VICE PRESIDENT, SCREENPLAY DEVELOPMENT
Bud Fleisher
VICE PRESIDENT, TRAVEL MANAGEMENT
Albert Cambata
VICE PRESIDENT, PUBLIC RELATIONS
Cecilia Korda-Bros
VICE PRESIDENT, SALES & MARKETING
Catherine White
GRAPHICS DIRECTOR
Juan Chavarria
BRANCHES
Washington, DC, New York, NY

Czar Productions, Inc.

39 Princeton St., West Hartford, CT 06110; (203) 233-2034.

PRESIDENT
Gene Czarnecki
MARKETING & SALES
Viviane Grady

H.W. Daily, Inc.

3409 Brinkman, Houston, TX 17018; (713) 861-9251, (800) 231-0591, (800) 392-5135. (TX)

PRESIDENT
Don Daily
MARKETING & SALES
David Bennett

Dawn's Video

519 W. Foothill, Suite C, Rialto, CA 92376; (714) 874-1414. Organized 1980. (Video specialty store.)

OWNER
Gregory C. George
BRANCHES
2085 E. Highland Ave., San Bernadino, CA 92404; (714) 864-3113
9725 Sierra, Fontana, CA 92335; (714) 350-8833
267 E. 40th, San Bernadino, CA 92404; (714) 883-5737
1330 Massachusetts Ave., Riverside, CA 92507; (714) 784-1414

Direct Cinema Limited

P.O. Box 69589, Los Angeles, CA 90069; (213) 656-4700. Organized 1974. (Specialized distributor of short videos and films, documentaries, independent features, animation.)

PRESIDENT
Mitchell W. Block
VICE PRESIDENTS
Michael Pulitzer III
Betsy A. McLane
COMPTROLLER
Sharon Levine

Discount Video Tapes, Inc.
371 W. Clark Ave., Suite B, Burbank, CA 91505;, (818) 843-3366. Organized 1979. (Specializing in rare and unusual pre-recorded videos. Retail and wholesale.)

PRESIDENT
Woody Wise

Walt Disney Educational Media Co.
500 S. Buena Vista St., Burbank, CA 91521; (818) 840-1000. (Division of Walt Disney Productions.)

MARKETING COORDINATOR
Linda Capuano

EDC Publishing
8141 E. 44th St., Tulsa, OK 74105; (918) 622-4522. Subsidiary of Educational Development Corp.

PRESIDENT
John O. Whitney
MARKETING & SALES
Jim Roginski

Eagle Productions, Ltd
7860 Mission Center Court, Suite 106, San Diego, CA 92108; (619) 297-8870.

East Texas Distributing
7171 Grand Blvd., Houston, TX 77504; (713) 748-2520, (800) 231-6648; 2732 W. McDowell, Phoenix, AZ 85009; (602) 233-3741, (800) 231-3218.

PRESIDENT
Ron Eisenberg
MARKETING & SALES
Jan Moore (Houston)
Janet Wheeler (Phoenix)

Eastin Phelan Corp.
P.O. Box 4528, Davenport, IA 52808; (319) 323-9735.

PRESIDENT
Robert Evans

Enter-Tel Inc.
25200 Chagrin Blvd., Beachwood, OH 44122; (216) 831-6940.

MARKETING
Rick Zenobi

Entertainment America Inc.
One Kaiser Plaza, Suite 1035, Oakland, CA 94612; (415) 839-4411.

PRESIDENT
Lawrence W. Jenkins
MARKETING & SALES
John Taggart

Environmental Video, Inc.
1116 8th St., Room B, P.O. Box 577, Manhattan Beach, CA 90266; (213) 546-4581. Organized 1981. (Manufactures and produces pre-recorded videocassettes for the home video market.)

PRESIDENT
James R. Spencer

Equestrian Video Library
712 Wilshire Blvd., Santa Monica, CA 90401; (213) 393-5800. Subsidiary of Mercedes Maharis.

PRESIDENT
Mercedes Maharis
NATIONAL SALES DIRECTOR
Sally Lasater

FJC-Intellimedia, Inc.
P.O. Box 6632, Syracuse, NY 13217-6632; (315) 472-3442.

PRESIDENT
Joseph Crisafulli
MARKETING & SALES
D. LoSurdo

Festival Films
2841 Irving Avenue South, Minneapolis, MN 55408; (612) 870-4744.

PRESIDENT
Ron Hall

First Movie Exchange of Colorado
3011 W. 74th Ave., Westminster, CO 80030; (303) 427-7788. Subsidiary of Wickman Ltd.

PRESIDENT
Dianne Lynn Wickman

First Video Exchange
17503 S. Figueroa, Gardena, CA 90248; (213) 516-6422, (800) 247-2351. Organized 1981. (National movie exchange, stock rotation specialist for video movie dealers.)

PRESIDENT
Jeff Leyton

G.G. Communications, Inc.
111 French Ave., Braintree, MA 02184; (617) 843-4860, (800) 525-3503.

PRESIDENT
Nicholas Russo

Galaxy Express Distributors
2337 Haddonfield Rd., Pennsauken, NJ 08110; (609) 488-0400, (215) 364-1862.

PRESIDENT
Barry Gerber

Glenn Video Vistas
6924 Canby Ave., Suite 103, Reseda, CA 9133;, (818) 981-5506. Organized 1980. (Sale of videotapes.)

OWNER/MANAGER
Murray Glass
AFFILIATIONS
Glenn Photo Supply

Grand Award Video Inc.
2170 W. Broadway, Room 526, Anaheim, CA 92801; (714) 995-0707. Organized 1983. (Manufacturer of video pre-recorded software and TV's wide screen.)

PRESIDENT
Jeffrey M. Scheirer
VICE PRESIDENT
Harry F. Scheirer
BOARD OF DIRECTORS
Jeffrey Scheirer, Harry F. Scheirer

Hartley Film Foundation
Cat Rock Rd., Cos Cob, CT 06807; (203) 869-1818.

PRESIDENT
Elda Hartley

Hearst Marine Books
105 Madison Ave., New York, NY 10016; (212) 889-3050. (Division of William Morrow, Inc.)

Home Entertainment Distributors
9549 Pen Ave. S., Minneapolis, MN 55431; (612) 887-9500, (800) 328-2960, (800) 352-2802 (MN). (Division of Lieberman Enterprises.)

PRESIDENT
Robert Okinow
MARKETING
Jeff Abrams
BRANCHES

1631 Deramus Rd., Kansas City, MO 64120.
2781 Peterson Place, Norcross, GA 30071.
3014 N. Wygant St., Portland, OR 97217.

Home And Industrial Distributors

300-1 Rte. 17S., Lodi, NJ 07644; (202) 777-4700, (800) 213-1586.

PRESIDENT
Alfred Goldberger

How To Video Corp.

606 N. Main St., Ashland City, TN 37015; (615) 792-4417, (615) 792-4472.

PRESIDENT
Jerry Hooker

IFEX Films/International Film Exchange Ltd.

201 West 52 St., New York, NY 10019; (212) 582-4318. Organized 1959. (Domestic and international distribution of feature films, documentaries, shorts and video programs.)

CHAIRMAN OF THE BOARD
Arthur "Skip" Steloff
PRESIDENT
Gerald J. Rappoport
SENIOR VICE PRESIDENT
Richard Grisar
EXECUTIVE VICE PRESIDENT
Christopher Wood
VICE PRESIDENT, THEATRICAL SALES
Jefrey Jacobs
VICE PRESIDENT, INTERNATIONAL SALES
Joy Pereths

Image Entertainment

6311 Romaine St., Hollywood, CA 90038; (213) 468-8867.

VICE PRESIDENT, MARKETING
Lee Kasper

Image Magnetic Associates Inc. (I.M.A.)

5514 Satsuma Ave., North Hollywood, CA 91601; (818) 762-3993.

PRESIDENT
David Allen
MARKETING & SALES
Steve Allen

Important Records

149-03 Guy R. Brewer Blvd., Jamaica, NY 11434; (718) 995-9200.

VICE PRESIDENT, MARKETING & SALES
Howie Gabriel

Ingram Video

347 Reedwood Dr., Nashville, TN 37217; (615) 361-5000, (800) 251-5902. (Subsidiary of Ingram Industries, Inc.)

PRESIDENT
Dick Fontaine
VICE PRESIDENT
Megan Burrows

Innovations in Video

8448 Reseda Blvd., Suite 101, Northridge, CA 91324; (818) 701-1423, (800) 624-9327, (800) 227-1586 (CA). Subsidiary of Video Distribution International Ltd.

Inter-Global Communications

(div. Radio's Reliable Resources)
630 Park La., 2nd floor, Philadelphia, PA 19144-3713; (215) 849-3997. Organized 1962. (International film/tape program buying service for television stations and small videolers of home video.)

GENERAL MANAGER
F.O. Pease
OFFICE MANAGER
A.E. Pease
FOREIGN MANAGER
A.P. Taylor
BUYER
B.P. Weber
SALES MANAGER
J.K. Sperling
AFFILIATIONS
Inter-Global News div.

International Audio-Visual, Inc.

100 Northill Dr. #23, Brisbane, CA 94005; (415) 467-103, 467-4663. (Chinese videos.)

PRESIDENT
S.S. Ling

International Historic Films, Inc.

3015 W. 59th St., Chicago, IL 60629; (312) 436-8051. Organized 1976. (Distribution and production of military and political features and documentaries. Also distribution of Eastern European films. Provides stock footage to producers. Sales and rental of films on videocassette through store and direct mail internationally. Videocassettes available on NTSC, PAL and SECAM videostandards.)

PRESIDENT
Peter Bernotas
AFFILIATIONS
Lithuanian Historical Society

International Home Video

431 N. Figueroa, Wilmington, CA 90744; (213) 513-1149. Organized 1983. (Manufactures and distributes pre-recorded videocassettes.)

CHAIRMAN
Irving Katzef
PRESIDENT
Russell Greene
EXECUTIVE VICE PRESIDENT
Marion Martelli
SECRETARY & TREASURER
Wayne Jones
BOARD OF DIRECTORS
Russell Greene, Irving Katzef, H.B. Meyers
BRANCHES
Video Latino, Country Video USA

International Home Videoclub, Inc.

220 Shrewsbury Ave., Red Bank, NJ 07701; (201) 741-7800, (800) 458-3000.

PRESIDENT
Joseph DeGraw

International Sailing Products

P.O. Box 355, Oyster Bay, NY 11771; (516) 922-5182, (800) 645-7676.

PRESIDENT
Steve Benjamin
VICE PRESIDENT
Paul Dickey

JEF Films Inc.

Film House, 143 Hickory Hill Circle, Osterville, MA 02655; (617) 428-7198. Organized 1973. (Production and distribution of films, TV shows and video programs throughout the world.)

PRESIDENT
Jeffrey H. Aikman
VICE PRESIDENT
Elsie Aikman
SECRETARY & TREASURER
Donald Aikman
MARKETING MANAGER
Jo-Anne Polak
SALES
Janie Barber
BOARD OF DIRECTORS
Jeffrey H. Aikman, Elsie Aikman, Donald Aikman
BRANCHES
Film Classic Exchange, Los Angeles, CA
JEF Films Inc.—England, Canada, Australia, Japan, China, Netherlands, New Zealand, Scandinavia, Norway, Denmark, Germany, Swe-

den, Hong Kong, Iceland, Fiji, Ireland, Scotland, Wales
AFFILIATIONS
Owner of Film Classic Exchange (founded 1916), VIP Video, XTC Video, JEF Video Line

Stefaan Janssen Studio

4615 N. Lincoln Ave., Chicago, IL 60625; (312) 728-9277. Organized 1983. (Sells and produces special interest programs for the home video market.)

OWNER
Stefaan Janssen
AFFILIATIONS
Member: VSDA; Center for New Television; AIFV

Jem Records

3619 Kennedy Rd., South Plainfield, NJ 07080; (201) 753-6100. (Distributes and manufactures records, tapes, compact discs, music video.)

PRESIDENT
Marty Scott
VICE PRESIDENT
Ed Grossi
TREASURER
Jeff Tenenbaum
BRANCHES
Grand Prairie TX; Reseda, CA

Journal Films, Inc.

930 Pitner Ave., Evanston, IL 60202; (312) 328-6700. Organized 1955. (Distributor of educational videos and films for the school and library markets.)

PRESIDENT
Joe Farragher
CHAIRMAN
Joel Altschul
EXECUTIVE VICE PRESIDENT
Esther Altschul
VICE PRESIDENT
Bruce Colling
NATIONAL SALES MANAGER
John Kelly

K-Video Productions

157 Wiltshire Rd., Claymont, DE 19703; (302) 798-2229. Organized 1980. (Educational tapes, corporate and private videos.)

PRESIDENT
John Kay
VICE PRESIDENT
Stan Kay
SECRETARY & TREASURER
Charmaine Imburgia
AFFILIATIONS
DBE, GWVCB, Delaware State Chamber of Commerce

Kalmbach Publishing Co.

1027 N. 7th St., Milwaukee, WI 53233; (414) 272-2060.

PRESIDENT
James J. King
MARKETING & SALES
Tom D'Amico

Kartes Video Communications, Inc.

10 E. 106th St., Indianapolis, IN 46280; (317) 844-1403, (800) 582-2000.

Kennen Publishing

150 Shoreline Highway, Bldg. E., Mill Valley, CA 94941; (415) 332-5828. (Subsidiary of Dudkowski-Lynch Assoc. Inc.)

PRESIDENT
Ed Dudkowski

Key Video

1211 Avenue of the Americas, New York, NY 10036; (212) 819-3200, (619) 459-0500. (Subsidiary of CBS/Fox Video.)

PRESIDENT
Herb Fischer
DIRECTOR OF PROD. MANAGEMENT
Joseph Annechino

King of Video, Inc.

3529 S. Valley View Blvd., Las Vegas, NV 89103; (800) 634-6143, (702) 362-2520. Organized 1979. Public: 1981. (Manufacture and wholesale distribution of pre-recorded videocassette tapes.)

PRESIDENT & CHIEF EXECUTIVE OFFICER
Steve Vincent
DIRECTOR OF FINANCE, GENERAL MANAGER, SECRETARY & TREASURER
Nancy E. Kelly
VICE PRESIDENT
Marvin L. Tragerman
BOARD OF DIRECTORS
Steve Vincent, Nancy E. Kelly, Marvin L. Tragerman

Kultur

1340 Ocean Avenue, Sea Bright, NJ 07760; (201) 842-6693.

Life Video Gospel Association

1435 Central Ave., College Place, WA 99324; (509) 522-0784. Organized 1979. (Produces and distributes religious videotapes.)

PRESIDENT
Donald M. Vories
TREASURER
Walter Anderson
SECRETARY
Jeanne Vories
BOARD OF DIRECTORS
Donald M. Vories, Walter Anderson, Jeanne Vories, Fred E.J. Harder, Vernon Shafer, Paul Turpel, Frank Salt, D.K. Smith, James Hannum

MAS Productions

18434 Bermuda St., Northridge, CA 91326; (818) 360-0371.

MCA Distributing Corp.

70 Universal City Plaza, 3rd floor, Universal City, CA 91608; (818) 777-4000. (Distributor of pre-recorded videocassettes and records.) A division of MCA/Universal.

SENIOR VICE PRESIDENT, DISTRIBUTION
John Burns
VICE PRESIDENT, VIDEO DISTRIBUTION
Louis Feola
VICE PRESIDENT, VIDEO PRODUCTS
Neil Hartley
BRANCHES
REGIONAL VIDEO DIRECTOR (EAST)
Bill Hickman
REGIONAL VIDEO DIRECTOR (MIDWEST)
Janis Durr
REGIONAL VIDEO DIRECTOR (SOUTHEAST)
Roger Mill
REGIONAL VIDEO DIRECTOR (WEST)
Steve Garwood

MPI Home Video

15825 Rob Roy Drive, Oak Forest, IL 60452; (312) 687-7881. (Production and distribution of programming for home video.)

PRESIDENT
Waleed B. Ali
VICE PRESIDENT
Malik B. Ali
MARKETING DIRECTOR
Jaffer Ali
BOARD OF DIRECTORS
Waleed B. Ali, Malik B. Ali, Jaffer Ali

M.S. Distributing Co.

2060 Carboy, Mount Prospect, IL 60656; (312) 364-2888.

PRESIDENT
Tony Dalesandro
MARKETING & SALES
Rick Chrzan

MPA Video Distributors

4740 Cote Vertu St., Montreal, Quebec, Canada M45 IJ9; (513) 333-7555.

VICE PRESIDENT
Norman Purpas

M.S.V. Distributors
40 S. Carolina St., Baltimore, MD 21231; (301) 675-1400, (800) 992-7799, (800) 492-1443. (Subsidiary of Musical Sales.)
PRESIDENT
Michael J. Bereson
MARKETING & SALES
J. Anthony Ray

MZ Packaging Corp.
21 Abendroth Ave., Port Chester, NY 10573; (914) 937-5892.

Macmillan Video.
866 Third Ave., New York, NY 10022; (718) 702-2000.
EXECUTIVE PRODUCER
James Macguire

Major Video Concepts
8399 Zionsville Rd., Indianapolis, IN 46268; (317) 875-8000, (800) 428-1400, (800) 732-1452 (IN) (Subsidiary of ADI/Mayflower Corp.)
VICE PRESIDENT & GENERAL MANAGER
Paul Guhl

Maljack Productions, Inc.
15825 Rob Roy Dr., Oak Forest, IL 60452; (800) 323-0442.

The Market Place
4112 Marsh Ave., Rockford, IL 61111; (815) 877-1514. Organized 1985. (Videocassette distribution of inspirational programs to the home and church markets. Children's programs, music concert videos, financial planning seminar.)
PRESIDENT
Max Anderson

Mass Media Video Ministries
2116 North Charles St., Baltimore, MD 21218; (301) 727-3270. Organized 1964. (A nationwide agency providing the educational and religious communities and other service organizations with quality video programs.)
PRESIDENT
Clifford J. York
VICE PRESIDENT & TREASURER
Janice P. York
BOARD OF DIRECTORS
Clifford J. York, Janice P. York

Media Concepts, Inc.
559 49th St. S., St. Petersburg, FL 33707; (813) 321-2122.
PRESIDENT
Bob Skidmore
MARKETING & SALES
John P. Gallagher
Dan O'Neil

Metacom Audio Publishing Group
1401-B West River Road North, Minneapolis, MN 55427; (612) 588-2781. Organized 1970. (Manufactures and distributes — primarily through direct mail—audio and video cassettes of subliminal self-help and public domain movies.)
PRESIDENT
James I. McCann
EXECUTIVE VICE PRESIDENT/GENERAL MANAGER
Phillip T. Levin
VICE PRESIDENT OF FINANCE/CONTROLLER
David Benson

Metro Video Distributors, Inc.
430 W. 54 St., New York, NY 10019; (212) 489-8130.
PRESIDENT
Arthur Morowitz

Mid-America Distributors, Inc.
3329 Chapel Hill Blvd., P.O. Box 8800, Durham, NC 27707.
CONTROLLER
Ronald S. Slotter

Mid-Continental Electronics, Inc.
659 Executive Dr., Willowbrook, IL 60521; (312) 850-7070, (800) 323-3153.
PRESIDENT
Ron Rubin
DIRECTOR OF OPERATIONS
Gary Stallman

Morris Video
936 Hermosa Ave., First Floor, Hermosa Beach, CA 90254; (213) 374-4984. Organized 1984. (Produces and distributes quality information and entertainment videos.)
PRESIDENT & C.E.O
Dawn Morris
VICE PRESIDENT & C.F.O.
George Morris, Ph.D.
BOARD OF DIRECTORS
Dawn Morris, George Morris, Ph.D., George Bott, David Van Horn.
BRANCH
663 The Village, Redondo Beach, CA 90277; (213) 374-4984

Movie Buff Video
250 W. 95 St., New York, NY 10025; (212) 666-0331. (Subsidiary of Manhattan Movietime.)
MARKETING & SALES
Bruce Goldstein

Movie Mogul
101 Twin Oaks, Rochester, IL 62563; (217) 498-8517. (Subsidiary of Kesinger Auto.)
PRESIDENT
Marc Kesinger

Museum of Modern Art of Latin America
1889 F St., N.W., Washington, D.C. 20006; (202) 789-6021.
MARKETING & SALES
Angel Hurtado

NSI Video
736 Longfellow Ave., Hermosa Beach, CA 90254; (213) 374-7476. (Subsidiary of Native Son International.)
PRESIDENT
Gerard Ravel

N.T.A. Home Entertainment
12636 Beatrice St., Los Angeles, CA 90066; (213) 306-4040. (Subsidiary of Republic Pictures Home Video Co.)
SENIOR VICE PRESIDENT
Nick Draklich

Naidoff Associates
65 Richard Rd., Ivyland, PA 18974; (215) 674-5410.
PRESIDENT
Bert Naidoff
MARKETING & SALES
Michael Smeyene

National Film Board of Canada
1251 Avenue of the Americas, 16th floor, New York, NY 10020; (212) 586-5131. (Film agency of Canada. Produces and distributes motion pictures.)

National Geographic Society
Educational Services, Washington, DC 20036; (202) 857-7090.

MARKETING & SALES
Wendy Rogers

New Breed Music

P.O. Box 661, Pomona, CA 91768; (714) 623-1999.

PRESIDENT
Jesse Mac Lynum, Jr.

New Mode Media

1 Park Ave., Old Greenwich, CT 06870; (203) 637-3616. (Division of Listening Library, Inc.)

PRESIDENT
Anthony Ditlow

Nite Flite

19410 Business Center Dr., Northridge, CA 91324; (818) 993-6912; (800) 423-5277.

Norstar Instructional Video Corp.

1580 Old Bayshore Highway, San Jose, CA 95112; (408) 436-2882. Organized 1984. (Instructional "How To" distribution company.)

PRESIDENT
Stephen K. Troy
PARTNER
Ray Oltman
BOARD OF DIRECTORS
Stephen K. Troy, Ray Oltman

Nostalgia Merchant

6233 W. Sunset Blvd., Suite 1019, Hollywood, CA 90028; (800) 421-4495.

Nova Video Art

10583 Felton Way, Cupertino, CA 95014; (408) 725-0708. Organized 1983. (Produces instructional dance videotapes—e.g. "Learn Classical Ballet and Enjoy It."

OWNER/PRODUCER
Lilia Peloquin
MARKETING DIRECTOR
Mike Peloquin
GRAPHIC DESIGNER/NARRATOR
Katalin Maritza Balogh
AFFILIATIONS
Video Productions: Vertex Video Associates
Music: Silver Label Recording Co.

On-Site Video

32825 Groves Rd., Bremen, OH 43107; (614) 569-4601. Organized 1982. (Video distribution.)

OWNER
Allen P. Brand

Pacific Art Video Records

P.O. Box 22770, Carmel, CA 93922; (408) 624-4704.

PRESIDENT
David Bean

Pacific Trade Group

94-527 Puahi Street, Waipahu, HI 96782; (808) 671-6735. Organized 1977. (Publisher and distributor of books and video tapes.)

PRESIDENT & MANAGER
Richard E. Pultz
VICE PRESIDENT, SALES
David A. Jasper
SECRETARY
Jane W. Pultz
CONTROLLER
James Todd
BOARD OF DIRECTORS
Richard E. Pultz, David A. Jasper, Jane W. Pultz, Faith Higshiguchi

Palm Beach Home Video

1665 12th St., Santa Monica, CA 90404; (213) 450-2027.

PRESIDENT
Randi Freeman

Palmer Video Corporation

1767 Morris Avenue, Union, NJ 07083; (201) 686-3030. Organized 1981. (Franchisor—video stores.)

PRESIDENT
Peter Balner
VICE PRESIDENT
Peter Margaritondo
VICE PRESIDENT, FINANCE
Joseph Berger

Panic Distributing Co.

2999 Silver Dr., Columbus, OH 43224; (614) 267-1211.

Penguin Video Productions

P.O. Box 65157, Los Angeles, CA 90065; (213) 222-2707.

PRESIDENT
Kim Dunnahoo

Perennial Education, Inc.

930 Pitner Ave., Evanston, IL 60202; (312) 328-6700. (Distributor of educational videos and films for the school and social service markets.)

PRESIDENT
Joe Farragher
CHAIRMAN
Joel Altschul
EXECUTIVE VICE PRESIDENT
Esther Altschul
VICE PRESIDENT
Bruce Colling

Phoenix Films Inc.

468 Park Avenue South, New York, NY 10016; (212) 684-5910.

PRESIDENT
H. Gelles
MARKETING & SALES
Robert Dunlap

Picture Start, Inc.

204 W. John St., Champaign, IL 61820; (217) 352-7353.

PRESIDENT
Ron Epple
MARKETING & SALES
Jeff Hellyer

Plus A Video Ltd.

158 Godwin Ave., Midland Park, NJ 07482; (201) 447-1501, (800) 524-0195.

PRESIDENT
Lee Friedman

Polo Trade Corp.

688 Main St., New York, NY 10044; (212) 759-7779.

MARKETING & SALES
Bill O'Leary

Price/Stern/Sloan Publishers, Inc.

410 N. La Cienega, Los Angeles, CA 90048; (213) 657-6100.

EXECUTIVE VICE PRESIDENT
Mick Clemente

Prism Entertainment Corporation

1875 Century Park E., Suite 1010, Los Angeles, CA 90067; (213) 277-3270. Organized 1983. (Home video distribution.)

CHAIRMAN—DIRECTOR
Paul Levinson

PRESIDENT—DIRECTOR
Barry Collier
SENIOR VICE PRESIDENT—DIRECTOR
Robin Montgomery
VICE PRESIDENT—DIRECTOR
Earl Rosenstein
BOARD OF DIRECTORS
Robert Borcharnt

Producers Consortium

337 E. 1165 N., Orem, Utah 84057; (801) 224-5407, (801) 226-8209. Organized 1985. (Produces and distributes film and video productions.)

PARTNERS
R. Conrad Teichert
P. Michael J. Karr
BOARD OF DIRECTORS
R. Conrad Teichert, P. Michael J. Karr
AFFILIATIONS
Kappa Tan Alpha, AFI, IFPA, SMPTE

Professional Research, Inc. (PRI)

930 Pitner Ave., Evanston, IL 60202; (312) 328-6700. (Distributor of educational films and videos for the health care market.)

PRESIDENT
Joe Farragher
CHAIRMAN
Joel Altschul
EXECUTIVE VICE PRESIDENT
Esther Altschul
VICE PRESIDENT
Bruce Colling
NATIONAL SALES MANAGER
Margaret Dugan

Public Access Producers Association

2652 N. Winchell, Portland, OR 97217; (503) 289-2309.

DIRECTOR
R.S. Kolemaine
MARKETING & SALES
R.S. Kolemaine

Quality Life Video

2819 Third St., Boulder, CO 80302; (303) 443-9536.

PRESIDENT
Robin Sutherland

Quality Video Service

P.O. Box 2622, Redmond, WA 98052; (206) 788-6840.

PRESIDENT
James P. Kehoe

RKO Home Video

(Subsidiary of RKO Pictures)
1900 Avenue of the Stars, Suite #1562, Los Angeles, CA 90067; (213) 277-3133. Organized 1983. (Ancillary distribution—home video and cable.)

VICE PRESIDENT
Ellen S. Wander
NATIONAL MARKETING MANAGER, ANCILLARY DISTRIBUTION
Robert D. Lazarus
MARKETING COORDINATOR
Maggie Leatherman
BOARD OF DIRECTORS
C. Robert Manby (Chairman); Mark Seiler, (President)

RMI Media Productions, Inc.

2807 W. 47th St. Shawnee Mission, KS 66205; (913) 262-3974.

PRESIDENT
David L. Little

Reader's Digest

Pleasantville, NY 10570; (914) 769-7000.

Republic Pictures Corporation

12636 Beatrice St., Los Angeles, CA 90066; (213) 306-4040. Organized 1952. (Film and video distribution.)

PRESIDENT
A.W. Groskopf
VICE PRESIDENT
Nick Draklich
CONTROLLER
Alex Tovar
BOARD OF DIRECTORS
George Hatch (Chairman of the Board); Robert Magness (Board Member); Paul J. O'Brien (Treasurer)

Reel Images

Box 137, Monroe, CT 06468; (800) 243-9289.

Rehabfilm

1123 Broadway, New York, NY 10010; (212) 741-5160. (Subsidiary of Rehabilitation Int'l., U.S.A.)

DIRECTOR OF MEDIA
John F. Moses

Rhapsody Films Inc.

P.O. Box 179, New York, NY 10014; (212) 243-0152. Organized 1982. (Distributes jazz and blues films for all markets— television, home video and non-theatrical.)

PRESIDENT
Bruce Ricker

Richman Brothers

6935 Airport Highway Lane, Pennsauken, NJ 08109.

PRESIDENT
Jerry Richman
MARKETING & SALES
Charlene Engelbrecht

Henry Rosenberg ltd.

200 Fifth Ave., New York, NY 10010; (212) 620-6110.

PRESIDENT
Henry Rosenberg

SBI Video

4901 Forbes Blvd., Lanham, MD 20706; (202) 459-8000, (800) 638-0243, (800) 492-3193 (MD). (Subsidiary of Schwartz Bros. Inc.)

GENERAL MANAGER
Dan Rosenberg
SALES MANAGER
Mark Pernia

STG Distributing, Inc.

4974 E. Clinton Ave., Suite 112, Fresno, CA 93727; (209) 454-0800. Organized 1984. (Video distribution and rack jobber.)

PRESIDENT
Jerry Welch
EXECUTIVE VICE PRESIDENT & SECRETARY
James Daily
TREASURER
Fred Atchity, Jr.
CHIEF FINANCIAL OFFICER
Frank Ryason
BOARD OF DIRECTORS
Bernard Horton, Fred Atchity, Jr., Howard Freedland, John Engvall

Schwartz Brothers, Inc.

4901 Forbes Blvd., Lanham MD 20706; (301) 459-8000. Organized 1946. (Wholesale distributor of videocassettes, compact discs, records, blank tapes, pre-recorded tapes, and accessories.)

PRESIDENT
James Schwartz
CHAIRMAN OF THE BOARD & EXECUTIVE VICE PRESIDENT
Stuart Schwartz
VICE PRESIDENT, FINANCE
Melvin C. Davis
VICE PRESIDENT, SALES

Jerome Jacobs
BOARD OF DIRECTORS
Milton Lyons, Joseph R. Cassidy, Howard Kolodny
BRANCHES
1165 Marlkress Rd., Cherry Hill, NJ 08003; (609) 424-2211 (Richard Salvador, branch manager)
1129 Bloomfield Ave., W. Caldwell, NJ 07006; (201) 882-2955 (Andy Miele, sales manager)
2440 Lakeside Ave., Cleveland, OH 44114; (216) 696-2701 (Harvey Korman, branch manager)
AFFILIATIONS
National Association of Record Merchandisers
National Association of Video Distributors
Video Software Dealers Association
Country Music Association

2nd Play Video
2340 Sawtelle Blvd., W. Los Angeles, CA 90064; (213) 477-2986.
PRESIDENT
James R. Russo
MARKETING & SALES
M. Jones
T. Wolworth
Vic Boxwell

Select-A-Tape
8756 Holloway Drive, Los Angeles, CA 90069; (213) 657-2706, (800) 421-4465. (Distributes midnight videos [horror films] and adult films.)
PRESIDENT
Alan Roberts

Self Reliance Foundation
147 E. Devargas, Santa Fe, NM 87501; (505) 984-0080.
PRESIDENT
Jeff Kline

Sight and Sound Distributors
8233 Brentwood Industrial Dr., St. Louis, MO 63144; (314) 781-9312; (800) 325-9232.
DIRECTOR
Dan Thompson
BRANCH
1144 Booth St., Kansas City, KS 66103; (913) 371-8152.

Simon and Schuster Communications
108 Wilmot, Deerfield, IL 60015; (312) 940-1260. (Division of Simon and Schuster.)

Sound Video Unlimited
7000 N. Austin Ave., Niles, IL 60648; (312) 647-0800.

Source Video Distributing Co., Inc.
141 Belle Forest Circle, Nashville, TN 37221; (800) 251-1638, (800) 342-5014 (TN).
PRESIDENT
Lee Cowen
MARKETING & SALES
Fred W. Phister

Special Interest Video
1717 Darby Rd., Sebastopol, CA 95472; (707) 829-0127. Organized 1980. (Distribution of instructional and special interest video tapes.)
PRESIDENT
Michael Heumann
MARKETING VICE PRESIDENT
Faison Jordan
SECRETARY & TREASURER
Marcia Ludwig
AFFILIATION
VSDA

Spectrum Video
18121 Napa St., Northridge, CA 91325; (818) 886-8680, (800) 423-5599. (Acquisition and production of alternative non-theatrical, how-to programming for distribution to home video market place.)
PRESIDENT
Fred Hirsch
VICE PRESIDENT
Dwight Krizman
AFFILIATION
VSDA

Spinnaker Software Corp.
1 Kendall Square, Cambridge, MA 02139; (617) 494-1200.
VICE PRESIDENT
Prescilla Seuss

Star Video Entertainment, Inc.
550 Grand St., Jersey City, NJ 07302-4112; (201) 333-4600.
PRESIDENT
Bernard Herman

Star Video Productions
10701 Wilshire Blvd., Room 2001, Los Angeles, CA 90024; (213) 470-6522. Organized 1980. (Production and distribution of How-to home videos.)
PRESIDENT
Alfredo Ringel
EXECUTIVE VICE PRESIDENT
Deborah Taper Ringel

Superior Video
495 Ellis St., #2938, San Francisco, CA 94102; (800) 472-3000.
PRESIDENT
Dave Jennings
MARKETING & SALES
Jim Benson

Supervideo
417 Colorado Ave., Santa Monica, CA 90401; (213) 394-9696. (Subsidiary of Exploration in Video.)
PRESIDENT
Nissim Raphael

The TV Collector
P.O. Box 188, Needham, MA 02192; (617) 238-1179. Organized 1976. (TV nostalgia magazine/tape trading market-place.)
PUBLISHER
Stephen W. Albert
EDITOR
Diane L. Albert

TV Sports Scene, Inc.
(TVSS, Inc.)
5804 Ayrshire Blvd., Minneapolis, MN 55436, (612) 925-9661. Organized 1970. (TV program distribution, national and international.)
PRESIDENT & CHAIRMAN OF THE BOARD
Donald L. Herrick
VICE PRESIDENT
Robert C. Bruce
SECRETARY & TREASURER
Barbara Conley
BOARD OF DIRECTORS
Donald L. Herrick, Robert C. Bruce, Barbara Conley
AFFILIATIONS
Owner of U.S. Television Communications, Inc. (USTC)
Owner—Division Northwest Advertising & Marketing
Owner—Division MED TV
Owner—Division Consumer Products Division TV Sports Scene, Inc.

Tamarelle's French Film House
110 Cohasset Stage Rd., Chico, CA 95926, (916) 895-3429.
PRESIDENT
Claire Tamarelle

Target Video
8859 Wilbur Ave., Northridge, CA 91324, (818) 993-7669; (800) 222-7555. (Subsidiary of Essex Video.)

CUSTOMER CONTACT
Nancy Pera

Teaching Films, Inc.
930 Pitner Ave., Evanston, IL 60202, (312) 328-6700. (Distributor of educational films and videos for the professional medical and allied health markets.)

PRESIDENT
Joe Farragher
CHAIRMAN
Joel Altschul
EXECUTIVE VICE PRESIDENT
Esther Altschul
VICE PRESIDENT
Bruce Colling
MARKETING MANAGER
Beth Kon

Thunderbird Films
Box 65157, Los Angeles, CA 90065.

Trans World Entertainment
6430 Sunset Boulevard, Suite 505, Hollywood, CA 90028, (213) 461-0467. Organized 1983. (Production of feature films, sales of all media worldwide, domestic video distribution.)

CHAIRMAN
Moshe Diamant
PRESIDENT
Sunil R. Shah

United Entertainment, Inc.
4111 So. Darlington St., Suite 600, Tulsa, OK 74135, (918) 622-6460. Organized 1983. (Manufactures and distributes pre-recorded video.)

PRESIDENT
Bill Blair
EXECUTIVE VICE PRESIDENT
Robert Blair
NATIONAL DIRECTOR, SALES & MARKETING
Rick Buehler
BRANCHES
18178 Mollie Lane, Yorba Linda, CA 92686
245 Unquowa Rd. #133, Fairfield, CT 06430

Universal Home Video
919 N. Broad St., Philadelphia, PA 19123, (215) 232-1100. (Subsidiary of Universal Record Distributing Corp.)

PRESIDENT
Harold B. Lipsius
MARKETING & SALES
Tony Putnick
Lou Reeve

VC II Home Video
13402 Wyandotte Ave., North Hollywood, CA 91605, (800) 221-4274. Organized 1978. (Acquires program licensing for video distribution. Produces, manufactures and distributes [worldwide] theatrical, cable and video.)

CHIEF OPERATING OFFICER
Rudy Sutton
MARKETING DIRECTOR
Dave Stevens
ACQUISITIONS
Mike Fredrychs

VTR Distributors, Inc.
105 Broadway Ave., Carnegie, PA 15106, (412) 279-9100; (800) 245-1172.

PRESIDENT
Paul Pasquarelli
CHAIRMAN
Zack Pilossoph

VVI Distributors Inc.
5320 Old Pineville Rd., Charlotte, NC 28210, (704) 525-3600; (800) 438-8273.

PRESIDENT
Patricia Ridenhour
MARKETING
Christopher Bodmer

Vencompass, Inc.
155 W. 8th St., Erie, PA 16501, (814) 453-7704.

PRESIDENT
Pamela Venable

Vidcom
175 West 2700 South, Salt Lake City, UT 84115, (801) 487-8888. Organized 1983. (Video software distributor.)

VICE PRESIDENT, GENERAL MANAGER
Gary A. Chytraus
VICE PRESIDENT, SALES & MARKETING
Ronald E. Chytraus
AFFILIATIONS
VSDA, NAVD

VidAmerica
231 E. 55 St., New York, NY 10022; (212) 355-1600.

Video Action
708 W. First St., Los Angeles, CA 90012; (213) 687-8262. Organized 1981. (Video production and distribution.)

OWNER (PARTNER)
Leslie T. Hamasaki
OWNER (PARTNER)
Ruth Watanabe
OPERATIONS MANAGER
Gregg S. Yokoyama

Video Aided Instruction, Inc.
182 Village Rd., East Hills, NY 11577; (516) 621-6176. Organized 1983. (Produces instructional, educational videocassettes.)

PRESIDENT
Peter Lanzer
VICE PRESIDENT
Mona Lanzer
BOARD OF DIRECTORS
Peter Lanzer, Mona Lanzer

Video Cassette Marketing Corp.
137 Eucalyptus, El Segundo, CA 90245; (213) 322-1140, (800) 492-3548.

PRESIDENT
James Spencer

Video City Productions
4266 Broadway, Oakland, CA 94611; (415) 428-0202. Organized 1983. (Manufactures and distributes pre-recorded VHS and Beta film product.)

MARKETING DIRECTOR
Bob Brown
OTHER COMPANY OWNED LABELS:
Combat Video, Art House Video, Chop 'Em Ups Video

Video Connection
3123 Sylvania Ave., Toledo, OH 43613; (419) 472-7727.

PRESIDENT
John Day

Video Dimensions
110 E. 23 St., Suite 603, New York, NY 10010; (212) 533-5999.

Video Gems
731 North La Brea Ave., Los Angeles, CA 90038; (213) 938-

2385. Organized 1979. (Manufacturer and distributor of pre-recorded videocassettes.)

PRESIDENT
Joseph Infante
VICE PRESIDENT
Vivienne Infante

Video Home Library

75 Spring St., New York, NY 10012; (212) 925-7744.

PRESIDENT
Andre D'Apice

Video Library of Arts

716 S. Main, Broken Arrow, OK 74012; (918) 251-0466. (Division of Ken Meyer Productions.)

PRESIDENT
Ken Meyer

The Video Naturals Company

2590 Glen Green, Suite #6, Los Angeles, CA 90068; (213) 469-0019. Organized 1982. (Produces and distributes "mood videos" for the home video market.)

PRESIDENT/OWNER
Steve Siporin
AFFILIATIONS
Distributors: Videotakes; Norstar; Metro Video

Video One Video Inc.

1600 124 Ave. N.E. Suite E., Bellevue, WA 98005; (206) 454-5992.

VICE PRESIDENT, SALES
Jim Koch

Video Paradise, Inc.

115 W. Main St., Westboro, MA 01581; (617) 366-8890.

PRESIDENT
Donald Rogers

Video Products

2428 Glendale Lane, Sacramento, CA 95825; (916) 971-9111.

VICE PRESIDENT
Bill Lapkin
BRANCH
19226 66th Ave. S., Kent, WA 98032, Erin Morgan (manager)

Video Reel, Inc.

7009 Owensmouth Ave., Suite 201, Canoga Park, CA 91303; (818) 710-1823. Organized 1983. (Produces and duplicates how-to sports videos.)

PRESIDENT
Robert Mann
VICE PRESIDENT
Bonnie Krolop
TREASURER
Robert Mann
SECRETARY
Bonnie Krolop
BOARD OF DIRECTORS
Robert S. Mann, Bonnie L. Krolop
AFFILIATION
Recording Association of America

Video Releasing Co. of Hawaii

1370 Kapiolani Blvd., Room 101A, Honolulu, HI 96814; (808) 946-1000. Organized 1975. (Wholesale distribution of videocassette programs.)

GENERAL PARTNER
John Dobovan

Video Services of America

1296 N. Post Oak Rd., Houston, TX 77055; (713) 957-0050; (800) 231-1717.

PRESIDENT
Will Smith

MARKETING & SALES
Doug Donnell

Video Trend, Inc.

12900 Richfield Court, Livonia, MI 48150; (313) 591-0200. Organized 1979. (Distributor of pre-recorded video.)

PRESIDENT
Gene Silverman
VICE PRESIDENTS
Robert Tollini
Carol Kloster
BRANCHES
Detroit, Chicago, Tampa, Seattle, Salt Lake City, Sacramento, San Francisco

Video Update Inc.

1636 Gervais, St. Paul, MN 55109; (612) 770-3779.

PRESIDENT
John Bedard
MARKETING & SALES
Bruce Carlson

Video Vision Associates, Inc.

7 Waverly Place, Madison, NJ 07940; (201) 377-0302.

PRESIDENT
William Clark
MARKETING & SALES
Patrick Binns

Videobrary

3518 Cahuenga Blvd. West, Suite 301, Hollywood, CA 90068; (213) 851-5811.

PRESIDENT
Tom Corradine
MARKETING & SALES
Paul Lisy

Videocasa

3911 Ponce de Leon Blvd. #2, Coral Gables, FL 33134; (305) 443-1335 and 854-1141, (800) 835-7612. Organized 1984. (Distributes Spanish language videotapes for the home entertainment market.)

PRESIDENT
Dennis Chern
VICE PRESIDENT
Raquel Bardisa
SALES REPRESENTATIVE
Jose Arenal
SALES REPRESENTATIVE, N.Y. OFFICE
Neil Farbman
AFFILIATIONS
Cinelatino

Videocassette Marketing Corporation

137 Eucalyptus Drive, El Segundo, CA 90245; (213) 322-1140, (800) 332-1140. Organized 1984. (Distributes children's, environmental and subliminal pre-recorded videocassettes to video stores and consumers.)

GENERAL MANAGER
Cindy E. Greisdorf

Videofashion

One West 37 St., 5th floor, New York, NY 10018; (212) 869-4666. Organized 1976. (World's first "Videomagazine." Produces and distributes 40 programs each year of fashion and lifestyle videos.)

CHAIRMAN & PRESIDENT
Nicholas Charney
INTERNATIONAL DISTRIBUTION
Marlene B. McGinnis

Videolearning Systems, Inc.

354 W. Lancaster Ave., Haverford, PA 19041; (215) 896-6600.

PRESIDENT
Homer H. Hewitt, III

Videomarketing and Distributing Inc.

14001 Richdale Dr., #200, Minnetonka, MN 55343; (612) 544-8588, (800) 328-4815.

PRESIDENT
Mark Saliterman
VICE PRESIDENT, SALES
Sid Haskowitz

Videoplan, Inc.

1448 W. Rosecrans Ave., Gardena, CA 90249; (213) 532-9024.

PRESIDENT
Peter Jacobs

Videotakes, Inc.

220 Shrewsbury Ave., Red Bank, NJ 07701; (201) 747-2444. Organized 1982. (Marketing of non-feature film videocassettes.)

PRESIDENT
Joe Kennedy, 509 Fisk Ave., Brielle, NJ 08730
SECRETARY
Jenny Peters, 26 W. 83 St., NY, NY 10024

Videoways

10,000 N.W. 80th Ave., Hialeah Gardens, FL 33016; (305) 557-5262.

PRESIDENT
Angel Tamargo

WEA, Corp. (Warner/Elektra/Atlantic Corp.)

111 N. Hollywood, Way, Burbank, CA 91505; (818) 843-6311. (Subsidiary of Warner Communications, Inc.)

PRESIDENT
Henry Droz
MARKETING & SALES
Dave Mount

Wall of Fame

13240 N.E. 20, Bldg., 19, Bellevue, WA 98005; (206) 643-9038. (Subsidiary of Independent Video Source.)

PRESIDENT
Weston Nishimura
MARKETING & SALES
Covington Vego

Wax Works/Video Works National Distributor

325 East 3rd St., Owensboro, KY 42301;, (800) 626-1918. Organized 1979. (Video distributor of all national major lines. Also audio distributor.)

PRESIDENT
Terry Woodward
SALES MANAGER
Kirk Kirkpatrick
CREDIT MANAGER
Bill Burton
BUYER
Noel Clayton
BRANCHES
4011 Winchester Rd., Memphis, TN 38118; (800) 331-0993, (901) 366-4088

Weiss Global Enterprises

2055 Saviers Rd., Suite 12, Oxnard, CA 93033; (805) 486-4495. Organized 1974. (Distributes television and motion picture programming.)

PRESIDENT
Adrian Weiss
SECRETARY & TREASURER
Steven A. Weiss
VICE PRESIDENTS
Ethel L. Weiss
Laurie Weiss
OPERATIONS MANAGER
Patricia C. Sandoval
INFORMATION SERVICES
Alex Gordon

REPRESENTATIVES
Midwest: Century Broadcasting Corp., E. Melvin Pinsel, 875 North Michigan Ave., Chicago, IL 60611; (312) 922-1000
Southeast/Southwest: Hank Profenius, 3207 W. Friendly Ave., Greensboro, NC 27408; (919) 292-1434
Texas; Arkansas; Oklahoma; & Memphis, TN: A. Scott Lanken, 795 Walnut Hill La., Apt. 302, Dallas, TX 75230; (214) 696-0518
Top 50 Markets: Gray-Schwartz Enterprises, Inc., Marv Gray, 4764 Park Granada, Suite 207, Calabasas, CA 91302; (818) 702-9888
Ancillary Markets: Tom J. Corradine, 3518 Cahuenga W., Suite 301, Hollywood, CA 90068; (213) 851-5811
West: Hank Guzik, P.O. Box 15911, San Diego, CA 92115; (619) 693-1683
Home Video: Vistar International Productions, Richard S. Ellman, Myles Spector, 3790 Dunn Dr., Suite C, Los Angeles, CA 90034; (213) 204-3392
FOREIGN
Latin America and Caribbean: D.L. Taffner/Limited, Rick Karo 31 W. 56 St., New York, NY 10019; (212) 245-4680
Far East: D.L. Taffner Australia Pty. Ltd., Neville Van Dyke, Unit 20, Greenwich Square, 130-134 Pacific Highway, Greenwich N.S.W. 2065, Australia; (612) 439-5699
Canada: D.L. Taffner & Associates, Janice Currie, 9 Prince Arthur Ave., Toronto, Ontario M5R 1B2, Canada; (416) 928-2922
Australia & New Zealand: D.L. Taffner Australia Pty. Ltd., Brett Weinberg, Unit 20, Greenwich Square, 130-134 Pacific Highway, Greenwich N.S.W. 2065, Australia; (612) 439-5699
Europe and United Kingdom: D.L. Taffner UK Ltd., George Blaug, 10 Bedford Square, London WC1B 3RA, England; (441) 631-1184

West Glenn

1430 Broadway, New York, NY 10018; (212) 921-0968.

EXECUTIVE VICE PRESIDENT
Vincent Cappuzzi

Western Film & Video, Inc.

30941 W. Agoura Rd., #302, West Lake Village, CA 91361; (818) 889-7350.

PRESIDENT
Gary R. Guenot

Western Publishing Company, Inc.

1220 Mound Ave., Racine, WI 53404; (414) 633-2431. (Subsidiary of Mattel Inc.)

PRESIDENT
Joseph Marino
VICE PRESIDENT, SALES
James O'Donnell

Weston Woods Studio Inc.

389 Newton Tpk., Weston, CT 06883; (203) 226-3355.

PRESIDENT
Morton Schindel
DIRECTOR OF MARKETING
Jerri Shaler

Wilson World Wide Video Systems, Inc.

2525 N.E. Broadway, Portland, OR 97232; (503) 281-6300.

PRESIDENT
Michael DeSimone

Win Records and Video, Inc.

45-50 38th Street, Long Island City, New York, NY 11101; (800) 221-1220, (800) 851-2525 (NY state). Organized 1955. (Wholesale distribution of home entertainment products: video software [full line]; records: tapes; CD's; and specially selected accessories.)

PRESIDENT
Sam Weiss
VICE PRESIDENT
George Weiss

Women Make Movies, Inc.

225 Lafayette St., Room 212, New York, NY 10012; (212) 925-0606. Organized 1972. (Facilitates the production, exhibition and distribution of media by and about women.)

PRESIDENT
Linda Gibson
VICE PRESIDENT

Elizabeth Merena
TREASURER
Joanne Sandler
SECRETARY
Wendy Lidell
BOARD OF DIRECTORS
Linda Gibson, Elizabeth Merena, Joanne Sandler, Wendy Lidell, Carolyn Jung, Bienvenida Matias, Carol Clement, Janet Benn, Blanca Vasquez, Madeline Anderson, Emma Cohn
AFFILIATIONS
Association of Independent Video and Filmmakers
The Women's Funding Coalition

World Almanac Education

1278 West Ninth St., Cleveland, OH 44113; (216) 621-7300. (Subsidiary of United Media-A Scripps Howard.)

PRESIDENT
Robert Metz
MARKETING & SALES
George Earl

World Vision Home Video, Inc.

660 Madison Ave., 3rd floor, New York, NY 10021; (212) 832-3838. Organized 1980. (Domestic home video distribution, marketing and sales.)

VICE PRESIDENT & GENERAL MANAGER
Tom Devlin
EASTERN DIVISION MANAGER
Carl Sansarica
MIDWEST DIVISION MANAGER
Brian O'Sullivan
WESTERN DIVISION MANAGER
Kathy Rost
SOUTHERN DIVISION MANAGER
Bruce Knox
MANAGER, SALES ADMINISTRATION
Shari Nowak
BRANCHES
Midwest, 625 N. Michigan Ave., Suite 410, Chicago, IL 60611
Southern, 14 Perimeter Center East, Suite 1406, Atlanta, GA 30346
Western, 9465 Wilshire Blvd., Suite 628, Beverly Hills, CA 90212
AFFILIATION
Taft Broadcasting Company

Worldwide Tape Distributors

223 Keats Dr., Sicklerville, NJ 08081; (609) 228-0205.

PRESIDENT
Ted Klempner

Worldwide Video

320 Grove St., Williamsport, PA 17701; (717) 323-8756.

GENERAL MANAGER
Mittie Oberdorf

ZBS Industries

701 Beta Drive, Cleveland, OH 44143; (800) 321-8774. Organized 1979. (Distributes pre-recorded video.)

PRESIDENT
Larry Beyer
VICE PRESIDENT
Earl Stein
SECRETARY/TREASURER
Jay Schultz
BOARD OF DIRECTORS
Larry Beyer, Earl Stein, Jay Schultz

Major Video Retail Stores

Academy Video
18122 Brookhurst St., #B, Fountain Valley, CA 92708; (714) 964-1691. (Video independent.)

OWNERS
Andy Richman
Susan Richman

Acorn Sports, Inc.
5816 Shakespeare Rd., Suite D, Columbia, SC 29204; (803) 735-0733. (Golf videos.)

PRESIDENT
D. Swing Meyer

Adventure Land Video
811 W. 11th St., Coffeyville, KS 67337; (316) 251-6165. (Video franchise.)

OWNER
Tim Kilpatrick

Aero-Space Visuals Society
1720 130 Ave. N.E., Bellevue, WA 98005; (206) 881-9444.

GENERAL MANAGER
Greg Maes

Alice In Videoland Ltd.
738 Ulster Ave., P.O. Box 2000-H, Kingston, NY 12401; (914) 338-5288. Organized 1983. (Video sales/rentals—televisions, stereo, sales. Related products' sales.)

PRESIDENT
Paula DeCesare
BRANCHES
Kingston, NY (2 locations); Saugerties, NY; Phoenicia, NY; Great Barrington, MA

All American Video-Los Osos
· 950 Los Osos Valley Rd., Los Osos, CA 93402; (805) 528-2820. (Franchise.)

PRESIDENT
Keith Lilley

All-In-One-Video
2806 N. Highway 441-27, Fruitland, FL 32731; (904) 326-3633. (Video chain.)

PRESIDENT
Gayle Lazenby

American Box Office Video Inc.
40 E. Main St., Hopkinton, MA 01748; (617) 435-5174, (617) 435-4270. Organized 1984. (4 video stores, video rack jobbers.)

PRESIDENT
Rachel Dworkin
BUYER
Steve Dworkin
CLERK
Mellissa Dworkin
BRANCHES
Milford, MA; Westboro, MA; Clinton, MA; Hudson, MA.
AFFILIATES
Somerville, Fitchburg, Framingham

American Home Video Corp./ Video Concepts Stores
7600 E. Orchard Rd., Suite 200, P.O. Box 5040, Denver, CO 80217; (303) 771-1282. (Subsidiary of Jack Eckerd Corp.) Video chain—270.

PRESIDENT
William G. Kelly
SOFTWARE BUYER
Mary F. Donovan
HARDWARE BUYER
David Nedelman

American Video Tape
1116 Edgewater Ave., Ridgefield, NJ 07657; (201) 941-4404, (800) 645-7186. (Subsidiary of American Tape.) Video, independent.

VICE PRESIDENT, MARKETING & SALES
Marc Gottlieb

Arizona Peddler
790 S. Main, Cottonwood, AZ 86326; (602) 634-5565. Independent video chain (3).

PRESIDENT
Jack Poland

At the Movies
1312 Round Rock Ave., Round Rock, TX 78664; (512) 255-6021. Independent video.

Audio Visuals of Tampa, Inc.
4333 W. Kennedy Blvd., Box 10099, Tampa, FL 33609; (813) 876-8718. Independent audio/visual.

PRESIDENT
Murray Segal

Barnes & Noble Inc.
122 Fifth Ave., New York, NY 10003; (212) 206-8800. Bookstore—independent chain.

DIRECTOR OF MARKETING
Barry Denenberg
SOFTWARE BUYER
Susan Barkan

Bee Gee Records & Tapes, Inc.
10 Northway Lane N., Latham, NY 12110; (518) 785-1122. Video chain (11).

PURCHASING
Mike Raikowski

Norman Beerger Productions
3217-A29, Arville St., Las Vegas, NV 89102-7612, (702) 876-2328. Organized 1984. (Produces and distributes wilderness home video programs.)

OWNER
Norman Beerger

Beverly Hills Videocentre, Inc.
187 S. Beverly Drive, Beverly Hills, CA 90212, (213) 550-1092. Organized 1980. (Sale and rental of pre-recorded videocassettes.)

PRESIDENT
Emil Reisman
SECRETARY
Jane Hamilton
BOARD OF DIRECTORS
Emil Reisman
BRANCHES
West Hollywood, CA 90046

Blackhawk Films, Inc.
1 Old Eagle Brewery, Davenport, IA 52802, (319) 323-9736. Independent franchise.

PRESIDENT
Ted Ewing

Les Blank's Flower Films and Video
10341 San Pablo Ave., El Cerrrio, CA 94530, (415) 525-0942. Organized 1967. (Seeks out and documents America's vanishing minority cultures, their music and traditions.)

PRODUCER/DIRECTOR/CAMERA
Les Blank
DISTRIBUTION MANAGER

Susan Kell
FOLKLORIST/2nd CAMERA
Christine Simon
EDITOR
Maureen Gosling

Bradford Video

394 S. Main St., Bradford, MA 01830, (617) 372-3160. Independent video.

OWNER
David Court

Bridgeport Video

742 W. 31st St., Chicago, IL 60616, (312) 326-1467. Independent video.

Britannica Video/Encyclopaedia Britannica

425 N. Michigan Ave., Chicago, IL 60611, (312) 321-6841. Direct mail.

Broadway Video

168 South Lake St., Forest Lake, MN 55025, (612) 464-8231. Organized 1982. (Supplies pre-recorded video tapes to an undersupplied market.)

MANAGER/OWNER
Thomas M. Houle
OWNER
Stuart J. Houle
BRANCHES
Broadway Video, Rack Jobbing

Brookshire Brothers Inc.

P.O. Box 1688, Lufkin, TX 75901, (409) 634-8155. Video chain (50).

PRESIDENT
W. Eugene Brookshire
SOFTWARE & HARDWARE BUYER
M.L. Colmer

Budget Video Inc.

(D/B/A Hollywood Home Theatre)
1540 N. Highland Ave., Suite 110, Hollywood, CA 90028, (213) 446-0121; (213) 466-0127. Organized 1979. (Dealer, distributor, retailer of video cassettes and laser discs.)

PRESIDENT
Larry S. Fine
VICE PRESIDENT
Stephen Stumbris

Calypso Video, Inc.

2040 Reynolds Rd., Southwyck Center, Toledo, OH 43614, (419) 865-4169. Independent video.

PRESIDENT
C. Opfermann

Canadian Tire Corp. Ltd.

P.O. Box 770, Station K, Toronto, Ont., Canada M4P 2V8, (416) 480-3000. Mass merchant. Chain (400 stores).

SOFTWARE BUYER
Rob Taylor

Cape Video, Inc.

Town Plaza, Cape Girardeau, MO 63701, (314) 651-4316. Electronics, independent.

PRESIDENT
Duane Bates

Captain Video

1326 Broad St., Central Falls, RI 02863, (401) 724-1297. Video, independent.

PRESIDENT
Fred Kilsey
VICE PRESIDENT & TREASURER
Mark Feinstein

Christopher's Video West, Inc.

8 S. 101st St., Rt. 59, Napverville, IL 60540, (313) 369-8993. Video independent.

PRESIDENT
P.A. Christopher
SECRETARY & TREASURER
S.L. Christopher

Cinema Concepts, Inc.

2461 Berlin Turnpike, Newington, CT 06111; (203) 667-1251. Organized 1971. (Non-theatrical distribution of entertainment motion pictures in 16mm, Beta, VHS, U-Matic, 8mm to school, libraries and home market. Mail-order plus three retail stores.)

PRESIDENT
Joel G. Jacobson
VICE PRESIDENT
Susan G. Jacobson
BRANCHES
Porter Plaza, Main St., Old Saybrook, CT 06475; (203) 388-1481
Rt. 72 Plaza, 859 Mill St., East Berlin, CT 06023; (203) 828-1815
AFFILIATIONS
Video Software Dealers Association (Joel Jacobson is a Board Director of CT Chapter)

City Lights Video, Inc.

98 Front St. South, Issaquah, Washington, 98027; (206) 392-6700. Organized 1983. (Sales and rental of video software.)

PRESIDENT
Alan Ligda
AFFILIATIONS
VSDA, (National and Washington State)

The Copps Corp.

2828 Wayne St., Stevens Point, WI 54481; (715) 344-5900. (Food and non-food distribution.)

CHAIRMAN
Michael Copps
PRESIDENT
Tim Copps
VICE PRESIDENT, WHOLESALE DISTRIBUTION
Fred Copps
VICE PRESIDENT, MERCHANDISING
Don Copps
VICE PRESIDENT, PUBLIC AFFAIRS
Tom Copps
VICE PRESIDENT, RETAIL OPERATIONS
Darrell Scherwinski
COMPTROLLER
Tom Seivwright

B. Dalton Bookseller

7505 Metro Blvd., Minneapolis, MN 55435; (612) 893-7000. (Subsidiary of Dayton Hudson.) Bookstore, chain.

SOFTWARE BUYER
Lesli Casciaro

Dawn's Video

519 W. Foothill, Suite C, Rialto, CA 92376; (714) 874-1414. Organized 1980. (Video specialty store.)

OWNER
Gregory C. George
BRANCHES
2085 E. Highland Ave., San Bernadino, CA 92404; (714) 864-3113
9725 Sierra, Fontana, CA 92335; (714) 350-8833
267 E. 40th, San Bernadino, CA 92404; (714) 883-5737
1330 Massachusetts Ave., Riverside, CA 92507; (714) 784-1414

Discount Video Tapes, Inc.

3717 W. Clark Ave., Suite B, Burbank, CA 91505; (818) 843-3366. Organized 1979. (Specializing in rare and unusual pre-recorded videos. Retail and wholesale.)

PRESIDENT
Woody Wise

Dodd Camera & Video

27179 Chagrin Blvd., Woodmere, OH 44122; (216) 292-2825. (Subsidiary of The Dodd Co.) Electronics, video chain (10 stores).

PRESIDENT
Richard L. Greiner, Sr.
MANAGER & SOFTWARE BUYER
Don Carter
VICE PRESIDENT & HARDWARE BUYER
Rick Greiner
GENERAL MANAGER
Don Carter

Doubleday & Co., Inc.

245 Park Ave., New York, NY 10167; (212) 953-4916. Mail order.

VICE PRESIDENT
Bernard Schwartz

Downtown Video

3110 W. Peterson, Chicago, IL 60659; (312) 338-1600. (Subsidiary of Downtown Records Inc.) Video chain (6 stores).

PRESIDENT
Howard Rosen
DIRECTOR & SOFTWARE BUYER
Ronald W. Kehr
HARDWARE BUYER
Ron Fischell

Entertainment Specialties

7007 Bandera Rd. #6, San Antonio, TX 78238; (512) 647-1183. (Subsidiary of W.T.S. Enterprises.) Video, independent.

PRESIDENT
Les Bank
SOFTWARE BUYER
Linda M. Skinner

Entertainment Tonite Video

Route 340 E., Charlestown, WV 25414; (304) 725-1216. (Subsidiary of MSA, Inc.) Video, novelty, farmers, market/grocery independent.

SOFTWARE & HARDWARE BUYER
Cullen Rinaldi

Everybody's Records Tapes & Video

5279 N. Lombard, Portland, OR 97203; (503) 286-9841. Organized 1971. (Home entertainment software.)

PRESIDENT
Tom Keenan
AFFILIATIONS
VSDA

Family Video

740 Mt. View Dr., Rapid City, SD 57702; (605) 348-7572. Video independent.

PRESIDENTS & BUYERS
Richard Ireland
Christine Ireland

Flower Films & Video

(see Les Blank's Flower Films & Video.)

French & Spanish Book Corp.

115 Fifth Ave., New York, NY 10003; (212) 673-7400. Bookstore, independent.

PRESIDENT
Emanuel Molho

Fu Tech

444 Ferry St., S.E., Salem, OR 97301; (503) 371-0410. Electronics, independent.

PRESIDENT
Ronald G. Rubel
GENERAL MANAGER, SOFTWARE & HARDWARE BUYER
Ron Rubel

G&A Stores, Inc./d/b/a Curtis Mathes

2500 S. Center, Marshalltown, Iowa 50158; (515) 752-5541. Organized 1984. (Sells TVs, VCRs, video cameras, and movie rental.)

PRESIDENT & TREASURER
Glenn Stalzer
VICE PRESIDENT & SECRETARY
Ann Stalzer

Great American Movie Emporium

5055 S. Kipling St., Suite C-9, Littleton, CO 80127; (303) 972-8200. (Subsidiary of Charvin Enterprises, Inc.) Video, franchise.

PRESIDENT
Charles E. De Shazer
VICE PRESIDENT, SOFTWARE & HARDWARE BUYER
Garvin De Shazer

Greenleaf Video, Inc.

2049 Century Park East, Suite 5121, Los Angeles, CA 90067; (213) 557-2043. Organized 1984 (Sells alternative videos to consumers and libraries.)

PRESIDENT
Barbara K. Greenleaf
SECRETARY
Jon W. Greenleaf

Hearst Marine Books

105 Madison Ave., New York, NY 10016; (212) 889-3050. (Division of William Morrow, Inc.) Catalog sales.

Home Entertainment Emporium

2100 Sepulveda Blvd., Manhattan Beach, CA 90266; (213) 546-2501. Video independent.

PRESIDENT & SOFTWARE BUYER
Tom MacManus
SALES MANAGER & HARDWARE BUYER
Ken Stephens

Home Film Festival

305 Linden St., Scranton, PA 18503; (717) 342-2185; (800) 258-3456. Independent mail order, catalog.

PRESIDENT
Dan Jury
SOFTWARE BUYER
Arlene O'Malley

Home Movies, Inc.

1016 Juan Tabo N.E., Albuquerque, NM 87112; (505) 292-8578. Organized 1983. (Video sales and rentals.)

CHIEF EXECUTIVE OFFICER & PRESIDENT
Troy D. Richards
VICE PRESIDENT
Kent Richards
BRANCHES
Home Movies II, 1115 San Mateo S.E., Albuquerque, NM 87108
Home Movies LTD., 7120 Wyoming Blvd., Albuquerque, NM 87109
Home Movies, Downtown, 505½ Fifth St., Downtown Albuquerque, NM.

Home Theater Video

1504-A Wyoming N.E., Albuquerque, NM 87112; (505) 293-5784. Video independent.

PRESIDENT
David Baumgartner

Home Video Network, Inc.

Route 93, Conyngham, PA 18219; (717) 788-5211. Video, drugstores, independent.

PRESIDENT
Walter Haentjens, Jr.

HARDWARE & SOFTWARE BUYERS
Joseph Bayzick
Rick Haentjens

Home Video Northwest

P.O. Box 06600, 3717 S.E. 42nd Ave., Portland, OR 97206; (503) 775-3184. Video, bookstore independent.

PRESIDENT & SOFTWARE BUYER
Stewart Reif

IFEX FILMS/International Film Exchange Ltd.

201 W. 52 St., New York, NY 10019; (212) 582-4318. Organized 1959. (Domestic and international distribution of feature films, documentaries, shorts & video programs.)

CHAIRMAN OF THE BOARD
Arthur "Skip" Steloff
PRESIDENT
Gerald J. Rappoport
SENIOR VICE PRESIDENT
Richard Grisar
EXECUTIVE VICE PRESIDENT
Christopher Wood
VICE PRESIDENT, THEATRICAL SALES
Jefrey Jacobs
VICE PRESIDENT, INTERNATIONAL SALES
Joy Pereths

Innovations

110 Painters Mill Rd., Owings Mills, MD 21117; (301) 363-4300. Catalog sales, two retail stores.

CUSTOMER CONTACT
Sam Pripstein

International Home Videoclub, Inc.

220 Shrewsbury Ave., Red Bank, NJ 07701; (201) 741-7800, (800) 458-3000. Independent, mail order, catalog.

PRESIDENT
Joseph F. DeGraw

International Sailing Products

P.O. Box 355, Oyster Bay, NY 11771; (516) 922-5182, (800) 645-7676. Catalog, franchise (3 stores).

PRESIDENT
Steve Benjamin
VICE PRESIDENT
Paul Dickey

International Video

9576 Quivira Rd., Lenexa, KS 66215; (913) 492-2311. Organized 1983. (Retail video software.)

OWNER
Michael Rupani

JBC Video Vesting DBA Video Show

546 N. State College Blvd., Fullerton, CA 92631; (714) 871-0711. Organized 1981. (Sale and rental of video cassettes.)

OWNERS
Christine and Rudolph Neely

J&L Video Productions, Ltd.

195 S. Main #1, Longmont, CO 80501; (303) 772-8355. Video independent.

PRESIDENT
Lois Ann Jones

Stefaan Janssen Studio

4615 N. Lincoln Ave., Chicago, IL 60625; (312) 728-9277. Organized 1983. (Sells and produces special interest programs for the home video market. Mail order.)

OWNER
Stefaan Janssen

AFFILIATIONS
Member: VSDA; Center for New Television; AIFV

Kaleidoscope Home Video

700 E. Maple, Centerville, Iowa 52544; (515) 437-1674. Organized 1984. (Home video rental and sales.)

OWNERS
Russell K. Davis
Donna S. Davis
BRANCH
Albia Kaleidoscope, Albia, Iowa

King's Video Center

1325 West Warner, Santa Ana, CA 92704; (714) 662-2898. Organized 1982. (Retail video hardware and software, sales and rental.)
BRANCH
Video Palace, 1170 West Baker, Costa Mesa, CA 92626

Long Drug Stores

141 N. Civic Dr., Walnut Creek, CA 94596; (415) 937-1170. Drugstores, chain (192 stores).

MERCHANDISE MANAGER
Terry Sandin

MAS Productions

18434 Bermuda St., Northridge, CA 91326; (818) 360-0371. Mail order.

CUSTOMER CONTACT
Richard Stark

MSI Video

5020 Sunnyside Ave., Suite 112, Beltsville, MD 20705; (301) 474-2220. Organized 1981. (National mail order sales of videocassettes.)

PRESIDENT
Lee Masser

Manzi Video Sales, Inc.

261 Halstead Ave., Harrison, NY 10528; (914) 835-5005. (d/b/a The Video Connection #130.) Video franchise.

PRESIDENT & BUYER
Michael S. Manzi

Maui Video Center

55 Kaanumanu Ave., Kahului, HI 96732; (808) 871-7098. Organized 1981. (Video hardware and software, sales and rentals.)

OWNER
Donald A. Schwanborg
BRANCHES
Maui Mall, Kahului, HI 96732

Meredith Corp. Better Homes & Gardens Book Club

750 Third Ave., New York, NY 10017; (212) 551-7040. Mail order.

CUSTOMER CONTACT
Jane Hamada

Metaventures

1102 S. Buchanan St., Arlington, VA 22204; (703) 845-8635. Video independent.

PRESIDENT & BUYER
Philip Latasa

Montgomery Video Inc.

18268 Village Mart Dr., Olney, MD 20832; (301) 774-2014. Video chain (5 stores.)

PRESIDENT & BUYER
Lou Kaufman

Morris Video

936 Hermosa Ave., First Floor, Hermosa Beach, CA 90254; (213) 374-4984. Organized 1984. (Produces and distributes quality information and entertainment video. Mail order.)

PRESIDENT & C.E.O.
Dawn Morris
VICE PRESIDENT & C.F.O.
George Morris, Ph.D.
BOARD OF DIRECTORS
Dawn Morris, George Morris, Ph.D., George Bott, David Van Horn.
BRANCHES
663 The Village, Redondo Beach, CA 90277; (213) 374-4984.

The Movie Merchants

3254 Youngfield St., Wheat Ridge CO 80033; (303) 234-9282. Organized 1980. (Video retailer.)

PRESIDENT & TREASURER
Shelley Gooch
VICE PRESIDENT & SECRETARY
Patrick Gooch
BOARD OF DIRECTORS
William Rahmig, Ramon Morton
BRANCHES
3186 S. Parker Rd., Aurora, CO 80014
9868 W. Belleview Ave., Littleton, CO 80023
7562 S. University, Littleton, CO 80122
AFFILIATIONS
VSDA, Wheat Ridge Chamber of Commerce

Movies Tonite

935 E. Broad St., Columbus, OH 43205; (614) 253-0193. Video independent.

PRESIDENT
John Sandefur
VICE PRESIDENT, SOFTWARE BUYER
Debra Harrington
VICE PRESIDENT, HARDWARE BUYER
Jane Sandefur

Movies Unlimited

7421 Manchester, St. Louis, MO 63143; (314) 781-4111. (Subsidiary of Video Information Corp.) Video chain (4 stores).

PRESIDENT
Kevin R. Toal

Movies Unlimited

6736 Castor Ave., Philadelphia, PA 19149; (215) 722-8298. Retail stores, mail order.

GENERAL MANAGER
Mr. Weiss

Music Plus Video

2551 S. Alameda St., Los Angeles, CA 90058; (213) 234-3336. (Subsidiary of Show Industries d/b/a Music Plus.) Video chain (34 stores).

PRESIDENT
Lou Fogelman
SOFTWARE BUYER
Mitch Perlis

Musical Sales Company

40 S. Caroline St., Baltimore, MD 21231; (301) 675-1400. (One-stop record, tape, CD, video [pre-recorded], and related accessories.)

PRESIDENT
Milton I. Bereson
VICE PRESIDENT
Molly E. Bereson

Nantucket Video Inc.

42 Main St., Nantucket, MA 02554; (617) 228-0101. Video independent.

PRESIDENT & BUYER
Gene Mahon

National Video, Inc.

7325 NE 55th Ave., Portland, OR 97218; (503) 284-2965. Organized 1980. (Franchisor of retail video specialty stores.)

PRESIDENT
Ron Berger
EXECUTIVE VICE PRESIDENT
Troy Cooper
VICE PRESIDENT, FINANCE
F. Kim Cox
BOARD OF DIRECTORS
Ron Berger, William LeVine, Jack Silverman, L. Barton Alexander, Byron Boothe, Ken Koger, Peter Dal Bianco

New Breed Music

P.O. Box 661, Pomona, CA 91768; (714) 623-1999. Independent video.

PRESIDENT
Jesse Mac Lynum, Jr.

New Mode Media

1 Park Ave., Old Greenwich, CT 06870; (203) 637-3616. (Division of Listening Library, Inc.) Catalog sales.

PRESIDENT
Anthony Ditlow

New York Video

717 Lexington Ave., 2nd floor, New York, NY 10022; (212) 755-4640. Organized 1978. (Video retailer specializing in custom audio video installations.)

PRESIDENT
Giovanni Cozzi
VICE PRESIDENT
Louise Cozzi

Nightingale-Conant Corp.

7300 N. Lehigh Ave., Niles, IL 60648; (312) 647-0300. Catalog sales.

CUSTOMER CONTACT
John Graham

Opening Night Video

9007 Willowbrook Mall, Wayne, NJ 07470; (201) 890-0066. Video chain (3 stores).

PRESIDENT
Harold Rosenbaum
VICE PRESIDENT & SOFTWARE BUYER
Joyce Mendelowitz

Osco Drug Inc.

1818 Swfit Dr., Oak Brook IL 60521; (312) 887-5000. Drug, chain (400 stores).

ELECTRONICS BUYER
Dean Kelsey

Palmer Video Corporation

1767 Morris Avenue, Union, NJ 07083; (201) 686-3030. Organized 1981. (Franchisor—video stores.)

PRESIDENT
Peter Balner
VICE PRESIDENT
Peter Margaritondo
VICE PRESIDENT, FINANCE
Joseph Berger

Paradise Video, Inc.

1063 Lower Main St., Suite C-109, Wailuku, Maui, HA 96793; (808) 244-9790. Organized 1981.

PRESIDENT
Calvin H. Inouye
VICE PRESIDENT
Jeffrey K. Yamanishi
SECRETARY & TREASURER
Alfred Cantorna
BRANCHES
250 Alamaha St., Kahului, Maui, HA 96732

AFFILIATIONS
VSDA

Pathmark

301 Blaire Rd., Woodbridge, NJ 07095; (201) 499-3000. Supermarket chain. Rental only.

CUSTOMER CONTACT
Gordon Keil

Popingo Video, Inc.

257 N. Broadway, Suite 400, Wichita, KS 67202; (316) 263-3456. Video franchise.

PRESIDENT
Byron W. Boothe
SOFTWARE BUYER
Ron Penix

Public Access Producers Association

2652 N. Winchell, Portland, OR 97217; (503) 289-2309. Video, direct mail, independent.

DIRECTOR & SOFTWARE BUYER
R.S. Kolemaine

Publishers Central Bureau

1 Park Ave., New York, NY 10016; (212) 532-9200. Catalog, mail order. Independent video.

DIRECTOR
John Ward

Pueblo Home Video, Inc.

1302 N. Elizabeth, Pueblo, CO 81003; (303) 546-3555. Video, independent.

PRESIDENT & BUYER
Waren E. Lombard
VICE PRESIDENT & BUYER
Carol Lombard

Rare Bird Video, Inc.

482 Broome St., New York, NY 10013; (212) 334-8150. Video chain (3 stores).

PRESIDENT
Jack Morris
SOFTWARE & HARDWARE BUYERS
Jack Morris
Wayne Quackenbush

Record & Video Warehouse

3110 W. Peterson, Chicago, IL 60659; (312) 338-1600. (Subsidiary of Record & Video Warehouse Inc.) Video, chain (6 stores).

PRESIDENT
Howard Rosen
SOFTWARE BUYER & DIRECTOR
Ronald W. Kehr
HARDWARE BUYER
Ron Fischell

Red Fox Video

Route 209 E., Elizabethville, PA 17023; (717) 362-3391.

Rehabfilm

1123 Broadway, New York, NY 10010; (212) 741-5160. Non-profit, private organization. (Subsidairy of Rehabilitation Int'l, U.S.A.)

DIRECTOR OF MEDIA
John F. Moses

Rite Aid Corp.

Trindle Rd. and Railroad Ave. Shiremanstown, PA 17091; (717) 761-2633. Drug chain (315 stores).

DIRECTOR
Jerry Cardinale
VIDEO BUYER
Gwen Monn

Rizzoli/A.C. Video

597 Fifth Ave., New York, NY 10017; (212) 223-0100. Organized 1985. Bookstore chain.

DIRECTOR
John Brancati

S.K. Video Co.

2563½ Harrison Ave., Butte, MT 59701; (406) 782-8211. Video, independent.

BUYER
Robert C. Wilson

San Francisco Home Video

1629 Pine St., San Francisco, CA 94109; (415) 673-9595. Video chain (11 stores). (Subsidiary of Georano, Inc.)

PRESIDENT
James O. George
SOFTWARE BUYER
Maria Williamson
HARDWARE BUYER & SALES MANAGER
Peter Hope

Schnuck Markets, Inc.

12921 Enterprise Way, Bridgeton, MO 63044; (314) 344-9600. Food markets, chain.

PRESIDENT
Craig D. Schnuck
BUYER
Cynthia Parentin

Sears and Roebuck, Co.

Sears Tower, Dept. 40-15, Chicago, IL 60684; (312) 875-8306. Department store, chain (810 stores).

MARKETING MANAGER
Mike Mangan

Shows To Go Video Centers of America, Inc.

6702 N. Cedar, Suite 204, Fresno, CA 93710; (209) 299-4306. Video chain (92 stores).

PRESIDENT
Bernard Horton
EXECUTIVE VICE PRESIDENT, SOFTWARE & HARDWARE BUYER
Mike Sherlock

Sound Warehouse

P.O. Box 75879, Oklahoma, OK 73147; (405) 947-1131. Video chain (40 stores).

SOFTWARE BUYERS
Buster Bassett
Alan Ziegal

Stansbury Stereo and Video Center

6330 Frankford Ave., Baltimore, MD 21206; (301) 488-9600. Electronics, independent video.

PRESIDENT
Jim Disney
VICE PRESIDENT & SOFTWARE BUYER
Dale Bennett
HARDWARE BUYERS
Jim Disney and Dale Bennett

Studio Associates Video Division

2049 Reynolds St., Sarasota, FL 33581; (813) 921-3474. (Subsidiary of Studio Associates, Inc.) Photographic darkroom, and independent video retailer.

SOFTWARE & HARDWARE BUYER
Charles Cyphers

Sunset Software

2265 Westwood Blvd., #140, Los Angeles, CA 90064; (213) 474-2446. Video, mail order.

PRESIDENT & SOFTWARE BUYER
Will Swan

Supervideo
417 Colorado Ave., Santa Monica, CA 90401; (213) 394-9696. Independent, video. (Subsidiary of Exploration in Video.)
PRESIDENT & HARDWARE BUYER
Nissim Raphael
STORE MANAGER & SOFTWARE BUYER
Liz Cervantes

TV Collector
P.O. Box 188, Needham, MA 02192; (617) 238-1179. Organized 1976. (TV nosalgia magazine/tape trading marketplace.)
PUBLISHER
Stephen W. Albert
EDITOR
Diane L. Albert

Tele-Video Enterprises, Inc.
813 W. Main St., Suite 22, Battle Ground, WA 98604; (206) 687-7239 (d/b/a Video City USA) Independent.
PRESIDENT & BUYER
Dan Riley

Times Mirror Magazines-Book Division
380 Madison Ave., New York, NY 10017; (212) 687-3000. (Subsidiary of Times Mirror, Co.) Book club.
EDITORIAL DIRECTOR
Grace Mischkin

Toys "R" Us
395 W. Passaic St., Rochelle Park, NJ 07662; (201) 845-5033. Chain (199 stores). Children's programs.

Transworld Video Inc.
22761 Pacific Coast Highway, Malibu, CA 90265; (213) 456-7071. (Subsidiary of Video Connection of America.) National procurement office for Video Connection franchise stores.
NATIONAL SALES MANAGER
Peter Barry

United Video, Inc.
500 Church St. North, Concord, NC 28025; (704) 788-2012. Organized 1981.
PRESIDENT & SECRETARY
Margaret R. Flower
VICE PRESIDENT & TREASURER
Kenneth G. Flower

Universal Video
13228 Converse Rd., San Antonio, TX 78233; (512) 656-2558. Independent.
PRESIDENTS
Alice and Gordon Haskell
BRANCH
8723 FM 471 West, San Antonio, TX 78250; (512) 647-1096.

University of Southern California
Davidson Conference Center, University Park, Los Angeles, CA 90089-0871; (213) 743-5219. Independent.
EXECUTIVE DIRECTOR
Philip J. Rapa

Video #1
8611 W. 95th St., Hickory Hills, IL 60457; (312) 598-0001. Independent.
PRESIDENT
Carole Bartolini
SOFTWARE & HARDWARE BUYER
Dave Able

Video Action
708 W. First St., Los Angeles, CA 90012; (213) 687-8262. Organized 1981. (Video production and distribution.)
OWNER (PARTNER)
Leslie T. Hamasaki
OWNER (PARTNER)
Ruth Watanabe
OPERATIONS MANAGER
Gregg S. Yokoyama

Video Age, Inc.
4820 Excelsior Blvd., Suite 112, Minneapolis, MN 55416; (612) 927-7484. Mail order, telephone sales.
PRESIDENT
William J. Hudlow

Video Biz
113 S. Third St., Richmond, VA 23219; (804) 788-1902. Video chain (7 stores). (Subsidiary of Video Products, Inc.)
PRESIDENT & HARDWARE BUYER
Scott Moffett
SOFTWARE BUYERS
Scott Moffett
Sharon Krohn

Video Biz—North Shore, Inc.
50 Maplewood Ave., Gloucester, MA 01930; (617) 283-3721. Video, franchise.
PRESIDENT & BUYER
Sarah S. Wall

Video Boulevard, Inc.
241 Haverford Ave., Narberth, PA 19072; (215) 664-4136. Organized 1981. (Video rentals and sales.)
PRESIDENT
Steven J. Freid
BRANCH
Video Boulevard, Inc., 5425 Oxford Ave., Philadelphia, PA 19124; (215) 288-2250.

Video Center Stores
750 S. Solano, Las Cruces, NM 88001; (505) 523-8907. (Subsidiary of Pata Corp.) Video, chain (6 stores).
PRESIDENT & SOFTWARE BUYER
Pat Kilpatrick

Video Centre
P.O. Box 1982, Winter Park, FL 32790; (305) 682-3070. Video, independent.
PRESIDENT & SOFTWARE BUYER
Philip Lashinsky

Video Channel Inc.
20103 Saticoy St., Room 2, Canoga Park, CA 91306; (818) 993-8273. Organized 1984. (Video tape sales and rentals.)
PRESIDENT & BUYER
Jeff S. Dickel

The Video Circuit
11507 S.W. Pacific Hwy., Portland, OR 97223; (503) 246-8852. Video chain (3 stores). (Subsidiary of Video Futures, Inc.)
PRESIDENT & BUYER
Leo A. Jerman

Video City Productions
4266 Broadway, Oakland, CA 94611; (415) 428-0202. Organized 1983. (Manufactures and distributes pre-recorded VHS and Beta film product.) Video, chain (9 stores).
MARKETING DIRECTOR
Bob Brown
OTHER COMPANY OWNED LABELS:
Combat Video, Art House Video, Chop 'Em Ups Video

Video Club
220 Shrewsbury Ave., Red Bank, NJ 07701; (201) 741-7800, (800) 458-3000. Independent, adult catalog.

PRESIDENT
Joseph DeGraw

Video Concepts Stores
(See American Home Video.)

Video Connection
3123 Sylvania Ave., Toledo, OH 43613; (419) 472-7727. Video specialty, chain (8 stores independent).

PRESIDENT
John Day

Video Connection of America, Inc.
22761 Pacific Coast Highway, Malibu CA 90265; (213) 456-7071. National headquarters for 200 franchised video stores.

PRESIDENT
Bert Tenzer
DIRECTOR OF FRANCHISE SALES
John Barry

Video Corner
553 49th St. S., St. Petersburg, FL 33707; (813) 321-2122. Video, chain (3 stores).

PRESIDENT & HARDWARE BUYER
Bob Skidmore
VICE PRESIDENT & SOFTWARE BUYER
John P. Gallagher
GENERAL MANAGER & HARDWARE BUYER
Richard E. Smith

Video Cove
5047 E. Elliot Rd., Phoenix, AZ 85044; (602) 893-9609. Video, independent.

PRESIDENT & BUYER
Bob Mulvihill

Video Crossroads
5448 Beach Blvd., Buena Park, CA 90621; (714) 521-3870. Video, franchise.

PRESIDENT
Ralph Zink
SOFTWARE & HARDWARE BUYER
Corinne Zink

The Video Exchange, Inc.
198 Union Blvd., Room 100, Lakewood, CO 80228; (303) 988-8540, (800) 423-9357. Organized 1981. (Sale of video rental store franchises.) Chain (85 stores).

PRESIDENT
Allen Kenfield
VICE PRESIDENTS
David Kenfield
James Perry
BOARD OF DIRECTORS
Allen Kenfield, David Kenfield, James Perry, Martin Kenfield
AFFILIATIONS
Venture Capital backed by Allied Capital Corp., Wash., DC

Video Experience
401 I St., Suite B., Arcata, CA 95521; (707) 826-1105. Video, independent.

PRESIDENT & BUYER
Doug Simas

Video Flicks
141 Caldwell Blvd., Nampa, ID 83651; (208) 465-5773. Video, independent.

PRESIDENT & BUYER
Dale R. Durbin

Video Galore
4456 Lake St., Lake Charles, LA 70605; (318) 474-9791. Video, franchise.

OWNER & SOFTWARE BUYER
Michael K. O'Carroll

Video Island, Inc.
1645 Downtown West Blvd., Knoxville, TN 37919; (615) 694-8051. Video, independent.

PRESIDENT
Calvin E. Pippin
MANAGER & BUYER
Barbara Spence

Video Joe
1203 Eastridge Dr., Slidell, LA 70458; (504) 646-2482. Video, independent.

OWNER & BUYER
Joe B. Howard
BUYER
Rusty Howard

Video King
7360 N. Lincoln Ave., Lincolnwood, IL 60646; (312) 675-2910. Video, chain (14 stores).

MERCHANDISE MANAGER
Vance Frederico

The Video Library
4152 Woodruff Ave., Lakewood, CA 90713; (213) 420-8383. Organized 1982. (Rentals and sales of video tapes and VCRs.)

PRESIDENT
Steve Cantril
SECRETARY & TREASURER
Debbie Cantril
BOARD OF DIRECTORS
Richard Burdick, Kathleen Burdick
BRANCH
The Video Library, 6418 E. Spring St., Long Beach, CA 90815.

Video One
5055 Town North Dr., Shreveport, LA 71107; (318) 425-5652. Organized 1981. (Video software.)

OWNERS
Mary L. West
Samuel E. West
PURCHASING AGENT
Samuel L. West

Video Palace
4537 Duke St, Alexandria, VA 22304; (703) 823-5466. Video, independent.

PRESIDENT & BUYER
Rick Brooks
VICE PRESIDENT & BUYER
Doc Brooks

Video Paradise Inc.
115 W. Main St., Westboro, MA 01581; (617) 366-8890.

PRESIDENT
Donald Rogers

Video Playback
137 Route 516, Old Bridge, NJ 08857; (201) 679-4045. Video, independent chain (5 stores).

PRESIDENT & HARDWARE BUYER
Myron S. Kozak
SOFTWARE BUYER
Mary T. Kozak

Video Plus, Inc.
Box 526, Albuquerque, NM 87103; (505) 265-8801. Video, chain (2 stores).

PRESIDENT
Patrick Riley
SOFTWARE & HARDWARE BUYER
John Van Haverbeke

Video Product, Inc. T/A Video Biz

115 S. 3rd St., P.O. Box 5406, Richmond, VA 23220; (804) 788-1902. Organized 1980. (Retail video.)

PRESIDENT & TREASURER
Scott Moffett
VICE PRESIDENT
Tabetha Moffett
SECRETARY
Deborah J. Moffett
BOARD OF DIRECTORS
Scott Moffett, Deborah Moffett, Tabetha Moffett, Robert Moffett
BRANCHES
Richmond, VA—3 locations; Colonial Heights, VA; Roanoke, VA; Salem VA—1 location
AFFILIATIONS
Video Biz, Inc., VSDA

Video Replay

1668 Merriman Rd., Akron, OH 44313; (216) 836-9773. Video, chain (3 stores).

PRESIDENT & HARDWARE BUYER
J. Dwight Taylor
SOFTWARE BUYER
Jane Friedhoff

Video Revolution

20948 Mission Blvd., Hayward, CA 94541; (415) 481-2880. Video, independent.

OWNER & BUYER
Ole Nordhavn
BRANCHES
1339 Washington Ave., San Leandro, CA 94577; (415) 483-9620.

Video Shack, Inc.

1608 Broadway, New York, NY 10019; (212) 581-6260. Video, independent (14 stores).

Video Shaks-Video Marts

1010 N. State St., Orem, UT 84057; (801) 225-6906. Video, chain (28 stores).

PRESIDENT
Clyde Roper
VICE PRESIDENT & BUYER
Steve Roper

Video Shoppe

3507 U.S. 19, Suite D, Spring Hill, FL 33526; (904) 683-3561. Video, independent (2 stores).

MANAGER & BUYER
Bob Hall

Video Show

(See JBC Video Vesting)

Video Source

8618-A Menaul N.E., Albuquerque, NM 87110; (505) 292-8969. Video, independent.

PRESIDENT & BUYER
Mark Sanchez

Video Specialties Company

153 Town and Country, Houston, TX 77024; (713) 465-0702. Organized 1972. (Sale and rental of videocassettes.)

PRESIDENT
John F. Dinwoodie
VICE PRESIDENT
Ann C. Dinwoodie
BUYER
David C. Dinwoodie

Video Spectrum Inc.

1808 Willow Spring Rd., Baltimore, MD 21222; (301) 285-8273. Video, independent.

PRESIDENT & BUYER
Dennis M. Biedronski

Video Star

2413 E. Fifth St., Tyler, TX 75701; (214) 593-4166. (Subsidiary of Texas Rents/Movies, Etc.) Video, electronics, chain (34 stores).

PRESIDENT
R.E. Dietrick
OWNER & HARDWARE BUYER
Michael O. Byrne
SOFTWARE BUYER
Vicky Lynn Branan

Video Station

513 McDowell, St., Asheville, NC 28803; (704) 258-1145. Video, electronics, independent.

PRESIDENT
Mariano Raigo
SECRETARY/TREASURER & BUYER
Robin Raigo

Video Station

3689 Sheridan Dr., Amherst, NY 14226; (716) 835-2577. Video chain (500 stores). (Subsidiary of Rob-Mer Corp.)

PRESIDENT & HARDWARE BUYER
R.A. Lozinak
SOFTWARE BUYER & MANAGER
M. Lozinak

Video Station

19 S. Willson, Bozeman, MT 59715; (406) 587-8918. Organized 1981. (Video movie specialty store.)

OWNER
Steve Flagg

Video Station

240 E. 1300 South, Orem, UT 84058; (801) 226-6626. Organized 1981. (Video rental, duplication, and production.)

OWNER
Mark Greer
MANAGER
Anssanette Hulshoff
BRANCHES
346 W. 100 South, Orem, UT 84058

The Video Station

25401 Alicia Parkway, Suite G, Laguna Hills, CA 92653; (714) 768-2900. Video, affiliation.

PRESIDENT
Glen Powers
GENERAL MANAGER & BUYER
Laurie Powers

The Video Station

494A Main St., Woburn, MA 01801; (617) 933-1445. Organized 1980. (Consumer electronics, video retailing.)

PRESIDENT
Joseph V. Elia
VICE PRESIDENT
Peter Malamas
SECRETARY
Jeanne M. Elia
BOARD OF DIRECTORS
Joseph V. Elia, Jeanne M. Elia, Vincent I. Melendy, Peter Malamas

Video Station, Inc.

374 Springfield Ave., Summit, NJ 07901; (201) 273-0024. Organized 1980. (Sales and rental of videocassettes, recorders, TV's, cameras, record-a-calls, radios, CD's, records, telephones.)

PRESIDENT
Pauline Podell

VICE PRESIDENT
Nancy Podell
BOARD OF DIRECTORS
Pauline Podell, Nancy Podell, Barbara Marshall, Linda Bachrach, Craig Podell

Video Stop

1709 Mabry Dr., Clovis, NM 88101, (505) 763-7976. (Subsidiary of Let Us Entertain You.) Video, chain (5 stores).

PRESIDENT
Rex Webb
MANAGER & BUYER
Jay Warthen

Video Take #1

1750 Whitehorse Rd., Trenton, NJ 08619, (609) 587-2882. Video, independent.

PARTNERS
James Carlucci, Jr., Janet D. Carlucci

Video Time II

4227 W. Bell Rd., Phoenix, AZ 85023, (602) 864-0867. Video, independent. (Subsidiary of Bodic, Inc.)

PRESIDENT & BUYER
R.J. Handly

Video Today Inc.

63 East 8th, Holland, MI 49423, (616) 392-2877. Organized 1981. (Video sales, rental and mail order.) Chain (4 stores).

PRESIDENT
Al Wagenaar
GENERAL MANAGER
Jim Robbert
BRANCHES
228 Washington, Grand Haven, MI (616) 842-5253
977 Butternut, Holland, MI (616) 399-2092
9505 School St., Jenison, MI (616) 457-3150
755 Michigan, Holland, MI (616) 392-6210
2273 44th St., Kentwood, MI (616) 455-2722
AFFILIATIONS
VADA, NARM, SBA of Michigan

Video Trends

137 Winter Haven Mall, Winter Haven, FL 33880, (813) 293-0372. Video, electronics, independent.

PRESIDENT & BUYER
Gary E. Stewart

Video USA

13 W. Broadway, Derry, NH 03038, (603) 432-3236. Video.

PRESIDENT & HARDWARE BUYER
Donald Phelps
VICE PRESIDENT & SOFTWARE BUYER
Hollie Dustin

Video Vantage Inc.

1078 S. Gaylord St., Denver, CO 80209, (303) 777-0710. Organized 1983. (Supplies the Washington Park neighborhoods with their video needs.)

PRESIDENT
Hugh M. Boyd
VICE PRESIDENT
John D. Boyd
SECRETARY & TREASURER
Karen P. Taylor
AFFILIATIONS
Denver Chamber of Commerce, Video Software Dealers Association

Video Ventures, Inc.

471 West 9160 South, Sandy, UT 84070, (801) 255-0505. Video, 65 branches in drug and food chains.

PRESIDENT
Jerry Burke

Video Village

P.O. Box 38 (449 E. I-30), Rockwall, TX 75087, (214) 722-2222. Organized 1981. (VCR and television sales, movie rentals.)

MANAGER
Lisa Allen
BRANCHES
Rowlett, Texas

Video Village/The Video House

P.O. Box 2595, Canyon Country, CA 91351, (805) 252-3048. Video, chain (4 stores).

PRESIDENT & HARDWARE BUYER
David M. Smith
OPERATION MANAGER & SOFTWARE BUYER
Maureen Brown

Video Worx

3011 W. 74th Ave., Westminster, CO 80030 (303) 427-1237. Video, independent.

PRESIDENT & BUYER
Don Wickman

Video Yesteryear

Box C, Sandy Hook, CT 06482. Organized 1978. Independent, mail order.

PRESIDENT & MARKETING & SALES
Jon Sonneborn

Video's To Go

9348½ Corbin Ave., Northridge, CA 91324, (818) 701-1115. Video, independent.

PRESIDENT & BUYER
Neil H. Estrin

Video-Forum

96 Broad St., Guilford, CT 06437, (203) 453-9794. (Subsidiary of Jeffrey Norton Publishers, Inc.) Catalog sales.

Videoland

2161 Hutton St., Carrollton, TX 75006; (214) 243-5700. Video, electronics, chain (15 stores).

AUDIO/VIDEO BUYER
Carl Jameson

Videologue Marketing Corp.

3409 Ave. H, Brooklyn, NY 11210; (718) 377-3194, (800) 431-9003. Direct, mail order, independent.

CUSTOMER CONTACT
Jeff Goldman

Videon, Inc.

6443 Fairview, Boise, ID 83704; (208) 375-8899. Video, chain (3 stores).

PRESIDENT
Brent Estep
MARKETING DIRECTOR & SOFTWARE BUYER
Jeff Troup
HARDWARE BUYER
Russ Riley

Videospace

1324 N.E. 20, Bldg. 19, Bellevue, WA 98005; (206) 643-1900. Video, chain (10 stores).

PRESIDENT
Weston Nishimura
GENERAL MANAGER & BUYER
Gregg Thomas

Visions

P.O. Box 341, 110 Midland Ave., Rye, NY 10580; (914) 937-8601, (212) 824-7711. Mail order.

GENERAL MANAGER
Grace Babtist

Waldenbooks

201 High Ridge Rd., Stamford, CT 06904; (203) 356-7500. (Subsidiary of K Mart Corp.) Bookstore, chain (900 stores).

PRESIDENT
Harry Hoffman
MANAGER, MARKETING DEVELOPMENT & BUYER
George Hodgkins

Ric Webb's Video City

2610 W. Nob Hill Blvd., Yakima, WA 98902; (509) 248-4763. Video, independent. (Subsidiary of Webtana Inc.)

PRESIDENT, MANAGER & BUYER
Ric Webb

Wegmans Food Markets Inc.

1500 Brooks Ave., P.O. Box 844, Rochester, NY 14692; (716) 328-2550. Food stores, chain (37 stores).

ASSISTANT DIRECTOR, GENERAL MERCHANDISING
Kevin Kamholtz

Wilson's Video

213 E. Dakota, Pierre, SD 57501; (605) 224-0530. Video, independent.

PRESIDENT
Roger R. Wilson

Equipment Manufacturers

* VIDEO MONITORS
* VIDEOCASSETTE RECORDERS
* VIDEOTAPE

Video Monitors

Advanced Technology Division

(Subsidiary of Symbolized Systems, Inc.)
23950 Craftsman Rd., Calabasa, CA 91302; (818) 999-1393, (800) 232-2142, (800) 423-3641 (CA).

CORP. PRESIDENT
Jack G. Abbott
DIRECTOR, SALES & MARKETING
Jon N. Nagy
NATIONAL SERVICE MANAGER
Charlie Shade

Amtron Corp.

2260 De La Cruz Blvd., Santa Clara, CA 95050; (408) 748-8500.

VICE PRESIDENT, RESEARCH/DEVELOPMENT
W.G. Widera
VICE PRESIDENT, SALES
L. Hamner

Asaca/Shibasoku Corp. of America

12509 Beatrice St., Los Angeles, CA 90066; (213) 827-7144, (800) 423-6347, Telex 182089.

CORPORATE PRESIDENT
T. Shigezaki
VICE PRESIDENT & GENERAL MANAGER
Alan Davis

Ball Electronic Systems Division

(Subsidiary of Ball Corp.)
P.O. Box 589, 9300 W. 108 Circle, Broomfield, CO 80020-0589; (303) 457-5260.

CORPORATE PRESIDENT
Richard Ringeon
PRESIDENT
H. Robert Gill
VICE PRESIDENT, MARKETING
H. Jurgen Mammitzch
NATIONAL SALES MANAGER
Richard Scarle

Barco

(see Elector USA, Inc.)

Cetec Gauss

(Division of Cetec Corp.)
9130 Glenoaks Blvd., Sun Valley, CA 91352; (213) 875-1900. Telex 194989.

CORPORATE PRESIDENT
Robert A. Nelson
PRESIDENT
W. Mort Fujii
EXECUTIVE VICE PRESIDENT
J.R. Williams
SALES
Jacques Fleischmann

Cohu, Inc. Electronics Division

5755 Kearny Villa Rd., PO Box 85623, San Diego, CA 92138-5623; (619) 277-6700. Organized 1957. CCTV system equipment—manufacturer and distributor.

PRESIDENT & CHIEF EXECUTIVE OFFICER
James W. Barnes
VICE PRESIDENT
A. Mack Rodgers
VICE PRESIDENT, FINANCE
Charles A. Schwan
BOARD OF DIRECTORS
William S. Ivans, William N. Jenkins, Jack M. Keeney, Dr. Robert W. Kerns, Gene E. Leary, Raymond C. Sebold, Frank W. Davis, John E. Goode, Jr.
AFFILIATIONS
Delta Design; BMS, Inc.; FRL, Inc.

Conrac Division, Conrac Corporation

600 N. Rimsdale Ave., Covina, CA 91722; (818) 966-3511. Organized 1947. (Manufacturer and marketer of precision video display monitors for the broadcast, computer graphics, medical imaging, and process control industries.)
Conrac division executives:

PRESIDENT
Warren J. O'Buch
VICE PRESIDENT, MARKETING & SALES
Robert F. Griffith
VICE PRESIDENT, ENGINEERING
Peter Portoulas
DIRECTOR OF Q.A.
Robert Nichols
VICE PRESIDENT, OPERATIONS
James Costelloe
CONTROLLER
Michael Whitten
DIRECTOR OF PERSONNEL
Lou Tirapelle
GENERAL SALES MANAGER
William A. Ems
MARKETING SERVICES MANAGER
Gene D. Ornstead
PRODUCT MARKETING MANAGER
Richard V. Owoc
BOARD OF DIRECTORS (Conrac Corp.)
Donald H. Putnam, Arthur H. Thornhill, Jr., Frederick S. Wonham, Daniel T. Carroll, John C. Lowe, Thomas K. Denton, Paul E. Graf, Barry J. Gordon, J. Markham Green.

Electror USA, Inc.

P.O. Box 699, Pine Brook, NJ 07058; (201) 882-0584. Telex 172335.

MARKETING & SALES
C.E. Barlow

Electrohome Limited

809 Wellington St., N., Kitchener, Ont., Canada N2G 4J6; (519) 744-7111.

CHAIRMAN, PRESIDENT & CHIEF EXECUTIVE OFFICER
J.A. Pollock
VICE PRESIDENT, FINANCE
W.A. Janci
VICE PRESIDENT, OPERATIONS
H.H. LaPier
VICE PRESIDENT, ELECTROHOME LIMITED, & PRESIDENT, C A P COMMUNICATIONS LIMITED
W.D. McGregor
SECRETARY/TREASURER
H.I. Eby
CORPORATE CONTROLLER
J.G. Gingerich
GROUP GENERAL MANAGER, ELECTRONICS DIV.
W.M. Nobbs

GBC CCTV Corp.

315 Hudson St., New York, NY 10013; (212) 989-4433, (800) 221-2240.

CORPORATE PRESIDENT
Stephen Lefkowitz

Hitachi Denshi America, Ltd.

(Division of Hitachi Denshi, Ltd.)
175 Crossways Park W., Woodbury, NY 11797; (516) 921-7200.

CORPORATION PRESIDENT
Ryuzo Muto
GENERAL MANAGER
S. Hotta
NATIONAL SALES MANAGER
Jack Breitenbucher
NATIONAL SERVICE MANAGER
Ted Ohnishi

Ikegami Electronics (U.S.A.), Inc.

37 Brook Ave., Maywood, NJ 07607; (201) 368-9171. Organized 1964. (Manufactures and markets professional TV cameras and monitors.)

PRESIDENT
N. Nishi
SENIOR VICE PRESIDENT
S. La Conte
VICE PRESIDENT (DISPLAY MONITOR DIVISION)
Y. Sato
DIRECTOR, SALES & MARKETING
H. Winch
COMMUNICATIONS MANAGER
R. Estony
BRANCHES
Northeast: 37 Brook Avenue, Maywood, NJ 07607; (201) 368-9171. John Chow, regional sales manager.
Southeast: 6201 Johns Road, Suite #5, Tampa, FL 33614; (813) 884-2046. Bud Mills, regional sales manager.
Midwest: 747 Church Rd., Units C4 & C5, Elmhurst, IL 60126; (312) 834-9774. Bob Johnston, regional sales manager.
West Coast: 3445 Kashiwa St., Torrance, CA 90505; (213) 534-0050. Jerry Kraus, regional sales manager.
Southwest: 13721 Omega Rd., Dallas, TX 75234; (214) 233-2844. Glen Smith, regional sales manager.
Networks and Canada: 37 Brook Ave., Maywood, NJ 07607; (201) 368-9171. John Webb, regional sales manager.

JVC Co. of America/ Professional Video Division

(Subsidiary of US JVC Corp.)
41 Slater Dr., Elmwood Park, NJ 07407; (201) 794-3900.

PRESIDENT
N. Sakoda
VICE PRESIDENT, GENERAL MANAGER
Daniel D. Roberts
NATIONAL PARTS/SERVICE MANAGER
Paul Hurst

Javelin Electronics, Inc.

19831 Magellan Dr., Torrance, CA 90502; (213) 327-7440, (800) 421-2716. Telex 19-444860 JAVELIN TRNC.

PRESIDENT
Donald T. Heckel
SALES OPERATIONS MANAGER
Michael M. Burton
NATIONAL SALES MANAGER
J. David Bittner

Lectrotech, Inc.

5810 N. Western Ave., Chicago, IL 60659; (312) 769-6262.

PRESIDENT
William Grossman
VICE PRESIDENT
Barry Grossman

Lenco, Inc.

Electronics Division, 300 N. Maryland St., Jackson, MO 63755; (314) 243-3147. TWX 910-760-1382.

PRESIDENT
Andrew Perrin
GENERAL MANAGER
Bruce Blair
DIRECTOR, MARKETING
Ken Tiffany
NATIONAL SALES MANAGER
Robert Henson
NATIONAL SERVICE MANAGER
Gary Stephens

Link Electronics, Ltd.

North Way, Andover, Hants, SP10 5AJ, England 0264-61345. Telex 47132 LINK G.

MANAGER
D. Mann
DIRECTOR, MARKETING
J. Tanner
SALES DIRECTOR
J. Wilson

Matsushita Electric of Canada Ltd.

(Subsidiary of Panasonic Video Systems/Panasonic Audio Systems.)
5770 Ambler Dr., Mississauga, Ontario, L4W 2T3 Canada, (416) 624-5010.

PRESIDENT
Tak Urabe
MANAGER, INDUSTRIAL VIDEO DEPARTMENT
J. Howells
MANAGER, PROFESSIONAL AUDIO SYSTEMS DEPT.
T. Nakamura
NATIONAL PARTS MANAGER
A. Frield
NATIONAL SERVICE MANAGER
W. Horrocks

Mitsubishi Electronics of America, Inc.

(Division of Mitsubishi Electric.)
991 Knox St., Torrance, CA 90502, (213) 515-3993.

PRESIDENT
Takeshi Sakurai
NATIONAL SALES MANAGER
Don Arrons

NEC Home Electronics (USA) Inc.

(Video Products Division.)
1401 Estes Ave., Elk Grove Village, IL 60007, (312) 228-5900.

PRESIDENT
M. Tsukimoto
GENERAL MANAGER (VIDEO PRODUCTS DIVISION)
Nick Akagi
ASSISTANT GENERAL MANAGER
Gerald A. Tangney
NATIONAL SALES MANAGER
Dustin Vallaly

Panasonic Industrial Co.

(Subsidiary of Matsushita Electric Corp. of America.)
One Panasonic Way, Secaucus, NJ 07094, (201) 348-7000.

PRESIDENT
Ken Kurahashi
VICE PRESIDENT, GENERAL MANAGER
Koichi Sadlashige

Pioneer Video Inc.

200 W. Grand Ave., Montvale, NJ 07645, (201) 573-1122.

PRESIDENT
Ken Kai
DIRECTOR, SPECIAL MARKETS
Brew Merrill

Quasar Company

(Division of Matsushita Electric Corp. of America)
9401 W. Grand Ave., Franklin Park, IL 60131, (312) 451-1200. Organized 1974. (Marketer of broad line of consumer electronics products.)

PRESIDENT
Jack Pluckhan
EXECUTIVE VICE PRESIDENT
Keith Nishikawa

RCA Closed Circuit Video Equipment

(Division of RCA Corp., New York)
New Holland Ave., Lancaster, PA 17604, (717) 295-6000.

DIRECTOR
C.L. Rintz
MARKETING MANAGER
V.C. Houk

Sharp Electronics Corporation

P.O. Box 650, Sharp Plaza, Mahwah, NJ 07430, (201) 529-8200. Organized 1962 (in USA), 1912 (worldwide). (Manufacturer of quality electronics products for home, office, industrial and broadcast use.)

CHAIRMAN OF THE BOARD & DIRECTOR

Mr. K. Kubo
PRESIDENT & DIRECTOR
Mr. S. Hirooka
EXECUTIVE VICE PRESIDENT & DIRECTOR
Mr. C. Daigneault
EXECUTIVE VICE PRESIDENT & DIRECTOR
Mr. T. Nagai
EXECUTIVE VICE PRESIDENT & DIRECTOR
Mr. T. Toda
SENIOR VICE PRESIDENT
Mr. K. Yamada
BOARD OF DIRECTORS
Mr. K. Kubo, Mr. S. Hirroka, Mr. C. Daigneault, Mr. T. Nagai, Mr. T. Toda.
BRANCHES
Atlanta, Chicago, Los Angeles, Georgia, Illinois, California
AFFILIATIONS
Wholly owned subsidiary of Sharp Corporation, Osaka, Japan.

Sony Video Communications

(Division of Sony Corp. of America.)
Sony Dr., Park Ridge, NJ 07656, (201) 930-1000.
CORPORATE PRESIDENT
Kenji Tamiya
PRESIDENT
Philip J. Stack
VICE PRESIDENT, SALES
Robert Mueller
NATIONAL SERVICE MANAGER
Philip Hart

Tektronix, Inc.

P.O. Box 500, Beaverton, OR 97077, (503) 627-7111. TWX 910-467-8708.
CORPORATE PRESIDENT
Earl Wantland
GENERAL MANAGER
Larry Kaplan
MARKETING MANAGER
Steve Kerman
SALES MANAGER
Austin Basso

Toshiba America, Inc.

(Division of Toshiba Corp.)
82 Totowa Rd., Wayne, NJ 07470, (201) 628-8000. Telex 130309.
CHAIRMAN
Mikio Kuroshima
EXECUTIVE VICE PRESIDENT
J. Paul Michie
NATIONAL SERVICE MANAGER
John Newman

Videotek, Inc.

125 N. York St., Pottstown, PA 14964, (215) 327-2292. TWX 710-653-0125.
CORPORATION PRESIDENT
Philip G. Steyaert
VICE PRESIDENT, NATIONAL SALES MANAGER
Peter H. Choi
NATIONAL SERVICE MANAGER
Rick Hollowbush

Videocassette Recorders

Akai America Ltd.

(Subsidiary of Akai Electric Co., Ltd.)
800 W. Artesia Blvd., Compton, CA 90224; (213) 527-3880. TX 67-7494.

EXECUTIVE VICE PRESIDENT
Charles E. Phillips
VICE PRESIDENT, SALES
Mike Wiggins
NATIONAL SERVICE MANAGER
John Carpenter

Ampex Corp. Audio-Video Systems Division

(Subsidiary of The Signal Cos., Inc.)
401 Broadway, Redwood City, CA 94063; (415) 367-2011, TELEX 348464.

CORPORATE PRESIDENT
Roy Ekrom
GENERAL MANAGER
Mark L. Sanders
MARKETING DIRECTOR
Willie Scullion
NATIONAL PARTS MANAGER
Paul Krueger

Curtis Mathes

One Curtis Mathes Parkway, Athens, TX 75751; (800) 527-7646.

Hitachi Denshi America, Ltd.

(Division of Hitachi Denshi, Ltd.)
175 Crossways Park W., Woodbury, NY 11797, (516) 921-7200.

CORPORATION PRESIDENT
Ryuzo Muto
GENERAL MANAGER
S. Hotta
NATIONAL SALES MANAGER
Jack Breitenbucher
NATIONAL SERVICE MANAGER
Ted Ohnishi

Ikegami Electronics (U.S.A.), Inc.

(Subsidiary of Ikegami, Tsushinki Co., Ltd.)
37 Brook Ave., Maywood, NJ 07607; (201) 368-9171. ITT: 219034 ITC N.J.

PRESIDENT
H. Nishi
SALES MANAGER
Stuart Rauch
MARKETING, SALES
Herman Schkolnick
NATIONAL SERVICE MANAGER
Jeff Cohen

Instant Replay

2951 So. Bayshore Dr., Miami, FL 33133; (305) 448-7088. Organized 1976. (Manufactures specialized VCR's: RGB output, multistandard, built in caption decoder. VHS Hi Fi Multistd.)

PRESIDENT
Charles Azar
VICE PRESIDENT
Petra Azar

JVC Co. of America/Professional Video Division

(Subsidiary of US JVC Corp.)
41 Slater Dr., Elmwood Park, NJ 07407; (201) 794-3900.

CORPORATION PRESIDENT
N. Sakoda
VICE PRESIDENT, GENERAL MANAGER
Daniel D. Roberts
NATIONAL PARTS, SERVICE MANAGER
Paul Hurst

Sanyo Electric Inc.

1200 W. Artesia Blvd., Compton, CA 90220; (213) 537-5830

CORPORATE PRESIDENT
T. Takyama
EXECUTIVE VICE PRESIDENT, SALES & MARKETING
Jeff Berkowitz
NATIONAL SERVICE MANAGER
Jose Balbin

Sony Video Communications

(Division of Sony Corp. of America.)
Sony Dr., Park Ridge, NJ 07656; (201) 930-1000.

CORPORATE PRESIDENT
Kenji Tamiya
PRESIDENT
Philip J. Stack
VICE PRESIDENT, SALES
Robert Mueller
NATIONAL SERVICE MANAGER
Philip Hart

Toshiba America, Inc.

(Division of Toshiba Corp.)
82 Totowa Rd., Wayne, NJ 07470; (201) 628-8000. Telex 130309.

CHAIRMAN
Mikio Kuroshima
EXECUTIVE VICE PRESIDENT
J. Paul Michie
NATIONAL SERVICE MANAGER
John Newman

NEC Home Electronics (USA) Inc.

Video Products Division
1401 Estes Ave., Elk Grove Village, IL 60007; (312) 228-5900.

PRESIDENT
I. M. Tsukimoto
GENERAL MANAGER (Video Products Div.)
Nick Akagi
ASSISTANT GENERAL MANAGER
Gerald A. Tangney
NATIONAL SALES MANAGER
Dustin Vallaly

Panasonic Industrial Co.

(Subsidiary of Matsushita Electric Corp. of America)
One Panasonic Way, Secaucus, NJ 07094; (201) 348-7000.

CORPORATE PRESIDENT
Ken Kurahashi
VICE PRESIDENT, GENERAL MANAGER
Koichi Sadlashige

Quasar Co.

(Division of Matsushita Electric Corp. of America)
9401 W. Grand Ave., Franklin Park, IL 60131; (312) 451-1200. Organized 1974. (Marketer of broad line of consumer electronics products.)

PRESIDENT
Jack Pluckhan
EXECUTIVE VICE PRESIDENT
Keith Nishikawa

Videotape

Agfa-Gevaert, Inc.
(Magnet Tape Division)
275 North St., Teterboro, NJ 07608; (201) 288-4100.

CORPORATE PRESIDENT
Robert A. M. Coppenrath
DIRECTOR OF MARKETING
Maria A. Curry
VIDEO PRODUCTS MANAGER
Kenneth F. Wiedeman

Ampex Corp. Magnetic Tape Division
(Subsidiary of The Signal Cos., Inc.)
401 Broadway, Redwood City, CA 94063; (415) 367-2011, TELEX 348464.

CORPORATE PRESIDENT
Roy Ekrom
VICE PRESIDENT, GENERAL MANAGER
Stanley Faught
NATIONAL SALES MANAGER
Richard Antonio

Fuji Photo Film USA, Inc., Magnetic Tape Division
350 Fifth Ave., New York, NY 10018; (212) 736-3335. TELEX ITT 423298.

CORPORATE PRESIDENT
Bernie Yasanaga
NATIONAL SALES MANAGER
Stan Bauer

JVC Co. of America/ Professional Video Division
(Subsidiary of US JVC Corp.)
41 Slater Dr., Elmwood Park, NJ 07407; (201) 794-3900.

CORPORATION PRESIDENT
N. Sakoda
VICE PRESIDENT, GENERAL MANAGER
Daniel D. Roberts
NATIONAL PARTS, SERVICE MANAGER
Paul Hurst

Magnetic Media Video Corp.
500 Eastern Parkway, Farmingdale, NY 11735; (516) 293-1010, Telex 14-3223.

VICE PRESIDENT, GENERAL MANAGER
John Cristiano
VICE PRESIDENT, SALES MANAGER
Paul Mastroianni

Matsushita Electric of Canada Ltd.
(Subsidiary of Panasonic Video Systems/Panasonic Audio Systems)
5770 Ambler Dr., Mississauga, Ont., L4W 2T3 Canada; (416) 624-5010.

CORPORATE PRESIDENT
Tak Urabe
MANAGER, INDUSTRIAL VIDEO DEPT.
J. Howells
MANAGER, PROFESSIONAL AUDIO SYSTEM DEPT.
T. Nakamura
NATIONAL PARTS MANAGER
A. Field
NATIONAL SERVICE MANAGER
W. Horrocks

Maxell Corp. of America
(Subsidiary of Hitachi)
60 Oxford Dr., Moonachie, NJ 07074; (201) 440-8020. Telex 134538.

CORPORATE PRESIDENT
H. Matsumoto
VICE PRESIDENT, GENERAL MANAGER
Ted Ozawa
NATIONAL SALES MANAGER, PROFESSIONAL/INDUSTRIAL PRODUCTS
James J. Ringwood

Maxima Magnetics, Inc.
300 Bonair Ave., Hatboro, PA 19040; (215) 443-0700, (800) 3 MAXIMA. Organized 1982. (Sells blank video and audio tape to professional users.)

PRESIDENT
William R. Goss
EXECUTIVE VICE PRESIDENT
Susan R. Goss
VICE PRESIDENT, OPERATIONS
Carol M. Moore
BOARD OF DIRECTORS
W.R. Goss, president; S.R. Goss, secretary/treasurer.

PD Magnetics
(Joint venture of N.V. Philips & E.I. du Pont de Nemours & Co., Inc.)
600 Heron Dr., Pureland Industrial Complex, Bridgeport, NJ 08014; (609) 467-2500. Telex 835420 CL

VICE PRESIDENT
Richard Sinclair
NATIONAL SALES MANAGER
E. Richard Buckley

Panasonic Industrial Co.
(Subsidiary of Matsushita Electric Corp. of America)
One Panasonic Way, Secaucus, NJ 07094; (201) 348-7000.

CORPORATE PRESIDENT
Ken Kurahashi
VICE PRESIDENT, GENERAL MANAGER
Koichi Sadlashige

Sony Video Communications
(Division of Sony Corp. of America)
Sony Drive, Park Ridge, NJ 07656; (201) 930-1000.

CORPORATE PRESIDENT
Kenji Tamiya
PRESIDENT
Philip J. Stack
VICE PRESIDENT, SALES
Robert Mueller
NATIONAL SERVICE MANAGER
Philip Hart

Sunkyong International, Inc.
30 Congress Dr., Moonachie, NJ 07074; (201) 440-5006, Telex WU 642177.

VICE PRESIDENT, MARKETING
George T. Saddler

TDK Electronics Corp.
12 Harbor Park Dr., Port Washington, NY 11050; (516) 625-0100, Telex 144535.

CORPORATION PRESIDENT
R. Kawakami
VICE PRESIDENT, SALES & MARKETING
Terry Tsutsui

Thor Electronics Corp.
321 Pennsylvania Ave., Linden, NJ 07036; (201) 486-3300. Telex 138968 THORLIND

CORPORATE PRESIDENT
Angelo Crudele
GENERAL MANAGER
Roy Gettis
MARKETING & SALES
D. Delane
NATIONAL PARTS MANAGER
Frank Destefano

3M/Magnetic Media Division

223-5S-01, 3M Center, St. Paul, MN 55125; (612) 733-1387. (Manufactures and sells blank audio and video cassettes, floppy disks, systems care products and accessories.)

DIVISION VICE PRESIDENT
D. Drew Davis
MARKETING DIRECTOR
Robert F. Burnett
MARKETING OPERATIONS MANAGER
George F. Burr

Consumer and Trade Publications

Quigley Publishing Company

Publishers of Motion Picture Product Digest (25 times a year), Motion Picture Almanac (Annual), Television and Video Almanac (Annual).—Fame. 159 West 53 St., New York, NY 10019; (212) 247-3100. Cable: Quigpubco, New York.

PRESIDENT AND PUBLISHER
Martin Quigley, Jr.
EDITOR-IN-CHIEF
Richard Gertner
GENERAL MANAGER
Robert McDonald

LONDON BUREAU

William Pay, Manager and London Editor; 15 Samuel Road, Langdon Hills, Basildon, Essex, England; 0268-417-055.

FOREIGN CORRESPONDENTS

ARGENTINA: Natalio Bruski, Calle Paso 240 (8°C), Buenos Aires.
EGYPT: Ahmed Sami, 4 El Ommara St., Apt. 13, Abbassia, Cairo.
GREECE: Rena Velissariou, 8432, Kolokotroni Str., Agia Paraskevi, Attikis, Athens. (804).
HOLLAND: Philip de Schaap, 9 Henriette Bosmansstrant, Amsterdam (Zuid).
JAPAN: A C. Pinder, Whaley-Eaton, Service, Central P.O. Box 190, Tokyo, Japan.
SRI LANKA: Chandra perea, 437 Pethiygoda, Kelanuja, Sri Lanka, Ceylon.
SWITZERLAND: Gerda Goepfert-Klimisch, Film-Bild-Archiv, Ch 6933, Agnuzzo, Cas Vigne, Barbengo, Ticino.

Motion Picture Almanac

(Annually) 159 West 53 St., New York, NY 10019; (212) 247-3100; Cable: Quigpubco, New York.

EDITOR
Richard Gertner
ASSOCIATE EDITOR
William Pay
ADVERTISING AND DISTRIBUTION
Robert McDonald

Television & Video Almanac

(Annually) 159 West 53 St., New York, NY 10019; (212) 247-3100; Cable: Quigpubco, New York.

EDITOR
Richard Gertner
VIDEO EDITOR
Jane Klain
ASSOCIATE EDITOR
William Pay
ADVERTISING AND DISTRIBUTION
Robert McDonald

Fame

159 West 53 St., New York, NY 10019; (212) 247-3100; Cable: Quigpubco, New York.

EDITOR
Richard Gertner
ASSOCIATE EDITOR
William Pay

Back Stage

(Weekly dealing with theatrical and nontheatrical films, television shows and commercials, cassettes, radio, and theater, published Friday), 330 West 42 St., New York, NY 10036; (212) 947-0020. 5150 Wilshire Blvd., L.A. CA 90036; (213) 936-5200, 100 East Ohio St., Chicago, IL 60611; (312) 943-0051.

MANAGING EDITOR & PUBLISHER
Allen Zwerdling
ADVERTISING DIRECTOR & PUBLISHER
Ira Eaker
ASSOCIATE PUBLISHER
Steve Elish
EDITOR
Anthony Vagnoni

Back Stage Television, Film, Tape & Production Directory

(Annually, January), 330 West 42 St., New York, NY 10036; (212) 947-0020.

EDITOR
Allen Zwerdling

Billboard

(Weekly dealing with records, music, entertainment artists, video hardware and software, etc, published Saturdays), 9107 Wilshire Blvd., Beverly Hills, CA 90210; (213) 273-7040. 1515 Broadway, New York, NY 10036, (212) 764-7415; 150 N. Wacker Drive, Chicago, IL 60606; (313) 236-9818; 733 15 St., N.W. Washington, DC; (202) 393-2580.

PUBLISHER
Lee Zhito
EXECUTIVE VICE PRESIDENT
Jules Perel
MANAGING EDITOR
Adam White

Cable Advertising, Merchandising and Programming Report (CAMP)

(Bi-weekly dealing with advertising and merchandising activities on basic and pay cable.) Knowledge Industry Publications, Inc., 701 Westchester Ave., White Plains, NY 10604; (914) 328-9157.

Classic Images

Box 809, Muscatine, IA 52671; (319) 263-2331.

Coming Attractions

(Published monthly by Convenience Video Corp, a subsidiary of Star Video Entertainment, and distributed to 160 video stores.) 225 W. 34 St., New York, NY 10001; (212) 736-3035.

PRESIDENT
Bernard J. Herman

Daily Variety

(Motion picture, television, homevideo, pay-TV, cable, radio, theatre, night clubs, daily) 1400 N. Cahuenga Blvd., Hollywood, CA 90028; (213) 469-1141.

EDITOR
Thomas M. Pryor
ASSOCIATE PUBLISHER
Michael Silverman
MANAGING EDITOR
Peter Pryor
MARKETING DIRECTOR
Michael Malak
GENERAL MANAGER
F. Phil Turner
PRODUCTION MANAGER
Bob Butler

Electronic Media

(Weekly publication dealing with information on the broadcast TV market including radio, TV and video.) Crain Communications Inc., 740 N. Rush St., Chicago, IL 60611, (312) 649-6650.

Hollywood Reporter, The

(Film, TV, entertainment, daily) 6715 Sunset Boulevard, Hollywood, CA 90028; (213) 464-7411; and 1501 Broadway, New York, NY, 10036; (212) 354-1858.

PUBLISHER & EDITOR-IN-CHIEF
Tichi Wilkerson Kassel
EDITOR
Marcia Borie
BUREAUS
NEW YORK: Morna Murphy-Martel, 1501 Broadway, New York, NY 10036
WASHINGTON, D.C.: Theresa McMasters, Rm. 1234, National Press Bldg., Washington, DC 20045; (202) 737-2828.
LONDON: Paul Mungo, 57 Duke St., London W.1.
AUSTRALIA: John Hanrahan, 269 Annandale St., Annandale 2038, Sydney, NSW.

Home Video Publisher

(Bi-weekly, analyzing home video publishing opportunities for special interest programming and feature film.) Knowledge Industry Publications, Inc., 701 Westchester Ave., White Plains, NY 10604; (914) 328-9157.

In Motion Film & Video Production Magazine

(Film and video production trade magazine published 8 times a year.) 421 Fourth St., Annapolis, MD 21403; (301) 269-0605.

EDITOR & PUBLISHER
Steve Lehuray

Independent Film & Video Makers Guide

(Guidebook for the independent film and video maker.) Michael Wiese Film Productions, P.O. Box 406, Westport, CT 06881; (203) 226-6979.

Millimeter

(Published monthly. Motion picture and TV production industry magazine.) 826 Broadway, New York, NY 10003; (212) 477-4700.

Optic Music Inc.

(A bi-monthly international film and video production magazine.) Organized 1983. 800 S. Robertson Blvd., Suite 7, Los Angeles, CA 90035; (213) 652-2067.

PUBLISHER/PRESIDENT
David Swartz
SECRETARY/ASSOCIATE PUBLISHER/MANAGING EDITOR
Paula Swartz
VICE PRESIDENT/DIRECTOR OF ADVERTISING
Steven Rich

Panorama

(Published monthly.) 850 Third Ave., New York, NY 10022; (212) 759-8100.

Photo Business

(Photographic trade publication.) Organized 1956. Published by Billboard Publications, Inc., 1515 Broadway, New York, NY 10036; (212) 764-7415.

EDITOR & ASSOCIATE PUBLISHER
Willard Clark
ASSOCIATE PUBLISHER, MARKETING & SALES
Doris Burke
MANAGING EDITOR
Richard Brandes
PRODUCTION MANAGER
Phyllis Hall

Photo Weekly

(Published weekly by Billboard Publications.) 1515 Broadway, New York, NY 10036; (212) 764-7415.

The Producer's Masterguide

(Annual international reference guide for producers in the motion picture, television, commercials, cable and videotape industries in the U.S., Canada, and the United Kingdom.) Published by New York Production Manual, Inc., 611 Broadway, Suite 807, New York, NY 10012-2608; (212) 777-4002.

PUBLISHER & TREASURER
Shmuel Bension
SENIOR CONSULTANT FILM PRODUCTION
David Golden
SENIOR CONSULTANT PUBLICITY
Renee L. Ash

Professional Video Production

(Video production manual.) Published by Knowledge Industry Publications, Inc., 701 Westchester Ave., White Plains, NY 10604; (914) 328-9157.

Rockamerica Magazine

(Monthly magazine dealing with the music industry.) 27 E. 21st St., New York, NY 10010, (212) 475-5791.

Television Digest

(Published weekly. Television Digest with Consumer Electronics, TV & CATV Addenda, AM/FM Addenda; Annual Television Factbook, Annual Cable & Station Coverage Atlas, Weekly Satellite Week, Weekly Video Week, Biweekly Public Broadcasting Report, Monthly Early Warnings Report, Daily Communications) 1836 Jefferson Place, N.W., Washington, D.C. 20036; (202) 872-9200.

EDITOR & PUBLISHER
Albert Warren
EDITORIAL DIRECTOR
David Lachenbruch
EXECUTIVE EDITOR
Dawson B. Nail
SENIOR EDITOR
Paul L. Warren

Variety

(International entertainment business weekly, published Wednesdays) 154 West 46th Street, New York, NY 10036, (212) 869-5700; 1400 N. Cahuenga Blvd., Hollywood, CA 90028, (213) 469-1141; 1483 Chain Bridge Rd., McLean, VA 22101, (703) 448-0510; 400 North Michigan Ave., Chicago, IL 60611, (312) 337-4984; PARIS: France, 33 Champs Elysees, Paris 75008, France, Phone 720-19-56; ROME: VARIETY, Via Bissolati, 20, 00187, Rome, Italy; 463-290. LONDON: VARIETY, 49 St. James's St., London SW1A 1JX, England; 493-4561; MADRID, Spain, Calle Lagasca, 104, 28006; Phone 276-4262; SYDNEY, 2000, N.S.W. 1-7 Albion Place, Phone 61-3124.

PUBLISHER AND EXECUTIVE EDITOR
Syd Silverman
ADVERTISING MANAGER
Mort Bryer
MANAGING EDITOR
Frank Meyer
TV/RADIO EDITOR
John Lippman
PICTURES SECTION EDITOR
Larry Cohn
MUSIC EDITOR
Ken Terry
HOMEVIDEO EDITOR
Jim Melanson

Video

(Monthly consumer magazine covering hardware and programming.) Published by Reese Communications, 460 W. 34th St. 20th Floor, New York, NY 10001, (212) 947-6500. Organized 1978.

PUBLISHER
Jay Rosenfield
ASSOCIATE PUBLISHER
Debra Halpert
EDITOR
Doug Garr

Video Business

(Published monthly by parent company CES Publishing Corp. A business-to-business magazine for video dealers.) 345 Park Ave. South, 6th Floor, New York, NY 10010, (212) 686-7744. Organized 1981.

PUBLISHER
Bill O'Brien
EDITOR
John Hubach
PRESIDENT & CHIEF EXECUTIVE OFFICER
Stuart J. Horton
VICE PRESIDENT/CORP. EDITORIAL DIRECTOR
Art Levis
EASTERN ADVERTISING
Corey Freidman
WESTERN ADVERTISING
Mitchell Wallis

Video Insider

(Bi-weekly newsletter for video retailers, distributors, manufacturers and producers.) 223 Conestoga, Rd., Wayne, PA 19087, (215) 688-7030.

Video Marketing Newsletter

(24 issues a year. News service for marketers of consumer video programs and hardware.) 1680 Vine St., Suite 82, Hollywood, CA 90028, (213) 462-6350.

Video Movies

(Monthly guide including review of late breaking videos.) 3841 W. Oakton St., Skokie, IL 60076, (312) 676-3470.

The Video Register 1985-86

(Annual. Directory listing organizations using video—manufacturers, dealers, program distributors, consultants/producers, production facilities.) Published by Knowledge Industry Publications, Inc., 701 Westchester Ave., White Plains, NY 10604, (914) 328-9157.

Video Review Magazine

(Monthly. Home video consumer magazine.) Published by Viare Publishing, 902 Broadway, New York, NY 10010, (212) 477-2200.

The Video Source Book

(A listing of more than 40,000 programs available on video tape from more than 800 sources.) The National Video Clearinghouse, Inc., 100 Lafayette Dr., Syosset, NY 11791; (516) 364-3686.

Video Store Magazine

(Monthly. Provides information to video retailers nationally on new releases, trends in the industry, industry statistics and promotional ideas.) 1700 East Dyer Rd., #250, Santa Ana, CA 92705; (714) 250-8060. Organized 1979.

PRESIDENT OF PUBLICATIONS
Richard Moeller
GROUP PUBLISHER
Eileen Paulin
PUBLISHER
David Rowe
EDITOR
Tom Adams
NATIONAL ADVERTISING SALES MANAGER
Denis Cambruzzi
BRANCH
545 Fifth Ave., New York, NY 10017; (212) 503-2949.

Video Tape and Disc Guide to Home Entertainment

(Updated reference guide containing titles and descriptive information about 6000 available videocassettes and discs for the consumer market.) Published by National Video Clearinghouse, Inc., 100 Lafayette Dr., Syosset, NY 11791; (516) 364-3686.

Video Times

(Monthly. Contains reviews of current movies on video and a user's guide to equipment.) Organized 1984. Published by Publications International, 3841 W. Oakton St. Skokie, IL 60076; (312) 676-3470.

PUBLISHER
Jay Butler
EDITOR
Laurie Forman
MANAGING EDITOR
Deb Lovelien

Video Trade News

(Monthly—for manufacturers and dealers who sell professional video equipment.) Published by C.S. Tepfer Publishing Co. Inc., 51 Sugar Hollow Rd., Danbury, CT 06810; (203) 743-2120.

Video Week

(Weekly. News magazine covering the business of program sales and distribution for videocassettes, disc, pay TV and news media.) Published by Television Digest, Inc., 1836 Jefferson Pl., NW, Washington, D.C. 20036; (202) 872-9200.

Videography Magazine

(Monthly. Professional video production trade magazine.) Organized 1976. 50 West 23 St., New York, NY 10010; (212) 645-1000.

PUBLISHER
Chuck Colletti
EDITOR
John Rice
BRANCHES
Media Horizons, 360 N. Michigan Ave., Chicago, IL 60601.
Media Horizons, 5455 Wilshire Blvd., Los Angeles, CA 90036.

Trade Associations

Association of Independent Television Stations

1200 18th St., N.W., Suite 502, Washington, DC 20036; (202) 887-1970.

CHAIRMAN
Eugene McCurdy
VICE CHAIRMAN
Charles L. Edwards
PRESIDENT
Preston R. Padden
SECRETARY
Milton Maltz
TREASURER
Robert J. Wormington
VICE PRESIDENT, GOVERNMENT RELATIONS
James B. Hedlund
VICE PRESIDENT, MARKETING
Howard Kamin
BOARD OF DIRECTORS
Ted Baze, Steven A. Bell, L. Martin Brantley, Charles L. Edwards, Lewis Freifeld, Milton Maltz, Eugene McCurdy, Kevin O'Brien, Preston R. Padden, Harry J. Pappas, Leavitt J. Pope, Harold E. Protter, John A. Serrao, Robert J. Wormington

Association of Visual Communicators, Inc.

900 Palm Ave., Suite Room B, S. Pasadena, CA 91030, (818) 441-2274. (Promotes and encourages excellence in the informational audio-visual industry.)

EXECUTIVE DIRECTOR
Michael Andrio
NATIONAL PRESIDENT
Patricia Rye
DATE OF ORGANIZATION
1957

International Tape/Disc Association

10 Columbus Circle, Room 2270, New York, NY 10019; (212) 956-7110.

CHAIRMAN OF THE BOARD
Gordon W. Bricker
PRESIDENT
J. Philip Stack
SENIOR VICE PRESIDENT
Alfred Markim
VICE PRESIDENT OF PLANNING
George Ricci
VICE PRESIDENT OF AUDIO
Maria A. Curry
VICE PRESIDENT OF VIDEO
Tony Mirabelli
VICE PRESIDENT OF LASER MEDIA
Ken Kai
EUROPEAN VICE PRESIDENT
Arnold Norregaard
TREASURER
Larry Finley
EXECUTIVE VICE PRESIDENT
Henry Brief
BOARD OF DIRECTORS
Officers are the following: Richard Stofan, Frank Day, Donald Bogue, Jacques Carpentier, Howard Schwartz, F.E. (Gene) Hull, R. Patrick Leonard, Jr., Daniel Grynberg, Stan Bauer, Don Winquist, Michael Upton, Daniel Roberts, James Ringwood, John Povolny, William Gallagher, William den Tuinder, Stan Hametz, E. Richard Buckley, Gerald T. Sadler, Terry Tsutsui, Nicholas Santrizos, Reid Anderson
DATE OF ORGANIZATION
1970
EUROPEAN OFFICE
Denmark: Arnold Norregaard, Bellevue Studio A/S, Dortheavej 71, DK-2400, Copenhagen

International Communications Industries Association (ICIA)

3150 Spring St., Fairfax, VA 22031; (703) 273-7200. (Formed to serve its members by developing and promoting services which will enhance their ability to conduct business successfully and profitably and with integrity and competence. Promotes the concept of free enterprise, and, in so doing, preserves the rights and freedoms of all business people in the communications industry.)

CHAIRMAN OF THE BOARD
George R. Bacon
PRESIDENT
Jerome Raymond
PRESIDENT-ELECT
Henry L. Marsh
VICE PRESIDENT
Herbert H. Taylor
SECRETARY-TREASURER
Theresa Staal
EXECUTIVE VICE PRESIDENT
Harry R. McGee
DATE OF ORGANIZATION
1939

International Television Association

6311 N. O'Connor Rd., Suite 110-LB51, Irving, TX 75039; (214) 869-1112. (Furthers the development of the professional video communicator; has 85 chapters in USA and 10 affiliates in foreign countries.)

PRESIDENT 1986–87
Michael Schwarz
PRESIDENT ELECT 1986–87
Tim Donovan
VICE PRESIDENT 1986–87
Les Magsamen
EXECUTIVE DIRECTOR
Fred Wehrli
CHAIRMAN OF THE BOARD 1985–86
Kathy Morris
DATE OF ORGANIZATION
1973

National Cable Television Association

1724 Massachusetts Ave., N.W., Washington, DC 20036; (202) 775-3550. (Represents the cable TV industry.)

PRESIDENT
James P. Mooney
EXECUTIVE VICE PRESIDENT
Bert W. Carp
VICE PRESIDENT AND GENERAL COUNSEL
Brenda L. Fox
VICE PRESIDENT, SCIENCE AND TECHNOLOGY
Wendell H. Bailey
ACTING VICE PRESIDENT, RESEARCH AND POLICY ANALYSIS
Cynthia B. Brumfield
VICE PRESIDENT, PROGRAMMING AND MARKETING
Char A. Beales
EXECUTIVE COMMITTEE:
Edward M. Allen, chm.; William B. Strange, Jr., vice chm.; John W. Goddard, sec.; James S. Cownie, treas.; Monroe M. Rifkin, immediate past chm.; Dr. John C. Malone, Robert Miron, Trygve Myhren
BOARD OF DIRECTORS
Daniel Aaron, Edward M. Allen, Kenneth L. Bagwell, Gregory B. Blow, William J. Bresnan, James S. Cownie, Steven B. Dodge, Charles F. Dolan, Frank Drendel, John D. Evans, Michael J. Fuchs, Joseph Gans, Sr., John W. Goddard, James L. Gray, Amos B. Hostetter, Jr., Glenn R. Jones, F. Frederick Kennedy, Philip B. Lind, Jerry D. Lindauer, Richard W. Loftus, Craig O. McCaw, Terence F. McGuirk, Dr. John C. Malone, Robert Miron, Harry F. Murray, Trygve E. Myhren, Myron T. Pattison, James O. Robbins, Clive Runnells, Frank S. Scarpa, Gene W. Schneider, Roy A. Sheppard, Abe Sonnenschein, William B. Strange, June E. Travis, Larry W. Wangberg
DATE OF ORGANIZATION
1952

National Federation of Local Cable Programmers

906 Pennsylvania Ave., S.E., Washington, DC 20003; (202) 544-7272.

EXECUTIVE DIRECTOR
Sue Miller Busbe

Videotape Production Association, Inc.

236 East 46 St., New York, NY 10017; (212) 986-0289.

CHAIRMAN OF BOARD
Morton Dubin
PRESIDENT, NEW YORK CHAPTER
Joe DiBuono
EXECUTIVE DIRECTOR
Janet Luhrs

Video Services

* Animation
* Audio Mixing & Sweetening
* Cleaning & Evaluation of Tapes
* Duplication
* Editing & Post Production
* Equipment—Sales & Rental
* Equipment Repair
* Mobile Units
* Production Studios & Stages
* Screening Rooms
* Transfers—Film to Tape
* Transfers—Tape to Film

VIDEOTAPE ANIMATION

LOS ANGELES

ACCOLADE PRODUCTIONS, 8686 Franklin Ave., Los Angeles, CA 90069; (213) 656-0925.

AMERICAN VIDEO FACTORY, 4150 Glencoe Ave., Marina Del Rey, CA 90292; (213) 823-8622.

AMERICAN VIDEOGRAM INC., 2207 S. Colby Ave., Los Angeles, CA 90064-1504; (213) 477-1535.

BERC, BROADCAST EQUIPMENT RENTAL COMPANY, 4545 Chermak St., Burbank, CA 91505; (818) 841-3000, (213) 464-7655.

CAUSE & EFX, 1523 Crossroads of the World, Los Angeles, CA 90028; (213) 466-3939.

CALIFORNIA COMMUNICATIONS, INC., 6900 Santa Monica Blvd., Los Angeles, CA 90038; (213) 466-8511.

COTTON CANDY/EYE ON VIDEO, 224 N. Juanita Ave., Los Angeles, CA 90004; (213) 382-4048.

GLENDALE STUDIOS, 1239 S. Glendale Ave., Glendale, CA 91205; (818) 502-5300.

GORDON, ALAN, ENTERPRISES, INC., 1430 N. Cahuenga Blvd., Hollywood, CA 90078; (213) 466-3561.

IMAGE WEST, 11846 Ventura Blvd., Studio City, CA 91604; (818) 506-5577.

MULTI-MEDIA WORKS, 7227 Beverly Blvd., Los Angeles, CA 90036; (213) 939-1185.

MARSH INTERNATIONAL FILMS, 21029 Itasca St., Suites A & B, Chatsworth, CA 91311; (818) 998-2188.

PACIFIC VIDEO, 809 N. Cahuenga Blvd., Los Angeles, CA 90038; (213) 462-6266.

RUXTON LTD, 611 N. Orchard Dr., Burbank, CA 91506; (818) 845-3724.

SCHULMAN VIDEO CENTER, 861 Seward St., Hollywood, CA 90038; (213) 465-8110.

SUNBREAK PRODUCTIONS, 256 S. La Cienega Blvd., Beverly Hills, CA 90211; (213) 659-2324.

SYSTEMS, 248 Hollywood Way, Burbank, CA 91505; (818) 846-9772.

VARITEL VIDEO/JACK SCHAEFFER, 3575 Cahuenga Blvd. West., Los Angeles, CA 90068; (213) 822-8872.

VIDEO IMAGE, 13450 Maxella Ave., Suite 270, Marina Del Rey, CA 90292; (213) 822-8872.

VIDTRONICS INC., 855 N. Cahuenga Blvd., Los Angeles, CA 90038; (213) 805-1165.

NEW YORK

MODERN TELECOMMUNICATIONS INC., 1443 Park Ave., New York, NY 10029; (212) 722-1818.

SAN FRANCISCO

ONE PASS FILM & VIDEO, One China Basin Building, San Francisco, CA 94107; (415) 777-5777.

VIDEO AUDIO MIXING & SWEETENING

LOS ANGELES

ALDAN CO. INC, 355 S. Mansfield Ave., Los Angeles, CA 90036; (213) 936-1032.

ALTAVIDEO, 3501 Cahuenga Blvd. W., Los Angeles, CA 90068; (213) 876-8008.

AMERICAN VIDEO FACTORY, 4150 Glencoe Ave., Marina Del Rey, CA 90292; (213) 823-8622.

AUDIO-VIDEO CRAFT INC., 7000 Santa Monica Blvd., Los Angeles, CA 90038; (213) 466-6475.

AUDIO VISUAL HEADQUARTERS CORP., 361 N. Oak St., Inglewood, CA 90302; (213) 419-4040.

BRITANNIA SCORING SERVICES, INC., 3249 Cahuenga Blvd. W., Hollywood, CA 90068; (213) 851-1244.

BURBANK STUDIOS, 4000 Warner Blvd., Burbank, CA 91522; (818) 954-6000.

BUZZY'S RECORDING SERVICES, 6900 Melrose Ave., Los Angeles, CA 90038; (213) 931-1867.

CALIFORNIA COMMUNICATIONS INC., 6900 Santa Monica Blvd., Los Angeles, CA 90038; (213) 466-8511.

CALIFORNIA RECORDING & VIDEO, 5023 Sunset Blvd., Los Angeles, CA 90027; (213) 666-1244.

CALIFORNIA ZEPHYR, 9348 Santa Monica Blvd., Suite 101, Beverly Hills, CA 90210; (213) 653-4004.

COLLECT-A-SOUND INC., 21029 Itasca, Suite A & B, Chatsworth, CA 91311; (818) 998-2188.

COMPACT SOUND SERVICES, 2813 W. Alameda Ave., Burbank, CA 91505; (818) 840-7000.

COMPACT VIDEO SERVICES, INC., 2813 W. Alameda Ave., Burbank, CA 91505; (818) 840-7000.

CONSOLIDATED FILM INDUSTRIES, 959 Seward St., Los Angeles, CA 90038; (213) 462-3161.

COTTON CANDY/EYE ON VIDEO, 224 N. Juanita Ave., Los Angeles, CA 90004; (213) 382-4048.

CREATIVE VIDEO SERVICES, 500 Ventu Park Rd., Newbury Park, CA 91320; (818) 707-2424.

CREST NATIONAL FILM & VIDEOTAPE LABS, 1141 N. Seward St., Los Angeles, CA 90038; (213) 462-3073.

DEVONSHIRE SOUND STUDIOS, 10729 Magnolia Blvd., North Hollywood, CA 91601; (818) 985-1945.

EFP/EBSEN FISHER PRODUCTIONS, 9541 Cedarbrook Dr., Beverly Hills, CA 90210; (213) 273-2208.

FREEMAN, DOUG, SOUND & EDITORIAL, 6362 Hollywood Blvd., Suite 219, Hollywood, CA 90028; (213) 467-8742.

GLENN, GLEN SOUND CO., 900 Seward St., Los Angeles, CA 90038; (213) 469-7221.

GREAT AMERICAN CINEMA CO., 10711 Wellworth Ave., Los Angeles, CA 90024, (213) 475-0937.

GROUP W CABLE VIDEO PRODUCTION CENTER, 2939 Nebraska Ave., Santa Monica, CA 90404; (213) 829-2676.

HARMONY GOLD USA, INC., 8831 Sunset Blvd., Suite 300, Los Angeles, CA 90069; (213) 652-8720.

HARRIS, CRAIG (sound composer), P.O. Box 36A45, Los Angeles, CA 90036; (818) 508-8000.

HOLLYWOOD NATIONAL STUDIOS, 6605 Eleanor Ave., Los Angeles, CA 90038; (213) 467-6272.

HORIZONTAL EDITING STUDIOS, 2625 W. Olive Ave., Burbank, CA 91505; (818) 841-6750.

INSTITUTE OF AUDIO/VIDEO ENGINEERING, 1831 Hyperlon Ave., Hollywood, CA 90027; (213) 666-3003.

KWHY-TV, CHANNEL 22, 5545 Sunset Blvd., Los Angeles, CA 90028; (213) 466-5441.

KENDUN RECORDERS INC., 619 S. Glenwood Pl., Burbank, CA 91506; (818) 843-8096.

LAJON PRODUCTIONS INC. 2907 W. Olive Ave., Burbank, CA 91505; (818) 841-1440.

LION SHARE RECORDING STUDIOS, 8255 Beverly Blvd., Los Angeles, CA 90048; (213) 658-5990.

M.F.I. VIDEO CENTER, 1905 Grace Ave., Hollywood, CA 90068; (213) 851-0373.

MARSH INTERNATIONAL FILMS, 21029 Itasca St., Suites A & B, Chatsworth, CA 91311; (818) 998-2188.

MASTER DIGITAL INC., 1749 14th St., Santa Monica, CA 90404; (213) 452-1511.

MERIDIAN, P.O. Box 1941, Hollywood, CA 90028; (213) 874-4367.

METAVISION, 347 S. Ogden Dr., Suite 220, Los Angeles, CA 90036; (213) 936-8281.

METROTAPE (a division of Metromedia), 5746 Sunset Blvd., Los Angeles, CA 90028; (213) 856-1000.

MUSIC LAB INC., 1831 Hyperlon Ave., Hollywood, CA 90027; (213) 666-3003.

NOVASONIC DIGITAL PRODUCTION MUSIC LIBRARY, 444 S. Victory Blvd., Burbank, CA 91502; (213) 661-7777.

ONE INCH VIDEO PRODUCTIONS INC., 4710 W. Magnolia Blvd., Burbank, CA 91505; (818) 760-6900.

ONE PASS FILM & VIDEO, One China Basin Building, San Francisco, CA 94107; (415) 777-5777.

OUTRIDER VIDEO & FILM, 2907 W. Olive Ave., Burbank, CA 91505; (818) 841-1440.

PACIFIC VIDEO, 809 N. Cahuenga Blvd., Los Angeles, CA 90038; (213) 462-6266.

PARAMOUNT RECORDING STUDIOS, 6245 Santa Monica Blvd., Hollywood, CA 90038; (212) 461-3717.

POSITIVE MEDIA, 5422 A. Fair Ave., North Hollywood, CA 91601; (818) 761-5192.

THE POST GROUP, 6335 Homewood Ave., Los Angeles, CA 90028; (213) 462-2300.

PRECISION FOLEY & ADR., 6353 Homewood Ave., Hollywood, CA 90028; (213) 462-8235.

PREMORE INC., 5130 Klump Ave., North Hollywood, CA 91601; (818) 506-7714.

ROCK SOLID PRODUCTIONS, 801 S. Main St., Burbank, CA 91506; (818) 841-8220.

RUSK SOUND STUDIO, 1556 N. La Brea Ave., Hollywood, CA 90028; (213) 462-6477.

SALTY DOG RECORDING STUDIO, 14511 Delano St., Van Nuys, CA 91411; (818) 994-9973.

SCHULMAN VIDEO CENTER, 861 Seward St., Hollywood, CA 90038; (213) 465-8110.

SCORE ONE RECORDING INC., 5500 Cahuenga Blvd., North Hollywood, CA 91601; (818) 762-6902.

SCOTTSOUND INC., 6110 Santa Monica Blvd., Los Angeles, CA 90038; (213) 462-6981.

SKYLINE PRODUCTIONS, 6309 Eleanor Ave., Hollywood, CA 90038; (213) 856-0033.

SOUND IMAGE STUDIOS INC., 6556 Willkinson Ave., North Hollywood, CA 91606; (818) 762-8881.

SOUND MASTER, 10747 Magnolia Blvd., North Hollywood, CA 91601; (213) 650-8000.

SOUND SERVICES INC. (S.S.I.), 7155 Santa Monica Blvd., Los Angeles, CA 90046; (213) 874-9344, (818) 986-3255.

SPEAR, JACK PRODUCTIONS INC., 7243 Santa Monica Blvd., Hollywood, CA 90046; (213) 851-4123.

STEVENS, KRIS ENTERPRISES INC., 14241 Ventura Blvd., Suite 204, Sherman Oaks, CA 91423; (818) 981-8255.

SUNRISE CANYON VIDEO, P.O. Box 10968, Burbank, CA 91510; (818) 845-7473.

SUNSET POST INC., 1813 Victory Blvd., Glendale, CA 91201; (818) 956-7912.

SUNSET SOUND FACTORY, 6357 Selma Ave., Hollywood, CA 90028; (213) 467-2500.

SUNWEST STUDIOS, 5533 Sunset Blvd., Hollywood, CA 90028; (213) 463-5631.

SUPERIOR VIDEO SERVICES, 13423 Saticoy St., North Hollywood, CA 91605; (818) 786-7060.

THE SYSTEM LTD, 1054 N. Cahuenga Blvd., Hollywood, CA 90038; (213) 461-3000..

TAJ SOUNDWORKS, 8207 W. Third St., Los Angeles, CA 90048; (213) 655-2775.

TAV SOUND INC., 6200 W. 3rd St., Los Angeles, CA 90038; (213) 937-2460.

VIA VISION PRODUCTIONS, 5919 Franklin Ave., Los Angeles, CA 90028; (213) 460-4864.

VIDEO ADVENTURES, 1015 Cahuenga Blvd., Hollywood, CA 90038; (213) 461-3288.

VIDEOASIS, 317 S. Verdugo Rd., Glendale, CA 91205; (818) 507-1037.

THE VIDEO TAPE CO., 10545 Burbank Blvd., North Hollywood, CA 91601; (818) 985-1666.

VIDE-U PRODUCTIONS, 612 N. Sepulveda Blvd., Los Angeles, CA 90049; (213) 472-7023.

VIDTRONICS, INC., 855 N. Cahuenga Blvd., Los Angeles, CA 90038; (213) 856-8200.

THE VILLAGE RECORDER, 1616 Butler Ave., West Los Angeles, CA 90025; (213) 478-8227.

VITELLO & ASSOCIATES, 6353 Homewood Ave., Hollywood, CA 90028; (213) 462-8235.

VOICE OVER L.A. INC., 1717 N. Highland Ave., Suite 620, Hollywood, CA 90028; (213) 463-VOLA.

WESTLAKE STUDIOS, 8447 Beverly Blvd., Los Angeles, CA 90048; (213) 654-2155.

WILDER BROTHERS VIDEO, 10327 Santa Monica Blvd., Los Angeles, CA 90025; (213) 557-3500.

NEW YORK

EDITEL, NEW YORK, 222 E. 44 St., New York, NY 10017; (212) 867-4600.

MODERN TELECOMMUNICATIONS, 1 Dag Hammarskjold Plaza, New York, NY 10017; (212) 355-0510.

VCA/TELETRONICS, 231 E. 55 St., New York, NY 10022; (212) 355-1600.

WINDSOR TOTAL VIDEO, 565 Fifth Ave., New York, NY 10017; (212) 725-8080.

VIDEOTAPE CLEANING & EVALUATION

LOS ANGELES

BONDED SERVICES, 5260 Vineland Ave., North Hollywood, CA 91601; (818) 761-4058.
CREATIVE VIDEO SERVICES, 500 Ventu Park Rd., Newbury Park, CA 91320; (818) 707-2424.
THE EDITING COMPANY, 8300 Beverly Blvd., Los Angeles, CA 90048; (213) 653-3570.
FILM PROCESSING CORP., 3602 S. Crenshaw Blvd., Los Angeles, CA 90016; (213) 737-8273.
IMAGE TRANSFORM INC., 4142 Lankershim Blvd., North Hollywood, CA 91602; (818) 985-7566.
MARSH INTERNATIONAL FILMS, 21029 Itasca St., Suite A & B, Chatsworth, CA 91311; (818) 998-2188.
SOUND MASTER, 10747 Magnolia Blvd., North Hollywood, CA 91601; (213) 650-8000.
STUDIO FILM & TAPE INC. 6670 Santa Monica Blvd., Los Angeles, CA 90038; (213) 466-8101.
TAV/COMMAND, INC., 1541 N. Vine St., Los Angeles, CA 90028; (213) 466-2141.
THE VIDEO TAPE CO., 10545 Burbank Blvd., North Hollywood, CA 91601; (818) 985-1666.

NEW YORK

P.A.T. FILM SERVICES, 630 Ninth Ave., New York, NY 10036; (212) 247-0900.
T.F.I., TAPE-FILM INDUSTRIES, 619 W. 54 St., New York, NY 10019; (212) 708-0500. Branch offices: 941 N. Highland Ave., Los Angeles, CA 90038; (213) 461-3361; 640 N. La Salle St., Chicago, IL 60610; (312) 957-6700.
VCA/TELETRONICS, 231 E. 55 St., New York, NY 10022; (212) 355-1600.

VIDEOTAPE DUPLICATION SERVICES

LOS ANGELES

A.M.E. INC., 2921 W. Olive Ave., Burbank, CA 91505; (818) 841-7440.
ABBEY TAPE DUPLICATORS INC., 9525 Vassar Ave., Chatsworth, CA 91311; (818) 882-5210.
ABERDEEN VIDEO, 3349 Cahuenga Blvd. West, Suite 1A, Los Angeles, CA 90068; (213) 874-3050.
ALTAVIDEO, 3501 Cahuenga Blvd. West, Los Angeles, CA 90068; (213) 876-8008.
AMERICAN VIDEO FACTORY, 4150 Glencoe Ave., Marina Del Rey, CA 90292; (213) 823-8622.
AMPAC VIDEO, 3637 Cahuenga Blvd. West, Hollywood, CA 90068; (213) 851-7200.
APOLLO PRODUCTION FACILITY, 1503 Cahuenga Blvd., Hollywood, CA 90028, (213) 464-7871; (213) 464-9924.
AUDIO GRAPHIC FILMS AND VIDEO, 6509 De Longpre Ave., Hollywood, CA 90028, (213) 462-6596; (213) 467-1234.
AUDIO PLUS VIDEO INTERNATIONAL INC., 1438 N. Gower St., Hollywood, CA 90028; (213) 856-0152.
AUDIO-VIDEO CRAFT INC., 7000 Santa Monica Blvd., Los Angeles, CA 90038; (213) 466-6475.
AUDIO VISUAL HEADQUARTERS CORP., 361 N. Oak St., Inglewood, CA 90302; (213) 419-4040.
BONDED SERVICES, 5260 Vineland Ave., North Hollywood, CA 91601; (213) 761-4058.
CAL VISTA INTERNATIONAL LTD., 6649 Odessa Ave., Van Nuys, CA 91406; (818) 780-9000.
CALIFORNIA COMMUNICATIONS INC., 6900 Santa Monica Blvd., Los Angeles, CA 90038; (213) 466-8511.
CALIFORNIA ZEPHYR, 9348 Santa Monica Blvd., Suite 101, Beverly Hills, CA 90210; (213) 653-4004.
CINE CRAFT-HOLLYWOOD, INC., 13062 Saticoy St., North Hollywood, CA 91605; (818) 765-1414.
COAST FILM LAB CO., 837 N. Cahuenga Blvd., Los Angeles, CA 90028; (213) 464-7293.
COLLECT-A-SOUND INC., 21029 Itasca, Suite A & B, Chatsworth, CA 91311; (818) 998-2188.
COMPACT VIDEO SERVICES INC., 2813 W. Alameda Ave., Burbank, CA 91505; (818) 840-7000.
COMPOSITE IMAGE SYSTEMS, 815 N. Cahuenga Blvd., Hollywood, CA 90038; (213) 461-5734.
CONSOLIDATED FILM INDUSTRIES, 959 Seward St., Los Angeles, CA 90038; (213) 462-3161.
COTTON CANDY/EYE ON VIDEO, 224 N. Juanita Ave., Los Angeles, CA 90004; (213) 382-4048.
CREATIVE SOUND PRODUCTIONS, 6290 Sunset Blvd., Suite 1026, Hollywood, CA 90028; (213) 871-1010.
CREATIVE VIDEO SERVICES, 500 Ventu Park Rd., Newbury Park, CA 91320; (818) 707-2424.
CREST NATIONAL FILM & VIDEOTAPE LABS, 1141 N. Seward St., Los Angeles, CA 90038; (213) 462-3073.
CUSTOM DUPLICATION INC., 3404 Century Blvd., Inglewood, CA 90303; (213) 670-5575.
DELUXE LABORATORIES, INC., 1377 N. Serrano Ave., Hollywood, CA 90027; (213) 462-6171.
DEVONSHIRE SOUND STUDIOS, 10729 Magnolia Blvd., North Hollywood, CA 91601; (818) 985-1945.
ECONOMY PRODUCTION EDITING & AIR CHECKS, 7557 Hampton Ave., Los Angeles, CA 90046; (213) 850-5411.
EDITEL LOS ANGELES, 729 N. Highland Ave., Hollywood, CA 90038; (213) 931-1821.
THE EDITING COMPANY, 8300 Beverly Blvd., Los Angeles, CA 90048; (213) 653-3570.
EMC PRODUCTIONS, 6855 Santa Monica Blvd., Suite 308, Hollywood, CA 90038; (213) 463-3282.
ENVIRONMENTAL VIDEO INC., P.O. Box 577, Manhattan Beach, CA 90266; (213) 546-4581.
FILMCORE PRINT AND TAPE, 901 N. Seward St., Los Angeles, CA 90038; (213) 464-7303.
FOTO-KEM INDUSTRIES INC., 2800 W. Olive Ave., Burbank, CA 91505; (818) 846-3101.
FOTO-TRONICS SYSTEMS INC., 2800 W. Olive Ave., Burbank, CA 91505; (818) 846-3101.
GLENDALE STUDIOS, 1239 S. Glendale Ave., Glendale, CA 91205; (818) 502-5300.
GLOBAL VISION CORPORATION, 3255 Cahuenga Blvd., Hollywood, CA 90068; (213) 851-1190.
GOLDEN WEST VIDEOTAPE, 5800 Sunset Blvd., Loś Angeles, CA 90028; (213) 460-5866.
H.C.V., 3034 Glendale Blvd., Los Angeles, CA 90039; (213) 662-1112.
HORIZONTAL EDITING STUDIOS, 2625 W. Olive Ave., Burbank, CA 91505; (818) 841-6750.
HQI STUDIOS, 19347 Londellus St., Northridge, CA 91324; (818) 993-4778.
IMAGE TRANSFORM INC., 4142, Lankershim Blvd., North Hollywood, CA 91602; (818) 985-7566.
IMAGE TRANSFORM LABORATORY, 3611 N. San Fernando Rd., Burbank, CA 91505; (818) 841-3812.
IMAGE WEST, 11846 Ventura Blvd., Studio City, CA 91604; (818) 506-5577.
INTER VIDEO, 3220 Burbank Blvd., Burbank, CA 91505; (818) 843-3633.
INTERNATIONAL VIDEO CONVERSIONS, 818 N. Cahuenga Blvd., Hollywood, CA 90038; (213) 463-7884.
INSTANT REPLAY EQUIPMENT CO., 5520 Westlawn Ave., Los Angeles, CA 90066; (213) 870-1231.
J.P. VIDEO SERVICES, 9538 W. Pico Blvd., Los Angeles, CA 90035; (213) 271-1209.
KWHY-TV, CHANNEL 22, 5545 Sunset Blvd., Los Angeles, CA 90028; (213) 466-5441.
KRAMER, JERRY & ASSOCIATES, 1312 N. La Brea Ave., Hollywood, CA 90028; (213) 462-2680.
LION SHARE RECORDING STUDIOS, 8255 Beverly Blvd., Los Angeles, CA 90048; (213) 658-5990.
LIONEL TELEVISION PRODUCTIONS, 417 Colorado Ave., Santa Monica, CA 90401; (213) 394-9697.
MGS SERVICES, 10507 Burbank Blvd., North Hollywood, CA 91601; (818) 508-5488.
M.R.I. FILM & VIDEO, 1905 Grace Ave., Hollywood, CA 90068; (213) 851-0373.
McINTIRE-HOFFMAN, INC., 18149 Ventura Blvd., Tarzana, CA 91356; (818) 345-9677.
McKAY, CAMERON PRODUCTIONS, 1011 N.. Cole Ave., Los Angeles, CA 90038; (213) 463-6073.
MARSH INTERNATIONAL FILMS, 21029 Itasca St., Suite A & B, Chatsworth, CA 91311; (818) 998-2188.
MASTER DIGITAL INC., 1749 14th St., Santa Monica, CA 90404; (213) 452-1511.
MEDIA HOME ENTERTAINMENT INC., 5730 Buckingham Pkway, Culver City, CA 90230; (213) 216-7900.
METROTAPE (A division of Metromedia), 5746 Sunset Blvd., Los Angeles, CA 90028; (213) 856-1000.
MUSIC LAB INC., 1831 Hyperion Ave., Hollywood, CA 90027; (213) 666-3003.
ONE INCH VIDEO PRODUCTIONS INC., 4710 W. Magnolia Blvd., Burbank, CA 91505; (818) 760-6900.
PACIFIC FILM LAB INC., 5244 Santa Monica Blvd., Los Angeles, CA 90029; (213) 661-1144.
PACIFIC VIDEO, 809 N. Cahuenga Blvd., Los Angeles, CA 90038; (213) 462-6266.
PAL VIDEO, 19061 Tina Pl., Tarzana, CA 91356; (818) 344-1603.
POSITIVE MEDIA, 5422 A Fair Ave., North Hollywood, CA 91601; (818) 761-5192.
THE POST GROUP, 6335 Homewood Ave., Los Angeles, CA 90028; (213) 462-2300.
POST PLUS INCORPORATED, 6650 Santa Monica Blvd., Hollywood, CA 90038; (213) 463-7108.
PROFESSIONAL ARTISTS GROUP, 845 N. Highland Ave., Hollywood, CA 90038; (213) 871-2222.
PROJECT ONE, 6669 Sunset Blvd., Hollywood, CA 90028; (213) 464-2285.
QPT EDITORIAL CORPORATION, 629 N. La Brea Ave., Los Angeles, CA 90036; (213) 936-7181.
RED CAR EDITING, 1040 N. Las Palmas Ave., Los Angeles, CA 90038; (213) 466-4467.
ROCK SOLID PRODUCTIONS, 801 S. Main St., Burbank, CA 91506; (818) 841-8220.
ROLLING VIDEO, 18730 Oxnard, Tarzana, CA 91356; (818) 993-6912.
RUSK SOUND STUDIO, 1556 N. La Brea Ave., Hollywood, CA 90028; (213) 462-6477.
RUXTON LTD., 611 N. Orchard Dr., Burbank, CA 91506; (818) 845-3724.
SAWYER CAMERA & VIDEO SERVICE, 1208 W. Isabel St., Burbank; CA 91506, (818) 843-1781.
SCHULMAN VIDEO CENTER, 861 Seward St., Hollywood, CA 90038; (213) 465-8110.
SELL PICTURES INC., 9701 Wilshire Blvd., Beverly Hills, CA 90212; (213) 874-5402.

SKYLIGHT PRODUCTION INC., 6815 Willoughby, Suite 201, Los Angeles, CA 90038; (213) 464-4500.
SOUND MASTER, 10747 Magnolia Blvd., North Hollywood, CA 91601; (213) 650-8000.
SOUND SERVICES, INC. (S.S.I.), 7155 Santa Monica Blvd., Los Angeles, CA 90046; (213) 874-9344, (818) 986-3255.
SPALLA, RICK VIDEO PRODUCTIONS, 1622 N. Gower, Los Angeles, CA 90028; (213) 469-7307.
SPEAR, JACK PRODUCTIONS, INC., 7243 Santa Monica Blvd., Hollywood, CA 90046; (213) 851-4123.
STEVENS, KRIS ENTERPRISES INC., 14241 Ventura Blvd., Suite 204, Sherman Oaks, CA 91423; (818) 981-8255.
SUNRISE CANYON VIDEO, P.O. Box 10968, Burbank, CA 91510; (818) 845-7473.
SUNSET POST INC., 1813 Victory Blvd., Glendale, CA 91201; (818) 956-7912.
SUPERCINE INC., 2213 W. Olive Ave., Burbank, CA 91506; (818) 843-8260.
SUPERIOR VIDEO SERVICES, 13423 Saticoy St., North Hollywood, CA 91605; (818) 786-7060.
TAV/COMMAND, INC., 1541 N. Vine St., Los Angeles, CA 90028; (213) 466-2141.
TELEPRINT OF LOS ANGELES, 3779 Cahuenga Blvd., West, Studio City, CA 91604; (818) 760-3191.
TYLIE JONES & ASSOC. INC., 10718 Riverside Dr., North Hollywood, CA 91602; (818) 980-7300.
TRANS-AMERICAN VIDEO INC., 1541 N. Vine St., Los Angeles, CA 90028; (213) 466-2141.
TRANSWORLD VIDEO LAB INC., 3812 W. Magnolia Blvd., Burbank, CA 91505; (818) 841-2416.
TRITRONICS INC., 733 N. Victory Blvd., Burbank, CA 91502; (818) 843-2288, (800) 232-2141.
UCL VIDEO, 823 N. Seward St., Los Angeles, CA 90038; (213) 469-7291.
UDELL, BILL PRODUCTIONS, 6006 Vantage Ave., North Hollywood, CA 91606; (818) 985-6866.
UNITEL VIDEO, 5555 Melrose Ave., Studio G, Los Angeles, CA 90038; (213) 468-4606.
VCI DUPLICATION, 915 Hollywood Way, Burbank, CA 91505; (818) 841-8550.
V.M.G. INC, 16042 Ventura Blvd., Suite 206, Encino, CA 91426; (818) 905-5311.
VALLEY VIDEO, 4209 W. Burbank Blvd., Burbank, CA 91505; (818) 841-2387.
VECTOR PRODUCTIONS INC., P.O. Box 7000-645, Redondo Beach, CA 90277; (213) 316-6031, 757-0520.
VIA VISION PRODUCTIONS, 5919 Franklin Ave., Los Angeles, CA 90028; (213) 460-4864.
VIDEO ADVENTURES INC., 1015 Cahuenga Blvd., Hollywood, CA 90038; (213) 461-3288.
VIDEO ASSOCIATES AND CO., 5419 Sunset Blvd., Los Angeles, CA 90027; (213) 463-3255.
VIDEO CRAFTSMEN INC., 6311 Romaine St., Los Angeles, CA 90038; (213) 464-4351.
VIDEO-IT INC., 1016 N. Sycamore Ave., Hollywood, CA 90038; (213) 876-4055; (213) VID-EOIT.
THE VIDEO TAPE CO., 10545 Burbank Blvd., North Hollywood, CA 91601; (818) 985-1666.
VIDEO WEST, 6430 Sunset Blvd., Suite 908, Los Angeles, CA 90028; (213) 465-3153.
VIDTRONICS INC., 855 N. Cahuenga Blvd., Los Angeles, CA 90038; (213) 856-8200.
VIDE-U PRODUCTIONS, 612 N. Sepulveda Blvd., Los Angeles, CA 90049; (213) 472-7023.
WEISBARTH, JACOB & ASSOC. INC., 9903 Santa Monica Blvd., Suite 256, Beverly Hills, CA 90212; (213) 475-0668.
WESTERN FILM INDUSTRIES, 30941 W. Agoura Rd., Suite 302, Westlake Village, CA 91360; (818) 889-7350.
WILDER BROTHERS VIDEO, 10327 Santa Monica Blvd., Los Angeles, CA 90025; (213) 557-3500.

NEW YORK

A N S INTERNATIONAL VIDEO LTD., 396 Fifth Ave., New York, NY 10018; (212) 736-1007.
ACE AUDIO VISUAL CO., 118 E. 28 St., Fifth Floor, New York, NY 10016; (212) 685-3344; 33-49 55th St., Woodside, NY; (718) 458-3800.
AMERICAN INC., 717 Lexington Ave., New York, NY 10022; (212) 888-0888.
AMERICAN VIDEO—CHANNELS INC., 321 W. 44 St., New York, NY 10036; (212) 765-6324.
BOGAZICI VIDEO LTD., 460 Seventh Ave., New York, NY 10001; (212) 563-9022.
CALAMAR PRODUCTIONS, 254 Park Avenue South, New York, NY 10010; (212) 254-7086.
CINE MAGNETICS FILM & VIDEO LABORATOREIS, 50 W. 40 St., New York, NY 10018; (212) 542-0700.
DEVLIN PRODUCTIONS INC., 150 W. 55 St., New York, NY 10019; (212) 582-5572.
DOLPHIN PRODUCTIONS, 140 E. 80 St., New York, NY 10021; (212) 628-5930.
EDITEL, NEW YORK, 222 E. 44 St., New York, NY 10017; (212) 867-4600.
ELECTROTECH TRADING CORP., 40-10 67th St., Woodside NY;(718) 899-8388.
EXPRESS VIDEO INC., 244 W. 49 St., New York, NY 10019; (212) 246-2311.
FAMA II PRODUCTIONS, 2750 Richmond Terrace, Staten Island, NY 10303; (718) 273-1780.
FOTO-VIDEO TRANSFER CENTER, 1 Times Square, New York, NY 10036; (212) 302-1866.
GML VIDEO INC., 137 Varick St., New York, NY 10013; (212) 645-3700.
GLOBE VIDEO SERVICES, INC., 286 Fifth Ave., New York, NY 10001; (212) 695-6868.
HK VIDEO REPRODUCTIONS INC., 160 Sixth Ave., New York, NY 10013; (212) 431-3397.
HALLENDAL ENTERPRIZES, 10 W. 25 St., New York, NY 10010; (212) 620-7446.
INTERNATIONAL VIDEO SERVICES, 1501 Broadway, New York, NY 10036; (212) 730-1411.
JUPITER PRODUCTION SERVICES, 55 W. 45 St., New York, NY 10036; (212) 575-1066.
MPCS COMMUNICATIONS, 514 W. 57 St., New York, NY 10019; (212) 586-3690.
MEDIATECH EAST, 515 W. 57 St., New York, NY 10019; (212) 765-8720.
MODERN TELECOMMUNICATIONS INC., 1443 Park Ave., New York, NY 10029; (2312) 722-1818.
NATIONAL VIDEO INDUSTRIES, INC., 15 W. 17 St., New York, NY 10011; (212) 691-1300.
OCCASIONAL VIDEO, 534 E. 84 St., New York, NY 10028; (212) 737-3058.
P.A.T. FILM SERVICES, 630 Ninth Ave., New York, NY 10036; (212) 247-0900.
PICSONIC PRODUCTIONS CORP., 1466 Broadway, New York, NY 10036; (212) 575-1910.
POWER PLAY RECORDS INC., 198 Bloomfield Ave., Newark, NJ; (201) 481-0972.
REEVES TELETAPE, 304 E. 44 St., New York, NY 10012; (212) 573-8888.
ROSS-LEVINE, 594 Broadway, New York, NY 10003; (212) 925-2020.
S-T VIDEOCASSETTE DUPLICATION CORP., 500 Willowtree Rd., Leonia, NJ, (212) 239-4653.
SYNESTHETICS INC., 58 Walker St., New York, NY 10013; (212) 431-4112.
TFI, TAPE-FILM INDUSTRIES, 619 W. 54 St., New York, NY 10019, (212) 708-0500.
TABCO FILM & VIDEO SERVICES, 850 Seventh Ave., New York, NY 10019; (212) 315-3880.
TELETECHNIQUES, 40 W. 72 St., New York, NY 10023; (212) 580-9551.
UNI VISION, 481 Eighth Ave., New York, NY 10001; (212) 563-1320.
UNITEL VIDEO, 515 W. 57 St., New York, NY 10019; (212) 265-3600.
VCA TELETRONICS, 231 E. 55 St., New York, NY 10022; (212) 355-1600.
VIDEO CASSETTE TRANSFERS, 160 W. 46 St., New York, NY 10036; (212) 575-8433.
VIDEO CENTRAL INC., 225 W. 36 St., New York, NY 10018; (212) 947-6960.
VIDEO PLANNING INC., 250 W. 57 St., New York, NY 10019; (212) 582-5066.
VIDEO PORTFOLIOS, 142 W. 24 St., New York, NY 10011; (212) 989-3858.
VIDEO 3000, 1400 Broadway, Penthouse Loft, New York, NY 10018; (212) 302-1313.
VIDEOROOM, 1487 Third Ave., New York, NY 10028; (212) 879-5333.
WINDSOR TOTAL VIDEO, 565 Fifth Ave., New York, NY 10017; (212) 725-8080.

ILLINOIS

AV CENTER, 5153 N. Lincoln Ave., Chicago, IL 60659; (312) 275-7098.

TELEMATRON PRODUCTIONS, INC., 3200 W. West Lake Ave., Glenview, IL 60025; (312) 729-5215.

MT. VIEW CALIFORNIA

TELEVISION ASSOCIATES, INC., 2410 Charleston Rd., Mt. View, CA; (415) 967-6040.

WASHINGTON

VIDEO PRESENTATIONS, 2326 Sixth Ave., Room 230, Seattle, WA 98121; (206) 728-9241.

CANADA

MANTA VIDEO LABS, 311 Adelaide St. E., Toronto, Ont., Canada M5A IN2; (416) 863-9316.

VIDEOTAPE EDITING & POST PRODUCTION FACILITIES AND SERVICES

WEST COAST

—A—

A.M.E. Inc., 2921 W. Olive Ave., Burbank, CA 91505; (818) 841-7440.

ABERDEEN VIDEO, 3349 Cahuenga Blvd. West, Suite 1A, Los Angeles, CA 90068; (213) 874-3050.

ACCOLADE PRODUCTIONS LTD., 8480 Beverly Blvd., Suite 160, Los Angeles, CA 90048; (213) 651-5757.

ACE AND EDIE, 722 N. Seward St., Hollywood, CA 90038; (213) 462-2185.

ADVENTURES IN FILM & TAPE, 1027 N. Cole Ave., Hollywood, CA 90038; (213) 460-4557.

ALDAN CO. INC., 355 S. Mansfield Ave., Los Angeles, CA 90036; (213) 936-1032.

ALL WEST VIDEO, 11320 Chandler Blvd., North Hollywood, CA 91601; (818) 508-8500.

ALTAVIDEO, 3501 Cahuenga Blvd. West, Los Angeles, CA 90068; (213) 876-8008.

AMERICAN VIDEO FACTORY, 4150 Glencoe Ave., Marina Del Rey, CA 90292; (213) 823-8622.

AMERICAN VIDEOGRAM INC., 2207 S. Colby Ave., Los Angeles, CA 90064-1504; (213) 477-1535.

AQUARIUS THEATRE, 6230 Sunset Blvd., Hollywood, CA 90028; (213) 460-6700.

AMPAC VIDEO, 3637 Cahuenga Blvd. West, Hollywood, CA 90068; (213) 851-7200.

AUDIO GRAPHIC FILMS AND VIDEO, 6509 De Longpre Ave., Hollywood, CA 90028; (213) 462-6596; (213) 467-1234.

AUDIO-VIDEO CRAFT INC., 7000 Santa Monica Blvd., Los Angeles, CA 90038; (213) 466-6475.

—B—

BERC, 4545 Chermak St., Burbank, CA 91505; (818) 841-3000; (213) 464-7655.

BLUE RIDGE EDITORIAL, 1019 N. Cole Ave., Hollywood, CA 90038; (213) 461-2846

BOSUSTOW VIDEO, 2207 Colby Ave., West Los Angeles, CA 90064; (213) 478-0821.

BOWEN VIDEO FACILITIES, 619 S. Victory Blvd., Burbank, CA 91504; (818) 841-0295.

BROADCAST EQUIPMENT RENTAL COMPANY, 4545 Chermak St., Burbank, CA 91505; (818) 841-3000, (213) 464-7655.

—C—

CCR VIDEO CORPORATION, 6410 Santa Monica Blvd., Los Angeles, CA 90038; (213) 464-7151.

CALIFORNIA COMMUNICATIONS INC., 6900 Santa Monica Blvd., Los Angeles, CA 90038; (213) 466-8511.

CALIFORNIA VIDEO CENTER, 15303 Ventura Blvd., Sherman Oaks, CA 91403; (818) 789-5000.

CALIFORNIA ZEPHYR, 9348 Santa Monica Blvd., Suite 101, Beverly Hills, CA 90210; (213) 653-4004.

CHRIS CRAFT VIDEO TAPE CENTER, 915 N. La Brea Ave., Los Angeles, CA 90038; (213) 850-2236.

COMPACT VIDEO SERVICES INC., 2813 W. Alameda Ave., Burbank, CA 91505; (818) 840-7000.

COMPLETE POST INC., 6087 Sunset Blvd., Hollywood, CA 90028; (213) 467-1244.

THE COMPLEX, 2323 Corinth St., Los Angeles, CA 90064; (213) 477-1938.

COMPOSITE IMAGE SYSTEMS, 815 N. Cahuenga Blvd., Hollywood, CA 90038; (213) 461-5734.

CONSOLIDATED FILM INDUSTRIES, 959 Seward St., Los Angeles, CA 90038; (213) 462-3161.

CORNERSTONE PRODUCTIONS, 6430 Sunset Blvd., Suite 1013, Hollywood, CA 90028; (213) 871-2255.

COTTON CANDY/EYE ON VIDEO, 224 N. Juanita Ave., Los Angeles, CA 90004; (213) 382-4048.

CRAVEN PRODUCTIONS, 727 N. Victory Blvd., Burbank, CA 91502; (818) 843-6009.

THE CREATIVE PARTNERSHIP, 6815 Willoughby Ave., Suite 102, Hollywood, CA 90028; (213) 461-3548.

CREATIVE VIDEO SERVICES, 500 Ventu Park Rd., Newbury Park, CA 91320; (818) 707-2424.

CROSS CUTS, 8550 Hollywood Dr., Suite 302, West Hollywood, CA 90069; (213) 854-3308.

—D—

DEVONSHIRE SOUND STUDIOS, 10729 Magnolia Blvd., North Hollywood, CA 91601; (818) 985-1945.

—E—

EFP/EBSEN FISHER PRODUCTION, 9541 Cedarbrook Dr., Beverly Hills, CA 90210; (213) 273-2208.

ECONOMY PRODUCTION EDITING & AIR CHECKS, 7557 Hampton Ave., Los Angeles, CA 90046; (213) 850-5411.

EDITEL-LOS ANGELES, 729 N. Highland Ave., Hollywood, CA 90038; (213) 931-1821.

THE EDITING COMPANY, 8300 Beverly Blvd., Los Angeles, CA 90048; (213) 653-3570.

EMERALD STUDIOS INC., P.O. Box 1647, Orange, CA 92668; (714) 771-7394.

—F—

FALCON COMMUNICATIONS, 800 S. Date Ave., Alhambra, CA 91803; (818) 576-2906.

FILM CORE PRINT & TAPE, 849 N. Seward St., Los Angeles, CA 90038; (213) 464-7303.

THE FILM PLACE, 1311 N. Highland Ave., Los Angeles, CA 90028; (213) 464-0116.

FILMLAND CORPORATE CENTER, 10000 Washington Blvd., Culver City, CA 90232; (213) 558-0071.

FORSHER, JAMES, COLLECTION OF ARCHIVAL FOOTAGE & STILLS, Raleigh Studios, 650 N. Bronson Ave., Suite 108, Los Angeles, CA 90004; (213) 461-0178.

FREEMAN, DOUG, SOUND & EDITORIAL, 6362 Hollywood Blvd., Suite 219, Hollywood, CA 90028; (213) 467-8742.

—G—

GLOBAL TELEVISION, 1950 Cotner Ave., Los Angeles, CA 90025; (213) 479-8081.

GOLDSON, DAVE, EDITING, 2406 W. Olive Ave., Burbank, CA 91505; (818) 980-7872.

GREAT AMERICAN CINEMA CO., 10711 Wellworth Ave., Los Angeles, CA 90024; (213) 475-0937.

GROUP W CABLE VIDEO PRODUCTION CENTER, 2939 Nebraska Ave., Santa Monica, CA 90404; (213) 829-2676.

—H—

H.C.V., 3034 Glendale Blvd., Los Angeles, CA 90039; (213) 662-1112.

HQ1 STUDIOS, 19347 Londelius St., Northridge, CA 91324; (818) 993-4778.

HARRIS, KEN, VIDEO PRODUCTIONS INC., 3960 Laurel Canyon Blvd., Suite 379, Studio City, CA 91604; (818) 780-0320.

HOLLYWOOD NATIONAL STUDIOS, 6605 Eleanor Ave., Santa Fe Springs, CA 90038; (213) 467-6272.

HOLLYWOOD PACIFIC STUDIOS, 6290 Sunset Blvd., Hollywood, CA 90028; (213) 463-8118.

HORIZONTAL EDITING STUDIOS, 2625 W. Olive Ave., Burbank, CA 91505; (818) 841-6750.

—I—

IMAGE PRODUCTIONS, 1812 W. Victory Blvd., Burbank, CA 91506; (818) 846-2047.

IMAGE TRANSFORM INC., 4142 Lankershim Blvd., North Hollywood, CA 91602; (818) 985-7566.

INNOVATION UNLIMITED, 4444 Via Marina, Penthouse-81, Marina Del Rey, CA 90291; (213) 823-4251.

INSTITUTE OF AUDIO/VIDEO ENGINEERING, 1831 Hyperion Ave., Hollywood, CA 90027; (213) 666-3003.

INTERMIX INC., 2505 S. Robertson Blvd., Los Angeles, CA 90034; (213) 870-2121.

INSTANT REPLAY EQUIPMENT CO., 5520 Westlawn Ave., Los Angeles, CA 90066; (213) 870-1231.

—J—

JDH SOUND, 12156 W. Olympic Blvd., Los Angeles, CA 90064; (213) 820-8802.

JKR PRODUCTIONS/JIM RUXIN, 12140 W. Olympic Blvd., Suite 21, Los Angeles, CA 90064; (213) 826-3666.

J.P. VIDEO SERVICES, 9538 W. Pico Blvd., Los Angeles, CA 90035; (213) 271-1209.

—K—

KCET, 4401 Sunset Blvd., Los Angeles, CA 90027, (213) 666-6500.

KTEH VIDEOSERVICES, 100 Skyport Dr., San Jose, CA 95115; (408) 947-6654.

KWHY-TV, CHANNEL 22, 5545 Sunset Blvd., Los Angeles, CA 90028; (213) 466-5441.

KRAMER, JERRY & ASSOCIATES, 1312 N. La Brea Ave., Hollywood, CA 90028; (213) 462-2680.

—L—

LAJON PRODUCTIONS INC., 2907 W. Olive Ave., Burbank, CA 91505; (818) 841-1440.

LASER EDIT INC., 540 N. Hollywood Way, Burbank, CA 91505; (818) 842-0777.

LIONEL TELEVISION PRODUCTIONS, 417 Colorado Ave., Santa Monica, CA 90401; (213) 394-9697.

—M—

MDC/TELEPRODUCTIONS—McDONNELL DOUGLAS, 15282 Newsboy Circle, Huntington Beach, CA 92647; (714) 896-2495.

M.F.I. VIDEO CENTER, 1905 Grace Ave., Hollywood, CA 90068; (213) 851-0373.

MACPHERSON'S FILM CONTINUITY SERVICE, 13371 Gladstone Ave., Sylmar, CA 91342; (818) 367-4769.

MARSH INTERNATIONAL FILMS, 21029 Itasca St., Suites A & B, Chatsworth, CA 91311; (818) 998-2188.

MASTER DIGITAL INC., 1749 14th St., Santa Monica, CA 90404; (213) 452-1511.

MATCHFRAME VIDEO, 2433 28th St, Suite H, Santa Monica, CA 90405; (213) 450-5094.

MATHERS, JIM VIDEO/FILMS, 4739 Lankershim Blvd., North Hollywood, CA 91602; (818) 762-2214.

McINTIRE-HOFFMAN INC., 18149 Ventura Blvd., Tarzana, CA 91356; (818) 345-9677.

MEGA PRODUCTIONS INC., 1714 N. Wilton Pl., Hollywood, CA 90028; (213) 462-6342.

MELROSE STAGE, 4361 Melrose Ave., Los Angeles, CA 90029; (213) 660-8466.

MERIDIAN, P.O. Box 1941, Hollywood, CA 90028; (213) 874-4367.

METAVISION, 347 S. Ogden Dr., Suite 220, Los Angeles, CA 90036; (213) 936-8281.

METROTAPE, (division of Metromedia), 5746 Sunset Blvd., Los Angeles, CA 90028; (213) 856-1000.

MOBILEFAX, 710 N. Seward St., Hollywood, CA 90038, (213) 467-4000.

MODERN VIDEOFILM, 7165 Sunset Blvd., Hollywood, CA 90046; (213) 851-8070.

MUSIC LAB INC., 1831 Hyperion Ave., Hollywood, CA 90027; (213) 666-3003.

—N—

NATARNO'S, JAN, VIDEOTAPE EDITING, 6132 DeLongpre Ave., Hollywood, CA 90028; (213) 462-5511.

NATIONAL TELEVISION NEWS INC., 213A, 23480 Park Sorrento, Calabasas Park, CA 91302; (818) 883-6121.

—O—

OCEANAIR EDITING, 1237 7th St., Santa Monica, CA 90401; (213) 395-8474.

ONE INCH VIDEO PRODUCTIONS INC., 4710 W. Magnolia Blvd., Burbank, CA 91505; (818) 760-6900.

ONE PASS FILM & VIDEO, One China Basin Building, San Francisco, CA 94107; (415) 777-5777.

ORACLE FILM & VIDEO, 1820 14th St., Suite 202, Santa Monica, CA 90404; (213) 450-6637.

OUTRIDER VIDEO & FILM, 2907 W. Olive Ave., Burbank, CA 91505; (818) 841-1440.

—P—

PRC OF AMERICA (PLASTIC REEL CORPORATION), 7165 Willoughby Ave., Los Angeles, CA 90046; (213) 851-7532.

PACIFIC VIDEO, 809 N. Cahuenga Blvd., Los Angeles, CA 90038; (213) 462-6266.

POSITIVE MEDIA, 5422A Fair Ave., North Hollywood, CA 91601; (818) 761-5192.

THE POST GROUP, 6335 Homewood, Los Angeles, CA 90028; (213) 462-2300.

POST PLUS INC., 6650 Santa Monica Blvd., 2nd Floor, Hollywood, CA 90038; (213) 463-7108.

POST-PRODUCTION SYSTEMS, 2433 28th St., Suite H, Santa Monica, CA 90405; (213) 450-5094.

POST TIME EDITORIAL INC., 1777 N. Vine St., Suite 303, Los Angeles, CA 90028; (213) 462-6968.

PRECISION FOLEY & ADR, 6353 Homewood Ave., Hollywood, CA 90028; (213) 462-8235.

PREMORE INC., 5130 Klump Ave., North Hollywood, CA 91601; (818) 506-7714.

PRO VIDEO & CINETAPE, 801 N. La Brea Ave., Los Angeles, CA 90038; (213) 934-8836.

PROFESSIONAL ARTISTS GROUP, 845 N. Highland Ave., Hollywood, CA 90038; (213) 871-2222.

—Q—

QPT EDITORIAL CORPORATION, 629 N. La Brea Ave., Los Angeles, CA 90036; (213) 936-7181.

—R—

RANDKEN CORPORATION, 1041 N. Mansfield Ave., Hollywood, CA 90038; (213) 464-1682.

RED CAR EDITING, 1040 N. Las Palmas, Los Angeles, CA 90038; (213) 466-4467.

REEL MAGIC, 11684 Ventura Blvd., Suite 325, Studio City, CA 91604; (818) 762-5670.

RENCHER'S EDITORIAL SERVICE, 728 Cahuenga Blvd., Hollywood, CA 90038; (213) 463-9836.

ROCK SOLID PRODUCTIONS, 801 S. Main St., Burbank, CA 91506; (818) 841-8220.

ROLAND, GLENN FILMS, 10711 Wellworth Ave., Los Angeles, CA 90024; (213) 475-0937.

—S—

SCHULMAN VIDEO CENTER, 861 Seward St., Hollywood, CA 90038; (213) 465-8110.

SCOTTSOUND INC., 6110 Santa Monica Blvd., Los Angeles, CA 90038; (213) 462-6981.

SIERRA VIDEO, 4216 N. Maxson Rd., El Monte, CA 91732, (818) 579-7023.

SKYLIGHT PRODUCTION INC., 6815 W. Willoughby, Suite 201, Los Angeles, CA 90038; (213) 464-4500.

SOUND MASTER, 10747 Magnolia Blvd., North Hollywood, CA 91601; (213) 650-8000.

SPALLA, RICK VIDEO PRODUCTIONS, 1622 N. Gower, Los Angeles, CA 90028; (213) 469-7307.

SPEAR, JACK PRODUCTIONS INC., 7243 Santa Monica Blvd., Hollywood, CA 90028; (213) 851-4123.

SPECTRA IMAGE INC., 540 N. Hollywood Way, Burbank, CA 91505; (818) 842-1111.

SQUARE WHEEL PRODUCTIONS/THE CONSULTANCY, P.O. Box 675, Van Nuys, CA 91408-0675; (818) 508-0332.

STARFAX, 8157 Lankershim Blvd., North Hollywood, CA 91605; (818) 768-2905.

STARLIGHT EDITING SERVICES, 5250 Strohm, North Hollywood, CA 91601; (818) 769-3874.

STRUMPELL, KENT, 1316 Santa Monica Mall, Suite 102, Santa Monica, CA 90401; (213) 395-3875.

SULLIVAN & ASSOCIATES, 201 N. Occidental Blvd., Los Angeles, CA 90026; (213) 384-3331.

SUNSET & VINE, 6290 Sunset Blvvd., Suite 905, Hollywood, CA 90028; (213) 466-7272.

SUNSET POST INC., 1813 Victory Blvd., Glendale, CA 91201; (818) 956-7912.

SUNWEST STUDIOS, 5533 Sunset Blvd., Hollywood, CA 90028; (213) 463-5631.

SUPERIOR VIDEO SERVICES, 13423 Saticoy St., North Hollywood, CA 91605; (818) 786-7060.

—T—

TAJ SOUNDWORKS, 8207 W. 3rd St., Los Angeles, CA 90048; (213) 655-2775.

TELEMEDIA PRODUCTIONS, 18321 Ventura Blvd., Suite 660, Tarzana, CA 91356; (818) 708-2005.

TELE VIDICS, 2223 E. 223rd St., Long Beach, CA 90810, (213) 830-5296.

TELEPRINT OF LOS ANGELES, 3779 Cahuenga West, Studio City, CA 91604; (818) 760-3191.

TELEVISION MATRIX, 1438 N. Gower St., Hollywood, CA 90028; (213) 465-9616.

TRANS-AMERICAN VIDEO INC., 1541 N. Vine St., Los Angeles, CA 90028; (213) 466-2141.

TRITRONICS INC., 733 N. Victory Bl., Burbank, CA 91502; (818) 843-2288, (800) 232-2141.

TYLIE JONES & ASSOC. INC., 10718 Riverside Dr., North Hollywood, CA 91602; (818) 980-7300.

—U—

UCL VIDEO, 823 N. Seward St., Los Angeles, CA 90038; (213) 469-7291.

UDELL, BILL, PRODUCTIONS, 6006 Vantage Ave., North Hollywood, CA 91606; (818) 985-6866.

UNITEL VIDEO, 5555 Melrose Ave., Studio G, Los Angeles, CA 90038; (213) 468-4606.

—V—

VRA TELEPLAY PICTURES, P.O. Box 8471, Universal Plaza Station, North Hollywood, CA 91608; (213) 462-1099.

VTR SERVICE AND SALES, 3169 Barbara Ct., Suite D, Hollywood, CA 90068; (213) 851-9700.
VALLEY VIDEO, 4209 W. Burbank Blvd., Burbank, CA 91505; (818) 841-2387.
VARITEL VIDEO/JACK SCHAEFFER, 3575 Cahuenga Blvd. West, Los Angeles, CA 90068; (213) 805-1165.
VECTOR PRODUCTIONS INC., P.O. Box 7000-645, Redondo Beach, CA 90277; (213) 757-0520, (213) 316-6031.
VIA VISION PRODUCTIONS, 5919 Franklin Ave., Los Angeles, CA 90028; (213) 460-4864.
VIDCOM, 2426 Townsgate Rd., Suite K, Westlake Village, CA 91361; (818) 991-1974.
VIDEO ADVENTURES INC., 1015 Cahuenga Blvd., Hollywood, CA 90038; (213) 461-3288.
VIDEOASIS, 317 S. Verdugo Rd., Glendale, CA 91205; (818) 507-1037.
VIDEO ASSOCIATES AND CO., 5419 Sunset Blvd., Los Angeles, CA 90027; (213) 463-3255.
VIDEO CRAFTSMEN INC., 6311 Romaine St., Los Angeles, CA 90028; (213) 464-4351.
VIDEO EVENTS INC., 1741 N. Ivar, Suite 210, Hollywood, CA 90028; (213) 465-4197.
VIDEO-IT INC., 1016 Sycamore Ave., Hollywood, CA 90038; (213) 876-4055.
VIDEO SUPPORT SERVICES INC., 3473½ Cahuenga Blvd. W., Los Angeles, CA 90068; (213) 469-9000.
THE VIDEO TAPE CO., 10545 Burbank Blvd., North Hollywood, CA 91601; (818) 985-1666.
VIDEO TRANSITIONS INC., 910 N. Citrus Ave., Los Angeles, CA 90038; (213) 465-3333.
VIDEO WEST, 6430 Sunset Blvd., Suite 908, Los Angeles, CA 90028; (213) 465-3153.
VIDE-U PRODUCTIONS, 612 N. Sepulveda Blvd., Los Angeles, CA 90049; (213) 472-7023.
VILLAGE VIDEO, 1616 Butler Ave., Los Angeles, CA 90025; (213) 478-8227.
VITELLO & ASSOCIATES, 6353 Homewood Ave., Hollywood, CA 90028; (213) 462-8235.

—W—

WMW-BRZEZINSKI VIDEO PRODUCTIONS, 6253 Hollywood Blvd., Suite 1111, Hollywood, CA 90028; (213) 465-3520.
WEISBARTH, JACOB & ASSOC. INC., 9903 Santa Monica Blvd., Suite 256, Beverly Hills, CA 90212; (213) 475-0668.
WILDER BROTHERS VIDEO, 10327 Santa Monica Blvd., Los Angeles, CA 90025; (213) 557-3500.
WOLLIN PRODUCTION SERVICES INC., 666 N. Robertson Blvd., Los Angeles, CA 90069; (213) 659-0175.

NEW YORK

A N S INTERNATIONAL VIDEO LTD., 396 Fifth Ave., New York, NY 10018; (212) 736-1007.
ALL-MOBILE VIDEO, 630 Ninth Ave., New York, NY 10036; (212) 757-8919.
BNS VIDEO SERVICES, INC. (division of Broadcast News Service, Inc.), GPO 2360, Pier 62, West 23 St., New York, NY 10011; (213) 466-0234, (212) 223-0969.
BROADWAY VIDEO, 1619 Broadway, New York, NY 10019, (212) 265-7600; 713-0540.
DEVLIN PRODUCTIONS, INC., 150 W. 55 St., New York, NY 10019; (212) 582-5572.
EDITEL NEW YORK, 222 E. 44 St., New York, NY 10017; (212) 867-4600.
EDITING CONCEPTS, 214 E. 50 St., New York, NY 10022; (212) 980-3340.
FAMA II PRODUCTIONS INC., 2750 Richmond Terrace, Staten Island, NY 10303; (718) 273-1780.
IMAGE MIX, INC., 305 E. 46 St., New York, NY 10017; (212) 752-3010.
INTERNATIONAL VIDEO SERVICES, 1501 Broadway, New York, NY 10036; (212) 730-1411.
JUPITER PRODUCTION SERVICES, 55 W. 45 St., New York, NY 10019; (212) 575-1066.
MAGNO VIDEO, 212 W. 48 St., New York, NY 10019; (212) 757-8855.
MODERN TELECOMMUNICATIONS, 1 Dag Hammarskjold Plaza, New York, NY 10017; (212) 355-0510.
NATIONAL VIDEO INDUSTRIES, 15 W. 17 St., New York, NY 10011; (212) 691-1300.
OCCASIONAL VIDEO, 534 E. 84 St., New York, NY 10028, (212) 737-3058.
P.A.T. FILM SERVICES, 630 Ninth Ave., New York, NY 10036; (212) 247-0900.
PICSONIC PRODUCTIONS, 1466 Broadway, New York, NY 10036; (212) 575-1910.
PICTURE PERFECT PRODUCTIONS, 630 Ninth Ave., New York, NY 10036; (212) 333-5220.
POWER PLAY RECORDS INC., 198 Bloomfield Ave., Newark, NJ; (201) 481-0972.
PRIMA LUX VIDEO, 30 W. 26 St., New York, NY 10010, (212) 206-1402.
REEVES TELETAPE, 304 E. 44 St., New York, NY 10017, (212) 573-8888.
ROSS-GAFFNEY, 21 W. 46 St., New York, NY 10036; (212) 719-2744.
SYMMETRY VIDEO PRODUCTIONS, 518 E. 6 St., (Apt. 8), New York, NY 10019; (212) 673-7605.
TFI, TAPE-FILM INDUSTRIES, 619 W. 54 St., New York, NY 10019; (212) 708-0500.
TULCHIN STUDIOS, 240 E. 45 St., New York, NY 10017, (212) 986-8270.
UNITEL, 515 W. 57 St., New York, NY 10019; (212) 265-3600.
VCA TELETRONICS, 231 E. 55 St., New York, NY 10022, (212) 355-1600.
VIDEO CASSETTE TRANSFERS, 160 W. 46 St., New York, NY 10036; (212) 575-8433.
VIDEO MEDIA PRODUCTIONS, 1493-33 88th St., Howard Beach, NY; (718) 845-3709.
VIDEO PLANNING INC., 250 W. 57 St., New York, NY 10019; (212) 582-5066.
VIDEO PORTFOLIOS, 142 W. 24 St., New York, NY 10011, (212) 989-3858.
VIDEO 3000, 1400 Broadway, Penthouse Loft, New York, NY 10018; (212) 302-1313.
WINDSOR TOTAL VIDEO, 565 Fifth Ave., New York, NY 10017; (212) 725-8080.

CONNECTICUT

E.C.A. STUDIO, Wilton, CT 06897; (203) 762-338,; (212) 333-5656.

PENNSYLVANIA

VIDEOSMITH INC., 2006 Chancellor St., Philadelphia, PA 19103; (215) 864-0658.

WASHINGTON, DC

CAPITOL VIDEO COMMUNICATIONS, INC., 2121 Wisconsin Ave., N.W., Washington, DC 20007; (202) 965-7800.
CIRACE VIDEO/INTERNATIONAL, P.O. Box 3510, Arlington, VA 22203; (703) 486-1555.

CANADA

MANTA VIDEO LABS, 311 Adelaide St. E., Toronto, Ont., Canada M5A IN2; (416) 863-9316.

VIDEO EQUIPMENT, SALES & RENTAL

WEST COAST

ADL VIDEO, 3311 Rowena St., Suite 18, Los Angeles, CA 90027; (213) 662-8385.
AMERICAN VIDEO FACTORY, 4150 Glencoe Ave., Marina Del Rey, CA 90292; (213) 823-8622.
AMERICAN VIDEOGRAM INC., 2207 S. Colby Ave., Los Angeles, CA 90064-1504; (213) 477-1535.
AMETRON RENTS, 1200 N. Vine St., Los Angeles, CA 90038; (213) 466-4321.
AMPEX CORPORATION, 500 Rodier Dr., Glendale, CA 91201; (818) 240-5000.
AQUASTAR SYSTEMS, 3960 Laurel Canyon Blvd., #406, Studio City, CA 91604; (818) 880-5639.
ATLAS VIDEO, 1343 N. Highland Ave., Hollywood, CA 90028; (213) 871-0790..
AUDIO GRAPHIC FILMS AND VIDEO, 6509 De Longpre Ave., Hollywood, CA 90028; (213) 462-6596, (213) 467-1234.
AUDIO KINETICS INC., 4721 Laurel Canyon Blvd., Suite 209, North Hollywood, CA 91607; (818) 980-5717.
AUDIO-VIDEO CRAFT INC., 7000 Santa Monica Blvd., Los Angeles, CA 900381 (213) 655-3511.
AUDIO VISUAL HEADQUARTERS CORP., 361 N. Oak St., Inglewood, CA 903021 (213) 419-4040.
BERC (BROADCAST EQUIPMENT RENTAL COMPANY), 4545 Chermak St., Burbank, CA 91505; (818) 841-3000, (213) 464-7655.
BACKGROUND ENGINEERS INC., 1213 Flower St., Glendale, CA 91201; (213) 465-4161, (818) 500-0454.
BETACAM SPECIALISTS, 3917 Riverside Dr., Suite 9137, Burbank, CA 91505; (818) 845-6480.
BUDGET VIDEO, 1534 N. Highland Ave., Los Angeles, CA 90028; (213) 466-2431, (213) 464-7655.
CCR VIDEO CORPORATION, 6410 Santa Monica Blvd., Los Angeles, CA 90038; (213) 464-7151.
CALIFORNIA COMMUNICATIONS INC., 6900 Santa Monica Blvd., Los Angeles, CA 90038; (213) 466-8511.
CINEMA PRODUCTS CORPORATION, 2037 Granville Ave., Los Angeles, CA 90025; (213) 478-1711; (213) 477-1971.
CINE VIDEO, 948 N. Cahuenga Blvd., Hollywood, CA 90038; (213) 464-6200.
COMPREHENSIVE SERVICE CORPORATION, 914 N. Formosa, Los Angeles, CA 90046; (213) 462-0969.
CONTINENTAL CAMERA SYSTEMS, 7240 Valjean Ave., Van Nuys, CA 91406; (818) 989-5222.
CRAVEN PRODUCTIONS, 727 N. Victory Blvd., Burbank, CA 91502; (818) 843-6009.
THE CREATIVE PARTNERSHIP, 6815 Willoughby Ave., Suite 102, Hollywood, CA 90028; (213) 461-3548.
DAVIS, WALT ENTERPRISES, INC., 3439 Cahuenga Blvd. West, Hollywood, CA 90068; (213) 876-6400.
EFP/EBSEN FISHER PRODUCTION, 9541 Cedarbrook Dr., Beverly Hills, CA 90210; (213) 273-2208.
GORDON, ALAN ENTERPRISES INC., 1430 N. Cahuenga Blvd., Hollywood, CA 90078; (213) 466-3561.
H.C.V., 3034 Glendale Blvd., Los Angeles, CA 90039; (213) 662-1112.
HOFFMAN VIDEO SYSTEMS, 1945 S.. Figueroa St., Los Angeles, CA 90007; (213) 749-3311.
HORIZONTAL EDITING STUDIOS, 2625 W. Olive Ave., Burbank, CA 91505; (818) 841-6750.
ILLUMINATION, 20548 Pacific Coast Highway, Malibu, CA 90265; (213) 456-3423.
INTER VIDEO, 3220 Burbank Blvd., Burbank, CA 91505; (818) 843-3633.
INSTANT REPLAY EQUIPMENT CO., 5520 Westlawn Ave., Los Angeles, CA 90066; (213) 870-1231.
J.P. VIDEO SERVICES, 9538 W. Pico Blvd., Los Angeles, CA 90035; (213) 271-1209.
KRAMER, JERRY & ASSOCIATES, 1312 N. La Brea Ave., Hollywood, CA 90028; (213) 462-2680.
L.A. VIDEO, 3801 W. 3rd St., Los Angeles, CA 90020; (213) 487-0524.
LIONEL TELEVISION PRODUCTIONS, 417 Colorado Ave., Santa Monica, CA 90401; (213) 394-9697.
MAGNASYNC MOVIOLA, 5539 Riverton Ave., North Hollywood, CA 91601; (818) 763-8441.
MARSH INTERNATIONAL FILMS, 21029 Itasca St., Suite A & B, Chatsworth, CA 91311; (818) 998-2188.
MEGA PRODUCTIONS INC., 1714 N. Wilton Pl., Hollywood, CA 90028; (213) 462-6342.
MILES & COMPANY, 1418 Dodson Ave., San Pedro, CA 90732; (213) 548-0462.
MONTAGE COMPUTER CORPORATION, 870 N. Vine St., Suite A, Los Angeles, CA 90038; (213) 465-5501.
OCEANAIR EDITING, 1237 7th St., Santa Monica, CA 90401; (213) 395-8474.
P.D.S. VIDEO PRODUCTIONS, 1102 W. Chestnut St., Burbank, CA 91506; (818) 841-4711.
PRC OF AMERICA (PLASTIC REEL CORPORATION), 8140 Webb Ave., North Hollywood, CA 91605 (818) 504-0400.
PAL VIDEO, 19061 Tina Place, Tarzana, CA 91356; (818) 344-1603.
POSITIVE MEDIA, 5422A Fair Ave., North Hollywood, CA 91601; (818) 761-5192.
POST-PRODUCTION SYSTEMS, 2433 28th St., Suite H, Santa Monica, CA 90405; (213) 450-5094.
RANK PRECISION IND. INC., 13340 Saticoy, Unit F, North Hollywood, CA 91605; (818) 765-7265.
ROCK SOLID PRODUCTIONS, 801 S. Main St., Burbank, CA 91506; (818) 841-8220.
RUXTON LTD., 611 N. Orchard Dr., Burbank, CA 91506; (818) 845-3724.
SAWYER CAMERA VIDEO SERVICE, 1208 W. Isabel St., Burbank, CA 91506; (818) 843-1781.
SCHULMAN VIDEO CENTER, 861 Seward St., Hollywood, CA 90038; (213) 465-8110.
SHORELINE LTD., 3459 Cahuenga Blvd., Hollywood, CA 90068; (213) 851-1236.
STARFAX, 8157 Lakershim Blvd., North Hollywood, CA 91605; (818) 768-2905.
STEENBECK INC., 9554 Vassar Ave., Chatsworth, CA 91311; (818) 998-4033.
STUDIO & REMOTE VIDEO, 10650 Magnolia Blvd., North Hollywood, CA 91601; (818) 508-6010.
STUDIO SPECTRUM INC., 1056 N. Lake St., Burbank, CA 91502; (818) 843-1610.
SUNSET & VINE, 6290 Sunset Blvd., Suite 905, Hollywood, CA 90028; (213) 466-7272.
SUPERIOR VIDEO SERVICES, 13423 Saticoy St., North Hollywood, CA 91605; (818) 786-7060.
T.V.S. INC., 10153 Riverside Dr., Suite 1B, Toluca Lake, CA 91602; (818) 763-1295.
TELEMEDIA PRODUCTIONS, 18321 Ventura Blvd., Suite 660, Tarzana, CA 91356; (818) 708-2005.
TRITONICS INC., 733 N. Victory Bl., Burbank, CA 91502; (818) 843-2288; (800) 232-2141.
U.T. PHOTO SERVICE INC., 3088 N. Clybourn Ave., Burbank, CA 91505; (213) 245-6631.
VTR SERVICE AND SALES, 3169 Barbara Ct., Suite D, Hollywood, CA 90068; (213) 851-9700.
VECTOR ENGINEERING, P.O. Box 7000-645, Redondo Beach, CA 90277; (213) 757-0520; (213) 316-6031.
VIDEO ADVENTURES INC., 1015 Cahuenga Blvd., Hollywood, CA 90038; (213) 461-3288.
VIDEO-IT INC., 1016 N. Sycamore Ave., Hollywood, CA 90038; (213) 876-4055; (213) VID-EOIT.
VIDEO SUPPORT SERVICES INC., 3473½ Cahuenga Blvd. West, Los Angeles, CA 90068; (213) 469-9000.
VIDEOTAPE PRODUCTS INC., 320 N. Madison Ave., Los Angeles, CA 90004; (213) 664-1144.
WEISBARTH, JACOB & ASSOC. INC., 9903 Santa Monica Blvd., Suite 256, Beverly Hills, CA 90212; (213) 475-0668.
WESTERN FILM INDUSTRIES, 30941 W. Agoura Rd., Suite 302, Westlake Village, CA 91360; (818) 889-7350.

NEW YORK

ANS LABS, 396 Fifth Ave., New York, NY 10018; (212) 714-9880.
ALL-MOBILE VIDEO, INC., 630 Ninth Ave., New York, NY 10036; (212) 757-8919.
AMERICAN VIDEO EXPRESS, 17 E. 8 St., New York, NY 10003; (212) 260-1600; 1265 Madison Ave., New York, NY 10028; (212) 831-3880; 957 Park Ave., New York, NY 10028; (212) 879-2233.
AMERICAN VIDEO INC., 717 Lexington Ave., New York, NY 10022; (212) 888-0888.
AUDIO SALON INC., 1553 Second Ave., New York, NY 10028; (212) 249-4104.

BARGAIN SPOT, 64 Third Ave., New York, NY 10003; (212) 674-1188.
BIG APPLE VIDEO, 367 First Ave., New York, NY 10010; (212) 420-0370.
BOGAZICI VIDEO LTD., 460 Seventh Ave., New York, NY 10001; (212) 563-9022.
BRYCE AUDIO STEREO COMPONENTS CO., 115 W. 40 St., New York, NY 10018; (212) 575-8600.
CTL ELECTRONICS INC., 116 W. Broadway, New York, NY 10013; (212) 233-0754.
THE CAMERA MART, 456 W. 55 St., New York, NY 10019; (212) 757-6977.
CAMERA SERVICE CENTER, INC., 625 W. 54 St., New York, NY 10019; (212) 757-0906.
COLUMBUS TV & VIDEO CENTER, 529 Columbus Ave., New York, NY 10024; (212) 496-2626.
COSMOPHONIC SOUND INC., 1614 Second Ave., New York, NY 10028; (212) 734-0459.
CRAZY EDDIE'S, 1117 Kings Hwy., Brooklyn, NY; (718) 645-1196.
ELECTRONIC RESOURCE CENTER, 151 W. 72nd St., New York, NY 10023; (718) 769-1213.
FIRST RUN VIDEO INC., 1390 Third Ave., New York, NY 10021; (212) 772-3838.
FORTY-SEVENTH ST. PHOTO INC., 38 E. 19 St., New York, NY 10003; (212) 260-4410; 116 Nassau St., New York, NY 10038; (212) 608-6934; 67 W. 47 St., New York, NY 10036; (212) 398-1410; 115 W. 45 St., New York, NY 10036; (212) 398-1410.
G & R VIDEO, 300 Park Ave. South, New York, NY 10010; (212) 533-1887.
GRANADA TV RENTAL, 1069 Third Ave., New York, NY 10021; (212) 935-4410.
GRAND CENTRAL RADIO, 155 E. 45 St., New York, NY 10017; (212) 682-3869.
HARVEY ELECTRONICS, 2 W. 45 St., New York, NY 10036; (212) 575-5000.
INTERCONTINENTAL TELEVIDEO INC., 29 W. 39 St., New York, NY 10018; (212) 719-0202.
INTERNATIONAL ELECTRONICS CO., 211 Eighth Ave., New York, NY 10011; (212) 243-2362.
J & R MUSIC WORLD, 23 Park Row, New York, NY 10038; (212) 732-8600.
JEMS SOUND LTD., 785 Lexington Ave., New York, NY 10021; (212) 838-4716; 77 E. 42 St., New York, NY 10017; (212) 687-1333.
JONES STREET VIDEO, 23 Jones St., New York, NY 10014; (212) 206-0249.
K V L AUDIO VISUALS INC., 529 W. 46 St., New York, NY 10036; (212) 977-4488.
LAST STOP VIDEO INC., 4979 Broadway, New York, NY 10034; (212) 304-9311.
LAUMIC CO., 306 E. 39 St., New York, NY 10016; (212) 889-3300.
LONGWOOD VIDEO, 32 W. 22 St., New York, NY 10010; (212) 741-3733.
MPCS VIDEO INDUSTRIES, 514 W. 57 St., New York, NY 10019; (212) 586-3690.
MAR VIDEO INC., 10 W. 30 St., New York, NY 10001; (212) 683-7966.
MARTIN AUDIO-VIDEO CORP., 423 W. 55 St., New York, NY 10019; (212) 541-5900.
MAYA VIDEO PRODS. INC., 172 Madison Ave., New York, NY 10001; (212) 532-6206.
METRO ELECTRONICS CORP., 81 West Broadway, New York, NY 10007; (212) 406-2760.
MODERN TELECOMMUNICATIONS, INC., Dag Hammarskjold Plaza, New York, NY 10017; (212) 355-0510.
NATIONAL AUDIO & VIDEO, 241 Madison Ave., New York, NY 10016; (212) 370-1762.
NATIONAL TELE-RENT INC., 150-09 12th Road, Whitestone, NY 11357; (212) 829-1600.
NATIONAL VIDEO INDUSTRIES, 15 W. 17 St., New York, NY 10011; (212) 691-1300.
NEW YORK VIDEO, 717 Lexington Ave., New York, NY 10022; (212) 755-4640.
NORTHEAST ELECTRONIC & VIDEO STORES, 420 Lexington Ave., New York, NY 10017; (212) 972-1799.
OLDEN CAMERA VIDEO & COMPUTER STORE, 1265 Broadway, New York, NY 10001; (212) 725-1234.
PT IMPORTS INC., 1123 Broadway, New York, NY 10010; (212) 929-8600.
PARC VENDOME VIDEO, 348 W. 57 St., New York, NY 10019; (212) 757-8500.
PUBLIC SERVICE VIDEO, 454 W. 46 St., New York, NY 10036; (212) 315-4277.
REEVES TELETAPE, 304 E. 44 St., New York, NY 10017; (212) 573-8888.
RELIANCE AUDIO-VISUAL CORP., 623 W. 51 St., New York, NY 10019; (212) 586-5000.
RODNEY'S VIDEO WAREHOUSE, 128 Mamaroneck Ave., White Plains, NY; (914) 946-9696.
S RENTAL CO., 118 E. 28 St., Fifth Floor, New York, NY 10010; (212) 685-3344; 33-49 55th St., Woodside, NY; (718) 458-3800.
SAVEMART INC., 171 E. 86 St, New York, NY 10028; (212) 369-1455; 88 Chambers St., New York, NY 10007; (212) 267-8130; 7 E. 14 St., New York, NY 10003; (212) 243-8456; 599 W. 181 St., New York, NY 10033; (212) 928-2000.
SELECT AUDIO VISUAL INC., 902 Broadway, New York, NY 10010; (212) 598-9800.
SOUND & VISION INC., 83 Leonard St., New York, NY 10012; (212) 219-3007.
SOUNDVIEW AV CO., 347 W. 39 St., New York, NY 10018; (212) 594-0183.
TAPE CITY, 404 Park Ave. South, New York, NY 10016; (212) 684-1500.
TECHNISPHERE, 29 E 19 St., New York, NY 10003; (212) 777-5100.
TOWN VIDEO SALES, 21 Ann St., New York, NY 10038; (212) 267-9760.
VICOM COMMUNICATIONS, 248 W. 33 St., New York, NY 10001; (212) 685-5232.
VIDEO CENTRAL, 225 W. 36 St., New York, NY 10018; (212) 947-6960.
VIDEO OVERSEAS INC., 249 W. 23 St., New York, NY 10011; (212) 645-0797.
VIDEO POWER USA INC., 511 W. 54 St., New York, NY 10019; (212) 315-0810.
VIDEO STOP INC., 367 Third Ave., New York, NY (212) 685-6199.
VIDEO WAREHOUSE, 119 W. 57 St., New York, NY 10019; (212) 247-0069.
VISUAL WORD SYSTEMS INC., 17 E. 45 St., New York, NY 10017; (212) 661-3366.
WEST VILLAGE VIDEO, 128 Charles St., New York, NY 10014; (212) 691-7430.
WILLOUGHBYS, 110 W. 32 St., New York, NY 10001; (212) 564-1600.
WINDSOR TOTAL VIDEO, 565 Fifth Ave., New York, NY 10017; (212) 725-8080.
THE WIZ, 12 W. 45 St., New York, NY 10036; (212) 302-2000; 2577 Broadway, New York, NY 10025; (212) 662-9000; 17 Union Sq., New York, NY 10003; (212) 741-9500; 1922 Third Ave., New York, NY 10029; (212) 369-0600.
ZAZY INTERNATIONAL, 49 W. 24 St., New York, NY 10011; (212) 807-8060.

VIDEO EQUIPMENT REPAIR

LOS ANGELES

AMETRON RENTS, 1200 N. Vine St., Los Angeles, CA 90038; (213) 466-4321.
AMPAC VIDEO, 3637 Cahuenga Blvd. West, Hollywood, CA 90068; (213) 851-7200.
ATLAS VIDEO, 1343 N. Highland Ave., Hollywood, CA 90028; (213) 871-0790.
CINEMA PRODUCTS CORPORATION, 2037 Granville Ave., Los Angeles, CA 90025; (213) 478-0711; (213) 477-1971.
DAVIS, WALT ENTERPRISES, INC., 3439 Cahuenga Blvd. West, Hollywood, CA 90068; (213) 876-6400.
GORDON, ALAN ENTERPRISES INC., 1430 N. Cahuenga Blvd., Hollywood, CA 90078; (213) 466-3561.
H.C.V., 3034 Glendale Blvd., Los Angeles, CA 90039; (213) 662-1112.
HOFFMAN VIDEO SYSTEMS, 1945 S. Figueroa St., Los Angeles, CA 90007; (213) 749-3311.
INSTANT REPLAY EQUIPMENT CO., 5520 Westlawn Ave., Los Angeles, CA 90066; (213) 870-1231.
POSITIVE MEDIA, 5422A Fair Ave., North Hollywood, CA 91601; (818) 761-5192.
SAWYER CAMERA & VIDEO SERVICE, 1208 W. Isabel St., Burbank, CA 91506; (818) 843-1781.
STARLIGHT EDITING SERVICES, 5250 Strohm, North Hollywood, CA 91601; (818) 769-3874.
STEENBECK INC., 9554 Vassar Ave., Chatsworth, CA 91311; (818) 998-4033.
U.T. PHOTO SERVICE INC., 3088 N. Clybourn Ave., Burbank, CA 91505; (213) 245-6631.
VTR SERVICE AND SALES, 3169 Barbara Ct., Suite D, Hollywood, CA 90068; (213) 851-9700.
VIDEO SUPPORT SERVICES, 3473½ Cahuenga Blvd. West, Los Angeles, CA 90068; (213) 469-9000.
VIDEO SYSTEMS INC., 12530 Beatrice St., Los Angeles, CA 90069; (213) 871-0677.
Z & A SERVICE, 9701 W. Washington Blvd., Culver City, CA 90232; (213) 836-3194.

NEW YORK

AABCO CO., 1588 York Ave., New York, NY 10028; (212) 535-9578.
ABS TV LABS, 4071 Broadway, New York, NY 10032; (212) 568-0123.
AJ'S VIDEO INC., 205 E. Broadway, New York, NY 10002; (212) 477-4880.
ADLER ENTERPRISES, 344 Third Ave., New York, NY 10010; (212) 685-6285.
ADVISORY TV & RADIO LABS, 175 Seventh Ave., New York, NY 10011; (212) 243-0786.
ALL CITY ELECTRONICS SERVICE INC., 1 E. 36 St., New York, NY 10016; (212) 689-7180.
AMERICAN VIDEO SERVICE DEPT., 209 Columbus Ave., New York, NY 10023; (212) 724-4870.
AUDIO SALON INC., 1553 Second Ave., New York, NY 10028; (212) 249-4104.
BERRY CAMERA REPAIR, 152 Fourth Ave., New York, NY 10003; (212) 677-8407.
BOGAZICI VIDEO LTD., 460 Seventh Ave., New York, NY 10001; (212) 563-9022.
BRYCE AUDIO/VIDEO CENTER, 115 W, 40 St., New York, NY 10018; (212) 575-8600.
CTL ELECTRONICS, 116 W. Broadway, New York, NY 10013; (212) 233-0754.
COLUMBUS TV & VIDEO CENTER, 529 Columbus Ave., New York, NY 10024; (212) 496-2626.
COSMOPHONIC SOUND, INC. 1614 Second Ave., New York, NY 10028; (212) 734-0459.
E C ELECTRONICS, 840 Eighth Ave., New York, NY 10019; (212) 586-6156.
E & F ELECTRONICS INC., 3455 Jerome Ave., Bronx, NY, (212) 653-1400.
ELECTRONIC RESOURCE CENTER, 151 W. 72 St., New York, NY 10023; (718) 769-1313.
GENERAL VIDEO, 250 W. 57 St., New York, NY 10019; (212) 315-4541.
GERMAN HI-FI SERVICE, 1574 Third Ave., New York, NY 10128; (212) 369-3366.
GRANADA TV RENTAL, 1069 Third Ave., New York, NY 10021; (212) 935-4410; (800) GRANADA; (800) 472-6232.
HARVEY ELECTRONICS, 2 W. 45 St., New York, NY 10036; (212) 575-5000.
INTERNATIONAL ELECTRONICS CO., 211 Eighth Ave., New York, NY 10011; (212) 243-2362.
JAPANESE AMERICAN TRANSITOR SERVICE, 86 W. Broadway, New York, NY 10007; (212) 964-8286.
LUNAR VIDEO LTD., 138 E. 25 St., New York, NY 10010; (212) 686-4802.
MARTIN AUDIO-VIDEO CORP., 423 W. 55 St., New York, NY 10019; (212) 541-5900.
MERCURY VIDEO SERVICE, 301 W. 56 St., New York, NY 10019; (212) 246-6711.
MIDTOWN AUDIO REPAIR & SERVICES INC., 151 W. 72 St., New York, NY 10023; (213) 496-2170.
NATIONAL TELE-RENT INC., 150-09 12th Rd., Whitestone, NY 11357; (212) 829-1600.
PYRAMID ELECTRONICS INC., 353 E. 76 St., New York, NY 10021; (212) 628-6400.
RIDGE RADIO & TELEVISION SERVICE CO., 51 University Place., New York, NY 10003; (212) 674-2515.
SELECT AUDIO VISUAL INC., 902 Broadway, New York, NY 10010; (212) 598-9800.
SUPERIOR ELECTRONIC CO., 122 Madison Ave., New York, NY 10016; (212) 962-6274.
TAPE CITY, 404 Park Avenue South, New York, NY 10016; (212) 684-1500.
TECHNETRON ELECTRONICS INC., 43 E. 29 St., New York, NY 10016; (212) 725-8778.
TECHNISPHERE CORP., 29 E. 19 St., New York, NY 10003; (212) 777-5100.
TELETECHNIQUES, 40 W. 72 St., New York, NY 10023; (212) 580-9551.
TELEVIDEO ELECTRONIC CORP., 233 W. 77 St., New York, NY 10024; (212) 874-7722.
TRIBORO TELEVISION SERVICE, 1626 First Ave., New York, NY 10028; (212) 249-0327.
UNIVERSITY, 13 Third Ave., New York, NY 10003; (212) 477-5240.
VIDEO CENTRAL, 225 W. 36 St., New York, NY 10018; (212) 947-6960.
VIDEO INSTALLATIONS PLUS INC., 1155 Warburton Ave. 8-M, Yonkers, NY; (914) 968-3636.
WILLOUGHBY'S, 110 W. 32 St., New York, NY 10001; (212) 564-1600.

VIDEO MOBILE UNITS

LOS ANGELES

ABC TELEVISION CENTER, 4151 Prospect Ave., Los Angeles, CA 90027; (213) 557-7777.
ADL VIDEO, 3311 Rowena St., Suite 18, Los Angeles, CA 90027; (213) 662-8385.
AMBASSADOR TV PRODUCTION, 392 W. Green St., Pasadena, CA (818) 577-5400.
AMERICAN VIDEO FACTORY, 4150 Glencoe Ave., Marina Del Rey, CA 90292; (213) 823-8622.
AQUASTAR SYSTEMS, 3960 Laurel Canyon Blvd., #406, Studio City, CA 91604; (818) 880-5639.
BERC (BROADCAST EQUIPMENT RENTAL COMPANY), 4545 Chermak St., Burbank, CA 91505; (818) 841-3000; (213) 464-7655.
BENNETT PRODUCTIONS INC., 6922 E. Ocean Blvd., Long Beach, CA 90803; (213) 433-4478.
BETACAM SPECIALISTS, 3917 Riverside Dr., Suite 9137, Burbank, CA 91505; (818) 845-6480.
BOWEN VIDEO FACILITIES, 619 S. Victory Blvd., Burbank, CA 91504; (818) 841-0295.
CCR VIDEO CORPORATION, 6410 Santa Monica Blvd., Los Angeles, CA 90038; (213) 464-7151.
CALIFORNIA ZEPHYR, 9348 Santa Monica Blvd., Suite 101, Beverly Hills, CA 90210; (213) 653-4004.
COTTON CANDY/EYE ON VIDEO, 224 N. Juanita Ave., Los Angeles, CA 90004; (213) 382-4048.
ECONOMY PRODUCTION, EDITING & AIR CHECKS, 7557 Hampton Ave., Los Angeles, CA 90046.
GLOBAL TELEVISION, 1950 Cotner Ave., Los Angeles, CA 90025; (213) 479-8081.
GOLDEN WEST VIDEOTAPE, 5800 Sunset Blvd., Los Angeles, CA 90028; (213) 460-5866.
HOLLYWOOD NATIONAL STUDIOS, 6605 Eleanor Ave., Los Angeles, CA 90038; (213) 467-6272.
KCOP, 915 N. La Brea Ave., Los Angeles, CA 90038; (213) 851-1000.
KLCS, 1061 W. Temple, Los Angeles, CA 90012; (213) 625-6958.
KMEX-TV, 5420 Melrose Ave., Los Angeles, CA 90038; (213) 466-3434.
KNBC, 3000 W. Alameda St., Burbank, CA 91523; (818) 840-4444.
KNET, 6121 Sunset Blvd., Los Angeles, CA 90028; (213) 460-3000.
KTEH VIDEOSERVICES, 100 Skyport Dr., San Jose, CA 95115; (408) 947-6654.
KTTV, 5746 Sunset Blvd., Los Angeles, CA 90028; (213) 462-7111.
LIONEL TELEVISION PRODUCTIONS, 417 Colorado Ave., Santa Monica, CA 90401; (213) 394-9697.
MDC/TELEPRODUCTIONS—McDONNELL DOUGLAS, 15282 Newsboy Circle, Huntington Beach, CA 92647; (714) 896-2495.
M.F.I. VIDEO CENTER, 1905 Grace Ave., Hollywood, CA 90068; (213) 851-0373.
MOBILE IMAGE, 2944 W. Mountain Pine Dr., La Crescenta, CA 91214; (213) 873-5203, (818) 248-6905.
MOBILEFAX, 710 N. Seward St., Hollywood, CA 90038; (213) 467-4000.
ONE INCH VIDEO PRODUCTIONS INC., 4710 W. Magnolia Blvd., Burbank, CA 91505; (818) 760-6900.
ONE PASS MOBILE SERVICES, 729 N. Highland Ave., Hollywood, CA 90038; (213) 937-4095.
P.D.S. VIDEO PRODUCTIONS, 1102 W. Chestnut St., Burbank, CA 91506; (818) 841-4711.
POSITIVE MEDIA, 5422A Fair Ave., North Hollywood, CA 91601; (818) 761-5192.
RUXTON LTD., 611 N. Orchard Dr., Burbank, CA 91506; (818) 845-3724.
SCHULMAN VIDEO CENTER, 861 Seward St., Hollywood, CA 90038; (213) 465-8110.
SIERRA VIDEO, 4216 N. Maxson Rd., El Monte, CA 91732; (818) 579-7045; (818) 579-7023.
SOUND MASTER, 10747 Magnolia Blvd., North Hollywood, CA 91601; (213) 650-8000.
STARFAX, 8157 Lankershim Blvd., North Hollywood, CA 91605; (818) 768-2905.
STUDIO & REMOTE VIDEO, 10650 Magnolia Blvd., North Hollywood, CA 91601; (818) 508-6010.
SUNRISE CANYON VIDEO, P.O. Box 10968, Burbank, CA 91510; (818) 845-7473.
SUPERIOR VIDEO SERVICES, 13423 Saticoy St., North Hollywood, CA 91605; (818) 786-7060.
TELE VIDICS, 2223 E. 223 St., Long Beach, CA 90810; (213) 830-5296.
TELEVISION MATRIX, 1438 N. Gower St., Hollywood, CA 90028; (213) 465-9616.
TRITRONICS, INC., 733 N. Victory Bl., Burbank, CA 91502; (818) 843-2288; (800) 232-2141.
UNITEL VIDEO, 5555 Melrose Ave. Studio G, Los Angeles, CA 90038; (213) 468-4606.
VIDCOM, 2426 Townsgate Rd., Suite K, Westlake Village, CA 91361; (818) 991-1974.
VIDEO ADVENTURES INC., 1015 Cahuenga Blvd., Hollywood, CA 90038; (213) 461-3288.
VIDEOTAPE ENTERPRISES, 8610 Sunset Blvd., Los Angeles, CA 90069; (213) 659-4801.
VIDEO WEST, 6430 Sunset Blvd., Suite 908, Los Angeles, CA 90028; (213) 465-3153.
VIDE-U PRODUCTIONS, 612 N. Sepulveda Blvd., Los Angeles, CA 90049; (213) 472-7023.

NEW YORK

ALL MOBILE VIDEO, 630 Ninth Ave., New York; NY 10036, (212) 757-8919.
BNS VIDEO SERVICES (Division of Broadcast News Service, Inc.), GPO 2360, New York, NY 10116; Pier 62, West 23 St., New York, NY 10011; (212) 466-0234,; (212) 223-0969.
FAMA II PRODUCTIONS, 2750 Richmond Terrace, Staten Island, NY 10303; (718) 273-1780.
MTI TELEVISION CITY, 1443 Park Ave., New York, NY 10029; (212) 722-1818.
MANHATTAN BRIDGE STUDIO, 156 Tillery St., Brooklyn Heights, NY; (718) 330-0555.
MODERN TELECOMMUNICATIONS, 1 Dag Hammarskjold Plaza, New York, NY 10017; (212) 355-0510.
UNITEL VIDEO, 515 W. 57 St., New York, NY 10019; (212) 265-3600.
VIDEO PLANNING INC., 250 W. 57 St., New York, NY 10019; (212) 582-5066.
WINDSOR TOTAL VIDEO, 565 Fifth Ave., New York, NY 10017; (212) 725-8080.

VIDEO PRODUCTION FACILITIES

LOS ANGELES

ABC TELEVISION CENTER, 4151 Prospect Ave., Los Angeles, CA 90027; (213) 557-7777.
ADL VIDEO, 3311 Rowena St., Suite 18, Los Angeles, CA 90027; (213) 662-8385.
ALDAN CO INC., 355 S. Mansfield Ave., Los Angeles, CA 90036; (213) 939-1032.
AMBASSADOR TV PRODUCTION, 392 W. Green St., Pasadena, CA 91123; (818) 577-5400.
AMERICAN VIDEO FACTORY, 4150 Glencoe Ave., Marina Del Rey, CA 90292; (213) 823-8622.
APOLLO PRODUCTION FACILITY, 1503 Cahuenga Blvd., Hollywood, CA 90028; (213) 464-7871, (213) 464-9924.
AUDIO-VIDEO CRAFT INC., 7000 Santa Monica Blvd., Los Angeles, CA 90038; (213) 466-6475.
BERC (BROADCAST EQUIPMENT RENTAL COMPANY), 4545 Chermak St., Burbank, CA 91505; (818) 841-3000, (213) 464-7655.
BAKER-NISBET INC., 451 N. La Cienega Blvd., Suite 12, Los Angeles, CA 90048; (213) 657-5687.
BECK BROTHERS VIDEO DEN, 8480 Beverly Blvd., Suite 145, Los Angeles, CA 90048; (213) 652-2143.
BETACAM SPECIALISTS, 3917 Riverside Dr., Suite 9137, Burbank, CA 91505; (818) 845-6480.
BOSUSTOW VIDEO, 2207 Colby Ave., West Los Angeles, CA 90064; (213) 478-0821.
BOWEN VIDEO FACILITIES, 619 S. Victory Blvd., Burbank, CA 91504; (818) 841-0295.
CALIFORNIA ZEPHYR, 9348 Santa Monica Blvd., Suite 101, Beverly Hills, CA 90210; (213) 653-4004.
CENTRE FILMS INC., 1103 N. El Centro Ave., Los Angeles, CA 90038; (213) 466-5123.
CHELSEA VIDEO STUDIOS, 6534 Sunset Blvd., Hollywood, CA 90028; (213) 464-5360.
CHRIS CRAFT VIDEO TAPE CENTER, 915 N. La Brea Ave., Los Angeles, CA 90038; (213) 850-2236.
COMPACT VIDEO SERVICES INC., 2813 W. Alameda Ave., Burbank, CA 91505; (818) 840-7000.
CONSOLIDATED FILM INDUSTRIES, 959 Seward St., Los Angeles, CA 90038; (213) 462-3161.
COTTON CANDY/EYE ON VIDEO, 224 N. Juanita Ave., Los Angeles, CA 90004; (213) 382-4048.
CREATIVE VIDEO SERVICES, 500 Ventu Park Rd., Newbury Park, CA 91320; (818) 707-2424.
EFP/EBSEN FISHER PRODUCTION, 9541 Cedarbrook Dr., Beverly Hills, CA 90210; (213) 273-2208.
ECONOMY PRODUCTION, EDITING & AIR CHECKS, 7557 Hampton Ave., Los Angeles, CA 90046; (213) 850-5411.
EMERALD STUDIOS INC., P.O. Box 1647, Orange, CA 92268; (714) 771-7394.
FALCON COMMUNICATIONS, 800 S. Date Ave., Alhambra, CA 91803; (818) 576-2906.
FIESTA SOUND & VIDEO, 1655 S. Compton Ave., Los Angeles, CA 90021; (213) 748-2057.
50/50 PRODUCTIONS, 3217 Dona Emilia Dr., Studio City, CA 91604; (818) 708-8433, (213) 650-1685.
GLENDALE STUDIOS, 1239 S. Glendale Ave., Glendale, CA 91205; (818) 502-5300.
GLOBAL TELEVISION, 1950 Cotner Ave., Los Angeles, CA 90025; (213) 479-8081.
GOLDEN WEST VIDEOTAPE, 5800 Sunset Blvd., Los Angeles, CA 90028; (213) 460-5868.
GROUP W CABLE VIDEO PRODUCTION CENTER, 2939 Nebraska Ave., Santa Monica, CA 90404; (213) 829-2676.
HQI STUDIOS, 19347 Londelius St., Northridge, CA 91324; (818) 993-4778.
HOLLYWOOD NATIONAL STUDIOS, 6605 Eleanor Ave., Los Angeles, CA 90038; (213) 467-6272.
HOLLYWOOD PACIFIC STUDIOS, 62900 Sunset Blvd., Hollywood, CA 90028; (213) 463-8118.
IMAGE TRANSFORM INC., 4142 Lankershim Blvd., North Hollywood, CA 91602 (818) 985-7566.
IMAGE WEST, 11846 Ventura Blvd., Studio City, CA 91604; (818) 506-5577.
INTERMIX INC., 2505 S. Robertson Blvd., Los Angeles, CA 90034; (213) 980-2121.
J.P. VIDEO SERVICES, 9538 W. Pico Blvd., Los Angeles, CA 90035; (213) 271-1209.
KCET, 4401 Sunset Blvd., Los Angeles, CA 90027; (213) 666-6500.
KWHY-TV, CHANNEL 22, 5545 Sunset Blvd., Los Angeles, CA 90028; (213) 466-5441.
LMI PRODUCTIONS, c/o Lee Magid, Inc., P.O. Box 532, Malibu, CA 90265; (213) 463-7210.
LA BREA STUDIOS, 1028 N. La Brea Ave., Hollywood, CA 90038; (213) 462-7210.
LIGHT-HOUSE PRODUCTIONS, 427 Linnie Canal, Venice, CA 90291; (213) 827-1537.
LONE STAR PICTURES INTERNATIONAL INC., 6430 Sunset Blvd., Hollywood, CA 90028; (213) 463-3175.
MARSH INTERNATIONAL FILMS, 21029 Itasca St., Suites A & B, Chatsworth, CA 91311; (818) 998-2188.
McINTIRE-HOFFMAN, INC., 18149 Ventura Blvd., Tarzana, CA 91356; (818) 345-9677.
MDC/TELEPRODUCTIONS—McDONNELL DOUGLAS, 15282 Newsboy Circle, Huntington Beach, CA 92647; (714) 896-2495.
MEGA PRODUCTIONS INC., 1714 N. Wilton Place, Hollywood, CA 90028; (213) 462-6342.
METROTAPE, (Division of Metromedia), 5746 Sunset Blvd., Los Angeles, CA 90028; (213) 856-1000.
MILES & COMPANY, 1418 Dodson Ave., San Pedro, CA 90732; (213) 548-0462.
MORRIS VIDEO INC., 663 The Village, Redondo Beach, CA 90277; (213) 374-4984.
ONE PASS FILM & VIDEO, One China Basin Building, San Francisco, CA 94107; (415) 777-5777.
PALARDO PRODUCTIONS, 1807 Taft Ave., Suite 4, Hollywood, CA 90028; (213) 469-8991.
P.D.S. VIDEO PRODUCTIONS, 1102 W. Chestnut St., Burbank, CA 91506; (818) 841-4711.
POSITIVE MEDIA, 5422A Fair Ave., North Hollywood, CA 91601; (818) 761-5192.
THE PRODUCTION GROUP, 1330 N. Vine St., Hollywood, CA 90028; (213) 469-8111.
PROFESSIONAL ARTISTS GROUP, 845 N. Highland Ave., Hollywood, CA 90038; (213) 871-2222.
PROFESSIONAL MEDIA SERVICE, 18301 Pammey Lane, Huntington Beach, CA 92648; (714) 964-0542.
PREMORE INC., 5310 Klump Ave., North Hollywood, CA 91601; (818) 506-7714.
REN-MAR STUDIOS, 846 N. Cahuenga Blvd., Los Angeles, CA 90038; (213) 463-0808.
SCHULMAN VIDEO CENTER, 861 Seward St., Hollywood, CA 90036; (213) 465-8110.
SELLULOID VIDEO, 3620 Overland Ave., Los Angeles, CA 90034; (213) 202-8990.
SPEAR, JACK PRODUCTIONS INC., 7243 Santa Monica Blvd., Hollywood, CA 90046; (213) 851-4123.
STUDIO & REMOTE VIDEO, 10650 Magnolia Blvd., North Hollywood, CA 91601; (818) 508-6010.
SOUND MASTER, 10747 Magnolia Blvd., North Hollywood, CA 91601; (213) 650-8000.
SULLIVAN & ASSOCIATES, 201 N. Occidental Blvd., Los Angeles, CA 90026; (213) 384-3331.
SUNRISE CANYON VIDEO, P.O. Box 10968, Burbank, CA 91510; (818) 845-7473.
SUPERCOLOSSAL PICTURES CORP., 3413 Cahuenga Blvd. West, Los Angeles, CA 90068; (213) 876-6770.
SUPERIOR VIDEO SERVICES, 13423 Saticoy St., North Hollywood, CA 91605; (818) 786-7060.
TELEVISION MATRIX, 1438 N. Gower St., Hollywood, CA 90028; (213) 465-9616.
TRADEWIND VIDEO PRODUCTIONS, Santa Monica, CA 90403, (213) 397-2267.
TRANS-AMERICAN VIDEO INC., 1541 N. Vine St., Los Angeles, CA 90028; (213) 466-2141.
TRITRONICS INC., 733 N. Victory Bl., Burbank, CA 91502; (818) 843-2288, (800) 232-2141.
UNITEL VIDEO, 5555 Melrose Ave., Studio G, Los Angeles, CA 90038; (213) 468-4606.
VIA VISION PRODUCTIONS, 5919 Franklin Ave., Los Angeles, CA 90028; (213) 460-4864.
VIDEO ADVENTURES INC., 1015 Cahuenga Blvd., Hollywood, CA 90038; (213) 461-3288.
VIDEO IMAGE, 13450 Maxella Ave., Suite 270, Marina Del Rey, CA 90202; (213) 822-8872.
VIDEO-IT INC., 1016 N. Sycamore Ave., Hollywood, CA 90038; (213) 876-4055, (213) VID-EOIT.
VIDEO SYSTEMS NETWORK, INC., 12530 Beatrice St., Los Angeles, CA 90066; (213) 870-1231.

VIDEO WEST, 6430 Sunset Blvd., Suite 908, Los Angeles, CA 90028; (213) 465-3153.

VINE STREET VIDEO CENTER, P.O. Box 8471, Universal City Plaza, Universal City, CA 91608; (213) 462-1099.

WILDER BROTHERS VIDEO, 10327 Santa Monica Blvd., Los Angeles, CA 90025; (213) 557-3500.

WINTERS PRODUCTIONS, Box 920, Montrose, CA 91020; (818) 790-4201.

NEW YORK

ANS INTERNATIONAL VIDEO LTD., 396 Fifth Ave., New York, NY 10018; (212) 736-1007.

BROADWAY STUDIOS, 25-09 Broadway, Astoria, NY 11106; (718) 274-9121.

CALAMAR PRODUCTIONS, 254 Park Ave. South, Penthouse D, New York, NY 10010; (212) 254-7086.

CAMERA MART STAGES, INC., 460 W. 54 St., New York, NY 10019; (212) 757-6977.

FAMA II PRODUCTIONS, 2750 Richmond Terrace, Staten Island, NY 10303; (718) 273-1780.

KAUFMAN-ASTORIA STUDIOS, 34-12 36th St., Astoria, NY 11106; (718) 392-5600.

MPCS VIDEO INDUSTRIES, 514 W. 57 St., New York, NY 10019; (212) 586-3690.

MANHATTAN BRIDGE STUDIOS & VIDEO, 156 Tillary St., Brooklyn Heights, NY 11201; (718) 330-0555.

MODERN TELECOMMUNICATIONS INC., 1 Dag Hammarskjold Plaza, New York, NY 10017; (212) 355-0510.

MOTHERS SOUND STAGES, 210 E. 5 St., New York, NY 10003; (212) 260-2050.

NATIONAL VIDEO INDUSTRIES, INC., 15 W. 17 St., New York, NY 10011; (212) 691-1300.

PRIMA LUX VIDEO, 30 W. 26 St., New York, NY 10010; (212) 206-1402.

REEVES TELETAPE, 304 E. 44 St., New York, NY 10017; (212) 573-8888.

SILVER CUP STUDIOS, 42-25 21st St., Long Island City, NY 11101; (718) 784-3390.

TELETECHNIQUES, 40 W. 72 St., New York, NY 10023; (212) 580-9551.

UNITEL VIDEO, 515 W. 57 St., New York, NY 10019; (212) 265-3600.

VCA/TELETRONICS INTERNATIONAL, 231 E. 55 St., New York, NY 10022; (212) 355-1600.

VIDEO PLANNING INC., 250 W. 57 St., New York, NY 10019; (212) 582-5066.

VIDEO PORTFOLIOS, 142 W. 24 St., New York, NY 10011; (212) 989-3858.

VIDLO VIDEO, 40 E. 21 St., New York, NY 10010; (212) 475-4140.

WINDSOR TOTAL VIDEO, 565 Fifth Ave., New York, NY 10017; (212) 725-8080.

CONNECTICUT

ECA STUDIO, Wilton, CT 06897; (203) 762-3380, (212) 333-5656.

ILLINOIS

TELEMATRON PRODUCTIONS, INC., 3200 W. West Lake Ave., Glenview, IL 60025; (312) 729-5215.

VIDEO SCREENING ROOMS

LOS ANGELES

AMERICAN VIDEO FACTORY, 4150 Glencoe Ave., Marina Del Rey, CA 90292; (213) 823-8622.
AMPAC VIDEO, 3637 Cahuenga Blvd., Hollywood, CA 90068; (213) 851-7200.
AUDIO-VIDEO CRAFT INC., 7000 Santa Monica Blvd., Los Angeles, CA 90038; (213) 466-6475.
AUDIO VISUAL HEADQUARTERS CORP., 361 N. Oak St., Inglewood, CA 90302; (213) 419-4040.
BOSUSTOW VIDEO, 2207 Colby Ave., West Los Angeles, CA 90064; (213) 478-0821.
CALIFORNIA ZEPHYR, 9348 Santa Monica Blvd., Suite 101, Beverly Hills, CA 90210; (213) 653-4004.
CHELSEA VIDEO STUDIOS, 6534 Sunset Blvd., Hollywood, CA 90028; (213) 464-5360.
THE CREATIVE PARTNERSHIP, 6815 Willoughby Ave., Suite 102, Hollywood, CA 90028; (213) 461-3548.
CREATIVE VIDEO SERVICES, 500 Ventu Park Rd., Newbury Park, CA 91320; (818) 707-2424.
ECONOMY PRODUCTION, EDITING & AIR CHECKS, 7557 Hampton Ave., Los Angeles, CA 90046; (213) 850-5411.
THE EDITING COMPANY, 8300 Beverly Blvd., Los Angeles, CA 90048; (213) 653-3570.
FALCON COMMUNICATIONS, 800 S. Date Ave., Alhambra, CA 91803; (818) 576-2906.
FOTO-TRONICS SYSTEMS INC., 2800 W. Olive St., Burbank, CA 91505; (818) 846-3101.
GLOBAL VISION CORPORATION, 3255 Cahuenga Blvd., Hollywood, CA 90068; (213) 851-1190.
HORIZONTAL EDITING STUDIOS, 2625 W. Olive Ave., Burbank, CA 91505; (818) 841-6750.
IMAGE TRANSFORM, 4142 Lankershim Blvd., North Hollywood, CA 91602; (818) 985-7566.
IMAGE WEST, 11846 Ventura Blvd., Studio City, CA 91604; (818) 506-5577.
INTERMIX INC., 2505 S. Robertson, Los Angeles, CA 90034; (213) 870-2121.
INSTANT REPLAY EQUIPMENT CO., 5520 Westlawn Ave., Los Angeles, CA 90066; (213) 870-1231.
JDH SOUND, 12156 W. Olympic Blvd., Los Angeles, CA 90064; (213) 820-8802.
J.P. VIDEO SERVICES, 9538 W. Pico Blvd., Los Angeles, CA 90035 (213) 271-1209.
KWHY-TV, CHANNEL 22, 5545 Sunset Blvd., Los Angeles, CA 90028; (213) 466-5441.
LIONEL TELEVISION PRODUCTIONS, 417 Colorado Ave., Santa Monica, CA 90401; (213) 394-9697.
MARKET STREET SCREENING ROOM, 73 Market St., Venice, CA 90291; (213) 396-5937.
MARSH INTERNATIONAL FILMS, 21029 Itasca St., Suite A & B, Chatsworth, CA 91311; (818) 998-2188.
PACIFIC VIDEO, 809 N. Cahuenga Blvd., Los Angeles, CA 90038; (213) 462-6266.
POSITIVE MEDIA, 5422A Fair Ave., North Hollywood, CA 91601; (818) 761-5192.
THE POST GROUP, 6335 Homewood Ave., Los Angeles, CA 90028; (213) 462-2300.
POST PLUS INCORPORATED, 6650 Santa Monica Blvd., 2nd floor, Hollywood, CA 90038; (213) 463-7108.
QPT EDITORIAL CORPORATION, 629 N. La Brea Ave., Los Angeles, CA 90036; (213) 936-7181.
SOUND MASTER, 10747 Magnolia Blvd., North Hollywood, CA 91601; (213) 650-8000.
SPEAR, JACK PRODUCTIONS INC., 7243 Santa Monica Blvd., Hollywood, CA 90046; (213) 851-4123.
STARLIGHT EDITING SERVICES, 5250 Strohm, North Hollywood, CA 91601; (818) 769-3874.
SUPERIOR VIDEO SERVICES, 13423 Saticoy St., North Hollywood, CA 91605:;(818) 786-7060.
UNITEL VIDEO, 5555 Melrose Ave., Studio G, Los Angeles, CA 90038; (213) 468-4606.
VALLEY VIDEO, 4209 W. Burbank Blvd., Burbank, CA 91505; (818) 841-2387.
VARITEL VIDEO/JACK SCHAEFFER, 3575 Cahuenga Blvd. West, Los Angeles, CA 90068; (213) 805-1165.
VIDEO ADVENTURES INC., 1015 Cahuenga Blvd., Hollywood, CA 90038; (213) 461-3288.
VIDEO CRAFTSMEN INC., 6311 Romaine St., Los Angeles, CA 90038; (213) 464-4351.
THE VIDEO HOUSE, 201 N. Hollywood Way, Suite 202, Burbank, CA 91505; (818) 954-9559.
VIDEO-IT INC., 1016 N. Sycamore Ave., Hollywood, CA 90038; (213) 876-4055; (213) VID-EOIT.
THE VIDEO TAPE CO., 10545 Burbank Blvd., North Hollywood, CA 91601; (818) 985-1666.
VIDE-U PRODUCTIONS, 612 N. Sepulveda Blvd., Los Angeles, CA 90049; (213) 472-7023.
VINE STREET VIDEO CENTER, P.O. Box 8471, Universal City Plaza, Universal City, CA 91608; (213) 462-1099.
WILDER BROTHERS VIDEO, 10327 Santa Monica Blvd., Los Angeles, CA 90025; (213) 557-3500.

NEW YORK

DEVLIN PRODUCTIONS INC., 150 W. 55 St., New York, NY 10019; (212) 582-5572.
MPCS VIDEO INDUSTRIES, 514 W. 57 St., New York, NY 10019; (212) 586-3690.
MODERN TELECOMMUNICATIONS INC., 1 Dag Hammarskjold Plaza, New York, NY 10017; (212) 355-0510.
P.A.T. FILM SERVICES, 630 Ninth Ave., New York, NY 10036; (212) 247-0900.
VCA/TELETRONICS, 231 E. 55 St., New York, NY 10022; (212) 355-1600.
WINDSOR TOTAL VIDEO, 565 Fifth Ave., New York, NY 10017; (212) 725-8080.

VIDEOTAPE TRANSFER, FILM TO TAPE

LOS ANGELES

A.M.E. INC., 2921 W. Olive Ave., Burbank, CA 91505; (818) 841-7740.
ALTAVIDEO, 3501 Cahuenga Blvd. West, Los Angeles, CA 90068; (213) 876-8008.
AMPAC VIDEO, 3637 Cahuenga Blvd. West, Hollywood, CA 90068; (213) 851-7200.
ANDERSON, HOWARD A., CO., 1016 N. Cole Ave., Los Angeles, CA 90038; (213) 463-2336.
AUDIO GRAPHIC FILMS AND VIDEO, 6509 De Longpre Ave., Hollywood, CA 90028; (213) 462-6596, (213) 467-1234.
AUDIO PLUS VIDEO INTERNATIONAL INC., 1438 N. Gower St., Hollywood, CA 90028; (213) 856-0152.
AUDIO-VIDEO CRAFT INC., 7000 Santa Monica Blvd., Los Angeles, CA 90038; (213) 466-6475.
BONDED SERVICES, 5260 Vineland Ave., North Hollywood, CA 91601; (818) 761-4058.
BUDGET VIDEO, 1534 N. Highland Ave., Los Angeles, CA 90028; (213) 466-2431.
CAL VISTA INTERNATIONAL INC., 6649 Odessa Ave., Van Nuys, CA 91406; (818) 780-9000.
CALIFORNIA COMMUNICATIONS INC., 6900 Santa Monica Blvd., Los Angeles, CA 90038; (213) 466-8511.
CALIFORNIA ZEPHYR, 9348 Santa Monica Blvd., Suite 101, Beverly Hills, CA 90210; (213) 653-4004.
CHELSEA VIDEO STUDIOS, 6534 Sunset Blvd., Hollywood, CA 90028; (213) 464-5360.
COMPACT VIDEO SERVICES INC., 2813 W. Alameda Ave., Burbank, CA 91505; (818) 840-7000.
COMPLETE POST INC., 6087 Sunset Blvd., Hollywood, CA 90028; (213) 467-1244
COMPOSITE IMAGE SYSTEMS, 815 N. Cahuenga Blvd., Hollywood, CA 90038; (213) 461-5734.
CONRAD FILM DUPLICATING CO., 6750 Santa Monica Blvd., Hollywood, CA 90038; (213) 463-5614.
CONSOLIDATED FILM INDUSTRIES, 959 Seward St., Los Angeles, CA 90038; (213) 462-3161.
COTTON CANDY/EYE ON VIDEO, 224 N. Juanita Ave., Los Angeles, CA 90004; (213) 382-4048.
CREATIVE VIDEO SERVICES, 500 Ventu Park Rd., Newbury Park, CA 91320; (818) 707-2424.
CREST NATIONAL FILM & VIDEOTAPE LABS, 1141 N. Seward St., Los Angeles, CA 90038; (213) 462-3073.
DELUXE LABORATORIES, INC., 1377 N. Serrano Ave., Hollywood, CA 90027; (213) 462-6171.
EDITEL-LOS ANGELES, 729 N. Highland Ave., Hollywood, CA 90038; (213) 913-1821.
THE EDITING COMPANY, 8300 Beverly Blvd., Los Angeles, CA 90048; (213) 653-3570.
FILM TECHNOLOGY CO. INC., 6900 Santa Monica Blvd., Los Angeles, CA 90038; (213) 464-3456.
FOTO-KEM INDUSTRIES INC., 2800 W. Olive Ave., Burbank, CA 91505; (818) 846-3101.
FOTO-TRONICS SYSTEMS INC., 2800 W. Olive Ave., Burbank, CA 91505; (818) 846-3101.
GLOBAL TELEVISION, 1950 Cotner Ave., Los Angeles, CA 90025; (213) 479-8081.
H.C.V., 3034 Glendale Blvd., Los Angeles, CA 90039; (213) 662-1112.
IMAGE TRANSFORM INC., 4142 Lankershim Blvd., North Hollywood, CA 91602; (818) 985-7566.
INTERNATIONAL VIDEO CONVERSIONS, 814 N. Cahuenga Blvd., Hollywood, CA 90038; (213) 463-7884.
JDH SOUND, 12156 W. Olympic Blvd., Los Angeles, CA 90064; (213) 820-8802.
KWHY-TV, CHANNEL 22, 5545 Sunset Blvd., Los Angeles, CA 90028; (213) 466-5441.
LAJON PRODUCTIONS, INC., 2907 W. Olive Ave., Burbank, CA 91505; (818) 841-1440.
M.F.I. VIDEO CENTER, 1905 Grace Ave., Hollywood, CA 90068; (213) 851-0373.
McINTIRE-HOFFMAN INC., 18149 Ventura Blvd., Tarzana, CA 91356; (818) 345-9677.
METROTAPE (Division of Metromedia), 5746 Sunset Blvd., Los Angeles, CA 90028; (213) 856-1000.
MODERN VIDEOFILM, 7165 Sunset Blvd., Hollywood, CA 90046; (213) 851-8070.
MUSIC LAB INC., 1831 Hyperion Ave., Hollywood, CA 90027; (213) 666-3003.
ONE PASS FILM & VIDEO, One China Basin Building, San Francisco, CA 94107; (415) 777-5777.
PACIFIC VIDEO, 809 N. Cahuenga Blvd., Los Angeles, CA 90038; (213) 462-6266.
PAL VIDEO, 19061 Tina Pl., Tarzana, CA 91356; (818) 344-1603.
THE POST GROUP, 6335 Homewood, Los Angeles, CA 90028; (213) 462-2300.
RUBBER DUBBERS INC., 626 Justin Ave., Glendale, CA 91201; (818) 241-5600.
RUSK SOUND STUDIO, 1556 N. La Brea Ave., Hollywood, CA 90028; (213) 462-6477.
RUXTON LTD., 611 N. Orchard Dr., Burbank, CA 91506; (818) 845-3724.
SAWYER CAMERA & VIDEO SERVICE, 1208 W. Isabel St. Burbank, CA 91506; (818) 843-1781.
SIERRA VIDEO, 4216 N. Maxson Rd., El Monte, CA 91732; (818) 579-7023.
SOUND SERVICES INC. (S.S.I.), 7155 Santa Monica Blvd., Los Angeles, CA 90046; (213) 874-9344.; (818) 986-3255.
SOUND WEST, INC., 12166 Olympic Blvd., Los Angeles, CA 90064; (213) 826-6560.
STARFAX, 8157 Lankershim Blvd., North Hollywood, CA 91605; (818) 768-2905.
STUDIO TELEVISION SERVICE, 7550 W. Sunset Blvd., Los Angeles, CA 90046; (213) 851-7556.
SUPERCINE INC., 2214 W. Olive Ave., Burbank, CA 91506; (818) 843-8260.
SUPERIOR VIDEO SERVICES, 13423 Saticoy St., North Hollywood, CA 91605; (818) 786-7060.
TAV/COMMAND, INC., 1541 N. Vine St., Los Angeles, CA 90028; (213) 466-2141.
TAV SOUND INC., 6200 W. Third St., Los Angeles, CA 90038; (213) 937-2460.
TELEPRINT OF LOS ANGELES, 3779 Cahuenga Blvd. West, Studio City, CA 91604; (818) 760-3191.
TRANS-AMERICAN VIDEO INC., 1541 N. Vine St., Los Angeles, CA 90028; (213) 466-2141.
TRANSWORLD VIDEO LAB INC., 3812 W. Magnolia Blvd., Burbank, CA 91505; (818) 841-2416.
TRITRONICS INC., 733 N. Victory Bl., Burbank, CA 91502; (818) 843-2288, (800) 232-2141
U C L VIDEO, 823 N. Seward St., Los Angeles, CA 90038; (213) 469-7291.
UNITEL VIDEO, 5555 Melrose Ave., Studio G, Los Angeles, CA 90038; (213) 468-4606.
V C I DUPLICATION, 915 Hollywood Way, Burbank, CA 91505; (818) 841-8550.
VALLEY VIDEO, 4209 W. Burbank Blvd., Burbank, CA 91505; (818) 841-2387.
VECTOR PRODUCTIONS INC., P.O. Box 7000-645, Redondo Beach, CA 90277; (213) 757-0520, (213) 316-6031.
VIDEO ADVENTURES INC., 1015 Cahuenga Blvd., Hollywood, CA 90038; (213) 461-3288.
VIDEO ASSOCIATES AND CO. 5419 Sunset Blvd., Los Angeles, CA 90038; (213) 463-3255.
VIDEO CRAFTSMEN INC., 6311 Romaine St., Los Angeles, CA 90038; (213) 464-4351.
VIDEO EVENTS INC., 1741 N. Ivar, Suite 210, Hollywood, CA 90028; (213) 465-4197.
VIDEO IMAGE, 13450 Maxella Ave., Suite 270, Marina Del Rey, CA 90292; (213) 822-8872.
THE VIDEOTAPE CO., 10545 Burbank Blvd., North Hollywood, CA 91601; (818) 985-1666.
VIDEO VIEW, 1617 N. El Centro Ave., Hollywood, CA 90038; (213) 463-4179.
VIDE-U PRODUCTIONS, 612 N. Sepulveda Blvd., Los Angeles, CA 90049; (213) 472-7023.
WEISBARTH, JACOB & ASSOC., INC., 9903 Santa Monica Blvd., Suite 256, Beverly Hills, CA 90212; (213) 475-0668.
WILDER BROTHERS VIDEO, 10327 Santa Monica Blvd., Los Angeles, CA 90025; (213) 557-3500.
WILLIAM SOUND SERVICE, 1343 N. Highland Ave., Los Angeles, CA 90028; (213) 461-5321.
YALE LABS, 1509 N. Gordon, Los Angeles, CA 90028, (213) 464-6181.

NEW YORK

ANS INTERNATIONAL VIDEO LTD., 396 Fifth Ave., New York, NY 10018; (212) 736-1007.

ALL MOBILE VIDEO, 630 Ninth Ave., New York, NY 10036; (212) 757-8919.

BOGAZICI VIDEO LTD., 460 Seventh Ave., New York, NY 10001; (212) 563-9022.

CINE MAGNETICS FILM & VIDEO LABORATORIES, 650 Halstand Ave., Mamaroneck, NY; (212) 542-0700; 50 W. 40 St., New York, NY 10018; (212) 921-1299.

DEVLIN PRODUCTIONS, 150 W. 55 St., New York, NY 10019; (212) 582-5572.

DOLPHIN PRODUCTIONS, 140 E. 80 St., New York, NY 10021; (212) 628-5930.

EUE/SCREEN GEMS, 222 E. 44 St., New York, NY 10017; (212) 867-4030.

EDITEL—NEW YORK, 222 E. 44 St., New York, NY 10017; (212) 867-4600.

ELECTROTECH TRADING CORP., 40-10 67th St., Woodside, NY; (718) 899-8388.

FAMA II PRODUCTIONS, 2750 Richmond Terrace, Staten Island, NY 10303; (718) 273-1780.

FOTO-VIDEO TRANSFER CENTER, One Times Square, New York, NY 10036; (212) 302-1866.

INTERNATIONAL VIDEO MARKET, 926 Second Ave., New York, NY 10022; (212) 826-1996; 1121 First Ave., New York, NY 10021; (212) 223-4601; 991 First Ave., New York, NY 10022; (212) 826-8846.

INTERNATIONAL VIDEO SERVICE, 1501 Broadway, New York, NY 10036; (212) 730-1411.

LANDMARK VIDEO INC., 350 Fifth Ave., New York, NY 10001; (212) 947-8637.

MPCS VIDEO INDUSTRIES, 514 W. 57 St., New York, NY 10019; (212) 586-3690.

MODERN TELECOMMUNICATIONS INC., 1443 Park Ave., New York, NY 10029; (212) 722-1818; 1 Dag Hammarskjold Plaza, New York, NY 10017; (212) 355-0510.

PICSONIC PRODUCTIONS CORP., 1466 Broadway, New York, NY 10036; (212) 575-1910.

REEVES TELETAPE, 708 Third Ave., New York, NY 10017; (212) 573-8888; 1697 Broadway, New York, NY 10019; (212) 307-4880.

S/T VIDEOCASSETTE DUPLICATION CORP., 500 Willowtree Rd., Leonia, NJ; (212) 239-4653.

TFI (TAPE FILM INDUSTRIES), 619 W. 54 St., New York, NY 10019; (212) 708-0500.

UNITEL VIDEO, 515 W. 57 St., New York, NY 10019; (212) 265-3600.

VCA/TELETRONICS, 231 E. 55 St., New York, NY 10022; (212) 355-1600.

VIDBO VIDEO LTD. (affiliate of Bogazici Video Ltd.,) 460 Seventh Ave., New York, NY 10001; (212) 563-9022.

VIDEO CASSETTE TRANSFERS, 160 W. 46 St., New York, NY 10036; (212) 575-8433.

VIDEO CONNECTION, 1137 Second Ave., New York, NY 10022; (212) 593-1010; 2244 Broadway, New York, NY 10024; (212) 724-2727.

VIDEO DUB INC., 423 W. 55 St., New York, NY; (212) 757-3300; (212) 582-9550.

VIDEO MEDIA PRODUCTIONS, 149-33 88th St., Howard Beach, NY; (718) 845-3709.

VIDEO PLANNING INC., 250 W. 57 St., New York, NY 10019; (212) 582-5066.

VIDEO STOP, 367 Third Ave., New York, NY 10016; (212) 685-6199.

VIDEOROOM, 1487 Third Ave., New York NY 10028; (212) 879-5333; 2165 Broadway, New York, NY 10024; (212) 799-2100.

WINDSOR TOTAL VIDEO, 565 Fifth Ave., New York, NY 10017; (212) 725-8080.

CANADA

MANTA VIDEO LABS, 311 Adelaide St. E, Toronto, Ont., Canada M5A IN2; (412) 863-9316.

VIDEOTAPE TRANSFER, TAPE TO FILM

LOS ANGELES

AMERICAN VIDEO FACTORY, 4150 Glencoe Ave., Marina Del Rey, CA 90292; (213) 823-8622.
AUDIO GRAPHIC FILMS AND VIDEO, 6509 De Longpre Ave., Hollywood, CA 90028; (213) 462-6596, (213) 467-1234.
COMPACT VIDEO SERVICES INC., 2813 W. Alameda Ave., Burbank, CA 91505; (818) 840-7000.
CONSOLIDATED FILM INDUSTRIES, 959 Seward St., Los Angeles, CA 90038; (213) 462-3161.
CREATIVE VIDEO SERVICES, 500 Ventu Park Rd., Newbury Park, CA 91320; (818) 707-2424.
CREST NATIONAL FILM & VIDEOTAPE LABS, 1141 N. Seward St., Los Angeles, CA 90038; (213) 462-3073.
THE EDITING COMPANY, 8300 Beverly Blvd., Los Angeles, CA 90048; (213) 653-3570.
IMAGE TRANSFORM INC., 4142 Lankershim Blvd., North Hollywood, CA 91602; (818) 985-7566.
INTERNATIONAL VIDEO CONVERSIONS, 815 N. Cahuenga Blvd., Hollywood, CA 90038; (213) 463-7884.
KWHY-TV, CHANNEL 22, 5545 Sunset Blvd., Los Angeles, CA 90028; (213) 466-5441.
ONE PASS FILM & VIDEO, One China Basin Building, San Francisco, CA 94107; (415) 777-5777.
ROUZER STUDIO, 7022 Melrose Ave., Los Angeles, CA 90038; (213) 936-2494.
RVS—TAPE TO FILM TRANSFER SERVICES, 2408 W. Olive Ave., Burbank, CA 91506; (818) 954-8621.
SOUND SERVICES INC., 7155 Santa Monica Blvd., Los Angeles, CA 90038; (213) 874-9344.
TAV SOUND INC., 6200 W. Third St., Los Angeles, CA 90038; (213) 937-2460.
TELEPRINT OF LOS ANGELES, 3779 Cahuenga Blvd. West, Studio City, CA 91604; (818) 760-3191.
VECTOR PRODUCTIONS INC., P.O. Box 7000-645, Redondo Beach, CA 90277; (213) 757-0520, (213) 316-6031.
VIDEO VIEW, 1617 N. El Centro Ave., Hollywood, CA 90028; (213) 463-4179.
WEISBARTH, JACOB & ASSOCIATES, INC., 9903 Santa Monica Blvd., Suite 256, Beverly Hills, CA 90212; (213) 475-0668.
WESTERN FILM INDUSTRIES, 30941 W. Agoura Rd., Suite 302, Westlake Village, CA 91360; (818) 889-7350.

NEW YORK

MODERN TELECOMMUNICATIONS INC., 1443 Park Ave., New York, NY 10029; (212) 722-1818; 1 Dag Hammarskjold, Plaza, New York, NY 10017; (212) 355-0510.
POSITIVE TRANSFER LTD., 545 Fifth Ave., New York, NY 10017; (212) 370-1400.
WARREN ROSENBERG VIDEO SERVICES, 308 E. 79 St., New York, NY 10021; (212) 744-1111.
WINDSOR TOTAL VIDEO, 565 Fifth Ave., New York, NY 10017; (212) 725-8080.

The Home Video World Market

THE HOME VIDEO WORLD MARKET

AUSTRALIA

Estimates indicate that approximately 30 per cent of the households with television sets also have video cassette recorders.

The following figures showing the number of VCRs sold here each year since 1979 reveal the rapid penetration of the market:

1979	26,000
1980	72,000
1981	150,000
1982	350,000
1983	500,000
1984	685,000
1985	600,000

Major video distributors total nine, while there are some 20 smaller outfits. Nearly all the majors have links to other Australian media groups as well as to leading world-wide film distributors.

For example, the major VCR wholesalers include CBS-Fox, Warner Video, and RCA/Columbia/Hoyts (latter is a leading theatre circuit) as well as CIC Video (film distributor with links to Paramount), Syme Video (media conglomerate with ties to Disney), and PBV (TV station owners with ties to MGM and United Artists). Other distributors are Thorn-EMI Video, Video Classics and Roadshow.

CANADA

Canada had a VCR population of approximately 2,000,000 early in 1986, which represents an estimated 28 per cent of television homes. As of then some 1,237,151 machines had been imported into the country (Canada does not manufacture videocassette recorders) compared with 1,265,084 at the end of 1984 and 136,969 during 1981.

Estimates indicate that cassette sales for 1985 were way above—as much as one and one-half times—the theatrical motion picture gross revenue, which was about $380,000,000 (Canadian) for the year.

Other data recently compiled by A.C. Nielsen of Canada:

About 72 per cent VCRs are VHS format.

Films are the most prevalent programs recorded.

More than 50 per cent of the usage occurs while the TV set is off, and the same percentage eliminates commercials while recording.

More than 20 per cent of households watch more TV since purchase of a VCR.

Nearly 75 per cent of households sampled cited recording of programs that would otherwise be missed as the chief reason for use.

EGYPT

Number of companies working on recording and distribution of video tapes: 167

Number of fully registered video clubs: 1725. Besides these there are about 2000 more small shops who rent to viewers for 1.50 E.P. (Eypgtian pounds) for each print for a period of 48 hours.

Number of families who own video recorders: 4.5 million. The figure is growing very fast.

General: There's no doubt that video is spreading rapidly in Egypt and is beginning to have a serious effect on theatrical film business. The Indian public enjoys watching films in its own homes at inexpensive prices with all members of the family on hand and the ability to invite friends and neighbors if they wish. Going to a movie theatre is annoying to them for many reasons, including crowded streets, the cost of transportation, and the lack of parking areas.

AHMED SAMI

GREAT BRITAIN

In five years the home video market in the UK has developed from virtually zero to a multi-million pound business. With such a rapid growth business, in some respects the pace has been too fast and inevitably mistakes were made but the all-important video dealer is now losing his tainted image. Nowadays, he is more likely to be more professional and business-like in his dealings with the public and is developing the ability to attract an increasing number of distributors.

Moreover, the industry is recognising the need for continued promotion to attract back their viewers when the initial novelty of owning a video and renting tapes wears off.

Statistically, the home video business continues to expand with weekly software rentals having increased by a million in the past year. A report commissioned by the British Videogram Association (BVA) revealed that the number of VCR owners has also increased along with the number of sales transactions. VCR penetration has increased from 40 to 44 per cent and the number in UK homes is likely to rise to 9.5 million by the end of 1986.

Cassette rentals have jumped from 4.5 million a week to 5.5 million, an increase of 22 per cent, and for the first time the percentage of active renters increased over the previous quarter of 1986 by one per cent. Sales of cassettes to the public, primarily via the sell-through market, increased by £60,000 from £82,000 to £142,000 and the software spend—which at the end of 1985 rested at £306 million—looked like reaching a record £400 million by the end of 1986.

Domestic and export sales for UK video distribution totalled £26.75 million for the second quarter of 1986. BVA director general Norman Abbott claimed this record-breaking performance to "some particularly attractive titles," buoyant hardware sales and increasing professionalism among video retailers.

At the same time the average hire charge for a cassette rental has gone up. On average video library owners are charging £1.21 a night for cassette hire. These figures show that £1.2 million is being spent on video each day. It means that more people rent videos in a year (330 million) than play squash (130 million); attend all football league fixtures (40 million); read paperback books (50 million) or buy record albums (101 million).

Leading distributors of pre-recorded tapes include Warner, CIC, Cannon, RCA/Columbia, CBS/Fox, Rank, Entertainment in Video, Walt Disney, Virgin, Heron, MGM/UA and Guild.

Piracy of video cassettes has sharply diminished since the foundation of the Video Copyright Protection Society (VCPS)—set up jointly by the BBC, the Independent Television Companies' Association and the Society of Film Distributors—and of FACT—the Federation Against Copyright Theft. This has come about most notably since the penalties were greatly increased when the Copyright Act was amended in 1983.

Now the VCPS is turning its attention to piracy overseas. One of the things it wishes to see in a new Copyright Act is a means of curbing the losses which the film and television industry suffers through the illegal export of films and television programmes. Tapes are frequently recorded off-air in the UK and exported overseas where they are duplicated and sold. It is estimated that several millions of pounds are being lost by the film and television industries by lost royalties to writers and performers, to production companies, and in effect all off-shoots.

The VCPS wants the Copyright Act amended to make it an offence to export copies of film and television programmes without authority.

Nevertheless, as with cinemas, the video business is dependent on the studios producing good entertainment and, at the same time, making the consumer aware of the product. Given these factors, there is no reason why the current upsurge in home-video viewing—despite the threat of Cable, Pay TV and Satellite broadcasting—should not continue for some years yet.

GREECE

Home video has exploded in this country as of 1983, invading homes, cafés, and other places. More and more videocassettes are produced every year and new video clubs are constantly opening.

Number of TV sets: 1,800,000

Number of Video Cassettes: it is estimated that about 300 videocassettes are legally produced every month.

Price of a videocassette: It is sold to retailers by the wholesalers for about 4,000-8,000 drachmas who are lending it for 100-200 drachmas.

Number of Wholesalers: There are more than 100 legally-operating companies with a yearly total income of five billion drachmas ($33,300,000) who have libraries of many titles old and new.

Number of Video Clubs (Retailers): 1200

Video Cassette Piracy: There is an extended traffic of illegal video cassette operators who import masters illegally and/or duplicate imported titles or local ones and sell their inferior copies cheaper to regional places. As there was no law against this piracy an organization was established by several producers to protect their interests. It is called "Protection Society of Video Cassette Producers" with Yannius Adam as its president. However, by a recent decision of the Supreme Court of Athens, the illegal reproduction of a video cassette is considered a forgery and the culprits are sentenced to imprisonment and/or heavy fines.

Hardware and Software Dealers: There are many dealers selling hardware and software equipment representing or acting as agents of AKAI, ASA, BAUER, BLAUPUNKT, GRUNDIC, HITACHI, LOWE, MAGNASONIC, MITSUBISHI, NORDMENDE, ORION, PANASONIC, PHILIPS, SANUO, SIEMENS, TELEFUNKEN, SONY, SALORA, etc. Their prices vary from 105,000-320,000 drachmas.

Producers, Wholesalers, Agents: Home Video Hellas, 15 Adrianiou Str. Athens 115 25. MTC Video Aristotelous Str. Athens, 176 71. EGEE Home Video, 70 Omerou Str. Nea Symrni AVM Audio Video Magnetics, Vasileos Georguiou & Kifissias Halandri. Audio Visual Enterprises, 7 Sohou Str. Athens, 11525. Video Sonic 58 Grypari Str. Callithea. CBS Electronics 311 Mesoguion Str. Athens 152 31. Key Video, 9-13 Gravias Str. Athens, 106 78. and many others.

RENA VELISSARIOU

HOLLAND

In the autumn of 1985 1.2 million families possessed a recorder which is six times as much as in 1981. It is expected that in the future this will grow by 30 per cent. The Dutch population being about 14,400,000 now and assuming that each family consists of husband, wife and two children, it means that one third of the Dutch families has a video recorder. Purchase of a recorder is relatively high by those with a good income, mostly by those living in the West of the Netherlands (the most prosperous provinces), those who look often to TV, and by members of the most important TV organizations: A.V.R.O, T.R.O.S. and V.O.O. 70 per cent of the owners of a recorder rent a print of pictures for instance with video companies. There are many stores in many cities and villages. TV programs are often copied (recorded) by 86 per cent of the owners of a recorder.

Because it is so popular to rent a motion picture with a video store price f.5,— to f. 15,— (a Dutch guilder is $0.40, about), for one day, competition with motion pictures is very serious. As a rule the "performances" in homes are often attended by those not possesssing a recorder. Attention to TV programs is not influenced: owners of a recorder look more frequently to these programs. Night films on TV are often recorded enabling viewers to see such pictures later at normal hours.

Younger and more educated people are visiting cinemas more than older and less educated people. Younger people don't want to stay home. They prefer to go to a cinema making their own choice: action pictures in general.

Going less to cinemas than in the past has its motives. The owning of a video recorder is an important one. Also: the decision to buy a recorder is also influenced by efforts to reduce expenses—the cost, for instance, of visiting a cinema.

In spite of gross receipts of about 100 million guilders by the videothèques, there has been no growth. The number of them is the same as some years ago. The number of pictures offered to videothèques is enormous. This is the conclusion of a study group of the Rotterdam Erasmus University, in charge of Cannon Screen Entertainment.

The piracy problem is still big, an estimation of 100 to 150 million guilders has been made, gross receipts of piracy. The Dutch film federation Nederlandse Bond van Bioscoop- en Filmondernemingen has a close cooperation with the Stichting Video Veilig (=Safe).

On sale here Philips, Blaupunkt and Gründig (West Germany), Sharp, Japanese video recorders (Sony, Akai, Hitachi), practically all VHS system. Prices between 1,000 and 2,000 guilders.

If weather is good in summer it means bad business for videothèques. In May 1986 the Top Ten have been 1. "Rambo First Blood Part 2" (Thorn-EMI), 2. "A View To a Kill" (Warner Home Video), 3. "Beverly Hills Cop" (Esselte CIC Video), 4. "Mad Max" (Warner Home Video), 7. "Police Academy 2" (Warner Home Video), 8. "Return of the Jedi" (CBS/Fox Video), 9. "Desperately Seeking Susan" (RCA/Columbia) and 10. "Gremlins" (Warner Home Video), according to Nederlandse Videoverhuur-Top-50. Cassettes cost 13 to 30 guilders depending on playing time, of BETA, VHS and VCC.

Most of the figures and data are derived from research by NOS, Hilversum and from the magazine "Skoop".

PHILIP DE SCHAAP

INDIA

With the expansion of TV networks throughout the country an increasing number of VCRs have made their appearance in Indian homes. A rough estimate puts the total number of VCRs in the country around 700,000. There are well over 40,000 video libraries renting out cassettes. Besides, there are about 50,000 video parlours in the country. In the absence of legitimate cassettes, they have been screening only pirated prints, thus depriving the national exchequer and the film industry of millions of rupees. In addition, there are over 3,000 video coaches and 15,000 hotel rooms having closed circuit TV. Many metropolitan cities have now started haing closed circuit TV in buildings and housing societies. A number of clubs, schools, hospitals and other institutions also have regular screening of films on video.

Widespread video piracy has undoubtedly affected the film industry's export earnings. For example: UK, which had nearly a hundred cinema halls showing Indian films, now practically has none. Similar is the case in Canada and USA. In India, however, the situation is different. The number of feature films produced in 1985 shows a marked increase over the previous year. So also the number of film theatres has increased. Colour TV and Video (priced at around Rs. 25,000) has still not percolated down to the middle and lower classes who are the main patrons of Indian films.

Through the film industry's concerted efforts the government has now passed a law against video piracy. Any person who exhibits or permits the exhibition of a video film in any place without proper certification is liable for imprisonment for a period of three years and a fine which may extend to Rs. 100,000. Taking advantage of the stringent laws the producers are now selling the video rights of their films; thus a new source of revenue has been opened to them.

A New Delhi-based company is all set to franchise 10,000 video theatres all over the country. The plan envisages the construction of compact 300 seater theatres in towns and villages where there are no additional cinema halls. With the total capital outlay of less than half a million rupees per theatre, a population of 50,000 is enough to sustain such a theatre.

The government owned TV network Doordarshan has increased its revenue from advertisments and sponsored programmes from Rs. 320 million in 1984-85 to Rs. 550 million in 1985-86. Many of the programmes are 13 part to 104 part serials. Most are shot on video tape consequently giving rise to video studios in the major cities.

B. D. GARGA

JAPAN

The Latin word video, to see, has been adopted for use in our modern world as a term which covers a rather large field in the electronics sector including video cassette recorders (VCRs) or video tape recorders (VTRs), and the compact disks (CDs) using laser beam technology. The Japanese, who don't know one Latin word from another, but are the most skillful people in the world in adapting other peoples' ideas and improving on them, are the world leaders in video manufacturing. At present they make 90 per cent of the world VCRs or VTRs produced, have close to 90 per cent of the most lucrative American market, and perhaps 99 percent of the market in Japan, where the market consists of 38.5 million households.

Video has an important relationship with television as well as with the movie industry in the past decade in two ways: from legal sales of cassettes or solid disks of movies, and the adverse factor, illegal pirating of copyrighted material or sale to the public, which hurts both producers and exhibitors and is rampant in many countries.

In the past year a new factor has appeared in Japan, about which little has been written though it may affect the movie industry beneficially or adversely. Marubeni, one of Japan's largest companies, has pledged to sell 100 one-man video theatres in the Tokyo metropolitan area and already has 15 operating near supermarkets or train stations, while the Tohokushinsha has opened two 99-seat video theatres on the 7th floor of a leading department store. The laser equipment usually comes from Sony as does the 4.4 by 1.8 meter screen, because both picture resolution and sound is enhanced in comparison to cassettes. The entire system cost comes to $60,000 with construction charges about the same for a 100-seat theatre employing one person who acts as cashier, operator and popcorn seller, plus daily janitorial service. Admission, varying on age and quallity of feature, runs $3.10 to $9.35. Some of the earlier video theatres used cassettes.

Jusco Co. reports monthly attendance at their 60-seat Chiba Video Theatre at 5,600 which shows that they are already a threat to nearby legitimate movie theatres. Cinematic Japan Co. already has more than 30 operating in the Tokyo area.

Since film attendance in Japan rose 3.1 per cent to 155,130,000 in 1985 despite the effect of VTRs added to households, there have been no diatribes by cinema importers, distributors, producers and exhibitors in the press complaining of lost revenues due to black market or legal cassettes or compact disks. The reason is that both attendance and overall revenues increased on the whole so complaints would sound incongruous.

While Japan has flooded the world with video exports, the public's use has been nowhere near the enthusiaism engendered in America, and to a lesser extent, Europe. The answer to this lies in the Japanese character and customs. It is true that increasing numbers of Japanese have been resorting to setting a timer to tape TV shows they are liable to miss and want to view later, and there are smaller numbers who tape the shows to send to family members working outside Japan and wish to keep up with what goes on in their homeland. In Japan's cities 31 per cent of households have VTRs, 1 per cent compact disks.

Going to the movies in Japan is either a habit or compulsion for youngsters and a "ceremony" for others and a chance to get out of the home. In general, the average Japanese would hesitate to pay out a goodly sum to purchase a cassette or solid disk for showing at home for his family, though admittedly the male members of the household might invest in soft porn. A Japanese home is not meant for entertaining outsiders so there is no question of inviting neighbors or friends to a veiwing. Entertaining is done outside the home and in no way consists of running a VTR for outsiders.

Of course, one cannot say with certainty that in the future these customs may not change and there may be a revolution in the use of VTRs or CDs such as took place in America or Europe. Thus, if there is blame to be handed out regarding competition with movies it still goes to TV.

What then will be done by the cinema industry, especially the exhibitors, if there is an explosive spread of video theatres in the future? Will they fight them or come to some sort of compromise, or even join them? Thus far there appears to be no opposition to them but that could change if box office profits fall and they begin to hurt the movie theatres or any other branch of the industry. Since they normally use imported features, producers and importers from abroad seem not worried.

Japan is foremost in the world in production and export of video tape recorders (VTRs) which now have a diffiusion rate in households in the world's major market countries reaching 30 per cent (compared to 40 per cent in Japan's urban areas and 31 per cent nationwide), a phenomena which took only 20 years since introduction of black-and-white in 1964 by Sony and development of a color model in 1966, followed by introduction of its Betamax in 1975 for home use, but since the end of 1985 VTR production in Japan is expected to show a lower rate of gain, partly because of the introduction of laser disks (CDs) now present in only 1 per cent of Japanese households.

Here again is the example of how the Japanese lifted the technological knowhow and research of foreign companies such as RCA and Zenith in America, and Philips of Holland, estimated at costing as much as a billion dollars, and developed them to the advantage of Japanese business in the case of the CDs. The history of VTRs shows the same trends.

What Philips and the Japanese companies are working on now includes an erasible disk, a further improvement—which may control the future.

In 1984 VTR exports increased 44.8 per cent to 22.07 million units, while domestic sales rose 16.8 per cent to 4.27 million units, of which sales to America jumped 119 per cent to 11.90 million units (53.9 per cent of exports), while sales to Europe which are controlled by quotas were 30.5 per cent of export totals declined 19.2 per cent to 3.75 million VTRs. In 1985 total VTR production was 27,124,000.

As for the cassettes themselves used inside VTRs, global demand at present is estimated at 385 million a year of which the US-Canadian market take 131 million, West Europe 108 million, Japan 80 million, and other countries 66 million.

Japanese companies are said to be producing some 1.75 million VTRs in West Europe, in addition to exporting there some 2.2 million under voluntary quotas. What is left in the market goes largely to Philips.

As for the compact disks (CDs) 1985 showed a 5.4 per cent increase in sales numbers to 4,133,000 but in value numbers the increase was only 3.3 per cent since newer models introduced sold at a lower price per unit.

When any discussion of VTRs is made, it is necessary to mention the battle between Sony's Betamax system and the rival VHS systems which are incompatible in that the cassettes are not interchangeable on the other equipment. That battle has resulted in defeat by Sony with only an estimated 12 per cent of the market with 88 per cent for VHS (Video Home System) developed by Victor of Japan.

Sony replied to this by introducing the 8mm single-unit video system, whose recording time is 120 minutes, which VTR makers are already copying. It was also Sony who, when the large American companies decided against putting CDs in production because of the huge capital outlay despite the fact that they had paid for research, went into CD production, along with, on a much smaller scale, Philips of Holland.

In 1970 Sony discovered that Philips of Holland, as well as RCA and Zenith, both American, had spent hundreds of millions of dollars on research and development of a laser diode disk to record, and spent four years unsuccessfully trying to develop a system. In 1978 Philips, after the American companies had written off videodisks as risky because of the expense, came to them with their technological data in order to prevent a second Betamax-VHS video tape problem by producing two incompatible systems competing.

This move was regarded by some as foolish since Sony then picked the ball up and carried it from there, in 1982 producing their first CD system with picture for $800. Other firms followed and now Japan has gone on to dominate not only the American market but also a lion's share of the world market to such an extent that the average person thinks it was Sony and not Philips who invented it. Sony still dominates the US market for CDs with Matsushita Electronics second. Philips has a good piece of the European market, and a very small bit of the Japanese market with Zenith dropping out before production, while RCA only produces some esoteric disk systems for the US government. A third American company MCA sold its factories to Pioneer Electronics of Japan. Apparently no other American companies are interested in trying to buck the Japanese who produced 245,000 CDs last year and expect to produce over 500,000 this year, practically for the North American market. Philips has a subsidiary, Marantz Japan, making CDs in Japan.

In Japan a CD system now costs about $600 (though reports state that they are sold as low as $300 overseas) and the sale of disks (close to 2,000 different titles) increased nine-fold to $212 million as coffee shops, bars and some 300 households purchased movies or other types of programs at prices ranging from $28.95 to $58.35 depending on how many sides (1,2, or 3) were needed for the complete show, since long features require a 2-sided disk and a single-side disk. It is not clear whether the so-called video theatres existing in Japan are allowed these cheap prices or must pay more, but probably the latter case is true.

There is also the question of pirating video tapes to be considered but so far in Japan the police have only taken action against piracy against Japanese companies and have done nothing about piracy of imported tapes which surely must be taking place, perhaps on a more inconspicuous basis.

The quasi-governmental NHK radio and TV network differs a bit from commercial surveys, stating that 37 per cent of Japan's 38.5 million households now have VTRs or CDs and diffusion in the Tokyo and Osaka regions is at a 40 per cent rate and in rural districts 31 per cent, terming it "the video revolution in Japan."

A. C. PINDER

PAKISTAN

Video has reached almost all well-to-do houses throughout the country. Young generation and cinemas are the hardest hit by video, because there is no censorship of video films, which are smuggled in from different countries in large quantity. Indian films have the biggest viewerships, as their import has been banned in Pakistan for the last 30 years. From the movie fans, hardly one per cent goes to cinema, the remaining 99 per cent watch video films.

The Government is making laws to regulate the Video Cassette Shops (VCS) in the country. Registration of these shops will be made obligatory. The existing copyright act will also be given sharper teeth to prevent the people from "indulging in illegal and immoral practices".

The Government has rejected proposals to ban video businesses to protect the national film industry. There are about 40,000 VCS in Pakistan. Each of these shops has at an average 10 VCRs or VCPs for renting out to viewers, who pay between Rs.50 and Rs.1000 a rent for 24 hours. Every VCS has between 500 and 1,000 video prints of Indian and foreign films. Almost same number (400,000) VCRs are owned privately. There is a license fee of Rs.200 for domestic use of VCR and Rs.400 for commercial use per year. Earlier custom used to charge 80 per cent duty on the import of VCR/VCP; it was reduced to flat Rs.3,000/–per VCR in the current budget.

Following the Government decision to extend legal cover to VCRs, investment interest for putting up facilities to assemble and manufacture of VCRs in the country seems to have picked up momentum. Philips Electrical Industries of Pakistan Ltd. have already been granted permission for assembly/manufacture of 25,000 VCR units per annum. Producers of Sony TV, Hitachi TV and National TV have sponsored projects to undertake assembly of 80,000 VCRs per annum in addition to the 25,000 units already sanctioned to Philips. As against this, the official estimates have placed the present demand for VCRs at 40,000 sets which is projected to increase to around 60,000 by 1988. The Industrial Investment Schedule for the sixth Plan has earmarked an investment of Rs.24 million for the establishment of new industrial plants for assembly and manufacture of VCRs.

For the last five years, illegal exhibition of latest Indian and foreign films (uncensored) on VCRs remained the biggest opposition to Pakistan cinema for a number of reasons, including high rate of cinema tickets (Rs.10 and Rs.10 for a balccony seat), strict censorship, poor maintenance of cinema houses, transportation problems, etc.; whereas video prints of latest Indian and foreign films are freely available for Rs.5 and Rs.10 for 24 hours. In thickly populated areas of cities like Karachi, Hyderabad, Lahore, Peshaware, Quetta etc., LEADS are supplied to houses on monthly subscription of Rs.100 or so for one picture a day and two on holidays. Elderly people prefer to enjoy Indian films produced between the 1950s and 1960s, as they are clean and can be seen with family members and pictures made in Pakistan (also clean). Films produced in India in 1970s and 1980s are (self) censored with remote controller by the heads of families, als they possess lots of vulgar and sexy scenes.

Pakistan also exports video prints of her feature films through the National Film Development Corporation to various countries where populations from Pakistan and India work. We earned a foreign exchange of Rs.3,279,475 through the export 169 video prints during 1983/84 and 1984/85.

We also sell popular TV plays in video to a number of countries.

A. R. SLOTE

SWITZERLAND

Statistics on Home Video: Number of home video cassette recorders in Switzerland: Every fifth Swiss Germann household owns by now a recorder; in the French part of Switzerland every fourth and in the Italian part every tenth household has one. By the end of 1986, almost every third Swiss household will have bought one. The yearly sales rate of recorders is ciphered by the wholesalers with 170,000 units. Almost 100 per cent of the recorders sold are the Japanese type Video Home System (VHS). The European device, Video 2000, a co-production of Philips and Grundig, has completely vanished, as well as Sony's Beta-System.

As per a poll effectuated in September 1985 by the national Radio- and Television Corporationn (SRG) by means of a so-called Telecontrol-Panel, the most passionate video cassette viewers are the habitants of the French part of Switzerland, followed by the Italian speaking Swiss and finally the Swiss Germans. Three quarters of the households provided with a recorder view preferably self-recorded cassettes; around 50 per cent prefer action and crime movies. Only the Swiss Italians use their video recorder in the order of 49 per cent for videogames. In the remaining regions video games are only scarcely used. Video cassettes loaned by video shops have, in Switzerland, yet a rather small market: 35 per cent of all in the German part, 44 per cent in the French speaking part and only 11 per cent in the Italian part of the country. Almost non-existent so far: the projection on home video recorders of films shot by the recorder-owners.

Governmental subsidy: January 1, 1986, the Federal Department of Culture, Federal Bureau of Cultural Promotion has decided to extend subsidies on Video productions, too, i.e. this authority will grant contributions not only for national film productions but also for VHS- and U-matic video films which have artistic qualities.

Government Departments: Bundesamt fuer Kulturpflege, Sektion Film, Thunstrasse 20, 3000 BERNE 6.

Associations: Schweizerischer Video-Verband, Schwarztorstrasse 7, P.O. Box 2485, 3001 BERNE.

GABRIELLA BROGGI

Companies

* NETWORKS
* SET MANUFACTURERS
* MAJOR PRODUCERS
* MAJOR GROUP STATION OWNERS

Companies

British Broadcasting Corporation

630 Fifth Avenue, New York, NY 10111; (212) 581-7100.
HEAD OF OPERATIONS, NORTH AMERICA
Peter Woon
TELEVISION PROGRAM PRODUCTION
Anne Watson
CHIEF ENGINEER
Ed Goldberg
NEW YORK CORRESPONDENTS
James Cox, Bob Friend
UNITED NATIONS OFFICE
United Nations Building, New York; (212) 688-6266
CORRESPONDENT
Robin Dilks
WASHINGTON OFFICE
CBS Bldg., 2030 M St., N.W., Washington, DC 20036; (202) 223-2050
CORRESPONDENTS
Martin Bell, Tim Sebastian-TV
David Macneil-Radio

Capital Cities/ABC, Inc.

1330 Ave. of the Americas, New York, NY 10019; (212) 887-7777; 41 Prospect Ave., Los Angeles, CA 90027; (213) 557-7777.
CHM. OF BOARD & CHIEF EXECUTIVE OFFICER
Thomas S. Murphy
PRESIDENT & CHIEF OPERATING OFFICER
Daniel B. Burke
EXECUTIVE VICE PRESIDENT
Joseph P. Dougherty
EXECUTIVE VICE PRESIDENT: CHAIRMAN &
CHIEF EXECUTIVE OFFICER, FAIRCHILD PUBLICATIONS
John B. Fairchild
EXECUTIVE VICE PRESIDENT;
PRESIDENT, ABC NETWORK DIVISION
John B. Sias
SENIOR VICE PRESIDENT; CHIEF FINANCIAL OFFICER
Ronald J. Doerfler
SENIOR VICE PRESIDENT;
PRESIDENT BROADCASTING DIVISION
Michael P. Mallardi
SENIOR VICE-PRESIDENT:
PRESIDENT PUBLISHING DIVISION
Philip J. Meek
SENIOR VICE PRESIDENT & GENERAL COUNSEL
Stephen A. Weiswasser
VICE PRESIDENT & CONTROLLER
Allan J. Edelson
VICE PRESIDENT
Andrew E. Jackson
SECRETARY
Gerald Dickler
TREASURER
David J. Vondrak
ASSISTANT CONTROLLER & ASSISTANT SECRETARY
David S. Loewith
ASSISTANT SECRETARY
Philip R. Farnsworth
ASSISTANT TREASURER
James M. Goldberg
BOARD OF DIRECTORS
Robert P. Bauman, Warren E. Buffett, Daniel B. Burke, Frank T. Cary, Gerald Dickler, Joseph P. Dougherty, John B. Fairchild, Leonard H. Goldenson, Allen Greenspan, Leon Hess, George P. Jenkins, Thomas M. Macioce, John H. Muller Jr., Thomas S. Murphy, Frederick S. Pierce, John B. Poole, John B. Sias, William I. Spencer, M. Cabell Woodward Jr.

FINANCIAL (ALL CAPITAL CITIES/ABC, INC.)

SENIOR VICE PRESIDENT AND CHIEF FINANCIAL OFFICER
Ronald J. Doerfler
VICE PRESIDENT, CORPORATE PLANNING
Ann Maynard Gray
VICE-PRESIDENT OF MANAGEMENT INFORMATION SYSTEMS
Edward D. Williams
TREASURER
David S. Vondrak
COMPTROLLER
Allan J. Edelson
ASSISTANT COMPTROLLERS
David S. Loewith, Allen Bomes
VICE PRESIDENT, CORPORATE INTERNAL AUDIT
Joseph H. Lock
VICE PRESIDENT, TAXES
Arnold Agree

ADMINISTRATION

VICE-PRESIDENT, ADMINISTRATION,
CAPITAL CITIES/ABC, INC.
Robert T. Goldman
DIRECTOR, CORPORATE SERVICES
Robert Sammon
VICE PRESIDENT OF REAL ESTATE AND CONSTRUCTION, ABC
Richard Hockman
VICE PRESIDENT, ADMINISTRATION, WEST COAST, ABC
Roger Lund
VICE PRESIDENT, HUMAN RESOURCES,
CAPITAL CITIES/ABC, INC.
John Frisoli
VICE PRESIDENT, PERSONNEL, CAPITAL CITIES/ABC, INC.
Anita Hecht
VICE PRESIDENT, LABOR RELATIONS,
CAPITAL CITIES/ABC, INC.
Richard L. Freund

OFFICE OF COMMUNICATION

PRESIDENT, OFFICE OF COMMUNICATION
James E. Duffy
VICE PRESIDENT, OFFICE OF COMMUNICATION
John E. (Jack) Harr

PUBLIC RELATIONS

VICE PRESIDENT, PUBLIC RELATIONS, ABC BROADCAST GROUP
Richard J. Connelly
VICE PRESIDENT, PLANNING AND VISUAL COMMUNICATION
Rick Giacalone
VICE PRESIDENT, PROGRAM INFORMATION
Tom Mackin
DIRECTOR, NEWS PUBLIC RELATIONS, ABC
Carol Olwert
DIRECTOR, NEWS INFORMATION, WASHINGTON
Joyce Kravitz
DIRECTOR, BUSINESS INFORMATION
Jeffrey R. Tolvin
DIRECTOR, VISUAL COMMUNICATION, EAST COAST
Peter Murray
DIRECTOR, VISUAL COMMUNICATION, WEST COAST
Hal Garb
DIRECTOR, COMMUNITY RELATIONS
Jane Paley
MANAGER, NEWSPAPER, PUBLICITY
Vic Ghidalia
MANAGER, ENTERTAINMENT PUBLICITY
David Horowitz
MANAGER, MAGAZINE PUBLICITY
Anne Marie Riccitelli
DIRECTOR, SPORTS INFORMATION
Irv Brodsky
MANAGER, BROADCAST PUBLICITY
Regina DiMartino
MANAGER, NEWS PUBLIC RELATIONS
Tom Goodman
MANAGER, COMMUNITY RELATIONS
Janice Gretemeyer
DIRECTOR, MOTION PICTURE PUBLIC RELATIONS
Bob Wright
DIRECTOR, SERIES PUBLIC RELATIONS
Carol S. Greenberg
MANAGER, PRESS RELATIONS, WEST COAST
Joe Maggio
MANAGER, BUSINESS INFORMATION, WEST COAST
Jim Brochu
DIRECTOR, SPECIAL PROJECTS, WEST COAST
Jerry Hellard
MANAGER, SPECIAL PROJECTS, WEST COAST
Michael D. Geller

LEGAL

SENIOR VICE PRESIDENT AND GENERAL COUNSEL, ABC, INC.
Stephen A. Weiswasser
VICE PRESIDENT AND ASSISTANT LEGAL COUNSEL
John T. Dealy
VICE PRESIDENT AND GENERAL ATTORNEY, ABC
Robert J. Kaufman

VICE PRESIDENT, AND GENERAL ATTORNEY, ABC-OWNED TV STATIONS AND ABC RADIO NETWORKS
Douglas Land
VICE PRESIDENT, GENERAL ATTORNEY AND DIRECTOR OF BUSINESS AFFAIRS, ABC NEWS
Samuel Antar

CORPORATE COMMUNICATIONS

VICE PRESIDENT, CORPORATE COMMUNICATIONS, ABC, INC.
Patricia J. Matson
VICE PRESIDENT, CORPORATE PROJECTS
Julie Hoover
DIRECTOR, VIDEO ENTERPRISES AND CORPORATE COMMUNICATIONS
Roann Rubin

EXECUTIVE AND RESEARCH

VICE PRESIDENT, MARKETING AND RESEARCH SERVICES
Marvin Mord
VICE PRESIDENT ENTERTAINMENT RESEARCH
Roy Rothstein
VICE PRESIDENT, AUDIENCE AND AFFILIATE RESEARCH
Paul Sonkin
VICE PRESIDENT, PRIMARY AND SOCIAL RESEARCH
Henry Schafer
VICE PRESIDENT, MARKET PLANNING AND TECHNOLOGY RESEARCH
Richard Montesano

ABC TELEVISION NETWORK

PRESIDENT
Mark Mandola

AFFILIATE RELATIONS

VICE PRESIDENT IN CHARGE OF AFFILIATE RELATIONS
George H. Newi
VICE PRESIDENT AND DIRECTOR OF AFFILIATE OPERATIONS
Buzz Mathesius
VICE PRESIDENT & DIRECTOR OF STATION RELATIONS
Bryce Rathbone
DIRECTOR PLANNING AND FINANCIAL ANALYSIS
Arnold Marfoglia

NETWORK SALES

EXECUTIVE VICE PRESIDENT IN CHARGE OF SALES
H. Weller (Jake) Keever
SENIOR VICE PRESIDENT AND GENERAL MANAGER, SALES
Robert I. Silberberg
SENIOR VICE PRESIDENT AND NATIONAL SALES MANAGER
John Tiedemann, Jr.
VICE PRESIDENT, MARKETING
Madeline Nagel
VICE PRESIDENT, DAYTIME SALES
Alfred A. Smith
VICE PRESIDENT, SPORTS SALES
J. Larre Barrett
VICE PRESIDENT AND DIRECTOR, SPORTS SALES
James Wasilko
VICE PRESIDENT, NEWS AND EARLY MORNING SALES
Lawrence Fried
VICE PRESIDENT, SALES ADMINISTRATION
Charles C. Allen
VICE PRESIDENT, SPECIAL PROGRAM SALES
Robert Cagliero
VICE PRESIDENT, REVENUE, PLANNING & SALES ADMINISTRATION
Robert T. Wallen
VICE PRESIDENT, TELEVISION NETWORK SALES DETROIT
Richard C. Wozniak
VICE PRESIDENT, TELEVISION NETWORK SALES, WESTERN DIVISION
William A. Harmond
VICE PRESIDENT, TELEVISION NETWORK SALES, CENTRAL DIVISION
Edward J. Wollock
VICE PRESIDENT, NEWS SALES, CENTRAL DIVISION, CHICAGO
William C. Gillogly
VICE PRESIDENT, REGIONAL SALES
Ed Ryan
VICE PRESIDENT AND DIRECTOR OF EASTERN SALES
Marvin Goldsmith
VICE PRESIDENT AND DIRECTOR, DAYTIME SALES
Fred Cohen
DIRECTOR, SALES SERVICE, NIGHTTIME
Harold Geary
VICE PRESIDENT, PRIME TIME SALE PROPOSALS
Elaine Chin
VICE PRESIDENT, EASTERN SALES MANAGER
George Cain
DIRECTOR, SALES SERVICE
Tom Mahoney
DIRECTOR, SPORTS MERCHANDISING AND PROMOTION
Al Cohen
DIRECTOR, SALES PROPOSALS AND DEVELOPMENT, CENTRAL DIVISION
John Saddler
VICE PRESIDENT, SALES MANAGER, CENTRAL DIVISION
Michael R. Rubin

ADVERTISING & PROMOTION

VICE PRESIDENT AFFILIATE MARKETING SERVICES
Paul W. (Pete) Barrett
VICE PRESIDENT, SALES DEVELOPMENT AND CREATIVE SERVICES
Chuck Gabelmann
DIRECTOR, ADVERTISING
Russell Roney
DIRECTOR, STATION ADVERTISING SERVICES
Alan Morris
DIRECTOR, GRAPHIC DESIGN, SALES DEVELOPMENT & CREATIVE SERVICES
Bill Dueuell
DIRECTOR, SALES DEVELOPMENT
Allen Hirschman

ABC SPORTS, INC.

PRESIDENT, SPORTS
Dennis Swanson
SENIOR VICE PRESIDENT OF SPORTS PLANNING & ADMINISTRATION
Stephen J. Solomon
VICE-PRESIDENT, PROGRAM PRODUCTION
Chuck Howard
VICE PRESIDENT, PROGRAM PLANNING
Charles Lavery
VICE PRESIDENT, PRODUCTION COORDINATION
Dennis Lewin
VICE PRESIDENT OF ADMINISTRATION AND FINANCIAL CONTROLS
Bob Apter
VICE PRESIDENT, OLYMPICS OPERATIONS
Marvin Bader

ABC TELEVISION SPOT SALES, INC.

PRESIDENT
John B. Watkins
VICE PRESIDENT
Philip J. Sweenie
DIRECTOR EASTERN SALES
Joseph Cohen
EASTERN SALES MANAGER
Mike Colleran
SALES MANAGER, MIDWEST
Scott Thomas
SALES MANAGER, SAN FRANCISCO
Franklin Lowe
SALES MANAGER, DETROIT
Ed Pearson
EASTERN SALES MANAGER
Mary Webb Ellis
SALES MANAGER, DALLAS
Mike Irvine
SALES MANAGER, ATLANTA
Deborah Shay
SALES MANAGER, LOS ANGELES
Michael Jack
DIRECTOR, RESEARCH SYSTEMS & SALES PLANNING
Christine McCoughey

CAPITAL CITIES/ABC OWNED TELEVISION STATIONS DIVISION

PRESIDENT—EAST
Dennis Swanson
PRESIDENT—WEST
Kenneth M. Johnson
VICE-PRESIDENT, RESEARCH AND PLANNING
Walter Stein
DIRECTOR, BUSINESS & FINANCIAL PLANNING
Vin Polley
DIRECTOR, MARKETING
Keith Ritter
PRESIDENT AND GENERAL MANAGER, WABC-TV
Bill Fyffe
PRESIDENT AND GENERAL MANAGER, WLS-TV
Joseph Ahern
PRESIDENT AND GENERAL MANAGER, KABC-TV
John Severing
PRESIDENT AND GENERAL MANAGER, KGO-TV
Len Spagnoletti

ABC VIDEO ENTERPRISES

PRESIDENT, ABC VIDEO ENTERPRISES
Herbert Granath
VICE PRESIDENT
John Healy

VICE PRESIDENT AND GENERAL MANAGER
Archie Purvis
VICE PRESIDENT, INTERNATIONAL DEVELOPMENT
Phil Boyer
VICE PRESIDENT
Bruce Maggin
VICE PRESIDENT, FINANCIAL CONTROLS & PLANNING
Jerry Sullivan
VICE PRESIDENT, GENERAL ATTORNEY & DIRECTOR OF BUSINESS AFFAIRS
Larry M. Loeb
DIRECTOR OF FINANCIAL PLANNING
Robert Wong
DIRECTOR, TELEVISION AND SALES, ABC PICTURES INTERNATIONAL, INC.
William Vitale
DIRECTOR, ABC MERCHANDISING, INC.
Carole Francesa

ABC ENTERTAINMENT

PRESIDENT
Brandon Stoddard
VICE PRESIDENT, WORLDWIDE PRODUCTION ABC THEATRICAL MOTION PICTURES
Stu Samuels
VICE PRESIDENT, WEST COAST PRODUCTION, ABC MOTION PICTURES, INC.
Joshua Donen
VICE PRESIDENT, MARKETING
Candace Farrell
VICE PRESIDENT, MOTION PICTURES FOR TELEVISION
Bruce J. Sallan
VICE PRESIDENT
Seymour Amlen
VICE PRESIDENT AND ASSISTANT TO THE PRESIDENT, ABC ENTERTAINMENT
Gus Lucas
VICE PRESIDENT, PROGRAM PLANNING AND SCHEDULING
Ted Harbert
EXECUTIVE PRODUCER AND DIRECTOR, FEATURE FILM CREATIVE POST PRODUCTION
Andre de Szekely
DIRECTORS, DRAMATIC SERIES DEVELOPMENT
C. Z. Wick, Mirielle Soria
DIRECTOR, COMEDY SERIES DEVELOPMENT
Stephen Kurzfeld
VICE PRESIDENT, NOVELS AND LIMITED SERIES FOR TELEVISION
Christy Welker
EXECUTIVE PRODUCER, NOVELS & LIMITED SERIES
Nina Rosenthal
EXECUTIVE PRODUCERS, MOTION PICTURES FOR TELEVISION
Susan Sands, Scott Spiegel
DIRECTOR, CURRENT COMEDY PROGRAMS
Ellen Franklin
DIRECTOR, CURRENT DRAMA PROGRAMS
John Barber
DIRECTOR, ARTIST RELATIONS
Dottie Gagliano
VICE PRESIDENT, AND SENIOR EXECUTIVE IN CHARGE OF SPECIALS
Gary L. Pudney
VICE PRESIDENT, CASTING
John Crosby
DIRECTOR, CASTING, WEST COAST
Donna Rosenstein
VICE PRESIDENT, CASTING, MOTION PICTURES
Ina Bernstein
VICE PRESIDENT, ADVERTISING
Dennis Fitch
VICE PRESIDENT, LONG RANGE PLANNING AND CHILDREN'S TELEVISION
Squire D. Rushnell
DIRECTOR, CHILDREN'S PROGRAMS, EAST COAST
Dolores Morris
DIRECTOR, CHILDREN'S PROGRAMS, WEST COAST
Jennie Trias
VICE PRESIDENT, PRIMETIME SERIES DEVELOPMENT
Ann Daniel
VICE PRESIDENT, COMEDY AND VARIETY SERIES DEVELOPMENT
Stuart Bloomberg
VICE PRESIDENT, SPECIAL PROGRAMS
John Hamlin
VICE PRESIDENT, EARLY MORNING PROGRAMS
Philip R. Beuth
VICE PRESIDENT, DAYTIME PROGRAMS
Jo Ann Emmerich
VICE PRESIDENT, DAYTIME PROGRAMS, EAST COAST
Mary Alice Dwyer-Dobbin
VICE PRESIDENT, ON-AIR PROMOTION
Roy Polevoy
VICE PRESIDENT, CREATIVE SERVICES
Stuart Brower
DIRECTOR, PLANNING & SCHEDULING, ON AIR PROMOTION, EAST COAST
Frank Cuciti
VICE PRESIDENT IN CHARGE OF PRODUCTION, ABC ENTERTAINMENT & ABC MOTION PICTURES, INC.
Herbert Jellinek
VICE PRESIDENT, BUSINESS AFFAIRS & CONTRACTS
Ronald B. Sunderland
VICE PRESIDENT, BUSINESS AFFAIRS, EAST COAST
Anthony Farinacci
VICE PRESIDENT, BUSINESS AFFAIRS, WEST COAST
Barry Gordon
VICE PRESIDENT, BUSINESS AFFAIRS, MOTION PICTURE FOR TELEVISION
Al Kaplan
DIRECTOR, DAYTIME PROGRAMS, EAST COAST
Randi LeWinter
VICE PRESIDENT, DAYTIME PROGRAMS, WEST COAST
Wally Weltman
DIRECTOR, EARLY MORNING PROGRAMMING
Amy Dorn Kopelan
DIRECTOR, PROGRAM ADMINISTRATION
Stephen K. Nenno
DIRECTOR, PROGRAM SERVICES
Judy Ahlborg
DIRECTOR, PROGRAM ADMINISTRATION, WEST COAST
Hank Miller
DIRECTOR, PROGRAM ADMINISTRATION, EAST COAST
Jack Sharkey
DIRECTOR, POST PRODUCTION
Al Ludington
DIRECTOR, DAYTIME CASTING
Mari Lyn Henry

ABC NEWS

PRESIDENT, ABC NEWS & SPORTS
Roone Arledge
SR. VICE PRESIDENT
Richard Wald
EXECUTIVE VICE PRESIDENT & ASSISTANT TO THE PRESIDENT
David Burke
V.P. & EXECUTIVE PRODUCER, SPECIAL BROADCASTS
Jeff Gralnick
VICE PRESIDENT OF ABC NEWS FOR PROGRAM DEVELOPMENT, EXECUTIVE PRODUCER, "20/20"
Av Westin
VICE PRESIDENT & WASHINGTON BUREAU CHIEF
George Watson
VICE PRESIDENT AND EXECUTIVE PRODUCER OF ABC's "WORLD NEWS TONIGHT"
William Lord
VICE PRESIDENT, NEWS PRACTICES
Robert Siegenthaler
VICE PRESIDENT, EXECUTIVE PRODUCER, DOCUMENTARIES
Pamela Hill
EXECUTIVE PRODUCER, "NIGHTLINE"
Richard Kaplan
EXECUTIVE PRODUCER, "WORLD NEWS THIS MORNING" & "GOOD MORNING, AMERICA" NEWS
Bob Roy
EXECUTIVE PRODUCER, "THIS WEEK WITH DAVID BRINKLEY" AND WEEKEND REPORTS
Dorrance Smith
VICE PRESIDENT, TELEVISION NEWS COVERAGE
Robert Murphy

BROADCAST OPERATIONS AND ENGINEERING

PRESIDENT
Julius Barnathan
VICE PRESIDENT AND GENERAL MANAGER, BROADCAST OPERATIONS EAST COAST
Philip J. Levens
V.P., BROADCAST ENGINEERING
Max Berry
DIRECTOR, TELEVISION NETWORK OPERATIONS, New York
Richard W. Stubbe
VICE PRESIDENT AND GENERAL MANAGER, BROADCAST OPERATIONS & ENGINEERING Los Angeles
Jack Neitlich
VICE PRESIDENT AND DIRECTOR, TV OPERATIONS, Washington
James Truelove
VICE PRESIDENT & DIRECTOR, INTERNATIONAL TECHNICAL PRODUCTION AND BROADCAST OPERATIONS, Paris
Jacques Lesgards
DIRECTOR NETWORKING SERVICES, New York
John Gilmore
MANAGER, ALLOCATIONS AND LICENSING
John Serafin
DIRECTOR OF PRODUCTION SERVICES, New York
J. Deet Jonker
DIRECTOR OF FILM SERVICES, New York
Edward Messina
DIRECTOR OF TELECOMMUNICATIONS, NEW YORK
William Hynes

DIRECTOR OF TV OPERATIONS, Los Angeles
Randy Hooper
DIRECTOR OF FILM SERVICES, Los Angeles
Robert Hudson
DIRECTOR OF PRODUCTION SERVICES, Los Angeles
David Loring
DIRECTOR, EQUIPMENT PLANNING
Michael Fisher
DIRECTOR, AUDIO/VIDEO SYSTEMS
Ben Greenberg
DIRECTOR, ALLOCATIONS AND R.F. SYSTEMS
Tony Uyttendaele

BROADCAST STANDARDS, QUALITY CONTROL

VICE PRESIDENT, POLICY AND STANDARDS, CAPITAL CITIES/ABC, INC.
Alfred R. Schneider

BROADCAST STANDARDS & PRACTICES

VICE PRESIDENT, EAST COAST
Alan Wurtzel
DIRECTOR, EAST COAST
Harvey C. Dzodin
VICE PRESIDENT, WEST COAST
Thomas Kersey

ABC INTERNATIONAL TELEVISION, INC.

PRESIDENT
Mark Mandala

CBS Inc.

51 W. 52nd St., New York, NY 10019; (212) 975-4321; 7800 Beverly Blvd., Los Angeles, CA 90036; (213) 852-2345.

BOARD OF DIRECTORS
William Paley, Roswell L. Gilpatric, Franklin A. Thomas, Henry B. Schacht, Marietta Tree, Newton N. Minow, Harold Brown, James R. Houghton, James D. Wolfensohn, Michel Bergerac, Walter Cronkite, Laurence A. Tisch.
ACTING CHIEF EXECUTIVE OFFICER
Laurence A. Tisch
CHAIRMAN
William Paley
PRESIDENT, CBS/BROADCAST GROUP
Gene F. Jankowski
EXECUTIVE VICE PRESIDENT, CBS BROADCAST GROUP
Thomas F. Leahy
EXECUTIVE VICE PRESIDENT, CBS BROADCAST GROUP
Neal H. Pilson
PRESIDENT, CBS ENTERTAINMENT
B. Donald Grant
PRESIDENT, CBS TELEVISION STATIONS
Neil E. Derrough
PRESIDENT, CBS RADIO
Robert L. Hosking
PRESIDENT, CBS SPORTS
Peter A. Lund
PRESIDENT, CBS NEWS
Van Gordon Sauter
PRESIDENT, CBS TELEVISION NETWORK
Anthony C. Malara

CBS ENTERTAINMENT (HOLLYWOOD)

PRESIDENT
B. Donald Grant
VICE PRESIDENT PROGRAMS
Kim LeMasters
VICE PRESIDENT, CBS ENTERTAINMENT PRODUCTIONS
Tony Barr
VICE PRESIDENT MOTION PICTURES FOR TV
Nancy Bein
VICE PRESIDENT FEATURE FILMS & LATE-NIGHT PROGRAMS
George Berntsen
VICE PRESIDENT DRAMATIC SPECIALS
Marian Brayton
VICE PRESIDENT DAYTIME, CHILDREN'S AND LATE NIGHT PROGRAMS
Michael S. Brockman
VICE PRESIDENT PRESS INFORMATION, HOLLYWOOD
Michael Buchanan
VICE PRESIDENT, PRINT ADVERTISING, WEST COAST
Casey Maxwell Clair
VICE PRESIDENT FINANCE
John J. Collins
VICE PRESIDENT MINISERIES
Peter Frankovich
VICE PRESIDENT ON-AIR PROMOTION
Jerold Goldberg
VICE PRESIDENT PROGRAM PLANNING & CURRENT PROGRAMS
Herbert Gross
VICE PRESIDENT TALENT & CASTING
Jean Guest
VICE PRESIDENT BUSINESS AFFAIRS, MUSIC OPERATIONS
Harry Heitzer
VICE PRESIDENT BUSINESS AFFAIRS, MOTION PICTURES FOR TV, MINISERIES
Richard J. Katz
VICE PRESIDENT BUSINESS AFFAIRS
William B. Klein
VICE PRESIDENT BUSINESS AFFAIRS, CONTRACT NEGOTIATIONS
Sid Lyons
VICE PRESIDENT BUSINESS AFFAIRS, ADMINISTRATION
James F. McGowan
VICE PRESIDENT MOTION PICTURES FOR TV, MINISERIES
Steve Mills
VICE PRESIDENT COMEDY PROGRAM DEVELOPMENT
Greg Maday
VICE PRESIDENT ADVERTISING & PROMOTION
Morton J. Pollack
VICE PRESIDENT PRODUCTION OPERATIONS
Norman S. Powell
VICE PRESIDENT CHILDREN'S PROGRAMS & DAYTIME SPECIALS
Judy Price
VICE PRESIDENT VARIETY AND INFORMATIONAL SPECIALS
Fred Rappoport
VICE PRESIDENT CURRENT PROGRAMS
Charles Schnebel
VICE PRESIDENT CBS MOTION PICTURES FOR TV
Robert Silberling
DIRECTOR PROGRAM ADMINISTRATION
Howard Adamson
DIRECTOR MOTION PICTURES FOR TV
Rick Berger
DIRECTOR PRIMETIME FEATURE FILMS
Joe Bowem
DIRECTOR VARIETY & INFORMATONAL SPECIALS
Jill Bowman
DIRECTOR TALENT & CASTING
Margie Glucksman Clark
DIRECTOR TALENT & CASTING
Lisa Freiberger
DIRECTOR DRAMATIC PROGRAM DEVELOPMENT
Maddy Desmoni-Horne
DIRECTOR DAYTIME PROGRAMMING
Barbara Hunter
DIRECTOR TALENT & CASTING
Rick Jacobs
DIRECTOR MOTION PICTURES FOR TV
John Kander II
DIRECTOR MOTION PICTURES FOR TV
Larry Strickman
DIRECTOR DRAMATIC SPECIALS
Lauren Joy Sand
DIRECTOR STORY DEPARTMENT
Ernie Loewy
DIRECTOR COMEDY PROGRAM DEVELOPMENT
Carole M. Kirschner
DIRECTOR CHILDREN'S PROGRAMMING, WEST COAST
Michael Chase Walker
DIRECTOR MINISERIES
Bill Wells

CBS/BROADCAST GROUP (HOLLYWOOD)

VICE PRESIDENT NATIONAL TV RESEARCH
Arnold Becker
VICE PRESIDENT PROGRAM PRACTICES
Carol A. Altieri
VICE PRESIDENT OPERATIONS, TELEVISION CITY
Charles Cappelman
VICE PRESIDENT & GENERAL MANAGER
Robert Norvet

CBS ENTERTAINMENT (NEW YORK)

VICE PRESIDENT, PROGRAMS, NEW YORK
ROseanne Leto
VICE PRESIDENT PRESS INFORMATION
Barrie Richardson
VICE PRESIDENT OPERATIONS & CREATIVE SERVICES, ADVERTISING & PROMOTION, EAST COAST
Herman Aronson
VICE PRESIDENT AFFILIATE ADVERTISING & PROMOTION
Bruce Weiner
DIRECTOR DAYTIME PROGRAMS, NEW YORK
Laurence A. Caso
DIRECTOR CHILDREN'S PROGRAMS, NEW YORK
Carolyn Ceslik
DIRECTOR TALENT & CASTING, NEW YORK
Holly Powell
DIRECTOR CASTING, NEW YORK
Laura Marino
DIRECTOR PROGRAM DEVELOPMENT, NEW YORK
Michael Marden
DIRECTOR SPECIAL PROJECTS, MOTION PICTURES FOR TV, MINISERIES
Elly Sidel

Children's Television Workshop

1 Lincoln Plaza, New York, NY; (212) 595-3456. (Educational Broadcasting.)

PRESIDENT
Joan Ganz Cooney
EXECUTIVE VICE PRESIDENT
David V. B. Britt
VICE PRESIDENT, GENERAL COUNSEL AND SECRETARY
Christopher W. Congalton
VICE PRESIDENT AND EXECUTIVE PRODUCER
David D. Connell
VICE PRESIDENT, FINANCE
Kenneth J. Gruver
VICE PRESIDENT, COMMUNITY EDUCATION SERVICES
Evelyn P. Davis
VICE PRESIDENT, SENIOR RESEARCH FELLOW
Edward L. Palmer
VICE PRESIDENT, CORPORATE COMMUNICATIONS
Ellen Rodman
VICE PRESIDENT, PRODUCTION
Alfred Hyslop
VICE PRESIDENT, CTW MAGAZINE GROUP
Nina B. Link
VICE PRESIDENT AND TREASURER
Wayne W. Luteran
VICE PRESIDENT, INTERACTIVE TECHNOLOGY & SCHOOL MATERIALS
Robert L. Madell
VICE PRESIDENT, RESEARCH
Keith W. Mielke
PRESIDENT, CTW PRODUCTS AND INTERNATIONAL TELEVISION GROUP
William F. Whaley

Columbia Pictures Television Group

Columbia Plaza, Burbank, CA 91505; (818) 954-6000.

PRESIDENT
Herman Rush

COLUMBIA PICTURES TELEVISION

SENIOR VICE PRESIDENT
Michael J. Grossman
SENIOR VICE PRESIDENT—FINANCE
William J. Kwasniewski

COLUMBIA PICTURES TELEVISION

Columbia Plaza, Burbank, CA 91505; (818) 954-6000.

PRESIDENT
Barbara Corday
SENIOR VICE PRESIDENT—CREATIVE AFFAIRS
Steven H. Berman
SENIOR VICE PRESIDENT & EXECUTIVE PRODUCTION MANAGER
Seymour M. Friedman
SENIOR VICE PRESIDENT—COMEDY DEVELOPMENT
Richard M. Heller
VICE PRESIDENT—MUSIC
Bodie Chandler
VICE PRESIDENT IN CHARGE OF BUSINESS AFFAIRS
Robert L. Chasin
VICE PRESIDENT—SPECIAL PROJECTS
Carole J. Coates-West
VICE PRESIDENT—ADVERTISING, PUBLICITY AND PROMOTION
Steve Astor
VICE PRESIDENT—LIVE AND TAPE PRODUCTION
Al Simon
VICE PRESIDENT—TALENT AND CASTING
Tim Flack
VICE PRESIDENT—BUSINESS AFFAIRS
Gary E. Fogel
VICE PRESIDENT—POST PRODUCTION
Christina J. Friedgen
VICE PRESIDENT—ADMINISTRATION
H. Lee Hetherington
VICE PRESIDENT—MOVIES AND MINISERIES
Andrew Hill
VICE PRESIDENT—DAYTIME AND FIRST-RUN SYNDICATION
Susan A. Simons
VICE PRESIDENT—FINANCIAL ADMINISTRATION AND CONTROLS
Thomas A. Tardio
VICE PRESIDENT—CURRENT PROGRAMS
Lance B. Taylor
DIRECTOR—OFF-NETWORK PROGRAMMING
Joseph Abrams
DIRECTOR—BUSINESS AFFAIRS
Lorna Ray Bitensky
DIRECTOR—ADVERTISING
June Burakoff-Smith
DIRECTOR—PRODUCTION COST CONTROL
Michael B. Browne
DIRECTOR—VIDEOTAPE OPERATIONS
Michael Clark
DIRECTOR—BUSINESS AFFAIRS
Myron Dubow
DIRECTOR—FINANCIAL PLANNING & ANALYSIS
Anthony D. Friscia
DIRECTOR—LOCATION DEPARTMENT
Louis Goldstein
DIRECTOR—BUDGET, AUDIT AND COST CONTROL
Robert Gros
DIRECTOR—COMEDY SERIES DEVELOPMENT
Bob Gumer
DIRECTOR—BUSINESS AFFAIRS
M. Robert Gumer
DIRECTOR—CONTRACT ADMINISTRATION
Mariann R. Harris
DIRECTOR—LIVE AND TAPE PRODUCTION
David C. Holman
DIRECTOR—DRAMATIC SERIES DEVELOPMENT
Ellen I. Levine
DIRECTOR—MOVIES AND MINISERIES
Laurie Levit
DIRECTOR—MUSIC LICENSING
Linda Kohn
DIRECTOR—TALENT AND CASTING
Jeff Oshen
DIRECTOR—TV ADMINISTRATION
Elizabeth Rockhill
DIRECTOR—CURRENT PROGRAMS
Mireille Soria
DIRECTOR—CASTING ADMINISTRATION
Shirley Trahd
DIRECTOR—PRODUCTION MANAGEMENT
Jonathan G. Zimmerman
ASSOCIATE DIRECTOR—BUSINESS AFFAIRS
Jacqueline Mosher
OPERATIONS MANAGER—BUSINESS AFFAIRS
Bonnie Wrobel

COLUMBIA PICTURES TELEVISION DOMESTIC DISTRIBUTION

15250 Ventura Blvd., Sherman Oaks, CA 91403; (213) 995-1300.

PRESIDENT
Bob King
VICE PRESIDENT—ADVERTISING, PROMOTION AND PUBLICITY
Stephen M. Astor
VICE PRESIDENT—RESEARCH, SYNDICATION AND NETWORK TV DISTRIBUTION
David Mumford
VICE PRESIDENT—MARKETING
Dick Woollen
DIRECTOR—SPECIAL MARKETING
William L. Clark
DIRECTOR—SPECIAL MARKETING
Thomas W. Holland
DIRECTOR—SALES, FIRST-RUN PROGRAMS
Lawrence J. Lynch
DIRECTOR—SALES & CONTRACT ADMINISTRATION
Valerie Rohrer
DIRECTOR—RESEARCH
Douglas M. Roth
DIRECTOR—SALES, SCREEN GEMS DIVISION
Donald J. Toye
MANAGER—AUDIENCE PROMOTION
Cynthia Lieberman
MANAGER—CONTRACT ADMINISTRATION
Ann Stewart
COORDINATOR—SYNDICATED SALES ADMINISTRATION
Vida A. Besel

DOMESTIC DISTRIBUTION REPRESENTATIVES

Atlanta Office: (404) 256-3007, 5730 Glenridge Drive, N.E., Atlanta, GA 30328.
VICE PRESIDENT—SOUTH, SOUTHEAST SALES
William Donald Bryan
SOUTHEAST SALES EXECUTIVE
Timothy R. Overmyer

Chicago Office: (312) 329-1650, 303 East Ohio St., Suite 2702, Chicago, IL 60611.
MIDWEST SALES EXECUTIVES
Noranne Frisby
Joseph V. Silha

Dallas Office: (214) 696-5211, 5949 Sherry Lane, Suite 1460, Dallas, TX 75225.
SOUTHWEST—SALES EXECUTIVE
Kenneth J. Doyle

Los Angeles Office: (818) 954-6000, Columbia Plaza North, Burbank, CA 91505.

VICE PRESIDENT—WESTERN SALES
RICHARD J. R. CAMPBELL
WESTERN SALES EXECUTIVE
Mitchell Sallitt
WESTERN SALES REPRESENTATIVE
Marlynda Salas

New York Office: (212) 702-6600, 711 Fifth Avenue, New York, NY 10022.
VICE PRESIDENT—EASTERN SALES
Herbert O. Weiss
EASTERN SALES EXECUTIVES
David Jacquemin
Stephen J. Mulderrig

COLUMBIA PICTURES INTERNATIONAL

711 Fifth Avenue, New York, N.Y. 10022; (212) 751-4400.

PRESIDENT
Patrick W. Williamson
EXECUTIVE VICE PRESIDENT
Brian McGrath

INTERNATIONAL OFFICES AND AGENTS

Argentina—Columbia Pictures of Argentina, Inc., LaValle 1878, Buenos Aires, Argentina, Manager

Australia—Columbia Pictures Television Pty., Ltd., 45 MacQuarie St., Sydney, 2000 Australia, Hugh Broun, Vice President and Managing Director

Brazil—Screen Gems Columbia Pictures of Brazil, Inc. Rua Santa Isabel 160-7° Andar 01221 Sao Paulo, Brazil, Helios Alvarez, Vice President and General Manager

Canada—Columbia Pictures Television Canada Limited, 365 Bloor Street East, Suite 1602, Toronto, Ontario M4W 3L4, John Migicovsky, General Manager

Egypt—14 Gawad Hosni Street, 4th Floor, Apt. 47, Cairo, A.R.E., Galal Rizk, Agent

France—Columbia Pictures Television, 20 Rue Troyon, 75017 Paris, France, Jacques Porteret, Director of French Sales

Germany—Columbia Television Vertriebsgesellschaft, M.B.H., Ickstattstrasse 1, 8000 Munich 5, West Germany, Max Kimental, Managing Director

Israel—Albert D. Matalon Co. Ltd., 15 Hess St., Tel Aviv, Israel 61043, Amnon Matalon, Agent

Italy—TV Overseas S.R.L., Via Sicilia N. 50, 00187, Rome, Italy, Jimmy Manca, Agent

Japan—Japan International Enterprises, Inc., 4th Floor, Yoneda Building, 17-20 Shimbashi 6-chome, Minato-Ku, Tokyo Pref., 105 Japan, Toru Ohnuki, General Manager

Mexico—Columbia Pictures Television International, Darwin 68, Office 301, Mexico City, Mexico 5, D. F., Alvaro Mutis, Sales Representative

Philippines—Columbia Pictures Television International, 3rd Floor, Room 307, Philippine, President Lines Bldg., 1000 United Nations Avenue, P.O. Box 3373, Manila, Philippines, Conrado Javier, Sales Representative

Kuwait—Rawafid Commercial Company, Maher Al Shawwa, Agent

Turkey—Mag Television Ankara Caddesi, 40-Kat2, P.O. Box 1126, Istanbul, Turkey, Osman Karaca, Agent

U.K. and Eire—Columbia Pictures Television, St. Margaret's House, 19/23 Wells Street, London WIP, 3 FP, England, Nicholas Bingham, Vice President, Tim Vignoles, VP TV Production and UK Sales

COLUMBIA PICTURES PAY—CABLE AND HOME ENTERTAINMENT GROUP

Columbia Plaza, Burbank, CA 91505; (213) 954-6000.

VICE PRESIDENT
Arthur Goldblatt
DIRECTOR—OPERATIONS
Richard B. Elliott
DIRECTOR—PLANNING
Robert T. Fleming
MANAGER—PLANNING
Joseph A. Rakauskas
MANAGER—PLANNING
Jim Tribbey

COLUMBIA PICTURES PAY TELEVISION & NON-THEATRICAL

Columbia Plaza, Burbank, CA 91505; (213) 954-6000.

VICE PRESIDENT AND GENERAL SALES MANAGER
Richard A. Rosen
NATIONAL SALES MANAGER—NON-THEATRICAL
Dennis Doph
MANAGER—CLIENT SERVICES AND NON-THEATRICAL
Patricia Lippell
MANAGER—PLANNING
Elaine R. Brewer

Corinthian Broadcasting Corporation

280 Park Avenue, New York, NY 10017; (212) 949-3900. (Group station owner)

PRESIDENT
James M. King
VICE PRESIDENT FINANCE & PLANNING
Harold A. Lewis
VICE PRESIDENT MARKETING SERVICES
Elissa Lebeck
VICE PRESIDENT ADMINISTRATION & HUMAN RESOURCES
Juli Wilhelm
VICE PRESIDENT, GENERAL COUNSEL
Lee C. Kitchin
VICE PRESIDENT PROGRAMMING
John J. Dorkin
VICE PRESIDENT ADVERTISING & PUBLIC RELATIONS
Michael Grant

Walt Disney Productions

500 S. Buena Vista Street, Burbank, CA 91521; (818) 840-1000. (Programming producer.)

CHAIRMAN OF THE BOARD AND CHIEF EXECUTIVE OFFICER
Michael D. Eisner
PRESIDENT AND CHIEF OPERATING OFFICER
Frank G. Wells
EXECUTIVE VICE PRESIDENT & CHIEF FINANCIAL OFFICER
Gary L. Wilson
VICE CHAIRMAN OF BOARD
Roy E. Disney
CHAIRMAN OF THE EXECUTIVE COMMITTEE
Raymond L. Watson

TELEVISION DIVISION

PRESIDENT—NETWORK TELEVISION
Gary Krisel
SENIOR VICE PRESIDENT—PRODUCTION/DISNEY SUNDAY MOVIE
Gary Barton
VICE PRESIDENT—NETWORK TELEVISION DEVELOPMENT
Grant Rosenberg
SENIOR VICE PRESIDENT—DOMESTIC TELEVISION DISTRIBUTION
Robert Jacquemin
SENIOR VICE PRESIDENT—MOTION PICTURE & TELEVISION PRODUCTION
Marty Katz
SENIOR VICE PRESIDENT—BUSINESS & LEGAL AFFAIRS
Bill Kerstetter
SENIOR VICE PRESIDENT—VIDEO
Bill Mechanic
VICE PRESIDENT—EASTERN OPERATIONS
Peter Afee
VICE PRESIDENT—TELEVISION PRODUCTION
Mitch Ackerman
VICE PRESIDENT—PROGRAMMING AND PRODUCTION
Jamie Bennett
VICE PRESIDENT—DEVELOPMENT/NETWORK TV
Joyce Brotman
VICE PRESIDENT—INTERNATIONAL VIDEO & PAY TV
Richard B. Cohen
VICE PRESIDENT—MARKETING/DOMESTIC TV
Jay Finkelman
VICE PRESIDENT—GENERAL SALES MANAGER/DOMESTIC TV
Richard Goldman
VICE PRESIDENT—POST PRODUCTION, MOTION PICTURES & TV
Don Hall
VICE PRESIDENTS—BUSINESS AFFAIRS/DOMESTIC TV
John Huncke, John Reagan
VICE PRESIDENT—MOTION PICTURE & TV PRODUCTION
Jane Rosenthal
VICE PRESIDENT—TELEVISION ANIMATION
Michael Webster

Eastman Kodak Company

343 State Street, Rochester, NY 14650; (716) 724-4000; 1901 W. 22nd St., Oakbrook, IL 60521; (312) 654-5300; 6706 Santa Monica Boulevard, Hollywood, CA 90038; (213) 464-6131; 1133 Ave. of the Americas, New York, NY 10036; (212) 930-8000; 6300 Cedar Springs Road, Dallas, TX 75235; (214) 351-3221 (Motion Picture and Audiovisual Products Division offices.)

CHAIRMAN OF THE BOARD & CHIEF EXECUTIVE OFFICER
Colby H. Chandler

PRESIDENT & EXECUTIVE OFFICER
Kay R. Whitmore
VICE CHAIRMAN & EXECUTIVE OFFICER
J. Phillip Samper
GROUP VICE PRESIDENT & GENERAL MANAGER, PHOTOGRAPHIC PRODUCTS GROUP
Wilbur J. Prezzano
VICE PRESIDENT & GENERAL MANAGER, MOTION PICTURE & AUDIOVISUAL PRODUCTS DIVISION
William A. Koch
GENERAL MANAGER, MARKETING, AND VICE PRESIDENT, MOTION PICTURE & AUDIOVISUAL PRODUCTS DIVISION
Leonard F. Coleman

Embassy Communications

1901 Avenue of the Stars, Los Angeles, CA 90067; (213) 553-3600. (A unit of The Coca-Cola Company)

CHAIRMAN AND CHIEF EXECUTIVE OFFICER
Gary Leiberthal
PRESIDENT
Glenn Padnick
EXECUTIVE VICE PRESIDENT, BUSINESS AFFAIRS
Kelly Smith
SENIOR VICE PRESIDENT, DOMESTIC SYNDICATION
Barry Thurston
SENIOR VICE PRESIDENT INTERNATIONAL SALES
Ron V. Brown
VICE PRESIDENT, MOTION PICTURE SALES AND ACQUISITIONS
Leslie Z. Tobin
VICE PRESIDENT, MARKETING
Michael Zucker
VICE PRESIDENT SYNDICATION, SOUTHERN REGION
Meade Camp

Fox Broadcasting Company

10201 W. Pico Blvd., Los Angeles CA 90035; (213) 277-2211; New York office: 40 W. 57 St., New York, NY 10019; (212) 977-5500.

CHAIRMAN AND CHIEF EXECUTIVE OFFICER, FOX, INC.
Barry Diller
PRESIDENT AND CHIEF OPERATING OFFICER
Jamie Kellner
SENIOR VICE PRESIDENT, MARKETING
David Johnson
VICE PRESIDENT, NETWORK MANAGEMENT
Scott Sassa
VICE PRESIDENT, FINANCE, FOX, INC.
J. Mark Hattendorf
SENIOR VICE PRESIDENT, PROGRAMMING
Garth Ancier
VICE PRESIDENT, PRIMETIME/LATE NIGHT PROGRAMMING
Kevin Wendle
DIRECTOR, LATE NIGHT PROGRAMMING
Paul Colichman
DIRECTOR, MOVIES-FOR-TELEVISION
Charles Hirschhorn
SENIOR VICE PRESIDENT, BUSINESS AFFAIRS
Jess Wittenberg
VICE PRESIDENT, RESEARCH
Andy Fessel
VICE PRESIDENT, ADVERTISING, PROMOTION & PUBLICITY
Dennis Fitch
PUBLICITY
Michael Binklow

NEW YORK OFFICE

VICE PRESIDENT, AFFILIATE RELATIONS
David Hilton
VICE PRESIDENT, EASTERN REGION
Greg Gush
VICE PRESIDENT, ADVERTISING SALES
John Lazarus
VICE PRESIDENT, EASTERN SALES
Pat Mastrandrea
DIRECTOR, EASTERN SALES
David Cassaro
DIRECTOR, RESEARCH
Al Cohen

International Creative Management, Inc.

40 West 57 St., New York, NY 10019; (212) 556-5600. 8899 Beverly Blvd., Los Angeles, CA 90048; (213) 550-4000. (Representatives of performing and creative talent in the entertainment industry.) A subsidiary of Josephson International Inc.

PRESIDENT
Jeff Berg

Lorimar-Telepictures Corp.

One Dag Hammarskjold Plaza, New York, NY 10022; (212) 686-9200; 3970 Overland Ave., Culver City, CA; (213) 859-3366.

CHAIRMAN AND CHIEF EXECUTIVE OFFICER
Merv Adelson
OFFICE OF THE PRESIDENT
Michael Garin, Dick Robertson, David E. Salzman, Michael Jay Solomon

Lorimar-Telepictures Television

PRESIDENT
David Salzman

Network Television Group

SENIOR VICE PRESIDENT, BUSINESS AFFAIRS
Irv Sepkowitz
VICE PRESIDENT, CREATIVE AFFAIRS
Joanne Brough
VICE PRESIDENT, PUBLICITY & ADVERTISING
Robert Crutchfield
VICE PRESIDENT, SERIES DEVELOPMENT
David Goldsmith
VICE PRESIDENT, BUSINESS AFFAIRS
Wilton Haff
VICE PRESIDENT, DAYTIME & CHILDREN'S PROGRAMMING
Lucy Johnson
VICE PRESIDENT, MOVIES & MINISERIES
Leslie Moonves
VICE PRESIDENT, NEW YORK STORY DEPARTMENT
Susan Pollock
VICE PRESIDENT, PRODUCTION
Robert Rosenbaum

First-Run Television Group

SENIOR VICE PRESIDENT, FIRST-RUN COMEDY DEVELOPMENT
Bob Jacobs
VICE PRESIDENT, PROGRAMMING
Jay Feldman
VICE PRESIDENT, PRODUCTION
Scott Stone

Domestic Distribution Group

PRESIDENT, OFF-NETWORK SYNDICATION
Pat Kenney
PRESIDENT, FIRST-RUN SYNDICATION
Jim McGillen
EXECUTIVE VICE PRESIDENT, PERENNIAL SYNDICATION
Scott Carlin
EXECUTIVE VICE PRESIDENT, MEDIA SALES
Karl Kuechenmeister
SENIOR VICE PRESIDENT, FIRST-RUN COMEDY MARKETING
Bob Jacobs
SENIOR VICE PRESIDENT, FIRST-RUN MIDWESTERN SALES
Mark Robbins
VICE PRESIDENT, PERENNIAL EASTERN SALES
Rob Barnett
VICE PRESIDENT, OFF-NETWORK NORTHEASTERN SALES
Tom Byrnes
VICE PRESIDENT, PAY CABLE & FEATURE FILM SYNDICATION
Dalton Danon
VICE PRESIDENT, MEDIA SALES
James Engleman
VICE PRESIDENT, DISTRIBUTION SERVICES
Roslyn Fisch
VICE PRESIDENT, OFF-NETWORK SOUTHWESTERN SALES
Bruce Genter
VICE PRESIDENT, NETWORK, OFF-NETWORK & THEATRICAL RESEARCH
Garry Hart
VICE PRESIDENT, FIRST-RUN MIDWESTERN SALES
Jeff Hufford
VICE PRESIDENT, FIRST-RUN EASTERN SALES
Jeannie Kadow
VICE PRESIDENT, MEDIA SALES
Peter Kranzler

VICE PRESIDENT, OFF-NETWORK SOUTHEASTERN SALES
Maury Lanken
VICE PRESIDENT, CREATIVE SERVICES
Jim Moloshok
VICE PRESIDENT, FIRST-RUN, PERENNIAL & SPORTS RESEARCH
Bruce Rosenblum
VICE PRESIDENT, SPORTS MEDIA SALES
Marc Solomon
VICE PRESIDENT, FIRST-RUN WESTERN SALES
Tom Straszewski
VICE PRESIDENT
Peter Temple
VICE PRESIDENT, FIRST RUN EASTERN SALES
Alicia Windroth

International Distribution Group

SENIOR VICE PRESIDENT, INTERNATIONAL SALES
Stuart Graber, Jeff Schlesinger
VICE PRESIDENT, INTERNATIONAL DISTRIBUTION SERVICES
Bonnie Adamson
VICE PRESIDENT, INTERNATIONAL DISTRIBUTION ADMINISTRATION
Rosemary Mazzo

MCA Television

(Distributor a subsidiary of MCA, Inc. as is Universal Television, the production arm. See listing.) 445 Park Ave., New York, NY 10022; (212) 759-7500. 100 Universal Plaza, Universal City, CA 91608; (818) 985-4321.

PRESIDENT, MCA TELEVISION GROUP
Al Rush
PRESIDENT, MCA TV
Don Menchel
EXECUTIVE VICE PRESIDENT, MCA-TV
Shelly Schwab
MCA TV CONSULTANT
Lou Friedland
SENIOR VICE-PRESIDENT, SALES MANAGER
Carl A. Russell
SENIOR VICE-PRESIDENT, MCA TV ENTERPRISES
Chuck Gerber
VICE PRESIDENT, MARKETING
Marc Grayson
VICE PRESIDENT, CREATIVE SERVICES
Mort Slakoff
VICE PRESIDENT, MANAGER OF RESEARCH
Bert Herbert
VICE PRESIDENT, MIDWEST AREA
Paul Hoffman
SALES EXECUTIVE, MIDWEST AREA
Steve Saltman
SALES EXECUTIVE, SOUTHEAST AREA
Jeff McElheney
VICE PRESIDENT, SOUTHWEST AREA
Tom Maples
SALES EXECUTIVE, WESTERN AREA
Bill Smith
VICE PRESIDENT, NORTHEAST AREA
Jim Kraus
VICE PRESIDENT, WESTERN AREA
Richard Nailling
SALES EXECUTIVE
Robert Raleigh
VICE PRESIDENT, ADVERTISER SALES
David Brenner
VICE PRESIDENT, STATION CLEARANCES
Bobbi Fisher
SALES EXECUTIVE
Stephanie Beatty
DIRECTOR, ADVERTISER SALES/EAST
Karen Volkman
SALES EXECUTIVE
Steve Rosenberg
VICE PRESIDENT, RESEARCH & SALES DEVELOPMENT
Don Micallef
RESEARCH MANAGER/BARTER DIVISION
Nadine Tekula
RESEARCH MANAGER/CASH DIVISION
Tom Russo
DIRECTOR OF OPERATIONS, CREATIVE SERVICES
Kate Kelleher
DIRECTOR OF PROMOTION & PUBLICITY
Gerri Pare
DIRECTOR OF SALES SERVICES
Steve Teamkin
ASSISTANT DIRECTOR OF OPERATIONS
Kathy Fenus
SALES EXECUTIVE
John Carson
SALES EXECUTIVE
Charlotte Sweet
VICE PRESIDENT, DIRECTOR OF LEGAL & BUSINESS AFFAIRS
Ernie Goodman
VICE PRESIDENT, TV DISTRIBUTION
Fran Toll
VICE PRESIDENT, MCA TV ENTERPRISES
Lin Oliver
VICE PRESIDENT, SYNDICATION SERVICES
David Darley
ASSISTANT GENERAL COUNSEL
Sara Rutenberg
MANAGER OF SALES ADMINISTRATION
Kathleen Sichler
DIRECTOR, ADVERTISER SALES/MIDWEST
Inger Jensen
BRANCH OFFICES:
Atlanta, Chicago, Dallas, New York, Universal City; Montreal, Canada; Toronto, Canada; London, England; Paris, France; Amsterdam, Netherlands; Tokyo, Japan; Sydney, Australia; São Paulo, Brazil; Beirut, Lebanon.

MGM/UA Communications Co.

450 Roxbury Dr., Beverly Hills, CA 90210; (213) 281-4000. Consists of the following companies: United Artists Pictures, Inc., Metro-Goldwyn-Mayer Pictures, Inc., MGM/UA Television, MGM-UA Distribution Co., MGM/UA Home Entertainment Group

BOARD OF DIRECTORS: Fred Benninger, Willie D. Davis, Cary Grant, Edward A. Horrigan, Jr., Kirk Kerkorian, Alasn Ladd, Jr., Arthur G. Linkletter, Lee Rich, Frank Rothman, Sidney Sapsowitz, Walter M. Sharp, Stephen D. Silbert, Anthony D. Thomopoulous, Kenneth L. Trefftzs

EXECUTIVE COMMITTEE: Fred Benninger, Kirk Kerkorian, Alan Ladd, Jr., Frank Rothman, Sidney H. Sapsowitz, Walter H. Sharp, Stephen D. Silbert, Anthony D. Thomopoulos

OFFICERS

CHAIRMAN OF THE BOARD AND CHIEF EXECUTIVE OFFICER
Lee Rich
CHAIRMAN OF THE EXECUTIVE COMMITTEE
Stephen D. Silbert
SENIOR EXECUTIVE VICE PRESIDENT
Sidney H. Sapsowitz
EXECUTIVE VICE PRESIDENT—FINANCE AND ADMINISTRATION
Burton J. Morrison
SENIOR VICE PRESIDENT—FINANCE AND CHIEF FINANCIAL OFFICER
Thomas P. Carson
SENIOR VICE PRESIDENT AND GENERAL COUNSEL—ENTERTAINMENT
Karla Davidson
SENIOR VICE PRESIDENT, CORPORATE GENERAL COUNSEL AND SECRETARY
William Allen Jones
VICE PRESIDENT AND CONTROLLER
Kathleen A. Coughlan
VICE PRESIDENT—ADMINISTRATION
Philip L. Cuppett
VICE PRESIDENT AND TREASURER
Walter C. Hoffer
VICE PRESIDENT—MANAGEMENT INFORMATION SERVICES
John Sanders
VICE PRESIDENT—CORPORATE LEGAL AFFAIRS
Sally Suchil
VICE PRESIDENT—TAXES
Daniel Taylor
VICE PRESIDENT—CORPORATE BUSINESS AFFAIRS
Thomas J. Taylor

MGM/UA TELEVISION PRODUCTIONS

BOARD OF DIRECTORS: Fred Benninger, David Gerber, Lee Rich, Frank Rothman, Sidney H. Sapsowitz, Wilater M. Sharp, Stephen D. Silbert

EXECUTIVE COMMITTEE: David Gerber, Lee Rich, Sidney H. Sapsowitz

OFFICERS

PRESIDENT
David Gerber
SENIOR VICE PRESIDENT—FINANCE
Thomas P. Carson
SENIOR VICE PRESIDENT AND GENERAL COUNSEL—ENTERTAINMENT
Karla Davidson
SENIOR VICE PRESIDENT, CORPORATE GENERAL COUNSEL AND SECRETARY
William A. Jones

SENIOR VICE PRESIDENT—BUSINESS AFFAIRS
Joel Katz
SENIOR VICE PRESIDENT IN CHARGE OF PRODUCTION AND PROGRAMMING
Lynn Loring
SENIOR VICE PRESIDENT—TELEVISION PRODUCTIONS
Christopher Seitz
VICE PRESIDENT—BUSINESS AFFAIRS
J. A. "TED" BAER
VICE PRESIDENT AND CONTROLLER
Kathleen A. Coughlan
VICE PRESIDENT—ADMINISTRATION
Leslie H. Frends
VICE PRESIDENT—TALENT
Mary Goldberg
VICE PRESIDENT IN CHARGE OF DEVELOPMENT
Peter Greenberg
VICE PRESIDENT AND TREASURER
Walter C. Hoffer
VICE PRESIDENT—BUSINESS AFFAIRS—TELEVISION PRODUCTION
Steve Knisely
VICE PRESIDENT—POST PRODUCTION
Bruce Pobjoy
VICE PRESIDENT—TAXES
Daniel Taylor
VICE PRESIDENT, PROGRAMMING
John Ruskin
VICE PRESIDENT, PROGRAMMING
Ronna Wallace
CONTROLLER
Joel Klinger

LICENSING DIVISION

VICE PRESIDENT, BUSINESS AFFAIRS
Judith A. Bresler
VICE PRESIDENT, FINANCIAL PLANNING AND ADMINISTRATION
Bradford R. Campbell
VICE PRESIDENT, LICENSING AND MERCHANDISE
William F. Dennis
VICE PRESIDENT, LICENSING
Lois Sloane
CONTROLLER
Sal Ilardi

MTM Enterprises, Inc.

4024 Radford Avenue, Studio City, CA; (213) 760-5000. (TV program production)

CHAIRMAN OF THE BOARD
Mary Tyler Moore
PRESIDENT
Arthur Price
EXECUTIVE VICE PRESIDENTS
Mel D. Blumenthal, Stuart Erwin, Jr.
VICE PRESIDENTS
Laurence Bloustein, Tom Palmieri, Geri Windsor, Ted Rich, Patricia Ahmann, James Goodman, Bernie Oseransky
DATE OF ORGANIZATION
1970

The Magnavox Consumer Electronics Company

1700 Magnavox Way, Fort Wayne, IN 46804; (219) 432-6511. (Set manufacturer)

PRESIDENT
Kenneth Meinken
SENIOR VICE PRESIDENT
K. C. Ingram
VICE PRESIDENT
John M. Fauth
VICE PRESIDENT
Donald L. Hamilton
VICE PRESIDENT
Samuel H. Newman
VICE PRESIDENT, SECRETARY & GENERAL COUNSEL
Samuel J. Rozel
VICE PRESIDENT
James T. Smith
VICE PRESIDENT
Arthur P. Stern
VICE PRESIDENT
Frank Van Steenberg, Sr.
VICE PRESIDENT & TREASURER
James M. Whelan
ASSISTANT SECRETARY
Jacob Kanter

Modern Talking Picture Service

General offices: 5000 Park St., North, St. Petersburg FL 33709; (813) 541-7571. (Distributor of free-loan sponsored films and video-cassettes.)

PRESIDENT
William M. Oard
VICE PRESIDENT & GENERAL MANAGER
Dan Kater
VICE PRESIDENT, OPERATIONS
James D. McPoland
DATE OF ORGANIZATION
1937

Divisions

Modern TV—Distributor of free-loan programs for television stations
Modern MPV—Distributor of programs and series for Cable Television Stations.
Modern Satellite Network—Distributor of programs and services for Cable Television Stations.

Regional Sales Offices:

New York: 45 Rockefeller Plaza, New York, NY 10111; (212) 765-3100.
Chicago: 2020 Prudential Plaza, Chicago, IL 60601; (312) 337-3252.
Washington, DC: 1901 L. Street, N.W. Washington, DC. 20036; (202) 293-1222.
San Francisco: 149 New Montgomery St., San Francisco, CA 94105; (415) 777-3995.
Canada: 143 Sparks Ave., Willowdale, Ontario, Canada M2H 2S5; (416) 498-7290.

National Booking Offices:

St. Petersburg, FL 33709: 5000 Park St., North; (800) 237-8913. Patrick Swonger, TV Manager.

National Broadcasting Co., Inc.

30 Rockefeller Plaza, New York, NY 10112; (212) 664-4444. Registered Telegraphic Address: NAT-BROCAST, NY; West Coast: 3000 West Alameda Blvd., Burbank, CA 91523; (818) 840-4444.

PRESIDENT AND CHIEF EXECUTIVE OFFICER
Robert Wright
VICE CHAIRMAN
Irwin Segelstein
PRESIDENT NBC ENTERPRISES
Jerome Wexler
GROUP EXECUTIVE VICE PRESIDENT
Raymond Timothy
GROUP EXECUTIVE VICE PRESIDENT
Robert Butler
PRESIDENT NBC ENTERTAINMENT
Brandon Tartikoff
PRESIDENT NBC TELEVISION NETWORK
Pierson Mapes
EXECUTIVE VICE PRESIDENT OPERATIONS AND TECHNICAL SERVICES
Michael Sherlock
GROUP EXECUTIVE VICE PRESIDENT
Robert Walsh
PRESIDENT NBC RADIO
Randall Bongarten
PRESIDENT NBC TELEVISION STATIONS
Albert Jerome
PRESIDENT NBC NEWS
Lawrence Grossman
PRESIDENT NBC SPORTS
Arthur Watson
EXECUTIVE VICE PRESIDENT & GENERAL COUNSEL
Corydon Dunham
EXECUTIVE VICE PRESIDENT PERSONNEL AND LABOR RELATIONS
Eugene McGuire
EXECUTIVE VICE PRESIDENT CORPORATE COMMUNICATIONS
M. S. Rukeyser
SENIOR VICE PRESIDENT BUSINESS AFFAIRS AND EXECUTIVE VICE PRESIDENT, NBC PRODUCTIONS
John Agoglia
VICE PRESIDENT CORPORATE PLANNING
Ellen Agress
VICE PRESIDENT RESEARCH
William Rubens

EXECUTIVE DIVISION

PRESIDENT AND CHIEF EXECUTIVE OFFICER
Robert Wright
GROUP EXECUTIVE VICE PRESIDENT
Raymond Timothy
GROUP EXECUTIVE VICE PRESIDENT
Robert Butler
GROUP EXECUTIVE VICE PRESIDENT
Robert Walsh

VICE CHAIRMAN
Irwin Segelstein

Corporate Planning

VICE PRESIDENT
Ellen Agress
VICE PRESIDENT, BUSINESS PLANNING
Barbara Watson

NBC Enterprises

PRESIDENT
Jerome Wexler
VICE PRESIDENT FINANCE & ADMINISTRATION
John Daly
VICE PRESIDENT INTERNATIONAL SALES
Miguel Perez-Colon
VICE PRESIDENT BUSINESS AFFAIRS
Susan Beckett

NBC Entertainment

PRESIDENT
Brandon Tartikoff
VICE PRESIDENT PROGRAM PRODUCTION
Perry Massey, Jr.
VICE PRESIDENT, MOTION PICTURES FOR TV
Anthony Masucci
VICE PRESIDENT MINI-SERIES AND NOVELS FOR TV
Susan Baerwald
VICE PRESIDENT, STORY DEPARTMENT
Patrick Betz
SENIOR VICE PRESIDENT EAST COAST, PROGRAM AND PROGRAM PLANNING
Lee Currlin
VICE PRESIDENT PROGRAMS EAST COAST
David Wedeck
VICE PRESIDENT, COMEDY DEVELOPMENT
Perry Simon
VICE PRESIDENT PROMOTIONS PROJECTS
Charles Stepner
VICE PRESIDENT ADVERTISING OPERATIONS AND ADMINISTRATION
Paul Wang
VICE PRESIDENT, ON-AIR PROMOTION
John Luma
VICE PRESIDENT, PRINT ADVERTISING
Jenesse Brewer
VICE PRESIDENT AFFILIATE/PROMOTION SERVICES
Martha Stanville
VICE PRESIDENT CHILDREN'S AND FAMILY PROGRAMS
Phyllis Vinson
VICE PRESIDENT SPECIALS AND VARIETY PROGRAMS
Richard Ludwin
VICE PRESIDENT DAYTIME PROGRAMS
Brian Frons
VICE PRESIDENT GAME PROGRAMS
Michael Tauber
VICE PRESIDENT FINANCE & ADMINISTRATION CONTROL, WEST COAST
Joseph Cicero
VICE PRESIDENT, CREATIVE AFFAIRS, NBC PRODUCTIONS
Ivan Fecan
VICE PRESIDENT FILM PRODUCTION
Charles Goldstein
VICE PRESIDENT DRAMA DEVELOPMENT
Michele Brustin
VICE PRESIDENT, ENTERTAINMENT PRODUCTION
Timothy Quealy
SENIOR VICE PRESIDENT, SERIES PROGRAM ENT.
Warren Littlefield
VICE PRESIDENT CURRENT DRAMATIC PROGRAMS
John Litvak
VICE PRESIDENT, FAMILY PROGRAMS
Winifred White
VICE PRESIDENT TALENT
Joel Thurm
VICE PRESIDENT, FILM PRODUCTION
Charles Goldstein
VICE PRESIDENT, PROGRAM PLANNING
Alan Sternfeld

NBC Network

GROUP EXECUTIVE VICE PRESIDENT
Raymond Timothy
PRESIDENT NBC-TV NETWORK
Pierson Mapes
VICE PRESIDENT FINANCE AND ADMINISTRATION
David Bivins
VICE PRESIDENT NETWORK POLICY AND PLANNING
George Hiltzik
SENIOR VICE PRESIDENT SALES
Robert Blackmore
VICE PRESIDENT PART PROGRAM SALES
Ron Dobson
VICE PRESIDENT NATIONAL SALES
Larry Hoffmer
VICE PRESIDENT SALES DEVELOPMENT AND MARKETING
Diane Seamans
VICE PRESIDENT EASTERN SALES
Richard Plastine
VICE PRESIDENT SALES DEVELOPMENT
Robert Conrad
VICE PRESIDENT AND GENERAL SALES MANAGER, EAST
Jon Nesvig
VICE PRESIDENT MARKETING
Robert Niles
VICE PRESIDENT, SPORTS SALES AND MARKETING
James Burnette
VICE PRESIDENT, OLYMPIC SALES AND MARKETING
Bert Zeldin
VICE PRESIDENT SALES ADMINISTRATION
Joseph Iaricci
VICE PRESIDENT, WEST COAST AND SPECIAL PROGRAMS SALES
Carl Meyer
VICE PRESIDENT PLANNING AND PRICING
William Caulfield
VICE PRESIDENT SPORTS SALES
Arthur Miller
VICE PRESIDENT CENTRAL AND NATIONAL FIELD SALES
Richard Schade
VICE PRESIDENT DETROIT SALES
John Spain Jr.
VICE PRESIDENT AFFILIATE RELAIONS
Anthony Cervini
VICE PRESIDENT SALES/AFFILIATE SERVICES
Richard Quaekenboss
VICE PRESIDENT AFFILIATE RELATIONS AND OPERATIONS
William Kelley
VICE PRESIDENT AFFILIATE SERVICES
James Ritter
VICE PRESIDENT PLANNING/AFFILIATE SERVICES
John Damiano

Legal

EXECUTIVE VICE PRESIDENT AND GENERAL COUNSEL
Corydon Dunham
VICE PRESIDENT, WASHINGTON D.C.
Robert Hynes
VICE PRESIDENT, GOVERNMENT RELATIONS
Sallie Forman
VICE PRESIDENT, GOVERNMENT RELATIONS
Terence Mahony
VICE PRESIDENT, WASHINGTON OPERATIONS
Tom Sawyer
VICE PRESIDENT, LAW, NEW YORK
Steve Stander
VICE PRESIDENT, LAW, WEST COAST
Don Zachary
VICE PRESIDENT, LAW, WASHINGTON
Howard Monder
VICE PRESIDENT, LAW BROADCAST ADMINISTRATION
Alan Gerson
VICE PRESIDENT, BROADCAST STANDARDS
Ralph Daniels
VICE PRESIDENT, PROGRAM INFORMATION RESOURCES
Bettye Hoffman
VICE PRESIDENT BROADCAST STANDARDS, WEST COAST
Maurice Goodman
VICE PRESIDENT, BROADCAST STANDARDS, EAST COAST
Richard Gitter
VICE PRESIDENT, COMPLAINCE & PRACTICES, WEST COAST
Meryl Marshall

News Division

PRESIDENT, NBC NEWS
Lawrence K. Grossman
EXECUTIVE VICE PRESIDENT
John J. Lane
VICE PRESIDENT AND ASSISTANT TO THE PRESIDENT
Timothy J. Russert
VICE PRESIDENT, NEWS
Joseph J. Angotti
VICE PRESIDENT, AFFILIATE NEWS SERVICES
Jo Moring
VICE PRESIDENT, FINANCE AND ADMIN.
Natalie Parks Hunter
VICE PRESIDENT, NEWS EUROPE
Edward Planer (London)
VICE PRESIDENT, NEWS, WASHINGTON
Robert McFarland
VICE PRESIDENT, RADIO NEWS
James Farley
VICE PRESIDENT, EDITORIAL PROJECTS
Gordon Manning
VICE PRESIDENT, EDITORIAL PRODUCTION SERVICES
Thomas Wolzien

Operations & Technical Services

EXECUTIVE VICE PRESIDENT
Michael Sherlock

VICE PRESIDENT, PRODUCTION OPERATIONS PLANNING
Robert Galvin
VICE PRESIDENT ENGINEERING
Steve Bonica
VICE PRESIDENT OPERATIONS AND TECHNICAL SERVICES, WEST COAST
Joseph Ulasewicz
VICE PRESIDENT MATERIALS AND SERVICES, WEST COAST
Fred Kigerl
VICE PRESIDENT BROADCAST OPERATIONS AND TECHNICAL SERVICES
John Frishette
VICE PRESIDENT PROGRAM PRODUCTION OPERATIONS
Maurice Corwin
VICE PRESIDENT, OPERATIONS SYSTEMS SOFTWARE
Eric Koopmann
VICE PRESIDENT SYSTEMS DEVELOPMENT
Rachele Lowenbraun
VICE PRESIDENT, OPERATIONS AND TECHNICAL MAINTENANCE
Crawford McGill
VICE PRESIDENT, PRODUCTION AND SERVICES
Leonard Lucas
VICE PRESIDENT, PRODUCTION OPERATIONS
Steven Seidenfrau
VICE PRESIDENT, MANAGEMENT INFORMATION SERVICES
Maurice Greenfield
VICE PRESIDENT, MANAGEMENT INFORMATION SERVICES, WEST COAST
Gerald Reeves
VICE PRESIDENT FINANCE AND ADMINISTRATION, WC.
John O'Neill, Jr.
VICE PRESIDENT MATERIALS AND SERVICES
Anthony Pedalino
VICE PRESIDENT BROADCAST OPERATIONS
Dave Baylor
VICE PRESIDENT FINANCE AND ADMINISTRATION
Arthur Dignam
VICE PRESIDENT, OPERATIONS AND ENGINEERING, OLYMPICS
Jack Weir

Personnel & Labor Relations

EXECUTIVE VICE PRESIDENT
Eugene McGuire
VICE PRESIDENT PERSONNEL
Richard Porrello
VICE PRESIDENT, PERSONNEL OPERATIONS
Nelson Rosabal
VICE PRESIDENT PERSONNEL ADMINISTRATION
Roberta Romberg
VICE PRESIDENT PERSONNEL AND LABOR RELATIONS, WEST COAST
Stanley Klubeck
VICE PRESIDENT LABOR RELATIONS
Day Krolik III
VICE PRESIDENT, LABOR RELATIONS, WEST COAST
Bernard Gehan
VICE PRESIDENT STAFF LABOR RELATIONS
John Rogers

Corporate Communications

EXECUTIVE VICE PRESIDENT
M. Rukeyser, Jr.
VICE PRESIDENT CORPORATE AND MEDIA RELATIONS
Elizabeth Hudson
VICE PRESIDENT CORPORATE INFORMATION, WEST COAST
Jay Rodriguez
VICE PRESIDENT, MEDIA OLYMPICS
Alan Baker
VICE PRESIDENT, MEDIA RELATIONS, EAST COAST
Curtis Block
VICE PRESIDENT, MEDIA RELATIONS, WEST COAST
Gene Walsh
VICE PRESIDENT, CORPORATE AFFAIRS
Robert Cornet
VICE PRESIDENT, CORPORATE AND MEDIA RELATIONS
Jay Michelis

Research

VICE PRESIDENT
William Rubens
VICE PRESIDENT NEWS & SOCIAL RESEARCH
Ron Milavsky
VICE PRESIDENT BROADCAST RESEARCH
Alfred Ordover
VICE PRESIDENT RADIO RESEARCH
Nicholas Schiavone
VICE PRESIDENT PROGRAM RESEARCH
Edward Frank
VICE PRESIDENT AUDIENCE RESEARCH
George Hooper
VICE PRESIDENT RESEARCH PROJECTS
Gerald Jaffe
VICE PRESIDENT TV STATIONS RESEARCH
Kathryn Lenard

Sports

PRESIDENT
Arthur A. Watson
EXECUTIVE VICE PRESIDENT
Kenneth Schanzer
EXECUTIVE VICE PRESIDENT, OLYMPICS
Mike Estridge
VICE PRESIDENT PROGRAM PLANNING AND DEVELOPMENT
Sean McManus
VICE PRESIDENT SPORTS NEGOTIATIONS
Bertram Zeldin
VICE PRESIDENT, SPORTS NEGOTIATIONS
Jeff Cokin
VICE PRESIDENT OPERATIONS
Kenneth Aagaard
VICE PRESIDENT FINANCE AND ADMINISTRATION
E. James Greiner
VICE PRESIDENT SPORTS PROJECTS PLANNING AND BUSINESS DEVELOPMENT
Jarobin Gilbert, Jr.

Television Business Affairs

SENIOR VICE PRESIDENT, NBC BUSINESS AFFAIRS
John Agoglia
VICE PRESIDENT, PROGRAM AND TALENT CONTRACTS
Jay Goldberg

Television Stations

GROUP EXECUTIVE VICE PRESIDENT
Robert Walsh
PRESIDENT, NBC TELEVISION STATIONS
Al Jerome
VICE PRESIDENT FINANCE AND ADMINISTRATION
Robert Finnerty
VICE PRESIDENT TV OPERATIONS AND ENGINEERING
Duffy Sasser II
VICE PRESIDENT AND GENERAL MANAGER WNBC-TV
Carl Carey
VICE PRESIDENT, TV STATIONS OPERATIONS AND ENGINEERING
Mark Mousky
VICE PRESIDENT, NEWS, TV STATIONS
Paul Beavers
VICE PRESIDENT, PROGRAMS
Wes Harris
VICE PRESIDENT, ADVERTISING AND PROMOTION
Ann Berk
VICE PRESIDENT, SALES
Bud Hirsch
VICE PRESIDENT, SPOT SALES
James Zafiros
VICE PRESIDENT AND GENERAL MANAGER, WMAQ-TV
Richard Lobo
VICE PRESIDENT AND GENERAL MANAGER, KNBC-TV
John Rohrbeck
VICE PRESIDENT AND GENERAL MANAGER, WKYC-TV
John Llewellyn
VICE PRESIDENT AND GENERAL MANAGER, WRC-TV
Fred DeMarco

Orion Home Entertainment Corporation

1875 Century Park East, Los Angeles, CA 90067; (213) 557-8700. 711 Fifth Ave., New York, NY 10022; (212) 758-5100; 9 West 57 St., New York, NY 10019; (212) 980-1117.

CHAIRMAN OF THE BOARD, CHIEF EXECUTIVE OFFICER
Lawrence B. Hilford
EXECUTIVE VICE PRESIDENT
William Bernstein
SENIOR VICE PRESIDENT, GENERAL COUNSEL AND SECRETARY
Leonard B. Pack
SENIOR VICE PRESIDENT FOR BUSINESS AFFAIRS
Robert A. Mirisch
SENIOR VICE PRESIDENT, CHIEF FINANCIAL OFFICER & TREASURER
Melvin F. Woods
VICE PRESIDENT FOR BUSINESS AFFAIRS
Kimberle Aronzon
VICE PRESIDENT, CHIEF ACCOUNTING OFFICER
Joel Grossman
ASSISTANT SECRETARY
John W. Hester
ASSISTANT TREASURER
Richards T. Matthews

ORION TELEVISION SYNDICATION

1875 Century Park East, Los Angeles, Ca. 90067; (213) 557-8700
PRESIDENT
J. Scott Towle
SENIOR VICE PRESIDENT—SALES AND MARKETING
Larry Hutchings

VICE PRESIDENT—SOUTHERN DIVISION
James Ricks, Jr.
VICE PRESIDENT—WESTERN DIVISION
Rick Jacobson
VICE PRESIDENT—CENTRAL DIVISION
Donald Frehe
VICE PRESIDENT—EASTERN DIVISION
Thomas Cerio
VICE PRESIDENT OF ADVERTISING & PROMOTION
Robert Oswaks

ORION TELEVISION, INC.

CHAIRM OF THE BOARD
Eric Pleskow
PRESIDENT
Richard M. Rosenbloom
EXECUTIVE VICE PRESIDENT
William Bernstein
SENIOR VICE PRESIDENT
J. Fred Whitehead
VICE PRESIDENT, DEVELOPMENT
Gary A. Randall
VICE PRESIDENT
Robert A. Mirisch
VICE PRESIDENT & TREASURER
Melvin F. Woods
VICE PRESIDENT, BUSINESS AFFAIRS
Edward A. Hoffman
VICE PRESIDENT, CURRENT PROGRAMS
Ann Stitch
SECRETARY
Leonard B. Pack
ASSISTANT TREASURER
Richards T. Matthews

Paramount Television Group

(A Division of Paramount Pictures Corporation) 5555 Melrose, Hollywood, CA 90038; (213) 468-5000. One Gulf & Western Plaza, New York, NY 10023; (212) 333-7600.

TELEVISION GROUP

PRESIDENT
Melvin Harris
VICE PRESIDENT FINANCE
Robert Sheehan

NETWORK TV PRODUCTION & VIDEO DISTRIBUTION

EXECUTIVE VICE PRESIDENT VIDEO DISTRIBUTION
Robert Klingensmith
EXECUTIVE VICE PRESIDENT NETWORK TV PRODUCTION
John Pike
SENIOR VICE PRESIDENT BUSINESS AFFAIRS
Cecelia Andrews
SENIOR VICE PRESIDENT & GENERAL MANAGER HOME VIDEO
Timothy Clott
SENIOR VICE PRESIDENT CREATIVE AFFAIRS
Jeffrey Hayes
VICE PRESIDENT LEGAL AFFAIRS
Howard Barton
VICE PRESIDENT BUSINESS/LEGAL AFFAIRS
Dan Black
VICE PRESIDENT ADVERTISING & SALES PROMOTION
Hollace Brown
VICE PRESIDENT VIDEO DISTRIBUTION
Alan Cole-Ford
VICE PRESIDENT SALES & MARKETING
Eric Doctorow
VICE PRESIDENT FINANCE
Gerald Goldman
VICE PRESIDENT PRODUCTION
Michael Schoenbrun
VICE PRESIDENT, BUSINESS AFFAIRS
Shirley Stahdnke
VICE PRESIDENT, CURRENT PROGRAMMING
John Symes
VICE PRESIDENT, LONG FORM & SPECIAL PROJECTS
Richard Berman
VICE PRESIDENT, SERIES DEVELOPMENT
Paul Heller

DOMESTIC TV & VIDEO PROGRAMMING

PRESIDENT
Lucille Salhany
EXECUTIVE VICE PRESIDENT, SALES & MARKETING
Steve Goldman
SENIOR VICE PRESIDENT & GENERAL SALES MANAGER
Robert Meidel
SENIOR VICE PRESIDENT PROGRAMMING
Frank Kelly
VICE PRESIDENT NETWORK DAYTIME TV & SPECIAL PROJECTS
Thomas Daniels
VICE PRESIDENT, ADVERTISING & PROMOTION
Meryl Cohen
VICE PRESIDENT ADVERTISER PROGRAM SALES
Robert Dahill
VICE PRESIDENT WESTERN DIVISION SALES
Jim Martz
VICE PRESIDENT EASTERN REGIONAL SALES MANAGER & FEATURES PLANNING
Joel Berman
VICE PRESIDENT CENTRAL REGIONAL MANAGER
Richard Montgomery
VICE PRESIDENT, BUSINESS AFFAIRS/LEGAL
Vance Van Petten
VICE PRESIDENT, ADMINISTRATION-SALES/CONTRACTS
Howard Green

PARAMOUNT TELEVISION INTERNATIONAL DISTRIBUTION (NY)

PRESIDENT
Bruce Gordon
VICE PRESIDENT, OPERATIONS
Joseph Lucas

INTERNATIONAL SALES OFFICES

ENGLAND: Paramount TV Ltd., 23 Berkeley House, Hay Hill, London, W1X 8JB, England.
VICE PRESIDENT, EUROPEAN SALES
Peter Cary
AUSTRALIA: Paramount Pictures Pty., Ltd., Suite 3209, Australia Square, Box 4272 GPO, Sydney, 2001, N.S.W. Australia.
VICE PRESIDENT, FAR EAST SALES
George Mooratoff
CANADA: Paramount Pictures Corp. Ltd., 146 Bloor Street W., Toronto, Ontario M5S 1M4, Canada.
VICE PRESIDENT, TV SALES, CANADA
Malcolm Orme
LOS ANGELES:
VICE PRESIDENT, LATIN AMERICA
Ramon Perez

Public Broadcasting Service

Headquarters: 1320 Braddock Place, Alexandria, VA 22314; (703) 739-5000; New York Office: 609 Fifth Ave., New York, NY 10017; (212) 753-7373; Los Angeles office: 4401 Sunset Blvd., Suite 335, Los Angeles, CA 90027; (213) 667-9289. (A private non-profit corporation providing national programming, distribution, and related services for public TV stations.)

CHAIRMAN
Alfred R. Stern
PRESIDENT
Bruce L. Christensen
SENIOR VICE PRESIDENT, PROGRAM SUPPORT & DEVELOPMENT
M. Peter Downey
SENIOR VICE PRESIDENT, BROADCAST OPERATIONS & ENGINEERING
Richard R. Green
SENIOR VICE PRESIDENT, CORPORATE SECRETARY
Michael E. Hobbs
SENIOR VICE PRESIDENT, EDUCATION SERVICES
William T. Reed
SENIOR VICE PRESIDENT, PROGRAMMING
Suzanne S. Weil
VICE PRESIDENT, ADVERTISING AND PROMOTION
Daniel C. Agan
VICE PRESIDENT, ADULT LEARNING
Dee F. S. Brock
VICE PRESIDENT, NEWS & PUBLIC AFFAIRS
Barry O. Chase
SENIOR VICE PRESIDENT, CHIEF FINANCIAL OFFICER
Amy S. Fleishman
VICE PRESIDENT, PROGRAM ADMINISTRATION & INFORMATION
Lance W. Ozier
SENIOR VICE PRESIDENT, ADMINISTRATION & COMPUTER SERVICES
Eric L. Sass
VICE PRESIDENT, DEVELOPMENT
Michael B. Soper

RCA Consumer Electronics Division

Box 1976, Indianapolis, IN 46206; (317) 267-5000. (Set manufacturer.)

GROUP VICE PRESIDENT
Jack K. Sauter

DIVISION VICE PRESIDENT OPERATIONS
D. Joseph Donahue
DIVISION VICE PRESIDENT MARKETING
S. S. Stepnes
DIVISION VICE PRESIDENT PUBLIC AFFAIRS
F. V. McCann

RKO General, Inc.

1440 Broadway, New York, NY 10018; (212) 764-7000. (Group station owner)

CHAIRMAN OF THE BOARD
Thomas F. O'Neil
VICE CHAIRMAN AND CHIEF OPERATING OFFICER
Hubert J. DeLynn
PRESIDENT
Frank Shakespeare
RADIO DIVISION—PRESIDENT
Robert J. Williamson
TELEVISION DIVISION—PRESIDENT
Pat A. Servodidio

Republic Pictures Corporation

12636 Beatrice Street, P.O. Box 66930, Los Angeles, CA 90066-0930; (213) 306-4040; Telex/Twx: 910-343-7417.

CHAIRMAN OF THE BOARD
George C. Hatch
PRESIDENT
Aubrey "Bud" Groskopf
VICE PRESIDENT, NATIONAL SALES MANAGER
Dick Jolliffe
VICE PRESIDENT, INTERNATIONAL SALES
Joe Levinsohn
SENIOR VICE PRESIDENT, HOME VIDEO
Nick Draklich
MANAGER, SPECIAL MARKETING
Barry Bernard
NORTHEASTERN SALES MANAGER
Terez Kiely
MIDWEST SALES MANAGER
Hugh West
SOUTHEAST SALES MANAGER
Lisa Ann Woodcock
SOUTHWEST SALES MANAGER
Diana Foster

CANADA—Kaleidoscope Entertainment, Inc./Randy Zalken, pres., 101 Duncan Mill Road, Suite 102, Don Mills, Ontario, M3B 1Z3.

UNITED KINGDOM & SELECTED PORTIONS OF WESTERN EUROPE—TV Programmes International, Ltd./Bernard Shaw, sales repr., 21 Cherry Garden Lane, Folkestone, Kent, England. Telephone: 303-76897, Telex: 966560 SHAW TV.

GREECE AND BALKANS—46 King Constantine Avenue/Panos Spyropoulos, sales repr., Athens, 516 Greece. Telephone: 7224-243/7234-896; Telex: 221880 APOL GR.

TURKEY—Umut Sanat Urunleri/Seher Karabol, sales repr., Istiklal Caddesi Lale Han No. 87/6, Beyoglu, Istanbul, Turkey. Telephone: 149-77-35/143-44-39, Telex: 23359 BOTX TR.

AUSTRIA—Post Box 192, Postamt 1140, Vienna, Austria, Mounir J. Chammas, sales rep.

Sony Corp. of America

One Sony Drive, Park Ridge, NJ 07656; (201) 930-1000. (Set manufacturer)

PRESIDENT, SONY CORP. OF AMERICA
Neil Vander Dussen
PRESIDENT, SONY COMMUNICATIONS PRODUCTS CO.
J. Phillip Stack
PRESIDENT, SONY TAPE SALES CO.
John Hollands
PRESIDENT, SONY BROADCAST PRODUCTS CO.
William Connolly

Spanish International Network (SIN)

460 West 42 St., New York, NY 10036; (212) 502-1300. (Producers of Spanish-language programming for television; has 241 satellite interconnected TV affiliates and 6 non-connected TV affiliates)

PRESIDENT
Rene Anselmo
EXECUTIVE VICE PRESIDENT
William Stiles
VICE PRESIDENT/NATIONAL SALES MANAGER
John Pero
VICE PRESIDENT/SALES DEVELOPMENT
Robert Hitchens
DIRECTOR OF PROGRAMMING
Rosita Peru
DIRECTOR OF PROGRAMMING DEVELOPMENT
Luis de Llano

Storer Communications, Inc.

12000 Biscayne Blvd., P.O. Box 61-8000, Miami, FL 33181-2710; (305) 899-1000. (Group station owner.)

CHAIRMAN, PRESIDENT AND CHIEF EXECUTIVE OFFICER
Terry Lee
PRESIDENT, TELEVISION STATIONS DIVISION
Joseph C. Dimino
PRESIDENT, CABLE DIVISION
Kenneth Bagwell
VICE PRESIDENT, TREASURER AND CHIEF FINANCIAL OFFICER
Kenneth R. Mosher
VICE PRESIDENT, COUNSEL AND SECRETARY
Abiah A. Church
VICE PRESIDENTS
Bill Flynn, Paul Raymon, H. W. Ray, Warren Zwicky, James Long, Andy Potos, Henry Davis, Daniel Berkery, Walter L. Threadgill, Kenneth Danielson, Loraine H. Strait, James Hall, C. David Whitaker, Elaine Stout, Bill Fox.

Taft Broadcasting Co.

1718 Young St., Cincinnati, OH 45210; (513) 721-1414. (Group stations owner)

CHAIRMAN OF THE BOARD
Charles S. Mechem, Jr.
VICE CHAIRMAN
Dudley S. Taft
EXECUTIVE VICE PRESIDENT AND CHIEF OPERATING OFFICER
Geroge E. Castrucci
EXECUTIVE VICE PRESIDENT, TV GROUP
Jack Sander
VICE PRESIDENT, BUSINESS AFFAIRS
Terry Schroeder
VICE PRESIDENT, TELEVISION PROGRAMMING
Gregory Miller

Taft Entertainment Company, The

10960 Wilshire Blvd., 10th floor, Los Angeles, CA 90024; (213) 208-2000.

PRESIDENT & CHIEF EXECUTIVE OFFICER
Sy Fischer
EXECUTIVE VICE PRESIDENT
Karl Honeystein
SENIOR VICE PRESIDENT, CREATIVE
Joel Cohen

DIVISIONS INCLUDE:

Cine Guarantors, 10960 Wilshire Blvd., 10th floor, Los Angeles, CA 90024; (213) 208-2000.

Hanna-Barbera Productions, Inc., 3400 Cahuenga Blvd., Hollywood, CA 90068; (213) 851-5000.

Ruby-Spears Enterprises, 3459 Cahuenga Blvd., Hollywood, CA 90068; (213) 874-5100.

The Sy Fisher Company, Inc., 10960 Wilshire Blvd., Los Angeles, CA 90024; (213) 208-0455.

Taft Entertainment Motion Pictures/Keith Barish Prods., 1800 Century Park East, Los Angeles, CA 90067; (213) 551-1911.

Taft Entertainment Television Production, 14144 Ventura Blvd., Sherman Oaks, CA 91422; (818) 905-6644.

Taft Merchandising Group, 415 Madison Ave., New York, NY 10017; (212) 751-1057.

Titus Productions, 211 East 51 St., New York, NY 10022; (212) 752-6460.

Twentieth Century Fox Television, Inc.

P.O. Box 900, Los Angeles, CA 90213; (213) 277-2211. A division of Twentieth Century-Fox Film Corp.

PRESIDENT, TELEVISION
Harris Katleman
EXECUTIVE VICE PRESIDENT, CREATIVE AFFAIRS
Peter Grad
EXECUTIVE VICE PRESIDENT, DOMESTIC SYNDICATION
Michael J. Lambert
SENIOR VICE PRESIDENT, BUSINESS AFFAIRS
David Freedman

SENIOR VICE PRESIDENT, PRODUCTION MANAGEMENT
Mark Evans
VICE PRESIDENT, SERIES DEVELOPMENT
Dayna Kalins
VICE PRESIDENT, PROGRAM DEVELOPMENT
Michael D. Klein
VICE PRESIDENT, STUDIO BUSINESS AFFAIRS
Lee Zuckerman
VICE PRESIDENT, TV POST PRODUCTION
Skip Lusk
SR. VICE PRESIDENT, DOMESTIC SYNDICATION
Joe Greene
VICE PRESIDENT, CREATIVE SERVICES
Jerry Greenberg
VICE PRESIDENT, TELEVISION LEGAL AFFAIRS
Walter Swanson
VICE PRESIDENT, NATIONAL SALES—EAST
Harry Mulford
DIRECTOR OF BUSINESS AND SALES ADMINISTRATION SYNDICATION
Stanley DeCovnick
DIRECTOR OF SALES ADMINISTRATION
Harold Potter
TV BUDGET & COST ADMINISTRATOR
Ed Lahti
DIRECTOR OF OPERATIONS, INTERNATIONAL
Edwin Greenberg
DIRECTOR OF SERVICING, INTERNATIONAL
Lourdes Chaves
DIRECTOR OF PRODUCTION, DAYTIME & SYNDICATED TV
Bob Braithwaite
VICE PRESIDENT, BUSINESS AFFAIRS
Alan Duke
WESTERN DIVISION SALES MANAGER
Tony Bauer

BRANCH OFFICES

- NEW YORK OFFICE: 40 West 57th Street, New York, New York 10019 (212) 977-5500; Joseph Greene, Vice President, Domestic Syndication; James Puffer, Northeastern Division Sales Manager; Harry Mulford, Vice President, National Sales.
- CHICAGO OFFICE: 35 East Wacker Drive, Suite 1234, Chicago, Illinois 60601 (312) 372-1589; Dennis Juravic, Central Division Vice President.
- DALLAS OFFICE: 11551 Forest Central Drive, Suite 300, Dallas, Texas 75243 (214) 343-9252; Al Shore, Southwestern Division Vice President.
- ATLANTA OFFICE: 2200 Century Parkway, Suite 560, Atlanta, Georgia 30345 (404) 634-0011; Michael Newson, Southeastern Division Vice President.
- LOS ANGELES OFFICE: Box 900, Beverly Hills, California 90213 (213) 277-2211; Tony Bauer, Western Division Vice President.

FOREIGN SALES OFFICES:

Twentieth Century-Fox France, Inc., 114 Rue la Boetie, 75008, Paris, France. Gilles Meunier Sales Rep.

Twentieth Century-Fox Film Company, Ltd., 31-32 Soho Square, London W.1., England. Malcolm Vaughan, Vice President, United Kingdom, Europe Middle/Near East and Africa. Michael Doury, Sales Representative, United Kingdom, Scandinavia.

Twentieth Century-Fox Film Corp. (Australia), P.O. Box Q301, Queen Victoria Building, Sydney 2000, Australia. Peter Broome, Vice President, Australia Far East.

Twentieth Century-Fox Television Japan, Fukide Building, 1-13 Toranomon 4, Chome Minato-Ku, Tokyo 105, Japan. Goro Uzaki, Sales Representative, Japan.

Fox Interamericana, S.A., Apartado 6-1023, Mexico, D.F. 06600 Gustavo Montaudon, Sales Manager, Mexico and Specific Spanish Language Markets.

Fox Film do Brazil—TV Division, Rua Dr. Costa Jr. 230 C.E.P., 05002 Sao Paulo, Brazil. Elie Wahba, Vice President, Latin America.

Universal Television

(A division of Universal City Studios Inc, a subsidiary of MCA Inc.)

Universal City Studios, Universal City, CA 91608; (213) 985-4321. (Producer of TV programs)

PRESIDENT
Robert A. Harris
EXECUTIVE VICE PRESIDENT, ADMINISTRATION
Ed Masket
SENIOR VICE PRESIDENT, PRODUCTION
Earl Bellamy
SENIOR VICE PRESIDENT, SERIES PROGRAMMING
Richard Lindheim
VICE PRESIDENT, DRAMATIC DEVELOPMENT
Charmaine Balian
VICE PRESIDENT, PUBLICITY, PROMOTION AND ADVERTISING
Ben Halpern
VICE PRESIDENT, CURRENT PROGRAMMING
Jim Korris
VICE PRESIDENT, TALENT & CASTING
Milt Hamerman
VICE PRESIDENT, COMEDY DEVELOPMENT
Brad Johnson
VICE PRESIDENT, BUSINESS AFFAIRS
Robert Kelley, Stuart Mandel, Paul Miller, Arnold Shane
VICE PRESIDENT, COMEDY PROGRAMS
Barbara Romen
VICE PRESIDENT, TALENT DEVELOPMENT & ACQUISITIONS
Pete Terranova
VICE PRESIDENT, MOVIES FOR TELEVISION
Tom Thayer

Warner Bros. Television

4000 Warner Blvd., Burbank CA 91522; (818) 954-6000. 75 Rockefeller Plaza, New York, NY 10019; (212) 484-8000.

TELEVISION PROGRAMMING

PRESIDENT
Harvey Shephard
EXECUTIVE VICE PRESIDENT
Barry M. Meyer
VICE PRESIDENT, SPECIAL PROJECTS
Karen Cooper
SENIOR VICE PRESIDENT, BUSINESS AFFAIRS
Art Stolnitz
SENIOR VICE PRESIDENT, CREATIVE AFFAIRS
Larry Lyttle
VICE PRESIDENT, SENIOR ADVERTISING, PUBLICITY & PROMOTION EXECUTIVE
Doug Duitsman
VICE PRESIDENT, SENIOR EXECUTIVE IN CHARGE OF PRODUCTION
Gary Credle
VICE PRESIDENT, MOVIES FOR TELEVISION AND MINI-SERIES
Norman Stephens
VICE PRESIDENT CURRENT PROGRAMMING
David Sacks
VICE PRESIDENT, DRAMA DEVELOPMENT
Ron Taylor
VICE PRESIDENT, COMEDY DEVELOPMENT
Scott Kaufer
VICE PRESIDENT, TALENT
Phyllis Huffman
VICE PRESIDENTS, BUSINESS AFFAIRS
Beverly Nix, Joe Reilly, Art Horan
VICE PRESIDENT, LEGAL AFFAIRS
Milt Segal
VICE PRESIDENT, FILM & TAPE PRODUCTION
Steve Papazian
VICE PRESIDENT, POST PRODUCTION
Karen Pingitore
VICE PRESIDENT, PRODUCTION & OPERATIONS
Tom Treloggen
DIRECTOR, STORY & PROGRAM ADMINISTRATION
Gus Blackmon
DIRECTOR, FINANCIAL ADMINISTRATION
Rosalee Jeffries
DIRECTOR, TV ESTIMATING
Mike McKnight
DIRECTOR, LEGAL AFFAIRS
Dan Schiffer
DIRECTOR, TALENT
Kathleen Letterie

NETWORK FEATURES, PAY TV & ANIMATION (WARNER BROS. CARTOONS, INC.)

75 Rockefeller Plaza, New York, NY 10019; (212) 484-8000.

PRESIDENT & PRESIDENT, WARNER BROS. CARTOONS
Edward Bleier
VICE PRESIDENT, PAY TV SALES & ADMINISTRATION
Stanley Solson
VICE PRESIDENT, SALES PLANNING, PAY-TV & NETWORK
Jeffrey Calman
VICE PRESIDENT, MARKETING
Eric Frankel
DIRECTOR, FINANCIAL AFFAIRS
J. T. Shadoan
DIRECTOR, CLIENT SERVICES, PAY TV & NETWORK
Margaret Jelcich
MANAGER, RESEARCH & ADMINISTRATION
Charlotte Mulford
MANAGER, ACCOUNTING/DATA SYSTEMS
Anthony Cochi

DOMESTIC DISTRIBUTION

PRESIDENT WORLDWIDE DISTRIBUTION

Charles D. McGregor
EXECUTIVE VICE PRESIDENT, WORLDWIDE OPERATIONS
Mauro A. Sardi
VICE PRESIDENT, DOMESTIC SALES MANAGER
William S. Hart
VICE PRESIDENT, WESTERN SALES
Ed Donaldson
VICE PRESIDENT, SOUTHERN SALES
Bill Seiler
VICE PRESIDENT, MIDWESTERN SALES
John Louis
EASTERN SALES DIRECTOR
Gary Cozen
NORTH CENTRAL SALES DIRECTOR
John Laing
SOUTHERN SALES DIRECTOR
John Bryan
VICE PRESIDENT RESEARCH
Paul Simon
VICE PRESIDENT, ADVERTISING, PROMOTION AND PUBLICITY
Ken Fournier
VICE PRESIDENT, FINANCIAL ADMINISTRATION
John Chickering
DIRECTOR PRODUCT COORDINATION
Dee Eulberg
VICE PRESIDENT, DOMESTIC SALES CONTRACTS
Dan McRae
DIRECTOR PUBLICITY & PROMOTION
Sharon Kneller
DOMESTIC SALES ADMINISTRATION
Eleanor Liebs

WARNER BROS. CARTOONS, INC.

4000 Warner Blvd., Burbank, CA 91522; (818) 954-3713.

VICE PRESIDENT, GENERAL MANAGER
Steven Greene
VICE PRESIDENT, EXECUTIVE PRODUCER
Hal Geer
DIRECTOR, PRODUCTION/ADMINISTRATION
Kathleen Helppie

DOMESTIC BRANCHES

New York: 630 Ninth Avenue, New York, NY 10036; (212) 484-8000.

OFFICE MANAGER & TECHNICAL SERVICE DIRECTOR
Erwin Markisch
MANAGER, BOOKING SERVICES
Joe Kivlehan
MANAGER, PROGRAM INFORMATION
Louis B. Marino
ASSISTANT TECHNICAL SERVICE MANAGER
Bruce Hoffman

Covington, La.: Lowe Davis Rd., P.O. Box 999; (504) 892-2703.

VICE PRESIDENT, SOUTHEASTERN SALES DIRECTOR
Bill Seiler

Los Angeles: 143 Patricia Way, P.O. Box 2749, Grass Valley, CA 95945; (916) 272-5343.

VICE PRESIDENT, WESTERN SALES DIRECTOR
Ed Donaldson

Ft. Mitchell: 3058 Brookwood Circle, Ft. Mitchell, KY 41017; (606) 341-2585.

VICE PRESIDENT, MIDWESTERN SALES DIRECTOR
John H. Louis

Chicago: 4000 Warner Blvd., Burbank, CA 91522; (818) 954-6012.

NORTH CENTRAL SALES DIRECTOR
John Laing

Georgia: 9 Spoon Court, Alpharetta, GA 30201; (404) 998-7732.

SOUTHERN SALES DIRECTOR
John Bryan

Pennsylvania: 50 Belmont Ave., Apt. 316, Bala Cynwyd, PA 19004; (215) 664-7307.

EASTERN SALES DIRECTOR
Gary Cozen

FOREIGN DISTRIBUTION

Warner Bros. TV Distribution, 4000 Warner Blvd., Burbank, CA 91522.

PRESIDENT WORLDWIDE DISTRIBUTION
Charles D. McGregor
EXECUTIVE VICE PRESIDENT, WORLDWIDE OPERATIONS
Mauro A. Sardi
VICE PRESIDENT, INTERNATIONAL SALES AND ADMINISTRATION
John Whitesell
INTERNATIONAL SALES
John Laing
VICE PRESIDENT PRODUCT COORDINATION
Dee Eulberg
VICE PRESIDENT, RESEARCH
Paul Simon
VICE PRESIDENT, ADVERTISING, PROMOTION AND PUBLICITY
Ken Fournier
VICE PRESIDENT, FINANCIAL ADMINISTRATION
John Chickering
DIRECTOR, FOREIGN SALES CONTRACTS
Jaime Ruiz
INTERNATIONAL ADMINISTRATION
Carolyn Hewitt
DIRECTOR PUBLICITY & PROMOTION
Sharon Kneller
INTERNATIONAL RECORDS & DATA
Charlene Pollock

FOREIGN SALES OFFICES

EUROPE, MIDDLE EAST & AFRICA: 135/141 Wardour St., London W1V 4AP, England.

VICE PRESIDENT SALES & ADMINISTRATION
Bryan Hambleton
ASSISTANT DIRECTOR SALES & ADMINISTRATION
Gary Phillips

AUSTRALIA, NEW ZEALAND & SOUTHEAST ASIA: 154 Castlereagh St.—5th floor, Alfred Moss House, Sydney, N.S.W., 2000 Australia, Box 2661, G.P.O. Sydney, N.S.W., 2001 Australia.

SALES DIRECTOR
Matt Brown

FRENCH SPEAKING TERRITORIES: 20 Lue Troyon, 75017 Paris, France.

DIRECTOR TELEVISION
Michel Lecourt

JAPAN: P.O. box 762, Tokyo Central, Japan.

TELEVISION SALES
Ken Sugizaki

SPAIN & PORTUGAL: Warner Espanola, S.A., Gran Via, 70-4, Madrid 13, Spain.

TELEVISION SALES
Xavier Azpiroz

LATIN AMERICA: Acapulco 37, Mexico 7 D.F., Mexico.

VICE PRESIDENT SALES
Jorge Sanchez

BRAZIL: Warner Bros. (South) Inc., Rua Senador Dantas, 19-10 Andar, Rio de Janeiro, Brazil.

BRAZIL TELEVISION SUPERVISOR
Louremberg do Nascimento

ARGENTINA: Tucuman 1938, Buenos Aires, Argentina.

TELEVISION MANAGER
Luis D'Alterio

CANADA: Warner Bros. Distributing, (Canada) Ltd., 70 Carlton St., Toronto, Ontario, Canada, M5B 1L7; (416) 922-5145.

William Morris Agency, Inc.

1350 Avenue of The Americas, New York, NY 10019; (212) 586-5100. Beverly Hills Office: 151 El Camino, Beverly Hills, CA 90212; (213) 274-7451. Nashville Office: 2325 Crestmoor Road, Nashville, TN 37125; (615) 385-0310. Overseas offices: London, Rome*, Sydney* & Munich*. (Representatives for artists and all creative talent in the entertainment and literary worlds.) *Corresponding offices.

OFFICE OF THE CHAIRMEN
Norman Brokaw (Beverly Hills), Lou Weiss (New York)
PRESIDENT, CHIEF EXECUTIVE OFFICER
Lee Stevens (New York)
EXECUTIVE VICE PRESIDENTS
Roger Davis, Tony Fantozzi, Walt Zifkin

VICE PRESIDENT, TREASURER
Larry Lewis (New York)

MOTION PICTURE DEPARTMENT

Beverly Hills—Department Head, Leonard Hirshan
Chris Black, John Burnham, Jim Crabbe, Ames Cushing, Elaine Goldsmith, J. J. Harris, Jean-Pierre Henreaux, Andy Howard, Joan Hyler, Alan Iezman, Rick Jaffa, Ed Limato, Ron Mardigian, Fred Milstein, Mike Peretzian, John Ptak, Judy Scott-Fox, Mike Simpson, Bobbi Thompson, Peter Turner, Irene Webb, Cary Woods, Carol Yumkas, Scott Zimmerman, Mike Zimring

New York—Department Head, Boaty Boatwright
Peter Franklin, Kevin Huvane, Myrna Jacoby, George Lane, Owen Laster, Phyllis Levy, Biff Liff, Dan Mizell, Gilbert Parker, Johnnie Planco, Ed Robbins, Katy Rothacker, Risa Shapiro, Esther Sherman, Steven Starr, Jonathan Trumper

TELEVISION DEPARTMENT

Worldwide Head, Jerry Katzman
Larry Auerbach, Arthur Axelman, Bruce Brown, Beth Cannon, Aaron Cohen, Lee Cohen, Robert Crestani, Ruth Engelhardt, Steve Glick, Sam Haskell, Dick Howard, Mark Itkin, Sol Leon, Ken Lindner, Gary Loder, Bryan Lourd, Deborah Miller, Larry Noveck, Bonnie Owens, Marc Pariser, Pietragallo, Pam Prince, Leonard Rosenberg, Hal Ross, Mark Teitlebaum, Steve Weiss, Fred Westheimer, Jeff Witjas

New York—Co-Department Heads, Ron Yatter, Leo Bookman.
Lucy Aceto, Jeff Alpern, Jim Arnoff, Leo Bookman, Art Fuhrer, Jim Griffin, Stephen Lane, Michael Naso, David Segal

Zenith Electronics Corporation

1000 Milwaukee Ave., Glenview, IL 60025; (312) 391-8181.

(Consumer home entertainment products; electronic do-it-yourself kits, instruments, home study education materials; microcomputer systems, video display terminals, components, and cable and subscription TV and videotex products.)

PRESIDENT AND CHIEF EXECUTIVE OFFICER
Revone W. Kluckman
SENIOR VICE PRESIDENT AND GROUP EXECUTIVE, CONSUMER PRODUCTS
Robert B. Hansen
GENERAL MANAGER CATV/STV OPERATIONS
James Faust

Cable Television

* STATISTICS AND HISTORY
* MAJOR CABLE SYSTEM OPERATORS
* MAJOR PROGRAM SUPPLIERS

Cable Television

STATISTICS

HISTORICAL DATES

FIRST OVER-THE-AIR TOLL-TV EXPERIMENTS: 1950, Skiatron system tested over WOR-TV in New York City. 1951, Telemeter system tested over KTLA-TV, Los Angeles; Zenith tested its system over its own experimental station in Chicago.

FEBRUARY 10, 1955: Federal Communications Commission started proceedings to determine whether it should authorize TV stations to transmit programs paid for on a subscription basis. Study involved 92 docket volumes reflecting the views of over 25,000 persons on legal, technical and policy questions.

MAY 23, 1957: FCC concluded it had authority to authorize use of TV broadcast frequencies for subscription operations if it found it were in the public interest to do so. Did not define whether this service should be classified as "broadcasting" or some other.

OCTOBER 17, 1957: FCC adopted its first report on the proceedings and declared it would consider applications to conduct trial pay-TV operations over TV stations provided certain conditions were met.

MARCH 24, 1959: FCC issued third report saying it was ready to consider any pay-TV application by a commecial TV station conforming with requirements, among which were limitation of three-year trial authorizations to markets where there were at least four commercial TV stations (including the pay-TV one), and one trial system allowed per market.

JUNE 22, 1960: Hartford Phonevision Co. (later RKO General Phonevision Co.), a licensee of WHCT (Channel 18), Hartford, CT, applied for authority to conduct a three-year trial subscription-TV operation. Application granted February 23, 1961. Operations began June 29, 1962, and concluded in January, 1969.

JULY 3, 1967: FCC's subscription TV committee submitted a fourth report proposing an over-the-air subscription TV service. Rules were designed to integrate subscription TV into the total TV system so good programming would continue to be available over regular TV stations.

DECEMBER 12, 1968: FCC formally established over-the-air subscription TV as a regular broadcast service.

Statistics for 1981 (supplied by FCC)*

Operating revenues totaled over $3.5 billion, a 60 per cent increase over 1980 revenues. Total operating expenses were $2.4 billion, leaving an operating income of $1.2 billion or a 33.4 per cent operating margin before expenses of depreciation/amortization, interest and taxes.

Net income before taxes was approximately $40 million and the cable industry's total assets had a book value of $7.91 billion (up 78 per cent from 1980).

Pay cable services yielded revenues of $1.17 billion or 32.6% of total revenues. The percentage of total revenues attributable to pay cable operations increased by 6.9 per cent in 1981.

The national average monthly subscriber rate for basic service was $7.94 in 1981, ranging from an average low of $6.50 in Vermont to a high of $20.01 in Alaska. The national average cable television installation fee was $18.32, ranging from $11.45 in Rhode Island to $40.00 in the Virgin Islands. That national average montly rate for pay cable TV was $9.56, ranging from $6.00 in the Virgin Islands to $12.93 in Alaska.

In 1981, pay cable services were offered by 2,406 financial entities comprising 9,264 communities in nearly every state. California, New York and Pennsylvania were the leading states in terms of pay cable revenues.

Approximately 12,000 communities with over 23 million subscribers (households) were served by cable television in 1981. These 12,000 communities were consolidated into 3,600 financial entities for reporting purposes. A financial entity is defined as one or more cable TV community systems which report to the Commission as one business entity—upon meeting certain ownership and technological requirements.

Recent Statistics

In 1985 cable television added 4.5 million new homes, bringing the total to 60.4 million, or 71% of U.S. TV households. Pay-TV subscribers grew to 30 million, representing some 42% of U.S. TV homes. Revenues of cable systems had jumped to $8 billion by the end of 1984 and pre-tax profits were estimated at $800 million.

---

* The FCC ceased compiling financial data on the cable TV industry after 1981.

Cable System Operators

American Cablesystems Corporation

55 Tozer Rd., Beverly, MA 01915; (617) 921-0080

CHAIRMAN & CHIEF EXECUTIVE OFFICER
Steven B. Dodge
EXECUTIVE VICE PRESIDENT
William A. Devereaux
EXECUTIVE VICE PRESIDENT & CHIEF OPERATING OFFICER
Barry D. Lemileux
SENIOR VICE PRESIDENTS
George B. Douglas III
David S. Prescott

American TV & Communications Corp.

(A subsidiary of Time, Inc.) 160 Inverness Drive West, Englewood, CO 80112; (303) 799-1200.

CHAIRMAN OF THE BOARD & CHIEF EXECUTIVE OFFICER & PRESIDENT
Trygve E. Myhren
EXECUTIVE VICE PRESIDENTS
Thomas W. Binning, Gary S. Bryson, James H. Doolittle, June E. Travis, Kevin H. Rorke
SENIOR VICE PRESIDENTS
John F. Gault, Lawrence H. James, James P. Cottingham, Robert M. Rast, Henry J. Gerken

Cable TV Company

217 East 9th St., Hazelton, PA 18201; (717) 455-6851

PRESIDENT
Joseph Gans, Sr.

Cablevision Systems Corporation

One Media Crossways, Woodbury, NY 11797; (516) 364-8450.

CHAIRMAN & CHIEF EXECUTIVE OFFICER
Charles P. Dolan
PRESIDENT & CHIEF OPERATING OFFICER
John Tatta

Cardinal Communications, Inc.

120 S. Washington St., Crawfordsville, IN 47933; (317) 362-6161

PRESIDENT
James F. Ackerman
VICE PRESIDENT
Myron T. Pattison

Comcast Cable Communications, Inc.

1 Belmont Ave., Bala Cynwyd, PA 19004; (215) 667-4200.

PRESIDENT
Robert B. Clasen

Continental Cablevision, Inc.

The Pilot House, Lewis Wharf, Boston, MA 02110; (617) 742-9500.

CHAIRMAN & CHIEF EXECUTIVE OFFICER
Amos B. Hostetter, Jr.
PRESIDENT
Timothy P. Neher
VICE PRESIDENT, MARKETING
Frederick C. Livingston
VICE PRESIDENT, PROGRAMMING
Robert A. Stengel
VUCE ORESUDEBT AND TRESURER
Nancy Hawthorne

Cox Cable Communications, Inc.

1400 Lake Hearn Drive, Atlanta, GA 30319; (404) 843-5000.

PRESIDENT
James O. Robbins
SENIOR VICE PRESIDENT FINANCE & ADMINISTRATION
Robert C. O'Leary
SENIOR VICE PRESIDENTS—OPERATIONS
Barry R. Elson, Wayne D. Knighton and G. Lewis Davenport
VICE PRESIDENT MARKETING & PROGRAMMING
Ajit M. Dalvi
VICE PRESIDENT, TECHNICAL OPERATIONS
Alex B. Best
CORPORATE DIRECTOR OF PUBLIC RELATIONS
David C. Andersen

Group W Cable

(A subsidiary of Westinghouse Broadcasting and Cable Co.) 888 Seventh Ave., New York, NY 10106; (212) 247-8700.

CHAIRMAN AND CHIEF EXECUTIVE OFFICER
William J. Bresnan
PRESIDENT AND CHIEF OPERATING OFFICER
Burton B. Staniar
VICE PRESIDENT OF NEW MARKETING DEVELOPMENT
Jane Hartley
VICE PRESIDENT OF PROGRAMMING
Martin Lafferty
VICE PRESIDENT OF ADVERTISING SALES
Thomas McKinney
ICE PRESIDENT SALES MARKETING
Tom Schmitt
CONTROLLER
Richard Hilton

Heritage Communications, Inc.

2195 Ingersoll Ave., Des Moines, IA 50312; (515) 246-1440.

CORPORATE OFFICERS

PRESIDENT
James M. Hoak, Jr.
EXECUTIVE VICE PRESIDENT/PRESIDENT TELECOMMUNICATIONS GROUP
James S. Cownie
EXECUTIVE VICE PRESIDENT/TELECOMMUNICATIONS GROUP
Rod Thole

OFFICERS TELECOMMUNICATIONS GROUP

SENIOR VICE PRESIDENT/ENGINEERING
Doug Truckenmiller
VICE PRESIDENT/PUBLIC RELATIONS
William J. Riley
VICE PRESIDENT/OPERATIONS
Nile McDonald
VICE PRESIDENT/OPERATIONS
Kevin Rice
VICE PRESIDENT/MARKETING
Dale Parker
VICE PRESIDENT/DEVELOPMENT
David Oman
VICE PRESIDENT/CONTROLLER
Loran Schiltz

Liberty Communications, Inc.

Box 7009, Eugene, OR 97401; (503) 485-5611.

PRESIDENT
Donald Tykeson
EXECUTIVE VICE PRESIDENT/TREASURER
Carolyn S. Chambers
VICE PRESIDENT/FINANCE
Robert R. Vickers
VICE PRESIDENT/COUNSEL
Roger A. Seltzer
VICE PRESIDENT/ENGINEERING
Jerome E. Partch
DIRECTOR OF SALES & MARKETING
Ron Lederer

Midwest Video Corp.

860 Tower Bldg., Little Rock, AR 72201; (501) 375-8885.

PRESIDENT
G. R. Morrell
VICE PRESIDENT
Lloyd B. Sands

NewChannels Corp.

(A subsidiary of Newhouse Broadcasting Corp.) 112 Northern Concourse, North Syracuse, NY 13212; (315) 455-5826.

PRESIDENT
E. R. Vadeboncoeur
EXECUTIVE VICE PRESIDENT
Robert Miron
FIRST VICE PRESIDENT/GENERAL MANAGER
Leo A. Calistri

Newhouse Broadcasting Corporation

112 Northern Concourse, No. Syracuse, NY 13212; (315) 455-5973

Post-Newsweek Cable

2621 East Camelback Road, Suite 150, Phoenix, AZ 85016

PRESIDENT
Howard Wall

Prime Cable Corporation

One American Center, Suite 3000, 600 Congress Ave., Austin, TX 78701; (512) 476-7888

SENIOR VICE PRESIDENT
Jerry D. Lindauer
VICE PRESIDENT, OPERATIONS
C. Ronald Dorchester

Rogers U.S. Cablesystems, Inc.

Commerical Union Tower, Suite 2602, Toronto Dominion Center, Toronto, Ontario, Canada M5K 1J5; (416) 864-3222

CHAIRMAN
Philip B. Lind

Sammons Communications, Inc.

Box 225728, Dallas, TX 75265; (214) 742-9828.

PRESIDENT
James Whitson
VICE PRESIDENT/CORPORATE DEVELOPMENT
William B. Strange, Jr.
VICE PRESIDENT/OPERATIONS
Mark S. Weber

Service Electric Cable TV, Inc.

201 West Centre St., Mahanoy City, PA 17948; (717) 773-2585.

PRESIDENT/TREASURER
John Walson
SECRETARY
Margaret Walson

Storer Cable Communications

Box 61-8000, Miami, FL 33161; (305) 899-1000.

PRESIDENT/TV CABLE COMMUNICATIONS
Kenneth L. Bagwell
EXECUTIVE VICE PRESIDENT
Jim Hall

TeleCable Corp.

Box 2098, 740 Duke St., Norfolk, VA 23510; (804) 624-5000.

CHAIRMAN OF THE BOARD
Frank Batten
PRESIDENT AND CHIEF EXECUTIVE OFFICER
Richard D. Roberts
VICE PRESIDENTS
Gordon R. Herring, James S. Key
VICE PRESIDENT, FINANCE & TREASURER
Alfred F. Ritter, Jr.

Tele-Communications, Inc.

54 Denver Technological Center, Box 22595, Wellshire Station, Denver, CO 80222; (303) 771-8200.

CHAIRMAN
Bob Magness
PRESIDENT & CHIEF EXECUTIVE OFFICER
John C. Malone

Teleprompter Corporation

888 Seventh Avenue, New York, NY 10019; (212) 247-8700

CHAIRMAN OF THE BOARD & CHIEF EXECUTIVE OFFICER
William J. Bresnan
PRESIDENT & CHIEF OPERATING OFFICER
M. Christopher Derick
VICE PRESIDENT/NEW MARKETING DEVELOPMENT
Jane Hartley
VICE PRESIDENT/ADVERTISING SALES
Thomas McKinney
CONTROLLER
Richard Hilton

Texas Community Antennas Group

3027 S.E. Loop 323, Tyler, TX 75701; (214) 595-3701.

PRESIDENT
Robert Rogers
VICE PRESIDENTS
R. Don Cowan, Wayne McKinney

Times Mirror Cable Television, Inc.

2381 Morse Ave., Irvine, CA 92714; (714) 660-0500.

PRESIDENT & CHIEF EXECUTIVE OFFICER
Larry W. Wangberg
BOARD CHAIRMAN
Ralph J. Swett
EXECUTIVE VICE PRESIDENT/ENGINEERING
Gilbert L. Tash
SENIOR VICE PRESIDENT/TREASURER
James F. Guthrie
SENIOR VICE PRESIDENT/GROUP OPERATIONS
James "Trey" Smith
SENIOR VICE PRESIDENT/GROUP OPERATIONS
Kent D. Franke

UACC Midwest, Inc.

1430 Balltown Road, Schenectady, NY 12309; (518) 385-1229.

PRESIDENT
Marvin L. Jones
SENIOR VICE PRESIDENT
A.C. "Sam" Belanger
VICE PRESIDENT/GENERAL MANAGER
G.W. Oswald
ENGINEERING VICE PRESIDENT
Frank C. Baxter

United Artists Cablesystems Corp.

60 Craig Rd., Monvale, NY 07645; (201) 930-9191

PRESIDENT & CHIEF EXECUTIVE OFFICER
Marvin J. Jones

Viacom Cable

1211 Ave. of the Americas, New York, NY 10036; (212) 575-5175. P.O. Box 13, Pleasanton, CA 9 94566; (415) 463-0870. (A division of Viacom International.)

PRESIDENT
John W. Goddard
SENIOR VICE PRESIDENTS
Danny Radcliff, Garrett Girvan, Kurt Jorgensen, Bill Lilly
EXECUTIVE VICE PRESIDENT
Edward Bennett
EXECUTIVE MARKETING DIRECTOR
Ted Yorio

Vision Cable Communications, Inc.

270 Sylvan Ave., Englewood Cliffs, NJ 07632.

EXECUTIVE VICE PRESIDENT & GENERAL MANAGER
Joel Fleming
VICE PRESIDENT/ENGINEERING
Richard M. White
VICE PRESIDENTS/OPERATIONS
Ronald G. Sumrow, V. Mitchell Roberts
VICE PRESIDENT/PROGRAMMING
Pamela T. Hammond

Warner Amex Cable Communications, Inc.

75 Rockefeller Plaza, New York, NY 10019; (212) 484-8080. Cable address: Warncable.

CHAIRMAN & CHIEF EXECUTIVE OFFICER
Drew Lewis

Western Communications, Inc.

Suite 225, 2855 Mitchell Dr., Box 4610, Walnut Creek, CA; (415) 935-3055.

CHAIRMAN
Richard T. Thieriot
PRESIDENT
Edward M. Allen

Cable and Pay TV Program Suppliers

Arts & Entertainment Network (A&E)

555 Fifth Ave., New York, NY 10017. (212) 661-4500. (A joint venture of Hearst Corp., ABC Video Enterprises, and RCA Cable, Inc.)

PRESIDENT & CHIEF EXECUTIVE OFFICER
Nickolas Davatzes

Associated Press

50 Rockefeller Plaza, New York, 10020; (212) 262-4152.

DIRECTOR OF/COMMUNICATIONS
Richard G. Atkins
VICE PRESIDENT/BROADCASTING
Roy Steinfort

Black Entertainment Television (BET)

1232-31st Street, N.W., Washington, D.C. 20007; (202) 337-5260.

PRESIDENT
Robert L. Johnson
VICE PRESIDENT OF ADVERTISING
Janis P. Thomas
VICE PRESIDENT OF NETWORK OPERATIONS
Jeff Lee
VICE PRESIDENT OF FINANCE
Antonia O. Duncan
VICE PRESIDENT AND GENERAL COUNSEL
Debra L. Lee

Cable News Network

Turner Broadcasting System, 1050 Techwood Dr. NW, Atlanta, GA 30318; (414) 898-8500.

BOARD CHAIRMAN & PRESIDENT OF TBS
R. E. (Ted) Turner
CNN EXECUTIVE VICE PRESIDENT
Burt Reinhardt
CNN SENIOR VICE PRESIDENT
Ed Turner

Cable News Network Headline News

1050 Techwood Drive, N.W., Atlanta, GA 30318; (404) 898-8500.

BOARD CHAIRMAN & PRESIDENT
R. E. (Ted) Turner
PRESIDENT
Burt Reinhardt
VICE PRESIDENT—HEADLINE NEWS
Paul R. Amos

Cable Satellite Public Affairs Network (C-SPAN)

Suite 412, 400 N. Capitol, St., N.W., Washington, D.C.; (202) 737-3220.

PRESIDENT & CHIEF OPERATING OFFICER
Paul A. Fitzpatrick
CHAIRMAN AND CHIEF EXECUTIVE OFFICER
Brian P. Lamb

Christian Broadcasting Network

CBN Center, Virginia Beach, VA 24363; (804) 424-7777.

PRESIDENT & CHAIRMAN
M. G. (Pat) Robertson

Cinemax

1271 Avenue of the Americas, New York, NY 10020; (212) 484-1000. A second pay-TV service created by Home Box Office, Inc. and designed to complement the foundation HBO service.

PRESIDENT AND CHIEF OPERATING OFFICER
Michael Fuchs
SENIOR VICE PRESIDENT, CINEMAX
Larry Carlson
SENIOR VICE PRESIDENT, CINEMAX PROGRAMMING
Lee deBoer
SENIOR VICE PRESIDENT, CINEMAX MARKETING & SALES
Dick Beahrs
VICE PRESIDENT, CORPORATE AFFAIRS
David Pritchard

Columbia Pictures Pay Television

Columbia Plaza South, Burbank, CA 91505; (213) 954-6000.

VICE PRESIDENT, PAY, CABLE & HOME ENTERTAINMENT
Arthur M. Goldblatt
DIRECTOR, PAY TELEVISION SALES
Dennis Wood
MANAGER, CLIENT SERVICES & NON-THEATRICAL
Patti Lippel

Cooper Wireless Cable, Inc.

286 Eldridge Rd., Fairfield, NJ 07006; (201) 227-8700.

PRESIDENT
Brian Cooper
EXECUTIVE VICE PRESIDENT
Harold Brownstein
DIRECTOR OF MARKETING
Bruce DeCourt
DIRECTOR OF FINANCE
Richard Hummers
DIRECTOR OF OPERATIONS
Robert Frank
DIRECTOR OF ADMINISTRATION
Thomas McGoldrick
DIRECTOR OF ENGINEERING
Thomas Rice

The Disney Channel

500 Park Ave., New York, NY 10022; (212) 735-5393. (A subsidiary of Walt Disney Productions)

PRESIDENT
John Cooke

ESPN, Inc.

ESPN Plaza, Bristol, CT 06010, (203) 584-8477; and 355 Lexington Ave., New York, NY 10017, (212) 661-6040.

PRESIDENT & CHIEF EXECUTIVE OFFICER
J. William Grimes
EXECUTIVE VICE PRESIDENT/MARKETING
Roger L. Werner
SENIOR VICE PRESIDENT/PRODUCTION
Steven M. Bornstein
VICE PRESIDENT, BUSINESS & LEGAL AFFAIRS
Andrew P. Brillant
VICE PRESIDENT, ADVERTISING SALES
Jack S. Bonanni
VICE PRESIDENT, PRODUCTION
Allan B. (Scotty) Connal
VICE PRESIDENT, FINANCE & ADMINISTRATION
Thomas A. Conway

Financial News Network

2525 Ocean Park Blvd., Santa Monica, CA 90405; (213) 450-02412.

PRESIDENT
Norman W. Potter
VICE PRESIDENT, PRODUCTION AND OPERATIONS
Paul Stenie
VICE PRESIDENT, MARKETING AND AFFILIATES
Arnie Rosenthal
DIRECTOR AFFILIATE RELATIONS
Christopher Taylor

Home Box Office, Inc.

1100 Avenue of the Americas, New York, NY 10036; (212) 512-1000. (A subsidiary of Time, Inc.)

CHAIRMAN AND CHIEF EXECUTIVE OFFICER
Michael Fuchs
PRESIDENT
Joe Collins
SENIOR VICE PRESIDENT, MARKETING
John Billock
EXECUTIVE VICE PRESIDENT, AFFILIATE SALES & OPERATIONS
Peter Frame
SENIOR VICE PRESIDENT, NETWORK OPERATIONS AND CORPORATE DEVELOPMENT
Ed Horowitz
VICE PRESIDENT, CORPORATE AFFAIRS
David Pritchard

Home Entertainment Productions

165 Beverly Road, Huntington Station, NY 11746; (516) 271-8800.

PRESIDENT
James Nishimura
GENERAL MANAGER
Phil Staros

Home Theater Network, Inc.

465 Congress St., Portland, ME 04101; (207) 774-0300.

PRESIDENT
Peter M. Kendrick
VICE PRESIDENT AND GENERAL MANAGER
Peter A. Newman
VICE PRESIDENT/SALES
Jan Robert Pearce
VICE PRESIDENT/ADMINISTRATION AND AFFILIATE RELATIONS
Kathryn R. Petersonn

Lifetime

1211 Avenue of the Americas, New York, NY 10036; (212) 719-7230. (Hearst/ABC-Viacom Entertainment Services)

PRESIDENT & CHIEF EXECUTIVE OFFICER
Thomas F. Burchill
VICE PRESIDENT/PROGRAMS
Charles B. Gingow

MTV Networks, Inc.

1775 Broadway, New York, NY 10019; (212) 713-6510.

PRESIDENT & CHIEF OFFICER
Robert W. Pittman

MTV-VH-1 & NICKELODEON

1133 Ave. of the Americas, New York, NY 10036.

Modern Satellite Service

5000 Park St. N., St. Petersburg, FL 33709; (813) 541-7571. (A division of Modern Talking Picture Service)

MANAGER OF PRODUCTION
Patrick M. Swonger

The Nashville Network

Box 10210, Stamford, CT 06904; (203) 965-6000. (A service of Opryland USA, Inc. and Group W. Satellite Communications.)

PRESIDENT AND CHIEF EXECUTIVE OFFICER OF OPRYLAND USA
E.W. Wendell
SENIOR VICE PRESIDENT, BROADCASTING, OPRYLAND USA
Tom Griscom
PRESIDENT, GWSC
Harlan Rosenzweig

Prism

50 Monument Rd., Bala Cynwyd, PA 19004; (215) 668-2210.

VICE PRESIDENT AND GENERAL MANAGER
Donald L. Heller
VICE PRESIDENT AND ASSISTANT GENERAL MANAGER
Sam Schroeder

Rainbow Programming Services

150 Crossways Park West, Woodbury, NY 11797; (516) 364-2222. (Bravo, American Movie Classics, SportsChannel New York, Sports Channel New England, SportsVision Chicago, PRISM of Philadelphia)

PRESIDENT AMC/BRAVO
John Janas
PRESIDENT/SPORTS SERVICES
Jack Williams

Reuters News-View

Reuters Ltd., 1700 Broadway, New York, NY 10019; (212) 603-3575.

SATELLITE SALES
J. Outman

Satori Entertainment Corporation

330 West 42nd St., New York, NY 10036; (212) 563-2323.

PRESIDENT
Ernest G. Sauer
SENIOR VICE PRESIDENT
Gary P. Connor
VICE PRESIDENT/ACQUISITION & PRODUCTION
Jeffrey Sass
VICE PRESIDENT/ADMINISTRATION
Janice Demadona
DIRECTOR PUBLICITY/ADVERTISING/PROMOTION
Nicole Satescu

Showtime/The Movie Channel, Inc.

1633 Broadway, New York, NY 10019; (212) 708-1600.

CHAIRMAN AND CHIEF EXECUTIVE OFFICER
Neil Austrian
EXECUTIVE VICE PRESIDENT, FINANCE & ADMINISTRATION
Ron Bernard
SENIOR VICE PRESIDENT, MARKETING & CREATIVE SERVICES
Joshua Sapan
EXECUTIVE VICE PRESIDENT, ORIGINAL PROGRAMMING
Peter Chernin
EXECUTIVE VICE PRESIDENT, SALES & AFFILIATE MARKETING
Jack Heim
EXECUTIVE VICE PRESIDENT, PAY PER VIEW
Scott Kurnit
VICE PRESIDENT, GENERAL COUNSEL
Gwen Marcus
SENIOR VICE PRESIDENT, PROGRAM PLANNING
Jim Miller
SENIOR VICE PRESIDENT, FILM ACQUISITIONS

Fred Schneier
SENIOR VICE PRESIDENT, DIRECT BOARDCAST DEVELOPMENT
Stephan Wm. Schulte, Sr.
SENIOR VICE PRESIDENT, ORIGINAL PROGRAMMING
Allen Sabinson
VICE PRESIDENT, SPECIAL EVENTS
C. David Batalsky

Spanish International Network

460 West 42 St., New York, NY 10036; (212) 502-1300. (Galavision)

DIRECTOR OF PROGRAMMING
Rosita Peru

Spectradyne (Hotels/Motels)

1501 N. Plano Road, Richardson, TX 75081; (214) 234-2721.

PRESIDENT
Howard Buchanan
VICE PRESIDENT OF PROGRAMMING
Bill Coleman

Tempo Television Network

(Formerly SPN) 6918 S. Yorktown, Tulsa, OK 74136; (918) 496-3200

BOARD CHAIRMAN
Edward L. Taylor
PRESIDENT
R. B. Smith
VICE PRESIDENT/NATIONAL SALES & PROGRAMMING
Ray Klinge
VICE PRESIDENT/EASTERN DIVISION
Jim Trecek
VICE PRESIDENT, WESTERN DIVISION
Seth Kittay

Trinity Broadcasting Network

Box A, Santa, CA 92711; (714) 832-2950.

PRESIDENT
Paul F. Crouch
VICE PRESIDENT
Jane P. Duff
SECRETARY/TREASURER
Norman G. Juggert
DIRECTOR AFFILIATE SERVICES
Stan Hollon

Twentieth Century Fox Telecommunications, Inc.

Box 900, Beverly Hills, CA 90213. 10201 W. Pico Blvd., Los Angeles, CA 90035; (213) 227-2211.

EXECUTIVE VICE PRESIDENT DOMESTIC SYNDICATION
Michael J. Lambert

USA Cable Network

1230 Ave. of the Americas, New York, NY 10020; (212) 408-9100

PRESIDENT & CHIEF EXECUTIVE OFFICE
Kay Koplovitz
SENIOR VICE PRESIDENT/PROGRAMMING
David Kenin

The Weather Channel

2840 Mt. Wilkinson Parkway, Suite 200, Atlanta, GA 30039; (404) 434-6800.

PRESIDENT
Michael J. Eckert
VICE PRESIDENT, PERSONNEL
Hugh Eaton
VICE PRESIDENT, SPECIAL PROJECTS
Douglas S. Holladay
VICE PRESIDENT, ADVERTISING SALES
Ed Peters
VICE PRESIDENT/AFFILIATE SALES
Sandy McGovern

WTBS

Turner Broadcasting System, 1050 Techwood Drive, N.W., Atlanta, GA 30318; (404) 827-1700.

PRESIDENT
Robert Wussler
VICE PRESIDENT OF OPERATIONS & ADMINISTRATION
James Kitchell

Z Channel

2939 Nebraska Ave., Santa Monica, CA 90404; (213) 453-1985.

DIRECTOR OF PROGRAMMING
Jerry Harvey
GENERAL MANAGER
Louise Henry

Trade Names of Cable & Pay-TV Suppliers

(See company listings)

AP Newscable (Associated Press)
American Movie Classics (Rainbow)
BET (Black Entertainment Network
Bravo (Rainbow Programming Services)
CBN Cable (Christian Broadcasting Network)
CNN (Cable News Network—Turner Broadcasting)
Cinemax (Cinemax—Time, Inc.)
C-SPAN (Cable Satellite Public Affairs Network
The Disney Channel (Group W/Disney)
ESPN (Entertainment & Sports Programming Network—Getty Oil)
Escapade (Rainbow Programming Services)
FNN (Financial News Network)
Gala Vision (Spanish International Network)
Home Box Office (Home Box Office—Time, Inc.)
Lifetime (Hearst/ABC/Viacom)
MTV (Warner Amex Satellite Entertainment Co.)
Modern Satellite Network (Modern Talking Picture Service)
The Movie Channel (Showtime/The Movie Channel)
Nashville Network (NLT Corp.)
News-View (Reuters News Agency)
Nickelodeon (Warner Amex)
The Playboy Channel (Rainbow)
Private Screenings (Satori Entertainment)
Showtime (Showtime/The Movie Channel)
UPI Cable Newswire (United Press International)
USA Network (Rogers/UA)
The Weather Channel (Landmark Communications)
WTBS (Turner)

Producers-Distributors

* PROGRAMS
* COMMERCIALS
* FEATURE FILMS
* SHORTS

Producers and Distributors

ABC Pictures International

1330 Avenue of Americas, New York, NY 10019. (212) 887-5700.

- Series: Moonlighting.
- Out on A Limb, Amerika.
- Made-For-TV Films: A Bunny's Tale, California Girls, Embassy, The Hearst and Davies Affair, Jacqueline Bouvier Kennedy, The Jericho Mile; Long Time Gone, Love Lives On, The Midnight Hour.
- Sports.
- News Specials.
- Children's Programming.
- Academy Awards Special.

AFP Distributors, Inc.

1540 Broadway, New York, NY 10036; (212) 582-1900. Sheldon Abromowitz, pres.; Barbara Brazong, v.p.; Judy Simyak, controller; John Wengen, ag. liaison.

APA Studios, Inc.

230 West 10th St., New York, NY 10014; (212) 929-9436. Organized 1963. (Special effects motion picture firm working in commercials, features, industrials; stop-motion, 3-D Animation hi-speed, time-lapse, locals and graphics, total production). Lee Howard, pres.; David Rogers, art director; Robert Self, production mgr.

Academy Film Productions, Inc.

3918 West Estes Ave., Lincolnwood, IL 60645; (312) 674-2122. Bernard Howard, pres. (Produce live and filmed or video-taped shows and commercials, slides, animation, slide films and industrial films).

Alan Enterprises, Inc.

32234 Pacific Coast Highway, Malibu, CA 90265; (213) 457-8321. Alan L. Gleitsman, pres.; Cheri Rosche, v.p.; Christine Buchanan, ops. mgr.

- The Promotables (15 features); The Classics (28 features); Special Cinema (58 features); The Wizard of Oz (90-min. special); American Caesar (5-hr. mini-series); Vietnam—The Ten Thousand Day War (13 hrs.); Felix the Cat (260 color cartoons); Speed Racer (52 half-hrs.); The Abbott and Costello Show (52 half-hrs.).

Alden Films

7820-20th Ave., Brooklyn NY 11214; (718) 331-1045. Paul Weinberg, pres. (Film and video distributors for Jewish Chautauqua Society, Hadassah, Natl. Council of Jewish Women, Eternal Light Film Library, Jewish Natl. Fund, Womens American ORT, Pioneer Women/Namaat, United Jewish Appeal, American Red Magen David, American Society for Technion.)

Allend'or Productions, Inc.

15036 Valley Vista Blvd., P.O Box 5550, Sherman Oaks, CA 91413; (213) 872-1332. Algernon G. Walker, pres.; Irene J. Brooks, v.p.; Marcia J. Walker, secy., treas.; (Motion-picture and TV production.)

Almi Television Productions

1585 Broadway, New York, NY 10036. (212) 315-8600. Dan Harrison, pres.

- Theatrical feature packages: Almi Film Festival (10); Children's Cinema Classics (65); Kung-Fu (13); She's A Lady (19); Hot Rocks (8); Thriller (18); Almi Passport (33); Great Comedy—Volume I (32); Great Comedy—Volume II (15); ½ hour animated special: Kitten's Christmas.

American Film Production

1540 Broadway, NY 10036; 582-1900. Sheldon Abromowitz, pres.; Barbara Brazong, v.p.: (Produce and distribute film and videotape TV commercials, industrial, public relations, sales, educational training, medical, merchandising and documentary program films.)

Amrit Productions, Inc.

206 West 99 St., Suite 5-D, New York, NY 10025; (212) 663-6933. Tirlok Malik, pres.; Chander Malik, v.p. (Producer and arranger of production and co-production of films for TV and video; arranges casting for Indian actors; also distributes video films.)

Animated Productions, Inc.

1600 Broadway, New York, NY 10019; Columbus 5-2942. Al Stahl, pres.; Richard Stahl, v.p.; Shirlee Debrier, production dir.; Peter Puzzo, exec. dir. (Producers of programs, television commercials, cartoons and shorts, industrial films, specialists in animation, stop motion, and fotomation.) Fully-animated—with punched tape—animation stand, precision Super 8 blowup optical bench, Super 8 with opticas.)

Arlington Film Studios

120–37 101st Ave. No., Seminole, FL 33542. Organized 1962. (Produce all types sound and silent motion picture films.) Producer: Frank Ruzz.

Arztco Pictures, Inc.

15 East 61st Street, New York, NY 10021; (212) 753-1050. Organized 1967. (Production of motion pictures, commercials, industrials, also editing services including negative matching.) Tony Arzt, pres., prod./dir.

Associated Press Broadcast Services

1825 K Street, N.W., Suite 615, Washington, D.C. 2007; (202) 955-7243. Roy Steinfort, v.p. of Broadcast Services. (TV Direct, the first nonexclusive video news service available to all TV news operations, including Washington Direct, BeatChecks, and AP Videographs; APTV Wire, the AP's high-speed selectable wire for TV stations.)

Astoria Pictures Corporation

34–31 35 St., Astoria, NY 11106; (212) 753-1484. Nelson Morris. (Producer of feature motion pictures.)

Atlantic Television, Inc.

Operational Headquarters, sales and distribution office: 8255 Sunset Blvd., Los Angeles, CA 90046; (213) 650-2500. Jonathan M. Dana, pres., m.p. & TV; Patricia Furnare, v.p., worldwide operations.

Audio Productions

(A division of Reeves Teletape, Inc.) 227 East 45 St., N.Y., NY 10017. (212) 573-8656. Peter J. Mooney, pres.; (Producers of Educational-Documentary and Industrial Films).

Aurora General Entertainment Corp.

2000 West Commercial Blvd., Fort Lauderdale, FL 33309 (305) 492-8500. 545 Fifth Ave., New York, NY 10017. (212) 682-2323.

- War Chronicles, Judy Garland specials, The Littlest Angel, Raggedy Ann and Andy, feature film packages, James Michener Specials, Upstairs at Xenon, The Amazing World of Kreskin.

B

BBC Enterprises Limited

Head Office: Woodlands, 80 Woodlane, London W12 OTT. Tel.: (01) 743-5588. BRYON PARKIN, MANAGING DIRECTOR Tel.: (01) 576-0204. Australia, Basil Sands, BBC Westfield Towers, 100 William St., Sydney; Tel Sydney 3586411. Canada, Educational & Training Sales, Christine Warren, 214 King Street West, Toronto, Tel.: (416) 585-2583. BBC Enterprises distributes all types of BBC TV Programming, licenses BBC titles for merchandising including the BBC Microcomputer, produces BBC Video and BBC Records and provides facilities for other broadcasters.

BBI, A Service of Metromedia, Inc.

5 TV Place, Boston, MA 02192; (617) 449-0400. Robert M. Bennett, pres; Chet Collier, v.p.; Paul Rich, v.p., GM syndication; Bruce Marson, v.p. GM production; Jack Duffield, v.p., media sales; Carl Menk, v.p. station sales.

Bob Banner Associates, Inc.

Pacific Design Center, 8687 Melrose Ave., Suite M-20, Los Angeles CA 90069; (213) 657-6800. Bob Banner, pres.; J. William Hayes, first v.p.; Stephen Pouliot, v.p. (Production of television programs, motion pictures and theatrical productions.)

Barbre Productions, Inc.

Div. of Combined Communications Corporation, P.O. Box 5667, 1089 Bannock Street, Denver, CO 80217, (303) 266-3601. Alvin G. Flanagan, pres.; Jon D. Ackelson, producer/director. (Producer, distributor of filmed shows, producer of film commercials and business films.)

- Prairie World of the Kit Fox (1); Valley of the Standing Rocks (1); Harry Jackson—A Man and His Art; The Troopers Are Coming; Rocky Mountain Conquest.

Robert Baron & Associates

21 West 46 St., New York, NY 10036; (212) 302-1515. Robert Baron, pres., prod.; John Whited, director; West Coast studio facilities, Helen Miles, mgr. & Prod.; Jules Brenner & Gayne Rascher, cameramen; Angie Ross, supervising editor. (Producers of TV commercials, industrials, sales promotion film & multi-media presentations; complete video tape facilities.)

Barry & Enright Productions

1888 Century Park, E., Los Angeles, CA, 90067 (213) 277-3414. Dan Enright, principal.

Ben Barry & Associates, Inc.

10246 Briarwood Drive, Los Angeles, CA 90077; (213) 274-1523. Ben Barry, pres.

- Feature films, including The Family, Honey Comb, Sabra, Action Man, Assassination, I Killed Rasputin, Peking Blonde, Singapore, Singapore, Johnny Banco, Black Sun, Restless Breed, Magnificent Matador, Sword of Monte Cristo, One Russian Summer, etc.
- Feature films, under House of Horrors heading, including The She Beast, Death Dream, Fangs of the Living Dead, The Night Evelyn Came Out of the Grave, Murder Clinic, Children Shouldn't Play with Dead Things, Blood Spattered Bride, Don't Look in the Basement, Nightmare Hotel, Kiss of the Tarantula, Invisible Terror, Zombies. Science fiction features: Star Pilot, Invaders from Mars, Fantastic Invasion from Planet Earth, No Survivors Please, Electronic Monster, Fabulous World of Jules Verne. New: Swingin' Summer, Restless Breed, Magnificent Matador.

Beck, Alexander, Films, Inc.

1540 Broadway, New York, NY 10036; (212) 575-9494. Alexander Beck, president. (Distributes feature films, shorts and Westerns.)

The Behrens Company, Inc.

51 S.W. 9th St., Miami, FL 33130; (305) 371-6077. Robert A. Behrens, pres.; Elizabeth H. Behrens, secty.

Best Film & Video Corporation

98 Cutter Mill Road, Great Neck, NY 11021; (516) 487-4515. Roy Winnick, pres. (Cable, pay TV, free TV, cassette and disc distribution and production).

Milton Blackstone/Associates

P.O. Box 1892, La Jolla, CA 92038; (619) 459-8255. Milton H. Blackstone, exec. prod. (Talent, promotion and special events direction, true-life commercials, pr. films.)

- Comedians' Golf Classic; Comedy Hall of Fame (special); Wonderful World of Water (special); Beach Ball; (Pro) Am Team Golf Championship; Mother Goose Parade (special); Jr. World Golf Championship (special); Defending Champion (series); Let There Be Balls (special); Golf Derby; Show Biz Salutes (series and specials); Sports City (in preparation) '76 Andy Williams Open (90 min.); Feature Film: Cockeyed Charley; New Series in Development; Hobo; Pilot; Something to Celebrate; Days of Pleasure—Nights of Despair.

Blair Entertainment

(A division of John Blair & Co.) 1290 Ave. of Americas, New York, NY 10104; (212) 603-5990. Richard C. Coveny, pres.; Guy Mazeo, exec. v.p.; Tim Harrington, v.p., finance & admin.; Linda Prozeller, bus. mgr.; Leslie Lillien, dir. creative svcs. Domestic Sales: Tony Brown, sr. v.p., genl. sls. mgr.; Joe Middelburg, v.p., natl. sls. mgr.; Jim Weathers, v.p., rgl. sls. mgr.; Monte Lounsbury, rgl. sls. mgr.; Al Lanken, rgl. sls. mgr.; Tony Fasola, rgl. sls. mgr.; Steve Hackett, rgl. sls. mgr.; Joe mirabella, acct. exec.; Paul Franklin, acct. exec.; Rob Roberson, act. exec.; Ken Kagen, v.p., mktg./rsrch.; Ann Foran, rsrch. mgr.; Dorothy Hamilton, dir. sls. svcs.; Sherryl Servello, traffic coord. Advertiser-Supported Sales: Alan Berkowitz, v.p., media mktg.; Howard Levy, v.p., adv. sls.; Norman Lesser, acct. exec. media sls.; Michael Weiser, v.p., dir. stn. clearance; Catherine Morrow, stn. clearance rep.; Marlene Rochman, stn. clearance rep.

- First Run: Strike It Rich (52 week first-run strip series); Divorce Court (52 week first-run series).
- Comedy: SCTV (156 half-hours).
- Series: Death Valley Days (130 half-hours in color); The Cisco Kid (156 half-hours in color).
- Feature Films: Revenge Movie Package (12 features).
- Sports: Wake Up the Echoes (one-hour history of Notre Dame football); NFL Great Moments (50 program inserts for each NFL team); Great Plays from Glory Days (50 program inserts of NFL Super Bowls and World Championships); Legends of College Basketball (90 program inserts); College Football Scrapbook (400 program inserts of regional and specific team vignettes); You Make the Call (program inserts, ABC Network); NFL Classics (program inserts, ABC Network; Fantastic Finishes (program inserts, NBC Network).
- Children's: Beachcombers (130 half-hours in color); Keystone Komedies (79 various lengths).
- Specials: Road to the Superbowl '87 (one-hour major television sports special broadcast prior to the Superbowl); NFL Update '86 (one-hour sports special); The Lollipop Dragon (2 half-hour specials); Telephone Interactive Programs (local market).

Borden Productions

Great Meadows Road, Concord, MA 01742 (617) 369-5030. Dick Borden, pres.; William Sweney, Gordon M. Beck, v.p.

Braverman Productions, Inc.

6290 Sunset Blvd., Suite 905, Hollywood, CA 90028; (213) 466-4111. Charles Braverman, pres.; David Fudge, production mgr. (Producers of feature films, TV specials, documentaries, commercials, titles and special montages, specialists in kinestasis animation.)

Bray Studios, Inc.

19 Ketchum St., Westport, CT 06880; (203) 226-3777. Paul Bray, Jr., pres. (Producers and distributors of films, film strips, slides and multi-media presentations on wide variety of subject matter; services for producers include animation art and photography as well as location crews and equipment.

The Brickyard, Inc.

3487 W. 2100 S., Suite 112, Salt Lake City, UT 84119; (801) 973-3353. L. Dee Johnson, rental & sls. mgr. (Motion picture & television producer's services, equipment rentals, sales, lease & servicing. All facets of production equipment & services.)

Barry Brown Brillig Prod., Inc.

300 Central Park West, New York, NY 10024; (212) 595-5454. Organized 1959; Barry Brown, pres. (Feature motion pictures, industrial films & TV commercials.)

Buena Vista International, Inc.

(A subsidiary of Walt Disney Productions) 350 South Buena Vista St., Burbank, CA 91521; (818) 840-5414. Harold P. Archinal, pres.; Ivan Genit, exec. v.p., Latin Amer. & S. Africa; Dino Troni, v.p., U.K. Europe/Mid East; Rolf Mittweg, v.p. Far East/Australasia; Etienne de Villiers, pres. Buena Vista International TV.

C

Camelot Entertainment Sales, Inc.

1700 Broadway, New York, NY 10119; (212) 315-4747. Richard R. Levy, pres.; Steve Hirsch, v.p., sls.

• Wheel of Fortune; Jeopardy!; Little Rascals Specials; Nightlife with David Brenner; Rock 'n' Roll Evening News; True Confessions; The Oprah Winfrey Show; Women of the World.

Campaign Coaches of Long Island

(A division of F.L.A., Inc.) 80 Winifred Drive, Merrick, NY 11566; (516) 378-4627. Frank C. Beckert, creative director. Richard E. Stember, Miami office manager. (305) 751-4373. (Advertising/public relations/marketing & sales.)

Steve Campus Productions, Inc.

24 Depot Square, Tuckahoe, NY 10707; (914) 961-1900. Steve Campus, pres. (Producer of educational, industrial, medical, documentary films, and multi-media productions.)

Stephen J. Cannell Prods.

7083 Hollywood Blvd., Hollywood, CA 90028. (213) 465-5800.

• The A-Team (NBC); Hardcastle & McCormick (ABC); Hunter (NBC); Riptide (NBC); The Lost Precinct (NBC).

George Carlson & Associates

113 Battery St., Seattle, WA 98121; (206) 441-1466. George Carlson, producer. (Program producers.)

• The Traveler/Northwest Traveler series.

Carthay Sound Stage

5907 West Pico Blvd., Los Angeles, CA (213) 938-2101. (Complete film videotape services & rental center.) Contact: Helen Miles.

Castle Hill Television

1414 Ave. of the Americas, New York, NY 10019 (212) 888-0800; 815 Amherst Ave., Los Angeles, CA 90049 (213) 820-8139. (Distributor)

• Castle Hill–Volume 1 (12 color features); Going Hollywood–The 30's (series).

Centerpoint Productions, Inc.

3575 Cahuenga Blvd., West, Suite 455, Los Angeles, CA 90068. (213) 850-1250. 767 Third Ave., Floor 15, New York, NY 10017. (212) 355-3160. Bill Ellis, chief exec. officer.

Cinecraft, Inc.

2515 Franklin Blvd., Cleveland, OH 44113; (216) 781-2300. Neil McCormick, pres.; Maria Keckan, CEO; (Production facility and services for video and film, for broadcast and corporate.)

Cinema Shares International Television, Ltd.

450 Park Ave., New York, NY 10022; (212) 421-3161. Beverly J. Partridge, pres. (TV distribution.)

Cinetudes Film Productions, Ltd.

295 West 4th St., New York, NY 10014; (212) 924-0400. Christine Jurzykowski, pres.; Gale Goldberg, exec. prod.; Anita Cinnamon, mktg. dir.; Alex Gartner, dir. of devel., prod. & acquisition. (Production of TV programs, motion pictures and theatrical productions)

Cineworld Corporation

P.O. Box 61-276, North Miami, FL 33161; (305) 891-1181. John F. Rickert, pres.; Ildiko M. Rickert, secty./treas. (Distribution, production, international co-production, financing and packaging)

City Film Productions, City Film Center, Inc.

64-12 65th Place, Middle Village, Queens, NY 11379; (718) 456-5050; John R. Gregory, exec. prod. (Producers of 8 mm/16 mm/35 mm motion pictures, for the fields of business, industry, advertising, sales, science, religion, education, health, entertainment and TV. Creative, consultation and production facilities.)

Dick Clark Co.

3003 West Olive Ave., Burbank, CA 91505; (213) 841-3003. Dick Clark pres.; Francis La Maina, exec. v.p., in chg. prod.; Barry Adelman, v.p., television development; Al Schwartz, v.p., prod.; Gene Weed, v.p., prod.; Jeff Margolis, producer/director; Paul Brownstein, v.p., programs & sls.

Coast Productions

1001 N. Pointsettia Place, Hollywood, CA 90046 (213) 876-2021. Jack Yopp, chm.; Steve Dollinger, Tim Galfus, Michael Gottlieb, directors; George Ellison, exec. prod. (Producers of TV commercials).

Coast Special Effects

4907 North Lankershim Blvd, North Hollywood, CA 91601; (213) 762-1182. Phil Kellison, EFX dir.; Nancy Evelyn, Ron Seawright, exec. prods.; Special Effects Directors: Joe Rayner, Dennis Gelbaum; Rich Epstein, producer. (Special effects for TV commercials and feature films.)

Colbert Television Sales

1888 Century Park East, Los Angeles, CA 90067; (213) 277-7751.

• The Joker's Wild (260 half-hours); Tic Tac Dough (260 half-hours); Bullseye (game strip). Rifleman (168). Specials (1 hr. each): Frank Sinatra, Jr. in concert; Bert Convy, Juliet Prowse in Las Vegas; Pia Zadora, Fiesta in Mexico, Frank Sinatra, Jr. in Paradise; Sale of the Century (260); Lassie Half-Hours (192); Lassie Movies (15); Lone Ranger Half-Hours (182); Lone Ranger Features (2); Adventures of the Lone Ranger (13); Sgt. Preston of the Yukon (78); Jeff's Collie (103); Timmy & Lassie (156); Skippy and the Bush Kangaroo (91); The Magic of Lassie (100 min.); Lassie, the New Beginning (2 hrs.).

Columbia Pictures Television

A Division of Columbia Pictures Industries, Inc.—Columbia Plaza, Burbank, CA 91505; (818) 954-6000. (For officers and divisions see listing in Companies section.)

• Features: Features of the 80's, Volume 1 (29); Volume 3 (20); Features of the 70's Volume 1 (30 features); Volume 2 (27); Volume 3 (30); Post 60 Volume 1 (55 features); Volume 2 (50); Volume 3 (51); Volume 4 (33); Volume 5 (39); Volume 6 (26); Volume 7 (30); Post 50 Volume 1 (73); Volume 2 (58); Post 48 (210).
SERIES AVAILABLE: Benson; Fantasy Island; Hart to Hart; Police Woman (91); Soap; S.W.A.T (37); Charlies Angels (110); Starsky & Hutch (90); What's Happening!! (65); Carter Country (44); L.A.T.E.R. (65); Barney Miller (124); Fish (35); Special Edition (24); Partridge Family (96); Bewitched (252); I Dream Of Jeannie (139); Dennis The Menace (146); Father Knows Best (191); Farmer's Daughter (101); Here Come The Brides (52); Wackiest Ship In The Army (29); Gidget (32); Donna Reed Show (175); George Burns and Gracie Allen (239); Hazel (154); Monkees (58); 2 Reel Comedies (162); Serial Package (51); Three Stooges (190); Quick Draw McGraw (135); Batfink; Hanna-Barbera Cartoons; Ruff'n Reddy; Magilla Gorilla; Peter Potamus; Huckleberry Hound and Yogi Bear (276); Flintstones (166); Celebrity Charades (45); Dealer's Choice; Diamond Head Game Show; New Quiz Kids; Wild Bill Hickok; Jungle Jim; Circus Boy; Adventures of Seaspray; Casey Jones; Jet Jackson; Ivanhoe; Tales of the Texas Rangers; Manhunt; Rescue 8; Tightrope; Route 66 (116); Talahassee 7000; Two Faces West; Shannon; Behind Closed Doors; All Star Theatre; Award Theatre; Celebrity Playhouse; Showcase 39; Big Playbook; Decision (26); Conflicts of Harry S. Truman; Winston Churchill, The Valiant Years.

Communication Commission of National Council of the Churches of Christ in the USA.

475 Riverside Drive, New York, NY 10115; (212) 870-2575. William F. Fore, assistant general secretary for communication; D. Williams McClurken, executive director for broadcasting and film; David W. Pomeroy, director, media resources.

• Davey and Goliath (60 films for children); Davey and Goliath specials: Christmas, Lost and Found, Happy Easter, Hallowe'en Who-Dun-It, New Year Promise, To the Rescue, School—Who Needs It!, others (including information about network religious TV programs).

Company of Artists Productions, Inc.

3518 W. Cahuenga Blvd., Suite 301, Hollywood, CA 90068, (213) 851-5811; Tom J. Corradine, exec. prod.; Mark Deemer, v.p. & gen'l. mgr, prod. supervisor; Jay O. Lawrence & Paul Lisy, v.p. video cassette div.; Edward Reagen, v.p., sls. mktg. (Producers of motion pictures & commercials.)

Condor Pictures, Inc.

1536 Viewsite Terrace, Hollywood, CA 90069; (213) OL 2-7447. Milton Simon, gen. mgr. (TV pilot films. Films made to order.)

Contempo Communications Inc.

1841 Broadway, Suite 1111, New York, NY 10023; (212) 247-4444. Joan F. Marshall, pres., (Theatrical, business, documentary, award-winning live shows, mixed-media, motion pictures, video sales mtgs.)

Coproducers Corporation

P.O. Box 61-276 North Miami, FL 33161; (305) 891-1181. John F. Rickert, pres.; Ildiko M. Rickert, secty./treas. (Distribution, production, international co-production, financing and packaging.)

Corporation for Entertainment & Learning, Inc., The

515 Madison Ave., New York, NY 10022; (212) 421-4030. Merton Y. Koplin, chm., chief exec. officer; Sanford H. Fisher, pres., chief operating officer; Charles D. Grinker, vice chm., creative director. (Creators of The Videotape News Library, a visual encyclopedia of America in the 20th Century on motion picture film and tape)

- Series: Creativity with Bill Moyers (PBS); A Walk Thru the 20th Century with Bill Moyers (PBS); The Animal Express (hosted by Joan Embery—130 part series on Entertainment Channel), distributed worldwide by 20th Century Fox; Dining in France, 13 half-hours hosted by Pierre Salinger (PBS); Celebrity Pursuit, 130 thirty-second programs in question & answer format surrounding a thirty-second commercial (syndicated by Program Syndication Services).

Corradine, Tom J., & Associates

3518 W. Cahuenga Blvd., Suite 301, Hollywood, CA., 90068; (213) 851-5811. Branch office in New York. Tom Corradine, pres.; Mark Deemer, v.p.; Bob Morgan, head booker; Edward Reagan, v.p., marketing; Paul Lisy, v.p., video cassette dir. (Distribute filmed series, feature films. Western representative for Weiss Global Enterprises and Bloom Film Group. National reps for TV National Releasing Corp., Lippert Pictures, Inc., and Film Video Releasing Corp.)

- 700 feature films, 192 Westerns, 500 cartoons, 6 series.

William G. Cox Film Enterprises

9726 Edward Drive, Sun City, AZ 85351. William G. Cox, owner-producer. (Produce commercials, news clips informational & public relations films.)

Thomas Craven Film Corporation

114 East 25 St., New York, NY 10010; (212) 777-7433. Michael Craven, pres.; Ernest Barbieri, v.p.; Frynne Hamden, secty. (Producers of films and videotapes. Producers of educational, informational, training, fund-raising, documentary, public relations and television films and tapes for corporate, non-profit and governmental clients. Producers of commercials and public service announcements. Producers of international films and tapes, with extensive overseas production experience. Brochure and additional info available on request.)

- Representative Credits: Recruiting films for Peace Corps; training and promotion films for Volkswagen, Porsche, Peugeot and Audi; training and informational tapes and films for several United Nations agencies; television specials on David Lean; Dylan Thomas and Samuel Taylor Coleridge; numerous films and tapes for U.S. military and governmental agencies.

Bing Crosby Productions, Inc.

6311 Romaine St., Hollywood, CA. 90038; (213) 465-3114. J. R. Rodgers, v.p., finance & business affairs; Ray Tucker, v.p. & secty.; John Boyette, treas. (Motion pictures, television (film & tape) syndication.)

Crossover Programming Company

6290 Sunset Blvd., Suite 905, Hollywood, CA 90028; (213) 466-4111. Charles Braverman, pres. (Producers of pay television series, specials, variety shows. Specialists in kinestasis animation.)

Crystal Pictures, Inc.

1560 Broadway, New York, NY 10036; (212) 757-5130. Joshua Tager, president; S. Tager, dir. of sls. (Distribute features, Westerns, packages & reissue TV series.) Telex: 620852

- 60 features; 200 short subjects; comedies (Charlie Chaplin & other old time comedies) (112); TV series (one hr. and ½ hrs.) (410).

Cummings Productions

℅ C. N. Weber, 5 Whitelaw Place, Baltimore, MD 21236. Ralph Waldo Cummings. (Creation and production of musical commercials, backgrounds, scores for promotional & entertainment projects.)

D

Depicto Films Corp.

504-A Aspen Lane, Wyckoff, NY 07481. J. R. von Maur, president. (Producers of filmed commercials and industrial motion pictures. Sales meeting and conventions, road shows.)

Walt Disney Productions

500 So. Buena Vista, Burbank, CA., 91521; (818) 840-1000; 500 Park Ave., New York, NY, 10022; (212) 593-8900. (For officers and personnel see listing under Companies.)

Documentary Films, Inc.

201 West 52 Street, New York, NY 10019; (212) 582-4318. NY Telex: 420748. Gerald J. Rappoport, Christopher Wood, exec. officers. (Distributor of feature and short documentary films to theatres, television, and non-theatrical markets.)

Dubie-Do Productions, Inc.

New York City (212) 765-4240 or 1 Laurie Drive, Englewood Cliffs, NJ 07632; (201) 568-4214. Richard S. Dubelman, pres. (TV and theatrical productions.)

Dunn Cal. Studios, Inc.

229 West Illinois St., Chicago IL 60610; (312) 644-7600. Deborah Rezzardi, pres. (Producers of motion pictures, multi-screen presentations, TV commercials, slidefilms for sales, training, promotion, indoctrination.)

E

Ralph Edwards Productions

1717 N. Highland Ave., Hollywood, CA 90028. Ralph Edwards, owner. (Creator, packager, producer television shows.)

- The People's Court-syndication.
- This is Your Life-syndication.
- Truth or Consequences—syndication

Ralph Edwards/Stu Billett Productions

1717 N. Highland Ave., Hollywood, CA 90028. (Creator, packager, producer television shows.)

- Superior Court—syndication.

Embassy Communications

1901 Avenue of the Stars, Suite 1600, Los Angeles, CA 90067; (213) 553-3600. (For officers see listing under Companies)

- Current Network Series: Who's the Boss?; The Facts of Life; 227; Sweet Surrender.
- Mini-Series/Features: Kane & Abel; A Greater Alarm; A Place to Call Home; Justice Delayed: The Lenell Geter Story; The Berlin Wall.
- Syndicated Series: The Jeffersons, Diff'rent Strokes; Maude; Sanford & Son; The Facts of Life; Good Times; One Day at a Time; Silver Spoons; Archie Bunker's Place; Square Pegs.

Empire Television

1551 N. LaBrea Ave., Los Angeles, CA 90028; (213) 850-6110. Telex: 4790597 EMPIREINC.

- Theatrical features: Ghoulies; The Dungeonmaster; Walking the Edge; Trancers; The Alchemist; Zone Troopers; Ghost Warrior; Re-Animator; Troll; Mutant Hunt.
- Heroes, Pirates, and Warriors: 14-picture adventure package.

F

Family Films

14622 Lanark Street, Panorama City, CA, 91402. Iris Austin, mgr.

Doris Faye Productions

325 W. 45 St., New York, NY 10036; (212) 246-0430. Organized 1959; Doris Faye, pres. (TV and film packagers; specialists in "educating through comedy" programs.)

Don Fedderson Productions

16255 Ventura Blvd., Suite 1117, Encino, CA 91436; (818) 986-3118. Don Fedderson, chairman of the board.

- My Three Sons (network); Family Affair (network).

The Film Company

111 Barrow St., New York, NY 10014; (212) 620-5654. Peter Bergmann, Anthony Lidelicato, Ronald Saland. (Motion picture production.)

Filmack Studios

1327 S. Wabash Ave., Chicago, IL 60605; (312) 427-3395. Joseph R. Mack, pres.; Robert Mack, v.p. (Motion picture film producer for TV and industry, as well as filmstrips and slides for education.)

Film/Jamel Productions, Inc.

195 So. Beverly Drive, Suite 412, Beverly Hills, CA 90212; (213) 273-7773. Gil Cates, pres. (Producers theatre, films, TV.)

Films Five, Inc.

42 Overlook Rd., Great Neck, NY 11020; (516) 487-5865. Walter Bergman, head of studio oper. (Producers of industrials, documentaries, commercials, live film, videotape & animation. Editorial department & massprint distribution on premises.)

Films of the Nations

7820 20th Ave., Brooklyn, NY 11214; (718) 331-1045. Jerome Schpiro, mgr. (Distributors of TV, industrial and educational free sponsored films.) Color and b/w.

Fima Noveck Productions

321 West 44 St., New York, NY 10036. (212) 315-4220. Fima Noveck, pres. (Production and post-production; commercials; features; MTV.)

Format Productions

4253 Reyes Drive, Tarzana, CA 91356; (818) 987-2390. Herbert Klynn, pres.; Marvin L. Klynn, exec. v.p. Selma Klynn, v.p.; Ruth Page, secty./treas. (Animation films for TV commercials, TV programming, theatrical shorts, feature and industrial films.)

Four Star International, Inc.

2831 W. Alameda Ave., Burbank, CA 91505-4455; (818) 842-9016. Alfred Markim, CEO; Richard Cignarelli, pres., Four Star Distribution.

- Series: Big Valley; Wanted Dead or Alive; Achievers (13½ hrs.).
- Movies: Star Two (15 new films); Star One (15 new films); No Restrictions (13 new films); Cisco Kid Features (13 features); Dick Tracy (8 features); 200 feature films.

Sandy Frank Film Syndication, Inc.

115 East 57 St., Suite 1410, New York, NY 10022; (212) 759-9199. Sandy Frank, pres.

Fries Distribution Company

(A subsidiary of Fries Entertainment, Inc.), 6922 Sunset Blvd., Los Angeles, CA 90028; (213) 466-2266. Telex: 3781675. Regional offices: New York (212) 593-2220; Atlanta (404) 231-0119. (Production and distribution of features and series for TV, cable & home video.)

- TV movie packages: Fries Frame I—27 made-for-TV movies including Adam, Bill, The Burning Bed, The Jayne Mansfield Story and the two-part Dempsey; Fries Frame 2—20 made-for-TV movies including Do You Remember Love, Toughlove, Bitter Harvest, Rosie: The Rosemary Clooney Story and the two-part Martian Chronicles.
- First-run series: Cover Story (26 half-hours of celebrity interviews); Off the Wall (26 half-hours; a weekly comedy magazine).

G

Galaxie Productions, Inc.

P.O. Box 1933, Washington, D.C. 20013; (202) 638-5595. Edward Jasen, president; Dr. Edward von Rothkirch, exec. v.p. & exec. prod.; S. McCormick, secty.-treas.; Paul Malec, chief engineer (Produce & distribute films for non-theatrical motion pictures & television: commercials, travelogues, documentaries, language dubbing on film, complete sound stage for audio recording, custom recording on tape or disk. Fully equipped audio visual, motion picture, & VTR remote truck for sound motion picture, VTR, & still photography. Branch offices: ℅ A. L. Weintraub, 5th Floor, 2250 S.W. 3rd Ave., Miami, FL 33129 & C.P.O. Box 1711, Tokyo 100-91 Japan; ℅ V.J. Pandhi, Suite 6G, 102–45 62nd Rd., Rego Park, NY 11375.

Gilson International

9200 Sunset Blvd., Los Angeles, CA 90069.

- Series: Hill Street Blues, Remington Steele, St. Elsewhere, Newhart, White Shadow, WKRP in Cincinnati, Last Resort, MTM Variety Hour, Paris, Duck Factory, Betty White Show, Doc, Three for the Road, Tony Randall Show, We've Got Each Other, Phyllis, Mary.
- Films: Boy Who Drank Too Much, Fighting Back, First You Cry, In Defense of Kids, Nowhere to Run, Something for Joey, Thornwell, Vampire, Critical List (4-hr. mini-series).

Glen Glenn Sound Co. (Todd-Ao Corp.)

900 North Seward Street, Hollywoodm CA 90038; (213) 469-7221. Robert Knudson, pres.; Ron Ward, opns. (Complete film and video-tape sound recording services for feature motion pictures and television programs).

Glenar Studios

211 S. Rose, Burbank, CA, 91505; (213) 848-0408. Sid Glenar, owner. (Produces films, commercials & animation.)

Melvin L. Gold Enterprises

301 East 48 St., New York, NY; (212) 688-0897. Mel Gold, pres. (Consultant, producer and packager of live and film TV programs, industrial films, commercials, features.)

Goodson-Todman Productions

375 Park Ave., New York, NY 10152; (212) 751-0600. 6430 Sunset Blvd., Hollywood, CA 90028; (213) 464-4300. Mark Goodson, owner; Giraud Chester, exec. v.p., Alan R. Sandler, v.p., finance; Gil Fates, exec. prod.; Howard Felsher, Frank Wayne, Chester Feldman, Jonathan Goodman, Mimi O'Brien, producers; Paul Alter, Marc Breslow, directors.

- The Rebel (film); The Richard Boone Show, Branded (film); Beat the Clock; To Tell The Truth; What's My Line; Password; The Price Is Right; Match Game PM; Tattletales; I've Got A Secret (all tape); Family Feud; Card Sharks; Match Game; Mind Readers; Password Plus; Child's Play; Body Language; Trivia Trap; Super Password.

Goulding-Elliott-Greybar Productions, Inc.

420 Lexington Avenue, New York, NY 10017; (212) 532-9014. Organized 1955. Ray Goulding pres./secty.; Bob Elliott, v.p./treas. (Production of radio and TV commercials and radio & TV programs.)

Granada Television International

1221 Avenue of Americas, Suite 3468, New York, NY 10020.

- First Among Equals; Game, Set and Match; Lost Empires; Floodtide; Death of the Heart; Man and Music; 27 Up; The Jewel in the Crown; The Return of Sherlock Holmes.

Sherry Grant Enterprises

17915 Ventura Blvd., Suite 208, Encino, CA 91316; (818) 705-2535.

Gray-Schwartz Enterprises, Inc.

Teleflix Division, 4764 Park Granada, #207, Calabasas, CA 91302; (818) 702-9888. Marv Gray, pres.

Greatest Fights of the Century, Inc.

9 East 40th St., New York, NY 10016; William D. Cayton, pres.; Jim Jacobs, dir. (Produce and distribute fight films.)

- Big Fights of the Decades Series (formerly titled Greatest Fights of the Century) 500 quarter-hour programs from 1900–1985, featuring all the world champions, each in his greatest, and most memorable fight, including George Foreman, Joe Frazier, Mohammad Ali, Floyd Patterson, Rocky Marciano, Joe Louis, Jack Dempsey, Sugar Ray Robinson, Rocky Graziano, Archie Moore, Larry Holmes, Marvin Hagler, Boom Boom Mancini, etc.

Group W Productions (Westinghouse Broadcasting Company)

3801 Barham Blvd., Los Angeles, CA 90068; (213) 850-3800. Edwin T. Vane, pres. & CEO; George E. Resing Jr., sr. v.p.; Kevin Tannehill, v.p., sls. & mktg.; Owen S. Simon v.p., creative services. Leonard T. Giarraputo, v.p., sls.; Carol Strond, v.p., research; Gerard Farrell, v.p., sls. research; Nancy Hamilton, v.p., operations; Jeff Snetiker, v.p., controller; Dan Cosgrove, v.p., media sls.; Tony Dwyer, v.p., domestic sls.; Fred Kuperberg, v.p., business affairs; Christine Foster, v.p., pgm. devel.

- Hour Magazine (5 shows weekly, 60 mins.); PM Magazine Program Service; He-Man and the Masters of the Universe (130 half hrs.); Bill Cosby's Adventures of Fat Albert (90 half hrs.); She-Ra: Princess of Power (93 half-hrs.); BraveStarr (65 half-hours).

Gutman, Leo A., Inc.

230 Park Ave., New York, NY; (212) 682-5652.

- Hennessey—96 half-hours (b & w), starring Jackie Cooper and a host of guest stars.

Guymark Studios, Inc.

3019 Dixwell Ave., Hamden, CT 06518. Anthony Guarino, Jr., pres.; Guy Guarino, v.p., chg. of photo; Mark Guarino, v.p., chg. of audio & video. (Producers facilities and technical services for sound film video animation, product photography. 1200 sq. ft. sound stage w/ cyclorama complete ¼″ & 16 mm sound studios, all format still photography studio, 16 mm animation studio, slide to film transfer, film to video transfer, ¾″ video editing, Time Code, digital video effects, character & graphics generator.)

H

H-R Productions, Inc.

159 West 53 St., New York, NY 10019; (212) 541-8015. Herbert Rosen, president. (Producer of films, package shows.)

Handel Film Corporation

8730 Sunset Blvd., W. Hollywood, CA 90069; (213) 657-8990. Leo A. Handel, pres.; Peter Mertens, producer. (Produces filmed series.)

- Magic of the Atom (10); The Age of the Atom (color special); Sweden-Vikings Today Style (color special); (color special); Police Dog; 1-hr TV special (1972); Art in America (series 1983–10); Thailand 1983; Phillipines 1984; Computer Series 1983–; Measuring Things (series 3) 1985; Singapore 1986.

Hanna-Barbera Productions, Inc.

(A Division of The Taft Entertainment Company) 3400 Cahuenga Blvd., Hollywood, CA 90068; (213) 851-5000. Joseph Barbera, pres.; William Hanna, sr. v.p.; Richard Sigler, v.p. bus. affairs; Jean MacCurdy, v.p., children's programs; John Michaeli, v.p. communications; Ross Sutherland, v.p. dir., personnel & labor relations; Iwao Takamoto, v.p. creative design; Maurice Morton, v.p. & gen. mgr; Joseph Taritero, v.p., creative affairs; Sam Edwing, v.p., development; Paul DeKorte, v.p. music; Jayne Barbera, v.p., animation production.

- Animated Series: The 13 Ghosts of Scooby-Doo (ABC); The Super Powers Team Galactic Guardians (ABC); The Snorks (NBC); The Jetsons (SYN); Challenge of the Gobots (SYN); Paw Paws (SYN); Funtastic Treasure Hunt (SYN); Galtar and the Golden Lance (SYN); The Greatest Adventure: Stories from the Bible (SYN).
- Animated Specials: Star Fairies (SYN); Pound Pupplies (SYN).

Larry Harmon Pictures Corp.

650 North Bronson Ave., Hollywood, CA 90004 (213) 463-2331. Larry Harmon, pres.

Harmony Gold U.S.A.

8831 Sunset Blvd., Los Angeles, CA 90069; (213) 652-8720. (Producer-distributor)

- Animated cartoon series: Captain Harlock (65 half-hr. episodes); Robotech (85 half-hr. episodes).
- Shaka Zulu (10 hour mini-series).
- Raggedy Ann & Andy (3 holiday specials).
- Bonzai Theater (19 90-min. features).
- Family Animation Showcase (20 animated features.
- 2-Part Classics (six 2-part, 4-hour series).
- Harmony Golden I (mini-package of 5 first-run features).
- Ghosts & Gold (26 half-hours, hosted by Robert Stack).
- Eye on Hollywood (65 half-hours).

Harris-Tuchman Productions, Inc.

4293 Sarah St., Burbank, CA 91505; (818) 841-4100. Ralph G. Tuchman, pres. & gen. mgr.; Fran Harris, v.p. & creative dir. (Producers of sales, training and industrial films.)

Harriscope Broadcasting Corporation

10889 Wilshire Blvd., Suite 1240, Los Angeles, CA 90024. Burt I. Harris, pres.; Jack Rosenthal, exec. v.p. & pres., broadcast div.; Harvey Simpson, finance dir.; Ruth Bender, exec. asst. (Production distribution of filmed programs and radio & TV broadcasting and CATV.)

- Jalopy Races From Hollywood (26); Main Event Wrestling (65); Beyond The Yukon (13); All Girl Wrestling (26); Blackstone, The Magician (39); So This Is Hollywood (24).

Hartley Film Foundation Inc.

59 Cat Rock Road, Cos Cob, CT 06807; (203) 869-1818. Elda Hartley, pres. (Producer of films and video tapes on philosophy, psychology, religion, and health.)

Henley, Arthur, Productions

234 Fifth Avenue, New York, NY 10001; (212) 263-0136. Arthur Henley, president. (Production, writing consultation, live and film.)

- Make Up Your Mind.

I

ITC Entertainment, Inc.

115 East 57 St., New York, NY 10022; (212) 371-6660. West Coast offices: 1271 Ventura Blvd., Studio City, CA 91604; (213) 760-2110. Arthur Kananack, pres.

Domestic Distribution: James C. Stern, exec. v.p. & gen. sls. mgr.; Charles Keys, v.p., western div. sls. mgr.; John Herrin, v.p. southern div. sls. mgr.; Reid Davis, v.p., midwestern sls. mgr.

International Distribution: Armando Nuñez, exec. v.p., foreign sales; Doralea Rosenberg, gen. mgr., ITC of Canada.

Acquisitions: Elliott Abrams, exec. v.p., acquisitions.

Creative & Production Services: Murray Horowitz, exec. v.p., advertising-public relations.

- Series: The Muppet Show (120 half-hours, color); Thunderbirds 2086 (24 half-hours, color); The Saint (114 hrs., 43 color); Return of The Saint (22, color); Edward The King (13 one-hours, color); When Havoc Struck (12 half-hours, color); The Protectors (52 half-hours); My Partner the Ghost (26 hours); Department S (28 hours); The Persuaders (22 hours); The Adventurer (26 half-hours); The Baron (26 hours); Man in a Suitcase (28 hours); The Prisoner (17 hours); Secret Agent (45 hours); Fury (114 half-hours); Space: 1999 (40 hours, color).
- Features: Entertainment Volume Six (16 features in color, including "Amos," "Not My Kid," & "Malice in Wonderland"); Entertainment Volume Five (16 features in color, including "All of Me," "Halloween," & "Sophie's Choice"); Entertainment Volume Four (16 features in color, including "On Golden Pond," "The Great Muppet Caper," & "The Elephant Man"); Entertainment Volume Three (16 features in color including "The Muppet Movie," All Quiet on the Western Front," & "The Jazz Singer"); Entertainment Volume Two (16 features in color, including "The Boys from Brazil," "Capricorn One," & "Movie, Movie"); Entertainment, Volume One (14 features in color, including "The Return of the Pink Panther," "The Eagle Has Landed," and "Great Expectations"); The Thrillers (43 made-for-television movies, color). SST: Super Space Theatre (13 science fiction films); Hammer House of Horror Double Feature (6 double features or 12 one-hr. features); Cinema 12 (12 features).

- Specials: Superlative Seven (musical-variety hour specials, color, starring Julie Andrews, Steve Lawrence, Eydie Gorme, Ethel Merman, etc.); The Very Special Seven (musical-variety hour specials, color, starring Julie Andrews, Peggy Lee, Dick Van Dyke, etc.)

Independent-International Pictures Corp.

Executive Plaza, 223 Route 18, East Brunswick, NY 08816; (201) 249-8982. Samuel M. Sherman, pres.; Dan Q. Kennis, chmn.; Al Adamson, exec. v.p. (Television distributor and packager-producer of feature film packages, TV specials, TV series.)

- Feature packages: Scream Showcase: Beyond the Living, Demons of the Dead, Doctor Dracula, Exorcism at Midnight, In Search of Dracula, Man with the Synthetic Brain, Midnight, Ship of Zombies, Terror of Frankenstein, Vampire Men of the Lost Planet, Hand of Power, Night Fiend, Horror of the Werewolf, Voice from the Grave; Action Group: The Gun Riders, Mission to Death, The Fakers, Queen of Sheba, The Barbarians, Submarine Attack, Fighting Rats of Tobruk, Money; Drive In Theatre: The Murder Gang, Intrigue in the Orient, Blazing Stewardesses, The Naughty Stewardesses, Trapped in the Desert, The Smiling Maniacs, Syndicate Sadists.

Independent Network, Inc.

11150 Olympic Blvd., West Los Angeles, CA 90064; (213) 479-6755. Irv Holender, pres.; Irving D. Ross, Dir. of U.S. sls. (Distribution & syndication; producers of films.)

- 26 hours of G.L.O.W. (Gorgeous Ladies of Wrestling).
- 16 feastures—Movie Madness #1.
- 14 features—Ninja/KungFu Theatre.
- 20 hours—Delta Heat (action adventure).

Interlingual Television, K.K.

Mori Building No. 7, No. 2 Nishikubo Tomoecho, Shiba, Minato-Ku Tokyo, Japan. Tel.: 434-2506; Cable Interlingual Tokyo; Telex: J22862, Interlin, Tokyo. Largest independent distributor of Television films in the the Far East, with affiliate offices in Australia, USA, Europe. Sub-licenses in Japan and other countries over 4,000 half-hours of telecasting film of U.S., European and Australian origin.

- Adventures of Long John Silver; Space Angel Cartoons; Four Seasons of Japan; Speed and Action; Big Challenge; Golf Around the World; Wings to Adventure; Let's Travel; World's Great Adventures; Pilopat and Pitafil; Popeye the Sailor; Funny Company; Joe & The Bees; New Avengers; Spunky & Tadpole; The Living Ocean; In the Kingdom of the Dolphin; Wild World of the East; The Lighthouse; Alburria—A Trip to Remember; Here Comes the Grump; Texas Jack and His Pals; Famous Fairytales; Wonderful World of Brother Buzz; Feature films (color, 27 titles); George; Color Classics—The Best of the Past.

International Film Bureau Inc.

332 S. Michigan Ave., Chicago, IL 60604; (312) 427-4545. Wesley Greene, pres. (Distributes live action, animated shorts, documentaries. Curriculum and general audience films for television.)

International Film Exchange, Ltd. (A Heritage Entertainment Co., Inc.)

201 West 52 Street, New York, NY 10019; (212) 582-4318; Cable: IFEXREP—New York; Telex: 420748. FAS: (212) 956-2257. Gerald J. Rappoport, Christopher Wood, Beulah Rappoport, Joy Pareths, exec. officers. (International distributors and producers of theatrical, non-theatrical, educational and television films.)

K

Stacy Keach Productions

5216 Laurel Canyon Blvd., North Hollywood, CA 91607; (213) 877-0472. Stacy Keach, Sr., pres.; Mary Keach, v.p.; Andrew J. Davis, secty. (Producer of films, commercials, public information films.)

- Properties: The Living Constitution Of The United States; The Declaration Of Independence; Your Living Bill of Rights As Interpreted By The U.S. Supreme Court; Living Proof; Back In Action; Approved Exercises for Senior Citizens; Approved Exercises for The Heart Patient.

M. A. Kempner, Inc.

4699 North Federal Highway, Pompano Beach, FL 33064; (305) 946-7660. Marvin A. Kempner, pres.

Killiam Shows, Inc.

6 E. 39 St., New York, NY 10016; (212) 679-8230. Paul Killiam, pres.; John Rogers, v.p. (Produces and distributes programs about silent films.)

King Features Entertainment Inc.

235 East 45 St., New York, NY 10017; (212) 682-5600. Telex: 7105812391. J. F. D'Angelo, chm.; Bruce L. Paisner, pres.; William E. Miller, exec. v.p.; Leonard Soglio, v.p, domestic sls. mgr.; Samuel Gang, intl. sls. mgr.

King International Corporation

124 Lasky Drive, Beverly Hills, CA 90212; (213) 274-0333. Frank King, pres.; Herman King, v.p. (Produces TV series.)

- Maya

King World Productions, Inc.

1700 Broadway, New York, NY 10010; (212) 315-4000. 150 El Camino Dr., Suite 305, Beverly Hills, CA 90212; (213) 858-1833. 980 N. Michigan Ave., Suite 1400, Chicago, IL 60611; (312) 337-6765. Roger M. King, bd. chm.; Michael G. King, pres.; Sid Cohen, sr. v.p., sls.

- Properties: ½ hr. strips: Wheel of Fortune, Jeopardy!, Headline Chasers. Movie Packages: Classic Detectives (34); Epics (5); Spotlight 10 (10); Popcorn Theatre (15). Off-net: Topper, Guns of Will Sonnett, Branded. Specials: Drug Wars (1 hr.), Wards of the Street (1 hr.).

Walter J. Klein Company, Ltd.

6311 Carmel Road, Box 2087, Charlotte, NC 28211-2087; (704) 542-1403. Walter J. Klein, pres.; Richard A. Klein, v.p. sales; David Jordan, controller; Betsy Klein, print sales dir.; Roxanne Mason, distribution dir.; Terry Losardo, production dir.; David Sherwin, editorial dir.; Charles Shedd, Dan Boyd, Charles Merzbacher, Joe Schumacher, Terry Shield, Julie Johnston, directors; Brady Brandwood, editor; Elizabeth Norkum, Lisa Wood, Barbara Cade, distribution assts.; Denise Joseph, Sandra Newton, Betty Stephens, Mary Babcock, John Edwards, administration. (Production and free distribution of sponsored films for industry, TV, government, associations for 38 years. complete film facilities on 2-acre lot. Member CINE, SMPTE, PRSA, AFI, AVC, IABC, CPRS.)

L

LBS Communications, Inc.

875 Third Ave., New York, NY 10022; (212) 418-3000; 9220 Sunset Blve., Suite 101-A, Los Angeles, CA (213) 859-1055; 625 N. Michigan Ave., Suite 1200, Chicago, IL 60611 (312) 943-0707. Phil Howort, pres., LBS Broadcast Group; Roger Lefkon, pres., LBS Entertainment; Mort Marcus, pres., Colex Enterprises; Paul Siegel, pres., LBS Enterprises.

- Children's Animation: Mask (75 episodes); Inspector Gadget (86); Heathcliff (86); Kideo TV (49); Kideo Theatre (8—90 min.)
- First-Run & Off-Network Syndication: The New Gidget (44 episodes); Strictly Business; Father Murphy (35); Tales from the Darkside (92)

The Landsburg Co., Inc.

11811 West Olympic Blvd., Los Angeles, CA 90064; (213) 478-7878. Alan Landsburg, chm. of bd.; Howard Lipstone, pres; Kay Hoffman, exec. v.p.; Joan Barnett, v.p., movies & mini-series; Jane Lipstone, v.p., pub.; Mark Pedowitz, v.p., business affairs; Bob Ames, controller. (Producer for TV and theatrical films and TV film and tape series.)

Don Lane Pictures, Inc.

35 West 45 St., New York, NY 10036; (212) 840-6355. Donald J. Lane, pres.; John Armstrong, producer/director; Carol Laufer, prod. mgr. (Produces commercial motion pictures, slide films and video cassettes; news films.)

Herbert S. Laufman & Company

8140 Rideway, Skokie, IL 60076; (312) 675-4578. Herbert S. Laufman,. pres. (Producers and distributors of live & film programs.)

- It's Baby Time (52).

Robert Lawrence Enterprises, Inc.

305 Madison Avenue, New York, NY 10165; (212) 996-2836. Robert L. Lawrence.

Herbert Leonard Enterprises, Inc.

5300 Fulton Ave., Van Nuys, CA 91401; (818) 783-0457. Herbert B. Leonard, pres.; Walter Bernstein, v.p.; James P. Tierney, Esq., secty. (Producers of filmed series and feature films.)

- Herbert B. Leonard produced Rin Tin Tin (164); Naked City (138); Route 66 (116); Popi (U.A.); produced and directed Going Home (MGM); Ladies Man (series); Breaking Away (pilot).

Liberty Studios, Inc.

238 East 26th Street, New York, NY 10010; (212) 532-1865. Organized 1961. Anthony Lover, pres., producer-director; David Bruce, George Apostol, directors. (Complete live action and special effects production, including motion control graphics, blue screen. Owns and operates fully equipped sound stages, editing/optical facilities, camera lighting, grip and sound equipment, equipment transfer trucks for sound stage as well as location shooting. Video production includes off-line room and on-line Beta.)

Jack Lieb Productions, Inc.

200 East Ontario St., Chicago, IL 60611. Warren H. Lieb, pres.; Charles Kite, editor; Sharon Lloyd Spence, prod. mgr. (Audiovisual producers).

Lorimar-Telepictures Television

3970 Overland Ave., Culver City, CA 90230; One Dag Hammarskjold Plaza, New York, NY 10017; (212) 735-1500. (For officers see listing under Companies)

- Network series: Dallas; Falcon Crest; Knots Landing; Valerie; Perfect Strangers; Better Days; Our House.
- First-run syndication: Mama's Family; One Big Family; It's a Living; ThunderCats; $1 Million Chance of a Lifetime; Love Connection; The People's Court; SilverHawks; Superior Court.
- Mini-series: The Two Mrs. Grenvilles.
- Movies: Baby Talk; Ghost of a Chance; Here a Thief, There a Thief.
- **Worldwide Product**
- Theatrical Features: Fire and Ice; Little Lord Fauntleroy; Dead and Buried; Final Countdown; Jaguar Lives; A Change of Seasons; The Hideaways; A Pleasure Doing Business; Riding Tall; The Savage Is Loose; Matilda; Phobia; The Silent Flute; O'Hara's Wife; Ride in the Wind; Smash Palace; The Wanderers; Phantasm; The Shooting; St. Helen's; Baltimore Bullet; City on Fire; Apprenticeship of Duddy Kravits; Smash Palace; Young Doctors in Love; etc. The Guys at Max's Bar; The Boat; Death Ship.
- Television Features: All the Kind Strangers; Angel City; Before and After; Better Late Than Never; Born to Be Sold; A Christmas Without Snow; Dark Night of the Scarecrow; The Daybreakers; Death of a Princess; Desperate Voyage; Exploring the Unknown; The Great American Traffic Jam; A Gun in the House; "Hey Abbott!"; The Last Giraffe; The Last Song; Look Back in Anger; Mark I Love You; The Pride of Jesse Hallam; A Private Battle; The Promise of Love; Reunion; Rivkin: Bounty Hunter; Another Story; The Suicide's Wife; 300 Miles for Stephanie; Vincent; They All Laughed; Daredevil Drivers; Coming Out of the Ice; The Sins of Dorian Gray; The Flight of the Drapers; The Wind in the Willows; High Rolling; etc.
- Mini-series: Alcatraz: The Whole Shocking Story; The Golden Moment; Guyana Tragedy: The Story of Jim Jones; Murder in Texas; The Sacketts; A Whale for the Killing; World War III.
- Series: Caribbean Nights; The Challengers; Detective School; Fridays; Games People Play; Here's Lucy; Look at U*S; My Favorite Martian; The People's Court; 24 Days of Christmas; The Game of the Century; Real People.
- Documentaries: Footsteps of Giants; Lost Treasure of the Concepcion; Princess; Americas in Transition; Five American Guns.
- Specials: The Beach Boys Rockin' at the Queen Mary; Boo; Alabama and Friends; "Freddie the Freeloader's Christmas Dinner"; "The Last Great Vaudeville Show"; Debby Boone; The Third Annual National Cheerleading Championship; The Fourth Annual National Collegiate Cheerleading Championship; James Clavell's "The Children's Story"; An Evening with Quentin Crisp; The Grammy Hall of Fame; Grandpa; Will You Run With Me?; The Heisman Trophy Special; David Sheehan's Hollywood; Lorette Lynn—The Lady and the Legend; The Manhattan Transfer; The Sound of Applause; Simon and Garfunkel Reunion Concert; Victor Borge in Concert; 1981 World Open Pocket Billiards Championships; 100 Years of Golden Hits; Three Animated Holiday Specials.
- Children's Series: The Little Kids' All-Star Band; The Magic Star Traveler; Memoirs of a Fairy Godmother; Mr. Moon's Magic Circus; Gepetto's Music Shop; The Great Space Coaster; The Waterville Gany.
- News Service: N.I.W.S. (News Information Weekly Service)

Lott Video Productions

The Lott Building, P.O. Box 1107, Santa Monica, CA; (213) 397-4217. D. N. Lott, owner. (Producers of film commercials.)

M

MCA Television

445 Park Ave., New York, NY 10022; (212) 759-7500. West Coast: 100 Universal Plaza, Universal City, CA 91608; (818) 985-4321. (For officers see listing under Companies)

- Latest product: Charles in Charge (52 half-hr. episodes); Kate & Allie (96 half-hrs.); Knight Rider (90 hrs. or 90 half-hrs.); Universal Pictures Prestige 13 (features, including Hitchcock's Rope and The Trouble with Harry); Universal Pictures Exploitable 13 (films including Repo Man, Terror in the Aisles, Streets of Fire, etc.); The A Team (128 hrs.); Harper Valley (52 half-hrs.); Operation Petticoat (152 half-hrs.); Blinkins (3 half-hr. specials); Universal's Marvelous Ten (movies, including Captain America, Munster's Revenge, etc.); Puttin' on the Hits Year 3 (36/16 half-hrs.); Universal Pictures Debut Network II (25 features, including Mask, The Breakfast Club, Fletch, The River, Scarface, etc.); Street Hawk/The Insiders (52 hrs.).
- Series: One-hour: Simon & Simon (125); Black Sheep Squadron (35); Magnum (129); The Columbo/McCloud/McMillan Mystery Movies (124); Quincy (148); Buck Rogers (37 1-hr. or 25 1-hrs. & 6 two-hrs.); Kojak (118); The Rockford Files (125); BJ/Lobo Show (86 half-hrs. or 86 hrs.); The Incredible Hulk (85); Emergency! (136); Olivia Newton-John Let's Get Physical (1 hr. music special); Half-hours: Gimme a Break (112); That's Incredible (165); House Calls (57); Leave It to Beaver (234); McHale's Navy (138); The Munsters (70); 90-min.: Banacek (16).
- Features: Universal Pictures Debut Network (33 features); Universal's Most Wanted List (23); The Hit List (36); Universal Network Movies 85 (52 two-hr., 33 1½ hrs.); Battlestar Galactica (12 two-hr. movies or 24 one-hrs.); Champagne Movies 34 (34); Ninety Minute Movies (49); Universal Grand 50 (48); Universal Star Spangled 33 (48); Universal World Premieres (35 two-hr movies); Comedy Festival I (26); Comedy Festival II (26); Universal 40 (39); :Universal 49 (49); Universal 52 (52); Universal 50 (45); Paramount Pre '48 (496); Paramount 100 Select (100); Universal 53 (52); Universal 123 (116); Universal 260 Select List (260 features, 90 color); Universal Color One Hundred (99); Universal 36 Black and White Elite (36); 77 Horror Greats (77); Western Roundup (26); Reserve (259); Diabolic Dozen (12).
- Encore Programs: All 1-hr. shows except where indicated: Baretta (82); Alias Smith & Jones (43); The Six Million Dollar Man (108); The Bionic Woman (58); Switch (70); Five Star Myster (87); The Bold ONes (98); Ironside (198); It Takes a Thief (65); The Name of the Game (76 1½ hrs.); Rod Serling's Night Gallery (97 half-hrs.); Run for Your Life (85); Rich Man, Poor Man Book 1 (12 hrs. in 1-hr., 2-hrs. or 90-min.); Best Sellers II (33); The Deputy (76 half-hrs.); Mickey Spillane's Mike Hammer (78 half-hrs.); Thriller (67); Men fro Shilo(23 ninety-min. movies); Wagon Train (32 ninety-min. episodes); Dead End Kids Movies (7 movies).

MCA Television International

100 Universal City Plaza, Universal City, CA 91608; (818) 777-1000. Robert E. Bramson, pres.; Colin P. Davis, exec. v.p. Foreign Offices: Brazil: Rua Said Aiach, 305, São Paulo, Brazil; 884-0166. Wanderley Fucciolo, v.p. Australia: Universal House, Poplst & Pelican St., Sydney, NSW, Australia 2000; 267-0944. Pat Cleary, v.p. Japan: Maison Kirakawa Bldg., 2-5-2 Hirakawa-cho, Chiyoda-ku; 265-5726. Keinosuke Kuragaki, v.p. Canada: 2450 Victoria Park Ave., Willowdale, Toronto, Ontario M2J 4A2, Canada; (416) 491-3000. Peter Hughes, v.p. Beirut, Lebanon: 1324 Mme. Curie St., Sammakieh Bldg., Beirut; 369-175. Kamal Sayegh, v.p. France: 8 Rue La Boetie, Paris 75008, France; 265-9780. Claude Perrier, v.p. Hendrik van Daalen, v.p. England: 139 Piccadilly, London W.1, England. 629-7211; Don Gale, v.p., U.K.

- Properties: Airwolf (47 one-hrs.); Alfred Hitchcock Presents (22 half-hrs.); All the News (2-hr pilot; 5 one-hr. episodes); Amen (13 half-hrs.); The A-Team (108 one hrs.); Blacke's Magic (14 one-hrs.); Blinkins (3 half-hrs.); Dalton (6 one-hrs.); The Equalizer (44 one-hr.); Fast Times (17 half-hrs.); George Burns Comedy Week (13 half-hrs.); Gimme a Break (134 half-hrs.); He's the Mayor (13 half-hrs.); The Insiders (13 one-hrs.); Knight Rider (90 one-hrs.); Leo & Liz in Beverly Hills (6 half-hrs.); Magnum (151 one-hrs.); Miami Vice (68 one-hrs.); Misfits of Science (17 one-hrs.); Murder She Wrote (70 one-hrs.); The New Leave It to Beaver (27 half-hrs.); Outlaws (1 two-hrs., 5 one-hrs.); Puttin' on the Hits (113 half-hrs.); Simon & Simon (129 one-hrs.); Still the Beaver (39 half-hrs.); Together We Stand (13 half-hrs.).

MGM/UA Television Distribution

1350 Avenue of the Americas, New York, NY 10019; (212) 708-0300. (For officers and personnel see listing under Companies.)

MGS Services

A subsidiary of Viacom International Inc., New York, NY, 619 W. 54 St., 10019; (212) 765-4500. Chicago, IL: 201 E. Erie St., 60611; (312) 337-3761; Los Angeles, CA: 10507 Burbank Blvd., N. Hollywood, CA 91601; (818) 508-5488.

MPO Videotronics, Inc.

619 West 54 St., New York, NY 10019; (212) 708-0560. Judd Pollock, pres.; 640 N. La Salle St., Chicago, IL 60610 (312) 527-3680; Hal Thompson, mgr.; Dallas, TX (214) 348-2728; Atlanta, GA (404) 875-0015; 2580 Turquoise Circle, Newbury Park, CA 91320; (805) 499-8513. Larry Kaiser.

MRC Films & Video

71 West 23rd Street, New York, NY 10010; (212) 989-1754. Lawrence Mollot, exec. producer. (Producer of industrial, documentary and television films and videocassettes. Also sound slide and filmstrip presentations and multi media productions.)

Madison Square Garden Network

2 Pennsylvania Plaza, New York, NY 10121; (212) 563-8000. Robert Gutowski, pres.; Bill Hyland,, sr. v.p./business affairs; John Taliaferro, pres., Hughes Television; sr. v.p., MSG Network; gen. mgr., Cablevision; Phil Harmon, sr. v.p./programming and production; James J. Cavazzini, exec. v.p.; Linda Burns, v.p./marketing; Doug Moss, v.p./advertising sls.; Pete Silverman, v.p./exec. producer; Karen Metsky, dir. public relations.

- Live Events: New York Knickerbockers basketball; New York Rangers hockey; College football and basketball, pro wrestling, pro boxing, track and field, tennis.

Manley Productions, Inc.

111 West 57 St., New York, NY 10019; (212) 541-7733. Walter H. Manley, gen. mgr.; Pat Hart, sls. mgr. Cable: Waltmanly Telex: 421832. (Producers and distributors.)

Manson International/Manson Television

11355 West Olympic Blvd., Los Angeles, CA 90064; (213) 208-8899. Telex: 188198 (TRT), 691242 (WUI). FAX: (213) 479-4729. Michael F. Goldman, pres.; Michael J. Werner, v.p. intl. sls. (Distributors of feature films, documentaries and entertainment specials to the international theatrical, video, cable TV and broadcast TV markets) Member NAPTE.

- 250-plus feature films, including three packages: Gallery of Terror, Galaxy Collection, Family Classics.

Marathon International Productions, Inc.

211 East 51 St., New York, NY 10022; (212) 688-1130. Konstantin Kalser, pres. and exec. producer. (Produce & distribute motion pictures and public information films.)

Medallion TV Enterprises, Inc.

8831 Sunset Blvd., W. Hollywood, CA 90069; (213) 652-8100. Telex: 910-490-1139. John A. Ettlinger, production. (Producers and distributors of film programs for TV, commercials, packages of live programs, lòcal and network.)

- Celebrity Billiards (30); Wrestling Stars of the 60s; High Road To Danger (39); Kingdom of the Sea (41); Wonders of the World (117); Star Route (26); Creeping Terror Package—Volumes I, II, III & IV, 20/20 Feature Package; Las Vegas Fight of the Week (26); The New Roller Derby (26 hrs.); Wrestling Spectacular (26 hrs.); Man Who Skied Down Mt. Everest (90 min. special); Dinah East (95 min. special); Something Else (39 half hrs.); Scrooge 'n' Jud; The Making of ... (26 half-hrs.); Action I-Action II (60 min. specials).

Milner-Fenwick, Inc.

2125 Greenspring Drive, Timonium, MD 21093; (301) 252-1700. David Milner, pres.; Richard Milner, v.p.; Michael Quitt, sales mgr., v.p. (Producers of medical, educational, training and documentary films and video-tapes—16mm, Super 8mm, ¾" and ½" video. Full motion picture services including sound recording, animation, live photography and editing.

Mode-Art Pictures

3075 West Liberty Avenue, Pittsburgh, PA 15216; (412) 343-8700. Robert L. Stone, gen. mgr.; James M. Seng, mgr. (Producers of documentary and industrial sales and safety films and television commercials. Also owns and operates a 930-seat theatre for motion pictures, live stage, teleconferences, meetings & seminars.)

Mode 2 Productions

3075 West Liberty Avenue, Pittsburgh, PA 15216; (412) 343-8700. Robert L. Stone, pres.; James M. Seng, v.p. (Producers of documentary and industrial sales and safety films and television commercials.)

Modern Sound Pictures, Inc.

1402 Howard St., Omaha, Nebraska, 68102; (402) 341-8476. Keith T. Smith, pres. (Distributor of over 200 feature films and 300 shorts.)

Modern Talking Picture Service, Inc.

General Offices: 5000 Park St., North, St. Petersburg, FL 33709; (813) 541-7571. (Distributor of free-loan sponsored films and video-cassettes, and collateral materials.)

Divisions

Modern TV: Distributor of free-loan 16mm-sound and color motion pictures and videocassettes, and TV spot newsclips and public service announcements for television stations.
Modern Video Programs: Distributor of programs and series for Cable Television Stations.
Modern Satellite Network: Distributor of programs and services.

Affiliations

Modern Telecommunications, Inc.
One Dag Hammarskjold Plaza, New York, NY 10017; (212) 355-0510. Robert Weisgerger, pres. (A post-production company specializing in videotape services).

Motion Picture Service Co., Inc.

125 Hyde St., San Francisco, CA 94102; (415) 673-9162. Lino Kwong, operations mgr. (Theatre advertising, special trailers, animated film strips, optical sound services, color film lab, computer graphics.)

Movietonews, Inc. (20th Century-Fox Film Corp.)

460 W. 54 St., New York, NY 10019; (212) 977-5500. (Stock film library, international newsreels.)

Multimedia Entertainment of Tennessee

3401 West End. Bldg., Suite 260 W., Nashville, TN 37203; (615) 298-1425. Richard C. Thrall, sr. v.p./gen. mgr.

N

NBC International, Ltd.

30 Rockefeller Plaza, New York, NY 10112; (212) 664-4444. Jerome Wexler, pres.; Mike Perez, v.p., intl. sls.; Eric J. Stanley, dir., intl. sls.; Lesley Gallo, mgr. intl. sls.

- Movies, mini-series, children's shows, comedy and drama series, sporting events, information programs, news programs, etc.

New World Television

1440 So. Sepulveda Blvd., Los Angeles, CA 90025; (213) 444-8100.

Ed Gradinger, pres. & CEO; Jon Feltheimer, exec. v.p.; Gerald Ament, sr. v.p., bus. affairs & prod.; Jim Begg, sr.

v.p., prod.; Freyda Rothstein, sr. v.p., creative affairs; James McNamara, v.p., intl. TV sls.; Neil Shenker, v.p. prod.

O

Odyssey Productions, Inc.

24 E. 51 St., New York, NY 10022; (212) 421-9595. Lowell Thomas, pres.

- Lowell Thomas Television series, High Adventure (color-11); World of Lowell Thomas (half-hour-41).

Lillian Okun Productions

307 East 44 St., New York, NY 10017; (212) 661-3958, ext. 311N. (Live shows—children and teen-age, women's.)

Orion Pictures Television, Inc.

9 West 57 St., New York, NY 10010; (212) 980-1117; Los Angeles, CA 90067; (213) 557-8700. (For officers see listing under Companies)

- Films: Orion III Film Package, including Back to School.
- Series: Cagney & Lacey.

Earl Owensby Studios

P.O. Box 184, Shelby, NC 28150; (704) 482-0611. Earl Owensby, pres.; Linda Comer, secty.

P

P.A.T. Film Services Inc.

630 Ninth Ave., New York, NY 10036; (212) 247-0900. Peter M. Piech, pres.; Ervin Rosenfeld, exec. v.p.; Charles Haydon, v.p. secretary; Andrew Cuomo, v.p., gen. mgr.; Michael Rosenfeld, video mgr. (Produces and distributes TV shows and commercials; ¾", VHS & Beta cassettes for distribution.)

Pakula Productions, Inc.

330 West 58 St., Suite 5H, New York, NY 10019; (212) 664-0640. (Motion picture and TV production) Alan J. Pakula, pres.: Hannah C. Pakula, v.p.; Eric Weissmann, secty.

Paramount Television

5555 Melrose St., Hollywood, CA 90038: (213) 468-5000. For officers and personnel see listing under Companies.

- Features & Specials: Portfolios I-XII; The Jesse Owens Story; Star Trek Memories; Paramount First-Run Network II: Concerts starring Sinatra, Cher, Diana Ross, etc.
- Operation Prime-Time (OPT) Projects: Solid Gold '79 (2 hrs.); The Girl, The Gold Watch & Everything (2 hrs.); The Top of the Hill (4 hrs.); The Way They Were (2 hrs.); Golda (4 hrs.); Smiley's People (6 hrs.); Solid Gold (48 hrs.); The Girl, The Gold Watch & Dynamite (2 hrs.)
- Series: Entertainment Tonight (first-run, live, 52 wks.); Taxi (66 half-hrs.); Solid Gold (48 hrs.); Laverne & Shirley (134 half-hrs.); Happy Days Again (189 half-hrs.); Make Me Laugh (195 half-hrs.); The Odd Couple (114 half-hrs.); The Brady Bunch (117 half-hrs.); Star Trek (79 hrs.); Love, American Style (224 half-hrs.); Star Trek Animated (22 half-hrs.); The Brady Kids (22 half-hrs.); Mission: Impossible (171 hrs.); The Untouchables (114 hrs.); The Lucy Show (156 half-hrs.); The Best of the West (13 half-hrs.); Bosom Buddies (19 half-hrs.); The Brady Brides (10 half-hrs.); Fonz & The Happy Days Gang (13 half-hrs.); Foul Play (10 hrs.); The Greatest American Hero (8 hrs.); Mean Jeans (13 half-hrs.); Nero Wolfe (14 hrs.); Happy Days (189 half-hrs.); Here's Boomer (24 half-hrs.); Mork & Mindy (73 half-hrs.); Number 96 (6 hrs.); Taxi (66 half-hrs.).
- Mini-Series: (hours in parentheses): A Town Like Alice (60); Backstairs at the White House (90); Evita Peron (4); Flesh and Blood (4); Golda (4); The Last Outlaw (8); The Moneychangers (6); Shogun (12); Smiley's People (6); The Timeless Land (8); Tinker, Tailor, Soldier, Spy (6); The Top of the Hill (4); Washington: Behind Closed Doors (12); Winds of War (16).
- Movies of the Week (hrs. in parentheses): An Act of Love (2); The Greatest American Hero (2); Midnight Offerings (2); Tenspeed and Brown Shoe (2); A Time for Love (2); Act of Violence (2); The Alternative (1½); Assault on the Wayne (1½); Big Bob Johnson (2); Call to Danger (1½); Barbary Coast (2); The Caper (1½); Case for the Defense (1½); Chopper Squad (1½); Cindy (2); Clone Master (2); The Cops and Robin (2); The Deadly Game (2); Death in the Family (1½); The Defection of Simas Kudirka (2); Delancey Street (1½); and others.

Tom Parker Theatrical Productions

18653 Ventura Blvd., Tarzana, CA 91536; (818) 342-9115. Telex: 858964. Tom Parker, dir. of prod. & sls. (Buying and distributing service for intl. TV and home video.)

Pathe Pictures, Inc.

141 West 54 St., New York, NY 10019; (212) 247-4767. Joseph P. Smith, pres.; Samuel A. Costello, v.p., secty. & treas.; James J. Harrington, v.p. & gen. counsel.; Joseph A. Volatile, dir. opns. (Producer of documentaries, educational films and children's programs.

- Milestones of the Century (365); Men of Destiny (130); Pathe Educational Shorts (103); Showtime at the Apollo (13); Musical Parade of Stars (1100); Captain David Grief (39); Showtime (39); When the Music's Over (hr. musical variety special).

John Pearson International

2980 Beverly Glen Circle, Suite 302, Los Angeles, CA 90077; (213) 933-5879. Arnie Frank, pres. (Distribution of TV series, features, specials, etc.)

- Series: (all half-hour and in color); That Girl (136).
- Cartoons: Animation Wonderland (18 5–14 minute episodes) Mini-Musical Cartoons (14).
- Features: Cry to the Wind, Flight to Holocaust, Minstrel Man, New Adventures of Heidi, Panic in Tokyo, Shinbone Alley, Bongo Man, California Girls, Communion, Femme Fidele, Red Nights of the Gestapo, Werewolf in Washington.
- Sports Programs: (all half-hour and in color) Andy at Indy (13 episodes); Chase the Wind, King Richard the Racer, Iron Men Steel Machines, Rodeo Cowboy, Twilight Cheat, Wings of the Wind. Hour programs in color: Roller Super Stars (26 eps.); World Championship Kick-Boxing (26 eps.); Salute to Baseball, The Winning Blow; Soul of Karate (40 mins.)
- Family Programs: (all half-hour and in color) Trick and Treat (130 episodes).
- Children's Programs: The Fabulous Storybook Lady (13 half-hours); Domingo (30 half-hour episodes).
- Entertainment Specials: Lucille Ball Specials (7); Bell Telephone Jubilee Spectacular (90 min.); Something Special (22 eps.—60 mins.); Soul to Soul (60 min.); Rock and Roll Revival (67 min.); Count Basie at the Hollywood Palladium (60 min.); Televisa Musical Specials (4—60 min.); Superstars—Las Vegas! including The Ben Vereen Special (86 min.); The John Davidson Special (70 min.); The Strange Case of Alice Cooper (72 min.); 11th World Popular Song Fest (60 min.); Average White Band (90 min.); An Evening with Charles Aznavour (60 min.); Susan George—Naturally (30 min.); Military Music Pageant (60 min.); Nazareth . . . Live! (60 min.); A Night in Las Vegas (60 min.); Today's Jazz (3—30 min.); Tina Turner—Queen of Rock & Roll (30 or 60 min.)
- Dramatic Specials: The Going Up of David Lev (90 min.); Macbeth (107 min.); The Shadow (30 min.); Teacher, Teacher (90 min.); The Trial of Sir Walter Raleigh (60 min.); Angel Dust (60 min.)
- Documentary Specials: Karate, Kung-Fu (60 min.); Sharks (60 min.); To America (97 min.); Giants of the Deep (60 min.), Other Roads, Other Ways (30 min.); Dolphin (60 min.); Shanghai Shadows (60 min.); And the Winner Is . . (45 min.); Energy—The Alternatives (30 min.); Ghosts and Gold (30 min.); Great American Hobo (30 min.); Great American Lumberjack (60 min.); Living with Grace (30 min.); The Wilson Crisis (30 min.); Voyage to Understanding (60 min.).
- Special Interest Programs: Baja Giants (30 min.); Ghosts & Gold (30 min.); Lucy in Disguise (60 min.). Country Rhapsody (7 films—various): B.F.A. Film/Video Catalogue (700 films—various).

Pohlman Film Productions, Inc.

527 N. 27th St., Milwaukee, WI 53208; (414) 342-6363. (Produces industrial motion pictures, multi-media slide shows; slide product.)

Premier Film, Video & Recording Corp.

3033 Locust St., St. Louis, MO 63103; (314) 531-3555. Wilson Dalzell, pres. (Producers of motion pictures, TV spots, strip films & carts, recording and record pressings and video productions, film to video transfer, etc.)

Prime T.V. Films, Inc.

509 Madison Avenue, New York, NY 10022; (212) 421-2170. Elsa Jane Campbell, pres.; Eduardo La Madrid, treas.

- Features: March of the Wooden Soldiers, When Comedy Was King, Golden Age of Comedy, Lady Take a Chance, D'Jango (color, western), Day the Sky Exploded, Incredible Petrified World, Teenage Zombies, Ape Man, Corpse Vanishes, Limping Man, White Fire, Memory of Love, Orient Express, Stars Look Down, Spotlight Scandals, Nine East Side Kids: East Side Kids, Boys of the City, That Gang of Mine, Flying Wild, Bowery Blitzkrieg, Mr. Wise Guy, Let's Get Tough, Smark Alecks, Neath Brooklyn Bridge.
- Series: Charlie Chaplin Comedy Theatre (26 half-hrs.); The Goldbergs; Courageous Cat (130 episodes, color, 5½ mins.).

Program Syndication Services, Inc.

405 Lexington Ave., New York, NY 10174; (212) 532-1560.

ProServ Television

1540 Eastgate Dr., Suite 200, Garland, TX 75041; (214) 270-7601. Bob Briner, pres.; Dennis Spencer, sr. v.p.; Herb Swan, v.p. of intl. sls. (Producers of live events, made-for-TV specials, weekly series, industrials, and home videocassettes.)

Q

Quality Program Sales, Inc.

824 Rome Drive, Los Angeles, CA 90065; (213) 222-8803. Kyle C. Thomas, pres. (Distributes films for TV.)

R

Radio and Television Packagers, Inc.

9 East 40 St., New York, NY 10016; (212) 532-1711. William Cayton, pres.; Mary Gretchen Limper, dir. of sls. (Producer and distributor of filmed series.)

- Jungle: (59 ¼-hr. programs); Cartoon Classics—The Amazing Gift, Beauty and the Beast, The Brave Duckling, The Ice Witch, The Enchanted Princess, The Fisherman and the Fish, Tale of the Northern Lights, Gunnar the Sailor, The Valiant Knight, The Magic Antelope, The Tiny Oxen, Omar and the Ogres, The Strange Circus, Wanda and the Wicked Princess, The Wild Swans, The Woodcutter's Wish, The Frog Princess, The Fire Bird, The Space Explorers, New Adventures of the Space Explorers, Mr. E. from Tau Ceti, The Underseas Explorers, Journey to the Beginning of Time (also available in episode form); Treasure Island Revisited; The Adventures of Mutt & Jeff and Bugoff; When Funnies Were Funny (42 full-color cartoons from the geniuses of early animation); Animations (32 language arts subjects).

Carl Ragsdale Associates, Ltd.

4725 Stillbrooke, Houston, TX 77035; (713) 729-6530. Carl V. Ragsdale, pres. (Producer of documentaries and industrial motion pictures, television commercials, and theater short subjects.)

- Branches: Suite 200, 2120 "L" St. NW, Wash., DC 20037; (202) 347-7095, Arthur Neuman, exec. prod. in charge; 12522 Argyle Dr., Los Alamitos, CA 90720; (213) 598-4201, Frank Coghlan, exec. prod. in charge.

Harry Rasky Productions, Inc.

(Production of feature films and TV specials.) CBC, P.O. Box 500, Terminal A, Toronto, Canada; (416) 925-3311. (World-wide co-productions.)

Redlin Productions, Inc.

19116 Lanark, Reseda, CA; (213) 885-8462. William A. Redlin, pres.; Emil F. Redlin, secty., treas. (Producer live and film programs, features.)

Republic Pictures Corporation

12636 Beatrice St., P.O. Box 66930, Los Angeles, CA 90066-0930; (213) 306-4040. Telex/Twx: 910-343-7417. (For officers see listing under Companies.)

- Hour Series: Americans (17); Bonanza (430); Cameo Theatre (26); Dean Martin (260); Dr. Kildare (142); Flip Wilson (96); High Chaparral (98); I Spy (82); Laramie (124); Laredo (56); My Friend Tony (16); Outlaws (50); Richard Boone Show (25); Seven Greatest (7); Shirley Temple Theater (14); Temple Houston (26); Theatre of Stars (53).
- Half Hour Series: Acapulco (8); Accidental Family (16); African Patrol (39); Animal Secrets (24); Bill Cosby (52); Bill Dana (26); Blue Angels (39); Boots & Saddles (39); Byline: Steve Wilson (39); Californians (69); Captain Nice (15); Captured (26); Car 54, Where Are You? (60); Commando Cody (12); Continental Classroom (160); Dr. Kildare (58); Falcon (39); Fibber McGee & Molly (26); Fireside Theatre (100); Frontier Doctor (39); Get Smart (138); Glencannon (39); Golddiggers (22); Grand Jury (39); Great Gildersleeve (39); H.R. Pufnstuf (17); Happy (26); Hero (16); How To Marry A Millionaire (52); Huck Finn, The New Adventures of (20); International Playhouse (26); Jim Backus Show (39); Kentucky Jones (26); Klondike (18); Let Them Live (13); Lilli Palmer Quality Theatre (36); Loretta Young (187); Man From Cochise (156); Man Without A Gun (52); Mantovani (38); Michael Shayne (32); Mr. Wizard (300); My World And Welcome To It (26); National Velvet (58); Not For Hire (39); Official Detective (39); Panic (31); People Are Funny (150); Pony Express (39); Red Skelton (24); Search & Rescue (26); Silent Service (78); Steve Donovan, Western Marshal (39); Stories of the Century (39); Stryker of Scotland Yard (13); T.H.E. Cat (26); Tab Hunter (32); The Third Man (77); This Is Alice (39); Union Pacific (39); Victory At Sea (26); Walter Winchell File (39).
- Specials: Alice Through The Looking Glass; All About Me; Herb Alpert (3); America and the Americans; Anne Bancroft, The Woman in the Life of a Man; Bill Cosby Fourth Special Or!?; Billie Jean King (5); 500+ Cartoons and Paramount Short Subjects, including Betty Boop, Little Lulu, Puppetoons and others; Children's Letters to God (Gene Kelly); Christie Comedies (107); Experiment In TV—Music; Fabulous Funnies; Funny Manns (104); Gumby (22); Hans Brinker; Heidi; Hot Dog (46); It Couldn't Be Done; Loving You (Elvis Presley Feature); Make Your Own Kind Of Music (8); The New Lion of Sonora (High Chaparral feature); A Picture of US; Republic Serials (chapters and feature versions); Ride The Wind (Bonanza feature); Super Plastic Elastic Goggles; TVI Acts (198); Flip Wilson; Currier & Ives (90-min. video music Christmas album).
- Film Packages: The Champions—152 features; Cary Grant—6 features; John Wayne Theatre—17 features; John Wayne Classic Theatre—29 features; Roy Rogers' "Great Movie Cowboys"—21 features; Horror—35 features; Science Fiction—34 features; Storybook Theatre—5 features; plus, over 500 short subjects; and, more than 1000 feature films.

Ring-Ting-A-Ling Productions

161 West 54 St., Suite 403, New York, NY 10019; (212) 245-8298. Robert Weiner, pres. (Producer of films and TV programs; casting director and talent coordinator.)

Riviera Productions

31628 Saddletree Dr., Westlake Village, CA 91361; (213) 462-8585. F. W. Zens, exec. producer; Leif Rise, assoc. producer, docums., shorts. (Produces filmed series, commercials, features.)

- Punch and Trudy (6); Teletunes (15); Aqua-Lung Adventures (13).

Richard H. Roffman Associates

697 West End Avenue, New York, NY 10025; (212) 749-3647. Richard H. Roffman, pres.; Malvina Cohn, John Bowman, v.p.s. (Producers and distributors of shows also do Public Relations and publicity and promotion for shows—also do casting for shows, etc.; also use guests and feature information on numerous cable TV and UHF-TV and AM-FM radio shows in N.Y.C. areas.)

Jack Rourke Productions

Box 1705 Burbank, CA 91507. Jack Rourke, pres.; William Hagens, v.p.; Jim Rourke, v.p., productions; sales; Hank Edwards, v.p., promotion.

Ruby-Spears Enterprises, Inc.

(A division of The Taft Entertainment Co.) 3255 Cahuenga Blvd., Hollywood, CA 90068; (213) 874-5100. Joseph Ruby, bd. chm.; Kenneth Spears, pres.

- Series: Punky Brewster (NBC); Lazer Tag (NBC); The Chipmunks (NBC); The Puppy's Great Adventures (CBS); The Centurions (syn.); Rambo (syn.); Chuck Norris Karate Kommandos (syn.)

S

SFM Entertainment

1180 Ave. of Americas, New York, NY 10036; (212) 790-4800.

- SFM Holiday Network (package of family feature films.) Mobil Showcase Network Documentary Network, March of Time series, Jayce and the Wheeled Warriors, Photon, Zoobilee Zoo; The Hugga Bunch, Rainbow Brite, Rose Petal Place.

Schaefer/Karpf/Eckstein Productions

3500 W. Olive Ave., Suite 730, Toluca Lake, CA 91505; (818) 953-7770.

Slesinger, Stephen, Inc.

1111 N. Westshore Blvd., Tampa, FL 33607; (813) 879-6968 or (813) 837-8773. Shirley A. Lasswell, pres. (Produces films.)

Southbrook Entertainment Corp.

9601 Wilshire Blvd., #M-100 , Beverly Hills, CA 90210; (213) 274-8021. Thomas J. McDermott, pres. (Producers & distributor of film series). Subsidaries include Lassie Television, Inc. and Lone Ranger Television, Inc.

- Lassie; Lone Ranger; Lone Ranger Cartoon, Sgt. Preston; Skippy the Bush Kangaroo; Magic of Lassie; Lassie the New Beginning.
- America at the Movies; An American Christmas Carol; Antonio and the Mayor; Aunt Mary; Bushido Blade; Chu Chu and the Philly Flash; City in Fear; Coffee, Tea or Me; Crime Club; Crisis in Mid-Air; Cutter's Trail; Daddy, I Don't Like It Like This; Deadly Harvest; Death of Innocence; Dr. Max; Escape; Face of Fear; Family Rico; The Four Feathers; Goodbye Raggedy Ann; Graduation Day; Horror at 37,000 Feet; Hunter; I Want to Keep My Baby; Legend of Walks Far Woman; Migrants; Mongo's Back in Town; Mother and Daughter; My Bodyguard; Nightmare; On the Right Track; Orphan Train; Relentless; Revenge of the Stepford Wives; The Seduction of Miss Leona; Something Evil; Thaddeus Rose and Eddie; That Lucky Touch; Travis Logan, D.A.; Visions of Death; When She Was Bad; Zorro the Gay Blade.

Rick Spalla Video Productions

Subsidiaries: Hollywood Newsreel Syndicate, Inc., and Rick Spalla Production, Inc.

1622 North Gower St., Hollywood, CA 90028 (213); 469-7307; 301 W. 45 St., New York, NY 10036; (212) 765-4646. Organized 1957. Rick Spalla, pres.; Anthony J. Spalla, v.p.; Jeff Spalla, prod. supvr.; Mike Spalla, music dir.; Maralee Spalla, p.r. (Film and video tape production-producer and packager of TV programs, commercials and industrial films.)

- Syndicated TV shows: Portrait of a Star; Hollywood Backstage; High Road to Danger; Hollywood Guest Shot; Hobby Nobbing . . . with the Stars; Century of Fashion; The Open Road, Hollywood's Fantastic Artists' and Models' Ball; Hollywood Star Newsreel, Holiday on Wheels, Portrait: The New Breed; Century of Fashion . . . in Motion Pictures; The Great Getaway; Live two-hr. special: California State network hook-up. Miss California International Beauty Pageant (2 hours) (Annual Competition in April.); The Wild . . . Wild . . . World of Spirit; Kay Crawford's Peparts Training Series (14 hrs.).

Aaron Spelling Productions, Inc.

132 So. Rodeo Drive, Beverly Hills, CA 90212; (213) 858-2000. Aaron Spelling, pres. (Production of motion pictures and television).

Survival Anglia Ltd.

420 Lexington Avenue, New York, NY 10017; (212) 867-6979 . John F. Ball, pres.; James T. de Kay, senior v.p.; Victor Simpkins, v.p., business affairs & corporate communications.

- *Properties:* Tales of the Unexpected (66 half-hrs., bizarre, mystery-suspense anthology with international stars); Tales of the Unexpected, Series Three (22 half-hrs.); World of Survival (21 half-hr. wildlife episodes hosted by John Forsythe); For a Better World (6 one-hr. wildlife/natural history adventures from around the world); Lions of Etosha (one-hr. special on lions filmed by cinematographer Des Bartlett); Warriors of the Gods (one-hr. special on Asian elephants by Dieter Plage).

T

TFI (Tape Film Industries)

619 West 54 Street, New York, NY 10019; (212) 708-0500; 941 N. Highland Avenue, Los Angeles, CA 90038; (213) 461-3361; 640 N. LaSalle St., Chicago, IL; (312) 951-6700. Charles A. Ahto, pres. (Duplication and distribution of TV commercials, film and video tape, complete storage facilities in N.J. & Delaware, post-production services; fulfillment services.)

D. L. Taffner/Limited

31 West 56 St., New York, NY 10019; (212) 245-4680. Donald L. Taffner, pres. (Distributor).

- Comedy: Benny Hill (85 half hrs.); Thames Comedy Originals (156 half hrs.); After Benny (40 half hrs.); Robins Nest (48 half hrs.); Man About the House (39 half hrs.); George & Mildred (38 half hrs.); Keep it in the Family (31 half hrs.)
- Feature Films: Best of Benny (90 mins.).
- Mini-Series: Blood & Honor (5 hrs.).
- Series/First Run: Too Close for Comfort (104 weeks); Check It Out (52 weeks); Ted Knight Show (52 weeks).
- Documentaries: Hollywood (13 hrs.); World at War (36 hrs.); Destination America (9 hrs.).
- Series/Off Network: Three's Company (222 half hrs.); Too Close for Comfort (107 half hrs.); The Ropers (26 half hrs.); Three's A Crowd (22 half hrs.).
- Specials: Benny Hill Specials I (5 hrs.).
- Animation: Danger Mouse (50 half hrs.).

Telecine Film Studios, Inc.

P.O. Box 613, Park Ridge, IL 60068; (312) 823-6405. Byron L. Friend, pres. (Producers of motion pictures, TV series, TV commercials, videotape.)

- Zoo Parade; Magic Ranch.

Telemated Motion Pictures

P.O. Box 176 Prince Sta., New York, NY 10012; (212) 475-8050. Saul Taffet, producer-director. (Producer of documentaries, commercials, industrial, corporate image, public relations, training, sales promotion, and educational films.

Telemount Pictures, Inc.

P.O. Box 1106, Santa Monica, CA 90406. Henry B. Donovan, pres. and producer. (Producers of Cowboy G-Men film series.)

- 39 Westerns; 13 shorts.

Teleworld, Inc.

245 West 55 St., New York, NY 10019; (212) 489-9310. Robert Seldelman, pres.; Noah Jacobs, v.p. sls. West Coast: 11340 W. Olympic Blvd., Los Angeles, CA 90064; (213) 478-2561. Donal Joannes.

Foreign Offices: United Kingdom: Dandelion, 49 St. Peter's St., London N1 8JP, England; 354-2472. Noel Cronin, sls. rep. Mid East: Transworld Television Corp., 81 Piccadilly, London, W1V 9HB, England; 499-7419. Issam Hamaoul, sls. rep. Spain: Apartdao 33009, Madrid-23, Spain; 637-5540. Antoniette Brughera Miranda, sls. rep. Australia: Telepix Pty. Ltd., 1/155 Alexander St., Crows Nest NSW, 2065 Australia; 439-7377. Robert Lapthorne, sls. rep. Latin America: Tel-Com Address: 23241 Ventura Blvd., Suite 209, Woodland Hills, CA 91364; (818) 882-2744. Mel Giniger, sls. rep.

- Mini-Series: Chiefs (6 hrs.); Kennedy (USA only; 7 hrs.); Mistral's Daughter (USA only; 8 hrs.)
- Features/Packages: Spiderman (USA only—7 live-action features); Teleworld's Top 50 (chiller & action features).
- Series/First Run: The Turning Point (24 half-hrs.); Powerhouse (16 half-hrs.).
- Series: The History Makers, Vol. I (13 half-hrs.); The History Makers, Vol. II (265 half-hrs.); International Award Theater (14 half-hrs.); Witness to Yesterday (26 half-hrs.); Star Maidens (USA only—13 half-hrs.); Castaway (USA only—13 half-hrs.); Heritage Civilization & the Jews (intl. only; 9 hrs.).

Telic

317 West 89 St., New York, NY 10024; (212) 874-0295. Woody Siegel, exec. director. (Directors, co-producers, consultants.)

Michael R. Terr Productions

2473 Crestview Dr., Hollywood, CA 90046; (213) 654-7506. John

Rienhardt, director; Michael Terr, producer. (Film programs and commercials.)

- Wildcat Rider (26); Dancing Age (13); Native Son; Gods of Bali; Black Man in the White World; Lolita Go Go; Here Comes the Sexy; Aliki; Two Kids That Stole a Moon; Songs of Siberia (Musical); The Enemies; Jazz at Its Level Best (13 one-half hour color musical); Jazz on Stage (13) one-half hour color-musical; A Tribute to Louis Armstrong and Mahalia Jackson (2½ hrs. Show); Manchurian Massacre (1976); Opium War Atom Boy (90 min.); (1976); Animation; The Open Heart; Mauricette; Cry in the Wind; Our Soviet Sister. New Films: Aba—The Black Superman, Walk the Walk, Deadwood 76, Eegah, Spies-a-Go-Go, The Face of Terror, Fallguy, The Choppers, A Fourth for Marriage.

Bob Thomas Productions

60 East 42 St., New York, NY 10165; (212) 221-3602. Robert G. Thomas, pres. (Motion picture and TV producer; program syndication & satellite services to reach 270 independent television stations.)

Titus Productions, Inc.

211 E. 51 St., New York, NY 10022; (212) 752-6460. Herbert Brodkin, pres.; Robert Buzz Berger, v.p. (Producers of motion pictures, television series and specials.)

Herb Tobias and Associates, Inc.

1901 Avenue of the Stars, Suite 840, Century City, Los Angeles, CA 90067; 277-6211. (Talent Agency.)

Tower Productions

11541 Landale St., No. Hollywood, CA 91602. H. G. and Barbara J. Rhinelander, owners. (Live programs.)

- Space Patrol (live, plus 300 half-hr. and 200 15-min. kinescopes).

Transvue TV International Co.

A Division of Transvue Pictures Corp., 5131 Colbath Ave., Sherman Oaks, CA 91423; (818) 990-5600. Herbert B. Schlosberg, pres.; K. Galloway, secty.

Tribune Entertainment Company

(A subsidiary of Tribune Broadcasting Co., Inc.) 435 North Michigan Ave., Room 1429, Chicago, IL 60611; (312) 222-4484. Sheldon Cooper, pres.; Donald Hacker, exec. v.p.; Joseph Antelo, v.p., exec. prod., At the Movies; William Kunkel, v.p. mktg. & sls.; Clark Morehouse, v.p., media sls.; Charles E. Hinds, v.p., admin.; Peter R. Marino, dir. pgm. development; Jack Devlin, dir. creative svcs.; Allan I. Grafman, dir. business affairs; Anne Rodgers, dir. sta. sls., media programming; Nancy Trainor, dir. sta. reltns.; Carol Forace, dir. prog. sls. dev. & rsch.; Dale Laackman, prod. mgr. (Producer-distributor)

- Series: Dempsey & Makepeace (1 hr.); At the Movies (weekly movie review); U.S. Farm Report (weekly); Soul Train (weekly); Ghostbusters (65 animated half hrs.)
- Mini-Series: A Married Man.
- Features: The Smurfs and the Magic Flute; Nadia.
- Specials: Rocker '85 (2 hrs.); Free at Last (2 hrs.); The Mystery of Al Capone's Vaults (2 hrs.).

Turn of the Century Fights, Inc.

9 East 40 St., New York, 10016; (212) 532-1711. William D. Cayton, pres.; Jim Jacobs, dir. (Produce and distribute fight films.)

- Knock-Out (now total of 500 subjects, from 1897 through 1985).
- The Legendary Champions (90-min. feature)

Twentieth Century Fox Television, A Division of Twentieth Century Fox Film Corp.

P.O. Box 900, Beverly Hills, CA 90213; (213) 277-2211. (For officers and personel see listing in Companies.)

- Series Available: Hours and Half Hours: Adventures in Paradise (91); The Barry Farber Show; The Best of the Midnight Special (52); Bracken's World (41); Bus Stop (25); Cade's County (24); Century Theatre—The Fortunes of Nigel 5, A Little Princess (3), The Pathfinder (5), Daniel Boone (165); The Fall Guy (112); Five Fingers (16); Follow the Sun (30); Jackie Gleason (100); Hagen (9); Ben Hall (13); Hong Kong (26); How Green Was My Valley (6); Husbands, Wives and Lovers (11); Jack the Ripper (6); Jessica Novak (7); Judd for Defense (50); Lancer (51); Land of the Giants (51); Legend of Custer (17); The Long Hot Summer (26); Lost in Space (83); The Monroes (26); The Monte Carlo Show (24); Nashville 99 (4); The New Perry Mason (15); The Paper Chase (51); Quiller (13); Roots of Rock 'N Roll (6); The Starlost (16); The Time Tunnel (30); Trapper John, M.D.; 12 O'clock High (78); Voyage to the Bottom of the Sea (110); Web (6); Young Daniel Boone (8); Anna & the King (13); Arnie (48); Audubon Wildlife Theatre (78); Batman (120); Billy Liar (7); Broken Arrow (72); Circus! (52); Dance Fever (94); Dobie Gillis (147); Doctor Dolittle (17); Double Deckers (17); Fantastic Voyage (17); The Felony Squad (73); The Ghost and Mrs. Muir (50); The Green Hornet (26); The Hardy Boys (17); Journey to the Center of the Earth (17); Julia (86); Ladies' Man (16); The Legend of Jesse James (34); The Loner (26); M*A*S*H (255); That's Hollywood (74); The Incredible World of Adventure (31); Masquerede Party; My Friend Flicka (39); Nanny and the Professor (54); 9 to 5 (39); Orson Welles Great Mysteries (26); Peyton Place (514); Return to the Planet of the Apes (animated) (13); Roll Out! (13); Room 222 (113); Run, Joe, Run!; Salty (26); Valentine's Day (34); On & Off Camera (6); Manimal (7); Trauma Center (13); Medstar; AfterMash (31); It's Not Easy (10); Emerald Point, N.A.S. (22); Fall Guy; Trapper John M.D. (132); Animal Express (130).
- Specials: An Unauthorized Biography: In Search of Howard Hughes; Christmas Gold; Fox Fanfare; Edith Piaf; Jacqueline Susann's Valley of the Dolls (5); Prime of Miss Jean Brodie; The Rules of Marriage (4); Time Tunnel Movies; Tomorrow's Child (2); Tourist (5); TV and the Fabulous 50's, Blood Feud (4); Helen Keller . . . The Miracle Continues (2); Sentimental Journey (2); Pygamlion (2); Charles Dickens' Classics (8).
- First Run Syndication: 9 to 5; Dream Girl USA; 100,000 Pyramid; Small Wonder; Dance Fever.
- Features: Big 36; Century 5 (35); Century 6 (32); Century 7 (25); Century 8 (25); Century 9 (30); Century 10 (30); Century 11 (23); Century 12 (23); Charlie Chan Features (34); Fox I (50); Fox II (50); Fox III (50); Golden Century (50); Laurel and Hardy (6); Mark One (11); Planet of the Apes (5); Premiere One (20); Shirley Temple (20); Special 42; Super 66; Fox Hollywood Theatre (2); Fox Mystery Theatre (15); Century 13; Big 36; Premiere 2.

Twyman Films, Inc.

4409 Forest Park Plaza, Dayton, OH 45405; (513) 276-5941. John F. Heck, pres. (Distributor of feature films from Warner Bros., Disney, Fox, Learning Corp., Columbia, Rank & the Rohauer Collection).

- A Paris; Josef von Sternberg's Anatahan; Louis Malle's Calcutta; Jean Luc Godard's Le Gai Savior; The Fables of Jean de la Fontaine (33) (in French or English); Frederic Rossif's A Wall In Jerusalem; Tristana, Nosferatu, Merveilleuse Visit, Miracle of Intervale Avenue Heureux Anniversarie, Codine, The Mad Adventures of "Rabbi" Jacob La Caza, Kwaidan, Das Tagebuch Elner Veriorenen (Diary of a Lost Girl), Un Chien Andalou.

U

UPA Productions of America

1875 Century Park East, Suite 2140, Los Angeles, CA 90067; (213) 556-3800. Henry G. Saperstein, pres.; (Distributes Mr. Magoo, Dick Tracy, Gerald McBoing-Boing color cartoons, family specials, and features, Godzilla, Rodan, sci-fi features etc. Produces animated commercials, theatrical films, industrial & TV programs.)

United Press International

1400 I St., NW, Washington, DC 20005; (202) 898-8000. Mario Vasquez-Rama, chm,; Maxwell McCrohon, v.p. & editor. (Distributes news, audio and information services.)

United States Productions, Inc.

47 East 88 St., New York, NY 10028; (212) 876-3774. Francis C. Thayer, pres.; Stowe C. Phelps, exec. prod.; Bert Shapiro, prod.-dir.; David Sawyer, prod.-dir.; Thomas Phipps, script editor. (Producers of theatrical, educational films, documentaries, industrials, commercials.)

Universal Television

A Division of Universal City Studios, Inc. Universal City, CA 91608, (213) 985-4321. (For officers see listing under companies.)

- '85–'86 season: Amazing Stories; Miami Vice; Knight Rider; Magnum P.I.; Simon & Simon Airwolf; and half-hrs.: Fast Times, Leo & Liz in Beverly Hills.

V

Valiant International Pictures

4774 Melrose Ave., Hollywood, CA 90029; (213) 665-5257. Harry Novak, pres.; Ivan Levitan, v.p.; Carmen Novak, secty./treas. (Distributor.)

Van Praag Productions, Inc.

135 E. 55 St., New York, NY 10022; (212) 838-2111. William van Praag, exec. dir., Eugene van Pragg, Anita Palumbo, Ray van Praag, Don O'Mara, staff directors.

Veritas Productions, Inc.

1 Laurie Drive, Englewood Cliffs, NJ 07632; (201) 568-4214 or New York City (212) 765-4240. Richard S. Dubelman, pres.; Joan D. Morley, asst. to pres. (TV and motion picture production)

Versatile Television Production, Inc.

324 Broadway, Cape Girardeau, MO 335-8816. TWX Cape Girardeau 968; Robert O. Hirsch, press.; Jerry Hollis, mgr. (Producers of animated, live action film and video tape commercials and industrial.)

Viacom International Inc.

1211 Avenue of the Americas, New York, NY 10036; (212) 575-5175.

Corporate personnel: Ralph M. Baruch, chm.; Terrence A. Elkes, pres. & CEO; Kenneth Gorman, chm., Viacom Cable Networks Group, & exec. v.p., Viacom International Inc.; Bud Getzler, chm., Viacom Entertainment Group; Jules Haimovitz, pres., Viacom Entertainment Group.; Gus Lucas, exec. v.p., Viacom Entertainment Group; Ronald Lightstone, sr. v.p., corporate & legal affairs; George Castell, v.p., corporate development; Kenneth Meyer, v.p., Human Resources; Gordon E. Belt, v.p. & CFO, treas.; Dennis Ellis, v.p., controller; John Brady, sr. v.p., finance/Viacom Entertainment Group; David Fluhrer, dir., corporate communications.

Viacom Enterprises Personnel: Joseph D. Zaleski, pres., domestic syndication; Dennis Gillespie, sr. v.p., mktg; Michael H. Gerber, sr. v.p.; Paul Kalvin, v.p., natl mktg. mgr.; Toby Martin, v.p., programs; Charles Tolep, v.p. & gen. mgr., licensing & merchandising; Eric Veale, v.p., sls. opns; Elissa Lebeck, v.p., res. & mktg. svcs.; Tony Guido, v.p., bus. affairs; Katherine Hogan, v.p., counsel entertainment; Kenneth Werner, dir., bus. affairs; Gerald Pinks, dir., domestic sls. svc.; Lisa Merians, dir, creative svcs.; Betsy Vorce, dir, public rels.; George Faber, dir, communications (L.A. office); Kim Schlotman, dir., mkt. strategy; Richard Dorfman, dir, advertiser sls.; Sean Deneny, mgr., Mid-Atlantic domestic sls.; Joe DiSalvo, sls. mgr., Northeastern div.

Viacom Productions: Tom Tannenbaum, pres., Viacom Productions.

Viacom World Wide: Willard Block, pres., Viacom World Wide Ltd.; Neil McHugh, v.p., new business & admin.; Raul Lefcovich, v.p., international; James Marrinan, v.p., international marketing, Viacom Latino Americana; Noreen Brittenham, assoc. dir., sls. admin., Viacom Latino Americana

Regional Offices: New York: 1211 Avenue of the Americas, New York, NY 10036; (212) 575-5175. Joseph DiSalvo, mgr., Northeast div.; Sean Deneny, mgr.; Mid-Atlantic domestic sls.; Los Angeles: 10900 Wishire Blvd., Los Angeles, CA 90024; (213) 208-2700. Brooks Carroll, v.p., sls., Western div.; Al Miller, acct. exec., Western div.; Atlanta: 400 Perimeter Center Terrace, Suite 982, Atlanta, GA 30346; (404) 395-7795; Frank Flanagan, v.p., Southeastern div.; Mary Crescas, acct. exec., Southeastern div.; Irving: 433 East Las Colinas Blvd., Suite 1160, Irving, TX 75039; (214) 556-2255; David Campbell, mgr., Southwestern div.; Gloria Martin, acct. exec., Southwestern div.; Chicago: 10 South Riverside Plaza, Suite 316; Chicago, IL 60606; (312) 648-5858; Dennis Emerson, v.p., Midwest; Dennis Boyle, mgr., Central Western div.

International Offices: London: Viacom International Limited, 40 Conduit St., London, W1R 9FB, England; (441) 434-4483; Cable: VIACOM London; Telex: 851-919122. Martha Burke-Hennessy, man. dir., Viacom S.A. & Viacom International Ltd. New York: Viacom Latino Americana, 1211 Ave. of the Americas, New York, NY 10028; (212) 575-5175; Telex: 620-235 VIA. James Marrinan, v.p., gen. mgr., Viacom Latino Americana; Sydney: Viacom International Pty. Ltd., 16th floor, St. Martins Tower, 31 Market St., Sydney, N.S.W. 2000, Australia; (612) 29-4391; Cable: TELECAST, Sydney; Telex: 790-20698; Peter Press, v.p., man. dir.; Lloyd Fryer. All mail to: P.O. Box 0342, Queen Victoria Bldg., Sydney, N.S.W. 2000, Australia. São Paulo: Viacom Video Audio Communicacoes Ltda., Alameda Jau', 1742, Il Andar, Caixa Postal 51521, 01499 São Paulo, Brazil; (55-11) 853-4633; Cable: NEWSHOWS, São Paulo; Telex: 391-01131773. Contact: Ivan Aragon, gen. mgr. Tokyo: Viacom Japan, Inc., 4F, Mitsuwa Bldg., 7-2 Ginza 6-Chome, Chuo-Ku, Tokyo 104, Japan; (81-3) 573-0551; Cable: VIACOMINTL, Tokyo; Telex: 781-24204. Jiro Sugiyama, pres., Viacom Japan, Inc. Toronto: Viacom Enterprises Canada Ltd., 45 Charles St., East, Toronto 5, Ont., Canada M4Y 1S2; Phone: (416) 925-3161; Cable: VIACOMCAN, Toronto; Telex: 369-06219596. Alastair Banks, v.p., gen. mgr. Zug: Viacom S.A., Chamerstrasse 18, 6300 Zug, Switzerland; Phone: 41-42-21-8122; Cable: VIACOM, Zug; Telex: 845-868-750. Contact: Manfred Metzger.

- Series, first-run: What a Country! (26 half-hr. originals); MTV top 20 Video Countdown (52 hour originals); The New Honeymooners (68 discovered half-hrs.); Newly-Released Perry Mason (26 hr. episodes not seen since original airdates); Bizarre (130 half-hrs.)
- Ad Hoc Network (offered jointly with Tribune Entertainment): TV Net (one per month: first-run primetime features never before seen on broadcast television.)
- Animated Series: Terrytoons (689 cartoon units); Harlem Globetrotters (22 half-hrs.); The Alvin Show (26 half-hrs.)
- Series, Off-Network: All in the Family (207 half-hrs.); Andy Griffith (249 half-hrs.); The Best of the Beverly Hillbillies (168 half-hrs.); The Bob Newhart Show (142 half-hrs.); Cannon (124 half-hrs.); Circus (24 half-hrs. & 1 1-hr. special); Clint Eastwood in Rawhide (217 half-hrs.); December Bride (154 half-hrs.); Dick Van Dyke (158 half-hrs.); Family Affair (138 half-hrs.); Family Feud (260 half-hrs.); Gomer Pyle (226 hrs.); Gunsmoke (226 hrs.); Have Gun Will Travel (156 half-hrs.); Hawaii Five-O (200 hrs.); Hogan's Heroes (168 half-hrs.); The Honeymooners (107 half-hrs.; 68 newly-recovered, 39 that have been in syndication); I Love Lucy (179 half-hrs.); I Spy (6 hrs.); The Life and Times of Grizzly Adams (35 hrs., 2 90-min. specials); Marshall Dillon (233 half-hrs.); The Mary Tyler Moore Show (168 half-hrs.); Millionaire (188 half-hrs.); My Three Sons (160 half-hrs.) Our Miss Brooks (127 half-hrs.); Perry Mason (271 hrs; 26 newly -recovered, 50 seen twice since their original airdates, 195 that have been in syndication); Petticoat Junction (148 half-hrs.); The Rookies (90 hrs.); Trackdown (71 half-hrs.); The Twilight Zone (168 half-hrs. & hrs.); The Wild, Wild West (104 hrs.); You Are There (65 half-hrs.)
- Packages/Features: Viacom I, II, III,IV, V, VI, VII, VIII, IX, V, XI; Viacom Movie Greats; The Legend Group; The Exploitables; The Explodables; Gasp; Thematics; Young and Reckless.

Vidistrib, Inc.

4209 Troost Avenue, Studio City, CA 91604; Tel.: (818) 762-3535. John P. Ballinger, pres.; Rita Cross, v.p.-treas. (TV show sales & distribution syndication, barter, consultation).

Viking Films, Inc.

1600 Broadway, New York, NY 10019; (212) 255-8858. Israel M. Berman, pres., exec. producer. (Produce educational, children's subjects, sciences, cartoons & puppets.)

W

WW Entertainment

(A division of World Northal Corporation) 205 East 42 St., New York, NY 10017; (212) 661-3350. George Hankoff, pres.; Louis S. Israel, sr. v.p. sls.; Tony Elmaleh, v.p., prod.; Marcia Skolnick, v.p., dir. research; Sylvia Delia, dir. sls./home video/cable TV.

- Feature Films—Martial Arts Feature Films: Black I (13 titles); Black Belt II (26 titles); Black Belt III (13 titles); Black Belt IV (29 titles); Black Belt V (13 titles); Action Flicks (7 titles); WW Entertainment I (16 titles).
- Series—The Best of Groucho (130 half-hrs.); Skyways (130 hrs.)
- Co-productions-BBC: 24 feature films.

Roger Wade Productions, Inc.

15 W. 44 St., New York, NY 10036; (212) 575-9111. Roger W. Wade, pres. (Producers of motion pictures for industry, sound slide films, multi-media, slides.)

Warner Bros. Television

4000 Warner Blvd., Burbank, CA 91522; (818) 954-6000. (For officers and personnel, see listing under Companies.)

Series and specials available for domestic sales as of July, 1986 (all color unless otherwise indicated)

- Miniseries: "V" (10 hrs.); Bare Essence (4 hrs. or 4½ hrs.); The Thorn Birds (10 hrs.); Pearl (6 hrs.); Scruples (6 hrs.); Roots

(12 hrs.); Roots: The Next Generation (14 hrs.)

- Series/Off Network: Growing Pains (half-hrs.); Night Court (half-hrs.); Matt Houston (68 hours); Private Benjamin (39 half-hrs.); The Dukes of Hazzard (147 hrs.); Alice (202 half-hrs.); Welcome Back, Kotter (95 half-hrs.); Chico and the Man (88 half-hrs.); F-Troop (65 half-hrs., 31 color); Superman (104 half-hrs., 52 color); Batman/Superman/Aquaman (69 animated half-hrs.) Harry-O (44 hrs.); Wonder Woman (61 hrs); Kung Fu (62 hrs.); The Waltons (221 hrs.); The FBI (234 hrs.); Tarzan (57 hrs.); Maverick (124 hrs.)
- Specials: The Phenomenon of Roots (1 hr.); David L. Wolper Specials of the Seventies (30 one-hr. specials)
- Features/Packages: Volume 26 (24 features); TV3 (13 features); Volume 25 (24 features); TV2 (13 feature titles); Volume 24 (18 features); 13 Classic Thrillers II (13 features); TVI (13 features); Volume 23 (20 features); Volume 22 (38 features); Volume 21 (26 features); The FBI Story (4 features); Volume 20 (30 features); Volume 19 (29 features, 28 in color); Volume 18 (28 features, 25 in color); Volume 17 (23 features, 21 in color); Volume 16 (18 features, 16 in color); Volume 14-15 (13 features, 12 in color); Volume 13 (25 features, 17 in color); Volume 2-A (22 features, 13 in color); Volume 1-A (24 features, 17 in color); 13 Classic Thrillers (13 features); Tarzan Features (32 features, 9 in color); The Bowery Boys (48 features); Starlite 6 (26 features, 12 in color); Starlite 5 (28 features, 18 in color); Starlite 4 (30 features, 16 in color); Starlite 3 (30 features, 19 in color); Special Features (17 features).
- Cartoons: Bugs Bunny & Friends (100 cartoons); Porky Pig & Friends (156 cartoons)

INTERNATIONAL

- Cartoons: Bugs Bunny & Friends (100 cartoons); Bugs Bunny cartoons (234 cartoons); Looney Toons (190 cartoons, 78 color, 112 black-and-white)
- Features/Packages: International 21 (51); International 21 (34); International 30 (66); International 29 (44); International 28 (7); International 27 (5); International 26 (11); International 25 (32); International 24 (80); International 23 (99); International 22 (135); International 21 (56); International 20 (3); International 19 (28); International 18 (26); International 17 (28); International 16 (92); International 15 (33); International 14 (36); International 13 (35); International 12 (36); International 11 (36); International 9 (1); International 5 (48); International 4 (127)
- Miniseries: Dream West (7 hrs.); Crossings (6 hrs.); Dress Gray (4 hrs.); North and South—I (12 hrs.); North and South—II (12 hrs.); Hollywood Wives (6 hrs.); The Thorn Birds (10); "V" (10); Roots (12); Roots: The Next Generation (14); The Mystic Warrior (5); Bare Essence (4); Scruples (6); Pearl (6); The Phenomenon of Roots (1); The Awakening Land (7); Born to the Wind (4); Hanging by a Thread (4); Haywire (4); Moviola (6); Night the Bridge Fell Down (4); Pirate (4); Salem's Lot (4)
- One-Hour Series: Scarecrow and Mrs. King; Hotel; The Colbys; Spenser: For Hire; Shell Game; Shadow Chasers (12); Hollywood Beat (14); "V" (19); Matt Houston (68); The Dukes of Hazzard (147); Harry O (44); Kung Fu (62); Tarzan (57); I Had Three Wives (6); MacGruder & Loud (13); Eye to Eye (6); Double Dare (6); Finder of Lost Loves (23); Glitter (13); The Yellow Rose (22); The Mississippi (23); Bare Essence (11); The Alaskans (36); Banyon (15); Bourbon Street Beat (39); Bret Maverick (16); Bronco (68); California Fever (10); Casablanca (5); Cheyenne (107); Code R (13); The Dakotas (19); Delphi Bureau (8); Dial M for Murder (13); Drama (42); Enos (17); The F.B.I. (238); Fitzpatricks (13); Freebie and the Bean (9); Gallant Men (25); Hawaiian eye (134); High Performance (4); Life on Earth (13); Maverick (124); The New Land (13); Nichols (24); Notorious Woman (7); Rafferty (13); Roaring 20's (45); Search (23); 77 Sunset Strip (205); The Streets of San Francisco (119); Sugarfoot (69); Superfriends (93); Challenge of Superfriends (16); Surfside Six (74); Time Express (4); The Tribal Eye (7); The Waltons (219); Wizards and Warriors (8); Wonder Woman (13); New Adventures of Wonder Woman (46); The Yeagers (4); Young Maverick (6)
- Half-Hour Series: Night Court; Growing Pains; Life with Lucy; My Sister, Sam; Head of the Class; Welcome Back, Kotter (95); Love, Sidney (44); Porky Pig Show (26); Private Benjamin (39); Roadrunner Show (26); Superman (104); Tarzan, Lord of the Jungle (34); Alice (202); Rubik, the Amazing Cube (13); Off the Rack (7); A.E.S Hudson Street (5); Another Day (13); Aquaman (18); At Ease (14); Batman (17); New Adventures of Batman (16); B.C. Archaelogy of Bible Lands (12); Bugs Bunny Show (78); Chicago Teddy Bears (13); Chico and the Man (88); Colt .45 (67); The Cowboys (12); Dorothy (4); The Dukes—Animated (20); Fat Albert and the Cosby Kids (60); Flo (29); F Troop (65); Goodnight, Beantown (8); Jimmy Stewart Show (24); Lassie's Rescue Rangers (17); Lawman (156); Little People, The Brian Keith Show (46); Marine Boy (78); Me and Maxx (10); Merrie Melodies Show (24); Mr. Roberts (30); New Adventures of Superman (34); No Time for Sergeants (34); Park Place (5); Shazam! (28); TV Funnies (16)

Weiss Global Enterprises

2055 South Saviers Road, Suite 12, Oxnard, CA 93030; (805) 486-4495. Cable: WEISSPICT. Adrian Weiss, pres.; Steven A. Weiss, secty./treas.; Ethel L. Weiss, v.p.; Laurie Weiss, v.p.; Patricia C. Sandoval, opns. mgr.; Alex Gordon, information services.

- Features: Galaxy "15": fifteen features including Ginger in the Morning, Molly and Promises! Promises!, Golden Showmanship "9": nine features including Cattle Queen of Montana, Slightly Scarlett; Westerns: 60 action features starring Johnny Mack Brown, Harry Carey, Fred Kohler, Jr., Rex Lease, Buddy Roosevelt and Bob Steele; Vintage Flicks: 24 features from the '30's and '40's; One-Hour Documentaries: The Brave Rifles (51 mins.), Our Time in Hell (51 mins.); Those Crazy Americans (54 mins.); Impact "120": 120 films produced by Robert L. Lippert, including Baron of Arizona, I Shot Jesse James, King Dinosaur, etc; Parade "4": 4 features of the '60's.
- Serials: Custer's Last Stand (15 episodes); The Black Coin (15 episodes); The Clutching Hand (15 episodes).
- Series, First-Run: America Confidential (5 half-hr. episodes per week); The Stan Kann Show (52 half-hrs.); Kids Say the Darndest Things (600 episodes, 5 min. each).
- Series, Off-Network: Make Room For Daddy (161 half-hr. programs); Canine Comments (13 quarter-hr. short subject); I Married Joan (98 half-hr. sit-coms); The Bill Dana Show (42 half-hrs.); Craig Kennedy, Crimonologist (26 half-hr. mysteries); Good Morning World (26 half-hr. sit-coms); Thrill of Your Life (13 half-hrs.); My Little Margie (126 half-hrs.); Rocky Jones, Space Ranger (39 half-hrs.); Waterfront (78 half-hrs.).
- Comedy Shorts: The Chuckle Heads (150 five-min. slapstick comedy shorts).
- Cartoons: Alice by Walt Disney (10 ten-min. cartoons); Krazy Kid Kartunes (4 six-min. cartoons); Nursery Rhymes (6 1½-min. cartoons).
- Specials: Glitter, Glamour & Gags—That Beauty Contest (1-hr. first run)

Worldvision Enterprises, Inc.

660 Madison Avenue, New York, NY 10021; (212) 832-3838. Kevin O'Sullivan, chm. & CEO; Neil Delman, pres. & COO; Lawrence Gottlieb, exec. v.p., finance; Bert Cohen, sr. v.p., intl. sls.; John D. Ryan, sr. v.p., domestic sls.; Jerry Rettig, sr. v.p., creative services; Randy Hanson, v.p., western div. mgr.; Jesse S. Weatherly, acct. exec. western div.; Jim Thomson, v.p., southern div. mgr.; Reggie Jester, acct. exec., southern div.; Paul Danylik, v.p., central div. mgr.; Victoria Lynn Quoss, acct. exec., central div.; Bill Baffi, v.p., eastern div. mgr.; Tim Davis, acct. exec. eastern div.; Burton Rosenburgh, v.p., Evergreen Programs, Inc. (sub. of Worldvision); Martin Weisman, acct. exec., Evergreen Programs, western div.; Carl Sansaricq, dir. sls. & mktg., Worldvision Home Video, Inc., (sub.); Dan Willis, v.p., intl. sls. admin.; Steve Blank, v.p., finance admin.; Ben De Augusta, v.p., ops.; Jerry Kaufer, v.p. creative svcs.; Rita Scarfone, v.p. adv. & promo.; Gerard Bixenspan, dir. of research & sls. develop.; Brian O'Sullivan, central div. mgr., Worldvision Home Video; Tom Devlin, v.p. & gen. mgr., Worldvision Home Video; Tim Newman, acct. exec., Evergreen Programs, central div.; Kathy Rost, western div. mgr., Worldvision Home Video. Bruce Knox, south. div., Worldvision Home Video; Karl Middleburg, acct. exec., south. div. Domestic Offices: New York, NY 10021, 660 Madison Ave.; (212) 832-3838. Chicago, IL 60611, 625 N. Michigan Ave.; (312) 642-2650. Beverly Hills, CA 90210, 9401 Wilshire Blvd.; (213) 273-7667. Atlanta, GA 30346, 14 Perimeter Terrace, Suite 105; (404) 394-7444.

- Hour Series: Barnaby Jones (177); Ben Casey (153); Breaking Point (30); Combat (152); Don Lane Show (130); Fugitive (120); The Invaders (43); Little House on the Prairie (216.5); Love Boat I (140); Love Boat II (115); Mod Squad (124 1-hr.); Man from Atlantis (13 1-hr;, 3 2-hr., 1 1½-hr.); Return to Eden (22)
- Half-Hour Series: Annie Oakley (80); Buffalo Bill, Jr. (40); Champion, the Wonder Horse (26); Come Along (13); Dark Shadows (780); Dickens & Fenster (32); Doris Day Show (128); Douglas Fairbanks Presents (115); F.D.R (25 ½-hr., 1 1-hr.); High Road (36); It Pays to Be Ignorant (39); Mickey Rooney (17); Next Step Beyond (24); N.Y.P.D. (49); On the Mat (52); One Man Show (26); One Step Beyond (94); People's Choice (104); Range Rider (76); The Rebel (76); Starring the Actors (13); Take My Word for It (130); That Girl (136); Throb (24); Wendy and Me (34); Wonders of the Wild (26).
- Mini-Series: Return to Eden (6 hours); Holocaust (10 hours); Against the Wind (13 hours).
- Features: Prime VII (25 color features); Prime VI (19); Prime V (26); Prime IV (26); Prime II (16); Prime II (16); Prime I (10).
- Animated & Children's Programming: Fun World of Hanna-Barbera (84 half-hrs.); H-B's World of Super Adventure (129 half-

hrs.); Banana Splits & Friends (125 half-hrs.); Saturday A.M. at the Movies (6 specials); Top Cat (30 half-hrs.); Wait Till Your Father Gets Home (48); Josie & The Pussycats (16); Josie & the Pussycats in Outer Space (16); Casper, the Friendly Ghost & His Friends (244 cartoons) The Jackson Five (23 half-hrs.); The Jerry Lewis Show (17 half-hrs.); King Kong (26 half-hrs.); Lancelot Link-Secret Chimp (17 half-hr.); Milton the Monster (26 half-hrs.); The Wonderful World of Professor Kitzel (104 cartoons); The Reluctant Dragon & Mr. Toad (17 half-hrs.); Smokey the Bear (51 half-hrs.); George of the Jungle (17 half-hrs.); The Funtastic World of Hanna-Barbera (weekly first-run 90-min. block); The Jetsons (65 episodes); Rambo (65 half-hrs.); Centurions (66 half-hrs.); Chuck Norris (5 half-hrs.); Sectaurs (66 half-hrs.).

- Specials: Jack Nicklaus at the Home of Golf (3 hrs.); The Fabulous Sixties (10 one-hrs.); The Bay City Rollers (1 hr.); Echo 1 (17 hrs.); Herbie Mann/Rahsaan Roland Kirk (half-hr.); Is It Christ? (1 hr.); The Last Nazi (90 mins.); Raphael (1 hrs.); Robert Flack/Donny Hathaway (half-hr.); The World of Miss World (1 hr.); The New Fangled Wandering Minstrel Show (1 hr.); The Musical Ambassadors, Kenny Rogers & The First Edition in New Zealand (1 hr.); Ron Luciano's Lighter Side of Sports (half-hr.); A Christmas Carol (animated half-hr.); An Evening with Irish Television (1 hr.); Russian Festival of Music and Dance; The Bobby Vinton Show (1 hr.); A Shark's Paradise (1 hr.); Amahl & the Night Visitors (1 hr.); Children of the Gael (1 hr.) Irish Rovers Special (1 hr.); The Night the Animals Talked (1 hr.).

Worldvision International:

AUSTRALIA: Worldvision Enterprises of Australia Pty. Ltd., 5–13 Northcliff St., Milsons Point 2061, Sydney; Tel.: 922-4722. Brian Rhys-Jones, mgr. dir., Australia & Far East.

BRAZIL: Worldvision Filmes do Brasil Ltd., Rua Macedo Sobrinho 50, Botafogo, CEP 22271, Rio de Janeiro; Tel.: 286-8992. Raymund Lopes Rodgigues, mgr. dir., Brazil.

CANADA: Worldvision Enterprises of Canada, 1200 Bay St., Suite #203, Toronto M4R 2A5, Canada; Tel.: (416) 967-1200. Mel Watson, v.p. sls., Canada

ENGLAND: Worldvision Enterprises, U.K. Ltd., 54 Pont St., London, S.W. 1, England, Tel.: 584-5357. William Peck, mng. dir., England.

FRANCE: Worldvision Enterprises S.A.R.L., 28, rue Bayard 75008, Paris, France; Tel.: 4273-3995. Mary Jane Fourniel, mng. dir., France & French-speaking countries.

GERMANY: Worldvision GmbH, Postfach 906, 8 München 33, Germany; Tel.: 26-4091. Mex Hartmann, mng. dir.

ITALY: Worldvision Enterprises, Inc., Via Del Corso, 22/Int. 10, 00186, Rome, Italy; Tel.: 67-87-056. Martin Michael Kiwe, v.p., European operations.

JAPAN: Worldvision Enterprises, Inc., Tsukiji Hamarikyu Bldg., 7th floor, 5-3-3, Tsukiji, Chou-ku, Tokyo 104, Japan; Tel.: 545-3977. Mie Horasawa, sls. rep., Japan and Korea.

- New Releases: The Last Frontier (Linda Evans, Jason Robards, Jack Thompson, CBS, 4-hr. mini-series); Shark's Paradise (2-hr. made-for-TV movie); Uncle Tom's Cabin (2-hr. movie, Showtime); You Again? (Jack Klugman, NBC, half-hr. series); Throb (Diana Canova, half-hr. series); On Wings of Eagles (Burt Lancaster, Richard Crenna, NBC, 5-hr. mini-series); AFI Life Achievement Award/Billy Wilder (NBC, 90 mins.); When the Bough Breaks (Ted Danson, NBC, 2-hr. movie); The Christmas Gift (John Denver, CBS, 2-hr. movie); Night of Courage (ABC, 2-hr. movie); Stranger in My Bed (Lindsay Wagner, NBC, 2-hr. movie); Gone to Texas (CBS, 3-hr. movie); Sam's Son (Michael Landon, Eli Wallach, Anne Jackson, Timothy Patrick Murphy, NBC, 2 hr.); Town of the 80's (Showtime, 4 one-hr. specials); Return to Eden (Rebecca Gilling, James Smille, one-hr. series); Dallas (CBS, 9th year, one-hr.); Highway to Heaven (NBC, 3rd year, one-hr.); Love Boat (ABC, 10th year, 6 hr.); Starring the Actors (13 half-hr. superstar interviews); That Girl (Marlo Thomas, ABC, 136 half-hr. series); Centurions (65 animated half-hrs.); Jetsons (65 animated half-hrs.); Funtastic World of Hanna-Barbera (consisting of: "Paw Paws," "Yogi's Treasure Hunt," "Galtar and the Golden Lance," each 21 animated half-hrs.); Chuck Norris (5 animated half-hrs.); The Flintstone Kids (ABC, 26 animated half-hrs.); Wildfire (CBS, 13 animated half-hrs.); Berenstain Bears (CBS, 13 animated half-hrs.); The Flintstones 25th Anniversary (one-hr. special); Jonny Quest (13 animated half-hrs.); Alvin & the Chipmunks (NBC, 8 half-hrs.); The Smurfs (NBC, 39½ animated half-hrs., available only in U.K., Ireland, and Canada.)
- Series (U.S. Networks, 1985/86): Sins (starring Joan Collins, CBS, 7-hr. mini-series); The Key to Rebecca (4-hr. mini-series starring Cliff Robertson, David Soul); Highway to Heaven (starring Michael Landon, NBC, one-hr. series); Double Take (mini-series, CBS, 4 hrs. starring Richard Crenna); Santa Barbara (starring Dame Judith Anderson, NBC, one-hr. serial); Welcome Home Bobby (2 hrs., made-for-TV movie, CBS); Dallas (hour, CBS); The Love Boat (hour, ABC); General Hospital (serial/hour/color, ABC); One Life to Live (serial/hour/color, ABC); All My Children (serial/hours/color, ABC); The Smurfs (24 animated half-hrs.); The 13 Ghosts of Scooby Doo (13 animated half-hrs., ABC); Alvin and the Chipmunks (10 animated half-hrs., NBC); Mr. T (6 animated half-hrs., NBC).
- Special Presentation Programming: Three Little House on the Prairie Special Presentations—Look Back to Yesterday (2 hrs.), Bless All the Dear Children (2 hrs.), The Last Farewell (2 hrs.); An Act of Love: The Patricia Neal Story (2 hrs.); Worldvision Dramatic Specials (10 one-hr. specials); Holocaust (9½ hrs.); Against the Wind (13 hrs.); The Ordeal of Patty Hearst (3 hrs.); The Trial of Lee Harvey Oswald (4 hrs.); The Last Nazi (90 min.); Russian Festival of Music and Dance (1 hr.); Reincarnation (2 hrs.); Little Mo (3 hrs.); Freedom Road (4 hrs.); Candid Camera Special (5 one-hrs.); Maximum Security (half-hr. series); Remember Me (2 hrs.).
- Feature Films: More than 200 titles—Prestige Package; 21 features in color including: "Night Watch," "A Touch of Class," "Hedda," "Baker's Hawk," "Black Market Baby," "Breakthrough," "Book of Numbers," "Fingers," "Cry For Me Billy," "Sweet Hostage," "Nasty Habits," and "Thieves"; Paragon Features; over 80 features in color. Stars include Robert Preston, Patty Duke Astin, Valerie Perrine, Dom DeLuise, Patricia Elliott, Gary Coleman, Mickey Rooney, George C. Scott, Henry Fonda, James Whitmore, Dennis Weaver, David Janssen, James Woods, Lee Majors, James Earl Jones, Ed Asner, Suzanne Pleshette, William Devane; Prime I, II, III, IV and V; 84 made-for-TV movies, all in color. Among the stars: Alan Alda, Fred Astaire, Ernest Borgnine, Walter Brennan, LeVar Burton, Sammy Davis Jr., Helen Hayes, Susan Hayward, Hal Holbrook, Janet Leigh, Ray Milland, Agnes Moorehead, Ryan O'Neal, Jack Palance, Lee Remick, Burt Reynolds, Jill St. John, Gloria Swanson, Barbara Stanwyck, Shelley Winters; Selznick Classics; 22 films including "Intermezzo," "Duel in the Sun," "Notorious," "Spellbound," "Rebecca," "The Spiral Staircase," "Portrait of Jenny," "The Farmer's Daughter," "The Garden of Allah," "Bill of Divorcement," "Made For Each Other," and "The Wild Heart"; ABC Pictures; including "Cabaret," "They Shoot Horses Don't They?," "Charly," "Take the Money and Run," "Straw Dogs," "For Love of Ivy," "Song of Norway," "The Killing of Sister George," and "Krakatoa, East of Java" (all in color).
- Children's Programming: Hanna-Barbera/Ruby-Spears; representing thousands of half-hours of animated programming; Casper the Friendly Ghost; Milton the Monster; Jerry Lewis Show; Jackson 5; Lancelot Link.
- Holiday Specials: The Cabbage Patch Kids' First Christmas; Smurfily Ever After (Smurfs Valentine Special, U.K., Ireland & Canada only); I Love the Chipmunks Valentine Special; Alvin & The Chipmunks Reunion (Easter); A Flintstone Christmas; Yogi's First Christmas; Casper's First Christmas; Christmas Comes to Pacland; Smurfs Christmas Special (U.K., Ireland, Canada only); My Smurfy Valentine (U.K., Ireland & Canada only); Smurfs Springtime Special/Easter (U.K., Ireland & Canada only); The Gathering; The Gathering II; Casper Halloween Special; The Pumpkin Who Couldn't Smile; The Thanksgiving Visitor; The Thanksgiving That Almost Wasn't; The Great Santa Claus Caper; A Christmas Story; A Christmas Carol; The Night the Animals Talked; Amahl and the Night Visitors; A Little Bit of Irish; Russian Festival of Music and Dance.
- Series: Little House on the Prairie (216 one hr., starring Michael Landon); Eight is Enough 112 one-hr. comedy-drama, starring Dick Van Patten); Kaz (22 one hr., starring Ron Liebman, Patrick O'Neal); Project UFO (26 fact-based action-adventure, one-hr.); The Andros Targets (starring James Sutorius, 13 one hr.); Spencer's Pilots (starring Christopher Stone, 11 one-hr.); Man From Atlantis (starring Patrick Duffy, 20-½ hrs.); Married: The First Year (starring Leigh McCloskey, 4 one-hr. drama); Pruitts of Southampton (starring Phyllis Diller, 130 half-hr. comedy); The Doris Day Show (128 half hrs.); Hunter (starring James Franciscus, Linda Evans, 13 one hr.); Mod Squad (starring Michael Cole, Peggy Lipton, 124 hr.); The Invaders (starring Roy Thinnes, 43 hrs.); The Fugitive (starring David Janssen, 120 hrs., 30 in color); The Next Step Beyond (John Newland, 24 half hr.); Thunder (12 half hrs.); Garrison's Gorillas (World War II drama, 26 hrs.); Cowboy in Africa (starring Chuck Connors, 26 hrs., color) Ben Casey (153 one-hr., b/w); Lucie Arnaz Show (6 half-hr.)

Worldwide Television News

1926 Broadway, New York, NY 10023; (212) 787-0842. Kenneth Coyte, v.p. & CEO; Roy Berke, U.S. manager. (Produces and distributes newsfilm, Roving Report documentary films, industrail and education documentaries, and industrail film clips.

FILM LIBRARY: 321 W. 44th Street, New York, NY 10036; (212) 265-4520. Vincent O'Reilly, library mgr.

Wrightwood Entertainment, Ltd.

8383 Wilshire Blvd., Suite 770, Beverly Hills, CA 90211; (213) 658-1020. W. P. Donnelly, pres.; Michael Childers, v.p., mktg.; Frank Molloy, v.p., business affairs.

- Feature film packages, including The Twelve Chairs (Mel Brooks), Together (Jacqueline Bisset), etc.; specials, including An Evening with Mel Brooks; plus animated programming including features, series & shorts.

Wright, Carter, Enterprises

6533 Hollywood Blvd., Hollywood, CA 90028; (213) 469-0944. Carter Wright, pres.; June Wright, talent coordinator. (Live and film shows, commercials).

Ziv International

1875 Century Park East, Suite 1610, Los Angeles, CA 90067; (213) 277-9064. Telex: 698619.

- Series: Angel (50), Animator's Film Library (60), Candy Candy (65), Captain Future (52), Captain Harlock (42), Captain Nemo (15), Fables of the Green Forest (52), Gumby (34), King Arthur, (44), Robot Festival, (130), Space Angel (52), Spunky & Tadpole (15), Villa Alegre (260), Man from Buttonwillow (52), Children of the World (13).
- Specials: Tom Jones Live in Vegas, Tony Bennett/Nancy Wilson, Crystal Gayle, Bal Du Moulin Rouge, Peter Cottontail, Silent Knight, Les Miserables.
- Feature length films: 300.
- Merchandising and licensing.

Television Stations

* CHANNEL ALLOCATIONS
* PERSONNEL

TELEVISION STATIONS

[A listing of television stations in the United States. All stations are authorized by and operate under the approval of the Federal Communications Commission, Washington, DC]

ALABAMA

Anniston

WJSU-TV (Channel 40) CBS

P.O. Box 40, Anniston, AL 36202 (205) 237-8651.

Harry E. Mabry, gen. mgr.; David Atchison, prog. dir.; Bill Hagler, gen. sales mgr.; James A. Hudson, chief eng.

Operation: 1969.

Birmingham

WBMG (Channel 42) CBS

Birmingham Television Company, Box 6146, Birmingham, AL 35209 (205) 252-9821.

Roy H. Park, pres.; Hoyle S. Broome, v.p. & gen. mgr.; Joyce Ross, gen. sls. mgr.; Fred Vinson, chief eng.; Ray White, news dir.; Linda McCarty, traffic dir.

Operation: 1965. TV homes in area: 541,000.

WBRC-TV (Channel 6) ABC

Taft Broadcasting Company, P.O. Box 6, Birmingham, AL 35201 (205) 322-6666.

Nick Bolton, gen. mgr.; Bob Fanning, gen. sales mgr.; Jerry Thorn, chief eng.; Telerep Agency, nat'l rep.

Operation: 1949; TV sets in area: 695,500.

WCAZ (Channel 68)

Celtic Media, Inc., 800 Lakeshore Dr., Sanford U., Birmingham, AL 35209 (205) 933-1830.

Sid Burgess, gen. mgr.; Harry Lawson, chief eng.

Operation: 1986.

WTTO (Channel 21)

2021 Golden Crest Dr., Birmingham, AL 35029 (205) 251-2100.

Byron H. Lasky, pres.; Charles B. Rountree, gen. mgr.

Operation: 1982.

WVTM-TV (Channel 13) NBC

WVTM-TV, Inc., P.O. Box 10502, Birmingham, AL 35202 (205) 933-2720.

Wayne Thomas, vice-pres. and genl. mgr.; Stan Bradley, sales mgr.; Paul D. Gross, chief eng.; Everett Holle, prog. dir.; Robert E. Smith, promo. dir.; nat'l reps.: Major Market Television.

Operation: 1949; TV sets in area: 593,000.

Dothan

WDHN (Channel 18) ABC

Southeast Alabama Broadcasting Co., P.O. Box 6237, Dothan, AL 36302 (205) 794-2651.

F. D'Addario, pres.; Betty Marshall-Walker, v.p. & gen. mgr.; Ruth McCullough, asst. mgr.; Shawn Ward, prgm. dir.; David Kirkland, prodn. mgr.; Dan Billings, dir. of eng.

WTVY (Channel 4) CBS

WTVY, Inc., P.O. Box 1089, Dothan, AL 36302; (205) 792-3195.

Charles Woods, owner-mgr.; Reginald Mitchell, prgm. dir.; Jerry Vann, news dir.; Jerry Finn, prodn. mgr.; John Gause, sales mgr.; Carl Blackmon, natl. sls. mgr.; Bill Lyster, chief eng.; regional rep., nat'l rep.: Seltel, Inc.

Operation: 1955; TV sets in area: 587,300.

Florence

WOWL-TV (Channel 15)

Television Muscle Shoals, Inc., 840 Cypress Mill Road, P.O. Box 2220, Florence, AL 35630 (205) 764-7711.

Dick Biddle, chm. of bd. & CEO; Jack Worley, pres.; Lincoln Williams, operations mgr.; Michael Jackson, chief eng.; Sara Biddle, community relations dir.; Donna Kelley, women's program dir.; Cathy Coggin, news desk mgr.

Operation: 1957; TV homes in area: approx. 234,000.

WTRT (Channel 26)

Alabama Mgr. Co., 4600 Jackson Hwy., Sheffield, AL 35660.

Larry M. DeArman, pres.

Huntsville

WAAY-TV (Channel 31)

Rocket City Television, Inc., 1000 Monte Sano Blvd., S.E.; Huntsville, AL 35801 (205) 539-1783.

M.D. Wmith IV, pres.; Dan Whitsett, vp. & sls. mgr.; Robert A. Gay, chief eng.

Operation: 1959.

WAFF-TV (Channel 48) NBC

American Valley Corp., Huntsville, AL 35801 (205) 533-4848.

Joe Goleniowski, v.p. & gen. mgr.; Lee Brantley, station operations mgr.; Harvey Libow, sls. mgr.; Bishop Ellison, chief eng.

Operation: 1954.

WHNT-TV (Channel 19) CBS

The Times Alabama Broadcasting, Inc., 960 Monte Sano Blvd., P.O. Box 19, Huntsville, AL 35804 (205) 533-1919.

Ray Gill, v.p. & gen. mgr.; Bill Ambrose, v.p. & sls. mgr.; Dick Wright, v.p. & opns. mgr.; Dan Roden, chief eng.; Glenn Bracken, news dir.

Operation: 1963.

WZDX (Channel 54)

Community Svc. Broadcasting, Suite 600, Osborne Office Center, Chattanooga, TN 37411 (615) 894-4980.

David Godbout, gen. mgr.; Chris Bailey, gen. sls. mgr.

Operation: April, 1985.

Mobile

WALA-TV (Channel 10) NBC

Universal Communications Corp., 210 Government St., Mobile, AL 36602, P.O. Box 1548 (205) 433-3754. TWX 810 741-2642. FAX-FFB.

Robert F. Finke, v.p. & gen. mgr.; Joe Cook, gen. sls. mgr.; Larry Pate, prog. dir., John Long, chief eng.; Mike Bourgeois, prod. mgr.; Stu Kellogg, news dir.; Ron Gollnick, sports dir.; Steve Johnson, pro. mgr.; Karen Smith, traffic mgr.; nat'l rep.: MMT Sales.

Operation: 1953; TV sets in area: 425,900.

WKRG-TV (Channel 5) CBS

WKRG-TV, Inc., 555 Broadcast Drive, Mobile, AL 36606 (205) 479-5555.

Kenneth R. Giddens, chm; Zelma K. Giddens, vice chm. and treas.; Toulmin Greer, vice chm.; C.P. Persons, Jr., pres. & gen. mgr.; D.H. Long, exec. v.p.; Thomas W. Diamond, senior v.p.; Carl Huag, v.p.; Mary Hutcheson, secret.; Curtis Willard, chief eng.; nat'l rep.: Katz Agency.

Operation: 1955; TV sets in area: 422,400.

WMPV-TV (Channel 21)

120 Zeigler Circle East, Mobile, AL 36608 (205) 633-2100.

Ed Bowlds, pres.

Operation: December, 1985.

WPMI (Channel 15)

P.O. Box 2766, Mobile, AL 36652.

Jim Hester, gen. mgr.; Sherry Blain, asst. gen. mgr.; Dan Bradley, gen. sls. mgr.; Betty Gurley, prog. dir.; Marshall Hart, opns. mgr.; Jerry McCook, chief eng.; nat'l rep.: Seltel.

Operation: 1982.

Montgomery

WCOV-TV (Channel 20) CBS

WCOV, Inc., P.O. Box 2505, Montgomery, AL 36196 (205) 288-7020.

H. Barfield, pres.; Karl Richards, v.p. & gen. mgr.; Phil Witt, chief eng.; nat'l rep.: Seltel.

Operation: 1953; TV sets in area, 172,300.

WKAB-TV (Channel 32) ABC

Montgomery Alabama Channel 32, P.O. Box 3236, Montgomery, AL 36109 (205) 272-5331.

Joseph D. Tydings, pres.; John Rogers, gen. mgr.; Don Darby, gen. sls. mgr.; Judy Motowicki, Operations mgr.; David L. Brown, chief eng. nat'l rep., H.R. Television.

Operation: March 24, 1962; TV households: 156,000.

WMCF-TV (Channel 45)

Life Anew Ministries, Inc., 6261 Atlanta Hwy., Montgomery, AL 36117 (205) 272-0045.

John Stalls, pres.

WSFA-TV (Channel 12) NBC

Cosmos Broadcasting Corp., 10 E. Delano, P.O. Box 2566, Montgomery, AL 36105 (205) 281-2900.

Macon G. Patton, chm. of bd. & pres.; Charles Whitshurst, v.p. & gen. mgr.; Bill Byrd, gen. sls. mgr., Richard Payne, chief eng.; natl. rep., Harrington, Righter & Parsons.

Operation: 1954; TV sets in area: 367,300.

Selma

WAKA-TV (Channel 8) CBS

Central Alabama Broadcasters, Inc., Box 1888, Selma, AL 36701 (205) 875-2240.

George Singleton, gen. mgr.; Randall Johns, prog. dir.; Mike Reynolds, opns. mgr.; Doug Dansby, chief eng.

Operation: 1960.

Tuscaloosa

WCFT-TV (Channel 33) NBC, CBS

Service Broadcasters, Inc.

Stan Siegal, gen. mgr.; Jim Caruthers, sls. mgr.; Tommy Ray, operations mgr.; John Fletcher, chief eng., Eva Rozier, promo. dir.; nat'l rep.: Adam Young Inc.

Operation: Oct. 29, 1965; TV households: 79,900.

WDBB (Channel 17)

Channel 17 of Tuscaloosa, Inc., Box 1006, Tuscaloosa, AL 35403; (205) 345-1117.

David R. Dubose, pres. & gen. mgr.; D. Mike Hood, gen. sls. mgr.; Linda Triplett, prog. dir. & film buyer; Sheryl Mallory, promo. mgr.; Al Whitaker, news dir.; John Batson, chief eng.

Operation: October, 1984.

ALASKA

Anchorage

KIMO (Channel 13) ABC

ABC Alaska Broadcasting, Inc. 2700 E. Tudor Road, Anchorage, AK 99507; (907) 561-1313.

Duane L. Triplett, pres. & gen. mgr.; Richard M. Zook, sr. v.p. & station mgr.; Larry Hogue, gen. sls. mgr., Steve Goodwin, chief eng.; Nat'l rep., Seltel.

Operation: 1967.

KTBY (Channel 4)

Totem Broadcasting Corp., 510 L St., Anchorage, AK 99501.

Robert C. Ely, sec.; Huntly Gordon, treas.

Operation: 1983.

KTUU-TV (Channel 2) NBC

P.O. Box 2880, Anchorage, AL 99501; (907) 276-0202.

Jessica Longston, pres.; Al Bramstedt, Jr., gen. & nat'l sls. mgr.; Coleen Quisenberry, lcl. sls. mgr.; Nancy Johnson, dir. mktg.; Gary O'Guinn, chief eng.; natl. rep.: Avery Knodel.

Operation: 1953; TV sets in area: 99,800.

KTVA (Channel 11) CBS

Northern Television, Inc., Box 10-2200, Anchorage, AK 99510; 272-3456.

A. G. Hiebert, chm.; Ron Moore, pres., Anchorage Div.; Bruce Sloan, operations mgr.; nat'l rep., Art Moore, Inc., Adam Young, Inc.

Operation: 1953; TV sets in area: 70,000.

Fairbanks

KATN-TV (Channel 2) ABC, NBC

Fairbanks TV, Inc., Box 74730, Fairbanks, AK 99707.

Duane L. Triplett, pres.; David L. Geesin, v.p., sta. mgr.; Larry Hogue, gen. sls. mgr.; Ralph Gillette, chief eng.; nat'l rep: Katz.

Operation: 1955; TV sets in area: 23,000.

KTVF (Channel 11) CBS

Northern Television, Inc., Box 950, Fairbanks, AK 99707 (907) 452-5121.

A. G. Hiebert, chm.; Henry Hove, pres.; nat'l rep., Art Moore, Inc.

Operation: 1955; TV sets in area: 27,000.

Juneau

KJUD (Channel 8) ABC, CBS, NBC

1107 Eighth St., Suite 2, Juneau, AK 99801 (907) 586-3145.

Duane Triplett, pres.; Ken Martin, v.p. & gen. mgr.; Rob Kewer, chief eng.; Bob Scot, news dir.; nat'l rep.: Seitel, Tacher.

Operation: 1956.

Sitka

KTNL (Channel 13) CBS

Box 2668, Sitka, AK 99835. (907) 747-6626.

Dr. Dan Etulain, pres. & gen. mgr.; William Ball, sta. mgr.; Charles Clark, prog. dir.; Garth Kanen, chief eng.

Operation: 1966.

ARIZONA

Flagstaff

KNAZ-TV (Channel 2) NBC

Grand Canyon TV Co., Box 1843, Flagstaff, AZ 86002 (602) 526-2232.

Dan Modisett, v.p. & gen. mgr.; Ed Bouchard, chief engr.

Operation: 1970.

Nogales-Tucson

KMSB (Channel 11)

Mountain States Broadcasting, 2445 N. Tucson Blvd., Tucson, AZ 85716; (602) 795-0311.

Randy Cantrell, v.p. & gen. mgr.; Harry West, prog. dir. & film buyer; Larry Lominac, prom. mgr.; Rich Heatley, chief eng.; nat'l rep.: Seltel.

Operation: February, 1967; TV households: 275,000.

Phoenix

KNXV-TV (Channel 15)

New Television Corp., 3722 E. Chipman Rd., Phoenix, AZ 85040. (602) 243-4151.

Byron H. Lasky, bd. chmn.; Edwin Cooperstein, pres. & gen. mgr.; Robert L. Oppenheim, v.p. & gen. counsel; Stanley Pesner, v.p. & treas.; Bruce Sherman, chief eng.; sls. rep.: Katz.

Operation: 1979.

KPAZ (Channel 21)

Trinity Broadcasting of Arizona, Inc., 3351 E. McDowell Rd., Phoenix, AZ 85008 (602) 273-1477.

Paul F. Crouch, pres.

Operation: December, 1969; TV households: 310,000.

KPHO-TV (Channel 5)

Broadcasting Division, Meredith Corporation, 4016 N. Black Canyon, Phoenix, AZ 85017 (602) 264-1000.

Richard Q. DeAngelis, v.p. & gen. mgr.; Don Pauly, gen. sls. mgr.; Bob Galle, natl. sls. mgr.; Charles Alvey, prgm. mgr.; George Hillis, promo. mgr.

Operation: 1949; Total TV Homes: in survey area, 693,000; metro area, 569,600.

KTSP-TV (Channel 10) CBS

KTSP-Taft Television & Radio Co., Inc., 511 W. Adams St., Phoenix, AZ 85003; (602) 257-1234.

Jack Sander, pres. & gen. mgr.; Gary Rockey, prog. mgr.; Tony Twibell, gen. sls. mgr.; Al Hillstrom, chief eng.; Donna Vogt, ad. & prom. mgr.; Sherree Lucas, bus. mgr.; Bill Miller, news dir.; nat'l rep.: HRP.

Operation: 1953; TV households in total survey area: 1,475,800.

KTVK (Channel 3) ABC

Arizona Television Company, 3435 North 16th St., P.O. Box 5068, Phoenix, AZ.

Delbert F. Lewis, pres. & gen. mgr.; Bill Lawrence, chief eng.; James G. Tuton, bus. mgr.; nat'l rep.: Edward Petry Co., Inc.

Operation: 1955; TV homes in area: 480,000.

KTVW (Channel 33)

Seven Hills TV Co., 3019 E. Southern Ave., Phoenix, AZ 85040. (602) 243-3333.

Jose C. Cancela, gen. mgr.; Barry Levisohn, ops. mgr.; Lawrence Beckman, chief eng.

Operation: 1979.

KUTP (Channel 45)

United Television, Inc., 4630 S. 33 St., Phoenix, AZ 85040 (602) 268-4500.

Jerry Braet, v.p. & gen. mgr.; Mike Durand, gen. sls. mgr.; Tom Foy, chief eng.; natl. rep.: Petry.

Operation: December, 1985.

Phoenix-Mesa

KPNX-TV (Channel 12) NBC

KPNX Broadcasting Co., 1101 N. Central Ave., P.O. Box 711, Phoenix, AZ 85001; (602) 257-1212.

C. E. Cooney, pres., gen. mgr.; Bob Allingham, v.p., prog. dir.; Leon Anglin, v.p., eng.; nat'l rep., Blair Television.

Operation: 1954; TV sets in area: 795,300.

Prescott

KUSK (Channel 7)

3211 Tower Rd., Prescott, AZ 86301; (602) 778-6770.

William H. Sauro, pres.; Rich Howe, gen. mgr. & sls. mgr.; Patricia Gray, opns. mgr.; Thayne Higgins, chief eng.

Operation: 1982.

Tucson

KGUN-TV (Channel 9)

May Broadcasting Co., P.O. Box 5707, Tucson, AZ 85703 (602) 792-9933.

Jack Parris, v.p. & gen. mgr.; Bruce Franzen, prog. mgr.; Bob Tobey, gen. sls. mgr.; John Sawyer, chief acct. Phil Aaland, chief eng.; nat'l rep.: Katz Continental.

Operation: 1956; TV sets in area: 238,970.

KOLD-TV (Channel 13) CBS

Universal Communications Corp., 115 W. Drachman St., Tucson, AZ (602) 624-2511.

Jay Watson, v.p. & gen. mgr.; Paul Cassidy, gen. sls. mgr.; Tom Foos. mgr.-programming/pro.; Phil Dunton, chief eng.; Gerald Jensen, news dir.; natl rep., MMT.

Operation: 1953; TV sets in area, 190,000.

KPOL (Channel 40)
2475 Jack Rabbit Ave., Tucson, AZ 85745; (602) 884-9001.
Julius Polan, pres.; David M. Reaban, v.p., gen. mgr. & film buyer; Frank C. Idaspe, v.p. & gen. sls. mgr.; David J. Polan, sta. mgr.; nat. rep.: Avery-Knodel.
Operation: December, 1984.

KVOA-TV (Channel 4) NBC
Channel 4-TV, Inc., P.O. Box 5188, 209 W. Elm, Tucson, AZ 85703 (602) 792-2270.
Jon F. Ruby, exec. v.p. & gen. mgr.; Jim Joslyn, station mgr.; Dave Kerrigan, prod. mgr.; Steve Ruppe, news dir.; Dave Hatfield, prog. dir.; Ralph Turk, chief eng.; Renee Bear, controller, nat'l. rep., Petry.
Operation: 1953; TV sets in area: 274,500.

Yuma

KYEL-TV (Channel 13) NBC
Beam Broadcasters, Ltd., Box 592, Yuma, AZ 85364; (602) 782-5113.
Joe Provenzano, v.p. & gen. mgr.; Frank Jacobs, sls. mgr.; Ed Corn, chief eng.; Frank Etherington, chief eng.; nat'l rep.: Katz.
Operation: December 1963; TV households, 755,900.

ARKANSAS

El Dorado

KTVE (Channel 10) NBC
KTVE, Inc., 2909 Kilpatrick Blvd., Monroe, LA 71201; (318) 323-1300.
James H. Gray, pres.; Hugh V. Roche, v.p. gen. & sis. mgr.; Pete Sparks, chief eng.
Operation: 1955.

Fayetteville-Springdale

KTVP (Channel 29) ABC, CBS
Sigma Broadcasting (An Arkansas partnership), P.O. Box 4150, Fort Smith, AR 72901 (501) 783-4105.
Robert Hernreich, pres.; Darrel Cunningham, gen. mgr.; Cliff Walker, sta. mgr.; Grayson Tobler, local sls. mgr.; Don Vest, chief eng.
Operation: December, 1977; TV households: 41,300.

Ft. Smith

KFSM-TV (Channel 5) NBC, ABC
Buford TV Inc. of Ft. Smith, 318 N. 13th St., Ft. Smith, AR 72901 (501) 783-3131.
Robert Browning, exec. v.p. & gen. mgr.; Gene Graham, gen. sls. mgr.; James Anhalt, chief eng.
Operation: 1956.

KHBS (Channel 40) ABC
Sigma Broadcasting (An Arkansas partnership), 2415 N. Albert Pike, Ft. Smith, AR 72901 (501) 783-4105.
Robert E. Henreich, pres.; Darrel Cunningham, gen. mgr.; Jarrel Wyatt, gen. sls. mgr.; Keith Fry, prog. dir.; Don Vest, chief eng.
Operation: 1971.

KPOM-TV (Channel 24)
Box 1867, 4624 Kelley Highway, Ft. Smith, AR 72902 (501) 785-2400.
Joe Edgell, gen. mgr. & film buyer; David Woods, news dir.; Jan Pearce, chief eng.; nat'l rep.: Seltel.
Operation: 1978.

Jonesboro

KAIT-TV (Channel 8) ABC
Channel Communications of Arkansas, Inc., P.O. Box 790, Jonesboro, AR 72403.
Bill McDonald, v.p. & gen. mgr.; Roberta Tate, natl. sls. mgr.; Al Banks, sls. mgr.; nat'l rep., Katz Continental.
Operation: July, 1963; TV households: 157,600.

Little Rock

KARK-TV (Channel 4) NBC
Mullins Broadcasting Co., 201 West Third, Little Rock, AR 72203 (501) 376-2481; TWX 910-722-7417.
A subsidiary of Combined Communications Corp., Phoenix, AZ.
David J. Jones, pres. & gen. mgr.; Ray V. Brown, gen. sls. mgr.; Jim Tuley, pgm. dir.; David A. Course, promo. dir.; Dean Howard, v.p. & chief eng.; nat'l rep., Blair Television.
Operation: 1954; TV sets in area: 546,310.

KLRT (Channel 16)
11711 West Markham, Little Rock, AR 72211 (501) 375-1616.
Allen S. Feuer, v.p. & gen. mgr.; Jerry D. Garrett, sls. mgr.; John Schweiger, opns. mgr.; Joe Swaty, prom. mgr.; Bill Powell, news & sports dir.; Dexter Merry, chief eng.
Operation: June, 1983.

KTHV (Channel 11) CBS
Arkansas Television Co., 8th & Izard Sts., P.O. Box 269, Little Rock, AR 72203 (501) 376-1111.
Robert L. Brown, pres. & gen. mgr., KTHV, Channel 11; C. S. Berry, chm. of bd., ARK Television Co.; Marcus George, pres. & treas., ARK Television Co.; Lonnie Gibbons, sales mgr.; Bob Hicks, prog. mgr.; nat'l rep: Katz.
Operation: 1955; TV sets in area: 647,500.

Little Rock-Pine Bluff

KATV (Channel 7) ABC
Leake Industries, Inc. 401 Main Street, Little Rock, AR 72203 (501) 372-7777. Also: Jefferson Square Shopping Center, Pine Bluff, AR 71603 (501) 535-7630; Suite 104, Meyer Bldg., Hot Springs, AR 71901 (501) 624-5777; McIlroy Bank, Fayetteville, AR 72701 (501) 442-0324.
James C. Leake, chmn.; John G. Leake, pres.; Dale Nicholson, v.p. & gen. ad. mgr.; Rod Holliday, secty.-treas.; Cal Dring, natl. sls. mgr.; Richard Smith, local sls. mgr.; A. R. Garrett, v.p. eng'.; Eric Nelson, prgm. dir.; nat'l rep.: Edward Petry & Co., Inc.
Operation: 1953; TV sets in area; 647,500.

CALIFORNIA

Anaheim

KDOC-TV (Channel 56)
1730 Clementine St., Anaheim, CA 92806 (714) 999-5000.
Pat Boone, pres.; Mike Volpe, gen. mgr.; Calvin Brack, dir. bus. affairs; Hoshang Moedeli, prog. dir; Bill Welty, chief eng.
Operation: 1982.

Bakersfield

KBAK-TV (Channel 29) ABC
Harriscope Broadcasting Corp., Box 2929, Bakersfield, CA 93303 (805) 327-7955.
Burt I. Harris, pres.; Wayne Killmer, v.p. & gen. mgr.; Bob Banks, chief eng'.; nat'l rep.: Katz.
Operation: 1953; TV sets in area: 560,100.

KERO-TV (Channel 23) CBS
McGraw-Hill Bdctg. Co., Inc., 321 21 Street, Bakersfield, CA 93303 (805) 327-1441. P.O. Box 2367.
John Proffitt, v.p. & gen. mgr.; Thomas Krol, prog. dir.; Norman Hall, dir. of eng.; Walt Brown, news dir.
Operation: 1953; TV sets in area: 280,000.

KGET-TV (Channel 17) CBS
Ackerley Communications, Inc., P.O. Box 1700, Bakersfield, CA 93301 (805) 327-7511.
Raymond A. Watson, pres. & gen. mgr.; Tom Randour, gen. sls. mgr.; Shirley Sanford, prog. dir.; Gene Ross, news dir.; Tom Ballew, chief eng.
Operation: 1959; TV sets in area: 105,000.

Chico

KCPM (Channel 24) NBC
Chico Broadcasting Co., Box 4406, Chico, CA 95927.
Melvin Querio, pres. & gen. mgr.; Ron Gittelson, gen. sls. mgr.; Donna O'Connor, prom. mgr.; Dan McGrath, prod. mgr.; Jack Koonce, chief eng.
Operation: September, 1985.

KHSL-TV (Channel 12) CBS
Golden Empire Broadcasting Co., Box 489, Chico, CA 95927 (916) 342-0141.
C. H. Kinsley, Jr., exec. v.p.; Dino Corbin, gen. mgr.; Bill Meyer, gen. sls. mgr.; Steve Sorenson, prod. mgr.; Russell B. Pope, dir. of eng.; Ernie Fellerson, chief eng. nat'l rep.: Seltel.
Operation: 1953; TV sets in area: 101,460.

Concord

KFCB (Channel 42)
First Century Bcstg., Inc. 5101 Port Chicago Hwy., Concord, CA 94520 (415) 676-8969.
Ronald C. Haus, pres.; Lloyd E. Miller, gen. mgr., prog. dir., & film buyer; Debra C. Fraser, prom. mgr.; Bob McAvoy, chief eng.
Operation: June, 1983.

Cotati

KRCB-TV (Channel 22)
Rural California Broadcasting Corp., Box 2638, Rohnert Park, Cotati, CA 94928; (707) 585-8522.
John F. Kramer, pres.; Nancy Dobbs-Dixon, gen. mgr.; Edward Kiscam, asst. mgr. & prog. dir.; Barbara Leger, promo. mgr.

El Centro

KECY-TV (Channel 9) ABC
Pacific Media Corporation, 646 Main Street, El Centro, CA 92243; P.O. Drawer 741, El Centro, CA 92244.
Bob Martins, vice pres./gen. mgr.; Bill Glenn, prog. dir.; nat'l rep.: Seltel.
Operation: Dec. 1968; TV Households: 436,300.

Eureka

KIEM (Channel 3) CBS, NBC
Precht Communications, Inc., 5650 S. Broadway, Eureka, CA (707) 443-3126.
Robert Precht, pres.; Mike Stocklin, v.p. & gen. mgr.; Peter McNair, sta. mgr.; Donald King, operations mgr.; Marsha Daly, gen. sls. mgr.; nat'l rep.: Avery-Knodel.
Operation: 1953.

KVIQ (Channel 6)
California Northwest Broadcasting Co., P.O. Box 1019, Eureka, CA 95501 (707) 443-3061.
Carl R. McConnel, pres.; Lynn F. Olsen, gen. mgr.; Sallie Gentry, prog. dir.; Mike Fiest, chief eng.
Operation: 1958.

Fontana (Los Angeles)

KTBN-TV (Channel 40)
Trinity Broadcasting Network, P.O. Box A, Santa Ana, CA 92711 (714) 832-2950.
Paul F. Crouch, pres.; Terrency Hickey, prog. dir.; Ben Miller, dir. of eng.; Stan Hollon, dir. sls.
Operation: 1967.

Fresno

KAIL (Channel 53)
Trans-America Broadcasting Corp., P.O. Box 5188, Fresno, CA 93755 (209) 299-9753.
John Lockhart mgr.
Operation: 1961.

KFSN-TV (Channel 30) CBS
Capital Cities Communications, Inc., 1777 G. St., Fresno, CA 93706. (209) 442-1170.
Mark Edwards, v.p. & gen. mgr.; Dudley Few, gen. sls. mgr.; Mark Arminio, lcl. sls. mgr.; Robert Billeci, chief eng.; Fernando Grando, prog. dir.
Operation: 1956.

KJEO (Channel 47) ABC
Retlaw Broadcasting Co., Box 5455, Fresno, CA (209) 222-2411.
Joseph C. Drilling, pres.; William A. Sawyers, v.p. & gen. mgr.; Walter Davis, local sls. mgr.; Jay Hill, chief eng.; Gary Vautin, prog. & promo, dir.; Andrew Mastoras, v.p.-bus. mgr.; Janice Crosby, v.p.-brdct. stnd.; Frances Hernandez, traffic mgr.; nat'l rep.: Peters, Griffin, Woodward.
Operation: 1953; Sets in area: 577,300.

KMPH (Channel 26)
Pappas Telecasting, Inc., 5111 McKinley Ave., Visalia, CA 93727 (209) 733-2600.
Harry J. Pappas, pres. & gen. mgr.; Edward G. Aiken, v.p./TV; Michael Granados, sta. mgr.; Joseph Shaffer, v.p./prog.; Lise Markham, natl. sls. mgr.; Joel Cheatwood;, news dir.; Dale Kelly, chief eng.
Operation: October, 1971.

KSEE (Channel 24) NBC
San Joaquin Communications Corp., 1544 Van Ness Ave., Fresno, CA 93721 (209) 268-6666.
Jim Thompson, pres. & gen. mgr.; Edgar Deatherage, gen. sls. mgr.; Robert Hess, chief engineer.
Operation: 1953; TV sets in area: 261,740.

Hanford-Fresno

KFTV (Channel 21)

Spanish International Communications Corp., 8515 E. Lacey Blvd., Hanford, CA 93230 (209) 584-3362.

August Ruiz, gen. mgr.; Ray Carrasco, gen. sls. mgr.; Mac McKenzie, chief eng.

Operation: 1962.

Los Angeles

KABC-TV (Channel 7) ABC

American Broadcasting Companies, Inc., ABC Television Center, Hollywood, CA 90027 (213) 557-7777.

Thomas K. Van Amburg, v.p. & gen. mgr.; Norman H. Sloane, dir. of admin.; Randall W. Hooper, dir., network prog. operations; Stephen L. Schaefer, sls. service mgr.; William F. Dryer, dir. of eng.; Martin Kirschen, dir. of finance & business affairs; Dennis Swanson, news dir.; natl. rep.: ABC Television Spot Sales, Inc.

Operation: 1949.

KBSC-TV (Channel 52)

Oak Broadcasting Systems, Inc., 1901 Ave. of Stars, Los Angeles, CA 90067 (213) 240-6820.

Andrew Jerrold Perenchio, pres. & gen. mgr.; John Mohr, station mgr.; Bill Morrison, sls. mgr.; Joe Hannigan, chief eng.; Alan Maretsky, traffic mgr.; Joni Penncok, pub. affairs dir.

Operations: 1966.

KCBS (Channel 2) CBS

CBS, Inc. 6121 Sunset Blvd., Los Angeles, CA 90028

James S. Bennett, v.p. & gen. mgr.; John Sutton, sls. dir.; Jay Strong, dir. prog.; Alan Ludlum, mgr. film svcs.; Michael Mischler, dir. comms.; Andrew Fisher, news dir.

Operation: 1950; TV sets in area: 5,028,100.

KCOP (Channel 13)

KCOP Television Inc., a Chris Craft Industries, station, 915 N. La Brea Ave., Hollywood, CA 90038 (213) 851-1000.

Bill Frank, pres. & gen. mgr.; Rick Feldman, gen. sls. mgr.; Peter Mathes, natl. sls. mgr.; Ellen Sambor & Michael Durand, lcl. sls. mgrs.; Win Korabell, dir. of eng.; Jane Clark, bus. mgr.; Peter Schlesinger, dir. of prgm. opns.; Carol Myers Martz, prgm. mgr.; Gary David, dir. of adv./promo.

Operation: 1948; TV sets in area: 4,132,100.

KHJ-TV (Channel 9)

KHJ-TV (Division of RKO General, Inc.), 5515 Melrose Avenue, Hollywood, CA 90038 (213) 467-5459.

Chuck Velona, gen. mgr., KHJ-TV; Sandy Rahimi, gen. sls. mgr.; Walt Baker, program dir.; Dick Paradise, promo. dir.; Buck Evans, chief eng.; Alan Timpson, controller, KHJ Division; nat'l rep., Blair.

Operation: 1948; TV sets in area: 3,511,000.

KMEX-TV (Channel 34)

Spanish International Bcstg. Co., 5420 Melrose Ave., Los Angeles, CA 90038 (213) 466-8131.

Daniel Villanueva, gen. mgr.; Robert Porter, v.p., eng'.; Louis Sweeney, v.p., nat'l sls.; Charles Barry, sls. mgr.; rep., Spanish International Network Sales Inc.

Operation: September, 1962; TV households: 1,500,000.

KNBC (Channel 4) NBC

National Broadcasting Co., Inc., 3000 W. Alameda Ave., Burbank, CA 91523 (213) 840-4444.

Thomas M. Straszewski, NBC v.p. & KNBC gen. mgr.; Bud Carey, sta. mgr.; David Ingraham, dir., business affairs; Robert Kennedy, mgr. adv. & promo.; Richard Askin, dir. sales; Petar Sardelich, mgr. production & operations; Warren Baker, dir. programs; Howard D. Sturm, mgr. public affairs; Saundra Willia, mgr. community relations/press & publicity; Jim Brooks, chief engineer; Rep: NBC Spot Sales.

Operation: Jan. 1949.

KTLA (Channel 5)

Golden West Television, Inc., 5800 Sunset Blvd., Hollywood, CA 90028.

Anthony B. Cassara, pres. & chief exec.; Steve Bell, v.p. & gen. mgr., KTLA.

Operation: 1947; TV sets in area: 4,138,000.

KTTV (Channel 11)

5746 Sunset Blvd., Hollywood, CA 90028 (213) 462-7111.

Charles D. Young, v.p. & gen mgr.; Martin Bergman, v.p. & gen. sls. mgr., Ron Tillman, v.p. and programming dir.; Bob Qudeen, nat'l sls. mgr.; Ted Bending, commercial operations dir.; Lew Schatzer, dir. of promo. and pub.; Ray Green, exec. prod.; Lee Pardee, v.p. & chief eng.; Walter R. Kalb, dir. of bus. affairs; Larry Attebery, news dir. Owned and operated by Metromedia Television, Inc. Rep., Metro TV Sales.

Operation: Jan. 1949.

KWHY-TV (Channel 22)

Harriscope of Los Angeles,Inc., 5545 Sunset Blvd., Los Angeles, CA 90028 (213) 466-5441.

Burt I. Harris, pres.; Burt I. Harris, Jr., v.p. & gen. mgr.; Mike Wagner, acct. exec.; John H. Nelson, acct. exec.; Eugene A. Harris, David J. Zulli, chief eng.

Operation: 1963.

Modesto

KCSO (Channel 19) Spanish language

Sainte Broadcasting Corp., P.O. Box 3689, Modesto, CA 95352 (209) 578-1900.

Chester Smith, pres.; Naomi L. Smith, comptroller.

Monterey

KMST-TV (Channel 46)

Retlaw Broadcasting Co., P.O. Box 1938, Monterey, CA 93940 (408) 649-0460.

Joseph Drilling, pres.; Ben Tucker, gen. mgr.; Cindy Lindsay, sls. mgr.; Kathy Nash, public affairs dir.; Mark Walker, prod. mgr.; Ken Warren, chief eng.; Bob Stock, pro. dir.; Michelle McCullouch, traffic mgr.; Bill Piggott, news dir.

Operations: February, 1969. TV households: 184,800.

Oxnard

KTIE (Channel 63)

KTIE-TV, Inc., 663 Maulhardt, Oxnard, CA 93030; (213) 278-4274.

Donald Sterling, pres.; Bob Bradley, gen. mgr.; Larry Scott, opns. mgr.; Bill Welty, chief eng.

Operation: December, 1984.

Palm Springs

KESQ-TV (Channel 42, Cable 3) ABC

P.O. Box 4200, Palm Springs, CA 92263. Owned by Gulf, Tampa, FL; (619) 328-8881.

Scott Vaughan, gen. mgr.; John S. Sloan, gen. sls. mgr.; nat'l rep.: Katz.

Operation: October 1968; TV households: 63,700.

KMIR-TV (Channel 36) NBC

Desert Empire TV Corp., P.O. Box 1506, Palm Springs, CA 92263 (619) 568-3636.

John Conte, pres. & gen. mgr.; Bob Lancaster, chief exec. & opns. mgr.; John Harrod, news dir. rep.: Avery Knodel.

Operation: Oct. 1968; TV households: 54,900.

Redding

KRCR TV (Channel 7) ABC

Sacramento Valley Television, Inc., 755 Auditorium Dr., Redding (Shasta Co.), CA 96001 (916) 243-7777.

Richard W. Green, pres. & gen. mgr.; William B. Smullin, v.p., dir. of operations; Doreeta Domke, operations mgr.; nat'l rep., Blair.

Sacramento

KCRA-TV (Channel 3) NBC

Kelly Broadcasting Co., 310 10th St., Sacramento, CA 95814 (916) 444-7300.

Robert E. Kelly, partner; Jon S. Kelly, partner; Nina N. Kelly, partner; Don Saraceno, gen. mgr.; nat'l rep.; Blair Television, Inc.

Operation: 1955; TV sets in area: 558,900.

KRBK-TV (Channel 31)

Koplar Communications, Inc., 220 N. Kings Hwy., St. Louis, MO 63108. (916) 929-0300.

Ted Koplar, pres.; Hal Protter, exec. v.p. & chief operations officer.

Operation: 1974.

KTXL (Channel 40)

Camellia City Telecasters, Inc., P.O. Box 40, Sacramento, CA 95801 (916) 452-8221.

Jack F. Matranga, pres., gen. mgr. & film buyer; Robert Parente, natl. sales mgr.; Bill Kreutzer, chief eng.; Cal Bollwinkel, operations & prog. mgr.

Operation: 1968.

KXTV (Channel 10) CBS

Belo Broadcasting Corp., 400 Broadway, Sacramento, CA 95818 (916) 441-4041.

Ward Huey, pres.; Allan Howard, v.p. & gen. mgr.; Michael Fiorile, gen. sls. mgr.; Kurt Eichsteadt, prog. mgr.; Michael Grant, mktg./promo. mgr.; natl. rep.: MMT.

Operation: 1955; TV sets in area: 648,500.

Salinas

KCBA (Channel 35) SIN

Sainte Broadcasting Corp., Box 3560, Salinas, CA 93912; (408) 422-3500.

Chester Smith, pres. & gen. mgr.; Hal Larson, gen. sls. mgr.; Phil Linn, chief eng.

Operation: November, 1981

KSBW-TV (Channel 8) NBC

Blair Broadcasting of California, Inc., P.O. Box 81651, 238 John St. Salinas, CA 93912 (408) 758-8888. (Affiliated with KSBY-TV, San Luis Obispo, CA)

Keith H. Moon, pres.; Rickie Ellis, nat'l sls. mgr.; Teresa Burgess, prog. mgr.; nat'l reps.: Blair.

Operation: 1953; TV homes in area: 188,900.

San Bernardino

KAGL (Channel 30)

Marantha Broadcasting Co., Box 10070, Anaheim, CA 92802 (714) 535-5456.

Robert Billman, pres.; Timothy Waisanem, gen. mgr.; Vera Waisanem, gen. sls. mgr.; Will Welty, prog. dir.

Operation: March, 1986.

KSCI (Channel 18)

Global Television, Inc., 1954 Cotner Ave., West Los Angeles, CA 90025; (213) 479-8081.

Thomas Headley, pres.; Paul Niedermeyer, gen. mgr.; Michael Adachi, gen. sls. mgr.; Christopher Hargrove, prog. dir.; Alfonso Araya, Spanish prog. dir.

Operation: June, 1977.

San Diego

KCST-TV (Channel 39) NBC

KCST-TV, Inc., 8330 Engineer Rd., San Diego, CA 92111 (619) 279-3939.

Bill L. Fox, v.p. & gen. mgr.; Bill Peterson, asst. gen. mgr.; Bruce Stein, dir. sls.; Tom Wimberly, dir. of tech. svcs.; Ken Nelson, news dir.; Ric Schwartz, prod. mgr.; Penny Martin, prog. mgr.

Operation: 1965.

KFMB-TV (Channel 8) CBS

Midwest Television, Inc., 7677 Engineer Road, San Diego, CA 92101 (714) 292-5362.

August C. Meyer, Jr., pres.; Robert L. Myers, vice-pres. & gen. mgr.; Bill Moylan, v.p., operations; John Weigand, chief eng.; nat'l rep.. Petry.

Operation: 1949, TV sets in area: 1,015,800.

KGTV (Channel 10) ABC

McGraw-Hill Broadcasting Co., P.O. Box 85347, San Diego, CA 92138 (619) 237-1010.

Clayton H. Brace, v.p. & gen. mgr.; William Christensen, dir. of eng.; Howard Oleff, local sls. mgr.; Joan Carson, gen. sls. mgr.; Helen Hutchings, dir., business affairs; Don Lundy, prog. dir.

Operation: 1953.

KTTY (Channel 69)

San Diego Family TV, Inc., 1696 Frontage Rd., Chula Vista, CA 92016; (619) 575-6969.

James M. Harmon, pres.; George F. Stanis, exec. v.p. & gen. mgr.; Walter Davis, gen. sls. mgr.; Gene Wilkin, prog. consult. & film buyer; Linda Fox, promo mgr.; Jan Garrett, new dir.; natl. rep.: Seltel.

Operation: October, 1984.

KUSI-TV (Channel 51)

7377 Convoy Ct., San Diego, CA 92111 (619) 571-5151.

William Rust, pres.; Michael McKinnin, gen. mgr.; William E. Moore, sta. mgr.; Joy Ollred, gen. sls. mgr.; nat'l rep.: Katz.

Operation: 1982.

XETV (Channel 6) Independent

Bay City Television, Inc., 8253 Ronson Road, Television Heights, San Diego, CA 92111 (619) 279-6666.

Martin M. Colby, v.p. & gen. mgr.; Louis J. Meiers, treas./bus. mgr.; Joan O'Laughlin, sta. mgr. and gen. sls. mgr.; Carol Healey, prog. & promo. dir.; Felipe Fernandez, chief eng.; Julian Kaufman, consultant; nat'l rep., Blair Television.

Operation: 1953; TV sets in area: 582,450.

XEWT-TV (Channel 12) Spanish language

Televisora de Calimex, S.A., P.O. Box 12, Tijuana, Baja California, Mexico (706) 685-9201 and 685-9202.

Jose Marquez, gen. mgr.; Carlos H. Luna, prog. prom. mgr.; Roberto Espinoza, business mgr.

San Francisco

KBHK-TV (Channel 44)

UTV of San Francisco Inc., 420 Taylor St., San Francisco, CA 94102 (415) 885-3750.

Robert Qudeau, v.p. & gen. mgr.; Heather Farnsworth, gen. sls. mgr.; Chris Jenkins, lcl. sls. mgr.; Richard Jones, natl. sls. mgr.; Nancy Graham, news & pub. affairs mgr.; Ed Hipps, eng. mgr.; Jo Russell, prod. mgr.

Operation: January, 1968. TV households: 3,953,400.

KDTV (Channel 14) Spanish language

Bahia de San Francisco TV Co., 2200 Palou Ave., San Francisco 94124, an affiliate of SIN Television Network.

Reynold V. Anselmo, pres.; Emilio Nicolas, Jr., v.p. & gen. mgr.; Jorge Belon, prod. & programming dir.; Sharon Michelucci, bus. mgr.; Kenneth Schreiner, chief eng.

Operation: 1975.

KGO-TV (Channel 7) ABC

American Broadcasting Companies, Inc., 277 Golden Gate Ave., San Francisco, CA 94102 (415) 863-0077.

Jim Osborn, v.p. & gen. mgr.; Bob Young, gen. sls. mgr.; Bob Woodruff, prog. dir.; Dave Kenworthy, dir. of adv. prom. & pub.; Pet Jacobus, news dir.; Jim Von Striver, chief eng.; Rose Guilbault, comm. affairs dir.; nat'l rep.: ABC Spot Sales.

Operation: 1949; TV homes in area: 1,575,000.

KPIX (Channel 5) CBS

Group W (Westinghouse Broadcasting Co.), 855 Battery St., San Francisco, CA 94111 (415) 362-5550.

Arthur Kern, v.p. & gen. mgr.; Fred Eppinger, natl. sls. mgr.; Marty Edelman, lcl. sls. mgr.; Ann Miller, prog. dir.; Bruno Cohen, news dir.

Operation: 1948; TV households in area: 1,894,000.

KRON-TV (Channel 4) NBC

Chronicle Broadcasting Co., subsidiary of The Chronicle Publishing Company, 1001 Van Ness Avenue, San Francisco, CA (415) 441-4444.

F.A. Martin III, pres. and chief exec. officer; James H. Smith, v.p. and gen. mgr.; G.E. "Tom" Pickell, v.p. of finance and admin.; Ron Collins, gen. sls. mgr.; David Wilson, prog. mgr.; Mike Ferring, news dir.; Bruce Lindgren, dir., creative services; nat'l rep.: Petry Television.

Operation: 1949; TV households in area: 2,068,000.

KTSF-TV (Channel 26)

Lincoln Broadcasting Co., 185 Berry St., San Francisco, CA 94107 (415) 495-4995.

Lillian L. Howell, owner; Brian Holton, sta. mgr.

KTVU (Channel 2)

San Francisco-Oakland Television, No. 2 Jack London Square, Oakland, CA 94607 (415) 834-1212.

Alan J. Bell, v.p. & gen. mgr.; Richard Goldman, gen. sls. mgr.; Michael Liff, natl. sales mgr.; Jay Sondheim, local sls. mgr.; Thomas A. Breen, prog. dir.; Marlene Holderbaum, contr.; Dick Weise, promo. mgr.; Ian Zellick, dir. of pub. affairs; Jay Finkelman, station mgr.; Ray Jacobs, dir. of operations; Fred Zehnder, news dir.; Ray Swenson, chief eng.

Operation: 1958.

KTZO (Channel 20)

Pacific FM Inc., 2500 Marin St., San Francisco, CA 94124. (415) 285-6420.

James J. Gabbert, pres.; Michael P. Lincoln, gen. mgr.; Bob Swisher, sls. mgr.

Operation: 1968; TV households, 770,300.

KWBB (Channel 38)

West Coast United Bdcstg. Inc., 4041 Rusont Way, Tacoma, WA 98102 (206) 756-0924.

Huntly Gordon, pres. & gen. mgr.; Doug Davis, gen. sls. mgr.; David Ratener, chief eng.; natl. rep.: Adam Young.

Operation: 1986.

Sanger

KMSG-TV (Channel 59)

Sanger Telecasters, Inc., Box 59, Sanger, CA 93657 (209) 435-5900.

Diane D. Cocola, pres.; James K. Zahn, gen. mgr.; Gary M. Cocola, gen. sls. mgr.; Jeff Wiedenhoeff, prog. dir.; Steve Weber, chief eng.

Operation: July, 1985.

San Jose

KICU-TV (Channel 36)

Ralph C. Wilson Industries, Inc., 1585 Schallenberger Rd., San Jose, CA 95109. (408) 298-6676. Studio: 1536 Kerley Dr., San Jose, CA 95112. (408) 298-6676.

William Hirshey, pres.; John Davidson, v.p. & gen. mgr.; Dan Romanelli, sta. mgr. & dir. of sls.; Brent Scheiner, gen. sls. mgr., Jim Kraenzel, chief eng.

Operation: 1967.

KNTV (Channel 11)

Gill Industries, 645 Park Avenue, San Jose, CA 95110; (408) 286-1111.

Robert M. Hosfeldt, v.p. & gen. mgr.; Stewart B. Park, prog. director & film buyer; John Yearwood, gen. sls. mgr.; Lee Schell, news dir.; Lou Bell, chief engr.; Barbara Smith, contr.; nat'l rep., Katz Television.

Operation: 1955.

KSTS (Channel 48)

National Group TV, Inc., 2349 Bering Dr., San Jose, CA 95131 (408) 946-3400.

N. John Douglas, chm. & news dir.; John Rohrbach, Jr., pres. & gen. mgr.; Mike Maze, opns. mgr.; Mike Kelley, gen. sls. mgr.; John Rohrbach, film buyer; Karl Kauffman, chief eng.

Operation: 1981.

San Luis Obispo

KSBY-TV (Channel 6)

Blair Broadcasting of California, Inc., 476 Hill St., San Luis Obispo, CA 93401 (805) 543-0920.

David Cox., v.p./gen. mgr.; John Grimes, operations mgr.; Ken Reid, chief eng.

Operation: 1953.

Santa Barbara

KEYT (Channel 3) ABC

Shamrock Broadcasting, P.O. drawer X, Santa Barbara, CA 93102.

Jack McWeeny, gen. mgr.; Steve Lakey, promo. mgr.; Renee Foley, prog. supvr.; King Harris, news dir.; Frank Goddard, chief eng.; nat'l rep.: Seltel.

Operation: 1953; TV sets in area: 200,000.

Santa Maria

KCOY-TV (Channel 12) CBS

Stauffer Communications, Inc., 1503 N. McClelland, Santa Maria, CA 93454 (805) 922-0505.

Charles Stauffer, gen. mgr.; Tom Murphy, prod. mgr.; Bill Pierce, news dir.; Dennis Bornhoft, chief eng. Rep.: Katz.

Operation: 1964; TV households: 193,000.

Santa Rosa

KFTY (Channel 50)

Sonoma Broadcasting, Inc., Box 1150, Santa Rosa, CA 95402.

James D. Johnson, exec. v.p. & gen. mgr.; Frank Savage, v.p., sls. & mktg.; Joe Perez, v.p., engineering; Rod Sherry, news dir.

Operation: 1981.

Stockton/Sacramento

KOVR (Channel 13)

Outlet Broadcasting, 225 E. Miner Ave., Stockton, CA 95202 (209) 466-6981. Sacramento Studio and Main Business Office: 1216 Arden Way, Sacramento, CA 95815 (916) 927-1313.

Chas. F. Kennedy, pres. & gen. mgr.; Doug Grant, sls. mgr.; Robert Hess, chief eng.; Henry Urick, prog. mgr.; nat'l rep: Katz Agency.

Operation: 1954; TV sets in area (Sacramento/Stockton Mkt.) 769,700.

COLORADO

Colorado Springs—Pueblo

KKTV (Channel 11) CBS

KKTV Inc., P.O. Box 2110, 80901; 3100 N. Nevada Ave., Colorado Springs, CO (303) 634-2844.

Barry Ackerley, pres.; James Lucas, v.p./gen. mgr.; nat'l rep.: Katz, West.

Operation: 1952; TV households in area: 367,300; Total households in survey area: 375,200.

KOAA-TV (Channel 5) NBC

Sangre de Cristo Communications, Inc., 2200 7th Avenue, Pueblo, CO 81003 (303) 544-5782.

John O. Gilbert, pres. & gen. mgr.; Kenneth Renfrow, chief eng.; Jack Sinclair, prog. dir.; Flo Isringhausen, natl. sls. mgr.; Marcy Cannon & Jim Schaeffer, lcl. sls. mgrs.; Dave Ross, dir. opns. news.

Operation: 1953; TV sets in area: 296,700.

KRDO-TV (Channel 13) ABC

Pikes Peak Broadcasting Co., P.O. Box 1457, Colorado Springs, CO 80901 (303) 632-1515.

Harry W. Hoth, Jr., pres.; Neil O. Klocksiem, gen. mgr.; Charles H. Upton, chief eng.

Operation: 1953; TV sets in area: 199,500.

KXRM-TV (Channel 21)

KXRM, Inc., 5050 Edison Ave., Colorado Springs, CO 80915.

Larry W. Douglas, pres., gen. mgr., prog. dir. & film buyer; Chip Lusko, gen. sls. mgr.; Roger G. Meyer, promo. mgr.; Jack Connelly, Sr., chief eng.

Operation: December, 1984.

Denver

KCNC (Channel 4) NBC

General Electric Broadcasting Company of Colorado, Inc., 1044 Lincoln Street, P.O. Box 5012 T.A., Denver, CO 80217 (303) 861-4444.

Robert L. Ogden, pres./gen. mgr.; J.H. MacDermott, v.p./sta. mgr.; David Layne, mgr. engineering; Jay Rabin, gen. sls. mgr.; Marv Rockford, v.p./news dir.; Lon Lee, v.p./prm. mgr.; Tom Edwards, production mgr.; Marv Danielski, promotion mgr.

KDVR (Channel 31)

Centennial Bcstg. Corpl., 100 Speer Blvd., Denver, CO 80203; (303) 831-8831.

George M. Sandoval, v.p. & sta. mgr.; Sid Gurkin, gen. sls. mgr.; John Schnick, promo.mgr.; Steve Coulam, eng. dir.; natl. rep.: MMT.

Operation: August, 1983.

KMGH-TV (Channel 7) CBS

McGraw-Hill Co., Inc., 123 Speer Blvd., Denver, CO 80203 (303) 832-7777.

Edward T. Reilley, pres.; Bob Wjite, v.p. & gen. mgr.; Robert Barron, gen. sls. mgr.; Mary Carole McDonnell, dir. of prog.; Robert A. Chernet, dir. of adv. & promo.; Shirley Thompson, traffic mgr.; Arta Boley, news dir.; Lary Pozzi, dir. of eng.

Operation: 1953.

KUSA (Channel 9) ABC

Gannet Broadcasting., 1089 Bannock St., Denver, CO 80204 (303) 893-9000.

Larry Deutsch, v.p. & gen. sls. mgr.; Charles T. Leasure, pres. & gen. mgr.; Darla Ellis, v.p. & prog. dir.; Lee Minard, promo. mgr.; Richard Mallary, news dir.; Tim Dietz, prod. mgr.

Operation: 1952; TV sets in area: 713,300.

KWGN (Channel 2)

WGN of Colorado, Inc., 6160 S. Wabash Way, Englewood, CO (303) 740-2222.

Robert A. Innes, v.p. & gen. mgr.; Mel Smith, prog. mgr.; Tanette Maffei, promo. mgr.; Lorrie Shilling, on-air promo. mgr.; Tarey Thornburg, film dir.; Ron Peters, chief eng.; Jack Brennan, v.p. & dir. of mktd.

Operation: 1952; TV sets in area: 568,400.

Durango

KREZ-TV (Channel 6) NBC, CBS

(Satellite of KREX-TV, Grand Junction, CO)

XYZ TV Inc., Box 789, Grand Junction, CO 81502 (303) 247-0820.
Larry Keenan, gen. mgr.
Operation: Nov., 1963.

Glenwood Springs

KCWS (Channel 3)
Western Slope Communications, Ltd., 6916 State Hwy. 82, Glenwood Springs, CO 81601 (303) 945-7333.
David B. Sontag, pres. & prog. dir.; Harlan Reams, gen. & gen. sls. mgr.; Bob Blauvelt, chief eng.
Operation: December, 1983.

Grand Junction

KJCT-TV (Channel 8) ABC, P.O. Box 3788, Grand Junction, CO 81502
Harry W. Hoth, pres.; Steve Robinson, sta. mgr.; Roger Hightower, chief eng.
Operation: 1979; TV households: 49,400

KREX-TV (Channel 5) CBS, NBC
XYZ Television, Inc., Hillcrest Manor, Grand Junction, CO (303) 242-5000.
Larry Keenan, gen. mgr. nat'l rep.: Katz.
Operation: 1954; TV sets in area: 61,000 (ARB).

Montrose

KREY-TV (Channel 10) NBC, CBS
(Satellite of KREX-TV, Grand Junction, CO)
XYZ Television Inc., Box 789, Grand Junction, CO 81502 (303) 249-9601.
Larry Keenan, gen. mgr.; Joe Reichman, sta. mgr.; nat'l rep.: Katz.
Operation: 1956.

Sterling

KTVS (Channel 3) CBS, ABC
(Satellite of KYCU-TV, Cheyenne, WY)
Wyneco Communications, Inc., 2923 E. Lincolnway, Cheyenne, WY 82001.
Carl J. Occhipinti, gen. mgr.; Gene Huston, res. mgr.; Jerry Homer, chief eng.; nat'l rep.: Katz.
Operation: Dec. 1963.

CONNECTICUT

Bridgeport

WBCT (Channel 43)
101 Ansonia Rd., Woodbridge, CT 06525.
L. Vlock, pres.; H. O'Neill, gen. mgr.
Operation: July, 1984

Hartford

WFSB-TV (Channel 3)
Post-Newsweek Stations, Connecticut, Inc., 3 Constitution Plaza, Hartford, CT 06115 (203) 525-0801.
G. William Ryan, pres. & gen. mgr.; Barry Barth, v.p. & sta. mgr.; Cathy Nierle, v.p., admin.; Dick Ahles, v.p. news.; Mike Dorsey, v.p. sls.
Operation: 1957; TV sets in area: 1,151,447.

WHCT (Channel 18)
A Division of Faith Center, Inc., 580 Deercliff Rd., Avon, CT 06001; (203) 677-2281.
Dr. Eugene Scott, pres.; Terry Wood, gen. mgr. & chief eng.
Operation: 1959.

WTIC (Channel 61)
Arch Communications, Inc., One Corporate Center, Hartford, CT 06103; (203) 527-6161.
Arnold L. Chase, pres.; Bruce C. Mayer, v.p. & gen. mgr.; Lew Krause, gen. sls. mgr.; David J. Uhrich, opns. mgr.; Neil Portnoy, chief eng.; natl. rep.: Katz.
Operation: September, 1984.

New Britain

WVIT (Channel 30) NBC
1422 New Britain Ave., West Hartford, CT 06110 (203) (203) 521-3030.
Pat Brady, v.p./gen. mgr.; Al Bova, v.p./sta. mgr.
Operation: 1953; TV sets in area: 820,000.

New Haven-Hartford

WTNH-TV (Channel 8) ABC
Capital Cities Communications, Inc., 135 College St., New Haven, CT (203) 777-3611.
Peter K. Orne, gen. mgr.; Marc Edwards, gen. sls. mgr.; Will Mebrane, prog. mgr.; O. Lyle Koch, promo. mgr.; Tom Kirby, news dir.; Bruce Lawrence, sls. mgr.; Steve Perler, bus. mgr.; Bill Ellison, dir. pub. aff.; Larry Curtis, chief eng.; nat'l rep.: Blair TV, Inc.
Operation: 1948; TV sets in area: 1,949,200.

New London

WLCT (Channel 26)
CTV of Connecticut, 216 Broad St., New London, CT 06320; (203) 444-2626.
Neil A. Denenburg, pres.; Jim Kontoleon, gen. mgr., prog. dir., film buyer & promo. mgr.; John Hysler, gen. sls. mgr.; Steven Ellis, chief eng.
Operation: March, 1985.

Waterbury

WTXX (Channel 20) IND
Channel 20 Enterprises, 414 Meadow St., Waterbury, CT 06702 (203) 575-2020.
Michael Finkelstein, pres.; Geoffrey Rose, gen. mgr.; Harvey Adelberg, gen. sls. mgr.; Melanie Gerig, prog. dir.; Charles Allen, chief eng.; nat'l rep.: MMT, Inc.
Operation: 1953: TV sets in area: 813,000.

DISTRICT OF COLUMBIA

Washington

WDCA-TV (Channel 20)
Channel 20 Inc., 5202 River Rd., Washington, DC 20016.
Milton Grant, v.p. & gen. mgr.; Joseph Girard, gen. sls. mgr.; Jim Reid, prog. mgr.; Don A. Doughty, dir. of engineering; Dan O'Brian, operations mgr.; Raymond E. Simko, bus. mgr.; rep.: PGW.
Operation: April, 1966; TV households: 1,724,500.

WDVM-TV (Channel 9) CBS
A division of the Evening News Association, Inc., 4001

Brandywine St., NW, Washington, DC 20016.
Edwin W. Pfeiffer, v.p./gen. mgr.; Ronald Townsend, station mgr.; Edward P. Jones, prgm. mgr.; Henry K. Yaggi III, dir. of sls.; Lawrence P. Herbster, dir. of bus. affairs; Henry Owen, dir. of eng.; Rep: MMT Sales.
Operation: 1949; TV households in ADI area: 1,390,300.

WFTY (Channel 50)
Hill Broadcasting, Inc., 6507 Chillum P.N.W., Washington, DC 20012 (202) 723-1040.
Gerald M. Liss, gen. mgr.; Angela Holmes, bus. mgr.; Gary W. Gillis, opns. mgr.
Operation: 1981.

WJLA-TV (Channel 7) ABC
Allbritton Communications Co. 4461 Connecticut Avenue, N.W. Washington, DC 20008.
Thomas B. Cookerly, pres. & gen. mgr.; James E. Griffin, Jr., v.p., dir. bdcst. opns.; Thursa C. Thomas, dir. public affairs; John Tollefson, v.p., eng.; John C. Long, v.p., dir. sls.; nat'l rep.: Petry Co.

WRC-TV (Channel 4) NBC
National Broadcasting Co., 4001 Nebraska Ave., N.W., Washington, DC 20016 (202) 885-4000.
Frederick DeMarco, v.p. & gen. mgr.; David Nuell, station mgr.; Lawrence Tompkins, dir. sls.; Larry Spero, mgr. sls.; Kathy McCampbell, dir. prog.; Jim Van Messel, news dir.; William Johnston, dir. oper. & eng.; Bill Scholz, dir. plant facilities & purchasing; Bob Casazza, promo. mgr.
Operation: June, 1947; TV households: 4,637,400.

WTTG (Channel 5)
Metromedia Television, a division of Metromedia, Inc., 5151 Wisconsin Ave., N.W. Washington DC 20016 (202) 244-5151.
Bob O'Connor, v.p. & gen. mgr.; Ed Shea, v.p. & gen. sls. mgr.; Richard Pfister, v.p. chg. of eng.; Sandra Pastoor, v.p. prog. dir.; Richard Kantor, v.p. bus. mgr.; Lindy Spero, dir. adv./promo.; nat'l rep.: Katz.
Operation: 1947; TV sets in area: 2,647,100.

FLORIDA

Clearwater

WCLF (Channel 22)
Christian Television Corp., Inc., 6922 142nd Ave., N., Largo, FL 33541 (813) 535-5622.
Robert D'Andrea, gen. mgr.; Lori Branham, prog. dir.; Carl Berger, chief eng.
Operation: 1979.

Cocoa

WTGL-TV (Channel 52)
Box 1852, 26 forrest Ave., Cocoa, FL 32922 (305) 631-2730.
Robert D'Andrea, pres.; J. Brock Lesperance, gen. mgr.; Phil Grace, v.p.; Jim Goodling, treas.; Gene Polino, secty.; Ken Mikesell, opns. dir.; Dale Wright, prog. dir.; Bill Bryan, chief eng.
Operation: 1982.

Daytona Beach-Orlando

WESH-TV (Channel 2)
WESH-TV Broadcasting, Inc., P.O. Box 1551, Daytona Beach, FL 32015; (904) 252-2222.
Tom Reiff, exec. v.p. & gen. mgr.; Jack Hitchcock, v.p. & sta. mgr.; Robert Fowler, gen. sls. mgr.; Kenneth Smith, oper. mgr.; nat'l rep.: Petry.
Operation: 1956; TV households: 1,516,000.

Fort Lauderdale

WSCV (Channel 51)
Oak Television of Fort Lauderdale, Inc., 4035 N. 29th Ave., Hollywood, FL 33022 (305) 920-9400.
Julio Rumbaut, pres. & gen. mgr.; Bruce Dunn, opns. mgr.
Operation: 1980.

Fort Myers

WBBH-TV (Channel 20) NBC
Waterman Broadcasting Corp. of Texas, 3719 Central Ave., Fort Myers, FL 33901 (813) 939-2020.
Howard L. Hoffman, v.p. & gen. mgr.; Bob Cleveland, chief eng.; Rosie Rose, compt.; Doug Kight, sales & mgr.; Jim Bradley, news admin.
Operation: December, 1968; TV households: 173,900.

WEVU (Channel 26) ABC
P.O. Box 06260, Fort Myers, FL 33906 (813) 332-0076.
Ray Karpowicz, gen. mgr.; Hank Douglas, sls. mgr.; Sue Caswell, prog. dir.
Operation: 1974.

WINK-TV (Channel 11) CBS
Fort Myers Broadcasting Co., 2824 Palm Beach Blvd., Fort Myers, FL 33902 (813) 334-1331.
Edward J. McBride, pres.; Robert F. Doty, v.p. & gen. mgr.; Jr.; Mike Dixon, gen. sls. mgr.; Clarence Mosley, dir. eng.; Jim Bennett, news dir.; Fred Greene, public affairs dir.; nat'l rep.: Blair Television.
Operation: 1954.

Fort Pierce

WTVX (Channel 34) CBS
WTVW, Inc., Box 3434, Ft. Pierce, FL 33450 (305) 464-3434.
Frank K. Spain, pres.; Lynwood N. Wright, gen. mgr.; Joan van Dyke, prog. dir.; Jay Oliver, promo. dir.; Max Berryhill, chief, eng.; nat't rep.: Avery-Knodel.
Operation: April 5, 1966; TV households: 69,400.

Fort Walton Beach

WPAN (Channel 53)
Ft. Walton Beach Broadcasting, 11 Tupelo Ave., S.E., Ft. Walton Beach, FL 32548; (904) 244-5353.
Elbert R. Davis, pres. & gen. mgr.; Hank Taylor, sta. mgr., prog. dir. & film buyer; Jim Riggs, gen. sls. mgr.; Patty Vogt, promo. mgr.; Jerry O'Laughlin, news dir.; Richard Gilbert, chief eng.; natl. rep.: Adam Young.
Operation: February, 1984.

Gainesville

WCJB (Channel 20) ABC
Gainesville Television, Inc., P.O. Box WCJB, Gainesville, FL 32602 (904) 372-3543.

Garry H. Ritchie, v.p. & gen. mgr.; Michael A. Sherrill, chief eng.
Operation: 1971.

Jacksonville

WAWS-TV (Channel 30)

Malrite of Jacksonville, Inc., 8675 Hogan Rd., Jacksonville, FL 33216 (904) 642-3030.

Lynn Fairbanks, sta. gen. mgr.; Dan Gasby, gen. sls. mgr.; Joe Gersh, natl. sls. mgr.; Richard M. Sullivan, dir. of prog. & operations.; nat'l rep.: I.N.T.V.
Operation: 1981.

WJKS-TV (Channel 17) NBC

9117 Hogan Rd., Box 17000, Jacksonville, FL 32216 (904) 641-1700.

John Radeck, v.p. & gen. mgr.; Karen Heniger, gen. sls. mgr.; Russ Myerson, prgm. mgr.; Harold Johnson, chief engr.
Operation: Feb. 1966.

WJXT (Channel 4) CBS

WJXT, operated by the Post-Newsweek Stations, Florida Inc., P.O. Box 5270, 1851 Southampton Road, Jacksonville, FL 32207 (904) 399-4000.

Gus Bailey, Jr., v.p. & gen. mgr.; Ann Pace, prog. dir.; Christy Birong, dir. community affairs; Don Carmichael, gen. sls. mgr.; Mel Martin, v.p./news dir.; Cindy Hass, op. mgr.; Jim Biggers, eng. mgr.; nat'l rep.: Petry.
Operation: 1949; TV sets in area: 546,000.

WNFT (Channel 47)

North Florida 47, Inc., 2117 University Blvd., So., Jacksonville, FL 32216 (904) 725-4700.

Ray Davis, v.p. & gen. mgr.; Larry Jacobs, prom. mgr.; Raymond Firment, sls. mgr.; Mark E. Cook, prog. opns. mgr.; Virginia McNulty, news dir.; Charles McHan, chief eng.
Operation: 1980.

WTLV (Channel 12) ABC

Television 12 of Jacksonville, Inc., Television P.O. Box TV-12, Jacksonville, FL 32231 (904) 354-1212.

Howard Kelley, gen. mgr.; Ken Bauder, gen. sls. mgr.; Steve Rabb, natl. sls. mgr.; Dave Richardson, news dir.; Harry Alexander, prod. dir.; Rosemary Shouldice, promo. dir.; Clyde Smith, chief eng.
Operation: 1957.

Lakeland

WTMV (Channel 32)

646 Boca Ceiga Isle Dr., St. Petersburg Beach, FL 33706; (813) 376-4224.

Dan L. Johnson, gen. mgr.; Betty Jo Johnson, sta. mgr.; Robert Hughes, promo. mgr.; Henry Ruiz, news dir.; Dan Lunin, chief eng.
Operation: January, 1985.

Leesburg

WIYE (SuperChannel 55)

Sharp Communications, Inc., Box 777, Leesburg, FL 32749-0777 (904) 787-2287.

Claud Bowers, pres. & gen. sls. mgr. & prog. dir.; Sylvia Bryan, film buyer; Carol Gentry, office mgr.; Gary Hawkins, chief eng.
Operation: 1982.

Melbourne

WMOD (Channel 43)

Southern Broadcasting Copr., 4450L Enterprise Ct., Melbourne, FL 32935(305) 254-4343.

Lou Frey, Jr., pres.; Michael Starr, gen. mgr.; Lon Mirolli, gen. sls. mgr.; Bert Golub, prog. dir. & film buyer; Sydelle Golub, promo. mgr.; Robert Delaney, news dir.; Carlo McDaniel, chief eng.; nat'l rep.: Adam Young.
Operation: 1982.

Miami

WBFS (Channel 33)

Ch. 33, Inc., 16550 N.W. 52 Ave., Miami, FL 33014; (305) 621-3333.

Milt Grant, pres.; Douglas Knight, sta. mgr.; Dilley Dekle, prog. dir.; Skip Moss, gen. sls. mgr.; Bill Faun, chief eng.
Operation: December, 1984.

WCIX-TV (Channel 6)

Taft Television and Radio Co., Inc., 8900 NW 18th Terrace, Miami, FL; (305) 593-0606.

Elliott Troshinsky, v.p. & gen. mgr.; Robert Furlong, gen. sls. mgr.; Mike Stopnick, promo. mgr.; Bernie Wimmers, dir. eng.; Dan Neumann, bus. mgr.; nat'l rep.: Telerep.
Operation: Sept. 1967; TV households: 1,164,000.

WDZL (Channel 39)

39 BCSTG. Ltd., 2055 Lee St., Hollywood, FL 33020 (305) 925-3939.

Odyssey Partners, owner; Harvey Cohen, exec. v.p. & gen. mgr.; Cyrus Russell, gen. sls. mgr.; Henry Hirsch, promo. mgr.; Robert Castillo, chief eng.; nat'l. rep.: Katz.
Operation: October, 1982.

WHFT-TV (Channel 45)

Lester Sumrall Evangelistic Assn. Inc., Box 12, South Bend, IN 46624 (305) 624-1700.

Lester Sumrall, pres.; Robert R. Brown, v.p. & gen. mgr.
Operation: 1975.

WLTV (Channel 23)

Spanish International Communications Corp., 695 N.W. 199th St., Miami, FL 33169 (305) 856-2323 (sales) (305) 652-4000 (operations).

Joaquin Blaya, v.p. & gen. mgr.; Harold M. Parks, nat'l sls. mgr.; Vivian Quevedo, sta. mgr.; Tony Segredo, sls. mgr.
Operation: 1954.

WPLG (Channel 10) ABC

(Formerly WLBW-TV) Post-Newsweek Stations of FA Inc., 3900 Biscayne Blvd., Miami, FL 33137.

Alan Perris, v.p. & gen. mgr.; Tom Weems, chief eng.; Dick Wexo, gen. sls. mgr.; Paul Nugent, nat'l sls. mgr.; Rufus Devane, local sls. mgr.; Norman A. Davis, area v.p.
Operation: November 1961; TV households: 1,925,000.

WSVN (Channel 7) NBC

Sunbeam Television Corp., 1401 79th Street Causeway, Miami, FL 33141 (305) 751-6692.

Edmund N. Ansin, pres.; Robert W. Leider, v.p. & gen. mgr.; John Fenwick, sls. mgr.; Neil Murphy, contr.; Merlin Haynie, chief eng.; David Bieber, ops. mgr.; Frank Struzzieri, prog. acquisition mgr.; Charmaine Meyer, creative services mgr.; Myrna Sonora, pub. affairs dir.; nat'l rep.: harrington, Righter & Parsons, Inc. Southern: Clem & Lowrance.
Operation: 1956; TV Households: 1,156,700.

WTVJ (Channel 4) CBS

Wometco Enterprises, Inc., 316 N. Miami Ave., Miami, FL 33128 (305) 377-8241.

Anthony Cassara, pres.; Alan Perris, gen. mgr.; Doug Barker, sta. mgr.; Al Buch, news dir.; Tom Beauchamp, dir. of tech. opns.; Al Rothstein, gen. sls. mgr.; Barry Allentuck, natl. sls. mgr.; Jim Paratone, dir. pgrm.; Lee Speckerman, dir. adv./promo.; nat'l rep.: MMT Sales, Inc.

Operation: 1949; TV homes in area: 1,390,500.

Naples

WEVU (Channel 26) ABC

Caloosa TV Corp., 28950 Old 41 Rd., SE, Bonita Springs, FL 33923 (813) 332-0076.

Ray Karpowicz, pres. & gen. mgr.; W.T. Roof, v.p. & asst. gen. mgr.; Hank Douglas, gen. sls. mgr.; Terry Murphy, prom. dir.; Sue Caswell, prog. dir.; Rick Snyder, news dir.; Jerry Blevins, chief eng.; nat'l. rep.: Avery-Knowel.

Operation: 1974.

Ocala

WBSP (Channel 51)

Big Sun TV, Inc., Box 3985, Ocala, FL 32678 (904) 351-5551.

Robert Ware, pres.

Operation: January, 1983.

Orlando

WCPX-TV (Channel 6) CBS

The Outlet Co., P.O. Box 66000, Orlando, FL 38253 (305) 843-0006.

Bruce G. Sundlun, pres.; David E. Henderson, pres.; & Outlet Bcst. Div.; Michael Schweitzer, v.p. & gen. mgr.; Jim Donnelley, gen. sls. mgr.; Everett H. Hughes, prog. dir.; Robert Diehl, chief eng.; nat'l rep.: Katz.

Operation: 1954; TV homes in area: 1,087,500.

WFTV (Channel 9) ABC

Channel Nine of Orlando, 639 W. Central, Orlando, FL 32802 (305) 841-9000.

Walter M. Windsor, gen. mgr.; Clifton L. Conley, gen. sls. mgr.; Bruce Baker, local sls. dir.; Clifford S. Pine, opns. mgr.; Paul Warnock, chief eng.; Ramon Parramore, film dir.; Richard Flynn, bus. mgr.

WOFL-TV (Channel 35)

Meredith Corp., 2300 S. Orange Blossom Trail, Orlando, FL 32805; (305) 422-0035.

Norris Reichel, v.p. & gen. mgr.; Martin Ross, gen. sls. mgr.; Sharon DeLuca, natl. sls. mgr.; Jim Miotke, lcl. sls. mgr.; Kate McSweeny, prog. mgr.; nat'l. rep.: MMT Sales.

Operation: 1979.

Palm Beach

WPTV (Channel 5) NBC

Scripps-Howard Bcastg. Co., P.O. Box 510, Palm Beach, FL 33480. Studio: 622 N. Flagler Drive, West Palm Beach, FL (305) 655-5455.

William J. Brooks, gen. mgr.; Jim Knight, asst. gen. mgr. & gen.sls. mgr.; Arvo O. Katajisto, ops. dir.; Ed Roos, chief eng.; nat'l rep.: Blair.

Operation: Aug. 1954. TV households: 1,152,800.

Panama City

WJHG-TV (Channel 7) NBC

WJHG-TV, P.O. Box 2349, Panama City, FL 32401 (904) 234-2125.

James H. Gray, pres.; Ray H. Holloway, v.p. & gen. mgr.; Roger Jones, sales mgr.; Jack Crusan, prod. mgr.; Scott Clark, chief eng.; nat'l rep.: Katz.

Operation: 1953; TV households: 293,700.

WMBB (Channel 13) ABC

Octagon Broadcasting Co., Box 1340, Panama City, FL 32401 (904) 769-2313.

Anthony C. Kupris, pres; John A. Kupris, v.p.; Mary R. Kupris, secty.-treas.; Rob Doll, gen. mgr.; Patti Clements, prog. dir.; Steve Cook, prod. mgr.; Les Waters, chief eng.

Operation: October, 1973; TV households: 255,200.

Pensacola

WEAR-TV (Channel 3) ABC

Rollins Telecasting, Inc., Box 12278, Pensacola, FL 32581 (904) 455-7311.

Rick Hubbell, group v.p., media; J. R. Robinette, v.p. & dir. TV; M. J. Groothand, gen. mgr. & film buyer; Bob Shields, gen. sls. mgr.; Joe Smith, op. mgr.; Harry Babb, chief eng.

Operation: 1954; TV households: 483,400.

WJTC (Channel 44)

Carnex, TV, Inc., 700 S. Palafox St., Pensacola, FL 32504; (904) 438-4444.

Joseph E. Carney, Jr., pres.; Hugh Robinson, gen. sls. mgr. & film buyer; Tom Eaton, film buyer.

Operation: November, 1984.

Sarasota

WXLT-TV (Channel 40) ABC

Sarasota-Bradenton Florida TV Co., Inc., P.O. Box 21239, Sarasota, FL 33583 (813) 922-0777.

Robert R. Nelson, pres. & gen. mgr.; Mike Burham, chief eng. & prod. mgr.; Tom Johnson, sls. mgr.

Operation: 1971.

Tallahassee

WTWC (Channel 40) NBC

Holt-Robinson TV, Inc., 8440 Deerlake Rd., Tallahassee, FL 32312 (904) 893-4140.

Stan Lightsey, pres.; Don Neil, gen. mgr.; John Burns, gen. sls. mgr.; Tina Johnson, prog. coor.; Mike Brown, chief eng.; nat'l. rep.: Young.

Operation: April, 1983.

WTXL-TV (Channel 27) ABC

Tallahassee 27 Ltd. Partnership, P.O. Box 13899, Tallahassee, FL 32317; (904) 898-3127.

Joseph D. Tydings, pres.; Mack Keoun, gen. mgr.; Chris Aldridge, gen. sls. mgr. & dir. opns.

Operation: September, 1976.

Tampa

WFTS (Channel 28)

Tampa Bay TV, Inc., 4501 E. Columbus Dr., Tampa, FL 33605; (813) 623-5234.

Lew Friefeld, gen. mgr.; Tom Watson, gen. sls. mgr.; Mike

Stephen, promo. mgr.; Walt Youmans, chief eng.; natl. rep.: Blair.
Operation: November, 1981.

WTVT (Channel 13) CBS
Gaylord Broadcasting Co., 3213 West Kennedy Blvd., Box 22013, Tampa, FL 33622; Transmitter, Route 1, Box 767, Riverview, FL 33569 (813) 876-1313.
Harry M. Apel, v.p., Gaylord Broadcasting Co. and gen. mgr., WTVT; Roger Ashley, asst. gen. mgr.; Don Wargo, gen. sls. mgr.; Carol Mountain, prod. mgr.; Dick A'Hearn, oper. mgr.; Jim West, news dir.; Lowell Otto, chief eng.; nat'l rep.: Tele Rep.
Operation: 1955; TV sets in area: 1,131,400.

WXFL (Channel 8) NBC
905 East Jackson St., P.O. Box 1410, Tampa, FL 33601 (305) 229-7781.
Robert T. Sutton, pres.; Frank De Tillio, v.p. & gen. mgr.; Jan De Camp, prod. mgr.; Diana Richards, promo. mgr.; Jack Lyons, gen. sls. mgr.; Joe Burns, natl. sls. mgr.; Doug Duperrault, prog. dir.; Ardell Hill, dir. of eng. & opns. mgr.
Operation: 1955; TV sets in area: 1,077,600.

St. Petersburg

WTOG (Channel 44)
Hubbard Broadcasting Inc., 365-105th Terrace, N.E. St. Petersburg, FL 33702 (813) 576-4444.
David A. Olmstead, v.p. & gen. mgr.; Ron Inman, gen. sls. mgr.; John Kays, chief eng.
Operation: 1968.

WTSP-TV (Channel 10) ABC
WTSP-TV, St. Petersburg/Tampa, FL, P.O. Box 10,000, St. Petersburg, FL 33733.
Lawrence M. Clamage, gen. mgr.; Paul Siracuse, gen. sls. mgr.; Larry Cazavan, prgm. mgr.; Ken Middleton, news dir.; Peter Ford, chief eng.; Cyndie Reynolds, promo. mgr.

W. Palm Beach

WFLX (Channel 29)
4130 Blue Heron Blvd., West Palm beach, FL 33404 (305) 845-2929.
Carl Hirsch, pres. & chief oper. officer; John C. Chaffee, pres., TV div.; nat'l rep.: Petry.
Operation: 1982.

WPEC-TV (Channel 12) ABC
Fairfield Drive, West Palm Beach, FL 33407 (305) 844-1212.
Alex W. Dreyfoos, Jr., pres.; Robert C. Wiegand, gen. mgr.; Thom Moody, prog. dir.
Operation: 1955.

GEORGIA

Albany

WALB-TV (Channel 10) NBC)
Gray Communications Systems, Inc., P.O. Box 3130, Albany, GA 31708 (912) 883-0154.
James H. Gray, pres.; Dorothy A. Zimmerman, secty.; Raymond E. Carow, v.p. & gen. mgr.; Barbara Jones, treas.; William N. Williams, chief eng.; nat'l rep.: Katz.
Operation: 1954.

WTSG (Channel 31)
Gordon Communications, Inc., Box 450, Albany, GA 31706 (912) 453-3100.
Carl Gordon, Jr., pres.; Fred L. Procise, gen. mgr.; Cynthia Hunkele, prog. & promo. mgr.; Tony Gainous, chief eng.
Operation: 1982.

Atlanta

WAGA-TV (Channel 5) CBS
Storer Communications, Inc., 1551 Briarcliff Rd. N.E., P.O. Box 4207, Atlanta, GA 30302 (404) 875-5551.
Paul Raymon, v.p. & gen. mgr.; J. Marc Doyle, dir. prog. opns.; Mary Stimmel, edit. dir.; Gene Adams, dir. tech. svcs.; Greg Gunn, prod. mgr.; Dick Goss, dir. creat. svcs.; Peter Schruth, dir. sls.; Victor Brust, natl. sls. mgr.; Diane Harnell, lcl. sls. mgr.; Chuck Lipton, mktg. dir.; nat'l rep.: Storer TV sales.
Operation: 1949.

WATL-TV (Channel 36)
WATL-TV, 575 Ponce de Leon Ave., Atlanta, GA 30308 (404) 892-3636.
David Henderson, pres.; John Serrao, gen. mgr.; Gene McHugh, gen. sls. mgr.; Don Hess, prog. dir.; Tom Vardase, prod. mgr.; David Jones, chief eng.; nat'l. rep.: Katz.
Operation: 1954.

WGNX-TV (Channel 46)
Tribune Broadcasting Co., 1810 Briarcliff Rd., P.O. Box 98097, Atlanta, GA 30359 (404) 325-4646.
Herman Ramsey, v.p. & gen. mgr.; Wayne Spracklin, gen. sls. mgr.
Operation: 1971.

WSB-TV (Channel 2) NBC
Cox Broadcasting Corporation, 1601 W. Peachtree Street, N.E., Atlanta, GA 30309 (404) 897-7000.
Clifford M. Kirtland, Jr., pres., Cox; Stanley G. Mouse, exec. v.p., Cox; William A. Schwartz, pres. bdstg. div., Cox; Don Elliot Heald, v.p. & gen. mgr., WSB-TV; Dale Smith, station mgr., WSB-TV; Ed Godfrey, news dir., WSB-TV; A. R. Van Cantfort, prgm. mgr., WSB-TV; John Carpenter, gen. sls. mgr., WSB-TV; William Powers, dir. of engineering, WSB-TV.
Operation: 1948.

WTBS (Channel 17)
Superstation, Inc., 1050 Techwood Dr., N.W., Atlanta, GA 30318 (404) 892-1717.
R. E. Turner, chm.; R.J. Wussler, pres.; Jack Petrik, v.p. pgrmng.; Jim Kitchell, v.p. opns.; Gerry Hogan, v.p. sls.; Jeff Grimshaw, promo. mgr.; Jack Verner, chief eng.
Operation: 1967.

WVEU (Channel 69)
Broadcasting Corp. of Georgia, 2700 N.E. Expressway, Bldg. A, Phoenix Business Park, Atlanta, GA 30345 (404) 325-6929.
Prentiss Q. Yancey, pres.; Vance L. Eckersley, v.p. & gen. mgr.; Willard L. Dougherty, gen. sls. mgr.; Joseph A. Everett, opns. mgr.; Larry Wood, prod. mgr.; Anthony Cox, chief eng.; Larry Upton, prog. mgr.; Peter L. Mandell, promo. mgr.
Operation: 1981.

WXIA-TV (Channel 11) ABC
Pacific & Southern Broadcasting Co., Inc., 1611 W. Peachtree St., N.E., Atlanta, GA 30309.

Jeff Davidson, pres. & gen. mgr.; Neil Kuvin, prgm. dir.; Howard Kaufman, gen. sls. mgr.; Elliot Bass, nat'l sls. mgr.; Russ Artz, chief eng.; Dick Williams, news dir.; Ben Perry, community affairs dir.; Jon Beacher, promo. mgr.; nat'l rep.: PGW-TV.

Operation: Sept., 1951; TV households: 1,568,400.

Augusta

WAGT-TV (Channel 26) NBC

P.O. Box 1526, Augusta, GA 30903 (404) 722-0026.

Nick Evans, Jr., gen. mgr.; Lee Sheridan, sta. mgr.; James Halpin, gen. sls. mgr.; Al Van Dinteren, chief eng.

Operation: Dec. 24, 1968; TV households: 183,700.

WJBF (Channel 6) ABC, NBC

Fuqua Television, Inc., Box 1404, Augusta, GA 30903 (803) 722-6664.

J. B. Fuqua, chm. of bd.; John Radeck, pres & gen. mgr.; John Wright, treas.; Walter Campbell, Jr., v.p. sales; Terry Sams, v.p. prog.; John Jopling, v.p. eng.; James E. Davis, v.p. news, nat'l rep.: H/R Television.

Operation: 1953; TV sets in area: 556,000.

WRDW-TV (Channel 12)

Television Station Partners, Drawer 1212, Augusta, GA 30903.

Ralph E. Becker, pres.; Jack West, v.p. & gen. mgr.; William J. Kemple, gen. sls. mgr.; C. Don Smith, chief eng.; Steve Johnston, program mgr.

Operation: Feb. 1954; TV households: 678,600.

Columbus

WLTZ (Channel 38) NBC

Columbus TV, Inc., Box 12289, Columbus, GA 31995; (404) 561-3838.

J. Curtis Lewis, Jr., pres.; Bob Walton, v.p. & gen. mgr.; Tom Breazeale, gen. sls. mgr.; R.C. Bartlett, prog. dir.; Dottie McMichael, promo mgr.; Tim Espar, news dir.; Bob Hoor, chief eng.; natl. rep.: Seltel.

Operation: October, 1970.

WRBL-TV (Channel 3) CBS

Columbus Broadcasting Co., Inc., 1350 13th Ave., Columbus, GA 31902 (404) 322-0601.

J. Barnett Woodruff, pres.; George Gingell, v.p. & gen. mgr.; Paul T. Berry, v.p. prgm. & op.; Robert Walton, v.p.-sales; Lacy Worrell, chief eng.

Operation: 1953; TV sets in area: 600,000.

WTVM (Channel 9) ABC

SFN Communications of Columbus, Inc., 1909 Wynnton Rd., Columbus, GA (404) 324-6471.

Gary Anderson, pres. & gen. mgr.; W. Carroll Ward, prod. dir.; Wayne Dougherty, sls. mgr.; Steve Faust, news dir.; David Williams, chief eng.; Jerry Bahr, prod. mgr.; nat'l rep.: Blair Television.

Operation: 1953; TV sets in area: 719,900.

WXTX (Channel 54)

Columbus Family TV, Inc., 6524 Buena Vista Rd., Box 12188, Columbus, GA 31907; (404) 561-5400.

Stephen Kent, gen. mgr.; Wade Griffith, gen. sls. mgr.; Kathy Barker, prog. dir. & promo. mgr.; Art Hook, film buyer; Norman Easterday, film mgr.; Jim Taylor, news dir.; John Terry, chief eng.

Operation: June, 1983.

Macon

WGXA (Channel 24) ABC

Russell Rowe Communications, box 340, Macon, GA 31297 (912) 745-2424.

Ken Gerdes, v.p. & gen. mgr.; Jim Wilcox, gen. sls. mgr.; Dale Stafford, opns. mgr.; Kelly Causey, promo. mgr.; Ron Wildman, news dir.; Richard Blanton, chief eng.; nat'l rep.: Blair.

Operation: 1982.

WMAZ-TV (Channel 13) CBS

Multimedia Broadcasting Company, Box 5008, Macon, GA 31213 (912) 746-1313.

James T. Lynagh, pres.; Don McGouirk, v.p. & gen. mgr.; Mim Crowley, gen. sls. mgr.; Sydney Thum, prog. dir,; Jim Lawhon, chief eng.; Lacy Worrell, dir. of eng.; nat'l rep.: Katz Agency, Inc.

WMGT (Channel Channel 41) NBC

Morris Network, Inc., Box 4328, Macon, GA (912) 745-4141.

Dean Hinson, pres.; Charles Morris, chmn.; Aubrey Wood, gen. sls. mgr.; Lisa Hill, prom. mgr.; John Gimlin, news dir.; Joe Sears, chief eng.; nat'l. rep.: Seltel.

Operation: 1968.

Savannah

WJCL (Channel 22) ABC

Lewis Bcstg. Corp., 10001 Abercorn St., Extension, Savannah, GA 31406 (912) 925-0022.

J. Fred Pierce, exec. v.p. & gen. mgr.; Christopher A. Barbieri, v.p., sls. & prgm.; Mary Poythress, opns. dir.

Operation: 1970.

WSAV (Channel 3) NBC

WSAV-TV, P.O. Box 2429, 1430 East Victory Drive., Savannah, GA 31402 (912) 236-0303. Station is owned by News-Press & Gazette Co., St. Joseph, MO; David R. Bradley, Jr., pres.

David R. DeArmand, gen. mgr.; Robert B. Beall, gen. sls. mgr.; David A. Kirby, news dir.; Cecil K. Daniel, Jr., prod. mgr.; Byron Strong, chief eng.; nat'l rep.: Blair.

Operation: 1956; TV sets in area: 206,500.

WTOC-TV (Channel 11) CBS

American Savannah Broadcasting Co., 516 Abercorn St., Savannah, GA 31401 (912) 234-1111.

Jess Mooney, v.p. & gen. mgr.; Bud Bradbury, prom. dir.; LaVaughn Thompson, chief eng.; nat'l rep.: Katz Agency Inc.

Operations: 1954; TV sets in area: 394,800.

Thomasville-Tallahassee (Fla.)

WCTV (Channel 6) CBS

John H. Phipps, P.O. Box 3048, Tallahassee, FL 32315 (904) 893-6666.

John E. Phipps, chm.; Dennis O. Boyle, pres.; Frank J. Flynn, Jr., v.p. & gen. mgr.; Jerry L. Williams, prm. mgr.; Melvin Blank, opns. mgr.; nat'l rep.: Blair TV.

Operation: 1955; TV sets in area: 416,500.

Toccoa

WNEG-TV (Channel 32)

Stephens County Broadcasting Co., 100 Blvd., Box 970, Toccoa, GA 30577; (404) 886-0032.

Roy E. Gaines, pres. & gen. mgr.; David Austin, gen. slsl. mgr.; Connie Gaines, prog. dir. & film buyer; Koejke Dutton, promo. mgr.; Mitch Dutton, prod. mgr.
Operation: September, 1984.

Valdosta

WVGA (Channel 44) ABC

Hi-Ho Broadcasting, Inc., Box 1588, Valdosta, GA 31601 (912) 242-4444.
Douglas L. Jones, gen. mgr. & sls. mgr.; Karen Evans, traf. mgr.; Bill Taylor, chief eng.; nat'l rep.: Adam Young.
Operation: 1980.

HAWAIIAN ISLANDS

Hilo, Hawaii

KGMD-TV (Channel 9) CBS

(Satellite of KGMB-TV, Honolulu)
Heftel Television-Hilo, Inc., P.O. Box 581, 1534 Kapiolani Blvd., Honolulu, HI 96814.
Operation: 1955.

KHAW-TV (Channel 11) NBC

(Satellite of KHON-TV, Honolulu)
KHON-TV, Inc., 1170 Auahi St., Honolulu, HI 96814.
Personnel same as KHON.
Operation: Nov. 1961.

KHVO (Channel 13) ABC

(Satellite of KHVH-TV, Honolulu)
Western Telestations Inc., Naniloa Hotel, Hilo, HI 96814 935-8289, Hilo; rep: The Katz Agency; 935-8289.
Operation: May, 1960; TV sets in area.

KOHA-TV (Channel 2)

Oceanic Bcstg. Co., Inc., Box 1006, Hilo, HI 96720.
Charles R. Henry, T.M. Henry, owners.
Operation: August, 1983.

Honolulu, Oahu

KGMB TV (Channel 9) CBS

Lee Enterprises, Incorporated 1534 Kapiolani Blvd., Honolulu, HI 96814 P.O. Box 581, Honolulu, HI 96809 (808) 944-5200.
Richard A. Weiner, gen.. mgr.; Robert B. Fox, prod. mgr.; Phil Arnone, prgm. mgr.; Robert W. Sevey, news dir.; James Doney, dir. of community svcs.; Barry Albright, chief eng.; John Funk, sls. mgr.; Ed Wong, contr.; nat'l Rep.: Katz Agency.
Operation: 1952. TV households (State): 261,170.

KHAI (Channel 20)

Media Central, Inc., 735 Sheridan St., Honolulu, HI 97814 (808) 943-1169.
Morton J. Kent, owner.
Operation: December, 1983.

KHNL-TV (Channel 13)

Mid-Pacific Television Associates, 150-B Puuhale Road, Honolulu, HI 96819
Richard J. Blangiardi, gen. mgr.; Shirley Feliciano, bus. mgr.
Operation: July, 1962; TV homes: 320,000.

KHON-TV (channel 2) Honolulu
KAII-TV WAILUKU SATELLITE
KHAW-TV HILO SATELLITE

KHON-TV, Inc. 615 Piikoi St., Honolulu HI 96814.
William S. Snyder, pres. & gen. mgr.; nat'l rep.: Blair TV
Operation: 1952; TV sets in area: 323,720.

KITV (Channel 4) ABC

Shamrock Broadcasting Co., 1290 Ala Moana Blvd., Honolulu, HI 96814; 537-3991.
Dick Grimm, pres.; Richard Schaller, gen. mgr.; Dave Moore, dir. of eng.; Muneo Hamada, bus. mgr.; Paul Udell, news dir.; Bob Turner, prog. dir.; Charlie Riley, prod. mgr.
Operation: 1954.

KSHO

Mauna Kea Bcstg. Co., 970 No. Kalaheo C314, Honolulu, HI 96734 (808) 254-5826.
Bill Kline, gen. mgr.; Tom Hagner, gen. sls. mgr.; Garrett Nakahodo, opns. dir.; Tom White, chief eng.; natl. rep.: Adam Young.
Operation: December, 1982.

Wailuku, Maui

KAII-TV (Channel 7) NBC

(Satellite of KHON-TV, Honolulu) KHON-TV, Inc., 1170 Auahi St., Honolulu, HI 96814.
Personnel: same as KHON-TV, Honolulu.
Operation: Nov. 1958.

KGMV-TV (Channel 3) CBS

(Satellite of KGMB-TV; Honolulu, Heftel Broadcasting-Maui, Inc., P.O. Box 1574, Kahului, HI 96732.
Cecil Heftel, pres., treas. & gen. mgr.; Earl McDaniel, gen. mgr.; Thomas Yoshida, chief eng. & sta. mgr.
Operation: 1955.

KMAU (Channel 12) ABC

(Semi-satellite of separately-owned, KITV, Honolulu)
Maui Publishing Co., Ltd., Box 550, Wailuku, HI 96814.
Operation: Dec., 1955.

IDAHO

Boise

KBCI-TV (Channel 2) CBS

Eugene Television, Inc., 1007 Jefferson St., Boise, ID 83707 (208) 336-5222.
Robert Booth, pres., Glenn Nickell, v.p.; Mary E. Miller, Jr., mgr.; Jack Flynn, sls. mgr.; Paul Greene, prog. dir.; nat'l rep.: Katz Television, Art Moore & Associates, Inc. (Pacific Northwest).
Operation: 1953; TV sets in area: 212,000.

KTVB-TV (Channel 7) NBC, ABC

KTVB, Inc. 5407 Fairview Ave., P.O. Box 7 Boise, ID 83701 (208) 375-7277.
Georgia M. Davidson, bd. chm. & dir.; Robert E. Krueger, pres. & gen. mgr.; Sal Celeski, news dir.; nat'l rep.: Avery-Knodel, Inc.

Idaho Falls

KIDK-TV (Channel 3) CBS

Idaho Falls Broadcasting Co., Inc., P.O. Box 2008, Idaho

Falls, ID 83403; (208) 522-5100.
Richard E. Carr, v.p. & gen. mgr.; Barbara Henricksen, prog. dir.; Kim Southwick, opns. dir.; Gary Smith, chief eng.; natl. rep.: Katz.
Operation: 1953; TV sets in area: 107,900.

KIFI-TV (Channel 8)
The Post Company, P.O. Box 2148, Idaho Falls, ID 83401 (208) 523-1171.
Jim Brady, v.p. & gen. mgr.; Herman G. Haefele, sta./natl. sls. mgr.; Cecil Cope, chief eng.; nat'l rep.: Seltel.
Operation: 1961.

Lewiston

KIVI (Channel 6) ABC
Sawtooth Communications, Inc., 1866 East Chisholm Dr., Nampa, ID 83651 (208) 336-0500.
Larry J. Chase, pres./gen.mgr.; Don Long, ops. mgr.; Rex. L. McArthur, gen. sls. mgr.; Ken Ritchie, local sls. mgr.; Dan Smede, news dir.; Andy Suk, chief eng.; nat'l. rep.: Seltel; regional rep.: Tacher.
Operation: 1974.

KLEW-TV (Channel 3) CBS
NWG Broadcasting Co., 2626 17th St., Lewiston, ID 83501; (208) 746-2636.
Gerry Cornwell, mgr.; Marlin Jackson, chief eng.; Vanessa Gerwells, news dir.; nat'l. rep.: H.R.
Operation: 1955.

Nampa

KTRV (Channel 12)
679 Sixth St., Nampa, ID 83651 (208) 466-1200.
Cary Jones, v.p./gen. mgr.; Diane Frisen, prog. dir.; Francis Wilson, chief eng.; Jim Barto, bus. mgr.; nat'l rep.: Petry.
Operation: 1981.

Pocatello-Blackfoot

KPVI (Channel 6) ABC
Futura Titanium Corp., 1866 E. Chisholm Dr., Nampa, ID 83702 (208) 233-6667.
Robert V. Hansberger, pres.; Michael W. Gee, gen. mgr.; James Barto, ops. mgr.; Brian Hogan, sta. mgr.; Joe Emig, gen. sls. mgr.; Jean Morand, chief eng.; Gregg Licht, news dir.; nat'l rep.: Seltel.
Operation: 1974; TV households: 89,900.

Twin Falls

KMVT (Channel 11) NBC, CBS, ABC
KMVT Broadcasting, Inc., 1100 Blue Lakes Blvd., N., Twin Falls, ID 83301 (208) 733-1280.
Jim Underwood, pres.; Lee Wagner, gen. mgr.; George Brown, ops. mgr.; George Brown, prog. dir.; Dennis Lowe, chief eng.; nat'l rep.: Katz.
Operation: 1955; TV sets in area: 45,830.

ILLINOIS

Aurora

WPWR-TV (Channel 60) FNN
Metrowest Corp., 4255 Westbrook Dr., Aurora, IL 60507 (312) 851-7515.
Fred Euchaner, pres.; Brent Stephenson, opns. mgr.; Elizabeth Hertel, pub. svc. mgr.; Neal Sabin, corp. prog. mgr.; Mike Dunlop, gen. sls. mgr.
Operation: April, 1982.

Bloomington

WYZZ (Channel 43)
Bloomington Comco, Inc., 1328 E. Empire, Bloomington, IN 61701 (309) 662-4373.
G.J. Robinson, pres.; Larry Halcomb, gen. mgr.; Bob Bechir, sls. mgr.; Tony Dinkins, prog. dir.; Neil Burk, chief eng.
Operation: 1982.

Champaign

WCIA (Channel 3) CBS
Midwest Television, Inc., 509 S. Neil St., Champaign, IL 61820 (217) 356-8333.
A. C. Meyer, Jr., pres.; Guy Main, exec. v.p.; Jack B. Everette, exec. v.p. & treas.; Gerald P. Johnson, sls. mgr.; Leonard Davis, natl. sales mgr.; Ed Mathais, prod. mgr.; Sheila Hickman, prog. dir. & film buyer; nat'l rep.: Petry.
Operation: 1953; TV sets in area: 329,000.

WICD-TV (Channel 15) NBC
Plains Television Partnership, 250 Country Fair Dr., Champaign, IL 61820 (217) 352-7673.
Elmer Balaban, partner; Joe Norris, stn. mgr; Ginger Rush, natl. sls. mgr. Ed Mason, local sales mgr.; David Boyer, chief eng.; Larry Waters, ops. mgr.; nat'l rep., Katz Television Continental.
Operation: 1959.

Chicago

WBBM-TV (Channel 2) CBS
CBS, Inc., 630 N. McClurg Court, Chicago, IL 60611 (312) 944-6000.
Guy Cummings, v.p. & gen. mgr.; Ed Spray, dir. of bdcst'.; Lilly Eide, dir. of communications; Aretha Marshall-Mills, dir. of community affairs; Jay Newman, news dir.; Edward A. Spray, prgm. mgr.; Lillian Courtney-Katz, sls. traffic mgr.; Dana Hart, dir. of research.
Operation: 1946; TV sets in area: 2,679,260.

WCFC (Channel 38)
Christian Communications of Chicagoland, Inc., 20 N. Wacker Dr., Chicago, IL 60606. (312) 977-3838.
Jerry K. Rose, pres. & gen. mgr.; Harold Wheat, sta. mgr.; Allan Winters, promotions, p.r. mgr.
Operation: 1976.

WCIU-TV (Channel 26)
Weigel Bdg. Co., Board of Trade, Chicago, IL 60604.
Howard Shapiro, pres. & gen. mgr.; Peter Zomaya, asst. gen. mgr. & sls. mgr.; Merri Houser, film dir.; Dick Ashenfelter, chief eng.; Ben Larson, Don Aguirre.
Operation: 1964.

WFLD-TV (Channel 32)
Metromedia, Inc., 300 North State St., Chicago, IL 60610.
Derk Zimmerman, v.p. & gen. mgr.; Al DeVaney, v.p. & gen. sls. mgr.; Robert Simone, prog. dir.; Dwain Spoonover, eng. mgr.; nat'l rep: Katz Independent Sales.
Operation: Jan., 1966; TV households: 3,138,000.

WGN-TV (Channel 9)
WGN, Continental Broadcasting Company, 2501 W. Bradley Pl., Chicago, IL 60618 (312) 528-2311.
Joseph T. Loughlin, v.p./gen. mgr.; Daniel D. Calibraro, v.p., corporate affairs; Bob Hoffman, dir. sls.; Gary Simcox, opns. mgr.; Ron McCoy, dir. creative svcs.; Paul Davis, news dir.; Charlotte O'Brien, mgr. of community affairs; Harry Q. Trigg, mgr. of film.

WLS-TV (Channel 7) ABC
American Broadcasting Companies Inc., 190 N. State St., Chicago, IL 60601 (312) 263-0880.
Peter B. Desnoes, v.p. & gen. mgr.; Richard Taylor, gen. sls. mgr.; Michael Velazquez, natl. sls. mgr.; Robert Hoffman, local sls. mgr.; Clar W. Heider, admin. asst.; Jeffrey M. McGrath, dir. of programming; Ernst Ledebuhr, contr.; Thomas Kuelbs, news dir.; Sharon McGill, research dir.; Joseph Kresnicka, dir. of eng.; Timothy J. Bennett, adv. promo. dir.; na'l. rep.: ABC TV Spot Sales.
Operation: Oct., 1943; TV homes: 2,995,000.

WMAQ-TV (Channel 5) NBC
National Broadcastg. Co., Merchandise Mart, Chicago, IL 60654 (312) 861-5555.
Monte Newman, v.p. & gen. mgr.; Dick Daggett, dir. sls.; Fred DeMarco, sta. mgr.; Rillon Smith, prgm. dir.; Gene Cartwright, dir. op.; Bill Marshall, dir., eng'.; Paul Beavers, News dir.; Carole Cartwright, mgr., Community Programs; Gail Sikevitz, exec. prod., prog. dept.; nat'l rep.: NBC Spot Sales.
Operation: 1949; TV sets in area: 3,530,230

WSNS-TV (Channel 44)
Video 44, a Joint Venture, 430 W. Grant Pl., Chicago, IL 60614 (312) 929-1200.
Burt I. Harris, pres., Harriscope (L.A.); Alan Silverman, pres., Essaness Theatre Corp.; Richard S. Plotkin, v.p. & gen. mgr.; Kevin Murphy, chief eng.; John Dickinson, ops. mgr.
Operation: April, 1970.

Decatur

WAND (Channel 17) ABC
(Serving Decatur, Springfield & Champaign)
WAND-Television, Inc. (subsidiary of Lin Broadcasting Corp., Inc.), 904 Southside Drive, Decatur, IL 62525 (217) 424-2500.
B. Geoghegan, pres. & gen. mgr.; T. J. Vaughan, v.p. sta. mgr.; Larry Katt, v.p. sls.; Nat'l Rep.: Blair.
Operation: 1953; TV sets in area: 569,506.

WFHL (Channel 23)
Decatur Foursquare Broadcasting, 2510 Parkway Ct., Decatur, IL 62526; (217) 428-2323.
James Houpt, Jr., pres.; Joel Sanchez, gen. mgr. & prog. dir.; Terry Reich, gen. sls. mgr.; Paul Osborne, news dir.; Dave Beck, chief eng.
Operation: May, 1984.

Harrisburg

WSIL-TV (Channel 3) ABC Primary
21 W. Poplar St., Harrisburg. IL; 62946.
Mel Wheeler, pres.
Operation: 1953.

Joliet

WGBO-TV (Channel 66)
Grant Bcstg. Co., 875 N. Michigan Ave., Chicago, IL 60611 (312) 751-6666.
Douglas F. Ruhe, pres.; Robert Ramirez, gen. mgr.; Wayne Smith, chief eng.
Operation: 1981.

Marion

WTCT-TV (Channel 27)
Tri-State Christian TV, Rt. 37, Marion, IL 62959 (618) 997-9333.
Garth Coonce, pres. & gen. mgr.; Carl O. Brady, v.p. eng.; W. Jean Brady, prog. dir.; nat'l. rep.: Spot Time Ltd.
Operation: 1981.

Moline

WQAD-TV (Channel 8)
3003 Park 16 St., Moline, IL 61625 (309) 764-8888.
H. Oliver Gillespie, pres. & gen. mgr.; Gene Smith, gen. sls. mgr.; Lloyd Bolkcom, dir. of comm. affairs; Peggy Vyncke, v.p. & sta. & business mgr.; Joh Riches, news dir.; Jeff Swanson, prog. dir.; Rick Serre, chief eng.
Operation: 1963.

Mount Vernon

WCEE (Channel 13)
Pyramid Broadcasting Corp. of Ill., Box 1300, Mount Vernon, IL 62864 (618) 822-6900.
William Varecha, pres.; Karen Lupke, gen. sls. mgr.; Steve Schrader, chief eng.
Operation: 1983.

Peoria

WEEK-TV (Channel 25) NBC
Eagle Broadcasting Corporation, 2907 Springfield Rd., E. Peoria, IL 61611 (309) 698-2525.
Frank J. Bussone, pres./gen. mgr.; Jeff Hawkinson, v.p./prog. & develop.; Ken Tofanelli, v.p./eng. & tech. svcs.; Dennis Upah, creative svcs. dir.; nat'l rep.: Katz Agency.
Operation: 1953; TV sets in area: 475,000.

WHOI-TV (Channel 19) ABC
Forward of Illinois, Inc. 500 N. Stewart St., Creve Coeur, IL 61611 (309) 698-1919.
Charles E. Sherman, pres. & gen. mgr.; William Thorson, sr. v.p. & gen. sls. mgr.; nat'l. rep.: Seltel.
Operation: Oct. 1953; TV households; 475,300.

WMBD (Channel 31) CBS
Midwest Television, Inc., 3131 N. University, Peoria, IL 61611 (309) 688-3131.
August C. Meyer, Jr., pres.; Guy F. Main, exec. v.p.: Gene Robinson, v.p. and gen. mgr.; Gene C. Robinson, stat. mgr.; Lloyd Peterson, op. mgr.; Walter Konetsco, chief eng.; nat'l rep.; Petry
Operation: 1958; TV sets in area: 338,300.

Quincy

WGEM-TV (Channel 10) NBC
Quincy Broadcasting Co., 513 Hampshire, P.O. Box 80, Quincy, IL 62306 (217) 228-6600.
T. A. Oakley, pres.; Richard Herbst, v.p. & gen. mgr.;

Fred Colgan, op. mgr.; Ben Stewart, v.p.-sls.; Jim Martens, chief eng.; nat'l rep.: Blair.

Operation: 1953; TV sets in area: 372,400.

Rockford

WIFR-TV (Channel 23) CBS

WIFR Television, Inc., 2523 N. Meridian Rd., Rockford, IL 61103.

Dennis Blake West, pres.; Jack Keefe, news dir.; Jim Brady, opns. mgr.; Doug Warkenthien, prod. mgr.; Roy Bilsbarrow, cont.; Barbara Schobinger, prog. supvr.

Operation: 1965.

WQRF-TV (Channel 39)

Orion Broadcasting Group, Inc., 128 Kishwaukee St., Rockford, IL 61104 (815) 987-3950.

Kim A. Carlson, gen. mgr.; Dean Turman, chief eng.; Ken Staaf, ops. mgr.; John Ongena, lcl. sls. mgr.

Operation: 1978.

WREX-TV (Channel 13) ABC

WREX-TV, West Auburn at Winnebago Rds., Rockford, IL 61105 (910) 642-0770.

Member of The Gilmore Broadcasting Corp.

James S. Gilmore, owner; John McWeeny, gen. mgr.; Jim Smith, dir. of natl. sls.; Warren A. Anderson, local sls. mgr.; Gene Hines, film mgr.; natl. rep.: Seltel.

Operation: September, 1953; TV households: 401,600.

WTVO (Channel 17) NBC

Winnebago Television Corp., N. Meridian Rd. & State, Rockford, IL 61105 (910) 963-5413.

Harry Balaban, pres.; Hal Froelich, mgr.; Richard McDaniel, prgm. dir.; Tom Anderson, sales mgr.; Al Petzke, chief eng.; Frank Sanders, film dir.; nat'l rep.: Adam Yound, Inc.

Operation: 1953; TV sets in area: 580,300.

Rock Island

WHBF-TV (Channel 4) CBS

Rock Island Broadcasting Co., Telco Bldg., 231 18 St., Rock Island, IL 61201 (309) 786-5441.

Anne Potter DeLong, pres.; Edward E. DeLong III, exec. v.p.; Charles F. Harrison, v.p. & gen. mgr.; Dewey L. Nelsen, asst. gen. mgr. & v.p. sls.; Wesley C. Hoots, chief eng. ; nat'l rep.: Petry Television, Inc.

Operation: 1950; TV sets in area: 486,000.

Springfield

WICS (Channel 20) NBC

2680 East Cook St., Springfield, IL 62703 (217) 753-5620.

John DiMatteo, pres.; Robert L. Gilbertson, exec. v.p.; Milton D. Friedland, gen. mgr.; Don Squires, gen. sls. mgr.; Virginia Rush, natl. sls. mgr.; Jerrold Merritt, chief eng.; Gary Spears, prog. mgr.; Steven Lane, creative svcs. dir.; H.K. Springer, comtr.; nat'l rep.: Katz Agency.

Operation: 1953: TV sets in area: 762,700.

WRSP (Channel 55)

Springfield Independent TV Co., 3440 Clearlake Ave., Springfield, IL 62702; (217) 523-8855.

Bruce Fleming, gen. mgr.; Bill Harper, gen. sls. mgr.; Ken Myers, chief eng.; natl. rep.: Seltel.

Operation: June, 1979.

INDIANA

Angola

WBKZ (Channel 63)

401 W. Broad St., Angola, IN 46703; (219) 665-7387.

James Chase, pres. & gen. mgr.; J.T. Flywheel, prog. dir.; Jerry Clark, chief eng.; natl. rep.: Spot-time.

Operation: April, 1983.

Bloomington-Indianapolis

WTTV (Channel 4) Independent

Teleco Indiana, Inc., 3490 Bluff Road, Indianapolis, IN 46217 (217) 787-2211.

Elmer C. Snow, pres. & gen. mgr.; Mike Davis, prgm. mgr.; Clyde Dutton, gen. sls. mgr.; Bernie Souers, asst. gen. sls. mgr.; Paul Bohrer, chief engineer.

Operation: 1949; TV sets in area; 650,000.

Elkhart-South Bend

WSJV (Channel 28) ABC

WSJV, Inc. (owner)—Subsidiary of Quincy Newspapers (Illinois) Inc., Box 1646, Elkhart, IN 46515 (219) 293-8616; South Bend (219) 674-5106.

Thomas A. Oakley, pres.; Don E. Fuller, v.p. & gen. mgr.; Jon Hart, gen. sls. mgr.; natl rep., Blair.

Operation: 1954; TV sets in ADI: 281,300.

Evansville

WEHT-TV (Channel 25) CBS

Gilmore Broadcasting Corp., P.O. Box 25, Evansville, IN 47701 (812) 424-9215.

James S. Gilmore, Jr., pres.; Ernest D. Madden, gen. mgr.; Dave Blythe, gen. sls. mgr.; Jenny Gager, div. contrl.; Larry Lufsey, chief eng.; nat'l rep.: Katz.

Operation: 1953; TV sets in area: 290,600.

WEVV (Channel 44) NBC

Ohio Valley TV, Inc., 629 Walnut St., Evansville, IN 47708; (812) 424-9201.

Michael Brooks, gen. mgr.; William Hight, gen. sls. mgr.; Bob Ramsey, prog. dir.; Frank Hertel, chief eng.; natl. rep.: Adam Young.

Operation: November, 1983.

WFIE (Channel 14) NBC

WFIE, Inc., 1115 Mt. Auburn Rd., Evansville, IN 47712 (812) 426-1414.

Conrad L. Cagle, pres. & gen. mgr.; Ralph S. Jackson, exec. v.p.; Bob West, dir. ops; Bill Hollander, news dir.

Operation: 1953; TV sets in area: 214,000.

WTVW (Channel 7)

Evansville Television, Inc., 405 Carpenter St., Evansville, (812) 422-1121.

Ken Schreiber, gen. mgr.; nat'l rep.: Seltel.

Operation: 1956; TV sets in area: 247,480.

Fort Wayne

WANE-TV (Channel 15) CBS

Indiana Broadcasting Corp., 2915 W. State Blvd., Fort Wayne, IN 46808 (219) 424-1515.

Robert A. Fishman, pres. & gen. mgr.; Meredith Smith, fin. mgr.; Dianne Adjan, prog. dir.; Tom Weber, chief eng.; nat'l rep.: Katz.

Operation: 1954; TV sets in area: 253,000.

WFFT-TV (Channel 55)

Ontario Corp., c/o Robert W. Faull, Box 2255, Fort Wayne, IN 46801 (219) 424-5555.

Van P. Smith, pres.; Robert W. Faull, gen. mgr.; Richard J. Stawicki, prog. dir.; James E. Jump, sls. mgr.; James E. Miller, chief eng.

Operation: December, 1977.

WKJG-TV (Channel 33) NBC

Thirty-Three, Inc., 2633 W. State Blvd., Ft. Wayne, IN 46808 (219) 422-7474.

Anton Hulman, Jr., pres.; Joseph R. Cloutier, exec. v.p. & treas.; Hilliard Gates, gen. mgr.; Calo Mahlock, asst. gen. mgr.; William Kline, sls. mgr.; Eugene A. Chase, chief eng.; nat'l rep., Blair Television.

Operation: 1953; TV sets in area: 280,000.

WPTA (Channel 21) ABC

WPTA-TV, Inc, 3401 Butler Road, Ft. Wayne, IN 46808 (219) 483-0584.

Edwin C. Metcalfe, v.p./gen. mgr.; Marvin Gottlieb, gen. sls mgr.; Barbara Wigham, v.p. dir. of prgm. & promo.; Bill MacDonald, sls. mgr.; Jack Maurer, news dir.; Ray Krueger, chief eng.; nat'l rep.: Blair Television.

Operation: 1956.

Indianapolis

WHMB-TV (Channel 40)

LeSea Bldg., Co., Box 12, South Bend, IN (317) 773-5050.

Lester Sumrall, pres.; Doug Garlinger, chief eng.; Wanda Linville, traffic mgr.

Operation: 1971.

WISH-TV (Channel 8) CBS

Indiana Broadcasting Corp., 1950 N. Meridian St., Indianapolis, IN 46207 (317) 924-4381.

Bill Stough, pres. & gen. mgr.; Eric Land, gen. sls. mgr.; Terry VanBibber, chief eng.; Karen Miller, prog. mgr.; Phil Michael, promo. mgr.; R. Lee Giles, news dir.; Tracey Cole, exec. prod.; Hallie Crombaugh, community affairs dir.; Joe Wertenberger, fin. mgr.; nat'l. rep.: Katz.

Operation: 1954; TV sets in area: 1,250,000.

WRTV (Channel 6) ABC

McGraw-Hill Broadcasting Company, Inc., 1330 North Meridian St., Indianapolis, IN 46206 (317) 635-9788.

Jerry Chapman, v.p. & gen. mgr.; Sharon Chalfin, gen. sls. mgr.; Ken Ladage, prog. dir.; Robert Flanders, v.p./dir. bus. systems develop. & eng.; Diane Alexander, promo. dir.; Beverly May, bus. mgr.; Bob Gamble, news dir; .nat'l. rep.; MMT Sales, Inc.

Operations: 1949.

WTHR (Channel 13) NBC

Video Indiana, Inc., 1000 N. Meridian St., Indianapolis, IN 46204 (317) 639-2311.

Michael J. Corken, gen. mgr.; Mary Maxwell, publ. affairs coord.; Robert Shire, gen. sls. mgr.; Tom Rose, prog. dir.; Steve Walton, chief eng.; Bob Campbell, news dir.; Mark Dillon, bus. mgr.; nat'l rep.: John Blair & Co.

Operation: 1957; Ownership change: 1975. TV sets in area: 1,284,200.

WXIN (Channel 59)

Outlet Communications, Inc., 1440 N. Meridian St., Indianapolis, IN 46202; (317) 632-5900.

Chris Duffy, pres.; John Newcomb, sta. mgr.; Beth Sullivan, gen. sls. mgr.; Jim Borgioli, chief eng.

Operation: February, 1984.

Lafayette

WLFI-TV (Channel 18)

WLFI-TV, Inc., 2605 Yeager Rd., West Lafayette, IN 47906; (Studio); P.O. Box 7018, Lafayette, IN 47906 (mailng). (317) 463-3516.

Robertr A. Ford, gen. mgr.; Thomas C. Combs, sls. mgr.; Ken Gardner, chief eng.; Nina Hart, prog. mgr.

Operation: May, 1953; TV households: 319,900.

Richmond

WKOI (Channel 43)

Trinity Broadcasting of Indiana, 1702 S. Ninth St., Richmond, IN 47374 (317) 935-2390.

Paul Crouch, pres.; Charles Quinn, gen. mgr.; Mary L. Laird, supvr.; Joe Hoyer, prog. dir.; Merle Rummel, chief eng.

Operation: 1982.

South Bend

WHME-TV (Channel 46)

Lester Sumrall Evangelistic Assn. Inc., Box 12, South Bend, IN 46624 (219) 291-8200.

Lester Sumrall, pres.; Steve Sumrall, group v.p.; Peter Sumrall, v.p. & gen. mgr.

Operations: July, 1974.

WNDU-TV (Channel 16) NBC

Michiana Telecasting Corp., Juniper Road, Box 1616, South Bend, IN 46634.

Bazil O'Hagan, pres. & gen. mgr.; Paul Walton, Jr., dir. prog. operations; nat'l rep.; Adam Young, Inc.

Operation: 1955; TV homes in area: 270,000.

WSBT-TV (Channel 22) CBS

WSBT, Inc., 300 W. Jefferson Blvd., South Bend, IN 46601 (219) 233-3141.

E. Berry Smith, pres. & gen. mgr.; Jerry Bleck, nat. sales mgr.; N. J. Gassensmith, program dir. & film dir.; Robert Bell, chief eng.; nat'l rep.; Katz Agency.

Operation: 1952; Sets in area: 327,200.

Terre Haute

WBAK-TV (Channel 38) ABC

WBAK Television Co., P.O. Box 719, Terre Haute, IN 47808 (812) 238-1515.

Cy N. Bahakel, pres.; Hal Edwards, gen. mgr.; David Pierce, chief eng.; Barry Sinnock, prod. mgr.; nat'l rep.: Seltel.

Operation: 1973.

WTHI-TV (Channel 10) CBS

Wabash Valley Broadcasting Corp., 918 Ohio St., Terre Haute, IN 47808 (812) 232-9481.

J. R. Cloutier, exec. v.p. & tres.; Russ Arnold, v.p. & gen. mgr.; Dave Bailey, gen. sls. mgr.; Ruth Baker, prgrm. dir.; nat'l rep. Katz Agency.

Operation: 1954; TV sets in area: 449,300.

WTWO (Channel 2) NBC

Indiana Telecasting Corp., P.O. Box 299, Terre Haute, IN 47808.

Mark Prather, exec. v.p. & gen. mgr.; Jerry Tiller, sls. mgr.;

Jim Bell, oper. mgr.; nat'l. rep.: Blair.
Operations: Sept., 1965.

IOWA

Ames

WOI-TV (Channel 5) ABC

Iowa State Univ. of Science & technology, Ames, IA 50011(515) 294-5555.

W. Robert Parks, pres.; Keith Ketcham, gen. mgr.; Ted Tostlebe, comm. mgr.; Bob Helmers, promo. mgr.; Keith Kethcam, chief eng.: Wilma Leason, film dir.; nat'l rep.: Katz.

Operation: 1950; TV sets in area: 458,000.

Cedar Rapids

KCRG-TV (Channel 9) ABC

Cedar Rapids Television Co., 2nd Ave. at 5th St. S.E., Cedar Rapids, IA 52401 (319) 398-8422.

Joseph F. Hladky, Jr., pres.; Ed Lasko, v.p. & gen. mgr.; Ron Stack, gen. sls. mgr.; Edna A. Herbst, v.p. & promotion dir.; Walt Alliss, chief eng. & ops. dir.; Paul Dicker, prog. dir.; James Laymon, bus. mgr.; nat'l rep.: H-R.

Operation: 1953; TV homes in area: 493,300.

KGAN-TV (Channel 2) CBS

KGAN-TV, Broadcast Park, Box 3131, Cedar Rapids, IA 52406 (319) 395-9060.

Mike Bock, gen. mgr.; Dick Aune, gen. sls. mgr.; Tim Noonan, prog. dir.; Bob Burns, chief eng.; nat'l rep.: The Katz Agency, Inc.

Operation: 1953; TV sets in area: 373,800.

Davenport

KLBJ-TV (Channel 18)

937 East 53 St., Suite D, Davenport, IA 52807 (319) 386-1818.

Lee Hanna, pres.; Gary Brandt, gen. mgr.; Bridget Bowen, gen. sls. mgr.; Sue Passe, Don Bargmann, chief engs.; natl. rep.: ITS.

Operation: July, 1985.

WOC-TV (Channel 6) NBC

WOC Broadcasting Co., 805 Brady St., Davenport, IA 52808 (319) 324-1661.

William Ryan, pres.; Kenneth H. MacQueen, v.p./gen. mgr.; Joseph Lentz, sls. mgr.; John Hegeman, chief eng.; nat'l rep.: Blair.

Operation: 1949; TV sets in area: 670,200.

Des Moines

KCCI-TV (Channel 8) CBS

Cowles Broadcasting, Inc., 9th & Pleasant St., P.O. Box 10305, Des Moines, IA 50306 (515) 247-8800.

Nolan Quam, pres. & gen. mgr.; Guy Koenigsberger, v.p., programs/community affairs; John Leifheit, gen. sls. mgr.; Paul Fredericksen, v.p./treas.; Bill Huey, v.p. & chief eng.; Paul Rhoades, v.p./news & public affairs; John Pascuzzi, dir. of development; Robert Day, adv./promo. mgr.; Pete Taylor, sport dir.; Max Rauer, local sls. mgr.

Operation: 1955; TV sets in area: 529,200.

KDSM-TV (Channel 17)

KCBR-TV, Inc., 5160 Park Ave., Des Moines, IA 50321 (516) 284-1717.

Rolland Johnson, pres.; Donald O'Connor, v.p. & gen. mgr.; Dan Havens, gen. sls. mgr.; Vicki Harbert, prom. mgr.; Bill Brister, chief eng.

Operation: January, 1983.

WHO-TV (Channel 13) NBC

WHO Broadcasting Co., 1801 Grand Ave., Des Moines, IA 50308 (515) 288-6511.

Daniel J. McCarthy, gen. mgr.; William H. Jackson, prgm. dir. & film buyer; Ray Johnson, gen. sls. mgr.; Brink Chipman, news dir.; Holly Lowe, promo. mgr.; Charles Myers, Chief Eng.; nat'l rep.: Blair Television.

Operation: 1954; households: 364,840.

Dubuque

KDUB-TV (Channel 40) ABC

Birney Imes, Jr., One Dubuque Plaza, Dubuque, IA 52001; (319) 556-4040.

Charles Cyberski, gen. mgr.; John Sloan, gen. sls. mgr.; Dave Lange, news dir.; Gary Haverland, chief eng.

Operation: June, 1970.

Kirksville, Mo.-Ottumwa, IA

KTVO (Channel 3) ABC

P.O. Box 949, Highway 63 N, Kirksville, MO 63501; (816) 665-7781.

Frank Jonas, gen. mgr.; Lowell Johnson, sls. mgr.; Keith Reynolds, chief eng.; Dean Weitenhogen, dir. pub. info.; nat'l rep.: Seltel.

Operation: 1955: TV sets in area: 146,600.

Mason City

KIMT-TV (CHANNEL 3) CBS

Spartan Radiocasting, Inc., Second & Pennsylvania, Mason City, IA 50401; 423-2540.

Earl Schoborg, gen. mgr.; Miles Moore, gen. sls. mgr.; Dale Byre, chief eng.; nat'l rep.: Katz Agency.

Operations: 1954; TV sets in area: 449,000.

Sioux City

KCAU-TV (Channel 9) ABC-TV

Forward of Iowa, Inc., 7th & Douglas Sts., Sioux City, IA 51101 (712) 277-2345.

William F. Turner, pres. & gen. mgr.; Jack Gilbert, sr. v.p. & news dir.; Ray Cole, v.p. & sls. mgr.; Al Kirts, prod. svcs. dir.; Paul O'Bryan, natl. sls. mgr.; Dave Slater, prog. dir.; Mark LeValley, tech. opns. mgr.; Jim Henry, promo. dir.; natl. rep.: Seltel.

Operation: 1953; TV homes in area: 378,600.

KMEG-TV (Channel 14) CBS

Medallion Broadcasters Inc., Box 657, 7th & Floyd Blvd., Sioux City, IA 51105 (712) 277-3554.

A. James Ebel, pres.; Bruce Lewis, gen. mgr.; Carl Keller, gen. sls. mgr.; Lyle Johnson, chief eng.; Greg Funk, bus. mgr.

Operation: Sept., 1967; TV homes: 152,900.

KTIV (Channel 4) NBC

KTIV Television Co., 3135 Floyd Blvd., Sioux City, IA 51105; (712) 239-4100.

Jim Waterbury, pres.; Mike Smith, v.p. & gen. mgr.; Mary Bracken, v.p./programming; Dale Russell, v.p., eng.; Jack Baker, v.p. sls.; nat'l rep.: John Blair Co.

Operation: 1954; TV sets in area: 372,200.

Waterloo

KWWL-TV (Channel 7) NBC

Black Hawk Broadcasting Co., E. 4th & Franklin, Waterloo, IA 50703 (319) 291-1200.

Robert Buckmaster, chmn.; Harry G. Slife, pres.; William L. Bolster, v.p., gen. mgr.; Thomas E. Rodden, secty.-treas.; Thomas L. Trunnell, sect.; Edward M. Tink, v.p. & dir. eng.; James Waterbury, v.p., ops.; nat'l rep., Blair.

Operation: 1953; TV sets in area: 412,700.

KANSAS

Colby

KLBY (Channel 4) ABC

999 S. Range, Colby, KS 67701; (913) 462-7535.

W.J. Kochtermann, gen. mgr.; Daniel J. McKenrick, sta. mgr.; Mike Morrison, film dir.; Dixie Thompson, promo. mgr.; Walt Ward, chief eng.

Operation: July, 1984.

Ensign

KTVC (Channel 6) CBS

Southwest Kansas Television Co., Box 157, Dodge City, KS 67801.

Sid Warner, pres.; W. H. Bailey, gen. mgr.;

Operation: 1957.

Garden City

KSNG-TV (Channel 11) NBC

(Satellite of KSNW-TV, Wichita, KS
Part of Kansas State Network)

Kansas State Network, Inc., South Highway 83, Garden City, KS 67846 (316) 276-2311. Rep.: Katz.

Stan Orth, sta. mgr.

Operation: Nov. 1958.

KUPK-TV (Channel 13) ABC

Satellite of KAKE-TV, Wichita, KS)

KAKE-TV & Radio Inc., Box 10, Wichita, KS 67201.

Martin Umansky, pres. & gen. mgr.; Bob Surber, v.p. & sta. mgr.; George Sides, news dir.; Paul Hinderliter, chief eng.; John Strauss, prog. dir.

Operation: Oct., 1964.

Goodland

KLOE-TV (Channel 10) CBS

Kays, Inc., Broadcast Plaza Box 569, Goodland, KS 67735 (913) 899-2321.

Kay Melia, gen. mgr.; natl. rep.: Blair.

Operation: 1958.

Great Bend

KSNC (Channel 2) NBC

(Satellite of KARD-TV, Wichita, KA)

Kansas State Network, Inc., P.O. Box 689, Great Bend, KS 67530 (316) 793-7868. Bill Ranker, gen. mgr.; Gary Gore, sls. mgr.; Tim McQuade, news. dir.; Jim Bowers, chief eng.

Operation: November, 1954.

Hays

KAYS-TV (Channel 7) CBS, ABC

(Satellite KLOE-TV Goodland, KS)

KAYS Inc., Box 817, Hays, KS, 67601.

Bernard Brown, sta. mgr.; Dannia Massier, chief engineer; Ken Fitch, prod. mgr.

Operation: Sept., 1958; TV households: 97,000.

Pittsburg

KOAM-TV (Channel 7) NBC

Mid-Continent Telecasting, Inc., P.O. Box 659, Pittsburg, KS 66762 (316) 231-0400.

Lester L. Cox, chm.; Bill Bengston, v.p. & gen. mgr.; Mildred Cox & H. Lang Rogers, v.p.; Fred Hughes, secty.; Louis R. Martin, V.P., prgm'. & op.; Jack Lawrence, chief eng.; nat'l rep.: Blair.

Operation: 1953.

Topeka

KLDH-TV (Channel 49) ABC

Mid-America Bcstg. of Topeka, 101 S.E. Monroe, Topeka, KS 66603 (913) 234-4949.

Larry D. Hudson, pres.; James C. Thompson, gen. mgr.; John Colyer, gen. sls. mgr.; Dennis Czechanski, prog. dir. & film buyer; Monica Frank, prom. mgr.; Bob Totten, news dir.; Gary Krohe, chief eng.; nat'l. rep.: Avery-Knodel.

Operation: June, 1983.

KSNT (Channel 27) NBC

Studio Broadcasting System Div., Highwood Service Inc., P.O. Box 2700, Topeka, KS 66601 (913) 582-4000.

Ralph C. Wilson, Jr., pres.; Wm. R. Hirshey, v.p.-bdcst'.; Harry L. Strader, station mgr.; Jim Evers, dir. of prodn. and op.; Scott McIver, dir. of acct'.; Herbert L. Brown, gen. sls. mgr.; William S. Beeman, dir. of eng'.; Bob Totten, dir. of news.

Operation: 1967; TV households: 737,390.

WIBW-TV (Channel 13) CBS

Stauffer Communications, Inc., Box 119, Topeka, KS 66601 (913) 272-3456.

Stanley H. Stauffer, pres.; Jerry Holley, v.p., brdgt.; George Logan, gen. mgr.; Vince Frye, gen. sls. mgr.; Carlos Fernandez, opns. mgr./prog. dir.; natl. rep.: Blair.

Operation: November, 1953; TV households: 514,800.

Wichita

KAKE-TV (Channel 10) ABC

KAKE-TV and Radio, Inc., 1500 North West St., Box 10, Wichita, KS (316) 943-4221.

Mark H. Adams, chmn. bd.; Charles E. Jones, treas.; Martin Umansky, pres. & gen. mgr.; Harold Newby, v.p. & chief eng.; John Froome, v.p. and asst. gen. mgr.; Bryce Benedict, v.p. and gen. sales mgr.; Paul Threlfall, v.p. & news mgr.; nat'l rep.: Katz Agency, Inc.

Operation: 1954.

KSAS-TV (Channel 24)

Channel 24 Ltd., 316 N. West St., Wichita, KA 67203 (316) 942-2424.

Alan Rudy, pres.; Harlan Reams, gen. & prom. mgr.; John Friend, gen. sls. mgr.; Mac MacShane, chief eng.; natl. rep.: ITS.

Operation: August, 1985.

KSNW-TV (Channel 3) NBC

(Satellites—KSNC-TV, Great Bend, KS, Ch. 2; KSNG-

TV, Garden City, KS, Ch. 11; KSNK-TV, McCook, NB, Ch. 8)

Kansas State Network, Inc., P.O. Box 333; 833 North Main St., Wichita, KS 67201 (316) 265-5631.

Robert C. Waddill, v.p. & gen. mgr.; Ralph Butler, dir. of sls.; Bill Andrews, creative services dir.; Jack McKain, dir. eng.; natl. rep.: Katz

Operation: 1955; TV sets in area: 417,000.

Wichita-Hutchinson

KWCH (Channel 12) CBS

Kansas Broadcsting System, 2815 E. 37th St., North, P.O. Box 12, Wichita, KS 67201 (316) 838-1212; 1800 N. Plum St., Hutchinson, KS (316) 665-5503.

Ronald J. Bergamo, v.p. & gen. mgr.; Steve Merren, gen. sls. mgr.; John Mileham, v.p./admin.; Jay Zacharias, chief eng.; Steve Ramsey, news dir.; Robert Wine, contr.

Operation: 1953; TV sets in area: 420,560.

KENTUCKY

Ashland

WTSF (Channel 61)

Tri-State Family Bcstg., Inc., 3100 Bath Ave., Ashland, KY 41101 (606) 329-2700.

Claude H. Messinger, gen. mgr. & chief exec. off.; Anne Bledsoe, prog. dir.; Virgil Adkins, chief eng.

Operation: April, 1983.

Beattyville

WLJC-TV (Channel 65)

North Route 11, Beattyville, KY 41311 (606) 464-3600.

Forest Drake, pres. & chief eng.; Nathaniel Drake, gen. mgr. & news dir.; Margaret Drake, gen. sls. mgr.; Bonnie West, promo. mgr.

Operation: 1982

Bowling Green

WBKO (Channel 13) ABC

Bluegrass Television, Inc., 537 E. 10th St., Box 1198, Bowling Green, KY 42101.

Clyde Payne, v.p. & gen. mgr.; Rich Dubose, lcl. sls. mgr.; Gene Prather, prog. dir.; Dave Chumley, chief eng.; Roy Brassfield, news dir.; nat'l rep.: Katz.

Operation: June, 1962; TV households: 265,600.

Campbellsville

WGRB (Channel 34)

Green River Bcstg., Inc., Box 400, Campbellsville, KY 42718 (502) 384-4738.

Linda L. Lynch, gen. mgr.; Dave L. Lynch, sta. mgr.; Greg Thomas, prog./promo. dir.; Larry Nelson, chief eng.; natl. rep.: Spot Time Ltd.

Operation: April, 1983.

Hazard

WYMT-TV (Channel 57) NBC

Kentucky Central TV, Inc., P.O. Box 929, Hazard, KY 41701 (606) 436-4444, 436-2522.

Terry Blosser, gen. sls. mgr.; Tammy Stacy, prog. dir.; Darwin Singleton, stn. mgr. & news dir.; Kathy Clark, traf. mgr.; Kenneth Combs, chief eng.

Operations: Oct., 1969.

Lexington

WKYT-TV (Channel 27) CBS

Kentucky Central Television Inc., Box 5037, Lexington, KY 40505; Offices: Rt. 4, Winchester Rd.; (606) 299-0411.

Ralph Gabbard, v.p. & gen. mgr.; Al Taylor, v.p., op.; Jere Pigue, v.p. sls.; Hall Schumacher, dir. of eng'.

Operation: June 1967; TV households: 409,800.

WLEX (Channel 18) NBC

WLEX-TV, Inc., P.O. Box 1457, Russell Cave Road, Lexington, KY 40591 (606) 255-4404.

Harry C. Barfield, pres. & gen. mgr.; Wm. B. Gess, v.p.; John G. Atchison, secty.; Joe Oliver, v.p. & natl. sls. dir.; Hays McMakin, local sales; L. Neuzel, chief prog.; Al Scheer, v.p. & chief eng.; nat'l rep.: Blair.

Operation: 1955; TV households in area: 585,000.

WTVQ-TV (Channel 36) ABC

Shamrock Broadcasting Co., P.O. Box 5590 Lexington, KY 40555 (606) 233-3600.

William L. Service, v.p. & gen. mgr.; Dave White, news dir.; Jerry Fox, prog. mgr.; Jerry W. Fox, sta. mgr.; Jack Lackey, chief eng.; Rep.: Katz TV.

Operation: 1968; TV households: 212,100.

Louisville

WAVE-TV (Channel 3) NBC basic

Cosmos Broadcasting Corp., P.O. Box 32970, Louisville, KY 40232; 725 S. Floyd Street, Louisville, KY 40203 (502) 585-2201.

Jim Keelor, v.p. & gen. mgr.; S. Wheeler Rudd, gen. sls. mgr.; John R. Karem, natl. sls. mgr.; Anne Coleman, prgm. dir.; J. Harold Culver, dir. of eng'. & op; Ed Godfrey, news dir.; David Taylor, prom. supvr.; nat'l. rep.: Katz Agency.

Operation: 1948; TV sets in area: 950,400.

WDRB-TV (Channel 41)

Independence Television Co., Independence Square, Louisville, KY 40203 (502) 584-6441.

Elmer F. Jaspan, pres. & gen. mgr.; Arch Chapman, gen. sls. mgr.; Wilson Hatcher, news dir.; Bob Jeu Devine, chief eng.

Operation: 1971.

WHAS-TV (Channel 11) CBS

WHAS, Inc., P.O. Box 1084, Louisville, KY 40201; 582-7840.

Barry Bingham, Sr., bd. chmn.; Barry Bingham, Jr., pres.; Bob Morse, exec. v.p. & gen. mgr.; Donna Zapata, sta. mgr.; Richard Sweeney, prog. dir.; Steve Steinberg, dir. of brdg.; Bill Bratton, dir. eng.; Mike Lerner, promo. dir.; Don Hoover, film dir.; nat'l. rep., Harrington, Righter and Parsons, Inc.

Operation: 1950; TV sets in area: 782,900.

WLKY-TV (Channel 32) ABC

Pulitzer Broadcasting Co., 1918 Mellwood Ave., P.O. Box 6205, Louisville, KY 40206 (502) 893-3671.

William W. Campbell, v.p. & gen. mgr.; Dick Polgreen, gen. sls. mgr.; Jack Shafer, prog. dir.; Tom Becherer, news dir.; Paul Kelley, v.p. & chief eng.; Lora Bradshaw, community affairs dir.

Operation: September, 1961; households: 610,900.

Madisonville

WLCN (Channel 19)

Life Anew Ministries, Inc., Box 1087, 721 Princeton Pike, Madisonville, KY 42431; (502) 821-2204.
John Stalls, pres.; John Price, v.p.
Operation: September, 1983.

Paducah

WPSD-TV (Channel 6) NBC

Paducah Newspapers, Inc., P.O. Box 1197, 100 Television Lane, Paducah, KY 42001 (502) 442-8214.
Fred Paxton, pres. & mgring dir.; John Williams, gen. mgr.; nat'l rep., Blair.
Operation: 1957; TV sets in area: 325,000.

LOUISIANA

Alexandria

KALB-TV (Channel 5) NBC

Lanford Telecasting Co., Inc., 605-11 Washington St., Alexandria, LA 71301 (318) 445-2456.
Robert E. Miller, v.p. & gen. mgr.; Berton Chaudoir, natl. sls. mgr.; Dowell Bushnell, sls. mgr.; Lesley Solmon, gen. serv. mgr.; Tom Webb, news dir.; Jimmy Fox, mgr. creative svcs.; nat'l rep.: The Katz Agency.
Operation: 1954; TV sets in area; 507,900.

KLAX-TV (Channel 31)

Cypress Comm. Corp., 1811 England Dr., Alexandria, LA 71301 (318) 473-2231.
James C. Richards, pres. & gen. mgr.; John Boyle, opns. mgr.; Charles Tarver, chief eng.
Operation: 1982.

Baton Rouge

WAFB-TV (Channel 9) CBS

Guaranty Broadcasting Corp., 844 Government St., Baton Rouge, LA 70821.
George A. Foster, Jr., bd. chmn.; Tom E. Gibbens, pres. & gen. mgr.; James D. Russell, secty. & treas.; Ed Lamy, v.p. & prog. dir.; Mervyn Rhys, v.p. & comm. mgr.; Mervyn Rhys, v.p., asst. gen. mgr.; Steve Ackerman, opns. mgr.; Margie Larson, promo. dir.; William Comeaux, chief eng., oper. mgr.; Grace McElveen, promo.-mdsing. dir., nat'l rep.: Katz Television.
Operation: 1953; TV sets in area: 460,000.

WBRZ (Channel 2) ABC

Louisiana Television Broadcasting Corp., P.O. Box 2906, Baton Rouge, LA 70821; 387-2222.
Douglas L. Manship, pres.; Charles Manship, treas.; Richard Manship, secty. & gen. mgr.; Jules L. Mayeux, gen. mgr.; Barbara Bree, prog. mgr.; William R. Yordy, chief eng.; Robert J. Headlee, asst. gen. sls. mgr.; Jim Primeaux, promo. mgr.; John Spain, news dir.; Jamie Politz, pub. affairs & personnel dir.; Pat Cheramie, local sls. mgr.; nat'l rep.: Blair Television.
Operation: 1955; TV sets TSA; 556,700; TV sets ADI 200,600.

WRBT (Channel 33) NBC

WRBT Television, Inc., P.O. Box 14685, Baton Rouge, LA 70808 (504) 766-3233.
Cyril E. Vetter, pres. & sta. mgr.; Bill Hathorn, gen. sls. mgr.
Operations: 1971.

Lafayette

KADN (Channel 15)

KADN Broadcasting, Inc., 1506 Eraste Landry Rd., Lafayette, LA 70506 (318) 237-1500.
Mike Mitchell, gen. mgr.; Eddie Blanchard, prog. dir.; Clark White, gen. sls. mgr.; Dave Pierce, sls. mgr.; Keith Towndsin, chief eng.; natl. rep.: Adam Young.
Operation: 1980.

KATC (Channel 3) ABC

Acadian Television Corp., 1103 Eraste Landry Rd., Lafayette, LA 70501 (318) 232-6111.
Mrs. Frances T. Kurzeg, pres.; William A. Patton, v.p. & gen. mgr.; Roy K. Rhodes, sls. mgr.; reps: The Meeker Co.; James S. Ayers Co., Inc. (Southeast); Busby, Finch & Woods (Southwest).
Operation: 1962; TV households: 357,600.

KLFY-TV (Channel 10) CBS

Texoma Broadcasters, Inc., Box 90665, Lafayette, LA 70509 (318) 981-4823.
M. N. Bostick, pres.; Thomas G. Pears, gen. mgr.; Terry Dover, op. mgr.; Dave Hebert, chief eng.; Dan Coleman, prod. spvsr.; nat'l rep.: Seltel.
Operation; 1955; TV sets in area: 321,000.

Lake Charles

KPLC-TV (Channel 7) NBC

Calcasieu TV & Radio, Inc., 320 Division St., P.O. Box 1488, Lake Charles, LA 70601 (318) 439-9071.
G. R. Chambers, owner; Rita S. Chambers, pres. & gen. mgr.; Jerry Goos, gen. sls. mgr.; Al Smith, exec. v.p., eng.; nat'l rep.: Katz.
Operation: 1954; TV sets in area: 247,800.

KVHP (Channel 29)

Lake Charles Electronic Media, 129 W. Prien Lake Rd., Lake Charles, LA 70601; (318) 474-1316.
Herschell Hardesty, pres.; Larry Campbell, gen. mgr. & gen. sls. mgr.; Scott Rogers, prog. dir.; Arthur Hixon, traffic mgr.; John High, chief eng.; natl. rep.: Seltel.
Operation: December, 1982.

Monroe

KARD (Channel 14) ABC

Woods TV Corp., 701 Parkwood Dr., West Monroe, LA 71291 (318) 388-0114.
Charles Woods, pres.; David Woods, gen. mgr.; Rodney Evans, chief eng.
Operation: August, 1967; TV households: 92,200.

KNOE-TV (Channel 8) CBS

Noe Enterprises Inc., 1400 Oliver Rd., P.O. Box 4067, Monroe, LA 71211 (318) 322-8155.
James A. Noe, Jr., pres. & gen. mgr.; Allen Jones, natl. sls. mgr.; Jack McCall, prog. dir.; Raymond Boyd, dir. of eng.; Lloyd Voorhees, mgr. regional/local sls. mgr.; Ansel Smith, ops. mgr.; rep.: Katz.
Operation: 1953; TV sets in area: 800,000.

KTVE (Channel 10) NBC

(A Gray Communications System Station)
KTVE, Inc., 400 West Main, El Dorado, AR 71730 (318) 321-1300; 2909 Kilpatrick Blvd., Monroe, LA.
H.V. Roche, v.p. & gen. mgr.; Mike Caruso, chief eng.;

John McCutcheon, reg. sls. mgr.; Frank Rogers, nat'l traffic dir.; Helen Johnson, prog. dir.; rep.: Katz.
Operation: 1955; TV sets in area: 298,200.

New Orleans

WDSU-TV (Channel 6) NBC

Cosmos Broadcasting Corp., 520 Royal St., New Orleans, LA 70130 (504) 527-0666.
Bob McRaney, Jr., v.p. & gen. mgr.; Evan Wiggins, opns. mgr.; Tano Compagno, prod. dir.; Richard Herd, gen. sls. mgr.; Larry Price, news dir.; Shelley Hobson, mktg. dir.; Joyce Eves, community affairs dir.; Steve Mohammed, bus. mgr.; Earle Connors, chief eng.; nat'l. rep.: Blair Television.

WGNO-TV (Channel 26) IND

Tribune Broadcasting Co., 2912 ITM Bldg., 2 Canal St., New Orleans, LA 70130; (504) 581-2600.
James Dowdle, pres.; Dennis Fitzsimmons, v.p. & gen. mgr.; Robert Gremillion, sta. mgr.; Randy Davis, chief eng.; sales rep.: Petry.
Operation: 1967; TV households: 425,800.

WNOL-TV (Channel 38)

Channel 38 Associates, 1661 Canal St., New Orleans, LA 70112; (504) 525-3838.
Gail C. Brekke, v.p. & gen. mgr.; Steve Firedham, v.p. & gen. sls. mgr.; Rod Cartier, v.p., prog. dir.; Jim Gonex, chief eng.; natl. rep.: Seltel.
Operation: March, 1984.

WVUE-TV (Channel 8) ABC

Gaylord Broadcasting Co., 1025 S. Jefferson Davis Pkwy., New Orleans, LA 70125 (504) 486-6161; TWX 810-951-6090.
Robert Olson, v.p. & gen. mgr.; Jack Long, asst. gen. mgr. & gen. sls mgr.; Donald B. Wilburn, prgm.; Rich Brase, prom. mgr.; Michael Caruso, chief eng.; nat'l. rep.: TeleRep.
Operation: 1959: TV sets in area: 2,000,000.

WWL-TV (Channel 4) CBS

Loyola University, 6363 St. Charles Ave., New Orleans, LA 70118.
J. Michael Early, v.p., bdcst'. & gen. mgr.; Maurice Guillerman, asst. gen. mgr. & gen. sls. mgr.; John Pela, dir. of creative svcs. & film buyer; Jerrold Whaley, nat'l. sls. mgr.; James Daboval, local sls. mgr.; Phil Johnson, news dir.; Hugh Burney, chief eng.; nat'l. rep.: Katz TV.
Operation: September, 1957; TV households: 684,000.

Shreveport

KMSS-TV (Channel 33)

Media South of Shreveport, Inc., Box 30033, Shreveport, LA 71130 (318) 631-5677.
Grey Teekell, pres.; Paul F. Bankston, gen. mgr.; Donna Calvert-Smith, gen. sls. mgr.; John Schweiger, prog. dir. & film buyer; Tim Price-Roberts, prom. mgr.; Don Adams, chief eng.; natl. rep.: ITS.
Operation: October, 1985.

KSLA-TV (Channel 12) CBS basic

USC Communications, Inc., P.O. Box 4812, Shreveport, LA 71104 (318) 222-1212.
Dan Bates, v.p. & gen. mgr.; Mike Armstrong, sls. mgr.; John Renshaw, prog. dir.; Tony Williams, promo. dir.; Tony Guess, chief eng.; nat'l. rep.: Harrington, Righter & Parsons.
Operation: 1954; TV sets in area: 657,800.

KTAL-TV (Channel 6) NBC

KTAL-TV, Inc., 3150 No. Market St., Shreveport, LA 71104 (318) 425-2422. Texas: 3227 Summerhill Rd., Texarkana; (214) 793-1133.
W. E. Hussman, pres.; H. Lee Bryant, v.p. for bdcst'.; Doug Yoder, nat'l. sls. mgr.; Kenny Gardner, sta. mgr.; Jean Byrd, prog. dir.; George Tracy, dir. of eng.
Operation: 1953; TV sets in area: 490,900.

KTBS-TV (Channel 3) ABC

KTBS, Inc., 312 E. Kings Highway, Shreveport, LA 868-3644.
E. Newton Wray, pres. & gen. mgr.; George D. Wray, Jr., vice-pres.; Charles W. Wray, secy-treas.; Edwin Wray, sta. mgr. & promo. mgr.; Marvin L. Perry, Jr., film dir.; Dave Hendricks, chief eng.; nat'l rep.: Katz Agency.
Operation: 1955; TV sets in area: 732,300.

MAINE

Bangor

WABI-TV (Channel 5) CBS

Community Broadcasting Service, 36 Hildreth St., Bangor, ME 04401 (207) 947-8321.
George J. Gonyar, v.p. & gen. mgr.; Dale Carter, chief eng.; nat'l rep.: Blair.
Operation: 1953; TV sets in area: 140,000.

WLBZ-TV (Channel 2) NBC

WLBZ Television, Inc., Box 934, Mt. Hope Ave., Bangor, ME 04401 (207) 942-4822.
Fred Thompson, pres.; Bruce McGorrill, exec. v.p.; Margo Cobb, v.p./gen. mgr.; Bruce Scott, chief eng.; nat'l. rep.: Katz Agency.
Operation: 1954; TV sets in area: 125,000.

WVII-TV (Channel 7) ABC

Bongor Communications, Inc., 41 Farm Rd. Bangor, ME 04401 (207) 945-6457.
Barbara J. Cyr, sta. mgr. & gen. sls. mgr.; Michele Morse, lcl./Canadian sls. mgr.; Gary Kasparek prod. mgr.; Jeff Barnd, news dir.; Judy Cooper, prog. dir.; reps.: Avery-Knodel, Creed Assoc., Metrospot of Canada.
Operation: 1965, TV households: 220,000.

Poland Spring

WMTW-TV (Channel 8)

Mt. Washington TV, a division of Harron Communications Corp., Inc., Auburn, ME 04210; (207) 782-1800. Sales dept., Portland; (207) 775-1800.
Paul Harron, pres.; Al Ritter, v.p. & gen. mgr.; Claus Wiese, sta. mgr.; John Ricker, chief eng.; nat'l rep.; Petry.
Operation: 1954.

Portland

WCSH-TV (Channel 6) NBC

Maine Radio and TV Co., 579 Congress St., Portland, ME 04101.
Mary R. Thompson, pres.; Jack S. Atwood, gen. mgr.; Don Powers, sta. mgr.; Arthur Leavitt, chief eng.; Bruce McGorill, sls. mgr., Lew Colby, promo. dir.; George Bowler, film dir.; nat'l rep.: Katz Agency.
Operation: 1953; TV sets in area: 210,000.

WGME-TV (Channel 13) CBS
Guy Gannett Broadcasting Services, Northport Plaza, Portland, ME 04104 (207) 797-9330.
Jean Gannett Hawley, pres.; Robert L. Gilbertson, exec. v.p.; David King, v.p. & gen. mgr.; Fred Desjardins, chief eng.; Jerry Senger, treas. nat'l rep., Blair TV assoc.
Operation: 1954; TV sets in area: 288,000.

Presque Isle

WAGM-TV (Channel 8)
Aroostook Broadcasting Corp., P.O. Box 1149, Presque Isle, ME 04769 (207) 764-4461.
W. L. Dickson, pres.; Norm Johnson, v.p. & gen. mgr.
Operation: 1956.

MARYLAND

Baltimore

WBAL-TV (Channel 11) NBC
The Hearst Corp., 3800 Hooper Ave., Baltimore, MD 21211 (301) 467-3000.
John C. Conomikes, v.p. & gen. mgr., Hearst Broadcasting Stations; Malcolm D. Potter, v.p. & gen. mgr., WBAL-TV; Lynn McIntyre, prog. dir.; Jack Gilmore, v.p. sls.; Robert Morgan, natl. sls. mgr.; David Elmore, lcl. sls. mgr.; nat'l. rep.: Blair.
Operation: March, 1948; TV households: 2,613,200.

WBFF (Channel 45)
Chesapeake TV Inc., 3500 Parkdale Ave., Baltimore, MD 21211 (301) 462-4500.
Julian S. Smith, gen. mgr.; Frederick M. Himes, Jr., op. mgr.; Robert Simmons, gen. sls. mgr.; Brock Abernathy, natl. sls. mgr.; William LeFevre, prog. mgr.; Dwight Weems, prod. mgr.; Augustine Levero, mkt. mgr.; Sharon Christopher Wylie, public affairs mgr.; Dennis Winters, chief eng.; Brad Foltyn, promo. mgr.
Operation: 1971.

WJZ-TV (Channel 13) ABC
Westinghouse Broadcasting Co., Inc., 3725 Malden Ave., Baltimore, MD 21211 (301) 466-0013.
Daniel L. Ritchie, pres. & chief exec. off., Westinghouse Broadcasting Co.; Paul Yates, v.p. & gen. mgr.; H. Brian O'Neill, creative svcs. mgr.; Stan Rudick, prgm. mgr.; Steven Engles, gen. sls. mgr.; Glenn Lahman, chief eng.; Richard Reingold, news dir.; Harold Murphy, bus. mgr.
Operation: 1948; TV sets in area: 2,653,500.

WKJL-TV (Channel 24)
Family Media Inc., 4820 Seton Dr., Baltimore, MD 21215 (301) 358-2400.
Ken Buschman, v.p. & gen. mgr.; Jay Cleaver, gen. sls. mgr.; Don May Sr., opns. mgr.; Patty Wecker, prom. mgr.; Pat Lardner, traf. mgr.; Jim Vest, chief eng.
Operation: December, 1985.

WMAR-TV (Channel 2) NBC
WMAR, Inc., 6400 York Road, Baltimore, MD 21212 (301) 377-2222.
Arnold J. Kleiner, v.p. & gen. mgr.; Joseph Bruno, chief eng.; William O. Gallagher, bus. mgr.; Barry M. Friedly, prod. mgr.; Charles Horich, v.p. & dir. of bdcst'.; Janet B. Covington, dir. of pub. affairs.
Operation: 1947; TV sets in area: 2,390,600.

WNUV-TV (Channel 54)
New Vision, Inc., 3001 Druid Park Dr., Baltimore, MD 21215 (301) 462-5400.
Samuel S. Kravetz, pres. & gen. mgr.; Mark Salditch, prog. dir. & film buyer; Paul Garnet, chief eng.
Operation: July, 1982.

Hagerstown

WHAG-TV
Great Trails Broadcasting Corp., 13 East Washington Street, Hagerstown, MD 21740 (301) 797-4400.
George J. Wymer, v.p. & gen. mgr.; Hugh J. Breslin III, gen. sls. mgr.; Chuck Noland, prog. dir.; Chris Thomas, acting chief eng.; Scot L. Freeman, bus. mgr.; Rep.: Katz.
Operation: 1970.

Salisbury

WBOC-TV (Channel 16) CBS, NBC
WBOC-TV, Inc., 17291 N. Salisbury Blvd., Salisbury, MD 21801; (301) 749-1111.
William Kenton, v.p. & gen. mgr.; Carol Hess, prog. dir.; Robert Getz, gen. sls. mgr.; Sally Cannon, news dir.; Vincent Donovan, chief eng.
Operation: 1954; TV sets in area: 139,150.

WMDT (Channel 47) ABC, NBC
Delmarra Broadcast Svc. Genl. Partnership. P.O. Box 4990, Salisbury, MD 21801; (301) 742-4747.
Frank Pilgrim, gen. mgr.; Sam Taylor, reg. & natl. sls. mgr.; Rich Dipilla, lcl. sls. mgr.; Clay Spurrier, chief eng.; Karen Adams, news dir.; natl. rep.: Seltel.
Operation: 1980.

MASSACHUSETTS

Adams-Pittsfield

WCDC (Channel 19) ABC
(Satellite of WTEN, Albany, NY)
Knight-Ridder Broadcasting, Inc. 341 Northern Blvd., Albany, NY 12204 (518) 436-4822.
Terence McGuirk, gen. mgr.; Archie Goodbee, gen. sls. mgr.; Gene Collins, prog. dir.; Tom Bryson, news dir.

Boston

WBZ TV (Channel 40) NBC
Westinghouse Broadcasting Co., Inc., 1170 Soldiers Field Road, Boston, MA 02134 (617) 787-7000.
Sy Yanoff, v.p. & gen. mgr.; John Spinola, sta. mgr.; Dan Lawlor, gen. sls. mgr.; Jeff Rosser, news dir.; George St. Andre, dir. of eng.; Dick Kurlander, prog. mgr.; Jolen Schmauss, creative services dir.; Terri Park, information services mgr.; Bob Houghton, cont.; Karen Huggins, human resources mgr.; Bob Hayes, traffic mgr.; Bill Ferrick, ops. mgr.
Operation: 1948; TV sets in area: 2,700,000.

WCVB-TV (Channel 5) ABC
Metromedia, Inc., 5 TV Place, Needham, MA 02192.
S. James Coppersmith, v.p. & gen. mgr.; Deborah Sinay, v.p., gen. sls. mgr.; Paul La Camera, v.p. prog. & public affairs; Philip Balboni, v.p. news; Burt Peretsky, pub. rel. mgr.; Ann Karelitz, mktg. mgr.; Donna Latson-Gittens, v.p. comm. prog.
Operation: 1972.

WNEV-TV (Channel 7) CBS

New England TV Corp., 7 Bulfinch Pl., Government Center, Boston, MA 02114 (617) 725-0777.

Seymour Yanoff, pres.; Vic Lai, v.p.-admin. fin.; Bill Ranson, v.p. & sls. mgr.; Jeff Schiffman, v.p.-prog.; Therese Park, v.p.-pub. rel.; Jeff Rosser, v.p.-news; Richard Weisberg, v.p.-mktg. & creative svcs.; Karl Renwanz, v.p.-eng.; nat'l. rep.: Telerep.

Operation: June, 1948; homes in area: 2,034,200.

WQTV (Channel 68)

1660 Soldier Field Rd., Boston, MA 02135 (617) 787-6868.

Byron H. Lasky, chmn.; Edwin Cooperstein, pres.; J. Clifford Curley, v.p. & gen. mgr.; William Cunningham, bus. mgr.; Alison Cooperstein, prog. dir.; Jeannie MacDonald, prom. mgr.; Robert Pierce, chief eng.; natl. rep.: Seltel.

Operation: January, 1979.

WSBK-TV (Channel 38) NBC, ABC, CBS

New Boston TV, Inc., 83 Leo Birmingham Pkwy, Brighton, MA 02135 (617) 783-3838.

Joseph C. Dimino, gen. mgr.; Daniel J. Berkery, sta. mgr.; B. J. Anderson, promo. mgr.; William B. Knight, compt.; John Anderson, dir. of sls. develop.; Stuart Tauber, natl. sls. mgr.; Ron Pulera, local sls. mgr.; Dick Beach, op. mgr. promo. mgr.; Doug Henderson, chief eng.

Operation: 1964.

WXNE-TV (Channel 25)

CBN Continental Broadcasting Network, Inc., 100 Second Ave., Needham Heights, MA 02194 (617) 449-4200.

M. G. Robertson, pres.; Robert E. Johnson, sr. v.p.; Tim B. Robertson, gen. mgr.; B. Randy Seiler, chf. eng.

Operation: 1977.

Boston-Cambridge

WLVI-TV (Channel 56)

Gannett Massachusetts Broadcasting, Ind., 75 Morrissey Bldg., Boston, MA 02125; (617) 265-5656.

Gerald R. Walsh, gen. mgr.; Victoria Gregorian, prog. mgr.; Kevin J. Dunn, gen. sls. mgr.; Thom Neeson, natl. sls. mgr.; Derick Dalton, lcl. sls. mgr.; Jack Fitzgerald, news dir.; Andrew M. Seyffert, v.p. & contrl; Gail Satz, prod. mgr.; Elizabeth Wrublin, promo. mgr.; Natalie McIver, news & pub. affairs mgr.

Operation: 1953.

Marlborough

WVJV-TV (Channel 66)

111 Speen St., Framingham, MA 01701; (617) 879-6666.

John H. Garabedian, CEO; Arnold Ginsburg, gen. mgr.; David Beadle, prog. dir.

Operation: March, 1983.

Springfield-Holyoke

WGGB-TV (Channel 40) ABC

The WHYN Stations Corp., 1300 Liberty Street, Springfield, MA 01101 (413) 785-1911.

Clifford Lefkovich, gen. mgr.; Dick Wylie, natl sls. mgr.; Rep.: Katz Agency.

Operation: 1953; TV sets in area: 1,213,500.

WWLP (Channel 22) NBC

Adams TV of Springfield, Inc., Box 2210, Springfield, MA 01102-2210 (413) 786-2200.

William M. Pepin, pres., gen. mgr.; John E. LaFleur, bus. mgr.; Louis Chenevert, chief eng.; E. Holland Low, v.p., natl. sls.; Daniel T. Sullivan, Jr., v.p., lcl. sls. mgr.; nat'l rep.: Blair.

Operation: 1953; TV sets in area: 714,900.

Vineyard Haven

WCVX-TV (Channel 58)

720 Main St., Suite 23, Vineyard Haven, MA 02601 (617) 775-4242.

Donald P. Moore, pres.; Edmond R. Nickerson, gen. mgr., prog. dir. & film buyer; Charles W. Holmes III, gen. sls. mgr.; Josh Violette, prom. mgr.; Francis I. Broadhurst, news dir.; John H. Rath, chief eng.; natl. rep.: Creed Assoc.

Operation: July, 1985.

Worcester

WHLL-TV (Channel 27)

Central Mass. TV, Inc., 15 Parker Rd., Shewsbury, MA 01545.

Lisa M. Protter, gen. mgr.; Greg Lano, gen. sls. mgr.; Thomas Powers, prod. mgr.; Bob Parmenter, traffic mgr.; Mike Krasner, news dir.; Jerry Gerrits, chief eng.

Operation: 1970; TV households: 2,416,500.

MICHIGAN

Alpena-Oscoda

WBKB-TV (Channel 11) CBS

Thunder Bay Broadcasting Co., 1390 Bagley St., Alpena, MI 49707 (517) 356-3434.

Stephen Marks, pres. & gen. mgr.; Pete Misiak, v.p.; Kelly Schulz, news dir.; Kevin Schalkofski, prod. mgr.; Mark Nowak, chief eng.; Debbie McKenney, prog. dir.

Operation: 1975.

Ann Arbor

WIHT (Channel 31)

Satellite Television Systems, Inc., Box 2267, Ann Arbor, MI 48106; (313) 973-7900.

Kip Farmer, v.p. & gen. mgr.; David B. Horowitz, prog. dir., Alfred Lile, chief eng.

Operation: 1981.

Battle Creek-Kalamazoo

WUHQ-TV (Channel 41) ABC

Channel 41, Inc., 5200 West Dickman Road, Battle Creek, MI 49016 (616) 968-9341.

John W. Lawrence, pres.; William J. Lawrence, Jr., bd. chmn.; Jerry Colvin, exec. v.p. & gen. mgr.; Linda Rosh, prog. & prom. mgr.; Michael J. Laemers, chief eng. & ops. mgr.; Phillip R. Ranns, controller; John Hampel, film dir.

Operation: 1971; Receivers in area: 938,000.

Bay City-Saginaw

WNEM-TV (Channel 5) NBC

WNEM-Television; Broadcasting div./Meredith Corp.; Offices and studios, 107 N. Franklin, Saginaw, MI (517) 755-8191. Sales office & studio: G-3426 Miller Road, Flint, MI (313) 732-2050.

Todd Holmes, v.p. & gen. mgr.; Bill Avery, prog. dir.;

Paul Virciglio, gen. sls. mgr.; Greg Surma, chief eng.; Fred Ertz, news dir.; nat'l. rep.: MMT Sales, Inc.
Operation: 1954; TV households in area: 421,200.

Cadillac

WWTV (Channel 9) CBS

Wilson Communications, Inc. P.O. Box 627; Cadillac, MI 49601 (616) 775-3478.
Ralph C. Wilson, Jr., chmn.; William R. Hirshey, pres.; J.A. Skip Simms, v.p. & gen. mgr.; nat'l rep.: Blair.
Operation: Jan. 1, 1954; TV sets in area: 1,234,200.

Cheboygan

WTOM (Channel 4) NBC

WTOM-TV, Inc., Box 546, Traverse City, MI 49684 (616) 947-7770.
Manuel Leitao, Jr., pres.; Donald R. Cote, v.p. & gen. mgr.; Bill Blaker, lcl. sls. mgr.; Leon Bush, chief eng.; nat'l rep.: Katz.
Operation: 1959.

Detroit

WDIV-TV (Channel 4) NBC

Post-Newsweek Station, Michigan, Inc. 550 Lafayette Blvd., Detroit, MI 48231 (313) 222-0444.
Amy S. McCombs, pres. & gen. mgr.; Robert Warfield, v.p. & news dir.
Operation: 1947; TV sets in area; U.S. total survey area: 3,182,00, total coverage area (inc. Canada): 3,448,000.

WGPR-TV (Channel 62)

WGPR, Inc., 3140-6 E. Jefferson Ave., Detroit, MI 48207 (313) 259-8862.
Dr. William V. Banks, pres. & gen. mgr.; James W. Panagos, v.p. & gen. sls. mgr.; Tenicia Gregory, v.p./cont. & sta. mgr.; Joe Spencer, acting prog. dir.; Ulysses W. Boykin, v.p. public affairs.
Operation: 1975.

WJBK-TV (Channel 2) CBS

Storer Broadcasting Company, Number Two Storer Place, Southfield, MI 48075 (313) 557-9000.
Bill Michaels, chm.; Peter Storer, pres.; Terry Lee, ex. v.p.; Jay Watson, v.p., gen. mgr.; Robert J. McBride, sta. mgr.; Mike Von Ende, news dir.; Tom Fox, community affairs dir.; James F. Major, prgm. dir.; Timothy J. Rocha, promo. mgr.
Operation: 1948; TV sets in area: 2,034,000.

WKBD-TV (Channel 50)

Field Communications, P.O. Box 359, Southfield, MI 48037.
George H. Williams, v.p. & gen. mgr.; George J. Kapel, gen. sls. mgr.; Jock L. Fritz, sls. mgr.; William P. Castleman, prog. mgr.; G. R. Fitzgerald, business mgr.; Al Martin, dir. of eng.; Edward Printz, prod. mgr.
Operation: 1965.

WXON-TV (Channel 20)

27777 Franklin Rd., Suite 708, Detroit, MI 48034 (313) 355-2900.
Aben E. Johnson Jr., pres.; Doug Johnson, v.p., gen. mgr. & prog. dir.; A.J. Schweizer, opns., mgr.; Walter Rodman, chief eng.; Tracey Nichol, news dir.; natl. rep.: Blair.
Operation: September, 1968.

WXYZ-TV (Channel 7) ABC

WXYZ, Inc., Broadcast House, 20777 W. Ten Mile Rd., Detroit. MI 48231 (313) 444-1111.
Jeanne Findlater, v.p. & gen. mgr.; Walter Rodammer, chief eng.; Francis L. Gannon, gen. sls. mgr.; Jan Coil, natl. sls. service mgr.; Milda Skorupskas, traffic mgr.; Larry Alt, prog. dir.; Christine McCaughey, research dir.; Ruth Whitmore, creative services dir.; Ed Pearson, natl. sls. mgr.; Barbara Shively, bus. mgr.; nat'l rep.: ABC Television Spot Sales, Inc.
Operation: 1948; TV sets in area: 1,823,423.

Detroit-Windsor (Canada)

CBET (Channel 9) CBC

Canadian Bdg. Corp., 825 Riverside Drive West, Windsor, Ont. N9A 5K9 (519) 254-2831.
H. L. Hackney, location mgr.; Fred Stecher, mgr. TV opns.; R. Kryger, mgr., TV tech. svcs.; J. Molnar, communications.
Operation; 1954.

Escanaba

WJMN-TV (Channel 3) ABC

(Satellite of WFRV-TV, Green Bay, WI)
WFRV Inc., P.O. Box 19055, Green Bay, WI 54307.
Rep.: Telerep.
Operation: 1969.

Flint

WJRT-TV (Channel 12) ABC

Knight-Ridder Broadcasting, Inc., 2302 Lapeer Rd., Flint MI 48502 (313) 233-3130.
P. Thomas Bryson, pres. & gen. mgr.; nat'l rep.; Blair.
Operation: 1958; TV households in area: 1,156,700.

Grand Rapids

WOTV-TV (Channel 8) NBC basic

Lin Central Broadcasting Corp., 120 College Ave., P.O. Box B, Grand Rapids, MI 49501; (616) 456-8888.
James Saunders, pres. & gen. mgr.; Lilliane Clary, bus. mgr.; Judy McDonald, prom. mgr.; Donald P. Gallagher, chief eng.; Sue McDonnell, gen. sls. mgr.; nat'l rep.: The Katz Agency, Inc.
Operation: 1951; TV sets in area: 532,500.

WXMI-TV (Channel 17)

3117 Plaza Drive, N.E., Grand Rapids, MI 49505; (616) 364-8722.
Richard Shively, , pres. & gen. mgr.; Richard J. Stawicki, opns. dir.; Pat Mullen, sls. dir.; Mark Krause, prog. mgr.; Bonnie Hunter, dir. of off.; Gary Beier, prom. dir.; Nancy Shirley, news; Dale Scholten, dir. of eng.; natl. rep.: Blair.
Operation: March, 1982.

WZZM (Channel 13)

Wometco WZZM Inc., P.O. Box Z, 645 Three Mile Rd., N.W., Grand Rapids, MI 49501.
George U. Lyons, pres. & gen. mgr.; Michael Seagly, ops. mgr.; Buss Kunst, gen. sls. mgr.

Kalamazoo

WWMT-TV (Channel 3) CBS

Gillett Bcstg., Inc., 590 W. Maple St., Kalamazoo, MI 49008 (616) 345-2101.

John E. Fetzer, chmn.; Carl E. Lee, pres. & gen. mgr.; Gordon Anderson, sr. v.p. & sta. mgr.; Jerrold M. Raffel, sls. mgr.; James Garrett, chief eng.; nat'l rep.: Avery-Knodel.
Operation: 1950; TV sets in area: 798,060.

Lansing

WLNS-TV (Channel 6) CBS

Backe Communications, Inc., 2820 E. Saginaw, Lansing, MI 48912 (517) 372-8282.
James M. King, pres. & gen. mgr.; Phillip E. Sherck, gen. sls. mgr.; Carl Onken, chief eng.; natl rep.: Harrington, Righter & Parsons.
Operation: 1950; TV homes in area: 1,063,100.

WSYM-TV (Channel 47)

600 West St. Joseph St., Lansing, MI 48933 (517) 484-7747.
Dale Parker, v.p. & gen. mgr.; Ken Laruick, gen. sls. mgr.; John M. Colmack, natl. sls. mgr.; Larry Getlack, chief eng.; rep.: MMT Sales.
Operation: December, 1982.

Lansing-Onondaga

WILX-TV (Channel 10) NBC

Adams TV of Lansing, Inc., P.O. Box 30380, Lansing, MI 48909 (517) 483-2621.
Ronald J. Kwasnick, gen. mgr./pres.; Joseph P. Murphy, sta. mgr.; Thomas M. Hartman, gen. sls. mgr.; Robert L. Serre, natl. sls. mgr.; Steven L. Reynolds, prod. mgr.; Nancie Gee, prog./promo. mgr.; William C. Hineman, chief eng.; Ross P. Woodstock, news dir.; Linda L. Murphy, v.p./finance; Timothy T. Staudt, sports dir.; Judith M. Keely, dir. comm. rels.; nat'l rep.: Katz.
Operation: 1959.

Marquette

WLUC-TV (Channel 6) CBS, NBC

WLUC Partners, P.O. Box 460, Marquette, MI 49855
Guy Spitsberg, gen. mgr.; Bob Ganzer, gen. sls. mgr.; Jack LaForest, prog. mgr.; Jack Truitt, chief eng.; Larry Deloria, promo. mgr.; Ed Kearney, news dir.; Steve Asplund, assign. mgr.; Dave Bradbury, film dir.; natl. rep.: Seltel.
Operation: 1956.

Saginaw-Bay City

WEYI-TV (Channel 25) CBS

Ziff-Davis Broadcasting Co., 2225 W. Willard Rd., Clio, MI 48420 (313) 687-1000.
Robert B. Farrow, gen. mgr.; George Leh, prog. mgr.; John E. Grandon, bus. mgr.; Ernest Hill, gen. sls. mgr.; Robert Volz, chief eng.
Operation: 1953.

Sault Ste. Marie

WGTQ (Channel 8) ABC

Michigan Television Network, Inc., 201 East Front St., Traverse City, MI 49684
Operation: 1976

WWUP-TV (Channel 10) CBS

Wilson Communications, Inc., Box 627, Cadillac, MI 49601.
Personnel: See WWTV, Cadillac.
Operation: 1962.

Traverse City

WGTU (Channel 29) WGTQ (Channel 8) ABC

Michigan Television Network, 201 E. Front St., Traverse City, MI 49684; (616) 946-2900.
Harry Calcutt, pres.; Gene Ellerman, exec. v.p. & gen. mgr.; Pat Mullen, sls. mgr.; Paul Baumgartner, chief eng.; Brad Graham, prog. & news dir.
Operation: 1971.

WPBN-TV (Channel 7) NBC

WPBN-TV, Inc., P.O. Box 546, Traverse City, MI 49685-0546 (616) 947-7770.
Henry V. Schones, Jr., pres.; Donald R. Cote, v.p. & gen. mgr.; Bill Blacker, lcl. sls. mgr.; Leon Bush, chief eng.
Operation: 1954.

MINNESOTA

Alexandria

KCMT (Channel 7)

Central Minnesota Television Co., Box 612, Alexandria, MN 56308 (612) 763-5166.
Tom Barnes, Jr., pres.; Glenn Flint, v.p. & gen. mgr.; Kenneth Bechtel, sta. mgr.; John Gunther, sls. mgr.; Carl Iverson, chief eng.; rep. Avery-Knodel, Inc., Harry Hyett Co. (Minn.).
Operation: 1958.

Austin

KAAL-TV (Channel 6) ABC

News Press & Gazette Co., P.O. Box 577, Austin, MN 55912 (507) 433-8836.
Clark Cipra, pres. & gen. mgr.; Janet Anderson, prog. dir.; Jerald Jones, v.p./eng.; Bill Wagman, news dir.; Greg Grimley, prod. mgr.

Duluth-Superior (Wis.)

KBJR-TV (Channel 6) NBC

RJR Communications, Inc., KBJR Building, Duluth MN 55802 (218) 727-8484.
Robert J. Rich, pres. & gen. mgr.; R. W. Pearson, v.p.; Steven Rich, prog. dir.; Bob Wilmers, chief eng.; Julie Nippet, pub. aff. dir.; nat'l rep.: Katz Agency.
Operation: 1954; TV sets in area: 336,500.

KDLH-TV (Channel 3) CBS

Beneder Broadcasting of Minnesota, Inc., 425 West Superior St., Duluth, MN 55802 (218) 727-8911.
John LaForge, gen. mgr.; Steve Hasskamp, chief eng.; Joe Golden, sls. mgr.; James Cuzzo, prog. dir.; nat'l rep.: Blair (Minneapolis).
Operation: 1954; TV sets in area: 326,090.

WDIO-TV (Channel 10) ABC

Channel 10, Inc., 10 Observation Road, Duluth, MN 55811 (218) 727-6864.
Frank P. Befera, pres. & gen. mgr.; George Couture, gen. sls. mgr.; Dave Poirier, prog. mgr.; George W. Woody, chief eng.; Joel Anderson, news dir.; Robin Buell, promo. mgr.
Operation: 1966.

Hibbing

WIRT (Channel 13) ABC

Channel 10, Inc., 10 Observation Rd., Duluth, MN 55811 (218) 727-6864.

Satellite of WDIO-TV, Duluth.

Operation: 1967.

Mankato

KEYC-TV (Channel 12) CBS

Mankato Broadcasting Corp., P.O. Box 128, Mankato, MN 56001 (507) 625-7905.

Howard J. Brown, pres.; Hap Halligan, v.p. & gen. mgr.; Eugene W. Schulte, v.p.-secty.-treas.; Lloyd Miller, sls. mgr.; Charles Pasek, prog. dir.; David Hooge, chief eng.

Operation: October, 1960; TV households: 202,200.

Minneapolis-St. Paul

KITN (Channel 29)

7325 Aspen Lane N., Minneapolis, MN 55428 (612) 424-2929.

Robert C. Fransen, gen. mgr.; Chris Westerkamp, gen. sls. mgr.; Mel House, stn. mgr. & film buyer; Robert Thaman, prom. mgr.; Don Kirby, chief eng.; natl. rep.: Seltel.

Operation: October, 1982.

KMSP-TV (Channel 9)

United Television, Inc. 6975 York Ave. So., Minneapolis, MN 55435 (612) 926-9999.

Evan Thompson, pres.; Stuart Swartz, sta. mgr.; Jim Clark, gen. sls. mgr.; Joe Carney, op. mgr.; Penny Parrish, news dir.; Glenn Smith, dir. of eng.; nat'l rep.: Telerep.

Operation: 1955; TV sets in area: 1,838,700.

KSTP-TV (Channel 5) ABC

Hubbard Broadcasting, Inc., 3415 University Ave., Minneapolis, MN 55414 (612) 646-5555.

Stanley S. Hubbard, pres.; Ralph J. Dolan, v.p. & sta. mgr.; James E. Blake, v.p. & gen. sls. mgr.; John Degan, ops. mgr.; Bob Sears, prod. mgr.; Terry Dolan, prog. mgr.; nat'l rep.: Petry Television, Inc.

Operation: 1948.

KTMA-TV (Channel 23)

Buford-Beaudoin Television of Minnesota, 620 Taft St., N.E., Minneapolis, MI 55413 (612) 623-0200.

John McNally, gen. mgr.; Wendell Nelson, chief eng.

Operation: September, 1982.

WCCO-TV (Channel 4) CBS

Midwest Communications, Inc. 90 South 11th St., Minneapolis, MN 55403 (612) 330-2400.

W. T. Doar, Jr., pres.; James M. Rupp. exec. v.p.; Loren Lucke, treas.; Robert McGann, sls. mgr.; Tom Cousins, community affairs/pub. relations dir.; Ronald Handberg, gen. mgr.; Everett Klosterman, contr.; nat'l rep.: TeleRep, Inc.

Operation: 1949; TV sets in area 1,683,400.

W*USA-TV (Channel 11)

WTCN-TV, Inc., 441 Boone Ave. No., Minneapolis, MN 55427 (612) 546-1111.

Joe H. Franzgrote, gen. mgr.; Elliot Bass, gen. sls. mgr.; Diane Mignone, lcl. sls. mgr.; Steven Thaxton, promo. mgr.; Tom Kirby, news dir.; Hillis Aldrich, chief eng.; natl. rep.: Blair.

Operation: 1965; TV homes in area: 1,711,700.

Rochester

KTTC-TV (Channel 10) NBC

KTTC Television, Inc., 601 First Ave., S.W., Rochester, MN 55901.

Ed Hutchings, v.p. & gen. mgr.; Jack Connors; sta. mgr. & natl. sls. mgr.; Ronald E. Gruber, op. mgr.; C. H. Sanders, chief eng.; natl. rep.: Seltel.

Operation: July, 1953; TV households: 363,300.

St. Cloud

KXLI (Channel 41)

L.E.O. Bcstg., Inc., 800 St. Germain, St. Cloud, MN 56301 (612) 252-0110.

N. Walter Goins, pres. & gen. mgr.; Liz Dennis, sta. mgr.; Roland King, gen. sls. mgr.; Jeffrey Stickels, prog. dir.; Larry Entner, chief eng.; nat'l. rep.: Adam Young.

Operation: November, 1982.

Walker

KNMT (Channel 12) NBC, ABC

Central Minnesota TV Co., Box 612, Alexandria, MN 56308.

Tom Barnes, Jr., pres.; Glenn W. Flint, v.p. & gen. mgr.; Kenneth Bechtel, sta. mgr.; Carl Iverson, chief eng.; rep.: Avery-Knodel Inc.

Operation: 1964.

MISSISSIPPI

Biloxi-Gulfport-Pascagoula

WLOX-TV (Channel 13) ABC

WLOX Broadcasting Co., DedBuys Rd., Biloxi, MS 39531 (601) 896-4778.

T. B. Majure, ex. v.p. & gen. mgr.; Earl Blessey, gen. sls. mgr.; Jas. O. Ray, chief eng.; Ray Williams, pgm. dir.; rep.: Avery-Knodel.

Operation; 1962; TV households: 369,100.

Columbus

WCBI-TV (Channel 4) CBS

Columbus Television, Inc., owner, P.O. Box 271, Columbus, MS 39701 (601) 327-4444.

Frank Imes, gen. mgr.; Brett Smith, prod. mgr.; Bill Morehead, chief eng.; Vallory Williamson, prog. dir.; nat'l rep.: Seltel.

Operation: 1956; TV sets in area: 237,200.

Greenville

WXVT (Channel 15) CBS

Big River Broadcasting Co., 3015 E. Reed Rd., Greenville, MS 38701. (601) 334-1500.

Joseph George, Jr., gen. mgr.; Pat Moose, gen. sls. mgr.; Ed Stopke, chief eng.

Operation: 1980.

Greenwood

WABG-TV (Channel 6) ABC

Mississippi Telecasting Co., Inc., P.O. Drawer 720, Greenwood, MS 38931 (601) 453-4001

Cy N. Bahakel, pres.; Ralph Robinson, sta. mgr.; Ada Mitchell, office mgr.; Robert Askew, chief eng.

Operation: 1959; TV households: 336,700.

Gulfport

WXXV-TV (Channel 25)

Four-O of Gulfport, Inc., Rt. 1, Box 150, Brandon, MS 39042; (601) 825-5721.

Robert Ratcliff, pres. & gen. mgr.

Operation: January, 1985.

Jackson

WAPT (Channel 16) ABC

Clay Broadcasting of Mississippi, Inc., Box 10297, Jackson, MS 39209 (601) 922-1607.

Ben Strickland, v.p. & gen. mgr.; Joe Root, station mgr.; Danny Bardin, dir. of eng.

Operation: 1970; TV household: 538,600.

WDBD (Channel 40)

Jackson Family TV, Inc., 3545 Edgewood Circle, N.E., Cleveland, TN 37311.

Brenda Harrison, pres.

Operation: November, 1984.

WJTV (Channel 12) CBS

Capitol Broadcasting Co., P.O. Box 8887, Jackson, MS 39204 (601) 372-6311.

Owens F. Alexander, exec. v.p. & gen. mgr.; Alan Axtell, gen. sls. mgr.; C. A. Perkins, chief eng.; Gen Ward, prog. dir.; Joe Lesem, news dir.; Phyllis Brooks, dir. of pub. affairs; Glenn Dear, prod. supvr.; nat'l rep.: The Katz Agency, Inc.

Operation: 1954; TV sets in area: 434,600.

WLBT (Channel 3) NBC

TV-3, Inc., 715 South Jefferson, Jackson, MS 39205 (601) 948-3333.

Frank E. Melton, gen. mgr. & CEO; Brad Streit, sta. mgr.; Dan Modisett, gen. sls. mgr.; Floyd Kinard, chief eng.; Larry Keeler, prod. mgr.; natl. rep.: Blair.

Operation: 1953; TV sets in area: 342,000.

Laurel-Hattiesburg

WDAM-TV (Channel 7)

Beam Communications Corp., P.O. Box 1978, Hattiesburg, MS 39401.

Frank L. Beam, pres.; Marvin Reuben, exec. v.p. & gen. mgr.; Cliff Brown, sta. mgr.; Ken Hawkins, sls. mgr.; Bobby Smith, chief eng. and oper. mgr.; Ann Daley, prog. mgr.; nat'l rep.: Katz.

Operation: 1956; TV set in area: 204,500.

Meridian

WHTV (Channel 24) ABC, NBC

Central TV, Inc., Box 5185, Meridian, MS 39301 (609) 693-2933.

Ronald E. Hale, pres. & gen. mgr.; Bob Horton, sta. mgr.

Operation: June, 1968; TV households: 60,900.

WLBM-TV (Channel 30) NBC

TV-3, Inc., 4608 Skyland Dr., Meridian, MS 39201 (601) 485-3030.

Frank Melton, CEO & pres.; Glenn Rose, gen. mgr. & sls. mgr.; Bert Case, news dir.; Floyd Kinard, chief eng.; natl. rep.: Katz.

Operation: October, 1982.

WTOK-TV (Channel 11) ABC

Southern Television Corp., Southern Bldg., Box 2988, Meridian, MS 39402 (601) 693-1441.

Channel 11 Television Co., Robert Ward, exec. v.p. & gen. mgr; John L. Buffington, sta. mgr.; Cecil Germany, nat'l. sls. mgr.; nat'l rep.: Petry.

Operation: 1953; TV sets in area: 151,900.

Tupelo

WTVA (Channel 9) NBC

WTWV, Inc., Beech Springs Rd., Box 350, Tupelo, MS 38801 (601) 842-7620.

Frank K. Spain, pres.; Mark Ledbetter, exec. v.p. & gen. mgr.; Bob Leech, dir. natl. sls; Charles Ed Bishop, prog. dir.; Wendell Robionson, chief eng.

Operation: 1957; TV sets in area: 433,900.

West Point

WVSB-TV (Channel 27) ABC

Venture Systems, Inc., Box 777, West Point, MS 39773 (601) 494-8327.

David C. Hopper, pres. & gen. mgr.; Kathy Poulin, gen. sls. mgr.; Lynda Mize, prom. mgr.; Chuck Govan, news dir.; Terry Smith, chief eng.; nat'l. rep.: Avery-Knodel.

Operation: May, 1983.

MISSOURI

Cape Girardeau

KFVS-TV (Channel 12) CBS

American Hirsch Broadcasting Co., Box 310 Broadway, Cape Girardeau, MO 63701 (314) 335-1212.

Walter H. McCroba, pres.; Joe Goleniowski, v.p. & gen. mgr.; George W. Jeter, sect-treas.; nat'l rep.: Katz Agency.

Operation: 1954.

Columbia

KMIZ-TV (Channel 17) ABC

Stauffer Communications, Inc., 501 Business Loop 70 East, Columbia, MO 65201 (314) 449-0917.

Rush Evans, gen. mgr. & film buyer; Robert Calvert, gen. sls. mgr.; Judy Pulliam, prog. dir.; Tina Vaudrin, prom. mgr.; Diana Meyer, news dir.; Tom Koenig, chief eng.; natl. rep.: Blair.

Operation: 1971.

KOMU-TV (Channel 8) ABC

The Curators of the University of Missouri, Highway 63, South, Columbia, MO 65201 (314) 442-1122.

Thomas R. Gray, gen. mgr.; Don Ruggles, sales mgr.; Robert Austin, dir. of prog.; William J. Reagan, chief eng.; John Quarderer, dir. of news; nat'l rep., Avery-Knodel, Inc.

Operation: 1953; TV sets in area: 505,200.

Hannibal, Mo.-Quincy, Ill.

KHQA-TV (Channel 7) CBS, ABC

Lee Enterprises, Inc., 510 Main St., Quincy, IL 62301.

Merritt Milligan, v.p.; John Phillips, gen. mgr.; Robert Fruehe, natl. sales mgr.; Jack Rose, local sls. mgr.; Lee Ellis, tech. dir.; Tom Robey, prgm. dir.; Gene Terry, news dir.; nat'l rep.: H-R TV Inc.

Operation: 1953; TV sets in area: 212,000.

Jefferson City

KRCG-TV (Channel 13) CBS

Box 659, Jefferson City, MO 65102 (314) 896-5144. Owned by Price Communications, Inc.

Robert Price, pres.; Bill Bengston, gen. mgr./natl. sls.; Bill Ward, lcl.-reg. sls. mgr.; Cleon Crum, chief eng.; Lee Gordon, prgm. dir.; Don Shinkle, news dir.; natl. rep.: Katz.

Joplin

KODE-TV (Channel 12) ABC

Gilmore Broadcasting Corp. (licensee), 1928 W. 13th St., Joplin, MO (417) 623-7260.

Douglas A. Padgett, v.p./gen. mgr.; Randy Collard, gen. sls. mgr.; Gayle Kirchner, dir. comm. affairs/promo. mgr.; natl. rep.: Seltel.

Operation: 1954; TV sets in area: 440,900 TV households per May '81 ARB.

KSNF (Channel 16) NBC

Mid-American Bcstg. Inc., P.O. Box 1393, Joplin, MO 64801 (417) 781-2345.

Don Long, v.p. & gen. mgr.; Ron Bormaster, gen. sls. mgr.; Wayne Boyd, lcl. sls. mgr.; Mel Brooks, chief eng.; Bill Brothers, prod. dir.; Don Gross, news dir.; Karen Long, opns. mgr. & prog. dir.; Mark Current, prom. dir.

Operation: September, 1967; TV households: 290,600.

Kansas City

KCTV (Channel 5) CBS

4500 Johnson Drive, Fairway, KS 66205 (913) 677-5555.

Philip A. Jones, v.p. & gen. mgr.; Pat North, gen. sls. mgr.; Erv Parthe, prog. dir.; Owen Uridge, promo. dir.; nat'l rep.: MMT Sales.

Operation: 1953.

KMBC-TV (Channel 9) ABC

Division—The Hearst Corp., 1049 Central, Kansas City, MO 64105 (816) 221-9999.

Paul Dinovitz, v.p. & gen. mgr.; Bill Lind, gen. sls. mgr.; Cheryl Craigie Parker, natl. sls. mgr.; Robert Twibeli, lcl. sls. mgr.; Deb McDermott, prog. dir.; Gerald Golden, resident controller; Michael Sullivan, news dir.; Joe Todaro, creative svs. dir.

Operation: August, 1953; TV households; 2,098,000.

KSHB-TV (Channel 41)

Scripps-Howard Broadcasting, 4720 Oak St., Kansas City, MO 64112 (816) 753-4141.

Bob Wormington, gen. mgr.; Peter D. Broke, asst. gen. mgr. & film buyer; Harold DeGood, chief eng.

Operation: September, 1970; TV households: 1,225,400.

KYFC (Channel 50)

Kansas City Youth for Christ., Inc. 4715 Rainbow Blvd., Shawnee Mission, KS 66205 (913) 262-1700.

Dr. Al Metsker, exec. dir.; David Lewis, gen. mgr.

Operation: 1978.

KZKC-TV (Channel 62)

Media Central, Inc., 2111 Blue Summit Dr., Kansas City, MO 64126 (816) 254-6262.

Steven M. Friedheim, gen. mgr.; Gayle Garrett, gen. sls. mgr.; Rebecca Rucker, prog. dir., film buyer & prom. mgr.; Karen Underwood, news dir.; Jim Cambron, chief eng.; nat'l. rep.: Seltel.

Operation: December, 1983.

WDAF-TV (Channel 4) NBC

Taft Broadcasting Company, Signal Hill, Kansas City, MO 64108 (816) 753-4567.

Dudley Taft, pres.; Earl Beall, v.p. & gen. mgr.; Randy Smith, gen. sales mgr.; Buddy Turner, operations mgr.; James Schmidt, chief eng.; nat'l rep.: Telerep.

Operation: 1949; TV sets in area: 1,510,400.

Poplar Bluff

KPOB-TV (Channel 15) ABC

(Satellite of WSIL-TV, Harrisburg, IL)

Mel Wheeler, Inc., 1710 Westminster, Suite F, Denton, TX 76205; natl. rep.: Seltel.

Operation: 1961.

St. Joseph

KQTV (Channel 2) ABC

Elba Development Corp., 311 Ridge Rd., E., Rochester, NY 14621. (816) 364-2371.

George Loar, v.p. & gen. mgr.; Mark Prather, gen. sls. mgr.; Lauren Hudson, news dir.

Operation: 1953.

St. Louis

KDNL-TV (Channel 30)

Evans Broadcasting Corp., 300 Park Ave., New York, NY 10036 (314) 436-3030.

Jack Petrik, pres. & gen. mgr.; Len Ziegel, v.p., sls.; Michael Gilham, gen. sls. mgr.; W. E. Anderson, chief eng.

Operation: 1969.

KMOX-TV (Channel 4) CBS

CBS, Inc. One Memorial Drive, St. Louis, MO 63102 (314) 621-2345.

Allan Cohen, v.p., gen. mgr.; Bob Finkel, dir. planning & admin.; Don Merl, prog. dir.; Eglon Simon, dir. sls.; John Lee, lcl. sls. mgr.; Jim Rothschild, dir. creative svcs.; Wally Wesley, dir. tech. oper.; Fred Burrows, news dir.; nat'l rep.: CBS-TV STNS.

Operation: 1959; est. TV sets in area: 1,037,390.

KPLR (Channel 11)

Koplar Communications, Inc., 4935 Lindell Blvd., St. Louis, MO. 63108 (314) 367-7211.

Marie Koplar, bd. chmn.; Edward Koplar, pres.; Barry Baker, exec. v.p. & gen. mgr.; Gregory Filandrinos, v.p./sls.; Larry Marcus, v.p. admin. & planning; Jim Wright, ops. mgr.; Denny Van Valkenburgh, natl. sls. mgr.; Howard Stevens, prog. mgr.; nat'l rep.: TeleRep.

Operation: 1959; TV sets in area: 1,000,000.

KSDK (Channel 5) NBC

Multimedia Broadcasting Co. Div. Multimedia Inc., 1000 Market St., St. Louis, MO 63101 (314) 421-5055.

Wm. J. Katsafanas, gen. sls. mgr.; Edward J. Piette, dir. bdgst. opns.; Richard Brase, dir. creative svcs.; Maryanne Brandmeier, lcl. sls. mgr.; Terry Doll, dir. pub. rels.; Steve Antoniotti, news dir.

Operation: 1947; TV households in area: 1,000,000.

KTVI (Channel 2) ABC

Times Mirror Broadcasting, 5915 Berthold Ave., St. Louis, MO 63110 (314) 647-2222.

Jon Petrovich, gen. mgr.; Steve Pontius, dir. sls.; Noble Redmon, dir. eng.; Vic Skaggs, dir. prog.; natl. rep.: Har-

rington, Righter, & Parsons.
Operation: 1953; TV sets in area: 1,498,000.

Springfield

KDEB-TV (Channel 27) ABC

Charles Woods Stations, 3000 Cherry St., Springfield, MO 65804 (417) 862-2727.

Charles Woods, pres.; Deborah Corbett, gen. mgr. & film buyer; Rick Lipps, gen. sls. mgr. & prog. dir.; Bill Leary, chief eng.; natl. rep.: Seltel.

Operation: 1968.

KOLR-TV (Channel 10) CBS

Independent Broadcasting Co., P.O. Box 1716 S.S.S., Springfield, MO 65805 (417) 862-1010.

J.H. Cooper, pres.; Ellis Shook, v.p. & gen. mgr.; John O. Cooper, treas.; Howard Frost, chief eng.; Bill Watts, gen. & natl. sls. mgr.; Mike Freeman, lcl. sls. mgr.; nat'l rep., Katz.

Operation: 1953; TV sets in area: 494,300.

KSPR (Channel 33)

Telepictures Broadcasting KSPR Corp., 3754 S. Glenstone St., Springfield, MO 65804 (417) 887-1333.

Jack Stuart, gen. mgr.; Mike McMellon, opns. mgr.; Malcolm Hukriede, sls. mgr.; Paul Katona, chief eng.

Operation: January, 1983.

KYTV (Channel 3) NBC

KY-3, Inc., P.O. Box 3500, Springfield, MO 65808 (417) 866-2766.

Donald S. Moeller, pres. & gen. mgr.; Houston Harte, v.p.; Robert G. Harbut, v.p.; Larry D. Franklin, v.p. & asst. secty.; John P. Zanotti, sect.; A. L. Hall, treas.-asst. secty.

Operation: 1953; TV sets in area: 459,600.

MONTANA

Billings

KTVQ (Channel 2) CBS

SJL, Inc., 3203 3rd Ave. N., P.O. Box 2557, Billings, MT (406) 252-5611.

Vic Miller, gen. mgr.; Lee Lareva, opers. dir.; Bob Collins, sales mgr.; Vic Miller, film buyer; Ron Jacobson, chief eng.; nat'l rep.: Blair.

Operation: 1953; TV sets in area: 105,350.

KULR-TV (Channel 8) ABC

Harriscope Broadcasting, Inc., P.O. Box 23909, Billings, MT 59104.

Burt Harris, pres.; E. D. "Bob" Merrill, v.p. & gen. mgr.

Operation: 1958; TV households: 100,300.

Butte

KTVM (Channel 6) ABC, NBC

(Satellite of KECI-TV, Missoula, MT)

Eagle Communications Inc., 750 Dewey Blvd., Butte MT 59701.

Bob Precht, chm.; Michael Stocklin, gen. mgr.; Charlie Cannaliato, chief eng.

KXLF-TV (Channel 4) ABC, CBS

KXLF-TV, Inc., 1003 S. Montana St., Butte, MT 59701 (406) 792-9111.

George Lilly, pres.; Ron Cass, v.p. & gen. mgr.; Ros Cass, natl. sls. mgr.; Marla Wilkin, local sls. mgr.; Vernon Hogge, chief eng.

Operation: 1953; TV households: 65,600.

Glendive

KXGN-TV (Channel 5) CBS, NBC

Glendive Broadcasting Corp., Broadcast Bldg., 210 South Douglas, Glendive, MT 59330 (406) 365-3377.

Lewis W. Moore, pres.; Dan Frenzel, mgr.; Mikel Huseby, chief eng.; Winnifred Norton, office mgr.

Operation: 1957.

Great Falls

KFBB-TV (Channel 5) ABC, NBC, CBS

KFBB Corp., P.O. Box 1139, Great Falls, MT (406) 453-4377.

Stan Whitman, gen. mgr.; Jack Fisher, gen. sls. mgr.; Ted Schroeder, ops./prog. mgr.; Don Ayers, prod./promo. mgr.; Joyce Stele, acct. supvr.; Ron Schlosser, chief eng.; Dick Pompa, news dir.; natl. rep.: Katz.

Operation: 1954; TV homes in area: 92,700.

KRTV (Channel 3) CBS, NBC

SJL, Inc., P.O. Box 1331, Great Falls, MT 59403.

Peter B. Friden, gen. mgr.

Operation: 1958.

Hardin

KOUS-TV (Channel 4) NBC

KOUS-TV, Inc., Drawer D. Hardin, MT (406) 665-3320.

Daniel W. Coon, pres.; Thom Curtis, gen. mgr.; Debbie Stoddard, prog. dir.; Vicki Stern, traffic mgr.; natl. rep.: Seltel.

Operation: 1980.

Helena

KTVH-TV (Channel 12) NBC

KTVH, Inc., Box 6125, Helena, MT 59604 (406) 443-5050.

Donald G. Bradley, pres. & gen. mgr.; Don Powers, chief eng.; rep.: Spot Time.

Operation: Jan., 1958; TV households; 91,200.

Kalispell

KCFW-TV (Channel 9) ABC, NBC

(Satellite of KECI-TV: Missoula, MT)

401 First Ave. E., P.O. Box 857, Kalispell, MT 59901.

Bob Precht, chr.; Mike Stocklin, v.p. & gen. mgr.; Mark Holston, news dir.; Mike Stocklin, sls. mgr.; Chris Neuhausen, chief eng.

Operation: June, 1968.

Miles City

KYUS-TV (Channel 3)

KOUS-TV, Inc., Box 1074, Miles City, MT 59301 (406) 232-3540.

Thom Curtis, gen. mgr.; Jim Furry, sta. mgr., sls. mgr.; Steve Easley, chief eng.

Operation: Sept., 1969.

Missoula

KECI-TV (Channel 13) ABC, NBC

Eagle Communications, 340 West Main, Missoula, MT (406) 721-2063.

Bob Precht, chmn.; Mike Stocklin, gen. mgr.; Jean Crepeau, prog. dir.; Sharikay Hettick, traffic dir.

TV households in area: 140,000 (ARB).

KPAX-TV (Channel 8) ABC, CBS

Garryowen Corp., Box 3500, Butte, MT 59701.

Pete Friden, gen. mgr.; Sarah Etchart, natl. sls. mgr.; Bill Moller, news dir.; Don Bradley, film buyer; Louis Tischer, chief eng.

Operation: May, 1970.

NEBRASKA

Albion

KBGT-TV (Channel 8)

Amaturo Group, Inc., Rt. 1, Box 31A, Genoa, NE 68640.

Frank E. Brosseau, pres.; Wayne Lansche, v.p./gen. mgr.; Glenda McCutcheon, prog. dir. & film buyer; Shawn Meister, prom. mgr.; Ray Gearhart, news dir.; Jerry Fuehrer, chief eng.

Operation: December, 1964.

Grand Island

KGIN-TV (Channel 11) CBS

(Satellite of KOLN-TV, Lincoln, NE)

Cornhusker Television Corp., KOLN Lincoln, NE. Studio: 231 S. Locust St., Grand Island, NE 68801.

Operation: Oct., 1961.

Hastings

KHAS-TV (Channel 5) NBC

Nebraska Television Corp., Highway 281, Box 578, Hastings, NE 68901 (402) 463-1321.

John T. Benson, gen. mgr.; Donald R. Seaton, v.p.; James D. Conway, secty.-treas.; Randy Nicholson, film dir.; nat'l rep.: Seltel.

Operation: 1956; TV sets in area: 116,000.

Hay Springs

KDUH (Channel 4) ABC

(Satellite of KOTA-TV).

Duhamel Enterprises, Inc., P.O. Box 1760, Rapid City, SD 57709.

Mrs. Helen S. Duhamel, chmn., William F. Duhamel, pres. & gen. mgr.; Monte Loos, opns. dir.; Jerry Dishong, sta. mgr.; Wes Haugen, sls. mgr.; Don Larsen, chief eng.; nat'l. rep.: Katz Agency.

Operation: 1958.

Hayes Center

KWNB-TV (Channel 6) ABC

(Satellite of KHGI-TV, Kearney, NE)

Same personnel as KHGI-TV; nat'l. rep.: Katz.

Operation: 1956; TV sets in area; 52,000.

Kearney

KHGI-TV (Channel 13) ABC

NTV Network, Kearney, NE (308) 743-2494. (Also Operates KWNB-TV, Hayes Center, NE; KSNB-TV, Superior, NE.)

Frank E. Brosseau, pres.; Peggy Huss, v.p. & gen. sls. mgr.; Jerry Fuehrer, chief eng.; natl. rep.: Katz.

Operation: 1953; TV households in area 615,800.

Lincoln

KOLN-TV/KGIN-TV (Channels 10 & 11) CBS

Cornhusker Television Corp., Box 30350, Lincoln, NE 68503 (402) 467-4321.

John E. Fetzer, chm.; A. James Ebel, pres. & gen. mgr.; Paul Jensen, v.p. & mgr.; Wes Maser, sls. mgr.; Lyle Kaufman, chief eng.; nat'l rep.: Harrington, Righter & Parsons.

Operation: 1953; TV sets in area: 371,000.

McCook-Oberlin

KSNK (Channel 8) NBC

(Satellite of KARD-TV, Wichita, KS)

Kansas State Network Inc., P.O. Box 238, Oberlin, KS 67749. Rep.: Katz.

Operation: November, 1959.

North Platte

KNOP-TV (Channel 2) NBC

North Platte Television, Inc., Box 749, North Platte, NE 69101. (308) 532-2222.

Ulysses A. Carlini, gen. mgr.; Jim Harmon, news dir.; Mark Himmler, chf. eng.

Operation: 1958.

Omaha

KETV (Channel 7) ABC

Channel 7, 27th & Douglas Sts., Omaha, NE 68131 (402) 345-7777.

Gary R. Nielsen, v.p. & gen. mgr.; Howard Shrier, sls. mgr.; Richard S. Spark, bus. mgr.; nat'l. rep.: Blair TV.

Operation: 1957; TV sets in area: 578,100.

KMTV (Channel 3) NBC

May Broadcasting Co., 10714 Mockingbird Dr., Omaha, NE 68131 (402) 592-3333.

Edward W. May, pres.; Owen L. Saddler, bd. chmn.; Jim Shaum, secty.; Frances M. Rankin, treas.; Norman W. Williams, exec. v.p., KMTV; Edward M. May, Jr., John R. Kidd, Bryce R. Pringle, v.p.s.; Roger C. Ottenbach, v.p. & gen. mgr., KMTV; Don Browers, prog. mgr.; Jeannette Bendtsen, promo. mgr.; Larry Steele, chief eng.; Art Jacobson, op. mgr.; Jay B. Maxey, gen. sls. mgr.; nat'l rep.: Katz.

Operation: 1949; TV sets in area: 415,000.

WOWT (Channel 6) CBS

3501 Farnam St., Omaha, NE 68131 (402) 346-6666.

Ed Zachary, pres. & gen. mgr.; John Dowd, sls. mgr.; John Dixon, prog. dir.; Steve Murphy, news dir.; Judy Horan, dir. promo. & merch.; Roger Moody, lcl. sls.; nat'l rep.: Petry.

Operation: 1949; TV sets in area 573,900.

Scottsbluff

KDUH-TV (Channel 4) NBC

Duhamel Bcstg. Enterprises, 1523 1st Ave., Scottsbluff, NE 69341 (308) 632-3071.

William F. Duhamel, pres.; Jerry Dishong, gen. mgr.; Wes Haugan, gen. sls. mgr.; Monte Loos, prog. dir., prom. mgr.

& film buyer; Richard Rose, news dir.; Dale Brye, chief eng.; natl. rep.: Katz.
Operation: March, 1958.

KSTF (Channel 10) CBS, ABC
(Satellite of KYCU-TV, Cheyenne, WY.)
Wyneco Comm., Inc., Inc., 2923 E. Lincolnway, Cheyenne, WY (307) 634-7755.
Carl J. Occhipinti, gen. mgr.; Bill Brennan, res. mgr.; Jerry Homer, chief eng.; mat'l rep.: Katz.
Operation: 1955.

Superior

KSNB-TV (Channel 4) ABC
(Satellite of KHGI-TV, Kearney, NE.)
Same personnel as KHGI-TV.; nat'l rep.: Katz.
Operation: October, 1965.

NEVADA

Henderson-Las Vegas

KVVU-TV (Channel 5)
KVVU Broadcasting Corp., 1900 E. Flamingo Road, Las Vegas, NV 89119 (702) 735-3191.
Herbert Kaufman, pres.; Forrest Chu, v.p.; Rusty Durante, v.p. & gen. mgr.; Bill Utton, gen. sls. mgr.; Jackie Smith, dir. of eng.
Operation: Sept., 1967; TV households: 155,000.

Las Vegas

KLAS-TV (Channel 8) CBS
3228 Channel 8 Dr., P.O. Box 15047, Las Vegas, NV 89114 (702) 733-8850.
Mark Smith, v.p./Gen. Mgr.; Ed Tabor, gen. sls. mgr.; Tony Malone, loc. sls. mgr.; Tom Franklin, dir. of eng'.; Lisa Nolan, promo. mgr; John Nelson, chief eng.; nat'l rep.: Katz Television.
Operation: 1953; TV sets in area: 213,000.

KRLR (Channel 21)
Dres Media, Inc., Box 26815, Las Vegas, NV 89126; (702) 382-2121.
Charlene Scott, pres.; Rick Scott, gen. mgr.; Gary Richie, gen. sls. mgr.; Jack Daniels, prog. dir.; John Sheridan, promo. mgr.; Tom Foy, chief eng.
Operation: July, 1984.

KTNV-TV (Channel 13) ABC
KTNV-TV, 3355 S. Valley View, Las Vegas, NV 89102 (702) 876-1313.
Ed Quinn, v.p. & gen. mgr.; Nancy Hunt, nat'l sls. mgr.; Jean Hites, local sls. mgr.; Sara Ohlson, prog. coordinator; George Maupin, sports dir.; Michael Williams, production mgr.; Matt James, news dir.; Ken Miller, chief eng.; William A. Kellogg, controller; Sherri Tolar, promotions mgr.
Operation: 1956; TV households: TSA 213,000, ADI 177,800.

KVBC (Channel 3) NBC
Valley Broadcasting Co., Box 44169, Las Vegas, NV 89116 (702) 649-0500.
Rolla D. Cleaver, gen. mgr.; Buzz Floyd, prog. mgr.; natl. rep.: Blair TV.
Operation: 1955.

Reno

KAME-TV (Channel 21)
Page Enterprises, 4920 Brookside Ct., Reno, NV 89502 (702) 786-2121.
Bill Andrews, pres. & gen.mgr.; Hermie Lopez, sls. mgr.; B.J. Andrews, sta. mgr.; Maggie Verhoef, promo. mgr.; Mike Andrews, news dir.; Al Ruch, chief eng.; nat'l rep.: Seltel.
Operation: October, 1981.

KCRL-TV (Channel 4) NBC
Circle L. Inc., 1790 Vassar St., Reno, NV 89510 (702) 322-9145.
Charles E. Cord, pres. & gen. mgr.; Jim Elliott, sta. mgr.; Norvel Seyler, chief eng.; Dick DeWitt, news dir.; rep.: Avery-Knodel, Inc.
Operation: 1962; TV households: 111,100.

KOLO-TV (Channel 8) ABC
Nevada Radio-Television, Inc., Box 10,000, Reno, NV 89510 (702) 786-8880.
Donald W. Reynolds, pres.; James C. Herzig. v.p. & gen. mgr.; Jack Hartman, gen. sales mgr.; W. I. Hopper, prog./operations mgr.; Earl Ling, film dir.; Robert Northam, chief eng. ; nat'l reps.: Peters, Griffin, Woodward.
Operation: 1953; TV sets in area: 110,000.

KREN-TV (Channel 27)
Sainte Broadcasting Corp., Box 3131, Reno, NV 89505 (209) 578-1900.
Chester Smith, pres.; Jerry Nichols, mgr.
Operation: November, 1985.

KTVN (Channel 2) CBS
Sarkes Tarzian, Inc., 4925 Energy Way, Reno, NV 89502 (702) 786-2212.
Dennis Slewert, gen. mgr; John Richardson, sta. & gen. sls. mgr.; Al Richards, chief eng.; Jim Ogle, news editor; rep.: Katz.
Operation: 1967; TV households: 71,000.

Winnemucca

KQJA (Channel 7)
Matlock Communications, Inc., Box 328, Eagle, ID 83616 (208) 939-0723.
Stephen J. Matlock, owner.

NEW HAMPSHIRE

Concord

WNHT (Channel 21)
NHTV 21, Inc., Box 2100, Concord, NH 03301 (603) 225-2100.
Frances Shaine, pres.; J.A. Skip Simms, gen. mgr.; Bob Joyce, prog. dir.; Bob J. Devine, chief eng.
Operation: November, 1983.

Derry

WNDS (Channel 50)
CTV of Derry, Inc., TV-50 Place, Derry, NH 03038 (603) 434-8850.
Dr. William H. Smith, pres.; James L. Lannin, gen. mgr.; Susane Newell, prog. dir.; Karri Rushlow, prom. mgr.; Thomas Howe, news dir.; Gregg Chadwick, chief eng.
Operation: September, 1983.

Manchester

WMUR-TV (Channel 9) ABC

United Television Co. of New Hampshire, Inc., 1819 Elm St., Manchester, NH 03104 (603) 623-8061.

Richard Eaton, prs.; Sam Phillips, gen. mgr.; Ray Harris, program dir.; nat'l rep.; UBC Sales.

Operation: 1954; TV sets in area: 965,576.

NEW JERSEY

Atlantic City

WWAC-TV (Channel 53)

Atlantic City TV Corp., 530 Atlantic Ave., Atlantic City, NJ 08401.

Frank J. Siracusa, pres.; Robert L. Bryan, gen. mgr.; George Campiss, gen. sls. mgr.; Mike Crawley, news dir.; Dan Merlo, chief eng.; nat'l rep.: Spot Time.

Operation: August, 1981.

Wildwood

WMGM-TV (Channel 40) NBC

South Jersey Broadcasting Corp., 15 Shore Rd., Linwood, NJ 08221 (609) 927-4440.

Howard Green, pres.; Jane B. Stark, sta. mgr. & gen. sls. mgr.; Kim Dougherty, prgm. prod. mgr.; Michael Schurman, news dir.

Operation: 1966; TV households: 400,000.

NEW MEXICO

Albuquerque

KGGM-TV (Channel 13) CBS

New Mexico Broadcasting Co., Inc., 1414 Coal Ave., S.W., Albuquerque, NM 87104 (505) 243-2285.

Bruce A. Hebenstreit, pres.; Paul Thorne, v.p. & sls. mgr.; Jack Mahoney, gen. mgr.; Brenda Yager, promo, dir.; Dick Doyle, chief eng.; Bud Holgerson, operations mgr.

KGSW (Channel 14)

Mountain States Broadcasting/Providence Journal Broadcasting, Box 25200, Albuquerque, NM 87125 (505) 842-1414.

Erick B. Steffens, gen. mgr.; Shirley Mix, sls. mgr.; Dudley Bullock, chief eng.; natl. rep.: Seltel.

Operation: 1981

KNAT (Channel 23)

Carson Communications, 1510 Coors Blvd., N.W., Albuquerque, NM 87105 (505) 836-1992.

Neil Simon, pres.; Rusty Durante, v.p. & gen. mgr.; Bob Brewer, sta. mgr.; M.A. Stoneking, gen. sls. mgr.; Sandie Bosley, prog. dir.; Bill Frost, chief eng.

Operation: 1975.

KOAT-TV (Channel 7) ABC

KOAT-TV, Inc., Box 25982, Albuquerque, NM 87125 (505) 884-7777.

Max A. Sklower, gen. mgr.; Elvin Smith, natl. sls. & op. mgr.; James Sharman, chief eng.; Monty Salisbury, news dir.; nat'l rep.: Blair.

Operation: 1953, TV homes in area: 276,000.

KOB-TV (Channel 4) NBC

Hubbard Broadcasting, Inc., 4 Broadcast Plaza, S.W., Albuquerque, NM (505) 243-4411.

Stanley S. Hubbard, pres.; Jerry Danziger, gen. mgr.; Dave Herman, sls. mgr.; Fern Bibeau, chief eng.; nat'l rep.: Edward Petry Co.

Operation: 1948; TV sets in area: 442,700.

Carlsbad

KAVE-TV (Channel 6) ABC

Box 12277, El Paso, TX 79912.

John Walton, pres.; Jerry Wright, gen. mgr.; Jack Harrel, chief eng.

Operation: 1956; TV sets in area: 15,600.

Clovis

KMCC (Channel 12) ABC

McAlister TV Enterprises, Box 2049, Clovis, NM 88130 (505) 769-1932.

Nick Brady, gen. mgr.; Herbert Compton, chief eng.

Operation: 1956.

Farmington

KOBF (Channel 12) NBC

P.O. Box 1620, Farmington, NM 87499. (505) 326-1141.

Bettie Cleveland, gen. mgr.; Bill Hirshey, prod. mgr.; Dan Bibeau, chief eng.

Operation 1972.

Las Cruces

KASK (Channel 48)

Las Cruces Full Power Television, Inc., 900 First National Tower, Las Cruces, NM 88001; (505) 524-2103.

Logan D. Matthews, pres. & gen. mgr.; Albert F. Gabalis, gen. sls. mgr.; Christopher Jackson, opns. mgr.; Gary Worth, news dir.; Keith Peterson, chief eng.; natl. rep.: Spot Time.

Operation: October, 1984.

Roswell

KBIM-TV (Channel 10) CBS

Caprock Telecasting, Inc., Box 910, Roswell, NM 88201 (505) 622-2120.

Joseph A. Carriere, pres.; Marc Reischman, sta. mgr.; E.C. Rader, dir. of eng.; Dave Brown, v.p., news; natl. rep.: Katz.

Operation: 1966; TV homes: 113,300.

Santa Fe

KCHF (Channel 11)

Son Broadcasting, Inc., Box 4338, Alburquerque, NM 87106; (505) 983-1111.

Belarmino R. Gonzales, pres. & gen. mgr.; Susan Stein, gen. sls. mgr.; Mary Kay Gonzales, opns. & promo. mgr.; Luther Kent, chief eng.

Operation: November, 1983.

KNMZ-TV (Channel 2)

Channel Two Associates, 2009 Pacheco St., Santa Fe, NM 87501 (505) 473-2002.

Michael A. Liff, gen. mgr. & prog. dir.; Mikele Meyers-Jennings, gen. sls. mgr.; Massoud Salarvand, dir. eng. & opns.; natl. rep.: ITS.

Operation: October, 1983.

NEW YORK

Albany

WNYT (Channel 13) NBC

Viacom Broadcasting Corp., P.O. Box 4035, Albany, NY 12204 (518) 436-4791.

Paul D. Arnzen, v.p. & gen. mgr.; Tom Burke, sta. mgr.; Frederick E. Lass, Chief eng.; Laurence J. Reilly, dir. of prod. sls.; Cynthia Williams, promo. dir.; Joseph Krone, promo. mgr.; Larry Price, news dir.; Richard Herd, gen. sls. mgr.; Fred Malbone, natl. sls. mgr.; Linda Cummings, traffic mgr.

Operation: 1954.

WRGB (Channel 6) CBS

WRGB, Inc., 1400 Balltown Rd., Schenectady, NY 12309; (518) 346-6666.

James J. Delmonico, pres. & gen. mgr.; David Lynch, v.p. & sta. mgr.; Terry Walden, mgr. prog.; Beverly Wittner, mgr. pub. affairs; Donald J. Decker, v.p., news; Donald Cohen, mgr., prom.

Operation: 1947.

WTEN (Channel 10)

Knight-Ridder Broadcasting Company, Incorporated, 341 Northern Blvd., Albany, NY 12204 (518) 436-4822.

WUSV (Channel 45)

Union St. Video, Inc., 165 Freemans Bridge Rd., Scotia, NY 12502.

Bruce Jackson, Steven Tocco, Joseph Motto, Keith Wheeler, owners.

Operation: 1984.

WXXA-TV (Channel 23)

Albany TV 23, Inc., P.O. Box 6423, Albany, NY 12206 (518) 438-8700.

James Boaz, pres., gen. mgr. & prog. dir.; David Low, gen. sls. mgr. & sta. mgr.; Janet Gray, prom. mgr.; Catherine Castracane, bus. mgr.; Sargent Cathrall, chief eng.; nat'l. rep.: Petry.

Operation: July, 1982.

Binghamton

WBNG-TV (Channel 12) CBS

Gateway Communications, Inc., 50 Front Street, Binghamton, NY 13902 (607) 723-7311.

Donald F. Snyder, gen. mgr.; John Mucha, pgm. dir.; Monty Pinker, gen. sales mgr.; Michael LaMonica, eng.

WICZ-TV (Channel 40)

Stainless, Inc., 70 Henry St., Binghamton, NY 13902 (607) 723-8251.

Jesse Pevear, v.p. & gen. mgr.; G. Ricciardelli, tech. dir.; nat'l rep.: Katz.

WMGC-TV (Channel 34) ABC

Pinnacle Communications, Inc., Box 813, Binghamton, NY 13902.

Philip Marcella, pres. & gen. mgr.; Roy Sova, gen. sls. mgr. & sta. mgr.; James Fetter, bus. mgr.; Frank Plessinger, prog. dir.; Paul Giarell, news dir.; natl. rep.: Seltel.

Operation: 1962; TV households: 224,300.

Buffalo

WGRZ-TV (Channel 2) NBC

WGRZ-TV, Inc., 259 Delaware Ave., Buffalo, NY 14202 (716) 856-1414.

Richard Tarr, pres.; Lyn P. Stoyer, sr. v.p. & gen. mgr.; Raymond P. Maselli, v.p. & gen. mgr.; Sue Pearce, v.p. & bus. mgr.; Tom Cochran, lcl. sls. mgr.; Joe Rape, prog. & mktg. mgr.; Pam Curtis, prom. mgr.; Gary Legters, opns. mgr.; Tim Rudell, news dir.; Richard Westlund, chief eng.; Joe Lentini, dir. community reltns.; nat'l. rep.: TeleRep.

Operation: August, 1954.

WIVB-TV (Channel 4) CBS

Buffalo Broadcasting Co., Inc., 2077 Elmwood Ave., Buffalo, NY 14207; (716) 874-4410.

Leslie G. Arries, Jr., pres.; Patricia K. Sroka, sta. mgr.; Sandy DiPasquale, gen. sls. mgr.; Ralph Thompsom, dir. of eng. nat'l rep.: Harrington, Righter & Parsons, Inc.

Operation: 1948; TV households in area: 1,038,700; U.S. & Canada: 2,700,300.

WKBW-TV (Channel 7)

WKBW-TV, Capital Cities Communications, Inc., 7 Broadcast Plaza, Buffalo, NY 14202.

Philip R. Beuth, v.p. & gen. mgr.; Richard Shepard, gen. sales mgr.; Rom Martzolf, program mgr.; Kathleen McGarry, promo. mgr.; Don Holland, Schief engineer; rep.: Blair TV.

Operation: 1958.

WUTV (Channel 29)

Whitehaven Entertainment Corp., 951 Whitehaven Road, Buffalo, NY 14072 (716) 773-7531

Herman Pease, pres. & gen. mgr.; Albert M. Benz, dir. of adm.; Ray Felckowski, dir. of eng.; Robert Jay, gen. sls. mgr.; Donna Rodriquez, prgm. dir.

Operation: December, 1970; TV households: 1,213,100.

Carthage-Watertown

WWNY-TV (Channel 7) CBS, ABC, NBC

Watertown/Carthage Television Corp., 120 Arcade St., Watertown, NY 13601 (315) 788-3800.

Howard J. Brown, pres.; Eugene W. Schulte, v.p.; David J. Alteri, acting gen. mgr. & sls mgr.; David N. Cummings, dir. ops.; Donald Morehouse, chief eng.; nat'l rep.: Katz TV.

Operation: 1954; TV sets in area: 156,920.

Elmira

WENY-TV (Channel 36) ABC

WENY, Inc., P.O. Box 208, Elmira, NY 14902 (707) 739-3636.

Howard L. Green, exec. v.p.; Michael C. Steele, gen. mgr.; C. Robert Edwards, sta. mgr.; John Herrick, prog. mgr.; Carl C. Egolf, dir. of eng.

Operation: Nov., 1969.

WETM-TV (Channel 18) NBC

(Satellite of WSTM-TV, Syracuse, NY)

WETM-TV, Inc., Box 1207, Elmira, NY 14902 (607) 733-5518.

Jon Wingate, v.p. & gen. mgr.; Larry Taylor, chief eng.

Operation: 1956; TV sets in area: 83,600.

New York City

WABC-TV (Channel 7) ABC

American Broadcasting Company, 7 Lincoln Square, New York, NY 10023 (212) 887-7777.

William C. Fyffe, v.p. & gen. mgr.; John S. Bonnani, v.p./sta. mgrl; Brooke Bailey, pgm. dir.; Cliff Love, editorial dir.; Howard Rothstein, bus. mgr.; Tim Miller, dir. of creative services; John Watkins, local sls. mgr.

Operation: 1948; TV sets in area: 6,000,000.

WCBS-TV (Channel 2) CBS

CBS Television Stations, Division of Columbia Broadcasting System, Inc., 524 West 57 Street, New York, NY 10019 (212) 975-4321.

Thomas F. Leahy, Sr. broadcast v.p., CBS/Broadcst Group; Neil E. Derrough, pres., CBS Television Stations Division; Edward M. Joyce, v.p. & gen. mgr. WCBS-TV; Peter Temple, sta. mgr., WCBS-TV; John J. Rafferty, dir. of sls.; Laurie Weng, gen. sls. mgr.; Joan Zenker, loc. sls. mgr.; Eglon Simons, nat'l. sls. mgr.; Michael Dainard, retail/developmental sls. mgr.; Renee Isely, dir. of planning & admin.; Steve Cohen, news dir.; Kirk Varner, mgr. adv. & promo.; Ann Levine May, dir. of broadcasting; Toni Johnson, oper. mgr.; William C. Lacey, director of broadcast admin.; Joseph Passarella, dir. of communications; Phil Shimkin, dir. of programming; Gary Cummings, dir. of editorials & station services

Operation: 1941; TV sets in area: 6,000,000.

WNBC-TV (Channel 4) NBC

WNBC-TV, 30 Rockefeller Plaza, New York, NY 10020 (212) 664-4444.

Albert T. Jerome, v.p. & gen. mgr.; Richard L. Lobo, sta. mgr.; Hilary Hendler, dir. sls.; Karen L. Copeland, dir. programs; Ron Kershaw, dir. news; Peter Sang, mgr., adv. & promo.; Joseph Michaels, dir., editorials; Charles Licaneli, mgr., broadcast standards; Spencer Wiles, mgr., community relations.

Operation: 1941; TV sets in area: 6,000,000.

WNEW-TV (Channel 5)

Metromedia Television, a division of Metromedia, Inc. 205 East 67th Street, New York, NY 10021 (212) 535-1000.

Robert E. O'Connor, v.p. & gen. mgr.; John von Soosten, v.p. & prgm. mgr.; William D. Kelly, v.p. & chief eng.

Operation: 1944; TV households in area: 6,471,396.

WOR-TV (Channel 9) Secaucus, NJ

RKO General Inc., 1440 Broadway, New York, NY 10018 (212) 564-8000.

Peter A. Leone, v.p. & gen. mgr.; Thomas Ryan, v.p./gen. sls. mgr.; Peter Ingrassia, natl. sls. mgr.; Cam Pardo, cont.

WPIX (Channel 11)

WPIX Inc., 11 WPIX Plaza, New York, NY 10017; (212) 949-1100.

Leavitt J. Pope, pres.; David Polinge, sr. v.p. asst. to pres.; Gerald Mulderring, sr. v.p. sls.; Otis Freeman, sr. v.p., eng.; John Corporon, sr. v.p. news; Pat Austin, sr. v.p., finance; Julie Nunnari, v.p. prog.; Paul Bisonette, v.p. creative svcs.; Bob Murch, v.p., eng.; Rosemary Durkin, v.p. acctg.; Jane Perlman, v.p. rsrch.; Claudia Gasparini, v.p., personnel; Martin Appel, v.p. pub. reltns.; Don Carney, v.p. spts. & spec. events; Kathleen Shephert, v.p. prod. & community affairs; Laurence Linehan, Gerard Puccio, John McGowan, v.p., sls.

Operation: 1948; TV sets in area: 8,702,000 (ARB).

New York-Newark (N.J.)

WNJU-TV (Channel 47)

1020 Broad St., Newark, NJ 07102; (201) 643-9100.

Carlos Barba, v.p. & gen. mgr.; Thomas Johansen, gen. sls. mgr.; Julio Omana, sta. mgr.; Morris Marotta, controller; George Csahanin, chief eng.; Manolo Garcia Oliva, public affairs; Sylvia Pascual, traffic mgr.

Operation: May, 1965; TV households: 2,300,000.

WWHT-TV (Channel 68/60)

WWHT, Inc., 390 W. Market St., Newark, NJ 07107.

Herb Lefkowitz, gen. mgr.; Joe Giardina, v.p. of engineering; Lia Afriat, mgr. of programming.

Operation: July, 1977.

New York-Paterson (N.J.)

WXTV (Channel 41)

Spanish International Communications Corp., 24 Meadowland Parkway, Secausus, NJ 07094.

Ivan Egas, gen. mgr.; George Kraus, chief eng.; rep.: Blair TV.

Operation: 1968.

Plattsburgh-Burlington (Vt.)

WPTZ (Channel 5) NBC

Rollins Telecasting Inc., P.O. Box 647, Atlanta, GA 30301.

W. P. Eaton, Jr., gen. mgr.; Lincoln Dixon, chief eng.; nat'l rep.: Blair Television.

Operation: 1956; TV homes in area: 252,600 (U.S.); 954,880 (Canada).

Poughkeepsie

WTBY (Channel 54)

Trinity Broadcasting of New York, Box 534, Fishkill, NY 12524 (914) 896-4610.

Paul Crouch, pres. & gen. mgr.; Stan Hollin, gen. sls. mgr.; Terry Hickey, prog. dir. & film buyer; Lindy Dressler, promo. mgr.; Dale Osborn, chief eng.

Operation: April, 1981.

Riverhead

WLIG (Channel 55)

Life Broadcasting Network, Inc., 175 Crossways Park, W., Woodbury, NY 11797 (516) 364-1500.

Michael Pascucci, pres.; Michael Hurley, v.p. & gen. mgr.; Bruce Georgi, gen. sls. mgr.; Lawrence Casey, promo. mgr.

Operation: January, 1985.

Rochester

WHEC-TV (Channel 10) CBS

WHEC, Inc., 191 East Avenue, Rochester, NY 14604 (716) 546-5670.

Arnold Klinsky, v.p. & gen. mgr.; Alan Cartwright, sls. dir.; John Walsh, chief eng.; Al Holzer, news dir.; natl. rep.: Telerep.

Operation: 1953; TV sets in area, 453,500.

WOKR (Channel 13) ABC

Flower City Television Corp., 4225 W. Henrietta Rd., Rochester, NY 14623 (716) 334-8700.

Vincent T. DeLuca, pres./gen. mgr.; Donald J. Loy, prog. dir.; James Ryan, cont.; Michael Coombs, prom. dir.; Clyde Parker, eng. mgr.; Kent Beckwith, gen. sls. mgr.; Robert Weinstein; natl. sls. mgr.; natl. rep.: MMT.

Operation: 1962; TV households: 1,191,800.

WROC-TV (Channel 8) NBC

Television Station Partners, 201 Humboldt St., Rochester, NY 14610 (716) 235-9136.

Thomas F. Kennedy, v.p. & gen. mgr.; Anne Lent, natl. sls. mgr.; Alicia Rodriguez, prog. dir.; Denise Marquart, prom. mgr.; David Nolan, news dir.; John Coon, chief eng.

Operation: 1949; TV sets in area: 479,000.

WUHF (Channel 31)

Mairite TV of New York, Inc., 360 East Ave., Rochester, NY 14604 (716) 232-3700.

Carl E. Hirsch, pres.; Jerry Carr, v.p. & gen. mgr.; Rick Rambaldo, sta. mgr. & gen. sls. mgr.; natl. rep.: Blair TV.

Operation: 1980.

Smithtown

WSNL-TV (Channel 67)

Wometco WWHT Corp., 3200 Expressway Dr., S., Central Islip, NY 11722 (516) 582-6700.

Herb Lefkowitz, v.p. & gen. mgr.; Joan May, news prod.; Joe Giardina, v.p., eng.

Operation: November, 1973.

Syracuse

WIXT-TV (Channel 9) ABC

WIXT-TV, Inc., 5904 Bridge St., East Syracuse, NY 13057 (315) 446-4780.

Steve Kronquest, v.p. & gen. mgr.; Frank Arkinson, lcl. sls. mgr.; Dave Krause, natl. sls. mgr.; John King, chief eng.

Operation: 1962.

WSTM-TV (Channel 3) NBC

WSTM-TV, Inc., 1030 James St., Syracuse, NY 13203 (315) 474-5100.

David J. Shurtleff, v.p. & gen. mgr.; Norman Cissno, gen. sls. mgr.; Marnie Blount, prom. dir.

Operation: 1950; TV sets in area: 525,000.

WTVH-TV (Channel 5) CBS basic

Meredith Corp. 980 James St., Syracuse, NY 13203 (315) 425-5555.

Larry Rhodes, v.p. & gen. mgr.; Robert Stettner, gen. sls. mgr.; Edward F. Merritt, dir. of eng.; nat'l rep.: MMT Sales Inc.

Operation: 1948 as WHEN-TV; TV sets in area: 480,000.

Utica

WKTV (Channel 2) NBC

Harron Communications Corp., P.O. Box 2, Utica, NY 13504 (315) 733-0404.

Shell Storrier, sr. v.p. & gen. mgr.; Paul Harron, Jr., pres.; Daniel German, program. dir. & promo. mgr. & film dir.; Marie Zumpano, traffic mgr.; Shaun Fitz-Gerald, merch. mgr.; Merv Ainsworth, chief eng.; nat'l rep.: Katz.

Operation: 1949; TV homes in area: 340,100.

WTUV (Channel 33)

Mohawk Valley Broadcasting Association, Box 95, Syracuse, NY 13250 (315) 472-0200.

Craig Fox, Joel Friedman, Kevin O'Kane, owners.

Operations: January, 1986.

WUTR (Channel 20) ABC

Roy H. Park Bdcst'. of Utica-Rome Inc., P.O. Box 20, Utica, NY 13503 (315) 797-5220.

Edward Bizzell, exec. v.p. & gen. mgr.; John S. Mucha, oper. mgr.; Wayne Perry, chief eng.; rep.: Blair Television.

Operation: Feb., 1970.

NORTH CAROLINA

Asheville

WHNS-TV (Channel 21)

Pappas Telecasting of the Carolinas, 521 College Ave., Asheville, NC 28813; (704) 258-2100.

Harry J. Pappas, pres.; Edward G. Aiken, v.p./TV; Joseph A. Shaffer, v.p./prog.; Ken Glover, gen. sls. mgr.; Tom Post, natl. sls. mgr.; Dale Kelly, dir. eng.

Operation: 1953; TV sets in area: 40,000.

WLOS-TV (Channel 13) ABC

Wometco Skyway Broadcasting Co., Box 2150, Asheville, NC 28802 (704) 255-0013. 7 Laurens Court, P.O. Box 2363, Greenville, SC 29602 (803) 242-6091.

Herry Birdwell, v.p./gen. mgr.; Buz Buzogany, prog. mgr./ promo. mgr.; Jack Long, gen. sls. mgr./natl. sls. mgr.; Gary Ferrell; natl. rep.: Telerep.

Operation: 1954; TV households in area: 1,254,300 TSA.

Burlington

WRDG (Channel 16)

Box 16, Burlington, NC 27215 (919) 376-9868.

Robert Kearn, pres.; Fred Wuenschel, gen. mgr. & chief eng.; Steve Rehburg, prog. dir.; Ronald Helms, prom. mgr.

Operations: August, 1984.

Charlotte

WBTV (Channel 3) CBS

Jefferson Pilot Broadcasting Co., One Julian Price Place, Charlotte, NC 28208 (704) 374-3500.

Joseph M. Bryan, chm. bd.; Wallace J. Jorgenson, pres.; James G. Babb, Jr., exec. v.p.; John A. Edgerton, v.p. & man. dir.; Stephen H. Greenwald, news and info. mgr.; John H. Hutchinson, Jr., broadcast oprs. mgr.; Mark D. deCastrique, program oprs. mgr.; Donald L. Baxter, gen. sls. mgr.; George K. Reynolds, tech. op. mgr.; Jim Thacker, sports dir.; Mrs. Tommi L. Jones, v.p./personnel; Joseph B. Young, v.p./research & planning; Gerald W. King, v.p./treas.; George B. Grills, Jr., dir. of eng.; Larry M. Harding, v.p./public aff.

Operation: 1949; TV sets in area; 1,150,540.

WCCB-TV (Channel 18)

WCCB-TV, Inc., 1 Television Place, Charlotte, NC 28205 (704) 372-1800.

Cy N. Bagakel, pres.; Lorraine Lancaster, sr. v.p.; Mike Kassner, v.p.; Carl Bruce, gen. mgr.; William Riordan, gen sls. mgr.; Howard Trivette, prog. dir.; Steward Albert, chief eng.; natl. rep.: Katz.

Operation: Dec., 1953.

WPCQ-TV (Channel 36)

Channel 36 Partners, Channel 36, Inc., General Partner, P.O. Box 18665, Charlotte, NC 28218 (704) 536-3636.

Stanley A. Rudick, v.p. & gen. mgr.; Jill H. Krasner, dir. bdcst. op.; Harlan Mumme, chief eng.

Operation: 1967; TV households: 2,165,200.

WSOC-TV (Channel 9) NBC

Carolina Broadcasting Company, P.O. Box 34665, Charlotte, NC 28234 (704) 335-4999.

Grey Stone, v.p., gen. mgr.; Jack Callaghan, sta. mgr.; Jerry Pelletier, gen. sls. mgr.; Martin Fenton, lcl. sls. mgr.; F. Robert McCourt, progr./opns. mgr.; A. Bruce Chastine, contr.; Alan Batten, dir., adv./promo.; Richard Moore, news dir.; Merle Thomas, chief eng.; natl. rep.: Telerep.

Operation: 1957; TV sets in area. 2,892,800.

Durham

WTVD (Channel 11) ABC

Capital Cities Communications Inc., Box 2009, 411 Liberty St., Durham, N.C. 27702 (919) 683-1111.

Paul Bures, pres./gen. mgr.; Denis O'Connor, gen. sls. mgr.; Jon L. Miller, prog. mgr.; Chrystie Swain, dir. of public affairs.; Ned Warwick, news dir.; William Higgs, bus. mgr.; Edward Wall, chief eng.

Operation: 1954; TV homes in area: 521,700 (ADI).

Durham-Raleigh

WPTF-TV (Channel 28) NBC

Durham Life Broadcasting Service, Inc., Box 1511, 410 S. Salibury St., Durham, NC 27602 (919) 832-8311.

Felton P. Coley, pres.; Robert B. Butler, v.p. & gen. mgr.; Robert Wolfe, prog. dir.; Kalen Johnson, promo. mgr.; Joe Glennon, asst. new dir.; nat'l rep.: TeleRep, Inc.

Operation: November, 1968; TV households, 598,000.

Fayetteville

WFCT (Channel 62)

Fayetteville Cumberland Telecasters, Inc., Drawer 62, Lumber Bridge, Fayetteville, NC 28357 (919) 843-3884.

Art Malendoski, gen. mgr.; Chuck Epier, gen. sls. mgr.; Brenda Robinson, prog. dir. & Film Buyer; George Johnson, chief eng.; natl. rep.: Adam Young.

Operation: March, 1985.

WKFT (Channel 40)

Central Carolina Television, Inc., 230 Donaldson St., Fayetteville, NC 28301 (919) 323-4040.

Thomas Scanlan, pres. & gen. mgr.; Dick Armfield, gen. sls. mgr.; John Koch, dir. of eng.

Operation: 1981.

Greensboro

WFMY-TV (Channel 2) CBS

WFMY Television Corp., P.O. Box TV2, Greensboro, N.C. 27420 (919) 379-9639.

Mike Conly, v.p. & gen. mgr.; Jack Foreitand, prog. dir.; nat'l. rep.: Blair

Operation: 1949; TV homes in area: 797,800.

WGGT (Channel 48)

Guildford Telecasters, Inc., 330 S. Greene St., Greensboro, NC 27401 (919) 274-4848.

Mark Conrad, v.p. & gen. mgr.; Kenny Gonzalez, prod. mgr.; LaRhe Vestalk, prog. opns. mgr.; Richard Nailling, prog. dir.; Becky Smith, promo. mgr.; John Bishop, chief eng.; nat'l rep.: Seltel.

Operation: May, 1981.

WLXI-TV (Channel 61)

Box TV-61, Greensboro, NC 27420 (919) 855-5610.

Gary S. Smithwick, pres.; Richard C. Snowden, gen. mgr.; Jeff Johnson, prog. dir.

Operation: January, 1983.

Greenville

WNCT-TV (Channel 9) CBS

Roy A. Park Broadcasting, Inc., P.O. Box 898, Greenville, NC 27834 (919) 756-3180.

Roy H. Park, pres. treas.; Mrs. Dorothy D. Park, secretary; T. B. Maxfied, asst. secretary: K. B. Skinner, asst. treas., asst. secretary; Blake C. Lewis, Jr., gen. mgr.; Hank Tribley, gen. mgr.; Dr. John D. Caldwell and William S. Wellons, dir.; John G. Clark, Jr., gen. sls. mgr.; Malcom Nicholson, prod. mgr.; Ed Fields, prog. mgr.; Heber Adams, chief eng.; nat'l rep.: Blair TV.

Operation: 1953; TV sets in area: 476,300.

Hickory

WHKY-TV (Channel 14)

Catawba Valley Bcstg. Co., Box 1059, Hickory, NC 28603 (704) 322-5115.

Thomas E. Long, sta. mgr. & sls. mgr.; Jeffrey B. Long, prog. dir.

Operation: 1968; TV households: 125,700.

High Point

WGHP-TV, Inc.

P.O. Box TV 8, Greensboro, NC 27420; (919) 889-0888.

John Purcell, v.p./gen. mgr.; Frank Terry, bus. mgr.; Robert Herron, gen. sls. mgr.; Gary Curtis, news dir.

Operation: October, 1963; TV households: 1,618,000.

Lexington

WEJC (Channel 20)

Koinonia Ministries, Inc., Box 2020, Lexington, NC 27293 (704) 246-2020.

William P. Register, pres. & gen. mgr.; Billy Register, stn. mgr.; Steve Anderson, prog. dir.; Steve Moore, opns. mgr.; Ray Vice, chief eng.

Operation: October, 1985.

New Bern

WCTI-TV (Channel 12) ABC

Malrite of North Carolina, P.O. Box 2325, New Bern, NC 28560.

B. T. Jenkins, v.p. & gen. mgr.

Raleigh

WLFL-TV (Channel 22)

Family Television Corp., 2410 Broad St., Raleigh, NC 27704 (919) 471-4461.

Grant Cotton, pres. & gen. mgr.; L.L. Leathers, exec. v.p.; Lon Mirolli, v.p./gen. sls. mgr.; Mike Cotton, prog. dir.; Lee Collins, prom. mgr.; John Todd, news dir.; Dallas Lloyd, chief eng.; natl. rep.: Seltel.

Operation: December, 1981.

WRAL-TV (Channel 5) ABC

Capitol Broadcasting Co., P.O. Box 12,000, Raleigh, NC 27605 (919) 821-8500.

James F. Goodman, pres. & chief exec. off.; John M. Brennan, sr. v.p. & treas.; John L. Greene, sr. v.p.; Louise S.

Stephenson, secty.; Neil Kuvin, opns. mgr.; Paul Quinn, gen. sls. mgr.; Wilbur Brann, chief eng.; nat'l rep.: Katz Television American.
Operation: 1956; TV sets in area: 950,000.

Washington

WITN-TV (Channel 7) NBC

WITN-TV Inc., U.S. 17 South, Box Office 468, Washington, NC 27889 (919) 946-3131.
Howard W. Meagle, Jr., v.p./gen. mgr.; David Jernigan, gen. sls. mgr.; Frank Brady, reg./lcl. sls. mgr.; Paul Oughton, opns. mgr.; Al Manning, eng.; Glen Denny, promo. mgr.; Fran Williams, bus. mgr.; Greg Albrecht, news dir.; Dick Jones, farm. dir.; nat'l. rep.: Seltel.
Operation: Sept. 1955; TVHH: 724,000.

Wilmington

WECT-TV (Channel 6) NBC, CBS

Atlantic Telecasting Corp., 322 Shipyard Blvd., Wilmington, NC 28401 (919) 791-8070.
Dan D. Cameron, pres.; Wayne Jackson, sta. mgr.; Bill Elks, Oper. dir.; C. D. Martin, Jr., sls. mgr.; Paul A. Brissette, Jr., exec. v.p. & gen. mgr.; Mike Loizides, chief eng.; Ernie Whitmeyer, prod. dir.; nat'l rep.: Adam Young.
Operation: 1954; TV sets in area: 325,000.

WJKA (Channel 26) CBS

Wilmington Telecasters, Inc., 1926 Oleander Dr., Wilmington, NC 28403 (919) 343-8826.
Kathrine Everett, pres.; John E. Shine, gen. mgr.; John Peck, gen. sls. mgr.; Christy Faughn, prog. & news dir., film buyer; Hattie Neas, prom. mgr.; Larry W. White, chief eng.; natl. rep.: Adam Young.
Operation: September, 1984.

WWAY (Channel 3) ABC

Clay Broadcasting Corp., Box 2068, 615 N. Front St. Wilmington, NC (919) 762-8581.
George Diab, pres.; Ty Watts, sls. mgr.; Mitchell Saieed, v.p./gen. mgr.; George Allen, sta. mgr.; Elliott Hunter, chief engineer; rep., Seltel.
Operation: 1964; TV households: 570,450.

Winston-Salem

WNRW-TV (Channel 45)

Television Corp. of N.C., 3500 Myer-Lee Dr., Winston-Salem, NC 27101 (919) 722-4545.
Tim McDonald, pres. & film buyer; Charles McFadden, v.p. & gen. mgr.; John Walsen, gen. sls. mgr.; Cathy Ball, prog. dir.; nat'l. rep.: Seltel.
Operation: September, 1979.

WXII-TV (Channel 12) NBC

700 Coliseum Drive, Winston-Salem, NC 27106 (919) 721-9944.
Reynard A. Corley, v.p. & gen. mgr.; Sally Cartwright, pub. svc. & prog. dir.; David L. Summers, gen. sls. mgr.; David C. Emery, news dir.; (Mrs.) Jerry Kenion, promo. mgr.; Henry Hunt, dir. of engineering; nat'l rep.: Katz Television.
Operation: 1953; households: 1,603,900 (TSA-May '83 ARB).

NORTH DAKOTA

Bismarck

KFYR-TV (Channel 5) NBC

Meyer Broadcasting Co., Broadway at Fourth, Bismarck, ND 58501 (701) 223-0900.
William Ekberg, pres.; Judith Johnson, v.p.; Tom Barr, gen. mgr.; Jerry Hegel, gen. sls. mgr.; Claire Anne Holmberg, prog. & opns. mgr.; Jack Davis, dir. eng.; nat'l rep: Blair Television Associates.
Operation: 1953; TV sets in area: 123,900.

KXMB-TV (Channel 12) CBS-ABC

Bismarck Television, Inc., 1811 N. 15th, Bismarck, ND 58501 (701) 223-9197.
Steve Reiten, sta. mgr. & v.p.; John von Rheden, sls. mgr.; Dick Gottschald, news dir.; Keuin Brown, prod. mgr.; John Kranle, chief eng.; natl. rep.: Katz.
Operation: 1955; TV sets in area: 42,205.

Devil's Lake-Grand Forks

WDAZ-TV (Channel 8) ABC

(Satellite of WDAY-TV, Fargo, ND)
WDAY Inc., 301 So. 8th St. N, Fargo, ND 58102 (701) 237-6500.
Rep.: Katz; Andy McDermott Ltd. (Canada).
Operation: 1967.

Dickinson

KQCD-TV (Channel 7) NBC

Meyer Broadcasting Co., Broadway at Fourth St., Bismarck, ND 58501 (701) 225-5483.
William A. Ekberg, pres.; Penny Borg, mgr.; natl. rep.: Blair TV
Operation: 1980.

KXMA-TV (Channel 2) CBS

Reiten Television of Dickinson, Inc., Drawer B, Dickinson, ND 58602 (701) 227-1400.
David Reiten, pres. & gen. mgr. & sls. mgr.; Louis Tysver, chief eng.; nat'l. rep.: Katz.
Operation: 1956; TV sets in area: 52,000.

Fargo

KTHI-TV, (Channel 11) NBC

Spokane Television, Inc., Box 1878, Fargo, ND 58102 (701) 237-5211; Box 127, Grand Forks, ND 58201 (701) 772-3481.
John Hrubesky, v.p. & gen. mgr.; Greg Holder, gen. sls. mgr.; Scott Hildre, lcl. sls. mgr.; Dale Bosch, opr. mgr.; Carol Gillett, traffic mgr.; Roger Johnson, chief eng.

KVRR (Channel 15)

Fargo Broadcasting Co., Inc., 4015 Ninth Ave., SW Fargo, ND 58103 (701) 277-0515.
John W. Boler, dir.; Myron Kunin, dir.; Jane Gensheimer, gen. mgr.; Loren Newharth, gen. sls. mgr.; Kent Lien, prog. dir. & film buyer; Gary Goodrich, bctg. group coor.; Timothy Anderson, chief eng.
Operation: January, 1983.

WDAY-TV (Channel 6) ABC

WDAY, Inc., 301 So. 8th St., Fargo, ND 58102 (701) 237-6500.
William Marcil, pres.; Bill Burn, exec. vice-pres.; Sumner

Rassmussen, gen. mgr.; Robert Prowse, promo. mgr.; Norm Schrader, news dir.; nat'l rep.: Peters, Griffin, Woodward, Inc.

Operation: 1953; TV sets in area: 174,700.

Minot

KMOT (Channel 10) NBC, ABC

Meyer Broadcasting Co., Box 1120, Minot, ND 58701 (701) 852-4101.

W. A. Ekberg, pres.; Wayne L. Sanders, sta. mgr.

KXMC-TV (Channel 13) CBS, ABC

KXMC TV, Inc., KXMC Bldg., Minot, ND 58501 (701) 838-2104.

Chester Reiten, pres. & gen. mgr.; Henry Buechler, mgr.; Rod Romine, prog. dir.; Duane Aase, chief eng.; nat'l rep.: Avery Knodel.

Operation: 1953; TV sets in area: 129,000.

Valley City-Fargo

KXJB-TV (Channel 4) CBS

North America Communications Corp., 4302 13th Ave. So. Fargo, ND 58103 (701) 282-0444.

Tom Barnes, Jr., pres. & gen. mgr.; Paul Wickre, gen. sls. mgr.; Carl Iverson, chief eng.; nat'l rep., H&R Television.

Operation: 1954; TV sets in area: 186,000.

Williston

KUMV-TV (Channel 8)

Box 1287, Williston, ND 58801; Meyer Broadcasting Co., Fourth at Broadway, Bismarck, ND 58501

William A. Ekberg, pres.; Cherie Olson, sta. mgr.

Operation: 1957.

KXMD-TV (Channel 11) ABC, CBS

KXMC-TV, Inc., KXMC-TV Bldg., Minot, ND 58704.

John Blake, sta. mgr.; Ron Meyer, chief eng. natl. rep.: Avery Knodel.

Operation: 1969

OHIO

Akron

WAKR-TV (Channel 23) ABC

Summit Radio Corp., P.O. Box 1590, 853 Copley Rd., Akron, OH 44309 (216) 535-7831.

Roger G. Berk, pres.; Bob Bostiam, v.p. & sta. mgr.; "Chip" Fox, sales mgr.; Wm. F. O'Neil, Jr., prod. dir.; Leo Zody, film ed.; Earl Miller, chief eng.; nat'l rep.: Spot Time.

Operation: 1953; TV sets in area: 340,000.

Canton

WDLI (Channel 17)

David Livingston Missionary Foundation, Inc., 6600 Atlantic Blvd., Louisville, OH 44641 (216) 875-5542.

Denny Hazen, gen. mgr. & prog. dir.; Mike Tonges, opns. dir. & chief eng.

Operation: January, 1967.

WOAC (Channel 67)

Canton 67, 4867 Fulton Dr., NW, Canton, OH 44718 (216) 492-5267.

Morton Kent, pres.; Mike Larson, gen. mgr.; Robert Hippler, gen. sls. mgr.; Rick Worrell, prog. dir.; Scott Davis, news dir.; Les Carpenter, chief eng.

Operation: September, 1981.

Cincinnati

WCPO-TV (Channel 9) CBS

Scripps-Howard Broadcasting Co., 500 Central Ave., Cincinnati, OH 45202 (513) 721-9900.

Robert R. Regalburo, v.p. & gen. mgr., Al Schottelkotte, v.p. & sta. dir.; Rick Reeves, dir. of ops.; J.B. Chase, gen. sls. mgr.; Jeff Sales, nat'l. sls. mgr.; Michael L. Burke, news dir.; Marilyn J. Scrupps, dir. of community affairs; Ruth Ackerman, lcl. sls. mgr.; Robbin Holliday, bus. mgr.; Burnie Wayner, chief eng.; nat'l rep.: Blair-TV, Inc.

Operation: 1949; TV sets in area: 1,000,000.

WIII (Channel 64)

5177 Fishwick Dr., Cincinnati, OH 45216; (513) 641-3220.

John Wyant, pres.; Lanny Pogue, exec. v.p.; J. Pat Foley, chief eng.

Operation: 1980.

WKRC-TV (Channel 12) ABC

Taft Broadcasting Company, 1906 Highland Avenue, Cincinnati, OH 45219 (513) 651-1200.

Dudley S. Taft, pres.; John Rose, gen. mgr. & v.p.; Ann Bryant, prog. dir.; John Dawson, gen. sls. mgr.; Carl Moorehead, chief eng.; Jim O'Shields, gen. sls. mgr.; Don North, news dir.; John Hill, film dir.

Operation: 1949; TV sets in area: 1,004,100.

WLWT (Channel 5) NBC

140 W. Ninth St., Cincinnati, OH 45202; (513) 352-5000.

Anthony H. Kiernan, v.p. & gen. mgr.; Thomas E. Kuelbs, news dir.; Thomas M. Lamarche, prog. dir.; Harry Schneider, controller; Florence Parker, dir. community svcs.; Edwin Dooley, chief eng.; Mickey Fisher, traf. mgr.; Thomas Storey, film dir.; natl rep.: Katz Television.

Operation: 1948; households: 2,221,800 (TSA—May '83 ARB).

Cleveland

WCLQ-TV (Channel 61)

Cleveland Associates Co., c/o Elmer Balaban, 190 N. State St., Chicago, IL 60601 (216) 524-6161.

Francis P. Brady, gen. mgr.; Gary Brandt, gen. sls. mgr.; J. Albert Callahan, ops. mgr.; Al Evans, chief eng.; natl. rep.: Adam Young.

Operation: 1981.

WEWS (Channel 5) ABC

Scripps Howard Broadcasting Co., 3001 Euclid Ave., Cleveland, OH 44115 (216) 431-5555.

Jack R. Howard, bd. chm.; Donald L. Perris, pres.; Edward D. Cervenak, v.p. & gen. mgr.; Jane Sherwin, lcl. sls. mgr.; Gary Stark, pgm. dir.; Clint Pace, gen. sls. mgr.; Albert A. Varga, chief eng.; Frederick Corrigan, dir. mktg.; Richard Tuininga, news dir.; Donald G. Webster, asst. gen. mgr.; rep. Blair-TV, Inc

Operation: 1947; Total TV househods: 1,824,400.

WJW-TV (Channel 8) CBS

Storer Communications, Inc., 5800 S. Marginal Rd., Cleveland OH 44103 (216) 431-8888.

C. David Whitaker, v.p. & gen. mgr.; Spencer Koch, dir. sls.; Mike Renda, natl. sls. mgr.; Louis Gattozzi, dir. opns.;

Robert Green, dir. tech. svcs.; Joann Stern, dir. creative svcs.; Tony Ballen, news dir.; Thomas Flavelle, controller; Virgil Dominic, sta. mgr.; Tony Ballow, dir. news.
Operation: 1949.

WKYC-TV (Channel 3) NBC

National Broadcasting Co., 1403 East Sixth Street, Cleveland, Ohio 44114 (216) 344-3333.
John Llewellyn, v.p. & gen. mgr.; Dan Klintworth, adv. & promo. mgr.; David Boylan, dir. of sls.; Raymond Smith, dir., tech. ops.; Kathleen McNulty, bus. mgr.; Gregory R. Stehlin, prog. dir.; Ron Bilek, news dir.; nat'l rep.: NBC Spot Sales.
Operation: 1948; TV sets in area: 3,663,800.

Columbus

WBNS-TV (Channel 10) CBS

Dispatch Printing Co., 770 Twin Rivers Drive, Columbus, OH 43216 (216) 460-3700.
Gene D'Angelo, pres. & gen. mgr.; Arnold Routson, v.p. sls.; William Orr, v.p., eng'.; John A. Haldi, vice pres., prgm.; Dale Laackman, prod. dir.; Gerald Cary, treas.; Larry Maisel, News dir.; Jay Scafone, dir. adv. & promo.; nat'l rep.:. Blair TV Inc.
Operation: 1949; TV sets in area: 557,400.

WCMH-TV (Channel 4) NBC

Outlet Broadcasting, 3165 Olentagny River Rd., Columbus, OH 43202 (614) 263-5441.
David E. Henderson, pres.; Gary Robinson, v.p. & gen. mgr.; Richard Lowe, gen. sales mgr.; Gary Lowell, nat'l sales mgr.; Dave Miller, prog. dir.; Darryl Moeller, community serv. dir.; Dave Smith, prom. mgr.; Richard Townley, news dir.; Bob Dye, chief eng.; Dave Goff, prod. mgr.; Juanita Mitchell, film dir., nat'l rep.: Petry Television Inc.
Operation: 1949; TV homes in area: 1,289,900.

WTTE (Channel 28)

Commercial Radio Institute, 6130 Sunbury Rd., Box 290, Columbus, OH 43216; (614) 695-2800.
Julian Smith, pres.; Frederick Himes, exec. v.p.; Robert Simmons, v.p.; William Rhodes, gen. mgr.; Robert Stegner, gen. sls. mgr.; natl. rep.: Seltel.
Operation: June, 1984.

WTVN (Channel 6) ABC

Taft Broadcasting Co., 1271 Dublin Road, Columbus, 43215 (614) 481-6666.
Charles Mechen, bd. chm.; Dudley S. Taft, pres.; Ro Grignon, exec. v.p.; Fred von Stade, v.p. & gen. mgr.; George Coles, gen. sls. mgr.; Mrs. Pat Cramer, prog. mgr.; Dave Parr, promo. dir.; Sue Swartz, pub. affairs dir.; John R. Owen, chief eng.; nat'l rep.: Harrington, Righter & Parsons, Inc.
Operation: 1949; TV sets in area: 727,000.

Dayton

WDTN (Channel 2) ABC

4595 South Dixie Ave., P.O. Box 741, Dayton, OH 45401.
Howard Ritchie, exec. v.p. & gen. mgr.; Ira Slakter, gen. sls. mgr.; Pat Baldwin, promo. & pub. mgr.; Steve Fisher, sta. mgr.; Ray Poland, chief eng.; nat'l rep.: Blair.
Operation: 1949; TV homes in area: 1,029,500.

WHIO-TV (Channel 7) CBS

Miami Valley Broadcasting Corp., 1414 Wilmington Avenue, Dayton, OH 45401 (513) 259-2111.
William A. Schwartz, pres. & CEO; Walter C. Liss, Jr., pres., bdgst. div.; Stanley G. Mouse, sr., v.p.; Neil Pugh, v.p. & sta. mgr.; John Hanley, cont.; Robert Wells, dir. of info. svcs.; John Clark, prog. dir.; Sim Kollinger, chief eng.; nat'l rep.: Tele-rep.
Operation: 1949; TV sets in area: 437,160.

WKEF (Channel 22) ABC

Springfield Television; Studio: 1731 Soldiers Home Road, Dayton, OH 45418 (513) 263-2662.
George J. Mitchell, pres., Ohio op.; Lon Mirolli, gen. sls. mgr.; Tim Coppock, prod. mgr.; Darrel Hunter, chief eng.; Berl Golub, prog. mgr. & film buyer; Sandy Patton, promo. dir.; Johnny Walker, dir. community affairs/special events; Kevin Kelly, news dir. rep.: H-R Television.
Operation: 1964; TV households: 1,399,000.

WRGT-TV (Channel 45)

Dayton Telecasting, Inc., 45 Broadcast Plaza, Dayton, OH 45408; (503) 263-4500.
Albert M. Holtz, pres.; Dave Miller, gen. mgr.; John Tamerlano, gen. sls. mgr.; George Boggs, opns. mgr.; Miles Ptacek, chief eng.; natl. rep.: Seltel.
Operation: September, 1984.

Lima

WLIO-TV (Channel 35) NBC, ABC

Lima Communications Corporation, 1424 Rice Ave., Lima, Ohio 45802 (419) 228-8835.
James C. Dages, pres. & gen. mgr.; Douglas A. Ferguson, sta. mgr. & prog. dir; Maurice Lamb, chief eng.; Bruce A. Opperman, sls. mgr.; nat'l rep.: The Katz Co.
Operation: 1952; TV sets in area: 333,900.

WTLW (Channel 44)

American Christian TV Services, Inc., 1844 Baty Rd., Lima, OH 45807; (419) 339-4444.
Larry Sheets, pres.; Ron Mighell, dir. & gen. sls. mgr.; Roger Rhodes, prog. dir. & film buyer; Keith Curtis, prod. dir.; Barb Mayer, prom. mgr.; David Morris, chief eng.
Operation: June, 1982.

Lorain-Cleveland

WUAB (Channel 43)

Gaylord Broadcasting Co. of Ohio, 8443 Day Dr., Parma, OH 44129 (216) 845-6043.
Ron St. Charles, asst. gen. mgr. & prog. dir.; Pat Murray, dir. of retail svcs.; Jim Weiss, contr.; Bill Scaffide, gen. sales mgr.; Harry Sykora, mgr. of engineering; Frank Fletcher, prom. mgr.

Newark

WSFJ (Channel 51)

Christian Television of Ohio, Inc., 10077 Jacksontown Rd., Thornville, OH 43076 (614) 833-0771.
Jean Rodabaugh, pres. & gen. mgr.; Betty J. Stanley, admin. asst.; David Glunt, exec. prod.; Charlotte Reichley, prog. dir.; natl. rep.: Hugh Wallace.
Operation: 1980.

Sandusky

WGGN-TV (Channel 52)

Christian Faith Bcstg., Box 247, Castalia, OH 44824 (419) 684-9496.

Shelby Gillam, pres.; Gene McClellan, gen. mgr.; Clyde Yost, chief eng.
Operation: December, 1982.

Shaker Heights

WOIO (Channel 19)

Channel 19, Inc., 2720 Van Aken Blvd., Cleveland, OH 44120; (216) 561-1919.
Hubert Payne, pres.; Dennis Thatcher, stn. & gen. sls. mgr.; Robert Affe, prog. dir. & film buyer; Craig Wright, prom. mgr.; Robert Thurber, chief eng.; Dave Smith, lcl. sls. mgr.; Val King, natl. sls. mgr.; natl. rep.: Petry.
Operation: May, 1985.

Springfield

WTJC (Channel 26)

Miami Valley Christian Television Inc., Box 26, Dayton, OH 45401 (513) 323-0026.
Marvin D. Sparks, v.p. & gen. mgr.; John Elliott, chief eng.; Rod Robison, promo, dir.
Operation: 1980

Steubenville

WTOV-TV (Channel 9) ABC, NBC

Ziff-Davis Broadcasting Co. Box 9999, Steubenville, OH 43952.
I. Martin Pompadur, pres.; Ziff Corp.; Ralph E. Becker, pres., Ziff-Davis Broadcasting Co.; Ray J. Chumley, vice pres./gen. mgr.; James McCreary, v.p./contr.; Tom Hansen, prgm. mgr.

Toledo

WDHO-TV (Channel 24) ABC

D. H. Overmyer Telecasting Co., Inc., 300 S. Byrne Rd., Toledo, OH 43615 (419) 535-0024.
William J. Shock, v.p./gen. mgr.; Garry Miller, gen. sls. mgr.; James Bowe, v.p. eng./ops.; rep.: Katz Television.
Operation: 1966; TV households: 1,775,100.

WTOL (Channel 11) CBS

Cosmos Broadcasting Corp., P.O. Box 715, Toledo, OH 43601 (419) 244-7411.
Guy W. Hempel, v.p. & gen. mgr.; Mel Stebbins, gen. sls. mgr.; Rob Wagley, natl. sls. mgr.; Paul Ladrow, lcl. sls. mgr.; Rick Gevers, news dir.; Steve Israel, prog. dir.; Wayne Thing, prod. mgr.; Sharon Newson, pub. affairs dir.; Jeff Bell, promo. mgr.; Paul Lentz, chief eng.; Nancy Gruhler, traffic mgr.; nat'l rep.: MMT Sales.
Operation: 1958; TV sets in area: 1,405,800.

WTVG-TV (Channel 13) NBC

Storer Communications, Inc., 4247 Dorr St., Toledo OH 436074 (419) 255-1313.
H. W. Ray, gen. mgr.; George Carlino. natl. sls. mgr.; Doug Sinn, gen. sls. mgr.; Chris States, promo. mgr.; nat'l rep.: Storer Television Sales, Inc.
Operation: 1948; TV sets in area: 751,100.

Youngstown

WFMJ-TV (Channel 21) NBC

The Vindicator Printing Co., 101 W. Boardman St., Youngstown, OH 44503 (216) 744-8611.
Betty J.H. Brown, pres.; Edward J. Adams, mgr.; Joan Harrison, film dir.; Larry Oleson, chief eng.; nat'l rep., Blair TV.
Operation: 1953; TV households in area: 280,500.

WKBN-TV (Channel 27) CBS

WKBN Broadcasting Corp., 3930 Sunset Blvd., Youngstown, OH 44501 (216) 782-1144.
W. P. Williamson, Jr., bd. chm.; Ruth L. Cruikshank, secty.; W. P. Williamson, III, pres. & gen. mgr.; David V. Stewart, treas.; W.F. Decker, sta. mgr.; C.R. Wade, sls. mgr.; Norm Berger, prog. dir.; nat'l rep.: Katz Agency.
Operation: 1953; TV sets in area: 514,000.

WYTV (Channel 33)

WYTV, Inc., 3800 Shady Run Rd., Youngstown, OH 44502.
Geoffrey Pearce, gen. mgr.

Zanesville

WHIZ-TV (Channel 18) NBC, ABC

Southeastern Ohio Television System, Downard Rd., Zanesville, OH 43701 (614) 453-0361.
Allan Land, group mgr.; Barbara Mitter, prog. dir.; Elmer Hartmeyer, chief eng.; Franklin Young, film oper. mgr.; nat'l rep.: Katz.
Operation: 1953; TV sets in area: 80,000.

OKLAHOMA

Ada

KTEN (Channel 10) ABC, CBS, NBC

Eastern Oklahoma Television Co., Inc., P.O. Box 728, Ada, OK 74820 (405) 332-3311.
Tom Johnson, pres. & gen. mgr.; Bill Green, chief eng.; Dan Hoover, v.p. & prog. dir.; nat'l rep.: Katz.
Operation: 1954; TV sets in area: 178,310.

Ardmore

KXII-TV (Channel 12)

Texoma Broadcasters, Inc., Box 1175, Sherman, TX.
M.N. Bostick, pres.; Richard R. Adams, gen. mgr.; Dennis Lite, chief eng.; Mike Leucke, prod. mgr.; nat'l rep.: Seltel.
Operation: 1956.

Bartlesville

KDOR (Channel 17)

Lea County TV, Inc., 4100 Adams Rd., Suite C-106, Bartlesville, OK 74006 (918) 335-3777.
Andy Graham, gen. mgr.; Jeanette Wise, gen. sls. mgr.; Miles Carter, chief eng.
Operation: February, 1984.

Lawton

KQOL-TV (Channel 45)

Great Plains Country TV Bcstg., 1605 Classen Choate Bldg., Oklahoma City, OK 73106 (405) 524-6625.
John I. Choate, pres. & sls. mgr.; William W. Choate, gen sls. mgr. & chief eng.
Operation: 1982.

KSWO-TV (Channel 7) ABC

KSWO Television Co., Inc., P.O. Box 708, Lawton, OK

73502 (405) 355-7000.
R. H. Drewry, pres.; Larry Patton, gen. mgr.; Jim Lockerd, chief eng.
Operation: 1953; TV sets in area: 225,000.

Oklahoma City

KAUT (Channel 43)

Rollins Telecasting of Oklahoma, Box 14843, Oklahoma City, OK 73113; (405) 478-4300.
Gene Autry, bd. chmn.; Don Richards, gen. mgr.; John Riggie, gen. sls. mgr.; Jack O'Meara, prom. mgr.; Dwaine Maggert, chief eng.; natl. rep.: Petry.
Operation: November, 1980.

KGMC (Channel 34)

Beverly Hills Hotel Corp., 1501 NE 85th, Oklahoma City, OK 73131 (405) 478-3434.
Ted Baze, gen. mgr.; T. Dan Loving, gen. sls. mgr.; Greg Mille, v.p & chief eng.; Paul Krimsier, v.p./asst. gen. mgr.; natl. rep.: Seltel.
Operation: 1979.

KOCO-TV (Channel 5) ABC

Ganett Broadcast Group, 1300 E. Britton, Oklahoma City, OK 73113.
Al Parsons, pres. & gen. mgr.; David Loveland, v.p. & gen. sls. mgr.; Ted Newcomb, v.p. & chief eng.; Lynette Unruh, compt.; Mike Palmer, v.p., bdcst. op.
Operation: 1954; TV households: 834,600.

KOKH (Channel 25)

Blair Broadcasting of Oklahoma, Inc., 1228 E. Wilshire Blvd., Oklahoma City, OK 73111 (405) 843-2525.
David Murphy, pres. & gen. mgr.
Operation: 1979.

KTBO-TV (Channel 14)

Trinity Bcstg. of Oklahoma, 3705 NW 63rd St., Oklahoma City, OK 73116 (405) 848-1414.
Paul F. Crouch, pres.; Al Brown, gen. mgr.; John Gordon, chief eng.
Operation: March, 1981.

KTVY (Channel 4) NBC

KTVY, Inc., 500 East Britton Road, Oklahoma City, OK 73114 (405) 478-1212.
Lee Allan Smith, v.p. & gen. mgr.; Bill Thrash, dir. opns.; Paul Wise, natl. sls. mgr.; Charles Andrew, promo. mgr.; John Bushnell, chief eng.
Operation: 1949; TV sets in area: 537,380.

KWTV (Channel 9) CBS

Griffin Television, Inc. P.O. Box 14159, Oklahoma City, OK 73113 (405) 843-6641.
John Griffin, owner; Jacques DeLier, pres. & gen. mgr.; Duane Harm, sta. mgr.; Jack Sallaska, prgm. dir.; Troy Brown, chief eng.; Charles Andrews, prom. & pub. dir.; nat'l rep.: HRP.
Operation: 1953; TV sets in area: 739,000.

Sayre

KVIJ-TV

(Satellite of KVII-TV, Amarillo, TX)
Marsh Media, Inc., One Broadcast Center, Amarillo, TX 79101 (405) 928-3233.
Rep.: Katz Television.
Operation: 1961.

Tulsa

KGCT-TV (Channel 41)

419 So. Main St., Tulsa, OK 74103 (918) 583-4100.
Ray L. Beindorf, pres. & Gen. mgr.; W. Randy Williams, prog. dir.; Tarica Myers, opns. dir.; Stan Friedman, promo. mgr. Dave Jones, chief eng.; nat'l rep.: Spot Time.
Operation: May, 1981.

KJRH-TV (Channel 2) NBC

Scripps-Howard Broadcasting Company, P.O. Box 2, Tulsa, OK 74101 (918) 743-2222.
Ben Hevel, gen. mgr.; William J. Donahue, asst. gen. mgr.; Tony Marino, news dir.; Michael J. Vrabac, gen. sls. mgr.; Art Bates, chief eng.; nat'l rep.; Blair Television.
Operation: 1954; TV sets in area: 460,300.

KOKI-TV (Channel 23)

Tulsa 23, 7422 E. 46 Place, Tulsa, OK 74135 (918) 663-6880.
James U. Lavenstein, pres. & gen. mgr.; Mike Braker, gen. sls. mgr.; Eugene Wilkin, prog. dir. & film buyer; Richard Enderwood, prom. mgr.; Robert G. Hardie, chief eng.; natl. rep.: Katz.
Operation: November, 1980.

KOTV (Channel 6) CBS

KOTV, Inc., 320 S. Frankfort St., Tulsa, OK 74120. (918) 582-6666.
John P. Irvin, v.p./gen. mgr.; Jim Bisagnni, gen. sls. mgr.; Bob Allen, prog. mgr.; Foster Morgan, news dir.; natl. rep.: Petry.
Operation: 1949

KTCT (Channel 47)

Television Communications, Inc., Box 54820, Tulsa, OK 74155; (918) 250-9402.
Jack Rehburg, pres. & gen. sls. mgr.; Randy Clark, gen. mgr.; Jeff Rehburg, v.p./prod.
Operation: April, 1985.

KTUL-TV (Channel 8) ABC

KTUL-TV, Inc., Box 8, Tulsa, OK 74101 (918) 446-3351.
James C. Leake, chmn.; John G. Leake, pres.; Thomas Goodgame, v.p. gen. mgr.; Robert Gregory, v.p., news.; Gary Ricketts, oper. mgr.; Edward Hunt, gen. sls. mgr.; Bill Shock, dir. eng.; Carl Barthlomew, promo. mgr.; nat'l rep.: Edward Petry & Co., Inc.
Operation: 1954; TV homes in area: 481,400.

OREGON

Bend

KTVZ (Channel 21) CBS, NBC

Ponderosa Television, Inc., Box 149, Bend, OR 97709 (503) 389-6511.
John Larkin, gen. mgr.; Cliff Williams, sls. mgr.; Teresa Bollard, ops. mgr.; natl. rep.: Katz.
Operation: 1977.

Coos Bay

KCBY-TV (Channel 11) CBS

(Satellite of KVAL-TV, Eugene, OR)
Eugene Television Inc., P.O. Box 1156, Coos Bay, OR 97420 (503) 269-1111.
Glenn Nickell, gen. mgr.; Bruce Bennett, sta. mgr.; Jerry Madsen, chief eng.

Eugene

KEZI-TV (Channel 9) ABC

Chambers Communications, Inc., P.O. Box 7009, Eugene, OR 97401 (503) 485-5611.
Carolyn S. Chambers, pres.; Bruce Liljegren, gen. mgr.; Dave Larson, asst. sta. mgr.; Beth Cookson, natl./reg. sls.; Joe Smeiser, prod. mgr.; Dennis Hunt, chief eng.
Operation: 1960; TV households: 226,200.

KMTR-TV (Channel 16) NBC

KMTR, Inc., Box 7365, Eugene, OR 97401 (513) 746-1600.
Robert W. Davis, pres. & gen. mgr.; Cam Wilson, v.p. & gen. sls. mgr. Judith Bell, prog. dir. & film buyer; Chris Pontrelli, promo. mgr.; Paul Riess, news dir.; John Bredesen, chief eng.; nat'l rep.; Seltel.
Operation: October, 1982.

KVAL-TV (Channel 13) Primary NBC

Eugene Television, Inc., Blanton Heights, P.O. Box 1313, Eugene, OR 97401 (503) 342-4961.
Glenn E. Nickell, v.p., gen. mgr.; John Doyle, news dir.; Bonnie Cole, natl sales; Gordon Bussey, lcl. sls. mgr.; Gregg McKay, film dir.; Jim Bowen, chief eng.; nat'l rep.: Katz Television, Inc.
Operation: 1954; TV sets in area: 263,800.

Klamath Falls

KOTI-TV (Channel 2)

Oregon Broadcasting Co., P.O. Box 2K, Klamath Falls, OR 97601 (503) 882-2222.
Wm. B. Smullin, pres.; Dick Good, station mgr.; nat'l rep.: Blair; reg. rep.: Art Moore & Associates.
Operation: 1956.

Medford

KDRV (Channel 12)

Sunshine TV, Inc., 1090 Knutson Ave., Medford, OR 97504 (503) 779-1212.
Dunbar Carpenter, pres.; Keith Lollis, gen. mgr; John Franz, chief eng.
Operation: January, 1984.

KOBI-TV (Channel 5) NBC

Oregon Broadcasting Co., P.O. Box 5M, Medford, OR 97501 (503) 779-5555.
William B. Smullin, pres.; Ed Zander, v.p. & gen. mgr.; Patricia D. Smullin, v.p.; Patricia C. Smullin, treas; Bill Kirk, chief eng.; nat'l rep.: Blair.
Operation: 1953.

KTVL-TV (Channel 10) NBC, ABC

Sierra/Cascade Communications, Inc., Box 10, Medford, OR 97501 (503) 773-7373.
J. L. DeArmond, pres.; Ray Johnson, exec. v.p. & gen. mgr.; John Larkin, mgr.; Art Chipman, natl. sales mgr.; Ellis Feinstein, dir. of eng'.; rep.: H-R Television, Simpson Reilly & Associates (Portland & Seattle).
Operation: 1961; TV households: 127,800.

Portland

KATU (Channel 2) ABC

Fisher Broadcasting, Inc., 2153 N.E. Sandy Blvd., Portland, OR 97232 (503) 231-4222.
Thomas R. Dargan, exec. v.p.; Fisher Bdcst.-Portland; Sherwood V. Hinman, v.p. & gen. mgr.; Robert D. Kalstad, sta. mgr.; Leland Petrik, prog. dir.; Robert Moore, chief eng.; Thomas Oberg, gen. sls. mgr.; Jim Rogers, natl. sls. mgr.; Joella Werlin, pub. affairs mgr.; rep.: Katz Television.
Operation: 1962; TV households: 814,800.

KGW-TV (Channel 8)

King Broadcasting Company, 1501 S. W. Jefferson St., Portland, OR 97201 (503) 226-5000.
Irwin P. Starr, v.p. & gen. man.
Operation: 1956.

KOIN-TV (Channel 6) CBS

KOIN-TV, Inc., 140 S. W. Columbia St., Portland, OR 97201 (503) 243-6666.
R. M. Schafbuch, gen. mgr.; Steve Currie, bdcst. opr. mgr.; Loren Neuharth, gen. sls. mgr.; Jane Hoyt, promo. mgr.; Lee Wood, chief eng.; nat'l rep.: Harrington, Righter & Parsons.
Operation: 1953; TV sets in area: 1,148,500.

KPTV (Channel 12)

Oregon Television, Inc., P.O. Box 3401, Portland, OR 97208; 735 S. W. 20th Place, Portland, OR (503) 222-9921.
Marty Brantley, pres. & gen. mgr.; Marty Brantley, station mgr.; Gordon White, prog. mgr. & film buyer; Craig A. Miller, promo. mgr.; Gene Phelps, chief eng.; rep.: Tele-Rep.
Operation: 1955; TV households: 814,100.

Roseburg

KPIC (Channel 4) CBS Primary

(Affiliate of KVAL-TV, Eugene, OR)
Southwest Oregon Television Broadcasting Corp., studio & office: 655 West Umpqua, Roseburg, OR 97470.
S. W. McCrenoy, pres.; Don Cithero, sta. mgr.; Glenn Nickell, gen. mgr.; natl. rep.: Katz.
Operation: 1956.

Salem

KECH (Channel 22)

Arnold Brustin & Christopher Desmond, managing partners; Bob Cook, sta. mgr.; Sherman Aldridge, lcl. sls. mgr.; Bob Ridgeway, chief eng.; natl. rep., Adam Young.
Operation: 1981.

PENNSYLVANIA

Allentown

WFMZ-TV (Channel 69)

Maranatha Broadcasting Co., Inc., E. Rock Rd., Allentown, PA 18103 (215) 797-4530.
Richard C. Dean, pres. & gen. mgr.; David G. Hinson, prog. dir.; Brad Rinehart, news dir.; Dean Dallmann, sls. mgr.; Kathy Craine, office mgr.; Barry Fisher, chief eng.
Operation: November, 1976.

Altoona

WOPC (Channel 23) ABC

John R. Powley, Box 2248, Altoona, PA 16603 (814) 943-2607.
John R. Powley, gen. mgr.
Operation: 1974.

WTAJ-TV (Channel 10) CBS

A Gateway Station; 5000 Sixth Avenue, Altoona, PA 16603 (814) 944-2031.
J. Thomas Conners, v.p. & gen. mgr.; George L. Walsh, gen. sls. mgr.; Douglas Parker, prog. mgr.; Jim Turcovsky, prod. mgr.; Richard Kline, chief eng.; Thomas F. Murphy, bus. mgr.; Gary L. Delph, promo. mgr.; George Tyll, news dir.
Operation: 1953.

Erie

WICU (Channel 12) NBC

Great Lakes Communications, Inc., 3514 State St. Erie, PA 16508 (814) 454-5201.
Arthur M. Ingram, pres.; Frederick Kalmbach, gen. mgr.; Clarence Paolella, gen. sls. mgr.; Mike Csop, chief eng.; Eric Johnson, prog. dir.; nat'l rep.: Katz TV Continental; Canadian rep.: Radio/Television Reps., Ltd. (Toronto).
Operation: 1949; TV sets in area: 274,000.

WJET-TV (Channel 24) ABC

JET Broadcasting Co., Inc., 8455 Peach St., Erie, PA 16509 (814) 864-4902.
Myron Jones, pres.; John Kanzius, exec. v.p./gen. mgr.; Ken Fanazini, opns. mgr./prog. dir.; Eric Johnson, news dir.; natl. rep.: Blair.
Operation: 1966; TV households: 160,500.

WSEE (Channel 35) CBS

Gillett Broadcasting of P.A., Inc., 1220 Peach St., Erie, PA 16501 (814) 455-7575.
Jerry Montgomery, pres. & gen. mgr.; Jack Rea, v.p./opns. mgr.; James Penna, chief eng.; nat'l. rep.: Peters, Griffin & Woodward.
Operation: 1954; U.H.F. sets in area 245,400.

Greensburg

WPCB-TV

Cornerstone TeleVision, Inc., Wall, PA, Greensburg, PA Greensburg, PA 15148 (412) 824-3930.
R. Rusell Bixler, pres.; David F. Kelton, exec. v.p.; Oleen Eagle, gen. mgr.; David Skeba, sta. mgr.; Jerry Foreman, chief eng.
Operation: April, 1979.

Harrisburg

WHP-TV (Channel 21) CBS-TV

WHP, Inc., P.O. Box 1507, Harrisburg, PA 17105 (717) 238-2100.
Donald C. Yeiser, gen. mgr.; Charlie Adams, gen. sls. mgr.; Maurice Gannaway, dir. eng.; nat'l rep.: Katz.
Operation: 1953; TV households in ADI: 508,900.

WHTM-TV (Channel 27) ABC

Box 2775, Harrisburg, PA 17105 (717) 236-2727.
John J. McCrory, pres.; C. Capps, v.p., gen. mgr. & film buyer; Nancy Tull, gen. sls. mgr.; Debra Adjan, prog. dir.; Joanne Alexis, prom. mgr.; Bob Janis, news dir.; Richard Kerlin, chief eng.; Joseph Fry, contrl.; nat'l. rep.: Harrington, Righter & Parsons.
Operation: June, 1953; TV sets in area: 503,000.

Johnstown

WFAT-TV (Channel 19)

P.O. Box 19, Johnstown, PA 14907–0019 (814) 266-1919.
Leon A. Crosby, owner; Timothy Lee Crosby, gen. mgr.; George S. Plenderleith, sta. mgr.; Michael D. Forosisky, sls. mgr.; William Caramana, chief eng.
Operation: 1953.

WJAC-TV (Channel 6) NBC

WJAC, Inc., Hickory Lane, Johnstown, PA 15905 (814) 255-7600.
James M. Edwards, Sr., pres.; Richard D. Schrott, v.p.; Philip A. Marcinek, prog. dir.; Arthur Vrooman, chief eng.; nat'l rep.: Harrington, Righter & Parsons.
Operation: 1949; TV sets in area, 1,372,860.

Lancaster

WGAL-TV (Channel 8) NBC

WGAL Television, Inc., 1300 Columbia Ave., Lancaster, PA 17604 (717) 393-5851.
David R. Dodds, v.p. & gen. mgr.; John Carpenter, gen. sls. mgr.; John Feeser, natl. sls. mgr.; Chic Kroll, lcl. sls. mgr.; Nelson Sears, prog. mgr.; Ed Wickenheiser, news dir.; natl. rep.: Blair.
Operation: March, 1949; TV households: 1,267,900.

Lancaster/Lebanon

WLYH-TV (Channel 15)

Television Hill, Lebanon, PA 17042 (814) 273-4551.
Licensee: Gateway Communications, Inc., Suite 612, Executive Building, Cherry Hill, NJ 08034 (609) 667-8100.
Robert W. Eolin, v.p. & gen. mgr.
Operation: May 2, 1957.

Philadelphia

KYW-TV (Channel 3) NBC

Group W (Westinghouse Broadcasting Co.), Independence Mall East, Philadelphia, PA 19106 (215) 238-4700.
James B. Thompson, vice pres. & gen. mgr.; Chuck Gingold, prgm. mgr.; Brian O'Neill, creative svcs. dir.; Allen Murphy, gen. sls. mgr.; Robert Fields, chief eng.; nat'l rep.: TVAR.
Operation: 1941; TV sets in area: 2,275,000.

WCAU-TV (Channel 10) CBS

WCAU-TV, Inc., City Ave. & Monument Rd., Philadelphia PA 19131 (215) 581-5510.
Steve Cohen, vice-pres. & gen. mgr.; Carol Netter, sls. dir.; Melvin D. Levine, dir. of labor relations & admin.; Jay Newman, news dir.; Gordon Hughes, dir. of bdcst.; John Byrne, dir. of opns. & eng.; Gordon W. West, mgr. of film & videotape services; nat'l rep.: CBS Television National Sales.
Operation: 1948; TV sets in area: 2,373,100.

WGBS-TV (Channel 57)

Channel 57 Corp., 420 N. 20th St., Philadelphia, PA 19130 (215) 563-5757.
Milton S. Grant, CEO & pres.; Albert Tedesco, gen. mgr., prog. dir., prom. mgr. & film buyer; Harry Jenny, chief eng.
Operation: June, 1981.

WPHL-TV (Channel 17)

WPHL-TV Inc., 5001 Wynnefield Ave., Philadelphia, PA 19131 (215) 878-1700.

Eugene McCurdy, pres. & gen. mgr.; Zvi Shoubin, sta. mgr. & prog. dir.; Gordon French, sls. dir.; John Ruzzi, gen. sls. mgr.; Joel Levitt, prod. mgr.; Walt Bundy, chief eng.; Bob DiMattina, dir. of finance.

Operation: July, 1960; TV households: 3,407,700.

WPVI (Channel 6) ABC

Capital Cities Communication, Inc., 4100 City Line Ave., Philadelphia, PA 19131 (215) 878-9700.

Lawence J. Pollock, v.p. & gen. mgr.; Arnie Kleiner, dir. sls.; Thomas K. Byrnes, gen. sls. mgr.; Art Moore, prom. mgr.; Alan Nesbitt, news dir.; Irwin L. Ross, chief eng.

Operation: 1947; TV sets in area: 4,556,200.

WTAF-TV (Channel 29)

Taft Broadcasting Co., 330 Market St., Philadelphia, PA 19106 (215) 925-2929

Randall E. Smith, gen. mgr.; Elliott Troshinsky, gen. sls. mgr.; Chuck Wing, lcl. sls. mgr.; Gregg Miller, prog. mgr.; Karen Corbin, prom. mgr.; Richard Owens, chief eng.; rep.: Telerep.

Operation: 1965; TV households: 3,037,000.

Pittsburgh

KDKA-TV (Channel 2) CBS

Westinghouse Broadcasting Co., Inc., 1 Gateway Center, Pittsburgh, PA 15222 (412) 392-2200.

Thomas L. Goodgame, v.p. & gen. mgr.; Carolyn Wean, sta. mgr.; Deb Zeyen, prog. mgr.; Joe Berwanger, gen. sls. mgr.; Jack Cvetic, chief eng.; Brad Crum, creative svcs. dir.; Carolyn McClair, info. svcs. dir.

WPGH-TV (Channel 53)

Broadcasting Group/Meredith Corporation, 750 Ivory Avenue, Pittsburgh, PA 15214 (412) 931-8600.

Bill Saltzgiver, v.p. & gen. mgr.; Nancy Palmer, prog. mgr.; Mark Albright, dir. eng.; Kathy Saunders, gen. sls. mgr.; Jim Lapiana, natl. sls. mgr.; Linda Blackburn, lcl. sls. mgr.; George Hillis, prod. mgr.; Terry Caywood, promo. mgr.

Operation under Meredith: Oct. 1978; Households (TV): 1,678,900.

WPTT-TV (Channel 22)

Commercial Radio Institute, Inc., 500 Seco Road, Pittsburgh, PA 15230 (412) 856-9010.

Julian S. Smith, pres.; Frederick M. Himes, exec. v.p. & gen. mgr.; Kenneth Buschman, sta. mgr.; Robert Simmons, v.p., sls.; Michael Silvert, sls. mgr.; natl. rep.: Adam Young.

Operation: 1978.

WPXI (Channel 11) NBC

WPXI Corp., 11 Television Hill, Pittsburgh, PA 15230 (412) 237-1100.

John A. Howell III, v.p. & gen. mgr.; Bruno M. Graziano, gen. sls. mgr.; Mark W. Barash, prog. dir.; Maureen Durkin, promo. mgr.; V. Byron Williams, news dir.; Glenn Romsos, chief eng.

Operation, 1957.

WTAE-TV (Channel 4) ABC

The Hearst Corp., 400 Ardmore Blvd., Pittsburgh, PA 15221 (412) 242-4300.

John G. Conomikes, gen. mgr. of bdcst' for Hearst; Fred Barber, v.p. & gen. mgr.; for WTAE-TV: Jack Shenkan, dir. of sls./brdgt. Hearst; Jerry Kalke, dir. of eng.; Paul Kilkullen, v.p./sls.; Judy Girard, dir. of prog.; B.J. Leber, dir. of promo. & creative svcs.; David Crantz, dir. of p.r. & spec. projects; Alan Sanford, prod. mgr.; Ray Coleman, community & station svcs. dir.; Joe Rovitto, news dir.; nat'l rep.: Katz Agency Inc.

Reading

WTVE (Channel 51)

Reading Broadcasting, Inc., Box 3248, Reading, PA 19604 (215) 921-9181.

Jeffrey D. Miller, gen. mgr.; Gibson White, chief eng.; Bruce Fox, sls. mgr.

Operation: 1980.

Red Lion

WGCB-TV (Channel 49)

Red Lion Television Inc., Box 88, Red Lion, PA 17356 (717) 246-1681.

John H. Norris, pres. & gen. mgr.; Fred W. Wise, v.p.; Jim Nicholls, prog. dir.; natl. rep.: Spot Time.

Operation: 1979.

Scranton/Wilkes-Barre

WDAU-TV (Channel 22) CBS

Scranton Broadcasters, Inc., 415 Lackawana Ave., Scranton, PA 18503 (717) 961-2222.

Eugene H. Bohi, pres./gen. mgr.; Kenny Gonzalez, prog. dir.; Kristin Long, gen. sls. mgr.; nat'l rep.: Blair.

Operation: 1953; TV sets in area: 751,710.

WNEP-TV (Channel 16) ABC

N.E.P. Communications, Inc., Wilkes-Barre/Scranton Airport, Avoca, PA 18641 (717) 826-1616.

Thomas P. Shelburne, bd. chmn.; Thomas Shelburne, Jr., pres.; Chester Saxwicki, v.p./eng.; Dean Hinson, v.p. mktg.; Peter P. Kozloski, treas.; Jay Newman, news dir.; nat'l rep.: Katz Agency, Inc.

Operation: 1954; TV sets in area: 352,375.

WOLF-TV (Channel 38)

Scranton TV Partners, Ltd., 916 Oak St., Scranton, PA 18508 (717) 347-9653.

Guyon Turner, CEO; T. Eugene Malone, gen. mgr.; Ron Evans, gen. sls. mgr.; Peter Rydell, prog. & news dir./film buyer; Joe Sokirka, prom. mgr.; Dave Swartz, chief eng.; natl. rep.: Seltel.

Operation: June, 1985.

Wilkes-Barre

WBRE-TV (Channel 28) NBC

Northeastern Television Investor, Ltd. Partnership, 62 S. Franklin St., Wilkes-Barre, PA 18773; (717) 823-3101.

Terry S. Baltimore, v.p. & gen. mgr.; Tom Rosing, gen. sls. mgr.; George Andresky, chief eng.; natl. rep.: Petry.

Operation: 1953; TV sets in area: 939,300.

York

WPMT (Channel 43) IND

Mohawk Bcstg., Inc., 2005 S. Queen St., York, PA 17403.

John A. Serrao, pres. & gen. mgr.; Donald M. Travis, gen. mgr.; Michael C. Conway, gen. sls. mgr.; Louis J. Castriota, prog. opns. & prom. mgr.; Jack M. Schuster, chief eng.; nat'l. rep.: Petry.

Operation: September, 1983; TV sets in area: 800,000.

RHODE ISLAND

Providence

WJAR-TV (Channel 10) NBC

Outlet Communications, Inc., 111 Dorrance St., Providence, RI 02903 (401) 751-5700.

Bruce G. Sundlun, chm. and CEO; David E. Henderson, pres. & COO; John Sawhill, v.p. & gen. mgr.; Fred Weiss, chief eng.; Jim Macfarlan, gen. sls. mgr.; Linda Sullivan, nat'l. sls. mgr.; nat'l. rep.: Katz.

Operation: 1949; TV sets in area: 1,891,000.

WLNE (Channel 6) CBS

430 County St., New Bedford, MA 02741; (617) 992-6666.

John D. Quinlan, gen. mgr.; B.W. Mayberry, opns. mgr.; Paul A. Karpowicz, gen. sls. mgr.; Doreen Dawson-Wade, sls. mgr.; Truman B. Taylor, prog. mgr.; George C. Wolf, news dir.; C. Robert Ogren, chief eng.; Robert B. Rieske, mgr. spec. projects.

Operation: 1963; TV households: 533,700.

WPRI-TV (Channel 12) ABC

Knight-Ridder Broadcasting, Inc., 25 Catamore Boulevard, East Providence, RI 02914 (401) 438-7200.

Robert E. Rice, pres. & gen. mgr.; Matthew L. Krein, gen. sls. mgr.; Hayden Williams, nat'l. sls. mgr.; Sandi Morvillo, reg. sls. mgr.; Edward Passarelli, bus. mgr.; T. Arthur Bone, v.p. & chief eng.; Cathy Perron, prog. mgr.; Jim Vescera, promo. mgr.; Edwin Hart, news dir.; Joseph Fogarty, admin. asst. to gen. mgr.; nat'l rep.: MMT Sales, Inc.

Operation: 1955; TV Households: 2,737,600 (ARB 5-81).

WSTG (Channel 64)

Channel 64 of New England, Inc., 8200 Greensboro Dr., Suite 1201, McLean, VA 22102 (617) 252-6935.

Paul B. Mowrey, v.p./bcstg.; George Costa, chief eng.

Operation: December, 1981.

SOUTH CAROLINA

Anderson

WAXA (Channel 40)

Mark III Bcstg. Co., P.O. Box 40, Anderson, SC 29622.

Anthony C. Kupris, pres.

Operation: October, 1984.

Charleston

WCBD-TV (Channel 2) ABC

State Telecasting Co. Inc., P.O. Box 879, Charleston, SC 29402.

W. Frank Harden, pres. & gen. mgr.; Virgil V. Evans, v.p.; Grange Cuthbert, asst. gen. mgr.; J. W. (Bill) Evans, III, dir. sls. & mktg.; Truman Kemp, lcl. sls. mgr.; James Abbott, dir. bdcst. ops.; Tessa Hooker, promo. mgr.; Don Feldman, news dir.; Walter Nelson, chif eng.

Operation: 1954.

WCIV (Channel 4) NBC

First Charleston Corp., Highway 703, Mt. Pleasant, SC 29464 (803) 884-8513.

Wm. E. Lucas, pres. & gen. mgr.; Frank Hunt, news mgr.; J. L. Edwards, sales mgr.; Carl Shaw, chief eng.

WCSC-TV (Channel 5) CBS

WCSC, Inc. 485 East Bay St., P.O. Box 186, Charleston, SC 29402 (803) 723-8371.

John M. Rivers, Sr., chmn. & treas. of WCSC, Inc.; John M. Rivers, Jr., pres.; Martha Rivers, 1st v.p. & secy.; Mark Pierce, v.p., gen. mgr.; WCSC-TV; Doug Atherton, gen. sls. mgr.; Eddie Bolling, natl./reg. sls. mgr.; Lovell Waugh, lcl. sls. mgr.; Jack Becknell, v.p., dir. of eng.; Bob Pettit, film dir.; Andy Hunt, promo. mgr.; Nat Ball, chief fin. officer; natl rep: Petry.

Operation: 1953; TV Households: 197,100.

Columbia

WCCT-TV (Channel 57)

Carolina Christian Bcgst. Inc., 1221 Sunset Blvd., W., Columbia, SC 29169 (803) 796-7757.

James H. Thompson, Paul B. Gorman, gen. mgr. & chief eng.; Ginger S. Bruce, sls. mgr. & pub. rel. dir.; Julie Brown, prog. dir.; Myra Campbell, traffic mgr.; Ginger S. Bryce, pub. rel. dir.

Operation: September, 1981.

WIS-TV (Channel 10) NBC

1111 Bull St., P.O. Box 367, Columbia, SC 29202; (803) 799-1010.

Dixon C. Lovvorn, sr. v.p. & gen. mgr.; Scott Parks, news dir.; Diane K. Bagwell, prog./promo./mgr.; C. Joseph Tonsing, gen. sls. mgr.; John Augustine, chief eng.

Operation: 1953; TV sets in area: 853,400.

WLTX-TV (Channel 19) CBS

Capital Communications, Inc., P.O. Drawer M, Columbia, SC 29250 (803) 776-3600.

Richard T. Laughridge v.p. & gen. mgr.; Donald M. Bryant, prog. dir.; Bill Aull, chief eng.; Richard T. Laughridge, natl. sls. mgr.; nat'l rep.: Katz Television.

Operation: 1953; TV sets in area: 289,800.

WOLO-TV (Channel 25) ABC

Columbia TV Broadcasters Inc., Box 4217, Columbia, SC 29240 (803) 754-7525.

Donald H. Krauss, gen. mgr.; Joe Mahan, sls. mgr.; Don Jones, chief eng.; rep.: Katz.

Operation: 1951; TV households in area: 259,600.

Florence

WBTW (Channel 13) CBS

Daily Telegraph Printing Co., 3430 N. TV Road, Florence, SC 29501 (803) 662-1565.

Joseph B. Foster, asst. v.p. & sta. mgr.; George L. Sansbury, sls. mgr.; Jim Griffin, news dir.; Russell Smith, prod. mgr.; Bernard E. Moore, techl. mgr.; nat'l rep.: Avery Knodel.

Operation: 1954; TV households: 353,400.

WPDE-TV (Channel 15)

Eastern Carolinas Broadcasting Co., Inc., Box F-15, Florence, SC 29501 (803) 665-1515.

Jerry Condra, pres. & gen. mgr.; Mark Manning, natl. sls. mgr.; Neal Morrison, lcl. sls. mgr.; Eric Sesit, creative svcs. dir.; Joyce Jordan, bus. mgr.; Timmy Gamble, chief eng.; natl. rep.: Seltel.

Operation: 1980.

Greenville

WYFF-TV (Channel 4) NBC

Pulitzer Broadcasting Co., 505 Rutherford St., Greenville, SC 29602.

Douglas A. Smith, sr. vice pres. & gen. mgr.; Bill Wheless, prgm. dir.; John Scott, sls. dir.; Bob King, chief eng.; David Foster, bus. mgr.; Andy Scott, promo. mgr.; nat'l rep.: Petry.
Operation: 1953; TV sets in area: 956,230.

Greenwood

WGCT-TV (Channel 48)
Metro Communications South, Inc., Box 3348, Greenwood SC 29648 (803) 227-8848.
Pete Stathakis, pres.; Ron Moore, v.p. & gen. mgr.
Operation: March, 1983.

Spartanburg

WSPA-TV (Channel 7) CBS
Spartan Radiocasting Co., Box 1717, Spartanburg, SC 29304 (803) 576-7777.
Walter J. Brown, pres.; K. James Yager, exec. v.p.; Joe Varholy, gen. mgr.; Walter Vieth, secty,-treas.; David Handy, prgm./stn. mgr.; Gil Anderson, dir. of eng'.; Richard Compton, chief eng.; Tom Ahner, trans. engineer; Jan Haswell, promo. mgr.; Ray Johnson, gen. sales mgr.; Bruce Miller, local/reg. sales mgr.; Al Kamhi, news dir.; nat'l rep.: Seltel.
Operation: 1956; TV sets in area: 2,300,000.

SOUTH DAKOTA

Aberdeen

KABY-TV (Channel 9) ABC
Sodak Broadcasting Co., North Highway 281, Box 1520, Aberdeen, SD 57401 (605) 225-9200.
Robert C. Matson, mgr.; Jim Paulson, news dir.; Earl Miller, chief eng.
Operation: 1958.

Florence

KDLO-TV (Channel 3) CBS
(Satellite of KELO-TV, Sioux Falls, SD)
Midcontinent Broadcasting Co., % KELO-TV, Phillips Ave. & 13th St., Sioux Falls, SD 57102 (605) 336-1100.
Joe Floyd, pres.; N. L. Benston, v.p.; E. R. Ruben, secty.-treas.; Evans Nord, pres. & gen. mgr. of KELO; Joe H. Floyd. v.p.; nat'l rep.: Seltel, Wayne Evans & Assoc. (Minneapolis).
Operation: 1955; TV sets in area: 375,500.

Lead

KHSD-TV (Channel 11) ABC
Duhamel Broadcasting Enterprises, Box 1760, Rapid City, S.D. 57709.
William F. Duhamel, pres. & gen. mgr.; Monte Loos, opns. dir.; Don Larsen, dir. of eng.; rep.; Katz.
Operation: November, 1966.

KIVV-TV (Channel 5) NBC
Dakota Broadcasting Co., Inc., Box 677, Rapid City, SD 57709 (605) 394-7777.
Ray Moser, gen. mgr.; Harvey Sachau, mgr. of eng.; Gerry Fenske, local sls. mgr.; Les Hofland, prod. mgr.; Robert Slocum, contr.; Dan Schillinger, news dir.; rep.: Blair.
Operation: July, 1976.

Pierre

KPRY-TV (Channel 4) NBC
(Satellite of KSF-TV, Sioux Falls)
South Dakota Broadcasting Co., 6th & Dakota Ave., Sioux Falls, SD 75102 (605) 336-1300.
Personnel: See KSFY-TV, Sioux Falls
Operation: 1976.

Rapid City

KEVN-TV (Channel 7) NBC
Dakota Broadcasting Co., Inc., Box 677, Rapid City, SD 57709 (605) 394-7777.
Ray Moser, gen. mgr.; Harvey Sachau, mgr. of eng.; Gerry Fenske, lcl. sls. mgr.; Les Hofland, prod. mgr.; Robert Slocum, contr.; Dan Schillinger, news dir.; rep.: Blair.
Operation: July, 1976.

KOTA-TV (Channel 3) ABC
KDUH Channel 4, KHSD Channel 11, KSGW Channel 12 (satellites).
Duhamel Broadcasting Enterprises, Duhamel Bldg., 6th & St. Joe Streets, P.O. Box 1760, Rapid City, SD 57709 (605) 342-2000.
Mrs. Helen S. Duhamel, chm.; William F. Duhamel, pres. & gen. mgr.; Monte Loos, opns. mgr.; Don Larsen, dir. of engineering; Verne Sheppard, farm dir.; nat'l rep: Katz Agency; Omaha rep., The Soderlund Company.
Operation: 1955; TV sets in area: 80,200.

Reliance

KPLO-TV (Channel 6) CBS
(Satellite of KELO-TV, Sioux Falls, SD)
Midcontinent Broadcasting Co., c/o KELO-TV., Phillips Ave. & 13th St., Sioux Falls, SD 57102 (605) 336-1100.
Joe Floyd, pres.; N. L. Bentson, v.p.; E. R. Ruben, secty.-treas.; Evans A. Nord, pres. & gen. mgr. of KELO; Joe H. Floyd, v.p.; nat'l rep.: Seltel, Wayne Evans & Assoc. (Minneapolis).
Operation: 1957; TV sets in area, 375,500.

Sioux Falls

KDLT-TV (Channel 5) NBC
Dakotaland Broadcasting, Inc. P.O. Box 1200, Mitchell SD 57301; (605) 996-7501.
Hal Greene, gen. mgr.; Jim Brady, chief eng.
Operation: 1983; TV households: 235,000.

KELO-TV (Channel 11) CBS
Midcontinent Broadcasting Co., Phillips at 13th, Sioux Falls, SD 57102 (605) 336-1100.
Joe Floyd, pres.; N. L. Bentson, v.p.; E. R. Ruben, secty.-treas.; Evans A. Nord, pres. & gen. mgr. of KELO; Joe H. Floyd, v.p.; Tom Sheeley, news, prgm. v.p.; Jack Townsend, sls. devel. dir.; Scott Burri, prod. mgr.; Connie Hodgen, promo. mgr.; nat'l rep.: Seltel, Wayne Evans & Assoc. (Minneapolis).
Operation: 1953; TV sets in area: 375,500.

KSFY-TV (Channel 13)
South Dakota Broadcasting Co., 6th & Dakota, Sioux Falls, SD 57102.
Jim Dunham, v.p. & gen. mgr.; Warren Murray, dir. of eng.; Gar Kellogg, prod. dir.; John Dunnicliff, prom. mgr.; Marge Hokenstad, prog. dir.; Jim Paulson, news dir.; sales rep.: Katz.
Operation: July, 1960; TV households: 309,300.

TENNESSEE

Chattanooga

WDEF-TV (Channel 12) CBS

Roy H. Park, Broadcasting of Tennessee, Inc., Broadcast Center, 3300 Broad St., Chattanooga, TN 37402 (615) 267-3392.

Roy H. Park, pres.; Robert G. Lee, v.p. & gen. mgr.; D. Michael Hood, gen. sls. mgr.; Doris A. Ellis, prog. dir.; William M. Christman, chief eng.; Charles Wilkie, bus. mgr.; nat'l rep.: Blair Television.

Operation: 1954; TV sets in area: 300,000.

WDSI (Channel 61)

WDSI Limited Partnership, 2401 E. Main St., Chattanooga, TN 37404 (615) 697-0661.

Mike Starr, gen. partner; Clifford Pine, gen. mgr. & prog. dir.; Cal Cass, gen. sls. mgr.; Cheryal Morgan, prog. asst.; Jeff Gregory, chief eng.; natl. rep.: ITS

Operation: January, 1972.

WRCB-TV (Channel 3) NBC

WRCB-TV, Sarkes Tarzian, Inc. 900 Whitehall Road, Chattanooga, TN 37405 (615) 267-5412.

Tom Tolar, gen. mgr.; Lawson Fox, prog. dir.; Doug Short, sls. mgr.; Patti Smith, promo, mgr.

Operation: 1956; TV sets in area: 571,800.

WTVC (Channel 9) ABC

WTVC, Inc., Box 1150, Chattanooga, TN 37401 (615) 266-4151.

F. Lewis Robertson, v.p., gen. mgr. & progr. mgr.; Dennis Brown, chief eng.; natl. rep.: Petry.

Operation: 1958; TV homes in area: 466,100.

Crossville

WINT-TV (Channel 20)

Cumberland Communications Corp., Box 608, Crossville, TN 38555; (615) 484-8424.

John A. Cunningham, gen. mgr. & chief eng.; James P. Young, sls. mgr.; Rita L. Young, prog. mgr.; Helen L. Cunningham, office mgr.; Wilda Golob, news & pub. affairs dir.; Robin Cunningham, film dir.

Operation: October, 1976.

Jackson

WBBJ-TV (Channel 7) ABC

Jackson Telecasters Inc.; Box 2387, Muse Street, Jackson, TN 38301 (901) 424-4515.

Phil Brassie, gen. mgr.; Ron Evans, sls. mgr.; Edward Ward, chief eng.; Cathy Goodrich, traffic mgr.; nat'l rep.: Katz.

Operation: 1965; TV homes in area: 426,200.

WJWT (Channel 16)

Goldeon Circle Broadcasting, Inc., 364 N. Royal, Jackson, TN 38301; (901) 424-1600.

Bud Borchert, gen. mgr. & prog. dir.; Bill King, gen. sls. mgr.; Pat McKnight, prom. mgr.

Operation: April, 1985.

Johnson City

WJHL-TV (Channel 11) CBS-ABC

Roy H. Park Broadcasting of the Tri-Cities, Inc., 338 East Main St., Johnson City, TN 37602 (615) 926-2151.

Roy H. Park, pres.; W. H. Lancaster, Jr., v.p. & gen. mgr.; Jack Dempsey, sls. mgr.; Al Gregory, prog. dir.; K. B. Skinner, treas.; Mrs. Dorothy Park, secy.; Carl E. Dickenson, chief eng.; nat'l rep.: Blair-TV.

Operation: 1953; TV sets in area: 556,100.

Kingsport-Johnson City-Bristol

WKPT-TV (Channel 19) ABC

Holston Valley Broadcasting Corp., 222 Commerce, Kingsport, TN 37660.

George DeVault, Jr., exec. v.p. & gen. mgr.; Ray Walker, v.p. & gen. sls. mgr.; Harold T. Dougherty, v.p. & chief eng.; rep.: Avery-Knode.

Operation: 1969; TV homes in ADI: 233,000.

Knoxville

WATE-TV (Channel 6) ABC

Nationwide Communications Inc., 1306 Broadway, N.E. Knoxville, TN 37917 (615) 637-9666.

Clark Pollock, pres.; Jim Mikels, gen. mgr.; Jim Abbott, sta. mgr.; Bob Williams, chief eng.; Steve Slack, gen. sls. mgr.; Bob King, prod. dir.; John Baldwin, promo. dir.; nat'l rep.: Blair.

Operation: 1953; TV sets in area: 420,500.

WBIR-TV (Channel 10) CBS

Multimedia Broadcasting Co., 1513 Hutchinson, Knoxville, TN 37901 (615) 637-1010.

Wilson C. Wearn, pres.; Neal Branch, v.p. & gen. mgr.; Peter Fennelly, prog. dir. & film buyer; Robert E. Horton, chief eng.; Lynn Leopper, sls. mgr.; nat'l rep.: The Katz Agency.

Operation: 1956; TV sets in area: 384,800.

WTVK (Channel 26) NBC

South Central Broadcasting Corp., Box 1388, Knoxville, TN 37901; Memorial Park Road on Sharps Ridge, Knoxville, TN 37901 (615) 687-2312.

John D. Engelbrecht, pres.; George F. Stoltz, v.p.; Leighman D. Groves, secty.-treas.; Duane V. Eastvold, gen. mgr.; Jerry Whitener, sls. mgr.; Robert Glenn, chief eng.; nat'l rep.: Seltel.

Operations: 1953; TV sets in ara: 302,700.

Memphis

WHBQ-TV (Channel 13) ABC

RKO General Inc. (NY), 485 So. Highland Ave., P.O. Box 11407, Memphis, TN 38111 (901) 320-1313.

Alex Bonner, v.p. & gen. mgr.; Jack Bolton, v.p. & gen. sls. mgr.; Dick Kvale, natl. sls. mgr.; Jimmie Mitchell, lcl. sls. mgr.; Robert Lewis, prog. dir.; Larry Caughlan, chief eng.; nat'l rep.: Harrington, Righter & Parsons.

Operation: 1953; TV households in area: 554,400.

WMC-TV (Channel 5) NBC

Scripps-Howard Broadcasting Co., 1960 Union Ave., Memphis, TN 38104 (901) 274-8515.

M. E. Greiner, Jr., v.p. & gen. mgr.; Edw. F. Greaney, Jr., asst gen. mgr. news & public affairs; J. P. Tucker, asst. gen. mgr. sls.; Ron Klayman, dir. bdcst. svcs.; Mason Granger, news dir.; Robert A. Frase, dir. eng.; Jay Perkins, prod. mgr.; Olivia Holmes, promo. mgr.; nat'l rep.: Blair-TV, Inc.

Operation: 1948; TV sets in area: 649,280.

WMKW-TV (Channel 30)

Television Corp. of Memphis, Box 30030, Memphis, TN

38130 (901) 346-3030.
Tim McDonald, pres.; Timothy M. Lynch, v.p. & gen. mgr.; Jeffery L. Feyes, gen. sls. mgr.; DeShon Darnell, natl. sls. mgr.; Doug Gillen, lcl. sls. mgr.; Janet L. Harris, dir. finance; Jean Anders, dir. promotions; Megan Wright, prog. dir.; Jim Mattson, dir. of eng.
Operation: April, 1983.

WPTY-TV (Channel 24)
WPTY Television, a Ltd. Partnership, 2225 Union Ave., Memphis, TN 38104; (901) 278-2424.
Margaret A. Ragsdale, gen. mgr.; Steve Barry, gen. sls. mgr.; George D. Causey, chief eng.; natl. rep.: Petry Television.
Operation: 1978.

WREG-TV (Channel 3) CBS
New York Times Broadcasting Service, Inc., 803 Channel 3 Drive, Memphis, TN 38103 (901) 525-1313.
Charles B. Brakefield, pres. & gen. mgr.; Jack Michael, v.p. & prog. dir.; Frank Roberts, natl. sales mgr.; Olin Morris, dir. pub. affairs; nat'l rep.: The Katz Agency, Inc.
Operation: 1956; TV sets in area: 515,000.

Nashville

WCAY-TV (Channel 30)
Television Corporation Stations, 300 Peabody St., Nashville, TN 37210 (615) 256-3030.
Tim McDonald, pres.; John Walser, gen. mgr.; Jerry Staggs, gen. sls. mgr.; Jenny Zoeller, prog. dir.; Kevin Kolbe, prog. mgr.; Carl Wolfe, chief eng.; natl. rep.: Telerep.
Operation: February, 1984.

WKRN-TV (Channel 2) ABC
441 Murfreesboro Rd., Nashville, TN 37210 (615) 248-7222.
Art Elliot, gen. mgr.; Gene Parker, opns. mgr.; Mike Sullivan, news dir.; nat'l. rep.: HRP.
Operation: 1953; TV sets in area: 634,500.

WSMV-TV (Channel 4) NBC
WSMV-TV, Inc., P.O. Box 4, Nashville, TN 37202 (615) 749-2244.
Mike Kettenring, pres. & gen. mgr.; Dan Akens, sta. mgr.; Brenda Jordan, prog. coord.; Lee Whitehurst, chief eng.; natl. rep.: MMT Sales.
Operation: 1950; TV homes in area: 1,083,200.

WTVF-TV (Channel 5) CBS
Channel Five Television Co., 474 James Robertson Pkwy., Nashville, TN 37219 (615) 244-5000.
Jock Harris, pres.; Harold Crump, v.p. & gen. mgr.; Thomas Erwin, v.p. & sta. mgr.; Chris Clark, v.p. & news div.; Bill Bumpers, v.p., opers. nat'l rep.: The Katz Agency, Inc.
Operation: 1954; TV sets in area: 813,000.

WZTV (Channel 17)
Reel Broadcasting Co., Inc., Multimedia, Inc., P.O. Box 90764, Nashville, TN 37209 (615) 244-1717.
Dan F. Maslan, gen. mgr.; Bill Walters, lcl. sls. mgr; Jim Crowley, natl. sls. mgr; Judy Jenkins, dir., prog.; Ray McInturff, chief eng.
Operation: March, 1976.

TEXAS

Abilene

KRBC-TV (Channel 9) NBC
Abilene Radio & Television Co., 4510 S. 14th St., Abilene, TX (915) 692-4242; TWX: 910-897-5414.
Dale Ackers, pres. & gen. mgr.; Ken Knox, sta. mgr.; Jerry Shackelford, prog. mgr.; Bob Lloyd, chief eng.; nat'l rep.: Blair Television.
Operation: 1953; TV sets in area: 200,000.

KTAB-TV (Channel 32) CBS
Big Country Television Co., Box 5676, Abilene, TX (915) 695-2777.
Bill Terry, sta. & sls. mgr.; Bryan Mundy, ops. mgr.; Jerry Marshall, lcl. sls. mgr.; Bob Bartlett, news dir.; Leland Ohlhausen, chief eng.; natl. rep.: Katz Television.
Operation: 1979; sets in area: 138,000.

Abilene-Sweetwater

KTXS-TV (Channel 12) ABC
Catclaw Communications, Co., U.S. Hwy. 83 Bypass No., Abilene, TX 79604 (915) 677-2281.
S.M. Moore, Jr., gen. mgr., pres. & CEO; Moe Strout, chief eng.; natl. rep.: Seltel.

Amarillo

KAMR-TV (Channel 4) NBC
Cannan Communications, Inc., P.O. Box 1224, Wichita Falls, TX 76307 (806) 376-5804.
Darrold A. Cannan, Jr., pres.; Ray Poindexter, v.p. & gen. mgr.; Irl Brown, sls. mgr.; John Schnabel, bus. mgr.; Ken High, chief eng.; Joe Sherrill, op. mgr.; Bruce Whiteaker, news dir.
Operation: 1953

KFDA-TV (Channel 10) CBS
Bass Broadcasting Company, P.O. Box 1400, Amarillo, TX 79105; (806) 383-2226.
Melvin L. Wheeler, pres.; Earle H. Rast, Jr., v.p. & gen. mgr.; Jack Byrd, oper. mgr.; Ron Slover, news director; Roy McCoy, weather director; Dave Coons, ch. eng.; Larry S. Faller, sales mgr.; Bedford Forrest, farm dir.
Operation: 1953; TV sets in area: 222,200.

KVII (Channel 7) ABC
Marsh Media, Inc., One Broadcast Center, Amarillo, TX 79101 (806) 373-1787.
James R. McCormick, pres. & gen. mgr.; John Patrick, gen. sales mgr.
Operation: 1957.

Austin

KBVO (Channel 42)
Drawer 2728, Austin, TX 78768.
Steve Beard, gen. & gen. sls. mgr.; John Martin, prog. dir. & film buyer; Rich Greene, prom. mgr.; George Taylor, chief eng.; nat'l. rep.: Katz.
Operation: November, 1983.

KTBC-TV (Channel 7) CBS
The Texas Broadcasting Corp., Box 2223, Austin, TX 78767 (512) 472-2424.
R. K. Evans, pres. & gen. mgr.; Gus Stewart, sls. mgr.; Al

Mustin, natl/reg. sls. mgr.; Wally Pryor, mgr.; Arthur Riley, chg. eng.

KTVV (Channel 36) NBC

Kingstip Communications, Inc., P.O. Box 490, Austin TX 78767 (512) 476-3636.

Jane Wallace, pres. & gen. mgr.; Steve McDonald, gen. sls. mgr.; Bill Hutchison, chief eng.

Operation: 1965.

KVUE (Channel 24) ABC

KVUE-TV, Inc. Box 9927, Austin TX 78766 (512) 459-6521.

Joe Jerkins, v.p. & gen. mgr.; Andy Lee, sta. mgr.; Al Helton, prog. mgr.; Michael J. Wenglar, chief eng.

Operation: 1971.

Beaumont

KBMT-TV (Channel 12) ABC

Texas Telecasting, Inc., Box 1550, Beaumont, TX 77706 (713) 883-7512.

Michael D. McKinnon, pres. & gen. mgr.; Wm. E. Moore, v.p., sta. mgr.; George Gould, v.p., gen. sales mgr., Earl Conner, chief eng.; nat'l rep.: Blair Television.

Operation: 1961.

KFDM-TV (Channel 6) CBS

Freedom TV Sub, Inc., P.O. Box 7128, 2955 Interstate 10 East, Beaumont, TX 77706 (409) 892-6622.

Larry Beaulieu, v.p. & sta. mgr.; Richard Kihn, chief eng.; nat'l rep., Petry & Co.

Operation: 1955; TV sets in area: 241,000.

Big Spring

KWAB-TV (Channel 4) CBS, ABC

Grayson Enterprises, Inc., 2500 Kentucky Way, Big Spring, TX 79720 (915) 267-6325.

Pat Hales, gen. mgr.; Joe Hull, natl. sls. rep.: Tony Radican, prod. mgr.

Operation: 1956. TV sets in area: 82,200.

Brownsville

KVEO (Channel 23) NBC

394 N. Expressway, Brownsville, TX 78520 (512) 544-2323.

Earl Noel, gen. mgr.; Mike Noel, natl. & reg. sls. mgr.; Sara Skaggs, gen. sls. mgr.; Yolanda Cortez, prog. dir.; Gilbert Resendez, chief eng.; natl. rep.: Seltel.

Operation: 1981.

Bryan

KBTX-TV (Channel 3) CBS

Brazos Broadcasting Co., E. 29th St., P.O. Drawer 3730, Bryan, TX 77801 (409) 846-7777.

M. N. Bostick, pres.; Harry L. Gillam, v.p. & sta. mgr.; John M. Lawrence, III, secty.-treas.; nat'l rep.: Seltel.

Operation: May, 1957; TV sets in area: 116,900.

Corpus Christi

KIII (Channel 3) ABC

South Texas Telecasting Co., Inc., 4750 S. Padre Island Dr., Corpus Christi, TX 78404.

Michael D. McKinnon, pres. & gen. mgr.; W. G. Heneger, auditor; Leonard Ropar, station & sls. mgr.; Billy Brotherton, sls. mgr.; rep.: Blair Television.

Operation: 1964; TV households: 318,900.

KORO (Channel 28)

Telecorpus, Inc., 102 N. Mesquite, Corpus Christi, TX 78401 (512) 883-2823.

Servando Caballero, gen. mgr.; Felipe Franco, chf. eng.

Operation: 1977.

KRIS-TV (Channel 6) NBC

Gulf Coast Broadcasting Co., Box 840, Corpus Christi, TX 78404 (512) 883-6511.

T. Frank Smith, pres. & gen. mgr.; Van Johnson, 1st v.p. & natl sales.; Charlie Barte, sls. mgr.; Marvin Born, dir. of eng.; nat'l rep.: Katz.

Operation: 1956; TV sets in area: 116,780.

KZTV (Channel 10) CBS

K-Six Television, Inc., Wilson Bldg., Corpus Christi, TX; 78401.

Vann M. Kennedy, pres. & gen. mgr.; Eugene Looper, prog. dir.

Operation: 1956.

Dallas-Fort Worth

KDFI-TV (Channel 27)

Box 270427, Dallas, TX 75247; (214) 637-2727.

John McKay, pres.; Thoren Schroeck, v.p., sls.; Mitch Keniston, chief eng.

Operation: January, 1981.

KDFW-TV (Channel 4) CBS

400 North Griffin St., Dallas, TX 75202 (214) 744-4000.

John McKay, v.p. & gen. mgr.; D. Demirjian, gen. sls. mgr; J. Martin, prog. dir.; Warren Farrar, chief eng.; national rep.: Harrington, Righter & Parsons.

Operation: 1949; TV sets in area: 1,351,600.

KRLD-TV (Channel 33)

Metromedia, 8001 Carpenter Freeway, Dallas, TX 75247; (214) 634-8833.

Raymond J. Schonbak, gen. mgr.; Katy Ellitt-Atteberry, gen. sls. mgr.; Tony deHaro, news dir.; Charles Smith, chief eng.; natl. rep.: Katz.

Operation: 1980.

KTXA (Channel 21)

Channel 21, Inc., 1712 E. Randol Mill Rd., Arlington, TX (817) 265-2100. Owned by Taft Bdcst. Co.

William P. Castleman, v.p./gen. mgr.; Dirk Brinkerhoff, gen. sls. mgr.; Kathy Daume, lcl. sls. mgr.; Glen P. Dyer, prod. mgr.; Jerry Stretch, mgr. bus. affairs.

Operation: 1981.

KXAS-TV (Channel 5) NBC

North Texas Broadcasting Corp., 3900 Barnett St., Ft. Worth, TX 76101 (817) 429-1550.

Blake Byrne, pres. & gen. mgr.; Russ Thornton, dir., admin. & devel.; Manny Munoz, dir. of bus. affairs; Patty Parker, gen. sls. mgr.; Sue McDonnell, sta. sls. mgr.; Tom Bedford, eng. dir.

Operation: 1948.

KXTX-TV (Channel 39)

Christian Broadcasting Network, Inc., Box 19307, Dallas TX 75219 (214) 521-3900.

M. G. Robertson, pres.; Bob Johnson, v.p. & gen. mgr.; Roger Baerwolf, sta. mgr.; Harold Wheat, op. mgr.; Dick Bove, gen. sls. mgr.; Art Runyon, chief eng.; Bill Dunn, prod. mgr.; sales rep.: Adam Young, Inc.
Operation: February, 1968; TV households: 2,006,100.

WFAA-TV (Channel 8) ABC
A. H. Belo Corp. (parent organization of The Dallas Morning News, WFAA-KZEW Radio and WFAA-TV), Communications Center, Dallas, TX 75202 (214) 748-9631.
Ward Huey, pres. & CEO, David T. Lane, v.p. & gen. mgr.; Phillip Keller, sta. mgr.; Chris Westerkamp, gen. sls. mgr.; Bob Turner, prod. & oper. mgr.; John Miller, news dir.; Charles Martin, chief eng.; Lee Minard, dir. creative svcs.; Aubrey Jenkins, controller; Petry Television, Inc., nat'l rep.
Operation: 1949; TV sets in area: 1,345,300.

El Paso

KCIK (Channel 14)
Cristo Rey Corp., 3100 N. Stanton St., El Paso, TX 79903 (915) 533-1414.
Robert Munoz, genl mgr.; Andy Austin, chief eng.; natl. rep: Adam Young.
Operation: 1979; sets in area: 283,200.

KDBC-TV (Channel 4) CBS
El Paso Television Co., 2201 Wyoming Ave., El Paso, Texas 79903 (915) 532-6551.
Sam Kobren, gen. mgr.; Richard Morales, bus. mgr.; Charles Maly, prog. dir.; Jim Tucker, chief eng.; Don Caparis, sls. dir.; natl. rep.: Seltel.
Operation: 1953; TV sets in area: 222,000.

KINT-TV (Channel 26)
Paso Del Norte Bcstg. Corp., 5426 N. Mesa Dr., El Paso, TX 79912 (916) 581-1126.
Richard A. Najera, pres.; Leopoldo L. Ramos, v.p./gen. mgr.; Walt Dalton, gen. sls. mgr.; Marty Otero, promo. & prog.; Alfredo Durand, chief eng.
Operation: January, 1984.

KTSM-TV (Channel 9) NBC
Tri-State Broadcasting Co., Inc., 801 N. Oregon St., El Paso, TX 79903 (915) 532-5432.
Karl O. Wyler, pres. & gen. mgr.; Jack Rye, exec. v.p. & progs.; John Phelan, v.p., sls.; W. T. McGill, v.p., eng'.; nat'l rep.: Avery-Knodel.
Operation: 1953; TV households in area: 172,500.

KVIA-TV (Channel 13)
KVIA-TV Marsh Media—El Paso, Box 12277, El Paso, TX 79912.
Wayne M. Roy, gen. mgr.; Don Guill, ops-mgr/prog. dir.; Fred Witt, gen. sls. mgr.; George Taylor, chief eng.; natl rep.: Katz Television.
Operation: 1956; TV sets in area: 168,600.

XEJ-TV (Channel 5) (Mexican Border—Juarez)
Television de la Frontera, S.A., Box 9555, El Paso, TX; 79903.
Pedro Meneses Hoyos, pres.; Maria Dolores Heredia, gen. mgr.; Guadalupe Ramirez, sls. mgr.; Ramon Hurtado, prog. mgr.; Hector Noriega, prod. mgr.; Esteban Guerrero, chief eng.; nat'l rep.: Spanish International Network Sales.
Operation: 1954.

XEPM-TV (Channel 2) (Juarez)
XEPM-TVTelevision Inc. Apdo. No. 271, Juarez, Mexico.
Pedro Meneses, Jr., owner; M. D. Heredia, gen. mgr.; Sergio D. Molinar, Jr., sales mgr.
Operation: 1961.

Fort Worth

KTVT (Channel 11)
Gaylord Broadcasting Co., 5322 Bridge St., Fort Worth, TX 76103 (817) 738-1951; Branch office: 10111 N. Central Expressway, Dallas, TX 75231.
Charles L. Edwards, v.p. & gen. mgr.; Harry J. Delanmey, sta. mgr.; natl. rep.: Telerep.

Harlingen

KGBT-TV (Channel 4) CBS
Harbenito Broadcasting Company, P.O. Box 711, Harlingen, TX 78551 (512) 423-3910.
McHenry Tichenor, bd. chmn.; McHenry T. Tichenor Jr., pres.; Mal Kasanoff, exec. v.p.; David Lykes, v.p./station mgr.; Frank Ogden, chief eng.; nat'l. rep.: Katz.
Operation: 1953. TV sets in area: 177,500.

Houston

KHOU-TV (Channel 11) CBS
Gulf Television Corp., P.O. Box 11, Houston, TX 77001 (713) 526-1111.
Terrence S. Ford, pres. & gen. mgr.; Jack O'Leen, gen. sls. mgr.; Robin Prince, prog. mgr.; David Earnhardt, opns. mgr.; Alan Parcell, news dir.; natl. rep.: Major Market TV.
Operation: March, 1953; TV households: 1,326,000.

KHTV (Channel 39)
KHTV, 7700 Westpark Drive, P.O. Box 1439, Houston, TX 77001 (713) 781-3930.
WKY Television System, Inc., E. L. Gaylord, pres.; Gene R. Jacobsen, gen. mgr.
Began operating 1/6/67.

KPRC-TV (Channel 2) NBC
Channel Two TV Co., 8181 Southwest Freeway, Houston, TX 77074 (713) 771-4631.
William P. Hobby, bd. chmn.; Harold Crump, pres.; Jeffrey H. Lee, exec. v.p. & gen. mgr.; John Buffington, prog. dir.; Paul Huhndorff, v.p. & op. mgr.; Bill Goodman, news dir.; Larry Shrum, gen. sls. mgr.; Jeff Kurtz, natl. sls. mgr.; Bruce Bryant, creative svcs. dir.; natl. rep.: Petry.
Operation: 1949; TV sets in area: 1,409,530.

KRIV-TV (Channel 26)
Metromedia Television, P.O. Box 22810, 3935 Westheimer, Houston, TX 77027 (713) 626-2610..
M. Jerry Marcus, v.p. & gen. mgr.; Mike Polatschek, gen. sls. mgr.
Operation: August, 1971; TV households: 1,115,900.

KTRK-TV (Channel 13) ABC
Capital Cities Communications, Inc.; mailing address: P.O. Box 12, Houston, TX 77001; offices and studios: 3310 Bissonnet, Houston, TX (713) 666-0713; TWX: 910-881-1511; Transmitter: Alameda, TX.
Thomas S. Murphy, pres. & chmn.; Kenneth Johnson, v.p. & gen. mgr.; Jim Mascusi, oper. dir.; Larry Autry, prod. dir.; Nancy K. Duke, bus. mgr.; Charles Wolf, prom. dir.; Walt Hawver, news oper. mgr.; Jess Mitchell, chief studio eng.; Jim

Keeley, gen. sls. mgr.; Robert Sutton, chief transmitter eng.; spot sales rep., Blair TV.
Operation: 1954; TV homes in area: 944,000.

KTXH (Channel 20)
Taft TV & Radio Co., Inc., 8950 Kirby Drive, Houston, TX 77054 (713) 661-2020.
Vincent F. Barresi, v.p. & gen. mgr.; Matt Reiff, gen. sls. mgr.; Patty Duncan, prog. dir.; Jeff Sohinki, promo. dir.; Don Johnson, bus. mgr.; Thomas Daniels, chief eng.; natl. rep.: Seltel.
Operation: November, 1982.

Irving

KLTJ (Channel 49)
Cela, Inc., 1957 E. Irving Blvd., Irving, TX 75060 (214) 721-0104.
Eldred Thomas, pres. & gen. mgr.; Mario Montes, prog. dir.; Richie Martin, prom. mgr.; Steve Fjordbak, news dir.; Tom Long Jr., chief eng.
Operation: April, 1984.

Laredo

KGNS-TV (Channel 8) NBC, ABC
Gulf Coast Broadcasting Co., Box 2829, Laredo, TX 78041 (512) 727-8888.
Bill McDonald, v.p. & gen. mgr.; Velia Herrera, asst. to gen. mgr.
Operation: 1956; TV sets in area: 23,000

KLDO (Channel 27) ABC
Panorama Broadcasting Co., 1600 Water St., Riverdrive Mall, Laredo, TX 78040; (512) 727-0027.
Jerry Morris, gen. mgr. & film buyer; Hugo Alcocer, gen. sls. mgr.; Elia Johnston, prog. dir.; Cindy Rodriguez, promo. mgr.; Randy Kent, news dir.; Merlin Miller, chief eng.; natl. rep.: Adam Young.
Operation: December, 1984.

KVTV (Channel 13) CBS
K-SIX TV Inc., Wilson Bldg., 601 Leopard St., Corpus Christi, TX 78401 (512) 723-2923.
Vann M. Kennedy, pres. & gen. mgr.; Richard M. King, sta. mgr.; Nicholas Sanchez, news dir.; Matt Sanderford, chief eng.; Frank Montgomery, resident eng.: sls. rep.: H-R TV.
Operation: December, 1973.

Longview

KLMG-TV (Channel 51) CBS
East Texas TV Network, 701 N. Access Rd., Box 5151, Longview, TX 75608.
Clara J. McLaughlin, pres. & CEO; J. Wesley Ferns, v.p. & gen. mgr.; Ron Cooke, gen. sls. mgr.; Cathy Smith, prog. dir.; Mary Hobbs, promo mgr., Steve Walker, news dir.
Operation: September, 1984.

Lubbock

KAMC-TV (Channel 28) ABC
McAlister TV Enterprises Inc., Box 2805, Lubbock, TX 79408 (806) 745-2828.
Bob Nash, pres. & gen. mgr.; Bill Maddox, sls. mgr.; Bill Baker, chief eng.; A. C. Wimberly, prog. dir.
Operation: 1968; TV homes in area: 147,180.

KCBD-TV (Channel 11) NBC
Caprock Telecasting Co., Inc., Box 2190, Lubbock, TX 79408 (806) 744-1414.
Carl Minor, gen. mgr.; Bill deTournillon, sta. mgr.; Peggy Sullivan, prog. dir.; Sherrell Lambert, dir. of eng.; Craig Wells, sls. mgr.; natl. rep.: Katz.
Operation: 1953: TV sets in area: 224,00.

KJTV (Channel 34)
Box 3757, Lubbock, TX, 79452 (806) 745-1134.
Ray Moran, gen. mgr.; Brad Moran, gen sls. mgr.; Jim Arnold, prog. dir.; Guy Smith, chief eng.; natl. rep.: Seltel.
Operation: January, 1982.

KLBK-TV (Channel 13) CBS, ABC
Charles Woods TV Corp., 7400 University Ave., Lubbock, TX 79408 (806) 744-2345.
Charles Woods, gen. mgr.; David Underwood, sta. mgr.; Larry Lee, sls. mgr.; John Harris, news dir.; Don King, chief eng.; natl. rep.: Blair.
Operation: 1952; TV sets in area: 188,000.

Lufkin

KTRE-TV (Channel 9) ABC
Buford Television Inc. of Lufkin, Box 729, Lufkin, TX 75901 (409) 853-5873.
Tom Ramey, gen. mgr.; Mark Logan, sta. mgr.; nat'l rep.: Katz.
Operation: 1955.

Midland

KMID-TV (Channel 2) ABC
Telepictures Broadcasting Corp., Inc., KMID-TV, Midland, TX 79711 (915) 563-2222.
John Foster, gen. mgr.; John Orr, gen. sls. mgr.; natl. rep.: Katz.
Operation: 1953; TV sets in area: 166,7000.

Monahans

KTPX-TV (Channel 9) ABC
Permian Basin Television Corp., Box 6699, Midland, TX 79711.
Bill Ritchie, gen. mgr.; Diana Dixon, sls. mgr.; Grady Woodward, dir. of eng.; Sandy McIntosh, prog. dir.
Operation: 1958; TV homes in area: 173,800.

Odessa

KOSA-TV (Channel 7) CBS
Forward Communications of Texas, Inc., 1211 N. Whitaker, Odessa, TX 79760 (915) 337-8301.
Doyce Elliott, pres. & gen. mgr.; T. Hughes, v.p. & sta. mgr.; Vic Luddington, natl. sls. mgr.; Ed Costello, local sls. mgr.; Bob Stephens, chief eng.; George Duesler, film dir. ; nat'l rep.: Seltel.
Operation: 1956; TV homes in area: 119,500.

Port Arthur

KJAC-TV (Channel 4) NBC
Southeast Texas Television Corp., P.O. Box 3257, 1748 Woodworth Blvd., Port Arthur, TX 77643 (409) 985-5557.
Geo Diab, pres.; Roy D. Shotts, v.p.-gen. mgr.; Gary Powers, comm. mgr.; Charles Ravell, chief eng.; nat'l rep.: Katz.
Operation: 1957; TV sets in area: 167,000.

San Angelo

KACB-TV (Channel 3) NBC

(Satellite of KRBC-TV, Abilene)

Abilene Radio & TV Co., 4510 14th St., P.O. Box 178, Abilene, TX 79604 (915) 692-4242.

Dale Ackers, pres.; Ken Knox, sta. & sls. mgr.; Jerry Shackelford, prog. dir.; Glen Welch, chief eng.; rep.: Blair TV.

Operation: 1962.

KIDY (Channel 6)

Sage Bcstg. Co., 3901 W. Heimer, Suite 190, Houston, TX 77027.

Raymond Schindler, pres.

Operation: July, 1983.

KLST (Channel 8) CBS

Jewell Television, 2800 Armstrong, San Angelo, TX 76903 (915) 655-7383.

Thomas Gresham, executor; John McGee, gen. mgr.; Gordon Hay, prog. dir. & film buyer; Lou Kordek, news dir.; Eddy Smith, chief eng.; nat'l. rep.: Katz.

Operation: June, 1983; sets in area: 69,900.

San Antonio

KENS-TV (Channel 5) CBS

5400 Fredericksburg Rd., San Antonio, TX 78229; P.O. Box TV5, 78299; (512) 366-5000.

William Moll, pres. bdcst./chm. bd.; Linda Brook, v.p. & gen. mgr.; Dave Sankovich, gen. sls. mgr.; Jerry Nordsiek, chief eng.; natl. rep.: Blair.

Operation: 1950; TV sets in area: 1,112,600.

KMOL-TV (Channel 4) NBC

United TV, Inc., P.O. Box 2641, San Antonio, TX 78205 (512) 226-4251.

Edward V. Cheviot, v.p. & gen. mgr.; Morton A. Barrett, gen. sls. mgr.; Kevin Donohue, lcl. sls. mgr.; Jack Carroll, prog. dir.; Don McMullin, news dir.; David Karbach, dir. of eng.; Bob Garcia, film dir.; rep.: Blair Television.

Operation: 1949; TV homes: 442,300.

KSAT-TV (Channel 12)

Outlet Communications, Inc., Box 2478, San Antonio, TX 78298 (512) 226-7611.

Bruce G. Sundlun, bd. chm. & CEO; David E. Henderson, pres. & COO; James Schiavone, v.p. & gen. mgr.; Rick Andrycha, prog. mgr.

Operation: 1957; TV homes in area: 945,300.

KWEX-TV (Channel 41)

The Spanish International Communications Corp., 411 E. Durango Blvd., San Antonio, TX 78204; (512) 227-4141.

Emilio Nicolas, v.p. & gen. mgr.; Julius Germano, Jr., v.p. & gen. sls. mgr.; Armando Solis, v.p. & bus. mgr.; James Meek, v.p. & chief eng.; Amparo Ortiz, oper. mgr.; Rick Sowa, network oper.

Temple-Waco

KCEN-TV (Channel 6) NBC

Channel 6, Inc., P.O. Box 188, Temple, TX 76501 (817) 773-6868; Waco office, 815 Professional Bldg., Waco, TX 76710 (817) 756-6605; TWX 910-890-4870.

Frank W. Mayborn, pres.; Dan Lesmeister, v.p. & gen. mgr.; Ken Smith, chief eng.; nat'l rep.: Blair TV.

Operation: 1953; TV sets in area: 210,900.

Tyler-Longview

KLTV (Channel 7) NBC, CBS, ABC

Channel 7, Inc., Box 957, Tyler, TX 75710 (214) 592-3871.

Robert P. Buford, Gerald B. & Geoffrey R. Buford, owners; Robert P. Buford, pres.; Frank E. Melton, exec. v.p. & gen. mgr.; Bob Way, chief eng.; Gayle Helms, prog. dir.; nat'l rep.: Katz Agency.

Operation: 1954; TV sets in area: 178,500.

Victoria

KAVU-TV (Channel 25) NBC

Community Bcstg. of Coastal Bend, Inc., Box 4929, Victoria, TX 77903 (512) 576-5288.

Doug McDougal, pres. & gen. mgr.; Bob Hesse, gen. sls. mgr.; Helen Villarreal, prog. dir.; Mike Burch, news dir.; Fred Berrad, tech. eng.; nat'l. rep.: Adam Young.

Operation: July, 1982.

KVCT (Channel 19) ABC

Victoria Communications Corporation, P.O. Box 1879, Victoria, TX 77902.

Dewey T. Acker, pres. & gen. mgr.; K. Layton Miller, gen. sls. mgr.; Doris Littles, prog. dir.; Tom Eastland, news dir.

Operation: 1969.

Waco

KWTX-TV (Channel 10) CBS, ABC

KWTX Broadcasting Company, 4520 Bosque Blvd., P.O. Box 7528, Waco, TX 76710 (817) 776-1330.

M. N. Bostick, pres. & gen. mgr.; Thomas Stribbling, v.p.; Robert Levy, secty.-treas.; John M. Brinegar, sls. mgr.; Barbara DeVeny, natl-regl. sls. contact; Jesse Dove, chief eng.; Ralph Webb, prog. dir.; nat'l rep.: H-R Television, Inc.

Operation: 1955; TV sets in area: 204,300.

Weslaco

KRGV-TV (Channel 5) ABC

Mobile Video Tapes, Inc., 900 E. Expressway Avenue, Weslaco, TX 78596 (512) 968-5555.

Douglas L. Manship, pres.; Ray Alexander, gen. mgr.; Jim Cook, lcl. sls. mgr.; Larry Taylor, gen. sls. mgr.; Julian Adame, prgm. dir.; Rick Diaz, news dir.; nat'l rep.: Blair Television.

Operation: 1954; TV sets in area: 218,000.

Wichita Falls

KAUZ-TV (Channel 6) CBS

Adams TV of Wichita Falls, P.O. Box 2130, Wichita Falls, TX 76307.

Hal Sundberg, gen. mgr.; Leon S. Hoeffner, chief eng.; nat'l. rep.: Blair Television.

KFDX-TV (Channel 3) NBC

Clay Broadcasting Corp. of Texas; Box 4000, Wichita Falls, TX 76308 (817) 692-4530.

Lyell Clay, chmn.; George Diab, pres.; John McGee, secty-treas.; Warren Silver, gen. mgr.; Tom Witherspoon, oper. mgr.; Chuck Howard, gen. sales mgr.; William Enloe, dir. of eng.; Peggy Edgar, film ed.; nat'l rep.: Katz.

Operation: 1953; TV sets in area: 250,000.

KJTL (Channel 18)

Thornberry TV Ltd., Box 4865, Wichita Falls, TX 76308 (817) 691-1808.

Max M. Andrews, pres., gen. mgr., prog. dir. & film buyer; Peter D'Acosta, stn. mgr.; Nancy Andrus, prom. mgr.; Karen Dickins, sls. mgr.; William A. Barber, chief eng.; natl. rep.: Seltel.

Operation: May, 1985.

UTAH

Salt Lake City

KSL-TV (Channel 5) CBS

KSL, Inc., Broadcast House, Salt Lake City, UT 84180 (801) 575-5500.

Jay W. Lloyd, pres. & gen. mgr.; William R. Murdock, v.p., gen. sls. mgr.; Alan Henderson, v.p.-mktg.; J. Talmage Ball, chief eng.; J. Spencer Kinard, v.p./news dir.; David Manookin, dir. prog.; nat'l rep.: Petry

Operation: 1949; TV homes in area: 841,900.

KSTU (Channel 20)

Adams TV of Salt Lake City, Inc., 5020 W. Amelia Earhart Dr., Salt Lake City, UT 84116 (801) 539-1220.

Vickie Street, gen. mgr./prog. dir.; Susan Adams, natl. sls. mgr.; Bonnie Nangle, lcl. sls. mgr.; natl. rep.: Blair.

Operation: 1978.

KTVX (Channel 4) ABC

United TV, Inc., 1760 Fremont Dr., Minneapolis, MN 84104.

Evan Thompson, pres.; David J. Woodcock, v.p. & gen. mgr.; Robert Galle, gen. sls. mgr.; Gordon Acker, prog. dir.; Handy Hoffman, promo. mgr.; Jim McDermaid, tech dir.

Operation: 1948; TV sets in area: 548,400.

KUTV (Channel 2) NBC

KUTV Inc., 2185 S. 3600 West, Salt Lake City, UT 84119 (801) 973-3000.

George C. Hatch, pres.; Al Seethaler, v.p. & gen. mgr.; John Mason, prog. dir.; Dick Thiriot, film buyer, nat'l rep.: katz.

Operation: 1954; TV set in area: 771,200.

VERMONT

Burlington

WCAX-TV (Channel 3) CBS

Mt. Mansfield Television, Inc., 100 Market Sq., Burlington, VT 05451 (802) 862-5761.

S. T. Martin, pres., gen. mgr. & prog. dir.; Phil Waterman, v.p. & gen. sls. mgr.; Stuart Hall, v.p. & prod. mgr.; Peter R. Martin, v.p., news-pub. affairs; Charles Liese, chief eng.; A. Sherman Rutter, film mgr.; nat'l rep., Avery-Knodel, Inc.

Operation: 1954; TV sets in area: U.S. 150,000, Canada 270,000.

WVNY-TV (Channel 22) ABC

Champlain Communications Corp., 100 Market Square, Burlington, VT 05401 (802) 658-8022.

Philip J. Lombardo, pres./gen. mgr.; William Bradley, sta. mgr./v.p.; George Rousseau, dir. bdct. opns.; Greg O'Connor, lcl. sls. mgr.; Ralph McClintock, chief eng.

Operation: 1968.

Hartford-Hanover

WNNE-TV (Channel 31)

WNNE-TV, Inc., Box 906, White River Junction, VT 05001 (802) 295-3100.

Charles E. Webb, gen. mgr.; Brad Worthen, sls. mgr.; Dave French, dir. of eng.; Mike Harding, news & ops. dir.

Operation: 1978.

VIRGINIA

Bristol

WCYB-TV (Channel 5) NBC, ABC

Appalachian Broadcasting Corporation, 101 Lee St., Bristol, VA 24201 (703) 669-4161.

Robert H. Smith, Jr., v.p. & gen. mgr.; Jack Shaver, v.p. sls.; Echel Edens, chief eng.; Charles Lineberger, prog. mgr.; Sandhi Kozsuch, dir. prod./creative svcs.; Steve Hawkins, news dir.; natl. rep.: Katz.

Operation: 1956; TV sets in area: 1,100,900.

Charlottesville

WVIR-TV (Channel 29) NBC

Virginia Broadcasting Corp., P.O. Box 769, Charlottesville, VA 22902 (804) 977-7082.

Lloyd T. Smith, Jr., pres.; Harold B. Wright, Jr., v.p. & gen. mgr.; Jim Fernald, gen. sls. mgr.

Operation: March, 1973; TV households: 82,000.

Hampton-Norfolk

WVEC-TV (Channel 13) ABC

1930 E. Pembroke Ave., Hampton, VA 23663; 613 Woodis Ave., Norfolk, VA 23510; (804) 625-1313.

J. William Beindorf, v.p. & gen. mgr.; Rick Keilty, gen. sls. mgr.; Meyer Davis, opns. & prog. mgr.; Cil Frazier, adv./promo. mgr.; Dick Cannon, chief eng.; natl. rep.: Petry.

Operation: 1953; TV sets in area: 502,900.

Harrisonburg

WHSV-TV (Channel 3) ABC

Shenandoah Valley Television Systems, Inc. P.O. Box TV 3, Highway 33 West, Harrisonburg, VA 22801 (703) 433-9191.

Michael Lennon, gen. mgr.; Bob Bolyaro, lcl. sls. mgr.; Christopher Jones, opns. mgr.; Bill Clausius, news dir.; David Orr, chief eng.

Operation: 1953; TV households: 293,500.

Lynchburg

WSET-TV (Channel 13) ABC

WSET, Inc. 2320 Langhorne Rd., P.O. Box 11588, Lynchburg, VA 24506 (804) 528-1313.

David F. McAtee, pres. & gen. mgr.; Beve Lutz, business mgr., Jack Tackett, v.p. & sls. mgr.; Willis Little, chief eng.; nat'l rep.: Katz Agency.

Operation: 1953; TV households in area: 350,630.

Manassas

WTKK (Channel 66)

National Capital Christian Broadcasting, Inc., 9008 Center St., Manassas, VA 22110 (703) 369-3400.

Lester R. Raker, pres.; John Parker, chief eng.; Lynda Drane, traffic mgr.

Operation: 1978.

Norfolk

WTKR-TV (Channel 3) CBS

WTKR-TV, Inc., 720 Boush St., Norfolk, VA 23510 (804) 446-1000.

Thomas F. Hartman, pres.; Joe Perkins, dir. of opns.; Bob McCall, sta. mgr.; Jim Graham, gen. sls. mgr.; Marti Daughtry, promo. coord.; Lou Paris, dir. of news; Julie McCollum, dir. of community affairs/personnel; Gene Gildow, dir. of eng..

Operation: 1950; TV sets in area: 485,900.

WTVZ (Channel 33)

TV Corp. of Virginia, Box 148, Norfolk, VA 23501 (804) 622-3333.

Richard Kitelyn, v.p. & gen. sls. mgr.; Timothy Lynch, gen. mgr.

Operation: 1979.

Norfolk-Portsmouth-Newport News

WAVY-TV (Channel 10) NBC

WAVY Television, Inc. (Division of LIN Broadcasting Corporation), 801 Wavy St., Portsmouth, VA 23704 (804) 393-1010.

Mike McGrew, pres. & gen. mgr.; Bill Logan, sta. mgr.; Jack Paris, gen. sls. mgr.; Paul Hecht, chief eng.; nat'l rep: Blair Television.

Operation: 1957.

Portsmouth

WYAH-TV (Channel 27)

CBN-Continental Broadcasting Network, Box 1338, Portsmouth, VA 23704 (804) 393-2501.

M. G. Robertson, pres.; Thomas Smith, v.p. & gen. mgr.; Ken Reichenbach, chief eng.; David Whitener, prog. mgr.; Larry Harris, prod. mgr.; Harry Styles, mgr., p.r.

Operation: 1961; TV homes in area: 535,000.

Richmond

WRLH-TV (Channel 35)

TV Corp. of Richmond, 1925 Westmoreland St., Richmond, VA 23230 (804) 359-3510.

Tim McDonald, pres.; Stephen M. Peskin, v.p. & gen. mgr.; Brendell Dezivra, gen. sls. mgr.; Jim Jacobs, prog. dir. & prom. mgr.; Jim Dugger, chief eng.; nat'l. rep.: Seltel.

Operation: February, 1982.

WTVR (Channel 6) CBS

Roy H. Park Broadcasting of Virginia, Inc., 3301 W. Broad St., P.O. Box 11064, Richmond, VA 23201 (804) 254-3600.

Ronald W. Philips, exec. v.p. & gen. mgr.; Richard Pegram, gen. sls. mgr.; Wanda Lewis, lcl. sls. mgr.; Bill Vay Scyoe, chief eng.; Terry Bynum, news dir.; Natl. rep.: Blair-TV, Inc.

Operation: 1948; TV sets in area: 665,900.

WWBT (Channel 12) NBC

Jefferson Pilot Broadcasting Company of Virginia, P.O. Box 12, 5710 Midlothian Pike, Richmond, VA 23201 (804) 233-5461.

W. J. Jorgenson, pres.; John H. Hutchinson, Jr., v.p. & gen. mgr.; Ellen Shulu, gen. sales mgr.; Dave Frasier, tech. op. mgr.; Rae Maupin, prgrm./oper. mgr.; nat'l rep.: Petry.

Operation: 1956; TV sets in area: 498,700.

Richmond-Petersburg

WXEX-TV (Channel 8) ABC

Nationwide Communications, Inc. 21 Buford Rd., Richmond, VA 23235 (804) 320-3201.

H. Joseph Lewin, gen. mgr.; Joe Killigrew, natl. sls. mgr.; Gene Walsh, prgm. dir.; Dan Vanko, chief eng.; nat'l rep.: Katz.

Operation: 1955.

Roanoke

WDBJ-TV (Channel 7) CBS

WDBJ Television, Inc. Mailing Address: P.O. Box 7, Roanoke, VA 24022; Street Address: 2001 Colonial Ave., S.W., Roanoke, VA 24015 (703) 344-7000.

C. H. McKeever, pres. & gen. mgr.; Kay Hall, prog. dir.; Tom Burkhart, dir.–sls. mktg.; Carl Guffey, dir. of opns.; Lorraine Snebold, promo. dir.; Al Dyson, chief eng.; nat'l rep.: Harrington, Righter & Parsons, Inc.

Operation: 1955; TV homes in area: 985,100.

WEFC (Channel 38)

612 Bullitt Ave., S.E., Roanoke, VA 24013.

C. Kenneth Wright, pres.; R.B. Stewart, Sr., gen. mgr.; E.T. Griffis, prog. dir.; Andrew Wright, chief eng.

Operation: November, 1984.

WSLS-TV (Channel 10) NBC

Roy H. Park Broadcasting of Roanoke, Inc., Church Ave. & Third Street, Roanoke, VA 24011 (703) 981-9110.

W. Randy Odil, v.p./gen. mgr.; Pete Watkins, gen. sls. mgr.; Mike Berkey, chief eng.; nat'l rep.: Blair TV.

Operation: 1952; TV sets in area: 680,900.

WASHINGTON

Bellingham

KVOS-TV (Channel 12) CBS

KVOS Television Corp., 1151 Ellis St., Bellingham, WA 98225 (206) 671-1212.

William Brazzil, pres.; Frank Jank, v.p. & gen. mgr.; John Price, chief eng.; Doug Davis, sls. mgr.; nat'l rep.: Adam Young, (U.S.); Metrospot (Canada).

Operation: 1953; TV sets in area: 1,250,000.

Pasco

KEPR-TV (Channel 19) CBS

Satellite of KIMA-TV, Yakima, WA)

NWG Broadcasting Co., P.O. Box 702, Yakima, WA 98907 (509) 452-9111.

John J. Noel, Jr., pres.; Dale Hazen, gen. mgr.; Dale Hall, sta. mgr.; Mike Rastovich, dir. of eng.; nat'l rep.: HR Television, Inc.; northwest: Art Moore & Associates, Inc.

Operation: 1954; TV sets in area: 334,400.

Richland-Pasco-Kennewick

KNDU (Channel 25) NBC

(Associated with KNDO, Yakima, WA)

Columbia Empire Broadcasting Corp., 1608 S. 24th Ave., Yakima, WA 98901; P.O. Box 2523, Tri-Cities, WA 99302 (509) 783-6151.

Hugh E. David, pres.; Elliott Kleeman, gen. mgr. & film buyer; Lee Maddon, gen. sls. & sta. mgr.; David Lloyd, news dir.; Ed Lyon, chief eng.; natl. rep.: Katz.

Operation: 1961.

KVEW (Channel 42) ABC

(A Satellite of KAPP, Yakima, WA)

Apple Valley Broadcasting, Inc., 601 N. Edison, Kennewick, WA 99336 (509) 735-8369.

Gary Pierone, v.p. & gen. mgr.; J. Marcus Wood, sta. mgr.; John McDaniel, chief eng.
Operation: 1970.

Seattle

KCPQ (Channel 13)

Kelly TV Co., Box 98829, 4400 Steilacoom Blvd., SW, Tacoma, WA 98499 (206) 582-8613.
Robert E. Kelly, gen. mgr.; Thomas French, bus. mgr.; Roy Albertson, gen. sls. mgr.; Dan Jensen, opns. dir.; Robert Galvin, prom. mgr.; Steve Hess, news dir.; Lee Pinski, chief eng.; nat'l. rep.: Seltel.
Operation: 1954.

KING-TV (Channel 5) NBC

King Broadcasting Co., 320 Aurora Avenue North, Seattle, WA 98109 (206) 223-5000.
Ancil H. Payne, pres.; Payson Hall, v.p., finance & planning; Jim Kime, v.p. op. & dev.; George V. Willoughby, Jr., v.p. & cor. cnl.; John Orose, treas.; Eric S. Bremner, v.p. & gen. mgr.; Robert Guy, prog. dir.) Don LaCombe, prod. dir.; Linda Clark, oper. dir.; Norm Heffron, news dir.; Emory Bundy, pub. affairs dir.; Nancy Gullick, promo. dir.; Sturges Dorrance, sls. mgr.; Jack Shawcroft, chief eng.; nat'l rep.: Blair TV, Inc.
Operation: 1948; TV sets in area: 941,600.

KIRO-TV (Channel 7) CBS

KIRO, Inc., Broadcast House, Third & Broad, Seattle, WA. 98121 (206) 624-7077.
Kenneth L. Hatch, pres.; Al F. Mladenich, sen. v.p.; Glenn C. Wright, v.p. & sta. mgr.; Michael Poth, local sls. mgr.; Charles Morris, eng. dir.; Judy Law, prog. dir.; natl. rep.: Petry Television, Inc.
Operation: February, 1958; TV households: 976,800.

KOMO-TV (Channel 4) ABC

Fisher Broadcasting Inc., 100 Fourth Ave., N., Seattle WA 98109.
W. W. Warren, chm., Fisher Bdcstg.; John F. Behnke, pres. & CEDO, Fisher; Jay W. Giesa, exec. v.p./bdcstg., Seattle; Monty D. Grau, v.p. & gen. mgr., KOMO; Patrick M. Scott, v.p. & sta. mgr.; Don Wilkinson, dir. of eng.; Fisher; Ed J. Lackner, v.p., corporate affairs, Fisher; nat'l rep.: The Katz Agency.
Operation: 1953; TV sets in area: 1,133,700.

KTZZ-TV (Channel 22)

Alden Television, 945 Dexter Ave., N., Seattle, WA 98109 (206) 282-2202.
Ted Minsky, pres.; Dean H. Woodring, v.p./gen. mgr.; Terri Williams, stn. & natl. sls. mgr.; Bill Hall, prog. dir. & film buyer; Cathy Keller, prom. mgr.; Sandy DeLainey, lcl. sls. mgr.; Karl Paulsen, chief eng.; natl. rep.: Seltel.
Operation: June, 1985.

Spokane

KAYU-TV (Channel 28)

KAYU-TV Partners, Ltd., Box 8115, Spokane, WA 99203 (509) 448-2828.
Robert Hamacher, gen. mgr. & film buyer; Lane Guinn, gen. sls. mgr.; Mark Flaherty, film buyer; Louise Hanson, promo. mgr.; Ronald Valley, eng. dir.; natl. rep.: TeleRep.
Operation: October, 1982.

KHQ-TV (Channel 6) NBC

KHQ, Inc., 4202 S. Regal, Spokane, WA 99203 (509) 448-4666.
J. Birney Blair, pres. & gen. mgr.; Robt. L. Busse, contr.; John V. Reber, v.p., gen. sls. mgr.; Scott Eymer, lcl. sls. mgr.; Michael Gee, sls. mgr.; Larry W. Gants, dir. prog. & promo.; Don Carmichael, opns. mgr.; William Isbel, chief eng.; natl. rep.: Katz Agency.
Operation: 1952; TV sets in area: 528,800 ARB.

KREM-TV (Channel 2) CBS

King Broadcasting Co., S-4103 Regal St., Spokane, WA 99203 (509) 448-2000.
Dennis Williamson, v.p. & gen. mgr.; John Rowland, sls. mgr.; Meg Antonius, prog. dir.; Warren P. Pritchard, chief eng.; nat'l rep.: Blair.
Operation: 1954; TV sets in area: 393,200.

KXLY-TV (Channel 4) ABC

KXLY-TV (Spokane Television, Inc.) W. 500 Boone Ave., Spokane, WA 99201 (509) 328-9084.
Elizabeth M. Burns, pres.; Stephen R. Herling, v.p. & gen. mgr.; Darrel Blue, opns. mgr.; Ted Bravakis, sls. mgr.; Don Pope, chief eng.; nat'l rep: HRP.
Operation: 1953; TV sets in area: 358,600.

KZZS-TV (Channel 22)

Spokane Ltd. Partnership, East 4022 Broadway, Spokane, WA 99202 (509) 534-5756.
Lee Schulman, pres. & gen. mgr.; Dick Wagschal, gen. sls. mgr.; Robert Wyatt, chief eng.; nat'l. rep.: Seltel.
Operation: December, 1983.

Tacoma

KSTW (Channel 11)

Gaylord Bdg. Co., Box 11411, Tacoma, WA 98411 (206) 572-5789.
Charles Edwards, v.p. & gen. mgr.; Bob Hamacher, gen. sls. mgr.; Paul Crittenden, chief eng.
Operation: 1953; TV households: 1,038,500.

KTBW-TV (Channel 20)

Trinity Bcstg. of Washington, 1909 W. 341 St., Tacoma, WA 98003 (206) 927-7720.
Paul F. Crouch, pres.; Paul A. Gray, gen. mgr.; Kenneth Hydron, acting chief eng.
Operation: March, 1984.

Vancouver

KPDX (Channel 49)

Columbia River TV, Inc., One Columbia River, Vancouver, WA 98660 (206) 254-4949.
Jack F. Matranga, pres.; Edward C. Branca, sta. mgr.; Ray Heacox, gen. sls. mgr.; Denny Moore, prog. dir.; Bob Nelson, chief eng.
Operation: October, 1983.

Yakima

KAPP (Channel 35)

Apple Valley Bcstg. Co., 1610 South 24th Ave., Yakima, WA 98902 (509) 453-0351.
Wayne McNulty, v.p.; R. Scott Marriner, sta. mgr.; Paul Bateman, chief eng.; T. O. Jorgenson, eng. supvr.; Bob Ivers, news dir.; rep.: Peters, Griffin, Woodward, Inc.
Operation: September, 1970; TV households: 148,700.

KIMA-TV (Channel 29) CBS

NWG Broadcasting Co., P.O. Box 702, Yakima, WA 98907 (509) 575-0029. Affiliated stations: KEPR-TV, Pasco, WA; KLEW-TV, Lewiston, ID.

John J. Noel, Jr., pres.; Dale Hazen, gen. mgr.; Stu Seibel, prog. dir.; Mike Rastovich, dir. of eng.; nat'l rp.: Selter; Pacific Northwest, Art Moore & Associates, Inc.

Operation: 1953; TV sets in area 768,900.

KNDO (Channel 23) NBC

(Operates associated station KNDU, Richland-Pasco-Kenewick, WA)

Columbia Empire Broadcasting Corp., 1608 S. 24th Ave., Box 10028, Yakima, WA 98909 (509) 248-2300.

Hugh E. Davis, pres.; Scott Hayner, gen. mgr.; Ben Shronshire, natl. sls. mgr.; Ronald Krons, eng'. dir.; Opal Laurent, compt., office mgr.; Larry Baker, news dir.

Operation: 1959.

WEST VIRGINIA

Bluefield

WVVA (Channel 6) NBC

WVVA Television, Inc., 130-138 S. Fifth St., Quincy, IL 62301 (304) 325-5487.

Al Marra, gen. mgr.; Erlene Branch, pgm. dir.; Jack De Lisi, sls. mgr.; Kenneth Dick, chief eng.; natl. rep.: Avery-Knodel.

Operation: 1955; TV sets in area: 635,700.

Charleston

WCHS-TV (Channel 8) CBS

WCHS AM-TV Corp., 1111 Virginia St. E., Charleston, WV (304) 346-5358.

O. Wayne Rollins, bd. chm.; R. Randall Rollins, pres.; Robert O. Paxson, gen. mgr.; Jo Corey, prog. mgr.; Dennis Adkins, gen. sls. mgr.; Robert Roush, chief eng.; Richard Cantner, news dir.; nat'l rep.: Petry.

Operation: 1954.

WVAH-TV (Channel 23)

W.V. Telecasting, Inc., 23 Broadcast Plaza, Hurricane, WV 25526 (304) 757-8823.

Albert M. Holtz, pres.; Gary Dreispul, sta. mgr.; William White, gen. sls. mgr.; George Panicza, chief eng.

Operation: September, 1982.

Clarksburg

WBOY-TV (Channel 12)

912 West Pike Street, Clarksburg, WV 26301 (304) 623-3311.

B. Imes, pres.; Stan Siegel, v.p. & gen. mgr.; Joe Wright, chief eng.; nat'l rep.: Seltel.

Operation: 1957.

WLYJ (Channel 46)

Christian Communication Center, 775 West Pike St., Clarksburg, West VA 26302 (304) 623-5784.

Joseph Rose, pres.; Jack L. Kincaid, mgr.; Wayne Fast, chief eng.

Operation: February, 1981.

Huntington-Charleston

WOWK-TV (Channel 13) ABC

Gateway Communications, Inc., 625 Fourth Ave., Huntington, WV 25701 (304) 525-7661.

Leo M. MacCourtney, v.p. & gen. mgr.; Paul N. Dicker, prog. dir.; Billie Sue Graybeal, natl. sls. mgr.; Mike Ferko, lcl. sls. mgr.; Jacqui Mullen, news dir.; Robert Willis, promo. dir.; Charles Goode, chief eng.; sls. rep.: Blair TV.

Operation: October, 1955; TV households: 877,300.

WSAZ-TV (Channel 3) NBC

Lee Enterprises, Inc., 645 Fifth Avenue, Huntington, WV 25701 (304) 697-4780.

Lloyd G. Schermer, pres. & treas.; George R. Andrick, sr. mgr.; Howard Kennedy, gen. mgr.; Harold B. Hall, sls. mgr.; Ron Ray, natl. sls. mgr.; Robert Harris, Charleston operations mgr.; George M. Curry, prog. dir.; Loren Tohia, news dir.; John P. Clay, chief eng.

Operation: 1949; TV sets in area: 684,700.

Oak Hill

WOAY-TV (Channel 4) ABC, Primary

Thomas Broadcasting Co., Box 251, Oak Hill, WV 25901 (304) 469-3361.

Robert R. Thomas III, pres.; Curtis W. Butler, v.p. & gen. mgr.; Don Watkins, prod. mgr.; Bob Cannon, oper. mgr.; nat'l. rep.: Katz.

Operation: 1954; TV sets in area: 377,820.

Parkersburg

WTAP (Channel 15) NBC

Benedek Broadcasting Inc., 121 W. 7th St., Parkersburg, WV 26102 (304) 485-4588.

Sherman A. Grimm, gen. mgr.; Glenn Wilson, prog. dir.; Charles Helmick, chief engineer; nat'l rep.: Seltel.

Operation: 1953; TV households in area: 70,620.

Weston-Clarksburg

WDTV (Channel 5) CBS

Withers Broadcasting Co. of WV P.O. Box 480, Bridgeport, WV 26330 (304) 842-3558.

W. Russell Withers, Jr., Pres.; Dusty Wayman, gen. mgr.; Nick Pelligrin, prog. dir. & traffic dir.; rep.: Avery-Knodel.

Operation: 1960; TV households, 798,200.

Wheeling

WTRF-TV (Channel 7) NBC, ABC

96 16th St., Wheeling, WV 26003 (304) 232-7777.

Charles E. Sherman, pres./gen. mgr.; Robert McFarland, chief eng.; George Carroll, oper. mgr.; Frank Curtis, v.p., asst. gen. mgr./sls. mgr.; Jim Squibb, lcl. sls. mgr.; William Ney, film dir.; Pat Gaughan, pub. affairs dir.; Don Murdock, continuity dir.; Janice Webster, promo. dir.; George Caroll, prog. dir.; Mark Davis, news dir.

Operation: 1953; TV sets in area: 523,000.

WISCONSIN

Appleton

WXGZ-TV (Channel 32)

Appleton Midwestern TV Ltd., 3025 N. Marshall Rd., Appleton, WI 45915 (414) 731-3232.

Bill Le Monds, gen. mgr.; Mark J. Jollie, gen. sls. mgr.; Sam Hutchison, prog. dir.; Art Hook, film buyer; Jim Radman, chief eng.

Operation: December, 1983.

Eau Claire

WEAU-TV (Channel 13) NBC

WEAU-TV Inc., 1907 South Hastings Way, Eau Claire, WI 54701.

Clark Wideman, gen. mgr.; Dick Dionne, opr. mgr.; Robert Fallis, chief eng.; nat'l rep.: Seltel; Hurley Co. (Minneapolis).

Operation: 1953; TV households: 421,640.

WQOW-TV (Channel 18) ABC

(A satellite of WXOW-TV, LaCrosse, WI) TAK Communications, Inc., 2881 S. Hastings Way, Eau Claire, WI 54701 (715) 835-1881.

Chuck Roth, gen. mgr.; Bill Anderson, opns. mgr.; Dave White, chief eng.; Bob Braun, sls. mgr.; Dick Hoffman, news dir.

Operation: 1980.

Greenbay

WBAY-TV (Channel 2) CBS

A division of Nationwide Communications Inc., 115 So. Jefferson St., Green Bay, WI 54301 (414) 432-3331.

Ted Kohl, gen. mgr.; Gary Andrich, gen. sls. mgr.; Richard Millhiser, prog. dir.; nat'l rep.: Blair, Inc.

Operation: 1953; TV sets in area: 707,700.

WFRV-TV (Channel 5) ABC

WFRV Inc., P.O. Box 19055, Green Bay, WI 54307 (414) 437-5411.

Robert B. Forrow, gen. mgr.; Mitch Lambert, gen. sls. mgr.; Mike O'Rourke, dir. opns. & prog.; Harry Hill, chief eng.; nat'l rep.: TeleRep.

Operation: 1955; TV households in area: 485,040.

WGBA (Channel 26) IND

TV 26 Inc., Box 26, 1145 Pine St., Green Bay, WI 54305 (414) 437-2626.

Robb Gray, gen. sls. mgr.; Hal Pontius, prog. dir.; William Cole, prom. dir.; Larry Burbey, chief eng.; natl. rep.: Avery Knodel.

Operation: 1980.

WLUK-TV (Channel 11) NBC

WLUK-TV, Inc., P.O. Box 19011, Green Bay, WI 54307 (414) 494-8711; TWX 910 263-1267.

Phil Nye, gen. mgr.; Rob Krieghoff, gen. sls. mgr.; Maryann Wiedemann, prgm. mgr.; Jim Steffey, chief eng.; nat'l rep.: HPR.

Operation: 1954.

LaCrosse

WKBT (Channel 8) CBS

Gross Telecasting of Wisconsin, Inc., 141 So. 6th St., La Crosse WI 54601 (608) 782-4678.

Peter S. Good, vice president & gen. mgr.; Edith S. Harris, natl. sls. mgr.; Al Leeman, chief eng.; nat'l rep.: Avery-Knodel, Inc.; Harry S. Hyett Co.—Rameland, Inc. (Minneapolis).

Operation: 1954; TV homes: 241,100 (NSI).

WXOW-TV (Channel 19) ABC

(Satellite of WKOW-TV, Madison, WI)

TAK Communications, Wisconsin TV Network Associates, P.O. Box 100, Madison, WI 53701.

Sharad Tak, gen. partner; William Gayman, v.p.; rep.: H-R Television; Katz.

Operation: March, 1970; TV households: 151,400.

Madison

WISC-TV (Channel 3) CBS

7025 Raymond Road, Madison, WI 53711 (608) 271-4321.

Elizabeth Murphy Burns, pres.; Gary DeHaven, gen. mgr.; Donna Kirner, natl. sls. mgr.; Curt Lundgren, chief eng.; nat'l rep.: HRP.

Operation: 1956; TV sets in area: 635,000.

WKOW-TV (Channel 27) ABC

TAK Communications, Wisconsin TV Network Associates, 5727 Tokay Blvd., Madison WI 53701 (608) 274-1234.

Sharad Tak, pres.; Phillip Keller, gen. mgr.; nat'l rep.: Katz Agency.

Operation: 1953; TV households in area: 194,800.

WMTV (Channel 15) NBC

Forward Television Inc., 615 Forward Dr., Madison, WI 53711 (608) 274-1515.

Laurie Leonard, pres. & gen. mgr.; Fred Sole, opns. mgr.

Operation: 1953; TV households in area: 203,000.

Milwaukee

WCGV-TV (Channel 24)

B&F Broadcasting, Inc., 5445 N. 27th St., Milwaukee, WI 53209 (414) 527-2424.

James P. Behling, v.p./gen. mgr.; Mitch Nye, gen. sls. mgr.; Betty Hertz, prog. mgr.; Larry Drydyk, chief eng.; natl. rep.: Katz.

Operation: 1980.

WISN-TV (Channel 12) ABC

WISN Division—The Hearst Corp., 759 No. 19 St., Milwaukee, WI 53233 (414) 342-8812.

C. Wayne Godsey, v.p. & gen. mgr.; Rick Henry, gen. sls. mgr.; John Stewart, natl. sls. mgr.; Thomas Gaertner, lcl. sls. mgr.; Eric Stearman, prod. mgr.; Stan Marinoff, dir. of bdcst. ops.; Tim Morrisey, news dir.; James Wagner, promo. mgr.; Noel Enders, resident cont.

Operation: 1954; TV sets in area: 675,600.

WITI-TV (Channel 6) CBS

Storer Broadcasting Co., 9001 North Green Bay Road, Milwaukee, WI 53209 (414) 355-6666.

Andrew P. Potos, vice-pres. & gen. mgr.; Raymond Engelhart, bus. mgr.; Allen Haushalter, prog. dir.; Robert Truscott, dir. of eng.; Donald Roering, chief eng.; Ted Sidelko, promo. mgr.

Operation: 1956; TV sets in area: 1,380,400.

WTMJ-TV (Channel 4) NBC

WTVM Inc., 720 East Capitol Drive, Milwaukee, WI 53201 (414) 332-9611.

Michael McCormick, pres.; Wayne Barnett, v.p. & gen. mgr.; Norb Ryan, gen. sls. mgr.; Mark Le Grand, lcl. sls. mgr.; James Wulliman, mgr. of eng.; Gerald McGrath, prgm. mgr.; Ed Hinshaw, ed. dir. & mgr. of pub. affairs; Tom Luljak, news dir.; Mike Stutz, mng. editor; Gerry Skowronski, film supvr.; Rod Synnes, comm. rel. dir.

Operation: 1947; TV households in area: 700,000.

WVTV (Channel 18)

Gaylord Broadcasting Co., P.O. Box 1818, Millwaukee, WI 53201 (414) 442-7050.

Mike Schuch, gen. mgr.; Al Leitl, asst. gen. mgr. & gen. sls. mgr.; Tom Chiakulus, prod. mgr.; Lori Wucherer, promo.

mgr.; William Witt, chief eng.; Bill Franks, prog. dir.; rep.: Telerep.
Operation: 1966; TV homes: 694,400.

Rhinelander (Wausau)

WAEO-TV (Channel 12) NBC

Northland TV Inc., Box 858, Rhinelander, WI 54501 (715) 369-4700.

Dr. Jasper F. Williams, M.D., bd. chm. John W. Swain, pres.; Carl R. Hilstrom, asst. v.p.; & gen. mgr.; Ned Westman, chief eng.; rep.: Spot Time Ltd.

Operation: 1966; TV homes in area: 230,000.

Wausau

WAOW-TV (Channel 9) ABC

(Outlet of The Wisc. TV Network)

Horizons Communication Corp. of Wis., 1908 Grand Ave., Wausau WI 54401 (715) 842-2251.

Terry Shockley, exec. v.p.; Bruce Liljegren, gen. mgr.; Dennis Lerch, op. mgr.; Don Stenz, chief eng.; rep.: Katz Television.

Operation: 1965; TV households: 170,310.

WSAW-TV (Channel 7) CBS

Forward Communications Corp., 1114 Grand Ave., Wausau, WI 54401 (715) 845-4211.

Richard D. Dudley, chmn./pres., Forward Comm.; Bart Kellenhauser, pres. WSAW-TV; Gene R. Anderson, sr. v.p., finance; Bill Jones, lcl. sls. mgr.; Jack Crowley, v.p., prog.; Mark Zelich, v.p., news; Joe Kamenick, chief eng.; natl. rep.: Seltel.

Operation: 1954.

WYOMING

Casper

KCWY-TV (Channel 14) CBS

Chrysostom Corp., Box 170, Casper, WY 82602 (307) 234-1111.

Robert J. Zipay, v.p. & gen. mgr.; Peter Sieler, gen. sls. & pgm. mgr.

Operation: 1980.

KTWO-TV (Channel 2) NBC, ABC, CBS

Harriscope Broadcasting Corp., 4200 E. Second Street, Casper, WY 82601 (307) 237-3711.

Burt I. Harris, pres.; Jack Rosenthal, exec. v.p.; Bob Price, v.p. and gen. mgr.; Steve Broomell, chief eng.; Byron Dunbar, film dir.; Dave Borino, prog. dir.; Debbie Hales, traffic dir.; nat'l rep.: Katz; regional rep.: Jonn McGuire, Denver.

Operation: 1957; TV homes in area: 109,200.

KXWY (Channel 20) ABC, NBC

Channel 20 Casper, Inc., 7020 Salt Creek Hwy., Casper, WY 82601 (307) 237-2020.

A.J. Stanton, pres.; Pete Sieler, gen. mgr.; Tracy Lee, news dir.; Don J. Powers, chief eng.; natl. rep.: Avery Knodel, Bob Hix Co.

Operation: October, 1984.

Cheyenne

KLWY (Channel 1 27)

Heart of Wyoming TV, Inc., 7020 Salt Creek Rte., Box 5, Casper, WY 82601 (307) 237-2020.

Daniel Burke, pres.; Peter C. Sieler, gen. mgr.; natl. rep.: Adam Young.

Operation: December, 1985.

KYCU-TV (Channel 5) CBS, ABC, NBC

Burke Broadcasting of Cheyenne, 2923 East Lincolnway, Cheyenne, WY; 82601 (307) 634-7755.

Jack R. Donahue, v.p. & gen. mgr.; Dusty Thein, gen. sls. mgr.; John Field, news dir.; nat'l rep.: Katz.

Operation: 1954; TV sets in area: 82,776.

Lander

KOWY (Channel 5) ABC, CBS

Chrysostom Corp., Box 170, Lander, WY 82601 (307) 234-1111.

Daniel Burke, pres.; Peter Sieler, sta. mgr. & film buyer; Mike Sullivan, prom. mgr.; Bea Birch, news dir.; Louie Tsyuer, chief eng.; nat'l. rep.: Seltel, Hix.

Operation: September, 1982.

Riverton-Worland-Thermopolis-Lander

KFWY-TV (Channel 10) NBC

Hi-Ho Broadcasting of Wyoming, 7020 Salt Creek Rd., Box 5, Casper, WY (307) 237-2020.

Peter G. Sieler, gen. mgr.

Operation: 1980; Households: 17,800.

Rock Springs

KWWY (Channel 13) CBS

Chrysostom Corp., Box 170 Rock Springs, WY 82601 (307) 234-1111.

Daniel Burke, pres.; Peter Sieler, gen. mgr.; Mike Sullivan, promo. mgr.; natl. rep.: Seltel.

Operation: 1977.

Sheridan

KSGW-TV (Channel 12) ABC

(A satellite of KOTA-TV, Rapid City, SD) Duhamel Broadcasting Enterprises, Box 1760, Rapid City, SD 57709.

Personnel: See KOTA-TV, Rapid City, SD

Operation: 1977.

Public Broadcasting Service Station Affiliates

Alabama
Birmingham . . . . . WBIQ
Cheaha State Park . . . . . WCIQ
Demopolis . . . . . WIIQ
Dozier . . . . . WDIQ
Florence . . . . . WFIQ
Huntsville . . . . . WHIQ
Louisville . . . . . WGIQ
Mobile . . . . . WEIQ
Montgomery . . . . . WAIQ

Alaska
Anchorage . . . . . KAKM
Bethel . . . . . KYUK-TV
Fairbanks . . . . . KUAC-TV
Juneau . . . . . KTOO-TV

Arizona
Phoenix . . . . . KAET
Tucson . . . . . KUAT

Arkansas
Arkadelphia . . . . . KETG
Fayetteville . . . . . KAFT
Jonesboro . . . . . KTEJ
Little Rock . . . . . KETS
Mountain View . . . . . KEMV
Newark . . . . . KLEP

California
Cotati . . . . . KRCB-TV
Eureka . . . . . KEET
Fresno . . . . . KMTF
Huntington Beach . . . . . KOCE-TV
Los Angeles . . . . . KCET
Los Angeles . . . . . KLCS
Redding . . . . . KIXE
Sacramento . . . . . KVIE
San Bernardino . . . . . KVCR-TV
San Diego . . . . . KPBS-TV
San Francisco . . . . . KQED
San Francisco . . . . . KQEC
San Jose . . . . . KTEH
San Mateo . . . . . KCSM-TV

Colorado
Broomfield . . . . . KBDI-TV
Denver . . . . . KRMA-TV
Pueblo . . . . . KTSC

Connecticut
Bridgeport . . . . . WEDW
Hartford . . . . . WEDH
New Haven . . . . . WEDY
Norwich . . . . . WEDN

Delaware
Seaford . . . . . WDPB
Wilmington . . . . . WHYY-TV

District of Columbia
Washington . . . . . WETA-TV
Washington . . . . . WHMM

Florida
Cocoa . . . . . WRES
Ft. Myers . . . . . WSFP-TV
Gainesville . . . . . WUFT
Jacksonville . . . . . WJCT
Miami . . . . . WPBT
Miami . . . . . WLRN-TV
Orlando . . . . . WMFE-TV
Pensacola . . . . . WSRE
Tallahassee . . . . . WFSU-TV
Tampa . . . . . WUSF-TV
Tampa . . . . . WEDU
Tampa/St. Petersburg . . . . . WEDU
West Palm Beach . . . . . WXEL-TV

Georgia
Athens . . . . . WGTV
Atlanta . . . . . WPBA
Chatsworth . . . . . WCLP-TV
Cochran . . . . . WDCO-TV
Columbus . . . . . WJSP-TV
Dawson . . . . . WACS-TV
Pelham . . . . . WABW-TV
Savannah . . . . . WVAN-TV
Valdosta . . . . . WTKV
Waycross . . . . . WXGA-TV
Wrens . . . . . WCES-TV

Guam
Agana . . . . . KGTF

Hawaii
Honolulu . . . . . KHET
Wailuku . . . . . KMEB-TV

Idaho
Boise . . . . . KAID
Moscow . . . . . KUID-TV
Pocate . . . . . KISU-TV

Illinois
Carbondale . . . . . WSIU-TV
Chicago . . . . . WTTW
Chicago . . . . . WYCC
Jacksonville . . . . . WJPT
Macomb . . . . . WIUM-TV
Moline . . . . . WQPT
Olney . . . . . WUSI-TV
Peoria . . . . . WTVP
Quincy . . . . . WQEC
Urbana . . . . . WILL-TV

Indiana
Bloomington . . . . . WTIU
Evansville . . . . . WNIN
Indianapolis . . . . . WFYI
Muncie . . . . . WIPB
St. John . . . . . WCAE
South Bend . . . . . WNIT
Vincennes . . . . . WVUT

Iowa
Council Bluffs . . . . . KBIN
Des Moines . . . . . KDIN-TV
Fort Dodge . . . . . KTIN
Iowa City . . . . . KIIN-TV
Mason City . . . . . KYIN
Red Oak . . . . . KHIN
Sioux City . . . . . KSIN
Waterloo . . . . . KRIN

Kansas
Hays . . . . . KOOD
Hutchinson . . . . . KPTS
Topeka . . . . . KTWU

Kentucky
Ashland . . . . . WKAS
Bowling Green . . . . . WKGR
Covington . . . . . WCVN
Elizabethtown . . . . . WKZT
Hazard . . . . . WKHA
Lexington . . . . . WKLE
Louisville . . . . . WKPC-TV
Louisville . . . . . WKMJ
Madisonville . . . . . WKMA
Morehead . . . . . WKMR
Murray . . . . . WKMU
Owensboro . . . . . WKOH
Owenton . . . . . WKON
Paducah . . . . . WKPD
Pikeville . . . . . WKPI
Somerset . . . . . WKSO

Louisana
Alexandria . . . . . KLPA-TV
Baton Rouge . . . . . WLPB-TV
Layfette . . . . . KLPB-TV

Lake Charles . . . KLTL-TV
Monroe . . . KLTM
New Orleans . . . WYES-TV
Shreveport . . . KLTS-TV

Maine
Augusta . . . WCBB
Biddeford . . . WMEA
Calais . . . WMED-TV
Orono . . . WMEB-TV
Presque Isle . . . WMEM-TV

Maryland
Annapolis . . . WAPB
Baltimore . . . WMPB
Hagerstown . . . WWPB-TV
Salisbury . . . WCPB

Massachusetts
Boston . . . WGBH-TV
Boston . . . WGBX-TV
Springfield . . . WGBY-TV

Michigan
Alpena . . . WCML-TV
Cadillac . . . WCMV
Detroit . . . WTVS
East Lansing . . . WKAR-TV
Flint . . . WFUM
Grand Rapids . . . WGVC
Kalamazoo . . . WGVK
Manistee . . . WCMW
Marquette . . . WNMU-TV
Mt. Pleasant . . . WCMU-TV
University Center . . . WUCM-TV

Minnesota
Appleton . . . KWCM-TV
Austin . . . KSMQ-TV
Bemidji . . . KAWE
Duluth-Superior, Wis. . . . WDSE-TV
Minneapolis-St. Paul . . . KTCA-TV
St. Paul . . . KTCI-TV

Mississippi
Biloxi . . . WMAH
Booneville . . . WMAE
Bude . . . WMAU
Greenwood . . . WMAO
Jackson . . . WMAA
Meridian . . . WMAW
Oxford . . . WMAV
State College . . . WMAB

Missouri
Jefferson City . . . KBBM-TV
Kansas City . . . KCPT
St. Louis . . . KETC
St. Louis . . . KUCU-TV
Sedalia-Warrensburg . . . KMOS-TV
Springfield . . . KOZK

Montana
Bozeman . . . KUSM

Nebraska
Aliance . . . KTNE-TV
Bassett . . . KMNE-TV
Hastings . . . KHNE-TV
Lexington . . . KLNE-TV
Lincoln . . . KUON-TV
Merriman . . . KRNE-TV
Norfolk . . . KXNE-TV
North Platte . . . KPNE-TV
Omaha . . . KYNE-TV

Nevada
Las Vegas . . . KLVX
Reno . . . KNPV

New Hampshire
Durham . . . WENH
Keene . . . WEKW-TV
Littleton . . . WLED-TV

New Jersey
Camden . . . WNJS
Montclair . . . WNJM
New Brunswick . . . WNJB
Trenton . . . WNJT

New Mexico
Albuquerque . . . KNME-TV
Las Cruces . . . KRWG
Portales . . . KENW

New York
Binghamton . . . WSKG
Buffalo . . . WNED-TV
Buffalo . . . WNEQ-TV
Garden City . . . WLIW
New York . . . WNYC-TV
New York . . . WNYE-TV
New York . . . WNET
Norwood . . . WNPI-TV
Plattsburgh . . . WCFE-TV
Rochester . . . WXXI
Schenectady . . . WMHT
Syracuse . . . WCNY-TV
Watertown . . . WNPE

North Carolina
Asheville . . . WUNF-TV
Chapel Hill . . . WUNC-TV
Charlotte . . . WTVI
Columbia . . . WUND-TV
Concord . . . WUNG-TV
Greenville . . . WUNK-TV
Linville . . . WUNE-TV
Wilmington . . . WUNJ-TV
Winston-Salem . . . WUNL-TV

North Dakota
Bismarck . . . KBME
Dickinson . . . KDSE
Fargo-Moorhead, Minn. . . . KFME
Grand Forks . . . KGFE
Minot . . . KSRE
Williston . . . KWSE

Ohio
Akron . . . WEAO
Aliance . . . WNEO
Athens . . . WOUB-TV
Cambridge . . . WOUC-TV
Cincinnati . . . WCET
Cleveland . . . WVIZ-TV
Columbus . . . WOSU-TV
Dayton . . . WPTD
Lima-Bowling Green . . . WBGU-TV
Oxford . . . WPTO
Portsmouth . . . WPBO-TV
Toledo . . . WGTE-TV

Oklahoma
Cheyenne . . . KWET
Claremore . . . KXON
Eufaula . . . KOET
Oklahoma City . . . KETA
Tulsa . . . KOED-TV

Oregon
Bend . . . KOAV-TV
Corvallis . . . KOAC-TV
La Grande . . . KTVR
Medford . . . KSYS
Portland . . . KOAP-TV

Pennsylvania
Bethlehem-Allentown . . . WLVT-TV
Clearfield . . . WPSX-TV
Erie . . . WQLN
Hershey . . . WITF-TV
Philadelphia . . . WXBE
Pittsburgh . . . WQED
Pittsburgh . . . WQEX
Scranton-Wilkes-Barre . . . WVIA-TV

Puerto Rico
Aguadilla . . . WKKU
Caquas . . . WUJA
Mayaguez . . . WIPM-TV
Ponce . . . WQTO
San Juan . . . WIPR-TV

Rhode Island
Providence . . . . WSBE-TV

South Carolina
Allendale . . . . WEBA-TV
Beaufort . . . . WJWJ-TV
Charleston . . . . WITV
Columbia . . . . WRLK-TV
Conway . . . . WHMC
Florence . . . . WJPM-TV
Greenville . . . . WNTV
Greenwood . . . . WNEH
Rock Hill . . . . WNSC-TV
Spartanburg . . . . WRET-TV
Sumter . . . . WRJA-TV

South Dakota
Aberdeen . . . . KDSD-TV
Brookings . . . . KESD-TV
Eagle Butte . . . . KPSD-TV
Lowry . . . . KQSD-TV
Martin . . . . KZSD-TV
Pierre . . . . KTSD-TV
Rapid City . . . . KBHE-TV
Vermillion . . . . KUSD-TV

Tennessee
Chattanooga . . . . WTCI
Cookeville . . . . WCTE
Lexington . . . . WLJT-TV
Memphis . . . . WKNO-TV
Nashville . . . . WDCN-TV
Sneedville . . . . WSJK-TV

Texas
Austin-San Antonio . . . . KLRN-TV
Austin . . . . KLRU-TV
Beaumont . . . . KITU
Belton . . . . KNCT
College Station . . . . KAMU-TV
Corpus Christi . . . . KEDT
Dallas . . . . KERA-TV
El Paso . . . . KCOS
Ft. Worth . . . . NEW-TV
Harlingen . . . . KLUJ
Harlingen . . . . KMBH
Houston . . . . KHBU
Houston . . . . KUHT
Lubbock . . . . KTXT
Odessa . . . . KOCV-TV
San Antonio . . . . KLRN-TV

Utah
Ogden . . . . KWBR
Provo . . . . KBYU-TV
Salt Lake City . . . . KUED

Vermont
Burlington . . . . WETK
Rutland . . . . WVER
St. Johnsbury . . . . WVTB
Windsor . . . . WVTA

Virginia
Fairfax . . . . WNVC
Goldvein . . . . WNVT
Marion . . . . WMSY-TV
Norfolk . . . . WHRO-TV
Norton . . . . WSBN-TV
Richmond . . . . WCVE-TV
Richmond . . . . WCVW
Roanoke . . . . WBRA-TV
Staunton . . . . WVPT

Virgin Islands
Charlotte Amalie . . . . WTJX-TV

Washington
Centralia . . . . KCKA
Pullman . . . . KWSU-TV
Seattle . . . . KCTS-TV
Spokane . . . . KSPS-TV
Tacoma . . . . KTPS
Yakima . . . . KYVE-TV

West Virginia
Grandview . . . . WSWP-TV
Huntington . . . . WPBY-TV
Morgantown . . . . WNPB-TV

Wisconsin
Green Bay . . . . WPNE
La Crosse . . . . WHLA
Madison . . . . WHA-TV
Menomoine-Colifax . . . . WHWC
Milwaukee . . . . WMVS
Milwaukee . . . . WMVT
Park Falls . . . . WLEF-TV
Wausau . . . . WHRM-TV

Wyoming
Lander . . . . KCWC-TV

Advertising Agencies

* STATION REPRESENTATIVES

Advertising Agencies

A. D. ADAMS ADVERTISING, 9 East 38th St., New York, NY 10016; (212) 685-9060.
A. D. ADAMS, pres.

WILLIAM HART ADLER, INC., One Concourse Plaza, 4711 Golf Road, Skokie, IL 60076.
WILLIAM HART ADLER, pres. and treas.

ALLIED ADVERTISING AGENCY, INC., 830 Statler Office Building, Boston, MA 02116; (617) 482-4100.
HOWARD SHAMBAN, TV dir.; MARC F. SHAMBAN, TV time buyer.

ANDERSON DAVID & SEEDS, INC., Colonial Building, Clinton, NY 13323; (212) 853-6141.
JAY C. ANDERSON, pres.; MARK ANDERSON, acct. exec.

ARNOLD & COMPANY, INC., Park Square Building, Boston, MA 02116.
GERARD GOLDEN, pres.; ARNOLD Z. ROSOFF, chairman & treasurer; LEN KARSAVOL, creative dir.; DENNIS LEE, copy chief; MARIE KACHINSKI, media dir.; STAVROS COSMOPULOS, exec. v.p., creative services; FRED SIEGEL, media; PHYLLIS MAYNARD, media; ANNE GOTZ, JOAN BENNETT, GINNY MEANEY, media.

N. W. AYER INCORPORATED, 1345 Ave. of the Americas, New York, NY 10105; (212) 974-7400.
MARCELLA ROSEN, sr. v.p. & media dir.; DAVID LEHMKUHL, group media dir., planning; JANE TWYON, group media dir., planning; RICHARD WELSH, group media dir., network & negotiation; DIANE ZGONC, group media dir., planning; SUSAN BELL, mgr. spot buying.

BBDO CHICAGO, INC., 410 N. Michigan Ave., Chicago, IL 60611; (312) DElaware 7-7860.
ARTHUR E. MEYERHOFF, chmn. of the bd.; ROGER J. MOHR, pres.; MICHAEL PARADISE, radio/TV dir.

TED BATES ADVERTISING/NEW YORK, 1515 Broadway, New York, NY 10036; (212) 869-3131.
ROBERT E. JACOBY, Chm.; ROBERT A BRUNS, Pres.; WALTER E. REICHEL, Sr. v.p.-Exec. Dir. Media & Programs Dept.; JOEL M. SEGAL, Sr. V.P.-Dir. TV/Radio Div. Division of TED BATES WORLDWIDE, INC. (same address) with affiliates in Fort Lauderdale, Chicago, Minneapolis, San Francisco, Los Angeles, Canada, Mexico, Argentina, Brazil, Chile, Colombia, Ecuador, Peru, Venezuela, United Kingdom, Norway, Sweden, Denmark, West Germany, Austria, Netherlands, Belgium, France, Spain, Italy, Greece, South Africa, Malaysia, Thailand, Singapore, Hong Kong, Japan, Philippines, Australia, New Zealand.

BEHRENDS & COMPANY, INC., P.O. Box 2556, 101 W. Green Drive, High Point, NC 27261.
RICHARD D. BEHRENDS, pres.; RICHARD FURMANSKI, v.p. & senior art dir.; ROBERT A. BODLE, JR., v.p. & exec. creative dir.; SYLVIA Y. PASSAVANT, secty.-treas.; JERRY BLACKWELDER, media dir.

HERBERT S. BENJAMIN ASSOCIATES, INC., 2736 Florida St., Baton Rouge, LA 70802; (504) 387-0611.
LEE HERZBERG, JR., chm./pres.; MARGARET S. WEBB, exec. v.p.; PATTI HASSELL, treas.; JACKLYN ROBBINS, secty.; LENORE USHER, v.p., acct. exec.; GUS WALES, v.p./creative dir.; RICHARD J. BARRA, v.p.; mgr. Lafayette branch office; ELISE GANETT, asst. v.p., exec. admin.

WALTER F. BENNETT CO., 20 N. Wacker Drive, Chicago, IL 60606; (312) 372-1131.
FRED DIENERT, pres.; TED DIENERT, exec. v.p.; JAN KLUTS, media dir.-time buyer. Other offices: 1634 Spruce St., Philadelphia, PA 19103; (215) 545-2003; 16479 Dallas Pkwy., Dallas, TX 72348; (214) 380-1122.

BENTON & BOWLES 909 Third Avenue, New York, NY 10022; (212) 758-6200.
JOHN S. BOWEN, pres. & chief exec. officer; VICTOR G. BLOEDE, chm. of bd. & chm., Benton & Bowles International; GEORGE SIMKO, sr. v.p. & group exec.

RALPH BING ADVERTISING CO., 16109 Selva Dr., San Diego, CA 92128; (714) 487-7444.
RALPH BING, TV dir.

FRANK BLOCK ASSOC., The Chase, 10th Floor, St. Louis, MO 63108; (314) 367-9600.
DAVID STOBLE, dir. mktg.

BOTSFORD, KETCHUM, INC., 55 Union St., San Francisco, CA 94111.
DENIS HITCHMOUGH, senior v.p., media; MORTY BARAN, dir. broadcast prod.; PATTY MORAN, v.p. mgr. broadcast business affairs.

LEO P. BOTT, JR., ADVERTISING, 111 E. Chestnut St., Chicago, IL 60611; (312) 787-7890.
LEO P. BOTT, JR., TV dir.; ED MORGAN, time buyer.

BRAVERMAN-MIRISCH INC., 1517 Schuyler Rd., Beverly Hills, CA 90210; (213) 274-5204.
MILLICENT BRAVERMAN, pres.

BURLINGAME/GROSSMAN, INC., 6160 N. Cicero Ave., Chicago, IL 60646; (312) 777-0610.
S. J. BRICHTA, TV dir.

LEO BURNETT COMPANY, INC., Prudential Plaza, Chicago, IL 60601; (312) 565-5959
JOHN J. KINSELLA, pres. & CEO; NORM L. MUSE, chm. of the board; WAYNE A. (AL) WIGGINS, vice chm., chief administrative officer; THOMAS D. HEATH, vice chm., corporate development; JOHN C. (JACK) KRAFT, exec. v.p., administration & finance.; HALL (CAP) ADAMS, Chm. & CEO, Leo Burnett U.S.A.; RICHARD (RICK) FIZDALE, pres. & chief creative officer, Leo Burnett, U.S.A.; HENRY J. (HANK) FEELEY, chm. & CEO, Leo Burnett International; MICHAEL CONRAD, pres. & chief creative officers, Leo Burnett International.

HAROLD CABOT & CO., INC., One Constitution Plaza, Boston, MA 02129; (617) 242-6200.
WILLIAM H. MONAGHAN, pres.; PETER CROWELL, media dir.; LOUIS STAMOULIS, dir. radio-TV.

CALDWELL-VAN RIPER, INC., 701 S. Clinton St., Fort Wayne, IN 46802; (219) 422-7495.
LESLEY HUNTLEY, media director.

CAMPBELL-EWALD CO., 30400 Van Dyke, Warren, MI; (313) 574-3400.
RICHARD D. O'CONNOR, chm.; PETER A. DOW, pres.; LOUIS M. SCHULTZ, exec. v.p., media dir.
Branch Offices: Atlanta, Chicago, Los Angeles, New York, San Francisco, Dallas, Washington, Miami, Pittsburgh.

CAMPBELL-MITHUN, INC., Northstar Center, Minneapolis, MN 55402; (612) 339-7383; and 111 East Wacker Drive, Chicago, IL 60601; (312) 565-3800.
WILLIAM D. DUNLOP, chm.-exec. comm. & CEO (Mpls.); WILLIAM E. STEIN, pres. & COO (Chicago); RAYMOND L. SACHS, vice chm. & vice chm./exec. comm. (Mpls.); EARL HERZOG, v.p., media dir. (Mpls.); ART EDELSTEIN, v.p., media dir. (Chicago); ALAN GERSTEN, v.p., media planning services dir. (Mpls.); LORNA TWEED, v.p., spot buying bdcst. mgr. (Mpls.); GAIL BURCH, assoc. media dir., (Mpls.); JANET BAK, v.p., assoc. media dir. (Chicago); JEANNE O'NEILL, assoc. media dir. (Chicago); TESS ZYCH, assoc. media dir. (Chicago).

THE CRAMER-KRASSELT CO., 733 N. Van Buren St., Milwaukee, WI 53202; (414) 276-3500.
ROBERT L. CHRISTIANSEN, chmn. of bd. & treas.; TED WING, pres; C. ROSS LITTIG, vice chm. of bd.; DONALD E. POM, media dir.-TV/radio; CAROL WALCZAK, buyer/planner; KATHY HARRISON, buyler/planner; CATHY POCHERT, bdcst. svs. mgr.

CRESWELL, MUNSELL, FULTZ & ZIRBEL, INC., 4211 Signal Ridge Road, N.E., Cedar Rapids, IA 54202; (319) 395-6500.
R. D. MEYOCKS, pres.; G. ANDERSON, F. BAKER, B. CLINE, W. FRITZ, R. HOWES, J. MEEKS, I. WAY and M. WHITE, sr. v.p.'s-radio/TV producers; T. F. TAYLOR, v.p. exec. prod.; M. MURRAY, S. MAYS.

CUNNINGHAM & WALSH, CHICAGO INC., 875 Michigan Ave., Chicago, IL 60611; (312) 943-9400.
CHARLES C. HATCHER, sr. v.p. dir. operations & bdcst. prod.; GREGG DEARTH, sr. v.p. dir. creative svcs; JOHN DOHERTY, pres. & CEO.

D'ARCY MASIUS BENTON & BOWLES, INC., 909 Third Ave., New York, NY 10022; (212) 758-6200.
New York: MICHAEL MOORE, sr. v.p., corporate media dir.; RICHARD LEVENSON, sr. v.p., exec. creative dir. Atlanta: REGIS C. NAPOLITANO, sr. v.p., media dir.; B.A. ALBERT, sr. v.p., creative dir. Bloomfield Hills: GEORGE M. ROGERS,

JR., sr. v.p. dir. of media services; STEPHEN C. KOPCHA, exec. v.p., creative dir. Chicago: JOSEPH P. ZELLER, sr. v.p. dir. media services; GARY J. HORTON, deputy mng. dir., chief creative officer. Houston: HEIDI ASKEW, v.p., media dir.; KEN THOREN, sr. v.p., creative dir.; Los Angeles: RON LAWRENCE, v.p., media dir.; KEN BERRIS, sr. v.p., creative dir. Minneapolis-St. Paul: GEORGE C. SCOTT, v.p., media and research dir.; DICK BRINER, v.p. creative dir.; St. Louis: JAMES PORCARELLI, sr. v.p., dir. of media services; ALBERT LERMAN, chief creative officer/deputy mng. dir. San Francisco: ROGER BARON, v.p. media dir.; SCOTT YOUNG, v.p., exec. creative dir.

DAVIS, JOHNSON, MOGUL & COLOMBATTO, INC., 3435 Wilshire Blvd., Los Angeles, CA 90010; (213) 388-3332.
ROBERT DAVIS, co-chm. & CEO; ROBERT COLOMBATTO, co-chm. & COO; BRAD BILL, pres.; LARRY WITTER, v.p. corp. media dir.

DIENER/HAUSER/BATES CO., INC., 116 N. Robertson Blvd., Suite 210, Los Angeles, CA 90048; (213) 855-1900.
EUGENE B. COFSKY, pres. West Coast div., BILL ISENBERGER, sr. v.p.; HICKEY SHAPIRO, v.p.

W. B. DONER & CO., 26711 Northwestern, Southfield, MI 48034; (313) 354-9700; also 2305 N. Charles Street, Baltimore, MD 21218; (301) 338-1600.
W. B. DONER, chm. of exec. comm.; HERBERT D. FRIED, chm. of bd.; STANLEY T. BURKOFF, pres.; SEYMOUR (SKIP) ROBERTS, exec. v.p.; M. KEVIN WIXTED, treas.; JAMES DALE, sr. v.p./exec. creative dir.

DOREMUS & COMPANY (Subsidiary of BBDO Intl., Inc.), 120 Broadway, New York, NY 10005; (212) 964-0700.
FRANKLIN E. SCHAFFER, chairman; G. BARRY McMENNAMIN, president; WILLIAM B. PALMER, creative dir.; LOUIS CROSSIN, media dir.
Branch offices; Boston, Chicago, San Francisco, Washington, Los Angeles, Miami, Minneapolis, Rockford, London.
Corresp. offices: Akron, Denver, Baltimore, Detroit, Cleveland, Pittsburgh, Dallas, Hartford, Houston, Atlanta, Kansas City, St. Louis.

DOYLE DANE BERNBACH INC., 437 Madison Avenue, New York, NY 10022; (212) 826-2000.
GEORGE NILES, v.p., media; JOSEPH R. DALY, chm. of the bd.; ROBERT LEVENSON, vice chm., creative; BARRY LOSGHRANE, pres. & CEO.

EISNER & ASSOCIATES, INC., 12 W. Madison St., Baltimore, MD 21201; (301) 685-3390.
H. W. EISNER, chm.; STEVE EISNER, pres.; GEORGE NILES, v.p., media.

MIKE FADELL ADVERTISING AGENCY, 6101 York, S. Minneapolis, MN 55410; (612) 922-5606.
MIKE FADELL, SR., TV dir. & timebuyer.

FAHLGREN & FERRISS, INC., 120 E. 4th St., Cincinnati, OH 45202; (513) 241-9200.
CHRIS CLEMENTS, sr. v.p. media & mktg. svcs.; WILLIAM FARSON, treas.

FAIRFAX INC., ADVERTISING, 635 Madison Ave., New York, NY 10022; (212) 350-1800.
STANLEY I. FISHEL, dir. of television; ROBERT McQUADE, producer; RICHARD MIRENDA, art director; MIKE COHN, media dir.

FOOTE, CONE & BELDING COMMUNICATIONS, INC., 101 Park Avenue, New York, NY 10178; (212) 907-1000; 401 North Michigan Ave., Chicago, IL 60611; (312) 467-9200.
JOHN O'TOOLE, chm. (New York); NORMAN W. BROWN, pres. & CEO (Chicago).
ADVERTISING OFFICES: Chicago, New York, San Francisco, Los Angeles, Greenwich, CT, Philadelphia, Toronto, Montreal, Mexico City, Kingston (Jamaica), San Juan (Puerto Rico), Caracas, Port of Spain (Trinidad), São Paulo (Brazil), Buenos Aires, Stockholm, Gothenburg (Sweden), Oslo, Copenhagen, Hamburg, Berlin, Amsterdam, Rotterdam, London, Nottingham, Brussels, Paris, Marseille, Lisbon, Madrid, Barcelona, Frankfurt-am-Main, Zurich, Vienna, Milan, Rome, Athens, Johannesburg, Durban, Cape Town, Tokyo, Hong Kong, Kuala Lumpur, Singapore, Jakarta, Sydney, Melbourne.

FOSTER & DAVIES, INC., Hanna Building, Cleveland, OH 44115; (216) 241-0711.

ALBERT FRANK-GUENTHER LAW, INC., 71 Broadway, New York, NY 10006; (212) 248-5200.
STEPHEN J. WITT, chm.; JOHN F. COWELL III, pres.
Branch office: San Francisco.

GERBER ADVERTISING AGENCY, 209 S.W. Ozk Ave., Portland, OR 97204; (503) 221-0100.
BETTY CHIMENTI, media dir.; CATHY MACDONALD, assoc. med. dir.; KAREN ANDRUS-HUGHES, media buyer.

GILLHAM ADVERTISING INC., Fifth Floor, Deseret Plaza Bldg., 15 East First South, Salt Lake City, UT 84111; (801) 328-0281.
LON RICHARDSON, JR. pres.; CRAIG OGAN, sr. v.p.; NANCY MOWER, v.p. finance; PENNY KISER, media dir.; CHARLES ELEGANTE, prod. mgr.; GAIL FRANKOSKI, traffic mgr.

GREY ADVERTISING, INC., 777 Third Ave., New York, NY 10017; (212) 546-2000.
EDWARD H. MEYER, pres. & chief exec. officer; ALEC GERSTER, v.p., dir. of media & programming.
Branch offices: Amsterdam-Baarn, Auckland, Brussels, Buenos Aires, Caracas, Chicago, Copenhagen, Detroit, Dusseldorf, Glasgow, Gothenburg, Hong Kong, Johannesburg, London, Los Angeles, Madrid, Malmoe, Milan, Minneapolis/St. Paul, Montevideo, Montreal, New York, Oslo, Paris, Rio de Janeiro, San Francisco, Santiago, Singapore, Stockholm, Sydney, Tokyo, Toronto, Vienna.

GRISWOLD, INC., 12th Floor—55 Public Square, Cleveland, OH 44113; (216) 696-3400.
PATRICK J. MORIN, pres.; BETTY LANDERS, chm.; TOM GILDAY, vice chm.; EDMOND FREHLICH, exec. v.p.; NEAL DAVIS, exec. v.p.; WILLIAM BROKAW, creative dir.; JAMES ZIEGLER, media dir.

GRUBB, GRAHAM & WILDER, INC., Century 21 Plaza, Champaign, IL 61820; (217) 344-4334.
ROBERT F. GRUBB, chm.; JOHN A. GRUBB, pres.; PATRICK CHELF, media dir.

ART GRUBER ASSOCIATES, ADVERTISING, 4407 East Lake Street, Minneapolis, MN 55406; (612) 722-6338.
ARTHUR R. GRUBER, pres. & treas.; E. M. GRUBER, sec.

HARRIS & LOVE, INC./ADVERTISING, 136 East So. Temple, Salt Lake City, UT 84111; (801) 532-7333.
DONALD G. WARE, pres.

HART-CONWAY CO., INC., 300 Triangle Bldg., Rochester, NY 14604; (716) 232-2930.
PETER B. WHITCOMBE, pres.; WILLIAM WESTERFELD, exec. v.p.

HENDERSON ADVERTISING, INC., 60 Pelham Pointe, Greenville, SC 29615; P.O. Box 2247, Greenville, SC 29602 (Mailing Address); (803) 271-6000.
RALPH W. CALLAHAN JR., chm. & pres.; BOB REUSCHLE, sr. v.p. media dir.

HICKS AND GREIST, INC., 220 E. 42 St., New York, NY 10036; (212) 370-9600.
CHARLES V. SKOOG, JR., chm.; D. EDWARD RICCHIUTO, pres.; S. PARKER, media dir.; DEMETRI KONTUPOULOS, TV prod. dir.

WM. F. HOLLAND CO., 252 Ludlow Ave., Cincinnati, OH 45220; (513) 221-1252
MARK S. HOLLAND, pres.

HOUCK ADVERTISING, 1402 Grandin Rd., Roanoke, VA 24015; (703) 989-6655.
WILLIAM B. HOUCK, chm.; WILLIAM B. HOUCK, JR., pres.; CYNTHIA G. CALDWELL, media buyer.

HUTCHINS/YOUNG & RUBICAM INC., 400 Midtown Tower; Rochester, NY 14604; (716) 546-6480.
FRANK M. HUTCHINS, chm.; JAMES N. MOREY, pres. & chief exec. officer; ROBERT H. MAHARRY, v.p., creative dir.; CHARLES E. RELLER, v.p. finance & adm., treasurer; OWEN J. CRUMB, v.p. & gen. mgr., pub. rel. div.; HARVEY J. BOZZI, JR., v.p./director of special projects.

HENRY J. KAUFMAN & ASSOCIATES, INC., 2233 Wisconsin Ave., N.W., Washington, DC 20007; (202) 333-0700.
STUART E. KARU, chm. & CEO; MICHAEL G. CARBERRY, pres. & COO; LISA JONES, media dir.; PHILIP SABATINO, v.p., graphic svcs.; FRED SELLERS, v.p., assoc. creative dir.; J. ROGER VILSACK, v.p. creative svcs.; ROD DAUSCH, v.p., finance & admin.

KELLY, ZAHRNDT & KELLY INC., 10805 Sunset Office Dr., St. Louis, MO 63127.
ROBERT W. KELLY, dir.; WILLIAM A. WILSON, MARY HOPPER, CHARLES CROWE, DAVE ERICH, acct. execs.

KERR, WEST & GISH, INC., 104 Kenner Ave., Suite 203, Nashville, TN 37205; (615) 297-9770.
AL KERR, pres.

KETCHUM COMMUNICATIONS, INC., Six PPG Place, Pittsburgh, PA 15222; (412) 456-3500.

Pittsburgh: WILLIAM H. GENGE, chm.; GERALD J. VOROS, pres.; HERBERT D. GORDON, sr. v.p., media services; JUDITH HOFSCHER, v.p., media dir.; RICHARD SLEEMAN, v.p. & broadcast services mgr.
New York office: Ketchum New York. THOMAS MILLER, pres.; JIM McHUGH, v.p., dir. media network, res. (N.Y.).

KEYES, MARTIN, 841 Mountain Ave., Springfield, NJ; (201) 376-7300.
Specialist: ROBYN GREEN-TAYLOR, media director.

KRUPNICK & ASSOCIATES, INC., 135 N. Meramec, St. Louis, MO 63105; (314) 862-9393.
WILLIAM W. QUADE, TV production.

KUTTNER & KUTTNER, INC., 646 N. Michigan Ave., Chicago, IL 60611; (312) 787-7940.

LEWIS, GILMAN & KYNETT, INC., 1700 Market St., Philadelphia, PA 19103; (215) 568-3775.
ROBERT G. WILDER, CEO, pres. & chm.; CARL E. CASSELMAN, exec. v.p., exec. creative dir.; EDWIN R. BATES, v.p., creative dir.; STEPHEN J. BARCUS, v.p., group supervisor; WESLEY G. HOTCHKISS, v.p.; CHESTER D. HARRINGTON, v.p. & exec. dir. of media services, MICHAEL A. WALSH, v.p., media dir.; FREDERIC C. MOFFATT, media acct. mgr.; GLORIA PEDALINO, media acct. mgr.; RICHARD BONDS, media acct. mgr.; GLORIA F. HARTMAN, media acct. mgr.; GUY S. MOSS, media acct. mgr.; JAMES J. SLOAN, media acct. mgr.

THE W. E. LONG ADVERTISING AGENCY, 309 W. Washington St., Chicago, IL 60606; (312) RA6-4606.
PAUL FRANK, gen. mgr. & creative dir.; THOMAS E. RADIKE, dir. mktg.; ANITA RAUH, media supervisor.

LOWE & HALL ADVERTISING, INC., 215 East Stone Ave., P.O. Box 3357, Greenville, SC; (803) 242-5350.
EDWARD E. BROWER, JR., pres.; KENNETH BROWER, exec. v.p.; W. T. HALL, v.p.; VALERIE VURNAKES, v.p.

McCANN-ERICKSON, 485 Lexington Avenue, New York, NY 10017; (212) 697-6000.
JOHN M. OTTER, sr. v.p. dir., natl. bdcast.; JOHN MATTIMORE, v.p., network supvsr.; WILLIAM SHERMAN, v.p., network supvsr.; CLARE SIMPSON, v.p., dir., Coca-Cola natl. bdcast.; ANN KOHL, network supvsr.; RICHARD FORESTER, LORI ISOLA, WENDY RICH, buyers.

EDWARD J. McELROY ADV., INC., 3600 Wilshire Blvd., Los Angeles, CA 90005; (213) 381-3045.
E. D. BROTSOS, pres. & acct. sup.; VICKI PANAGIOTIS, media dir.; LISA C. MOLLER, acct. exec./prod. mgr.

McKENZIE, KING & GORDON, 1800 N. Argyle, Hollywood, CA 90028; (213) 466-3421.
MARIE McKENZIE, pres.; DON McKENZIE, creative dir., MARIE SELTZER, media dir.; KEVIN MCKENZIE, assoc. creative dir.

MELDRUM & FEWSMITH, INC., 1220 Huron Rd., Cleveland 15, OH; (216) 241-2141.
CHRIS PERRY, v.p. creative dir., BRUCE S. CHILDERS, mkt. services.

NEEDHAM & GROHMANN, INC., 30 Rockefeller Plaza, New York, NY 10020; 245-6200.
H. A. HEINSIUS, president; WILLIAM R. HOGAN, art dir.; JOHN L. GILLESPIE, N. ROBERT LORMAN, ANTHONY E. F. CORNWELL, v.p.'s.

NEEDHAM, HARPER & STEERS ADVERTISING, INC., 909 Third Avenue, New York, NY 10022; (212) 758-7600.
PAUL C. HARPER, JR., chmn. of the bd. & chief exec. officer; JOEL P. BAUMWOLL, pres. NH&S New York; BARRON Z. BIEDERMAN, pres. NH&S/Issues & Images; LOIS KOREY, exec. v.p. & creative dir.; 303 E. Wacker Dr., Chicago, IL 60601 (312) 861-0200. B. BLAIR VEDDER, JR.; chief op. officer; KEITH L. REINHARD, pres. NH&S Chicago; JOEL M. HOCHBERG, sr. v.p. & creative dir.; 10889 Wilshire Blvd., Los Angeles, CA 90024 (213) 208-5000. BRADLEY H. ROBERTS, pres. NH&S West; RICHARD KELLEY, sr. v.p. & creative dir.

NOWAK BARLOW JOHNSON, 117 Highbridge St., Fayetteville, NY 13066; (305) 637-9895.
DONALD G. NOWAK, pres. & CEO; Ed Gabriel, audio-visual dir.

OHLMEYER ADVERTISING, 9 West 57 St., New York, NY 10019; (212) 418-6900.
DON OHLMEYER, chm.; PHIL HOWERT, pres.; LEE PRATT, v.p., media dir.; DEAN HEITLER, v.p. mgr. supvsr.; PETER CHRISANTHUPOULUS, v.p. bdcst. supvr.

THE PITLUK GROUP, 45 N.E. Loop 410, San Antonio, TX 78216; (512) 366-3100.
LOUIS H. PITLUK, pres.; JACK N. PITLUK, JR., v.p.; HELEN THOMPSON, med. dir.; ED GORI, creative dir.

ROCKLIN, IRVING & ASSOCIATES, 65 E. South Water St., Chicago, IL 60601; (312) 726-2324.
ROBERT ROCKLIN, pres.; LEAH ROCKLIN, v.p.; PATTY JO WONG, creative dir.; DICK NEFF, writer; JOSEPH LUTZKE, sr. acct. exec.; KARL RAACK, art dir.; JEAN CARMOSINO, comptroller; YVONNE CURRAN, traffic mgr.; MARC ROCKLIN, radio time buyer.

RUDER, FINN & ROTMAN, INC., 110 East 59th St. New York, NY 10022; (212) 593-6400.
DAVID FINN, chmn. of bd.; WILLIAM RUDER, pres.; DICK CUNNINGHAM, bdcst. communications dept.

RUMRILL-HOYT, INC., 60 Corporate Woods, Rochester, NY 14623.
JOSEPH M. VALERIO, chm.; RICHARD THOMPSON, pres. & CEO; DONNA BIEDENBACH, R-TV spvr.; WILLIAM J. MACKEY, v.p. and media dir.

LOWE RUNKLE CO., 6801 N. Broadway, Oklahoma City, OK 73114 (405) 848-6800.
OSCAR HEUSER, pres. & CEO; MARK BAUSKE, dir. bdcst. prod.

SAATCHI & SAATCHI COMPTON, INC., 625 Madison Ave., New York, NY 10022.
O. MILTON GOSSETT, pres. & CEO; C. CAPUANO, v.p. art & TV commercial production; BRUCE COX, sr. v.p./dir. bdcst. programming. Branch offices: Los Angeles, CA; Southfield, MI.

SHOTWELL AND PARTNERS, INCORPORATED, 801 East Blvd., Charlotte, NC 28203; (704) 372-8880
ED BEAM, producer.

SIMONS MICHELSON ZIEVE INC., 3250 West Big Beaver Road, Troy, MI 48084; (313) 649-5600.
MORTON ZIEVE, JAMES A. MICHELSON, officers; JON KATZ, TV dept. dir.

SPIRO & ASSOCIATES, INC., 100 S. Broad St., Phila., PA; (215) WAlnut 3-5400.
HERB SMITH, sr. v.p., media dir.

SPITZ ADVERTISING INC., 530 Oak St., Syracuse, NY; (315) 479-5581.
WILLIAM SPITZ, president; CHRIS SLATER, radio-TV dir.; NICK BIBKO, acct. exec.; FAN SPITZ, single sls. & prod.

TATHAM-LAIRD & KUDNER, 980 N. Michigan Avenue, Chicago, IL 60611; (313) 337-4400.
CHICAGO: CHARLOTTE BEERS, chm. & CEO; WILLIAM YOUNGCLOUS, pres. & COO; JOHN J. VALVERDE, sr. partner, chief financial officer; PHILIP GERBER, sr. partner, media opns. dir.; LEONARD F. MATERNA, media svcs. dir.; WERNER WOLFF, mgr. broadcast business affairs.

J. WALTER THOMPSON COMPANY, 466 Lexington Ave., New York, NY 10017; (212) 210-7000.
DON JOHNSON, bd. chm. & chief exec. officer; JOSEPH W. O'DONNELL, chm.-elect. DENIS LANIGAN, vice-chm. & chief operating officer; JACK CRONIN, vice-chm.; BURT MANNING, vice chm.—Creative Resources, JACK PETERS, pres.
J. Walter Thompson USA Inc., (subsidiary of J. Walter Thompson Co.) offices: Atlanta, Chicago, Detroit, Los Angeles, New York, San Francisco, Washington, DC.
Service offices: Charlotte, Dallas, Denver, Houston, Indianapolis, Kansas City, Memphis, Miami, New Orleans, Oklahoma City, Omaha, Philadelphia, Phoenix, Rochester, Salt Lake City, St. Louis.
J. Walter Thompson Co. International offices: Buenos Aires, Sydney, Melbourne, Perth, Brisbane, Vienna, Brussels, São Paulo, Rio de Janeiro, Toronto, Montreal, Vancouver, Santiago, Copenhagen, Santo Domingo, Quito, Guyaquil, Helsinki, Lyon, Paris, Frankfurt, Dusseldorf, Hamburg, Athens, Guatemala City, Hong Kong, Milan, Rome, Osaka, Tokyo, Kuala Lumpur, Mexico City, Amsterdam, Wellington, Auckland, Zug, Lima, Manila, Lisbon, San Juan, Singapore, Johannesburg, Cape Town, Madrid, Barcelona, Colombo, Stockholm, Zurich, Asuncion, Bangkok, Istanbul, Izmir, Dubai, London, Manchester, Caracas, Montevideo.

TRACY-LOCKE ADVERTISING INC., Plaza of the Americas, South Tower, P.O. Box 50129, Dallas, TX 75250; (214) 742-3131.
MORRIS HITE, bd. chm.; NORM CAMPBELL, pres.; BOB BELTON, v.p. bdcst prod.; LARRY SPIEGEL, sr. v.p. dir. media & research; WALT ATKINSON, v.p., media serv. dir.; CLAUDE CAYLOR, v.p., media dir.; JUDY MILLER, v.p., media buying director; GINA BURKS, dir. of network; CAROL CASTELLANO, dir. of spot.

VAN BRUNT & CO., ADVERTISING-MARKETING INC., 300 E. 42nd Street, New York, NY 10017; (212) 949-1300.
EDWIN VAN BRUNT, chm. bd.; ALBERT VAN BRUNT, pres.;

HOWARD KARP, creative dir.; WILLIAM BUCKLEY, dir. of broadcast.

VICTOR VAN DER LINDE CO., INC., 381 Broadway, Westwood, NJ 07675; (201) 664-6830.
A. K. KINGSLEY, v.p.

MORTON DENNIS WAX AND ASSOCIATES, 1560 Broadway, New York, NY 10036; (212) 302-5360
MORTON DENNIS WAX, pres.; SANDRA WAX, v.p./gen. mgr.

WEBSTER & HARRIS ADVERTISING AGENCY, 1313 Broadway, Lubbock, TX 79401; (806) 747-2588.
REX WEBSTER & LEON HARRIS, acct. execs. partners; JIMMY GRAY, prod. mgr.

WILLIS/CASE/HARWOOD, INC., 3411 Office Park Drive, Dayton, OH 45439; (513) 299-7394.
MICHEAL G. HEALY, pres.; SANDRA MAGEE, dir. of media.

YOUNG & RUBICAM INC., 285 Madison Ave., New York, NY 10017; (212) 953-2000.
EDWARD N. NEY, chm., pres. & chief exec. officer; ALEXANDER KROLL, exec. v.p.; pres. Y&R USA div.; JOSEPH W. OSTROW, exec. v.p., dir. communications svcs.; RICHARD H. LOW, exec. v.p., dir. bdcst, programming & purchasing.
Y&R USA OFFICES: Cedar Rapids, IA & Des Moines; Chicago; Cincinnati, OH; Denver, CO; Detroit, MI; Houston, TX; Kansas City, MO; New York, NY; Los Angeles, San Diego & San Francisco, CA; Rochester, NY; St. Petersburg, FL.
Y&R International Offices: Adelaide, Melbourne & Sydney, Australia; Madrid, Spain; Berne & Zurich, Switzerland; Brussels, Belgium; Buenos Aires, Argentina; Copenhagen, Denmark; Frankfurt & Munich, Germany; Stockholm & Gothenburg, Sweden; Hong Kong; London, England; Mexico City, Mexico; Milan, Italy; Montreal & Toronto, Canada; Oslo, Norway; Paris, France; San Juan, Puerto Rico; Santo Domingo, Dominican Republic; São Paulo, Brazil; Singapore; Tokyo, Japan; Vienna, Austria; Amsterdam, The Netherlands; Santigo, Chile.

Station Representatives

ABC-TV TELEVISION SPOT SALES, INC., 1345 Ave. of the Americas, New York, NY 10019 (212) 887-7777.
JOHN B. WATKINS, pres.; PHILIP J. SWEENIE, v.p.; JOSEPH COHEN, east. sls. mgr.; MICHAEL COLLERAN, est. sls. mgr.; MARY WEBB ELLIS, east. sls. mgr.
Branch Offices: Chicago 60601, Two Illinois Center; (312) 750-7777, SCOTT THOMAS, sls. mgr.; Los Angeles 90067, 2040 Ave. of Stars; (213) 557-6241, MICHAEL JACK; San Francisco 94111, 900 Front St.; (415) 863-0077, FRANKLIN LOWE; Southfield, MI (Detroit) 48075, 3000 Town Center, (313) 355-4490., ED PEARSON; Dallas 75251, 2 Forest Plaza/12201 Merit Dr.; (214) 960-7981, MICHAEL IRVINE; Atlanta 30339, 200 Galleria Parkway, NW; (404) 956-0822, DEBBIE SHAW.

AVERY-KNODEL TELEVISION, 437 Madison Avenue, New York, NY 10022 (212) 421-5600.
J. W. KNODEL, chmn.; ROBERT J. KIZER, pres.; F. ROBERT KALTHOFF, exec. v.p.
Branch Offices: Chicago 60601, 2600 Prudential Plaza; (312) 467-6111, F. ROBERT KALTHOFF; San Francisco 94104, 155 Montgomery Street; (415) 986-8082, JOSEPH FRIEDMAN; Los Angeles 90005, 633 South Shatto Place; (213) 385-6394; Atlanta 30326, 3340 Peachtree Road, N.E.; (404) 233-4474, JAMES GOSSETT; Dallas 75219, 3626 North Hall St., Suite 608; (214) 528-1741 WALLIS S. IVY; Detroit, 48084, DAVID BRANGAN; St. Louis 63102, 410 Mansion House Center; (314) 241-5051, FRED W. JOHNSON; Minneapolis, St. Paul: toll free exchange, 929-1300, Edna, MN 55435, 6700 France Ave., Suite 155, MAUREEN KVAM; Denver 80206, 280 Columbine Ave.; (303) 321-1086, BOB HIX; Portland 97204, 620 SW 5th Suite 907; (503) 223-5980, RON HILLBURY; Seattle 98109, P.O. Box 19417; (206) 624-9200, JACK DAVIES; Haddonfield 08033, 537 Mt. Vernon Avenue, TOM WOOD.

BLAIR TELEVISION, 1290 Ave. of Americas, New York, NY 10104; (212) 603-5000.
HARRY B. SMART, chairm/CEO; WALTER A. SCHWARTZ, pres./COO; PATRICK J. DEVLIN, exec. v.p./dir. of sls. operations; JAMES R. KELLY, sr. v.p./dir. of client services; WILLIAM E. BREDA, JR., sr. v.p./dir. of affiliate/IND sls.; FLOYD J. GELINI, sr. v.p./dir. of regional sls.; SANFORD S. ACKERMAN, v.p./dir. of finance/planning/admin.; KENNETH P. DONNELLON, v.p.; STEVEN A. MURPHY, v.p./management systems & services.
Branch offices: Chicago, Atlanta, Boston, Charlotte, Cleveland, Dallas, Detroit, Houston, Jacksonville, Los Angeles, Miami, Minneapolis, Philadelphia, St. Louis, San Francisco, Seattle.

CBS TELEVISION STATIONS NATIONAL SALES, 51 West 52nd St., New York, NY 10019 (212) 975-4321.
RHODERIC H. PERTH, v.p. & gen. mgr.; GARY MONTANUS, dir. eastern sales; Branch offices: Chicago, 630 North McClurg Court, (312) 944-6000, INGER JENSON, dir., midwest sales; Detroit, 26877 Northwest Hwy., (313) 352-2800, CHET COLLINS, mgr.; San Francisco, 1 Embarcadero Center, (415) 433-0500, FRANKLIN WHEELER, mgr.; Los Angeles, Sunset Blvd., (213) 460-3000, ROBERT BERGLUND; Atlanta: 6 Piedmont Center, (404) 261-2227, SAM STOLWORTH, mgr.

CREED ASSOCIATES, INC., Park Square Bldg., Boston, MA 02116 (617) 482-4845.
R. A. KEATING, R. P. LUETTERS, IRENE KELLEHER.

GROUP W TELEVISION SALES, 90 Park Ave., New York, NY 10016 (212) 883-6100.
ROBERT KUNATH, pres.; JOEL SEGALL, v.p., natl. sls. mgr.; ARMA E. ANDON, v.p.; EDWARD GOLDMAN, v.p. NY sls. mgr.; JEFF OSBORNE, v.p., admin. sls. & mktg.; DANA S. FITZGERALD, NY group sls. mgr.; RUDY TAYLOR, NY group sls. mgr.; ANTHONY DeTHOMAS, controller; JOSEPH PICCIRILLO, dir. research.
Branch offices: Atlanta, GA 30326, 3330 Peachtree Rd. NE, Suite 345; (404) 885-5336; Boston, MA 02134, 1170 Soldiers Field Rd.; (617) 787-7220, DAVID BIGGS; Chicago, IL 60611, 625 N. Michigan Ave., Suite 400; (312) 454-6910, RICHARD KURZAWSKI; Dallas, TX 75251, 12221 Merit Drive, Suite 620; (214) 458-9767, JERRY DANFORD; Detroit (Oak Park), MI 48237, 25900 Greenfield Rd., Suite 243; (313) 968-2160, ROBERT E. NEWSHAM; Los Angeles, CA 90048, 6420 Wilshire Blvd., Suite 1150; (213) 655-3556, ALAN BUCKMAN; Philadelphia, PA 19106, Independence Mall East; (215) 238-4966, THOMAS HOLLINGSHEAD; San Francisco, CA 94111, 825 Battery St.; (415) 765-8793, E. JAMES HODGETT.

KATZ COMMUNICATIONS, INC., One Dag Hammarskjold Plaza, New York, NY 10022; (212) 572-5500.
JAMES L. GREENWALD, chm., CEO; RICHARD D. MENDELSON, pres., COO; MICHAEL I PACKMAN, SR., v.p., chief finan. off.; LUCILLE F. LUONGO, v.p., corp. relations.
KATZ TELEVISION: PETER GOULAZIAN, pres.; DICK GOLDSTEIN, SR., v.p.; PAUL D. ARNZEN, v.p., dir. new business; JOHN VON SOOSTEN, v.p. & dir; prg.; GEORGE FELDMAN, v.p., dir. mgt. serv.; LAURA NILON, mgr., TV admn.; DICK WEINSTEIN, v.p., planning & devel.; BOB EINHORN, v.p., sls. research.
KATZ AMERICAN TELEVISION: JAMES E. BELOYIANIS, pres.; MICHAEL HUGGER, v.p. & gen. sls. mgr.; MAURY WIND, v.p., reg'l offices.; ROBERT BLAGMAN, v.p., sr. natl. sls. mgr., RED; CHICKIE BUCCO, N.Y. team mgr., RED; IBRA MORALES, v.p., natl. sls. mgr., & NY sls. mgr, EAGLES: SWAIN WEINER, NY Team mgr., EAGLES; KEN PERREN, v.p., natl. sls. mgr., BLUE; JAY ZEITCHIK, NY team mgr., BLUE; RUSS WHITE, v.p., natl. sls. mgr., WHITE; KEITH J. GREEN, N.Y. team mgr., WHITE; MARK SHOTTLAND, v.p., natl. sls. mgr., STARS; T.C. SHULTZ, NY team mgr., STARS; BILL CARROLL, dir. prog.; DICK WILLIAMS, v.p., dir., natl. sls. devel.; BUB BOWLIN, dir., Response Sls. supervisor; LISA SCHOENBACK, v.p., dir, American Research.
KATZ TELEVISION CONTINENTAL: TOM OLSON, pres.; JACK HIGGINS, v.p., gen. mgr.; JAY FRIESEL, v.p., gen. sls. mgr.; BOB LEVENSTEIN, v.p., gen. sls. mgr.; JERRY CIFARELLI, natl. sls., mgr., EAST; CHRIS JORDAN, NY sls. mgr., EAST: DAN LUCCI, v.p., natl. sls. mgr., EAST CENTRAL; MARGARET TJEPKEMA, NY sls. mgr., EAST CENTRAL; HERB KING, v.p., natl. sls. mgr., SOUTHEAST; MIKE SPIESMAN, NY sls. mgr. SOUTHEAST; EARL OVERTON, v.p., natl. sls. mgr., SOUTH CENTRAL; MARK RYAN, NY sls. mgr., SOUTH CENTRAL; JOHN WALL, v.p., natl. sls. mgr., WEST CENTRAL; MARTY McHALE, NY sls. mgr., WEST CENTRAL; ARDIE BIALEK, v.p., natl. sls. mgr. WEST; CAREY MOLEY, NY sls. mgr. WEST; MITCHELL PRAVER, v.p. prog. dir.; BUB BOWLIN, dir. response sls. spvr.; MICHAEL STEINBERG, dir., continental research.
KATZ INDEPENDENT TELEVISION: MARTY OZER, pres.; MICKY COLEN, v.p,. regnl. sls. mgr.; PAT GARVEY, v.p., natl. sls. mgr., LANCERS; JOANNA HEMLEB, NY team mgr., LANCERS; MICHAEL RAOUNAS, v.p. natl sls. mgr., SABERS; JILL NOVORRO, NY team mgr., SABERS; SUSAN ZILLER BRAZELL, v.p., natl. sls. mgr., SWORDS; STUART ZUCKERMAN, v.p., mgr. SWORDS; JOE WHITE, team mgr., SWORDS; CATHY EGAN, v.p., dir. of mktg.; SERGE VALLE, v.p., programming; ANDI-POCH, dir., sports sponsorship sls.; JOAN RUTMAN, dir., independent research.

ART MOORE INC., 220 W. Mercer, Seattle, WA 98119 (206) 282-3400.
GREG SMITH, EARLE BAKER, SANDY RUNNION, RICK STAEB, RUTH HALLETT. Branch: Portland, OR 97214, 516 S.E. Morrison; (503) 228-2451, DARRELL RUTTER, BRUCE WORKMAN, TEDDI JONES, LYNN THORSEN.

NBC SPOT SALES, NATIONAL BROADCASTING COMPANY, INC., 30 Rockefeller Plaza, New York, NY 10020 (212) 247-8300.
RICHARD H. CLOSE, v.p.; BYRON GOODELL, dir. of TV spot sales; RICHARD BERGH, eastern TV mgr. BILL FROMM, dir. of new business & prom.

NATIONAL TIME SALES, 9 East 41 St., New York, NY 10016 (212) 661-6550.
H. FRANKLIN, sales mgr.
Branch offices: Chicago, 60645, 3322 W. Peterson Ave.; (312) 478-5544, HOOPER JONES; Atlanta, 30309, 1819 Peachtree Rd. N.E.; (404) 355-7961, BERNARD OCHS; Dallas, 75202, 1407 Main St.; (214) 748-2172, JACK RILEY; San Francisco, 94133, 559 Pacific Ave.; SAM POSNER; Beverly Hills, 90028, 111 N. La Cienega Blvd.; CHUCK DWYER; San Jose, 95129, 4320 Stevens Creek Blvd.; (408) 249-5287, GENE BERNALD.

THE BERNARD I. OCHS CO., 805 Longleaf Dr., N.E., Atlanta, GA 30342 (404) 262-1200.
BARNEY OCHS; PAT CASTLEBERRY, sec.

PETRY TELEVISION, INC., 3 East 54 St., New York, NY 10022 (212) 688-0200.
DAVID S. ALLEN, pres.; D.W. SCHELLENGER, sr. v.p., finance & admin; HARRY STECKER, sr., v.p., dir. of mktg.; JOHN SCOGNAMILLO, v.p., controller; TOM BELVISO, v.p., admin.
PETRY TELEVISION: WILLIAM FAGAN, pres.; George Blinn, sr. v.p., gen. sls. mrg.; JERRY LINEHAN, v.p., dir. of sls.; STEVE EISENBERG, v.p., dir. of sls.; KATHY CLINTON, v.p.., dir. of regnl. sls.; ROBERT MIGGINS, v.p., regnl. area (West Coast); GREG MOLOZNIK, v.p., regnl. area (Midwest); PAT McNEW, v.p., regnl. area (North); LAVERNE COLE, v.p., regnl. area (Southeast); GEORGE DENNIS, dir. of manpower devel.; PATRICK TWYON, dir. of sports; ALAN SCHLOSS-

BERG, dir. of sports; TEDDY S. REYNOLDS, dir. or research; CHERYL SOUCY, dir. of mktg.; JOANNI DIPRISCO, dir. of mktg.; DICK KURLANDER, dir. of programming; JOHN DORKIN, assoc. dir. of programming; KEVIN NUGENT, group sls. mgr., FALCONS; BILL SHAW, group sls. mgr., HAWKS; PAUL MORRISEY, group sls. mgr., RAVENS; ROB FRIEDMAN, group sls. mgr., ROADRUNNERS; BILL BURKE, group sls. mgr., THUNDERBIRDS.
PETRY NATIONAL: MICHAEL T. MEMBRADO, pres.; WILILAM WIEHEl, v.p.; JOHN HEISE, v.p., dir. of sales; ROBERT HEBENSTREIT, dir. of research; JACK FENTRESS, v.p., dir. of programming; JOSEPH LYONS, v.p. group mgr., RED; CHUCK HANRAHAN, group sales mgr., WHITE; AL WESTERMANN, v.p., sr. group mgr., BLUE.
BRANCH OFFICES: CHICAGO, 410 Michigan Ave., Suite 1180, 60611; Greg Moloznick, v.p. regnl. area mgr. (Midwest); James Ottolin, group sls. mgr., RED; Stu Strizak, group sls. mgr., BLUE; Kent Francis, dir. of agri mktg.; LOS ANGELES, 8383 Wilshire Blvd., Suite 626, Beverly Hills, CA 90211; Bob Muggins, v.p., regnl. area mgr., (West Coast); Jime Valice, group sls. mgr., RED; ATLANTA, 400 Colony Sq., Suite 1605, 30361; Chris Teter, group sls. mgr.; BOSTON, 419 Boylston St., 02116; Diane Gosdanian, v.p., sls. mgr.; Charlotte Two Fairview Plaza, 5950 Fairview Rd., Suite 804, 28210; STOCKTON HOLT, sls. mgr.; CLEVELAND, 1111 Superior Ave., Suite 7A, 44114; Craig Mc Murray, sls. mgr.; DALLAS, 3811 Turtle Creek Blvd., Suite 520, 75219; Laverne Cole, v.p., regnl. area mgr. (Southeast); Cliff Hahne, mgr.; Cynthia Grimm, group sls mgr.; DENVER 6025 South Quebec, Suite 250, Englewood, CO 80111; Kathy Crawford Gilbert, sls. mgr.; DETROIT, 3221 W. Big Beaver Rd., Troy, MI 48084; Patrick McNew, v.p., regnl. sls. mgr., (North); HOUSTON, 2100 West Loop South, Suite 707, 77027; Chuck Sitta, sls. mgr.; MINNEAPOLIS, 706 Second Ave. S., 55402; Tom Vannelli, sls. mgr.; PHILADELPHIA, Two Penn Center Plaza, Suite 406, 19102; Dave Bell, sls. mgr.; ST. LOUIS, Ten South Broadway, 63102, Pat Carroll-Lee, sls. mgr.; SAN FRANCISCO, 909 Montgomery St., Suite 402, 94133; Don Brownstein, sls. mgr.; SEATTLE, 200 W. Mercer, Suite 505, 98119; MARC F. MEAHL, sls. mgr.; TAMPA, 9400 Fourth St. N., Suite 114, St. Petersburg, FL 33792; JUDY OBERNIER, sls. mgr.

RADIO-TELEVISION REPRESENTATIVES LIMITED, 10 Price Street, Toronto, Ontario. M4W 1Z4 (416) 962-3221.
ROBERT H. QUINN, pres. & gen. mgr.; LEN MOORE, v.p., mktg.; MARK BURKO, v.p./tv sls. mgr.
Branch offices: Montreal: 1118 St. Catherine St., W., Room 201, Montreal, Que. H3B 1H5; (514) 866-3466, MARK BURKO; Calgary: 300–5th Ave., SW, Suite 2050, Calgary, Alta. T2P 3C4; (403) 269-3496, GARY DIETRICK; Vancouver: 6–969 West Broadway, Vancouver, B.C. V5Z 1K3; (604) 736-6634, FRANK JOBES; Winnipeg: 802–288 Notre Dame Ave., Winnipeg, Man. R3B 1N7; (204) 943-9574, HENRY BOSCHMAN.

SELTEL, INC., 750 Third Ave., New York, NY 10017; (212) 697-0944. TWX: 710-581-3801/3791/5065/6768/2512.
JACK MULDERRIG, pres. & CEO/ RAYMOND J. JOHNS, exec. v.p.; STEVE BOUTIS, SR., v.p, finance; JOSEPH CUSENZA, sr. v.p., affiliate operations; DAVID SCHWARTZ, sr. v.p., independent operations; C. WILLIAM COLDWELL, v.p., natl. sls. mgr., affiliate Red & Blue Teams; JUDY KLEINBERGER, v.p., natl. sls. mgr., affiliate White Team; PHYLLIS TAORMINE, v.p., natl. sls. mgr., Indy-Raiders Team; DAN PARISI, natl. sls. mgr., Indy-Rangers & Rebels Team; JANEEN BJORK, v.p., dir. of programming; DOUGLAS DARFIELD, v.p., research dir.
Chicago: 211 E. Ontario, Suite 700, Chicago, IL 60611; (312) 642-2450. TWX: 910-221-0241, 0242, 5195. MARTY MILLER, sr. v.p., central region mgr.; JIM PARKET, v.p., sls. mgr. affiliate Red Team; RANDY BROWN, sls. mgr. affiliate White Team; TODD ROHDE, sls. mgr. Indy-Raiders Team; DAN POPRAVAK, sls. mgr., Indy-Rangers Team.
Atlanta: 1819 Peachtree Road, N.E. Atlanta, GA 30309; (404) 355-7701. TWX: 810-751-3101. PAUL BREWER, mgr.
Boston: 545 Boylston St., 7th Floor, Boston, MA 02116; (617) 236-8666. TWX: 710-321-0016. PETER DURAN, mgr.
Charlotte: 5821 Park Rd., Suite 112, Charlotte, NC 28209; (704) 554-7124. SUZY PLETTNER, mgr.
Dallas: 3010 LBJ Freeway, Suite 1130, Dallas, TX 75234; (214) 484-4871.. TWX: 910-861-4210. MICHAEL CUSTARDO, mgr.
Denver: 222 Milwaukee St., Suite 210, Denver, CO; (303) 333-4845. Telex: 100-230-450296. CHRIS MATTHEWS, mgr.
Detroit: 26211 Central Park Blvd., Suite 202, Southfield, MI 48076-4107; (313) 354-3611. TWX: 810-224-4502. JESS CHALKER, v.p., mgr.
Houston: 4848 Loop Central Dr., Suite 710, Houston, TX 77081. (713) 660-8881. TWX: 910-881-0063. SABRINA LEONARD, mgr.
Los Angeles: 5757 Wilshire Blvd., Los Angeles, CA 90036; (213) 930-2450. TWX: 910-321-4124. LAVADA HEALTH, v.p., mgr.; DAVE WARE, sls. mgr. Indy-Raiders; ED TINNEY, sls. mgr. Indy-Rangers; JUDY MALCOLM-GRAGG, sls. mgr. affiliate team; RALPH CLAUSSEN, sls. mgr. affiliate White Team.
Miami: 6101 Blue Lagoon Dr., Suite 460, Miami, FL 33126; (305) 266-4066. TWX: 810-848-0197. ENID BLUESTONE, mgr.
Minneapolis: 623 Second Ave. South, Suite 408, Minneapolis, MN 55402; (612) 338-7707. TWX: 910-576-3419. MIKE CLEARY, mgr.
Philadelphia: 1411 Walnut St., Suite 1125, Philadelphia, PA 19103; (215) 563-5400. TWX: 710-670-1017. JOSEPH PEDRI, mgr.
Portland: 1512 S.W. 18th Ave., Portland, OR 97201; (503) 226-2911. EASY LINK: 629-275-56+. RICHARD GOHLMAN, mgr.
St. Louis: St. Louis Place, 200 N. Broadway, Suite 1125, St. Louis, MO 63102; (314) 241-4193. TWX: 910-761-0400. RICHARD J. QUIGLEY III, v.p., mgr.
San Francisco: 50 Francisco St., San Francisco, CA 94133; (415) 391-8890. TWX: 910-372-7361. EDWARD OUTLAND, mgr.
Seattle: 701 Dexter Ave., North, Suite 216, Seattle, WA 98109; (206) 285-1913. EASY LING: 627-625-31. BOB TACHER, mgr.

STAUFFER COMMUNICATIONS, Inc., 100% owner of WIBW-TV, Box 119, Topeka, KA 66601 (913) 272-3456.
JERRY HOLLEY, v.p.; GEORGE LOGAN, TV station mgr.; R. C. SENATE, natl. sls. mgr. Represented nationally by The Katz Agency, Inc., New York, Chicago, Dallas, Detroit, Atlanta, San Francisco, Los Angeles, Seattle, Charlotte, Cleveland, Memphis, Portland, Boston, Jacksonville, Minneapolis, St. Louis, Philadelphia.

STORER TELEVISION SALES, INC., 800 Third Ave., New York, NY 10022 (212) 935-6000.
FRANCIS BARRON, pres.; PETER E. MURRAY, exec. v.p., sales; PETER STORER, JR., research director.
Branch Offices: Chicago: 410 No. Michigan Ave., (312) 329-1930; CHARLES LIEBER, v.p., Midwest sales; Detroit: Number Two Storer Place, (313) 557-0300; ELAINE CARPENTER, Det. sls. mgr.; Atlanta: Three Piedmont Ctr., (404) 233-9935; RICHARD GOLDSTEIN, Southern sls. mgr.; San Francisco: 150 Lombard Street, (415) 981-8860, SHAWN McGREEVY, v.p., S.F. sls.; Los Angeles, 6420 Wilshire Blvd., (213) 651-0841, JOSEPH MERTENS, v.p., West Coast sls.

ADAM YOUNG, INC., 3 E. 54th St., New York, NY 10022 (212) 688-5100.
ADAM YOUNG, chm. of bd.; VINCENT J. YOUNG, pres.; ARTHUR W. SCOTT, exec. v.p.; AJOAN M. BARRON, v.p. & gen. sales mgr.
BRANCH OFFICES: ATLANTA, GA 30329; 57 Executive Park South; (404) 633-1735; LARRY FINCH, mgr.; CHICAGO 60611, 444 No. Michigan Ave.; (312) 744-1313; LOIS HAMELIN, mgr.; DALLAS 75219; 3626 No. Hall St.; (214) 522-0816; SUSAN CLAIR WAGNER, mgr.; DETROIT: 2855 Coolidge, Troy, MI 48084; (313) 649-3999, ALLAN ABUR, mgr.; DENVER, 80206, P.O. Box 61498; (303) 377-6526; BOB HIX, mgr.; LOS ANGELES 90010, 4929 Wilshire Blvd., (213) 938-2081; KEITH ERLING THOMPSON, v.p., west. sls.; PHILADELPHIA/PITTSBURGH: See N.Y. address; RICHARD GOLDEN, acct. exec.; ST. LOUIS, MO 63105; P.O. Box 50269; (314) 991-5249; BRUCE W. SCHNEIDER, mgr.; SAN FRANCISCO 94104; 425 California St.; (415) 986-5366; KEITH BAINBRIDGE, mgr.

Programs

* NETWORK
* SYNDICATED

1986–87 Prime Time Shows

Series titles are listed alphabetically by network, along with time slots, suppliers, production staff heads (executive producer: EP; executive supervising producer, ESP; supervising producer: SP; senior producer: Sr. P; producer: P; co-producer: CP; director: D), cast regulars and semi-regulars.

ABC-TV

Series Title	Day	Hr.	Mins.	Supplier	Production Principals	Cast Regulars & Semi-Regulars
ABC Sunday Night Movie	Sun	9:00	120	Various		
Colbys, The	Thu	9:00	60	Richard & Esther Shapiro Prods.-Aaron Spelling Prods.	EP: Richard & Esther Shapiro, Aaron Spelling, Douglas S. Cramer SP: E. Duke Vincent, Robert & Eileen Pollock P: William Bast, Paul Huson, Dennis Hammer	Charlton Heston, John James, Katharine Ross, Emma Samms, Maxwell Caulfield, Tracy Scoggins, Claire Yarlett, Stephanie Beacham, Ricardo Montalban, Kim Morgan Greene, Kevin McCarthy, James Houghton, Adrian Paul
Disney Sunday Movie, The	Sun	7:00	120	Walt Disney TV		Michael Eisner
Dynasty	Wed	9:00	60	Richard & Esther Shapiro Prods.-Aaron Spelling Prods.	EP: Richard & Esther Shapiro, Aaron Spelling, Douglas S. Cramer SP: E. Duke Vincent, Robert & Eileen Pollack, Elaine Rich P: Edward DeBlasio, Laurence Heath	John Forsythe, Linda Evans, Gordon Thomson, Jack Coleman, Michael Nader, Heather Locklear, Ted McGinley, Wayne Northrop, Christopher Cazenove, Keren Cellini, Diahann Carroll, Joan Collins, Troy Beyer, Richard Lawson, Leanne Hunley
Ellen Burstyn Show, The	Sat	8:30	30	Ellen Burstyn Prods.-P.S. 235 Prods.-Touchstone Films	EP: Norman Steinberg SP: David Frankel, Howard Gewirtz P: Ronald E. Frazier	Ellen Burstyn, Elaine Stritch, Megan Mullally, Jesse Tender, Barry Sobel
Growing Pains	Tue	8:30	30	Warner Bros. TV	EP: Michael Sullivan, Dan Guntzelman, Steve Marshall	Alan Thicke, Joanna Kerns, Kirk Cameron, Tracey Gold, Jeremy Miller
Head of the Class	Wed	8:30	30	Eustis Elias Prods.-Warner Bros. TV	EP: Rich Eustis & Michael Elias P: Gary Gilbert, Alan Rosen, Gayle Maffeo	Howard Hesseman, William G. Schilling, Jeanetta Arnette, Leslie Bega, Dan Frischman, Robin Givens, Khrystyne Haje, Jory Husain, Tony O'Dell, Brian Robbins, Kimberly Russell, Daniel J. Schneider, Tannis Vallely
Heart Of The City	Sat	9:00	60	American Flyer Films-20th Fox TV	EP: Michael Zinberg SP: E. Arthur Kean P: David H. Balkan	Robert Desiderio, Jonathan Ward, Christina Applegate, Dick Anthony Williams, Kario Salem, Branscombe Richmond
Hotel	Wed	10:00	60	Aaron Spelling Prods.	EP: Aaron Spelling, Douglas S. Cramer SP: E. Duke Vincent P: Henry Colman, Andrew Laskos & James Fritzhand, Tom Swale & Duane Poole	James Brolin, Connie Sellecca, Nathan Cook, Michael Spound, Heidi Bohay, Shari Belafonte-Harper, Efrem Zimbalist Jr., Michelle Phillips, Ralph Bellamy
Jack & Mike	Tue	10:00	60	David Gerber Co.-MGM/UA TV	EP: David Gerber SP: Jack Bender, Liz Coe P: Christopher Chulack CP: David Braff	Shelley Hack, Tom Mason, Kevin Dunn, Holly Fulger, Jacqueline Brookes
Life With Lucy	Sat	8:00	30	Lucille Ball Prods.-Aaron Spelling Prods.	EP: Aaron Spelling, Douglas S. Cramer, Gary Morton SP: E. Duke Vincent P: Madelyn Davis, Bob Carroll Jr. CP: Vic Rauseo, Linda Morris	Lucille Ball, Gale Gordon, Ann Dusenberry, Larry Anderson, Jenny Lewis, Philip J. Amelio II, Donovan Scott
MacGyver	Mon	8:00	60	Henry Winkler/-John Rich Prods.-Paramount TV	EP: Henry Winkler, John Rich, Steve Downing SP: Mark Lisson, Bill Froehlich P: Kevin Inch CP: Stephen Kandel	Richard Dean Anderson, Dana Elcar
Monday Night Football	Mon	9:00	120+	ABC Sports	EP: Roone Arledge P: Ken Wolfe D: Chet Forte	Al Michaels, Frank Gifford
Moonlighting	Tue	9:00	60	Picturemaker Prods.-ABC Circle Films	EP: Glenn Gordon Caron, Jay Daniel SP: Artie Mandelberg, Karen Hall P: Ron Osborn, Jeff Reno, Roger Director	Cybill Shepherd, Bruce Willis, Allyce Beasley, Curtis Armstrong
Mr. Belvedere	Fri	8:30	30	Lazy B/F.O.B. Prod.-20th Fox TV	EP: Frank Dungan & Jeff Stein, Tony Sheehan P: Patricia Rickey CP: Jeff Ferro, Ric Weiss	Christopher Hewett, Ilene Graff, Rob Stone, Brice Beckham, Bob Uecker

Series Title	Day	Hr.	Mins.	Supplier	Production Principals	Cast Regulars & Semi-Regulars
Our World	Thu	8:00	60	ABC News	EP: Av Westin Sr. P: Pete Simmons, Susan Lester, Ellen Rossen	Linda Ellerbee, Ray Gandolf
Perfect Strangers	Wed	8:00	30	Miller-Boyett Prods.-Lorimar Telepictures	EP: Thomas L. Miller, Robert L. Boyett, Dale McRaven SP: William Bickley & Michael Warren P: Mark Fink CP: James O'Keefe, Paula A. Roth	Bronson Pinchot, Mark Linn-Baker, Ernie Sabella, Lise Cutter
Sidekicks	Fri	9:30	30	Motown Prods.-Walt Disney TV	EP: Bill Dial, Richard Chapman, Michael L. Weisbarth P: Ric Rondell CP: Bob Comfort, Sally Baker	Gil Gerard, Nancy Stafford, Keye Luke, Ernie Reyes Jr., Frank Bonner
Sledge Hammer	Fri	9:00	30	New World TV	EP: William P. D'Angelo P: Alan Spencer D: Martha Coolidge	David Rasche, Anne-Marie Martin, Harrison Page
Spenser: For Hire	Sat	10:00	60	Warner Bros. TV-Jadda Prods.-John Wilder	EP: Juanita Bartlett SP: William R. Yates, Stephen Hattman, Michael J. Maschio P: Cleve Landsberg	Robert Urich, Avery Brooks, Carolyn McCormick, Ron McLarty, Richard Jaeckel
Starman	Fri	10:00	60	Michael Douglas Prods.-Henerson/Hirsch Prods.-Columbia Pictures TV	EP: Michael Douglas, James Henerson, James Hirsch SP: Leon Tokatyan P: John B. Mason, Mike Gray	Robert Hays, C. B. Barnes, Michael Cavanaugh
20/20	Thu	10:00	60	ABC News	EP: Av Westin	Hugh Downs, Barbara Walters, Robert Brown, Lynn Sherr, Stone Phillips, Tom Jarriel, John Stossel
Webster	Fri	8:00	30	Georgia Bay Prods.-Emmanuel Lewis Entertainment-Paramount TV	EP: Bruce Johnson, Ken Hecht & Bob Brunner SP: Fred Rubin P: Nancy Steen, Neil Thompson CP: Clare Witt	Susan Clark, Alex Karras, Emmanuel Lewis, Jack Kruschen, Henry Polic II
Who's The Boss?	Tue	8:00	30	Embassy TV	EP: Blake Hunter, Martin Cohan SP: Robert Sternin, Prudence Fraser P: Ellen Guylas	Tony Danza, Judith Light, Alyssa Milano, Danny Pintauro, Katherine Helmond, Robin Thomas

CBS-TV

Series Title	Day	Hr.	Mins.	Supplier	Production Principals	Cast Regulars & Semi-Regulars
Better Days	Wed	8:30	30	Magnum/Thunder Road Prods.-Lorimar-Telepictures	EP: Stuart Sheslow, Jeff Freilich, Arthur Silver P: Marty Nadler, Ron Rubin D: Bill Bixby	Rafael Sbarge, Chip McAllister, Guy Killum, Randee Heller, Dick O'Neill
CBS Sunday Night Movies	Sun	9:00	120		Various	
CBS Tuesday Night Movies	Tue	9:00	120		Various	
Cagney & Lacey	Mon	10:00	60	Mace Neufeld Prods.-Barney Rozenzweig Prods.-Orion TV	EP: Barney Rosenzweig SP: Shelley List, Jonathan Estrin P: Georgia Jeffries, Ralph Singleton CP: P.K. Knelman	Sharon Gless, Tyne Daly, Al Waxman, Carl Lumbly, Martin Kove, Harvey Atkin, John Karlen, Robert Hegyes, Stephen Macht, Tony LaTorre, Troy Slaten, Paul Mantee
Dallas	Fri	9:00	60	Lorimar-Telepictures	EP: Leonard Katzman SP: Calvin Clements Jr. P: David Paulsen	Barbara Bel Geddes, Patrick Duffy, Linda Gray, Larry Hagman, Susan Howard, Steve Kanaly, Howard Keel, Ken Kercheval, Priscilla Beaulieu Presley, Victoria Principal, Dack Rambo, Steve Forrest
Designing Women	Mon	9:30	30	Bloodworth/Thomason Mozark Prods.-Columbia Pictures TV	EP: Harry Thomason, Linda Bloodworth-Thomason SP: E. Jack Kaplan P: Emily Marshall D: Jack Shea	Delta Burke, Dixie Carter, Annie Potts, Jean Smart
Downtown	Sat	8:00	60	Ron Samuels Prods.-Tri-Star TV	EP: Ron Samuels, Reuben Leder SP: Art Schaefer P:Christopher Beaumont CP: Phil Combest	Michael Nouri, Robert Englund, Millicent Martin, Blair Underwood, Mariska Hargitay, Virginia Capers
Equalizer, The	Wed	10:00	60	Universal TV	EP: James McAdams SP: Ed Waters P: Alan Barnette CP: Coleman Luck, Scott Shepherd, Daniel Lieberstein, Peter A. Runfolo	Edward Woodward, Robert Lansing, William Zabka, Ron O'Neal
Falcon Crest	Fri	10:00	60	Amanda Prods.-Lorimar-Telepictures	EP: Joanne Brough, Jeff Freilich, Michael Filerman SP: Ernie Wallengren, Greg Strangis P: John F. Perry CP: Richard Gollance	Jane Wyman, Robert Foxworth, Lorenzo Lamas, David Shelby, Ana-Alicia, William R. Moses, Margaret Ladd, Laura Johnson, Edward Albert, John Callahan, Abby Dalton, Dana Sparks, Susan Sullivan, Cesar Romero, Kim Novak, John Saxon, Brett Cullen, Jane Badler, Chao-L Chi, Marjoe Gortner

Series Title	Day	Hr.	Mins.	Supplier	Production Principals	Cast Regulars & Semi-Regulars
Kate & Allie	Mon	8:00	30	Mort Lachman & Associates-Reeves Entertainment Group	EP: Merrill Grant, Mort Lachman P: Bill Persky, Bob Randall D: Bill Persky	Susan Saint James, Jane Curtin, Ari Meyers, Frederic Koehler, Allison Smith
Kay O'Brien	Thu	10:00	60	William Asher Prods.-Orion TV	EP: William Asher P: Peter Katz CP: Bryce Zabel & Brad Markowitz	Patricia Kalember, Lane Smith, Priscilla Lopez, Brian Benben, Tony Soper, Keone Young, Jan Rubes
Knots Landing	Thu	9:00	60	Roundelay/MF Prods. Lorimar-Telepictures	EP: David Jacobs, Michael Filerman P: Larry Kasha, Mary-Catherine Harold	Teri Austin, Hunt Block, Tonya Crowe, William Devane, Kevin Dobson, Julie Harris, Michele Lee, Constance McCashin, Donna Mills, Pat Petersen, Ted Shackelford, Steve Shaw, Douglas Sheehan, Nicollette Sheridan, Joan Van Ark
Magnum, P.I.	Wed	9:00	60	Belisarius Prods.-GlenA. Larson Prods.-Universal TV	EP: Donald P. Bellisario, Charles Floyd Johnson SP: Chris Abbott-Fish P: Rick Weaver, Jay Huguely	Tom Selleck, John Hillerman, Roger E. Mosley, Larry Manetti
Murder, She Wrote	Sun	8:00	60	Universal TV	EP: Peter S. Fischer P: Robert F. O'Neill	Angela Lansbury, Tom Bosley, William Window
My Sister Sam	Mon	8:30	30	Pony Prods.-Warner Bros. TV	EP: Diane English SP: Tom Cherones P: Karyl Geld Miller, Korby Siamis D: Ellen Chast Falcon	Pam Dawber, David Naughton, Rebecca Schaeffer, Joel Brooks, Jenny O'Hara
New Mike Hammer, The	Sat	9:00	60	Jay Bernstein Prods.-Columbia Pictures TV	EP: Jay Bernstein SP: Sam Rolfe P: Jon Andersen, B. W. Sandefur, Ed Scharlach	Stacy Keach, Lindsay Bloom, Don Stroud, Kent Williams
Newhart	Mon	9:00	30	MTM Enterprises	EP: Douglas Wyman, David Mirkin CP: Arnie Kogen, Michael loman	Bob Newhart, Mary Frann, Peter Scolari, Julia Duffy, Tom Poston, William Sanderson, Tony Papenfuss, John Voldstad
Scarecrow & Mrs. King	Fri	8:00	60	Shoot The Moon Enterprises-Warner Bros. TV	EP: George Geiger, Robert W. Gilmer P: Sascha Schneider, Tom Chehak CP: Ronald G. Smith, Dennis Duckwall	Kate Jackson, Bruce Boxleitner, Beverly Garland, Mel Stewart, Martha Smith, Paul Stout, Greg Morton
Simon & Simon	Thu	8:00	60	Universal TV	EP: John G. Stephens SP: David Moessinger P: Mark A. Burley, Stephen A. Miller CP: Thomas & Jo Perry	Jameson Parker, Gerald McRaney, Mary Carver, Tim Reid
60 Minutes	Sun	7:00	60	CBS News	EP: Don Hewitt Sr. P: Phillip Scheffler D: Arthur Bloom	Mike Wallace, Morley Safer, Harry Reasoner, Ed Bradley, Diane Sawyer, Andy Rooney
Together We Stand	Wed	8:00	30	Al Burton Prods.-Sherwood Schwartz Co.-Universal TV	EP: Al Burton, Sherwood Schwartz P: Michael Jacobs D: Will MacKenzie	Elliott Gould, Dee Wallace Stone, Ke Huy Quan, Scott Grimes, Katie O'Neill, Natasha Bobo
Twilight Zone, The	Sat	10:00	60	CBS Entertainment-Persistence Of Vision	EP: Philip DeGuere SP: Anthony & Nancy Lawrence P: Harvey Frand, Ken Swor	
Wizard, The	Tue	8:00	60	BSR Prods.-20th Fox TV	EP: Michael Berk, Douglas Schwartz SP: Paul B. Radin P: Peter H. Hunt, Rick Mittleman	David Rappaport, Douglas Barr, Fran Ryan, Roy Dotrice

NBC-TV

Series Title	Day	Hr.	Mins.	Supplier	Production Principals	Cast Regulars & Semi-Regulars
ALF	Mon	8:00	30	Alien Prods.	EP: Tom Patchett, Bernie Brillstein SP: Thad Mumford P: Paul Fusco CP: Laurie Gelman D: Peter Bonerz	Max Wright, Anne Schedeen, Benji Gregory, Andrea Elson, ALF
A-Team, The	Fri	8:00	60	Stephen J. Cannell Prods.-Universal TV	EP: Stephen J. Cannell, Frank Lupo, John Ashley SP: Jo Swerling Jr. P: Tom Blomquist	George Peppard, Dirk Benedict, Dwight Schultz, Mr. T., Robert Vaughn, Eddie Velez
Amazing Stories	Mon	8:30	30	Amblin Entertainment-Universal TV	EP: Steven Spielberg P: David Vogel	
Amen	Sat	9:30	30	Carson Prods.	EP: Ed. Weinberger, David Lloyd SP: Jack Michon CP: Reuben Cannon, Ken Johnston	Sherman Hemsley, Clifton Davis, Anna Maria Horsford, Barbara Montgomery, Roz Ryan, Maria McDonald, Jester Hairston, Franklyn Seales
Cheers	Thu	9:00	30	Charles/Burrows/Charles Prods.-Paramount TV	EP: Glen & Les Charles, James Burrows P: David Angell, Peter Casey & David Lee CP: Tim Berry D: James Burrows	Ted Danson, Shelley Long, Rhea Perlman, John Ratzenberger, Woody Harrelson, Kelsey Grammer, George Wendt

Series Title	Day	Hr.	Mins.	Supplier	Production Principals	Cast Regulars & Semi-Regulars
Cosby Show, The	Thu	8:00	30	Carsey-Werner Co.-Bill Cosby	EP: Marcy Carsey, Tom Werner, John Markus SP: Caryn Sneider Mandabach P: Carmen Finestra, Matt Williams	Bill Cosby, Phylicia Rashad, Sabrina LeBeauf, Lisa Bonet, Malcolm-Jamal Warner, Tempestt Bledsoe, Keshia Knight Pulliam, Clarice Taylor, Earle Hyman
Crime Story	Tue	9:00	60	Michael Mann Co.-New World TV	EP: Michael Mann P: Peter McIntosh	Dennis Farina, Anthony Denison, Stephen Lang, Darlanne, Fluegel, William Smitrovich, John Santucci, Paul Butler, William Campbell, Steve Ryan
Easy Street	Sun	8:00	30	Viacom Prods.	EP: Sheldon Bull, Andy Borowitz P: Max Tash	Loni Anderson, Jack Elam, Lee Weaver, Dana Ivey, James Cromwell, Arthur Malet
Facts Of Life, The	Sat	8:00	30	Embassy Communications	EP: Richard Gurman P:Rita Dillon D: John Bowab	Cloris Leachman, Lisa Whelchel, Mindy Cohn, Kim Fields, Nancy McKeon, MacKenzie Astin
Family Ties	Thu	8:30	30	UBU Prods.-Paramount TV	EP: Gary David Goldberg SP: Alan Uger P: Ruth Bennett, Marc Lawrence, Carol Himes CP: June Galas	Meredith Baxter Birney, Michael Gross, Michael J. Fox, Justine Bateman, Tina Yothers, Brian Bonsall, Marc Price
Gimme A Break	Wed	9:00	30	Mort Lachman & Associates-Reeves Entertainment Group	EP: Rod Parker, Hal Cooper, Mort Lachman P: Arthur Julian D: Hal Cooper	Nell Carter, Telma Hopkins, John Hoyt, Joey Lawrence, Matthew Lawrence
Golden Girls, The	Sat	9:00	30	Witt-Thomas-Harris Prods.-Touchstone Films	EP: Paul Junger Witt, Tony Thomas P: Kathy Speer, Terry Grossman CP: Winifred Hervey, Mort Nathan, Barry Fanaro, Marsha Posner Williams	Bea Arthur, Betty White, Rue McClanahan, Estelle Getty
Highway To Heaven	Wed	8:00	60	Michael Landon Prods.	EP: Michael Landon P: Kent McCray D: Michael Landon, Victor French	Michael Landon, Victor French
Hill Street Blues	Thu	10:00	60	MTM Enterprises	EP: Jeffrey Lewis, David Milch, Jeff Melvoin, John Litvack SP: Scott Brazil P: Michael Vittes CP: Steve Bello	Daniel J. Travanti, Michael Warren, Bruce Weitz, Robert Prosky, James B. Sikking, Joe Spano, Tauren Blacque, Kiel Martin, Betty Thomas, Dennis Franz, Charles Haid, Veronica Hamel, Robert Clohessy, Megan Gallagher
Hunter	Sat	10:00	60	Stephen J. Cannell Prods.	EP: Roy Huggins SP: Jo Swerling Jr. P: Stuart Segall	Fred Dryer, Stepfanie Kramer, Charles Hallahan, Garrett Morris
L.A. Law	Fri	10:00	60	20th Fox TV	EP: Steven Bochco, Gregory Hoblit SP: Terry Louise Fisher P: Ellen S. Pressman	Harry Hamlin, Richard Dysart, Corbin Bernsen, Jill Eikenberry, Michele Green, Alan Rachins, Michael Tucker, Jimmy Smits, Susan Ruttan, Susan Dey
Matlock	Tue	8:00	60	InterMedia Entertainment-Strathmore Prods.-Viacom Prods.	EP: Fred Silverman, Dean Hargrove SP: Richard Collins P: Joel Steiger, Robert Schlitt	Andy Griffith, Linda Purl, Kene Holliday
Miami Vice	Fri	9:00	60	Michael Mann Co.-Universal TV	EP: Michael Mann SP: Kerry McCluggage P: Richard Brams CP: Dennis Cooper, Dick Wolf	Don Johnson, Philip Michael Thomas, Saundra Santiago, Michael Talbott, John Diehl, Olivia Brown Williamson, Edward James Olmos
NBC Monday Night At The Movies	Mon	9:00	120	Various		
NBC Sunday Night At The Movies	Sun	9:00	120	Various		
Night Court	Thu	9:30	30	Starry Night Prods.-Warner Bros. TV	EP: Reinhold Weege SP: Jeff Melman P: Bob Stevens CP: Tim Steele	Harry Anderson, Markie Post, John Larroquette, Richard Moll, Charles Robinson, Marsha Warfield
1986	Tue	10:00	60	NBC News	EP: Ed Fouhy Sr. P: Joan Carrigan, Sid Feders D: Joe Cortina	Roger Mudd, Connie Chung, Ed Rabel, Lucky Severson, Maria Shriver, Peter Kent
Our House	Sun	7:00	60	Blinn/Thrope Prods.-Lorimar-Telepictures	EP: William Blinn, Jerry Thorpe P: Jerry McNeely CP: Parke Perine	Wilford Brimley, Deidre Hall, Shannen Doherty, Chad Allen, Keri Houlihan, Gerald S. O'Loughlin, John McCook
St. Elsewhere	Wed	10:00	60	MTM Enterprises	EP: Bruce Paltrow SP: Mark Tinker P: John Masius, Tom Fontana	Ed Flanders, Norman Lloyd, Ed Begley Jr., Stephen Furst, Eric Laneuville, Howie Mandel, David Morse, Christine Pickles, Denzel Washington, William Daniels, Jamie Rose, Bruce Greenwood, France Nuyen
227	Sat	8:30	30	Embassy Communications	EP: Dick Bensfield, Jack Elinson P: Bill Boulware, Ron Bloomberg CP: Roxie Wenk-Evans	Marla Gibbs, Hal Williams, Alaina Reed, Jackee Harry, Regina King, Helen Martin, Curtis Baldwin, Kia Goodwin
Valerie	Sun	8:30	30	Miler-Boyett Prods.-Lorimar-Telepictures	EP: Thomas L. Miller, Robert L. Boyett, Tony Cacciotti SP: Steve Pritzker, Chip & Doug Keyes	Valerie Harper, Jason Bateman, Danny Ponce, Jeremy Licht, Josh Taylor, Edie McClurg

Series Title	Day	Hr.	Mins.	Supplier	Production Principals	Cast Regulars & Semi-Regulars
					P: Judy Pioli, Rick Mitz, Laura Schrock CP: Rick Correll	
You Again?	Wed	9:30	30	Taft Entertainment TV-Lawson Group-Sweater Prods.	EP: Bernie Orenstein, Saul Turteltaub P: Liz Sage CP: Al Aidekman	Jack Klugman, John Stamos, Elizabeth Bennett

Syndicated Shows, 1986–87

Half-Hour Off-Network Shows

Title	No. of Episodes	Distributor
Alice	202	Warner Brothers
All In The Family	207	Viacom
Andy Griffith	249	Viacom
Angie	37	Paramount
Archie's Place	97	Embassy
Barney Miller	170	Columbia
Batman	120	20th Fox
Benson	120	Columbia
Best Of Dating Game	175/85	Bel-Air
Best Of Groucho	130	WW Ent.
Beverly Hillbillies	168	Viacom
Bewitched	252	DFS
BJ/Lobo	86	MCA
Bosom Buddies	37	Paramount
Brady Bunch	117	Paramount
Branded	48	King World
Carol Burnett Show	150	Burnett
Carson Comedy	130	Columbia
Diff'rent Strokes	144	Embassy
Donny & Marie Show	65	Osmond Ent.
Family Feud	65	Viacom
Family Feud	260	Viacom
Fantasy Island	200	Columbia
Flying Nun	82	Colex
Gidget (avail. after barter)	32	Colex
Gilligan's Island	98	MGM/UA
Gimme A Break	85	MCA
Good Times	133	Embassy
Guns of Will Sonnett	50	King World
Happy Days	255	Paramount
Harper Valley P.T.A.	29	MCA
Here's Lucy	144	Telepictures
Hitchcock Presents	265	MCA
Hogan's Heroes	168	Viacom
Honeymooners	39	Viacom
I Dream Of Jeannie	139	DFS
I Love Lucy	179	Viacom
Jeffersons	207	Embassy
Lassie	192	Colbert
Laugh In	130	Lorimar
Laverne & Shirley	178	Paramount
Leave It To Beaver	234	MCA
M*A*S*H I	197	20th Fox
M*A*S*H/Renewal	255	20th Fox
Maude	142	Embassy
Mayberry RFD	78	Telepictures
Mork & Mindy	95	Paramount
My Favorite Martian	107	Telepictures
Night Gallery	97	MCA
One Day At A Time	187	Embassy
Operation Petticoat	32	MCA
Partridge Family	96	DFS
Pvt. Benjamin	39	Warner Bros.
Real People	195	Telepictures
Rifleman	168	Colbert

Sanford & Son	136	Embassy
Saturday Night Live	102	Orion
SCTV	156	Blair
Show Of Shows	65	ZIV
Soap	92	Columbia
Square Pegs	20	Embassy
Tattletales	260	Victory
Taxi	93	Paramount
That's Incredible	165	MCA
That's My Mama	39	Columbia
The Ropers	26	Taffner
Three'a A Crowd	22	Taffner
Three's Company	174	Taffner
Too Close For Comfort	107	Taffner
Topper	78	King World
What's Happening	65	Columbia
WKRP In Cincinnati	90	Victory

Hour Off-Network Shows

Title	No. of Episodes	Distributor
12 O'Clock High	78	20th Fox
ABR Collection	12	ABR
Avengers	83	Orion
Barnaby Jones	177	Worldvision
BJ/Lobo Show	86	MCA
Black Sheep Squadron	35	MCA
Blue Knight	23	Lorimar
Buck Rogers	37	MCA
Cannon	124	Viacom
Charlie's Angels	115	Columbia
Chips Patrol	138	MGM/UA
Dallas	161	Lorimar
Dick Clark Presents	13	Syndicast
Dukes Of Hazzard	143	Warner Bros.
Dynasty	118	Metromedia
Eight Is Enough	112	Lorimar
Eischeid	13	Colex
Family	86	LBS
Fantasy Island	130	Columbia
Flamingo Road	37	Lorimar
Ghost Story/Circle of Fear	13/9	Colex(LBS)
Greatest American Hero	42/42/21	Lexington
Hart To Hart	112	Columbia
Hawaii 5-O	200	Viacom
Hawk	17	Colex
Hitchcock Hour	93	MCA
Incredible Hulk	85	MCA
Knots Landing	128	Lorimar
Kojak	118	MCA
Little House On The Prairie	216	Worldvision
Lost In Space	83	20th Fox
Lou Grant	114	Victory
Love Boat	140	Worldvision
Mannix	130	Paramount
Matt Houston	65 (est.)	Warner Bros.
Mission Impossible	171	Paramount
Mystery Movies	124	MCA
Police Story	84	Columbia
Police Woman	91	Columbia

Quincy	148	MCA
Rockford Files	125	MCA
Roller Derby	56	ABR
Route 66	52	Colex
Saturday Night Live	102	Orion
Star Trek	79	Paramount
Street Hawk	13	MCA
Switch	26	MCA
That's Incredible	107	MCA
The Man From U.N.C.L.E.	132	MGM
The Prisoner	17	ITC
Thriller	67	MCA
Tom Jones	24	ABR
Trapper John, M.D.	132	20th Fox
Vegas	68	MPC
Very Special Events	13	Bel-Air
Voyage To The Bottom Of The Sea	110	20th Fox
Voyagers/Whiz Kid	34/18	MCA
Waltons	221	Warner Bros.
Wonder Woman	61	Warner Bros.

1985–86 Mini-Series

CROSSINGS

Aaron Spelling Prods. P: Howard W. Koch. Exec. P: Spelling, Douglas S. Cramer. D: Karen Arthur. W: Bill & Jo LaMond, based on Danielle Steel's novel. Shown on ABC Feb. 23, 24 & 25, 1986. (6 hrs.)

Cast: Cheryl Ladd, Lee Horsley, Christopher Plummer, Jane Seymour, Garrick Dowhan, Stewart Granger, Joan Fontaine, Joanna Pacula, Horst Buchholz, Zach Galligan, Jan Rubes, Carl Stevens, Herta Ware, Tony Steedman.

DREAM WEST

Sunn Classic Pictures. P: Hunt Lowry. Exec. P: Chuck McLain. D: Dick Lowry. W: Evan Hunter, based on David Nevin's novel. Shown on CBS April 13, 14, 15 & 20, 1986. (7 hrs.)

Cast: Richard Chamberlain, Alice Krige, Claude Akins, John Anderson, Lee Bergere, Jeff East, Michael Ensign, Mel Ferrer, Burton Gilliam, John Harkins, Gayle Hunnicutt, Matt McCoy, Cameron Mitchell, Nobel Willingham, F. Murray Abraham, Rene Enriquez, Ben Johnson, Jerry Orbach, G.D. Spradlin, Rip Torn, Fritz Weaver, Anthony Zerbe, Bill Campbell, Jamie Cromwell, Lee de Broux, Jonathan Frakes, John Francis, Stefan Geirasch, Richard Hamilton, William Hare, Dave Lowry, Kip Niven, John Quade.

IF TOMORROW COMES

CBS Entertainment Prods. P: Carmen Culver, Nick Gilliott. Exec. P: Bob Markell. Spvr. P-D: Jerry London. W: Culver, based on Sidney Sheldon's novel. Shown on CBS March 16, 17 & 18, 1986. (7 hrs.)

Cast: Madolyn Smith, Tom Berenger, David Keith, Liam Beeson, Jack Weston, Richard Kiley, Joe Cortese, George DiCenzo, Susan Hess, Jeffrey Jones, John Laughlin, Susan Tyrrell, Harold Sylvester, Lane Smith, C.C.H. Pounder, Frank Dent, Alice Hirson, Barry Jenner, James Ry, Anne Schedeen, Lois Foraker.

KANE & ABEL

Schreckinger Communications; Embassy TV. P: Fern Field, Stan Kallis. Exec. P: Jud Kinberg, Michael Grade, Jinny Schreckinger. D: Buzz Kulik. W: Robert W. Lenski, based on Jeffrey Archer's novel. Shown on CBS Nov. 17, 18 & 19, 1985. (7 hrs.)

Cast: Peter Strauss, Sam Neill, Ron Silver, David Dukes, Fred Gwynne, Tom Roberts Byrd, Alberta Watson, Reed Birney, Vyto Ruginis, Jim Eikenberry, Richard Anderson, Kate McNeil, Veronica Hamel, Lisa Banes, Christopher Cazenove, Sheree J. Wilson, Kent Broadhurst, Debra Engle, Harry Groener, Jan Rubes, Richard Seff.

LORD MOUNTBATTEN: THE LAST VICEROY

George Walker Prods. P: Judith dePaul. Exec. P: Walker. D. Tom Clegg. W: David Butler. Shown on PBS Jan.26–March 2, 1986, on Sundays once a week. (6 hrs.)

Cast: Nicol Williamson, Janet Suzman, Ian Richardson, Sam Dastor, Vladek Sheybal, Wendy Hiller, Nigel Davenport, A.K. Hangal, Minnie Boga, Zia Mohyeddin, Protap Roy, Sumant Mustaker, Patrick Allen, Malcolm Terris, Owen Holder, Frederick Treves, John Rolfe.

MUSSOLINI: THE UNTOLD STORY

Trian Prods. P: Stirling Silliphant, Hal Polaire. Exec. P: Raymond Katz, Bernie Sofronski. D: William A. Graham. W: Silliphant. Shown on NBC Nov. 24, 25 & 26, 1985. (7 hrs.)

Cast: George C. Scott, Lee Grant, Mary Elizabeth Mastrantonio, Virginia Madsen, Raul Julia, Gabriel Bryne, Robert Downey, Gunnar Moeller, Vernon Dobtcheff, Anne Louise Lambert, Gina Bellman, Kenneth Colley, Michael Aldridge, Annabel Leventon.

NORTH & SOUTH, BOOK II

David L. Wolper Prods.; Robert A. Papazian Prods.; Warner Bros. TV. P: Papazian. Exec. P: Wolper. D. Kevin Connor. W: Richard Fielder, based on John Jakes' novel, "Love & War." Shown on ABC May 4, 5, 6, 7, 8 & 11, 1986. (12 hrs.)

Cast: Kirstie Alley, David Carradine, Phillip Casnoff, Mary Crosby, Lesley-Anne Down, Jonathan Frakes, Genie Francis, Teri Garber, Wendy Kilbourne, Kate McNeil, Jim Metzler, James Read, Lewis Smith, Parker Stevenson, Patrick Swayze, Lloyd Bridges, Olivia de Havilland, Linda Evans, Morgan Fairchild, Hal Holbrook, Lee Horsley, Nancy Marchand, Wayne Newton, Jean Simmons, James Stewart, David Ogden Stiers, Inga Swenson, Anthony Zerbe.

ON WINGS OF EAGLES

Edgar J. Scherick Associates; Taft Entertainment. P: Lyn Raynor. Exec. P: Scherick. D: Andrew V. McLaglen. W: Sam H. Rolfe, based on Ken Follett's book. Shown on NBC May 18 & 19, 1986. (5 hrs.)

Cast: Burt Lancaster, Richard Crenna, Paul LeMat, Louis Giambalvo, Jim Metzler, Lawrence Pressman, Robert Wightman, Cyril O'Reilly, Esai Morales, Martin Doyle, Bob Delegall, Bill Bumiller, James Sutorius, Richard Crenna Jr., Constance Towers, Alan Fudge, Parviz Sayyad, Patti McCormack.

PETER THE GREAT

PTG Prods.; NBC Prods. P: Marvin J. Chomsky. D: Chomsky, Lawrence Schiller. W: Edward Anhalt. Shown on NBC Feb. 2, 3, 4 & 5, 1986. (8 hrs.)

Cast: Maximilian Schell, Vanessa Redgrave, Laurence Olivier, Omar Sharif, Jan Niklas, Trevor Howard, Lilli Palmer, Hanna Schygulla, Renee Soutendijk, Elke Sommer, Ursula Andress, Mel Ferrer, Helmut Griem, Jeremy Kemp, Natalya Andreichenko, Boris Plotnikov, Jan Malmsjo, Geoffrey Whitehead, Graham McGrath, Mike Gwilyn, Gunther-Maria Halmer.

SINS

Grief-Dore Co.; Collins-Holm Prods.; New World TV. P: Steve Krantz. Exec. P: Joan Collins, Peter Holm, Bonny Dore, Leslie Greif. D: Douglas Hickox. W: Laurence Heath, based on Judith Gould's novel. Shown on CBS Feb. 2, 3, & 4, 1986. (7 hrs.)

Cast: Joan Collins, Jean-Pierre Aumont, Marisa Berenson, Steven Berkoff, Joseph Bologna, Elizabeth Bourgine, Judi Bowker, Capucine, Neil Dickson, Arielle Dombasle, James Farentino, Paul Freeman, Allen Garfield, Giancarlo Giannini, Lauren Hutton, Gene Kelly, Catherine Mary Stewart, William Allen Young, Timothy Dalton, Feodor Atkine, Faith Brook, John McEnery, Regine, Alexandra Stewart, Peter Vaughan.

TENDER IS THE NIGHT

BBC; Showtime-The Movie Channel. P: Betty Willingale. Exec P: Jonathan Powell. D: Robert Knights. W: Dennis Potter, based on F. Scott Fitzgerald's novel. Shown on Showtime Oct. 27, Nov. 5, 12, 19 & 26, 1985. (6 hrs.)

Cast: Peter Strauss, Mary Steenburgen, John Heard, Sean Young, Edward Asner, Piper Laurie, Jurgen Brugger, Erwin Kohlund, Joris Stuyck, Kate Harper, Nancy Paul, Astrid Frank, Francois Guetary, Rosario Serrano, Richard Kinford, Keith Edwards.

1985–86 Motion Pictures Made for Television

Listed herewith are new films especially made for television and shown for the first time during the 1985–86 season. Key for credits: P is Producer; Exec. P: Executive Producer; D: Director; W: Writer. Running time indicated includes commercials.

ACCEPTABLE RISKS

ABC Circle Films. P: R.W. Goodwin. D: Rick Wallace. W. Norman Strum. Shown on ABC March 2, 1986. (2 hrs.)

Cast: Brian Dennehy, Kenneth McMillan, Christine Ebersole, Beah Richards, Richard Gilliland, Vic Polizos, Peter Jurasik, Cicely Tyson, Patti Cohoon, Steve Eastin, Richard McKenzie, Tom Simcox.

ACT OF VENGEANCE

Telepix Canada Corp. Prods. P: Jack Clements. Exec. P: Frank Konigsberg, Larry Sanitsky. Co-P: Iris Sawyer. D: John Mackenzie. W: Scott Spencer, based on Trevor Armbrister's book. Shown on HBO April 20, 1986. (110 mins.)

Cast: Charles Bronson, Ellen Burstyn, Wilford Brimley, Hoyt Axtim, Ribert Schenkkan, Ellen Barkin, Maury Chaykin, Caroline Kava, Peg Murray, William Newman, Alan North, Raynor Scheine, Tom Harvey, Alf Humphreys, Joseph Kell.

ADVENTURES OF HUCKLEBERRY FINN

American Playhouse; the Great Amwell Co.; WGBH Boston; WGBY-TV, Springfield, MA. P: Jane Iredale. Exec. P-Music: William Perry. D: Peter H. Hunt. W: Guy Gallo, adapted from Mark Twain's novel. Shown on PBS March 10, 17, 24, 1986. (4 hrs.)

Cast: Patrick Day, Anne Shropshire, Sada Thompson, Eugene Oakes, Samm-Art Williams, Frederic Forrest, Lillian Gish, Richard Kiley, Jim Dale, Barnard Hughes, Butterfly McQueen, Geraldine Page, Jason Hankins, Richard Niehaus, Bill Chamness, David Watters, Harriet Cartmell, Amy Shouse, Omer W. Johnson.

ALEX: THE LIFE OF A CHILD

Mandy Films. P: Nigel McKeand. Exec. P: Leonard Goldberg. D: Robert Markowitz. W: Carol Evan McKeand and Nigel McKeand, based on Frank Deford's book. Shown on ABC April 23, 1986. (2 hrs.)

Cast: Craig T. Nelson, Bonnie Bedelia, Gennie James, Danny Corkill, Mark Withers, Melonie Mazman, Brenda Bazinet, Lindsey Cook Amelio, Harley Cross.

ALICE IN WONDERLAND

Irwin Allen Prods.; P&G Prods.; Columbia Pictures TV. P: Allen. D: Harry Harris. W: Paul Zindel, based on Lewis Carroll's "Alice's Adventures in Wonderland" and "Through the Looking Glass." Shown on CBS Dec. 9 & 10, 1985. (4 hrs.)

Cast: Natalie Gregory, Sheila Allen, Scott Baio, Red Buttons, Sid Caesar, Imogene Coca, Sammy Davis, Jr., Sherman Hensley, Arte Johnson, Roddy McDowall, Jayne Meadows, Robert Morley, Anthony Newley, Donald O'Connor, Martha Raye, Telly Savalas, Ringo Starr, Shelley Winters, Steve Allen, Ernest Borgnine, Beau Bridges, Lloyd Bridges, Carol Channing, Patrick Duffy, George Gobel, Eydie Gorme, Merv Griffin, Ann Jillian, Harvey Korman, Steve Lawrence, Karl Malden, Donna Mills, Pat Morita, Louis Nye, John Stamos, Sally Struthers, Jack Warden, Jonathan Winters.

AMOS

The Bryna Co.; Vincent Pictures. P: Bill Finnegan, Sheldon Pinchik. Exec. P: Peter Douglas. D: Michael Tuchner. W: Richard Kramer, based on the novel by Stanley West. Shown on CBS Sept. 29, 1985. (2 hrs.)

Cast: Kirk Douglas, Elizabeth Montgomery, Dorothy McGuire, Pat Morita, Kay Walston.

THE ANNIHILATOR

Universal TV. Exec. P: Roderick Taylor. Spvr. P: Alex Beaton. D: Michael Chapman. W: Roderick & Bruce A. Taylor. Shown on NBC April 7, 1986. (2 hrs.)

Cast: Mark Lindsay Chapman, Susan Blakely, Lisa Blount, Brion James, Earl Boen, Geoffrey Lewis, Catharine Mary Stewart, Nicolle Eggert, Paul Brinegar, Barry Pearl, Barbara Townsend, Glen Vernon, Christopher Johnson, Channing Chase.

ASSASSIN

Sankan Prods. Inc. P: Neil T. Maffeo. Exec. P-D-W: Sandor Stern. Shown on CBS March 19, 1986. (2 hrs.)

Cast: Robert Conrad, Karen Austin, Richard Young, Jonathan Banks, Robert Webber.

BADGE OF THE ASSASSIN

Daniel H. Blatt/Robert Singer Prods. Exec. P: Blatt & Singer, Robert K. Tanenbaum. D: Mel Damski. W: Lawrence Roman, based on the book by Tanenbaum & Phillip Rosenberg. Shown on CBS Nov. 2, 1985. (2 hrs.)

Cast: James Woods, Yaphet Kotto, Alex Rocco, David Harris, Steven Keats, Larry Riley, Pam Grier, Rae Dawn Chong, Richard Bradford, Kene Holliday, Toni Kalem, Tamu Blackwell, Richard Books.

BEHIND ENEMY LINES

TVS Prods.; MTM Enterprises. P: Gareth Davies. Exec. P-W: Stephen McPherson. D: Larry Sheldon. Shown on NBC Dec. 29, 1985. (2 hrs.)

Cast: Hal Holbrook, Ray Sharkey, Maryam D'Abo, Lucy Hornak, Alun Lewis, Tom Isbell, Peter Whiteman, Anne Twomey, Stephen Shellen, David McCallum, Renee Soutendijk, Benedict Taylor, Patricia Hodge.

BETRAYED BY INNOCENCE

Inter Planetary Prods. P: Micheline H. Keller. Exec. P: Max A. Keller, Robert Lloyd Lewis. D: Elliot Silverstein. W: Ken August, Stanford Whitmore. Shown on CBS March 1, 1986. (2 hrs.)

Cast: Barry Bostwick, Lee Purcell, Cristen Kauffman, Isaac Hayes, Craig Richard Nelson, Joel Collodner, Thom Christopher, Paul Sorvino, Susan Marie Synder, Philip Bruns, Dendrie Allyn Taylor, Jim Townsend, Vincent Pandoliano, Joe d'Angelo

BETWEEN TWO WOMEN

Jon Avnet Co. P: Carol Schreder. Exec. P-D: Avnet. W: Larry Grusin & Avnet, based on Gillian Martin's novel "Living Arrows." Shown on ABC March 10, 1986. (2 hrs.)

Cast: Farrah Fawcett, Colleen Dewhurst, Michael Nouri, Bridgette Andersen, Danny Corkill, Steven Hill, Terry O'Quinn, Kenneth Danziger, Carmen Argenziano, Bronson Pinchot.

BEVERLY HILLS COWGIRL BLUES

The Leonard Goldberg Co. P-W: Rick Husky. Exec. P: Goldberg. D: Corey Allen. Shown on CBS Oct. 5, 1985. (2 hrs.)

Cast: James Brolin, Lisa Hartman, David Hemmings, Irena Ferris, Michael C. Gwynne, Alexa Hamilton, Lane Smith, Drake Hogestyn, Stuart Whitman.

BEVERLY HILLS MADAM

NLS Prods.; Orion TV. P: Everett Chambers. Exec. P-W: Nancy Sackett. D: Harvey Hart. Shown on NBC April 6, 1986. (2 hrs.)

Cast: Faye Dunaway, Melody Anderson, Donna Dixon, Terry Farrell, Robin Givens, Louis Jourdan, Marshall Colt, William Jordan, Nicolas Coster, William Traylor, Gary Hershberger, Aki Aleong, Rod McCary, Beulah Quo.

BLIND JUSTICE

CBS Entertainment Prods. P: Andrew Gottlieb. D: Rod Holcomb. W: Josephine Cummings & Richard Yalem. Shown on CBS March 9, 1986 (2 hrs.)

Cast: Tim Matheson, Mimi Kuzyk, Philip Charles MacKenzie, Tom Atkins, Lisa Eichhorn, John Kellogg, Marilyn Lightstone, Anne Haney, David Froman, John M. Jackson, Linda Thorson, Jack Blessing, Ann Ryerson, Sam Dalton, Daniel Davis, Leonardo Donato.

BLOOD & ORCHIDS

Lorimar Prods. P: Andrew Adelson. Exec. P: Malcolm Stuart. D: Jerry Thorpe. W: Norman Katkov, based on his novel. Shown on CBS Feb. 23 & 24, 1986. (4 hrs.)

Cast: Kris Kristofferson, Jane Alexander, Sean Young, Jose Ferrer, Susan Blakely, David Clennon, George Coe, Richard Dysart, Elizabeth Lindsey, Haunani Minn, William Russ, James Saito, Matt Salinger, Madeline Stowe, Arthur Rosenberg.

THE BLUE LIGHTNING

Alan Sloan Inc.; Seven Network; Coote-Carroll Australia. P: Ross Matthews. Co-P-W: William Kelly. D: Lee Phillips. Shown on CBS May 7, 1986. (2 hrs.)

Cast: Sam Elliott, Rebecca Gilling, John Meillion, Robert Coleby, Max Phipps, Robert Culp, Ralph Cotterill, Jack Davis, Ray Meagher, Michael Carman, Norm Erskine.

BRASS

Carnan Prods. Inc.; Orion TV. P: T.J. Castronova. Exec. P: Jerry Golod. D: Corey Allen. W: Roy Baldwin, Matt Harris. Shown on CBS Sept. 10, 1985. (2 hrs.)

Cast: Carroll O'Connor, Lois Nettleton, Larry Atlas, Samuel E. Wright, Jimmy Balo, Paul Shenar, Begona Plaza, Pauline Meyers, Vincent Gardenia, Anita Gillette.

BRIDGE ACROSS TIME

Fries Entertainment. P: Jack Michon, Richard Maynard. Exec. P: Charles Fries, Irv Wilson. D: E.W. Swackhamer. W: William F. Nolan. Shown on NBC Nov. 22, 1985. (2 hrs.)

Cast: David Hasselhoff, Stepfaine Kramer, Randolph Mantooth, Adrienne Barbeau, Clu Gulager, Lindsay Bloom, Ken Swofford, Rose Marie, Lane Smith, David Fox-Brenton, Barbara Bingham, Michael Boyle, Paul Rossilli.

BROTHERHOOD OF JUSTICE

Margot Winchester Prods. Inc.; Taper Media Enterprises; Guber-Peters Entertainment Co.; Phoenix Entertainment Corp. P: Judith R. James, Winchester. Exec. P: Guber, Peters. D: Charles Braverman. W: Noah Jubelirer, Jeffrey Bloom. Shown on ABC May 18, 1986. (2 hrs.)

Cast: Keanu Reeves, Lori Loughlin, Kiefer Sutherland, Joe Spano, Darren Dalton, Evan Mirand, Don Michael Paul, Gary Riley, Billy Zane, Danny Nucci, Danny De La Paz, Jim Haynie.

A CASE OF DEADLY FORCE

Telecom Entertainment. P: Bruce Pustin. Exec. P: Michael Lepiner, Ken Kaufman. D: Michael Miller. W: Dennis Nemac, based on Lawrence O'Donnell Jr.'s novel, "Deadly Force." Shown on CBS April 9, 1986. (2 hrs.)

Cast: Richard Crenna, John Shea, Lorraine Toussaint, Frank McCarthy, Tom Isbell, Tate Donovan, Michael O'Hare, Dylan Baker, Beth Fowler, Tracy Fitzpatrick, Kristin Rhose, Paul O'Brien, Ken Cheeeman, Anthony Heald.

CHARLEY HANNAH

A. Shane Co. P: Roger Bacon. Exec. P: Joan Conrad. D: Peter H. Hunt. W: David J. Kinghorn. Shown on ABC April 5, 1986. (2 hrs.)

Cast: Robert Conrad, Shane Conrad, Christian Conrad, Joan Leslie, Red West, Kelly Minter, B. Miko Machalski, Antoni Corone, Mario Sanchez, Stephen J. Cannell, James Deuter, Alex Paez.

CHASE

CBS Entertainment Prods. P: Sam Strangis. D: Rod Holcomb. W. David E. Peckinpah. Shown on CBS Nov. 23, 1985. (2 hrs.)

Cast: Jennifer O'Neill, Robert S. Woods, Michael Parks, Terence Knox, John Philbin, Kathleen York, J.E. Freeman, Cooper Huckabee, Richard Farnsworth, Michol Sullivan, John Walter Davis, Douglas Newell, Dick Arnold, Rich Hawkins.

CHILD'S CRY

Shoot the Moon Enterprises; Phoenix Entertainment Group. P-D: Gilbert Cates. Exec. P: Kate Jackson, Gerald I. Isenberg. W: Jonathan B. Rintels, Jr. Shown on CBS Feb. 9, 1986. (2 hrs.)

Cast: Lindsay Wagner, Peter Coyote, Tallesin Jaffe, Gerald S. O'Loughlin, Guy Boyd, Brent Jennings, Vic Polizos, Marlene Warfield, Jack Radar, E.J. Castillo, Peter Hobbs, Davis A. Penhale, Kathelen Garrarrett, Anne Cee Byrd.

CHILDREN OF THE NIGHT

Robert Guenette Prods. P: Conrad Holzgang. Exec. P: Guenette. D: Robert Markowitz. W: Vickie Patik, Guenette. Shown on CBS Oct. 26, 1985. (2 hrs.)

Cast: Kathleen Quinlan, Nicholas Campbell, Mario Van Peebles, Lar Park-Lincoln, Wally Ward, Eddie Velez, David Crowley, Donald Hotton, Marta Kober, Laura Esterman, Sherri Stone, Michael Shaner, Vincent J. Isaac.

THE CHILDREN OF TIMES SQUARE

Gross-Weston Prods.; Fries Entertainment. P: Marcy Gross, Ann Weston. D-W: Curtis Hanson. Shown on ABC March 3, 1986. (2 hrs.)

Cast: Howard E. Rollins Jr., Joanna Cassidy, Brandon Douglas, David Ackroyd, Larry B. Scott, Jason Bernard, Danny Nucci, Silvana Gallardo, Gregory Martin, Annie Oringer, Selma Archerd, Guy Christopher, Ysamine Delawari, Cecelia Garcia, Jacob Vargas, Terry Wills.

CHOICES

Robert Halmi Prods. P: Halmi. D: David Lowell Rich. W: Judith Parker. Shown on ABC Feb. 17, 1986. (2 hrs.)

Cast: George C. Scott, Jacqueline Bisset, Melissa Gilbert, Laurie Kennedy, Steven Flynn.

CLASSIFIED LOVE

CBS Entertainment Prods. P-D: Don Taylor. W: Diane English, suggested by Sherri Foxman's book. Shown on CBS March 8, 1985. (2 hrs.)

Cast: Michael McKean, Stephanie Faracy, Dinah Manoff, Franc Luz, Paula Trueman, Chevi Colton, Matt Craven, Barrett Heins, Jack Anthony Rose, Michele Seyler, Tom Cuff, Jesse Bradford, Keith Langsdale, Michael Ayr, Ron Guttman, Dee Ann Allen.

CLUB MED

Lorimar Prods. P: Ervin Zavada. Exec. P: Karen Mack. D: Bob Giraldi. W: Judith Paige Mitchell, Jeff Freilich. Shown on ABC Jan. 19, 1986. (2 hrs.)

Cast: Jack Scalia, Linda Hamilton, Patrick Macnee, Janie Lee Burns, Jeff Kaake, Traci Lin-Gaui, Bill Maher, Adam Mills, SinBad, Timothy Williams, Allison Argo, Lorraine Chanel.

CONVICTED

Larry A. Thompson Prods. P: Paul Pompian. Exec. P: Thompson. D: David Lowell Rich. W: Jonathan B. Rintels Jr. Shown on ABC May 12, 1986. (2 hrs.)

Cast: Lindsay Wagner, John Larroquette, Carroll O'Connor, Gary Grubbs, Jenny Lewis, Gabriel Damon, Alyson Craft, Jamie McEnnan, Glen Morrissey, Charles Bartlett, Patricia Gaul, Laurie O'Brien, Caitlin O'Heanrey, Burton Gilliam, Paul Comi, Peter Jason.

COPACABANA

Dick Clark Cinema Prods.; Stiletto Ltd. P: R.W. Goodwin. Exec. P: Clark, Dan Paulson. D: Waris Hussein. W: James Lipton, based on the characters in the song, "Copacabana," by Barry Manilow, Bruce Sussman, Jack Feldman. Shown on CBS Dec. 3, 1985. (2 hrs.)

Cast: Barry Manilow, Annette O'Toole, Ernie Sabella, Estelle Getty, James T. Callahan, Andra Akers, Silvana Gallardo, Joe Bologna, Cliff Osmond, Dwier Brown, Stanley Brock, Clarence Felder, Hamilton Camp.

CRIME OF INNOCENCE

Ohlmeyer Communications. P: Paul Radin. Exec. P: Don Ohlmeyer, Karen Danaher. W: Michael Berk, Douglas Schwartz. D: Michael Miller. Shown on NBC Oct. 27, 1985. (2 hrs.)

Cast: Andy Griffith, Ralph Waite, Diane Ladd, Shawnee Smith, Tammy Lauren, Jordan Charney, Brian Robbins, Michael Champion, Oceana Marr, Michelle Rogers, Belita Moreno.

DALLAS: THE EARLY YEARS

Lorimar-Telepictures. P: Joseph B. Wallenstein. Exec. P: David Jacobs, Malcolm Stuart. D: Larry Elikann. W: Jacobs. Shown on CBS March 23, 1986. (3 hrs)

Cast: David Grant, Dale Midkiff, Molly Hagan, David Wilson, Hoyt Axton, Larry Hagman, Bill Duke, Geoffrey Lewis, Diane Franklin, Marshall Thompson, William Frankfather, Liz Keifer, Wendel Meldrum, Matt Mulhern, Bernie Moore.

DALTON: CODE OF VENGEANCE II

Universal TV. Exec. P: Lou Shaw. D: Alan Smithee. W: Luther Murdoch, Aiken Woodruff. Shown on NBC May 11, 1986. (2 hrs.)

Cast: Charles Taylor, Ed Bruce, Tony Frank, Alex Harvey, Karen Landry, Belinda Montgomery, Mitch Pileggi, Donnelly Rhodes, William J. Sanderson, Shannon Stein.

DEAD MAN'S FOLLY

Warner Bros. TV. P: Neil Hartley. D: Clive Donner. W: Rod Browning, based on the novel by Agatha Christie. Shown on CBS Jan. 8, 1986. (2 hrs.)

Cast: Peter Ustinov, Jean Stapleton, Constance Cummings, Tim Pigott-Smith, Jonathan Cecil, Kenneth Cranham, Susan Wooldridge, Christopher Guard, Jeff Yagher, Nicolette Sheridan.

A DEADLY BUSINESS

Thebaut/Frey Prods.; Taft Entertainment TV. P: Harry R. Sherman. Exec. P: Jim Thebaut. D: John Korty. W: Al Ramrus. Shown on CBS March. 4, 1986. (2 hrs.)

Cast: Alan Arkin, Armand Assante, Jon Polito, Raymond Serra, George Morfogen, Michael Learned, James Rebhorn, John Seitz, Marx Gomes, Stephen Pearlman, Dave Nichols, Doug Lennox, Marcia Diamond, Marilyn Boyle, Bernard Behrens.

DEATH OF A SALESMAN

Roxbury and Punch. P: Robert F. Colesberry. D: Volker Schloendorff. W: Arthur Miller. Shown on CBS Sept. 15, 1985. (3 hrs.)

Cast: Dustin Hoffman, Kate Reid, John Malkovich, Stephen Lang, Charles Durning, Louis Zorich, David S. Chandler, Jon Polito, Kathy Rossetter.

THE DELIBERATE STRANGER

Stuart Phoenix Prods.; Lorimar-Telepictures. P-D: Marvin J. Chomsky. Exec. P: Malcolm Stuart. W: Hesper Anderson, based on Richard W. Laren's book. Shown on NBC May 4 and 5, 1986. (4 hrs.)

Cast: Mark Harmon, Frederic Forrest, George Grizzard, Ben Masters, Glynnis O'Connor, M. Emmet Walsh, John Ashton, Bonnie Bartlett, Frederick Coffin, Deborah Goodrich, Billy Green Bush, Lawrence Pressman, Macon McCalman, Jeanetta Arnette.

DIARY OF A PERFECT MURDER

InterMedia Entertainment; Strathmore Prods.; Viacom Prods. P: Joel Steiger. Exec. P: Fred Silverman, Dean Hargrove. D: Robert Day, W: Hargrove. Shown on NBC March 3, 1986. (2 hrs.)

Cast: Andy Griffith, Lori Lethin, Alice Hirson, Kene Holiday, Steve Inwood, Jack Bannon, James McEachin, Lawrence Pressman, Dennis Lipscomb, Katherine Cannon, Jeanette Nolan, Al Ruscio, Erica Yohn, Terence Ford, Irene Arranga.

DOUBLETAKE

Titus Prods.; Worldvision Enterprises. P: Thomas DeWolfe. Exec. P: Herbert Brodkin, Robert Berger. D: Jud Taylor. W: John Gay, based on the novel by William Bayer called "Switch." Shown on CBS Nov 24 & 26, 1985. (4 hrs.)

Cast: Richard Crenna, Beverly D'Angelo, Vincent Baggetta, Paul Gleason, Cliff Gorman, Drew Snyder, Lee Richardson, Julie Bovasso, Eddie Jones, Lois Smith, Tom Aldredge, Priscilla Lopez, Jeffrey DeMunn, Hansford Rowe, Concetta Tomei.

DRESS GRAY

Frank von Zerneck Films; Warner Bros. TV. P-D: Glenn Jordan. Exec. P: von Zerneck. W: Gore Vidal, based on Lucian K. Truscott IV's book. Shown on NBC March 9, 10, 1986. (4 hrs.)

Cast: Eddie Albert, Alec Baldwin, Lloyd Bridges, Patrick Cassidy, Susan Hess, Hal Holbrook, Alexis Smith, Lane Smith, James B. Sikking, Albert Salmi, Ron Rifkin, Tim Van Patten, Cameron Dye, Peter Nelson, Louise Latham, Jason Beghe, Gary Kasper, Joseph Kell, David Harum, Steve Kosko, Patricia Herd, Rick Goldman, Arthur French, Richard Doyle, Alma Martinez.

AN EARLY FROST

NBC Prods. P: Perry Lafferty. Co-P: Art Seider. D: John Erman. W: Ron Cowen, Daniel Lipman. Shown on NBC Nov. 11, 1985. (2 hrs.)

Cast: Aidan Quinn, Gena Rowlands, Ben Gazzara, Sylvia Sidney, D.W. Moffett, John Glover, Sydney Walsh.

THE EXECUTION OF RAYMOND GRAHAM

Alliance Entertainment; Jozak/David W. Rintels Prods. P: Rintels. Exec. P: Gerald I. Isenberg, Hans Proppe, Robert Lantos. D: Daniel Petrie. W: Mel Frohman. Shown on ABC Nov. 17, 1985. (2 hrs.)

Cast: Graham Beckel, George Dzundza, Jeff Fahey, Morgan Freeman, Linda Griffith, Laurie Metcalf, Kate Reid, Alan Scarfe, Josef Sommer, Philip Sterling.

EWOKS: THE BATTLE FOR ENDOR

Lucasfilm Ltd. P: Thomas G. Smith. Exec. P: George Lucas. D-W: Jim & Ken Wheat. Shown on ABC Nov. 24, 1985. (2 hrs.)

Cast: Wilford Brimley, Warwick Davis, Aubree Miller, Sian Phillips, Carel Struycken, Niki Bothelo, Erick Walker, Marianne Horine, Daniel Frishman, Tony Cox, Pam Grizz, Roger Johnson, Johnny Weismuller Jr., Michael Pritchard.

THE FIFTH MISSILE

Bercovici/St. Johns production; MGM/UA TV. P: Arthur Fellows. Exec. P-W: Eric Bercovici, based on the novel "The Gold Crew" by Thomas N. Scortia and Frank M. Robinson. D: Larry Peerce. Shown on NBC Feb. 23, 1986. (3 hrs.)

Cast: Robert Conrad, Sam Waterston, David Soul, Richard Roundtree, Yvette Mimieux, Art LeFleur, Bruce McGuire, Jonathan Banks.

A FIGHTING CHOICE

Walt Disney TV. P: Nelle Nugent. D: Ferdinand Fairfax. W: Craig Buck. Shown on ABC April 13, 1986. (2 hrs.)

Cast: Beau Bridges, Karen Valentine, Patrick Dempsey, Frances Lee McCain, Lawrence Pressman, Danielle von Zerneck, Allan Arbus, Alice Hirson, Parker Jacobs, Allen Williams, Phillip Linton, Robin Thomas, Charles Lanyer, Nina Henderson.

FINAL JEOPARDY

Frank von Zerneck Films. P: Robert M. Sertner. Exec. P: von Zerneck. D: Michael Pressman. W: Shirl Hendryx. Shown on NBC Dec. 8, 1985. (2 hrs.)

Cast: Richard Thomas, Mary Crosby, Jeff Corey, Jonathan Goldsmith, Michael Cavanaugh, Joey Sagal, Jaime Alba, Travis McKenna, Johnny Venocura, Jordan Charney, John Malloy, Lycia Naff.

FORTRESS

HBO Premiere Films. Crawford Prods. P: Raymond Menmiur. Exec. P: Hector & Ian Crawford, Terry Stapleton. D: Arch Nicholson. W: Everett DeRoche, based on the novel by Gabrielle Lord. Shown on HBO Nov. 24, 1985. (90 mins.)

Cast: Rachel Ward, Sean Garlick, Rebecca Rigg, Robin Mason, Marc Gray, Beth Buchanan, Asher Keddie, Bradley Meehan, Anna Crawford, Richard Terrill, Peter Hehir, Roger Stephen.

THE GIRL WHO SPELLED FREEDOM

Knopf/Simons Prods.: ITC Prods.; Walt Disney TV. P: R.W. Goodwin. Exec. P: Judith A. Palone, D: Simon Wincer. W: David A. Simons, Christopher Knopf. Shown on ABC Feb. 22, 1986. (2 hrs.)

Cast: Wayne Rogers, Mary Kay Place, Kieu Chinn, Kathleen Sisk, Margot Pinvidic, Susan Walden, Blue Mankuma, Jade Chin, Diana Ung, Linda Wong, Jasmin Tam, Wilson Lo, Raymond Lau.

THE GLADIATOR

Walker Bros. Prods.; New World TV. P: Robert Lovenheim. Exec. P: Jeffrey Walker, Michael Chase Walker, Tom Schulman. Co-P-W: William Bleich. D: Abel Ferrara. Shown on ABC Feb. 3, 1986. (2 hrs.)

Cast: Ken Wahl, Nancy Allen, Robert Culp, Stan Shaw, Rosemary Forsyth, Brian Robbins, Rick Dees.

HAREM

Highgate Pictures. P: Michael Dryhurst. Exec. P: Martin Manulis. D. Billy Hale. W: Karol Ann Hoeffner. Shown on ABC Feb. 9 & 10, 1986. (4 hrs.)

Cast: Nancy Travis, Art Malik, Sarah Miles, Yaphet Kotto, Julian Sands, Cheri Lunghi, Omar Sharif, Ava Gardner, Shirley Cain, George Camiller, David Gant, Michael Gwilym, Barrie Houghton, Stephen Jenn, Ian Gentile, Robert Lang.

HELP WANTED: KIDS

Stan Rogow Prods.; Walt Disney TV. P-W: Stephen Black, Henry Stern. Exec. P: Rogow. D: David Greenwalt. Shown on ABC Feb. 2, 1986. (2 hrs.)

Cast: Cindy Williams, Bill Hudson, Chad Allen, Hillary Wolf, John Dehner, Joel Brooks, Miriam Flynn, Billie Bird, Carol Morley, Ebbe Roe Smith, Cecily Thompson.

HOSTAGE FLIGHT

Shooting Star Prods. P: James Hay. Exec. P: Frank von Zerneck, Robert M. Sertner. D: Steven Hilliard Stern. W: Stephen Zito, Felix Culver. Shown on NBC Nov. 17, 1985. (2 hrs.)

Cast: Ned Beatty, Dee Wallace Stone, Rene Enriquez, Barbara Bosson, Ina Balin, Mitch Ryan, John Sanderford, Jack Gilford, Kim Ulrich, John Karlen, Frank McRae, Kabir Bedi, Kristina Wayborn, Frank Annese, Frank M. Bernard.

INTIMATE STRANGERS

Nederlander TV & Film Prods.; Telepictures Prods. P: Kenneth Utt. Exec. P: John Bard Manulis, Gladys Rackmil. D: Robert Ellis Miller. W: Norman McLeod Morrill. Shown on CBS Jan 1, 1986. (2 hrs.)

Cast: Teri Garr, Stacy Keach, Cathy Lee Crosby, Priscilla Lopez, Justin Deas, Max Gail, Max Barabas, Tresa Hughes, Bob E. Hannah, Robert Goodman, Ray Forchion, Manny Bronz.

INTO THIN AIR

Tony Ganz Prods.; Major H Prods. P: Joseph Stern. Exec.P: Ganz, Irv Wilson, Ron Howard. D: Roger Young. W: George Rubino. Shown on CBS Oct. 29, 1985. (2 hrs.)

Cast: Ellen Burstyn, Robert Prosky, Sam Robards, Nicholas Pryor, John Dennis Johnston, Patricia Smith, Tate Donovan, Caroline McWilliams, J.P. Bumstead, Bill Calvert, Britt Leach, Ebbe Roe Smith.

IZZY AND MOE

Robert Halmi Inc. P: Robert Halmi Sr. D: Jackie Cooper. W: Robert Boris. Shown on CBS Sept. 23, 1985. (2 hrs.)

Cast: Jackie Gleason, Art Carney, Cynthia Harris, Zohra Lampert, Dick Latessa, Thelma Lee, Drew Snyder, Jesse Doran.

I DREAM OF JEANNIE: 15 YEARS LATER

Can't Sing Can't Dance Prods.; Columbia Pictures TV. P: Hugh Benson. Exec. P: Barbara Corday. D: Bill Asher. W: Irma Kalish. Shown on NBC Oct. 20, 1985. (2 hrs.)

Cast: Barbara Eden, Wayne Rogers, Bill Daily, Hayden Rorke, MacKenzie Astin, Dori Brenner, Andre De Shields, John Bennett Perry, Dody Goodman, Michael Fairman, Belita Morena, Ronalda Douglas, Lee Taylor-Allan, Dierk Torsek.

JENNY'S WAR

Louis Rudolph Prods: HTV Ltd.; Columbia Pictures TV. P: Robert Chenault. Exec. P: Rudolph. D: Steven Gethers. W: Gethers, based on the novel by Jack Stoneley. Shown on Operation Prime Time stations in October 1985. (4 hrs.)

Cast: Dyan Cannon, Elke Sommer, Hartmut Becker, Robert Hardy, Nigel Hawthorne, Christopher Casenove, Sion Tudor Owen, John Moulder-Brown, Patrick Ryecart, Nicholas Courtney, Oscar Quitak, Hugh Grant.

JOHN & YOKO: A LOVE STORY

Carson Prods. P: Aida Young. Exec. P: John J. McMahon. D-W: Sandor Stern. Shown on NBC Dec. 2, 1985. (3 hrs.)

Cast: Mark McGann, Kim Miyori, Kenneth Price, Peter Capaldi, Philip Walsh, Richard Morant, Rachel Laurence, Joe Randall, Cutler, Samuel Wetmore, Paul Lockwood, Catherine Wrigley.

JOHNNY BULL

Herbert Brodkin Prod. for Titus Prods. P: Thomas De Wolfe. Exec. P: Brodkin. D: Claudia Weill. W: Kathleen Betsko Yale. Shown on ABC May 19, 1986. (2 hrs.)

Cast: Jason Robards, Colleen Dewhurst, Peter MacNicol, Kathy Bates, Suzanna Hamilton, Bill Cobbs, Tom Wright, Thomas Martell Brimm, Daniel R. Butler, Richard Cowl, E. Brian Dean, Cherie Elledge, Pat Fuleihan.

KILLER IN THE MIRROR

Litke-Grossbart Prods.; Warner Bros. TV. P Michael S. McLean. Exec. P: Jack Grossbart. D-W: Frank De Felitta. Shown on NBC March 31, 1986. (2 hrs.)

Cast: Ann Jillian, Len Cariou, Max Gail, Allen Garfield, Christopher North, Jessica Walter, Andra Akers, Parley Baer, Eileen Barrett, Joseph Chapman, Barney Martin.

KUNG FU: THE MOVIE

Lou-Step Prods.; Warner Bros. TV. P: Skip Ward. Exec. P: Paul R. Richard. Co-P: David Carradine. D: Richard Lang. W: Durrell Royce Crays. Shown on CBS Feb. 1, 1986. (2 hrs.)

Cast: David Carradine, Kerrie Keane, Mako, William Lucking, Luke Askew, Keye Luke, Benson Fong, Brandon Lee, Martin Landau, Ellen Geer, Robert Harper, Paul Rudd, John Alderman.

THE LAST DAYS OF FRANK AND JESSE JAMES

A Joe Cates production. P: Phillip Cates. Exec. P: Joe Cates. D: William A. Graham. W: William Stratton. Shown on NBC Feb. 17, 1986. (2 hrs.)

Cast: Johnny Cash, Kris Kristofferson, June Carter-Cash, Willie Nelson, Margaret Gibson, Gail Youngs, Ed Bruce, Marcia Cross, Darrell Wilks.

A LETTER TO THREE WIVES

Michael Filerman Prods.; 20th Fox TV. P: Karen Moore. Exec. P: Filerman. D: Larry Elikann. W: Sally Robinson, based on a story by John Klempner, adaptation by Vera Caspary and a screenplay by Joseph L. Mankiewicz. Shown on NBC Dec. 16, 1985. (2 hrs.)

Cast: Loni Anderson, Michele Lee, Stephanie Zimbalist, Ben Gazzara, Charles Frank, Michael Gross, Doris Roberts, Ann Sothern, Whitney Kershaw, James Staley, David Garrison, Stephen Shellen, Nancy Warren.

LONG TIME GONE

Picturemaker Prods.: ABC Circle Films. P: Jay Daniel. Exec. P-W: Glenn Gordon Caron. D: Robert Butler. Shown on ABC May 23, 1986. (2 hrs.)

Cast: Paul LeMat, Wil Wheaton, Ann Dusenberry, Ray Giradin, Barbara Stock, Richard Sarafian, Deborah Wakeham, Eddie Zammit, Bill Marcus.

LOVE IS NEVER SILENT

Marian Rees Associates. P: Dorothea G. Petrie. Exec. P: Rees, Julianna Field. D: Joseph Sargent. W: Darlene Craviotto, based on the novel, "In This Sign," by Joanne Greenberg. Shown on NBC Dec. 9, 1985. (2 hrs.)

Cast: Mare Winningham, Phyllis Frelich, Ed Waterstreet, Frederic Lehne, Cloris Leachman, Sid Caesar, Susan Ann Curtis, Mark Hildreth, Lou Fant, Julianna Field, Jeremy Christall.

LOVE, MARY

CBS Entertainment Prods. P: Ellis A. Cohen. D: Robert Day. W: Clifford Campion. Shown on CBS Oct. 8, 1985. (2 hrs.)

Cast: Kristy McNichol, Matt Clark, David Paymer, Rachel Ticotin, Piper Laurie, Leslie Wing.

LOVE ON THE RUN

NBC Prods. P: Jay Benson. Exec. P-W: Sue Grafton, Steve Humphrey. D: Gus Trikonis. Shown on ABC Oct. 21, 1985. (2 hrs.)

Cast: Stephanie Zimbalist, Alec Baldwin, Constance McCashin, Ernie Hudson, Madison Mason, Howard Duff, Matthew Cowles, Kit Lefever, Savannah Smith Boucher, David Hayward, Burke Byrnes, Beau Staff, Arnold Turner, Eric Server.

THE LONG HOT SUMMER

Leonard Hill Films. P: Dori Weiss. Exec. P: Hill, John Thomas Lenox. D: Stuart Cooper. W: Rita Mae Brown (Part I); Brown and Dennis Turner (Part II), based on the novel by William Faulkner and a screenplay by Irving Ravetch and Harriet Frank Jr. Shown on NBC Oct. 6 & 7, 1985. (4 hrs.)

Cast: Don Johnson, Jason Robards, Ava Gardner, Cybill Shepherd, Judity Ivey, William Russ, William Forsythe, Wings Hauser, Alexandra Johnson, Stephen Davies, Charlotte Stanton, Albert Hall.

LOST IN LONDON

Emmanuel Lewis Entertainment; D'Angelo Prods; Group W. Prods. P: Peter Manley. Exec. P: Bill D'Angelo. D: Robert Lewis. W: Ron Rubin. Shown on CBS Nov. 20, 1985. (2 hrs.)

Cast: Emmanuel Lewis, Lynne Moody, Ben Vereen, Freddie Jones, Basil Hoskins, Courtney Roper, Bobby Collins, Horace Oliver, Amber Jane Raab, Michelle Welch, Wayne Goddard, Peter Hughes, Deidre Costello.

MAFIA PRINCESS

Jack Farren Prods.; Group W. Prods. P: Lew Gallo. Exec. P: Farren. D: Robert Collins. W: Robert W. Lenski, based on the book by Antoinette Giancana & Thomas C. Renner. Shown on NBC Jan. 19, 1986. (2 hrs.)

Cast: Susan Lucci, Kathleen Widdoes, Tony Curtis, Chuck Shamata, Louis DiBanco, David McIlwraith, Tony DeSantis, Marsha Moreau, Albert Schultz, Norma Edwards, Ken Pogue, Tom Harvey, Bill Lake, Laurie Waller-Benson, John MacKenzie.

MASTER HAROLD . . . AND THE BOYS

Lorimar Prods.: WNET, New York. P: Iris Merlis. Exec. P: Michael Brandman, Emanuel Azenberg. D: Michael Lindsay-Hogg. W: Athol Fugard. Shown on PBS in November, 1985. (90 mins.)

Cast: Matthew Broderick, Zakes Mokae, John Kani.

A MASTERPIECE OF MURDER

20th Fox TV. P: Terry Morse. Exec. P: Andrew J. Fenady. D: Charles S. Dubin. W: Fenady, Terry Nation. Shown on NBC Jan. 27, 1986. (2 hrs.)

Cast: Bob Hope, Don Ameche, Kevin McCarthy, Jayne Meadows, Anne Lloyd Francis, Frank Gorshin, Stella Stevens, Clive Revill, Claudia Christina, Jamie Farr, Yvonne DeCarlo.

THE MIDNIGHT HOUR

ABC Circle Films. P: Ervin Zavada. D: Jack Bender. W: Bill Bleich. Shown on ABC Nov. 1, 1985. (2 hrs.)

Cast: Shari Belafonte-Harper, LeVar Burton, Peter DeLuise, Jonna Lee, Kevin McCarthy, Lee Montgomery, Dick Van Patten, Jonelle Allen, Dedee Pfeiffer, Cindy Morgan.

MIRACLE OF THE HEART: A BOYS TOWN STORY

Larry White Prods,; Columbia Pictures TV. P: Hugh Benson. Exec. P: White. D: Georg Stanford Brown. W: B.E. Sandefur, William Putnam. Shown on SYN stations April 3, 1986. (2 hrs.)

Cast: Art Carney, Casey Siemaszko, Jack Bannon, Darrell Larson, Reginald T. Dorsey, Lisa Sloan, Shashawnee Hall, Jacob Vargas, Anne Pitoniak, Kristy Swanson.

MRS. DELAFIELD WANTS TO MARRY

Schaefer/Karpf Prods.; Gaylord Prod. Co. P-D: George Schaefer. Exec. P: Merrill H. Karpf. Co.-P-W: James Prideaux. Shown on CBS March 30, 1986. (2 hrs.)

Cast: Katharine Hepburn, Bibi Besch, Denholm Elliott, Brenda Forbes, Charles Frank, Harold Gould, Suzanne Lederer, John Pleshette, David Ogden Stiers, Kathyrn Walker, Babs Chula, Daphne Goldrick, Tom Heaton, Antony Holland.

MURDER: BY REASON OF INSANITY

LS Entertainment, Inc. P: Lawrence Schiller. D: Anthony Page. W: Scott Swanton, based on an article by Marilyn Goldstein. Shown on CBS Oct. 1, 1985. (2 hrs.)

Cast: Candice Bergen, Jurgen Prochnow, Hector Elizondo, Eli Wallach, Alison LaPlaca, Lee Kessler.

MURROW

HBO Premiere Films; Titus Prods.; TVS. P: Dickie Bamber. Exec. P: Herbert Brodkin, Robert Berger. D: Jack Gold. W: Ernest Kinoy. Shown on HBO Jan. 19, 1986. (2 hrs.)

Cast: Daniel J. Travanti, Dabney Coleman, Edward Herrmann, Jack McMartin, Robert Vaughn, David Suchet, Harry Ditson, Bob Sherman, Kathryn Leigh Scott, Christopher Muncke.

MY TWO LOVES

Alvin Cooperman Prods; Taft Entertainment TV. Exec. P: Cooperman. D: Noel Black. W: Reginald Rose, Rita Mae Brown. Shown on ABC April 7, 1986. (2 hrs.)

Cast: Mariette Hartley, Lynn Redgrave, Barry Newman, Sada Thompson, Sarah Inglis, Robert L. Leonard, Eve Roberts, Arturo Tamaez, Thee Swan, Rachel Fey, Ray Loberto, Edwin Neal, Diane Perella, Lee Connally.

NEWS AT ELEVEN

Turman/Foster Co. Prods.; Finnegan Associates. P: Bill Finnegan. Exec. P: Lawrence Turman, David Foster. D-W: Mike Robe. Shown on CBS April 2, 1985. (2 hrs.)

Cast: Martin Sheen, Peter Riegert, Barbara Babcock, David S. Sheiner, Christopher Allport, Susan Krebs, Christa Denton, Mandy Ingber, Sydney Penny, Sheree J. Wilson, Brooke Bundy, Sandy McPeak, Tina Caspart, Carlos Lacamara.

NOBODY'S CHILD

Joseph Feury Prods.; Gaylord Prod. Co. P: Feury. Exec. P: Dyson Lovell. Co-P: Milton Justice. D: Lee Grant. W: Mary Gallagher, Ara Watson. Shown on CBS April 6, 1986. (2 hrs.)

Cast: Marlo Thomas, Ray Baker, Caroline Kava, Kathy Baker, Anna Maria Horsford, Madeleine Sherwood, Jackson Davies, Michael Higgins, Blanche Baker, Vanessa Santos, Donna Ford, William Nunn, Stefania de Stefanis, Karen Austin, Garwin Sanford, Joseph Golland, Sheila Moore.

NORTH BEACH & RAWHIDE

CBS Entertainment Prods. P: Roni Weisberg. D: Harry Falk. W: Jimmy Sangster, John Beard, George Yanok. Shown on CBS Nov. 12 & 13, 1985. (2 hrs.)

Cast: William Shatner, Tate Donovan, James Olson, Ron O'Neal, Lori Loughlin, Conchata Ferrell, C.W. Bailey, Grace Zabriski, Gretchen Corbett, Christopher Penn, Geoffrey Blake.

ONE TERRIFIC GUY

CBS Entertainment Prods. P: Mike Merrick, Joseph Siegman. D: Lou Antonio. W: Cynthia Whitcomb. Shown on CBS Feb. 18, 1986. (2 hrs.)

Cast: Mariette Hartley, Wayne Rogers, Laurence Luckinbill, Geoffrey Blake, Brian Robbins, Susan Rinell.

THE OTHER LOVER

Larry Thompson Prods.; Columbia Pictures TV. P: Hugh Benson. Exec. P: Thompson. D: Robert Ellis Miller. W: Judith Parker, Susan Titus. Shown on CBS Sept. 24, 1985. (2 hrs.)

Cast: Lindsay Wagner, Jack Scalia, Max Gail, Millie Perkins, John Bennett Perry, Shannen Doherty, Jaime Lyn Hart.

OUT OF THE DARKNESS

Grosso-Jacobson Prods.; Centerpoint Prods. P: Sonny Grosso, Larry Jacobson. D: Jud Taylor. W: T.S. Cook. Shown on CBS Oct. 12, 1985. (2 hrs.)

Cast: Martin Sheen, Hector Elizondo, Matt Clark, Jennifer Salt, Eddie Egan, Robert Trebor, Val Avery, Joe Spinell, Victor Arnold, Ann Talman, VInce Grand, Bernie McInerney, Paul Jabara, Dick Latessa, Sam MacMurray.

OUTRAGE!

Irwin Allen Prods.; Columbia Pictures TV. P: Allen. D: Walter Grauman. W: Henry Denker, based on his novel. Shown on CBS March 2, 1986. (2 hrs.)

Cast: Robert Preston, Beau Bridges, Burgess Meredith, Linda Purl, Anthony Newley, William Allen Young, Mel Ferrer, Sheila Allen, Nick Angotti, Selma Archerd, Paul Cloud, Bill Dearth, Robert Dowdell, Greg Finley, Seth Foster.

PASSION FLOWER

Doris Keating Prods.; Columbia Pictures TV. P: Andrew Gottlieb. Exec. P: Keating. D: Joseph Sargent. W: Richard A.

Guttman. Shown on CBS Jan. 19, 1986. (2 hrs.)
Cast: Bruce Boxleitner, Barbara Hershey, Nicol Williamson, John Waters, Dick O'Neill, Carolyn Nelson, Moshe Kedem, Jenny Ong, Peggy Williamson, Jane Mason, Lindsay Jones, Kathleen Watson.

PERRY MASON RETURNS
InterMedia Entertainment; Strathmore Prods.; Viacom. P: Barry Steinberg. Exec. P: Fred Silverman, Dean Hargrove. D: Ron Satlof. W: Hargrove. Shown on NBC Dec. 1, 1985. (2 hrs.)
Cast: Raymond Burr, Barbara Hale, William Katt, Holland Taylor, Richard Anderson, Kerri Keane, Al Freeman Jr., David McIlwraith, Robert Weiss, Cassie Yates, Patrick O'Neal.

PERRY MASON: THE CASE OF THE NOTORIOUS NUN
Intermedia Entertainment Co.; Strathmore Prods.; Viacom. P: Barry Steinberg. Exec. P: Fred Silverman, Dean Hargrove. D: Ron Satlof. W. Joel Steiger. Shown on NBC May 25, 1986. (2 hrs.)
Cast: Raymond Burr, Barbara Hale, William Katt, Timothy Bottoms, Michele Green, Jon Cypher, Arthur Hill, David Ogden Stiers, William Prince, Barbara Parkins, Tom Bosley. James McEachin, Ed Winter, Gerald S. O'Loughlin, Hagan Beggs.

PICKING UP THE PIECES
CBS Entertainment Prods. P: Dorothea G. Petrie. D: Paul Wendkos. W: Gordon Cotler. Shown on CBS Oct. 22, 1985. (2 hrs.)
Cast: Margot Kidder, David Ackroyd, Ari Meyers, Barbara Rhoades, Joyce Van Patten, Len Birman, Herbert Edelman, Robin Gammell, Stephen Young, James Farentino, Jack Higgins, C.B. Barnes, Christianne Hirt, Tom Heaton.

PLEASURES
Catalina Prod. Group; Columbia Pictures TV. P: Peter Katz. Exec. P: Franklin R. Levy, Gregory Harrison, Matthew Rushton. Co-P: Jon Andersen. D: Sharron Miller. W: Jill Gordon. Shown on ABC March 31, 1986. (2 hrs.)
Cast: Joanna Cassidy, Linda Purl, Tracy Nelson, Rick Moses, Pamela Segall, David Paymer, Sasha Mitchell, Barry Bostwick, Pamela Dunlap, Elizabeth Kerr, Richard Gates.

PRINCE OF BEL AIR
Leonard Hill Films. P: Albert J. Salzer. Exec. P: Hill. D: Charles Braverman. W: Dori Pierson, Marc Rubel. Shown on ABC Jan. 20, 1985. (2 hrs.)
Cast: Mark Harmon, Kirstie Alley, Robert Vaughn, Patrick Laborteaux, Bartley Braverman, Deborah Harmon, Katherine Moffat, Scott Getlin, Michael Horton, Jonathan Stark, Sherry Hursey, Lisanne Falk, Dean Cameron, Don Swayze.

PROMISES TO KEEP
Sandra Harmon Prods.; Green/Epstein Prods.; Telepictures Prods. P: Harmon. Exec. P: Jim Green, Allen Epstein. D: Noel Black. W: Phil Penningroth. Shown on CBS Oct. 15, 1985. (2 hrs.)
Cast: Robert Mitchum, Christopher Mitchum, Bentley Mitchum, Claire Bloom, Tess Harper, Merritt Butrick, Jane Sibbett, Hugh Gillian, Peter Hobbs, Paul Mantee, Thomas Oglesby, Andy Romano, Richard Partlow.

RESTING PLACE
Hallmark Hall of Fame. D: John Korty. W: Walter Halsey Davis. Shown on CBS April 27, 1986. (2 hrs.)
Cast: John Lithgow, Richard Bradford, Morgan Freeman, C.C.H. Pounder, G.D. Spradlin, Frances Sternhagen, M. Emmet Walsh, John Philbin, Brian Tarantia, Richard Brooks, Tegan West, Buck Herron, Bob Hannah, Mert Hatfield, Hugh Jarrett, Denise Mickelbury, Wallace Wilkinson, Charles Kahlenberg, Marc Clement.

THE RETURN OF MICKEY SPILLANE'S MIKE HAMMER
Jay Bernstein Prods.: Columbia Pictures TV. P: Gray Frederickson. Exec. P: Bernstein. D: Ray Danton. W: Larry Brody, Janie Hendler, James M. Miller. Shown on CBS April 18, 1986. (2 hrs.)
Cast: Stacy Keach, Don Stroud, Lindsay Bloom, Kent Williams, Lauren Hutton, John Karlen, Frank McRae, Mike Preston, Leo Penn, Mickey Rooney, Stephen Macht, Vincent Edwards, Bruce Boxleitner, Dabney Coleman, Dionne Warwick.

RETURN TO MAYBERRY
Viacom. P: Robin S. Clark. Exec. P: Andy Griffith, Richard O. Linke, Dean Hargrove. D: Bob Sweeney. W: Harvey Bullock, Everett Greenbaum. Shown on NBC April 13, 1986. (2 hrs.)
Cast: Andy Griffith, Ron Howard, Don Knotts, Jim Nabors, George Lindsey, Jack Dodson, Hal Smith, Howard Morris, Betty Lynn, Aneta Corsault, Denver Pyle, Maggie Peterson, Doug Dillard, Rodney Dillard, Dean Webb, Mitch Jayne.

THE RICHEST CAT IN THE WORLD
Les Alexander Prods.; Walt Disney TV. P: Andy Rose, Alex Gorby. Exec. P: Alexander. D: Gregg Beeman. W: Alfa-Betty Olsen, Marshall Efron, Rose, Gorby. Shown on ABC March 9, 1986. (2 hrs.)
Cast: Ramon Bieri, Steven Kampmann, Caroline McWilliams, Steve Vinovich, Jesse Welles, George Wyner, Brandon Cali, Kellie Martin, Palmer the Cat, J.A. Preston, Christina Cocek.

THE RIGHT OF THE PEOPLE
Big Name Films; Fries Entertainment. P: Thomas Fries. Exec. P: Charles Fries. W-D: Jeffrey Bloom. Shown on ABC Jan. 13, 1986. (2 hrs.)
Cast: Michael Ontkean, Jane Kaczmarek, Billy Dee Williams, John Randolph, M. Emmet Walsh, Jamie Smith Jackson, Janet Carroll, Jeffrey Josephson, Joanne Linville.

ROCKABYE
Peregrine Producers Group Inc,; Bertinelli Prods. Inc. P: Jack Grossbart, Marty Litke. Exec. P: Roger Gimbel, Freyda Rothstein. D: Richard Michaels. W: Laird Koenig. Shown on CBS Jan. 12, 1986. (2 hrs.)
Cast: Valerie Bertinelli, Rachel Ticotin, Jason Alexander, Ray Baker, Jo Henderson, Roderick Cook, James Rebhorn, Jonathan Raskin.

SAMARITAN: THE MITCH SNYDER STORY
Levine-Robins Prods. Ltd. in association with Fries Entertainment, Inc. P: Deborah Joy LeVine, Debbie Robins. Exec. P: Charles Fries, Irv Wilson. D: Richard T. Heffron. W: Clifford Campion. Shown on CBS May 19, 1986. (2 hrs.)
Cast: Martin Sheen, Roxanne Hart, Joe Seneca, Stan Shaw, Cicely Tyson, James Avery, Guy Boyd, Janet Carroll, Jordan Charney, Brett Cullen, Conchata Ferrell, Dorothy Fielding, James Handy, Matthew Laurence, John McLiam, Dey Young, Gail Youngs.

SECOND SERVE
Linda Yellen Prods.; Lorimar-Telepictures Prod. Exec. P: Yellen. D: Anthony Page. W: Stephanie Liss, Gavin Lambert, based on "The Renee Richards Story: Second Serve" by Richards with John Ames. Shown on CBS May 13, 1986. (2 hrs.)
Cast: Vanessa Redgrave, Martin Balsam, William Russ, Alice Krige, Kerrie Keane, Richard Venture, Reni Santoni, Louise Fletcher, Jeff Corey, Alan Feinstein, Nina Van Pallandt, Michael Cavanaugh, Kenneth Tigar, Alison LaPlace.

SHATTERED SPIRITS
Sheen/Greenblatt Prods; Robert Greenwald Prods. P-D: Robert Greenwald. Exec. P: Paul Pompian. W: Gregory Goodell. Shown on ABC Jan. 6, 1986. (2 hrs.)
Cast: Martin Sheen, Melinda Dillon, Matthew Laborteaux, Lukas Haas, Roxana Zal, Jill Schoenlen, Jenny Gago, Gaby Mandelik, Lenny Hicks, Dyana Ortelli, John Herzfeld, John Miranda.

SIN OF INNOCENCE
Renee Valente Prods.; Jeremac Prods.; 20Th Fox TV. P: Valente. Exec. P: Valente, Jerry McNeely. D: Arthur Allan Seidelman. W: McNeely. Shown on CBS March 26, 1986. (2 hrs.)
Cast: Bill Bixby, Dee Wallace Stone, Megan Follows, Dermot Mulroney, James Naughton, Loren Peele, Darlene Wheatley, John Morrow, Cary Silver, Jerry McNeely, Steve Coleman, Jane Bruns, John Archie, Sandra Patton, Barry Hober.

STAGECOACH
Raymond Katz Prods.; Heritage Entertainment. P: Hal W. Polaire, Jack Thompson. Exec. P: Katz, Willie Nelson. D: Ted Post. W: James Lee Barrett. Shown on May 18, 1986. (2 hrs.)
Cast: Johnny Cash, Willie Nelson, Kris Kristofferson, Waylon

Jennings, John Schneider, Elizabeth Ashley, Anthony Newley, Tony Franciosa, Mary Crosby, Merritt Butrick, June Carter Cash, Jesse Colter, Alex Kubic, David Allan Coe.

STARK: MIRROR IMAGE

CBS Entertainment Prods. P-W: David H. Balkan. D: Noel Nossek. Shown on CBS May 14, 1986. (2 hrs.)

Cast: Nicolas Survoy, Kirstie Alley, Pat Corley, Ben Murphy, Michelle Phillips, David Ackroyd, Barry Gordon, Belinda Montgomery, Dennis Hopper, Jeffrey Alan Chandler, Gina Gershon, Peter Boyden, Thomas Ryan, Jeffrey Josephson, Diane Delano, Sly-Ali Smith.

STONE PILLOW

Schaefer/Karpf Prods.; Gaylord Prod. Co. P-D: George Schaefer. Exec. P: Merrill H. Karpf. W: Rose Leiman Goldemberg. Shown on CBS Nov. 5, 1985. (2 hrs.)

Cast: Lucille Ball, Daphne Zuniga, William Converse-Roberts, Stephen Lang, Susan Batson, Anna Marie Horsford, Stefan Schnable, Rebecca Schull, Imogene Bliss, Michael Champagne.

STREETS OF JUSTICE

Universal TV. P: Alan Barnette. Exec. P-D-W: Christopher Crowe. Shown on NBC Nov. 10, 1985. (2 hrs.)

Cast: John Laughlin, Robert Loggia, Lance Henriksen, Jack Thibeau, John Hancock, William Sanderson, Douglas Dirkson, Robin Gammell, Cristina Raines, Paul Shenar, Kate Charleson.

SILENT WITNESS

Robert Greenwald Prods. P-W: Conrad Bromberg. Exec. P: Greenwald, Joe Wizan. D: Michael Miller. Shown on NBC Oct. 14, 1985. (2 hrs.)

Cast: Valerie Bertinelli, John Savage, Chris Nash, Melissa Leo, Pat Corley, Steven Williams, Jacqueline Brooks, Alex McArthur, Katie McCombs, Tom Signorelli.

13 AT DINNER

Warner Bros. TV. P: Neil Hartley. D: Lou Antonio. W: Rod Browning, based on the novel by Agatha Christie. Shown on CBS Oct. 19, 1985. (2 hrs.)

Cast: Peter Ustinov, Faye Dunaway, David Suchet, Bill Nighy, Diane Keen, John Stride, Benedict Taylor, Jonathan Cecil, Allan Cuthbertson, Lee Horsley.

THIS CHILD IS MINE

Beth Polson Prods.; Finnegan Associates; Telepictures Prods. P: Pat Finnegan. Exec. P: Polson. D: David Greene. W: Charles Rosin. Shown on NBC Nov. 4, 1985. (2 hrs.)

Cast: Lindsay Wagner, Chris Sarandon, Michael Lerner, John Philbin, Kathleen York, Frank Dent, Joan McMurtrey, Matthew Faison, Nancy McKeon, Carolyn Coates.

THOMPSON'S LAST RUN

Cypress Point Prods.; Phoenix Entertainment Group. P: Jennifer Faulstich. Exec. P: Gerald W. Abrams. D: Jerrold Freedman. W: John Carlen. Shown on CBS Feb. 16, 1985. (2 hrs.)

Cast: Robert Mitchum, Wilford Brimley, Kathleen York, Guy Boyd, Royce Wallace, Susan Tyrrell, Daniel McDonald, Benjamin Gregory, Helena Humann.

TIME FLYER

Three Blind Mice Prods. P: Annette Handley, Susan B. Landau, Alan Shapiro. D-W: Mark Rosman. Shown on ABC Feb. 9, 1986. (2 hrs.)

Cast: Peter Coyote, Huckleberry Fox, Art Carney, Dennis Lipscomb, Joe Flood, Mittie Smith, Frank Simons, Stu Klitsner, Morgan Upton, Bennett Cale.

A TIME TO LIVE

Blue Andre Prods.; ITC Prods. P: Andre. Exec. P: Judith A. Polone. D: Rick Wallace. W: John McGreevey. Shown on NBC Oct. 28, 1985. (2 hrs.)

Cast: Liza Minnelli, Jeffrey DeMunn, Swoosie Kurtz, Scott Schwartz, Corey Haim, Henry Sanders, Janine Manatis, Karen Shallo, Kurt Reis, Trevor Smith, Francois Klanfer, Ken Pogue, Samantah Langevin.

A TIME TO TRIUMPH

Billos/Kaufman Prods.; Phoenix Entertainment Group. P: Fran Billos, Judy Kaufman. Exec. P: Ethel Winant. D: Noel Black. W: Lavina Dawson, George Yanok. Shown on CBS Jan. 7, 1986. (2 hrs.)

Cast: Patty Duke, Joseph Bologna, Julie Bovasso, Denise B. Mickelbury, Dara Modglin, Jackie Welch, Keign Colbert, Mert Hatfield, Mike McGehee, Charlotte Dillon, Lucy Ann Dow.

T.J. HOOKER: BLOOD SPORT

Spelling/Goldberg Prods.; Columbia Pictures TV. P: Kenneth R. Koch, Don Ingalls. Exec. P: Leonard Goldberg. D: Vincent McEveety. W: Rudolph Borchert, Ingalls, Stan Berkowitz, Bruce Reisman, Rick Husky. Shown on CBS May 21, 1986. (2 hrs.)

Cast: William Shatner, Heather Locklear, James Darren, Don Murray, Kim Miyori, Nobu McCarthy, Henry Darrow, Tim O'Connor, James Pax, Keye Luke, Hugh Farrington, Yuji Okumoto, Soon-Teck Oh, Randy Hamilton, Buck Taylor.

TOUGHLOVE

Fries Entertainment. P: Ervin Zavanda. Exec. P: Charles Fries, Irv Wilson. D: Glenn Jordan. W: Karen Hall. Shown on ABC Oct. 13, 1985. (2 hrs.)

Cast: Lee Remick, Bruce Dern, Jason Patric, Eric Schiff, Deedee Pfeiffer, Dana Elcar, Beth Miller, Piper Laurie, Erica Yohn, Sean Frye, Jim Haynie, Janet MacLachlan.

TRAPPED IN SILENCE

Reader's Digest Entertainment. P: Jeff Grant, Dick Atkins. D: Michael Tuchner. W: Pat A. Victor, based on "Murphy's Boy" by Torey Hayden. Shown on CBS May 11, 1986. (2 hrs.)

Cast: Marsha Mason, Kiefer Sutherland, John Mahoney, Stephen Pearlman, Ron Silver, Amy Wright, Harsh Nayyar, Karen Shallo, John McCurry, Rebecca Schull, Joan Pape, Frances Foster, Jason Brill, Robert L. Bell.

TRIPLECROSS

Tisch-Avnet Prods.; ABC Circle Films. P-W: Dusty Kay. Exec. P: Steve Tisch, Avnet. D: David Greene. Shown on ABC March 17, 1986. (2 hrs.)

Cast: Ted Wass, Markie Post, Gary Swanson, Shannon Wilcox, Barbra Horan, Robert Costanzo, Ric Mancini, Mike Genovese, Christopher McDonald, Donald Hotton, Tony Longo, Sandy Simpson, Steven Williams, Anthony Holland, Rex Ryon.

UNDER SIEGE

Ohlmeyer Communications; Telepictures Prods. P: Karen Danaher. Exec. P: Don Ohlmeyer. D: Roger Young. W: Bob Woodward, Christian Williams, Richard Harwood, Alfred Sole. Shown on NBC Feb. 9, 1986. (3 hrs.)

Cast: Peter Strauss, Mason Adams, Lew Ayres, George Grizzard, Hal Holbrook, E.G. Marshall, David Opatoshu, Thaao Penghlis, Stan Shaw, Beatrice Straight, Ann Sweeny, Victoria Tennant, Fritz Weaver, Paul Winfield.

VANISHING ACT

P: Robert Cooper. Exec. P: Richard Levinson, William Link. D: David Greene. W: Levinson, Link. Shown on CBS May 4, 1986. (2 hrs.)

Cast: Mike Farrell, Margot Kidder, Fred Gwynne, Graham Jarvis, Elliott Gould.

VITAL SIGNS

CBS Entertainment Prods. P-D: Stuart Miller. W: Les Hutson. Shown on CBS Feb. 11, 1986. (2 hrs.)

Cast: Edward Asner, Gary Cole, Kate McNeil, John Randolph, James Sloyan, Barbara Barrie, Phillip Sterling, Mary Ann Thebus.

WELCOME HOME, BOBBY

Titus Prods., Inc. P: Thomas De Wolfe, Cyma Rubin. Exec. P: Herbert Brodkin, Robert Berger. D: Herbert Wise. W: Conrad Bromberg. Shown on CBS Feb. 22, 1986. (2 hrs.)

Cast: Tony Lo Bianco, Timothy Williams, Gisela Caldwell, Nan Woods, Adam Baldwin, Stephen James, John Karlen, John Pleshette.

WILD HORSES

Wild Horses Prods.; Telepictures Prods. P: Hunt Lowry. Exec. P: Ken Kragen, Dick Lowry. D: Rick Lowry. W: Roderick Taylor, Daniel Vining. Shown on CBS Nov. 12, 1985. (2 hrs.)

Cast: Kenny Rogers, Pam Dawber, Ben Johnson, David Andrews, Richard Masur, Karen Carlson, Richard Farnsworth.

A WINNER NEVER QUITS

A Blatt/Singer Production; Columbia Pictures TV. P: James Keach, Lynn Raynor. D: Mel Damski. W: Burt Prelutsky. Shown on ABC April 14, 1986. (2 hrs.)

Cast: Keith Carradine, Mare Winningham, Dennis Weaver, G.W. Bailey, Fionulla Flanagan, Ed O'Neill, Jack Kehoe, Huckleberry Fox, Charles Hallahan, Jary Jo Deschanel, Dana Delany, David Haid, Steve Rees, Andrew Lubeskie.

YOUNG AGAIN

Sharmill Prods.; Walt Disney TV. P-D: Steven H. Stern. W: Barbara Hall. Shown on ABC May 11, 1986. (2 hrs.)

Cast: Lindsay Wagner, Robert Urich, Jack Gilford, K.C. Reeves, Jessica Stern, Jason Nicoloff, Peter Spence, Jeremy Ratchford, Jonathan Welsh, Louise Vallance, Vincent Murray.

Organizations

* NATIONAL GROUPS
* REGIONAL UNITS
* GUILDS & UNIONS

ORGANIZATIONS

Academy of Television Arts and Sciences

3500 West Olive Ave., Suite 700, Burbank, CA 91505; (818) 953-7575. (Formed in 1948 to advance the arts and sciences of television.) Awards Emmys for nighttime programming and publishes Emmy Magazine, Hank Rieger, editor.

PRESIDENT
Richard Frank
FIRST VICE PRESIDENT
Doug Duitsman
SECOND VICE PRESIDENT
Larry Gershman
VICE PRESIDENT, LOS ANGELES
Walt Baker
SECRETARY
Mel Sawelson
TREASURER
Meryl Marshall
IMMEDIATE PAST PRESIDENT
Diana Muldaur
EXECUTIVE DIRECTOR
James Loper
AWARDS ADMINISTRATOR
John Leverence
BOARD OF GOVERNORS
Stu Berg, Barbara Brogliatti, Hazel Catmull, Patrick Collins, Fred Chulack, Robert Crutchfield, Marc Danields, William Finnegan, Preston Fischer, Ian Fraser, John Furia, Lee Gabler, Mike Gavin, Dan Gingold, Bill Hargate, Tom Huth, Jerry Immel, Jordan Kerner, Herb Klynn, A. Richard Larson, Linda Lavin, Sydney Litwack, Margaret Loesch, Ellis Marcus, Mina Mittelman, Richard Mulligan, J.H. Rowland Perkins II, Sally Powers, Jeane Renick, Phil Roman, Stu Rosen, Peter Schlesinger, Howard Schwartz, Jan Scott, Gary Shaffer, Susan Simons, Howard Smit, Jerry Smith, Jim Smith, Jay Strong, Bob Sweeney, Russ Tinsley, Ed Vane, Harry Wolf

Actor's Equity Association (AAAA-AFL-CIO-CLC)

(Organized May 16, 1913; Membership, 35,000) 165 West 46th St., New York, NY 10036, (212) 869-8530.

PRESIDENT
Colleen Dewhurst
FIRST VICE-PRESIDENT
Barbara Colton
SECOND VICE-PRESIDENT
Mary Lou Westerfeld
THIRD VICE-PRESIDENT
Patrick Quinn
FOURTH VICE PRESIDENT
Ellen Burstyn
TREASURER
Casper Roos
RECORDING SECRETARY
Lynn Archer
EXECUTIVE SECRETARY
Alan Eisenberg
EXECUTIVE CONSULTANT
Willard Swire
COUNSEL
Cohn, Glickstein, Lurie
MIDWEST REGIONAL V.P.
Madeline Fallon
WESTERN REGIONAL V.P.
Joseph Ruskin

Advertising Council, The

825 Third Avenue, New York, NY 10022; (212) 758-0400.

CHAIRMAN
John Elliott, Jr.
PRESIDENT
Robert P. Keim
VICE PRESIDENT OF PUBLIC AFFAIRS
William F. Rhatican
BRANCH OFFICES
The Advertising Council, 1717 North Highland Ave., Los Angeles CA; The Advertising Council, 1930 Rhode Island Ave., N.W., Washington DC 20036.

Advertising Research Foundation

3 E. 54th St., New York, NY 10022; (212) PLaza 751-5656.

CHAIRMAN
John H. Kofron
VICE CHAIRMAN
George S. Fabian
PRESIDENT
Michael J. Naples
SENIOR VICE PRESIDENT, DIRECTOR OF OPERATIONS
James H. Moore
SECRETARY
John C. Welbber
GENERAL COUNSEL
Gilbert H. Weil

American Advertising Federation

1400 K St., NW, Suite 1000, Washington, DC 20005; (202) 898-0089.

CHAIRMAN OF THE BOARD
Bernard Flanagan
PRESIDENT
Howard H. Bell

American Association of Advertising Agencies

666 Third Avenue, New York, NY 10017; (212) 682-2500.

CHAIRMAN OF THE BOARD
Louis T. Hagopian, N W Ayer Incorporated, New York
VICE CHAIRMAN
Robert E. Jacoby, Ted Bates Worldwide, Inc., New York
SECRETARY-TREASURER
Ronald Stone, Stone, August & Company, Birmingham, Michigan
PRESIDENT
Leonard S. Matthews, A.A.A.A., New York
WASHINGTON REPRESENTATIVE
Bradley H. Roberts, Executive Vice President
WESTERN OFFICE REPRESENTATIVE
Robert P. Stephens, Vice President, Beverly Hills, CA
EXECUTIVE VICE PRESIDENT
Harry Paster
SENIOR VICE PRESIDENTS
Tony Gruber
VICE PRESIDENTS
Donald Ambuhl, Marilyn Bockman, Robert J. Finn, Jerry Graniero, Gloria A. Lanza-Bajo, Donald C. Lewis, Bernard Ryan, James C. Martucci

American Cinema Editors

(Organized November 28, 1950; Membership: 2500) 4416½ Finley Avenue, Los Angeles, CA 90027; (213) 660-4425.

PRESIDENT
Bob Bring
VICE PRESIDENT
Eve Newman
SECRETARY
Bernie Balmuth
TREASURER
Ernest V. Milano
BOARD OF DIRECTORS
Scott C. Eyler, Robert L. Kimble, Frederic L. Knudtson, Alan C. Marks, Chuck Montgomery, Millie Moore, Peter Parasheles

American Federation of Musicians (AFL-CIO)

(Organized October, 1896; Membership: 280,000) Suite 600, Paramount Bldg., 1501 Broadway, New York, NY 10036; (212) 869-1330.

PRESIDENT
Victor W. Fuentealba, Suite 600, Paramount Bldg., 1501 Broadway, New York, NY 10036; (212) 869-1330.
VICE PRESIDENT
John Glasel, 5020 Stacey Avenue, Las Vegas, NV 89108.
CANADA VICE PRESIDENT
J. Alan Wood, 25 Overlea Blvd., Toronto, Ont., Canada M4H 1B1.
SECRETARY-TREASURER
Kelly L. Castleberry II, Suite 600, Paramount Bldg.,1501 Broadway, New York, NY 10036.
EXECUTIVE BOARD
Eugene Frey, Harold Dessent, Sam Folio, John Glasel, Richard Q. Totusek.

American Federation of Television and Radio Artists (AAAA-AFL-CIO)

(Organized August, 1937; Membership 60,000) 1350 Avenue of the Americas, New York, NY 10019; (212) 265-7700.

PRESIDENT
Frank Maxwell
FIRST VICE PRESIDENT
Ann Loring
SECOND VICE PRESIDENT
Len Dresslar
VICE PRESIDENTS
K.T. Stevens, Peter Hackes, Belva Davis, Shelby Scott, Kenneth Barry, Chris Ward, Lee Lawson
TREASURER
Kenneth Roberts
RECORDING SECRETARY
Mike Botula
NATIONAL EXECUTIVE DIRECTOR
John C. Hall Jr.
DIRECTOR, CENTRAL REGION
Herbert Neuer
DIRECTOR, WESTERN REGION
Donald S. Tayer
DIRECTOR, EASTERN REGION
Dan Mallinger
CONTROLLER
Dan Friedenreich
NATIONAL REPRESENTATIVES
Harold Kocin, Walter Grinspan, Louis Santillana, Jr.

American Guild of Musical Artists (AFL-CIO), Branch of Associated Actors and Artistes of America

(Organized 1936; Membership 6,000) 1841 Broadway, Suite 911, New York, NY 10023; (212) 265-3687.

PRESIDENT
Nedda Casei
FIRST VICE PRESIDENT
Eileen Schauler
SECOND VICE PRESIDENT
Elinor Harper
THIRD VICE PRESIDENT
Robert Manno
FOURTH VICE PRESIDENT
Muriel Costa-Greenspon
FIFTH VICE PRESIDENT
Betty Baisch
TREASURER
Lawrence Davidson
RECORDING SECRETARY
Yolanda Antoine
NATIONAL EXECUTIVE SECRETARY
Gene Boucher
ASSOCIATE EXECUTIVE SECRETARY
Alan Olsen
ASSISTANTS TO THE EXECUTIVE SECRETARY
Thomas Jamerson, Alexander Dube
COUNSEL
Becker and London
DIRECTOR OF MEMBERSHIP
Annelise Kamada
FINANCIAL SECRETARY
Catherine Thomas
DIRECTOR OF PUBLIC RELATIONS
Michael Rubino

CANADA: Graham Spicer, 615 Yonge Street, Toronto, Ontario M4Y 2T4, (416) 967-4252; CHICAGO: Herbert Neuer, 307 North Michigan Ave., Chicago, IL 60601, (312) 372-8081; LOS ANGELES: Dennis Moss, 12650 Riverside Drive, Suite 205, North Hollywood, CA 91607, (213) 877-0683; NEW ENGLAND: Robert M. Segal, 11 Beacon Street, Boston, MA 02108, (617) 742-0208; NEW ORLEANS: Rosemary Le Boeuf, 619 N. Hennessy, New Orleans, LA, (504) 486-9410; NORTHWEST: Carolyn Carpp, 5051 148 Ave., NE, Bellevue, WA 98007, (206) 881-7235; PHILADELPHIA: Mark P. Muller, Lafayette Building, 8th Floor, 5th and Chestnut Street, Philadelphia, PA 19106, (215) 925-8400; SAN FRANCISCO: Harry Polland/Donald Tayer, 100 Bush Street, Suite 1500, San Francisco, CA 94104, (415) 986-4060; TEXAS: Benny Hopper, 3915 Fairlakes Drive, Dallas, TX 75149, (214) 279-4720; WASHINGTON/BALTIMORE: Joshua J. Kaufman, 918 16th St., NW, Suite 503, Washington, DC 20006, (202) 466-3030.

American Guild of Variety Artists (AAAA-AFL-CIO)

(Organized July 14, 1939; Registered Membership: 35,000; Active Membership: 5,000) 184 Fifth Ave., New York, NY 10010; (212) 675-1003.

HONORARY PRESIDENT
George Burns
HONORARY FIRST VICE PRESIDENT
Rod McKuen
HONORARY THIRD VICE PRESIDENT
Ann Corio
EXECUTIVE PRESIDENT
Alan Jan Nelson
EXECUTIVE VICE PRESIDENT
Will Aherne
SECRETARY TREASURER
Jack London
REGIONAL VICE PRESIDENTS
Dick Martin, Margie Coate, Ronald Puckett, Stanley Burns, Bob Freed, Tommy Spencer, Harry Lewis, Thomas Merriweather, Tina Marie, Steve Stephens, Ted Monson, Bobby Faye, Don George, Etta Rollins, Ralph Shaw.

American Humane Association

(Organized 1877) Hollywood office: 14144 Ventura Blvd., Sherman Oaks, CA 91423; (818) 501-0123; National Headquarters: 9725 East Hampden, Denver, CO 80231; (303) 695-0811. (Liaison with the television and motion picture industry as supervisors of animal action in television and motion picture production.)

PRESIDENT
Art Slade
VICE PRESIDENT
Hortense Landau
TREASURER
Charles W. Ennis
DIRECTOR—HOLLYWOOD OFFICE
Carmelita Pope

American Society of Cinematographers, Inc.

(Organized 1919; Membership: 286) 1782 North Orange Drive, Hollywood, CA 90028; (213) 876-5080.

PRESIDENT
Stanley Cortez
FIRST VICE PRESIDENT
Leonard South
SECOND VICE PRESIDENT
Harry Wolf
THIRD VICE PRESIDENT
Ted Voigtlander
SECRETARY
Joseph Westheimer
TREASURER
Linwood G. Dunn

American Society of Composers, Authors and Publishers (ASCAP)

(Organized February 13, 1914; Membership: 19,000

Music Writers, 8,700 Publishers) One Lincoln Plaza, New York, NY 10023, (212) 595-3050; 6430 Sunset Blvd., Hollywood, CA 90028.

PRESIDENT
Hal David
VICE PRESIDENTS
Arthur Hamilton, Irwin Z. Robinson
SECRETARY
Morton Gould
TREASURER
Leon J. Brettler
ASSISTANT SECRETARY
John Green
ASSISTANT TREASURER
Sidney Herman
COUNSEL
Bernard Korman
MANAGING DIRECTOR
Gloria Messinger
WESTERN REGIONAL DIRECTOR
Todd Brabec, ASCAP, 6430 Sunset Boulevard, Hollywood, CA 90028
SOUTHERN REGIONAL EXECUTIVE DIRECTOR
Connie Bradley, ASCAP, Two Music Square West, Nashville, TN37203

Associated Actors and Artistes of America (AAAA-AFL-CIO)

(Organized July 18, 1919; Membership: 85,000) 165 West 46th St., New York, NY 10036; (212) 869-0358.

PRESIDENT
Frederick O'Neal
VICE PRESIDENTS
Ken Orsatti, Willard Swire, Gene Boucher, Rod McKuen
TREASURER
Harold M. Hoffman
EXECUTIVE SECRETARY
John C. Hall, Jr.
AFFILIATES
Actors' Equity Association, American Federation of Television and Radio Artists, American Guild of Musical Artists, American Guild of Variety Artists, Asociacion Puertorriqueña de Artistas y Tecnicos del Espectaculo, Hebrew Actors Union, Italian Actors Union, Screen Actors Guild, Screen Extras Guild.

Association of Independent Video and Filmmakers, Inc.

625 Broadway, New York, NY 10012; (212) 473-3400. (Membership: over 5,000 independent professionals, including producers, directors, writers and technicians in film and video; publishes The Independent Magazine.)

PRESIDENT
Lawrence Sapadin

Association of National Advertisers, Inc.

155 East 44th St., New York, NY 10017; (212) 697-5950.

PRESIDENT
DeWitt F. Helm, Jr.
SENIOR VICE PRESIDENT, WASHINGTON, D.C.
Daniel L. Jaffe
VICE PRESIDENTS
Peter Eder, Clark Holt, Anthon C. Lunt, Bob Taber
COMPTROLLER
James R. Cosgrove

Association of Talent Agents

(Organized July, 1937; Membership: 180) (Official Organization of Talent Agents in Hollywood.) 9255 Sunset Boulevard, Suite 318, Los Angeles, CA 90069; (213) 274-0628.

EXECUTIVE DIRECTOR
Chester L. Migden
FIRST VICE PRESIDENT
Roger Davis
VICE PRESIDENT
Sid Craig
VICE PRESIDENTS
Carter Gibson, Eric Klass
SECRETARY-TREASURER
Sandra L. Joseph

Authors' Guild, Inc.

(Membership: 6,000) 234 West 44th St., New York, NY 10036; (212) 398-0838.

PRESIDENT
Madeleine L'Engle
VICE PRESIDENT
Robert K. Massie
SECRETARY
Gerold Frank
TREASURER
Barbara W. Tuchman
EXECUTIVE SECRETARY
Peter Heggie

The Authors League of America, Inc.

(Membership: 12,000) Authors League, 234 West 44th St., New York, NY 10036; (212) 391-9198.

PRESIDENT
Garson Kanin
VICE PRESIDENT
Robert Anderson
SECRETARY
Toni Morrison
TREASURER
Garson Kanin
COUNSEL
Irwin Karp
ADMINISTRATOR
Nancy Weidner

Banff Television Festival

P.O. Box 1020, Banff, Alberta, Canada, T0L 0C0; (403) 762-3060. (Honors excellence in world TV)

EXECUTIVE DIRECTOR
Carrie Hunter
FESTIVAL DIRECTOR
Jerry Ezekiel
MARKETING & MEDIA RELATIONS
Barbara A. Moss
BUSINESS MANAGER
Jim Bertram

Broadcast Music, Inc.

320 West 57th Street, New York, NY 10019; (212) 586-2000. 6255 Sunset Boulevard, Hollywood, CA 90028; (213) 465-2111. 10 Music Square, East, Nashville, TN 37203; (615) 259-3625. 5105 Tollview Drive, Suite 240, Rolling Meadows, IL 60008; (312) 870-8060. 1320 S. Dixie Highway, Coral Gables, FL 33146; (305) 666-6122. 1650 Borel Place, San Mateo, CA 94402; (415) 349-9590. 1325 S. Dairy Ashford, Suite 260, Houston, TX 77077; (713) 558-3500. Shovel Shop Square 3A, North Easton, MA 02356; (617) 238-0174. 275 Broadhollow Road, Melville, NY 11747; (516) 293-6664. 255 Ponce de Leon Ave., Pan Am Bldg., Hato Rey, Puerto Rico 00917; (809) 754-6490.

BOARD CHAIRMAN
Robert Pratt
PRESIDENT
Edward M. Cramer
SENIOR VICE PRESIDENT, SPECIAL COUNSEL AND ASSISTANT TO THE PRESIDENT
Theodora Zavin
SENIOR VICE PRESIDENT, PERFORMING RIGHTS ADMINISTRATION
Frances Preston
VICE PRESIDENT, NASHVILLE
Roger Sovine
VICE PRESIDENT, CALIFORNIA
Ronald M. Anton
VICE PRESIDENT, FOREIGN PERFORMING RIGHTS ADMINISTRATION
Helmut Guttenburg
VICE PRESIDENT, LICENSING

Lawrence P. Sweeney
VICE PRESIDENT, ADMINISTRATION
Alan H. Smith
VICE PRESIDENT, SECRETARY, AND GENERAL COUNSEL
Edward W. Chapin
CONTROLLER
Thomas Curry

Broadcast Pioneers

320 West 57th Street, New York, NY 10019; (212) 586-2000.

PRESIDENT
Jack G. Thayer
FIRST VICE PRESIDENT
Sol Paul
VICE PRESIDENT
James Delmonico
EXECUTIVE DIRECTOR
Edward J. DeGray

Catholic Actors Guild of America

(Organized April, 1914; Membership: 550) 1501 Broadway, New York, NY 10036; (212) 398-1868.

PRESIDENT
William J. O'Malley
FIRST VICE PRESIDENT
Frederick O'Neal
SECOND VICE PRESIDENT
Hildegarde
TREASURER
Martin Kiffel
EXECUTIVE SECRETARY
Suzanne Richardson
CHAIRMAN OF EXECUTIVE BOARD
Lisa Di Julio

Catholic Broadcasting Office

(See Office for Film & Broadcasting)

Catholic Communications Foundation

Ste. 198, Box 9000, Carlsbad, CA 92008; (714) 942-1120. Established by the Catholic Fraternal Benefit Societies to assist the national, regional and local radio and television activities of the Catholic Church in the United States. The Foundation awards communications training scholarships to the Institute for Religious Communications. The CCF's board of directors is composed of Bishops of the Catholic Church, fraternal benefit society executives and representatives from the communications industry.

CHAIRMAN
Most Reverend Anthony G. Bosco, Auxiliary Bishop of Pittsburgh
PRESIDENT
Most Reverend Kenneth Povish, Bishop of Lansing, MI.
EXECUTIVE DIRECTOR
James R. Bastis

Catholic Conference (U.S.), Department of Communication

Suite #1300, 1011 First Ave., New York, NY 10022; (212) 644-1898.

SECRETARY OF COMMUNICATION
Richard H. Hirsch

The Department of Communication of the U.S. Catholic Conference (the public policy agency of the Catholic Bishops of America) addresses the Church's apostolate in and through the print and electronic media. It provides advice and technical assistance on more than 100 radio and 50 network television programs a year.

The Department also publishes a weekly guide to current films and television programs that appear in 100 plus papers of the Catholic Press in the United States. In this activity the Department reviews all current nationally-released 35mm films, and provides information about resources for film utilization and education (16mm films, books, magazines, festivals). The critical reviews are addressed to the moral, as well as the aesthetic, dimensions of motion pictures, and are the result of a consensus based on the reactions of the Department's professional staff and Board of Consultors. All films reviewed are also classified according to the Department's rating system. In addition, this weekly service carries information and evaluative studies on trends and issues pertinent to television, with an emphasis on educational material.

The Department also plays a liaison role for the USCC with the film and broadcasting industries, national media, and religious agencies and organizations. It is a member of OCIC and UNDA, the international Catholic organizations for film and broadcasting, respectively. Consultation and information services are also provided for the Pontifical Commission for Social Communications and the communication offices of national episcopal offices throughout the world.

The Department includes the National Catholic News Service. For more than 60 years this agency has been the primary source of news about the Church worldwide for the American Catholic and secular press. NC News also produces a weekly television newscast and "Origins," the well-known documentary service with subscribers throughout the United States and the world.

With staff assistance, the episcopal members of the Communication Committee administer funds raised through the Catholic Communication Campaign, an annual collection. These funds are used to support a variety of media programs, projects, and studies in this country and the Third World.

Clear Channel Broadcasting Service

1776 K St., N.W., Washington, DC 20006; (202) 429-7020.

PRESIDENT
Thomas S. Glade, KSL, Salt Lake City, Utah
SECRETARY & TREASURER
Daniel C. Calibraro, WGN, Chicago
LEGAL COUNSEL
R. Russell Eagan of Wiley & Rein, Washington, DC.

Communication Commission of National Council of Churches of Christ in the USA

475 Riverside Dr., New York, NY 10027; (212) 870-2567.

CHAIRPERSON
Richard Anderson
ASSISTANT GENERAL SECRETARY FOR COMMUNICATION, NCC
William F. Fore
EXECUTIVE DIRECTOR FOR BROADCASTING AND FILM
D. Williams McClurken
DIRECTOR FOR MEDIA RESOURCES
David W. Pomeroy

Corporation for Public Broadcasting

1111 16th St., N.W. Washington, DC 20036; (202) 293-6160.

PRESIDENT
Sonia Landau
VICE CHAIRMAN
Ken Towery
VICE PRESIDENT, TELECOMMUNICATIONS
David J. Brugger
VICE PRESIDENT, TREASURER
Donald E. Ledwig

VICE PRESIDENT, CORPORATE COMMUNICATIONS
Ronald E. Weber
ACTING GENERAL COUNSEL AND SECRETARY
Paul Symczak

Directors Guild of America, Inc. (DGA)

National office: 7950 Sunset Blvd., Hollywood, CA 90046; (213) 656-1220. 110 West 57th St., New York, NY 10019; (212) 581-0370. Chicago: 520 N. Michigan Ave., Suite 400, Chicago, IL 60611; (312) 644-5050.

PRESIDENT
Gilbert Cates
NATIONAL VICE PRESIDENT
Tom Donovan
NATIONAL EXECUTIVE DIRECTOR
Michael H. Franklin
VICE PRESIDENTS
Daniel Petrie, Lawrence Auerbach, Gene Reynolds, Max Schindler, Arthur Hiller, Elia Kazan
SECRETARY/TREASURER
Sheldon Leonard
ASSISTANT SECRETARY/TREASURER
Marilyn Jacobs

The Dramatists Guild, Inc.

(Membership: 896 Active; 7,000 Associate; 537 Subscribing) 234 West 44th St., New York, NY 10036; (212) 398-9366.

PRESIDENT
Peter Stone
VICE PRESIDENT
Terrence McNally
SECRETARY
Sheldon Harnick
TREASURER
Ruth Goetz
EXECUTIVE DIRECTOR
David E. LeVine
COUNSEL
Irwin Karp

Electronic Industries Association

2001 Eye Street, N.W., Washington, DC 20006; (202) 457-4900.

CHAIRMAN OF THE BOARD
Bruce Carswell, GTE Corp.
PRESIDENT
Peter F. McCloskey
TREASURER
C. Travis Marshall, Vice President, Motorola, Inc.
VICE PRESIDENT PUBLIC AFFAIRS
Mark V. Rosenker

Episcopal Actors Guild of America, Inc.

(Organized 1926; 750 members) 1 East 29th St., New York, NY 10016; (212) 685-2927.

HONORARY PRESIDENTS PRESIDING BISHOP
The Right Rev. Edmond L. Browning
BISHOP OF NEW YORK
The Right Reverend Paul Moore, Jr., S.T.D.
RETIRED BISHOP OF NEW YORK
The Right Reverend Horace W. B. Donegan, D.D.
PRESIDENT EMERITUS
Ray Heatherton
PRESIDENT
Barnard Hughes
VICE PRESIDENTS
Rev. Norman J. Catir, Jr., Warden of the Guild Walter Abel, Joan Fontaine, Rex Harrison, Mike Mearian
RECORDING SECRETARY
Michelle Trudeau
TREASURER
Frederic Langford
EXECUTIVE SECRETARY
Lon C. Clark

Federal Communications Commission

1919 M Street, N.W., Washington, DC 20054.

CHAIRMAN
Mark Fowler
COMMISSIONERS
James H. Quello, Mimi Weyforth Dawson, Dennis R. Patrick
CHIEF, OFFICE OF PLANS AND POLICY
Peter Pitsch
CHAIRMAN, REVIEW BOARD
Joseph A. Marino
CHIEF JUDGE, OFFICE OF ADMINISTRATIVE LAW JUDGES
Thomas B. Fitzpatrick
GENERAL COUNSEL
Jack D. Smith
MANAGING DIRECTOR
Edward Minicel
CHIEF/MASS MEDIA BUREAU
James C. McKinney
CHIEF, COMMON CARRIER BUREAU
Albert Halpern
CHIEF, FIELD OPERATIONS BUREAU
Richard M. Smith
CHIEF, PUBLIC INFORMATION OFFICE
William A. Russell, Jr.

The Harry Fox Agency

205 East 42 St., New York, NY 10017; (212) 370-5330.

(Music Licensing Bureau)

PRESIDENT
Edward P. Murphy

Girls Friday of Show Business

(See Women in Show Business)

Institute of Electrical and Electronics Engineers, Inc.

345 East 47th Street, New York, NY 10017 (212) 705-7900.

PRESIDENT
Dr. Bruno O. Weinschel
PRESIDENT-ELECT
Henry L. Bachman
EXECUTIVE VICE PRESIDENT
Dr. Emerson W. Pugh
VICE PRESIDENT—EDUCATIONAL ACTIVITIES
Dr. Cyrill J. Tunis
VICE PRESIDENT—PROFESSIONAL ACTIVITIES
Carleton A. Bayless
VICE PRESIDENT—PUBLICATION ACTIVITIES
Charles H. House
VICE PRESIDENT—REGIONAL ACTIVITIES
Dennis Bodson
VICE PRESIDENT—TECHNICAL ACTIVITIES
Merlin G. Smith
SECRETARY/TREASURER
Dr. Michiyuko Uenohara
TREASURER
Edward J. Doyle
GENERAL MANAGER AND EXECUTIVE DIRECTOR
Eric Herz

International Alliance of Theatrical Stage Employes & Moving Picture Machine Operators of the U.S. and Canada (AFL-CIO)

(Organized nationally, July 17, 1893; internationally, October 1, 1902.) 1515 Broadway, New York, NY 10036; (212) 730-1770.

INTERNATIONAL PRESIDENT
Alfred W. Ditolla
INTERNATIONAL PRESIDENT EMERITUS
Walter F. Diehl
GENERAL SECRETARY-TREASURER
James J. Riley
FIRST VICE PRESIDENT
Frank A. Hobbs, Niles, IL
SECOND VICE PRESIDENT
Adrian J. Short, Jr., Cleveland
THIRD VICE PRESIDENT
John J. Nolan, Paramus, NJ
FOURTH VICE PRESIDENT

J. E. Johnson, Karnack, TX
FIFTH VICE PRESIDENT
John J. Ryan, Burtonsville, MD
SIXTH VICE PRESIDENT
Gene Allen, Hollywood, CA
SEVENTH VICE PRESIDENT
Edward C. Powell, San Francisco
EIGHTH VICE PRESIDENT
Michael W. Proscia, New York City
NINTH VICE PRESIDENT
Alan L. Cowley, Hamilton, Ont.
TENTH VICE PRESIDENT
Nick Long, Burbank, CA
ELEVENTH VICE PRESIDENT
Alex B. Parizer, Woodbridge, CT
INTERNATIONAL TRUSTEES
William L. Daniel, Chamblee, GA; Ada Philpot, San Francisco; Nels L. Hansen, Las Vegas.

The Alliance is comprised of approximately 900 local unions covering the United States, Canada and Hawaii. Following is a list of the New York, Chicago and Hollywood locals:

PRODUCTION

AFFILIATED PROPERTY CRAFTSMEN LOCAL 44 (IATSE-AFL-CIO), HOLLYWOOD

(Organized May 15, 1939) 7429 Sunset Blvd., Hollywood, CA 90046; (213) 876-2320 and 838-7788.

ART DIRECTORS, LOCAL 876 (IATSE) HOLLYWOOD

(Chartered January 7, 1960) 14724 Ventura Blvd., Sherman Oaks, CA 91403; (818) 905-0599.

BROADCASTING STUDIO EMPLOYEES, LOCAL 782 (IATSE), NEW YORK

(Chartered Jan. 5, 1945) 41 Nottingham Rd., Glen Rock, NJ 97452; (201) 445-7372.

FIRST AID EMPLOYEES, LOCAL 767 (IATSE), LOS ANGELES

(Chartered Oct. 80, 1942) 8736 Swinton Ave., Sepulveda, CA 91343; (213) 894-3781.

INTERNATIONAL PHOTOGRAPHERS OF THE MOTION PICTURE INDUSTRIES (Cameramen) IPMPI LOCAL 666, CHICAGO

(Chartered Jan. 1, 1929) Suite 1122, 327 S. La Salle St., Chicago, IL; (312) 341-0966.

IPMPI, LOCAL 659 (IATSE), LOS ANGELES

(Organized 1928) 7715 Sunset Blvd., Hollywood, CA 90046; (213) 876-0160.

IPMPI, LOCAL 644 (IATSE), NEW YORK

(Organized Nov. 15, 1926) 250 W. 57th St., New York, NY 10019; (212) 247-3860.

INTERNATIONAL SOUND TECHNICIANS OF THE MOTION PICTURE BROADCAST AND AMUSEMENT INDUSTRIES, LOCAL 695 (IATSE-AFL), LOS ANGELES

(Organized Sept. 15, 1930) 15840 Ventura Blvd., Encino, CA 91436; (213) 872-0452 and 981-0452.

LABORATORY TECHNICIANS, LOCAL 780 (IATSE), CHICAGO

(Chartered Nov. 10, 1944) 327 S. La Salle St., Room 1720, Chicago, IL; (312) 922-7105.

LABORATORY TECHNICIANS, LOCAL 683 (IATSE-AFL-CIO), LOS ANGELES

(Organized Sept. 29, 1919) 6721 Melrose Ave., Hollywood, CA 90038; (212) 935-1123.

LABORATORY TECHNICIANS, LOCAL 702 (IATSE-AFL), NEW YORK

(Organized September, 1937) Room 1405, 165 West 46th Street, New York, NY 10036; (212) 869-5540.

MAKE-UP ARTISTS & HAIR STYLISTS, LOCAL 706 (IATSE), HOLLYWOOD

11519 Chandler Blvd., No. Hollywood, CA 91601.

MAKE-UP ARTISTS AND HAIR STYLISTS, LOCAL 798 (IATSE), NEW YORK

(Chartered Feb. 18, 1949) 1790 Broadway, New York, NY 10019; (212) 757-9120.

MOTION PICTURE COSTUMERS, LOCAL 705 (IATSE-AFL), HOLLYWOOD

(Chartered Nov. 1, 1937) 1427 N. La Brea Ave., Hollywood, CA 90028; (213) 851-0220.

MOTION PICTURE EDITORS GUILD, LOCAL 776 (IATSE), LOS ANGELES

(Chartered Aug. 2, 1944) Secretary's Address: 7715 Sunset Blvd., Hollywood, CA 90046; (213) 876-4770.

MOTION PICTURE FILM & VIDEO TAPE EDITORS, LOCAL 771 (IATSE), NEW YORK

(Chartered Aug. 18, 1943) 353 West 48 St., New York, NY 10036; (212) 765-1069.

MOTION PICTURE SCRIPT SUPERVISORS AND PRODUCTION OFFICE COORDINATORS LOCAL 161

250 W. 57 St., Room 1202, New York, NY 10019; (212) 245-4562.

MOTION PICTURE SET PAINTERS, LOCAL 729 (IATSE), HOLLYWOOD

(Chartered Aug. 1, 1953) 11650 Riverside Dr., North Hollywood, CA 91602; (213) 877-0671.

MOTION PICTURE STUDIO CINETECHNICIANS, LOCAL 789 (IATSE), HOLLYWOOD

(Chartered April 16, 1945) 1635 Vista Del Mar, Hollywood, CA 90028; (213) 462-7288.

MOTION PICTURE SCREEN CARTOONISTS, LOCAL 839 (IATSE), HOLLYWOOD

(Chartered Jan. 18, 1952) 4729 Lankershim Blvd., North Hollywood, CA 91602; (213) 766-7151.

MOTION PICTURE SCREEN CARTOONISTS, LOCAL 841 (IATSE), NEW YORK

(Chartered April 16, 1952) 127 E. 35 St., New York, NY 10016; (212) 684-0760.

MOTION PICTURE STUDIO ELECTRICAL TECHNICIANS, LOCAL 728 (IATSE), AND M.P.M.O. OF U.S. AND CANADA-AFL-CIO

(Chartered May 15, 1939) 3400 Barham Blvd., Hollywood, CA 90068; (213) 851-3300.

MOTION PICTURE CRAFTS SERVICE, LOCAL 727 (IATSE), HOLLYWOOD

(Organized May 15, 1939) 12754 Ventura Blvd., Suite 205, North Hollywood, CA 91604.

MOTION PICTURE STUDIO ART CRAFTSMEN, (Illustrators and Matte Artists) LOCAL 790 (IATSE), HOLLYWOOD

(Chartered April 17, 1945) Suite 210, 7715 Sunset Blvd., Los Angeles, CA 90046; (213) 876-2010.

MOTION PICTURE STUDIO GRIPS, LOCAL 80 (IATSE), HOLLYWOOD

(Organized May 15, 1939) 6926 Melrose Ave., Los Angeles, CA 90038; (213) 931-1419.

MOTION PICTURE STUDIO TEACHERS AND WELFARE WORKERS, LOCAL 884 (IATSE) HOLLYWOOD

(Chartered September 1, 1960) 9617 Haas Avenue, Los Angeles, CA 90047; (213) 754-8419.

PUBLICISTS, LOCAL 818 (IATSE), HOLLYWOOD

(Chartered July 11, 1955) 1427 N. La Brea Ave., Hollywood CA 90028.

RADIO AND TELEVISION SOUND EFFECTS, LOCAL 844 (IATSE), NEW YORK

(Chartered July 17, 1952), Box 637, Ansonia Station, New York, NY 10023.

SCENIC & TITLE ARTISTS, LOCAL 816 (IATSE) LOS ANGELES

(Chartered March 31, 1949) 7429 Sunset Blvd., Hollywood, CA 90046; (213) 876-1440.

SCRIPT SUPERVISORS, LOCAL 871 (IATSE), HOLLYWOOD

(Chartered January 1, 1958) 14274 Ventura Blvd., Sherman Oaks, CA 91403; (213) 784-6885.

SET DESIGNERS AND MODEL MAKERS, LOCAL 847 (IATSE), HOLLYWOOD

(Chartered Nov. 14, 1952) Suite 210, 7715 Sunset Blvd., Los Angeles 46, CA; (213) 876-2010.

STORY ANALYSTS, LOCAL 854 (IATSE), HOLLYWOOD

(Chartered Oct. 18, 1954) 7715 Sunset Blvd., Los Angeles, CA 90046; (213) 876-2010.

MOTION PICTURE STUDIO MECHANICS, LOCAL 476 (IATSE), CHICAGO

(Chartered Feb. 2, 1931) Room 1743; 327 S. La Salle St., Chicago, IL 60604; (312) 922-5215.

STUDIO MECHANICS, LOCAL 52 (IATSE-AFL), NEW YORK

(Organized 1924) 221 W. 57th St., New York, NY 10019; (212) 765-0741.

STUDIO PROJECTIONISTS AND VIDEO PROJECTION TECHNICIANS, LOCAL 165 (IATSE), HOLLYWOOD

(Chartered May 15, 1939) 14724 Ventura Blvd., Sherman Oaks, CA 91403; (213) 462-6385.

TELEVISION BROADCASTING STUDIO EMPLOYEES, LOCAL 794 (IATSE), NEW YORK

(Chartered June 7, 1945) 144 Aster Ave., Hawthorn, New York, NY 10532.

DISTRIBUTION

FILM EXCHANGE EMPLOYEES, BACK ROOM, LOCAL B-45 (IATSE), CHICAGO

(Chartered May 1, 1937)

FILM EXCHANGE EMPLOYEES, BACK ROOM, LOCAL B-61 (IATSE), LOS ANGELES

(Chartered May 1, 1937) 7715 Sunset Blvd., Room 226, Hollywood, CA 90046.

FILM EXCHANGE EMPLOYEES, FRONT OFFICE, LOCAL F-45 (IATSE), CHICAGO

(Chartered Sept. 4, 1942) c/o G. R. Kuehnl, Apt. 1611, 5455 Sheridan Rd., Chicago, IL 60640.

In addition to the above, there are 34 locals of Back Room Employees and 29 locals of Front Office Employees in the other exchange cities.

MOTION PICTURE HOME OFFICE AND FILM EXCHANGE EMPLOYEES, LOCAL H-63 (IATSE), NEW YORK

(Chartered Mar. 19, 1945) 29 East 49 St., New York, NY 10017; (212) 759-0686.

EXHIBITION

AMUSEMENT AREA EMPLOYEES, LOCAL B-192 (IATSE) LOS ANGELES

(Chartered Oct. 1, 1965) 7715 Sunset Blvd., Room 226, Los Angeles, CA 90046.

EXHIBITION EMPLOYEES, LOCAL 829 (IATSE), NEW YORK

(Chartered December 11, 1950) 150 E. 58 St., New York, NY 10022; (212) 752-4427.

PROJECTIONISTS LOCAL 110 (IATSE), CHICAGO

(Chartered Feb. 4, 1915) 875 N. Michigan Ave. Suite 4160, Chicago, IL 60611; (312) 787-0220.

PROJECTIONISTS LOCAL 150 (IATSE), LOS ANGELES

(Chartered July 16, 1908) 1800 S. Vermont Ave., Los Angeles, CA 90006; (213) 733-1191.

PROJECTIONISTS LOCAL 306 (IATSE), NEW YORK

(Organized July, 1913) 745 7th Ave., New York, NY 10019; (212) 586-5157, and 55 Flatbush Ave., Brooklyn, NY; (212) 852-2700.

STAGE EMPLOYEES, LOCAL 4 (IATSE), BROOKLYN

(Chartered April 8, 1888) 2917 Glenwood Rd., Brooklyn, NY 11210; (212) 252-8777.

STAGE EMPLOYEES, LOCAL 2 (IATSE), CHICAGO

(Chartered July 17, 1893) 222 W. Adams St., Room 1345, Chicago, IL 60606.

STAGE EMPLOYEES, LOCAL 33 (IATSE), LOS ANGELES

(Chartered Mar. 1, 1896) 4605 Landershim Blvd. Suite 833, N. Hollywood, CA 91602; (213) 985-0633-4.

STAGE EMPLOYEES, LOCAL 1 (IATSE), NEW YORK

(Chartered July 17, 1893) 1775 Broadway, New York, NY 10019; (212) 489-7710.

THEATRE EMPLOYEES, LOCAL B-46 (IATSE), CHICAGO

(Chartered May 1, 1937) 875 N. Michigan Ave. Suite 4160, Chicago, IL 60611; (312) 787-0220.

THEATRE EMPLOYEES, LOCAL B-183 (IATSE), NEW YORK

(Chartered May 6, 1942) 235 W. 46th St., Rm. 320, New York, NY 10036; (212) 245-2331, 2332.

THEATRICAL WARDROBE ATTENDANTS, LOCAL 769 (IATSE), CHICAGO

3314 Lake Shore Drive, Apt. 805, Chicago, IL 60657.

THEATRICAL WARDROBE ATTENDANTS, LOCAL 768 (IATSE), LOS ANGELES

(Chartered Dec. 3, 1942) 5909 Melrose Ave. Suite 17, Los Angeles, CA 90038.

THEATRICAL WARDROBE ATTENDANTS, LOCAL 764 (IATSE), NEW YORK

(Chartered Sept. 4, 1942) 1501 Broadway, Room 1604, New York, NY; (212) 221-1717.

TREASURERS AND TICKET SELLERS & CASHIERS, LOCAL 750 (IATSE), CHICAGO

(Chartered Aug. 1, 1941) 188 W. Randolph St., Room 1920, Chicago, IL 60601.

TREASURERS AND TICKET SELLERS, LOCAL 857 (IATSE), LOS ANGELES

(Chartered June 1, 1955) 6513 Hollywood Blvd., Room 204, Hollywood, CA 90028.

TREASURERS AND TICKET SELLERS, LOCAL 751 (IATSE), NEW YORK

(Chartered Aug. 1, 1941) 257 West 52 St., New York, NY 10019; (212) 315-0544.

Outside the three cities covered by the above listings, there are over 900 IATSE locals in the exhibition field.

International Brotherhood of Electrical Workers (AFL)

(Organized November 28, 1891; Membership over 1,000,000) 1125 15th Street, N.W., Washington, DC 20005; (202) 833-7000.

INTERNATIONAL PRESIDENT
Charles H. Pillard, 1125 15th St., N.W., Washington, DC 20005
INTERNATIONAL SECRETARY
Jack F. Moore, 1125 15th St., N.W., Washington, DC 20005
INTERNATIONAL TREASURER
Thomas Van Arsdale, Jr., 158-11 Jewel Ave., Flushing, NY 11365
DISTRICT OFFICES
Willowdale, Ontario: 45 Sheppard Ave. East, Suite 401; K. G. Rose
Braintree, MA: Battery March Park, Quinay, MA 02169, John E. Flynn
White Plains, NY: 222 Mamaroneck Ave., J. J. Barry
Cincinnati, OH: 7710 Reading Rd., Suite 9, B. G. Williamson
Birmingham, AL: No. 2 Metroplex Dr., Suite 113, D. H. Waters
Carol Stream, IL: 373 Schmale Road, Suite 201, James P. Conway
Arlington, TX: 2701 Ave. E. East, Suite 412, Orville A. Tate, Jr.
Idaho Fall, ID 83402: P.O. Box 1216, Jon Walters
Walnut Creek, CA: 150 N. Wiget Lane, Suite 700, S. R. McCann
Rosemont, IL: 10400 W. Higgins Rd., Suite 400, A. M. Ripp
Springfield, MO: 300 So. Jefferson, Suite 300, Ray Edwards
Chattanooga, TN: Franklin Bldg., Suite 515, John A. Hightower

IBEW LOCAL 349 (FILM)

(Organized April 24, 1904) 1657 N.W. 17th Avenue, Miami, FL 33125; (305) 325-1330.

BUSINESS MANAGER
Art Fernandez

IBEW LOCAL 40 (FILM)

(Organized March 5, 1923) 5643 Vineland Ave., No. Hollywood, CA 91601; (213) 877-1171.

BUSINESS MANAGER
Russell J. Bartley

International Radio and Television Society Inc.

420 Lexington Avenue, Suite 531, New York, NY 10170; (212) 867-6650.

PRESIDENT
James L. Greenwald
FIRST VICE PRESIDENT
Betty Hudson
VICE PRESIDENTS
Frank J. Biondi Jr., Mark H. Cohen, Roy Danish, Gordon H. Hastings, Tony C. Malara, David H. Polinger
SECRETARY
Jerome S. Boros

TREASURER
Gerald Hassell
EXECUTIVE DIRECTOR
Stephen B. Labunski

Musicians Union Local 47 American Federation of Musicians (AFL-CIO)

(Organized October 30, 1894; Membership: 15,000) 817 Vine Street, Hollywood 38, CA; (213) HOllywood 2-2161.

PRESIDENT
Bernie Fleischer
VICE PRESIDENT
Vince DiBari
SECRETARY
Serena Kay Williams
TREASURER
Bill Douglass
TRUSTEES
Buddy Collette, Peggy Gilbert, Cliffie Stone
DIRECTORS
Jeanne Aiken, Garnett Brown, Chase Craig, Frank (Chico) Guerrero, Lyle (Spud) Murphy, Ann Patterson

National Academy of Television Arts and Sciences, The

National Office: 110 West 57th St., New York, NY 10019; (212) 586-8424. (Formed to advance the arts and sciences of television.) (Organized 1957.) Awards Emmys for daytime, children's, religious, sports and news documentary programming.

CHAIRMAN OF THE BOARD
Richard R. Rector
PRESIDENT
John Cannon
VICE CHAIRMAN
Richard Schneider
VICE PRESIDENT
Paul Rich
SECRETARY
J. Subler

National Association of Broadcasters

1771 N St., N.W., Washington, DC 20036; (202) 429-5300. (Organized 1922 to foster and promote the development of the arts of aural and visual broadcasting in all its forms; to protect its members in every lawful and proper manner from injustices and unjust exactions; to do all things necessary and proper to encourage and promote customs and practices which will strengthen and maintain the broadcasting industry to the end that it may best serve the public.)

CHAIRMAN
Ted L. Snider
PRESIDENT
Edward O. Fritts
TELEVISION BOARD OF DIRECTORS
Leslie G. Arries, Margo Cobb, Frank Flynn, Tom Goodgame, Wallace Jorgenson (vice chm.), Peter Kizer, Michael McCormick, Ben McKeel, Robert Munoz, Leavitt Pope, Harold Protter, Gregory Stone, Donna Zapata, Derk Zimmerman. Networks: Eugene S. Cowen (ABC), Robert D. Hynes (NBC), Robert McConnell (CBS).

National Association of Television Program Executives, Inc.

342 Madison Avenue, Suite 933, New York, NY 10173; (212) 949-9890.

PRESIDENT
David Simon, Fox Television Stations
EXECUTIVE DIRECTOR
A. Philip Corvo

National Music Publishers' Association, Inc.

205 East 42 St., New York, NY 10017; (212) 370-5330.

CHAIRMAN
Irwin Z. Robinson
PRESIDENT
Edward P. Murphy
VICE PRESIDENTS
Wesley H. Rose, Ralph Peer II, Leon J. Brettler
SECRETARY
Samuel Trust
TREASURER
Sidney B. Herman

Permanent Charities Committee of The Entertainment Industries

Samuel Goldwyn-Permanent Charities Building, 463 N. La Cienega Blvd., Los Angeles, CA 90048; (213) 652-4680. (A donor federation within the entertainment industries supporting community wide charities.)

FIRST VICE PRESIDENT
J. Nicholas Counter III
SECOND VICE PRESIDENT
Daniel E. Slusser
SECRETARY
William K. Howard
TREASURER
Robert S. Colbert, CPA
PRESIDENT & CEO
Paul C. Masterson
VICE PRESIDENT, OPERATIONS AND DEVELOPMENT
Irwin J. Kaplan

Producer-Writers Guild of America Pension Plan

310 North San Vicente Boulevard, Suite 305, Los Angeles, CA 90048; (213) 659-6430.

CHAIRMAN
Donald Sanford
VICE CHAIRMAN
George Malko
SECRETARY
Judith Gordon
VICE SECRETARY
John McLean

SESAC, INC.

(One of the world's foremost music licensing organizations. A special projects department handles scoring for motion pictures, slide films, syndicated TV series and agency produced commercials; programming for background music and premium albums.)

The Coliseum Tower, 10 Columbus Circle, New York, NY 10019; (212) 586-3450.

CHAIRMAN
A. H. Prager
PRESIDENT
W. Robert Thompson
TREASURER
R. C. Heinecke
EXECUTIVE VICE PRESIDENT
Vincent Candilora

Screen Actors Guild (AAAA-AFL-CIO)

(Organized July, 1933; Membership: 58,000) 7750 Sunset Blvd., Hollywood, CA 90046; 876-3030. Branches—New York, 1700 Broadway, New York, NY 10019, John T. McGuire; Chicago, 307 N. Michigan Ave., Herbert H. Neuer; Boston, 11 Beacon Street, Robert M. Segal; Lathrup Village, MI 48076, 28690 Southfield Rd., Jane Ford, Dallas, TX 75204, 3220 Lemmon Ave., Clinta Dayton; San Francisco, CA 94104, 100 Bush St., Don Tayer; FL. 3266 Ponce de

Leon Blvd., Coral Gables, FL, Melvin B. Karl.

PRESIDENT
Patty Duke
PRESIDENT EMERITUS
Leon Ames
FIRST VICE PRESIDENT
Christopher Mitchum
SECOND VICE PRESIDENT
Maureen Donnelly
THIRD VICE PRESIDENT
Dean Santoro
FOURTH VICE PRESIDENT
F.J. O'Neal
FIFTH VICE PRESIDENT
Reed Farrell
SIXTH VICE PRESIDENT
Dan Caldwell
VICE PRESIDENTS
Bruce McLaughlin, Patricia Pellows, William Schallert, Larry Keith, Marie Windsor, Eugene Francis
RECORDING SECRETARY
Sumi Haru
TREASURER
Yale Summers

NATIONAL EXECUTIVE STAFF

NATIONAL EXECUTIVE SECRETARY
Ken Orsatti
ASSOCIATE NATIONAL EXECUTIVE SECRETARY
John McGuire
PUBLIC RELATIONS DIRECTOR
Mark Lockner
COUNSEL
Leo Germer
CONTROLLER
Gerald Wilson

Society of Motion Picture and Television Engineers

(Organized 1916; Membership: 8,800) 595 Hartsdale Ave., White Plains, NY 10607; (914) 761-1100.

PRESIDENT
Harold J. Eady
EXECUTIVE VICE PRESIDENT
M. Carlos Kennedy
PAST PRESIDENT
Leonard Coleman
ENGINEERING VICE PRESIDENT
Richard G. Streeter
FINANCIAL VICE PRESIDENT
Blain Baker
CONFERENCE VICE PRESIDENT
Maurice L. French
SECTIONS VICE PRESIDENT
Sherwin H. Becker
SECRETARY
Stephen D. Kerman
TREASURER
Roderick T. Ryan
EXECUTIVE DIRECTOR
Lynette Robinson

The Songwriters Guild

276 Fifth Ave., Suite 306, New York, NY 10001; (212) 686-6820; California Office: 6430 Sunset Blvd., Hollywood, CA 90028; (213) 462-1108. Nashville Office: 50 Music Square West, Nashville, TN 37203; (615) 329-1782.

PRESIDENT
George David Weiss

Station Representatives Association, Inc.

230 Park Avenue, New York, NY 10017; (212) 687-2484.

PRESIDENT
Dave Allen
VICE PRESIDENT/RADIO
Dick Sharpe
VICE PRESIDENT/TV
Steve Herson
SECRETARY
Mike Bellantoni
TREASURER
Ed Kiernan
MANAGING DIRECTOR
Jerry Feniger
ADMINISTRATIVE ASSISTANT
Audrey Tanzer
DIRECTORS
(Radio board) Dick Sharpe, Bill Fortenbaugh, Jerry Schubert, Bob Ferraro, Jack Masla, Edward Kiernan, Mike Bellantoni. (TV board) William Bee, Wally Schwartz, Neil Kennedy, Peter Ryan, Pete Goulazian, Steve Herson, Dave Allen.

Television Bureau of Advertising

477 Madison Ave., New York, NY 10022; (212) 486-1111. (Organized 1954.); 3060 Mercer University Drive, Suite 310, Atlanta, GA 30341; (404) 451-2727; 8585 N. Stemmons Freeway/Suite 507 Dallas, TX 75247; (214) 631-0796; 155 No. Michigan Ave., Suite 360, Chicago, IL 60601; (312) 565-4496; 3155 West Big Beaver Road, Suite 217, Troy, MI 48084; (313) 649-6688; 6380 Wilshire Blvd., Los Angeles, CA 90048; (213) 653-8890.

PRESIDENT
Roger D. Rice
CHAIRMAN OF THE BOARD
E. Blake Byrne
VICE PRESIDENT
Robert Kunath
SECRETARY
Ward L. Huey Jr.
TREASURER
Walter A. Schwartz
CHAIRMAN EX-OFFICIO
William G. Moll
EXECUTIVE VICE PRESIDENT OPERATIONS
Rogert Baker
EXECUTIVE VICE PRESIDENT SALES
Robert A. Lefko
SENIOR VICE PRESIDENT RESEARCH & MARKETING
Harvey Spiegel
SENIOR VICE PRESIDENT NATIONAL SALES
Richard D. Severance
SENIOR VICE PRESIDENT, CREATIVE SERVICES
Beverly Keene
VICE PRESIDENT, COMMUNICATIONS
Robert M. Grebe
VICE PRESIDENT, MEMBER SERVICES
Barbara Zeiger
VICE PRESIDENT, MEMBERSHIP
C. Joseph Gavin
VICE PRESIDENT, LOCAL SALES MANAGER
Wallace Westphal
VICE PRESIDENT CENTRAL DIVISION
David Michaels
VICE PRESIDENT, DETROIT
Richard O'Donnell
VICE PRESIDENT, WESTERN DIVISION
Arthur Trudeau
VICE PRESIDENT, SOUTHWESTERN DIVISION
Chuck Hanson
VICE PRESIDENT, SOUTHEASTERN DIVISION
Perry Bascom
VICE PRESIDENT, WESTERN DIVISION
Robert Fairbanks

Television Information Office

745 Fifth Avenue, New York, NY 10022; (212) 759-6800.

DIRECTOR
Roy Danish
MANAGER OF CREATIVE SERVICES
Bert Briller
MANAGERS, STATION SERVICES
Henry Levinson, Lynne Grasz
MANAGER, RESEARCH SERVICES
James Poteat

Theatre Authority, Inc.

(Organized May 21, 1934) 485 Fifth Avenue, New York, NY 10017; (212) 682-4215.

PRESIDENT
Harold M. Hoffman

RECORDING SECRETARY
Sandford I. Woff
TREASURER
Joan Greenspan
COUNSEL
Jacob I. Goodstein

United Nations—Radio and Visual Services Division, Department of Public Information

United Nations, New York, NY 10017; (212) 754-6945.

DIRECTOR, RADIO AND VISUAL SERVICES DIVISION
Georges Leclère
CHIEF OF VISUAL SERVICE
Peter Hollander

Women in Film

(Non-profit organization formed in 1973 by professional women in the motion picture and television industries; purpose is to serve as a support group and act as a clearing house and resource of information on qualified professional women in those industries, 6464 Sunset Blvd., #660, Los Angeles, CA; (213) 463-6040. Branches in New York, Washington, D.C. and Atlanta, GA

PRESIDENT EMERITUS—FOUNDER
Tichi Wilkerson
PRESIDENT
Barbara Klein
BOARD OF DIRECTORS
Pat Davies, Fern Field, Irma Kalish, Bonnie Karrin, Marcy Kelly, Judith Gerians, Betsy Pollock, Patricia Price, Marilyn Shanker, Sue Terry, Maxine Thomas, Molly Wilson, Annett Wolf, Cathy Zheutlin
EXECUTIVE ADMINISTRATOR
Debbie Supnik

Women in Show Business

(A philanthropic organization composed of women in the entertainment industry dedicated to providing funds for reconstructive and restorative surgery for children) P.O. Box 2535, North Hollywood, CA 91602; (818) 762-4669.

PRESIDENT
Sherry Tischler
EXECUTIVE VICE PRESIDENT/WAYS & MEANS
Linda Desiante
FIRST VICE PRESIDENT/PROGRAM
Jeanne Taylor
EXECUTIVE VICE PRESIDENT
Lynn Helsel
SECOND VICE PRESIDENT/MEMBERSHIP
Anne Parlapiano
RECORDING SECRETARY
Frances Wright
CORRESPONDING SECRETARY
Janet Taylor
TREASURER
Margaret Weiner

Writers Guild of America

NATIONAL CHAIRMAN
Frank Pierson

WRITERS GUILD OF AMERICA, EAST, INC.

555 West 57th Street, New York, NY 10019; (212) 245-6180.

PRESIDENT
Edward Adler
VICE PRESIDENT
Art Wallace
SECRETARY-TREASURER
Ken Gaughran
EXECUTIVE DIRECTOR
Mona Mangan

WRITERS GUILD OF AMERICA, WEST, INC.

8955 Beverly Boulevard, Los Angeles, CA 90048; (213) 550-1000.

PRESIDENT
Ernest Lehman
VICE PRESIDENT
Irma Kalish
SECRETARY-TREASURER
William Ludwig
EXECUTIVE DIRECTOR
Brian Walton

State Associations of Broadcasters

ALABAMA BROADCASTERS ASSOCIATION
Ben K. McKinnon, exec. dir.; Bill Dunnavant, pres.
Box 43525, Birmingham 35243; (205) 942-4571.

ALASKA BROADCASTERS ASSOCIATION
Peter Van Nort, pres.
%KIAK, Box 73410, Fairbanks 99707; (907) 452-1931.

ARIZONA BROADCASTERS ASSOCIATION
Tommy Vascocu, pres.; Ken Heady, exec. dir.; Mike Cutchall, v.p.; Jack Sander, secty. & treas.
Box 654, Scottsdale 85252; (602) 991-1700.

ARKANSAS BROADCASTERS ASSOCIATION
Jim Howe, pres.; Pat Willcox, exec. dir.
2024 Arkansas Valley Drive, Suite 201, Little Rock 72212; (501) 227-7564.

CALIFORNIA BROADCASTERS ASSOCIATION
Victor J. Biondi, exec. dir.; Karmi A. Speece, exec. asst.
1127 11th St., Suite 730, Sacramento 95814; (916) 444-2237.

CENTRAL ALASKA BROADCASTING INC.
Duane L. Triplett, pres.; Richard M. Zook, secty.-treas.
2700 E. Tudor Rd., Anchorage 99507; (907) 276-1313.

COLORADO BROADCASTERS ASSOCIATION
Cliff Dodge, exec. dir.; Judy Gaughan, admin. asst.
2620 S. Parker Rd., Suite 340, Aurora 80014; (303) 337-7373.

CONNECTICUT BROADCASTERS ASSOCIATION
Michael Hanson (WNLK/WLYQ, Norwalk) pres.; Geoffrey Rose (WTXX-TV, Waterbury), v.p.; Lee Manson (WRCH/WRCQ, Hartford), secty.-treas.; Barry Barth (WFSB-TV, Hartford) asst. secty./treas.
15 Highland Park Rd., North Haven 06473; (203) 239-5724.

FLORIDA ASSOCIATION OF BROADCASTERS, INC.
Gayle Swofford, pres.; Harry Smith, pres.-elect; Bob Foss, exec. v.p.; James Colley, v.p., radio,; Douglas Barker, v.p., TV; Frank Watson, secty.-treas.
Box 2514, Sarasota 33577; (904) 681-6444.

GEORGIA ASSOCIATION OF BROADCASTERS, INC.
William G. Sanders, exec. v.p.; Eve Moffa, asst. v.p.
6065 Roswell Rd., Suite 604, Atlanta 30328; (404) 252-0964.

HAWAIIAN ASSOCIATION OF BROADCASTERS
Dick Schaller (KIKU-TV, Honolulu), pres.
Station KIKI-TV, 150 B Puhale Rd., Honolulu 96819; (808) 847-1178. % KNUI Radio, Box 35, Kahului 96732; (808) 877-5566.

IDAHO STATE BROADCASTERS ASSOCIATION
Connie Searles, exec. dir.; Lee Wagner (KMVT-TV Twin Falls), pres.; R.C. Weisenberger (KGEM/KJOT Boise), v.p.; Brian Hogan (KPVI-TV Pocatello), secty.-treas.
Box 994, Boise 83701; (208) 345-3072.

ILLINOIS BROADCASTERS ASSOCIATION
Wally Gair, exec. dir.
6 Drawbridge Rd., Springfield 62704; (217) 787-6503.

INDIANA BROADCASTERS ASSOCIATION, INC.
Joyce Martello, exec. dir.; Edwin C. Metcalf, pres.
310 N. Alabama, Suite A, Indianapolis 46204; (317) 638-1332.

IOWA BROADCASTERS ASSOCIATION
William F. Sanders (KICD, Spencer), pres.; Nolan Quam (KCCCI-TV, Des Moines), v.p.; Glenn Olson (KQWC, Webster City), treas.; Jack Shelley, exec. secty.
1230 Marston Ave., Ames 50010; (515) 232-1449.

KANSAS ASSOICATION OF BROADCASTERS
Harriet J. Lange, exec. dir.
818 Merchants Nat'l Bank Bldg., Topeka 66612; (913) 235-1307.

KENTUCKY BROADCASTERS ASSOCIATION
J.T. Whitlock, exec. dir. & treas.; Dr. Charles Anderson, pres.
Box 680, Lebanon 40033; (502) 692-3126.

LOUISIANA ASSOCIATION OF BROADCASTERS
Gene Dickerson, pres.; Hugh Hyman, exec. dir.
732 North Blvd., Suite C, Baton Rouge 70802; (504) 383-7486.

MAINE ASSOCIATION OF BROADCASTERS
Claude Wiese, pres.; Helen Dudman, pres.-elect; Norman G. Gallant, exec. dir.
Box PI, 385 Western Ave., Augusta 04330; (207) 623-3870.

MARYLAND-DISTRICT OF COLUMBIA-DELAWARE BROADCASTERS ASSOCIATION, INC.
Thomas J. Miles (WCTD, Federalsburg, MD), pres.; Edward Wetter (WABS, Arlington, VA), v.p.; Malcolm D. Potter (WBAL-TV, Baltimore), secty.; C. Robert Taylor (WDEL/WSTW, Wilmington, Del.), treas.; Robert B. Cochrane, exec. dir.
Route 1-Box 559, St. Michaels, MD 21663; (301) 745-5155.

MASSACHUSETTS BROADCASTERS ASSOCIATION
Joseph C. Rayball, exec. dir.; Claire B. Freeman, admin. asst.
7 North Main St., Suite 302, B. Attleboro 02703; (617) 222-0170.

MICHIGAN ASSOCIATION OF BROADCASTERS
William C. Robbins (Fetzer Broadcasting) pres.; Richard S. Sommerville, (WSMA, Marine City) v.p.; Thomas J. Cleary, exec. dir.
Box 16015, Lansing 48901; (517) 371-1729.

MINNESOTA BROADCASTERS ASSOCIATION
Mel Paradis (KLGR, Redwood Falls), pres.; Don Wohlenhaus (KWRC, Buffalo), 1st v.p.; Ned Goodwin (KBUN/KBHP, Bemidji); Ray Foslid, exec. dir.
7400 Metro Blvd., Suite 113, Minneapolis 55435; (612) 835-1980.

MISSISSIPPI BROADCASTERS ASSOCIATION
Eddie Hallady, pres.; Robert Ward, pres.-elect; Bob O'Brien, v.p.; Don Furr, secty. & treas.; Jackie Lett, exec. dir.
Box 4561, Jackson 39216; (601) 362-5444.

MISSOURI BROADCASTERS ASSOCIATION
Joe Embser (KSOZ, Point Lookout), pres.; John Monick (WSUI-KSUI, Iowa City, IA), v.p.; Jeffrey Stoll (KUMR, Rolla), secty.-treas.
1800 Southwest Blvd., Jefferson City 65101; (314) 636-6692.

MISSOURI PUBLIC RADIO ASSOCIATION
Arlen Diamond, pres.; Joe Embser, v.p.
%KSMU, 901 S. National, Springfield 65804; (417) 836-5878.

MONTANA BROADCASTERS ASSOCIATION
Robert W. Hoene, exec. dir.
Box 503, Helena 59624; (406) 442-3961.

NEBRASKA BROADCASTERS ASSOCIATION
Ed Zachary (WOWT, Omaha), pres.; Gene Koehm (KNEN, Norfolk) pres.-elect; Jana Pentz-McBride (KMAZ-KWBE, Beatrice) v.p.; Larry Walkin (KRNU, Lincoln), secty.-treas.; Eric Brown (KRVN-AM-FM, Lexington), past pres.; Ed Schafer, exec. dir.
7101 Mercy Rd., Suite 419, Omaha 68106; (402) 391-8236.

NEVADA BROADCASTERS ASSOCIATION
Bill Andrews (KAME-TV, Reno), pres.; Dennis Siewart (KTVN (TV), Reno) v.p., TV; Nancy Reynolds (KENO-KOMP, Las Vegas), v.p., radio; Ruth Uhls (KLVX, Las Vegas), secty.-treas.; Al King, exec. dir.
4987 S. Wrightview, Las Vegas 89120; (702) 456-5020.

NEW HAMPSHIRE ASSOCIATION OF BROADCASTERS
Richard Osborne, pres.; B. Allan Sprague, exec. dir.
Box 900, Manchester 03105; (603) 669-5144.

NEW JERSEY BROADCASTERS ASSOCIATION
Arnold Zucker, exec. dir.; John Morris, pres.; Joe Knox Jr., v.p.
Room 205, Johnston Hall, Rutgers University, New Brunswick 08903; (201) 247-3337.

NEW MEXICO BROADCASTERS ASSOCIATION
Joe Carriere (KBIM-TV, Roswell), pres.; Kenny Kendrick, pres.-elect.; Ms. Dee Schelling, exec. dir.
790-9D Tramway Lane NE, Albuquerque 87122; (505) 299-6908.

NEW YORK STATE BROADCASTERS ASSOCIATION, INC.
Lawrence Levite (WBEN-AM-FM, Buffalo), chmn.; Walter Maxwell (WGHQ (AM)-WBPM (FM), Kingston), v.p.; James Champlin (Beck-Ross Communications, Rockville Center), secty.; Ronald Pulera (WTEN-TV, Albany), treas.
90 State St., Suite 530, Albany, 12207; (518) 434-6100.

NORTH CAROLINA ASSOCIATION OF BROADCASTERS
Don Curtis, pres.; Wade H. Hargrove, exec.-dir.
Box 627, Raleigh 27602; (919) 821-7300.

NORTH DAKOTA BROADCASTERS ASSOCIATION
Paul Wickre, pres.; David E. Beach.
Box 8116, Grand Forks 58202; (701) 777-2577.

OHIO ASSOCIATION OF BROADCASTERS, INC.
Dale V. Bring, exec. dir.
100 E. Broad St., Suite 1206, Columbus 43215; (614) 228-4052.

OKLAHOMA ASSOCIATION OF BROADCASTERS
Carl Smith (KRAV/KGTO, Tulsa), pres.; Linda Saunders, exec. dir.
4545 N. Lincoln, Oklahoma City 73105; (405) 528-2475.

OREGON ASSOCIATION OF BROADCASTERS
Burns Nugent, pres.; John Larkin (KTVZ-TV, Bend), v.p.; Vern Mueller, gen. mgr.
Box 20037, Portland 97220; (503) 257-3041.

PENNSYLVANIA ASSOCIATION OF BROADCASTERS
Fred Young (Hearst Corp., Pittsburgh), pres.; Harry Haas (WFLN-FM, Philadelphia), v.p., radio; Robert Eolin Jr. (WLHY-TV, Lancaster), v.p., TV; Brian Danzis (WCBM (AM)-WSFM (FM), Harrisburg), treas.; Robert Zimmerman (WRSC (AM)-WQWK (FM)), past-pres.
407 N. Front St., Harrisburg 17101; (717) 233-3511.

RHODE ISLAND BROADCASTERS ASSOCIATION
Roger E. Bouchard, pres.; John Quinlin, v.p.
%Roger E. Bouchard, WNRI Radio, 786 Diamond Hill Rd., Woonsocket 02895; (401) 769-0600.

ROCKY MOUNTAIN BROADCASTERS ASSOCIATION
Bernard J. Bustos, pres.; Henry Fletcher, exec. dir.
Box 220, Pocatello, Idaho 83204; (208) 233-5020.

SOUTH CAROLINA BROADCASTERS ASSOCIATION
Nicholas Frangias, pres.; Dr. Richard M. Uray, exec. mgr.
Univ. of South Carolina College of Journalism, Columbia 29208; (803) 777-6783.

SOUTH DAKOTA BROADCASTERS ASSOCIATION
Joe H. Floyd, pres.; Bob Reimers, v.p.; Lenore Thomson, secty.-treas.; Verl Thomson, exec. dir.
4609 W. 12th St., Sioux Falls 57106; (605) 336-7110.

TENNESSEE ASSOCIATION OF BROADCASTERS
Thomas R. King, exec. dir.; Ken Maness (WJCW/WQUT, Johnson City) pres.
Box 40185, Nashville 37204; (615) 331-4535.

TEXAS ASSOCIATION OF BROADCASTERS
Dudley Waller (KEBE/KOOI-FM, Jacksonville) pres.; John Barger (WOAI/KAJA (FM), San Antonio) v.p.-pres. elect; Bonner McLane, exec. v.p.; David Lane, secty.-treas.
Box 14787, Austin 78761; (512) 459-0656.

UTAH BROADCASTERS ASSOCIATION
James Burgoyne (KBLQ) pres.; Earl J. Glade Jr., exec. dir.
Box 401, Provo 84603; (801) 226-3094.

VERMONT ASSOCIATION OF BROADCASTERS
Mark Brady, pres.
%WFAD, Middlebury; (802) 388-2490.

VIRGINIA ASSOCIATION OF BROADCASTERS
Peter Easter, exec. dir.
301 E. Market St., Charlottesville 22901; (804) 977-3716.

VIRGINIA PUBLIC RADIO ASOCIATION
Jim Miskimen, pres.; Jerry Glass, treas.
%WMRA Radio, Harrisonburg 22607; (703) 568-6221.

WASHINGTON STATE ASSOCIATION OF BROADCASTERS
James A. Murphy, pres.; Harold Greenberg, chmn. of the bd.; Val E.E. Limburg, secty.-treas.
2300 Westin Bldg., Seattle 98121; (206) 488-4100.

WEST VIRGINIA BROADCASTERS ASSOCIATION
William A. O'Brien (WJLS/WBKW, Beckley), pres.; Marilyn Fletcher, exec. dir.
2120 Weberwood Dr., South Charleston 25303; (304) 344-3798.

WISCONSIN BROADCASTERS ASSOCIATION
Lee Davis (WCUB/WKKB, Manitowoc), pres.; Bart Kellnhauser (WSAW-TV, Wausau), secty.; Robert J. Bodden, exec. dir.
Box 701, Platteville 53818; (608) 348-6238.

WYOMING ASSOCIATION OF BROADCASTERS
Kim Love, pres.; Dave Montgomery, pres.; Jeff Kehl, 1st v.p.; Roy Maple, 2nd v.p.; Ray Lansing, exec. secty.-treas.
Box 1873, Cheyenne 82003; (307) 632-7622.

The Press

* TRADE PUBLICATIONS
* NEWSPAPER LISTING

Trade Publications

Quigley Publishing Company

Publishers of Motion Picture Product Digest (25 times a year), Motion Picture Almanac (Annual), Television Almanac (Annual). – Fame. 159 West 53rd St., New York, NY 10019; (212) 247-3100; Cable: Quigpubco, New York.

PRESIDENT AND PUBLISHER
Martin Quigely, Jr.
EDITOR-IN-CHIEF
Richard Gertner
GENERAL MANAGER
Robert McDonald

LONDON BUREAU

William Pay, Manager and London Editor; 15 Samuel Road, Langdon Hills, Basildon, Essex, England. Tel.: 0268-417-055.

FOREIGN CORRESPONDENTS

ARGENTINA: Natalio Bruski, Calle Paso 240 (8°_C), Buenos Aires.
EGYPT: Ahmed Sami, 4 El Ommara St., Apt. 13, Abbassia, Cairo.
GREECE: Rena Velissariou, 8432, Kolokotroni Str., Agia Paraskevi, Attikis, Athens. (804).
HOLLAND: Philip de Schaap, Wimbledon Park 99, XL Amstelveen, Netherlands.
INDIA: B. D. Garga, 55 Anita, Mt. Pleasant Rd., Bombay 400006, India.
JAPAN: A. C. Pinder, Whaley-Eaton Service, Central P.O. Box 190, Tokyo, Japan.
SRI LANKA: Chandra Perera, 437 Pethiygoda, Kelanuja, Sri Lanka, Ceylon.
SWITZERLAND: Gabriella Broggi, Via E. Maraini 20B, 6900 Massagna, Switzerland.

Motion Picture Almanac

(Annually) 159 West 53rd St., New York, NY 10019; 247-3100; Cable: Quigpubco, New York.

EDITOR
Richard Gertner
ASSOCIATE EDITOR
William Pay
ADVERTISING AND DISTRIBUTION
Robert McDonald

Television & Video Almanac

(Annually) 159 West 53rd St., New York, NY 10019; 247-3100; Cable: Quigpubco, New York.

EDITOR
Richard Gertner
ASSOCIATE EDITOR
William Pay
VIDEO EDITOR
Jane Klain
ADVERTISING AND DISTRIBUTION
Robert McDonald

Fame

159 West 53rd St., New York, NY 10019; 247-3100; Cable: Quigpubco, New York.

EDITOR
Richard Gertner
ASSOCIATE EDITOR
William Pay

Advertising Age

(Weekly) 740 Rush St., Chicago, Il. 60611; 649-5200; 220 East 42nd St., New York, NY 10017; (212) 210-0100.

CHAIRMAN
Mrs. G. D. Crain
CHAIRMAN, EXECUTIVE COMMITTEE
S. R. Bernstein
PUBLISHER
Louis F. Demarco
PRESIDENT & EDITOR-IN-CHIEF
Rance Crain

The American Cinematographer

(Monthly on the 1st—Semi-technical) Published by American Society of Cinematographers, Inc., 1782 North Orange Drive, Hollywood, CA 90028; (213) 876-5080.

EDITOR
George Turner
ASSISTANT EDITOR
Jean Turner
ADVERTISING
Angie Gollmann
CIRCULATION MANAGER
Patty Armacost

Back Stage

(Weekly dealing with theatrical and nontheatrical films, television shows and commercials, cassettes, radio, and theater, published Friday), 330 West 42 St., New York, NY 10036, (212) 947-0020; 5150 Wilshire Blvd., L.A. CA 90036, (213) 936-5200; 100 East Ohio St., Chicago, IL 60611, (312) 943-0051.

MANAGING EDITOR & PUBLISHER
Allen Zwerdling
ADVERTISING DIRECTOR & PUBLISHER
Ira Eaker
ASSOCIATE PUBLISHER
Steve Elish
EDITOR
Anthony Vagnoni

Back Stage Television, Film, Tape & Production Directory

(Annually, March), 330 West 42 St., New York, NY 10036; (212) 947-0020.

EDITOR
Allen Zwerdling

Billboard

(Weekly dealing with records, music, entertainment artists, video hardware and software, etc., published Saturdays), 9107 Wilshire Blvd., Beverly Hills, CA 90210, 273-7040; 1 Astor Plaza, New York, NY 10036, 764-7300; 150 N. Wacker Drive, Chicago, IL 60606; Central 6-9818; 733 15 St., N.W., Washington 5, D.C.; 393-2580.

PUBLISHER
Lee Zhito
EXECUTIVE VICE PRESIDENT
Jules Perel
MANAGING EDITOR
Adam White

Broadcasting—The News Magazine of the Fifth Estate

(Weekly on Monday; also publishes Broadcasting Yearbook every March.) Washington Headquarters: 1735 DeSales Street, N.W. 20036, (202) 638-1022; New York: 630 Third Ave., 10017, (212) 599-2830; Hollywood: 1680 No. Vine St. 90028,. (213) 463-3148.

PRESIDENT AND PUBLISHER
Lawrence B. Taishoff
VICE PRESIDENT/OPERATIONS

David N. Whitcombe
SENIOR EDITORIAL CONSULTANT
Edwin H. James
MANAGING EDITOR
Donald V. West

Celebrity Bulletin

(A chronicle of the day to day activities of celebrities in New York, Hollywood, London, Paris and Rome. Published daily.) 1780 Broadway, New York, NY 10019; (212) 757-7979.

PUBLISHERS
Celebrity Service, Inc.

Celebrity Register

(A biographical index, published every two years) 1780 Broadway, Suite 300, New York, NY 10019; (212) 245-1460; 1 (800) FOR CELEBS.

PUBLISHER
Celebrity Service, Inc.
EDITOR
Earl Blackwell

Contact Book

(An entertainment industry directory, published annually) 1780 Broadway, New York, NY 10019; (212) 245-1460.

PUBLISHER
Celebrity Service, Inc.
EDITOR
Donnali Shor

Daily Variety

(Motion picture, television, homevideo, pay-TV, cable, radio, theatre, night clubs, daily) 1400 N. Cahuenga Blvd., Hollywood, CA 90028; (213) 469-1141.

EDITOR
Thomas M. Pryor
ASSOCIATE PUBLISHER
Michael Silverman
MANAGING EDITOR
Peter Pryor
MARKETING DIRECTOR
Michael Malak
GENERAL MANAGER
F. Phil Turner
PRODUCTION MANAGER
Bob Butler

Electronics

(Design, production and application bi-weekly for engineers and management) McGraw-Hill Information Systems Co., 1221 Avenue of the Americas, New York, NY 10020. Tel.: (212) 512-2645.

PUBLISHER
Laurence Altman
EDITOR-IN-CHIEF
Robert W. Henkel
EXECUTIVE EDITORS
Arthur Erikson, News
Samuel Weber, Technical

Facts, Figures, Film & TV

(Magazine for syndicated programming). 100 Lafayette Drive, Syosset, NY 11791; (516) 496-3355.

PUBLISHER
Harvey Seslowsky
VICE PRESIDENT-EDITOR-IN-CHIEF
Miss Avra Fliegelman

Film News

Pub 4 times in the year by Film News Company. (Spring, Summer, Fall, Winter) The international review of AV materials and equipment. Editoral and business office: Box 619, LaSalle, IL 61301.

EDITOR
J. Paul Carvico

Film Quarterly

(Quarterly; published Fall, Winter, Spring and Summer. A critical journal of motion pictures and their related arts; successor to *The Quarterly of Film, Radio and Television and the Hollywood Quarterly.*) Editorial, Sales, and Advertising office: University of California Press, Berkeley, CA 94720; (415) 642-6333.

EDITOR
Ernest Callenbach
Published by University of California Press

Hollywood Report

(Quarterly) 917 So. Tremaine Avenue, Hollywood, 90019, CA; (213) 939-2345.

EDITOR
Syd Cassyd

Hollywood Reporter, The

(Film, TV, Entertainment, Daily) 6715 Sunset Boulevard, Hollywood, CA 90028; (213) 464-7411; and 1501 Broadway, N.Y., N.Y., 10036; (212) 354-1858.

PUBLISHER & EDITOR-IN-CHIEF
Tichi Wilkerson Kassel
MANAGING EDITOR
Paul Wilner
BUREAUS
NEW YORK: 1501 Broadway, N.Y.C. 10036; (212) 354-1858.
WASHINGTON D.C.: Rm. 1139, National Press Bldg., Washington D.C. 20045; (202) 737-2828.
LONDON: 57 Duke St., London W.1.; 01-629/6765, 6766.

I.A.T.S.E. Official Bulletin

(Quarterly) 1515 Broadway, New York, NY 10036. Tel.: (212) 730-1770.

EDITOR
James J. Riley

International Photographer

(Monthly, on the 5th) 7715 Sunset Boulevard, Hollywood, CA 90046; 876-0160.

PUBLISHER
International Photographer
EDITOR
George Toscas

International Motion Picture Almanac

(See Quigley Publications)

Journal of the Society of Motion Picture and Television Engineers

(Technical monthly) 595 West Hartsdale Ave., White Plains, NY 10607; (914) 761-1100.

EDITOR
Jeffrey B. Friedman
ADVERTISING MANAGER
Janice Baio

The Producer's Master-Guide

(Annual) 611 Broadway, Suite 807, New York, NY 10012; (212) 777-4002. International reference guide for producers in the motion picture, television, commercials, cable and videotape industries in the U.S., Canada, the Caribbean Islands, Bermuda, Ireland, and the United Kingdom.

PUBLISHER AND TREASURER
Shmuel Bension
SENIOR CONSULTANT PUBLICITY
Renee L. Ash

Radio-Electronics

(Monthly dealing with technical aspects of electronics, including TV, radio, computers, and electronic service technicians, high-fidelity enthusiasts and experimenters) 500B Bicounty Blvd., Farmingdale, NY 11735 (516) 293-3000.

PUBLISHER
Larry Steckler
EDITORIAL DIRECTOR
Art Kleiman
MANAGING EDITOR
Brian Fenton

Teletales, The News Letter of the National Academy of Television Receiver Owners of America

(Quarterly) 917 So. Tremaine, Hollywood 90019, CA; WE 9-2345.

EDITOR
Syd Cassyd

Television Digest

(Published weekly. Television Digest with Consumer Electronics, TV & Cable Action Update, AM/FM Addenda; Annual Television & Cable Factbook, Annual Cable & Station Coverage Atlas, Weekly Satellite Week, Weekly Video Week, Biweekly Public Broadcasting Report, Monthly Early Warning Report, Daily Communications) 1836 Jefferson Place, N.W., Washington, DC 20036; (202) 872-9200.

EDITOR & PUBLISHER
Albert Warren
EDITORIAL DIRECTOR
David Lachenbruch
EXECUTIVE EDITOR
Dawson B. Nail
SENIOR EDITOR & ASSOCIATE PUBLISHER
Paul L. Warren

Television Factbook

(Published annually by Television Digest, Inc.) 1836 Jefferson Place, N.W., Washington, DC 20036.

EDITOR & PUBLISHER
Albert Warren
MANAGING EDITOR
Michael C. Taliaferro
EDITORIAL DIRECTOR
Mary Appel

Television Index

4029 27 St., Long Island City, NY 11101, (718) 937-3990.

EDITOR & PUBLISHER
Jerry Leichter

Television/Radio Age

(Bi-weekly trade magazine) 1270 Sixth Ave., New York, NY 10020; PL 7-8400.

PUBLISHER
Sol J. Paul
EDITOR
Sanford Josephson
EXECUTIVE EDITOR
Alfred J. Jaffe
MANAGING EDITOR
Ed Rosenthal
ASSISTANT EDITORS
Bob Sobel, George Swisshelm, David Halliday
PRODUCTION DIRECTOR
Marvin Rabach
BRANCH OFFICES
1607 N. El Centro, #25, Hollywood, CA 90028, (213) 464-3553; Commerce House, 6 London St., London, W21HR, England

Variety

(International entertainment business weekly, published Wednesdays) 154 West 46 Street, New York, NY 10036, (212) 869-5700; 1400 N. Cahuenga Blvd., Hollywood, CA 90028, (213) 469-1141; 1483 Chain Bridge Rd., McLean, VA 22101, (703) 448-0510; 400 North Michigan Ave., Chicago, IL 60611, (312) 337-4984; PARIS: France, 33 Champs Elysees, Paris 75008, France; Phone 720-19-56; ROME: VARIETY, Via Bissolati, 20, 00187, Rome, Italy; 463-290. LONDON: VARIETY, 49 St. James's St., London SW1A 1JX, England; 493-4561; MADRID, Spain, Calle Lagasca, 104, 28006; Phone 276-4262; SYDNEY, 2000, N.S.W. 1-7 Albion Place, Phone: 61-3124; TORONTO, 74 Albany Ave.; (416) 531-1600; SCANDINAVIA, Copenhagen 18 Skenderade; Phone: 91-0040.

PUBLISHER AND EXECUTIVE EDITOR
Syd Silverman
ADVERTISING MANAGER
Mort Bryer

Great Britain

Image Technology

(Technical monthly) Journal of the British Kinematograph, Sound and Television Society. 549 Victoria House, Vernon Place, London, WC1B 4Dj, england. Tec.: 01 242-8400.

Screen International

Published by King Publications Ltd. Weekly, covering news, reviews, comment and pictures of the film and television industries. 6-7 Great Chapel Street, London, W.1. Tel.: 01 43 5741.

PUBLISHER
Peter King
EDITOR
Peter Noble

NEWSPAPERS IN PRINCIPAL MARKETS OF THE U.S.

Arranged alphabetically by states, this list gives the names and addresses of newspapers in cities and market areas of over 100,000 population which maintain regular motion picture and television departments.

Alabama

Birmingham, The News, 2200 North 4th Ave., 35202.
Birmingham, Post-Herald, 2200 North 4th Ave., 35202.
Huntsville, Times, 2317 Memorial Pkway., 35807.
Mobile, Mobile Press Register., 304 Government St., 36602.
Montgomery, Advertiser, 107 South Lawrence, 36104.

Arizona

Phoenix, Republic, 120 East Van Buren St., 85004.
Tucson, Arizona Star, 208 North Stone, 87501.

Arkansas

Little Rock, Democrat, Capitol Ave. & Scott., 72203.
Little Rock, Arkansas Gazette, 112 West Third St., 72203.

California

Anaheim, Bulletin, 232 South Lemon St., 92805.
Berkeley, Berkeley Gazette, 2048 Center St., 94704.
Burbank, Daily Review, 220 E. Orange Grove Ave., 91502.
Culver City, Evening Star News, 4043 Irving Place., 90230.
Fresno, Bee, 1559 Van Ness Ave., 93721.
Glendale, News Press, 111 North Isabel, 91209.
Long Beach, Independent Press-Telegram, 604 Pine Ave., 90801.
Huntington Park, Daily Signal, 6414 Rugby Ave., 90255.
Los Angeles, Herald-Examiner, 1111 S. Broadway, 90054.
Los Angeles, Times Mirror Co., Times Mirror Sq., 90053.
Oakland, The Tribune Publishing Co., 401-13th St., 94612.
Pasadena, Star News, 525 East Colorado St., 91109.
Riverside, Press-Enterprise Co., 3512-14th St., 92502.
Sacramento, Bee, 21st & Q Streets, 95813.
Sacramento, Sacramento Union Inc., 301 Capitol Mall., 95812.
San Bernardino, Sun, 399 "D" St., 92401.
San Diego, DBA Union-Tribune, 940 Third Ave., 92112.
San Francisco, Chronicle, 901 Mission St., 94119.
San Francisco, The Examiner, 110 5th Ave., 94119.
San Gabriel Valley, The Tribune, 2037 W. San Bernardino Rd., 91790.
San Jose, Mercury-News, 750 Ridder Park Dr., 95131.
San Pedro, News Pilot, 356 W. 7th Street., 90733.
Santa Ana, Register, 625 North Grand Ave., 92711.
Santa Monica, Evening Outlook, 1540 Third, 90406.
Stockton, Stockton Daily Record, 530 E. Market St., 95202.
Torrance, South Bay Breeze, 5215 Torrance Blvd., 90503.
Van Nuys, Van Nuys News & Valley News & Green Sheet, 14539 Sylvan St., 91408.

Colorado

Denver, The Post, 650 15th St., 80202.
Denver, Rocky Mt. News, 400 West Colfax Ave., 80204.

Connecticut

Bridgeport, Post, 410 State St., 06602.
Hartford, Courant, 285 Broad St., 06101.
Hartford, The Times, 10 Prospect St., 06101.
New Haven, The Journal-Courier, 367 Orange St., 06503.
New Haven, The Register, 367 Orange St., 06503.
Waterbury, American-Republican, Inc., 389 Meadow St., 06702.

Delaware

Wilmington, News-Journal Co., 831 Orange St., 19899.

District of Columbia

Washington, Post, 1515 "L" St., N.W., 20005.

Florida

Fort Lauderdale, News, 101 North New River Drive East., 33302.
Jacksonville, Florida Times-Union, One Riverside Ave., 32201.
Miami, Herald, 1 Herald Plaza, 33101.
Miami, The News, 1 Herald Plaza, 33101.
St. Petersburg, Times, P.O. Box 1121, 33731.
Tampa, Tribune, 505 East J. F. Kennedy Blvd., 33602.

Georgia

Atlanta, Journal-Constitution, 10 Forsyth St., N.W., 30302.
Columbus, Ledger-Enquirer Newspapers, 17 West 12th St., 31902.
Macon, Telegraph, 120 Broadway, 31201.
Savannah, Savannah News-Press, 105-111 West Bay St., 31402.

Hawaii

Honolulu, Advertiser, P.O. Box 3110, 96802.
Honolulu, Honolulu Star-Bulletin, Inc. 605 Kapiolani Blvd., 96813.
Honolulu, Hawaii Hochi, 917 Kokea St., 96817.
Honolulu, Hawaii Times, 916 Nuuana Ave., 96807.

Illinois

Chicago, Chicago Today, 445 N. Michigan Ave., 60611.
Chicago, Daily Calumet, 9120 Baltimore, 60617.
Chicago, The News, 401 North Wabash, 60611.
Chicago, The Sun-Times, Field Enterprises, Inc., Newspaper Div., 401 North Wabash, 60611.
Chicago, Tribune, 435 North Michigan Ave., 60611.
Joliet, Herald News, 78 No. Scott St., 60431.
Moline, Daily Dispatch, 1720-5th Ave., 61265.
Peoria, Peoria Journal Star Inc., 1 News Plaza, 61601.
Rock Island, Argus, 1724-4th Ave., 61202.
Rockford, Register-Star, 99 East State St., 61105.
Waukegan, News-Sun, 100 W. Madison St., 60085.

Indiana

Evansville, Courier & Press, 201 N.W. 2nd St., 47701.
Fort Wayne, Journal-Gazette, 701 S. Clinton St., 46802.
Fort Wayne, News Sentinel, 600 West Main St., 46802.
Gary, Post-Tribune, 1065 Broadway, 46402.
Hammond, Times, 417 Fayette St., 46320.
Indianapolis, Star & News, 307 North Pennsylvania St., 46206.
South Bend, Tribune, 225 West Colfax, 46626.

Iowa

Cedar Rapids, Gazette, 500-3rd Ave., S.E., 52401.
Davenport, Times Democrat, 124 E. 2nd St., 52808.
Des Moines, Register & Tribune, 715 Locust St., 50304.
Sioux City, Journal, 5th & Douglas St., 51102.
Waterloo, Courier, 501 Commercial St., 50704.

Kansas

Kansas City, Kansas, 901 North 8th St., 66101.
Topeka, Capital-Journal, 6th & Jefferson, 66607.
Wichita, The Eagle and Beacon, 825 E. Douglas St., 67201.

Kentucky

Louisville, The Courier-Journal & Times, 525 West Broadway, 40202.

Louisiana

Baton Rouge, Advocate, 525 Lafayette St., 70821.
New Orleans, The Times-Pacayune, 3800 Howard Ave., 70140.
Shreveport, Journal-Times, 222 Lake St., 7110?.

Maryland

Baltimore, News American, Lombard & South Sts., 21230.
Baltimore, Sun, Calvert & Center Sts., 21230.

Massachusetts

Boston, Christian Science Monitor, One Norway St., 02115.
Boston, Globe, 135 Morrissey Blvd., 02107.
Boston, Boston-Herald Traveler, 300 Harrison Ave., 02106.
Boston, Record American, 5 Winthrop Square, 02106.
New Bedford, Standard-Times, 555 Pleasant St., 02742.
Springfield, Republican, 1860 Main St., 01101.
Worcester, Worcester Telegram & Gazette, 20 Franklin St., 01601.

Michigan

Ann Arbor, News, 340 E. Huron St., 48106.
Detroit, Free Press, 321 West Lafayette Blvd., 48231.
Detroit, Evening News, 615 Lafayette Blvd., 48231.
Flint, The Journal, 200 East 1st St., 48502.
Grand Rapids, The Press, Press Plaza, Vandenberg Center, 49502.
Kalamazoo, Kalamazoo Gazette, 401 S. Burdick St., 49003.
Lansing, State Journal, 120 East Lenawee St., 48919.
Muskegon, Chronicle, 981 Third St., 49443.
Pontiac, Press, 48 W. Huron St., 48056.
Royal Oak, Tribune, 210 E. Third St., 48068.
Sagniaw, News, 203 South Washington Ave., 48605.

Minnesota

Duluth, Herald, 424 West 1st., 55801.
Minneapolis, Star & Tribune, Fifth and Portland Ave., 55415.
St. Paul, Dispatch, 55 East 4th St., 55101.

Mississippi

Biloxi-Gulfport, Herald, De Buys Rd., 39501.
Jackson, Clarion Ledger-News, Box 40, 39205.

Missouri

Kansas City, Star, 1729 Grand Ave., 64108.
St. Louis, Globe-Democrat, 12th Blvd. at Delmar, 63101.
St. Louis, The Post-Dispatch, 1133 Franklin Ave., 63101.
Springfield, Springfield News & Leader, 651 Boonville, 65801.

Nebraska

Lincoln, Journal-Star, 926 "P" Street, 68501.
Omaha, World-Herald, 14th & Dodge, Sts., 68102.

Nevada

Las Vegas, Review-Journal, 737 North Main St., 89101.
Las Vegas, Sun, 121 S. Highland Ave., 89104.

New Hampshire

Manchester, Union Leader, 35 Amherst St., 03105.

New Jersey

Camden, Courier-Post, 08101.
Elizabeth, Journal, 295-299 North Broad St., 07207.
Jersey City, Journal, 30 Journal Square, 07306.
Newark, Evening News, 215-221 Market St., 07101.
Newark, Newark Morning Ledger, 1 Star Ledger Plaza, 07101.
Passaic-Clifton, Herald-News, 988 Main Ave., 07055.
Paterson, News, News Plaza & Straight St., 07509.
Trenton, Times, 500 Perry St., 08605.

New Mexico

Albuquerque, Journal, 7th & Silver, S.W., 87101.

New York

Albany, Times-Union, 645 Albany-Shaker Road, 12201.
Buffalo, The Evening News, 218 Main St., 14240.
Buffalo, Courier-Express, 787 Main St., 14240.
Long Island, Newsday, 500 Stewart Ave., Garden City, 11530.
New York City:
Brooklyn Daily, Inc., 2427 Surf Ave., Brooklyn, 11224.
The News, 220 East 42nd St., 10017.
The Post, 210 South St., 10002.
The Times, 229 West 43rd St.,10036.
Wall St. Journal, 30 Broad St., 10004.
Niagara Falls, Gazette, 310 Niagara St., 14302.
Rochester, Times-Union, 55 Exchange St., 14614.
Syracuse, The Post-Standard, Clinton Square, 13202.
Utica, Observer-Dispatch, 221 Oriskany Plaza, 13503.
Yonkers, The Herald Statesman, Larkin Plaza, 10702.

North Carolina

Charlotte, Observer, 600 South Tryon St., 28201.
Durham, Herald, 115-19 Market St., 27702.
Greensboro, The News, 200-04 North Davie St., 27402.
Raleigh, News & Observer, 215 S. McDowell St., 27601.
Winston-Salem, Journal-Sentinel, 416-20 North Marshall, 27102.

North Dakota

Fargo, Forum, 101-5th St., 58102.

Ohio

Akron, The Beacon Journal, 44 East Exchange St., 44309.
Canton, The Repository, 500 Market Ave., South, 44702.
Cincinnati, The Enquirer, 617 Vine St., 45201.
Cincinnati, Post & Times-Star, 800 Broadway St., 45202.
Cleveland, The Plain Dealer, 1801 Superior Ave., 44114.
Cleveland, The Press, 901 Lakeside Ave., 44114.
Columbus, The Citizen-Journal, 34 South Third St., 43216.
Columbus, The Dispatch, 34 South Third St., 43216.
Dayton, Journal-Herald, 4th & Ludlow Sts., 45401.
Toledo, The Toledo Blade, 541 Superior St., 43604.
Youngstown, The Vindicator, Vindicator Square, 44501.

Oklahoma

Oklahoma City, Oklahoma Journal, 7430 S.E. 15th St., 73110.
Oklahoma City, Oklahoman, 500 North Broadway, 73125.
Tulsa, The World & Tribune, 315 South Boulder Ave., 74102.

Oregon

Portland, The Oregon Journal, 1320 Southwest Broadway, 97201.
Portland, The Oregonian, 1320 Southwest Broadway, 97201.

Pennsylvania

Allentown, The Call, 6th & Linden Sts., 18105.
Erie, The Times, 20 East 12th St., 16501.
Philadelphia, The Bulletin, 30th & Market Sts., 19101.
Philadelphia, The Inquirer, 400 North Broad St., 19101.
Philadelphia, The News, 400 N. Broad St., 19101.
Pittsburgh, Post Gazette, 50 Blvd. of Allies, 15222.
Pittsburgh, Pittsburgh Press Co., 34 Blvd. of Allies, 15222.
Reading, The Eagle, 345 Penn St., 19601.
Scranton, Tribune, 338 North Washington Ave., 18501.
Scranton, The Times, Penn & Spruce, 18501.

Rhode Island

Providence, The Journal, 75 Fountain St., 02902.

South Carolina

Columbia, The State-Record, P.O. Box 1333, 29202.

Tennessee

Chattanooga, The News-Free Press, 400 E. 11th St., 37401.
Chattanooga, Times, 117 E. 10th St., 37401.
Knoxville, The Journal, 210 W. Church Ave., 37901.
Knoxville, The News-Sentinel, 240 West Church Ave., 37901.
Memphis Press-Scimitar, 495 Union Ave., 38101.
Nashville, The Banner, 1100 Broadway, 37203.
Nashville, The Tennessean, 1100 Broadway, 37203.

Texas

Abilene, Reporter News, North 2nd & Cypress Sts., 79604.
Amarillo, The Globe-Times, 900 Harrison St., 79105.
Austin, American-Statesman, 308 Guadalupe, 78767.
Beaumont, The Enterprise, 380 Walnut St., 77704.
Corpus Christi, The Caller-Times, 820 Lower Broadway, 78401.
Dallas, The News, Communications Center, 75222.

Dallas, The Times Herald, 1101 Pacific, 75202.
El Paso, Times, 401 Mills St., 79999.
Fort Worth, The Press, 507 Jones, 76102.
Fort Worth, The Star-Telegram, 400 West 7th St., 76101.
Houston, The Chronicle, 512-20 Travis St., 77002.
Houston, The Post, 4747 Southwest Freeway, 77001.
Lubbock, The Avalanche-Journal, 8th St. & Avenue "J", 79408.
San Antonio, The Express, Avenue "E" & 3rd St., 78205.
San Antonio, The Light, McCullough & Broadway, 78206.
Waco, Tribune-Herald, 900 Franklin, 76703.
Wichita Falls, The Times, 1301 Lamar St., 76307.

Utah

Salt Lake City, Desert News, 34 East 1st St., South, 84110.
Salt Lake City, The Tribune, 143 South Main St., 84101.

Virginia

Alexandria, Gazette, 717 No. St. Asaph St., 22313.
Arlington, Northern Va. Sun, 3409 Wilson Blvd., 22210.
Newport News-Hampton, The Daily Press, 7505 Warwick Blvd., 23607.
Norfolk, Virginian-Pilot, 150 West Brambleton Ave., 23501.
Richmond, Times-Dispatch, 333 East Grace St., 23213.
Roanoke, Times-World, 201-09. W. Campbell Ave., 24010.

Washington

Seattle, The Post-Intelligencer, 6th & Wall, 98121.
Seattle, The Times, Fairview Ave. N & John, 98111.
Seattle, Daily Journal of Commerce, 83 Columbia St., 98104.
Spokane, Chronicle, W. 927 Riverside, 99210.
Tacoma, The Tribune, 711 Helens Ave., 98401.

Wisconsin

Madison, Capital-Times, 115 South Carroll St., 53701.
Milwaukee, The Journal, 333 West State, 53201.
Milwaukee, Sentinel, 918 N. 4th St., 53201.

The Industry in Great Britain and Ireland

* INDUSTRY DEVELOPMENTS
* PROGRAM CONTRACTORS
* SERVICES
* AD AGENCIES
* COMPANIES AND PERSONNEL
* ORGANIZATIONS
* STUDIOS AND LABORATORIES

BRITISH YEAR IN REVIEW

1985–86 was another buoyant period for British commercial television with revenue increases of plus ten per cent. Two factors influencing this trend were the boost in advertising income from the World Cup transmissions and several major stock exchange flotations.

In one month during the summer of 1986, the Independent Television companies' advertising revenue was more than £94 million, an increase of 28 per cent compared to the same period the previous years. Two examples of successful stock market flotations were Thames Television—the London weekday ITV contractors—and TV-am, commercial television's breakfast television service.

With television in 98 per cent of homes here, it has been estimated that British viewers watch more than any nation except Japan and America. Indeed, there is almost saturation in viewing. Research shows that the public on average spend some 28 hours each week watching television.

On the non-commercial front, the British Broadcasting Corporation (BBC) which is funded by an annual tax on owners of TV sets, continues to maintain its high standard of programmes and compete at all levels with a diversified schedule. As an example, the BBC's "Eastenders" series at times draws upwards of 23 million viewers compared to ITV's "Coronation Street" audience of 19 million. The BBC's Breakfast Television and ITV's TV-am have reached audiences of 7.5 million and 9.9 million, respectively. During peak time an average of 9.6 million people tune in to ITV, one million up on the BBC's 8.6 million.

At the same time, the vast majority of overseas material on British telelvision originates in the USA. ITV's and Channel 4's quota of overseas material is 14 per cent of total programme output. This comprises theatrical motion pictures, TV films and series such as "The A Team," "Airwolf," "Benson," "Cheers," "Hill Street Blues," "Dallas," and "Dynasty." Estimates of the prices paid by local contractors and the BBC for American TV shows are around $13,000 for half-hour episodes to between $50,000 and $3 million for a feature film.

Traditional broadcast television is a very important user of feature films. In terms of total audience, four billion individual film viewings a year is a reasonable estimate. Much film buying for the independent television companies is carried out centrally and this, taken with the BBC, means that the demand side of the market is essentially a duopoly.

During the first half of 1986, however, there was a fall-off in the audiences for feature films with none among the Top 20 most popular programmes. The three highest feature film screenings during this period, all on the ITV network, were "You Only Live Twice" with a 17.3 million audience, "From Russia With Love" with 17.25 million, and "An Officer and a Gentleman" with 16.35 million. This compares to the British soap opera "Coronation Street" with 19.25 million. It has resulted in a competitive struggle for audiences between the ITV and BBC with the emphasis being put on home-produced dramas.

While the CEA (Cinematograph Exhibitors' Association) maintains its three year TV holdback and a one year cable TV holdback, it has conceded that there will be an automatic exclusion (in addition to that for short and foreign films) which will apply to any cinema film made for an audited production cost not exceeding £1.25 million.

It is a decision prompted by the increasing involvement of the BBC and ITV Programme Contractors to produce material, sometimes in cooperation with the independent production sector, which is indistinguishable from feature films. More and more production companies make both films and television programmes.

Also, it is claimed, this CEA holdback or "window" before a cinema film is seen on television or video, is in the interests of all concerned. This theory is based on the publicity value, for all media, of a high profile cinema release before any other distribution but also to the maximization of revenue from each market in turn. This is essential for the preservation of a healthy production sector which the television and video industries need as much as the cinema.

Satellite Broadcasting, Cable and Pay TV are still in the development stages. Financial and managerial problems have delayed Cable's impact on Britain's viewing habits. The original 11 companies and consortia granted licenses to provide full wideband cable networks are in varied states of development. The IBA (Independent Broadcasting Authority) hopes to make decisions about DBS (Direct Broadcasting by Satellite) before the end of 1986 with the possibility of the service coming into operation by 1990.

The Superchannel pan-European satellite TV service, however, is expected to be launched by the end of 1986. It will be operated by ITV stations and the Virgin group.

On the other hand, the growth of home video continues apace with over nine million VCRs currently in use with an estimated software spend of between £350 and 400 million in 1986.

Perhaps the best summing up of the present state of television in the U.K. is made in the IBA's annual report which states: "Even though technological change has been occurring less rapidly than some observers predicted a few years agò, the 1980s are likely to be seen in retrospect as a transitional period in the history of British broadcasting. The four public service television channels as yet face little competition from other television services."

Also, Channel 4 has been a success story—not least in the rapid build-up of its coverage at a considerably faster rate than for any other U.K. or European television channel. For five years the Independent Broadcasting Authority has concentrated a considerable part of its resources, including almost £50 million on this work. The target is that, as soon after 1987 as possible, complete parity will be achieved with ITV.

PROGRAMME TRANSMISSIONS ON ITV*

Weekly average, year ended 30th March 1986

	Duration Hrs. Min.	Percentage %
News and news magazine	11:01	10½
Current affairs and general factual	10:54	10¼
Arts	0:42	¾
Religion	2:31	2½
Adult education	1:51†	1¾
School programmes	6:50	6½
Pre-school	3:35	3½
Children's informative programmes	2:12	2
INFORMATIVE	39:36	37¾
Plays, series, TV movies	26:21	25
Feature films	8:18	8
NARRATIVE	34:39	33
Children's drama and entertainment	7:24	7
Entertainment and light music	14:29	13¾
Sport	9:00	8½
TOTAL ALL PROGRAMMES	105:15‡	100

Source: IBA Annual Report

*Excluding TV-am's 21 hours per week.

†To this total should be added 13 minutes per week of general factual material shown at peak time which was accepted by the IBA as educationally valuable and supported by educational material and activities.

‡Opening captions totalling 7 minutes per week are not specified above, but are included in the total.

Government Units and Program Contractors

HOME OFFICE

Queen Anne's Gate, London, SW1H 9AT. Tel: 01-213-3000.

The Secretary of State for the Home Department is empowered to licence persons or corporate bodies to operate broadcasting stations as laid down in the Wireless Telegraphy Act, 1949. The BBC is incorporated by Royal Charter and operates under this and a License and Agreement granted on the 2nd April 1981. The provisions of the Charter and the License Agreement run to 31st December 1996. The Independent Broadcasting Authority operates under the Broadcasting Act 1981 which extends the life of the Authority until 31st December 1996 and under a licence that runs to the same dates.

BRITISH BROADCASTING CORPORATION TELEVISION SERVICE

Television Centre, Wood Lane, London W.12. Tel: 01-743 8000.

CHAIRMAN OF GOVERNORS: Stuart Young
ADMINISTRATION
Director General: Alasdaire Milne
Managing Director, Television: Bill Cotton
Controller BBC-1: Michael Grade
Controller BBC-2: Graeme McDonald
Chief Accountant: Dick Bates
Controller, Resource Operations: Charles Paton
Controller Personnel: Roger Chase
General Manager Administrative and Accommodation Services, Television: Roger Pugh
PROGRAMME DEPARTMENTS
Presentation
Head of Presentation Department: Malcolm Walker
Community Programmes
Editor: Michael Fentiman
Drama Group
Head of Plays: Peter Goodchild
Head of Series and Serials: Jonathan Powell
Light Entertainment Group
Head of Comedy: Gareth Gwenham
Head of Variety: James Moir
Current Affairs Group
Head of Current Affairs Programmes: Peter Pagnamenta
Outside Broadcasts Group
Head of Group: Cliff Morgan
Head of Sport: Jonathan Martin
Head of Entertainment & Events Programmes: Phil Lewis
Science and Features
Head of Science and Features: Mick Rhodes
Music and Arts
Head of Music and Arts: Alan Yentob
Documentary Programmes
Head of Documentary Features: Will Wyatt
Children's Programs
Head of Children's Programmmes: Anna Home
School Broadcasting
Head of School Broadcasting: Eurfron Gnaynne Jones
Continuing Education
Head of Continuing Education: David Hargreaves
Open University
Head of Open University Production Centre: John Radcliffe
Religious Broadcasting
Head of Religious Programmes: Dr. Colin Morris
NEWS AND CURRENT AFFAIRS
Editor Television News: Ron Neil
PROGRAMME SERVICES
Studio Management
Head of Studio Management: Harry Cottrell
Scenic Services Group
General Manager, Design and Scenic Services: Peter Donnelly
Scenic Operations
Head of Scenic Operations: W. O. Parkinson
Television Design
Head of Television Design Department: Peter Seddon
Visual Effects
Head of Visual Effects Department: J. O'Hara
Graphic Design
Head of Graphic Design: Brian Tregidden
Costume
Head of Costume Department: Miss M. E. McPherson
Make-Up
Head of Make-Up Department: Jean Shardlow
Film Operations and Services
General Manager, Film Operations and Services: Ray Mobsby
Script Unit
Head of Television Script Unit: A. J. Henderson
Artists Bookings
Head of Artists' Contracts: Glyn Martin
Co-Productions
Programme Acquisition
General Manager, Programme Acquisition: Alan Howden
ENTERPRISES LTD.
BBC Enterprises Ltd. Managing Director: Byron Parkin
INFORMATION SERVICES
Chief Press & Publicity Officer: Keith Samuel
LIAISON UNIT
Head of Television Liaison: Brian Denney
ENGINEERING
Chief Engineer: Bob Longman
Controller, Resource Development and Engineering TV: Duncan Thomas
Assistant Controller, Resource Development and Engineering, TV: Tony Stanley
Controller, Resource Operations, TV: Charles Paton
Assistant, Controller, Resource Operations, TV: Norman Taylor
Head of Engineering, Television Studios: D. McGregor
Head of Engineering, Television Outside Broadcasts: J. Hughes
Head of Engineering, Television Network: A. Manners
INTERNATIONAL UNIT
Head of International Unit: Hugh Sheppard

INDEPENDENT BROADCASTING AUTHORITY

70 Brompton Road, London, SW3 1EY. Tel: 01-584 7011.

The Authority was created by Parliament in 1954 as the Independent Television Authority, to provide a comprehensive television service additional to that of the BBC. Under the terms of the Sound Broadcasting Act, 1972, the Authority was renamed the Independent Broadcasting Authority and its functions were extended to cover the provision of Independent Local Radio.

The Broadcasting Act 1980 provided for the setting up of the Channel Four Television Company as a subsidiary of the IBA; it started broadcasting in England, Scotland and Northern Ireland on November 2, 1982. A separate Welsh Fourth Channel Authority was also established by this Act; broadcasting on November 1, 1982. The Broadcasting Act 1981 has consolidated a number of Acts relating to the IBA.

The Authority selects and appoints the ITV & ILR programme companies; supervises the programmes provided by the contractors—and the Channel Four Television Company—and their scheduling; controls advertising, and builds, owns and operates transmitting stations. Fifteen ITV programme companies provide programmes in 14 regions of the United Kingdom (two companies operate in London). As a part of its review of the ITV system, the Authority, in December 1980, offered a contract to broadcast a new national breakfast-time television service, which started in February 1983, to TV-AM. In addition, changes were made to some ITV companies.

By July 1985, 44 Independent Local Radio contractors were providing a programme service in areas of the United Kingdom (two companies operating in London).

Both ITV and ILR are financed mainly by the sale of advertising time.

The Members of the Authority are appointed by the Home Secretary and consist of a Chairman and Deputy Chairman and ten other members, of whom three make the interests of Scotland, Wales and Northern Ireland, respectively, their special care.

Chairman: The Rt. Hon. the Lord Thomson of Monifieth
Director General: J. Whitney
Director of Administration: Lady Littler
Director of Television: David Glencross
Director of Engineering: Dr. J. R. Forrest
Director of Radio: John Thompson, C.B.E.
Director of Finance: P. Rogers
Head of Advertising Control: H. Theobalds
Dep. Director of Television: Miss C. Mulholland
Head of Research: Dr. R. Towler
Head of DBS Services: Bernard Green

INDEPENDENT BROADCASTING AUTHORITY GENERAL ADVISORY COUNCIL

Drawn from various walks of life, the Council is appointed to give the IBA impartial advice on the general pattern and content of ITV programmes.

Chairman: Mrs. D. D. Jackson, A.C.I.S.

INDEPENDENT BROADCASTING AUTHORITY ADVERTISING ADVISORY COMMITTEE

The Committee, under the terms of the Broadcasting Act 1981, must be representative of organizations, authorities and persons concerned with standards of conduct of advertising including, in particular, the advertising of medical or surgical goods or services, and the public as consumers.
Chairman: Prof. A. L. Diamond

INDEPENDENT BROADCASTING AUTHORITY SCOTTISH COMMITTEE

Chairman: J. R. Purvis

INDEPENDENT BROADCASTING AUTHORITY NORTHERN IRELAND COMMITTEE

Chairman: Mrs. J. McIvor

INDEPENDENT BROADCASTING AUTHORITY WELSH COMMITTEE

Chairman: G. R. Peregrine.

INDEPENDENT TELEVISION NEWS LTD.
ITN House, 48 Wells Street, London, W1P 4DE. Tel: 01-637 2424.
Directors: Lord Buxton (Chairman), Sir Alastair Burnett, Richard Dunn, Paul Fox, William Hodgson, Alex Mair, David McCall, Paul McKee, Daniel Moloney, David Nicholas (Editor and Chief Executive), Robert Phillis, David Plowright, Brian Tesler, Ron Wordley.

PROGRAM CONTRACTORS

(Appointed by the Independent Broadcasting Authority).

ANGLIA TELEVISION LTD.
Head office: Anglia House, Norwich, NR1 3JG. Tel: Norwich 615151. Telex: Telanglia 97424; London Office: Brook House, Park Lane, London. Tel: 01-408 2288. Telex: 25353.
EAST OF ENGLAND TRANSMITTERS:
Chairman: Lord Busxon.
Directors: The Lord Buxton, M.C.DL., D. S. McCall, D. T. Puttnam, P. C. Garner, P. W. Gibbings, Mrs. J. Nutting, P. G. Sharman, T. P. Wootton.
Programme Controller: P. C. Garner
Sales Director: T. P. Wootton
Company Secretary: G. M. Rae

BORDER TELEVISION
The Television Centre, Carlisle, CA1 3NT, Cumbria. Tel: 0228 25101; London Office: 33 Margaret Street, London, W1N 7LA. Tel: 01-637 4363.
NORTHWEST ENGLAND—SOUTH SCOTLAND, NORTH NORTHUMBERLAND, AND ISLE OF MAN TRANSMITTERS
Directors: The Earl of Lonsdale (Chairman), James L. Graham (Managing), T. M. Glover (Sales Director), P. Brownlow (Financial Director), M. Bragg, J. R. Wills, P. Corlay, M. Sutherland, H. J. Brewis, Miss M. E. Burkett, O.B.E., B.A., F.M.A., J.I.M. Smail, O.B.E., M.C., T.D., D.L., J.C. Clucas, Dr. June Paterson-Brown, D.W. Trimble, M.A.
Secretary: P. Brownlow
Chief Engineer: R. Dale
Controller of Programmes: P. Gorley
Assistant Controller of Programmes (Planning): E. Hadwin
Editor: L. Howell

CENTRAL INDEPENDENT TELEVISION PLC
(Transmission Area—The Midlands. Period—All Week) West Midlands: Central House, Broad Street, Birmingham B1 2JP. Tel: 021 643 9898. *East Midlands:* TV Centre, Lenton Lane, Nottingham NG7 2NA. Tel: 0602 863322. *London:* 35/38 Portman Square, London W1H 9FH. Tel: 01-486 6688.
MIDLANDS TRANSMITTER
Chairman: Sir Gordon Hobday
Managing Director: Robert Phillis
Directors

Andy Allan	*(Director of Programmes)*
Cliff Baty	*(Director of Finance)*
Ellis Birk	
Charles Denton	*(Chief Executive Zenith)*
David Justham	*(Chairman, West)*
John Madocks, CBE DL	*(Chairman, East)*
Howard Perlin	
Robert Maxwell MC	
Dick Emery	*(Director of Sales)*
Alan Pankhurst	*(Director of Personnel & Industrial Relations)*
Jean Parker	
Sir Leo Pliatzky KCB	
John Jackson	
L. Murray Thomson	

Secretary: Colin A. Campbell
HEADS OF DEPARTMENTS
Director of Operations: Peter Gardner
Director of Personnel & Industrial Relations: Alan Pankhurst
Director of Programmes: Andy Allan
Director of Public Affairs: Marshall Stewart
Cable & Satellite Executive: Jeremy Taylor
Controller of Drama: Ted Childs
Controller, Education & Religion: Philip Grosset
Controller of Entertainment & Music: Jon Scoffield
Controller of Features Group: Richard Creasey
Controller of News & Current Affairs: Robert Southgate
Controller of Programme Planning & Presentation: John Terry
Controller of Sport: Billy Wright CBE
Controller of Young People' Programmes: Lewis Rudd
Controller of Public Affairs: Keith Smith
Studio Controller (West): Dave Davidovitz
Studio Controller (East): Peter Pearson
Chief of Press & Publicity Officer, West: John Palmer
Head of Production Planning: Tony Page
Head of Sport (West): Gary Newbon
Head of Rights Negotiations: Dorothy Viljoen
Chief of Engineering: Gerry Kaye
Chief Press Officer: Alan Deeley
Legal Adviser: Colin A. Campbell

CHANNEL FOUR TELEVISION
60 Charlotte Street, London W1P 2AX. Tel: 01-631 4444. Telex 892356 FOURTVG.
Chairman: R. Hon. Edmund Dell
Chief Executive: Jeremy Isaacs
Managing Director: Justin Dukes

CHANNEL TELEVISION
The Television Centre: Rouge Bouillon St. Helier, Jersey. Tel: Jersey 73999. Telex 4192265 (TVJYG).
Chairman: Major J. R. Riley.
Directors: Harold Fielding, Mrs. M. Kay Mouat, J. C. Rowe, D. le Marquand, G. R. Dorey.
Managing Director: Kenneth Killip, O.B.E.
Company Secretary: Rosie Tollow
Director of Programmes: John P. Henwood.
Director of Sales and Marketing: Michael J. Le Cocq
Controller of Finance: Euan MacGregor

GRAMPIAN TELEVISION LTD.
Queen's Cross, Aberdeen. AB9 2XJ: Scotland. Tel: 0224 646464; Albany House, 68 Albany Road, West Ferry. Dundee. DDS 1NW, Scotland. Tel: 0383 739363.
NORTH SCOTLAND TRANSMITTER
Directors: Iain M. Tennant, J.P. (Chairman); Douglas F. Hardie, C.B.E., J.P., Robert L. Christie; Fiona J. Lyall, M.B., C.H.B., D.P.H., Angus S. Macdonald, Alex Mair, M.B.E. (Chief Executive); The Lord Forbes, K.B.E., D.L. J.P.; Neil Paterson; Sir George Sharp, O.B.E., J.P.; Calum A. Macleod, M.A., LLB. (Deputy Chairman), Donald H. Waters, C.A., Neil R. Welling.
EXECUTIVES
Chief Executive: Alex Mair, M.B.E.; Director of Operations: Robert Christie; Programme Planning Controller: Alastair Beaton; Publicity and Promotions Executive: Michael J. McLintock, M.A.
Head of News and Current Affairs: Alistair Gracie
Head of Engineering: Alex Ramsay
Company Secretary: Donald H. Waters C.A.
Facilities Executive: Michael Stubbings
Production Executive: John Hughes
Head of Sales and Marketing: Neil R. Welling
Sales Controller: Christopher Kidd
Regional Sales Manager: Alan Blackburn
Sales Administration Manager: John Stacey
Financial Controller: Graham Good, C.A.
Administration Executive: Sydney M. Clark
Head of Documentaries: Edward Brocklebank

GRANADA TELEVISION LTD.
36 Golden Square, London, W.1. Tel: 01-734-8080. Granada TV Centre, Manchester 3. Tel: 061-832 7211.
LANCASHIRE TRANSMITTER
Directors: Sir Denis Forman (Chairman), A. Bernstein (Deputy Chairman), D. E. Plowright (Managing Director), Lord Evans of Claughton, A. H. Coe (Financial Director), D. H. Harker, B. L. Heads, W. Lloyd, N. Phillips, A. Quinn, M. Scott, S. Towneley, Mrs. J. Wooller, A. Mutch (Secretary).
Granada International: Barrie Heads (Managing Director)

HTV LTD.
London Sales Office: 99 Baker Street, London, W1-M 2AJ. Tel: 01-486 4311. The Television Centre, Cutverhouse Cross, Cardiff CF5 6XJ. Tel: Cardiff 590590. Television Centre, Bristol BS4 3HG. Tel: Bristol 778366. Scottish Life House, Bridge St., Manchester, Tel: 061-834 3765.
WALES AND WEST OF ENGLAND TRANSMITTERS
Chairman: G. E. McMatters
Managing Director: R. W. Wordley

Sales Director: C. D. Romaine
Research Executive: I. Platt
Secretary: G. S. Tovey, FCIS, FCA.

LONDON WEEKEND TELEVISION LTD.
South Bank Television Centre, Kent House, Upper Ground, London SE1 9LT. Tel: 01-261 3434.

LONDON TRANSMITTER—Friday 5:15 p.m. to Sunday closedown
Chairman and Managing Director: Brian Tesler
General Manager: Vic Gardiner
Director of Programmes: John Birt
Finance Director: Peter McNally
Sales Director: Ron Miller
Secretary: Judith T. Thomas
Controller Staff Relations: Roy van Gelder
Director of Production: Peter Cazaly
Chief Engineer: Roger Appleton

RADIO TELEFIS EIREANN
Donnybrook Dublin 4, Ireland: Tel: (01) 693111. London Office: Ireland House, 150 New Bond Street, London, W1Y OHD Tel: 01-493 8921 NATIONAL NETWORK OF THE REPUBLIC OF IRELAND.

Chairman: James P. Culliton
Director-General: Vincent Finn
Asst. Director-General: R. K. Gahan
Asst. Director-General: J. P. Sorohan
Director of Public Affairs: D. Holden
Director of Television Programmes: Bob Collins
Director of Radio Programmes: Michael Carroll
Director of News: Weslay Boyd

SCOTTISH TELEVISION, P.L.C.
Cowcaddens, Glasgow, Scotland. Tel: Glasgow 332 9999. Telex 77388.

CENTRAL SCOTLAND TRANSMITTER
Directors: Sir Campbell Fraser LL.D. D. Univ. *(Chairman),* William Brown C.B.E. *(Managing Director and Deputy Chairman),* Sir Kenneth Alexander, LL.D., D. Univ., Gavin Boyd C.B.E., Rev. Robin D. Buchanan-Smith, Ferdinando Coia, Mrs. Dorothy Dunnett, Charles A. Fraser C.V.O., D.L., Hugh W. Henry, David K. Johnstone, Angus J. MacDonald, Alan L. Montgomery.

TELEVISION SOUTH PLC
Television Centre, Southampton SO9 5HZ Tel: 0703 34211. Telex: 477217.
Television Centre, Maidstone ME14 5NZ Tel: 0622 54945

SOUTH & SOUTH-EAST OF ENGLAND TRANSMITTER
Directors: Lord Boston of Faversham QC *(Chairman),* David Quayle, James Gatward *(Chief Executive),* Anthony Brook FCA *(Managing Director, Television),* William Fernie, John Fox *(Director of Sales and Marketing),* Guy Libby, Mrs. Blanche Lucas, Frank Sanderson, Baroness Sharples, Malcolm Truepenny JP *(Director of Production Operations).*

TELEVISION SOUTH WEST LTD.
Derry's Cross, Plymouth, Devon PL1. Tel: 0752 663322.

SOUTH WEST ENGLAND TRANSMITTER
Directors:
Chairman: Sir Brian Bailey OBE
Vice-Chairman: Sir John Colfox DL
Deputy Programme Controller: Rosamund Davies
Director of Programmes: Michael Reinhold BSc
Financial Director: John Roberts, FCA, FCT, MIMC
Managing Director: Harry Turner
Fred Hain
Lt Cdr Douglas Hale, RN (Ret'd)
The Earl of Iddlesleigh
David Johnstone MA FCA
Gareth Keene, MA, LLB
John Peters, MBE
Norman Thompson
Peter Wayne FRTS
Bernard Webster BSc (Eng) C.ENG
FIEE FIERE
Officers:
Company Secretary: Patricia Stewart LLB
Head of News & Current Affairs: Donald Arkins
Head of Presentation & Publicity: David Sunderland, MRTS AMBIM
Director of Engineering: David Jenkin, T.ENG (CEI) MITE
Head of Religious Programmes: John Bartlett
Head of Office Services: Wendy Bowes
Chief Accountant: Michael Boddy, FCMA
Industrial Relations & Training Manager: Eric Kennaugh
Head of New Business: Martin Bowley
Regional Sales Manager—Bristol: Derek Prosser
Programme Planning Officer: Liz Mahoney

THAMES TELEVISION LTD.
Thames Television House, 306-318 Euston Road, London NW1 3BB. Tel: 01-287 9494. Teddington Lock, Teddington, Middlesex TW11 9NT. Tel: 01-977 3252. Norfolk House, Smallbrook Queensway, Birmingham B5 4LF. Tel: 021-643 9151.

LONDON TRANSMITTER
Directors:
H. S. L. Dundas, *(Chairman)*
Richard Dunn, *(Man. Dir.)*
Sir John Read, *(Dep. Chairman)*
Mrs. Mary Baker
Lord Brabourne
David Elstein (Director of Programmes)
R. M. Denny
P. Hayman, H. Moirgue
Ben E. Marr, *(Company Secretary & Director of Personnel)*
J. T. Davey
Derek Hunt, *(Director of Finance)*
Jonathan Shier, *(Sales & Marketing)*
C. S. Wills

THAMES INTERNATIONAL
(Wholly-owned subsidiary for programme sales)
149 Tottenham Court Road, London, W1P 9LL. Tel: 01-387 9494
Managing Director: M. Phillips

TV-am LIMITED
Breakfast Television Centre, Hawley Crescent, London NW1 8EF. Tel: 01-267-5483

Board of Directors:
Chairman: Mr. T. M. Aitken
Managing Director: Mr. B. Gyngell
General Manager: Mr. A. G. Moore
Director of Sales: Mr. A. C. Vickers
Mr. J. Aitken, MP
Mr. A. M. Davies
Mr. D. Frost
Mr. I.A.N. Irvine
The Lord Matthews
Executives:
Company Secretary: Mr. A. Ford
Director of Programmes: Mr. B. Gyngell
Controller, Programmes: Mr. J. McColgan
Controller, News and Current Affairs: Mr. B. Ludford
Financial Controller: Mr. S. Zographos
Company Lawyer: Miss Deborah Fosbrook
Editor, Features: Ms. Kathy Rowan
Controller, Operations: Mr. I. Stuart
Chief Engineer: Mr. C. Collingham
Sales Controller: Mr. P. Bushell
Manager, Press and Publicity: Mr. D. Keighley

TYNE TEES TELEVISION LTD.
Head Office: The Television Centre, City Road, Newcastle upon Tyne, NE1 2AL. Tel: 091-2610181. Middlesbrough Office: Corporation House, Corporation Road, Middlesbrough. Tel: 0642 219181. London Office: 15 Bloomsbury Square, London, WC1A 2LJ. Tel: 01-405 8474.

NORTH EAST TRANSMITTER
Directors:
D. W. Reay (Managing)
R. Eagle
D. S. Hellewell
C. W. Stoddart
A. J. Wonfor
Sir Ralph Carr-Ellison, TD, DL
R. H. Dickinson, MA
D. C. Eccles
Viscount Ridley, TD, DL
G. Oliver Worsley, TD, MA
Prof. Laurence W. Martin, MA, PhD
P. Nicholson, DL, FCA
D. Stevenson, CBE
J. Wilkinson, BA.Com.
G. E. Ward Thomas, CBE, DFC

ULSTER TELEVISION plc
Havelock House, Ormeau Road, Belfast BT7 1EB Tel: 228122. Telex: 74654. London Office: 6 York Street, London, W1H 1FA, Tel: 01-486-5211.

NORTHERN IRELAND TRANSMITTER
Directors: R. B. Henderson, C.B.E., M.A., F.R.T.S., DLitt, *(Chairman);* J. D. Smyth BSc ACA *(Managing);* J. B. McGuckian BSc (Econ.) *(Deputy Chairman);* H. R. C. Catherwood *(Vice Chairman),* Mrs. B. E. MacQuitty BsC (Econ) *(Vice Chairman);* P. C. J. Battle *(Sales);* J. A. Creagh *(Assistant Managing)*; J. B. Waddell *(Programme Controller)*; R. E. Benner, O.B.E.; Lord Dunluce FRSA; Captain O. W. J. Henderson, O.B.E., D.L., F.B.I.M.; G. C. Hutchinson; Mrs. A. B. McCollum, E. J. O'Driscoll.

WALES4CYMRU
Welsh Fourth Channel Authority, Sophia Close, Cardiff

CF19XY Tel: (0222) 43421. Telex: 497146.

YORKSHIRE TELEVISION LTD.
The Television Centre, Leeds, LS3 1JS Tel: 0532 438283 Telex: 557232. Television House, 32 Bedford Row, London, WC1R 4HE Tel: 01-242 1666. Charter Square, Sheffield, S1 4HS Tel: 0742 23262. 185 Ferensway, Hull, HU1 3PH Tel: 0482 24488. 2 Saltergate, Lincoln, LN2 1DH Tel: 0522 30738. 8 Bullring Lane, Grimsby, South Humberside, DN31 1DY Tel: 0472 57026. 88 Baifgate, Lincoln, LN1 3AR. Tel: 0522 30738.

YORKSHIRE TRANSMITTER
Directors: Sir Derek Palmar *(Chairman);* R. L. Fox *(Managing Director);* J. Fairley *(Director of Programmes);* P. R. McKee *(Deputy Managing Director);* G. J. A. Hardy *(Commercial Director);* C. W. Leach *(Sales and Marketing Director);* E. W. Wright *(Director and General Manager);* G. Brotherton-Ratcliffe; Mrs. P. M. David; S. H. Hall; J. G. S. Linacre,, N. G. W. Playne, A. A. Whitaker, F. S. K. Baron.
Executives:
David Cunliffe (Controller, Drama Programmes); John Fairley (Controller, Factual Programmes); V. Lawrence (Controller, Light Entertainment); R. Bairstow (Head of Programme Planning); K. Bellini (Head of Programme Purchasing); F. Cieslik (Contracts Manager); D. Dallas (Head of Science and Features); M. Drury (Head of Casting); B. Harris (Controller of Business Affairs); D. C. Bould (Assistant Commercial Director); R. Charles (Head of Sport and Outside Broadcasts); G. Ironside (Head of Local Programmes); C. Jelley (Head of Education and Religion); J. Q. Rogers (Chief Engineer); P. Rogers (Head of Production Operations); P. Smale (Head of Technical Operations); J. Smith (Head of Programme Administration); G. Brown Lee (Controller of Press and Publicity); D. Stephenson (Regional Sales Manager); M. Thornhill (Labour Relations Officer); C. Jelley (Head of Education and Religion); J. Willis (Editor of Documentaries and Current Affairs); E. Wright (General Manager); R. J. Coyle (Company Secretary).

TV Program Material—Producers and Distributors

ABACUS PRODUCTIONS LTD.
31 Shelton Street, London WC2; Tel: 01-240 1277; Cables: ABAFILMS LONDON.
Directors: John Mackey (Chairman), Ron Trainer (Managing), Betty J. Martin.
Producers of TV and cinema commercials on both film and video. Matte process, stop motion, model animation, own studios, 2 stages, cove, 2 cutting rooms, Preview Theatre. Rostrum techniques, front projection screen.

ADVISION LTD.
23 Gosfield Street, London, W1P 7HB. Tel: 01-580 5707. Telex: 28668.
(Sound recording facilities: music, video and film dubbing, also video editing and digital sound facilities.)

ABC SPORTS INTERNATIONAL INC.
215 Great Portland Street, London, W1N 5HD. Tel: 01-636 7366.

AEROFILMS
Gate Studios, Station Road, Boreham Wood, Herts: WD6 1EJ; Tel: 01-207 0666.

AIR-TIME PRODUCTIONS LTD.
50-Frith Street, London, W.1. Tel: 01-734 9304.
Director: Johnny Fielder.

AML INTERNATIONAL LTD.
6 Goodwins Court, St. Martins Lane, London WC2N 4LL. Tel: 01-836 0576. Cables: AMATEL. Telex: 267664.

JOHN ANDERSON HIRE
Court Lane, Iver, Bucks. Tel: Iver 653737 (production facilities).

ANDERSON BURR PICTURES
Bray Studios, Water Oakley, Windsor, Berks. Tel: 0628 22111 or 01-748 8323.

EAMONN ANDREWS STUDIOS LTD.
Television Club, 46/48 Harcourt Street, Dublin, Ireland. Tel: Dublin, 758891.
Directors: Eamonn Andrews, Dermod Cafferky, Lorlan Bourke. (Tape, disc-recording, filming, Radio & TV programme contractors.)

ANIMALS UNLIMITED
Careys Wood, Smallfield, Surrey: (Animal agency). Tel: 034 284.
(Animal agency.)

ANVIL FILM & RECORDING GROUP LTD.
Denham Studios, North Orbital Rd., Denham, Nr. Uxbridge, Middx. Tel: 0895 833522. Telex: 934704.
Directors: R.I.C.H. Warren (Chairman), R. W. Keen, K. Somerville, C. Eng. MIERE., Peter Gray, G. V. Manolescue, FCA.

ARMADA PRODUCTIONS
86/88 Wardour Street, London WIV 3LF. Tel: 01-734 6312.
Managing Director: J. D. Dooley.

ARTS INTERNATIONAL
32 Ecclestron Square, London, SW1V 1PB. Tel: 01-834 6811.

ATHOS FILM PRODUCTIONS LTD.
Athos House, Cambridge Rd., Hanwell, London, W.7. Tel: 01-579 4301-6. Telex: 28905 Ref. 325.
Directors: P. G. A. Bucknall, The Viscount Portman, D. B. Bucknall, R. Orr-Ewing.
(Production, video and film, 35/16mm cutting rooms, dubbing, recording studios.)

AUDIO INFILMS LTD.
7 Lexington Way, Barnet, Herts. EW5 2SN. Tel: 01-440 4322.

AUSTRALIAN BROADCASTING CORPORATION
54 Portland Place, London, WIN 4DY. Tel: 01-631 4456. Cables: Austcast, London. Telex: 263897 (News) 23494 (Admin.).
Gen. Manager for Europe: K. MacKriell.

AUSTRALIAN FILM COMMISSION
2nd Floor, Victory House, 99-101 Regent Street, London W1. Tel: 01-734 9383. Telex: 28711 Ausfilm. G.

AUTOCUE LTD.
Autocue House, 265 Merton Road, London, S.W.18 5JS. Tel: 01-870 0104. Telex: Autocue Telexir 885039 Autocu G.
Contact: Mick Gould
(Computer & closed circuit prompting facilities for film, TV and conferences; Aston Caption Charactor Generator Hire.)

BBC TELEVISION ENTERPRISES
Woodlands, 80 Wood Lane, London W12 OTT. Tel: 01-743 5588 & 01-576 0202. Cables: Telecentre London, Telex: 934678 & 265781; Overseas Sales Offices: Westfield Towers, 100 Williams Street, Sydney, New South Wales 2011, Australia; Distributors for U.S.A.: Lionheart Television International, 1762 Westwood Boulevard, Los Angeles, CA 90024, U.S.A.
Director of Programme Sales: Roy Gibbs.

BOULTON-HAWKER FILMS LTD.
Hadleigh, Ipswich, Suffolk 1P7 5BG. Tel: 0473 82 2235.
Directors: K. P. Boulton, M. J. Boulton, S. J. Boulton, N. H. L. Rea, D.A. Boulton.

BRENT WALKER FILM & THEATRE DIVISION
Knightsbridge House, 197, Knightsbridge, London SW7 1RB. Tel: 01-225 1941. Telex: 23639.

BRITISH TRANSPORT FILMS
British Railways Board, Audio Visual Services, 222 Marylebone Road, London NW1 6JJ. Tel: 01-262 3232.

CAMERA LOCATION SERVICES
16 St. James Close, St. John's Woking, Surrey. Tel: 04862 4645.
(Researchers, suppliers film and photographic locations.)

CANADIAN BROADCASTING CORPORATION
43-51 Great Tirchfield Street, London, W.1. Tel: 01-580 0336 Telex: 23771.

CARLTON TELEVISION LTD.
St. John's Wood Studios, St. John's Wood Terrace, London, NW8. Tel: 01-722 9255. Telex: 28177
Managing Director: Barry Johnstone

CAVALIER FILMS LTD.
34 Deacon's Hill Road, Elstree, Herts. Tel: 01-953 1403.
Directors: D. T. Rogers, A. V. Kimber.
(Specialized films, documentary, commercials.)

CBS NEWS
100 Brompton Rd., London, S.W.3. Tel: 01-584 3366. Telex: 916 319. Cables: Colnews London.
(News, radio and TV coverage.)

CENTRAL OFFICE OF INFORMATION
Hercules Road, London, SE1 7DU. Tel: 01-261 8495.
Films and Television Division: *Director:* John Hall.
Radio Services: *Head:* Eric Turnbull.

CBS/FOX VIDEO
Perivale Industrial Park, Greenford, Middx. UB6 7RU. Tel: 01-997 2552.

CHATSWORTH TELEVISION
97-99 Dean Street, London, W1V SRA. Tel: 01-734 4302. Telex: 28604 Ref. 890.

ROGER CHERRILL LTD.
65-66 Dean Street, London W1V 6PL. Tel: 01-437 7972.
(Post sync Dialogue, Dubbing and Effects, Film and TV Production, Post Production.)

CHESS VALLEY FILMS LTD.
Film House, Little Chalfont, Bucks: HP7 9PY. Tel: 02-404 2222 and 2020.

Directors: Ronald E. Haddock, F.I.I.P., V. G. Haddock, Heather M. Davies, MBKS.
(Production 35/16mm film broadcast and non-broadcast TV and allied services.)

CHRYSALIS VISUAL PROGRAMMING
12-13 Stratford Place, London, W1N 9AF. Tel: 01-408 2355. Telex: 21753.

CINE-LINGUAL SOUND STUDIOS LTD.
27-29 Berwick Street, London, W1V 3RF. Tel: 01-437 0136.

CINESOUND EFFECTS LIBRARY LTD.
Imperial Studios, Maxwell Road, Elstree Way, Boreham Wood, Herts WD6 IWE. Tel: 01-953 5837 and 5545, 1587, 4904.

(Sound effects.)

CINE VIDEO LTD.
245 Old Marylebone Road, London NW1 5QT. Tel: 01-402 8385.

CINEVISTA LTD.
Suite 4, 3 Bateman Street, London, W.1. Tel: 01-437 7187.

Directors: John Simmons, Cecilia Simmons.
(Entertainment and sponsored material.)

COLOUR FILM SERVICES LTD.
22-5 Portman Close, Baker Street, London, W1H 4BE. Tel: 01-486 2881.

Chairman: Roland Chase.
Managing Director: H. Manley.
(Advertising material.)

COLUMBIA PICTURES TELEVISION
A Division of Columbia Pictures Corporation Ltd. St. Margaret's House, 19/23 Wells Street, London, W1P 3FP. Tel: 01-637 8444. Telex: 263392 COLP1C G. Cables: Columfilm, London.

Vice President, European Production: Tim Vignoles.
Vice President, European Sales: Nicholas Bingham.
(Production and distribution TV film series.)

CRANEZOOM LTD.
28 Saint Mary le Park Court, Albert Bridge Road, London, S.W.11. 4QD. Tel: 01-223 0034.

CROWN INTERNATIONAL PRODUCTIONS PLC.
Crown Television Centre, Church Road, Claygate, Esher, Surrey KT10 0JP. Tel: 0372 69111. Telex: 8811232 GREENS G.

C.T.S. STUDIOS LTD.
The Music Centre, Engineers Way, Wembley, Middx: Tel: 01-903 4611. Telex: 923400.

Contact: Peter Harris.

CTVC
Hillside, Merry Hill Road, Bushey, Watford WD2 1DR. Tel: 01-950 4426.

(Production and postproduction, film and video library hire facilities.)

CUCUMBER STUDIOS LTD.
19/21 Heddon Street, London, W1. Tel: 01-437 0109.

CYGNET LTD.
Bilton Centre, Coronation Road, High Wycombe, Bucks HP12 3TA. Tel: 0494 450541. Telex: 83659 BIGGSC G.

Managing Director: D. N. Plunket.

GODFREY DAVIES PRODUCTIONS LTD.
8-10 Neals Yard, Covent Garden, London, W.C.2. Tel: 01-836 6538.

DE LANE LEA SOUND CENTRE
75 Dean Street, London, W.1. Tel: 01-439 1721.

(Sound Recording, Foreign Version Dubbing, editing facilities.)

DE WOLFE LTD.
80-88 Wardour Street, London, W1V 3LF Tel: 01-439 8481.

Directors: James Sylvester de Wolfe, Gordon Chambers.
(Library record music, original scores.)

DIFFUSION D'INFORMATIONS PAR LE FILM S.A.
Associate of Film Producers Guild Ltd.) 22 Rue de la Corraterie, Geneva, Switzerland.

Directors: N. C. B. Abbott, G. Busby, A. Marks.
(Documentary & industrial films.)

WALT DISNEY PRODUCTIONS LTD.
31–32 Soho Square, London, W1V 6AP. Tel: 01-734 8111. Telex: 21532. FAX 01-4398741.

DORLAND ADVERTISING LTD.
121-141, Westbourne Terrace, London, W.2. Tel: 01-262 5077.

DRAKE AUDIO VISUAL
89 St. Fagans Road, Fairwater, Cardiff CF5 3AE.

Managing Director: R. G. Drake.
Marketing Director: H. Drake.

DRUMMER FILMS LTD.
14 Haywood Close, Pinner HA5 3LQ.

Man. Dir.: Martin M. Harris (Producer).

DUCK LANE FILM PRODUCTIONS LTD.
8 Duck Lane, London, W1V1FL Tel: 01-439 3912. Telex: 25554.

Directors: R. Andrews.

EDUCATIONAL & TELEVISION FILMS LTD.
247a Upper Street, London, N1-1RU. Tel: 01-226 2298.

General Manager: Stanley Forman.

ELEPHANT VIDEO LTD.
15–17 Old Compton Street, London, W1V 6JR. Tel: 01-437 9541. Cables: Eaglepix, London, W.1. Telex: 928152 GALAFI G.

Directors: Barry Jacobs, A. Jacobs.

ENTERTAINMENT IN VIDEO LTD.
60–66 Wardour Street, London W.1. Tel: 01-437 1943. Telex: 27950.

Directors: Michael L. Green, Nigel Green, Trevor H. Green.

EPA INTERNATIONAL PROGRAMMERS LTD.
P.O. Box 228, London SW16 1BP. Tel: 01-677 7523.

EUREKA LOCATION MANAGEMENT
16 Broadwick St., London, W1V 1FH. Tel: 01-734 4100, 734 1787, 734 7451. Telex: 265 871, answerback MONREF G, quoting ref. 76:WJJ 106. Electronic mail—Telecom gold.

Head of Operations: Ian Lloyd

EUSTON FILMS LTD.
365 Euston Road, London, NW1 3AR. Tel: 01-387 0911

Executive Director of Production: Johnny Goodman.

EWART TELEVISION(STUDIO) LTD.
Wandworth Plain, London, SW18 1ET. Tel: 01-874 0131. Cables: Keithewart, London. Telex: 929509.

Managing Director: Keith Ewart.
(Full studio and post production television facility.)

EYELINE FILM AND VIDEO LTD.
77 Dean Street, London, W.1. Tel: 01-734 3391. Telex: 265351.

Directors: Harold Orton, Jacki Roblin, George H. Brown, Alfred Shaughnessy, Gordon Grimward.
(Ent. advertising material.)

FALKMAN FILMS & VIDEO
33 Gresse Street, London, W1P IPN. Tel: 01-636 1371.

Directors: B. Falk, L. Green, C. Thompson.

FIVE CITIES FILMS LTD.
Elite Studios. Toller Lane, Bradford 8. Tel: Bradford 46711/2/3.

Directors: D. Roebuck, S. J. Josephs.
(Commercials advertising and ind. films.)

FLAMINGO FILM PRODUCTIONS
P.O. Box 130, Hove, East Sussex BN3 6QU Tel: 0273 550088. Telex: 877050.

Directors: R. Kruger, J. S. Kruger.
(Producers of feature films, musical video films and advertising material.)

MARK FORSTATER PRODUCTIONS LTD.
42a, Devonshire Close, Portland Place, London, W.I. Tel: 01-631 0611.

FOWLER-CHAPMAN COMPANY LTD.
28 Saint Mary le Park Court, Albert Bridge Road, London, SW11 4QD. Tel: 01-223 0034.

FREMANTLE INTERNATIONAL, INC.
21–22 Poland Street, London, W.1. Tel: 01-437 2673.

President: Paul Talbot.
Chief Executive: Anthony Gwner.
(TV film Distributors.)

JAMES GARRETT & PARTNERS LTD.
25 Bruton Street, London, W1X 7DB. Tel: 499 6452. Telex: 261163. FAX: 408 1797.

Directors: J. L. M. P. Garrett (Chmn.); M. Gilmour (Managing); D. T. Peers (Dep'y. Chmn.); D. T. Cromwell (Prod. Dir.); M. Garrett; F. Bloom.
(Advertising film producers.)

GATEWAY AUDIOVISUAL/VIDEO
470–472 Green Lanes, Palmers Green, London, N. 13 5XF. Tel: 01-882 0177. Telex: 896462.

Directors: G. L. Smart, A.R.P.S., M.B.K.S., A. P. Gillet.
(Industrial, advertising, educational and training films.)

GENERAL SCREEN ENTERPRISES LTD.
Film House, 97 Oxford Road, Uxbridge, Middx. Tel: Uxbridge 31931. Telex: 934883.

Managing Director: Fred Chandler.
Scriptwriters: Tony Hill, Tony Church.
(Main titles, trailers, commercials, opticals, special effects.)

G.H.W. PRODUCTIONS LTD.
52 Queen Anne Street, London, W1M 9LA. Tel: 01-935 1186.

Directors: Peter Rogers, Betty E. Box, O.B.E.; D. G. Truscott.

GLOBAL TELEVISION SERVICES LTD.
159-165, Great Portland Street, London, W1N 6NR. Tel: 01-637 4041.

Directors: Ian R. Warren, T. L. Donald, I. L. Donald.
European Purchasing Agent for programmes for Australian Broadcasting Commission and Broadcasting Corporation of New Zealand. World Distributors for Portman Quintet Productions.

BOB GODFREY FILMS LTD
55 Neal Street, London, W.C.2 Tel: 01-240 1793/1889.

(Animation for television and cinema. Commercials. 16/35 mm camera service.)

GOLDCREST FILMS AND TELEVISION LTD.
180 Wardour Street, London, WIV 3AA. Tel: 01-437 8696. Telex: 267458 Goldcr. FAX: 01-437 4448.

GOLDEN COMMUNICATIONS (OVERSEAS) LTD
47 Greek Street, London, W1V 5LQ. Tel: 01-439 1431.

G.P.A. (FILMS) LTD.
22 Romily Street, London, W.1. Tel: 01-734 6994.

Director: Gerry Poulson.

GRANADA TELEVISION INTERNATIONAL LTD.
36 Golden Square, London, W1R 4AH Tel: 01-734 8080. Telex: 27937; 18 Rue Volney, 75002 Paris, France. Tel: (33 1) 42.61.79.10. Telex: 213008; 1221 Avenue of the Americas, Suite 3468, New York, NY 10020, U.S.A. Tel: (212) 869 8480. Telex: 62454 UW.

Managing Director: Barrie Heads.
(Overseas distributors of TV programmes made by Granada.)

GTO FILMS AND VIDEO INTERNATIONAL LTD.
36 Soho Square, London, W1V 5DG. Tel: 01-734 4334. Telex: 297648 GTO ARL.

ELAINE GREENE LTD.
31, Newington Green, London, N16 9PU. Tel: 01-249 2971.

Directors: Elaine Greene, Ilsa Yardley, Timothy Webb.
(Literary agency.)

GUILD HOME VIDEO
Crown House, 2 Church Street, Walton-on-Thames, Surrey KT12 2QS. Tel: 01-546 3377. Telex: 269651. Fax: 01 546 4568.

HALLIFORD STUDIOS LTD
Manygate Lane, Shepperton, Middx. TW17 9EG: Tel: Walton-on-Thames 226341.

Studio Manager: Allan d'Aguiar.

HAMMER FILM PRODUCTIONS LTD.
EMI Elstree Studios, Boreham, Herts. Tel: 01-953 1600.

Directors: Brian Lawrence, Roy Skeggs.

HAMPDEN GURNEY STUDIOS, LTD.
Hampden Gurney Street, London, W1H 5AL. Tel: 01-402 6255 and 01-258 0106. Cables: Jaksonfilm London W1. Telex: 896559 GECOMS-G.

STEWART HARDY FILMS LTD.
Manor Way, Boreham Wood, Herts. Tel: 01-953 3730/4743.

Director: J. R. Williams.
(Animation, diagram, cartoon films.)

HEMISPHERE PRODUCTIONS LTD.
105 Mount Street, London, W.1. Tel: 01-493 5041.

Managing Director: Barry Levinson (U.S.A.).

HERON HOME ENTERTAINMENT
A Heron International Company. Unit 4, Brunswick Industrial Park Road, New Southgate, London N11 1JL. Tel: 01-368 1226. Telex: (London) 897654LTBEST G.

GERARD HOLDSWORTH PRODUCTIONS LTD.
31 Palace Street, London, SW1E 5HW Tel: 01-828 1671.

Directors: Mary V. Holdsworth, P. H. Filmer-Sankey, Don Kelly.
(Documentaries, TV program material.)

I.F.A. (SCOTLAND) LTD.
1 North Claremont Street, Glasgow, C3. Scotland. Tel: 041-332 3620.

INCA FILMS LTD.
76 Brewer Street, London, W1R 4HU. Tel: 01-437 3877.

Directors: Anne Balfour Fraser, Timothy Burrill, Brian Little, Eric Falk, Frances Cockburn.
(Documentary, Advertising and Entertainment material.)

INDEPENDENT TELEVISION NEWS LTD.
ITN House, 48 Wells Street, London, W1P 4DE Tel: 01-637 2424.

(Production facilities.)

INTERNATIONAL TELEVISION ENTERPRISES LTD
27 Upper Brook Street, London WIY IPD. Tel: 01-491 1441.

INTERVISION VIDEO LTD.
Unit 1, McKay Trading Estate, Kensal Road, London, W10 5BX. Tel: 01-960 8211. Telex: 291877 Vision G.

ITC ENTERTAINMENT LTD.
45 Seymour Street, London, W1A 1AG. Tel: 01-262 8040.

ITN LTD.
ITN House, 48 Wells Street, London, W1P 4DE. Tel: 01-637 2424.

(Colour television film & sound facilities in central London.)

ISLAND PICTURES
22 St. Peter's Square, London W.6. Tel: 01-741 1511.

IVS ENTERPRISES LTD.
54 Warwick Square, London, SW1V 2AJ. Tel: 01-834 6012

BRIAN JACKSON FILMS LTD.
Hampden Gurney Studios. Hampden Gurney Street, London, W1H 5AL. Tel: 01-402 6255 and 01-258 0106. Cables: JAKSONFILM London, W1. Telex: 896559 GECOMS-G.

J & M
9 Clifford Street, London, W.I. Tel: 01-734 2181.

JARAS ENTERTAINMENTS LTD.
21 Cavendish Place, London, W1M 9DL. Tel: 01-580 5927.

CYRIL JENKINS PRODUCTIONS LTD.
7 Coniston Court, Carlton Drive, London SW15 2BZ. Tel: 01-788 2733.

Directors: Cyril G. Jenkins, J. M. Jenkins.
(Entertainment, docomentary and advertising material.)

KADEK VISION LTD.
Shepperton Studios Centre, Post 21, Studios Road, Shepperton, Middlesex, TW17 0QD. Tel: (09328) 66941. Telex: 24887 Vision G.

KRUGER LEISURE ORGANISATION (FILM, VIDEO & TV DISTRIBUTION) LTD.
P.O. Box 130, Hove, East Sussex BN3 6QU. Tel: 0273 550088. Telex: 877050.

Directors: J. S. Kruger, R. Kruger, H. R. Kruger.

KIMPTON WALKER LTD.
47/49 Acre Lane, London. SW2 5Tn. Tel: 01-737 3317. Telex: 27789.
(Theatre, film and television scenery.)

LEE ELECTRIC (LIGHTING) LTD.
128 Wembley Park Drive, Wembley, Middx. Tel: 01-903 9655 and 01-903 9811.

LEE FILTERS LTD.
Central Way, Walworth Industrial Estate, Andover, Hants. SP10 5AN. Tel: 0264-66245. Telex: 477259.

LE VIEN FILMS LTD.
15 Chesterfield Hill, London, W.1. Tel: 01-629 4545 Cables: Vienfilms London, W.1.
Executive Producer: Jack Le Vien.
(TV films and features.)

LIBRA PRODUCTIONS LTD.
Marl Cottage, Mark Cross, Crowborough, Sussex. Tel: Rotherfield 2172/2746.
Directors: Kevin Scott (U.S.A.), Thomas Kyffin.
(Producers of television programmes.)

LIMEHOUSE PRODUCTIONS LTD
Limehouse Studios, Canary Wharf, West India Docks, London E14 9SJ. Tel: 01-987 2090. Telex: 296149.
Group Managing Director: Ian Reed.

LITTLE KING PRODUCTIONS LTD.
13-14 Bateman Street, London, W.1. Tel: 01-437 9611.
Contacts: Dr. Simon C. Nicholas, M.B., B. Chir., Simon Manley-Cooper.
(Medical and Industrial Films for film & video.)

LONDON FILM PRODUCTIONS LTD
44a Floral Street, London WC2E 9DA. Tel: 01-379 3366. Telex: 896805.

LONDON MARKET
33 Southampton Street, London WC2E 7QH. Tel: 01-240 8676.
Contact: Karol Kulik.

LONDON WEEKEND TELEVISION INTERNATIONAL
Seymour Mews House, Semour Mews, Wigmore Street, London, W1H 9PE. Tel: 01-487 3975. Telex: 22872 TV film G.

LORIMAR DISTRIBUTION LTD.
16 Berkeley Street, London, W.1. Tel: 01-493 1566.
Managing Director: Ray Lewis.

LORIMAR-TELEPICTURES INTERNATIONAL LTD.
49 Berkeley Square, Londno, W1X 5Db. Tel: 01-409 1190. Telex: 25153 Lormar G. Fax: 01-629 2064 (2 or 3).
Managing Director: Stuart B. Graber.

MMA PRESENTATIONS LTD.
16 Neal's Yard, Monmouth Street, London, WC2H 9DP. Tel: 01-379 3595.
(Music and jingles, radio and TV producers, scripts, conference organisers.)

MARK I PRODUCTIONS LTD.
Lee International Studios, 128 Wembley Park Drive, Wembley, Middlesex, HA9 8JE. Tel: 01-902 1262.

MECCA LEISURE PRODUCTIONS LTD
76 Southwark Street, London SE1 0PP. Tel: 01-928 2323. Cables: Mecca World, London.

MEDIA RELEASING DISTRIBUTORS LTD.
60–66 Wardour Street, London, W.1. Tel: 01-437 2341. Telex: 943763 CROCOM G(MRD).
Directors: Trevor H. Green, J. Green.

MIRRORVISION
Holborn Circus, London, EC1P 1DQ. Tel: 01-822 3052. Telex: 27286.

THE MOVING PICTURE COMPANY
25 Noel Street, London, W.1. Tel: 01-434 3100. Telex: 27256.
(Production Facilities.)

NBC NEWS WORLDWIDE INC.
8 Bedford Avenue London, WC1. Tel: 01-637 8655.

NATIONAL FILM AND TELEVISION SCHOOL
Beaconsfield Studios, Station Road, Beaconsfield, Bucks. HP9ILG. Tel: 04946 71234.

NATIONAL SCREEN
Studios: 15 Wadsworth Road, Greenford, Middx. UB6 7JN Tel: 01-998 2851. Telex: 934522. London Office: Wedgewood Mews, Greek Street London, W1V 5LE. Tel: 01-437 4851.
Directors: John Mahony, F.C.M.A. (UK, Chairman, Chief Executive), Brian McIlmail (UK), Andrew Milne (UK), Sir James Carreras, K.C.V.O., M.B.E. (UK), Esther Harris, F.B.K.S. (UK), Burton Robbins (USA), Norman Robbins (USA), Robert Gruen (USA).
(Producers and distributors of publicity accessories; trailers, main titles, opticals, special effects and TV commercials.)

RICHARD NEED PRODUCTIONS LTD.
93-95 Wardour Street, London W.1. Tel: 01-437 1782.
Manageing Dierectors: N.C.B. Abbott, G. Busby.
(Commercials.)

NETWORK TELEVISION LTD.
47 Poland Street, London WIV 3DF. Tel: 01-734 0496.

NEW CENTRAL FILM SERVICES LTD.
97-99 Dean Street, London, W.1. Tel.: 01-734 5827-8.
(Editing equipment hire, cutting rooms, production offices, cutting room supplies.)

NICHOLAS CARTOON FILMS LTD.
Maidensgrove, Nr. Henley-on-Thames, Oxon. Tel.: Turville Heath 286.
Directors: D. N. Spargo, P. M. Spargo.
(Cartoon.)

NUMO PRODUCTIONS LTD.
3 Richmond Mews, London, W.1. Tel.: 01-439 4017.

NVC CABLE LTD.
32 Eccleston Square, London, SW1V 1PB. Tel: 01-834 2300. Telex: 893045 NVCG.

ORIGINAL ELECTRIC PICTURE COMPANY
65 Creffield Road, London, W3 9PS. Tel.: 01-993 7189.
Production: Stanley Dubens.
Account Executive: J. M. Drysdale . (Commercials, Documentaries, Video, AV Presentations.)

OVERSEAS FILM AND TELEVISION CENTRE LTD.
Overseas House, 19-23 Ironmonger Row, London, EC1. Tel.: 01-251 2793.
Directors: D. S. Bowden, P. Whale, A. Muscat, K. Minchell, C. G. E. Gover.
(Ent. and adv. producers.)

PADDINGTON AND COMPANY LTD.
22 Crawford Place, London, W.1.
Directors: Michael Bond, Karen Bond, Nicholas Durbridge, Linda Pooley.

DAVID PARADINE PRODUCTIONS LTD.
Breakfast Television Centre, Hawley Crescent, London NW1 8EF. Tel: 01-482 2898. Telex: 27613 TALKIN G. Fax: 01-482 0871.

PARAMOUNT TELEVISION
23 Berkeley House, Hay Hill, London, W.1. Tel.: 01-629 1150.
Managing Director: Peter Cary.
(TV film distributors.)

PAXTON RECORDS
Paxton Music Ltd., Borough Green, Sevenoaks, Kent. Tel.: Borough Green 3261.
(Music library on disc and tapes for films, TV and radio.)

PEARL & DEAN GROUP LTD.
Broadwick House, Broadwick Street, London, W1V 1FP. Tel: 01-434 2200.
Managing Director: Clive Landa.

PETROFILMS UK LTD
8 West Street, London W.C.2. Tel: 01-836 2112.

PIC PRODUCTIONS LTD
98 Wardour Street, London W1. Tel: 01-734 0243. Telex: COMGEN G 21135.
(Production of electronic news service kits; short films, interviews.)

PHOENIX FILMS LTD.
Manor Road, Goring-On-Thames, RG8 9DP. Tel: 04-918 72365.

Directors: B. G. Hanson, M. E. Hanson.
(Live-action, cartoon, stop motion.)

PIZAZZ PICTURESS
30 Berwick StreetLondon, W.1. Tel: 01-439 2681.

Producer: Pamela Dennis.
Directors: Eric Goldberg, Mario Cavalli.

PLATO FILMS LTD.
247A Upper Street, London, N1 IRU. Tel: 01-226 2298.

Managing Director: Stanley Forman.

POLYGRAM FILMS (UK) Ltd.
1 Rockley Road, London, W14 ODL. Tel: 01-743 3474. Telex: 298816.

(Producers, distributors, film and TV material.)

PORTMAN–QUINTET PRODUCTIONS LTD
159–165 Great Portland Street, London, W.I. Tel: 01-437 1164. Cables: Helpful, London, W.I.

RICHARD PRICE TELEVISION ASSOCIATES LTD
Seymour Mews House, Seymour Mews, London WIH 9PE. Tel: 01-935 9000. Fax: 01-487 3975.

PRIMROSE FILM PRODUCTIONS LTD.
61 Regents Park Road, London, N.W.1. Tel: 01-722 7475 and 01-340 9627.

Directors: Louis Hagen, Anne Hagen.
(Animation, live action, children's programmes.)

PRODUCTIONS ASSOCIATES (UK) LTD
The Stable Cottage, Pinewood Studios, Pinewood Road, Iver Heath, Bucks. SLO ONH. Tel: 01-486 9921.

PROSPECT STUDIOS LTD.
High Street, Barnes, London, SW13 9LE. Tel: 01-876 6284-5.

QUADRANT TELEVISION
Surrey House, Sutton, Surrey 5M14QQ Tel: 01-642 0924.

(Production and post-production facilities.)

QUIGLEY PUBLICATIONS
(Subsidiary of Quigley Publishing Co. Inc. of New York) 15 Samuel Road, Langdon Hills, Basildon, Essex. Tel: 0268 417055.

Manager: William Pay

RADIO LUXEMBOURG (LONDON) LTD.
38 Hertford Street, London, W1V 8BA. Tel: 01-493 5961.

Director of Sales and Marketing: Brian Mellor.
(Representatives of European television production group—Societe Internationale de Programmes Pour Telediffusion. British representatives of Radio Tele-Luxembourg.)

RANDOM FILM PRODUCTIONS LTD.
Unit 2, Cornwall Works, Cornwall Avenue, Finchley, London N3 1LD. Tel: 01-349 9155.

Directors: F. G. Woosnam-Mills, M. R. Woosnam-Mills, S.A. Tennant.
(Documentaries and educational.)

RANK ADVERTISING FILMS LTD.
127 Wardour Street, London, W.1. Tel: 01-439 9531.

Managing Director: Douglas Thomas.
Cinema, Video, Indoor and Outdoor Poster Contractors. Producers of Industrial cinema and video films, TV cinema and video commercials.

RANK VIDEO SERVICES LTD.
Phoenix Park, Great West Road, Brentford, Middlesex, TW8 9PL. Tel: 01-568 4311. Telex: 22345.

Managing Director: Nicholas Watkins.

RANK FILM DISTRIBUTORS LTD.
127 Wardour Street, London, WIV 4AD. Tel: 01-437 9020. Telex: 262556.

Managing Director: F. P. Turner.

REDIFFUSION P.L.C.
Carlton House, Lower Regent Street, London, SW1Y 4LS Tel: 01-629 8886.

Chairman: R. M. Denny

RKO PROGRAMMES INTERNATIONAL
19–20 Poland Street, London, WIV 3DD. Tel: 01-437 6808.

THE ROBERT STIGWOOD GROUP LTD.
118/120 Wardour Street, London, W.1. Tel: 01-437 2512. Telex: 264267.

REX ROBERTS STUDIOS LTD.
22, Glasthule Road, Dun Laoghaire, Co. Dublin, Ireland. Tel: Dublin 808305.

(Adv. material.)

SAGITTA PRODUCTIONS LTD.
℅Pamela Gillis Management, 46 Sheldon Avenue, London, N6 4JR. Tel: 01-340 7868.

Managing Director: John Hawkesworth
(TV and film series.)

SAMUELSON GROUP PLC
303-315 Cricklewood Broadway, Edgware Road, London, NW2 6PQ. Tel : 01-452 8090. Cables: Samcine London. Telex: 21430.

Directors: S. Samuelson C.B.E. (Chairman and Chief Executive), M. Samuelson, (Man. Dir.), N. Samuelson.
(Equipment supply.)

SATELLITE TELEVISION PLC
31/36 Foley Street, London w1P 7LB. Tel: 01-636 4077. Telex: 266943.

SCREENTEL ASSOCIATES LTD
1–2 John Princes Street, London, WIM 9HD. Tel: 01-491 4997.

SEVEN SEAS FILMS LTD.
83 Duke Street, Grosvenor Square, London, W.1. Tel: 01-629 0788.

Directors: J. Rayfield, Brian Everett.

THE SINCLAIR FILM COMPANY LTD.
Charton Manor, Farningham, Kent. Tel: 0322 862188

Managing Director: Ian Sinclair.
(Entertainment, documentary and TV films.)

SOUTHBROOK INTERNATIONAL TELEVISION COMAPNY PLC
55 South Audley Street, London, W1Y 5FA. Tel: 01-491 7024. Telex: 298369 CITY.

SOUTHERN TELEVISION LTD
P.O. Box 15, 2–4 New Road, Southampton SO9 7DF. Tel: 0703 28296/229666. Telex: 296149 LIMHSE G.

Managing Director: Frank Copplestone.

SOVEREIGN FILMS LTD.
Charton Manor, Farningham, Kent. Tel: 0322 862188

Directors: Ian Sinclair (Managing), Viscount Throwley.
(Entertainment, documentary, & TV films)

SURVIVAL ANGLIA LTD.
Brook House, Park Lane, London, W.1. Tel: 01-408 2288.

Executive Director: M. A. Hay

SWIFT FILM PRODUCTIONS
1 Wool Road, Wimbledon, London, S.W.20. Tel: 01-946 2040.

Director: T. Peter Hadingham, M.B.K.S.
(Industrial, advertising and documentary & TV 16mm films, filmstrips, AV programmes.)

SWINDON CABLE LTD.
Newcome Drive, Hawksworth Estate, Swindon, SN2 1TU. Tel: 0793 615601.

SYSTEM TWO LTD.
Film and Television Studios, No. 3. Woking Business Park, Albert Drive, Woking, Surrey GU21 SJY. Tel: 04862 27676.

Directors: Laurence R. Greetham, Simon D. Currey, Sue M. Greetham.

TALBOT TELEVISION LTD.
21–22 Poland Street, London, W1V 5AN. Tel: 01-437 2673.

President: Paul Talbot.
Chief Executive: Anthony Gruner.
(TV film distributors.)

TARA LTD.
35 Endell Street, London, W.C.2. Tel: 01-836 0213 and 01-836 9407.
Directors: Jack Saward, Charmian Saward.

TELE-PRODUCTIONS ASSOCIATES.
3rd Floor, 31 Great Queen Street, London, W.C.2. Tel: 01-405 5006.
Managing Director: Marcia Glassman.
(Supplies of artistes, voice-overs, commentators, announcers, personalities.)

TELEVISION INTERNATIONAL ENTERPRISES LIMITED
22 South Audley Street, London WIY GES. Tel: 01-499 9252.

TELEVISION REPORTERS INTERNATIONAL LTD.
THORN EMI Elstree Studios, Borehan Wood, Herts. Tel: 01-953 1600.
Directors: Robert S. Baker, Roger G. Moore, John Goodman.

THAMES TELEVISION INTERNATIONAL
149 Tottenham Court Road, London, W1P 9LL. Tel: 01-387 9494.

TITAN INTERNATIONAL PRODUCTIONS LTD
185A Newmarket Road, Norwich, Norfolk NR4 6AP. Tel: 0603 51139.
Directors: P. Newbrook, E. Newbrook.

TOONDER FILM (IRELAND) LTD.
18 Gardiner Place, Dublin, Ireland. Tel.: Dublin 874101.
(Ent. & advt. material.)

TOWN AND COUNTRY PRODUCTIONS LTD
Parry's Lodge, Threapwood, Malpas, Cheshire, SY14 7AW. Tel: 0948 309.
Directors: J. C. A. Minoprio, C. P. Minoprio.

TRANSATLANTIC FILMS
Albert House, 9 Holland Park, London WII 3TH. Tel: 01-727 0132.

TRANSWORLD INTERNATIONAL
14–15 Fitzhardinge Street, London, W1H 9PL. Tel: 01-486 9171. Fax: 01-935 5820.

TRIANGLE FILM PRODUCTIONS LTD.
15 Oslo Court, Prince Albert Road, London, N.W.8 Tel: 01-722 5656. Cables: Triphilms London N.W.8. Telex: 885493 WINBNK.

TRIBUNE PRODUCTIONS LTD.
THORN EMI Elstree Studios, Boreham Wood, Herts. Tel: 01-953 1600.
Directors: Robert S. Baker, A. Bailer, M. G. Mahoney, G. S. Barnett.

TRICKFILM STUDIOS LTD.
13 Charlotte Mews, London W.1. Tel: 01-580 0183.

TRILION VIDEO LTD.
36-44 Brewer Street, London, W.1. Tel: 01-439 4177.
Managing Director: Bill Hope.

TRIUMPH FILMS INC.
10 Blomfield Villas, London, W.2. Tel: 01-286 1711.
Director: Peter Hanmer.
(Producers of advertising film and shorts.)

TWICKENHAM FILM STUDIOS LTD.
Twickenham Studios, The Barons, St. Margarets, Twickenham, Middlesex. Tel: 01-892 4477.
Directors: G. Coen, G. Humphreys, M. Landserger, S. J. Mullens
Secretary: M. Darby

TYBURN PRODUCTION LTD.
Pinewood Studios, Iver Heath, Bucks. Tel: IVER 651700. Telex: 847505.
Directors: Kevin Francis, Gillian Garrow, M. J. Freeth, J. W. Malins, F.C.A.
Executive Producer: Kevin Francis
Head of Research & Development: Gillian Garrow
Music Supervisor: Philip Markell
(Producers and distributors of TV and home video programming).

UNICORN PICTURES LTD.
Suite 4, 3 Bateman Street, London, W.1. Tel: 01-437 7187.
Director: John Simmons.

UNITED VIDEO INTERNATIONAL
54 Warwick Square, London, SW1V 2AJ. Tel: 01-834 6012.

UNIVERSAL PICTURES LTD.
139 Picadilly, London, W1V 9FH. Tel: 01-629 7211.

VIRGIN VISION LTD.
328 Kensal Road, London, W10 5XJ. Tel: 01-968 8888. Telex: 892890 VIRGIN G. Fax: 01-968 8537.

VISCOM PRODUCTION LTD.
25-27 Farringdon Road, London, EUM 3HA. Tel: 01-404 5041. Telegraphic Address: Agavision London, W1. Telex: 24474 VISCOM G.
Directors: D. Kinglsey (chmn.), Patrick F. Friesner, Geoffrey J. Reeve, I. P. M. Phillips.
(Int. visual communications.)

VIKING FILMS LTD.
6A Rodway Road, Roehampton, London, SW15 5DS. Tel: 01-789 1532.
(Set construction facilities.)

VIEWSPORT LTD
21 Cavendish Place, London W1M 9DL. Tel: 01-580 5927.
Managing Director: Jarvis Astaire.

VISNEWS LTD.
Cumberland Avenue, London, NW10 7EH. Tel: 01-965 7733.
General Manager: Peter Marshall.
Company Secretary/Financial Controller: Barry MacDonald.
NEWS DIVISION:
Head of News: Tom Hudson.
Head of Broadcast Facilities: Chris Laid.

VISUAL PROGRAMME SYSTEMS LTD.
%S. B. Gilinsky & Co. 2 Promenade Chambers, Edgwarebury Lane, Edgware, Middlesex, HA8 7J2. Tel: 01-958 8236

VOICE OF LONDON LTD.
245 Old Marylebone Road, London, NW1 5RT. Tel: 01-402 8385.
Studio Manager: Miss Pat Smith.
(Studio facilities.)

WARNER BROS. TELEVISION LTD.
Warner House, Pinewood Studios, Iver Heath, Bucks. Tel: Iver 654 545.

WATERLOO PRODUCTIONS
1 Lower James Street, London, W.1. Tel: 01-734 8311.

JOSEF WEINBERGER LTD.
12–14 Mortimer Street, London, W1N 8EL. Tel: 01-580 2827.
(Representing Telemusic Library, France.)

RICHARD WILLIAMS ANIMATION LTD.
London Studio: 13 Soho Square, London, W1V 5FB. Tel: 01-437 4455. Cables: Animfilm, London W1V 5FB. Telex: 299556 Anfilm G. Hollywood Studio: 3193 Cahuenga Boulevard West Hollywood, CA 90068, U.S.A. Tel: (213) 851-8060.
Director: Richard Williams.

WORLD AUDIOVISUAL ENTERTAINMENT PLC
18 Great Marlborough Street, London, W1V 1AF. Tel: 01-439 9598. Telex: 264036 WAVE G.

WORLDMARK PRODUCTIONS LTD.
18 Middle Row, London W10 5AT. Tel: 01-960 3251. Telex: 946240 Cweasy G. (Reply ref. 19017530).
Directors: Tony Maylam, Drummond Challis.

WORLD MIRROR PRODUCTIONS LTD.
Denham Studios, North Orbitel Rd., Denham, Uxbridge, Middx. Tel: Denham 833522.
Managing Directors: Ken Cameron, R. I. C. H. Warren.
(Documentaries, travelogues.)

WORLD WIDE TELEVISION FILM SERVICES LTD.
21–25, St. Anne's Court, London, W1V 3AW. Tel: 01-434 1121.
Directors: C. Parris, P. Gilpin, Lord Willis, R. Aylott, F.C.A., R. King.

WORLDWIDE TELEVISION NEWS
WTN House, 31–36 Foley Street, London W1P 7LB. Tel: 01-323 3255. Telex: 23915; 1926 Broadway, New York, NY 10023, U.S.A. Tel: (212) 787-0842. Telex: 237853.

(Five daily satellite news services covering Europe, Atlantic and Pacific; weekly hour-long compilation of world news; weekly one-hour news feature service; world sports cassette service; comprehensive world news archives; broadcasting facilities centre; camera crew hire worldwide; special shooting and commercial productions.)

WYATT CATTANEO PRODUCTIONS LTD.
22 Charing Cross Rd., London, W.C.2. Tel; 01-379 6444.

SONNY ZAHL ASSOCIATES LTD.
57 Great Cumberland Place, London, W1H 7LJ. Tel: 01-724 3684 and 723 5699.

ZOOM PRODUCTION COMPANY
102 Dean Street, London, W1V 5RA. Tel: 01-434 3895. Fax: 01-734 2751.

Services for TV Producers

CAMERAS—ACCESSORIES FILM STOCK—TELE-CINE—VIDEO AND EDITING EQUIPMENT

ACMADE INTERNATIONAL
Oakside, (Division of Oakside International Holdings Ltd.), Oxford Road, Uxbridge, Middlesex. Tel: Uxbridge 36313. Telex: 8954606.

ADVANCED VIDEO HIRE LTD
51 The Cut, London, SE1 8LF. Tel: 01-928 1963. Telex: 8813278.

AGFA-GEVAERT LTD.
Great West Road, Brentford, Middlesex. Tel: 01-560 2131.

AMPEX GREAT BRITAIN LTD.
Acre Road, Reading, Berks. Tel: 0734 875200.

AUTOCUE LTD.
265 Merton Road, London. S.W.18 5JS. Tel: 01-870 0104. Telex: Autocue Telexir 885039 Autocu G.

F. W. O. BAUCH LTD.
49 Theobald Street, Boreham Wood, Herts. Tel: 01-953 0091. Telex: 27502. Cables: Bauch Borehamwood.

R. R. BEARD LTD.
f10 Trafalgar Avenue, London, SE15 6NR. Tel: 01-703 3136 and 9638.

BELL & HOWELL LTD.
Alperton House, Bridgewater Road, Wembley, Middlesex, HA0 1EG. Tel: 01-902 8812.

CINESOUND INTERNATIONAL LTD.
Imperial Studios, Maxwell Road, Boreham Wood, Herts. LWD6 1WE. Tel: 01-953 5387.

CINETECHNIC LTD.
169 Oldfield Lane, Greenford, Middlesex. Tel: 01-578 1011; and 35 Briardale Gardens, London, NW3 7PN. Tel: 01-435 2289.

JOE DUNTON CAMERAS LTD.
128 Wembley Park Drive, Wembley, Middlesex, HA9 8JE. Tel: 01-903 7933. Telex: 291843.

EDRIC AUDIO VISUAL LTD.
34-36 Oak End Way, Gerrard's Cross, Bucks. Tel: (02813) 84646/7/8.

ENGLISH ELECTRIC VALVE COMPANY LTD.
Waterhouse Lane, Chelmsford, Essex. Tel: 0245-61777. Telegrams: Enelectico, Chelmsford. Telex: 99103.

EVERSHED POWER-OPTICS LTD.
Bridge Wharf, Bridge Road, Chertsey, Surrey KT16 8LJ. (STD 09328) 61181, Telex: 929945 Epochy G. Cable: Lenservo Chertsey.

FRANSCOPE
Grove House, 551 London Road, Isleworth, Middx. TW7 4DS. Tel: 01-568 0131. Telex: 935054.

FUJI PHOTO FILM (UK) LTD.
Fuji Film House, 125 Finchley Road, London NW3 6JH. Tel: 01-586 5900, (Med. X-Ray Division 01-586 931) Telex: 8812995.

HAYDEN LABORATORIES LTD.
Hayden House, Chiltem Hill, Chalfront St. Peter, Gerrards Cross, Bucks. SL9 9EW. Tel: 02-813 88447/89221.

INTERNATIONAL VIDEO CORPORATION
10 Portman Road, Reading, Berkshire. RG3 1JR. Tel: 0734 585421. Telex: 847579.

ITN LTD.
ITN House, 48 Wells Street, London, W1P 4DE. Tel: 01-637 2424.

KEM ELECTRONIC LTD
24 Vivian Avenue, Hendon Central, London, NW4 3XP. Tel: 01-202 0244. Telex: 28303.

H. A. KINGSTON
34 Charlotte Street, London, W.1. Tel: Museum 5308.

K. G. M. VIDIAIDS LTD.
Clock Tower Road, Isleworth, Midd. Tel: 01-568 0151.

KODAK LTD. Motion Picture and Television Division
P.O. Box 66, Kodak House, Station Road, Hemel Hempstead, Herts. HP1 1JU. Tel: Hemel Hempstead 62331 (0442).

LEEVERS RICH EQUIPMENT LTD.
319 Trinity Road, London, SW18 3SL. Tel: 01-874 9054. Telex: 923455. Cables: Leemag. London.

LEE ELECTRIC (LIGHTING) LTD.
85 Barby Road, London W10 5HH. Tel: 01-969 2454. Telex: 924743.

LIPSNER-SMITH CO. LTD.
Unit 7, Longbridge Way, Cowley Mill Trading Estate, Uxbridge, UB8 2YG. Tel: Uxbridge 52191.

MARCONI COMMUNICATION SYSTEMS LTD.
Marconi House, Chelmsford, Essex, CM1 1PL. Tel: (0245) 353221.

ERNEST F. MOY LTD.
Unit 5, Brunswick Park Ind. Est., New Southgate, London, N11 1JF. Tel: 01-361 1211. Telegraphic Address: Movedor, London, N11.

NEILSON-HORDELL LTD.
Unit 11, Central Trading Estate, Staines, Middx. TW18 4UU. Tel: 0784 56456 and 54105.

FREDERICK G. PALMER LTD.
40 Frith Street, London, W.1 Tel: Gerrard 4796.

PHOTOGRAPHIC ELECTRICAL CO. LTD.
71, Dean Street, London, W1V 6 DE. Tel: 01-437 4633/4. Cables: Photoelect London. Telex: 25554.

PYE TELECOMMUNICATIONS LTD.
9 Priestley Way, Eldonwall Estate, Edgware Road, London, NW2 7AF. Tel: 01-452 6411. Head Office: St. Andrews Road, Cambridge. Tel: 0223 61222.

RANK AUDIO VISUAL LTD.
P.O. Box 70, Great West Road, Brentford, Middlesex, TW8 9HR. Tel: 01-568 9222. Telex: 27976.
Managing Director: Ronald Sharp.

RANK CINTEL
Watton Road, Ware, Herts. Tel: Ware 3939. Telex: 81415.
Managing Director: Chris Waldron.

RANK TAYLOR HOBSON
P.O. Box 36, 1 New Star Road, Thurmaston Lane, Leicester LE4 7JQ. Tel: 0533 763-771. Telex: 342338.
Managing Director: William Ramdsen.

RANK STRAND
P.O. Box 70, Great West Road, Brentford, Middlesex, TW8 9HR. Tel: 01-568 9222.

RCA LTD.
Lincoln Way, Windmill Road, Sunbury-on-Thames, Middlesex. Tel: Sunbury 85511. Telex: 27976.
Managing Director: Michael Lowe.

PHILIP RIGBY & SONS LTD.
14 Creighton Avenue, Muswell Hill, London, N10 1NU. Tel: 01-883 3703.

RONFORD-BAKER
Braziers, Oxhey Lane, Watford, Herts. WD1 4RJ. Tel: 01-428 5941.

RONFORD LTD.
Shepperton Studio Centre, Shepperton, Middx. TW17 0QD. Tel: Chertsey (09328) 64111/61423.

SAMUELSON GROUP PLC
303-315 Cricklewood Broadway, London, NW2 6PQ. Tel: 01-452 8090. Cables: Samcine London. Telex: 21430.

SHURE ELECTRONICS LTD.
Eccleston Road, Maidstone, Kent, ME15 6AU. Tel: 0622 59881.

TECHNOVISION CAMERAS LTD.
Unit 4, St. Margaret's Business Centre, Moore Mead Road, St. Margaret's, Twickenham, Middlesex. Tel: 01-891 5961. Telex: 917408 TECNOV G.

THORN EMI LTD.
Thorn House, Upper St. Martins Lane, London, WC2H 9ED. Tel: 01-836 2444.

W. VINTEN LTD.
Western Way, Bury St. Edmunds, Suffolk, IP33 3TB. Tel: Bury St. Edmunds 2121.

WESTAR SALES & SERVICES LTD.
Unit 1, Fairway Drive, Bilton Fairway Industrial Estate, Greenford, Middx. UB6 8PW Tel: 01-578 0957.

FILM & MUSIC LIBRARIES

ABBEY ROAD STUDIOS
3 Abbey Road, London NW8. Tel: 01-286 1161.

ACME FILM PRODUCTIONS LTD.
174 Wardour Street, London, W1V 3AB. Tel: 01-437 1572/1889.

BOOSEY & HAWKES MUSIC PUBLISHERS LIMITED
295 Regent Street, London, W1R 8JH. Tel: 01-580 2060. Telex: 8954613 Boosey G.

BOURNE MUSIC LTD.
34/36 Maddox Street, London, W1R 9PD. Tel: 01-493 6412 and 6583.

BRENT LABORATORIES LTD.
North Circular Road, Cricklewood, London, N.W.2. Tel: 01-452 4271.

C.T.S. STUDIOS LTD.
THE MUSIC CENTRE
Engineers Way, Wembley, Middlesex. Tel: 01-903 4611. Telex: 923400.

DE WOLFE LTD.
80-88 Wardour Street, London, W1V 3LF. Tel: 437 4933-4.

EMI MUSIC PUBLISHING CO. LTD.
138 Charing Cross Road, London, WC2HOLD. Tel: 01-836 6699.

FILM BOOKING OFFICES, LTD.
(Film Library Ltd.)
174 Wardour Street, London, W1V 3AB. Tel: 01-437 1572.

HARMONIC MUSIC LIBRARY LTD.
332a Regents Park Road, London, N3 2LN Tel: 01-349 4521.

ITN LTD.
ITN House, 48 Wells Street, London, W1P 4DE. Tel: 01-637 2424.

MOZART EDITION (GREAT BRITAIN) LTD.
Greenhill House, 90/93 Cowcross Street, London, E4M 6BH. Tel: 01-253 0949.

THE MUSIC CENTRE
Engineers Way, Wembley, Middlesex. Tel: 01-903 4611.

W. PAXTON & CO. LTD.
Paxton Music Ltd., Borough Green, Sevenoaks, Kent. Tel: Borough Green 3261.

PEER INTERNATIONAL LIBRARY LTD.
8 Denmark Street, London, WC2H 8LT. Tel: 01-836 4524.

PORTLAND RECORDING STUDIOS LTD.
35 Portland Place, London, W1N 3AG. Tel: 01-637 2111/4.

SOUTHERN LIBRARY OF RECORDED MUSIC LTD.
8 Denmark Street, London, WC2H 8LT. Tel: 01-836 4524.

STUDIO FILM VIDEO LABORATORIES LTD.
8-14 Meard Street, London, W.1. Tel: 437-0831.

JOSEF WEINBERGER LTD.
12-14 Mortimer Street, London, W1N 8EL. Tel: 01-580 2827.
(Representing Telemusic Library, France.)

LABORATORIES

BRENT LABORATORIES LTD.
North Circular Road, Cricklewood, London, NW2 7AT. Tel: 01-452 4271.

BUCK FILM & VIDEO LABORATORIES LTD.
Banbury Avenue, Slough, Berks. SL1 4LH. Tel: 0753 76611. Telex. 848393. BUCLAB G; and 89–91 Wardour Street, London, W1V 4EP. Tel: 01-437 5548.

COLOUR FILM SERVICES LTD.
22-25 Portman Close, Baker Street, London, W1A 4BE. Tel: 01-486 2881. Telex. 24672.

FILMATIC LABORATORIES LTD.
16 Colville Road, London, W11 2BS. Tel: 01-221 6081. Telex: 295046 FILMAT-G.

ITN LTD.
ITN House, 48 Wells Street, London, W1P 4DE. Tel: 01-637 2424.

HALLIFORD STUDIOS
Manygate Lane, Shepperton, Middlesex. Tel: Walton-on-Thames 26341. Cables: Hallifilms.

KAY/MGM LABORATORIES LTD.
22 Soho Square, London, W.1. Tel: 01-437-7811. Telex: 28463; 91/95 Gillespie Road, Highbury, London, N.5. Tel: 01-226 4422. Telex: 28463.
Managing Director: B. E. Compton.

KINGLY STUDIOS LTD.
17 Kingley Court, Kingley Street, London, W.1. Tel: Gerrard 6372.

LEE INTERNATIONAL FILM STUDIOS LTD.
128 Wembley Park Drive, Wembley, Middlesex. Tel: 01-902 1262.

LEEVERS-RICH & CO. LTD.
80/82 Wardour Street, London, W1V 3LF. Tel: 01-437 4161.

MORENO SOUND STUDIOS
35 Broadhurst Gardens, Hampstead, London, N.W.6. Tel: Maida Vale 1841.

PINEWOOD STUDIOS
Iver Heath, Bucks. Tel: Iver 651700. Telex: 847505 PINE W G. Cables: PINEWOOD Iver Heath.

PORTLAND RECORDING STUDIOS LTD.
35 Portland Place, London, W1N 3AG. Tel: 01-637 2111/4.

RANK FILM LABORATORIES LTD.
Denham, Uxbridge, Middx. UB9 5HQ. Tel: Denham (0895) 832323. Telex: 934704.
Managing Director: J.W. Downer.
Sales Controller: M.A. Levy.

RCA LTD.
Lincoln Way, Windmill Road, Sunbury-on-Thames, Middlesex. Tel: Sunbury 85511.

SAMUELSON FILM SERVICE LTD.
303-315 Cricklewood Broadway, London, N.W.2. 6PQ. Tel: 01-452 8090.

STUDIO FILM & VIDEO LABORATORIES LTD.
8-14 Meard Street, London, W1V 3HR. Tel: 01-437 0831.

TECHNICOLOR LTD.
P.O. Box 7, Bath Road, West Drayton, Middx. UB7 0DB. Tel: 01-759 5432. Fax: 01-897 2666.

TWICKENHAM FILM STUDIOS, LTD.
St. Margarets, Twickenham, Middlesex. TW1 2AW. Tel: 01-892 4477. Telex: 8814497.

UNITED MOTION PICTURES (LONDON) LTD.
3 and 36/38 Fitzroy Square, London, W.1. Tel: 01-580 1171 and 01-388 1234.

WORLD WIDE RECORDING STUDIOS
21-25, St. Anne's Court, London, W1V 3AW. Tel: 01-434 1121.

MARKET RESEARCH

BRITISH MARKET RESEARCH BUREAU LTD.

Saunders House, 53 The Mall, London, W.5. Tel: 01-567 3060.

EXCHANGE TELEGRAPH COMPANY LTD. (THE)
Extel House, East Harding Street, London, E.C.4. Tel: 01-353 1080.

MASS-OBSERVATION LTD.
229-243 Shepherds Bush Road, London, W.6. Tel: 01-748 9172.

MOTION PICTURE RESEARCH
Barnaby House, 19 Rathbone Street, London, W1P 1AF. Tel: 01-636 6128.

RESEARCH SERVICES LTD.
St. Martin's House, 110 St. Martin's Lane, London, WC2N. Tel: 01-240-2450. Telex. 21914.

TELLEX MONITORS LTD.
47 Gray's Inn Road, London, WUX 8PR. Tel: 01-405 7151.

RECORDING STUDIOS

ADVISION SOUND STUDIOS
23 Gosfield Street, London, W1P 7HB. Tel: 01-580 5707. Telex: 28668.

AIR STUDIOS
214 Oxford Street, London, W.1. Tel: 01-637 2758.

EAMONN ANDREWS STUDIOS LTD.
The Television Club, 46/48, Harcourt Street, Dublin, Ireland. Tel: Dublin 758891.

ANVIL FILM & RECORDING GROUP LTD.
Denham Studios, North Orbital Road, Denham, Bucks. Tel: 0895 833522. Telex: 934704.

AUDIO INTERNATIONAL RECORDING STUDIOS LTD.
18 Rodmarton Street, London, W1H 3FW. Tel: 01-486 6466.

BRENT LABORATORIES LTD.
North Circular Road, Cricklewood, London, N.W.2. 7AT. Tel: 01-452 4271.

CBS RECORDING STUDIOS
CBS Records. 31–37 Whitfield Street, London, W1P 5RE. Tel: 01-636 3434.

CINESOUND EFFECTS LIBRARY LTD.
Imperial Studios, Maxwell Road, Elstree Way, Boreham Wood, Herts, WD6 IWE. Tel: Elstree 5837 and 5545, 4904, 1587.

CLARENCE STUDIOS LTD.
7 College Approach, Greenwich, London, S.E. 109HY Tel: 01-858 3798 and 4910.

COLOUR FILM SERVICES LTD.
22–25 Portman Close, Baker Street, London, W1A 4BE. Tel: 01-486 2881.

C.T.S. STUDIOS LTD.
The Music Centre, Engineer's Way, Wembley, Middlesex. Tel: 01-903 4611. Telex: 923400.

DELTA SOUND SERVICES LTD.
Shepperton Studio Centre, Squires Bridge Road, Shepperton, Middx. TW17 0QD. Tel: Chertsey 62045/46.

ELSTREE STUDIOS LTD.
Boreham Wood, Herts. Tel: 01-953 1600. Telegrams: Emifilms, Boreham Wood. Telex: 922436 EFILMS G. Fax 01-207 0860.

MUSIC CENTRE SOUND STUDIOS
(C.T.S. STUDIOS LTD. and DE LANE LEA MUSIC LTD.) Engineers Way, Wembley, Middlesex. Tel: 01-903 4611. Telex: 923400.

NATIONAL SCREEN
15 Wadsworth Road, Greenford, Middlesex. Tel: 01-998-2851; 2. Wedgwood Mews, 12-13 Greek Street, London, W1V 5LE. Tel: 01-437 4851-6. Telex: 934522.

NEW CENTRAL FILM SERVICES LTD.
97–99 Dean Street, London W.1. Tel: 01-734 5827-8.

PORTLAND RECORDING STUDIOS LTD.
35 Portland Place, London, W1N 3AG Tel: 01-637 2111.

RANK FILM LABORATORIES LTD.
Denham, Uxbridge, Middlesex, UB9 5HQ. Tel: Denham (0895) 832323.

Managing Director: J. W. Downer.
Sales Controller: M. A. Levy.

STUDIO FILM & VIDEO LABORATORIES LTD.
8–12 Meard Street, London, W.1. Tel: 01-437 0831.

UNITED MOTION PICTURES (LONDON) LTD.
Boston House, 36/38 Fitzroy Square, London, W.1. Tel: 01-580 1171.

W.F.S. (FILM FACILITIES) LTD.
153 Wardour Street, London, W1V 3TB. Tel: 01-437 5532.

PRODUCTION SERVICES

AKA FILM SERVICES LTD.
60 Farringdon Road, London EC1R 3BP. Tel: 01-251 3885

ATLANTIS FILMS
36 Railwayside, Barnes, London SW13. Tel: 01-878 3766.

BARRY WESTWOOD LIMITED
206 West Street, Fareham, Hants., PO16 0HF. Tel: 0329-285941.

BENEDICT LINDAND LTD
1–2 Newman Passage, London W.1. Tel: 10-637 7808 & 01-580 6266. Telex: 23565 Chance G.

CAMERA EFFECTS
8–11 Bateman Street, London W.1. Tel: 01-437 9377.

CAPWORTH POST PRODUCTIONS LTD.
Lorrimer House, 47 Dean Street, London W.1. Tel: 01-437 3123.

CHERRILL, ROGER LTD.
65–66 Dean Street, London, W1V 5HD. Tel: 01-437 7972.

CINEBUILD LTD.
1 Wheatsheaf Hall, Wheatsheaf Lane, London S.W.8. Tel: 01-582 8750. Telex: 943763 Crocom G Cinebuild.

CINEFOCUS LTD
44 Mountfield Road, Ealing, London W.5. Tel: 01-997 2236 and 01-997 5835.

(Full crewing facilities, including transport.)

CINEVIDEO LTD.
Marylebone Cine Tape Studios, 245 Old Marylebone Road, London, NW1 5QT. Tel: 01-402 8385. Cable: Filmprod London.

CLAPP, NIKKI
56 Chertsey Road, St. Margarets, Twickenham, Middlesex. Tel: 01-891 0054.

Languages: Greek, Italian & French.

COMBINED PRINTS & PRODUCTION SERVICE LTD.
65–66 Dean Street, London, W1V 5HD. Tel: 01-437 7972.

CROW FILM & TV SERVICES LTD.
123 Askew Road, London, W12 9AU. Tel: 01-749 7271.

DEE & COMPANY
46 Potters Lane, New Barnet, Herts., EN5 5BE. Tel: 01-449 7553.

EDINBURGH FILM STUDIOS
Nine Mile Burn, by Penicuik, Midlothian, EH 26 9LX, Scotland. Tel: Penicuik 72131.

EDIT 142
1st Floor, 151–153 Wardour Street, London W.1. Tel: 01-439 7934.

FILM PRODUCTION SERVICES
"Shortend", 82 Holywell Road, Studham, Nr. Dunstable, Beds. Tel: 0582 873107.

FOCUS FILMS (LEEDS) LTD.
281 Meanwood Road, Leeds, LS7 2JR. Tel: 0532-625267.

GAZELLE FILM PRODUCTIONS LTD.
IPA House, Orange Street, Bristol, BS2 9HG. Tel: 421214/5.

GENERAL SCREEN ENTERPRIZES LTD.
97 Oxford Road, Uxbridge, Middlesex. Tel: 89-31931.

GODFREY DAVIES PRODUCTIONS LTD.
19 Calthorpe Road, Edgbaston, Birmingham, B15 1RP. Tel: 021-455 0818.

GOULD, MARTYN PRODUCTIONS
63 Dean Street, London, W1V 5HG. Tel: 01-734 0688. Telex: 22775.

KAUFMAN, MIKE (POST PRODUCTIONS) LTD.
80–82 Wardour Street, London, W1V 3LF. Tel: 01-734 8335. Telex: 264864 Answerback MKPPLN G.

LOUIS ELMAN + LEAH INTERNATIONAL PRODUCTIONS LTD.
Denham Studios, Denham, Nr. Uxbridge, Middlesex. Tel 0895 833036 & 853522. Telex: 934704.

MAGPIE FILM PRODUCTIONS LTD.
22 Bodenham Road, Northfield, Birmingham, B31 5DP, West Midlands. Tel: 021-475 6666 & 021-471 1396.

MARALL SMITH FILMS
15a The Mall, London, W5 2PJ. Tel: 01-567 9032/9065.

MERCURY PRODUCTION OFFICES
Tel: 01-734 5000 (Single Offices or Suites in Wardour Street, London).

MILLS, PETER FILM EDITING LTD.
75 Dean Street, London, W1V 5HA. Tel: 01-437 3003 & 01-439 1721.

NAP LTD.
22 Tavistock Street, London, W.C.2. Tel: 01-836 7608.

NORWOOD STUDIOS LTD.
147 Victoria Road, Leeds, LS6 1DU. Tel: 0532-787539.
(For rushes—35mm and 16mm optical and mags.)

N S & H CREATIVE PARTNERSHIP
13 John Street, London, W.C.1. Tel: 01-405 2324.

PEERLESS CAMERA CO.
15 Neals Yard, London, WC2H 9DP. Tel: 01-836 3367.

PLATYPUS FILMS LTD.
9 Grape Street, London, WC2H 8DR. Tel: 01-240 0351. See display advertisement.

POST HOUSE (POST PRODUCTIONS) LTD.
12 D'Arblay Street, London, W1V 3FP. Tel: 01-439 1705/6/7.

PRATER AUDIO VISUAL
139 Greenwich High Road, London S.E.10. Tel: 01-858 5715/3435.

RANK VIDEO SERVICES LTD.
Phoenix Park, Great West Road, Brentford, Middlesex, TW8 9PL. Tel: 01-568 4311. Telex: 22345.
Managing Director: Nicholas Watkins.

SAMUELSON GROUP PLC
303–315 Cricklewood Broadway, London, NW2 6PQ. Tel: 01-452 8090. Telex: 21430 Cables Samcine, London.

SIDHARTHA FILMS
Calton Studios, 24 Calton Road, Edinburgh, 3H8 8DP Scotland. Tel: 031-556 6218.

SOLUS ENTERPRISES
85 Marshall Street, London, W1V 1LL. Tel: 01-734 0645.

TABS
63 Stirling Court, Marshall Street, London W.1. Tel: 01-734 3356/7
EC: Janet Easton
(Specialities: Technicians answering and booking service.)

TATOOIST INTERNATIONAL LTD.
9 Lyme Steet, London N.W.1. Tel: 01-267 0242.

TELEVISUAL LTD.
58 Kew Road, Richmond, Surrey, TW9 2PQ. Tel: 01-940 8855.

THORN EMI VIDEO FACILITIES
39–45, Tohenham Court Road, London, W.1. Tel: 01-636 7694.

VISNEWS LIMITED
Cumberland Avenue, London, NW10 7EH. Tel: 01-965 7733. Telex: 22678 Cables Visnews, London.
(International production services supported by World-wide Communications Network).

WSTV PRODUCTION LTD.
159–163 Great Portland Street, London, W1N 5FD. Tel: 01-323 1144/8.
(Video tape production, TV cmml.)

WETFORD FILMS LTD.
Wetford Lodge, 163 Nightingale Lane, London S.W.12. Tel: 01-675 1333.

WOLFF PRODUCTIONS
6a Noel Street, London, W1V 3RB. Tel: 01-439 1838.

WOOD, PATRICK FILM SERVICES
13 South Road, Amersham, Bucks. Tel: 02403-4941.

TITLING—SPECIAL EFFECTS

BRENT LABORATORIES LTD.
North Circular Road, Cricklewood, London, N.W.2 7AT. Tel: 01-452 4271.

CINE-SOUND EFFECTS LTD.
(Soundefex Ltd., Lansdowne Vaults Ltd.) Imperial Studios, Maxwell Road Boreham Wood, Herts. Tel: 01-953 5837 and 1587, 4904, 5545.

ELECTROCRAFT CONSULTANTS LTD.
(Electrocraft Instruments Ltd.) Head Office: Coombeswell, Farnham Lane, Haslemere, Surrey. Hindhead 5190. Sales Office Works: Liss Mill, Mill Road, Liss, Hans. Tel: Liss 3444.

FILMTEXT LTD.
37 Kew Road, Richmond Surrez, TW9 2NQ. Tel: 01-940 5034.

GENERAL SCREEN ENTERPRISES LTD.
97 Oxford Road, Uxbridge, Middx. Tel: Uxbridge 31931.

KAY/MGM LABORATORIES LTD.
91/95 Gillespie Road, Highbury, London, N.5. Tel: 01-226 4422. Telex: 28463.

NATIONAL SCREEN
15 Wadsworth Road, Greenford, Middlesex, UB6 7JN. Tel: 01-998 2851; 2 Wedgwood Mews, Greek Street, London, W1V 5LE. Tel: 01-437 4851-6. Telex: 934522.

RANK FILM LABORATORIES LTD.
Denham Uxbridge, Middlesex, UB9 5HQ. Tel: Denham (0895) 832323.
Managing Director: J. W. Downer.
Sales Controller: M. A. Levy.

RANK PHICOM VIDEO GROUP
142 Wardour Street, London, W1V 4BU. Tel: 01-734 2235. Telex: 261237.

STUDIO FILM VIDEO LABORATORIES LTD.
8-12 Meard Street London, W.1. Tel: 01-437 0831.

TECHNICOLOR LTD.
(Subsidiary of Technicolor Inc.) P.O. Box No. 7 Bath Road, West Drayton, Middlesex, UB7 0DB5. Tel: 01-759 5432. Telegraphic and Cable Address: Technicolor, West Drayton. Telex: 22344.

UNIVERSAL FILM LABORATORY LTD.
Braintree Road, Ruislip, Middlesex. Tel: 01-841 5101.

STUDIOS

BRAY STUDIOS (Samuelson Group)
Windsor Road, Windsor, Berks. Tel: 0628 22111. Telex: 21430. Cables: Samcine London.
(4 stages, total 23,600 sq. ft. All depts. theatre, workshops, bar and catering.)

BUSHEY
(Cygnet Ltd.)
Melbourne Road, Bushey, Herts. Tel: 01-950 1621.
Studio Manager: Philip Lee
2 Stages (66′ × 33′ × 15 high with cycloroma backing; 30′ × 22′ × 12 high with video gallery)

CARLTON TELEVISION LTD.
St. John's Wood Studios, St. John's Wood Terrace, London, N.W.8. Tel: 01-722 9255. Telex: 28177.

Managing Director: Barry Johnstone.
Sound stage (63×32×25). Facilities for features and commercials, film or videotape.

CINEVIDEO LTD.
245 Old Marylebone Road, London, NW1 5QT. Tel: 01-402 8385.

CREATIVE FILM MAKERS LTD.
Pottery Lane House, Pottery Lane, Holland Park, London, W11 4LZ. Tel: 01-229 5131.

C.T.S. STUDIOS LTD.
The Music Centre, Engineers Way, Wembley, Middlesex. Tel: 01-903 4611. Telex: 923400.

ELSTREE STUDIOS LTD.
Boreham Wood, Herts. Tel: 01-953 1600. Telex: 436 EFILMS G. Fac: 01-207 0860.

Managing Director: Andrew Mitchell.
Nine sound stages (one 30,000 square feet, four 15,000 square feet, two 8,000 square feet, one 15,750 square feet, one 5,200 square feet.)
Theatres: Three viewing, one dubbing, one ADR and looping theatre. RCA sound. Complete Dolby installation in transfers, looping, re-recording and viewing for producing Dolby encoded optical sound tracks.

GATEWAY AUDIO/VIDEO
470–472 Green Lanes, London, NI3 5XF. Tel: 01-882 0177.

HALLIFORD FILM STUDIOS LTD.
Manygate Lane, Shepperton, Middlesex, TW17 9EG. Tel: Walton-on-Thames 226341 (5 lines).

Studio Manager: Allan d'Aguiar.
Two stages (60×60, 60×40) totalling 6,000 sq. ft.

ITN LTD.
ITN House, 48 Wells Street, London, WIP 4DE. Tel: 01-637 2424.

2 television studios, 7 Marconi colour cameras, VTR and telerecording, telecine, etc.

LEE INTERNATIONAL FILM STUDIOS SHEPPERTON
Studios Road, Shepperton, Middlesex, TW17 0QD. Tel: 09328 62611.

Contact: Cathy Bunce.
10 stages.

LIMEHOUSE STUDIOS
Canary Wharf, West Indian Docks, London, 314 9SJ. Tel: 01-987 2090.

MORENO FILM STUDIOS
35 Broadhurst Gardens, London, N.W.6. Tel: Maida Vale 0645.

Directors: George Moreno (Managing), Fred Thompson.

NATIONAL FILM STUDIOS OF IRELAND
Ardmore House, Bray, Co. Wicklow, Ireland. Tel: Dublin 862971. Telex: 30418.

PINEWOOD STUDIOS
Iver Heath, Bucks. Tel: Iver 651700. Telex: 847505 Pine w G.

Managing Director: Cyril Howard.
A. 165 ft.×110 ft.×35 ft. (with tank 40 ft.×30 ft.×8 ft.)
B. 110 ft.×80 ft.×34 ft.
C. 110 ft.×80 ft.×34 ft.
D. 165 ft.×110 ft.×35 ft. (with tank 40 ft.×30 ft.×8 ft.)
E. 165 ft.×110 ft.×35 ft. (with tank 40 ft.×30 ft.×8 ft.)
F. 100 ft.×75 ft.×35 ft. (with tank 20 ft.× 20 ft.×8 ft.)
G. 55 ft.×49 ft.×23 ft.
H. 90 ft.×37 ft.×28 ft.
LARGE PROCESS STAGE: 175 ft.×28 ft., including West Wing: 68 ft.×33 ft.
SMALL PROCESS STAGE: 75 ft.×32 ft.×17 ft.
SPECIAL EFFECTS STAGE (silent)—89 ft.×80 ft.×20 ft. and Glass Matte Dept.
J. 110 ft.×80 ft.×30 ft. (dual-purpose, film and TV).
K. 110 ft.×80 ft.×30 ft. (dual-purpose, film and TV).
L. 105 ft.×90 ft.×31 ft. (dual-purpose, film and TV).
M. 105 ft.×90 ft.×31 ft. (dual-purpose, film and TV).
Stage (silent) 336 ft.×139 ft.×40 ft.
SOUND & PROJECTION DEPARTMENT: Fisher booms. Fully staffed transfer section (tape/35mm/cassette/disc.)
Seven theatres, with arc illumination:
Theatre 1: Viewing—35mm Fedi reversible projectors. COMOPT, SEPOPT, SEPMAG. All formats including Scope.
Max. screen width 30ft. 50 seats.
Dubbing—Mono or Dolby stereo. Neve console. 14 dubbers.
Theatre 2: Viewing—35mm Westar reversible projectors. COMOPT, SEPOPT, COMMAG, SEPMAG. All formats including Scope.
Max. screen width 34ft; 50 seats.
Dubbing—Comprehensive stereo facility, utilising 3 6-track recorders for separated dialogue, effects and music. All Dolby formats, including divided surrounds. 60-input console with computer control of faders and panners. 16 dubbers.
Theatres 3 & 4: 15-seater viewing theatres with all formats, COMOPT, SEPOPT, SEPMAG.
Theatre 5: Post-sync and effects theatre, 47′×30′×18′. All surfaces, splash tank, instant props. Twin ADR or loops.
Theatre 6: Viewing—35mm Westar, reversible projectors. COMOPT, SEPOPT, SEPMAG. All formats including Scope.
Max. screen width 11ft; 15 seats.
Dubbing, post-sync and effects. 18-input console, 3-track reversible system. Dolby noise reduction.
Theatre 7: Luxury viewing room. 70/35/16mm projection. COMOPT, SEPOPT (including Dolby stereo), COMMAG, SEPMAG. Every screen and soundtrack format, including divided surrounds.
Max. screen width 31ft. 115 super seats. PA, Capability for audio-visual. Reception lounge available.
Theatres 1, 2 and 6 are equipped with Westrex variable area photo recorders.
CAMERA DEPARTMENT: Range of 35 mm cameras available, including studio reflexes, Mitchell standard and high speed, Arriflex. Lenses include Varotal and Angenieux zooms, Kowa primes. Wide choice of accessories: crystal motors, geared and fluid heads. Oxberry and Moviola dollies.
EDITING: 44 35mm cutting rooms available. Service staff.
SPECIAL EFFECTS: Fully equipped process projection dept., including front projection and 70m rear and foreground projection. Models of all kinds. Equipped for all effects.
STILLS: Stills studio. Dressing rooms. Production and Unit Offices: Many available.
EXTERIOR LOT: 72 acres with formal gardens, lake, woods and concrete service roads. Paddock tank 230 ft. wide narrowing to 110 ft. Backing 240 ft. × 60 ft. Another tank 75 ft. × 225 ft. Both tanks contain approximately 800,000 gallons. Props available and world's largest scenedock. Comprehensive catering dept.

PRODUCTION VILLAGE
(Samuelson Group Plc.)
100 Cricklewood Lane, London, NW2 2DS. Tel: 01-450 8969.

PROSPECT STUDIOS LTD.
High Street, Barnes, London, S.W.13. Tel: 876 6284/5.

SEEZERS TELEVISION STUDIOS
30, Upper Abbey Street, Dublin 1, Ireland. Tel: Dublin 48909 and 47079.

Stage sizes: 50×70; 20×12.

SHEPPERTON STUDIO CENTRE
Studios Road, Shepperton, Middlesex, TW17 0QD. Tel: 09328 62611. Telex: 929416 Movies G.

Five sound and one silent stages.

TELEVISION INTERNATIONAL OPERATIONS LIMITED
9–11 Windmill Street, London, W1P 1HF. Tel: 01-637 2477. Telex: 268208 TVIUK G. Cables: Incolour London.

Managing Director: Ian Reed
Sales Director: Peter Saxton
Studios: outside broadcasting, mobile VTR. All tone and colour standards; full technical crews and prod. VTR recording and editing. Network links. Digital Standards Conversion.

TWICKENHAM
St. Margaret's, Twickenham, Middlesex. Tel: 01-892 4477.

Owned by Twickenham Film Studios, Ltd.
Stage One: 7,192 square feet. Stage Two: 2,000 square feet, Stage Three: 5,700 square feet.
RCA Sound. Re-Recording and dubbing theatres with 36 input 6 track stereo Rock & Roll (High speed 6 times).
Directors: G. Coen, G. Humphreys, M. Landsberger, S. J. Mullens.

W.F.S. (FILM FACILITIES) LTD.
153 Wardour Street, London, W1V 3TB. Tel: 01-437 5532.

WORLD WIDE RECORDING STUDIOS
21–25 St. Anne's Court, London, W1V 3AW. Tel: 01-434 1121.

Director of Recording: P. Gilpin.

ZOOM TELEVISION LTD.
142 Wardour Street, London, W1V 4BU. Tel: 01-734 2235.
Chairman: G. F. Sadler

NEWS FILM SERVICE

CBS NEWS
100 Brompton Road, London S.W.3. Tel: 01-584 3366.

NBC NEWS WORLDWIDE INC.
8 Bedford Avenue, London W.C.1. Tel: 01-637 8655

VISNEWS LIMITED
Cumberland Avenue, London, N.W.10. Tel: 965 7733.
General Manager: Peter Marshall
NEWS DIVISION:
Head of News: Tom Hudson
Head of BROADCAST FACILITIES: Chris Laid

WORLDWIDE TELEVISION NEWS
WTN House, 31–36 Foley Street, London, W1P 7LB. Tel: 01-323 3255. Telex: 23915.

COSTUME SUPPLIERS

MORRIS ANGEL & SON LTD.
119 Shaftesbury Avenue, London W.C.2. Tel: 01-836 5678. (P.B.X.)

BERMAN AND NATHANS LTD.
Head Office: 18 Irving Street, Leicester Square, London, WC2H 7AX. Tel: 01-839 1651.
Main Store: 40 Camden Street, London, NW1 0EN. Tel: 01-387 0999.

BRITISH ADVERTISING AGENCIES

THE AB MARKETING & ADVERTISING GROUP LTD.
Gratton House, 9–13, Newton Road, Leeds, L57 4HU. Tel: Leeds 620351.
T.V. Executive: J. H. Murray.

APEX ADVERTISING LTD.
47 Cross Road, Coventry. Tel: Coventry 85151.
T.V. Executive: D. R. Harris.

A.P. SERVICES LTD.
186–8 Shaftesbury Avenue, London W.C.2. Tel: Covent Garden 3121.
TV Executive: A. I. Smith.

ARKS LTD.
17 Harcourt Street, Dublin 2, Ireland. Tel: Dublin 01-757981.
TV Executives: Brian Graham, John Canise.

BBDO BATTEN, BARTON, DURSTINE & OSBORN LTD.
25/27 St. George Street, London, W1R 0NT. Tel: 01-493 8455.
Head of Television: John C. Henderson.

B.B.P. ADVERTISING
(BOSWELL, BARRATT & PHILLIPS LTD.)
B.B.P. House, 117 John Bright Street, Birmingham, B1 IBQ.
T.V. Executive: H. Harms.

BENTON & BOWLES LTD.
197 Knightsbridge, London S.W.7. Tel: 01-589 1444.
Head of Television: Stephen Spencer.

ROBERT BRANDON & PARTNERS LTD.
10 Clifford Street, London W.1. Tel: 01-734 0511.

BRIDGE ADVERTISING LTD.
178–202 Great Portland Street, London, W1N 6AQ. Tel: 01-637 7481/5.
T.V. Executive: W. H. Pearson.

BROCKIE HASLAM AND ALLON LTD.
72–74 Brewer St., London W.1. Tel: 01-734 0491.

D.H. BROCKLESBY LTD.
Nicholsons House, Maidenhead, Berks. Tel: Maidenhead 29322. Telex: 84407.
T.V. Executive: Colin Lovejoy.

BROOKS PUBLICITY SERVICES
4, Seaford Court. 220/222, Great Portland Street, London, W1N 5HH. Tel: 01-388 2117. Telex: 21237G.

L. GRAHAM BROWNE (LONDON) LIMITED.
56/58, Gamage Building, Holborn Circus, London E.C.1. Tel: 01-405 6207.

BROWNE'S ADVERTISING LTD.
117 Piccadilly, London, W1V 0BL. Tel: 01-499 5351.
Creative Director: David Knight.

BRUNNING ADVERTISING & MARKETING LTD.
Brunning House, 100 Whitechapel Road, London E.1. Tel: 01-247 6525.
T.V. Executive: D. Walker.

BRUNNING ADVERTISING & MARKETING (LEEDS) LTD.
Apson House, 53 Margate, Leeds, LS9 7DR. Tel: Leeds 30054-5.

BRUNNING ADVERTISING & MARKETING (MANCHESTER) LTD.
57 Hilton Street, Manchester, M1 2EJ. Tel: 061-236 5636.

BUTLER DENNIS & GARLAND LTD.
153–155 Regent Street, London, W1R 7FD. Tel: 01-437 4377.
Creative Controller: A. D. Dell.

CAVENDISH PUBLICITY SERVICE LTD.
34, Oxford Street (4th floor), London W.1. Tel: 01-580 3377.
T.V. Executive: A. G. Howard.

CLARENDON ADVERTISING LTD.
57 Clarendon Road, Leeds 2. Tel: Leeds 35121.
T.V. Executive: John Somers.

COLLETT, DICKENSON PEARCE & PARTNERS LTD.
110 Euston Road, London N.W.[1]. Tel: 01-388 2424.

JOHN COLLINGS & PARTNERS LTD.
Nascreno House, Soho Square, London W.1. Tel: Regent 2141.
Media: A. J. Blair.
T.V.: D. Scott-Job.

COMMERCIAL ADVERTISING SERVICE LTD.
Silverwood House, 129 Barlow Moor Road, West Didsbury, Manchester, M20 8PP. Tel: 061-434 1211.
T.V. Executives: K. Greenhalgh, J. L. Richman, J. A. Gatcliffe, P. Newman, T. Lee.

CONNELL, MAY AND STEAVENSON LTD.
William Blake House, Marshall St., London W.1. Tel: 01-734 9041.

E. ALLAN COOPER & CO. LTD.
Waldorf House, 18 Exeter Street, London W.C.2. Tel: 01-836 3104.

S. V. COURT ADVERTISING LTD.
Chronicle House, 72–78 Fleet Street, London E.C.4 1HY. Tel: 01-353 2771.
T.V. Executive: Mrs. Diana Gibson.

W. S. CRAWFORD LTD.
141, Westbourne Terrace, London, W2 6JR. Tel: 01-723 3227.

DAVIDSON PEARCE LTD.
67, Brompton Road, London S.W.3. Tel: 01-589 4595.
Chairman & Managing Director: C. J. Hawes.

DOMAS LTD. ADVERTISING AND MARKETING
77 Ranelagh Road, Dublin 6, Ireland. Tel: Dublin 9710757.

DORLAND ADVERTISING LTD.
121–141 Westbourne Terrace, London W.2. Tel: 01-262 5077.

DOWNTOWN ADVERTISING
103 Wardour Street, London W.1. Tel: 01-439 7111.

DOYLE DANE BERNBACH LTD.
62–64 Baker Street, London W.1. Tel: 01-486 7122.
Media Director: T. Wheeler.

DRYDEN-ALLEN LTD.
4 Hills Road, Cambridge, CB2 1JP. Tel: Cambridge 65215/6.

DUNCAN ONGLEY ASSOCIATES LTD.
43–44 Windmill Street, London W.1. Tel: 01-437 8761.

EVERETTS LTD.
10 Grecoat Place, London, SW1P 1SE. Tel: 01-799 7822.
T.V. Director: Bernie Kay.

FARMER ADVERTISING LTD.
Stentor House, 16 Moncrieffe Road, Sheffield, PS7 1HS.
Chairman: J. C. H. McMillan; Joint.
Managing Directors: J. C. Wells, J. Wardle.
Directors: C. W. R. Guthrie, C. D. Farmer, V. Smith, J. L. Bradshaw, R. C. Milner.

FARMER ADVERTISING (HULL) LTD.
80 Beverley Road, Hull. Tel: Hull 29001.
T.V. Executive: D. N. Dean.

FOGARTY ADVERTISING LTD.
72 Haddington Road, Dublin 4, Ireland. Tel: Dublin 681455.

FOOTE, CONE & BELDING LTD.
82 Baker Street, London W.1. Tel: 01-935 4426.
T.V. Head: Ian Hoath.

FORBES KEIR LTD.
DuBarry Bldg., 58/64 Lime Street, Liverpool. Tel: 051-709 6162.
T.V. Directors: J. G. S. Furness, M.I.P.A., L. Hamblet, M.I.P.A., A. McDermott.
T.V. Executive: J. G. S. Furness.

FORDHAM SADLER ADVERTISING LTD.
West End House, Hills Place, London W.1. Tel: 01-437 8146.
T.V. Executive: Peter Rose.

GARRATT BAULCOMBE PARTNERS LTD.
Bolton House, 194 Old Brompton Road, London, SW5 0AS. Tel: 01-370 6781.

FRANK GAYTON ADVERTISING LTD.
156 Upper New Walk, Leicester. Tel: Leicester 26001.
T.V. Directors: Alan W. Gayton, Nigel Parry Williams.

GEE ADVERTISING LTD.
London, Leicester, Leeds, Manchester. T.V. Department: 19 Grafton Street, London W.1. Tel: Hyde Park 6827.

THE GENERAL ADVERTISING CO. OF LONDON LTD.
The Centre, 68 High Street, Weybridge, Surrey, KT13 8JF. Tel: Weybridge 40251.

G. S. GERRARD LTD.
10 Argyll Street, London W.1. Tel: 01-437 6816
T.V. Executive: W. Purvis.

GODBOLDS LTD.
99 Aldwych, London W.C.2. Tel: 01-242 9671.
T.V. Director: Geoffrey Godbold.

GOLLEY, SLATER & PARTNERS LTD.
42 Drury Lane, London W.C.2. Tel: 01-240 5131.
Media: S. Cullen.

GRAHAM & GILLIES & WARWICK LTD.
Ingestre Court, Ingestre Place, London, W1R 4AL. Tel: 01-437 9055.

GRANT ADVERTISING LTD.
2 Basil Street, London, SW3 1AA. Tel: 01-584 7050.
T.V. Executive: C. Coast.

GREAT GUNS! LTD.
79 New Cavendish Street, London, W1M 8AJ. Tel: 01-636 4020.
Executive Producer: J. G. Warner.

HERBERT GREAVES LTD.
26 Brown Street, Manchester, W2 1DL. Tel: 061-832 3841.
T.V. Executives: Derrick H. Greaves, Miss M. Greaves.

JAMES M. GREENWOOD ADVERTISING LTD.
100 Whitechapel Road, London E.1. Tel: 01-247 6525.

GREY ADVERTISING LTD.
50–51 Cenduit Street, London, W1R 0AR. Tel: 01-493 6700.

CREIGHTON GRIFFITHS ROYDS LTD.
30, Cathedral Road, Cardiff, Wales. Tel: Cardiff 397711.
Account Executives: R. Petersen, D. M. Creighton Griffiths, G. Huws.
T.V. Buyer: G. J. Hughes.

JOHN HALIFAX LTD.
84 Northampton Street, Leicester. Tel: Leicester 50841/2.
T.V. Executives: Gordon A. Penman, H. C. Clements.

HARDING, QUANTRILL, O'BRIEN LTD.
Byrom House, 21 Quay St., Manchester, M3 3HT. Tel: 061-832 2523.

HARWOOD PRESS (ADVERTISING) LTD.
21–51, West Street, Harrow, Middlesex. Tel: 01-422 5656.
T.V. Executive: R. B. F. Harwood.

HEWLAND, RUDER & FINN INTERNATIONAL LTD.
15 Albemarle Street, London W.1. Tel: 01-492 1143.
Film & T.V. Executive: V. A. Stump.

CHARLES F. HIGHAM LTD.
Hesketh House, Portman Square, London, W1H 0JH. Tel: 0-486 5041.
T.V. Executive: Peter King.
Creative Director: Brian Baldwin.

HOBSON BATES & PARTNERS LTD.
Hobson House, 155 Gower Street, London W.C.1. Tel: 01-387 4313.
T.V. Production Controller: R. Evans.

CHARLES HOBSON & GREY LTD.
12/13 Conduit Street, London W.1. Tel: Hyde Park 6700.
T.V. Executive: M. W. Reynolds.

HECTOR HUGHES & PARTNERS LTD.
Colquhoun House, Broadwick Street, London W.1. Tel: 01-437 0724.
T.V. Executives: R. C. Harrold, R. Collins.

HUNTER ADVERTISING LTD.
Royal Exchange Bldgs., Glasgow, C.1., Scotland. Tel: 041-221 1162.
T.V. Executive: A. Ferguson Hunter.

HUTCHINSON PUBLICITY LTD.
3, Fitzroy Square, London W.1. Tel: 01-388 7601.
T.V. Executive: Jeremy Cox.

GEORGE HYNES & PARTNERS LTD.
New Mercury House, 82 Farringdon Street, London E.C.4. Tel: 01-353 4030.

INDUSTRIAL PUBLICITY SERVICE LTD.
I.P.S. House, 38 Monmouth Street, London W.C.2. Tel: Covent Garden 1902.
T.V. Executive: P. M. Graham.

INTERLINK ADVERTISING LTD.
63/66 St. Martin's Lane, London, WC2N 4JK. Tel: 01-836 4466.
Managing Director: F. J. Josling, FIPA.

IRISH INTERNATIONAL ADVERTISING & MARKETING LTD.
9 Fitzwilliam Square, Dublin, Ireland. Tel: 760231.
Managing Director: Finbar P. Costello.

JAFFE & YOUNG ADVERTISING LTD.
43 South Street, London, W1Y 5PD. Tel: 01-409 0932.
Managing Director: R. C. Young.

WALTER JUDD LTD.
1A, Bow Lane, London E.C.4. Tel: 01-236 4541.

KINGSCOTT LTD.
18/20 St. Andrew Street, London E.C.4. Tel: 01-353 6316/9.
T.V. Executive: L. D. Conquest, M.I.P.A.

LINTAS LTD.
Lintas House, New Fetter Lane, London E.C.4. Tel: 01-

483 8030.
Creative Director: I. M. Drake.

LONGLEYS & HOFFMANN LTD.
60–61 Lionel Street, Birmingham, 83 1JF. Tel: 01-236 7532.
T.V. Executive; P. J. Niblett.
Time Buyer: R. D. Rawlinson.

LOVELL AND RUPERT CURTIS LTD.
30 Bouverie Street, London E.C.4. Tel: 01-353 0871.
T.V. Executive: A. C. Hind. M.I.P.A.

L.P.A. LTD.
2 Basil Street, London, SW3 1AD. Tel: 01-584 7050.

LUCIEN TELEVISION & SCREEN ADVERTISING LTD.
Hesketh House, Portmen Square, London W.1. Tel: 01-486 3161.
T.V. Executive: V. H. Rawlinson.

MACKAY & PARTNERS LTD.
36 Upper Brook Street, London W.1. Tel: 01-493 1343.
T.V. Executive: Walter Speight.

BARBOUR MacLAREN ADVERTISING LTD.
101, West Nile Street, Glasgow C.1., Scotland. Tel: 041 332 9211.
T.V. Executives: D. Sanderson, T. Willies.

MacLAREN, DUNKLEY, FRIEDLANDER LTD.
197 Oxford Street, London W.1. Tel: 01-437 9000.

McCALLUM ADVERTISING LTD.
7 Queen Street, Edinburgh, EH2 1JP, Scotland. Tel: 031-266 6441.
T.V. Executive: M. Gilderdale.

McCANN-ERICKSON ADVERTISING LTD.
McCann-Erickson House, 36 Howland Street, London W.1. Tel: 01-580 6690.

McCONNELL & CO. (ADVERTISING) LTD.
25 Princes Drive, Colwyn Bay, North Wales. Tel: Colwyn Bay 2889.
T.V. Executive: E. M. Roberts.

MASIUS, WYNNE-WILLIAMS & D'ARCY-MACMANUS LTD.
2 St. James's Square, London S.W.1. Tel: 01-839 3422.
Creative Directors: R. Greene, C. Sharpe.

MWK & P
37 Dean Street, London, W1V 5AP. Tel: 01-437 8644.

OGILVY, BENSON & MATHER LTD.
Brettenham House, Lancaster Place, London W.C.2. E 7EZ. Tel: 01-836 2466.
T.V. Manager: R. Barker.

MAYFAIR ADVERTISING LTD.
Cliffords Inn, London E.C.4. Tel: 01-242 8135.

MEARNS AND GILL ADVERTISING LTD.
7 Carden Place, Aberdeen, Scotland. Tel: Aberdeen 26311.
T.V. Executives: J. A. Graeme Mearns, J. D. Gill, J. Cardno, G. J. Scott.

PETER A. MENZIES ADVERTISING
2 Newton Place, Glasgow, C.3 7PT, Scotland.

MITCHELLS ADVERTISING SERVICE LTD.
420 Sauchiehall Street, Glasgow, C.2., Scotland. Tel: Douglas 2241/2.

JOHN NEWTON (Publicity), LTD.
198 Corn Exchange, Manchester 4. Tel: 061-834 1828.
T.V. Executives: T. D. Farmer, D. F. George.

NATIONAL ADVERTISING CORPORATION LTD.
150 Regent Street, London W.1. Tel: 01-437 7866 (20 lines).
T.V. Executive: Mike Storm.

NORMAN, CRAIG AND KUMMEL LTD.
Greater London House, Hampstead Road, London N.W.1. Tel: 01-387 9311.

O'KENNEDY-BRINDLEY LTD.
64-6 Lower Gardiner Street, Dublin, Ireland.
T.V. Executive: Niel O'Kennedy.

OMNIFIC ADVERTISING, LTD.
Astral House, 17–19 Maddox Street, London, W1R 0EY. Tel: 01-499 0477.

OSBORNE LTD.
Hesketh House, Portman Square, London, W1H 9FG. Tel: 01-486 5877.
Creative Director: Geoff Drew, AMIPA.
T.V. Director: P. King.

J. H. PARKER & CO. LTD.
Northern Bank Chambers, 114 Grafton Street, Dublin 2, Ireland. Tel: 771 371.
T.V. Executive: P. J. Dempsey.

PEERS ADVERTISING LTD.
Walton House, High Street, Bromley, Kent: Tel: 01-464 3661.
Media: A. M. Albinson.

ALFRED PEMBERTON LTD.
Pemberton House, 29 Marylebone Road, London, NW1 5JU. Tel: 01-486 1222.

PERARD FOX AND PARTNERS LTD.
9 Hillgate Street, London W.8. Tel: 01-727 3141.
T.V. Executives: Ruth Rose.

PICKERSGILL PUBLICITY SERVICE LTD.
Lavender Walk, Leeds 9. Tel: Leeds 29137.
T.V. Executives: L. Pickersgill, D. Walls.

REDHEAD ADVERTISING LTD.
11-17 Archbold Terrace, Newcastle-on-Tyne, NE2 1DW. Tel: 0632 815424; 20 Bride Lane, Fleet Street, London, EC4Y 8DX. Tel: 01-353 4691.
Directors: C. H. D. Redhead, R. D. Redhead, F. W. Watson.

REID WALKER LTD.
Hutton House, Hutton Street, London, EC4Y 8HP. Tel: 01-583 9371. Telex: 885857.
T.V. Executive: N. R. Field, F.I.P.A.

RICHMOND TOWERS LTD.
26 Fitzroy Square, London, W1P 6BT. Tel: 01-388 7421.
T.V. Executive: L. Carpenter.

ROBERTSON & SCOTT (ADVERTISING) LTD.
42 Charlotte Square, Edinburgh, EH2 4HJ, Scotland. Tel: 031-255 6602. Glasgow Office: 124 St. Vincent St., Glasgow. Tel: 041-221 9021.
Managing Director: D. J. Mackenzie, M.I.P.A.

ROE DOWNTON LTD.
103–109 Wardour Street, London, WIV 3TD. Tel: 01-439 7111.

F. JOHN ROE ASSOCIATES LTD.
20 St. Ann's Square, Manchester. Tel: 061 832 5111. & F. John Roe Advertising Ltd. 73 Grosvenor Street, London, W.1. Tel: 01-493 8501.
Directors: Derek J. Roe, Graham Roe.

ROLES & PARKER LTD.
Eagle Street, London W.C.1. Tel: 01-242 7744.
Media: J. V. Standish.

ROYDS LONDON LTD.
Royds House, Mandeville Place, London, W1M 6AE. Tel: 01-935 7733.
T.V., Film & Radio Dept. Director: Eve Samuel.

SAATCHI & SAATCHI COMPTON LTD.
81–84 Charlotte Street, London, W1A 1OP. Tel: 01-636 5060.

SAWARD, BAKER & CO. LTD.
79 New Cavendish Street, London, W1M 8AJ. Tel: 01-636 4020.
Media Director: D. J. Clark, AMIPA.
TV, Radio & Cinema Manager: J. G. Warner.

SCIENTIFIC ADVERTISING & MARKETING LTD.
Clifford's Inn, Fleet Street, London E.C.4. Tel: 01-242 8844.
T.V. Executives: R. C. Hilling, M.I.P.A., T. G. Hartshorne, M.A.A., M.I.P.A.

SEVERN-SMITH ADVERTISING LTD.
Mason Road, Kidderminster. Tel: Kidderminster 62876. Bradford Office: Rooley Lane, Bradford 1. Tel: Bradford

682344. Exeter Office: Southernhay East, Exeter. Tel: Exeter 70747.
T.V. Executive: N. Taner.

SHAW & UNDERWOOD (ADVERTISING SERVICES) LTD.
164 High Street, Bordesley, Birmingham, B12 OLF. Tel: 021-772 5001/2.
T.V. Executive: C. I. Randle.

SMEE'S ADVERTISING LTD.
3–5 Duke Street, Manchester Square, London W.1. Tel: 01-486 6644.
Media Controller: B. A. Jupp.

A. N. SPICER (ADVERTISING) LTD.
3 The Parsonage, Manchester 3.

THE SPIERS ADVERTISING LTD.
36 Southbourne Crescent, London, NW4 2JY. Tel: 01-346 4002.
T.V. Executive: B. X. Spiers.

STUART ADVERTISING AGENCY LTD.
22 Red Lion Street, London, WC1R 4PX. Tel: 01-831 7444.

TALBOT ADVERTISING
44-5 Fleet Street, London E.C.4. Tel: 01-353 5438.
T.V. Executive: P. J. Riley.

J. WALTER THOMPSON CO. LTD.
40 Berkeley Square, London, WIX 6AD. Tel: 01-629 9496.

OON & HEALTH LTD.
1266 Warwick Road, Knowle, Solihull, West Midlands. Tel: Knowle 4164/7.
Marketing and Television Manager: D. H. Langstone.

UNITED KINGDOM ADVERTISING CO. LTD.
Aspen House, 25 Dover Street, London W.1. Tel: 01-491 7621.
T.V. Executive: Mike Storm.

C. VERNON & SONS LTD.
178-202 Great Portland St., London W.1. Tel: 01-637 1488.
Head of T.V.: Roy A. Fowler.

C. P. WAKEFIELD LTD.
Wakefield House, 153 Fleet Street, London E.C.4. Tel: Fleet Street 4588 (3 lines) & 3521 (4 lines).
T.V. Executive: R. J. Wakefield, M.I.P.A.

WARWICK PARSONS JACKSON LTD.
14-16, Great Pulteney Street, London, W1R 4AR. Tel: 01-734 8951.
T.V. Executive; Production: G. N. Jackson.
Buying: L. Cowdrey.

WASEY CAMPBELL/EWAND LTD.
Williams House, Eastbourne Terrace, London, W.2 6LD. Tel: 01-262-3424.

JACK WHITE & ASSOCIATES
Stratford House, Moseley Road, Birmingham, B12 OHU. Tel: 021-772 4147-8-9.
T.V. Executives: H.J.V. White, M.I.P.A., M.A.A., H. G. Griffiths, A.M.I.P.A.

WHITES OF BRISTOL
Priory House, Marlborough Street, Bristol, BS1 3NY. Tel: Bristol 23053.

SIDNEY F. WICKS LTD.
21 Newton Street, Manchester, M1 1HJ. Tel: 061-236 0947.
T.V. Executive: David W. Wicks.

WILCOX ADVERTISING LTD.
10A, Chandos Street, London, W1M 9DE. Tel: Regent 1471-5.
T.V. Executives: W. E. Chester, A. Nicholas.

DAVID WILLIAMS AND KETCHUM LTD.
52, Bedford Row, London, WC1R 4LX. Tel: 01-242 8123.
T.V. Executive: Frank Gonella.

W.S. CRAWFORDS LTD.
141 Westbourne Terrace, London W.2. Tel: 01-723 3227.

WTV STUDIOS LTD.
112/114 Thorpe Road, Norwich, NOR 15T. Tel: Norwich 26721.

THE YELLOWHAMMER CO. LTD.
46 Wigmore Street, London, W1H 9DF. Tel: 01-486 7011.

YOUNG & RUBICAM LTD.
Greater London House, Hempstead Road, London N.W.1. Tel: 01-387 9366.
Creative Director: Dennis Auton.
Manager T.V. Dept.: Gilbert King.

ZETLAND ADVERTISING LTD.
6 Jerzis Court, Princes Street, London W.1. Tel: 01-409 2829.

PROFESSIONAL & TRADE ASSOCIATIONS

THE ADVERTISING ASSOCIATION
Abford House, 15 Wilton Road, London S.W.1. Tel: 01-828 2771.
(The Advertising Association is a federation of all trade associations with advertising interests: advertisers, media, agencies and services. It aims to ensure that everyone with a view or a voice in advertising—participants, supporters and critics—should understand the role of advertising in society and the economy, and the part it plays in creating prosperity and full employment.)
Director General: Roger Underhill.

THE ADVERTISING STANDARDS AUTHORITY
Brook House, 2–16 Torrington Place, London, WC1E 7HN. Tel: 01-580 5555 (9 lines).

ASSOCIATION OF BROADCASTING AND ALLIED STAFFS
Thorndike House, 70–76 Bell Street, London, NWI 6SP. Tel: 01-262 0162.
General Secretary: D. A. Hearn.

ASSOCIATION OF CINEMATOGRAPH, TELEVISION AND ALLIED TECHNICIANS
(Affiliated to Trades Union Congress and Labour Party). 111 Wardour Street, London W.1. Tel: 01-437 8506.
President: Bruce Anderson.
General Secretary: Alan Sapper.
(The Association is the recognized Trade Union for film, television and radio technicians and negotiates salaries and working conditions. It also controls the A.C.T.T. Employment Bureau as an agency exclusively for film and TV technicians.)

ASSOCIATIONS OF INDEPENDENT PRODUCERS
17 Great Pulteney Street, London W1. Tel: 01-437 9191.
Director: Sally Davies.

ASSOCIATION OF PROFESSIONAL RECORDING STUDIOS LTD.
23 Chestnut Avenue, Chorleywood, Herts, WD3 4HA. Tel: 0923 772907.
Secretary: E. L. Masek.

ASSOCIATION OF PROFESSIONAL VIDEO DEALERS LTD.
P.O. Box 25, Godalming, Surrey, GX7 1PL. Tel: 04868 23429.
Director and Secretary: Charles Potter.

BRITISH ACADEMY OF FILM AND TELEVISION ARTS
195 Piccadilly, London, W1V 9LG. Tel: 01-734 0022.
President: H. R. H. The Princess Anne.
Vice President: Sir Richard Attenborough, C.B.E.
Chairman: Graham Benson.
Hon. Treasurer: Richard Price.
Director: Reginald Collin.
The British Academy of Film and Television Arts exists in order to promote, improve and advance original and creative work amongst people engaged in film and television production.

BRITISH ACTORS' EQUITY ASSOCIATION
(Incorporating the Variety Artistes Fed.) 8 Harley Street, London, W1N 2AB. Tel: 01-637 9311 and 636 6367. Cables: Britequity, London.
Honorary Treasurer: Milton Johns.
General Secretary: Peter Plouviez.

BRITISH FILM DESIGNERS GUILD
26–28, Binney Street, London W.1. Tel: 01-499 4336.
Executive Consultant: John French

BRITISH FILM INSTITUTE
127 Charing Cross Road, London, WC2H 0EA., Tel: 01-437 4355.

Founded 1933. Principal object to encourage the development of the art of the film, to promote its use as a record of contemporary life and manners and to foster public appreciation and study of it from these points of view. The Institute has a similar role in relation to television. The Board of Governors is appointed by the Minister of the Arts. The National Film Archive and the National Film Theatre are departments of the Institute which publishes Sight and Sound, a quarterly film magazine and the Monthly Film Bulletin, and provides services for education, film availability regions and production.
Chairman: Sir Richard Attenborough, C.B.E.
Director: Anthony Smith.
Deputy Director & Secretary: Gerry Rawlinson.

BRITISH FILM & TELEVISION PRODUCERS ASSOCIATION LTD.
162–170 Wardour Street, London, W1V 4LA. Tel: 01-437 7700.

President: Kenneth Maidment.
Secretary: Andrew Patrick.

BRITISH KINEMATOGRAPH SOUND AND TELEVISION SOCIETY
110/112 Victoria House, Vernon Place, London, WC1B 4AD. Tel: 01-242 8400.

President: Dennis Boxall.
Secretary: William Pay.
Founded in 1931, the Society was incorporated in 1946 to service the industries of its title, encouraging technical and scientific progress. To further these aims, the Society disseminates to its Members information on technical developments within these industries, arranges technical lectures, international conferences, and demonstrations, and encourages the exchange of ideas. The broad nature of its purpose is made possible by the subscriptions of its Members and by its freedom from political or commercial bias. The *BKSTS Journal* is published monthly and is sent free to all members.

BRITISH MUSIC INFORMATION CENTRE
10 Stratford Place, London, W1N 9AE. Tel: 01-499 8567.

Centre Director: Roger W. Wright.
(Reference library of works by 20th Century British composers.)

THE BRITISH RADIO AND ELECTRONIC EQUIPMENT MANUFACTURERS' ASSOCIATION
Landseer House, 19 Charing Cross Road, London, WC2H OES. Tel: 01-930 3206. Telex: 296215 BREMA G.

Director: O. P. Surron, CBE.
Secretary: R. B. S. Purdy, OBE.

BRITISH SOCIETY OF CINEMATOGRAPHERS LTD.
% Tree Tops, 11 Croft Road, Chalfont St. Peter, Gerrards Cross, Bucks, SL9 9AE. Tel: 0753 888052.

Secretary and Treasurer: Frances Russell.
(To promote and encourage the pursuit of the highest standards in the craft of motion picture photography.)

BRITISH VIDEOGRAM ASSOCIATION LTD
21–22 Poland Street, London, W1V 3DD. Tel: 01-437 5722. Telex: 295101.

BROADCASTING AND ENTERTAINMENT TRADES ALLIANCE
181–185 Wardour Street, London, W1V 3AA. Tel: 01-439 7585.

Joint General Secretaries: D. A. Hearn, J. L. Wilson.

CABLE TELEVISION ASSOCIATION
Tex House, 62–64 Beresford Street, London, SE18 6BG. Tel: 01-316 7376.

Secretary: A. W. Brittain, A.C.I.S.

CENTRAL CASTING LTD.
162–170 Wardour Street, London, W1V 3AT. Tel: 01-437 1881.

Directors: O. Beuselinck, J. Goodman, B. J. Kingham, K. L. Maidment, J. A. Walton, B. T. Yeoman.
General Manager: B. T. Yeoman.
(Licensed annually by the Dept. of Employment.)

CHILDREN'S FILM & TELEVISION FOUNDATION LTD
Elstree Studios, Borehamwood, Herts., WD6 1JG. Tel: 01-953 1600. Cables: Chififo Borehamwood.

Chief Executive: S. T. Taylor, F.C.I.S.

CINEMA AND TELEVISION BENEVOLENT FUND
Royalty House, 72 Dean Street, London, W1V 6LT. Tel: 01-437 6567.

Executive Director: P. J. C. Ratcliffe, O.B.E.
Secretary: H. V. Hughes, F.C.A.
(The Fund gives relief by financial grants and allowances to needy members or ex-members of the film industry or independent TV, and their widows; maintenance and education of orphans and generally to assist those in distress due to sickness, injury, unemployment or old age. Convalescence is available to assist in recovery after illness or operations at "Glebelands," Wokingham, Berks. Admission to Convalescent Home free upon application to the Secretary.)

COMPOSERS' GUILD OF GREAT BRITAIN
10 Stratford Place, London, W1N 9AE. Tel: 01-499 4795.

General Secretary: Miss Elizabeth Yeoman.
(Objects: To further artistic and professional interests of its members.)

CONFEDERATION OF ENTERTAINMENT UNIONS
60-62 Clapham Road, London, SW9 0JJ.

President: Alan Sapper.
Vice-President: P. Plouviez.
Treasurer: P. Leech.
Secretary: J. Morton.
(Confederation of trades unions engaged in the entertainment industry.)

DIRECTORS GUILD OF GREAT BRITAIN
56 Whitfield Street, London W.1. Tel: 01-580 2256.

ELECTRICAL ELECTRONIC TELECOMMUNICATION AND PLUMBING UNION
Hayes Court, West Common Road, Bromley, BR2 7AU. Tel: 01-462 7755; London Area Office: 15 Abbeville Road, London, SW4 9LA. Tel: 01-675 2211.

(Representing electrical operatives engaged in studio production.)
General Secretary: Eric Hammond.

THE ENTERTAINMENT AGENTS' ASSOCIATION LTD.
403 Collingwood House, Dolphin Square, London, SW1V 3NE. Tel: 01-834 0515.

President: Bunny Lewis.
Secretary: Gordon Blackie.
(Founded in 1927 as the Agents' Assoc. and name changed to present one in February, 1966. The Association comprises the principal agencies in all branches of the entertainment industry.)

FEDERATION AGAINST COPYRIGHT THEFT (FACT)
19-23 Wells Street, London, W1P 3FP. Tel: 01-637 9567. Telex: 27428.

Director General: P. C. Duffy.

FILM ARTISTES' ASSOCIATION
F.A.A. House, 61 Marloes Road, London W.8. Tel: 01-937 4567-8.

General Secretary: Sean Branningan.

GENERAL MUNICIPAL BOILERMAKERS & ALLIED TRADES UNION
Thorne House, Ruxley Ridge, Claygate, Esher, Surrey. Tel: Esher 62081. Telex: 27428.

General Secretary: John Edmonds.

GUILD OF BRITISH CAMERA TECHNICIANS
303-315 Cricklewood Broadway, London, NW2 6PQ. Tel: 01-450 3821 and 450 0000.

Chairman. Lou Lavelly.

GUILD OF FILM PRODUCTION ACCOUNTANTS AND FINANCIAL ADMINISTRATORS (GFPA)
Pinewood Studios, Iver, Bucks., SL0 oNH. Tel: Iver 651700.

President: Cyril Howard
Hon. Secretary: Robin Busby

GUILD OF FILM PRODUCTION EXECUTIVES
Pinewood Studios, Iver Heath, Bucks. Iver Tel: 651700.

President: David Orton.
(The Guild is an association of many of the more experienced production executives in the UK film industry.)

THE INCORPORATED SOCIETY OF BRITISH ADVERTISERS LTD.
44 Hertford Street, London W1Y 8AE. Tel: 01-499 7502.

(Objects: The protection and advancement of the advertising interests of all member companies.)
Director: K. N. Miles.

INDEPENDENT PROGRAMME PRODUCERS' ASSOCIATION
50-51 Berwick Street, London, W1V 3LA. Tel: 01-439 7034.

INDEPENDENT TELEVISION COMPANIES ASSOCIATION, LTD.
Knighton House, 56 Mortimer Street, London, W1N 8AN. Tel: 01-636 6866. Telex: 262988.

(The Association exists to represent and promote the interests of the programme companies appointed by the Independent Broadcasting Authority. The members are Anglia Television Ltd., Border Television p.l.c., Central Independent Television, p.l.c., Channel Television, Grampian Television p.l.c., Granada Television Ltd., HTV Ltd., London Weekend Television Ltd., Scottish Television p.l.c., TVS p.l.c., TSW-Television South West Ltd., Thames Television Ltd., Tyne Tees Television Ltd., Ulster Television p.l.c., Yorkshire Television Ltd., TV-a.m. Ltd.)
General Secretary: David Shaw.

INSTITUTE OF PRACTITIONERS IN ADVERTISING
44 Belgrave Square, London, SW1X 8QS. Tel: 01-235 7020. Fax: 01-245 9904.

INSTITUTION OF ELECTRONIC AND RADIO ENGINEERS
99 Gower Street, London, WC1E 6AZ. Tel: 01-388 3071.

INTERNATIONAL TELEVISION ASSOCIATION (UK)
P.O. Box 47, 38 Great Queen Street, London, WC2B 5AE. Tel: 01-405 2244.

MECHANICAL COPYRIGHT PROTECTION SOCIETY LTD.
Elgar House, 41 Streatham High Road, London, SW16 1ER. Tel: 01-769 4400. Cables and Telegrams: Mecolico, London S.W.16. Telex: 946792 MCPSG.

(*Objects:* The Society has the authority of some ten thousand music copyright owners in the U.K. and Commonwealth, the U.S.A., Germany, Italy and other countries to licence the use of their works for all forms of mechanical reproduction, including sound synchronisation in cinematograph, television and advertising films.)
Managing Director: R. W. Montgomery
Company Secretary and Financial Controller: K. R. D. Lowde.
Commercial Operations Controller: G. J. Churchill.

MOTION PICTURE EXPORT ASSOCIATION OF AMERICA INC.
162-170 Wardour Street, London W.1. Tel: 01-437 2282.

MUSICIANS' UNION
60–62, Clapham Road, London, SW9 0JJ Cables: Amuse., London S.W.9. Tel: 01-582 5566.

General Secretary: John Morton.

NATIONAL TELEVISION ASSOCIATION
P.O. Box 47, 38 Great Queen Street, London, WC2B 5AE. Tel: 01-405 2244.

NATIONAL TELEVISION RENTAL ASSOCIATION LTD.
4th Floor, Rediffusion House, 8–12 Camden High Street, London NW1 0JJ. Tel: 01-387 5768.

Secretary: A. W. Brittain, A.C.I.S.

THE PERFORMING RIGHT SOCIETY LTD.
29–33 Berners Street, London, W1P 4AA. Tel: 01-580 5544. Telex: 892678 PRSLONG.

(An association of composers, authors and publishers of music.)

THE PERSONAL MANAGERS' ASSOCIATION LTD.
℅ Secretary: Alison Shelley: Redfern House, Woodside Hill, Chalfont St. Peter, Bucks.. SL9 9TF.

(An association of the principal personal managers who represent stars, feature players, authors, writers, producers, directors and technicians.)
President: Peter Dunlop.

PHONOGRAPHIC PERFORMANCE LTD.
Ganton House, 14/22 Ganton Street, London, W1V 1LB. Tel: 01-437 0311.

(A company founded by the British recording industry to own and exercise the public performance and broadcasting rights in sound recordings in the U.K. and to issue licences for public performances and broadcasting.)
General Manager: J. B. Love.

THE RADIO, ELECTRICAL AND TELEVISION RETAILERS' ASSOCIATION (RETRA) LTD.
RETRA House, 57-61 Newington Causeway, London, SE1 6BE. Tel: 01-403 1463.

Director: R. T. Edom

THE RADIO INDUSTRY COUNCIL
Landseer House, 19 Charing Cross Road, London, WC2H 0ES. Tel: 01-930 3206.

Director: O. P. Sutton, CBE.
Secretary: R. B. S. Purdy, OBE.

RADIO SOCIETY OF GREAT BRITAIN
Lambda House, Cranborne Road, Potters Bar, Herts., EN6 3JE. Tel: 0707 59015..

General Manager: David A. Evans.

ROYAL TELEVISION SOCIETY
Tavistock House East, Tavistock Square, London, WC1H 9HR, Tel: 01-387 1970.

Chairman: Peter Marshall.
Hon. Secretary: Tony Pilgrim.

SCREEN ADVERTISING WORLD ASSOCIATION LTD.
205 Wardour Street, London, W1V 3FA. Tel: 01-734 7621.

SOCIETY OF AUTHORS
84 Drayton Gardens, London, SW10 9SD. Tel: 01-373 6642.

(An independent trade union representing authors.)

SOCIETY OF AUTHORS BROADCASTING GROUP
84 Drayton Gardens, London, SW10 9SD. Tel: 01-363 6642.

(Representing film, TV and radio writers.)
(A subsidiary group within the Society of Authors.)

VARIETY CLUB OF GT. BRITAIN (TENT NO. 36)
32 Welbeck, Street, London, W1M 7PG.

Press Guy: David Jones.

VIDEO COPYRIGHT PROTECTION SOCIETY LIMITED
15–19 Cavendish Place, London W1M 0JA. Tel: 01-580 8152/3/4.

Chief Executive: Graham Wadsworth.

THE WRITERS GUILD OF GREAT BRITAIN
430 Edgward Road, London, W2 1EH Tel: 01-723 8074.

(The Writers Guild of Great Britain is the Trades Union Council-affiliated union which is the recognised representative body for negotiating agreements for writers in film, television, and radio as well as in the field of theatre and of publishing. As well as negotiating industrial agreements, the Guild represents writers wherever their interests need to be represented.)
President: Maureen Duffy.
Hon. Treasurer: Patrick Campbell.
Gen. Sec.: Walter J. Jeffrey.

EQUIPMENT & APPARATUS MANUFACTURERS

AMPEX INTERNATIONAL
Acre Road, Reading, Berks. Tel: 0734 85200.

ARRI (G.B.) LTD.
The Movie House, 2/3 Airlinks, Spitfire Way, Heston, Middlesex. Tel: 01-848 8881.

ARMSTRONG AMPLIFIERS LTD.
32A Blackhorse Lane, London, E17 6HJ. Tel: 01-523 0023.

BELLING AND LEE LTD.
Great Cambridge Road, Enfield, Middlesex. Tel: 01-363 5393. Telex: 263265.

(Electronic Components, RFI Shielding and Suppression)

ENGLISH ELECTRIC VALVE COMPANY LTD.
Waterhouse Lane, Chelmsford, Essex. Tel: 0245 61777. Telegrams: Enelctico, Chelmsford. Telex: 99103.

GENERAL ELECTRIC COMPANY, P.L.C. (THE)
1 Stanhope Gate, London, W1A 1EH. Tel: 01-493 8484.

ITT CONSUMER PRODUCTS (UK) LTD.
Chester Hall Lane, Basildon, Essex, SS14 3BW. Tel: 0268 3040.

MARCONI COMMUNICATION SYSTEMS LTD.
Marconi House, New Street, Chelmsford, Essex, CM1 1PL. Tel: 0245 353221.

PINEWOOD STUDIOS LTD.
Pinewood Road, Iver, Buckinghamshire, SL0 0NH. Tel: (Iver) 651700. Telex: 847505.

Managing Director: Cyril Howard
(Film and TV studios and also the sale of goods and services relating to the manufacture of cinematograph and television films)

PYE TVT LTD.
P.O. Box 41, Coldhams Lane, Cambridge, CB1 3JU. Tel: 0223 245115.
(The Broadcast Company of Phillips)

RANK ADVERTISING FILMS LTD.
127 Wardour Street, London, W1V 4AD. Tel: 01-439 9531. Telex: 262556.
Managing Director: Douglas Thomas
(Sale of advertising space in cinemas, theatres and bingo halls; selling of poster advertising space and the production of advertising, industrial and educational films and filmstrips)

RANK AUDIO VISUAL LTD.
P.O. Box 70, Great West Road, Brentford, Middlesex, TW8 9HR. Tel: 01-568 9222. Telex: 27976
Managing Director: Ronald Sharp
(Operation of video cassette library; producing and distributing internationally management training films)

RANK FILM LABORATORIES LTD.
North Orbital Road, Denham, Uxbridge, Middlesex, UB9 5HQ. Tel. (Denham) 832323. Telex 934704.
Managing Director: James Downer
(Processing of colour and black and white film for cinema and television)

RANK FILM DISTRIBUTORS LTD.
127 Wardour Street, London, W1V 4AD. Tel: 01-437 9020. Telex: 262556.
Managing Director: Frederick Turner
(Distribution of cinematograph films)

RANK THEATRES LTD.
439-445 Godstone Road, Whyteleafe, Surrey. Tel: (Upper Warlingham) 3355. Telex: 262305.
Operations Director (Acting): Stanley Fishman
(Management of cinemas)

RANK VIDEO SERVICES LTD.
Phoenix Park, Great West Road. Brentford, Middlesex, TW8 9PL.
Managing Director: Nicholas Watkins
(Operation of video and broadcast facilities and video cassette duplication)

Industrial Division

RANK CINTEL LTD.
Watton Road, Ware, Hertfordshire, SG12 0AE. Tel: (Ware) 3939. Telex: 81415.
Managing Director: Chris Waldron
(Manufacturer of telecine equipment for broadcast and film/tape transfer)

RANK TAYLOR HOBSON LTD.
P.O. Box 36, 1 New Star Road, Thurmaston Lane, Leicester, LE4 7JQ. Tel: (Leicester) 763771. Telex: 342338.
Managing Director: William Ramsden
(Manufacturer of precision measurement equipment, professional cine lenses and thermal imaging scanners)

RANK STRAND LTD. (UK Office)
P.O. Box 70, Great West Road, Brentford, Middlesex, TW8 9HR. Tel. 01-568 9222. Telex. 27976.
Managing Director: Michael Lowe
(Manufacturer and supplier of lighting and lighting control equipment)

RCA LTD. (Subsidiary of RCA Corporation)
Lincoln Way Windmill Road, Sunbury-on-Thames, Middlesex. Tel: Sunbury 85511.

SAMCINE SALES LTD.
303 Cricklewood Broadway, London, NW2 6PQ. Tel: 01-450 4557.

TECHNOVISION
Unit 4, St. Margaret's Business Centre, Twickenham, Middlesex, TW1 1JN. Tel: 01-891 5961.

THORN EMI LTD.
Thorn House, Upper St. Martins Lane, London, WC2H 9ED. Tel: 01-836 2444.

THORN EMI LAMPS & COMPONENTS LTD.
Miles Road, Mitcham, Surrey, CR4 37X. Tel: 01-640 1221.

WESTAR SALES & SERVICE LTD.
Unit 1, Fairway Drive, Bilton Fairway Industrial Estate, Greenford, Mddlesex, UB6 8PW. Tel: 01-578 0957. Telex: 923003.

WOTAN LAMPS LTD.
1 Gresham Way, Durnsford Road, London, SW19 8HU. Tel: 01-947 1261.

The World Market

* MARKET ANALYSES
* STATIONS
* OUTLOOK
* PROGRAM SOURCES

THE WORLD MARKET

AFGHANISTAN

People's Radio & Television Afghanistan, Post Office Box 544, Kabul; 8 stations, 13,000 sets.

ALBANIA

Radiodiffusion TV Albanaise, Tirana, government-owned experimental station, broadcasts sixteen hours weekly to some 204,000 sets, many of them located in public places so that segments of the populace not owning sets can view the programs.

ANGOLA

Television Popular de Angola, C.P. 2604, Luanda; 24,000 sets.

AUSTRALIA

Industry Make-Up: Australia has three commercial networks: The Seven Network (owned by the Fairfax Group); The Nine Web (Consolidated Press Holdings); and Network 10 (News Ltd. and others). Government-owned networks: Australian Broadcasting Corp., and Special Broadcasting Service. Total number of commercial stations is 50: ABC has 274 stations including regional transmitters and translators; Special Broadcasing covers nine territories.

Viewing Patterns: Total TV households: 4,798,000; families viewing (aggregate): 4,664,000; families viewing (percentage): 97.2%. Average viewing time per week of all age groups is 19 hours, 4 minutes.

National Top 10 Programs—1985–86: (in order) 60 Minutes; A Country Practice; Sale of the Century; News, Sports & Weather; It's a Knockout; Willesee; The Cosby Show; Sunday Movies; Current Affairs Programs; George & Mildred.

BAHRAIN

Bahrain TV, P.O. Box 1075, Manama, Bahrain, operates 1 channel and 1 relay for some 170,000 color sets.

BANGLADESH

Pilot station established in 1964 by government. Now includes originating station at Dacca with relay stations at Chittagong, Natore, Khulna, Sylhet, and Rangpur plus two under construction. Address Bangladesh TV, Television Bhaban, Rampura P.O. Box 456, Dacca. 290,000 sets.

BRAZIL

Brazil now has some 20,000,000 sets using PAL. The audience is estimated at about 80,000,000, which makes this country the highest selling and fastest growing market in Latin America.

Brazilian law requires that all owners of radio or TV stations be of Brazilian nationality. A further law stipulates that all foreign films shown on TV be dubbed, and that no station may transmit more than 22 half hours of foreign films for each 72 hours of weekly transmission time. Stations which transmit less than 12 hours per day have a corresponding lower quota. Seven sound studios, four in Rio de Janeiro and three in Sao Paulo take care of the dubbing of all American and some Italian, Argentine and Mexican films that come into the country.

Professional Association of Radio and TV Station Owners: Sindicato dos Proprietarios de Impresas de Radio Diffusao a Televisao, Avenida Presidente 'Churchill 97 Sala 606, Rio de Janeiro.

BRUNEI

Established 1975 by governmental Radio TV Brunei, Bander Seri Begawan, Brunei. Two channels; 54,000 sets.

BURMA

Burma Broadcasting Service, Prome Road, Kamayut Post Office, Rangoon. One station. 60,000 sets

CAMBODIA (Kampuchea)

Radio Kampuchea Television, 28 Ave Preah Mohaksatryany Kossonak, Phnom Penh City, broadcasts daily on Channel 8 with relay to Bokor. Sets are estimated at 50,000.

CANADA

Number of TV Sets: Of an estimated 8,857,000 private households, 88.4% in 1984 had at least one color TV set and 17.8% two or more. The latter figure was up from 15.6% in March of 1983.

Number of TV Stations: 211, including 30 Canadian Broadcasting Corp. outlets (owned and operated); 25 independent CTV member stations; and six French-tract TVA outlets based in Quebec.

Cable: 60% of all households, or 5,000,000, subscribe to basic cable TV services. Of those, 31.4% have cable converters rented in 1984 from cable operators or purchased outright. Compared to 1983 the former figure is constant; however, the latter is an increase of 26.3% over the previous year. Cable operators presently take in some $352,200,000 (Canadian) annually.

TV Corporations: Canadian Broadcasting Corporation, Box 500, Station A (416) 925-3311; (English and French networks) Radio-Canada CBC Enterprises/Les Entreprises, 1400 Dorchester Blvd., E., Montreal Quebec, Canada H2L 2M2; CTV-TV Network, Ltd., 42 Charles St. E., Toronto, Ontario, Canada M4Y 1T5 (416) 928-6000; Global Communications, Ltd., 81 Barber Green Road, Don Mills, Ontario, Canada M3C 2A2 (416) 446-5311; TV Ontario (educational network), 2180 Yonge St., Box 200, Station Q, Toronto, Ontario, Canada M4T 2T1 (416) 484-2600; Tele-Metropole (Quebec Network), 1600 de Maisonneuve, Montreal, Quebec, Canada H2L 4P6 (514) 526-9251.

Pay TV Corporations: First Choice Canadian Communications Corp., (covers eastern half of Canada from Ontario to Newfoundland), 1 Dundas St. W., Suite 1700, Toronto, Ontario, Canada M5G 1Z3 (416) 977-5485; Superchannel—Alarcom Pay TV Ltd., (covers Western half of Canada from Manitoba to British Columbia), 5324 Calgary Trail, Suite 200, Edmonton, Alberta T6H 4J8 (403) 437-7744; Super Ecran (French-language service in Quebec), 666 Sherbrook W., 15th Floor, Montreal, Quebec, Canada H3E 1E7 (514) 288-2188; MuchMusic (national), 99 Queen St. E., Toronto, Ontario, Canada M5C 2M1; The Sports Network (national), 1155 Leslie St., Don Mills, Ontario, Canada M3C 2J6 (416) 449-2244.

Government Organizations: The National Film Board of Canada, 150 Kent St., Ottawa, Ontario K1A 0M9 (613) 922-3615; Telefilm Canada, Banque Nationale Tower, 600 de la Gauchetiere St. W, Montreal, Quebec, H3B 4L2; National Film, Television and Sound Archives, 344 Wellington St., Ottawa, Ontario, K1A 0N3 (613) 995-1311.

Industry Organizations: The Federation of Canadian Guilds and Unions in Film and Television, 2239 Yonge St., Toronto, Ontario M4S 2B5 (416) 489-1311; Canadian Cable Television Association, 85 Albert St., Ontario, KIP 6A4 (613) 232-2631.

CHINA (Communist)

Peking TV, opened in 1969, consists of three networks, one purely local and the other two broadcasting by micro-wave to the rest of the country. Color broadcasts began in 1973. Shanghai, China's largest city, has two channels on the air for about 9 hours daily with some 50% of the programs listed as entertainment, 20% movies, news or documentaries, and 20% sports or children's programs, in addition to educational and foreign language-instruction programs. Chinese officials blame the Cultural Revolution for the slow growth of TV and say that after the Gang of Four was ousted in the following decade TV stations were opened in all 29 of China's provinces and private set ownership rose to 52 million tuned to 70 stations and 130 relays. With some 7 million sets being added annually, China is producing 800 TV dramas a year. Twenty percent of all households now have TV sets and by 1990 this number will be doubled.

CCTV began use of International Telecommunications Satellite Organization facilities to reach parts of China where reception is poor to non-existent but only until they set up their own satellite service for which they are setting up 50 ground stations. Some 62% of the country is covered already as far as reception is concerned.

A poll indicates 92% of Peking's residents watch TV regularly while in a nearby suburban area with only 6.7 sets per 100 households, 87% of residents watch TV. CTV broadcasts 30 hours weekly, programming news, instruction, cartoons, variety and drama. Audience estimated at 800 million.

China now manufactures some 7.1 million sets annually and it is estimated that the number of sets will soon reach 60 million, including sets open to the public audience. Total number of nation-wide stations (including micro-wave relay stations) is over 40. Black-and-white sets sell for the equivalent of $370 and color sets for about $1,335 and there is a waiting list for the former. Domestic and imported films are broadcast from time to time, including American feature films occasionally.

Central Broadcasting Administration, Hsin Men, Peking, now offers nation-wide TV commercials at rates ranging from about $625 for a 15-second spot to a full minute for $1,800.

CHINA (Taiwan)

Television began in 1962 by the Educational Television Station which later became the private China Television Service in 1971. There are now three networks: Taiwan Television Enterprise (1962), China Television Company (1969) and China Television Service. All three act as private corporations deriving revenues from commercials. These three stations have 24 transmitters with total broadcasts of about 265 hours weekly for some 5.3 million set owners who pay about $1.50 annually for a license. About 80% of the programs are domestic, with most of the imports from the U.S.A. Over one-third of the sets are color. Taiwan has two communication satellite stations. A new rule states that commercials must not exceed 15% total broadcast time. Movie theatre owners complain that the three imported feature films shown weekly on television hurt their box office.

All three networks broadcast in color, TTV and CTV 6 hours 25 minutes weekdays and 12 hours weekends and holidays while CTS broadcasts 10.15 hours weekdays, 15 hours on Saturday and 17 hours Sunday or holidays. News takes an average of 21%, public service over 10%, culture and education 20%, entertainment 48%. TTV has 10 transmitters, CTV 6, and CTS 8, plus an equal number of relay stations. Sets number 5,100,000.

New rules call for no commercials during programs of less than 30 minutes and all commercials to secure government approval. In the future, 80% of all programs must originate in Taiwan with entertainment programs taking up no more than 55% of broadcast time and 45% or more devoted to educational, cultural or news types.

With relay stations it is estimated that 100% of the island's population of 18 million receives TV reception. About 12% of programs are imports, mostly from America, and these are broadcast in the original English with Chinese captions, which has served to develop knowledge of the English language among the populace.

TV showings of full-length Chinese-language, feature films imported from Hong Kong were stopped following retaliatory action by local cinema interests but the government may step in later and permit such showings, except on Sundays and holidays when the theatres reap their largest harvest. Inquiries should be addressed: Ministry of Communications, Taipei, Taiwan, Republic of China, or to: China Radio/TV Assoc. 6-144 Hsin Shen (South) Rd., Section 1, Taipei, Taiwan, Republic of China.

CONGO

Radio-TV de Congo, B.P. 2241, Brazzaville. One station; 5,000 sets.

EGYPT

Television in Egypt is attached to the Ministry of Information. The President of Egyptian TV is Mrs. Samia Sadek.

The Central station in Cairo transmits about 150 hours a week through two channels. A third channel started on Oct. 6, 1985, transmitting about 30 hours a week. The three channels cover most of Egypt including Aswan, Luxor, the New Valley, Sinai, and Saudi Arabia.

Egyptian TV follows the European technical transmission with an image of 825 scansions.

The TV receivers in use number over 15 million. The Arabic Department shoots a movie news review weekly and it is sent to 35 stations all over the world with which Arab TV exchange cultural and documentary materials.

ETHIOPIA

Ethiopia Television, Post Office Box 544, Addis Ababa. Two stations; 48,000 sets.

FINLAND

Finland has a two-channel television system that differs considerably from the other countries. There is at present in Finland one radio and television operation licence which has been granted to the Finnish Broadcasting Company, Oy Yleisradio Ab. The existence of MTV, Oy Mainow-TV-Reklam Ab, which is a private commercial TV company, is acknowledged in the same licence.

The basis for official relations between the companies were laid down in more detail in the basic agreement concluded in 1976. Television broadcasting in Finland is under parliamentary control. The Administrative Council of the Finnish Broadcasting Company appointed by Parliament is the highest organ exercising programme policy. It has two functions. The Administrative Council exercises programme policy control over both companies. In addition, as its name implies, it is the highest administrative organ in the Finnish Broadcasting Company.

MTV has its own corresponding administrative council.

As a bilingual country Finland also has programmes in Swedish on both tv-channels.

Some 19 hours per week—out of the total of 75—are sold by Oy Yleisradio Ab to MTV. At the end of 1981 a one-year price agreement was signed, according to which MTV's levy to the Finnish Broadcasting Company is at least 191.2 million marks in 1982. MTV produces nearly 43% of its programmes.

Numbers of color sets is today about 0.9 million (57% of all sets).

The Finnish Broadcasting Company: Head Office, Kesäkatu 2, 00260 Helsinki 26 (Telephone 441141) Broadcasting Center, Yleisradiokeskus, Pasila 00240 Helsinki 24 (Telephone 418811) TV 2 Television Center, Tohloppi, 33270 Tampere 27 (Telephone 445455), MTV, Oy Mainos-TV-Reklam AB, Pasilankatu 44, 00240 Helsinki 24 (Telephone 15001).

FRANCE

Networks: France has three television networks, all state-operated, drawing funds from an annual tax on TV set owners and advertising. (Revenues from spot ads are limited to about 25% of the budget.)

The newtworks are TF-1, which was created first and led the field in audience numbers until the second channel, Antenne-2, overtook it in 1983. The third regional network is FR-3.

Networks are under the jurisdiction of the High Authority (HA) composed of nine members which has named their presents since 1982, before which the president of the republic made such selections.

Canal Plus has a concession to run for 12 years initially. Its largest investor (40%) is the government-controlled conglomerate Havas. Most of the rest of the shares are held by state companies.

Production Companies: Societé Française de Production is the largest production facility in Europe. It is state-owned and has 2,500 employees. It receives no funds from the TV set fee, deriving 80% of its revenues from work for the state networks.

GHANA

Ghana Broadcasting Corporation, Broadcast House, Post Office Broad Box 1633, Accra. Five stations, 145,000 sets.

GREECE

TV is nationwide and the most popular entertainment of the Greek public, to the detriment of all other kinds of recreation, particularly film theatres. There are two TV channels in Athens operated by the National Radio-Television Organization, ERT 1 and ERT 2. Both channels operate in color. TV, like sound broadcasting, is controlled by the state and responsibility for both services is invested in both of these state units. The ERT 1 has a TV relay station in Thessaloniki telecasting the news from northern Greece and another in Patras covering news bulletins from southern Greece. Both channels have many relay towers throughout the country. By a draft law, not debated by the Greek parliament at the time of writing, both channels will merge under one company under state control. The new company will be called Helliniki Radiophonia Tileorasi ERT (Greek Radio Television). It will serve as an enterprise of public benefit open to all trends of the medium.

Each channel airs seven to ten hours of programming on weekdays and ten hours on Sundays and holidays, which are mostly videotaped. About 60% of this programming is covered by news, educational subjects, discussion panels, local movies and series; the rest is covered by foreign films and series. ERT 1 is a full member of the E.B.U. and transmits all important international events via satellite.

It is estimated that more than 1,000,000 black and white sets have been sold in Greece; the number of color sets reaches 800,000, in a population of 10,000,000 people. The ERT 1 office and studio is located at 436 Mesoguion Str., Athens; its town house address is 16 Mourouzi Str., Athens. The president is Andreas Tsouderos and the director general is Theodore Halatsis.

ERT 2 channel is located at 136 Mesoguion Str. and Katehaki, Athens. The president is Alecos Papadopoulos and the program director is Andreas Antoniades.

TV Commercials: A great number of spots are sold daily by both channels to several advertising agencies. The price per minute varies according to the time and the popularity of the program. The highest price paid so far was before and after each telecast of the World Cup soccer games from Mexico transmitted directly via Eurovision.

Agencies: There are several agencies acting on behalf of various foreign TV companies: Hellas Television International, 96 Academias Str., Athens, representing MGM, Screen Gems, Warner Bros., RAI, Sacis, Paramount, Rank, Titanus, Egyptian TV, Austrialian TV, Spanish TV, Brazilian TV, World Vision, Romulus, World Fair Communications, Thames TV, Film Marketing Servicing, etc.; Apollon TV International Enterprises, 46 King Constantine Avenue, Athens, representing Anthony Morris, Children's Television Workshop, Embassy Telecommunications, Four Star Entertainment, Corp., Henson International Television, John Pearson International, Lassis Television, London Films, Marvin Goodman Associates, Metromedia Productions, NBC International NOS, NTA Associates, Orion, P.S.O Samuel Goldwyn, Strenghold Televideo, Mexican TV, Toho, Teleworld, Tristar, etc.; Yannis Triantifyllis, 8 Klisovis Str., Athens, agnet of ITV TV, etc.; and Dennis Petropoulos, agent of N.T.A. II Likavitou Str., Athens, Con. Trikoupis I Halkokondyli Str., Athens, etc.

Local TV Production: Both channels produce several telepictures and serials for local use and for export to foreign TV stations. ERT 1, in order to support local film production, is subsidizing some Greek pictures which are also shot as serials.

Other local TV producers are: Hellas TV Productions, 96 Academias

Str., Athens, manager Andreas Lappas; Dennis Petropoulos II, Licavitou Str., Athensl Panos Spyropoulos, 46 King Constantine Avenue, Athens; Andromesa Dyo Epe, 47 Lemnou Str.; Kinimatografiki Epe, 4 Tim Filimonos Tr., Athens; Basil Baros, 26 Democritou Str., Athens; N. Samaras, 14 Strat. Syndesmou Str., Athens; TVEM, 52 Skoufa Str., Athens; Aris Tsopanellis, 5–7 Kapodistriou Str., Athens; DYAS Film; ASTYR FILM; FINOS FILM, etc.

TV Studios: Television Enterprise S.A. Studios, head office, 28 Kapodistriou Str., Athens, manager Ch. Elmatzoglou. ATA Ltd. Studios, head office, 8 Homerou Str., Athens, Manager George Rallis. FIN Films Spata Attikis, Sklavis Studio, head office, 69 Zoodohou Piguis Str., Athens. Roussopoulos Bros. Studio Cinemagic, 53 Hiou Str., Athens, etc.

—RENA VELISSARIOU

GUAM (U.S. Possession)

Guam Television operates one station with two channels for 17 hours daily, servicing an estimated 153,000 sets in the hands of Americans and natives. Owner is Pacific Broadcasting Corp., Agana. Some color is broadcast. The Department of Education, Agana, operates Channel 12, some 14 hours daily.

GUINEA

Radio-Diffusion Guinienne, B.P. 391, Conraky. 7,600 sets.

HOLLAND

The number of TV sets as of Jan. 1, 1986, was 4,574,183. The market is practically saturated. The total Dutch population is almost 14,400,000. Practically every Dutch family has a TV set now; two sets per family is no longer an exception.

TV competition with motion picture theatres and video is strong; the situation in the film business is growing worse every year. In general TV competition is strongest in winter. Younger people usually do not stay home on Friday and Saturday nights.

German and Belgian TV is received well, especially German. (German and Belium border Holland.) The central antennae system is steadily growing in importance. A color TV set costs, depending on size, 51 cm, 56 cm, 66 cm, from 800 to 1,800 Dutch florins (one dollar was fl. 2.46 at the time of writing). Various shops sell at prices lower than the "official" ones. Philips latest 70 mm set costs fl. 3,000.

There are two channels, with commercials under the name of Ster-Televisie. Commercials are shown every night except Sunday on both channels. A program is never interrupted by a commercial. Sky Channel has been a tremendous success in Holland from the start. A new studio has been opened in the center of Amsterdam in a former cinema.

The Nederlandse Omroep Stichting (N.O.S.) is the central radio and TV organization, but there are eight main subdivision stations: a Roman-Catholic one (K.R.O.); two political ones (left): V.A.R.A. and V.P.R.O.; two Protestant sections, N.C.R.V. and E.O. (steadily growing in importance), and three neutral sections: A.V.R.O., T.R.O.S. and V.O.O. (with a large number of popular youth programs, pop and country music in particular). A.V.R.O. has the largest number of members, closely followed by T.R.O.S. The V.O.O. station is still growing in importance. There are also some minor TV organizations.

Although N.O.S. has an important part of the playing time, the eight stations are completely independent, as far as their activities are concerned. They are, with N.O.S., the most important buyers on the international market. Of the educational and religious stations TELEAC (a series of popular subjects, mathematics courses, etc.) and I.K.O.N. (religious) are the biggest.

A yearly contribution of fl. 158 is paid by the owner of a set to the government. This includes the the fee for a radio set.

On an average, feature films are programmed two nights a week, and, in summer, now and then, also on afternoons (films for all ages). On Wednesday nights only if there is no football match. The film industry organization (Nederlandse Bond van Bioscopen en Filmondernemingen—N.B.B. now) has an agreement with the TV authorities that pictures can be shown only on TV 40 months or more after the first release date in motion picture theatres; exceptions are possible. Although showings of motion pictures on TV on weekends are not included in that agreement, the attitude of the Bioscoopbond has become more flexible; there is a regular contact between the federation and TV authorities. The countries of origin of pictures on TV vary, but American and English films are shown mostly, in addition to TV series from these countries. Miami Vice, The Cosby Show, Lou Grant, Me and My Girl, Cheers, Dempsey and Makepeace, The A-team, Love Boat, and Man About the House (reissue) are very popular, as are German thrillers. The quality of programs is good; there are also many comments on the political news.

Radio and TV fall under the Ministry of Welfare, Social Health and Culture (W.V.C.). A conflict between this ministry and the TV companies has declined.

Due to the high standard of living many people can afford to buy a TV with cash. Buying by installment has never been popular since the war, though that system draws more clients gradually, mainly due to the economic situation and high costs of living. Dutch stations are in Hilversum, as is broadcasting. Philips is the most important manufacturer of TV sets. Big imports are from Germany and Japan. The address of the Nederlandse Omroep Stichting (N.O.S.)is 53, Emmastraat, P.O. Box 10, 1200 JB Hilversum, Holland.

Members of the organization of TV cable companies have to pay duties to the N.B.B. and to, among others, the main American companies: author rights of a producer, of a motion picture shown on cable TV.

The big problem is the piracy of motion pictures, which is still very much in evidence. There are also illegal stations regularly captured by the police.

—PHILIP DE SCHAAP

HONG KONG

Established 1957 by Rediffusion (HK) as closed circuit, converted to conventional TV in 1974. Asia Television (ATV) Central P.O Box 1414, Kowloon, Hong Kong. Additional outlets: Television Broadcast (HK-TVB), 77 Broadcast Drive, P.O. Box 100, Kowloon, Hong Kong; and, Radio TV Hong Kong, Kowloon Central P.O. Box 200, Hong Kong (governmental unit acting as producer for above).

INDIA

At present, there are eight full fledged TV stations located at Delhi, Bombay, Madras, Calcutta, Lucknow, Srinagar, Jullundur, and Amritsar, in addition to several relay stations all over the country.

Apart from these, there are seven relay stations which were set up for the SITE (Satellite Instructional Television Experiment) program which ran for one year, from August 1975. They are in Jaipur, Hyderabad, Gulbarga, Muzaffarpur, Sambalpur, Raipur and Pij, near Ahmedabad. At present, programs for Hyderabad and Gulbarga in Telugu and Kannada are recorded at Hyderabad. Cuttack records programs in Oriya and feeds Sambalpur. Jaipur, Muzaffarpur and Raipur are supplied with pre-recorded tapes in Hindi by Delhi. At Pij recording is done at the SAC (Space Application Centre) studios and telecast for one hour daily. Altogether, these terrestrial stations cover 40% of the viewers formerly covered by the SITE program.

The launching of the Indian National Satellite System (INSAT-IB) in 1984 has completely changed the electronic media scene, opening up new possibilities in mass communication. Already Doordarshan puts its programs over 132 low power and 47 high power transmitters covering 70% of the population. The new expansion program covers 480 million people (260 million rural and 220 million urban). Probably nowhere else in the world has a government undertaken TV expansion on such a vast scale in so short a time.

New installations will cover all towns with a population of 100,000 or above. INSAT-IB has facilitated the national linkage with HPTs and LPTs relaying national programs from the Centre (Delhi), and serves the states with educational and area specific programs.

There are an well over 5,000,000 TV sets in the country, with a nightly audience of nearly 60,000,000, in comparison to 13,000,000 viewers that go to the cinema daily. About half the TV sets are concentrated in metro towns but with LPTs now beaming to cover over half the country's population, the growth rate of TV sets is expected to be a staggering three million annually in the next two years. As part of its plan to extend TV coverage to remote parts of the country, the Government will shortly begin the installation of very low power transmitters (VLPT) with a range of about 20 km. These are ideal for relaying programs to hilly areas, remote locations and isolated island that are sparsely populated.

—B.D. GARGA

INDONESIA

The government-owned RRI-TV, on the air since 1962, banned commercials in 1981, and in 1984 banned the showing of foreign-made TV series from 1985 on the grounds that the people preferred domestic-made fare. Up to the time of the ban a single American-made TV show daily had averaged an estimated 24 million viewers, a fact that tends to contradict the governmental view.

At present stations are operated on 2 channels in Jakarta, Bandung, Jogakarta, Semarang and Tjiribon, with some 203 relays. Broadcasting hours average above 40 hours weekly with some programs in color to sets estimated to number over 2 million. Programs are 50% entertainment, 25% educational, 25% public service, live 60% of the time, and 40% video-taped. With the departure of imported shows, the government will increase educational shows based on national culture. Indonesia is building 50 relays under its fourth 5-year plan since its 203 relays now reach only 27% of its population of 114 million. Inquiries to TV Republic Indonesia (TVRI), Yayasan Televisi, Senayan Jakarta. 10 stations; 3,000,000 sets.

IRAN

Islamic Republic of Iran Broadcasting, Post Office Box 98-200, Teheran. Sixteen stations, 2.1 million sets.

IRAQ

Iraq Broadcasting & Television, Broadcasting House, Salihiya, Baghdad. Six stations, 725,000 sets.

IRELAND

Telefis Eireann is the official name of the television service in Ireland.

Television, like sound broadcasting, is run as an independent State Statuary body and responsibility for both services is vested in Radio Eireann, the Broadcasting Authority. This Authority, appointed by the Government, consists of nine members serving on a part-time basis under a chairman selected by the Government. The present chairman is T. Andrews.

The Minister for Posts and Telegraphs, who is responsible for the autonomously operated Authority, reserves to himself the duties of fixing and collecting license fees from domestic viewers, licenses transmitting stations, and has a veto on the appointment and conditions of the Authority's top executive. The Director-General, Kevin McCourt, is employed full-time.

The Television service began in 1962. It has five main high power transmitters and thirteen satellite "transposers," serving areas outside the range of the main transmitters. Its national coverage is estimated at 98 per cent of the population. The national technical standard is a 625 line one, but programs are also broadcast on a 405 line in the Eastern and Northwestern parts of the country.

The Authority, which has the responsibility of providing programs of suitable cultural and national content, transmits 44 hours per week, with occasional additional programs. In addition, educational programs for schools, two and a half hours per week, are broadcast for 33 weeks of the year on behalf of the Department of Education.

Of the 44 hours of weekly programs, 22 are of home origin. The balance are imported mainly from Great Britain and America.

There are about 350,000 receiving sets in operation, of which about 200,000 are able to receive programs from Great Britain's BBC-TV and Independent TV stations as well as Radio Telefis Eireann.

ISRAEL

Israel television broadcasts daily in Arabic and Hebrew. Arabic programs start at 6:00 p.m. and continue to 8 p.m. Programs include documentaries, round-ups, news, films, variety shows, discussions, games, etc. These programs include, as well, weekly interviews with individuals of the Arab Israeli population who can convey regards to their relatives in neighboring countries, such as Egypt, Syria, Lebanon, Jordan through this medium.

At 8:00 the Hebrew programs begin, offering the same variety of broadcast as the Arabic programs. Hebrew broadcasts continue up to 11:30 or midnight. The majority of Hebrew programs are subtitled in Arabic; and foreign language broadcasts, including films, are subtitled in both Hebrew and Arabic. Similarly, most of the Arabic programs have Hebrew subtitles.

Besides the above mentioned programs, television broadcasts every morning (except Saturday) educational programs beginning at 8:00 and continuing to 4:00. This is followed by children's programs which continue to 6:30 and include films, puzzles, games, cartoons, etc.

ITALY

From its inception the Italian television industry was dominated by a public network agency—RAI— but toward the end of the 1970's its dominance was finally challenged by private broadcasting. Prime networks are Canale-5, Italia-1 and Rete 4. The first two are part of the Silvio Berlusconi conglomerate while the third is owned by the Mondadori publishing group.

Overseeing RAI is a parliamentary commission which elects 10 of its 16 directors. The others are elected by IRI (Institute for Reconstruction of Industry) which owns 99.55% of RAI, the rest being held by a publishing association. RAI gets its operating authority from the Ministry of Post and Telecommuncations; its finances are reviewed by the Ministry of Finance. RAI is funded by license fees and advertising. (Ads are limited to 5% of airtime.)

RAI operates three TV networks: RAI-1, its main and most successful outlet; RAI-2, an alternate network; and RAI-3, whose viewers are few although it is the only one which does not carry advertising.

RAI has transmitters all over Italy and uses 21 regional offices. It has five production centers and provides the majority of its own programming, including that for a worldwide news service it operates.

Private TV companies are not subject to the same rule as RAI. For instance they carry up to 14–18% advertising in airtime.

Trends: TV in Italy has made tremendous advances in acquiring programming the last several years. It is reported public and private broadcasters have invested close to $500,000,000 in foreign films and TV programs to attract TV viewers.

IVORY COAST

TV Ivorienne, Television House, Latrille, BP 8883, Abidjan. Operates 11 stations. Sets estimated at 310,000.

JAPAN

Non-commercial TV broadcasting began in Tokyo Feb. 1, 1953, by the quasi-governmental Nippon Hoso Kyuokai (NHK) followed seven months later by the first commercial TV broadcast of Nippon Television Network (NTV). Broadcast time for NHK, which began with only 866 set-owners paying a fee of Yen 200 monthly, was 4 hours a day compared to 6 hours by NTV, which was affiliated with the Yomiuri newspapers. By 1960 NHK possessed 60 stations and there were 47 commercial stations broadcasting, while the number of sets had increased to about 7 million, topping the 10 million mark two years later.

Although commercial networks as they are established in the U.S. are legally forbidden, there came about a nationwide grouping of commercial stations with the Tokyo stations acting as pivotal points and providing tieups and programs. Thus in 1959, 16 commercial stations formed Japan News Network which soon spread to other programming areas, with JOKR in Tokyo, followed by three other such groupings centering on NTV, Nippon Educational Television (renamed Asahi National Broadcasting in 1977), and the Fuji TV key stations in Tokyo. It was then apparent that several newspapers with national sales systems, through capital tieups, were virtually in control of the national commercial networks.

Educational broadcasts were begun by NHK in 1959, followed three weeks later by Nippon Educational Television, which later dropped the "educational" pretense and became a regular broadcaster, as TV Tokyo (JOTX) did later, when it was found impossible to operate a private educational TV station in Japan for financial reasons.

The Tokyo Metropolitan area, which comprises almost 30% of Japan's population of 122.4 million, is served by Channel 1 NHK general network station, Channel 3 NHK educational network station, Channels 4, 6, 8 and 10 operated by NTV, TBS, Fuji, TV Asahi commercial network stations, respectively, and semi-independent TV Tokyo (JOTX) on channel 12 and TVK (UHF) 42 in Yokohama.

NHK's general programming lists 8 regional stations throughout the nation, 45 local stations and numerous relay stations in the VHF range to bring general programming to 3,492 outlets (2,851 UHF outlets). NHK educational facilities comprise 8 regional stations, 37 local stations, 2,207 relay stations for a total of 3,416 outlets of which 2,778 are UHF, including use of mini-satellite relays. It must be emphasized that in most cases (but not all) the general and educational services make use of the same facilities.

There are 42 companies operating both radio and TV stations and 63 operating only TV stations. In the VHF sector some 48 companies operate 486 stations; in UHF 55 companies operate 5,662 stations, plus 9 SHF stations, a total of 6,157.

These four "networks" operate in the 8 key areas of Japan—Tokyo, Osaka, Nagoya, Fukuoka, Sapporo, Hiroshima, Sendai, and Hokkaido—which are 4 commercial-station areas (plus NHK). Other stations located in less populous areas use a cross network arrangement by which programs from plural key stations are received. There is Asahi National Broadcasting with 18 stations, Fuji Telecasting with 27, Tokyo Broadcasting System with 25, and Nippon Television with 29 stations. In addition several independent stations have ties and non-commercial NHK covers 30 million of Japan's 37 million households.

In 1984 NHK launched its direct broadcasting satellite which beams two TV channels to people living in mountainous areas and remote islands who until then had had trouble receiving TV programs, bringing protests that an organization in the red would make so huge an expenditure for some 420,000 TV sets.

While NHK collects monthly fees from 31,400,000 registered sets, the Home Ministry estimates the total number is 62,495,000 (including households with more than one), of which 9,423,000 are black and white and 53,072,000 are color. Some 98.5% of registered households possess one or more color sets for which they are assessed a flat $6.50 a month versus $4.25 for black-and-white sets. Thus, it is no surprise that NHK is by far the wealthiest broadcasting corporation in the world with 16,000 employees, which it has promised to reduce to 15,000, and a 23-story headquarters in Tokyo. With revenues of over $2.113 and expenses of $2.053 billion, it predicts deficits in 1987.

With 36.2% of the national advertising budget, TV is the leading advertising medium with designated prime time from 7:00 to 11:00 p.m. and ad spot buying rates determined on the gross rating point though, with a seller's market, card rates are often disregarded. Top rate for a 60-second network shop is $48,000 and a 54-minute program for a month about $1.4 million; generally contracts are for 6 months but recently 3-month contracts became available, there being waiting lists for sponsors. Sporting events, especially baseball, in non-prime time bring top prices due to good results. Though rules call for not more than 18% of broadcast time be devoted to commercials, this rule is only loosely followed. In addition some stations persist in intensifying audio volume for favored commercials. TV ad expenditures increased 2.3% to $5.8 billion (this figure in dollars increased considerably because of the appreciation of the yen relative to the falling value of the dollar). Advertising for household appliances and supplies, automobiles, department stores, cosmetics and detergents gained while pharmaceuticals, and entertainment industries waned.

The largest TV advertiser, the food-beverage industry, which is allowed to advertise high alcohol beverages including whiskey, took 28% of TV ads.

Although an agreement was once reached to restrict broadcasting hours to 16.5 a day to conserve energy, many commercial station are broadcasting past the midnight deadline; NHK signs off by midnight. While TV is undoubtedly the most influential medium for both young and old, various polls disagree when attempts are made to determine the average daily time a Japanese watches the tube. NHK says the average Japanese spends 23 hours 19 minutes a week watching TV. Nielsen gives the Tokyo viewing time as 8 hours 12 minutes daily, taking into consideration the viewing by each household member. Favorite shows have veered from soap operas to various kinds of emceed shows, especially quiz shows. Men prefer sports shows, including baseball, sumo wrestling, golf, and, recently, American-style football, though old-type samurai dramas are still popular with both sexes. The younger audience spends much time watching cartoons before graduating to teen-age singing shows, contests or quizzes. In the past year some 800 full length feature films and some 300 Japanese-made films were broadcast, almost all from America and the rest from Italy, Britain, France, Germany, Hong Kong and other nations. These imports, especially those from the U.S. tend to be grade B films or films made in America especially for TV. These are almost always dubbed into Japanese but a few are available in the original language on a different wavelength for the benefit of TV sets equipped with multiplex receivers. Each network averages about 5 movies weekly and imports occasionally break into the top 30 weekly programs.

Current American TV shows, none shown in prime time, include "Kojak," "The Fugitive," "Hawaii Five-0," "Ironhorse," "T.J. Hooker," "60 Minutes," "The Little House on the Prairie," "The A-Team," "McCloud," "Lou Grant," "The Greatest American Hero," "Moonlighting," "The Hangman," "The Unexpected" and other oldies in which the Japanese audience has only mild interest, at best.

A survey indicated imported feature films shown on TV cost more than domestic movies but are shown more often so tend to dominate the medium, so it must be assumed their frequency on TV reflects a response to demand, even taking into consideration the reluctance of Japanese movie studios to contribute to the prosperity of what they consider a dangerous competitor to their own industry.

As with the old TV programs purchased from abroad, Japanese buyers insist on rock bottom prices, the result being a formidable collection of of full length feature films which, due to their age and caliber, are mostly trash. With few exceptions, they can only be characterized as mixed second- and third-rate. Despite that films are repeated year after year. Once dubbed into Japanese, some Japanese say, it does not make much difference if the film is good or not. Sellers abroad are advised when contracting to provide a special clause on re-runs without compensation.

NKH general stations average 18 hours daily, 37.3% devoted to news and commentaries, 21% to entertainment, 27% to culture, and 14% to education. Commercial stations average 20.3 hours with entertainment 40.6%, cultural 23.9%, news 16.4%, education 12.1%, sports 5.6% and announcements .6%. Of this broadcasting average over 17 hours consisted of sponsored programs and 3 hr. of sustaining programs. Although broadcasters claimed that advertising commercials (including a daily average of 241 spot announcements) took only 6% of total broadcasting time of each station on the average, anyone with a stop watch knows that this is not true. Over 60% of Japanese polled indicated an opinion that there were far too many commercials, while 50% objected to the ads shown in conjunction with kiddies' programs and thought such programs should carry no ads.

Sponsors of a 30-minute prime time show pay about $8,000 on a Tokyo station with other spots going for $3,500 per sponsor.

Production cost for a one-hour program is only $80,000, about one-fifth of the cost in the U.S. Payments for authoring a 30-minute script is $300 at NHK and as low as $150 at commercial stations. However, writers with a national reputation get much more.

A study of 107 commercial TV stations reveals that although the UHF outlets located in the periphery of the large cities are doing only moderately well as regards operating profits, the older-established VHF stations, particularly those affiliated with networks and in Tokyo or Osaka, enjoyed a good year.

Japan exports very few TV programs of its own but it is the world's largest exporter of TV sets and in addition sells TV equipment, complete broadcasting studios and nationwide setups abroad.

While a critic would rate Japanese TV in general as somewhat below the not very high American standard, and take umbrage at the great percentage of time taken by commercials on all stations except those of NHK, the average Japanese is satisfied with it. Lately, the government tried steps to prevent further intensification by stations of audio volume for commercials and limited them to 18% of total program time.

Quiz games have the highest average ratings followed by prime time cinema feature films. Then comes sports, samurai or home dramas, action dramas, kiddie and cartoon shows, musical, news, imported TV shows, and finally educational broadcasts.

There are no national cable TV systems but 38,221 cable TV stations feed to 4.3 million households where TV reception is poor or non-existent. In the cities, cable TV is piped to hotels (usually in English) and to some high-class apartment houses, and to a few private subscribers. In the suburbs some multi-storied housing complexes have their own cable TV. Very few dishes used for satellite reception now exist though the first private satellite broadcasting company promises it will be in full operation by 1980. Since 1985 NHK and private telecasters have had contracts to use Intelsat and a European satellite on a 24-hour basis but ordinarily they take only a few extra bits daily for inclusion on news broadcasts since they are not too interested in outside world news unless it affects Japan. In fact, this is also true as regards imported TV shows; they prefer their own, and imports are shown only on non-prime time and the late night hours. As for cinema features, usually each station shows one weekly on prime time. Most of the rest are late shows or late-late shows.

Addresses of the commercial networks can be found in the World TV Broadcasters list in this volume and additional information can be obtained from National Association of Commercial Broadcasters in Japan, Bungei Shunjusha Building, 3 Kioi-cho, Chiyoda-ku, Tokyo, All Japan TV Production Companies Assoc., Akasaka White House, 4-1-6 Akasaka, Minato-ku, Tokyo 107, or from Advertising Association of Broadcasters in Japan, 8-10 Nishi Ginza, Tokyo. For non-commercial TV information one should address Nippon Hoso Kyokai (NHK), 2-2-1 Jinnan, Shibuya-ku, Tokyo 150.

—A. C. PINDER

JORDAN

Jordan Television Corporation, Post office Box 1041, Amman. 310,000 sets; 12 stations.

KENYA

Voice of Kenya TV, Broadcasting House, P.O. Box 30456, Nairobi. One channel, 72,000 sets.

LIBERIA

Liberia Broadcasting Corporation, Post Office Box 594, Monrovia. One station, 36,000 sets.

MADAGASCAR

Television Madagascar, P.O. Box 442, Tanarive, Madagascar, operates a single station and three relays. 80,000 sets.

MALAYSIA

TV Malaysia was established in 1963 and now serves an estimated 885,000 sets on an average of 6 hours daily, half of broadcasts are in color. Originating station is at Kuala Lumpur, serving three networks on the main peninsula. One network extends to Sabah, where there is also a secondary station at Kota Kinabalu, which operates a small network of its own, extending to Sarawak. Inquiries to TV Malaysia (RIM), Broadcasting Dept., Kuala Lumpur 22-10.

Malaysia opened its first commercial TV channel in December, 1985.

MEXICO

Television began in 1950. It is estimated there are now 6,500,000 sets. In Mexico City there are six over-the-air channels, of which four are run by the privately-held Televisia under government concession on the other two by the government. There are five cable channels in Mexico City, all under control of Televisia. In addition there are 29 independent stations around the country.

MICRONESIA

Micronesia Broadcasting Corp., Taga Hotel, Saipan, Mariana Islands, comprises two stations broadcasting 16 hours daily on a commercial basis.

MONGOLIA

This Communist bloc nation established Radio-TV Mongolia in 1970 and now consists of two stations with satellite connection with Soviet Russia. Located in Ulan Bator, broadcasting to 30,000 sets.

NEW CALEDONIA

Societe Nationale de Radio-TV, P.O. Box G3 Cedex, Noumea, broadcasts on 4 channels in color to an estimated 40,000 sets.

NEW ZEALAND

The state-owned and operated Broadcasting Corp. of N.Z. television service operates two national networks in color—the TV1 network which originates programs from the Avalon television complex in Lower Hutt (near Wellington), and the TV2 network which originates programs from the Auckland studios. TV1 transmits some 88 hours of programs a week, and TV2 about 71 hours. Five days are commercial. Sundays are non-commercial on each network. Fridays are non-commercial on TV1, and Saturdays non-commercial on TV2.

Locally made programs are estimated at about 3,000 hours annually, which includes drama, news and current affairs, light entertainment, religion, service programs and sport. The balance of program output is purchased from overseas, mainly from Britain, the U.S. and Australia. Use of satellite links permits same-day presentation of world news items and live telecasts, particularly of sports. There are 956, 200 sets.

NIGERIA

Western Nigeria TV Service, Television House, Bompai Road, Kano. Ten stations, 4,200,000 sets.

NORTH KOREA

Experimental telecasting, using Russian equipment since 1960s, followed by establishment of a national network of 20 stations with regional stations and relays. Korean Central Broadcasting Committee, Television Section, Pyongyang, Democratic Peoples Republic of (North) Korea.

OMAN

Oman Color TV, Ministry of Information & Culture, P.O. Box 600, Muscat, Oman. Three stations and 1 relay for 150,000 sets.

PAKISTAN

Television came to Pakistan in November 1964, when the first station at Lahore went on the air. There were hardly 500 sets then. In May 1967, Pakistan Television Corporation Ltd., a public limited company was formed with an authorized capital of Rs. 5 crores and a paid-up capital of Rs. 3.19 crores. All shares of the corporation are held by the government of Pakistan. It now runs all five TV centers in the country. These stations are in Karachi, Lahore, Rawalpindi/Islamabad, Peshawar and Quetta and transmit five to eight hours of programming, including canned foreign films.

Out of 96 million, 77.11 million or 81.77% of the population of Pakistan sees PTV color programs, transmitted by 5 full-fledged production centers and 23 transmitters. When started in 1964, only 9.32% of the population could view black-and-white PTV programs.

There are at present approximately 1,815,804 licensed TV sets; the number of unlicensed sets is around 30%, or 544,741, or the sets in the country. Average viewership per TV set is estimated at 8 persons.

The area under the umbrella of TV signals has steadily risen from 8,029 square kilometers in 1964 to around 280,588 square kilometers by mid-1985, 35.25% of the total area of the country excluding the disputed territory of Jammu and Kashimir.

The amount of broadcasting is about an average of 56 hours a week, excluding special transmissions. Most of the programs are telecast on the national network. The main sources of income of PTV are commercials and license fees of Rs. 200 per year per domestic and Rs. 400 per commercial set, which comes to around Rs. 30 crore (license fees only).

A major breakthrough in the field of TV communication occurred in the mid-1970s when Pakistan was linked with the outside world through satellite. On July 24, 1981 PTV for the first time showed an interview with the Pakistani ambassador to Britain (in London) which was taken live from Karachi via satellite. Now all Pakistani viewers can see live programs (if PTV wishes) from abroad, as all TV stations have been linked with the national microwave network. Most of the international events, such as Islamic foreign ministers' conferences, cricket matches, tennis, soccer, boxing, the President and Prime Minister of Pakistan's foreign visits, Mehfil-e-Qiratl, Haj, important speeches at the United Nationas, reports from the war fronts of Lebanon, Iran, Iraq, Afghanistan, etc, are telecase with the cooperation of ABC, CBS, NBC, etc. live through satellite. Some Middle Eastern programs, including those from India, Oman, Dubai, Saudi Arabia, and Abu Dhabi, etc. are clearly visible in parts of Pakistan with the help of boosters in high antenna. Indian (Amritsar) TV is clearly seen in Lahore and surrounding areas even without the help of boosters.

One of the major goals of PTV has been to extend its service deeper into rural areas. PTV has been successful in achieving this to a high degree by setting up 23 powerful boosters/transmitters which act a rebroadcasting stations and are linked to the five main TV transmission centers. Meanwhile over 100 cities and town and thousands of villages are covered by telecast. As already mentioned, 81.77% of the population, or 77 million people, can see programs; nearly 62 million of these in electrified areas. Programs of special interest to rural folk such as waterlogging, fertilizer usage, improving seed methods, cooperative measures, etc. are regularly telecast. 14.73% of playing time goes to news; 13.45% is devoted to foreign films.

Surveys have showed that color TV has reached most well-to-do houses throughout Pakistan and black-and-white TVs have been installed in most average houses. PTV is run as a commercial service. Advertisements, which are shown in breaks and between programs, average 3.05% of broadcast time. The 15% increase in the rate of commercials under Islamic laws have slightly affected the business.

News readers and announcers (women) have to wear full sleeve shirts and cover their head and start the bulletin with the name of Almighty Allah and "Assalam-o-Alaikum" (Hello).

Pakistan manufactured 121,005 TV sets in 1984. At present PTV extends technical cooperation to Uganda, Libya, United Arab Emirates and International Telecommunications (ITC).

Color programs were introduced on PTV on December 20, 1976. Today there are five full-fledged color centers in Karachi, Lahore, Rawalpindi/Islamabad, Peshawar, and Quetta. The Quetta center covers the most territory. It also has a technical institute. Seven new boosters/rebroadcasting centers are scheduled to be installed in the next three years. These boosters will not only take TV signals in the less developed regions of the country, but will also meed the needs of remote areas of the NWFP, Baluchistan, Axad Kashmit, and Northern Areas. Most canned and domestic programs are telecast in color daily from all stations/centers. PTV has continued to add modern equipment to introduce new techniques. Electronic News Gathering (ENG) was adopted for action news and location coverage last year. Lately teleprompters frame synchronizer and character generator, having Arabic and English prints have been added at TV-Rawalpindi/Islamabad for news and the subtitling of progrms in Arabic.

There are estimated to be between 500,000 and 600,000 color sets throughout the country. The government charges an 80% duty on black-and-wnite and color TV sets brough into the country as personal baggage. Howver, there was no duty on locally manufactured balck-and-white or color sets. However, a 10% duty was introduced for the new budget for 1986–87.

A number of PTV programs have won international awards, including the Japan Prize Contest at Sapporo in 1972, the Shiraz Film Festival in Iran in 1973, the Federal Republic of Germany in 1974, the Hollywood Festival of World TV in 1974, Golden Prague, the Asia Pacific Broadcasting Union Prize Competition in Colombo, Sri Lanka in 1980, the "Special Commendation" Prix Futura in Berlin in 1981, the Asia Pacific Broadcasting Union in Manila in 1981, the Asia Pacific Broadcasting Union in Singapore in 1982, the Raduga Festival in Moscow in 1983, the "Transtel Prize" at the 8th Prix Futura in Berlin in 1983, the Seoul Prize at the International Television Programs Contest in Seoul in 1984 and in 1985.

PTV made a profit, for the first time, of Rs. 145 million during 1983–84, a remarkable achievement. Since then it has been a profit-making corporation.

PTV has important plans to increase coverage even further with special emphasis on remote and less developed areas and to establish a second channel for educational television during the current financial year. Highlights of the plan, expected to be completed during the next few years are:

1. To extend the range of TV signals to cover 95% of the population, 87% of the area.

2. To establish a second channel exclusively for the educational television service, initially from Karachi, Lahore, and Islamabad (by the end of 1986). At present one hour of educational programs is presented from Karachi and Lahore daily.

Currently about 2,500 creative technicians, including producers, cameramen, designers, editors, engineers and other technical staff, work for PTV. Artistes and performers are not on the permanent staff; they are paid daily wages according to their work in the programs. The highest remuneration paid to a performer is Rs. 26 a minute; the lowest, for a minor role, is Rs. 3 a minute. About 3,000 outside talents, including composers, singers, actors, announcers, instrumentalists, writers, etc. participate in PTV programs. A training institute for the artistes and technicians has been completed at Islamabad; a second is likely to start this year at Quetta.

The government of Pakistan has approved a project of Rd. 100 million for a ground receiving station to receive satellite pictures directly. Accepting the space age concept of viewing TV programs directly from satellites, official clearance has been given to a plan for manufacturing special sets for this purpose. Initially, only institutions and organizations involved in scientific academic work of the media will be allowed in this facility. The set, called Direct Broadcasting Satellite Receiver (DSBR), has been tested by SUPARCO, Pakistan's space agency. With the introduction of DBSR, Pakistan wil be the first country in the world to introduce this technology at an official level.

—A.R. SLOTE

PHILIPPINES

Broadcasts began in 1953 by DZAQ-TV then owned by Alto Broadcasting. At present 40 stations are on the air for commercial broadcasting and one government station; most are located in Manila. The number of sets is estimated at over 4,000,000. ABS-CBN was replaced by KBS. Others are Associated Broadcasting. Inter-Island Broadcasting, Metropolitan Broadcasting, Philippines Broadcasting. Radio Mindanao Network, Republic Broadcasting and Southern Broadcasting. More provincial outlets are planned.

Commercial ad revenues have averaged 30.8% gains over the past 10 years and now 46% of all advertising money spent is for TV compared to 29% for newspaper ads.

PUERTO RICO

Television started in 1954, and there are about 750,000 sets in

Puerto Rico. Most public places, such as restaurants and clubs, have television sets for their patrons; the medium is available in local hotels upon request.

Even though most Puerto Ricans know English, and the number of persons who will acquire a working knowledge of English will increase considerably through intensification of English instruction in public schools and the migration of Puerto Rican families to the United States, and workers who come back from the States with more knowledge of English. Television programming is in English and Spanish. WKAQ-TV, owned and operated by the newspaper El Mundo, on channel 4, has 30% of its programming in English of which 10% have Spanish sub-titles. There are 10 private stations in all.

Kinescope versions of top North American television shows are shown on both stations.

Cable television is on the rise here. The largest operator is Cable TV of Puerto Rico. It is owned by Harris Cable of Los Angeles, which bought the San Juan franchise in 1976, starting with some 8,000 customers.

Cable programming is also being expanded. At first the cable company offered only HBO and Virgin Islands stations. Receiving stations were built to bring in programs by satellite and by 1980 programs were being funneled from the states. Puerto Ricans now have a choice of 21 cable channels.

Cable TV charges its subscribers $11 a month for a basic package of 12 channels. HBO and Galavision cost $9.95 each additionally. Cable currently reaches greater San Juan, Bayamon, Carolina, Trujillo Alto and Guaynabo, which have an estimated 300,000 homes.

QATAR

Qatar TV Service (governmental), Ministry of Information, P.O. Box 1836 Doha, Qatar. Color since 1973. One station and relay; 120,000 sets.

SAMOA (AMERICAN)

Three TV stations serve some 42,000 sets on the American part of this Pacific island as well as a number of sets on the part administered by New Zealand. The station is also used daily for educational instructions to local schools. Address: Television of Samoa, Pago Pago. There are six channels.

SAUDI ARABIA

Established 1957, now 56 stations and 2 networks. General Directorate of TV, Ministry of Information, P.O. Box 570, Riyadh, Saudi Arabia; ARAMCO-TV, Box 96, Dhahran, Saudi Arabia. 1,900,000 sets.

SOUTH KOREA

Commercial TV broadcasting began in 1956, but the station burned three years later and it was not until 1961 when the government established the Korea Broadcasting Service (KBS-TV) network. The commercial network of Tongyang Broadcasting Co. (TBC) began in 1964 and was followed by the commercial Munwha Broadcasting Co. (MBC) in 1969. The American Forces Korea Network (AFKN-TV) was also established to serve American troops, and now comprises 6 stations.

KBS, which is entirely government-owned and collects a montly fee from each household with a TVset, is somewhat unique since its takes commerical advertising, unlike most governmental networks. Political opponents of the regime are rarely mentioned on broadcases; this one-sided coverage had led to a boycott by some of the public who refuse to pay fees. KBS also holds a controlling 65% interest in the only other commercial broadcaster, Munhwa Broadcasting. Under the present regime, Other stations were compelled by the government to merge with KBS, except for the Christian Broadcasting System which has been restricted since 1980 to broadcasting only religious programs. The government uses KBS profits from advertising revenues for education scholarships and expenses of newsmen traveling abroad.

KBS-TV has its key station in Seoul and 21 local stations, with other local stations, making a total of 33 TV stations, including those operated by MBC and the former TBC. Color broadcasting started in 1980. Almost 10 million sets are in operation, covering almost every household. If armed forces of USA are counted, the total stations number 33.

Korean broadcasts are limited to 6.5 hours of evening time and 4 hours mornings on weekdays, 11 hours on Saturday and 17 on Sunday. Monthly fees of about $1.00 are collected and advertisements are accepted.

On Saturdays and Sundays between 8 and 9 p.m. it is estimated that 60% or more of the population gather before their sets to view commercial station MBC's soap opera "Love and Truth" which is far beyond the average 30% viewing for such shows and above the 50% for previous "smash hits."

In 1981 the Republic of Korea "consolidated" all news media and took over the private stations, so daily listings read: KBS-1 TV (7 cities), KBS-2 TV (2), KBS-3 TV-UHF (6), MBC-TV (6). Korean Broadcasting Advertisement Corporation handles all TV and radio advertising.

SIERRA LEONE

Sierra Leone TV Service, New England, Private Mail Bag, Freetown. One station, 30,000 sets.

SINGAPORE

TV Singapore went on the air in 1963 and now serves an estimated 750,000 sets on four channels in four languages. One channel broadcasts 66 hours weekly the others 40 hours; of this total about 146 hours weekly are in color. Inquiries to Radio-TV Singapore, P.O. Box 1902, Singapore 11.

SOUTH AFRICA

South African Broadcasting Corp., P.O. Box 8606, Johannesburg 2000, started broadcasts in 1976 and now has over 80 stations with four services broadcasting 7 languages over 3 channels to over 2.2 million sets. From 1978 advertising was accepted.

Associated South West African Broadcasting, P.O. Box 321, Windhoek, Namibia, South West Africa, an autonomous statutory body, broadcasts 6 hours daily from Windhoek.

SPAIN

The first time Televisión Española—(now Radio-Televisión Española, RTVE)—transmitted on a regular basis was October 29, 1956, on a scan system of 625 lines at 25 frames per second. That program lasted three hours with a range of 70 kilometres, broadcasting for about 400 sets. The First Channel (VHF) was followed by a Second Channel (UHF) in 1967, complementary at first, but then somewhat competitive and with a clearer trend towards "culture." Channel 1 covers now all of Spain, including the Balearic and Canary Islands. Channel 2 reaches 80% of national territory. According to the Director of Television, Channel 2 has a ceiling of 85% of territory, since the investment costs double when the 70% level of coverage is reached.

RTVE is now an autonomous agency under the Ministry of Culture, Paseo de la Castellana 109, Madrid 16. All programs are controlled by a Censorship Board. Drama, films and episodes of series are classified according to ratings: "general" (no sign on the screen), "older than 14" (a small lozenge), "older than 18" (two small lozenges).

The official number of sets was 10,960,000 at the beginning of 1984. There are no official figures for color sets (German PAL system). They are gradually replacing old black-and-white ones which no factories produce now, except for small, portable battery sets.

In 1984 the production of programs will be entirely financed by advertising and tie-in merchandising, since the government withdrew the annual subsidy. Both channels carry ad spots. Due to nocturnal habits of Spaniards, the costliest time comes around 10:30 p.m. The ad spots appear on the screen at regular half-hour or one hour intervals, till 7 p.m. Later the spots rhythm accelerates, mainly during feature films in spite of audience and film directors' protests.

Staff and Studios: Director General of the Autonomous Agency RTVE (officially called "Ente", Italian style) is José María Calvinño, the target of constant attacks from the right-wing opposition party. Director of TVE is Antonio López.

The ruling Socialist Party controls the TVE Council, a multi-partisan body which applies the 1981 Statute of Television. Home rule in Catalonia and the Basque provinces opened the door to regional independent TV centers. Even the Andalusian parliament asked for a Third Channel covering the south of Spain.

RTVE built in Madrid a 210 meter high tower ("Torrespaña") for news and live broadcasts. This "Towerspain" is now one of the landmarks of the capital.

TVE has ten news broadcasting stations in provinces. The Canary Islands set up their own programming. National Headquarters are at Prado del Rey, Madrid 24, with general offices and nine studios with total area of 3,000 square meters. Additional studios are in Barcelona.

Fixed, salaried personnel is about 2,300, with other estimated 5,000 contributing freelancers. An important group of steady contributors got permanent status by sentence of the Supreme Labor Court.

Programming Schedule and Contents: Channel 1 broadcasts 76 h 45′ weekly, with accent on week-ends. Same happens with Channel 2, which broadcasts 46 h 45′ weekly. Total of weekly broadcasting time: 123 h 30′. Special programs such as prize boxing bouts, sports championships, bullfights, royal and political messages, etc., move or remove normal programming.

Many broadcasting hours consist in theater movies (about seven features weekly) and filmed foreign production, including American series as "Flamingo Road", "Winds of War", "Masada", "The Martian Chronicles", etc. TVE broadcasts too many debate and panel shows, too many heavy music meetings, but lacks comedy fare. From

1982 the Ente has invested in prestige Spanish features, which first are being shown in theaters and then will be adapted to television as miniseries. Many of them have won awards at international film festivals.

Price range for half hour of screening time is $1,500–$2,000. One-hour series generally brings twice the half-hour price. Price range for feature films is $7,800–$17,000, dubbed into Spanish at Madrid studios. Only "Film Society" screenings (Channel 2) accept foreign prints with Spanish subtitles.

Foreign Markets: The estimate of TVE foreign sales for 1985 surpasses $5 million, the estimate for 1984 is $3,860,000. The whole TVE sales team goes in force to world markets like MIP-TV. But the main problem in Spain is the proliferation of video-recorders and the underground market of bootleg cassettes, in spite of frequent raids by police and Justice officers. Cable TV is not even mentioned here, and for the time being the Socialist government has ruled out private TV networks.

SWITZERLAND

As of April 30, 1986, there were 2,205,713 TV sets in operation in Switzerland and 1295 transmitters and boosters on the air. The French language station schedules about 87 hours; the German language station about 78 hours; and the Italian lanaguage station about 66 hours of programming weekly (without Eurovision/European TV Programme exchanges).

Commerical TV was introduced on a limited basis on February 1, 1965. From January 1, 1974, 20 minutes weekly, only on workdays, were allowed; the cost per minute as of January 1, 1986, was 19,800 Swiss francs. On October 1, 1982, the cost of annual licenses was fixed at 174 Swiss francs for private sets. As of December 1985, 91.6% of all Swiss households had color TV sets.

Swiss Italians are the more fervid TV fans, with a daily 2 hour and 31 minute presence in front of their TV sets; Swiss French total 2 hours and 12 minutes, while Swiss Germans switch on the set only 2 hours and 6 minutes every day.

Swiss Italians only tune in a national channel 33% of the time their set is switched on; 67% of the time they watch foreign channels, especially Italian ones. The Swiss channels are more favored by Swiss Germans and Swiss French: 40% for the former, 41% for the latter. For the remaining 60%, Swiss Germans tune in the channels of neighboring German, while the French Swiss watch French channels.

Festival: In 1983, during the Interational Film Festival Locarno (August) for the first time about 100 TV movies from a great number of European and overseas countries were shown in a special section called "TV-movies." The 1986 edition of the TV-movies offered a program of 120 movies from 24 countries, 14 of which shared in a special award, The Eye of the Leopard.

—GABRIELLA BROGGI

TAHITI

Office of Radiodiff-Television Francaise, Papeete, operates four channels 34 hours weekly to serve the estimated 24,000 sets of this French possession. It is owned by the government and buys canned programs in Paris.

THAILAND

Thai Television Company (government-owned) opened its first station in 1955 and there are four stations (two using color) and 8 relays on a commercial basis. Stations are also operated under names of Bangkok Broadcasting & TV, Bangkok Entertainment Co. and Mass Communication Organization of Thailand, all located in Bangkok. Sets are estimated at 3,743,000, some color.

In 1980 a ban on broadcasts from 6:30 to 8:00 p.m., as a power-saving measure, allegedly improved "family relationships," so at present broadcasts are limited to 8 hours on weekdays, and 16 hours on weekends and holidays.

TURKEY

Turkish Radio Television Corp., P.O. Box 98, Kizilay-Ankara serves 5.5 million TV sets via 37 stations.

UNITED ARAB EMIRATES

Established 1969 by Thompson TV International and Abu Dhabi TV Service. In 1971 United Arab Emirates TV Service, P.O. Box 637 Abu Dhabi established separate facilities which now consist of three stations and three relays. Dubai Radio and Color TV, P.O. Box 1695, Kubai, now broadcasts on two channels from 1 station and 1 relay in Arabic, French and English. 100,000 sets.

VIETNAM

Since 1968 the Government Information Department of the Democratic Republic of Vietnam has operated one non-commercial station in Hanoi. Number of sets is about 760,000.

A second station was added in Saigon (now known as Ho Chi-Minh City) when South Vietnam was "liberated" and the divided country became one.

Hanoi has initiated use of a Russian satellite and 7 hours of color telecasts on weekdays and all day Saturday and Sunday, compared with the previous 4 hours a day in black and white.

WEST GERMANY

TV Households: Out of approximately 24,000,000 German households, 23,000,000 have at least one television set. Of these, about 16,000,000 have at least one color set. Some 23,000,000 households have at least one radio. Total TV set sales per year: about $2.2-billion.

TV Networks: Germany has no networks similar to those in the U.S. In fact, there are no privately-owned commercial TV stations; all telecommunication is state-owned. Basically, the two national TV outlets are: ARD, the national hookup of nine regional stations; and ZDF or second channel, a single nationally-beamed station based in Mainz near Frankfurt. ARD's nine stations each contribute to one joint national broadcasting operation, five regional channels and several radio channels. ARD has a budget of about $1,640-billion; ZDF, $556,000,000. Commercials are aired on both stations in sharply limited timeslots. Stations are supported largely by $6.50 monthly license fees paid by TV set owners.

YEMEN (Arab Republic)

San'a Television, Ministry of Information, San'a, established in 1977, currently broadcasts on 3 channels to some 120,000 sets.

YEMEN (People's Republic)

Established in 1964, People's Democratic Republic of Yemen, P.O. Box 1264, Aden, broadcasts on 3 channels to an estimated 55,000 sets.

ZIMBABWE

Established in 1960 as Rhodesia TV, and now named Zimbabwe Broadcasting Corp., P.O. Box H.G. 200, Highlands, Harare, its 6 stations serve some 560,000 sets.

WORLD TV BROADCASTERS

Europe

ALBANIA
RADIOTELEIZIONI SHQIPTAR
Rrga Ismail Qemali, Tirana.

AUSTRIA
OSTERREICHISCHER RUNDFUNK GmbH ORF
Argentinierstrasse 30a, 1041 Vienna Postfach 700.

BELGIUM
RADIODIFFUSION-TELEVISION BELGE (R.T.B.) (FRENCH)
Boulevard A. Reyers, 1040, Bruxelles.
BELGISCHE RADIO EN TELEVISIE (B.R.T.) (FLEMISH)
Omreopcentrum A. Reyerslaan, 1040, Brussel.

BULGARIA
BULGARIAN TELEVISION
Todor Strashimirov 2, Sofia 4.

CYPRUS
CYPRUS BROADCASTING CORPORATION
P.O. Box 4824, Nicosia.

CZECHOSLOVAKIA
CESKOSLOVENSKA TELEVIZIE
M. Gorkeho 29, Prague 1.

DENMARK
RADIO DENMARK
Television Service, Radio Denmark, Radiohuset, Rosenornsalle, Alle 22, Copenhagen.

FINLAND
FINNISH BROADCASTING CO.
Kesakatu 2, Helsinki 26.

FRANCE
TELEDIFFUSION DE FRANCE
116, avenue du President Kennedy. F-75790 Paris Cedex 16.

GERMANY

GERMAN FEDERAL REPUBLIC
DEUTSCHE RUNDFUNK-UND FERNSEHANSTALTEN
BAYERISCHER RUNDFUNK
Rundfunkplatz 1, 8 Munich 2.
HESSISCHER RUNDFUNK
Frankfurt (Main), Bertramstr. 8.
NORDEUTSCHER RUNDFUNK
Hamburg, 13, Rothenbaumchaussee 132/134.
RADIO BREMEN
Heinrich-Hertz-Str. 13, Bremen, 33.
SAARLANDISCHER RUNDFUNK
66 Saarbrucken, Funkhaus Halberg, Postfach 1050.
SENDER FREIES BERLIN
Berlin 19, Masurenallee 8-14.
SUEDDEUTSCHER RUNDFUNK
7000 Stuttgart 1, Neckarstr. 145.
SUEDWESTFUNK
757 Baden-Baden, Hans-Bredow-Strass.
WESTDEUTSCHER RUNDFUNK
Appellhofplatz 1, 5 Cologne 1. Postfach 101950.
ZWEITES DEUTSCHES FERNSEHEN
Essenheimer Landstrasse, 65 Mainz-Lerchenberg, Postfach 4040.

GIBRALTAR
GIBRALTAR BROADCASTING, LTD.
Television House, Wellington Front.
GIBRALTAR TELEVISION
28 John Mackintosh Square, Gibraltar.

HOLLAND
NEDERLANDSE OMROEP STICHTING (N.O.S.)
P.O. Box 10, Hilversum.

HUNGARY
MAGYAR RADIO ES TELEVIZIO
Television Direction, V. Szabadsagter, 17, Budapest.

IRELAND
RADIO EIREANN TELEFIS
Donnybrook, Dublin 4.

ITALY
RADIO-TELEVISIONE ITALIANA
Viale Mazzini 14, 00195, Rome.

LUXEMBOURG
TELE LUXEMBOURG
Villa Louvigny.

MALTA
THE MALTA TELEVISION SERVICE LTD.
Television House, P.O. Box 384, Gwardamanga.

MONACO
TELE MONTE CARLO
16, Blvd. Princesse Charlotte, Monte Carlo.

POLAND
POLSKIE RADIO I TELEWIZJA
Woronicza St., Warsaw.

PORTUGAL
RTP-RADIOTELEVISAO PORTUGUESA S.A.R.L.
Rua de S. Domingos (a Lapa) 26, Lisboa.

ROMANIA
RADIODIFUZIUNEA TELEVIZUNEA ROMANA
Calea Dorobantilor, 191, Bucarest O. Romania.

SPAIN
TELEVISION ESPANOLA
de Prado del Rey, Madrid.

SWEDEN
SVERIGES RADIO
AB S-105 10 Stockholm.

SWITZERLAND
SWISS BROADCASTING CORPORATION
Giacommettistrasse 3, CH-3000 Berne 15.

USSR
SOVJET TELEVISION
Akademika Koroljova 12, Moscow.

YUGOSLAVIA
TELEVISION YOUGOSLAVE
Boriso Kidrica 70/1 Belgrade.

Africa

ALGERIA
RADIODIFFUSION-TELEVISION ALGERIENNE
21 Blvd. des Martyrs, Algiers.

BOURKINA FASSO (Upper Volta)
TELEVISION NATIONALE DE BOURKINA
Post Office Box 7029, Ouagadougou.

BENIN
OFFICE DE RADIODIFFUSION ET DE TELEVISION DU BENIN
BP 366, Cotonou.

CAMEROUN
UNITE TC, RADIO DIFFUSION DU CAMEROUS
Ministry of Information, Yaonde.

CENTRAL AFRICAN REPUBLIC
TELEVISION CENTRAFRICAINE
Ministry of Information, B.P. 940, Bangui.

DJIBOUTI
RADIO TELEVISION DE DJIBOUTI
B.P. 97, Ave. St. Laurent du Var, Djibouti.

EGYPT
U.A.R. BROADCASTING CORPORATION OF CARIO
Television Bldg., Cornish Road, P.O. Box 1186, Cairo.

GABON
RADIO TELEVISION GABONAISE
B.P. 10150, Libreville.

GHANA
GHANA BROADCASTING CORPORATION
P.O. Box 1633, Accra.

KENYA
KENYA BROADCASTING SERVICE
P.O. Box 30456, Nairobi.

LIBYA
LIBYA JAMAHIRIAYH BROADCASTING TV
P.O. Box 33, Tripoli.

MOROCCO
RADIODIFFUSION TELEVISION MAROCAINE
1, Zankat al Brihi, Rabat.

NIGERIA
BROADCASTING COMPANY OF NORTHERN NIGERIA, LTD.
Television House, P.O. Box 250, Kaduna.
NIGERIAN BROADCASTING CORP.
P.M.B. 12005, Victoria Island, Lagos, Nigeria.
WESTERN NIGERIA RADIOVISION SERVICE
Television House, P.O. Box 1460, Ibadan.

SIERRA LEONE
SIERRA LEONA TV BROADCASTING
New England, Private Mail Bag, Freetown.

SUDAN
SUDAN TELEVISION
Box 1094, Omduran, Sudan (107,000 sets)

TANZANIA
TV ZANZIBAR
TV Zanzibar, P.O. Box 314, Zanzibar (7,500 sets)

TUNISIA
RADIODIFFUSION TV TUNISIA
71 Ave. de la Liberté, Tunis.

ZAIRE
ZAIRE TELEVISION
Box 3171, Kinhasa, Zaire (71,000 sets)

ZAMBIA
ZAMBIA TELEVISION
P.O. Box 50015, Lusaka, Zambia (70,000 sets)

Asia

NATIONALIST CHINA
TAIWAN TELEVISION ENTERPRISES LTD.
No. 10, Pa Te Road, Sec 3, Taipei.
CHINESE TELEVISION SERVICE
N. 100, Kuang Fu South Road, Taipei.

GUAM
KUAM TELEVISION
Pacific Broadcasting, Box 368, Agana, Guam.

HONG KONG
TELEVISION BROADCASTS, LTD.
77 Broadcast Drive, Hong Kong.

REDIFFUSION (Hong Kong Ltd.)
81 Broadcast Drive, Kowloon, Hong Kong.

INDIA
ALL INDIA TELEVISION
Television Centre, All India Radio, Akashwani Bhawan, 5th Floor, Parliament Street, New Delhi, 110001.

INDONESIA
JAJASAN TELEVISI RI (RRI-TV)
Senajan, Jakarta

IRAN
IRAN REPUBLIC BROADCASTING
P.O. Box 19395, Tehran 17-74.

IRAQ
TV-STATION OF THE REP. OF IRAQ
Ministry of Guidance, Broadcasting House, Salhiya, Baghdad.

JAPAN
NIPPON HOSO KYOKAI (NHK)
2-2-1 Jinnan, Shibuya-ku, Tokyo 150.

ASAHI BROADCASTING CO. LTD. (ABC) JOBX-TV
Osaka.

KANSAI TELEVISION CORP. (KTV) JONR-TV
Osaka.

MAINICHI BROADCASTING SYSTEM (MBS) JOQR-TV
Osaka.

FUJI TELECASTING CO.
7 Kawada-cho, Ichigaya, Shinjuku, Tokyo.

ASAHI NATIONAL BROADCASTING CO. (TV ASAHI or ANB) formerly Nippon Educational Television (NET)
6-4-10 Roppongi, Tokyo.

NIPPON TELEVISION NETWORK (NTV)
14 Niban-cho, Chiyoda-ku, Tokyo.

TOKYO BROADCASTING SYSTEM (TBS)
5-3-6, Akasaka, Minato-ku, Tokyo.

NATIONAL ASSOCIATION OF COMMERCIAL BROADCASTERS
Bungei Shunju Bldg., 3 Kioi-cho, Chiyoda-Ku, Tokyo.

MCA JAPAN LTD.
Maison Hirakawa, 2-5-2 Hirakawa-cho, Chiyoda-ku, Tokyo.

JAPAN (Audience Research) A.C. NIELSEN CO.
1-1-71 Naka-Meguro, Meguro-ku, Tokyo 153.

VIDEO RESEARCH CORP.
2-16-7 Ginza, Chuo-ku, Tokyo 104.

TOKYO CHANNEL 12 TV (JOTX)
4-4 Shiba Koen, Tokyo.

CABLE TELEVISION JCTV
c/o ANB, 6-4/10 Roppongi, Minato-ku, Tokyo.

TVK (UHF) CHANNEL 42
Yokohama, 231.

TELEVI OSAKA (JOBH)
2-2 Kyobashi, Higashi-ku, Osaka 530

YOMIURI TELEV (JOIX)
1-8-11 Higashi-Tenma, Osaka 530.

HOKKAIDO BUNKA HOSO (JOBM)
14-1-5 Nishi Kita-Ichijo, Sapporo 060.

HOKKAIDO BROADCASTING (JOHR)
5-2 Nishi Kita Ichijo, Chuo-ku, Sapporo 060.

HOKKAIDO TELEVI HOSO (JOHH)
4-13-10-17 Hiragishi, Toyohira-ku Sapporo.

SAPPORO TELEVI (JOKX)
8-1-1 Nishi Kita-Ichijo, Sapporo 060.

OKINAWA TELEVI (JOOF)
1-2-20 Kumoji, Naha 900.

RYUKU HOSO (JORR)
2-3-1 Kumoji, Naha 900.

RKB MAINICHI HOSO (JOFR)
4-1-10 Watanabe-dori Fukuoka 810

FUKUOKA HOSO (JOFH)
1-1-1 Watanabe-dori, Fukuoka 810.

KAGOSHIMA HOSO (JOTI)
4-31 Yamano-kuchi-machi, Kagoshima

SOUTH KOREA
KOREA BROADCASTING SYSTEM
33-3 ga, Namsan-Rong, Chung-Ku, Seoul.

KUWAIT
KUWAIT-TV
P.O. Box 621, Kuwait.

LEBANON
COMPAGNIE LIBANAISE DE TELEVISION
P.O. Box 4848, Beirut.

MALAYSIA
TELEVISION MALAYSIA
Dept. of Broadcasting, P.O. Box 1047, Kuala Lumpur.

PHILIPPINES
INTERCONTINENTAL BROADCASTING CORPORATION
P. Guevarra Ave., San Juan, Rizal.

KANLAON BROADCASTING SYSTEM, INC.
Broadcast Plaza, Bohol Ave., Quezon City.

REPUBLIC BROADCASTING SYSTEM
E de los Santos Avenue, Diliman, Quezon City.

SAUDI ARABIA
SAUDI ARABIAN TELEVISION
P.O. Box 570, Riyadh.

THAILAND
THAI TELEVISION CO. LTD.
Bangkhunprom, Bangkok.

THAI ARMY TELEVISION STATION
Pahol Youthin Road, Bangkok.

BANGKOK ENTERTAINMENT
2357 New Petchburi, Bangkok.

Pacific

AMERICAN SAMOA
TELEVISION OF SAMOA
Department of Education, Pago Pago, 96799.

AUSTRALIA
AUSTRALIAN BROADCASTING

COMMISSION

Government owned.
145 Elizabeth St., P.O. Box 487 G.P.O., Sydney, N.S.W. 2001.

AMALGAMATED TELEVISION SERVICES

Pty. Ltd. Television Station A.T.N., Channel 7
Television Centre, Epping, 2121, Sydney, N.S.W.

TELEVISION CORPORATION LIMITED

Television Station TCN, Channel 9
Artarmon Road, Willoughby, 2068, Sydney, N.S.W.

UNITED TELECASTERS LIMITED (Channel A-10)

Epping & Pittwater Rds., North Ryde 2113, N.S.W.

HERALD-SUN TV

Pty. Ltd. Television Station HSV Channel 7
Cnr. Dorcas and Wells St., South Melbourne, Victoria.

GENERAL TELEVISION COR.

Pty. Ltd. Television Station GTV, Channel 9
22-46 Bendigo Street, Richmond, Melbourne, Victoria.

AUSTRAMA TELEVISION (Channel 0)

ATC C/Ansett Transport Industries Ltd.
489 Swanston Street, Melbourne, Victoria.

CANBERRA TELEVISION LTD.

Television Station CTC, Channel 7
Canberra Television Centre, Black Mountain, ACT, P.O. Box 633, Canberra.

BRISBANE TV LIMITED

Sir Samuel Griffiths Drive, Mt. Coot-tha, Brisbane, Queensland.

QUEENSLAND TELEVISION LIMITED

Sir Samuel Griffiths Drive, Mt. Coot-tha, Brisbane, Queensland.

TELEVISION BROADCASTER LTD.

Television Station ADS, Channel 7
125 Strangeways Terrace, North Adelaide, South Australia.

SOUTHERN TELEVISION CORP. LTD.

Television Station NWS, Channel 9
202–208 Tynte Street, North Adelaide, South Australia.

TVW LIMITED

Television Station TVW, Channel 7
Osborne Park Road, Tuart Hill, Perth, W.A.

TASMANIAN TELEVISION LIMITED

TVT, Channel A-6
G.P.O. Box 1209M, Hobart (Tas.)

MARIANAS ISLANDS

KUAM TELEVISION

P.O. Box 368, Agana.

NEW CALEDONIA

RADIODIFFUSION TV, NOUMEA

Box 327, Noumea.

NEW ZEALAND

NEW ZEALAND BROADCASTING COUNCIL

P.O. Box 30, 355, Lower Hutt, New Zealand.

TAHITI

TELEVISION FRANCE L

Box 125, Papeete.

Central America

COSTA RICA

TELEVISORA DE COSTA RICA LTDA.

Apt. 3376, San Jose.

CUBA

CMQ-TV

Radiocentre, Habana.

CMBF-TV

Mazon y San Miguel, Habana.

DOMINICAN REPUBLIC

RAHINTEL TELEVISION

P.O. Box 1220, zone 7.

GUATEMALA

RADIO-TELEVISION GUATEMALA, S.A.

Apt. 1367, Guatemala.

HAITI

TELE-HAITI

P.O. Box 1126, Port-au-Prince.

HONDURAS (Rep.)

RADIO Y TELEVISION HONDURENA, S.A.

Tegucigalpa.

JAMAICA

JAMAICAN BROADCASTING CORP.

5–9 South Ocean Avenue., P.O. Box 100, Kingston.

MEXICO

TELEVISION DE LA FRONTERA, S.A.

Vincente Guerrero num. 704 Ciudad Juarez, Chih.

RADIO PANAMERICANA, S.A.

Av. Chapultepec num. 18 Mexico, D.F.

TELEVISION DEL NORTE, S.A.

Aparatado Postal num. 1833 Monterrey, N.L.

TELEVIMEX, S.A.

Av. Chapultepec num. 18 Mexico D.F.

RADIO TELEVISION S.A.

Calle Quinta num. 210 Desps. 14–16 Edificio Barbachano Tiajuana, B.C.

CADENA TELEVISION DEL NORTE, S.A.

Monterrey, N.L. (Dom. Av. Chapultepec num. 18 Mexico, D.F.)

RAFAEL TIJERINA CARRANZA

Aldama num. 2611 Nuevo Laredo, Tams.

TELEVISION TAPATIA, S.A. de C.V.

Circunvalacion num. 265 Guadalajara, Jal.

TELEVISORA DE LA LAGUNA, S.A.

Torreon, Coah. (Dom. Av. Chapultepec mun. 18, Mexico, D.F.)

TELEVISION PASO DE CORTES, S.A.

Av. Chapultepec num. 18 Mexico, D.F.

SERGIO R. MOLINAR FERNANDEZ

Apartado Postal num. 271 Ciudad Juarez, Chih.

TELEVISORA DE CHIHUAHUA, S.A.

Chihuahua, Chih. (Dom. Av. Chapultepec num. 18 Mexico, D.F.)

TELEVISORA DE HERMOSILLO, S.A.

Hermosillo, Son. (Dom. Av. Chapultepec num. 18 Mexico, D.F.)

TELEVISORA DE GUADALAJARA, S.A.

Guadalajara, Jal. (Dom. Av. Chapultepec num. 18 Mexico, D.F.)

TELEVISORA DE CALIMEX, S.A.

Tiajuana, B.C. (Dom. Av. Chapultepec num. 18 Mexico. D.F.)

TELEVISORA DE OCCIDENTE, S.A.

Guadalajara, Jal. (Dom. Av. Chapultepec num. 18, Mexico, D.F.)

TELEVISORA DEL NORTE, S.A.

Monterrey, N.L. (Dom. Av. Chapultepec num. 18 Mexico, D.F.)

TELEVISORA DE YUCATAN, S.A.

Merida, Yrc. (Dom. Av. Chapultepec num. 18 Mexico, D.F.)

TELEVISION DE GUANAJUATO, S.A.

Cerro del Zamorano, Qro. (Dom. Av. Chapultepec mun. 18 Mexico, D.F.)

TV DE CULIACAN, S.A.

Culiacan, Sin. (Dom. Av. Chapultepec num. 18 Mexico, D.F.)

TELEVISORA DE MEXICALI, S.A.

Apartado Postal num. 1356 Mexicali, B.C. (Dom. Av. Chapultepec num. 18 Mexico, D.F.)

TELEVISION DE COLIMA, S.A. de C.V.

Anillo Cirunvalacion num. 1080 Nte. Colima, Col.

FELIPE ARRIOLA GANDARA

Av. Alvaro Obregon num. 138 Nogales, Son.

CARLOS FERRAEZ MATOS

Calle Bolivar entre Diaz Miron y Boulevard Miguel Aleman Veracruz, Ver.

TELEVISION GONZALES CAMERENA, S.A.

Av. Chapultepec num. 18 Mexico, D.F.

TELEVISORA DEL GOLFO, S.A.

Ciudan Madero, Tams. (Dom. Av. Chapultepec num. 18 Mexico, D.F.)

TELEVISION DE MEXICO, S.A.

Av. Chapultepec num. 18 Mexico, D.F.

ANTONIO SUAREZ REYES

Av. Punta Banda y Eugenia, Frallion-Amiento Chapultepec Ensenada, B.C.

NETHERLANDS ANTILLES

TELECURACAO

P.O. Box 415, Curacao.

NICARAGUA

TELEVISION DE NICARAGUA, S.A.

Apdo 1505, Managua.

PANAMA

CIRCUITO RPC-TELEVISIÓN

Direccion de Correos y Telecommunicaciones, Ministerio de Gobierno y Justicia, Panama.

TELEVISORA NACIONAL S.A. PANAMA

Ric. Chiari, Panam.

PUERTO RICO

WKAQ-TV

Telemundo Inc., Box W.

WIPM-TV

Dept. of Education
Hato Rey, San Juan.

WAPA-TV

WAPA-TV Broadcasting Corp.
P.O. Box 2050, San Juan.

WORA-TV

Quality Telecasting Corp.
Box 43, Mayaguez.

WIPR-TV

Dept. of Education
Hato Rey, San Juan.

WRIK-TV

Ponce TV Corp.
Darlington Bldg.

WSUR-TV

American Colonial Broadcasting Corp.
Box 4189, San Juan.

WKBM-TV

American Colonial Broadcasting Corp.
Box 4189, San Juan.

WOLE-TV

Western Broadcasting Corp.
Box 415, Aguadilla.

TRINIDAD

TRINIDAD AND TOBAGO TELEVISION CO. LTD.

Television House
12a Maraval Road, Port-of-Spain.

VIRGIN ISLANDS

ISLAND TELERADIOSERVICE, INC.

P.O. Box 1947, St. Thomas.

South America

ARGENTINA

PRIMERA TELEVISION ARGENTINA

Av. Alem 735, Buenos Aires.

COMPANIA ARGENTINA DE TELEVISION, S.A.

Castex 3345, Buenos Aires.

PRODUCCIONES ARGENTINA DE TV

Lima 1261, Buenos Aires.

TELEONCE

Calle Pavon 2444, Buenos Aires.

RIO DE LA PLATA

San Juan, 1160, Buenos Aires.

DIFUSORA MARPLATENSE

Av. Luro 2907, Mar del Plata.

SOCIEDAD DIFUSORA MENDOZA

Garibaldi 7, Mendoza.

TELECOLOR, S.A.

Av. Gral Paz 266, Cordoba.

BRAZIL

TELEVISAO—TUPI

Av. Joao Luiz Alves, 13-Urca, Rio de Janeiro.

TELEVISAO—RIO

Av. Atlantica 4264, Rio de Janeiro.

EMISSORA DE TELEVISAO CONTINENTAL

Rue das Laranjeiras 291, Rio de Janeiro.

TELEVISAO MAYRINK VEIGA

Rio de Janeiro.

RADIO GLOBO DO RIO DE JANEIRO

Rua Irineau Marinho 35, Rio de Janeiro.

CHILE

TV CHILE

Bellavista 0990, Casilla Postal 16.104, Correo 9, Santiago.

COLOMBIA

R. TELEVISORA NACIONAL

Direccion General de la Radiotelevisora National de Colombia Apartado Nacional 1824, Bogota.

ECUADOR

LA VOZ DE LOS ANDES—TELEVISION

Cas: 691, Quito.

PRIMERA TELEVISION ECUATORIANA S.A.

Illingworth 114 y Pichincha, Guayaquil.

PERU

MINISTRY OF EDUCATION

Ministerio de Educacion Publica
Direccion de Cultera, Lima.

TELEVISORA AMERICA

Montero Rosas, Lima.

TELEVISORA PANAMERICANA

Ave. Arequipa 1110, Lima.

TELEVISORA VICTORIA

Av. Tacna 543, Lima.

TELEVISORA EXCELSIOR

Ave. Manco Capac, Lima.

TELEVISORA EL SOL

Jose Galvez 1040, Lima.

TELEVISORA SUR PERUANA

P.O. Box 514, Arequipa.

URUGUAY

TV MONTE CARLO

18 DE Julio 1855, Montevideo.

SAETA-TV

Lorenzo Carnelli 1234, Montevideo.

VENEZUELA

TELEVISORA NACIONAL

Apt. 3979, Caracas.

CORPORACION VENEZOLANA DE TELEVISION

Apartado 6674, Caracas.

R. CARACAS TV

Apartado 2057, Caracas.